CONTENTS

Saunders Nursing Drug Handbook 2008

BARBARA B. HODGSON, RN, OCN
Cancer Institute
St. Joseph's Hospital
Tampa, Florida

ROBERT J. KIZIOR, BS, RPh
Education Coordinator
Department of Pharmacy
Alexian Brothers Medical Center
Elk Grove Village, Illinois

SAUNDERS
ELSEVIER

SAUNDERS
ELSEVIER

11830 Westline Industrial Drive
St. Louis, Missouri 63146

ISBN: 978-1-4160-4063-7

SAUNDERS NURSING DRUG HANDBOOK 2008

NOTICE

Knowledge and best practice in this field are constantly changing. As new research and experience broaden our knowledge, changes in practice, treatment and drug therapy may become necessary or appropriate. Readers are advised to check the most current information provided (i) on procedures featured or (ii) by the manufacturer of each product to be administered, to verify the recommended dose or formula, the method and duration of administration, and contraindications. It is the responsibility of the practitioner, relying on their own experience and knowledge of the patient, to make diagnoses, to determine dosages and the best treatment for each individual patient, and to take all appropriate safety precautions. To the fullest extent of the law, neither the Publisher nor the Authors assume any liability for any injury and/or damage to persons or property arising out of or related to any use of the material contained in this book.

The Publisher

Library of Congress Control Number: 2007924248

Executive Vice President, Nursing & Health Professions: Sally Schrefer
Publishing Executive: Barbara Nelson Cullen
Executive Editor: Cindy Tryniszewski
Developmental Editors: Gina Hopf, Terri Greenberg
Publishing Services Manager: Melissa Lastarria
Senior Project Manager: Joy Moore
Designer: Mark Oberkrom

Printed in the United States of America

Last digit is the print number: 9 8 7 6 5 4 3 2 1

I dedicate this work to my daughter Lauren, a true friend, for her unconditional love; my daughter Kathryn, always supportive, always encouraging; and my son, Keith, a source of great pride to us all. This is also dedicated to my sons-in-law, Jim and Andy, who have added so very much to my family, and to my granddaughters, Jaime, Sarah, Andrea, Katie and the smallest members of my growing family, my granddaughter, Paige Olivia, and my grandsons, Logan James, Ryan James, and Dylan Boyd. I couldn't love you more.

BARBARA HODGSON, RN, OCN

To all health care professionals, who in the expectation of little glory or material reward dedicate themselves to the art and science of healing.

ROBERT KIZIOR, BS, RPh

AUTHOR BIOGRAPHIES

Barbara Hodgson, RN, OCN

Born and raised in Michigan, Barbara was married and raising a young family in Chicago when she decided to fulfill a lifelong dream and become a nurse. After graduation, she started her own business as author and publisher of **Medcards, The Total Medication Reference Guide,** the first of its kind. These drug cards were designed to assist nursing students in understanding drug information to give knowledgeable care to their patients.

In 1981, she met co-author Robert (Bob) Kizior, who was teaching a pharmacology class. After class, Barbara approached him and asked if he would be interested in working on **Medcards** with her. He agreed, and together they became so successful that a few years later Barbara was able to fulfill another dream and move to Florida.

By 1987, Barbara was approached by W.B. Saunders and asked to author the **Saunders Nursing Drug Handbook.** Since then, Barbara and Bob have worked together on this handbook and on two more drug resources, the **Saunders Electronic Nursing Drug Cards** and the **Saunders Drug Handbook for Health Professions.**

Barbara specializes in oncology at the Cancer Institute, St. Joseph's Hospital, in Tampa, Florida. Barbara's daughter Lauren; her son-in-law, Jim; and her son, Keith, are emergency nurses. Her daughter Kathryn is a research biologist and is presently attending nursing school.

Barbara's favorite interests are spending time with her very busy, tight-knit family and, when she has a rare moment, getting her hands full of dirt working in her garden.

Robert (Bob) Kizior, BS, RPh

Bob graduated from the University of Illinois School of Pharmacy and is licensed to practice in the state of Illinois. He has worked as a hospital pharmacist for more than 35 years at Alexian Brothers Medical Center in Elk Grove Village, Illinois—a suburb of Chicago. Bob is the Education Coordinator for the Department of Pharmacy, where he participates in educational programs for pharmacists, nurses, physicians, and patients. He plays a major role in conducting Drug Utilization Reviews and is a member of the Infection Control Committee and the Bariatric Committee. His hospital experience is diverse and includes participation in clinical pharmacy initiatives on inpatient units and in the surgical pharmacy satellite. Bob is a former adjunct faculty member at William Rainey Harper Community College in Palatine, Illinois. It was there that Bob first met Barbara and commenced their long-standing professional association.

An avid fan of Big Ten college athletics, Bob also has eclectic tastes in music that range from classical, big band, rock 'n' roll, and jazz to country and western. Bob spends much of his free time reviewing the professional literature to stay current on new drug information. He and his wife, Marcia, and their two Labrador retrievers—Zak and Callie—enjoy escape weekends at their year-round lake house in central Wisconsin.

CONSULTANTS

Katherine B. Barbee, MSN, ANP, F-NP-C
Kaiser Permanente
Washington, District of Columbia

Lisa Brown
Jackson State Community College
Jackson, Tennessee

Marla J. DeJong, RN, MS, CCRN, CEN, Capt.
Wilford Hall Medical Center
Lackland Air Force Base, Texas

Diane M. Ford, RN, MS, CCRN
Andrews University
Berrien Springs, Michigan

Denise D. Hopkins, PharmD
College of Pharmacy
University of Arkansas
Little Rock, Arkansas

Barbara D. Horton, RN, MS
Arnot Ogden Medical Center School of Nursing
Elmira, New York

Mary Beth Jenkins, RN, CCRN, CAPA
Elliott One Day Surgery Center
Manchester, New Hampshire

Kelly W. Jones, PharmD, BCPS
McLeod Family Medicine Center
McLeod Regional Medical Center
Florence, South Carolina

Autumn E. Korson
Western Michigan University Bronson School of Nursing
Kalamazoo, Michigan

Linda Laskowski-Jones, RN, MS, CS, CCRN, CEN
Christiana Care Health System
Newark, Delaware

Jessica K. Leet, RN, BSN
Cardinal Glennon Children's Hospital
St. Louis, Missouri

Denise Macklin, BSN, RNC, CRNI
President, Professional Learning Systems, Inc.
Marietta, Georgia

Nancy L. McCartney
Valencia Community College
Orlando, Florida

Judith L. Myers, MSN, RN
Health Sciences Center
St. Louis University School of Nursing
St. Louis, Missouri

Kimberly R. Pugh, MSEd, RN, BS
Nurse Consultant
Baltimore, Maryland

Regina T. Schiavello, BSN, RNC
Wills Eye Hospital
Philadelphia, Pennsylvania

Gregory M. Susla, PharmD, FCCM
National Institutes of Health
Bethesda, Maryland

Elizabeth Taylor
Tennessee Wesleyan College of Nursing
Fort Saunders Regional
Knoxville, Tennessee

REVIEWERS

Cheryl Andersen, LPN, BA (Psychology)
Private Duty Nurse
Kirkland, Washington

Darlene Baker, MSN, RN
Green Country Technology Center
Okmulgee, Oklahoma

Michelle Butler
LPN/RN Student
Bellevue, Nebraska

Nikki Cook, RN, BSN, ACLS, PALS, TNCC
Student Nurse
Medcenter One Health Systems College of Nursing
Bismarck, North Dakota

Cené L. Gibson, MSN, RN
LPN Instructor
Francis Tuttle Technology Center
Oklahoma City, Oklahoma

Robert E. Lamb, PharmD
Consultant Pharmacist
REL & Associates, LLC
Downingtown, Pennsylvania

Rachelle Loera
LVN
West Covina Medical Group
West Covina, California

Amber McKenzie, RN, BSN
PICU RNII
Memorial Hermann Children's Hospital
Houston, Texas
School Nurse
West Memorial Jr. High
Katy, Texas

Carolyn Reiter
Student Nurse
Penn Valley School of Nursing
Kansas City, Missouri

Dianne P. Robinson, RN, BSN
Centre Medical and Surgical Associates, P.C.
State College, Pennsylvania

Erica Seamon, PharmD
Natural Standard Research Collaboration
Cambridge, Massachusetts

Marci Lyn Slusser
Nursing Student
Reading Community College
Reading, Pennsylvania

Catherine Ulbricht, PharmD
Natural Standard Research Collaboration
Cambridge, Massachusetts

Shannon Wilson, RN, BS
Clinic
Sherman, Illinois

PREFACE

Nurses are faced with the ever-challenging responsibility of ensuring safe and effective drug therapy for their patients. Not surprisingly, the greatest challenge for nurses is keeping up with the overwhelming amount of new drug information, including the latest FDA-approved drugs and changes to already approved drugs, such as new uses, dosage forms, warnings, and much more. Nurses must integrate this information into their patient care quickly and in an informed manner.

Saunders Nursing Drug Handbook 2008 is designed as an easy-to-use source of current drug information to help the busy nurse meet these challenges. What separates this book from others is that it guides the nurse through patient care to better practice and better care.

This handbook contains the following:

1. **An IV Compatibility Chart.** This handy chart is updated in this edition and bound into the handbook to prevent accidental loss.
2. **The Classification Section.** The action and uses for some of the most common clinical and pharmacotherapeutic classes are presented. This section includes a classification that is new to this edition, medications that treat systemic fungal infections. Unique to this handbook, each class provides an at-a-glance table that compares all the generic drugs within the classification according to product availability, dosages, side effects, and other characteristics. Its purple full-page color tab ensures you can't miss it!
3. **An attractive four-color atlas of medications.** This section contains photographs of 158 of the most commonly used oral medications. The medications, both brand and generic, are shown in their different dosage forms. Just look for the glossy purple full-page color tab to help you identify those medications presented to you sans prescription bottle or order. A 💊 appears in the individual drug entries when there is a corresponding illustration in the atlas.
4. **An alphabetical listing of drug entries by generic name.** Purple letter thumb tabs help you page through this section quickly. New to this edition is information alerting you to drugs that should not be crushed. The icon, shown in the Availability section, identifies these non-crushable formulations. Tall Man lettering, with emphasis on certain syllables to avoid confusing similar sounding/looking medications, is shown in slim purple capitalized letters (e.g., *aceta**ZOLAMIDE**). High Alert drugs with a purple flag are considered dangerous by the Joint Commission on Accreditation of Healthcare Organizations (JCAHO) and the Institute for Safe Medication Practices (ISMP) because if they are administered incorrectly, they may cause life-threatening or permanent harm to the patient. The entire High Alert generic drug entry sits on a purple-shaded background so it's easy to spot! To make scanning pages easier, each new entry begins with a shaded box containing the generic name, pronunciation, trade name(s), fixed-combination(s), and classification(s).

5. **Herbal entries.** Included in this edition are 17 of the most commonly used herbs, each indicated with a purple leaf. In this edition, each herb is cross-referenced to the Herbal Therapies and Interactions (Appendix G) so that you have the most comprehensive view of herbal therapies related to patient care.
6. **Trade name cross-references in the A to Z section of the book.** We have over 400 of the most-prescribed trade name drugs with cross-references within the A to Z section! These entries are shaded in gray for easy identification.
7. **A comprehensive reference section.** Appendixes include vital information on calculation of doses, controlled drugs, cytochrome P450 enzymes, drip rates for critical care medications, drugs of abuse, equi-analgesic dosing, FDA pregnancy categories, herbal therapies and interactions, lifespan and cultural aspects of drug therapy, non-crushable drugs, normal laboratory values, orphan drugs, poison antidotes, recommended childhood and adult immunizations, signs and symptoms of electrolyte imbalance, sound-alike and look-alike drugs, Spanish phrases often used in clinical settings, and techniques of medication administration.
8. **Drugs by Disorder.** You'll find Drugs by Disorder in the front of the book for easy reference. It lists common disorders and the drugs often used for treatment.
9. **The index.** The comprehensive index is located at the back of the book on light purple pages. Undoubtedly the best tool to help you navigate the handbook, the comprehensive index is organized by showing generic drug names in **bold**, trade names in regular type, classifications in *italics,* drugs with expanded information on the Internet with an EVOLVE icon evolve, and the page number of the main drug entry listed first and in **bold.**
10. **A mini CD. Saunders Nursing Drug Handbook 2008** has a mini CD-ROM packaged in the back of the book. The software features 340 monographs for most commonly used medications. Users can customize and print these drug entries.

A DETAILED GUIDE TO THE SAUNDERS NURSING DRUG HANDBOOK

An intensive review by Consultants and Reviewers helped us to revise the **Saunders Nursing Drug Handbook** so that it is most useful in educational and clinical practice. The main objective of the handbook is to provide essential drug information in a user-friendly format. The bulk of the handbook contains an alphabetical listing of drug entries by generic name.

To maintain the portability of this handbook and meet the challenge of keeping content current, we have also included additional information for some medications on an EVOLVE Internet site. EVOLVE also includes drug alerts (e.g., medications removed from the market) and drug updates (e.g., new drugs, updates on existing entries). Information is periodically added, allowing the nurse to keep abreast of current drug information. The drug entries with EVOLVE enhancement are indicated with an EVOLVE icon evolve next to the generic drug name.

You'll also notice that some entries for infrequently used medications are condensed to reflect only the absolutely essential points the nurse should know when called upon to administer them.

We have incorporated the IV Incompatibilities heading. The drugs listed in this section are not compatible with the generic drug when administered directly by IV push, via Y-site, or via IV piggyback. We have highlighted the intravenous drug administration and handling information with a special heading icon and have broken it down by Reconstitution, Rate of Administration, and Storage.

We present entries in an order that follows the logical thought process the nurse undergoes whenever a drug is ordered for a patient:

- What is the drug?
- How is the drug classified?
- What does the drug do?
- What is the drug used for?
- Under what conditions should you **not** use the drug?
- How do you administer the drug?
- How do you store the drug?
- What is the dose of the drug?
- What should you monitor the patient for once he or she has received the drug?
- What do you assess the patient for?
- What interventions should you perform?
- What should you teach the patient?

The following are included within the drug entries:

Generic Name, Pronunciation, Trade Names. Each entry begins with the generic name and pronunciation, followed by the U.S. and Canadian trade names. Exclusively Canadian trade names are followed by a purple maple leaf ♣. Trade names that were most prescribed in the year 2006 are underlined in this section.

Do Not Confuse With. Drug names that sound similar to the generic and/or trade names are listed under this heading to help you avoid potential medication errors.

Fixed-Combination Drugs. Where appropriate, fixed-combinations, or drugs made up of two or more generic medications, are listed with the generic drug.

Pharmacotherapeutic and Clinical Classification Names. Each full entry includes both the pharmacotherapeutic and clinical classifications for the generic drug. When available, the page number of the classification description in the front of the book is provided in this section as well.

Action/Therapeutic Effect. This section describes how the drug is predicted to behave, with the expected therapeutic effect(s) under a separate heading.

Pharmacokinetics. This section includes the absorption, distribution, metabolism, excretion, and half-life of the medication. The half-life is bolded in purple for easy access.

Uses/Off-Label. The listing of uses for each drug includes both the FDA uses and off-label uses. The off-label heading is shown in bold purple for emphasis.

Precautions. This heading incorporates a discussion about when the generic drug is contraindicated or should be used with caution. The cautions warn the nurse of specific situations in which a drug should be closely monitored.

Lifespan Considerations. This section includes the pregnancy category and lactation data, as well as age-specific information concerning children and the elderly.

Interactions. This heading enumerates drug, food, and herbal interactions with the generic drug. As the number of medications a patient receives increases, awareness of drug interactions becomes more important. Also included is information about therapeutic and toxic blood levels in addition to the altered lab values that show what effects the drug may have on lab results.

Product Availability. Each drug monograph gives the form and availability of the drug. A new icon identifies non-crushable drug forms.
Administration/Handling. Instructions for administration are given for each route of administration (e.g., IV, IM, PO, rectal). Special handling, such as refrigeration, is also included where applicable. The routes in this section are always presented in the order IV, IM, Subcutaneous, PO, with subsequent routes in alphabetical order (e.g., Ophthalmic, Otic, Topical). **IV administration** is broken down by reconstitution, rate of administration (how fast the IV should be given), and storage (including how long the medication is stable once reconstituted).
IV Compatibilities/IV Incompatibilities . These sections give the nurse the most comprehensive compatibility information possible when administering medications by direct IV push, via a Y-site, or via IV piggyback. This edition includes information about lipids.
Indications/Routes/Dosage. Each full entry provides specific dosing guidelines for adults, the elderly, children, and patients with renal and/or hepatic impairment. Dosages are clearly indicated for each approved indication and route.
Side Effects. Side effects are defined as those responses that are usually predictable with the drug, are **not** life-threatening, and may or may not require discontinuation of the drug. Unique to this handbook, side effects are grouped by frequency listed from highest occurrence percentage to lowest so that the nurse can focus on patient care without wading through myriad signs and symptoms of side effects.
Adverse Effects/Toxic Reactions. Adverse effects and toxic reactions are very serious and often life-threatening undesirable responses that require prompt intervention from a health care provider.
Nursing Considerations. Nursing considerations are organized as care is organized. That is:

- What needs to be assessed or done before the first dose is administered? (Baseline Assessment)
- What interventions and evaluations are needed during drug therapy? (Intervention/Evaluation)
- What explicit teaching is needed for the patient and family? (Patient/Family Teaching)

Saunders Nursing Drug Handbook is an easy-to-use source of current drug information for nurses, students, and other health care providers. It is our hope that this handbook will help you provide quality care to your patients.

We welcome any comments you may have that would help us to improve future editions of the handbook. Please contact us via the publisher at *http://evolve.elsevier.com/SaundersNDH.*

Barbara B. Hodgson, RN, OCN
Robert J. Kizior, BS, RPh

ACKNOWLEDGMENTS

I offer a special heartfelt thank you to my co-author, Bob Kizior, for his continuing, superb work. Without Bob's effort in this major endeavor, this book would not have reached the par excellence it has achieved. Bob and I particularly and especially thank Cindy Tryniszewski, our Executive Nursing Editor, for her total dedication to making this edition one of Saunders' finest works. It has been a wonderful pleasure working with her through the years. We gratefully acknowledge Gina Hopf and Terri Greenberg, our Developmental Editors, in helping ease our workload. Our thanks also go to Dan Fitzgerald and the staff at Graphic World Publishing Services for their tenacious detail work. It takes many eyes to transform a book into a work of art. Without their efforts, this would not have happened. I thank my siblings, Jane Sperry and Milt, Bruce, Rich, Vance, and Greg Boyd, who have encouraged me through the years; Jim Witmer, BSN, CCRN, CEN, for the many hours he spent assisting me in this huge endeavor and the consistent support he offered; and Andrew Ross, who enlightens my family so dearly.

Barbara Hodgson, RN, OCN

BIBLIOGRAPHY

Briggs GG, Freeman RK, Yaffe SJ: *Drugs in Pregnancy and Lactation: A Reference Guide to Fetal and Neonatal Risk,* ed 7, Philadelphia, 2005, Lippincott Williams & Wilkins.

Drug Facts and Comparisons 2007, Philadelphia, 2006, Lippincott Williams & Wilkins.

Lacy CF, Armstrong LL, Goldman MP, Lance LL: *Lexi-Comp's Drug Information Handbook,* ed 14, Hudson, 2006, Lexi-Comp.

Mosby's Drug Consult 2006, ed 15, St. Louis, 2006, Mosby.

Natural Medicines Comprehensive Database, 2006.

Takemoto CK, Hodding JH, Kraus DM: *Lexi-Comp's Pediatric Dosage Handbook,* ed 12, Hudson, 2004, Lexi-Comp.

Trissel LA: *Handbook of Injectable Drugs,* ed 14, Bethesda, MD, 2006, American Society of Health-System Pharmacists.

USPDI Drug Information for the Health Care Professional, 2006.

ILLUSTRATION CREDITS

Kee JL, Hayes ER, McCuiston LE (eds): *Pharmacology: A Nursing Process Approach,* ed 5, Philadelphia, 2006, WB Saunders.

Mosby's GenRx, ed 12, St. Louis, 2004, Mosby.

DRUGS BY DISORDER

Note: Not all medications appropriate for a given condition are listed, nor are those not listed inappropriate.

Generic names appear first, followed by brand names in parentheses.

Allergy
Beclomethasone (Beclovent, Vanceril)
Betamethasone (Celestone)
Brompheniramine (Dimetane)
Budesonide (Pulmicort, Rhinocort)
Chlorpheniramine (Chlor-Trimeton)
Clemastine (Tavist)
Cyproheptadine (Periactin)
Desloratadine (Clarinex)
Dexamethasone (Decadron)
Dimenhydrinate (Dramamine)
Diphenhydramine (Benadryl)
Epinephrine (Adrenalin)
Fexofenadine (Allegra)
Flunisolide (AeroBid, Nasalide)
Fluticasone (Flovent)
Hydrocortisone (Solu-Cortef)
Loratadine (Claritin)
Prednisolone (Prelone)
Prednisone (Deltasone)
Promethazine (Phenergan)
Triamcinolone (Kenalog)

Alzheimer's disease
Donepezil (Aricept)
Galantamine (Reminyl)
Memantine (Namenda)
Rivastigmine (Exelon)
Tacrine (Cognex)

Angina
Amlodipine (Norvasc)
Atenolol (Tenormin)
Diltiazem (Cardizem, Dilacor)
Isosorbide (Imdur, Isordil)
Metoprolol (Lopressor)
Nadolol (Corgard)
Nicardipine (Cardene)
Nifedipine (Adalat, Procardia)
Nitroglycerin
Propranolol (Inderal)
Ranolazine (Ranexa)
Timolol (Blocadron)
Verapamil (Calan, Isoptin)

Anxiety
Alprazolam (Xanax)
Buspirone (BuSpar)
Diazepam (Valium)
Hydroxyzine (Atarax, Vistaril)
Lorazepam (Ativan)
Oxazepam (Serax)
Venlafaxine (Effexor)

Arrhythmias
Acebutolol (Sectral)
Adenosine (Adenocard)
Amiodarone (Cordarone, Pacerone)
Digoxin (Lanoxin)
Diltiazem (Cardizem, Dilacor)
Disopyramide (Norpace)
Dofetilide (Tikosyn)
Esmolol (Brevibloc)
Ibutilide (Corvert)
Lidocaine
Mexiletine (Mexitil)
Moricizine (Ethmozine)
Procainamide (Procan, Pronestyl)
Propafenone (Rythmol)
Propranolol (Inderal)
Quinidine
Sotalol (Betapace)
Tocainide (Tonocard)
Verapamil (Calan, Isoptin)

Arthritis, rheumatoid (RA)
Abatacept (Orencia)
Adalimumab (Humira)
Anakinra (Kineret)
Aspirin

Auranofin (Ridaura)
Aurothioglucose (Solganal)
Azathioprine (Imuran)
Betamethasone (Celestone)
Capsaicin (Zostrix)
Celecoxib (Celebrex)
Cyclosporine (Sandimmune)
Diclofenac (Cataflam, Voltaren)
Diflunisal (Dolobid)
Etanercept (Enbrel)
Hydroxychloroquine (Plaquenil)
Infliximab (Remicade)
Leflunomide (Arava)
Methotrexate
Penicillamine (Cuprimine)
Prednisone (Deltasone)
Rituximab (Rituxan)

Asthma
Albuterol (Proventil, Ventolin)
Aminophylline (Theophylline)
Arformoterol (Brovana)
Beclomethasone (Beclovent, Vanceril)
Budesonide (Pulmicort)
Cromolyn (Crolom, Intal)
Dexamethasone (Decadron)
Epinephrine (Adrenalin)
Flunisolide (AeroBid)
Fluticasone (Flovent)
Formoterol (Foradil)
Hydrocortisone (Solu-Cortef)
Ipratropium (Atrovent)
Levalbuterol (Xopenex)
Metaproterenol (Alupent)
Methylprednisolone (Solu-Medrol)
Mometasone (Asmanex)
Montelukast (Singulair)
Nedocromil (Tilade)
Prednisolone (Prelone)
Prednisone (Deltasone)
Salmeterol (Serevent)
Terbutaline (Brethine)
Theophylline (SloBid)
Zafirlukast (Accolate)

Attention deficit hyperactivity disorder (ADHD)
Atomoxetine (Strattera)
Bupropion (Wellbutrin)
Desipramine (Norpramin)
Dexmethylphenidate (Focalin)
Dextroamphetamine (Dexedrine)
Imipramine (Tofranil)
Methylphenidate (Ritalin)
Mixed amphetamine (Adderall)
Modafinil (Provigil)

Benign prostatic hypertrophy (BPH)
Alfuzosin (UroXatral)
Doxazosin (Cardura)
Dutasteride (Avodart)
Finasteride (Proscar)
Oxybutynin (Ditropan)
Tamsulosin (Flomax)
Terazosin (Hytrin)

Bladder hyperactivity
Darifenacin (Enablex)
Solifenacin (VESIcare)
Tolterodine (Detrol)
Trospium (Sanctura)

Bronchospasm
Albuterol (Proventil, Ventolin)
Bitolterol (Tornalate)
Epinephrine (Adrenalin)
Levalbuterol (Xopenex)
Metaproterenol (Alupent)
Salmeterol (Serevent)
Terbutaline (Brethine)

Cancer
Abarelix (Plenaxis)
Aldesleukin (Proleukin)
Alemtuzumab (Campath)
Alitretinoin (Panretin)
Altretamine (Hexalen)
Anastrozole (Arimidex)
Arsenic trioxide (Trisenox)
Asparaginase (Elspar)
Azacitadine (Vidaza)
BCG (TheraCys, Tice BCG)
Bevacizumab (Avastin)
Bexarotene (Targretin)
Bicalutamide (Casodex)
Bleomycin (Blenoxane)
Bortezomib (Velcade)
Busulfan (Myleran)
Capecitabine (Xeloda)
Carboplatin (Paraplatin)

Carmustine (BiCNU)
Cetuximab (Erbitux)
Chlorambucil (Leukeran)
Cisplatin (Platinol)
Cladribine (Leustatin)
Clofarabine (Clolar)
Cyclophosphamide (Cytoxan)
Cytarabine (Ara-C, Cytosar)
Dacarbazine (DTIC)
Dactinomycin (Cosmegen)
Dasatinib (Sprycel)
Daunorubicin (Cerubidine, DaunoXome)
Denileukin (Ontak)
Docetaxel (Taxotere)
Doxorubicin (Adriamycin, Doxil)
Epirubicin (Ellence)
Erlotinib (Tarceva)
Estramustine (Emcyt)
Etoposide (VePesid)
Fludarabine (Fludara)
Fluorouracil
Flutamide (Eulexin)
Fulvestrant (Faslodex)
Gefitnib (Iressa)
Gemcitabine (Gemzar)
Gemtuzumab (Mylotarg)
Goserelin (Zoladex)
Hydroxyurea (Hydrea)
Ibritumomab (Zevalin)
Idarubicin (Idamycin)
Ifosfamide (Ifex)
Imatinib (Gleevec)
Interferon alfa-2a (Roferon A)
Interferon alfa-2b (Intron A)
Irinotecan (Camptosar)
Letrozole (Femara)
Leuprolide (Lupron)
Lomustine (CeeNU)
Mechlorethamine (Mustargen)
Megestrol (Megace)
Melphalan (Alkeran)
Mercaptopurine (Purinethol)
Methotrexate
Mitomycin (Mutamycin)
Mitotane (Lysodren)
Mitoxantrone (Novantrone)
Nelarabine (Arranon)
Nilutamide (Nilandron)
Oxaliplatin (Eloxatin)
Paclitaxel (Taxol)
Panitumumab (Vectibix)
Pemetrexed (Alimta)
Pentostatin (Nipent)
Plicamycin (Mithracin)
Procarbazine (Matulane)
Rituximab (Rituxan)
Sorafenib (Nexavar)
Streptozocin (Zanosar)
Sunitinib (Sutent)
Tamoxifen (Nolvadex)
Temozolomide (Temodar)
Teniposide (Vumon)
Thioguanine
Thiotepa (Thioplex)
Topotecan (Hycamtin)
Toremifene (Fareston)
Tositumomab (Ber)
Trastuzumab (Herceptin)
Tretinoin (Vesanoid)
Valrubicin (Valstar)
Vinblastine (Velban)
Vincristine (Oncovin)
Vinorelbine (Navelbine)
Vorinostat (Zolinza)

Cerebrovascular accident (CVA)
Aspirin
Clopidogrel (Plavix)
Heparin
Nimodipine (Nimotop)
Ticlopidine (Ticlid)
Warfarin (Coumadin)

Chronic obstructive pulmonary disease (COPD)
Albuterol (Proventil, Ventolin)
Aminophylline (Theophylline)
Budesonide (Pulmicort)
Epinephrine (Adrenalin)
Formoterol (Foradil)
Levalbuterol (Xopenex)
Metaproterenol (Alupent)
Salmeterol (Serevent)
Theophylline (SloBid)
Tiotropium (Spiriva)

Congestive heart failure (CHF)
Bisoprolol (Zebeta)
Bumetanide (Bumex)
Candesartan (Atacand)

Captopril (Capoten)
Carvedilol (Coreg)
Digoxin (Lanoxin)
Dobutamine (Dobutrex)
Dopamine (Intropin)
Enalapril (Vasotec)
Fosinopril (Monopril)
Furosemide (Lasix)
Hydralazine (Apresoline)
Isosorbide (Isordil)
Lisinopril (Prinivil, Zestril)
Losartan (Cozaar)
Metoprolol (Lopressor)
Milrinone (Primacor)
Nitroglycerin
Nitroprusside (Nipride)
Quinapril (Accupril)
Ramipril (Altace)
Torsemide (Demadex)
Valsartan (Diovan)

Constipation
Bisacodyl (Dulcolax)
Docusate (Colace)
Lactulose (Kristalose)
Lubriprostone (Amitiza)
Methylcellulose (Citrucel)
Milk of magnesia (MOM)
Polyethylene glycol (Miralax)
Psyllium (Metamucil)
Senna (Senokot)
Tegaserod (Zelnorm)

Crohn's disease
Cyclosporine (Neoral)
Hydrocortisone (Cortenema)
Infliximab (Remicade)
Mesalamine (Asacol, Pentasa)
Olsalazine (Dipentum)
Sulfasalazine (Azulfidine)

Deep vein thrombosis (DVT)
Dalteparin (Fragmin)
Enoxaparin (Lovenox)
Heparin
Tinzaparin (Innohep)
Warfarin (Coumadin)

Depression
Amitriptyline (Elavil, Endep)
Bupropion (Wellbutrin)
Citalopram (Celexa)
Clomipramine (Anafranil)
Desipramine (Norpramin)
Doxepin (Sinequan)
Escitalopram (Lexapro)
Fluoxetine (Prozac)
Imipramine (Tofranil)
Maprotiline (Ludiomil)
Mirtazapine (Remeron)
Nefazodone
Nortriptyline (Aventyl, Pamelor)
Paroxetine (Paxil)
Phenelzine (Nardil)
Sertraline (Zoloft)
Tranylcypromine (Parnate)
Trazodone (Desyrel)
Venlafaxine (Effexor)

Diabetes mellitus
Acarbose (Precose)
Chlorpropamide (Diabinese)
Exenatide (Byetta)
Glimepiride (Amaryl)
Glipizide (Glucotrol)
Glyburide (Micronase)
Insulin
Metformin (Glucophage)
Miglitol (Glyset)
Nateglinide (Starlix)
Pioglitazone (Actos)
Pramlintide (Symlin)
Repaglinide (Prandin)
Rosiglitazone (Avandia)
Sitagliptin (Januvia)

Diabetic peripheral neuropathy
Amitriptyline (Elavil)
Bupropion (Wellbutrin)
Carbamazepine (Tegretol)
Citalopram (Celexa)
Duloxetine (Cymbalta)
Gabapentin (Neurontin)
Lamotrigine (Lamictal)
Lidocaine patch (Lidoderm)
Methadone (Dolophine)
Nortriptyline (Pamelor)
Oxcarbazepine (Trileptal)
Oxycodone (Oxycontin)

Paroxetine (Paxil)
Phenytoin (Dilantin)
Pregabalin (Lyrica)
Tramadol (Ultram)
Venlafaxine (Effexor)

Diarrhea
Bismuth subsalicylate (Pepto-Bismol)
Diphenoxylate and atropine (Lomotil)
Kaolin-pectin (Kaopectate)
Loperamide (Imodium)
Octreotide (Sandostatin)
Rifaximin (Xifaxan)

Duodenal, gastric ulcer
Cimetidine (Tagamet)
Esomeprazole (Nexium)
Famotidine (Pepcid)
Lansoprazole (Prevacid)
Misoprostol (Cytotec)
Nizatidine (Axid)
Omeprazole (Prilosec)
Pantoprazole (Protonix)
Rabeprazole (Aciphex)
Ranitidine (Zantac)
Sucralfate (Carafate)

Edema
Amiloride (Midamor)
Bumetanide (Bumex)
Chlorthalidone (Hygroton)
Ethacrynic acid (Edecrin)
Furosemide (Lasix)
Hydrochlorothiazide (HydroDIURIL)
Indapamide (Lozol)
Metolazone (Zaroxolyn)
Spironolactone (Aldactone)
Torsemide (Demadex)
Triamterene (Dyrenium)

Epilepsy
Acetazolamide (Diamox)
Carbamazepine (Tegretol)
Clonazepam (Klonopin)
Clorazepate (Tranxene)
Diazepam (Valium)
Fosphenytoin (Cerebyx)
Gabapentin (Neurontin)
Lamotrigine (Lamictal)
Levetiracetam (Keppra)
Lorazepam (Ativan)
Oxcarbazepine (Trileptal)
Phenobarbital
Phenytoin (Dilantin)
Primidone (Mysoline)
Tiagabine (Gabitril)
Topiramate (Topamax)
Valproic acid (Depakene, Depakote)
Zonisamide (Zonegran)

Esophageal reflux, esophagitis
Cimetidine (Tagamet)
Esomeprazole (Nexium)
Famotidine (Pepcid)
Lansoprazole (Prevacid)
Nizatidine (Axid)
Omeprazole (Prilosec)
Pantoprazole (Protonix)
Rabeprazole (Aciphex)
Ranitidine (Zantac)

Fever
Acetaminophen (Tylenol)
Aspirin
Ibuprofen (Advil, Motrin)
Naproxen (Aleve, Anaprox, Naprosyn)

Fibromyalgia
Acetaminophen (Tylenol)
Amitriptyline (Elavil)
Carisoprodol (Soma)
Citalopram (Celexa)
Cyclobenzapine (Flexeril)
Duloxetine (Cymbalta)
Fluoxetine (Prozac)
Pregabalin (Lyrica)
Tramadol (Ultram)
Venlafaxine (Effexor)

Gastritis
Cimetidine (Tagamet)
Famotidine (Pepcid)
Nizatidine (Axid)
Ranitidine (Zantac)

Gastroesophageal reflux disease (GERD)
Cimetidine (Tagamet)
Esomeprazole (Nexium)
Famotidine (Pepcid)

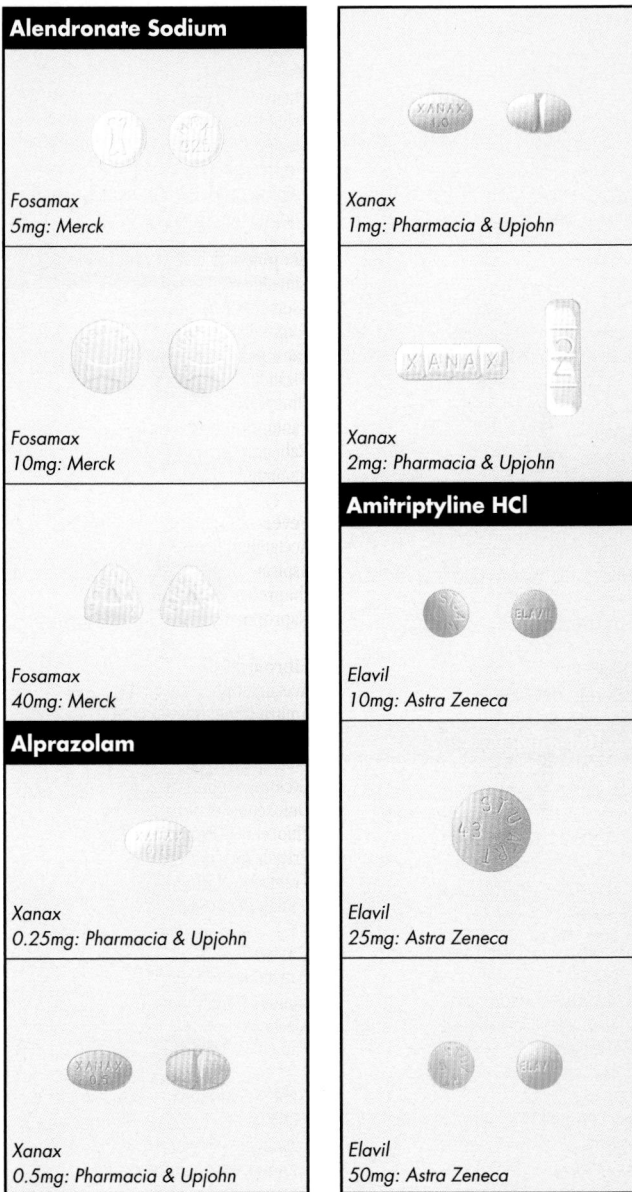

Alendronate Sodium

Fosamax
5mg: Merck

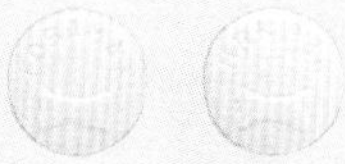

Fosamax
10mg: Merck

Fosamax
40mg: Merck

Alprazolam

Xanax
0.25mg: Pharmacia & Upjohn

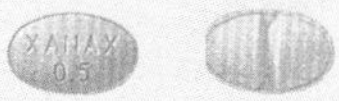

Xanax
0.5mg: Pharmacia & Upjohn

Xanax
1mg: Pharmacia & Upjohn

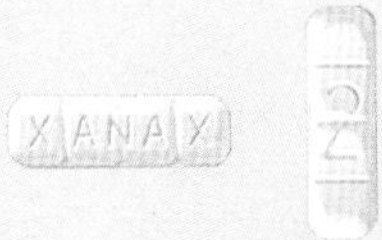

Xanax
2mg: Pharmacia & Upjohn

Amitriptyline HCl

Elavil
10mg: Astra Zeneca

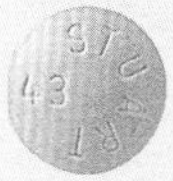

Elavil
25mg: Astra Zeneca

Elavil
50mg: Astra Zeneca

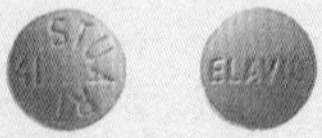

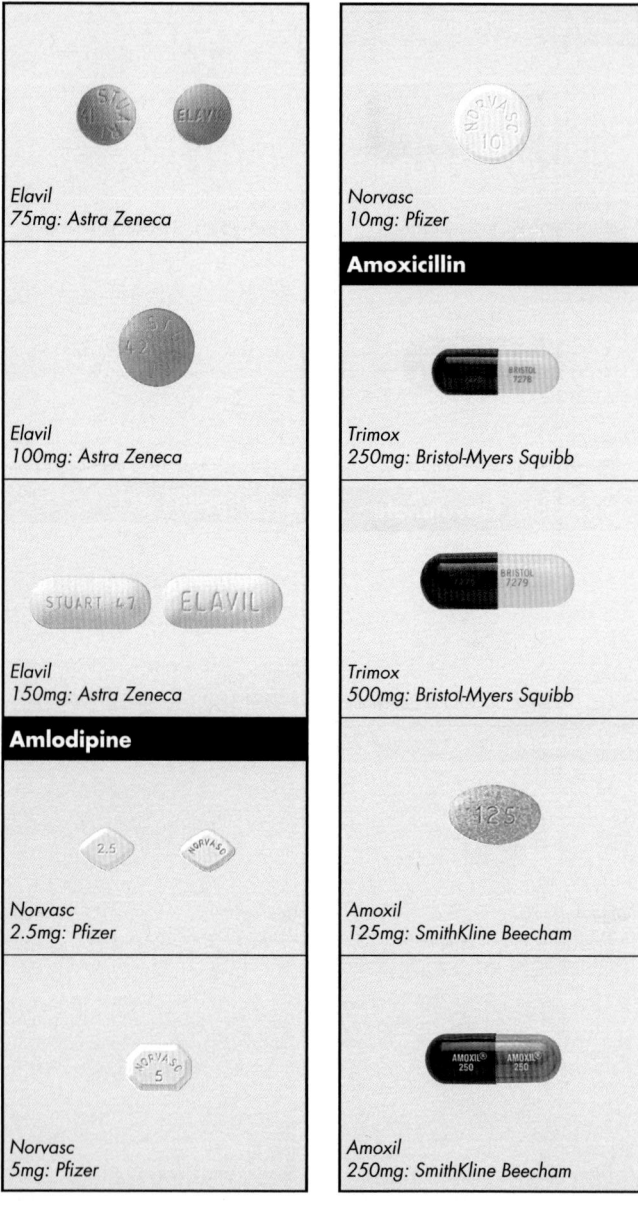

Elavil
75mg: Astra Zeneca

Elavil
100mg: Astra Zeneca

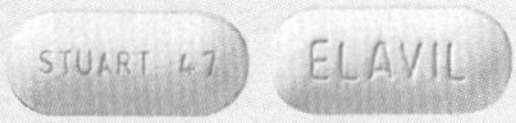

Elavil
150mg: Astra Zeneca

Amlodipine

Norvasc
2.5mg: Pfizer

Norvasc
5mg: Pfizer

Norvasc
10mg: Pfizer

Amoxicillin

Trimox
250mg: Bristol-Myers Squibb

Trimox
500mg: Bristol-Myers Squibb

Amoxil
125mg: SmithKline Beecham

Amoxil
250mg: SmithKline Beecham

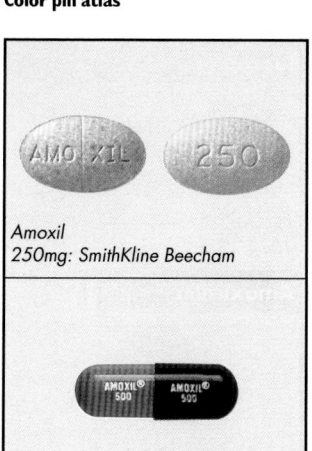

Amoxil
250mg: SmithKline Beecham

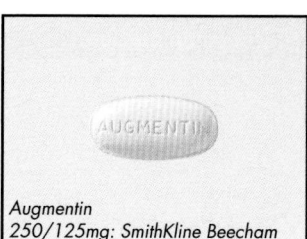

Amoxil
500mg: SmithKline Beecham

Amoxicillin; Clavulanate

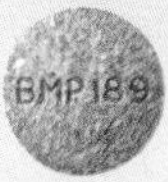

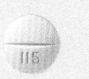

Augmentin
125/31.25mg: SmithKline Beecham

Augmentin
200mg: SmithKline Beecham

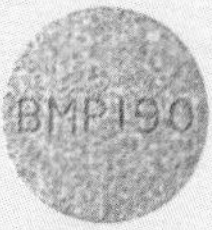

Augmentin
250/62.5mg: SmithKline Beecham

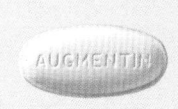

Augmentin
250/125mg: SmithKline Beecham

Augmentin
500/125mg: SmithKline Beecham

Augmentin
875/125mg: SmithKline Beecham

Atenolol; Chlorthalidone

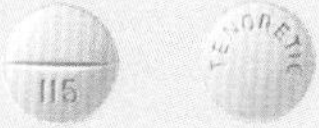

Tenoretic
50/25mg: Astra Zeneca

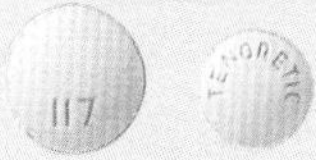

Tenoretic
100/25mg: Astra Zeneca

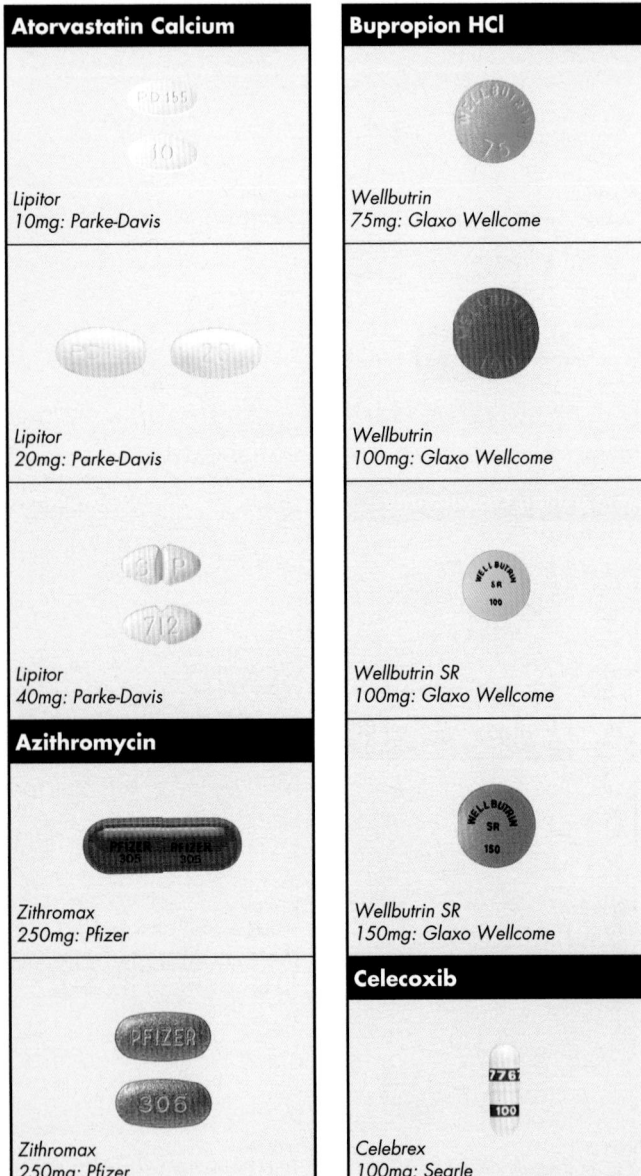

Atorvastatin Calcium

Lipitor
10mg: Parke-Davis

Lipitor
20mg: Parke-Davis

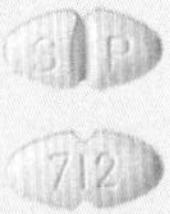

Lipitor
40mg: Parke-Davis

Azithromycin

Zithromax
250mg: Pfizer

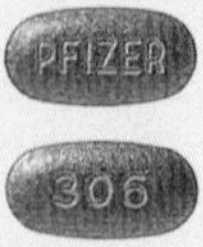

Zithromax
250mg: Pfizer

Bupropion HCl

Wellbutrin
75mg: Glaxo Wellcome

Wellbutrin
100mg: Glaxo Wellcome

Wellbutrin SR
100mg: Glaxo Wellcome

Wellbutrin SR
150mg: Glaxo Wellcome

Celecoxib

Celebrex
100mg: Searle

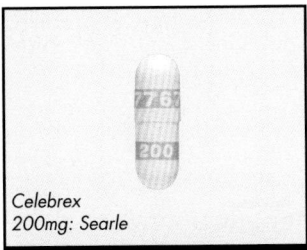

Celebrex
200mg: Searle

Cephalexin

Keflex
250mg: Dista

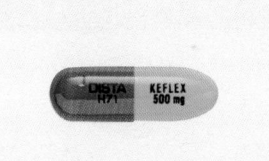

Keflex
500mg: Dista

Cetirizine

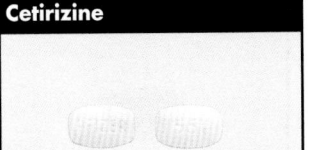

Zyrtec
10mg: Pfizer

Ciprofloxacin HCl

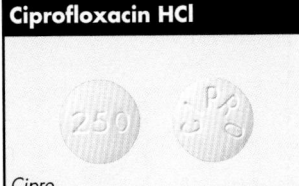

Cipro
250mg: Miles

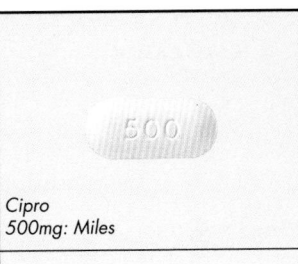

Cipro
500mg: Miles

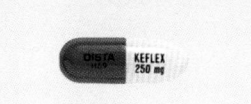

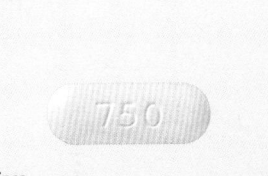

Cipro
750mg: Miles

Citalopram Hydrobromide

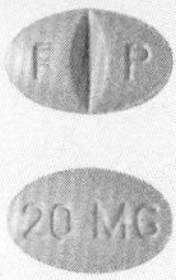

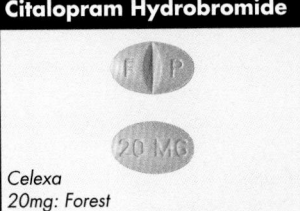

Celexa
20mg: Forest

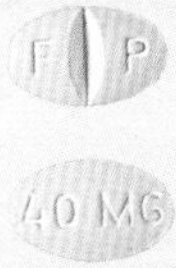

Celexa
40mg: Forest

Clonazepam

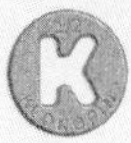

Klonopin
0.5mg: Roche

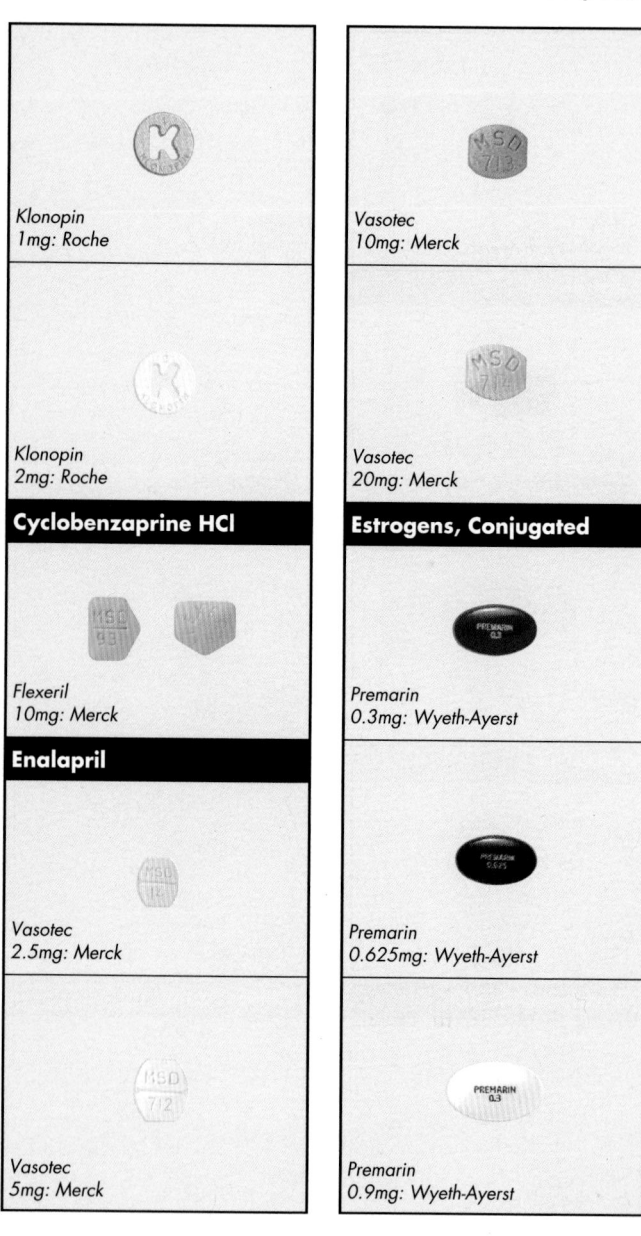

Klonopin
1mg: Roche

Klonopin
2mg: Roche

Cyclobenzaprine HCl

Flexeril
10mg: Merck

Enalapril

Vasotec
2.5mg: Merck

Vasotec
5mg: Merck

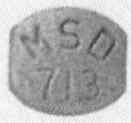

Vasotec
10mg: Merck

Vasotec
20mg: Merck

Estrogens, Conjugated

Premarin
0.3mg: Wyeth-Ayerst

Premarin
0.625mg: Wyeth-Ayerst

Premarin
0.9mg: Wyeth-Ayerst

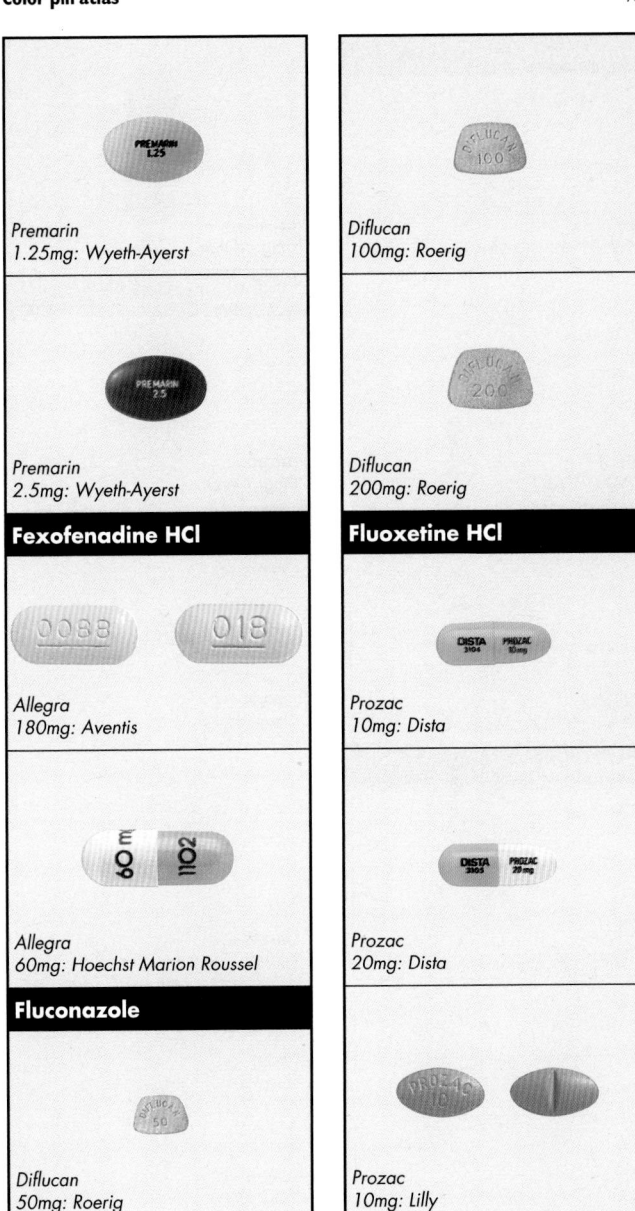

Premarin
1.25mg: Wyeth-Ayerst

Premarin
2.5mg: Wyeth-Ayerst

Fexofenadine HCl

Allegra
180mg: Aventis

Allegra
60mg: Hoechst Marion Roussel

Fluconazole

Diflucan
50mg: Roerig

Diflucan
100mg: Roerig

Diflucan
200mg: Roerig

Fluoxetine HCl

Prozac
10mg: Dista

Prozac
20mg: Dista

Prozac
10mg: Lilly

Furosemide

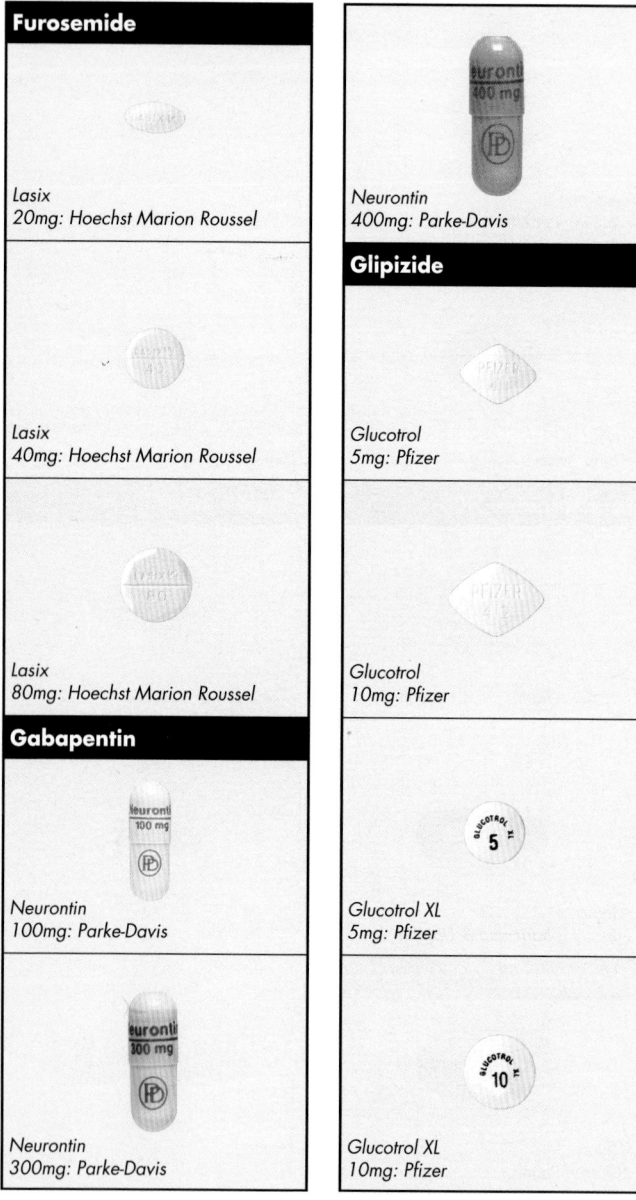

Lasix
20mg: Hoechst Marion Roussel

Lasix
40mg: Hoechst Marion Roussel

Lasix
80mg: Hoechst Marion Roussel

Gabapentin

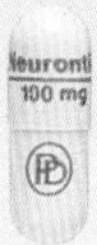

Neurontin
100mg: Parke-Davis

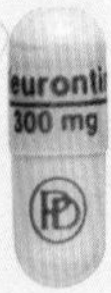

Neurontin
300mg: Parke-Davis

Neurontin
400mg: Parke-Davis

Glipizide

Glucotrol
5mg: Pfizer

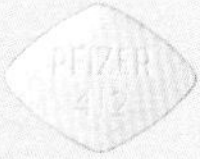

Glucotrol
10mg: Pfizer

Glucotrol XL
5mg: Pfizer

Glucotrol XL
10mg: Pfizer

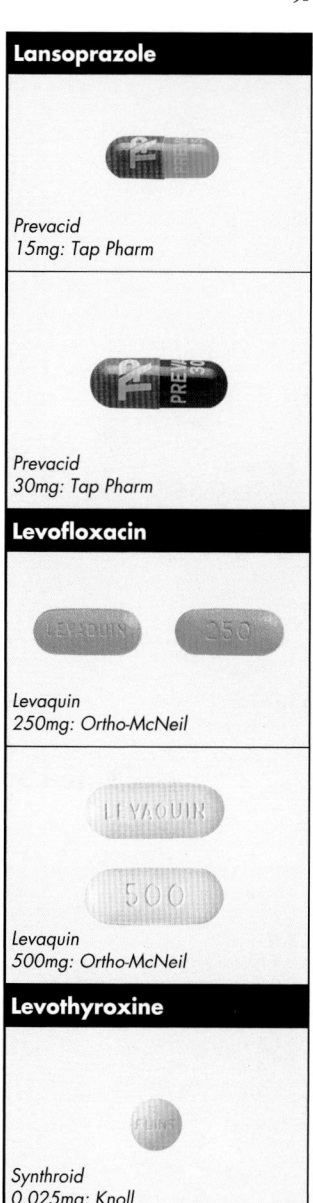

Hydrochlorothiazide

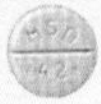

HydroDIURIL
25mg: Merck

HydroDIURIL
50mg: Merck

Ibuprofen

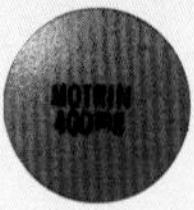

Motrin
400mg: Pharmacia & Upjohn

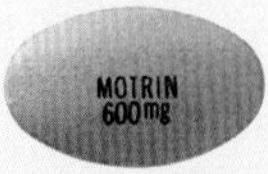

Motrin
600mg: Pharmacia & Upjohn

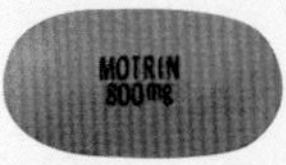

Motrin
800mg: Pharmacia & Upjohn

Lansoprazole

Prevacid
15mg: Tap Pharm

Prevacid
30mg: Tap Pharm

Levofloxacin

Levaquin
250mg: Ortho-McNeil

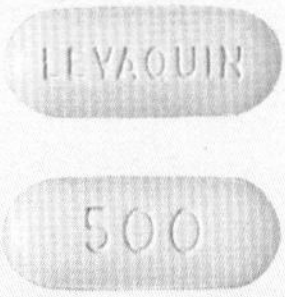

Levaquin
500mg: Ortho-McNeil

Levothyroxine

Synthroid
0.025mg: Knoll

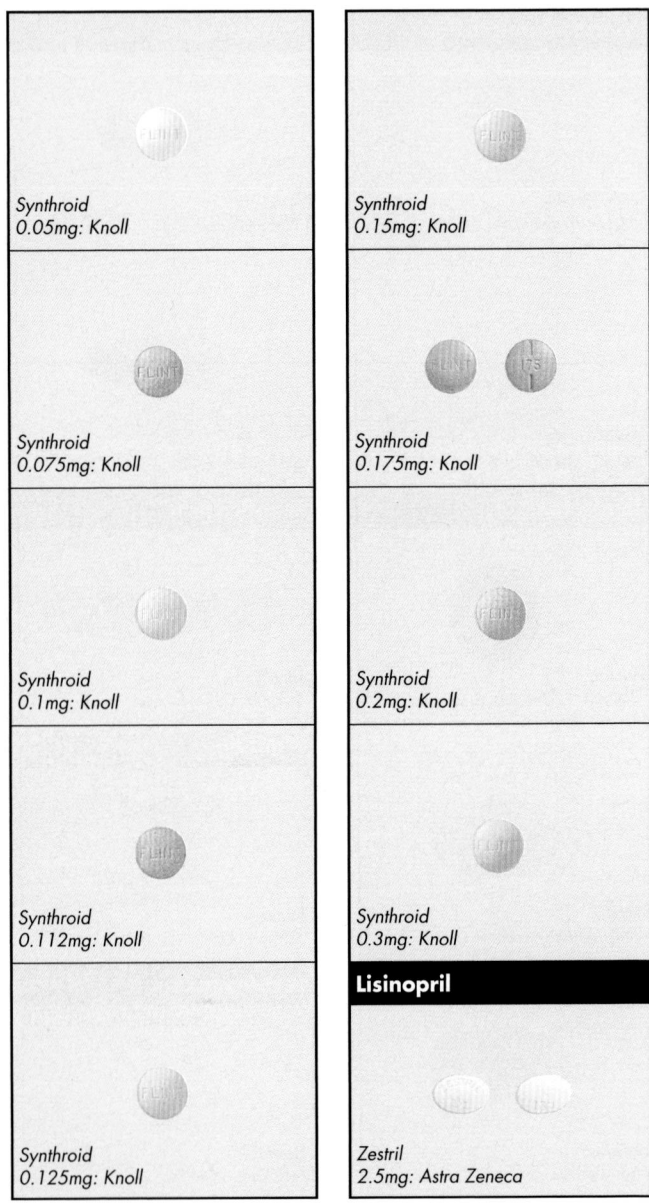

Synthroid
0.05mg: Knoll

Synthroid
0.075mg: Knoll

Synthroid
0.1mg: Knoll

Synthroid
0.112mg: Knoll

Synthroid
0.125mg: Knoll

Synthroid
0.15mg: Knoll

Synthroid
0.175mg: Knoll

Synthroid
0.2mg: Knoll

Synthroid
0.3mg: Knoll

Lisinopril

Zestril
2.5mg: Astra Zeneca

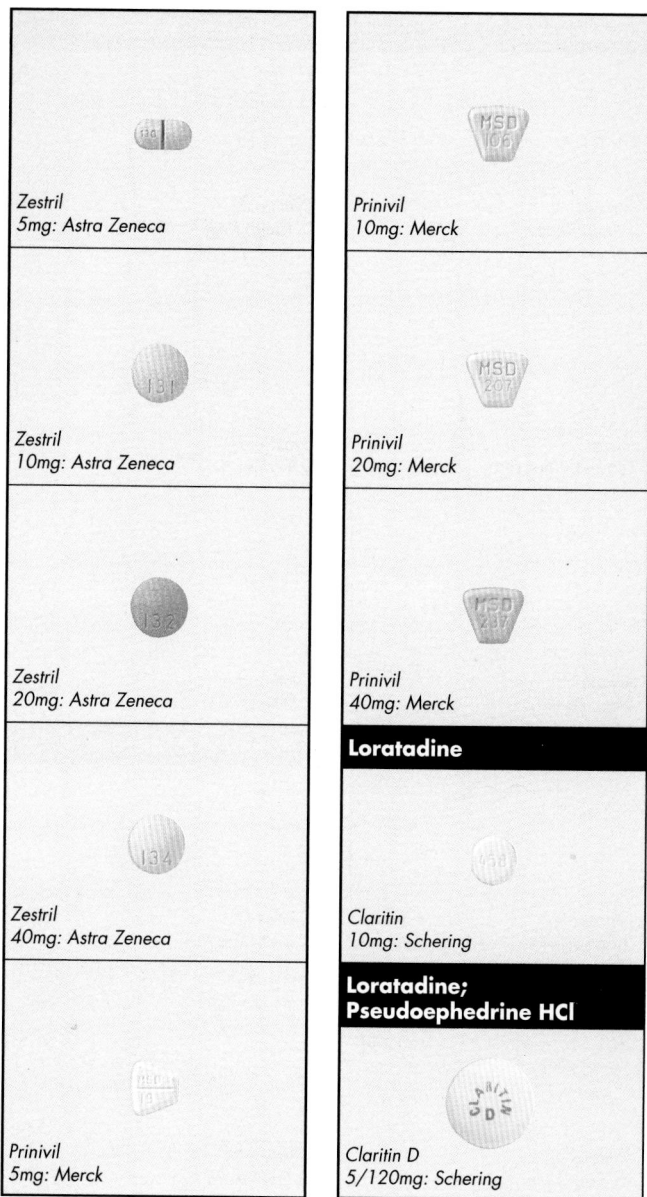

Zestril
5mg: Astra Zeneca

Zestril
10mg: Astra Zeneca

Zestril
20mg: Astra Zeneca

Zestril
40mg: Astra Zeneca

Prinivil
5mg: Merck

Prinivil
10mg: Merck

Prinivil
20mg: Merck

Prinivil
40mg: Merck

Loratadine

Claritin
10mg: Schering

Loratadine; Pseudoephedrine HCl

Claritin D
5/120mg: Schering

Lorazepam

Ativan
0.5mg: Wyeth-Ayerst

Ativan
1mg: Wyeth-Ayerst

Ativan
2mg: Wyeth-Ayerst

Metformin HCl

Glucophage
500mg: Lipha

Glucophage
850mg: Lipha

Metoprolol Succinate

Toprol XL
50mg: Astra Zeneca

Toprol XL
100mg: Astra Zeneca

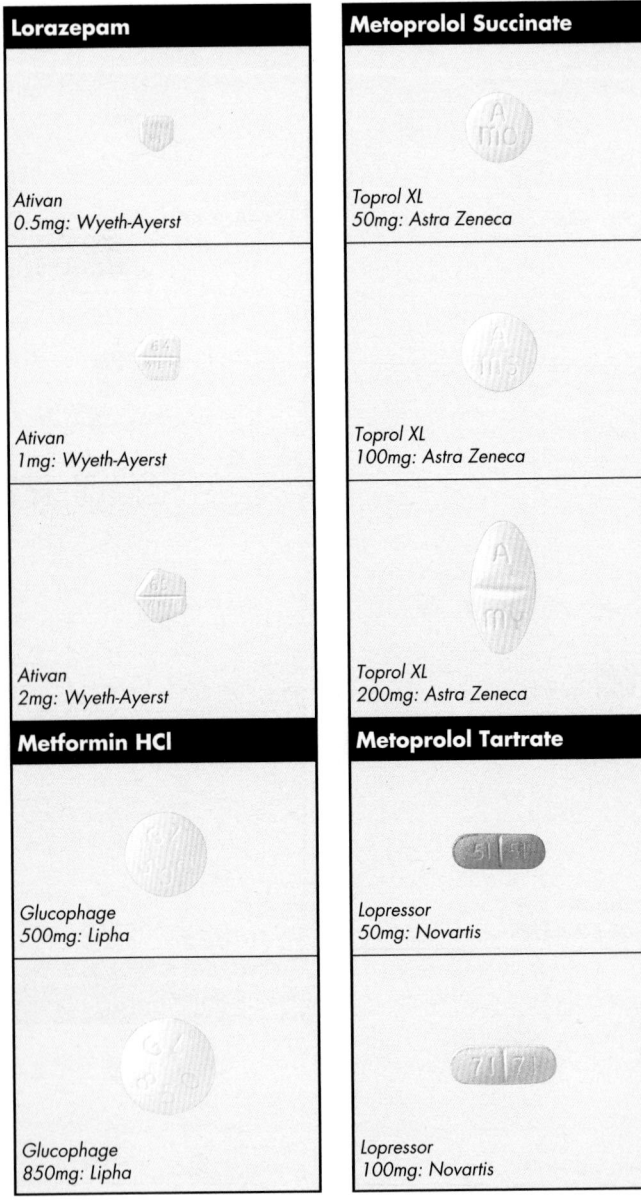

Toprol XL
200mg: Astra Zeneca

Metoprolol Tartrate

Lopressor
50mg: Novartis

Lopressor
100mg: Novartis

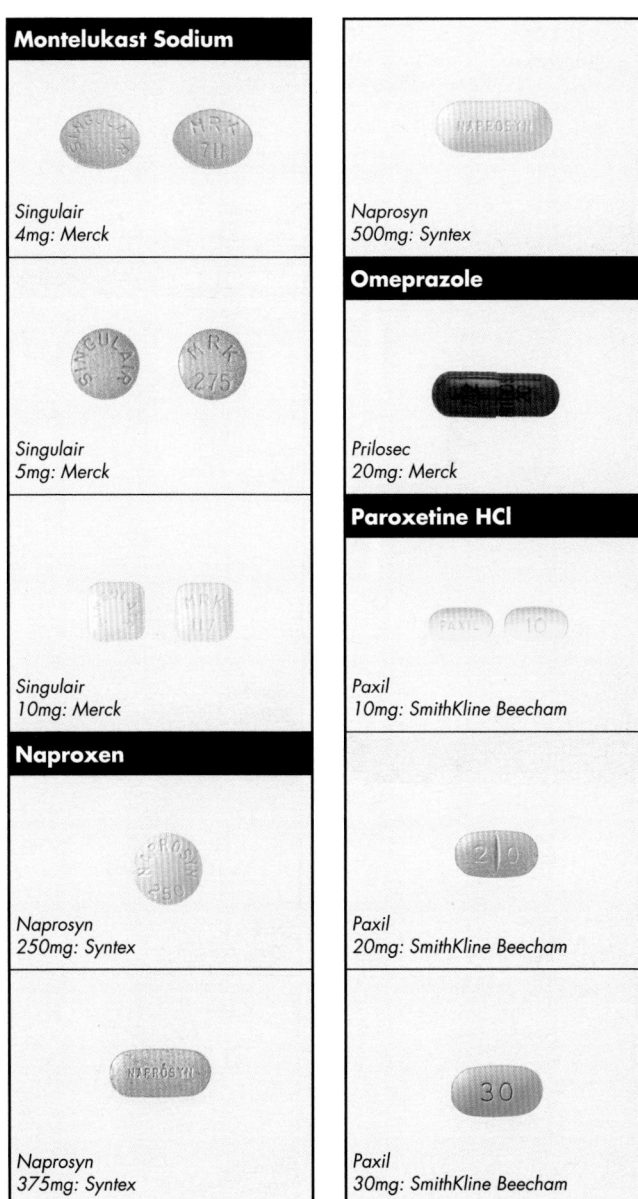

Montelukast Sodium

Singulair
4mg: Merck

Singulair
5mg: Merck

Singulair
10mg: Merck

Naproxen

Naprosyn
250mg: Syntex

Naprosyn
375mg: Syntex

Naprosyn
500mg: Syntex

Omeprazole

Prilosec
20mg: Merck

Paroxetine HCl

Paxil
10mg: SmithKline Beecham

Paxil
20mg: SmithKline Beecham

Paxil
30mg: SmithKline Beecham

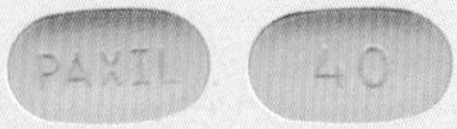

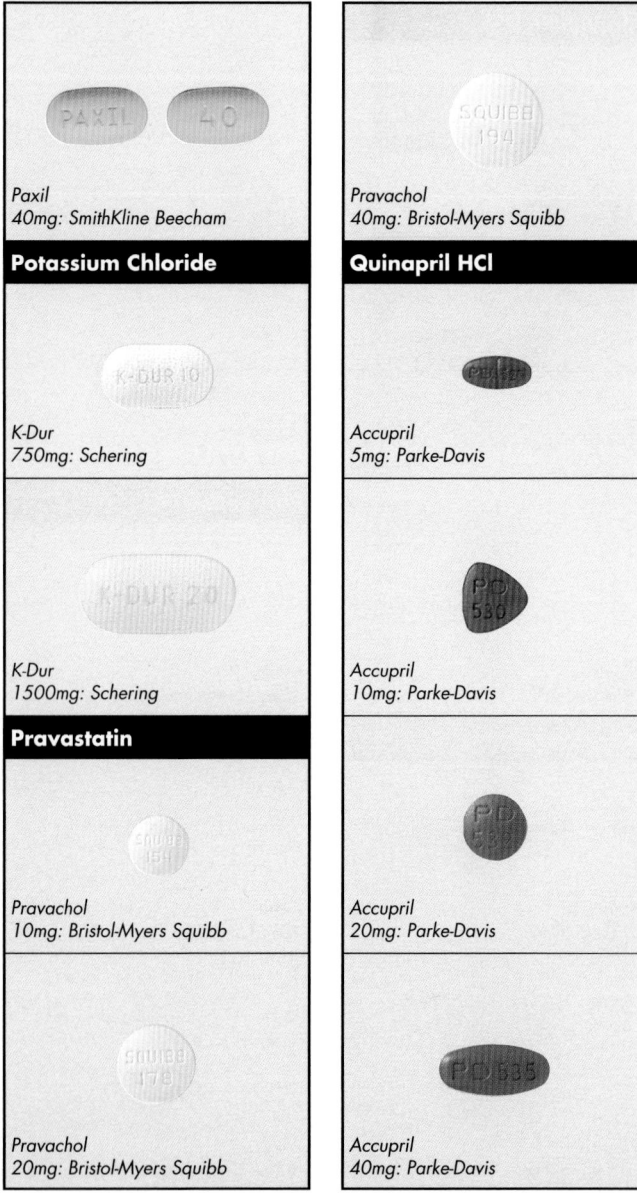

Paxil
40mg: SmithKline Beecham

Potassium Chloride

K-Dur
750mg: Schering

K-Dur
1500mg: Schering

Pravastatin

Pravachol
10mg: Bristol-Myers Squibb

Pravachol
20mg: Bristol-Myers Squibb

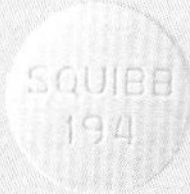

Pravachol
40mg: Bristol-Myers Squibb

Quinapril HCl

Accupril
5mg: Parke-Davis

Accupril
10mg: Parke-Davis

Accupril
20mg: Parke-Davis

Accupril
40mg: Parke-Davis

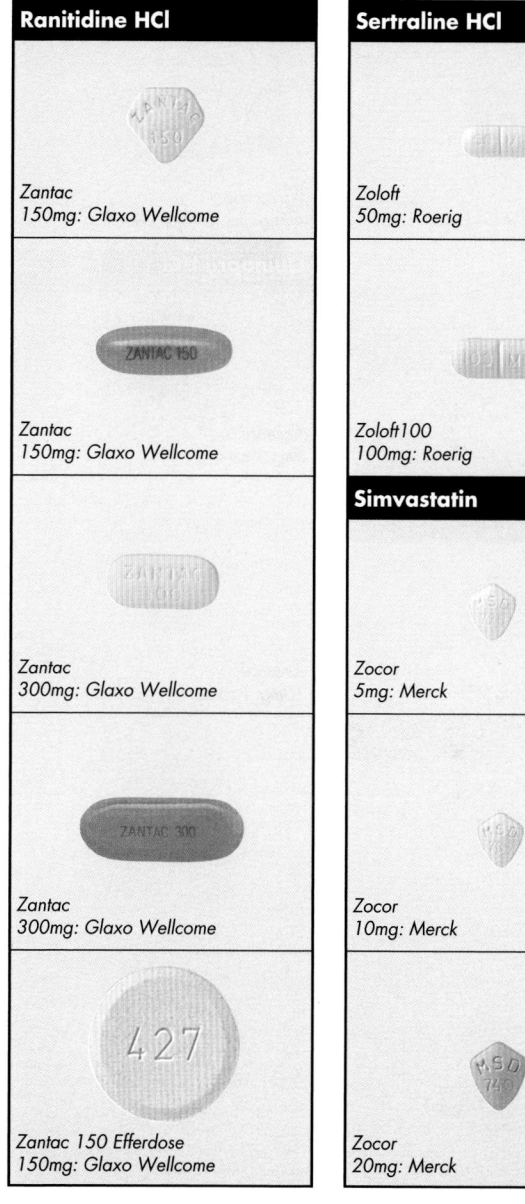

Ranitidine HCl

Zantac
150mg: Glaxo Wellcome

Zantac
150mg: Glaxo Wellcome

Zantac
300mg: Glaxo Wellcome

Zantac
300mg: Glaxo Wellcome

Zantac 150 Efferdose
150mg: Glaxo Wellcome

Sertraline HCl

Zoloft
50mg: Roerig

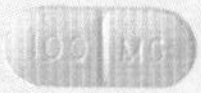

Zoloft100
100mg: Roerig

Simvastatin

Zocor
5mg: Merck

Zocor
10mg: Merck

Zocor
20mg: Merck

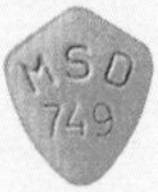

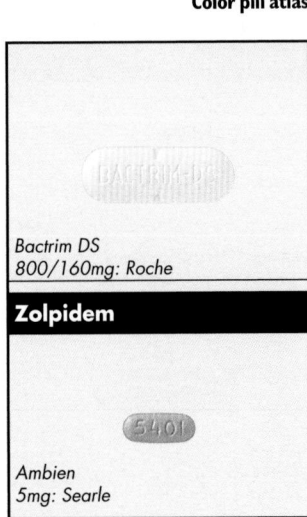

Zocor
40mg: Merck

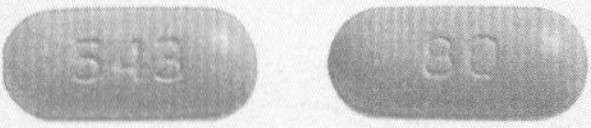

Zocor
80mg: Merck

Sulfamethoxazole; Trimethoprim

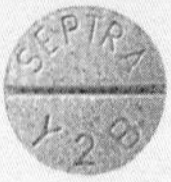

Septra
400/80mg: Glaxo Wellcome

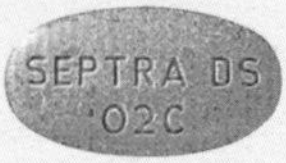

Septra
800/160mg: Glaxo Wellcome

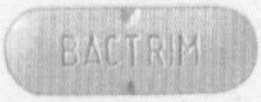

Bactrim
400/80mg: Roche

Bactrim DS
800/160mg: Roche

Zolpidem

Ambien
5mg: Searle

Ambien
10mg: Searle

Lansoprazole (Prevacid)
Metoclopramide (Reglan)
Nizatidine (Axid)
Omeprazole (Prilosec)
Pantoprazole (Protonix)
Rabeprazole (Aciphex)
Ranitidine (Zantac)

Glaucoma
Acetazolamide (Diamox)
Apraclonidine (Iopidine)
Betaxolol (Betoptic)
Bimatoprost (Lumigan)
Brimonidine (Alphagan)
Brinzolamide (Azopt)
Carbachol
Carteolol (Ocupress)
Dipivefrin (Propine)
Dorzolamide (Trusopt)
Echothiophate iodide (Phospholine)
Latanoprost (Xalatan)
Levobunolol (Betagan)
Metipranolol (OptiPranolol)
Pilocarpine (Isopto Carpine)
Timolol (Timoptic)
Travoprost (Travatan)
Unoprostone (Rescula)

Gout
Allopurinol (Zyloprim)
Colchicine
Indomethacin (Indocin)
Probenecid (Benemid)
Sulindac (Clinoril)

Human immunodeficiency virus (HIV)
Abacavir (Ziagen)
Amprenavir (Agenerase)
Atazanavir (Reyataz)
Darunavir (Prezista)
Delavirdine (Rescriptor)
Didanosine (Videx)
Efavirenz (Sustiva)
Emtricitabine (Emtriva)
Enfuvirtide (Fuzeon)
Indinavir (Crixivan)
Lamivudine (Epivir)
Lopinavir/ritonavir (Kaletra)
Nelfinavir (Viracept)
Nevirapine (Viramune)
Ritonavir (Norvir)
Saquinavir (Fortovase, Invirase)
Stavudine (Zerit)
Tenofovir (Viread)
Tipranavir (Aptivus)
Zalcitabine (Hivid)
Zidovudine (AZT, Retrovir)

Hypercholesterolemia
Atorvastatin (Lipitor)
Cholestyramine (Questran)
Colesevelam (Welchol)
Colestipol (Colestid)
Ezetimibe (Zetia)
Fenofibrate (Tricor)
Fluvastatin (Lescol)
Gemfibrozil (Lopid)
Lovastatin (Mevacor)
Niacin (Niaspan)
Pravastatin (Pravachol)
Rosuvastatin (Crestor)
Simvastatin (Zocor)

Hyperphosphatemia
Aluminum salts
Calcium salts
Lanthanum (Fosrenol)
Sevelamer (Renagel)

Hypertension
Amlodipine (Norvasc)
Atenolol (Tenormin)
Benazepril (Lotensin)
Bisoprolol (Zebeta)
Candesartan (Atacand)
Captopril (Capoten)
Clonidine (Catapres)
Diltiazem (Cardizem, Dilacor)
Doxazosin (Cardura)
Enalapril (Vasotec)
Eplerenone (Inspra)
Eprosartan (Teveten)
Felodipine (Plendil)
Fosinopril (Monopril)
Hydralazine (Apresoline)
Hydrochlorothiazide (HydroDIURIL)
Indapamide (Lozol)
Irbesartan (Avapro)
Isradipine (DynaCirc)

Labetalol (Normodyne, Trandate)
Lisinopril (Prinivil, Zestril)
Losartan (Cozaar)
Methyldopa (Aldomet)
Metolazone (Diulo, Zaroxolyn)
Metoprolol (Lopressor)
Minoxidil (Loniten)
Moexipril (Univasc)
Nadolol (Corgard)
Nicardipine (Cardene)
Nifedipine (Adalat, Procardia)
Nitroglycerin
Nitroprusside (Nipride)
Olmesartan (Benicar)
Perindopril (Aceon)
Pindolol (Visken)
Prazosin (Minipress)
Propranolol (Inderal)
Quinapril (Accupril)
Ramipril (Altace)
Spironolactone (Aldactone)
Telmisartan (Micardis)
Terazosin (Hytrin)
Timolol (Blocadren)
Trandolapril (Mavik)
Valsartan (Dovan)
Verapamil (Calan, Isoptin)

Hypertriglyceridemia
Atorvastatin (Lipitor)
Fenofibrate (Tricor)
Fluvastatin (Lescol)
Gemfibrozil (Lopid)
Lovastatin (Mevacor)
Niacin (Niaspan)
Omega-3 Acid Ethyl Esters (Omacor)
Pravastatin (Pravachol)
Rosuvastatin (Crestor)
Simvastatin (Zocor)

Hyperuricemia
Allopurinol (Zyloprim)
Probenecid (Benemid)

Hypotension
Dobutamine (Dobutrex)
Dopamine (Intropin)
Ephedrine
Epinephrine
Norepinephrine (Levophed)
Phenylephrine (Neo-Synephrine)

Hypothyroidism
Levothyroxine (Levoxyl, Synthroid)
Liothyronine (Cytomel)
Thyroid

Idiopathic thrombocytopenic purpura (ITP)
Cyclophosphamide (Cytoxan)
Dexamethasone (Decadron)
Hydrocortisone (SoluCortef)
Immune globulin intravenous
Methylprednisolone (SoluMedrol)
Prednisone
Rh_o(D) Immune globulin (RhoGam)
Rituximab (Rituxan)

Insomnia
Diphenhydramine (Benadryl)
Estazolam (ProSom)
Eszopiclone (Lunesta)
Flurazepam (Dalmane)
Ramelteon (Rozerem)
Temazepam (Restoril)
Triazolam (Halcion)
Zaleplon (Sonata)
Zolpidem (Ambien)

Migraine headaches
Almotriptan (Axert)
Amitriptyline (Elavil, Endep)
Dihydroergotamine
Eletriptan (Relpax)
Ergotamine (Ergomar)
Frovatriptan (Frovan)
Naratriptan (Amerge)
Propranolol (Inderal)
Rizatriptan (Maxalt)
Sumatriptan (Imitrex)
Zolmitriptan (Zomig)

Multiple sclerosis (MS)
Glatiramer (Copaxone)
Interferon beta-1a (Avonex, Rebif)
Interferon beta-1b (Betaseron)
Mitoxantrone (Novantrone)
Natalizumab (Tysabri)

Myelodysplastic syndrome
Azacitidine (Vidaza)
Decitabine (Dacagen)
Lenalinomide (Revlimid)

Myocardial infarction (MI)
Alteplase (Activase)
Aspirin
Atenolol (Tenormin)
Captopril (Capoten)
Clopidogrel (Plavix)
Dalteparin (Fragmin)
Diltiazem (Cardizem, Dilacor)
Enalapril (Vasotec)
Enoxaparin (Lovenox)
Heparin
Lidocaine
Lisinopril (Prinivil, Zestril)
Metoprolol (Lopressor)
Morphine
Nitroglycerin
Propranolol (Inderal)
Quinapril (Accupril)
Ramipril (Altace)
Reteplase (Retavase)
Streptokinase
Timolol (Blocadren)
Warfarin (Coumadin)

Nausea
Aprepitant (Emend)
Chlorpromazine (Thorazine)
Dexamethasone (Decadron)
Dimenhydrinate (Dramamine)
Dolasetron (Anzemet)
Dronabinol (Marinol)
Droperidol (Inapsine)
Granisetron (Kytril)
Hydroxyzine (Vistaril)
Lorazepam (Ativan)
Meclizine (Antivert)
Metoclopramide (Reglan)
Nabilone (Cesamet)
Ondansetron (Zofran)
Palonosetron (Aloxi)
Prochlorperazine (Compazine)
Promethazine (Phenergan)
Trimethobenzamide (Tigan)

Obesity
Benzphetamine (Didrex)
Diethylpropion (Tenuate)
Mazindol (Sanorex)
Orlistat (Xenical)
Phendimetrazine (Bontril)
Phentermine (Ionamin)
Sibutramine (Meridia)

Obsessive-compulsive disorder (OCD)
Citalopram (Celexa)
Clomipramine (Anafranil)
Fluoxetine (Prozac)
Fluvoxamine (Luvox)
Paroxetine (Paxil)
Sertraline (Zoloft)

Osteoarthritis
Acetaminophen (Tylenol)
Celecoxib (Celebrex)
Diclofenac (Cataflam, Voltaren)
Etodolac (Lodine)
Flavocoxid (Limbrel)
Flurbiprofen (Ansaid)
Ibuprofen (Motrin)
Ketoprofen (Orudis)
Meloxicam (Mobic)
Nabumetone (Relafen)
Naproxen (Naprosyn)
Oxaprozin (Daypro)
Piroxicam (Feldene)
Salicylates (Aspirin)
Sulindac (Clinoril)
Tramadol (Ultram)

Osteoporosis
Alendronate (Fosamax)
Calcitonin (Miacalcin)
Calcium salts
Conjugated estrogens (Premarin)
Estradiol (Estrace)
Ibandronate (Boniva)
Raloxifene (Evista)
Risedronate (Actonel)
Teriparatide (Forteo)
Vitamin D

Paget's disease
Alendronate (Fosamax)

Calcitonin (Miacalcin)
Etidronate (Didronel)
Pamidronate (Aredia)
Risedronate (Actonel)
Tiludronate (Skelid)

Pain, mild to moderate
Acetaminophen (Tylenol)
Aspirin
Celecoxib (Celebrex)
Codeine
Diclofenac (Cataflam, Voltaren)
Diflunisal (Dolobid)
Etodolac (Lodine)
Flurbiprofen (Ansaid)
Ibuprofen (Advil, Motrin)
Ketorolac (Toradol)
Naproxen (Anaprox, Naprosyn)
Propoxyphene (Darvon)
Salsalate (Disalcid)
Tramadol (Ultram)

Pain, moderate to severe
Butorphanol (Stadol)
Fentanyl (Sublimaze)
Hydromorphone (Dilaudid)
Meperidine (Demerol)
Methadone (Dolophine)
Morphine (MS Contin)
Nalbuphine (Nubain)
Oxycodone (OxyFast, Roxicodone)
Oxymorphone (Oprana)
Ziconotide (Prialt)

Panic attack disorder
Alprazolam (Xanax)
Clonazepam (Klonopin)
Paroxetine (Paxil)
Sertraline (Zoloft)
Venlafaxine (Effexor)

Parkinsonism
Amantadine (Symmetrel)
Apomorphine (Apokyn)
Bromocriptine (Parlodel)
Carbidopa/levodopa (Sinemet)
Diphenhydramine (Benadryl)
Entacapone (Comtan)
Pergolide (Permax)
Pramipexole (Mirapex)
Rasagiline (Azilect)
Ropinirole (Requip)
Selegiline (Eldepryl)
Tolcapone (Tasmar)

Peptic ulcer disease
Cimetidine (Tagamet)
Esomeprazole (Nexium)
Famotidine (Pepcid)
Lansoprazole (Prevacid)
Misoprostol (Cytotec)
Nizatidine (Axid)
Omeprazole (Prilosec)
Pantoprazole (Protonix)
Rabeprazole (Aciphex)
Ranitidine (Zantac)
Sucralfate (Carafate)

Pneumonia
Amoxicillin (Amoxil)
Amoxicillin/clavulanate (Augmentin)
Ampicillin (Polycillin)
Azithromycin (Zithromax)
Cefaclor (Ceclor)
Cefpodoxime (Vantin)
Ceftriaxone (Rocephin)
Cefuroxime (Kefurox, Zinacef)
Clarithromycin (Biaxin)
Co-trimoxazole (Bactrim, Septra)
Erythromycin
Gentamicin (Garamycin)
Levofloxacin (Levaquin)
Linezolid (Zyvox)
Moxifloxacin (Avelox)
Piperacillin/tazobactam (Zosyn)
Telithromycin (Ketek)
Tobramycin (Nebcin)
Vancomycin (Vancocin)

Pneumonia, *Pneumocystis carinii*
Atovaquone (Mepron)
Clindamycin (Cleocin)
Co-trimoxazole (Bactrim, Septra)
Pentamidine (Pentam)
Trimethoprim (Proloprim)

Posttraumatic Stress Disorder
Amitriptyline (Elavil)
Aripiprazole (Abilify)
Citalopram (Celexa)

Escitalopram (Lexapro)
Fluoxetine (Prozac)
Olanzapine (Zyprexa)
Paroxetine (Paxil)
Propranolol (Inderal)
Quetiapine (Seroquel)
Risperidone (Risperdol)
Sertraline (Zoloft)
Venlafaxine (Effexor)
Ziprasidone (Geodon)

Pruritus
Amcinonide (Cyclocort)
Brompheniramine (Dimetane)
Cetirizine (Zyrtec)
Chlorpheniramine (Dimetane)
Clemastine (Tavist)
Clobetasol (Temovate)
Cyproheptadine (Periactin)
Desloratadine (Clarinex)
Desonide (Tridesilon)
Desoximetasone (Topicort)
Diphenhydramine (Benadryl)
Fluocinolone (Synalar)
Fluocinonide (Lidex)
Halobetasol (Ultravate)
Hydrocortisone (Cort-Dome, Hytone)
Hydroxyzine (Atarax, Vistaril)
Prednisolone (Prelone)
Prednisone (Deltasone)
Promethazine (Phenergan)

Psychosis
Aripiprazole (Abilify)
Chlorpromazine (Thorazine)
Clozapine (Clozaril)
Fluphenazine (Prolixin)
Haloperidol (Haldol)
Olanzapine (Zyprexa)
Perphenazine (Trilafon)
Quetiapine (Seroquel)
Risperidone (Risperdal)
Thioridazine (Mellaril)
Thiothixene (Navane)
Ziprasidone (Geodon)

Pulmonary arterial hypertension
Bosentan (Tracleer)
Epoprostenol (Flolan)
Iloprost (Ventavis)
Sildenafil (Revatio)
Treprostinil (Remodulin)

Respiratory distress syndrome (RDS)
Beractant (Survanta)
Calfactant (Infasurf)
Poractant alfa (Curosurf)

Schizophrenia
Aripiprazole (Abilify)
Chlorpromazine (Thorazine)
Clozapine (Clozaril)
Fluphenazine (Prolixin)
Haloperidol (Haldol)
Olanzapine (Zyprexa)
Perphenazine (Trilafon)
Quetiapine (Seroquel)
Risperidone (Risperdal)
Thioridazine (Mellaril)
Thiothixene (Navane)
Ziprasidone (Geodon)

Smoking cessation
Bupropion (Zyban)
Clonidine (Catapres)
Nicotine (Nicoderm, Nicotrol)
Nortriptyline (Pamelor)
Varenicline (Chantix)

Thrombosis
Dalteparin (Fragmin)
Enoxaparin (Lovenox)
Heparin
Tinzaparin (Innohep)
Warfarin (Coumadin)

Thyroid disorders
Levothyroxine (Levoxyl, Synthroid)
Liothyronine (Cytomel)
Thyroid

Transient ischemic attack (TIA)
Aspirin
Clopidogrel (Plavix)
Ticlopidine (Ticlid)
Warfarin (Coumadin)

Tremor
Atenolol (Tenormin)

Chlordiazepoxide (Librium)
Diazepam (Valium)
Lorazepam (Ativan)
Metoprolol (Lopressor)
Nadolol (Corgard)
Propranolol (Inderal)

Tuberculosis (TB)
Ethambutol (Myambutol)
Isoniazid (INH)
Pyrazinamide
Rifabutin (Mycobutin)
Rifampin (Rifadin)
Rifapentine (Priftin)
Streptomycin

Urticaria
Cetirizine (Zyrtec)
Cimetidine (Tagamet)
Clemastine (Tavist)
Cyproheptadine (Periactin)
Diphenhydramine (Benadryl)
Hydroxyzine (Atarax, Vistaril)
Loratadine (Claritin)
Promethazine (Phenergan)
Ranitidine (Zantac)

Vertigo
Dimenhydrinate (Dramamine)
Diphenhydramine (Benadryl)
Meclizine (Antivert)
Scopolamine (Trans-Derm Scop)

Vomiting
Aprepitant (Emend)
Chlorpromazine (Thorazine)
Dexamethasone (Decadron)
Dimenhydrinate (Dramamine)
Dolasetron (Anzemet)
Dronabinol (Marinol)
Droperidol (Inapsine)
Granisetron (Kytril)
Hydroxyzine (Vistaril)
Lorazepam (Ativan)
Meclizine (Antivert)
Metoclopramide (Reglan)
Nabilone (Cesamet)
Ondansetron (Zofran)
Palonosetron (Aloxi)
Prochlorperazine (Compazine)
Promethazine (Phenergan)
Scopolamine (Trans-Derm Scop)
Trimethobenzamide (Tigan)

Zollinger-Ellison syndrome
Aluminum salts
Cimetidine (Tagamet)
Esomeprazole (Nexim)
Famotidine (Pepcid)
Lansoprazole (Prevacid)
Omeprazole (Prilosec)
Pantoprazole (Protonix)
Rabeprazole (Aciphex)
Ranitidine (Zantac)

Drug Classification Contents

Anesthetics: General

USES

IV anesthetic agents are used to induce general anesthesia. The general anesthetic state consists of unconsciousness, amnesia, analgesia, immobility, and attenuation of autonomic responses to noxious stimuli.

Volatile inhalation agents produce all the components of the anesthetic state but are administered through the lungs via an anesthesia machine. Agents for use include desflurane, sevoflurane, isoflurane, enflurane, and halothane.

General anesthetics are medications producing unconsciousness and a lack of response to all painful stimuli.

ACTION

IV anesthetic agents: Most agents produce CNS depression by action on the GABA receptor complex. GABA is the primary inhibitory neurotransmitter in the CNS. Ketamine produces dissociation between the thalamus and the limbic system.

Volatile inhalation agents: Not fully understood but may disrupt neuronal transmission throughout the CNS. These agents may either block excitatory or enhance inhibitory transmission through axons or synapses.

ANESTHETICS: GENERAL

Name	Availability	Uses	Dosage Range	Side Effects
Etomidate (Amidate)	**I:** 2 mg/ml	IV induction	0.2–0.6 mg/kg	Myoclonus, pain on injection, nausea, vomiting, respiratory depression
Ketamine (p. 652) (Ketalar)	**I:** 10 mg/ml, 50 mg/ml, 100 mg/ml	Analgesia, sedation, IV induction	1–4.5 mg/kg	Delirium, euphoria, nausea, vomiting
Methohexital (Brevital)	**Powder for injection:** 500 mg	IV induction, sedation	50–120 mg	Cardiovascular depression, myoclonus, nausea, vomiting, respiratory depression

Midazolam (p. 770) (Versed)	**I:** 1 mg/ml, 5 mg/ml	Anxiolytic, amnesic, sedation	1–5 mg titrated slowly	Respiratory depression
Propofol (p. 981) (Diprivan)	**I:** 10 mg/ml	Sedation IV induction Maintenance	0.5 mg/kg 2–2.5 mg/kg 100–200 mcg/kg/min	Cardiovascular depression, delirium, euphoria, pain on injection, respiratory depression
Thiopental (Pentothal)	**Powder for injection:** 2.5% (25 mg/ml)	IV induction	Titrate vs. pt response **Average:** 50–75 mg	Cardiovascular depression, nausea, vomiting, respiratory depression

I, Injection.

Anesthetics: Local

USES

Local anesthetics suppress pain by blocking impulses along axons. Suppression of pain does not cause generalized depression of the entire nervous system. Local anesthetics may be given topically and by injection (local infiltration, peripheral nerve block [axillary], IV regional [Bier block], epidural, and spinal).

ACTION

Most local anesthetics fall into one of two groups: esters or amides. Both provide anesthesia and analgesia by reversibly binding to and blocking sodium (Na) channels. This slows the rate of depolarization of the nerve action potential; thus, propagation of the electrical impulses needed for nerve conduction is prevented.

Anesthetics: Local *(continued)*

ANESTHETICS: LOCAL

Name	Uses	Onset (min)	Duration (hrs)	Side Effects
Esters				
Chloroprocaine (Nesacaine)	Local infiltrate, nerve block, spinal	6–12	0.5–1	Seizures, bradycardia, cardiac arrest, hypotension, arrhythmias, anxiety, dizziness, restlessness, erythema, pruritus, urticaria, blurred vision, allergic reaction
Procaine (Novocaine)	Local infiltrate, nerve block, spinal	2–5	0.5–1.5	Burning sensation/pain at site of injection, tissue irritation, CNS stimulation followed by CNS depression, chills
Amides				
Bupivacaine (Marcaine, Sensorcaine)	Local infiltrate, nerve block, epidural, spinal	5	2–9	Cardiac arrest, hypotension, bradycardia, palpitations, seizures, restlessness, anxiety, dizziness, nausea, vomiting, blurred vision, weakness, tinnitus, apnea
Lidocaine (p. 689)	Local infiltrate, nerve block, spinal, epidural, topical, IV regional	Less than 2	0.5–1	Bradycardia, hypotension, arrhythmias, agitation, anxiety, dizziness, seizures, pruritus, rash, nausea, vomiting, altered taste, visual changes, tinnitus, respiratory depression, allergic reaction

Mepivacaine (Carbocaine, Polocaine)	Local infiltrate, nerve block, epidural	3–20	2–2.5	Bradycardia, syncope, arrhythmias, anxiety, seizures, dizziness, restlessness, chills, pruritus, urticaria, nausea, vomiting, incontinence, blurred vision, tinnitus, allergic reaction
Ropivacaine (Naropin)	Local infiltrate, nerve block, epidural, spinal	1–15	3–15	Hypotension, bradycardia, headache, pruritus, nausea, vomiting, dizziness, anxiety, tinnitus, dyspnea, cardiac arrest, arrhythmias, seizures, syncope, chills.

Note: Most side effects are manifestations of excessive plasma concentrations.

Anesthetics: Local Topical

ANESTHETICS: LOCAL TOPICAL

Name	Indications	Peak Effect (min)	Duration (min)
Amides			
Dibucaine (Nupercainal)	Skin	Less than 5	15–45
Lidocaine (p. 689)	Skin, mucous membranes	2–5	15–45

(continued)

ANESTHETICS: LOCAL TOPICAL *(continued)*

Name	Indications	Peak Effect (min)	Duration (min)
Esters			
Benzocaine	Skin, mucous membranes	Less than 5	15–45
Cocaine (p. 281)	Mucous membranes	2–5	30–60
Tetracaine (Pontocaine)	Skin, mucous membranes	3–8	30–60

Angiotensin-Converting Enzyme (ACE) Inhibitors

USES

Treatment of hypertension (HTN), adjunctive therapy for congestive heart failure (CHF).

ACTION

Antihypertensive: Exact mechanism unknown. May be related to competitive inhibition of angiotensin I converting enzyme (ACE) activity causing decreased conversion of angiotensin I to angiotensin II, a potent vasoconstrictor. Reduces peripheral arterial resistance.

Congestive heart failure: Decreases peripheral vascular resistance (afterload), pulmonary capillary wedge pressure (preload), improves cardiac output, exercise tolerance.

ACE INHIBITORS

Name	Availability	Uses	Dosage Range (per day)	Side Effects
Benazepril (p. 125) (Lotensin)	**T:** 5 mg, 10 mg, 20 mg, 40 mg	HTN	**HTN:** 5–80 mg	Headaches, dizziness, fatigue, cough
Captopril (p. 183) (Capoten)	**T:** 12.5 mg, 25 mg, 50 mg, 100 mg	HTN CHF	**HTN:** 50–450 mg **CHF:** 12.5–450 mg	Insomnia, headaches, dizziness, fatigue, GI complaints, cough, rash
Enalapril (p. 411) (Vasotec)	**T:** 2.5 mg, 5 mg, 10 mg, 20 mg **IV:** 1.25 mg/ml	HTN CHF	**HTN:** 10–40 mg; (**IV:** 1.25 mg q6h) **CHF:** 5–20 mg	Chest pain, hypotension, headaches, fatigue, dizziness
Fosinopril (p. 520) (Monopril)	**T:** 10 mg, 20 mg, 40 mg	HTN CHF	**HTN:** 10–80 mg **CHF:** 20–40 mg	Hypotension, nausea, vomiting, cough
Lisinopril (p. 695) (Prinivil, Zestril)	**T:** 2.5 mg, 5 mg, 10 mg, 20 mg, 40 mg	HTN CHF	**HTN:** 10–40 mg **CHF:** 5–20 mg	Chest pain, hypotension, headaches, dizziness, fatigue, diarrhea
Moexipril (p. 787) (Univasc)	**T:** 7.5 mg, 15 mg	HTN	**HTN:** 7.5–30 mg	Dizziness, fatigue, diarrhea, cough
Perindopril (Aceon)	**T:** 2 mg, 4 mg, 6 mg	HTN	**HTN:** 4–16 mg	Hypotension, dizziness, fatigue, syncope, cough
Quinapril (p. 998) (Accupril)	**T:** 5 mg, 10 mg, 20 mg, 40 mg	HTN CHF	**HTN:** 10–80 mg **CHF:** 10–40 mg	Chest pain, hypotension, headaches, dizziness, fatigue, diarrhea, nausea, vomiting, cough
Ramipril (p. 1009) (Altace)	**C:** 1.25 mg, 2.5 mg, 5 mg, 10 mg	HTN CHF	**HTN:** 2.5–20 mg **CHF:** 1.25–10 mg	Hypotension, headaches, dizziness, cough
Trandolapril (p. 1168) (Mavik)	**T:** 1 mg, 2 mg, 4 mg	HTN CHF	**HTN:** 1–4 mg **CHF:** 1–4 mg	Dizziness, dyspepsia, cough, asthenia, syncope, myalgia

C, Capsules; ***CHF,*** congestive heart failure; ***HTN,*** hypertension; ***IV,*** intravenous; ***T,*** tablets.

Angiotensin II Receptor Antagonists

USES

Treatment of hypertension (HTN) alone or in combination with other antihypertensives. Treatment of heart failure (HF).

ACTION

Angiotensin II receptor antagonists (AIIRA) block vasoconstrictor and aldosterone-secreting effects on angiotensin II by selectively blocking the binding of angiotensin II to AT_1 receptors in vascular smooth muscle and adrenal gland, causing vasodilation and a decrease in aldosterone effects.

ANGIOTENSIN II RECEPTOR ANTAGONISTS

Name	Availability	Uses	Dosage Range (per day)	Side Effects
Candesartan (p. 179) (Atacand)	**T:** 4 mg, 8 mg, 16 mg, 32 mg	HTN HF	2–32 mg 4–32 mg	Headaches, upper respiratory tract infection, pain, dizziness
Eprosartan (p. 429) (Teveten)	**T:** 400 mg, 600 mg	HTN	400–800 mg	Headaches, upper respiratory tract infection, myalgia
Irbesartan (p. 635) (Avapro)	**T:** 75 mg, 150 mg, 300 mg	HTN	75–300 mg	Headaches, upper respiratory tract infection
Losartan (p. 709) (Cozaar)	**T:** 25 mg, 50 mg, 100 mg	HTN	25–100 mg	Dizziness, headaches, upper respiratory tract infection, diarrhea, fatigue, cough
Olmesartan (p. 864) (Benicar)	**T:** 5 mg, 20 mg, 40 mg	HTN	20–40 mg	Headaches, upper respiratory tract infection, flu-like symptoms, dizziness, bronchitis, rhinitis, back pain, pharyngitis, sinusitis, diarrhea, peripheral edema
Telmisartan (p. 1110) (Micardis)	**T:** 40 mg, 80 mg	HTN	20–80 mg	Upper respiratory tract infection, dizziness, back pain, sinusitis, diarrhea
Valsartan (p. 1200) (Diovan)	**T:** 80 mg, 160 mg	HTN HF	80–320 mg 80–320 mg	Dizziness, headaches, upper respiratory tract infection, diarrhea, fatigue

HF, Heart failure; ***HTN,*** hypertension; ***T,*** tablets.

Antacids

USES

Relief of symptoms associated with hyperacidity (e.g., heartburn, acid indigestion, sour stomach), hyperacidity associated with gastric/duodenal ulcers, treatment of pathologic gastric hypersecretion associated with Zollinger-Ellison syndrome, symptomatic treatment of gastroesophageal reflux disease (GERD), prevention and treatment of upper GI stress-induced ulceration and bleeding (esp. in ICU).

Aluminum carbonate and hydroxide in conjunction with a low-phosphate diet to reduce elevated phosphate in pts with renal insufficiency. Calcium for calcium deficiency, magnesium for magnesium deficiency.

ACTION

Act primarily in the stomach to neutralize gastric acid (increase pH). Antacids do not have a direct effect on acid output. The ability to increase pH depends on the dose, dosage form used, presence or absence of food in the stomach, and acid-neutralizing capacity (ANC). ANC is the number of mEq of hydrochloric acid that can be neutralized by a particular weight or volume of antacid.

Reduce elevated phosphate by binding with phosphate in the intestine to form an insoluble complex, which is then eliminated.

ANTACIDS

Antacid	Brand Names	Availability	Dosage Range	Side Effects
Aluminum				
Hydroxide (p. 45)	Amphojel, Alu-Tab, Dialume	**T:** 300 mg, 500 mg, 600 mg **C:** 500 mg	500–1,500 mg 3–6 times/day	Chalky taste, mild constipation, abdominal cramps *Long-term use:* Neurotoxicity in dialysis pts, hypercalcemia, osteoporosis *Large doses:* Fecal impaction, peripheral edema

(continued)

ANTACIDS *(continued)*

Antacid	Brand Names	Availability	Dosage Range	Side Effects
Calcium				
Carbonate (p. 175)	Tums	**T (chewable):** 500 mg, 750 mg, 1,000 mg	500–1,500 mg as needed	Chalky taste *Large doses:* Fecal impaction, peripheral edema, metabolic alkalosis *Long-term use:* Difficult/painful urination
Magnesium				
Hydroxide (p. 716)	Milk of Magnesia	**T (chewable):** 311 mg **L:** 400 mg/5 ml, 800 mg/5 ml	**T:** 622–1,244 mg up to 4 times/day **L:** 2.5–7.5 ml up to 4 times/day	Chalky taste, diarrhea, laxative effect, electrolyte imbalance (dizziness, irregular heartbeat, fatigue)
Oxide (p. 716)	Mag-Ox 400	**T:** 400 mg, 420 mg, 500 mg	400–800 mg/ day	Same as above

C, Capsules; ***L,*** liquid; ***T,*** tablets.

Antianxiety Agents

USES

Treatment of anxiety including generalized anxiety disorder (GAD), panic disorder, obsessive-compulsive disorder (OCD), social anxiety disorder (SAD), post-traumatic stress disorder (PTSD), and acute stress disorder. In addition, some benzodiazepines are used as hypnotics, anticonvulsants to prevent delirium tremors during alcohol withdrawal, and as adjunctive therapy for relaxation of skeletal muscle spasms. Midazolam, a short-acting benzodiazepine, is used for preoperative sedation and relief of anxiety for short diagnostic/endoscopic procedures (see individual monograph for midazolam).

ACTION

Benzodiazepines are the largest and most frequently prescribed group of antianxiety agents. The exact mechanism is unknown but may increase the inhibiting effect of gamma-aminobutyric acid (GABA), which inhibits nerve impulse transmission by binding to specific benzodiazepine receptors in various areas of the central nervous system (CNS).

◀ **ALERT** ▶ Refer to individual entries of non-benzodiazepine drugs for more information on uses and actions.

ANTIANXIETY AGENTS

Name	Availability	Uses	Dosage Range (per day)	Side Effects
Benzodiazepine				
Alprazolam (p. 39) (Xanax)	**T:** 0.25 mg, 0.5 mg, 1 mg, 2 mg **S:** 0.5 mg/5 ml, 1 mg/ml	Anxiety, panic disorder	0.75–10 mg	Drowsiness, weakness, fatigue, ataxia, slurred speech, confusion, lack of coordination, impaired memory, paradoxical agitation, dizziness, nausea
Chlordiazepoxide (p. 238) evolve (Librium)	**C:** 5 mg, 10 mg, 25 mg **T:** 10 mg, 25 mg **I:** 100 mg	Anxiety, alcohol withdrawal	5–300 mg	Same as alprazolam
Clorazepate (p. 276) evolve (Tranxene)	**C:** 3.75 mg, 7.5 mg, 15 mg **SD:** 11.25 mg, 22.5 mg	Anxiety, alcohol withdrawal, anticonvulsant	7.5–90 mg	Same as alprazolam
Diazepam (p. 350) (Valium)	**T:** 2.5 mg, 5 mg, 10 mg **S:** 5 mg/5 ml, 5 mg/ml **I:** 5 mg/ml	Anxiety, alcohol withdrawal, anticonvulsant, muscle relaxant	2–40 mg	Same as alprazolam

(continued)

ANTIANXIETY AGENTS ***(continued)***

Name	Availability	Uses	Dosage Range (per day)	Side Effects
Benzodiazepine *(continued)*				
Lorazepam (p. 707) (Ativan)	**T:** 0.5 mg, 1 mg, 2 mg **S:** 2 mg/ml **I:** 2 mg/ml, 4 mg/ml	Anxiety	0.5–10 mg	Same as alprazolam
Oxazepam (p. 880) (Serax)	**C:** 10 mg, 15 mg, 30 mg **T:** 15 mg	Anxiety, alcohol withdrawal	30–120 mg	Same as alprazolam
Nonbenzodiazepine				
Buspirone (p. 166) (BuSpar)	**T:** 5 mg, 10 mg, 15 mg, 30 mg	Anxiety	7.5–60 mg	Dizziness, light-headedness, headaches, nausea, restlessness
Hydroxyzine (p. 588) (Atarax, Vistaril)	**T:** 10 mg, 25 mg, 50 mg, 100 mg	Anxiety, rhinitis, pruritus, urticaria, nausea or vomiting	100–400 mg	Drowsiness; dry mouth, nose, and throat
Paroxetine (p. 904) (Paxil)	**S:** 10 mg/5 ml **T:** 10 mg, 20 mg, 30 mg, 40 mg **T(CR):** 12.5 mg, 25 mg, 37.5 mg	Anxiety, depression, obsessive-compulsive disorder, panic disorder	10–50 mg	Drowsiness; dry mouth, nose, and throat; dizziness; diarrhea; diaphoresis; constipation; vomiting; tremors
Trazodone (p. 1173) (Desyrel)	**T:** 50 mg, 100 mg, 150 mg, 300 mg	Anxiety, depression	100–400 mg	Drowsiness, dizziness, headaches, dry mouth, nausea, vomiting, unpleasant taste
Venlafaxine (p. 1209) (Effexor)	**C:** 37.5 mg, 75 mg, 150 mg	Anxiety, depression	37.5–225 mg	Drowsiness, nausea, headaches, dry mouth

C, Capsules; ***CR,*** controlled-release; ***I,*** injection; ***S,*** solution; ***SD,*** single dose; ***T,*** tablets.

Antiarrhythmics

USES

Prevention and treatment of cardiac arrhythmias, such as premature ventricular contractions, ventricular tachycardia, premature atrial contractions, paroxysmal atrial tachycardia, atrial fibrillation and flutter.

ACTION

The antiarrhythmics are divided into four classes based on their effects on certain ion channels and/or receptors located on the myocardial cell membrane. Class I is further divided into three subclasses (IA, IB, IC) based on electrophysiologic effects.

Class I: Block cardiac sodium channels and slow conduction velocity, prolonging refractoriness and decreasing automaticity of sodium-dependent tissue.

Class IA: Block sodium and potassium channels.

Class IB: Shorten the repolarization phase.

Class IC: No effect on repolarization phase, but slow conduction velocity.

Class II: Slow sinus and atrioventricular (AV) nodal conduction.

Class III: Block cardiac potassium channels, prolonging the repolarization phase of electrical cells.

Class IV: Inhibit the influx calcium through its channels, causing slower conduction through the sinus and AV nodes.

ANTIARRHYTHMICS

Name	Availability	Uses	Dosage Range	Side Effects
Class IA				
Disopyramide (p. 375) evolve (Norpace, Norpace CR)	**C:** 100 mg, 150 mg **C(ER):** 100 mg, 150 mg	AF, WPW, PSVT, PVCs, VT	400–800 mg/day	Dry mouth, blurred vision, urinary retention, CHF, proarrhythmia

(continued)

ANTIARRHYTHMICS ***(continued)***

Name	Availability	Uses	Dosage Range	Side Effects
Class IA *(continued)*				
Procainamide (p. 969) (Pronestyl, Procan-SR)	**T:** 250 mg, 375 mg, 500 mg **C:** 250 mg, 375 mg, 500 mg **T (SR):** 250 mg, 500 mg, 750 mg, 1,000 mg **I:** 100 mg/ml, 500 mg/ml	AF, WPW, PVCs, VT	**A (PO):** 250–500 mg q3h; **(ER):** 250–750 mg q6h	Hypotension, fever, agranulocytosis, SLE, headaches, proarrhythmia
Quinidine (p. 1000) (Quinidex, Quinaglute)	**T:** 200 mg, 300 mg **T (ER):** 300 mg, 324 mg **I:** 80 mg/ml	AF, WPW, PVCs VT	**A:** 200–600 mg q2–4h; **(ER):** 300–600 mg q8h	Diarrhea, hypotension, nausea, vomiting, cinchonism, fever, thrombocytopenia, proarrhythmia
Class IB				
Lidocaine (p. 689) (Xylocaine)	**I:** 300 mg for IM **IV Infusion:** 2 mg/ml, 4 mg/ml	PVCs, VT, VF	**IV:** 50–100 mg bolus, then 1–4 mg/min infusion	Drowsiness, agitation, muscle twitching, seizures, paresthesias, proarrhythmia
Mexiletine (Mexitil)	**C:** 150 mg, 200 mg, 250 mg	PVCs, VT, VF	**A:** 600–1,200 mg/day	Drowsiness, agitation, muscle twitching, seizures, paresthesias, proarrhythmia, nausea, vomiting
Tocainide (Tonocard)	**T:** 400 mg, 600 mg	PVCs, VT, VF	**A:** 1,200–1,800 mg/day	Drowsiness, agitation, muscle twitching, seizures, paresthesias, proarrhythmia, nausea, vomiting, diarrhea, agranulocytosis

Class IC

Flecainide (Tambocor)	**T:** 50 mg, 100 mg, 150 mg	AF, PSVT, life-threatening ventricular arrhythmias	**A:** 200–400 mg/day	Dizziness, tremors, light-headedness, flushing, blurred vision, metallic taste, proarrhythmia
Moricizine (Ethmozine)	**T:** 200 mg, 250 mg, 300 mg	Life-threatening ventricular arrhythmias	**A:** 600–900 mg/day	Nausea, dizziness, perioral numbness, euphoria
Propafenone (p. 979) (Rythmol)	**T:** 150 mg, 225 mg, 300 mg	PAF, WPW, life-threatening ventricular arrhythmias	**A:** 450–900 mg/day	Dizziness, blurred vision, altered taste, nausea, exacerbation of asthma, proarrhythmia

Class II (Beta-Blockers)

Acebutolol (p. 9) (Sectral)	**C:** 200 mg, 400 mg	AF, A flutter, PSVT, PVCs	**A:** 600–1,200 mg/day	Bradycardia, hypotension, depression, nightmares, fatigue, sexual dysfunction
Esmolol (p. 442) (Brevibloc)	**I:** 10 mg/ml, 250 mg/ml	AF, A flutter, PSVT, PVCs	**A:** 50–200 mcg/kg/min	Hypotension
Propranolol (p. 984) (Inderal)	**T:** 10 mg, 20 mg	AF, A flutter, PSVT, PVCs	**A:** 10–30 mg 3–4 times/day	Bradycardia, hypotension, depression, nightmares, fatigue, sexual dysfunction

(continued)

ANTIARRHYTHMICS ***(continued)***

Name	Availability	Uses	Dosage Range	Side Effects
Class III				
Amiodarone (p. 57) (Cordarone, Pacerone)	**T:** 200 mg, 400 mg **I:** 50 mg/ml	AF, PAF, PSVT, life-threatening ventricular arrhythmias	**A (PO):** 800–1,600 mg/day for 1–3 wks, then 600–800 mg/day **(IV):** 150 mg bolus, then IV infusion	Blurred vision, photophobia, constipation, ataxia, proarrhythmia
Dofetilide evolve **(Tikosyn)**	**C:** 125 mcg, 250 mcg, 500 mcg	AF, A flutter	**A:** Individualized	Torsades de pointes, hypotension
Ibutilide evolve **(Corvert)**	**I:** 0.1 mg/ml	AF, A flutter	**A (greater than 60 kg):** 1 mg over 10 min; **(less than 60 kg):** 0.01 mg/kg over 10 min	Torsades de pointes
Sotalol (p. 1080) (Betapace)	**T:** 80 mg, 120 mg, 160 mg, 240 mg	AF, PAF, PSVT, life-threatening ventricular arrhythmias	**A:** 160–640 mg/day	Fatigue, dizziness, dyspnea, bradycardia, proarrhythmia
Class IV (Calcium Channel Blockers)				
Diltiazem (p. 365) (Cardizem)	**I:** 25 mg/ml vials, **Infusion:** 1 mg/ml	AF, A flutter, PSVT	**A (IV):** 20–25 mg bolus, then infusion of 5–15 mg/hr	Hypotension, bradycardia, dizziness, headaches
Verapamil (p. 1211) (Calan, Isoptin)	**I:** 5 mg/2 ml	AF, A flutter, PSVT	**A (IV):** 5–10 mg	Hypotension, bradycardia, dizziness, headaches, constipation

A, Adults; ***AF,*** atrial fibrillation; ***A flutter,*** atrial flutter; ***C,*** capsules; ***CHF,*** congestive heart failure; ***ER,*** extended-release; ***I,*** injection; ***PAF,*** paroxysmal atrial fibrillation; ***PSVT,*** paroxysmal supraventricular tachycardia; ***PVCs,*** premature ventricular contractions; ***SLE,*** systemic lupus erythematosus; ***SR,*** sustained-release; ***T,*** tablets; ***VF,*** ventricular fibrillation; ***VT,*** ventricular tachycardia; ***WPW,*** Wolff-Parkinson-White syndrome.

Antibiotics

USES

Treatment of wide range of gram-positive or gram-negative bacterial infections, suppression of intestinal flora before surgery, control of acne, prophylactically to prevent rheumatic fever, prophylactically in high-risk situations (e.g., some surgical procedures or medical conditions) to prevent bacterial infection.

ACTION

Antibiotics (antimicrobial agents) are natural or synthetic compounds that have the ability to kill or suppress the growth of microorganisms.

One means of classifying antibiotics is by their antimicrobial spectrum. Narrow-spectrum agents are effective against few microorganisms (e.g., aminoglycosides are effective against gram-negative aerobes), whereas broad-spectrum agents are effective against a wide variety of microorganisms (e.g., fluoroquinolones are effective against gram-positive cocci and gram-negative bacilli).

Antimicrobial agents may also be classified based on their mechanism of action.

- Agents that inhibit cell wall synthesis or activate enzymes that disrupt the cell wall, causing a weakening in the cell, cell lysis, and death. Include penicillins, cephalosporins, vancomycin, imidazole antifungal agents.
- Agents that act directly on the cell wall, affecting permeability of cell membranes, causing leakage of intracellular substances. Include antifungal agents amphotericin and nystatin, polymixin, colistin.
- Agents that bind to ribosomal subunits, altering protein synthesis and eventually causing cell death. Include aminoglycosides.
- Agents that affect bacterial ribosome function, altering protein synthesis and causing slow microbial growth. Do not cause cell death. Include chloramphenicol, clindamycin, erythromycin, tetracyclines.
- Agents that inhibit nucleic acid metabolism by binding to nucleic acid or interacting with enzymes necessary for nucleic acid synthesis. Inhibit DNA or RNA synthesis. Include rifampin, metronidazole, quinolones (e.g., ciprofloxacin).
- Agents that inhibit specific metabolic steps necessary for microbial growth, causing a decrease in essential cell components or synthesis of nonfunctional analogues of normal metabolites. Include trimethoprim, sulfonamides.
- Agents that inhibit viral DNA synthesis by binding to viral enzymes necessary for DNA synthesis, preventing viral replication. Include acyclovir, vidarabine.

Antibiotics *(continued)*

SELECTION OF ANTIMICROBIAL AGENTS

The goal of therapy is to achieve antimicrobial action at the site of infection sufficient to inhibit the growth of the microorganism. The agent selected should be the most active against the most likely infecting organism, least likely to cause toxicity or allergic reaction. Factors to consider in selection of an antimicrobial agent include the following:

- Sensitivity pattern of the infecting microorganism
- Location and severity of infection (may determine route of administration)
- Pt's ability to eliminate the drug (status of renal and hepatic function)
- Pt's defense mechanisms (includes both cellular and humoral immunity)
- Pt's age, pregnancy status, genetic factors, allergies, CNS disorder, preexisting medical problems

CATEGORIZATION OF ORGANISMS BY GRAM STAINING

Gram-Positive Cocci	Gram-Negative Cocci	Gram-Positive Bacilli	Gram-Negative Bacilli
Aerobic	**Aerobic**	**Aerobic**	**Aerobic**
Staphylococcus aureus	*Neisseria gonorrhoeae*	*Listeria monocytogenes*	*Escherichia coli*
Staphylococcus epidermidis	*Neisseria meningitidis*	*Bacillus anthracis*	*Klebsiella pneumoniae*
Streptococcus pneumoniae	*Moraxella catarrhalis*	*Corynebacterium diphtheriae*	*Proteus mirabilis*
Streptococcus pyogenes		**Anaerobic**	*Serratia marcescens*
Viridans streptococci		*Clostridium difficile*	*Pseudomonas aeruginosa*
Enterococcus faecalis		*Clostridium perfringens*	*Enterobacter* spp.
Enterococcus faecium		*Clostridium tetani*	*Haemophilus influenzae*
Anaerobic		*Actinomyces* spp.	*Legionella pneumophila*
Peptostreptococcus spp.			**Anaerobic**
Peptococcus spp.			*Bacteroides fragilis*
			Fusobacterium spp.

Antibiotic: Aminoglycosides

USES

Treatment of serious infections when other less toxic agents are not effective, are contraindicated, or require adjunctive therapy (e.g., with penicillins or cephalosporins). Used primarily in the treatment of infections caused by gram-negative microorganisms, such as those caused by *Proteus, Klebsiella, Pseudomonas, Escherichia coli, Serratia, and Enterobacter*. Inactive against most gram-positive microorganisms. Not well absorbed systemically from GI tract (must be administered parenterally for systemic infections). Oral agents are given to suppress intestinal bacteria.

ACTION

Bactericidal. Transported across bacterial cell membrane; irreversibly binds to specific receptor proteins of bacterial ribosomes. Interfere with protein synthesis, preventing cell reproduction and eventually causing cell death.

ANTIBIOTIC: AMINOGLYCOSIDES

Name	Availability	Dosage Range	Side Effects
Amikacin (p. 50) **(Amikin)**	**I:** 50 mg/ml, 250 mg/ml	**A:** 15 mg/kg/day **C:** 15 mg/kg/day	Nephrotoxicity, neurotoxicity, ototoxicity (both auditory and vestibular), hypersensitivity (skin itching, redness, rash, swelling)
Gentamicin (p. 543) **(Garamycin)**	**I:** 10 mg/ml, 40 mg/ml	**A:** 3–5 mg/kg/day **C:** 6–7.5 mg/kg/day	Same as amikacin
Neomycin (p. 826)	**T:** 500 mg	**A:** 1 g for 3 doses as preop	Nausea, vomiting, diarrhea

(continued)

ANTIBIOTIC: AMINOGLYCOSIDES *(continued)*

Name	Availability	Dosage Range	Side Effects
Streptomycin	**I:** 1 g	**A:** 15 mg/kg/day **C:** 20–40 mg/kg/day **Maximum:** 1 g	Same as amikacin Peripheral neuritis (numbness), optic neuritis (any vision loss)
Tobramycin (p. 1153) (Nebcin)	**I:** 40 mg/ml,10 mg/ml	**A:** 3–5 mg/kg/day **C:** 6–7.5 mg/kg/day	Same as amikacin

A, Adults; ***C*** *(dosage),* children; ***I,*** injection; ***T,*** tablets.

Antibiotic: Cephalosporins

USES

Broad-spectrum antibiotics, which, like penicillins, may be used in a number of diseases, including respiratory diseases, skin and soft tissue infection, bone/joint infections, GU infections, prophylactically in some surgical procedures.

First-generation cephalosporins have good activity against gram-positive organisms and moderate activity against gram-negative organisms, including *Escherichia coli, Klebsiella pneumoniae, Proteus mirabilis.*

Second-generation cephalosporins have increased activity against gram-negative organisms.

Third-generation cephalosporins are less active against gram-positive organisms but more active against the Enterobacteriaceae with some activity against *Pseudomonas aeruginosa.*

Fourth-generation cephalosporins have good activity against gram-positive organisms (e.g., *Staphylococcus aureus*) and gram-negative organisms (e.g., *Pseudomonas aeruginosa*).

ACTION

Cephalosporins inhibit cell wall synthesis or activate enzymes that disrupt the cell wall, causing cell lysis and cell death. May be bacteriostatic or bactericidal. Most effective against rapidly dividing cells.

ANTIBIOTIC: CEPHALOSPORINS

Name	Availability	Dosage Range	Side Effects
First-Generation			
Cefadroxil (p. 200) (Duricef)	**C:** 500 mg **T:** 1 g **S:** 125 mg/5 ml, 250 mg/5 ml, 500 mg/5 ml	**A:** 1–2 g/day **C:** 30 mg/kg/day	Abdominal cramps/pain, fever, nausea, vomiting, diarrhea, headaches, oral/vaginal candidiasis
Cefazolin (p. 201) (Ancef, Kefzol)	**I:** 500 mg, 1 g, 2 g	**A:** 0.75–6 g/day **C:** 25–100 mg/kg/day	Same as cefadroxil
Cephalexin (p. 229) (Keflex, Keftab)	**C:** 250 mg, 500 mg **T:** 250 mg, 500 mg, 1 g	**A:** 1–4 g/day **C:** 25–100 mg/kg/day	Same as cefadroxil
Second-Generation			
Cefaclor (p. 198) (Ceclor)	**C:** 250 mg, 500 mg **T (ER):** 375 mg, 500 mg **S:** 125 mg/5 ml, 187 mg/5 ml, 250 mg/5 ml, 375 mg/5 ml	**A:** 250–500 mg q8h **C:** 20–40 mg/kg/day	Same as cefadroxil May have serum sickness–like reaction
Cefoxitin (p. 212) (Mefoxin)	**I:** 1 g, 2 g	**A:** 3–12 g/day	Same as cefadroxil
Cefpodoxime (p. 214) (Vantin)	**T:** 100 mg, 200 mg **S:** 50 mg/5 ml, 100 mg/5 ml	**A:** 200–800 mg/day **C:** 10 mg/kg/day	Same as cefadroxil
Cefprozil (p. 216) (Cefzil)	**T:** 250 mg, 500 mg **S:** 125 mg/5 ml, 250 mg/5 ml	**A:** 0.5–1 g/day **C:** 30 mg/kg/day	Same as cefadroxil

(continued)

ANTIBIOTIC: CEPHALOSPORINS ***(continued)***

Name	Availability	Dosage Range	Side Effects
Second-Generation *(continued)*			
Cefuroxime (p. 225) (Ceftin, Kefurox, Zinacef)	**T:** 125 mg, 250 mg, 500 mg **S:** 125 mg/5 ml, 250 mg/5 ml **I:** 750 mg, 1.5 g	**A (PO):** 0.25–1 g/day; **(IM/IV):** 2.25–9 g/day **C (PO):** 250–500 mg/day; **(IM/IV):** 50–100 mg/kg/day	Same as cefadroxil
Third-Generation			
Cefdinir (p. 203) (Omnicef)	**C:** 300 mg **S:** 125 mg/5 ml	**A:** 600 mg/day **C:** 14 mg/kg/day	Same as cefadroxil
Cefditoren (p. 205) (Spectracef)	**T:** 200 mg	**A:** 400–800 mg/day	Same as cefadroxil
Cefotaxime (p. 210) (Claforan)	**I:** 500 mg, 1 g, 2 g	**A:** 2–12 g/day **C:** 100–200 mg/kg/day	Same as cefadroxil
Ceftazidime (p. 218) (Fortaz, Tazicef, Tazidime)	**I:** 500 mg, 1 g, 2 g	**A:** 0.5–6 g/day **C:** 90–150 mg/kg/day	Same as cefadroxil

Ceftibuten (p. 220) (Cedax)	**C:** 400 mg **S:** 90 mg/5 ml, 180 mg/5 ml	**A:** 400 mg/day **C:** 9 mg/kg/day	Same as cefadroxil
Ceftizoxime (p. 221) (Cefizox)	**I:** 500 mg, 1 g, 2 g	**A:** 1–12 g/day **C:** 150–200 mg/kg/day	Same as cefadroxil
Ceftriaxone (p. 223) (Rocephin)	**I:** 250 mg, 500 mg, 1 g, 2 g	**A:** 1–4 g/day **C:** 50–100 mg/kg/day	Same as cefadroxil

Fourth-Generation

Cefepime (p. 207) (Maxipime)	**I:** 500 mg, 1 g, 2 g	**A:** 1–6 g/day	Same as cefadroxil

A, Adults; ***C,*** capsules; ***C*** *(dosage),* children; ***ER,*** extended-release; ***I,*** injection; ***S,*** suspension; ***T,*** tablets.

Antibiotic: Fluoroquinolones

USES

Fluoroquinolones act against a wide range of gram-negative and gram-positive organisms. They are used primarily in the treatment of lower respiratory infections, skin/skin structure infections, UTIs, and sexually transmitted diseases.

ACTION

Bactericidal. Inhibit DNA gyrase in susceptible microorganisms, interfering with bacterial DNA replication and repair.

Antibiotic: Fluoroquinolones *(continued)*

ANTIBIOTIC: FLUOROQUINOLONES

Name	Availability	Dosage Range	Side Effects
Ciprofloxacin (p. 253) (Cipro)	**T**: 250 mg, 500 mg, 750 mg **S**: 5 g/100 ml **I**: 200 mg, 400 mg	**A (PO)**: 250–750 mg q12h; **(IV)**: 200–400 mg q12h	Dizziness, headaches, anxiety, drowsiness, insomnia, abdominal pain, nausea, diarrhea, vomiting, phlebitis (parenteral)
Gemifloxacin (p. 540) (Factive)	**T**: 320 mg	**A**: 320 mg/day	Same as ciprofloxacin
Levofloxacin (p. 684) (Levaquin)	**T**: 250 mg, 500 mg, 750 mg **I**: 250 mg, 500 mg, 750 mg	**A (PO/IV)**: 250–750 mg/ day as single dose	Same as ciprofloxacin
Lomefloxacin (p. 699) (Maxaquin)	**T**: 400 mg	**A**: 400 mg/day	Same as ciprofloxacin
Moxifloxacin (p. 795) (Avelox)	**T**: 400 mg **I**: 400 mg	**A**: 400 mg/day	Same as ciprofloxacin; may prolong QT interval
Norfloxacin (p. 853) (Noroxin)	**T**: 400 mg	**A**: 400 mg q12h	Same as ciprofloxacin
Ofloxacin (p. 860) (Floxin)	**T**: 200 mg, 300 mg, 400 mg	**A**: 200–400 mg q12h	Same as ciprofloxacin

A, Adults; ***I,*** injection; ***S,*** suspension; ***T,*** tablets.

Antibiotic: Macrolides

USES

Macrolides act primarily against gram-positive microorganisms and gram-negative cocci. Azithromycin and clarithromycin appear to be more potent than erythromycin. Macrolides are used in the treatment of pharyngitis/tonsillitis, sinusitis, chronic bronchitis, pneumonia, uncomplicated skin/skin structure infections.

ACTION

Bacteriostatic or bactericidal. Reversibly bind to the P site of the 50S ribosomal subunit of susceptible organisms, inhibiting RNA-dependent protein synthesis.

ANTIBIOTIC: MACROLIDES

Name	Availability	Dosage Range	Side Effects
Azithromycin (p. 114) (Zithromax)	**T:** 250 mg, 600 mg **S:** 100 mg/5 ml, 200 mg/5 ml, 1-g packet **I:** 500 mg	**A (PO):** 500 mg once, then 250 mg days 2–5; **(IV):** 500 mg/day **C (PO):** 10 mg/kg once, then 5 mg/kg/day on days 2–5	**PO:** Nausea, diarrhea, vomiting, abdominal pain **IV:** Pain, redness, swelling at injection site
Clarithromycin (p. 262) (Biaxin)	**T:** 250 mg, 500 mg **T (XL):** 500 mg **S:** 125 mg/5 ml	**A:** 250–500 mg q12h **C:** 7.5 mg/kg q12h	Headaches, loss of taste, nausea, vomiting, diarrhea, abdominal pain/discomfort
Dirithromycin (Dynabac) evolve	**T:** 250 mg	**A, C (older than 12 yrs):** 500 mg/day as a single daily dose	Dizziness, nausea, vomiting, diarrhea, abdominal pain, headaches, weakness

(continued)

ANTIBIOTIC: MACROLIDES *(continued)*

Name	Availability	Dosage Range	Side Effects
Erythromycin (p. 438) (Ery-Tab, PCE, Eryc, EES, EryPed, Erythrocin)	**T:** 200 mg, 250 mg, 333 mg, 400 mg, 500 mg **C:** 250 mg **S:** 125 mg/5 ml, 200 mg/5 ml, 250 mg/5 ml, 400 mg/5 ml, 100 mg/2.5 ml	**A (PO):** 250–500 mg q6h **C (PO):** 30–50 mg/kg/day **A, C (IV):** 15–20 mg/kg/day **Maximum:** 4 g/day	**PO:** Nausea, vomiting, diarrhea, abdominal pain **IV:** Inflammation, phlebitis at injection site

A, Adults; ***C,*** capsules; ***C*** *(dosage),* children; ***I,*** injection; ***S,*** suspension; ***T,*** tablets; ***XL,*** long acting.

Antibiotic: Penicillins

USES

Penicillins may be used to treat a large number of infections, including pneumonia and other respiratory diseases, UTIs, septicemia, meningitis, intra-abdominal infections, gonorrhea and syphilis, bone/joint infection.

Penicillins are classified based on an antimicrobial spectrum:

Natural penicillins are very active against gram-positive cocci but ineffective against most strains of *Staphylococcus aureus* (inactivated by enzyme penicillinase).

Penicillinase-resistant penicillins are effective against penicillinase-producing *Staphylococcus aureus* but are less effective against gram-positive cocci than the natural penicillins.

Broad-spectrum penicillins are effective against gram-positive cocci and some gram-negative bacteria (e.g., *Haemophilus influenzae, Escherichia coli, Proteus mirabilis*).

Extended-spectrum penicillins are effective against *Pseudomonas aeruginosa, Enterobacter, Proteus* species, *Klebsiella,* and some other gram-negative microorganisms.

ACTION

Penicillins inhibit cell wall synthesis or activate enzymes, which disrupt the bacterial cell wall, causing cell lysis and cell death. May be bacteriostatic or bactericidal. Most effective against bacteria undergoing active growth and division.

ANTIBIOTIC: PENICILLINS

Name	Availability	Dosage Range	Side Effects
Natural			
Penicillin G benzathine (p. 916) (Bicillin, Bicillin LA)	**I:** 600,000 units, 1.2 million units, 2.4 million units	**A:** 1.2 million units/day **C:** 0.3–1.2 million units/day	Mild diarrhea, nausea, vomiting, headaches, sore mouth/tongue, vaginal itching/discharge, allergic reaction (including anaphylaxis, skin rash, urticaria, pruritus)
Penicillin G potassium (p. 917) (Pfizerpen)	**I:** 1, 2, 3, 5 million-unit vials	**A:** 2–24 million units/day **C:** 100–250,000 units/kg/day	Same as penicillin G benzathine
Penicillin V potassium (p. 919) (Apo-Pen-VK)	**T:** 250 mg, 500 mg **S:** 125 mg/5 ml, 250 mg/5 ml	**A:** 0.5–2 g/day **C:** 25–50 mg/kg/day	Same as penicillin G benzathine
Penicillinase-Resistant			
Cloxacillin (Tegopen)	**C:** 250 mg, 500 mg **S:** 125 mg/5 ml	**A:** 1–2 g/day **C:** 50–100 mg/kg/day	Same as penicillin G benzathine Increased risk of hepatic toxicity
Dicloxacillin (Dynapen, Pathocil)	**C:** 125 mg, 250 mg, 500 mg **S:** 62.5 mg/5 ml	**A:** 1–2 g/day **C:** 12.5–25 mg/kg/day	Same as penicillin G benzathine Increased risk of hepatic toxicity
Nafcillin (p. 808) (Unipen)	**C:** 250 mg **I:** 500 mg, 1 g, 2 g	**A (PO):** 1–6 g/day; **(IV):** 2–6 g/day **C (PO):** 25–50 mg/kg/day; **(IV):** 50 mg/kg/day	Same as penicillin G benzathine Increased risk of interstitial nephritis
Oxacillin (Bactocill)	**C:** 250 mg, 500 mg **S:** 250 mg/5 ml **I:** 250 mg, 500 mg, 1 g, 2 g	**A (PO/IV):** 2–6 g/day **C (PO/IV):** 50–100 mg/kg/day	Same as penicillin G benzathine Increased risk of hepatic toxicity, interstitial nephritis

(continued)

ANTIBIOTIC: PENICILLINS *(continued)*

Name	Availability	Dosage Range	Side Effects
Broad-Spectrum			
Amoxicillin (p. 63) (Amoxil, Trimox)	**T:** 125 mg, 250 mg, 500 mg, 875 mg **C:** 250 mg, 500 mg **S:** 50 mg/ml, 125 mg/5 ml, 250 mg/5 ml	**A:** 0.75–1.5 g/day **C:** 20–40 mg/kg/day	Same as penicillin G benzathine
Amoxicillin/clavulanate (p. 65) (Augmentin)	**T:** 250 mg, 500 mg, 875 mg **T (chewable):** 125 mg, 200 mg, 250 mg, 400 mg **S:** 125 mg/5 ml, 200 mg/5 ml, 250 mg/5 ml, 400 mg/5 ml	**A:** 0.75–1.5 g/day **C:** 20–40 mg/kg/day	Same as penicillin G benzathine
Ampicillin (p. 70) (Principen)	**C:** 250 mg, 500 mg **S:** 125 mg/5 ml, 250 mg/5 ml **I:** 125 mg, 250 mg, 500 mg, 1 g, 2 g	**A:** 1–12 g/day **C:** 50–200 mg/kg/day	Same as penicillin G benzathine
Ampicillin/sulbactam (p. 72) (Unasyn)	**I:** 1.5 g, 3 g	**A:** 6–12 g/day **C:** 100–200 mg/kg/day	Same as penicillin G benzathine
Extended-Spectrum			
Carbenicillin (Geocillin)	**T:** 382 mg	**A:** 382–764 mg 4 times/day	Same as penicillin G benzathine
Piperacillin/tazobactam (p. 942) (Zosyn)	**I:** 2.25 g, 3.375 g, 4.5 g	**A:** 2.25–4.5 g q6–8h **C:** 200–400 mg/kg/day	Same as penicillin G benzathine
Ticarcillin/clavulanate (p. 1137) (Timentin)	**I:** 3.1 g	**A:** 3.1 g q4–6h **C:** 200–300 mg/kg/day	Same as penicillin G benzathine

A, Adults; ***C,*** capsules; ***C*** *(dosage),* children; ***I,*** injection; ***S,*** suspension; ***T,*** tablets.

Anticoagulants/Antiplatelets/Thrombolytics

USES

Treatment and prevention of venous thromboembolism, acute MI, acute cerebral embolism; reduce risk of acute MI; reduce total mortality in pts with unstable angina; prevent occlusion of saphenous grafts following open heart surgery; prevent embolism in select pts with atrial fibrillation, prosthetic heart valves, valvular heart disease, cardiomyopathy. Heparin also used for acute/chronic consumption coagulopathies (disseminated intravascular coagulation).

ACTION

Anticoagulants: Inhibit blood coagulation by preventing the formation of new clots and extension of existing ones *but do not dissolve formed clots.* Anticoagulants are subdivided into two common classes. *Heparin:* Indirectly interferes with blood coagulation by blocking the conversion of prothrombin to thrombin and fibrinogen to fibrin. *Coumarin:* Acts indirectly to prevent synthesis in the liver of vitamin K–dependent clotting factors.

Antiplatelets: Interfere with platelet aggregation. Effects are irreversible for life of platelet. Medications in this group act by different mechanisms and are used in combinations to provide desired effect.

Thrombolytics: Act directly or indirectly on fibrinolytic system to dissolve clots (converting plasminogen to plasmin, an enzyme that digests fibrin clot).

ANTICOAGULANTS/ANTIPLATELETS/THROMBOLYTICS

Name	Availability	Uses	Side Effects
Anticoagulants			
Argatroban (p. 86)	**I:** 100 mg/ml	Prevent/treat VTE in pts with HIT or at risk for HIT undergoing PCI	Bleeding
Bivalirudin (p. 145) (Angiomax)	**I:** 250-mg vials	Pts with unstable angina undergoing PTCA	Bleeding
Dalteparin (p. 311) (Fragmin)	**I:** 2,500 units, 5,000 units, 7,500 units, 10,000 units	Hip surgery; abdominal surgery; unstable angina or non–Q-wave myocardial infarction	Bleeding, hematoma

(continued)

ANTICOAGULANTS/ANTIPLATELETS/THROMBOLYTICS *(continued)*

Name	Availability	Uses	Side Effects
Anticoagulants	*(continued)*		
Enoxaparin (p. 415) (Lovenox)	**I**: 30 mg, 40 mg, 60 mg, 80 mg, 100 mg, 120 mg, 150 mg	Hip surgery; knee surgery; abdominal surgery; unstable angina or non–Q-wave myocardial infarction; acute illness	Bleeding, thrombocytopenia, hematoma
Fondaparinux (p. 513) (Arixtra)	**I**: 2.5 mg	Hip surgery; knee surgery	Bleeding, thrombocytopenia, hematoma
Heparin (p. 568)	**I**: 1,000 units/ml, 2,500 units/ml, 5,000 units/ml, 7,500 units/ml, 10,000 units/ml, 20,000 units/ml	Prevent/treat VTE	Bleeding, thrombocytopenia, skin rash
Lepirudin (p. 674) (Refludan)	**I**: 50-mg vials	Prevent VTE in pts with HIT	Bleeding
Tinzaparin (p. 1146) (Innohep)	**I**: 20,000 units/ml vials	Treatment of VTE (with warfarin)	Bleeding, thrombocytopenia
Warfarin (p. 1230) (Coumadin)	**PO**: 1 mg, 2 mg, 2.5 mg, 3 mg, 4 mg, 5 mg, 6 mg, 7.5 mg, 10 mg **I**: 2 mg/ml	Prevent/treat VTE in pts; prevent systemic embolism in pts with heart valve replacement, valve heart disease, myocardial infarction, atrial fibrillation	Bleeding, skin necrosis

HIT, Heparin-induced thrombocytopenia; ***I,*** injection; ***PCI,*** percutaneous coronary intervention; ***PTCA,*** percutaneous transluminal coronary angioplasty; ***VTE,*** venous thromboembolism.

Name	Availability	Uses	Side Effects
Antiplatelets			
Abciximab (p. 5) (ReoPro)	**I:** 2 mg/ml	Adjunct to PCI to prevent acute cardiac ischemic complications (with heparin and aspirin)	Bleeding, hypotension, nausea, vomiting, back pain, allergic reactions, thrombocytopenia
Aspirin (p. 96)	**PO:** 81 mg, 165 mg, 325 mg, 500 mg, 650 mg	TIA in males; myocardial infarction prophylaxis; cardiac vascular disease	Tinnitus, dizziness, hypersensitivity, dyspepsia, minor bleeding, GI ulceration
Clopidogrel (p. 275) (Plavix)	**PO:** 75 mg	Reduce risk in pts with unstable angina, non–Q-wave myocardial infarction, recent myocardial infarction, CVA	Bleeding
Dipyridamole (p. 373) (Persantine)	**PO:** 25 mg, 50 mg, 75 mg	Prevent postoperative thromboembolic complications following cardiac valve replacement	Dizziness, GI distress
Eptifibatide (p. 430) (Integrilin)	**I:** 0.75 mg/ml, 2 mg/ml	Treatment of acute coronary syndrome	Bleeding, hypotension
Ticlopidine (p. 1138) (Ticlid)	**PO:** 250 mg	Reduce risk stroke in pts with CVA precursors, TIA	Neutropenia, agranulocytosis, thrombocytopenia, aplastic anemia, increased serum cholesterol/triglycerides, rash, diarrhea, nausea, vomiting, GI pain
Tirofiban (p. 1150) (Aggrastat)	**I:** 50 mcg/ml, 250 mcg/ml	Treatment of acute coronary syndrome	Bleeding, thrombocytopenia

CVA, Cerebrovascular attack; ***I,*** injection; ***PCI,*** percutaneous coronary intervention; ***PO,*** oral; ***TIA,*** transient ischemic attack.

(continued)

ANTICOAGULANTS/ANTIPLATELETS/THROMBOLYTICS *(continued)*

Name	Availability	Indications	Side Effects
Thrombolytics			
Alteplase (p. 43) (Activase)	**I:** 50 mg, 100 mg	Acute myocardial infarction, acute ischemic stroke, pulmonary embolism	Bleeding, cholesterol embolism, arrhythmias
Reteplase (p. 1019) (Retavase)	**I:** 10.4 units	Acute myocardial infarction	Bleeding, cholesterol embolism, arrhythmias
Streptokinase (p. 1087)	**I:** 250,000 units, 750,000 units, 1.5 million units	Myocardial infarction; venous thromboembolism; arterial thromboembolism	Bleeding, cholesterol embolism, arrhythmias, hypotension
Tenecteplase (p. 1114) (TNKase)	I: 50 mg	Acute myocardial infarction	Bleeding, cholesterol embolism, arrhythmias

I, Injection.

Anticonvulsants

USES

Anticonvulsants are used to treat seizures. Seizures can be divided into two broad categories: partial seizures and generalized seizures. *Partial seizures* begin focally in the cerebral cortex, undergoing limited spread. Simple partial seizures do not involve loss of consciousness but may evolve secondarily into generalized seizures. Complex partial seizures involve impairment of consciousness.

Generalized seizures may be convulsive or nonconvulsive and usually produce immediate loss of consciousness.

ACTION

Anticonvulsants can prevent or reduce excessive discharge of neurons with seizure foci or decrease the spread of excitation from seizure foci to normal neurons. The exact mechanism is unknown but may be due to (1) suppressing sodium influx, (2) suppressing calcium influx, or (3) increasing the action of GABA, which inhibits neurotransmitters throughout the brain.

ANTICONVULSANTS

Name	Availability	Uses	Dosage Range	Side Effects
Carbamazepine (p. 185) (Tegretol)	**S:** 100 mg/5 ml **T (chewable):** 100 mg **T:** 200 mg **T (ER):** 100 mg, 200 mg, 400 mg **C (ER):** 200 mg, 300 mg	Complex partial, tonic-clonic, mixed seizures; trigeminal neuralgia	**A:** 800–1,200 mg/day **C:** 400–800 mg/day	Dizziness, diplopia, leukopenia
Clonazepam (p. 271) (Klonopin)	**T:** 0.5 mg, 1 mg, 2 mg	Petit mal, akinetic, myoclonic, absence seizures	**A:** 1.5–20 mg/day	CNS depression, sedation, ataxia, confusion, depression

(continued)

ANTICONVULSANTS *(continued)*

Name	Availability	Uses	Dosage Range	Side Effects
Diazepam (p. 350) (Valium)	**T:** 2 mg, 5 mg, 10 mg **I:** 5 mg/ml **R:** 2.5 mg, 5 mg, 10 mg, 20 mg	Adjunctive therapy status epilepticus	**A (PO):** 4–40 mg/day; **(IM/IV):** 5–30 mg **C (PO):** 3–10 mg/day; **(IM/IV):** 1–10 mg	CNS depression, sedation, confusion, mental depression, respiratory depression
Fosphenytoin (p. 522) (Cerebyx)	**I:** 50 mg PE/ml	Status epilepticus, seizures occurring during neurosurgery	**A:** 15–20 mg PE/kg bolus, then 4–6 mg PE/kg/day maintenance	Burning, itching, paresthesia, nystagmus, ataxia
Gabapentin (p. 529) (Neurontin)	**C:** 100 mg, 300 mg, 400 mg	Partial seizures with and without secondary generalization	**A:** 900–1,800 mg/day	CNS depression, fatigue, drowsiness, dizziness, ataxia
Lamotrigine (p. 665) (Lamictal)	**T:** 25 mg, 100 mg, 150 mg, 200 mg	Partial seizures	**A:** 100–500 mg/day	Dizziness, ataxia, drowsiness, diplopia, nausea, rash
Oxcarbazepine (p. 881) (Trileptal)	**T:** 150 mg, 300 mg, 600 mg	Partial seizures	**A:** 900–1,800 mg/day	Drowsiness, dizziness, headaches
Phenobarbital (p. 928)	**T:** 30 mg, 60 mg, 100 mg **I:** 65 mg, 130 mg	Tonic-clonic, partial seizures; status epilepticus	**A (PO):** 100–300 mg/day; **(IM/IV):** 200–600 mg. **C (PO):** 3–5 mg/kg/day; **(IM/IV):** 100–400 mg	CNS depression, sedation, paradoxical excitement and hyperactivity, rash
Phenytoin (p. 934) (Dilantin)	**C:** 100 mg **T: (chewable):** 50 mg **S:** 125 mg/5 ml **I:** 50 mg/ml	Tonic-clonic, psychomotor seizures	**A (PO):** 300–600 mg/day; **IV:** 150–250 mg **C (PO):** 4–8 mg/kg/day; **(IV):** 10–15 mg/kg	Nystagmus, ataxia, hypertrichosis, gingival hyperplasia, rash, osteomalacia, lymphadenopathy

Primidone (p. 966) (Mysoline)	**T:** 50 mg; 250 mg **S:** 250 mg/5 ml	Complex, partial, akinetic, tonic-clonic seizures	**A:** 750–2,000 mg/day **C:** 10–25 mg/kg/day	CNS depression, sedation, paradoxical excitement and hyperactivity, rash, dizziness, ataxia
Tiagabine (p. 1135) (Gabitril)	**T:** 4 mg, 12 mg, 16 mg, 20 mg	Partial seizures	**A:** Initially, 4 mg up to 56 mg **C:** Initially, 4 mg up to 32 mg	Dizziness, asthenia, nervousness, anxiety, tremors, abdominal pain
Topiramate (p. 1157) (Topamax)	**T:** 25 mg, 100 mg, 200 mg	Partial seizures	**A:** 25–400 mg/day **C:** 1–9 mg/kg/day	Impaired concentration, speech impairment, fatigue
Valproic acid (p. 1198) (Depakene, Depakote)	**C:** 250 mg **S:** 250 mg/5 ml **Sprinkles:** 125 mg **T:** 125 mg, 250 mg, 500 mg **T (ER):** 500 mg **I:** 100 mg/ml	Complex partial, absence seizures	**A, C:** 15–60 mg/kg/day	Nausea, vomiting, tremors, thrombocytopenia, hair loss, hepatic dysfunction
Zonisamide (p. 1247) (Zonegran)	**C:** 100 mg	Partial seizures	**A:** 500 mg/day	Drowsiness, dizziness, anorexia, headaches, nausea

A, Adults; ***C,*** capsules; ***C*** *(dosage),* children; ***ER,*** extended-release; ***I,*** injection; ***PE,*** phenytoin equivalent; ***R,*** rectal; ***S,*** suspension; ***T,*** tablets.

Antidepressants

USES

Used primarily for the treatment of depression. Imipramine is also used for childhood enuresis. Clomipramine is used only for obsessive-compulsive disorder (OCD). Monoamine oxidase inhibitors (MAOIs) are rarely used as initial therapy except for pts unresponsive to other therapy or when other therapy is contraindicated.

ACTION

Antidepressants are classified as tricyclics, MAOIs, or second-generation antidepressants (further subdivided into selective serotonin reuptake inhibitors [SSRIs] and atypical antidepressants). Depression may be due to reduced functioning of monoamine neurotransmitters (e.g., norepinephrine, serotonin [5-HT], dopamine) in the CNS (decreased amount and/or decreased effects at the receptor sites). Antidepressants block metabolism, increase amount/effects of monoamine neurotransmitters, and act at receptor sites (change responsiveness/sensitivities of both presynaptic and postsynaptic receptor sites).

ANTIDEPRESSANTS

Name	Availability	Uses	Dosage Range (per day)	Side Effects
Tricyclics				
Amitriptyline (p. 59) (Elavil)	**T:** 10 mg, 25 mg, 50 mg, 75 mg, 100 mg, 150 mg	Depression	40–300 mg	Drowsiness, blurred vision, constipation, confusion, postural hypotension, cardiac conduction defects, weight gain, seizures
Clomipramine (p. 270) (Anafranil)	**C:** 25 mg, 50 mg, 75 mg	OCD	25–250 mg	Same as amitriptyline
Desipramine (p. 334) (Norpramin)	**T:** 10 mg, 25 mg, 50 mg, 75 mg, 100 mg, 150 mg	Depression	25–100 mg	Same as amitriptyline

Doxepin (p. 389) (Sinequan)	**C:** 10 mg, 25 mg, 50 mg, 75 mg, 100 mg, 150 mg **OC:** 10 mg/ml	Depression	25–300 mg	Same as amitriptyline
Imipramine (p. 606) (Tofranil)	**T:** 10 mg, 25 mg, 50 mg **C:** 75 mg, 100 mg, 125 mg, 150 mg	Depression, enuresis	30–300 mg	Same as amitriptyline
Nortriptyline (p. 854) evolve (Aventyl, Pamelor)	**C:** 10 mg, 25 mg, 50 mg, 75 mg **S:**10 mg/5 ml	Depression	25–100 mg	Same as amitriptyline
Protriptyline (Vivactil)	**T:** 5 mg, 10 mg	Depression	15–60 mg	Same as amitriptyline

Monoamine Oxidase Inhibitors

Phenelzine (p. 926) evolve (Nardil)	**T:** 15 mg	Depression	15–90 mg	Sedation, hypertensive crisis, weight gain, orthostatic hypotension
Tranylcypromine (p. 1170) evolve (Parnate)	**T:** 10 mg	Depression	30–60 mg	Same as phenelzine

Selective Serotonin Reuptake Inhibitors

Citalopram (p. 258) (Celexa)	**T:** 20 mg, 40 mg **S:** 10 mg/5 ml	Depression	25–60 mg	Insomnia or sedation, nausea, agitation, headaches
Escitalopram (p. 440) (Lexapro)	**T:** 5 mg, 10 mg, 20 mg	Depression	10–20 mg	Insomnia or sedation, nausea, agitation, headaches
Fluoxetine (p. 498) (Prozac)	**C:** 10 mg, 20 mg, 40 mg **T:** 10 mg **S:** 20 mg/5 ml	Depression, OCD, bulimia	10–80 mg	Akathisia, sexual dysfunction, skin rash, urticaria, pruritus, decreased appetite, asthenia, diarrhea, drowsiness, headaches, diaphoresis, insomnia, nausea, tremors
Fluvoxamine (p. 510) evolve (Luvox)	**T:** 25 mg, 50 mg, 100 mg	OCD	100–300 mg	Sexual dysfunction, fatigue, constipation, dizziness, drowsiness, headaches, insomnia, nausea, vomiting

(continued)

ANTIDEPRESSANTS *(continued)*

Name	Availability	Uses	Dosage Range (per day)	Side Effects
Selective Serotonin Reuptake Inhibitors *(continued)*				
Paroxetine (p. 904) (Paxil)	**T:** 10 mg, 20 mg, 30 mg, 40 mg **S:** 10 mg/5 ml	Depression, OCD, panic attack, social anxiety disorder	20–50 mg	Asthenia, constipation, diarrhea, diaphoresis, insomnia, nausea, sexual dysfunction, tremors, vomiting, urinary frequency or retention
Sertraline (p. 1057) (Zoloft)	**T:** 25 mg, 50 mg, 100 mg **S:** 20 mg/ml	Depression, OCD, panic attack	50–200 mg	Sexual dysfunction, dizziness, drowsiness, anorexia, diarrhea, nausea, dry mouth, abdominal cramps, decreased weight, headaches, increased diaphoresis, tremors, insomnia
Atypical				
Bupropion (p. 164) (Wellbutrin)	**T:** 75 mg, 100 mg **SR:** 100 mg, 150 mg	Depression	150–450 mg	Insomnia, irritability, seizures
Duloxetine (p. 401) (Cymbalta)	**C:** 20 mg, 30 mg, 60 mg	Depression, neuropathic pain	40–60 mg	Nausea, dry mouth, constipation, decreased appetite, fatigue, diaphoresis
Mirtazapine (p. 779) (Remeron)	**T:** 15 mg, 30 mg, 45 mg	Depression	15–45 mg	Sedation, dry mouth, weight gain, agranulocytosis, hepatic toxicity
Trazodone (p. 1173) (Desyrel)	**T:** 50 mg, 100 mg, 150 mg, 300 mg	Depression	50–600 mg	Sedation, orthostatic hypotension, priapism
Venlafaxine (p. 1209) (Effexor)	**T:** 25 mg, 37.5 mg, 50 mg, 75 mg, 100 mg **T (ER):** 37.5 mg, 75 mg, 150 mg	Depression, anxiety	75–375 mg	Increased blood pressure, agitation, sedation, insomnia, nausea

C, Capsules; ***ER,*** extended-release; ***OC,*** oral concentrate; ***OCD,*** obsessive-compulsive disorder; ***S,*** suspension; ***SR,*** sustained-release; ***T,*** tablets.

Antidiabetics

USES	ACTION
Insulin: Treatment of insulin-dependent diabetes (type 1) and non–insulin-dependent diabetes (type 2). Also used in acute situations such as ketoacidosis, severe infections, major surgery in otherwise non–insulin-dependent diabetics. Administered to pts receiving parenteral nutrition. Drug of choice during pregnancy.	*Insulin:* A hormone synthesized and secreted by beta cells of Langerhans' islet in the pancreas. Controls storage and utilization of glucose, amino acids, and fatty acids by activated transport systems/enzymes. Inhibits breakdown of glycogen, fat, protein. Insulin lowers blood glucose by inhibiting glycogenolysis and gluconeogenesis in liver; stimulates glucose uptake by muscle, adipose tissue. Activity of insulin is initiated by binding to cell surface receptors.
Sulfonylureas: Control hyperglycemia in type 2 diabetes not controlled by weight and diet alone. Chlorpropamide also used in adjunctive treatment of neurogenic diabetes insipidus.	*Sulfonylureas:* Stimulate release of insulin from beta cells; increase sensitivity of insulin to peripheral tissue. Endogenous insulin must be present for oral hypoglycemics to be effective.
Alpha-glucosidase inhibitors: Adjunct to diet to lower blood glucose in pts with type 2 diabetes mellitus whose hyperglycemia cannot be managed by diet alone.	*Alpha-glucosidase inhibitors:* Work locally in small intestine, slowing carbohydrate breakdown and glucose absorption.
Biguanides: Adjunct to diet to lower blood glucose in pts with type 2 diabetes mellitus whose hyperglycemia cannot be managed by diet alone.	*Biguanides:* Decrease hepatic glucose output; enhance peripheral glucose uptake.
Thiazolinediones: Adjunct in pts with type 2 diabetes currently on insulin therapy.	*Thiazolinediones:* Decrease insulin resistance.

Antidiabetics *(continued)*

Antidiabetics

INSULIN

Type	Onset	Peak	Duration	Comments
Rapid Acting				
Apidra, glulisine	10–15 min	1–1.5 hrs	3–5 hrs	Stable at room temp for 28 days Can mix with NPH
HumaLog, lispro (p. 618)	15–30 min	0.5–2.5 hrs	6–8 hrs	Stable at room temp for 28 days Can mix with NPH
NovoLog, aspart	10–20 min	1–3 hrs	3–5 hrs	Stable at room temp for 28 days Can mix with NPH
Short Acting				
Humulin R, Novolin R, regular	30–60 min	1–5 hrs	6–10 hrs	Stable at room temp for 28 days Can mix with NPH
Intermediate Acting				
Humulin N, Novolin N, NPH	1–2 hrs	6–14 hrs	16–24 hrs	Stable at room temp for 28 days Can mix with aspart, lispro, glulisine
Long Acting				
Lantus, glargine (p. 618)	1.1 hrs	No significant peak	24 hrs	Do NOT mix with other insulins Stable at room temp for 28 days
Levemir, detemir	0.8–2 hrs	Relatively flat	12–24 hrs (dose dependent)	Do NOT mix with other insulins Stable at room temp for 42 days

ORAL AGENTS

Name	Availability	Dosage Range	Side Effects
Sulfonylureas			
Chlorpropamide (Diabinese)	**T:** 100 mg, 250 mg	100–500 mg/day	Hypoglycemia, weight gain, skin rash, hemolytic anemia, GI distress, cholestasis
Glimepiride (p. 550) (Amaryl)	**T:** 1 mg, 2 mg, 4 mg	1–8 mg/day	Same as chlorpropamide
Glipizide (p. 552) (Glucotrol)	**T:** 5 mg, 10 mg **T (XL):** 5 mg	**T:** 2.5–40 mg/day **XL:** 5–20 mg/day	Same as chlorpropamide
Glyburide (p. 556) (DiaBeta, Micronase)	**T:** 1.25 mg, 2.5 mg, 5 mg **PT:** 1.5 mg, 3 mg	**T:** 1.25–20 mg/day **PT:** 1–12 mg/day	Same as chlorpropamide
Alpha Glucosidase Inhibitors			
Acarbose (p. 8) (Precose)	**T:** 25 mg, 50 mg, 100 mg	75–300 mg/day	Flatulence, diarrhea
Miglitol evolve **(Glyset)**	**T:** 25 mg, 50 mg, 100 mg	75–300 mg/day	Same as acarbose
Dipeptidyl Peptidase Inhibitors			
Sitagliptin (Januvia) (p. 1066)	**T:** 25 mg, 50 mg, 100 mg	25–100 mg/day	Nasopharyngitis, upper respiratory infection, headaches

(continued)

ANTIDIABETICS *(continued)*

Oral Agents *(continued)*

Name	Availability	Dosage Range	Side Effects
Biguanides			
Metformin (p. 743) (Glucophage)	**T:** 500 mg, 850 mg **XR:** 500 mg	**T:** 0.5–2.5 g/day **XR:** 1,500–2,000 mg/day	Nausea, vomiting, diarrhea, loss of appetite, metallic taste, metabolic acidosis (rare)
Meglitinides			
Nateglinide (p. 820) (Starlix)	**T:** 60 mg, 120 mg	60–120 mg 3 times/day	Hypoglycemia, weight gain
Repaglinide (p. 1017) (Prandin)	**T:** 0.5 mg, 1 mg, 2 mg	0.5–1 mg with each meal (**Maximum:** 16 mg/day)	Same as nateglinide
Thiazolidinediones			
Pioglitazone (p. 940) (Actos)	**T:** 15 mg, 30 mg, 45 mg	15–45 mg/day	Mild anemia, mild to moderate edema, weight gain
Rosiglitazone (p. 1042) (Avandia)	**T:** 2 mg, 4 mg, 8 mg	4–8 mg/day	Same as pioglitazone
Miscellaneous			
Exenatide (p. 462) (Byetta)	**I:** 5 mcg, 10 mcg	5–10 mcg 2 times/day	Diarrhea, dizziness, dyspnea, headaches, nausea, vomiting
Pramlintide (p. 955) (Symlin)	**I:** 0.6 mg/ml	15–60 mcg immediately prior to meals	Allergic reaction, hypoglycemia, abdominal pain, anorexia, arthralgia, headaches, nausea, vomiting

I, Injection; ***PT,*** Prestab; ***T,*** tablets; ***XL,*** extended-release; ***XR,*** extended-release.

Antidiarrheals

USES	ACTION	
Acute diarrhea, chronic diarrhea of inflammatory bowel disease, reduction of fluid from ileostomies.	*Systemic agents:* Act at smooth muscle receptors (enteric) disrupting peristaltic movements, decreasing GI motility, increasing transit time of intestinal contents.	*Local agents:* Adsorb toxic substances and fluids to large surface areas of particles in the preparation. Some of these agents coat and protect irritated intestinal walls. May have local anti-inflammatory action.

ANTIDIARRHEALS

Name	Availability	Type	Dosage Range
Bismuth (p. 142) **(Pepto-Bismol)**	**T**: 262 mg **C**: 262 mg **L**: 130 mg/15 ml, 262 mg/15 ml, 524 mg/15 ml	Local	**A**: 2 **T** or 30 ml **C (9–12 yrs)**: 1 **T** or 15 ml **C (6–8 yrs)**: 2/3 **T** or 10 ml **C (3–5 yrs)**: 1/3 **T** or 5 ml
Diphenoxylate (with atropine) (p. 372) **(Lomotil)**	**T**: 2.5 mg **L**: 2.5 mg/5 ml	Systemic	**A**: 5 mg 4 times/day **C**: 0.3–0.4 mg/kg/day in 4 divided doses **(L)**
Kaolin (with pectin) (p. 650) **(Kaopectate)**	**S**: 262 mg/15 ml 525 mg/15 ml	Local	**A**: 60–120 ml after each bowel movement **C (6–12 yrs)**: 30–60 ml **C (3–5 yrs)**: 15–30 ml
Loperamide (p. 702) (Imodium)	**C**: 2 mg **T**: 2 mg **L**: 1 mg/5 ml, 1 mg/ml	Systemic	**A**: Initially, 4 mg (**Maximum:** 16 mg/day) **C (9–12 yrs)**: 2 mg 3 times/day **C (6–8 yrs)**: 2 mg 2 times/day **C (2–5 yrs)**: 1 mg 3 times/day **(L)**

A, Adults; ***C,*** capsules; ***C*** *(dosage),* children; ***L,*** liquid; ***S,*** suspension; ***T,*** tablets.

Antifungals: Systemic Mycoses

Systemic mycoses are subdivided into opportunistic infections (*candidiasis*, *aspergillosis*, *cryptococcosis*, and *mucomycosis*) that are seen primarily in debilitated or immunocompromised hosts and nonopportunistic infections (*blastomycosis*, *histoplasmosis*, and *coccidioidomycosis*) that occur in any host. Treatment can be difficult because these infections often resist treatment and may require prolonged therapy.

ANTIFUNGALS: SYSTEMIC MYCOSES

Name	Indications	Side Effects
Amphotericin B (p. 67)	Potentially life-threatening fungal infections, including aspergillosis, blastomycosis, coccidioidomycosis, Cryptococcus, histoplasmosis, systemic candidiasis	Fever, chills, headache, nausea, vomiting, nephrotoxicity, hypokalemia, hypomagnesemia, hypotension, dyspnea, arrhythmias, abdominal pain, diarrhea, increased hepatic function tests.
Amphotericin B lipid complex (Abelcet) (p. 67)	Invasive fungal infections	Same as amphotericin B
Amphotericin B liposomal (AmBisome) (p. 67)	Empiric therapy for presumed fungal infections in febrile neutropenic pts, treatment of cryptococcal meningitis in HIV-infected pts, treatment of aspergillosis, candida, Cryptococcus infections, treatment of visceral leishmaniasis	Same as amphotericin B
Amphotericin colloidal dispersion (Amphotec) (p. 67)	Invasive aspergillosis	Same as amphotericin B
Anidulafungin (Eraxis) (p. 79)	Candidemia, esophageal candidiasis	Diarrhea, hypokalemia, increased hepatic function tests, headache

Caspofungin (Cancidas) (p. 197)	Candidimia, invasive aspergillosis, empiric therapy for presumed fungal infections in febrile neutropenic pts	Headache, nausea, vomiting, diarrhea, increased hepatic function tests
Fluconazole (Diflucan) (p. 487)	Treatment of vaginal candidiasis, oropharyngeal, esophageal candidiasis and cryptococcal meningitis. Prophylaxis to decrease incidence of candidiasis in pts undergoing bone marrow transplant receiving cytotoxic chemotherapy and/or radiation.	Nausea, vomiting, abdominal pain, diarrhea, dysgeusia, increased hepatic function tests, liver necrosis, hepatitis, cholestasis, headache, rash, pruritus, eosinophilia, alopecia.
Itraconazole (Sporanox) (p. 648)	Blastomycosis, histoplasmosis, aspergillosis, onychomycosis, empiric therapy of febrile neutropenic pts with suspected fungal infections, treatment of oropharyngeal and esophageal candidiasis	Congestive heart failure, peripheral edema, nausea, vomiting, abdominal pain, diarrhea, increased hepatic function tests, liver necrosis, hepatitis, cholestasis, headache, rash, pruritus, eosinophilia
Ketoconazole (Nizoral) (p. 653)	Candidiasis, chronic mucocutaneous candidiasis, oral thrush, candiduria, blastomycosis, coccidiodomycosis	Nausea, vomiting, abdominal pain, diarrhea, gynecomastia, increased hepatic function tests, liver necrosis, hepatitis, cholestasis, headache, rash, pruritus, eosinophilia
Micafungin (Mycamine) (p. 768)	Esophageal candidiasis, candida infections, prophylaxis in pts undergoing hematopoetin stem cell transplantation	Fever, chills, hypokalemia, hypomagnesemia, hypocalcemia, myelosuppression, thrombocytopenia, nausea, vomiting, abdominal pain, diarrhea, increased hepatic function tests, dizziness, headache, rash, pruritus, pain or inflammation at injection site, fever
Posaconazole (Noxafil) (p. 950)	Prevent invasive aspergillosis and candida infections in pts 13 yrs and older who are immunocompromised, treatment of oropharyngeal candidiasis	Fever, headaches, nausea, vomiting, diarrhea, abdominal pain, hypokalemia, cough, dyspnea
Voriconazole (Vfend) (p. 1227)	Invasive aspergillosis, candidemia, esophageal candidiasis, serious fungal infections	Visual disturbances, nausea, vomiting, abdominal pain, diarrhea, increased hepatic function tests, liver necrosis, hepatitis, cholestasis, headache, rash, pruritus, eosinophilia

Antifungals: Topical

USES

Treatment of tinea infections, cutaneous candidiasis (moniliasis) due to *Candida albicans.*

ACTION

Exact mechanism unknown. May deplete essential intracellular components by inhibiting transport of potassium, other ions into cells; alter membrane permeability, resulting in loss of potassium, other cellular components.

ANTIFUNGALS: TOPICAL

Name	Availability	Dosage Range	Side Effects
Butenafine (Mentax)	**C:** 1%	2 times/day	Burning, stinging, pruritus, contact dermatitis, erythema
Ciclopirox (Loprox)	**C:** 1% **L:** 1%	2 times/day	Irritation, pruritus, redness
Clioquinol (Vioform)	**C:** 3% **O:** 3%	2–3 times/day	Irritation, stinging, swelling
Clotrimazole (p. 278) (Lotrimin, Mycelex)	**C:** 1% **L:** 1% **S:** 1%	2 times/day	Erythema, stinging, blistering, edema, pruritus
Econazole (Spectazole)	**C:** 1%	1–2 times/day	Burning, stinging, irritation, erythema
Ketoconazole (p. 653) evolve (Nizoral)	**C:** 2%	1–2 times/day	Irritation, pruritus, stinging
Miconazole (p. 769) (Micatin, Monistat)	**C:** 2% **P:** 2%	2 times/day	Irritation, burning, allergic contact dermatitis

Nystatin (p. 856) (Mycostatin, Nilstat)	**C:** 100,000 g **O:** 100,000 g **P:** 100,000 g	2–3 times/day	Irritation
Oxiconazole (Oxistat)	**C:** 1% **L:** 1%	1–2 times/day	Pruritus, burning, stinging, irritation, pain, tingling
Sertaconazole evolve **(Ertaczo)**	**C:** 2%	2 times/day	Dry skin, burning, pruritus, erythema
Terbinafine (p. 1118) (Lamisil)	**C:** 1% **G:** 10 mg	1–2 times/day	Irritation, burning, pruritus, dryness
Tolnaftate (Tinactin)	**C:** 1% **G:** 1% **S:** 1%	2 times/day	Mild irritation
Triacetin (Fungoid)	**C:** 1% **S:** 1%	3 times/day	Irritation
Undecylenic acid (Desenex, Cruex, Caldesene)	**C, O, P**	As needed	None significant

C, Cream; ***G,*** gel; ***L,*** lotion; ***O,*** ointment; ***P,*** powder; ***S,*** solution.

Antiglaucoma Agents

USES

Reduction of elevated intraocular pressure (IOP) in pts with open-angle glaucoma and ocular hypertension.

ACTION

Medications that decrease IOP by increasing outflow of aqueous humor:

- *Miotics (direct acting):* Cholinergic agents or miotics stimulate ciliary muscles, leading to increases in contraction of the iris sphincter muscle.

Antiglaucoma Agents *(continued)*

ACTION *(continued)*

• *Miotics (indirect acting):* Primarily inhibit cholinesterase, allowing accumulation of acetylcholine, prolonging parasympathetic activity.
• *Sympathomimetics:* Increase the rate of fluid flow out of the eye and decrease the rate of aqueous humor production.

Medications that decrease IOP by decreasing aqueous humor production:
• *Alpha$_2$-agonists:* Activate receptors in ciliary body, inhibiting aqueous secretion and increasing uveoscleral aqueous outflow.
• *Beta-blockers:* Reduce production of aqueous humor.
• *Carbonic anhydrase inhibitors:* Reduce fluid flow into the eye by inhibiting enzyme carbonic anhydrase.
• *Prostaglandins:* Increase outflow of aqueous fluid through uveoscleral route.

ANTIGLAUCOMA AGENTS

Name	Availability	Dosage Range	Side Effects
Miotics			
Carbachol (Isopto-Carbachol)	**S:** 0.75%, 1.5%, 2.25%, 3%	1 drop 2 times/day	Ciliary or accommodative spasm, blurred vision, reduced night vision, diaphoresis, increased salivation, urinary frequency, nausea, diarrhea
Echothiophate (Phospholine Iodide)	**S:** 0.03%, 0.06%, 0.125%, 0.25%	1 drop 2 times/day	Headaches, accommodative spasm, diaphoresis, vomiting, nausea, diarrhea, tachycardia
Physostigmine (p. 938)	**O:** 0.25%	Apply up to 3 times/day	Blurred vision, eye pain
Pilocarpine evolve **(Isopto Carpine)**	**S:** 0.25%, 0.5%, 1%, 2%, 3%, 4%, 5%, 6%, 8%, 10%	1–2 drops 3–4 times/day	Same as carbachol

Sympathomimetics			
Dipivefrin (Propine)	**S:** 0.1%	1 drop q12h	Ocular congestion, burning, stinging
Epinephrine (p. 419)	**S:** 0.5%, 1%, 2%	1 drop 1–2 times/day	Mydriasis, blurred vision, tachycardia, hypertension, tremors, headaches, anxiety
Alpha$_2$-Agonists			
Apraclonidine (Iopidine)	**S:** 0.5%	1–2 drops 3 times/day	Hypersensitivity reaction, change in visual acuity, lethargy
Brimonidine (Alphagan)	**S:** 0.2%	1–2 drops 2–3 times/day	Hypersensitivity reaction, headaches, drowsiness, fatigue
Prostaglandins			
Bimatoprost (Lumigan)	**S:** 0.03%	1 drop daily in evening	Ocular hyperemia, eyelash growth, pruritus
Latanoprost (Xalatan)	**S:** 0.005%	1 drop daily in evening	Burning, stinging, iris pigmentation
Travoprost (Travatan)	**S:** 0.004%	1 drop daily in evening	Ocular hyperemia, eye discomfort, foreign body sensation, pain, pruritus
Unoprostone (Rescula)	**S:** 0.15%	1 drop 2 times/day	Iris pigmentations
Beta-Blockers			
Betaxolol (p. 133) (Betoptic-S)	**Suspension:** 0.25% **S:** 0.5%	1–2 drops 1–2 times/day	Transient irritation, burning, tearing, blurred vision
Carteolol evolve **(Ocupress)**	**S:** 1%	1 drop 2 times/day	Mild, transient ocular stinging, burning, discomfort

(continued)

ANTIGLAUCOMA AGENTS *(continued)*

Name	Availability	Dosage Range	Side Effects
Beta-Blockers *(continued)*			
Levobetaxolol (Betaxon)	**S:** 0.5%	1 drop 2 times/day	Transient irritation, burning, tearing, blurred vision
Levobunolol (Betagan)	**S:** 0.25%, 0.5%	1 drop 1–2 times/day	Local discomfort, conjunctivitis, brow ache, tearing, blurred vision, headaches, anxiety
Metipranolol (OptiPranolol)	**S:** 0.3%	1 drop 2 times/day	Transient irritation, burning, stinging, blurred vision
Timolol (p. 1142) (Istalol, Timoptic)	**S:** 0.25%, 0.5% **G:** 0.25%, 0.5%	**S:** 1 drop 2 times/day (Istalol): 1 drop daily **G:** 1 drop daily	Drowsiness, difficulty sleeping, fatigue, weakness
Carbonic Anhydrase Inhibitors			
Acetazolamide (p. 13) (Diamox)	**T:** 125 mg, 250 mg **C:** 500 mg	0.25–1 g/day	Diarrhea, loss of appetite, metallic taste, nausea, paresthesia
Brinzolamide (Azopt)	**Suspension:** 1%	1 drop 3 times/day	Blurred vision, bitter taste
Dorzolamide (Trusopt)	**S:** 2%	1 drop 2–3 times/day	Burning, stinging, blurred vision, bitter taste

C, Capsules; ***G,*** gel; ***O,*** ointment; ***S,*** solution; ***T,*** tablets.

Antihistamines

USES

Symptomatic relief of upper respiratory allergic disorders. Allergic reactions associated with other drugs respond to antihistamines, as do blood transfusion reactions. Used as a second-choice drug in treatment of angioneurotic edema. Effective in treatment of acute urticaria and other dermatologic conditions. May also be used for preop sedation, Parkinson's disease, and motion sickness.

ACTION

Antihistamines (H_1 antagonists) inhibit vasoconstrictor effects and vasodilator effects on endothelial cells of histamine. They block increased capillary permeability, formation of edema/wheal caused by histamine. Many antihistamines can bind to receptors in CNS, causing primarily depression (decreased alertness, slowed reaction times, somnolence) but also stimulation (restlessness, nervousness, inability to sleep). Some may counter motion sickness.

ANTIHISTAMINES

Name	Availability	Dosage Range	Side Effects
Azatadine (Optimine)	**T:** 1 mg	**A:** 1–2 mg q12h **C:** 0.05 mg/kg/day	Dry mouth, urinary retention, blurred vision, sedation, dizziness, paradoxical excitement
Brompheniramine (Brovex)	**T:** 4 mg **T (SR):** 4 mg, 6 mg **S:** 2 mg/5 ml	**A:** 4–8 mg q4–6h or **T (SR):** 8–12 mg q12–24h **C:** 0.5 mg/kg/day	Dry mouth, urinary retention, blurred vision
Cetirizine (p. 231) (Zyrtec)	**T:** 5 mg, 10 mg **S:** 5 mg/5 ml	**A:** 5–10 mg/day **C (6–12 yrs):** 5–10 mg/day **C (2–5 yrs):** 2.5–5 mg/day	Minimal CNS and anticholinergic side effects

(continued)

ANTIHISTAMINES *(continued)*

Name	Availability	Dosage Range	Side Effects
Chlorpheniramine (Chlor-Trimeton)	**T:** 4 mg **T (chewable):** 2 mg **T (SR):** 8 mg, 12 mg **S:** 2 mg/5 ml	**A:** 2–4 mg q4–6h or **SR:** 8–12 mg q12–24h **C:** 0.35 mg/kg/day	Same as brompheniramine
Clemastine (p. 264) (Tavist Allergy)	**T:** 1.34 mg, 2.68 mg **S:** 0.67 mg/5 ml	**A:** 1.34–2.68 mg q8–12h **C (6–12 yrs):** 0.67–1.34 mg q8–12h	Same as azatadine
Cyproheptadine evolve **(Periactin)**	**T:** 4 mg **S:** 2 mg/5 ml	**A:** 4 mg q8h **C:** 0.25 mg/kg/day	Same as azatadine
Dexchlorpheniramine (Polaramine)	**T:** 2 mg **S:** 2 mg/5 ml	**A:** 2 mg q4–6h **C:** 0.5–1 mg q4–6h	Same as brompheniramine
Dimenhydrinate (Dramamine)	**T:** 50 mg **L:** 12.5 mg/5 ml	**A:** 50–100 mg q4–6h **C:** 12.5–50 mg q6–8h	Same as azatadine
Diphenhydramine (p. 369) (Benadryl)	**T:** 25 mg, 50 mg **C:** 25 mg, 50 mg **L:** 6.25 mg/5 ml, 12.5 mg/5 ml	**A:** 25–50 mg q6–8h **C (6–11 yrs):** 12.5–25 mg q4–6h **C (2–5 yrs):** 6.25 mg q4–6h	Same as azatadine
Fexofenadine (p. 480) (Allegra)	**T:** 30 mg, 60 mg, 180 mg	**A:** 60 mg q12h or 180 mg/day; **C (6–11 yrs):** 30 mg q12h	Same as cetirizine
Hydroxyzine (p. 588) (Atarax)	**T:** 10 mg, 25 mg, 50 mg, 100 mg **C:** 25 mg, 50 mg, 100 mg **S:** 10 mg/5 ml, 25 mg/5 ml	**A:** 25 mg q6–8h **C:** 2 mg/kg/day	Same as azatadine

Loratadine (p. 705) (Claritin)	**T:** 10 mg **S:** 1 mg/ml	**A:** 10 mg/day **C (6–12 yrs):** 10 mg/day	Same as cetirizine
Promethazine (p. 977) (Phenergan)	**T:** 12.5 mg, 25 mg, 50 mg **S:** 6.25 mg/5 ml, 25 mg/5 ml	**A:** 25 mg at bedtime or 12.5 mg q8h **C:** 0.5 mg/kg at bedtime or 0.1 mg/kg q6–8h	Same as azatadine

A, Adults; ***C,*** capsules; ***C*** *(dosage),* children; ***L,*** liquid; ***S,*** syrup; ***SR,*** sustained-release; ***T,*** tablets.

Antihyperlipidemics

USES

Cholesterol management.

ACTION

Bile acid sequestrants: Bind bile acids in the intestine; prevent active transport and reabsorption and enhance bile acid excretion. Depletion of hepatic bile acid results in the increased conversion of cholesterol to bile acids.

HMG-CoA reductase inhibitors (statins): Inhibit HMG-CoA reductase, the last regulated step in the synthesis of cholesterol. Cholesterol synthesis in the liver is reduced.

Niacin (nicotinic acid): Reduces hepatic synthesis of triglycerides and secretion of VLDL by inhibiting the mobilization of free fatty acids from peripheral tissues.

Fibric acid: Increases the oxidation of fatty acids in the liver, resulting in reduced secretion of triglyceride-rich lipoproteins and increases lipoprotein lipase activity and fatty acid uptake.

Cholesterol absorption inhibitor: Acts in the gut wall to prevent cholesterol absorption through the intestinal villi.

Antihyperlipidemics *(continued)*

ANTIHYPERLIPIDEMICS

Name	Primary Effect	Dosage	Comments/Side Effects
Bile Acid Sequestrants			
Cholestyramine (Prevalite, Questran) (p. 243)	Decreases LDL	4 g once or twice daily	May bind drugs given concurrently. Take at least 1 hr before or 4–6 hrs after cholestyramine. **Side Effects:** Constipation, heartburn, nausea, vomiting, stomach pain
Colesevelam (Welchol) (p. 285)	Decreases LDL	6–7 625-mg tablets once daily or 2 divided doses with meals	Take with food. **Side Effects:** Constipation, dyspepsia, weakness, myalgia, pharyngitis
Colestipol (Colestid)	Decreases LDL	**T:** 2–16 g daily **G:** 5–30 g daily	Do not crush tablets. May bind drugs given concurrently. Take at least 1 hr before or 4–6 hrs after colestipol. **Side Effects:** Constipation, headache, dizziness, anxiety, vertigo, drowsiness, nausea, vomiting, diarrhea, flatulence
Cholesterol Absorption Inhibitor			
Ezetimibe (Zetia) (p. 463)	Decreases LDL	10 mg once daily	Administer at least 2 hrs before or 4 hrs after bile acid sequestrants. **Side Effects:** Dizziness, headache, fatigue, diarrhea, abdominal pain, arthalgia, sinusitis, pharyngitis

Fibric Acid

Fenofibrate (Antara, Lofibra, Tricor, Triglide) (p. 470)	Decreases TG	Antara: 43–130 mg/day Lofibra: 67–200 mg/day Tricor: 48–145 mg/day Triglide: 50–160 mg/day	May increase levels of ezetimibe. Concomitant use of statins may increase rhabdomyolysis, elevate CPK levels, and cause myoglobinuria. **Side Effects:** Abdominal pain, constipation, diarrhea, respiratory complaints, headache, fever, flu-like syndrome, asthenia
Gemfibrozil (Lopid) (p. 539)	Decreases TG	600 mg 2 times/day	Give 30 min before breakfast and dinner. Concomitant use of statins may increase rhabdomyolysis, elevate CPK levels, and cause myoglobinuria. **Side Effects:** Fatigue, vertigo, headache, rash, eczema, diarrhea, abdominal pain, nausea, vomiting, constipation

Niacin

Niacin, nicotinic acid (Niacor, Niaspan) (p. 832)	Decreases LDL, TG Increases HDL	**Regular-release (Niacor):** 1.5–6 g/day in 3 divided doses **Extended-release (Niaspan):** 375 mg to 2 g once daily at bedtime	Diabetics may experience a dose-related elevation in glucose. **Side Effects:** Increased hepatic function tests, hyperglycemia, dyspepsia, itching, flushing, dizziness, insomnia

(continued)

ANTIHYPERLIPIDEMICS *(continued)*

Name	Primary Effect	Dosage	Comments/Side Effects
Statins			
Atorvastatin (Lipitor) (p. 104)	Decreases LDL, TG Increases HDL	10–80 mg/day	May interact with CYP3A4 inhibitors (e.g., amiodarone, diltiazem, cyclosporine, grapefruit juice) increasing risk of myopathy. **Side Effects:** Myalgia, myopathy, rhabdomyolysis, headache, chest pain, peripheral edema, dizziness, rash, abdominal pain, constipation, diarrhea, dyspepsia, nausea, flatulence, increased hepatic function tests, back pain, sinusitis
Fluvastatin (Lescol) (p. 509)	Decreases LDL, TG Increases HDL	20–80 mg/day	Primarily metabolized by CYP2C9 enzyme system. May increase levels of phenytoin, rifampin. May lower fluvastatin levels. **Side Effects:** Headache, fatigue, dyspepsia, diarrhea, nausea, abdominal pain, myalgia, myopathy, rhabdomyolysis
Lovastatin (Mevacor) (p. 711)	Decreases LDL, TG Increases HDL	10–80 mg/day	May interact with CYP3A4 inhibitors (e.g., amiodarone, diltiazem, cyclosporine, grapefruit juice) increasing risk of myopathy. **Side Effects:** Increased CPK levels, headache, dizziness, rash, constipation, diarrhea, abdominal pain, dyspepsia, nausea, flatulence, myalgia, myopathy, rhabdomyolysis
Pravastatin (Pravachol) (p. 957)	Decreases LDL, TG Increases HDL	10–80 mg/day	May be less likely to be involved in drug interactions. Cyclosproine may increase pravastatin levels. **Side Effects:** Chest pain, headache, dizziness, rash, nausea, vomiting, diarrhea, increased hepatic function tests, cough, flu-like symptoms, myalgia, myopathy, rhabdomyolysis

(continued)

ANTIHYPERLIPIDEMICS *(continued)*

Name	Primary Effect	Dosage	Comments/Side Effects
Rosuvastatin (Crestor) (p. 1044)	Decreases LDL, TG Increases HDL	5–40 mg/day	May be less likely to be involved in drug interactions. Cyclosporine may increase rosuvastatin levels. **Side Effects:** Chest pain, peripheral edema, headache, rash, dizziness, vertigo, pharyngitis, diarrhea, nausea, constipation, abdominal pain, dyspepsia, sinusitis, flu-like symptoms, myalgia, myopathy, rhabdomyolysis
Simvastatin (Zocor) (p. 1063)	Decreases LDL, TG Increases HDL	5–80 mg/day	May interact with CYP3A4 inhibitors (e.g., amiodarone, diltiazem, cyclosporine, grapefruit juice) increasing risk of myopathy. **Side Effects:** Constipation, flatulence, dyspepsia, increased hepatic function tests, increased CPK, upper respiratory tract infection.

CPK, Creatine phosphokinase; ***G***, granules; ***HDL***, high-density lipoprotein; ***LDL***, low-density lipoprotein; ***T***, tablets; ***TG***, triglycerides.

Antihypertensives

USES

Treatment of mild to severe hypertension.

ACTION

Many groups of medications are used in the treatment of hypertension. In addition to the alpha-adrenergic central agonists, peripheral antagonists, and vasodilators listed in the following table, refer to the classifications of diuretics, beta-adrenergic blockers, calcium channel blockers, and ACE inhibitors or to individual drug monographs.

Alpha-agonists (central action): Stimulate alpha$_2$-adrenergic receptors in the cardiovascular centers of the CNS, reducing sympathetic outflow and producing an antihypertensive effect.

Alpha-antagonists (peripheral action): Block alpha$_1$-adrenergic receptors in arterioles and veins, inhibiting vasoconstriction and decreasing peripheral vascular resistance, causing a fall in B/P.

Vasodilators: Directly relax arteriolar smooth muscle, decreasing vascular resistance. Exact mechanism unknown.

ANTIHYPERTENSIVES

Name	Availability	Dosage Range	Side Effects
Alpha-Agonists: Central Action			
Clonidine (p. 273) (Catapres)	**T:** 0.1 mg, 0.2 mg, 0.3 mg **P:** 0.1 mg/hr, 0.2 mg/hr, 0.3 mg/hr	**PO:** 0.2–0.8 mg/day **Topical:** 0.1–0.6 mg/wk	Sedation, dry mouth, constipation, sexual dysfunction, bradycardia
Methyldopa (p. 752) evolve (Aldomet)	**T:** 125 mg, 250 mg, 500 mg	**PO:** 0.5–3 g/day	Same as clonidine Impaired memory, depression, nasal congestion

Alpha-Agonists: Peripheral Action

Doxazosin (p. 388) (Cardura)	**T:** 1 mg, 2 mg, 4 mg, 8 mg	**PO:** 2–16 mg/day	Dizziness, vertigo, headaches
Prazosin (p. 959) evolve (Minipress)	**C:** 1 mg, 2 mg, 5 mg	**PO:** 6–20 mg/day	Dizziness, light-headedness, headaches, drowsiness
Terazosin (p. 1117) (Hytrin)	**C:** 1 mg, 2 mg, 5 mg, 10 mg	**PO:** 1–20 mg/day	Dizziness, headaches, asthenia

Vasodilators

Hydralazine (p. 573) (Apresoline)	**T:** 10 mg, 25 mg, 50 mg, 100 mg	**PO:** 40–300 mg/day	Anorexia, nausea, diarrhea, vomiting, headaches, palpitations
Minoxidil (p. 777) (Loniten)	**T:** 2.5 mg, 10 mg	**PO:** 10–40 mg/day	Rapid/irregular heartbeat, hypertrichosis, peripheral edema

C, Capsules; ***P,*** patch; ***T,*** tablets.

Antimigraine (Triptans)

USES

Treatment of migraine headaches with or without aura in adults 18 yrs and older.

ACTION

Triptans are selective agonists of the serotonin (5-HT) receptor that inhibit neuropeptide release and vasodilation, causing vasoconstriction.

Antimigraine (Triptans) *(continued)*

TRIPTANS

Name	Availability	Dosage Range	Contraindications	Side Effects
Almotriptan (p. 37) (Axert)	**T:** 6.25 mg, 12.5 mg	6.25–12.5 mg; may repeat after 2 hrs	Ischemic heart disease, angina pectoris, arrhythmias, previous MI, uncontrolled hypertension	Drowsiness, dizziness, fatigue, hot flashes, chest pain/discomfort, paresthesia, nausea, vomiting
Eletriptan (p. 408) (Relpax)	**T:** 20 mg, 40 mg	**A:** 20–40 mg; may repeat after 2 hrs	Same as almotriptan	Asthenia, nausea, dizziness, drowsiness
Frovatriptan (p. 524) (Frova)	**T:** 2.5 mg	2.5 mg; may repeat after 2 hrs; no more than 3 **T**/day	Same as almotriptan	Hot/cold sensations, dizziness, fatigue, headaches, chest pain, skeletal pain, dry mouth, dyspepsia, flushing
Naratriptan (p. 818) (Amerge)	**T:** 1 mg, 2.5 mg	2.5 mg; may repeat once after 4 hrs	Same as almotriptan	Atypical sensations, pain, nausea
Rizatriptan (p. 1039) (Maxalt, Maxalt-MLT)	**T:** 5 mg, 10 mg **DT:** 5 mg, 10 mg	5 or 10 mg; may repeat after 2 hrs	Same as almotriptan	Atypical sensations, pain, nausea, dizziness, drowsiness, asthenia, fatigue
Sumatriptan (p. 1094) (Imitrex)	**T:** 25 mg, 50 mg **NS:** 5 mg, 20 mg **I:** 4 mg, 6 mg	**PO:** 25–100 mg; may repeat q2h **NS:** 5–20 mg; may repeat after 2 hrs **Subcutaneous:** 4–6 mg; may repeat after 1 hr	Same as almotriptan	*Oral:* Atypical sensations, pain, malaise, fatigue *Injection:* Atypical sensations, flushing, chest pain/discomfort, injection site reaction, dizziness, vertigo *Nasal:* Discomfort, nausea, vomiting, altered taste

Zolmitriptan (p. 1244) (Zomig)	**T:** 2.5 mg, 5 mg **DT:** 2.5 mg, 5 mg	2.5–5 mg; may repeat after 2 hrs	Same as almotriptan	Atypical sensations, pain, nausea, dizziness, asthenia, drowsiness

A, Adults; ***DT,*** disintegrating tablets; ***I,*** injection; ***NS,*** nasal spray; ***T,*** tablets.

Antipsychotics

USES

Primarily used in managing psychotic illness (esp. in pts with increased psychomotor activity). Also used to treat the manic phase of bipolar disorder, behavioral problems in children, nausea and vomiting, intractable hiccups, anxiety and agitation, as adjunct in treatment of tetanus, and to potentiate effects of narcotics.

ACTION

Effects of these agents occur at all levels of the CNS. Antipsychotic mechanism unknown but may antagonize dopamine action as a neurotransmitter in basal ganglia and limbic system. Antipsychotics may block postsynaptic dopamine receptors, inhibit dopamine release, increase dopamine turnover.

These medications can be divided into the phenothiazines and nonphenothiazines (miscellaneous). In addition to their use in symptomatic treatment of psychiatric illness, some have antiemetic, antinausea, antihistamine, anticholinergic, and/or sedative effects.

ANTIPSYCHOTICS

			Relative Side Effect Profile			
Name	Availability	Dosage	EPS	Anticholinergic	Sedation	Hypotension
Aripiprazole (p. 88) (Abilify)	**T:** 5 mg, 10 mg, 15 mg **DT:** 10 mg, 15 mg **I:** 9.75 mg	**PO:** 15–30 mg/day **I:** Up to 30 mg/day	Low	Low	Low	Low

(continued)

ANTIPSYCHOTICS ***(continued)***

Name	Availability	Dosage	Relative Side Effect Profile: EPS	Anticholinergic	Sedation	Hypotension
Chlorpromazine (p. 241) (Thorazine)	**T:** 10 mg, 25 mg, 50 mg, 100 mg, 200 mg **SR:** 30 mg, 75 mg, 100 mg **OC:** 30 mg/ml, 100 mg/ml	50–2,000 mg/day	Moderate	Moderate	High	High
Clozapine (p. 280) (Clozaril, FazaClo)	**T:** 25 mg, 100 mg **DT:** 25 mg, 100 mg	75–900 mg/day	Rare	High	High	High
Fluphenazine (p. 500) (Prolixin)	**T:** 1 mg, 2.5 mg, 5 mg, 10 mg **I:** 25 mg/ml **OC:** 5 mg/ml	**PO:** 2–40 mg/day **I:** 12.5–75 mg q2wk	High	Low	Low	Low
Haloperidol (p. 566) (Haldol)	**T:** 0.5 mg, 1 mg, 2 mg, 5 mg, 10 mg, 20 mg **I:** 5 mg/ml **OC:** 2 mg/ml	2–40 mg/day	High	Low	Low	Low
Loxapine (Loxitane)	**C:** 5 mg, 10 mg, 25 mg, 50 mg **OC:** 25 mg/ml **I:** 50 mg/ml	20–250 mg/day	High	Low	Moderate	Moderate
Mesoridazine (p. 739) (Serentil)	**T:** 10 mg, 25 mg, 50 mg, 100 mg **I:** 25 mg/ml **OC:** 25 mg/ml	100–400 mg/day	Low	High	High	High
Olanzapine (p. 862) (Zyprexa)	**T:** 2.5 mg, 5 mg, 7.5 mg, 10 mg, 15 mg, 20 mg **DT:** 5 mg, 10 mg **I:** 10 mg	10–20 mg/day	Low	Low	Moderate	Low

Quetiapine (p. 997) (Seroquel)	**T**: 25 mg, 100 mg, 200 mg, 300 mg	100–800 mg/day	Rare	Low	Moderate	Moderate
Risperidone (p. 1032) (Risperdal)	**T**: 0.25 mg, 0.5 mg, 1 mg, 2 mg, 3 mg, 4 mg **OC**: 1 mg/ml **I**: 25 mg, 37.5 mg, 50 mg	2–6 mg/day **IM**: 25–50 mg q2wk	Low	Low	Low	Moderate
Thioridazine (p. 1130) evolve (Mellaril)	**T**: 10 mg, 15 mg, 25 mg, 50 mg, 100 mg, 150 mg, 200 mg **OC**: 30 mg/ml, 100 mg/ml	50–800 mg/day	Low	High	High	High
Thiothixene (p. 1134) (Navane)	**C**: 1 mg, 2 mg, 5 mg	5–60 mg/day	High	Low	Low	Low
Trifluoperazine (p. 1183) (Stelazine)	**T**: 1 mg, 2 mg, 5 mg, 10 mg **I**: 5 mg/ml **OC**: 2 mg/ml	5–80 mg/day	High	Low	Low	Low
Ziprasidone (p. 1241) (Geodon)	**C**: 20 mg, 40 mg, 60 mg, 80 mg **I**: 20 mg	40–160 mg/day	Low	Low	Low to moderate	Low to moderate

C, Capsules; ***DT,*** disintegrating tablets; ***EPS,*** extrapyramidal symptoms; ***I,*** injection; ***OC,*** oral concentrate; ***SR,*** sustained-release; ***T,*** tablets.

Antivirals

USES

Treatment of HIV infection. Treatment of cytomegalovirus (CMV) retinitis in pts with AIDS, acute herpes zoster (shingles), genital herpes (recurrent), mucosal and cutaneous herpes simplex virus (HSV), chickenpox, and influenza A viral illness.

ACTION

Effective antivirals must inhibit virus-specific nucleic acid/protein synthesis. Possible mechanisms of action of antivirals used for non-HIV infection may include interference with viral DNA synthesis and viral replication, inactivation of viral DNA polymerases, incorporation and termination of the growing viral DNA chain, prevention of release of viral nucleic acid into the host cell, or interference with viral penetration into cells.

Antivirals *(continued)*

ANTIVIRALS

Name	Availability	Uses	Side Effects
Abacavir (p. 1) (Ziagen)	**T:** 300 mg **OS:** 20 mg/ml	HIV infection	Nausea, vomiting, loss of appetite, diarrhea, headaches, fatigue
Acyclovir (p. 17) (Zovirax)	**T:** 400 mg, 800 mg **C:** 200 mg **I:** 50 mg/ml	Mucosal/cutaneous HSV-1 and HSV-2, varicella-zoster (shingles), genital herpes, herpes simplex, encephalitis, chickenpox	Malaise, anorexia, nausea, vomiting, light-headedness
Adefovir (p. 21) (Hepsera)	**T:** 10 mg	Chronic hepatitis B	Asthenia, headaches, abdominal pain, nausea, diarrhea, flatulence, dyspepsia
Amantadine (p. 46) (Symmetrel)	**C:** 100 mg **S:** 50 mg/5 ml	Influenza A	Anxiety, dizziness, light-headedness, headaches, nausea, loss of appetite
Amprenavir (p. 74) (Agenerase)	**C:** 50 mg, 150 mg **OS:** 15 mg/ml	HIV infection	Hyperglycemia, rash, abdominal pain, nausea, vomiting, diarrhea
Cidofovir (p. 246) (Vistide)	**I:** 75 mg/ml	CMV retinitis	Decreased urination, fever, chills, diarrhea, nausea, vomiting, headaches, loss of appetite
Darunavir (p. 320) (Prezista)	**T:** 300 mg	HIV infection	Diarrhea, nausea, vomiting, headaches, skin rash, constipation
Delavirdine (p. 329) (Rescriptor)	**T:** 100 mg, 200 mg	HIV infection	Diarrhea, fatigue, rash, headaches, nausea
Didanosine (p. 357) (Videx)	**T:** 25 mg, 50 mg, 100 mg, 150 mg, 200 mg **C:** 125 mg, 200 mg **Powder for suspension:** 100 mg, 167 mg, 250 mg	HIV infection	Peripheral neuropathy, anxiety, headaches, rash, nausea, diarrhea, dry mouth

Efavirenz (p. 406) (Sustiva)	**C:** 50 mg, 100 mg, 200 mg	HIV infection	Diarrhea, dizziness, headaches, insomnia, nausea, vomiting, drowsiness
Famciclovir (p. 465) (Famvir)	**T:** 125 mg, 250 mg, 500 mg	Herpes zoster, genital herpes	Headaches
Foscarnet (p. 518) (Foscavir)	**I:** 24 mg/ml	CMV retinitis, HSV infections	Decreased urination, abdominal pain, nausea, vomiting, dizziness, fatigue, headaches
Ganciclovir (p. 532) (Cytovene)	**C:** 250 mg, 500 mg **I:** 500 mg	CMV retinitis, CMV disease	Sore throat, fever, unusual bleeding/bruising
Indinavir (p. 612) (Crixivan)	**C:** 200 mg, 400 mg	HIV infection	Blood in urine, weakness, nausea, vomiting, diarrhea, headaches, insomnia, altered taste
Lamivudine (p. 663) (Epivir)	**T:** 100 mg, 150 mg **OS:** 5 mg/ml, 10 mg/ml	HIV infection	Nausea, vomiting, abdominal pain, paresthesia
Lopinavir/ritonavir (p. 704) (Kaletra)	**C:** 133/33 mg **OS:** 80/20 mg	HIV infection	Diarrhea, nausea
Nelfinavir (p. 824) (Viracept)	**T:** 250 mg **Powder:** 50 mg/g	HIV infection	Diarrhea
Oseltamivir (p. 875) (Tamiflu)	**C:** 75 mg **S:** 12 mg/ml	Influenza	Diarrhea, nausea, vomiting
Ribavirin (p. 1022) (Virazole)	**Aerosol:** 6 g	Lowers respiratory infections in infants, children due to respiratory syncytial virus (RSV)	Anemia
Ritonavir (p. 1035) (Norvir)	**C:** 100 mg **OS:** 80 mg/ml	HIV infection	Weakness, diarrhea, nausea, decreased appetite, vomiting, altered taste

(continued)

ANTIVIRALS *(continued)*

Name	Availability	Uses	Side Effects
Saquinavir (p. 1048) (Invirase)	**C:** 200 mg	HIV infection	Weakness, diarrhea, nausea, oral ulcers, abdominal pain
Stavudine (p. 1086) (Zerit)	**C:** 15 mg, 20 mg, 30 mg, 40 mg **OS:** 1 mg/ml	HIV infection	Paresthesia, decreased appetite, chills, fever, rash
Tenofovir (p. 1116) (Viread)	**T:** 300 mg	HIV infection	Diarrhea, nausea, pharyngitis, headaches
Valacyclovir (p. 1194) (Valtrex)	**T:** 500 mg	Herpes zoster, genital herpes	Headaches, nausea
Valganciclovir (p. 1196) (Valcyte)	**T:** 450 mg	CMV retinitis	Anemia, abdominal pain, diarrhea, headaches, nausea, vomiting, paresthesia
Zalcitabine (p. 1234) (Hivid)	**T:** 0.375 mg, 0.75 mg	HIV infection	Paresthesia, arthralgia, rash, nausea, vomiting
Zanamivir (p. 1237) (Relenza)	**Inhalation:** 5 mg	Influenza	Cough, diarrhea, dizziness, headaches, nausea, vomiting
Zidovudine (p. 1239) (Retrovir)	**T:** 300 mg **C:** 100 mg **S:** 50 mg/5 ml	HIV infection	Fatigue, fever, chills, headaches, nausea, muscle pain

C, Capsules; ***I,*** injection; ***OS,*** oral solution; ***S,*** syrup; ***T,*** tablets.

Beta-Adrenergic Blockers

USES

Management of hypertension, angina pectoris, arrhythmias, hypertrophic subaortic stenosis, migraine headaches, MI (prevention), glaucoma.

ACTION

Beta-adrenergic blockers competitively block $beta_1$-adrenergic receptors, located primarily in myocardium, and $beta_2$-adrenergic receptors, located primarily in bronchial and vascular smooth muscle. By occupying beta-receptor sites, these agents prevent naturally occurring or administered epinephrine/norepinephrine from exerting their effects. The results are basically opposite to those of sympathetic stimulation.

Effects of $beta_1$-blockade include slowing heart rate, decreasing cardiac output and contractility; effects of $beta_2$-blockade include bronchoconstriction, increased airway resistance in pts with asthma or chronic obstructive pulmonary disease (COPD). Beta-blockers can affect cardiac rhythm/automaticity (decrease sinus rate, SA/AV conduction; increase refractory period in AV node). Decrease systolic and diastolic B/P; exact mechanism unknown but may block peripheral receptors, decrease sympathetic outflow from CNS, or decrease renin release from kidney. All beta-blockers mask tachycardia that occurs with hypoglycemia. When applied to the eye, reduce intraocular pressure and aqueous production.

BETA-ADRENERGIC BLOCKERS

Name	Availability	Selectivity	Dosage Range	Side Effects
Acebutolol (p. 9) (Sectral)	**C:** 200 mg, 400 mg	$Beta_1$	200–1,200 mg/day	Light-headedness, fatigue, weakness, decreased sexual function, insomnia
Atenolol (p. 100) (Tenormin)	**T:** 25 mg, 50 mg, 100 mg	$Beta_1$	50–100 mg/day	Same as acebutolol
Betaxolol (p. 133) (Kerlone)	**T:** 10 mg, 20 mg	$Beta_1$	10–20 mg/day	Same as acebutolol

(continued)

BETA-ADRENERGIC BLOCKERS ***(continued)***

Name	Availability	Selectivity	Dosage Range	Side Effects
Bisoprolol (p. 143) (Zebeta)	**T:** 5 mg, 10 mg	$Beta_1$	2.5–20 mg/day	Same as acebutolol
Carteolol (Cartrol)	**T:** 2.5 mg, 5 mg	$Beta_1$, $beta_2$	2.5–10 mg/day	Same as acebutolol
Carvedilol (p. 193) (Coreg)	**T:** 3.125 mg, 6.25 mg, 12.5 mg, 25 mg	$Beta_1$, $beta_2$, $alpha_1$	12.5–50 mg/day	Same as acebutolol
Esmolol (p. 442) (Brevibloc)	**I:** 10 mg/ml, 250 mcg/ml	$Beta_1$	50–200 mcg/kg/min	Same as acebutolol
Metoprolol (p. 763) (Lopressor)	**T:** 50 mg, 100 mg/ml **I:** 1 mg/ml	$Beta_1$	50–450 mg/day	Same as acebutolol Increased risk of CNS effects
Nadolol (p. 805) (Corgard)	**T:** 20 mg, 40 mg, 80 mg, 120 mg, 160 mg	$Beta_1$, $beta_2$	40–320 mg/day	Same as acebutolol
Penbutolol (Levatol)	**T:** 20 mg	$Beta_1$, $beta_2$	10–40 mg/day	Same as acebutolol
Pindolol (Visken)	**T:** 5 mg, 10 mg	$Beta_1$, $beta_2$	10–60 mg/day	Same as acebutolol
Propranolol (p. 984) (Inderal)	**T:** 10 mg, 20 mg, 40 mg, 60 mg, 80 mg, 90 mg **C (SR):** 60 mg, 80 mg, 120 mg, 160 mg **S:** 4 mg/ml, 8 mg/ml **I:** 1 mg/ml	$Beta_1$, $beta_2$	80–320 mg/day	Same as acebutolol Increased risk of CNS effects
Sotalol (p. 1080) (Betapace)	**T:** 80 mg, 120 mg, 160 mg, 240 mg	$Beta_1$, $beta_2$	160–640 mg/day	Same as acebutolol
Timolol (p. 1142) (Blocadren)	**T:** 5 mg, 10 mg, 20 mg	$Beta_1$, $beta_2$	10–60 mg/day	Same as acebutolol

C, Capsules; ***I,*** injection; ***S,*** solution; ***SR,*** sustained-release; ***T,*** tablets.

Bronchodilators

USES

Relief of bronchospasm occurring during anesthesia and in bronchial asthma, bronchitis, emphysema.

ACTION

Inhaled corticosteroids: Exact mechanism unknown. May act as anti-inflammatories, decrease mucus secretion.

Beta$_2$-adrenergic agonists: Stimulate beta-receptors in lung, relax bronchial smooth muscle, increase vital capacity, decrease airway resistance.

Anticholinergics: Inhibit cholinergic receptors on bronchial smooth muscle (block acetylcholine action).

Leukotriene modifiers: Decrease effect of leukotrienes, which increase migration of eosinophils, producing mucus/edema of airway wall, causing bronchoconstriction.

Methylxanthines: Directly relax smooth muscle of bronchial airway, pulmonary blood vessels (relieve bronchospasm, increase vital capacity). Increase cyclic 3,5-adenosine monophosphate.

BRONCHODILATORS

Name	Availability	Dosage Range	Side Effects
Anticholinergics			
Ipratropium (p. 633) (Atrovent)	**Neb:** 0.02% **MDI:** 18 mcg/actuation **Nasal:** 0.03%, 0.06%	**A (Neb):** 0.02% q3–4h **A (MDI):** 2 puffs 4 times/day **A (Nasal):** 2 sprays 2–4 times/day	Palpitations, anxiety, dizziness, headaches, pain, nausea, dry mucous membranes, dyspnea
Tiotropium (p. 1147) (Spiriva)	**Inhalation powder:** 18 mcg	**A:** Once/day	Dry mouth, tachycardia, constipation, blurred vision, urinary difficulty/ retention, upper respiratory tract infections

(continued)

BRONCHODILATORS *(continued)*

Beta-Agonists

Albuterol (p. 26) (Proventil, Ventolin, Volmax)	**T**: 2 mg, 4 mg **T (SR)**: 4 mg, 8 mg **S**: 2 mg/5 ml **MDI (Neb)**: 0.5%, 2.5 mg/3 ml, 1.25 mg/3 ml, 0.63 mg/3 ml	**A, C (MDI)**: 2 puffs q4–6h as needed **A, C (Rotacaps)**: 1–2 caps q4–6h as needed **A (Neb)**: 2.5 mg q4–6h as needed **C (Neb)**: 0.1–0.15 mg/kg q4–6h as needed **A [T (SR)]**: 4–8 mg q12h **C [T (SR)]**: 4 mg q12h	Tremors, tachycardia, palpitations, hypokalemia
Arformoterol (p. 85) (Brovana)	**Neb**: 15 mcg/2 ml	**A (Neb)**: 15 mcg q12h	Asthenia, fever, bronchitis, COPD, headache, vomiting, hyperkalemia, anxiety, tremors
Formoterol (p. 514) (Foradil)	**C**: 12 mcg	**A**: 1 capsule q12h	Same as arformoterol
Levalbuterol (p. 681) (Xopenex)	**Neb**: 0.63 mg/3 ml, 1.25 mg/3 ml	**A**: 0.63 mg q6–8h as needed	Same as albuterol
Metaproterenol (p. 741) (Alupent)	**MDI (Neb)**: 5% **S**: 10 mg/5 ml **T**: 10 mg, 20 mg		Same as albuterol
Piruterol (Maxair)	**MDI**	**A, C**: 2 puffs q4–6h as needed	Same as albuterol
Salmeterol (p. 1046) (Serevent)	**MDI** **C**: 50 mcg	**A (MDI)**: 2 puffs q12h **C**: 1–2 puffs q12h **A, C (C)**: 1 inhalation q12h	Same as albuterol
Terbutaline (p. 1120) (Brethine, Bricanyl)	**MDI** **T**: 2.5 mg, 5 mg	**A**: 2.5 mg 3–4 times/day **C**: 0.05 mg/kg/dose 3 times/day	Same as albuterol

Inhaled Anti-Inflammatory Agents

Beclomethasone (p. 124) (Beconase AQ, Qvar)	**MDI**	1–2 inhalations 2–4 times/day	Oropharyngeal candidiasis, dysphonia, hoarseness, cough
Budesonide (p. 158) (Pulmicort)	**MDI** **Neb**	**MDI (A):** 1–4 inhalations 2 times/day **D (older than 6 yrs):** 1–2 inhalations 2 times/day	Same as beclomethasone
Cromolyn (p. 296) (Intal)	**MDI** **Neb**	**MDI: C (older than 5 yrs):** 2 inhalations up to 4 times/day **Neb: C (older than 2 yrs):** 20 mg 4 times/day	Cough, urticaria, bronchospasm
Flunisolide (p. 494) (AeroBid)	**MDI**	**A:** 2–4 inhalations 2 times/day **C (6–15 yrs):** 1–2 inhalations 2 times/day	Same as beclomethasone
Fluticasone (p. 506) (Flovent)	**MDI** **Rotadisk**	**MDI: A, C (older than 12 yrs):** 2 inhalations 2 times/day **Rotadisk: A, C (older than 4 yrs):** 1 inhalation 2 times/day	Same as beclomethasone
Mometasone (p. 789) (Asmanex)	**MDI**	1 puff 2 times/day or 2 puffs once daily up to 4 puffs/day	Pharyngitis, sinusitus, upper respiratory tract infection, allergic rhinitis, dyspepsia, headache, fatigue
Nedocromil (p. 822) (Tilade)	**MDI**	**A, C (older than 6 yrs):** 2 inhalations 4 times/day	Altered taste, headaches, nausea
Triamcinolone (p. 1178) (Azmacort)	**MDI**	**A:** 2 inhalations 3–4 times/day or 4–8 inhalations 2 times/day **C:** 1–2 inhalations 3–4 times/day or 2–6 inhalations 2 times/day	Same as beclomethasone

(continued)

BRONCHODILATORS *(continued)*

Leukotriene Modifiers

Montelukast (p. 791) (Singulair)	T: 4 mg, 5 mg, 10 mg	**A**: 10 mg/day **C (6–14 yrs)**: 5 mg/day **C (2–5 yrs)**: 4 mg/day	Dyspepsia, increased hepatic function tests
Zafirlukast (p. 1233) (Accolate)	T: 10 mg, 20 mg	**A, C (12 yrs and older)**: 20 mg 2 times/day **C (5–11 yrs)**: 10 mg 2 times/day	Same as montelukast

A, Adults; ***C,*** capsules; ***C*** *(dosage),* children; ***MDI,*** metered dose inhaler; ***Neb,*** nebulization; ***S,*** syrups; ***SR,*** sustained-release; ***T,*** tablets.

Calcium Channel Blockers

USES

Treatment of essential hypertension, treatment of and prophylaxis of angina pectoris (including vasospastic, chronic stable, unstable), prevention/control of supraventricular tachyarrhythmias, prevention of neurologic damage due to subarachnoid hemorrhage.

ACTION

Calcium channel blockers inhibit the flow of extracellular Ca^{2+} ions across cell membranes of cardiac cells, vascular tissue. They relax arterial smooth muscle, depress the rate of sinus node pacemaker, slow AV conduction, decrease heart rate, produce negative inotropic effect (rarely seen clinically due to reflex response). Calcium channel blockers decrease coronary vascular resistance, increase coronary blood flow, reduce myocardial oxygen demand. Degree of action varies with individual agent.

CALCIUM CHANNEL BLOCKERS

Name	Availability	Dosage Range	Side Effects
Amlodipine (p. 62) (Norvasc)	**T:** 2.5 mg, 5 mg, 10 mg	2.5–10 mg/day	Abdominal pain, flushing, headaches
Diltiazem (p. 365) (Cardizem)	**T:** 30 mg, 60 mg, 90 mg **T (SR):** 120 mg, 180 mg, 240 mg **C (SR):** 60 mg, 90 mg, 120 mg, 180 mg, 240 mg, 300 mg, 360 mg **I:** 5 mg/ml	**PO:** 120–360 mg/day **I:** 20–25 mg IV bolus, then 5–15 mg/hr infusion	Dizziness, drowsiness
Felodipine (p. 468) (Plendil)	**T:** 2.5 mg, 5 mg, 10 mg	5–10 mg/day	Peripheral edema, headaches
Isradipine (p. 646) (DynaCirc)	**T:** 5 mg, 10 mg **C:** 2.5 mg, 5 mg	5–20 mg/day	Headaches
Nicardipine (p. 834) (Cardene)	**C:** 20 mg, 30 mg **C (ER):** 30 mg, 45 mg, 60 mg **I:** 2.5 mg/ml	**PO:** 60–120 mg/day	Flushing, feeling of warmth
Nifedipine (p. 838) (Adalat, Procardia)	**C:** 10 mg, 20 mg **T (ER):** 30 mg, 60 mg, 90 mg	30–120 mg/day	Peripheral edema, dizziness, flushed face, headaches, nausea
Nimodipine (p. 840) (Nimotop)	**C:** 30 mg	60 mg q4h for 21 days	Nausea
Verapamil (p. 1211) (Calan, Isoptin)	**T:** 40 mg, 80 mg, 120 mg **T (SR):** 120 mg, 180 mg, 240 mg	120–480 mg/day	Constipation, nausea

C, Capsules; ***ER,*** extended-release; ***I,*** injection; ***SR,*** sustained-release; ***T,*** tablets.

Cardiac Glycosides (Inotropic Agents)

USES

CHF, atrial fibrillation, atrial flutter, paroxysmal atrial tachycardia, treatment of cardiogenic shock with pulmonary edema.

ACTION

Direct action on myocardium causes increased force of contraction, resulting in increased stroke volume and cardiac output. Depression of SA node, decreased conduction time through AV node, and decreased electrical impulses due to vagal stimulation slow heart rate. Improved myocardial contractility is probably due to improved transport of calcium, sodium, and potassium ions across cell membranes.

CARDIAC GLYCOSIDES (INOTROPIC AGENTS)

Name	Availability	Dosage Range	Side Effects
Digoxin (p. 361) (Lanoxin)	**C:** 0.05 mg, 0.1 mg, 0.2 mg **T:** 0.125 mg, 0.25 mg **E:** 0.05 mg/ml **I:** 0.1 mg/ml, 0.25 mg/ml	**PO/IV:** 0.125–0.375 mg/day	Arrhythmias, blurred vision, confusion, hallucinations, nausea, vomiting, diarrhea, abdominal pain
Inamrinone	**I:** 5 mg/ml	**IV:** 0.75 mg/kg bolus, then 5–10 mcg/kg/min infusion	Arrhythmias, hypotension
Milrinone (p. 775) (Primacor)	**I:** 1 mg/ml	**IV:** 50 mcg/kg bolus, then 0.375–0.75 mcg/kg/min infusion	Arrhythmias, hypotension, headaches

C, Capsules; ***E,*** elixir; ***I,*** injection; ***T,*** tablets.

Chemotherapeutic Agents

USES

Treatment of a variety of cancers; may be palliative or curative. Treatment of choice in hematologic cancers. Often used as adjunctive therapy (e.g., with surgery or irradiation); most effective when tumor mass has been removed or reduced by radiation. Often used in combinations to increase therapeutic results, decrease toxic effects. Certain agents may be used in nonmalignant conditions: polycythemia vera, psoriasis, rheumatoid arthritis, or immunosuppression in organ transplantation (used only in select cases that are severe and unresponsive to other forms of therapy). Refer to individual monographs.

ACTION

Most antineoplastics inhibit cell replication by interfering with the supply of nutrients or genetic components of the cell (DNA or RNA). Some antineoplastics, referred to as *cell cycle–specific* (CCS), are particularly effective during a specific phase of cell reproduction (e.g., antimetabolites and plant alkaloids). Other antineoplastics, referred to as *cell cycle–nonspecific,* act independently of a specific phase of cell division (e.g., alkylating agents and antibiotics). Some hormones are also classified as antineoplastics. Although not cytotoxic, they act to depress cancer growth by altering the hormone environment. In addition, there are a number of miscellaneous agents acting through different mechanisms.

CHEMOTHERAPEUTIC AGENTS

Name	Availability	Side Effects
Abarelix (p. 2) (Plenaxis)	**I:** 100 mg	Fatigue, headaches, nausea, abdominal pain, hot flashes, menstrual disorders
Aldesleukin (p. 631) (Proleukin)	**I:** 22 million units	Hypotension, sinus tachycardia, nausea, vomiting, diarrhea, renal impairment, anemia, rash, fatigue, agitation, pulmonary congestion, dyspnea, fever, chills, oliguria, weight gain, dizziness
Alemtuzumab (p. 30) (Campath)	**I:** 30 mg/3 ml	Rigors, fever, fatigue, hypotension, neutropenia, anemia, sepsis, dyspnea, bronchitis, pneumonia, urticaria

(continued)

CHEMOTHERAPEUTIC AGENTS *(continued)*

Name	Availability	Side Effects
Alitretinoin (p. 34) (Panretin)	**Gel:** 0.1%	Burning, pain, edema, dermatitis, rash, skin disorders
Altretamine (Hexalen)	**C:** 50 mg	Nausea, vomiting, myelosuppression, peripheral neuropathy, altered mood, ataxia, dizziness, anxiety, vertigo
Aminoglutethimide (Cytadren)	**T:** 250 mg	Orthostatic hypotension, hypothyroidism, vomiting, anorexia, rash, drowsiness, headaches, fever, myalgia
Anastrozole (p. 78) (Arimidex)	**T:** 1 mg	Peripheral edema, chest pain, nausea, vomiting, diarrhea, constipation, abdominal pain, anorexia, pharyngitis, vaginal hemorrhage, anemia, leukopenia, rash, weight gain, diaphoresis, increased appetite, pain, headaches, dizziness, depression, paresthesias, hot flashes, increased cough, dry mouth, asthenia, dyspnea, phlebitis
Arsenic trioxide (p. 90) (Trisenox)	**I:** 10 mg/ml	AV block, GI hemorrhage, hypertension, hypoglycemia, hypokalemia, hypomagnesemia, neutropenia, oliguria, prolonged QT interval, seizures, sepsis, thrombocytopenia
Asparaginase (p. 94) (Elspar)	**I:** 10,000 units	Anorexia, nausea, vomiting, hepatic toxicity, pancreatitis, nephrotoxicity, clotting factor abnormalities, malaise, confusion, lethargy, EEG changes, respiratory distress, fever, hyperglycemia, depression, stomatitis, allergic reactions, drowsiness
Azacitadine (p. 110) (Vidaza)	**I:** 100 mg	Edema, hypokalemia, weight loss, myalgia, cough, dyspnea, upper respiratory tract infection, back pain, pyrexia, weakness
BCG (Tice BCG, TheraCys)	**I:** 50 mg, 81 mg	Nausea, vomiting, anorexia, diarrhea, dysuria, hematuria, cystitis, urinary urgency, anemia, malaise, fever, chills
Bevacizumab (p. 136) (Avastin)	**I:** 25 mg/ml	Increased B/P, fatigue, blood clots, diarrhea, decreased WBCs, headaches, decreased appetite, stomatitis
Bexarotene (p. 137) (Targretin)	**C:** 75 mg **Gel:** 1%	Anemia, dermatitis, fever, hypercholesterolemia, infection, leukopenia, peripheral edema
Bicalutamide (p. 139) (Casodex)	**T:** 50 mg	Gynecomastia, hot flashes, breast pain, nausea, diarrhea, constipation, nocturia, impotence, pain, muscle pain, asthenia, abdominal pain

Bleomycin (p. 147) (Blenoxane)	**I:** 15 units, 30 units	Nausea, vomiting, anorexia, stomatitis, hyperpigmentation, alopecia, pruritus, hyperkeratosis, urticaria, pneumonitis progression to fibrosis, weight loss, rash
Bortezomib (p. 149) (Velcade)	**I:** 3.5 mg	Anxiety, dizziness, headaches, insomnia, peripheral neuropathy, pruritus, rash, abdominal pain, decreased appetite, constipation, diarrhea, dyspepsia, nausea, vomiting, arthralgia, dyspnea, asthenia, edema, pain
Busulfan (p. 167) (Myleran)	**T:** 2 mg	Nausea, vomiting, hyperuricemia, myelosuppression, skin hyperpigmentation, alopecia, anorexia, weight loss, diarrhea, stomatitis
Capecitabine (p. 181) (Xeloda)	**T:** 150 mg, 300 mg	Nausea, vomiting, diarrhea, stomatitis, myelosuppression, palmoplantar erythrodysesthia syndrome, dermatitis, fatigue, anorexia
Carboplatin (p. 189) (Paraplatin)	**I:** 50 mg, 150 mg, 450 mg	Nausea, vomiting, nephrotoxicity, myelosuppression, alopecia, peripheral neuropathy, hypersensitivity, ototoxicity, asthenia, diarrhea, constipation
Carmustine (p. 192) (BiCNU)	**I:** 100 mg	Anorexia, nausea, vomiting, myelosuppression, pulmonary fibrosis, pain at injection site, diarrhea, skin discoloration
Cetuximab (p. 232) (Erbitux)	**I:** 2 mg/ml	Dyspnea, hypotension, acne-like rash, dry skin, weakness, fatigue, fever, constipation, abdominal pain
Chlorambucil (p. 236) (Leukeran)	**T:** 2 mg	Myelosuppression, dermatitis, nausea, vomiting, hepatic toxicity, anorexia, diarrhea, abdominal discomfort, rash
Cisplatin (p. 256) (Platinol-AQ)	**I:** 50 mg, 100 mg	Nausea, vomiting, nephrotoxicity, myelosuppression, neuropathies, ototoxicity, anaphylactic-like reactions, hyperuricemia, hypomagnesemia, hypophosphatemia, hypokalemia, hypocalcemia, pain at injection site
Cladribine (p. 261) (Leustatin)	**I:** 1 mg/ml	Nausea, vomiting, diarrhea, myelosuppression, chills, fatigue, rash, fever, headaches, anorexia, diaphoresis
Cyclophosphamide (p. 300) (Cytoxan)	**I:** 100 mg, 200 mg, 500 mg, 1 g, 2 g **T:** 25 mg, 50 mg	Nausea, vomiting, hemorrhagic cystitis, myelosuppression, alopecia, interstitial pulmonary fibrosis, amenorrhea, azoospermia, diarrhea, darkening skin/fingernails, headaches, diaphoresis

(continued)

CHEMOTHERAPEUTIC AGENTS *(continued)*

Name	Availability	Side Effects
Cytarabine (p. 305) (Cytosar, Ara-C)	**I:** 100 mg, 500 mg, 1 g, 2 g	Anorexia, nausea, vomiting, stomatitis, esophagitis, diarrhea, myelosuppression, alopecia, rash, fever, neuropathies, abdominal pain
Dacarbazine (p. 308) (DTIC)	**I:** 200 mg	Nausea, vomiting, anorexia, hepatic necrosis, myelosuppression, alopecia, rash, facial flushing, photosensitivity, flu-like symptoms, confusion, blurred vision
Dasatinib (p. 321) (Sprycel)	**T:** 20 mg, 50 mg, 70 mg	Pyrexia, pleural effusion, febrile neutropenia, GI bleeding, pneumonia, thrombocytopenia, dyspnea, anemia, cardiac failure, diarrhea
Daunorubicin (p. 323) (Cerubidine)	**I:** 20 mg	CHF, nausea, vomiting, stomatitis, mucositis, diarrhea, hematuria, myelosuppression, alopecia, fever, chills, abdominal pain
Daunorubicin (p. 323) (DaunoXome)	**I:** 50 mg	Nausea, diarrhea, abdominal pain, anorexia, vomiting, stomatitis, myelosuppression, rigors, back pain, headaches, neuropathy, depression, dyspnea, fatigue, fever, cough, allergic reactions, diaphoresis
Denileukin (p. 332) (Ontak)	**I:** 300 mcg/2 ml	Hypersensitivity reaction, back pain, dyspnea, rash, chest pain, tachycardia, asthenia, flu-like symptoms, chills, nausea, vomiting, infection
Docetaxel (p. 378) (Taxotere)	**I:** 20 mg, 80 mg	Hypotension, nausea, vomiting, diarrhea, mucositis, myelosuppression, rash, paresthesia, hypersensitivity, fluid retention, alopecia, asthenia, stomatitis, fever
Doxorubicin (p. 391) (Adriamycin)	**I:** 10 mg, 20 mg, 50 mg, 75 mg, 150 mg, 200 mg	Cardiotoxicity, including CHF; arrhythmias, nausea, vomiting, stomatitis, esophagitis, GI ulceration, diarrhea, anorexia, hematuria, myelosuppression, alopecia, hyperpigmentation of nail beds and skin, local inflammation at injection site, rash, fever, chills, urticaria, lacrimation, conjunctivitis
Doxorubicin (p. 391) (Doxil)	**I:** 20 mg, 50 mg	Neutropenia, palmoplantar erythrodysesthesia syndrome, cardiomyopathy, CHF
Epirubicin (p. 422) (Ellence)	**I:** 2 mg/ml	Anemia, leukopenia, neutropenia, infection, mucositis
Erlotinib (p. 434) (Tarceva)	**T:** 25 mg, 100 mg, 150 mg	Diarrhea, rash, nausea, vomiting

Estramustine (p. 448) (Emcyt)	**C:** 140 mg	Increased risk of thrombosis, gynecomastia, nausea, vomiting, diarrhea, thrombocytopenia, peripheral edema
Etoposide (p. 458) (VePesid)	**I:** 20 mg/ml **C:** 50 mg	Nausea, vomiting, anorexia, myelosuppression, alopecia, diarrhea, drowsiness, peripheral neuropathies
Exemestane (p. 461) (Aromasin)	**T:** 25 mg	Dyspnea, edema, hypertension, mental depression
Fludarabine (p. 489) (Fludara)	**I:** 50 mg	Nausea, diarrhea, stomatitis, bleeding, anemia, myelosuppression, skin rash, weakness, confusion, visual disturbances, peripheral neuropathy, coma, pneumonia, peripheral edema, anorexia
Fluorouracil (p. 496) (Adrucil, Efudex)	**I:** 50 mg/ml **Cream:** 1%, 5% **Solution:** 1%, 2%, 5%	Nausea, vomiting, stomatitis, GI ulceration, diarrhea, anorexia, myelosuppression, alopecia, skin hyperpigmentation, nail changes, headaches, drowsiness, blurred vision, fever
Flutamide (p. 505) (Eulexin)	**C:** 125 mg	Hot flashes, nausea, vomiting, diarrhea, hepatitis, impotence, decreased libido, rash, anorexia
Fulvestrant (p. 525) (Faslodex)	**I:** 250 mg/5 ml, 125 mg/2.5 ml syringes	Asthenia, pain, headaches, injection site pain, flu-like symptoms, fever, nausea, vomiting, constipation, anorexia, diarrhea, peripheral edema, dizziness, depression, anxiety, rash, increased cough, UTI
Gefitinib (p. 535) (Iressa)	**T:** 250 mg	Diarrhea, rash, acne, nausea, dry skin, vomiting, pruritus, anorexia
Gemcitabine (p. 537) (Gemzar)	**I:** 200 mg, 1 g	Increased hepatic function tests, nausea, vomiting, diarrhea, stomatitis, hematuria, myelosuppression, rash, mild paresthesias, dyspnea, fever, edema, flu-like symptoms, constipation
Gemtuzumab (p. 542) (Mylotarg)	**I:** 5 mg/20 ml	Anemia, hematuria, hepatic toxicity, pneumonia, herpes simplex, nausea, vomiting, dyspnea, headaches, hypotension, hypoxia, mucositis, myelosuppression, peripheral edema, tachycardia, thrombocytopenia
Goserelin (p. 560) (Zoladex)	**I:** 3.6 mg, 10.8 mg	Hot flashes, sexual dysfunction, erectile dysfunction, gynecomastia, lethargy, pain, lower urinary tract symptoms, headaches, nausea, depression, diaphoresis

(continued)

CHEMOTHERAPEUTIC AGENTS *(continued)*

Name	Availability	Side Effects
Hydroxyurea (p. 586) (Hydrea)	**C:** 500 mg	Anorexia, nausea, vomiting, stomatitis, diarrhea, constipation, myelosuppression, fever, chills, malaise
Ibritumomab (p. 593) (Zevalin)	**Injection kit**	Neutropenia, thrombocytopenia, anemia, infection, asthenia, abdominal pain, fever, pain, headaches, nausea, peripheral edema, allergic reaction, GI hemorrhage, apnea
Idarubicin (p. 597) (Idamycin PFS)	**I:** 5 mg, 10 mg, 20 mg	CHF, arrhythmias, nausea, vomiting, stomatitis, myelosuppression, alopecia, rash, urticaria, hyperuricemia, abdominal pain, diarrhea, esophagitis, anorexia
Ifosfamide (p. 599) (Ifex)	**I:** 1 g, 3 g	Nausea, vomiting, hemorrhagic cystitis, myelosuppression, alopecia, lethargy, drowsiness, confusion, hallucinations, hematuria
Imatinib (p. 602) (Gleevec)	**C:** 100 mg	Nausea, fluid retention, hemorrhage, musculoskeletal pain, arthralgia, weight gain, pyrexia, abdominal pain, dyspnea, pneumonia
Interferon alfa-2a (p. 623) (Roferon-A)	**I:** 3 million units, 6 million units, 9 million units, 18 million units	Anorexia, nausea, diarrhea, myelosuppression, pruritus, myalgia, dizziness, headaches, paresthesias, fatigue, fever, chills, dyspnea, flu-like symptoms, vomiting, coughing, altered taste
Interferon alfa-2b (p. 624) (Intron-A)	**I:** 3 million units, 5 million units, 10 million units, 18 million units, 25 million units, 50 million units	Mild hypotension, hypertension, tachycardia with high fever, nausea, diarrhea, altered taste, weight loss, thrombocytopenia, myelosuppression, rash, pruritus, myalgia, arthralgia associated with flu-like symptoms
Irinotecan (p. 636) (Camptosar)	**I:** 40 mg, 100 mg	Diarrhea, nausea, vomiting, abdominal cramps, anorexia, stomatitis, increased AST, severe myelosuppression, alopecia, diaphoresis, rash, weight loss, dehydration, increased serum alkaline phosphatase, headaches, insomnia, dizziness, dyspnea, cough, asthenia, rhinitis, fever, back pain, chills
Letrozole (p. 676) (Femara)	**T:** 2.5 mg	Hypertension, nausea, vomiting, constipation, diarrhea, abdominal pain, anorexia, rash, pruritus, musculoskeletal pain, arthralgia, fatigue, headaches, dyspnea, coughing, hot flashes

Leuprolide (p. 679) (Lupron)	**I:** 3.75 mg, 5 mg, 7.5 mg, 11.25 mg, 15 mg, 22.5 mg, 30 mg	Hot flashes, gynecomastia, nausea, vomiting, constipation, anorexia, dizziness, headaches, insomnia, paresthesias, bone pain
Lomustine (p. 701) (CeeNU)	**C:** 10 mg, 40 mg, 100 mg	Anorexia, nausea, vomiting, stomatitis, hepatic toxicity, nephrotoxicity, myelosuppression, alopecia, confusion, slurred speech
Mechlorethamine (Mustargen)	**I:** 10 mg/ml	Severe nausea and vomiting, metallic taste, diarrhea, myelosuppression, alopecia, phlebitis, vertigo, tinnitus, hyperuricemia, infertility, azoospermia, anorexia, headaches, drowsiness, fever
Megestrol (p. 726) (Megace)	**T:** 20 mg, 40 mg **Suspension:** 40 mg/ml	Deep vein thrombosis, Cushing-like syndrome, alopecia, carpal tunnel syndrome, weight gain, nausea
Melphalan (p. 729) (Alkeran)	**T:** 2 mg	Anorexia, nausea, vomiting, myelosuppression, diarrhea, stomatitis
Mercaptopurine (Purinethol)	**T:** 50 mg	Anorexia, nausea, vomiting, stomatitis, hepatic toxicity, myelosuppression, hyperuricemia, diarrhea, rash
Methotrexate (p. 748) (Rheumatrex)	**T:** 2.5 mg, 5 mg, 7.5 mg, 10 mg, 15 mg **I:** 5 mg, 50 mg, 100 mg, 200 mg, 250 mg	Nausea, vomiting, stomatitis, GI ulceration, diarrhea, hepatic toxicity, renal failure, cystitis, myelosuppression, alopecia, urticaria, acne, photosensitivity, interstitial pneumonitis, fever, malaise, chills, anorexia
Mitomycin-C (p. 782) (Mutamycin)	**I:** 20 mg, 40 mg	Anorexia, nausea, vomiting, stomatitis, diarrhea, renal toxicity, myelosuppression, alopecia, pruritus, fever, hemolytic uremic syndrome, weakness
Mitotane (Lysodren)	**T:** 500 mg	Anorexia, nausea, vomiting, diarrhea, skin rashes, depression, lethargy, drowsiness, dizziness, adrenal insufficiency, blurred vision, impaired hearing
Mitoxantrone (p. 784) (Novantrone)	**I:** 20 mg, 25 mg, 30 mg	CHF, tachycardia, ECG changes, chest pain, nausea, vomiting, stomatitis, mucositis, myelosuppression, rash, alopecia, urine discoloration (bluish green), phlebitis, diarrhea, cough, headaches, fever
Nelarabine (p. 823) (Arranon)	**I:** 5 mg/ml	Anemia, neutropenia, thrombocytopenia, nausea, vomiting, diarrhea, fatigue, fever, dyspnea, severe neurologic events (convulsions, peripheral neuropathy)

(continued)

CHEMOTHERAPEUTIC AGENTS ***(continued)***

Name	Availability	Side Effects
Nilutamide (p. 839) (Nilandron)	**T:** 50 mg	Hypertension, angina, hot flashes, nausea, anorexia, increased hepatic enzymes, dizziness, dyspnea, visual disturbances, impaired adaptation to dark, constipation, decreased libido
Oxaliplatin (p. 877) (Eloxatin)	**I:** 50 mg, 100 mg	Fatigue, neuropathy, abdominal pain, dyspnea, diarrhea, nausea, vomiting, anorexia, fever, edema, chest pain, anemia, thrombocytopenia, thromboembolism, altered hepatic function tests
Paclitaxel (p. 891) (Taxol)	**I:** 30 mg, 100 mg	Hypertension, bradycardia, ECG changes, nausea, vomiting, diarrhea, mucositis, myelosuppression, alopecia, peripheral neuropathies, hypersensitivity reaction, athralgia, myalgia
Panitumumab (p. 901) (Vectibix)	**I:** 20 mg/ml	Pulmonary fibrosis, severe dermatologic toxicity, infusion reactions, abdominal pain, nausea, vomiting, constipation, skin rash, fatigue
Pegaspargase (Oncaspar)	**I:** 750 international units/ml	Hypotension, anorexia, nausea, vomiting, hepatic toxicity, pancreatitis, depression of clotting factors, malaise, confusion, lethargy, EEG changes, respiratory distress, hypersensitivity reaction, fever, hyperglycemia, stomatitis
Pemetrexed (p. 912) (Alimta)	**I:** 500 mg	Anorexia, constipation, diarrhea, neuropathy, anemia, chest pain, dyspnea, rash, fatigue
Pentostatin (Nipent)	**I:** 10 mg	Nausea, vomiting, hepatic disorders, elevated hepatic function tests, leukopenia, anemia, thrombocytopenia, rash, fever, upper respiratory infection, fatigue, hematuria, headaches, myalgia, arthralgia, diarrhea, anorexia
Plicamycin evolve **(Mithracin)**	**I:** 2.5 mg	Anorexia, nausea, vomiting, stomatitis, diarrhea, clotting factor disorders, facial flushing, mental depression, confusion, fever, hypocalcemia, hypophosphatemia, hypokalemia, headaches, dizziness, rash
Procarbazine (p. 971) (Matulane)	**C:** 50 mg	Nausea, vomiting, stomatitis, diarrhea, constipation, myelosuppression, pruritus, hyperpigmentation, alopecia, myalgia, paresthesias, confusion, lethargy, mental depression, fever, hepatic toxicity, arthralgia, respiratory disorders

Rituximab (p. 1037) (Rituxan)	**I:** 100 mg, 500 mg	Hypotension, arrhythmias, peripheral edema, nausea, vomiting, abdominal pain, leukopenia, thrombocytopenia, neutropenia, rash, pruritus, urticaria, angioedema, myalgia, headaches, dizziness, throat irritation, rhinitis, bronchospasm, hypersensitivity reaction
Sorafenib (p. 1079) (Nexavar)	**T:** 200 mg	Fatigue, alopecia, nausea, vomiting, anorexia, constipation, diarrhea, neuropathy, dyspnea, cough, asthenia, pain
Streptozocin (Zanosar)	**I:** 1 g	May lead to insulin-dependent diabetes, nausea, vomiting, nephrotoxicity, renal tubular acidosis, myelosuppression, lethargy, diarrhea, confusion, depression
Sunitinib (p. 1096) (Sutent)	**C:** 12.5 mg, 25 mg, 50 mg	Hypotension, edema, fatigue, headache, fever, dizziness, rash, hyperpigmentation, diarrhea, nausea, dyspepsia, altered taste, vomiting, neutropenia, thrombocytopenia, increased ALT/AST
Tamoxifen (p. 1102) (Nolvadex)	**T:** 10 mg, 20 mg	Skin rash, nausea, vomiting, anorexia, menstrual irregularities, hot flashes, pruritus, vaginal discharge or bleeding, myelosuppression, headaches, tumor or bone pain, ophthalmic changes, weight gain, confusion
Temozolomide (p. 1112) (Temodar)	**C:** 5 mg, 20 mg, 100 mg, 250 mg	Amnesia, fever, infection, leukopenia, neutropenia, peripheral edema, seizures, thrombocytopenia
Teniposide (Vumon)	**I:** 50 mg/5 ml	Hypotension with rapid infusion, diarrhea, nausea, vomiting, mucositis, myelosuppression, alopecia, anemia, rash, hypersensitivity reaction
Thioguanine	**T:** 40 mg	Anorexia, stomatitis, myelosuppression, hyperuricemia, nausea, vomiting, diarrhea
Thiotepa (p. 1132) (Thioplex)	**I:** 15 mg	Anorexia, nausea, vomiting, mucositis, myelosuppression, amenorrhea, reduced spermatogenesis, fever, hypersensitivity reactions, pain at injection site, headaches, dizziness, alopecia
Topotecan (p. 1159) (Hycamtin)	**I:** 4 mg	Nausea, vomiting, diarrhea, constipation, abdominal pain, stomatitis, anorexia, neutropenia, leukopenia, thrombocytopenia, anemia, alopecia, headaches, dyspnea, paresthesia
Toremifene (p. 1161) (Fareston)	**T:** 60 mg	Elevated hepatic function tests, nausea, vomiting, constipation, skin discoloration, dermatitis, dizziness, hot flashes, diaphoresis, vaginal discharge or bleeding, ocular changes, cataracts, anxiety

(continued)

CHEMOTHERAPEUTIC AGENTS *(continued)*

Name	Availability	Side Effects
Tositumomab (p. 1164) (Bexxar)	**I:** 14 mg/ml	Headaches, rash, pruritus, abdominal pain, anorexia, diarrhea, nausea, vomiting, arthralgia, myalgia, cough, dyspnea, asthenia, chills, fever, infection
Trastuzumab (p. 1171) (Herceptin)	**I:** 440 mg	CHF, heart murmur (S3 gallop), nausea, vomiting, diarrhea, abdominal pain, anorexia, rash, peripheral edema, back or bone pain, asthenia, headaches, insomnia, dizziness, cough, dyspnea, rhinitis, pharyngitis
Tretinoin (p. 1176) (Vesanoid)	**C:** 10 mg	Flushing, nausea, vomiting, diarrhea, constipation, dyspepsia, mucositis, leukocytosis, dry skin/mucus membranes, rash, pruritus, alopecia, dizziness, anxiety, insomnia, headaches, depression, confusion, intracranial hypertension, agitation, dyspnea, shivering, fever, visual changes, earaches, hearing loss, bone pain, myalgia, arthralgia
Valrubicin (Valstar)	**I:** 200 mg/5 ml	Dysuria, hematuria, urinary frequency/incontinence/urgency
Vinblastine (p. 1214) (Velban)	**I:** 10 mg	Nausea, vomiting, stomatitis, constipation, myelosuppression, alopecia, peripheral neuropathy, loss of deep tendon reflexes, paresthesias, diarrhea
Vincristine (p. 1216) (Oncovin)	**I:** 1 mg, 2 mg, 3 mg	Nausea, vomiting, stomatitis, constipation, pharyngitis, polyuria, myelosuppression, alopecia, numbness, paresthesias, peripheral neuropathy, loss of deep tendon reflexes, headaches, abdominal pain
Vinorelbine (p. 1218) (Navelbine)	**I:** 10 mg, 50 mg	Elevated hepatic function tests, nausea, vomiting, constipation, ileus, anorexia, stomatitis, myelosuppression, alopecia, vein discoloration, venous pain, phlebitis, interstitial pulmonary changes, asthenia, fatigue, diarrhea, peripheral neuropathy, loss of deep tendon reflexes
Vorinostat (p. 1228) (Zolinza)	**C:** 100 mg	Diarrhea, fatigue, nausea, thrombocytopenia, anorexia, dygeusia

C, Capsules; ***I,*** injection; ***T,*** tablets.

Cholinergic Agonists/Anticholinesterase

USES

Paralytic ileus and atony of urinary bladder. Myasthenia gravis (weakness, marked fatigue of skeletal muscle). Terminates, reverses effects of neuromuscular blocking agents.

ACTION

Cholinergic agonists: Referred to as *muscarinics* or *parasympathetics* and consist of two basic drug groups: choline esters and cholinomimetic alkaloids. Primary action mimics actions of acetylcholine at postganglionic parasympathetic nerves. Primary properties include the following:

Cardiovascular system: Vasodilation; decreased cardiac rate; decreased conduction in SA, AV nodes; decreased force of myocardial contraction.

Gastrointestinal: Increased tone, motility of GI smooth muscle, increased secretory activity of GI tract.

Urinary tract: Increased contraction of detrusor muscle of urinary bladder, resulting in micturition.

Eye: Miosis, contraction of ciliary muscle.

Anticholinesterase (anti-ChE), also known as *cholinesterase inhibitors:* Inactivates cholinesterase, which prevents acetylcholine breakdown,-causing acetylcholine to accumulate at cholinergic receptor sites. These agents can be considered indirect-acting cholinergic agonists. Primary properties include action of cholinergic agonists just noted.

Skeletal neuromuscular junction: Effects are dose dependent. At therapeutic doses, increases force of skeletal muscle contraction; at toxic doses, reduces muscle strength.

CHOLINERGIC AGONISTS/ANTICHOLINESTERASE

Name	Availability	Uses	Dosage Range	Side Effects
Bethanechol (p. 135) (Urecholine)	**T:** 5 mg, 10 mg, 25 mg, 50 mg **I:** 5 mg/ml	Nonobstructive urinary retention	**PO:** 10–50 mg 3–4 times/day **Subcutaneous:** 2.5–5 mg 3–4 times/day	Increased urinary frequency, salivation, belching, nausea, dizziness

(continued)

CHOLINERGIC AGONISTS/ANTICHOLINESTERASE *(continued)*

Name	Availability	Uses	Dosage Range	Side Effects
Edrophonium (Tensilon)	**I:** 10 mg/ml	Diagnosis of myasthenia gravis, reverses tubocurarine	**IV:** 10 mg over 30 sec up to 40 mg	Bradycardia, nausea, vomiting, diarrhea, urinary frequency
Neostigmine (p. 827) (Prostigmin)	**T:** 15 mg **I:** 0.25 mg/ml, 0.5 mg/ml, 1 mg/ml	Symptomatic control of myasthenia gravis, neuromuscular blocker	**PO:** 15–365 mg/day **Subcutaneous, IM:** 0.5 mg **IV:** 0.5–2 mg	Diarrhea, diaphoresis, nausea, vomiting, abdominal cramps
Pyridostigmine (p. 993) (Mestinon)	**T:** 60 mg **T (ER):** 180 mg **S:** 60 mg/5 ml **I:** 5 mg/ml	Treats myasthenia gravis, reverses tubocurarine	**PO:** 60–1,500 mg/day **IM:** 0.5–1.5 mg/kg **IV:** 0.1–0.25 mg/kg	Diarrhea, diaphoresis, nausea, vomiting, abdominal cramps

ER, Extended release; ***I,*** injection; ***S,*** suspension; ***T,*** tablets.

Contraception

ACTION

Combination oral contraceptives decrease fertility primarily by inhibition of ovulation. In addition, they can promote thickening of the cervical mucus, thereby creating a physical barrier for the passage of sperm. Also, they can modify the endometrium, making it less favorable for nidation.

CLASSIFICATION

Oral contraceptives either contain both an estrogen and a progestin (combination oral contraceptives) or contain only a progestin (progestin-only oral contraceptives). The combination oral contraceptives have three subgroups:

Monophasic: Daily estrogen and progestin dosage remains constant.

Biphasic: Estrogen remains constant, but the progestin dosage increases during the second half of the cycle.

Triphasic: Progestin changes for each phase of the cycle.

Over the past several years, options have expanded to include a combined hormonal patch (Ortho Eva), vaginal ring (NuvaRing), and extended cycle contraceptives (e.g., Loestrin-24 FE, Seasonale, Seasonique, Yaz).

COMMON COMPLAINTS WITH THE ORAL CONTRACEPTIVES

Too much estrogen	Nausea, bloating, breast tenderness, increased B/P, melasma, headache
Too little estrogen	Early or mid-cycle breakthrough bleeding, increased spotting, hypomenorrhea
Too much progestin	Breast tenderness, headache, fatigue, changes in mood
Too little progestin	Late breakthrough bleeding
Too much androgen	Increased appetite, weight gain, acne, oily skin, hirsutism, decreased libido, increased breast size, breast tenderness, increased LDL cholesterol, decreased HDL cholesterol

CONTRACEPTIVES

Name	Estrogen Content	Progestin Content
Low-Dose Monophasic Pills		
Alesse Aviane Lessina Levlite Lutera	EE 20 mcg	Levonorgestrel 0.1 mg
Junel 1/20 Junel Fe 1/20 Loestrin 1/20, Fe 1/20 Microgestin 1/20, Fe 1/20	EE 20 mcg	Norethindrone 1 mg
Levlen Levora Nordette Portia	EE 30 mcg	Levonorgestrel 0.15 mg
Cryselle Lo/Ovral Low-Ogestrel	EE 30 mcg	Norgestrel 0.3 mg

(continued)

CONTRACEPTIVES ***(continued)***

Name	Estrogen Content	Progestin Content
Junel 1.5/30 Junel Fe 1.5/30 Loestrin Fe 1.5/30 Microgestin 1.5/30 Microgestin Fe 1.5/30	EE 30 mcg	Norethindrone acetate 1.5 mg
Apri Desogen Ortho-Cept Reclipsen Solia	EE 30 mcg	Desogestrel 0.15 mg
Yasmin	EE 30 mcg	Drospirenone 3 mg
Demulen 1/35 Kelnor 1/35 Zovia 1/35	EE 35 mcg	Ethynodiol diacetate 1 mg
Ortho-Cyclen Mononessa Previfem Sprintec	EE 35 mcg	Norgestimate 0.25 mg
Necon 1/50 Norinyl 1+50 Ortho-Novum 1/50	Mestranol 50 mcg	Norethindrone 1 mg
Ovcon-35 Ovcon-35 chewable	EE 35 mcg	Norethindrone 0.4 mg
Brevicon Modicon Necon 0.5/35 Nortrel 0.5/35	EE 35 mcg	Norethindrone 0.5 mg

Necon 1/35 Norethin 1/35 Norinyl 1+35 Nortrel 1/35 Ortho-Novum 1/35	EE 35 mcg	Norethindrone 1 mg
High-Dose Monophasic Pills		
Ovcon-50	EE 50 mcg	Norethindrone 1 mg
Ogestrel 0.5/50	EE 50 mcg	Norgestrel 0.5 mg
Demulen 1/50 Zovia	EE 50 mcg	Ethynodiol diacetate 1 mg
Biphasic Pills		
Mircette Kariva	EE 20 mcg x 21 days, placebo x 2 days, 10 mcg x 5 days	Desogestrel 0.15 mg x 21 days
Gencept 10/11 Necon 10/11 Ortho-Novum 10/11	EE 35 mcg	Norethindrone 0.5 mg x 10 days, 1 mg x 11 days
Triphasic Pills		
Estrostep Fe	EE 20 mcg x 5 days, 30 mcg x 7 days, 35 mcg x 9 days	Norethindrone 1 mg x 21 days
Ortho Tri-Cyclen Lo	EE 25 mcg x 21 days	Norgestimate 0.18 mg x 7 days, 0.215 mg x 7 days, 0.25 mg x 7 days
Cesia Cyclessa Velivet	EE 25 mcg x 21 days	Desogestrel 0.1 mg x 7 days, 0.125 mg x 7 days, 0.15 mg x 7 days

(continued)

CONTRACEPTIVES ***(continued)***

Name	Estrogen Content	Progestin Content
Enpresse Tri-Levlen Triphasil Trivora	EE 30 mcg x 6 days, 40 mcg x 5 days, 30 mcg x 10 days	Levonorgestrel 0.05 mg x 6 days, 0.075 mg x 5 days, 0.125 mg x 10 days
Ortho Tri-Cyclen Trinessa Tri-Previfem Tri-Sprintec	EE 35 mcg x 21 days	Norgestimate 0.18 mg x 7 days, 0.215 mg x 7 days, 0.25 mg x 7 days
Aranelle Leena Tri-Norinyl	EE 35 mcg x 21 days	Norethindrone 0.5 mg x 7 days, 1 mg x 9 days, 0.5 mg x 5 days
Ortho-Novum 7/7/7 Nortrel 7/7/7 Necon 7/7/7	EE 35 mcg x 21 days	Norethindrone 0.5 mg x 7 days, 0.75 mg x 7 days, 1 mg x 7 days

Extended-Cycle Pills

Loestrin-24 FE	EE 20 mcg	Norethindrone 1 mg
Seasonale	EE 30 mcg	Levonorgestrel 0.15 mg
Seasonique	EE 30 mcg x 84 days, 10 mcg x 7 days	Levonorgestrel 0.15 mg
Yaz	EE 20 mcg	Drospirenone 3 mg

Progestin-Only Pills

Camilia Errin Jolivette Micronor Nor-QD Nora-BE	N/A	Norethindrone 0.35 mg

Emergency Contraception

Plan B	N/A	Levonorgestrel 0.75 mg

Hormonal Alternative to Oral Contraception

Depo-Provera CI Medroxyprogesterone Acetate	None	Medroxyprogesterone 150 mg
Depo-SubQ Provera 104	None	Medroxyprogesterone 104 mg
Implanon	None	Etonogestrel (release rate varies over time)
Mirena	None	Levonorgestrel 20 mcg/day for 5 yrs
NuvaRing	Ethinyl estradiol 15 mcg/day	Etonogestrel 0.12 mg/day
Ortho Evra	Ethinyl estradiol 20 mcg/day	Noreigestromin 150 mcg/day

Corticosteroids

USES

Replacement therapy in adrenal insufficiency, including Addison's disease. Symptomatic treatment of multiorgan disease/conditions. Rheumatoid arthritis, osteoarthritis, severe psoriasis, ulcerative colitis, lupus erythematosus, anaphylactic shock, acute excacerbation of asthma, status asthmaticus, organ transplant.

ACTION

Suppress migration of polymorphonuclear leukocytes (PML) and reverse increased capillary permeability by their anti-inflammatory effect. Suppress immune system by decreasing activity of lymphatic system.

CORTICOSTEROIDS

Name	Availability	Route of Administration	Side Effects
Beclomethasone (p. 124) (Beconase)	**Inhalation, nasal:** 42 mcg/spray, 84 mcg/spray	Inhalation, intranasal	**I:** Cough, dry mouth/throat, headaches, throat irritation **Nasal:** Headaches, sore throat, intranasal ulceration
Betamethasone (p. 131) (Celestone, Diprolene)	**I:** 4 mg/ml	IV, intralesional, intra-articular	Nausea, vomiting, increased appetite, weight gain, insomnia
Budesonide (p. 158) (Rhinocort, Pulmicort)	**Nasal:** 32 mcg/spray	Intranasal	**Nasal:** Headaches, sore throat, intranasal ulceration
Cortisone (p. 291) (Cortone)	**T:** 5 mg, 10 mg, 25 mg	PO	Same as betamethasone
Dexamethasone (p. 339) (Decadron)	**T:** 0.5 mg, 1 mg, 4 mg, 6 mg **OS:** 0.5 mg/5 ml **I:** 4 mg/ml	PO, parenteral	Same as betamethasone
Fludrocortisone (p. 491) (Florinef)	**T:** 0.1 mg	PO	Same as betamethasone
Flunisolide (p. 494) (AeroBid, Nasalide)	**Inhalation, nasal:** 25 mcg/spray	Inhalation, intranasal	Same as beclomethasone
Fluticasone (p. 506) (Flonase, Flovent)	**Inhalation:** 44 mcg, 110 mg/220 mcg **Nasal:** 50 mg, 100 mcg	Inhalation, intranasal	Same as beclomethasone
Hydrocortisone (p. 579) (Solu-Cortef)	**T:** 5 mg, 10 mg, 25 mg **I:** 100 mg, 250 mg, 500 mg, 1 g	PO, parenteral	Same as betamethasone
Methylprednisolone (p. 756) (Solu-Medrol)	**T:** 4 mg **I:** 40 mg, 125 mg, 500 mg, 1 g, 2 g	PO, parenteral	Same as betamethasone
Prednisolone (p. 960) (Prelone)	**T:** 5 mg **OS:** 5 mg/5 ml, 15 mg/5 ml	PO	Same as betamethasone

Prednisone (p. 962)	**T:** 1 mg, 2.5 mg, 5 mg, 10 mg, 20 mg, 50 mg	PO	Same as betamethasone
Triamcinolone (p. 1178) (Azmacort, Kenalog)	**T:** 4 mg, 8 mg **Inhalation:** 100 mcg	PO, inhalation	Same as betamethasone **I:** Cough, dry mouth/throat, headaches, throat irritation

I, Injection; ***OS,*** oral suspension; ***T,*** tablets.

Corticosteroids: Topical

USES

Provide relief of inflammation/pruritus associated with corticosteroid-responsive disorders (e.g., contact dermatitis, eczema, insect bite reactions, first- and second-degree localized burns/sunburn).

ACTION

Diffuse across cell membranes, form complexes with cytoplasm. Complexes stimulate protein synthesis of inhibitory enzymes responsible for anti-inflammatory effects (e.g., inhibit edema, erythema, pruritus, capillary dilation, phagocytic activity).

Topical corticosteroids can be classified based on potency:

Low potency: Modest anti-inflammatory effect, safest for chronic application, facial and intertriginous application, with occlusion, for infants/young children.

Medium potency: For moderate inflammatory conditions (e.g., chronic eczematous dermatoses). May use for facial and intertriginous application for only limited time.

High potency: For more severe inflammatory conditions (e.g., lichen simplex chronicus, psoriasis). May use for facial and intertriginous application for short time only. Used in areas of thickened skin due to chronic conditions.

Very high potency: Alternative to systemic therapy for local effect (e.g., chronic lesions caused by psoriasis). Increased risk of skin atrophy. Used for short periods on small areas. Avoid occlusive dressings.

CORTICOSTEROIDS: TOPICAL

Name	Availability	Potency	Side Effects
Alclometasone (Aclovate)	**C, O:** 0.05%	Low	Skin atrophy, contact dermatitis, stretch marks on skin, enlarged blood vessels in the skin, hair loss, pigment changes, secondary infections
Amcinonide (Cyclocort)	**C, O, L:** 0.1%	High	Same as alclometasone
Betamethasone dipropionate (p. 131)	**C, O, G, L:** 0.05%	High	Same as alclometasone
Betamethasone valerate (p. 131)	**C:** 0.01%, 0.05%, 0.1% **O:** 0.1% **L:** 0.1%	High	Same as alclometasone
Clobetasol (Temovate)	**C, O:** 0.05%	High	Same as alclometasone
Desonide (Tridesilon)	**C, O, L:** 0.05%	Low	Same as alclometasone
Desoximetasone (Topicort)	**C:** 0.25%, 0.5% **O:** 0.25% **G:** 0.05%	High	Same as alclometasone
Dexamethasone (p. 339) (Decadron)	**C:** 0.1%	Medium	Same as alclometasone
Fluocinolone (Synalar)	**C:** 0.01%, 0.025%, 0.2% **O:** 0.025%	High	Same as alclometasone
Fluocinonide (Lidex)	**C, O, G:** 0.05%	High	Same as alclometasone

Flurandrenolide (Cordran)	**C, O, L:** 0.025%, 0.05%	Medium	Same as alclometasone
Fluticasone (p. 506) (Cutivate)	**C:** 0.05% **O:** 0.005%	Medium	Same as alclometasone
Halobetasol (Ultravate)	**C, O:** 0.05%	High	Same as alclometasone
Hydrocortisone (p. 579) (Hytone)	**C, O:** 0.5%, 1%, 2.5%	Medium	Same as alclometasone
Mometasone (p. 789) (Elocon)	**C, O, L:** 0.1%	Medium	Same as alclometasone
Prednicarbate (Dermatop)	**C:** 0.1%	—	Same as alclometasone
Triamcinolone (p. 1178) (Aristocort, Kenalog)	**C, O, L:** 0.025%, 0.1%, 0.5%	Medium	Same as alclometasone

C, Cream; ***G,*** gel; ***L,*** lotion; ***O,*** ointment.

Diuretics

USES

Thiazides: Management of edema resulting from a number of causes (e.g., CHF, hepatic cirrhosis); hypertension either alone or in combination with other antihypertensives.

Loop: Management of edema associated with CHF, cirrhosis of the liver, and renal disease. Furosemide used in treatment of hypertension alone or in combination with other antihypertensives.

Potassium-sparing: Adjunctive treatment with thiazides, loop diuretics in treatment of CHF and hypertension.

ACTION

Act to increase the excretion of water/sodium and other electrolytes via the kidneys. Exact mechanism of antihypertensive effect unknown; may be due to reduced plasma volume or decreased peripheral vascular resistance. Subclassifications of diuretics are based on their mechanism and site of action.

Thiazides: Act at the cortical diluting segment of nephron, block reabsorption of Na, Cl, and water; promote excretion of Na, Cl, K, and water.

Loop: Act primarily at the thick ascending limb of Henle's loop to inhibit Na, Cl, and water absorption.

Potassium-sparing: Spironolactone blocks aldosterone action on distal nephron (causes K retention, Na excretion). Triamterene, amiloride act on distal nephron, decreasing Na reuptake, reducing K secretion.

DIURETICS

Name	Availability	Dosage Range	Side Effects
Thiazide, Thiazide-related			
Chlorothiazide (Diuril)	**T:** 250 mg, 500 mg **S:** 250 mg/5 ml **I:** 500 mg	5–20 mg/day	Confusion, fatigue, muscle cramps, abdominal discomfort
Chlorthalidone evolve **(Hygroton)**	**T:** 15 mg, 25 mg, 50 mg, 100 mg	25–200 mg/day	Same as chlorothiazide

Hydrochlorothiazide (p. 574) (HydroDIURIL)	**T:** 25 mg, 50 mg, 100 mg **C:** 12.5 mg **Solution:** 50 mg/15 ml	25–100 mg/day	Same as chlorothiazide
Indapamide (p. 610) (Lozol)	**T:** 1.25 mg, 2.5 mg	2.5–5 mg/day	Loss of appetite, diarrhea, headaches, dizziness, light-headedness, insomnia, upset stomach
Metolazone (p. 761) (Zaroxolyn)	**T:** 2.5 mg, 5 mg, 10 mg	2.5–10 mg/day	Same as chlorothiazide

Loop

Bumetanide (p. 160) (Bumex)	**T:** 0.5 mg, 1 mg, 2 mg **I:** 0.25 mg/ml	5–10 mg/day	Orthostatic hypotension, cramps or pain, hypokalemia (dry mouth, fatigue, muscle cramps), blurred vision, headaches
Furosemide (p. 526) (Lasix)	**T:** 20 mg, 40 mg, 80 mg **OS:** 10 mg/ml, 40 mg/5 ml **I:** 10 mg/ml	**HTN:** 40–80 mg/day **Edema:** Up to 600 mg/day	Orthostatic hypotension, cramps or pain, hypokalemia (dry mouth, fatigue, muscle cramps), blurred vision, headaches
Torsemide (p. 1162) (Demadex)	**T:** 5 mg, 10 mg, 20 mg, 100 mg **I:** 10 mg/ml	**Edema:** 10–200 mg/day **HTN:** 5–10 mg/day	Constipation, dizziness, upset stomach, headache, hypokalemia (dry mouth, fatigue, muscle cramps)

Potassium-sparing

Amiloride (p. 52) (Midamor)	**T:** 5 mg	5–20 mg/day	Hyperkalemia
Spironolactone (p. 1082) (Aldactone)	**T:** 25 mg, 50 mg, 100 mg	25–100 mg/day	Hyperkalemia, nausea, vomiting, abdominal cramps, diarrhea
Triamterene (p. 1180) (Dyrenium)	**C:** 50 mg, 100 mg	Up to 300 mg/day	Same as amiloride

C, Capsules; ***HTN,*** hypertension; ***I,*** injection; ***OS,*** oral solution; ***S,*** suspension; ***T,*** tablets.

Fertility Agents

Infertility is defined as a decreased ability to reproduce as opposed to *sterility*, the inability to reproduce. Infertility may be due to reproduction dysfunction of the male, female, or both.

Female infertility can be due to disruption of any phase of the reproductive process. The most critical phases include follicular maturation, ovulation, transport of the ovum through the fallopian tubes, fertilization of the ovum, nidation, and growth/development of the conceptus. Causes of infertility include the following:

Anovulation, failure of follicular maturation: Absence of adequate hormonal stimulation; ovarian follicles do not ripen, and ovulation will not occur.

Unfavorable cervical mucus: Normally the cervical glands secrete large volumes of thin, watery mucus, but if the mucus is unfavorable (scant, thick, or sticky), sperm is unable to pass through to the uterus.

Hyperprolactinemia: Excessive prolactin secretion may cause amenorrhea, galactorrhea, and infertility.

Luteal phase defect: Progesterone secretion by the corpus luteum is insufficient to maintain endometrial integrity.

Endometriosis: Endometrial tissue is implanted in abnormal locations (e.g., uterine wall, ovary, extragenital sites).

Androgen excess: May decrease fertility (most common condition is polycystic ovary).

Male infertility is due to decreased density or motility of sperm or semen of abnormal volume or quality. The most obvious manifestation of male infertility is impotence (inability to achieve erection). Whereas in female infertility an identifiable endocrine disorder can be found, most cases of male infertility are not associated with an identifiable endocrine disorder.

ACTION

Antiestrogens: Nonsteroidal estrogen antagonist that increases follicle-stimulating hormone (FSH) and leutinizing hormone (LH) levels by blocking estrogen-negative feedback at the hypothalamus.

Gonadotropins: Produce ovulation induction in women with hypogonadotropic hypogonadism and polycystic ovarian syndrome (PCOS). Ovaries must be able to respond normally to FSH and LH stimulation.

Gonadotropin-releasing hormone (GnRH) agonists: Causes down-regulation of endogenous FSH and LH levels. GnRH agonists stimulate release of pituitary gonadotropins. Suppression of endogenous LH can decrease number of oocytes released prematurely, improve oocyte quality, and increase pregnancy rates.

Gonadotropin-releasing hormone (GnRH) antagonists: Suppress endogenous LH surges during ovarian stimulation. GnRH antagonists avoid initial flare-up seen with GnRH agonists, shortening the number of days needed for LH suppression and allowing ovarian stimulation to begin within the spontaneous cycle.

MEDICATIONS TO INDUCE OVULATION

Name	Category	Availability	Uses	Side Effects
Cetrorelix (Cetrotide)	GnRH antagonist	**I:** 0.25 mg, 3 mg	Inhibition of premature LH surges in women undergoing ovarian hyperstimulation	OHSS (ovarian hyperstimulation syndrome): Abdominal pain, indigestion, bloating, decreased urinary output, nausea, vomiting, diarrhea, rapid weight gain, shortness of breath, peripheral/dependent edema; headaches, pain/redness at injection site

(continued)

MEDICATIONS TO INDUCE OVULATION ***(continued)***

Name	Category	Availability	Uses	Side Effects
Chorionic gonadotropin (p. 245) (Humegon, Pregnyl, Profasi HP)	Gonadotropin	**I:** 5,000 units, 10,000 units, 20,000 units	In conjunction with clomiphene, human menotropins or urofollitropin to stimulate ovulation	OHSS (ovarian hyperstimulation syndrome): Abdominal pain, indigestion, bloating, decreased urinary output, nausea, vomiting, diarrhea, rapid weight gain, shortness of breath, peripheral/dependent edema; ovarian enlargement, ovarian cyst formation
Clomiphene (Clomid, Milophene, Serophene)	Antiestrogen	**T:** 50 mg	Anovulation, oligo-ovulation with intact pituitary/ovarian response and endogenous estrogen	Ovarian cyst formation, ovarian enlargement visual disturbances, premenstrual syndrome, hot flashes
Follitropin alpha (Gonal-F)	Gonadotropin	**I:** 37.5 international units FSH, 75 international units FSH, 150 international units FSH	In conjunction with human chorionic gonadotropin to stimulate ovarian follicular development in pts with ovulatory dysfunction not due to primary ovarian failure (e.g., anovulation, oligo-ovulation)	OHSS (ovarian hyperstimulation syndrome): Abdominal pain, indigestion, bloating, decreased urinary output, nausea, vomiting, diarrhea, rapid weight gain, shortness of breath, peripheral/dependent edema; flu-like symptoms, upper respiratory tract infections, bleeding between menstrual periods, nausea, ovarian enlargement, ovarian cysts, acne, breast pain/tenderness

Follitropin beta (Follistim AQ)	Gonadotropin	**I:** 75 international units FSH	In conjunction with human chorionic gonadotropin to stimulate ovarian follicular development in patients with ovulatory dysfunction not due to primary ovarian failure (e.g., anovulation, oligo-ovulation)	OHSS (ovarian hyperstimulation syndrome): Abdominal pain, indigestion, bloating, decreased urinary output, nausea, vomiting, diarrhea, rapid weight gain, shortness of breath, peripheral/dependent edema; flu-like symptoms, breast tenderness, dry skin, rash, dizziness, fever, headaches, nausea, fatigue
Ganirelex (Antagon)	GnRH antagonist	**I:** 250 mcg/0.5 ml	Inhibition of premature LH surges in women undergoing ovarian hyperstimulation	OHSS (ovarian hyperstimulation syndrome): Abdominal pain, indigestion, bloating, decreased urinary output, nausea, vomiting, diarrhea, rapid weight gain, shortness of breath, peripheral/dependent edema; headaches, nausea, pain/redness at injection site
Goserelin (p. 560) (Zoladex)	GnRH agonist	**Implant:** 3.6 mg, 10.8 mg	Endometriosis, adjunct to menotropins for ovulation induction	Hot flashes, amenorrhea, blurred vision, edema, headaches, nausea, vomiting, breast tenderness, weight gain
Leuprolide (p. 679) (Lupron)	GnRH agonist	5 mg/ml for subcutaneous injection	Endometriosis, adjunct to menotropins/human chorionic gonadotropin for ovulation induction	Hot flashes, amenorrhea, blurred vision, edema, headaches, nausea, vomiting, breast tenderness, weight gain

(continued)

MEDICATIONS TO INDUCE OVULATION *(continued)*

Name	Category	Availability	Uses	Side Effects
Menotropins (Pergonal)	Gonadotropin	75 units FSH, 75 units LH activity; 150 units FSH, 150 units LH activity	In conjunction with chorionic gonadotropin for ovulation stimulation in pts with ovulatory dysfunction due to primary ovarian failure	OHSS (ovarian hyperstimulation syndrome): Abdominal pain, indigestion, bloating, decreased urinary output, nausea, vomiting, diarrhea, rapid weight gain, shortness of breath, edema of lower extremities; ovarian enlargement, ovarian cyst formation
Nafarelin (p. 807) (Synarel)	GnRH	2 mg/ml nasal spray	Endometriosis, adjunct to menotropins/human chorionic gonadotropin for ovulation induction	Loss of bone mineral density, breast enlargement, bleeding between regular menstrual periods, acne, mood swings, seborrhea, hot flashes
Urofollitropoin (Fertinex, Metrodin)	Gonadotropin	75 units FSH activity, 150 units FSH activity	In conjunction with human chorionic gonadotropin for ovulation stimulation in pts with polycystic ovary syndrome who have elevated LH:FSH ratio and have failed clomiphene therapy	OHSS (ovarian hyperstimulation syndrome): Abdominal pain, indigestion, bloating, decreased urinary output, nausea, vomiting, diarrhea, rapid weight gain, shortness of breath, edema of lower extremities; ovarian enlargement, ovarian cyst formation, pain/redness at injection site, breast tenderness, nausea vomiting, diarrhea

I, Injection; ***T***, tablets.

H_2 Antagonists

USES

Short-term treatment of duodenal ulcer (DU), active benign gastric ulcer (GU), maintenance therapy of DU, pathologic hypersecretory conditions (e.g., Zollinger-Ellison syndrome), gastroesophageal reflux disease (GERD), and prevention of upper GI bleeding in critically ill pts.

ACTION

Inhibit gastric acid secretion by interfering with histamine at the histamine H_2 receptors in parietal cells. Also inhibit acid secretion caused by gastrin. Inhibition occurs with basal (fasting), nocturnal, food-stimulated, or fundic distention secretion. H_2 antagonists decrease both the volume and H_2 concentration of gastric juices.

H_2 ANTAGONISTS

Name	Availability	Dosage Range	Side Effects
Cimetidine **(p. 249)** **(Tagamet)**	**T:** 200 mg, 300 mg, 400 mg, 800 mg **L:** 300 mg/5 ml **I:** 150 mg/ml	**Treatment of DU:** 800 mg/at bedtime, 400 mg 2 times/day or 300 mg 4 times/day **Maintenance of DU:** 400 mg/at bedtime **Treatment of GU:** 800 mg/at bedtime or 300 mg 4 times/day **GERD:** 1,600 mg/day **Hypersecretory:** 1,200–2,400 mg/day	Headaches, fatigue, dizziness, confusion, diarrhea, gynecomastia

(continued)

H2 ANTAGONISTS ***(continued)***

Name	Availability	Dosage Range	Side Effects
Famotidine (p. 466) (Pepcid)	**T**: 10 mg, 20 mg, 40 mg **T (chewable)**: 10 mg **DT**: 20 mg, 40 mg **Gelcap**: 10 mg **OS**: 40 mg/5 ml **I**: 10 mg/ml	**Treatment of DU**: 40 mg/day **Maintenance of DU**: 20 mg/day **Treatment of GU**: 40 mg/day **GERD**: 40–80 mg/day **Hypersecretory**: 80–640 mg/day	Headaches, dizziness, diarrhea, constipation, abdominal pain, tinnitus
Nizatidine (p. 849) (Axid)	**T**: 75 mg **C**: 150 mg, 300 mg	**Treatment of DU**: 300 mg/day **Maintenance of DU**: 150 mg/day	Fatigue, urticaria, abdominal pain, constipation, nausea
Ranitidine (p. 1011) (Zantac)	**T**: 75 mg, 150 mg, 300 mg **C**: 150 mg, 300 mg **Syrup**: 15 mg/ml **Granules**: 150 mg **I**: 0.5 mg/ml, 25 mg/ml	**Treatment of DU**: 300 mg/day **Maintenance of DU**: 150 mg/day **Treatment of GU**: 300 mg/day **GERD**: 300 mg/day **Hypersecretory**: 0.3–6 g/day	Blurred vision, constipation, nausea, abdominal pain

C, Capsules; ***DT,*** disintegrating tablets; ***I,*** injection; ***L,*** liquid; ***OS,*** oral suspension; ***T,*** tablets.

Hematinic Preparations

USES	ACTION
Prevention or treatment of iron deficiency resulting from improper diet, pregnancy, impaired absorption, or prolonged blood loss.	Iron supplements are provided to ensure adequate supplies for the formation of hemoglobin, which is needed for erythropoiesis and O_2 transport.

HEMATINIC (IRON) PREPARATIONS

Name	Availability	Elemental Iron	Side Effects
Ferrous fumarate (p. 478) (Femiron, Feostat)	**T:** 63 mg, 200 mg, 324 mg **S:** 100 mg/5 ml **D:** 45 mg/0.6 ml	33	Constipation, nausea, vomiting, diarrhea, abdominal pain/cramps
Ferrous gluconate (p. 478) (Fergon)	**T:** 240 mg, 325 mg	12	Same as ferrous fumarate
Ferrous sulfate (p. 478) (Fer-In-Sol)	**T:** 325 mg **Syrup:** 90 mg/5 ml **E:** 220 mg/5 ml **D:** 75 mg/0.6 ml	20	Same as ferrous fumarate
Ferrous sulfate exsiccated (p. 478) (Slow-Fe)	**T:** 187 mg, 200 mg **T (SR):** 160 mg **C (ER):** 160 mg	30	Same as ferrous fumarate

C, Caplets; ***D,*** drops; ***E,*** elixir; ***ER,*** extended-release; ***S,*** suspension; ***SR,*** sustained-release; ***T,*** tablets.

Hormones

USES

Functions of the body are regulated by two major control systems: the nervous system and the endocrine (hormone) system. Together they maintain homeostasis and control different metabolic functions in the body.

Hormones are concerned with control of different metabolic functions in the body (e.g., rates of chemical reactions in cells, transporting substances through cell membranes, cellular metabolism [growth/secretions]). By definition, a hormone is a chemical substance secreted into body fluids by cells and has control over other cells in the body.

Hormones can be local or general:

- *Local hormones* have specific local effects (e.g., acetylcholine, which is secreted at parasympathetic and skeletal nerve endings).

Hormones (continued)

ACTION

- *General hormones* are mostly secreted by specific endocrine glands (e.g., epinephrine/norepinephrine are secreted by the adrenal medulla in response to sympathetic stimulation), transported in the blood to all parts of the body, causing many different reactions.

Some general hormones affect all or almost all cells of the body (e.g., thyroid hormone from the thyroid gland increases the rate of most chemical reactions in almost all cells of the body); other general hormones affect only specific tissue (e.g., ovarian hormones are specific to female sex organs and secondary sexual characteristics of the female).

Endocrine hormones almost never directly act intracellularly affecting chemical reactions. They first combine with hormone receptors either on the cell surface or inside the cell (cell cytoplasm or nucleus). The combination of hormone and receptors alters the function of the receptor, and the receptor is the direct cause of the hormone effects. Altered receptor function may include the following:

Altered cell permeability, which causes a change in protein structure of the receptor, usually opening or closing a channel for one or more ions. The movement of these ions causes the effect of the hormone.

Activation of intracellular enzymes immediately inside the cell membrane (e.g., hormone combines with receptor that then becomes the activated enzyme adenyl cyclase, which causes formation of cAMP).

◀ **ALERT** ▶ cAMP has effects inside the cell. It is not the hormone but cAMP that causes these effects.

Regulation of hormone secretion is controlled by an internal control system, the negative feedback system:

- Endocrine gland oversecretes.
- Hormone exerts more and more of its effect.
- Target organ performs its function.
- Too much function in turn feeds back to endocrine gland to decrease secretory rate.

The endocrine system contains many glands and hormones. A summary of the important glands and their hormones secreted are as follows:

The pituitary gland (hypophysis) is a small gland found in the sella turcica at the base of the brain. The pituitary is divided into two portions physiologically: the anterior pituitary (adenohypophysis) and the posterior pituitary (neurohypophysis). Six important hormones are secreted from the anterior pituitary and two from the posterior pituitary.

Anterior pituitary hormones:

- Growth hormone (GH)
- Adrenocorticotropin (corticotropin)
- Thyroid-stimulating hormone (thyrotropin) (TSH)
- Follicle-stimulating hormone (FSH)

ACTION *(cont.)*

- Luteinizing hormone (LH)
- Prolactin

Posterior pituitary hormones:

- Antidiuretic hormone (vasopressin)
- Oxytocin

Almost all secretions of the pituitary hormones are controlled by hormonal or nervous signals from the hypothalamus. The hypothalamus is a center of information concerned with the well-being of the body, which in turn is used to control secretions of the important pituitary hormones just listed. Secretions from the posterior pituitary are controlled by nerve signals originating in the hypothalamus; anterior pituitary hormones are controlled by hormones secreted within the hypothalamus. These hormones are as follows:

- Thyrotropin-releasing hormone (TRH) releasing thyroid-stimulating hormone
- Corticotropin-releasing hormone (CRH) releasing adrenocorticotropin
- Growth hormone-releasing hormone (GHRH) releasing growth hormone and growth hormone inhibitory hormone (GHIH) (same as somatostatin)
- Gonadotropin-releasing hormone (GnRH) releasing the two gonadotropic hormones LH and FSH
- Prolactin inhibitory factor (PIF) causing inhibition of prolactin and prolactin-releasing factor

Anterior Pituitary Hormones

All anterior pituitary hormones (except growth hormone) have as their principal effect stimulating target glands.

Growth Hormone (GH)

Growth hormone affects almost all tissues of the body. GH (somatopropin) causes growth in almost all tissues of the body (increases cell size, increases mitosis with increased number of cells, and differentiates certain types of cells). Metabolic effects include increased rate of protein synthesis, mobilization of fatty acids from adipose tissue, decreased rate of glucose utilization.

Thyroid-Stimulating Hormone (TSH)

Thyroid-stimulating hormone controls secretion of the thyroid hormones. The thyroid gland is located immediately below the larynx on either side of and anterior to the trachea and secretes two significant hormones, thyroxine (T_4) and triiodothyroxine (T_3), which have a profound effect on increasing the metabolic rate of the body. The thyroid gland also secretes calcitonin, an important hormone for calcium metabolism. Calcitonin promotes deposition of calcium in the bones, which decreases calcium concentration in the extracellular fluid.

Adrenocorticotropin

Adrenocorticotropin causes the adrenal cortex to secrete adrenocortical hormones. The adrenal glands lie at the superior poles of the two kidneys. Each gland is composed of two distinct parts: the adrenal medulla and the cortex. The adrenal medulla, related to the sympathetic nervous system, secretes the hormones epinephrine and norepinephrine. When stimulated, they cause constriction of blood vessels, increased activity of the heart, inhibitory effects on the GI tract, and dilation of the pupils. The adrenal cortex secretes corticosteroids, of which there are two major types: mineralocorticoids and glucocorticoids. Aldosterone, the principal mineralocorticoid, primarily

Hormones *(continued)*

ACTION *(cont.)*

affects electrolytes of the extracellular fluids. Cortisol, the principal glucocorticoid, affects glucose, protein, and fat metabolism.

Luteinizing Hormone (LH)

Luteinizing hormone plays an important role in ovulation and causes secretion of female sex hormones by the ovaries and testosterone by the testes.

Follicle-Stimulating Hormone (FSH)

Follicle-stimulating hormone causes growth of follicles in the ovaries before ovulation and promotes formation of sperm in the testes.

Ovarian sex hormones are estrogens and progestins. Estradiol is the most important estrogen; progesterone is the most important progestin.

Estrogens mainly promote proliferation and growth of specific cells in the body and are responsible for development of most of the secondary sex characteristics. Primarily cause cellular proliferation and growth of tissues of sex organs/other tissue related to reproduction. Ovaries, fallopian tubes, uterus, vagina increase in size. Estrogen initiates growth of breast and milk-producing apparatus, external appearance.

Progesterone stimulates secretion of the uterine endometrium during the latter half of the female sexual cycle, preparing the uterus for implantation of the fertilized ovum. Decreases the frequency of uterine contractions (helps prevent expulsion of the implanted ovum). Progesterone promotes development of breasts, causing alveolar cells to proliferate, enlarge, and become secretory in nature.

Testosterone is secreted by the testes and formed by the interstitial cells of Leydig. Testosterone production increases under the stimulus of the anterior pituitary gonadotropic hormones. It is responsible for distinguishing characteristics of the masculine body (stimulates the growth of male sex organs and promotes the development of male secondary sex characteristics, e.g., distribution of body hair, effect on voice, protein formation, and muscular development).

Prolactin

Prolactin promotes the development of breasts and secretion of milk.

POSTERIOR PITUITARY HORMONES

Antidiuretic Hormone (ADH) (Vasopressin)

ADH can cause antidiuresis (decreased excretion of water by the kidneys). In the presence of ADH the permeability of the renal-collecting ducts and tubules to water increases, which allows water to be absorbed, conserving water in the body. ADH in higher concentrations is a very potent vasoconstrictor, constricting arterioles everywhere in the body, increasing B/P.

Oxytocin

Oxytocin contracts the uterus during the birthing process, esp. toward the end of the pregnancy, helping expel the baby. Oxytocin also contracts myoepithelial cells in the breasts, causing milk to be expressed from the alveoli into the ducts so that the baby can obtain it by suckling.

ACTION *(cont.)*

PANCREAS

The pancreas is composed of two tissue types: *acini* (secrete digestive juices in the duodenum) and *islets of Langerhans* (secrete insulin/glucagons directly into the blood). The islets of Langerhans contain three cells: alpha, beta, and delta. Alpha cells secrete glucagon, beta cells secrete insulin, and delta cells secrete somatostatin.

Insulin promotes glucose entry into most cells, thus controlling the rate of metabolism of most carbohydrates. Insulin also affects fat metabolism.

Glucagon effects are opposite those of insulin, the most important of which is increasing blood glucose concentration by releasing it from the liver into the circulating body fluids.

Somatostatin (same chemical as secreted by the hypothalamus) has multiple inhibitory effects: depresses secretion of insulin and glucagon, decreases GI motility, decreases secretions/absorption of the GI tract.

Human Immunodeficiency Virus (HIV) Infection

USES

Antiretroviral agents are used in the treatment of HIV infection.

ACTION

Currently five classes of antiretroviral agents are used in the treatment of HIV disease. *Nucleoside reverse transcriptase inhibitors (NRTIs)* compete with natural substrates for formation of proviral DNA by reverse transcriptase inhibiting viral replication.

Nucleotide reverse transcriptase inhibitors (NtRTIs) inhibit reverse transcriptase by competing with the natural substrate deoxyadenosine triphosphate and by DNA chain termination.

Nonnucleoside reverse transcriptase inhibitors (NNRTIs) directly bind to reverse transcriptase and blocks RNA-dependent and DNA-dependent DNA polymerase activities by disrupting the enzyme's catalytic site.

Protease inhibitors (PIs) bind to the active site of HIV-1 protease and prevent the processing of viral gag and gag-pol polyprotein precursors resulting in immature, noninfectious viral particles.

Fusion inhibitors interfere with the entry of HIV-1 into cells by inhibiting fusion of viral and cellular membranes.

Human Immunodeficiency Virus (HIV) Infection *(continued)*

ANTIRETROVIRAL AGENTS FOR TREATMENT OF HIV INFECTION

Name	Availability	Dosage Range	Side Effects
Nucleoside Analogues			
Abacavir (p. 1) **(Ziagen)**	**T**: 300 mg **OS**: 20 mg/ml	**A**: 300 mg 2 times/day	Nausea, vomiting, malaise, rash, fever, headaches, asthenia, fatigue
Abacavir/lamivudine **(Epzicom)**	**T**: 600 mg abacavir/ 300 mg lamivudine	**A**: once/day	Allergic reaction, insomnia, headaches, depression, dizziness, fatigue, diarrhea, fever, abdominal pain, anxiety
Didanosine (p. 357) **(Videx)**	**T**: 25 mg, 50 mg, 100 mg, 150 mg, 200 mg **C**: 125 mg, 200 mg, 250 mg, 400 mg **OS**: 100 mg, 167 mg, 250 mg	**T (weighing more than 60 kg)**: 200 mg 2 times/day; **(weighing less than 60 kg)**: 125 mg 2 times/day **OS (weighing more than 60 kg)**: 250 mg 2 times/day; **(weighing less than 60 kg)**: 167 mg 2 times/day	Peripheral neuropathy, pancreatitis, diarrhea, nausea, vomiting, headaches, insomnia, rash, hepatitis, seizures
Emtricitabine (p. 409) **(Emtriva)**	**C**: 200 mg	**A**: 200 mg/day	Headaches, insomnia, depression, diarrhea, nausea, vomiting, rhinitis, asthenia, rash
Emtricitabine/tenofovir **(Truvada)**	**T**: 200 mg emtricitabine/ 300 mg tenofovir	**A**: once/day	Dizziness, diarrhea, headaches, rash, belching/flatulence, skin discoloration

Emtricitabine/efavirenz/ tenofovir (Atripla)	**T:** 200 mg emtricitabine/ 600 mg efavirenz/ 300 mg tenofovir	**A:** once/day	Lactic acidosis, headaches, dizziness, abdominal pain, nausea, vomiting, rash
Lamivudine (p. 663) (Epivir)	**T:** 100 mg, 150 mg **OS:** 5 mg/ml, 10 mg/ml	**A:** 150 mg 2 times/day **C:** 4 mg/kg 2 times/day	Diarrhea, malaise, fatigue, headaches, nausea, vomiting, abdominal pain, peripheral neuropathy, arthralgia, myalgia, skin rash
Stavudine (p. 1086) (Zerit)	**C:** 15 mg, 20 mg, 30 mg, 40 mg **OS:** 1 mg/ml	**A:** 40 mg 2 times/day (20 mg 2 times/day if peripheral neuropathy occurs)	Peripheral neuropathy, anemia, leukopenia, neutropenia
Zalcitabine (p. 1234) (Hivid)	**T:** 0.375 mg, 0.75 mg	**A (weighing more than 60 kg):** 0.75 mg 3 times/day; **(weighing less than 60 kg):** 0.375 mg 3 times/day	Peripheral neuropathy, stomatitis, granulocytopenia, leukopenia
Zidovudine (p. 1239) (Retrovir)	**C:** 100 mg **T:** 300 mg **Syrup:** 50 mg/5 ml, 10 mg/ml	**A:** 500–600 mg/day (100 mg 5 times/ day or 300 mg 2 times/day)	Anemia, granulocytopenia, myopathy, nausea, malaise, fatigue, insomnia
Zidovudine/lamivudine (AZT/3TC) (Combivir)	**C:** 300 mg AZT/150 mg 3TC	**A:** 1 capsule 2 times/day	Myelosuppression, peripheral neuropathy, pancreatitis
Zidovudine/lamivudine/ abacavir (AZT/3TC/ABC) (Trizivir)	**C:** 300 mg AZT/150 mg 3TC/ 300 mg ABC	**A:** 1 capsule 2 times/day	Myelosuppression, peripheral neuropathy, anaphylactic reaction

Nucleotide Analogues

Tenofovir (p. 1116) (Viread)	**T:** 300 mg	**A:** 300 mg/day	Nausea, vomiting, diarrhea

(continued)

ANTIRETROVIRAL AGENTS FOR TREATMENT OF HIV INFECTION *(continued)*

Name	Availability	Dosage Range	Side Effects
Nonnucleoside Analogues			
Delavirdine (p. 329) (Rescriptor)	**T:** 100 mg, 200 mg	**A:** 200 mg 3 times/day for 14 days, then 400 mg 3 times/day	Rash, nausea, headaches, elevated hepatic function tests
Efavirenz (p. 406) (Sustiva)	**C:** 50 mg, 100 mg, 200 mg	**A:** 600 mg/day **C:** 200–600 mg/day based on weight	Headaches, dizziness, insomnia, fatigue, rash, nightmares
Nevirapine (p. 830) (Viramune)	**T:** 200 mg	**A:** 200 mg/day for 14 days, then 200 mg 2 times/day	Rash, nausea, fatigue, fever, headaches, abnormal hepatic function tests
Protease Inhibitors			
Amprenavir (p. 74) (Agenerase)	**C:** 50 mg, 150 mg **OS:** 15 mg/ml	**A:** 1,200 mg 2 times/day **C (4–16 yrs, weighing less than 50 kg):** 20 mg/kg 2 times/day or 15 mg/kg 3 times/day	Rash, diarrhea, headaches, nausea, vomiting, numbness, abdominal pain, fatigue
Atazanavir (p. 98) (Reyataz)	**C:** 100 mg, 150 mg, 200 mg, 300 mg	**A:** 400 mg/day	Headaches, diarrhea, abdominal pain, nausea, rash
Darunavir (p. 320) (Prezista)	**T:** 300 mg	**A:** 600 mg 2 times/day	Diarrhea, nausea, vomiting, headaches, skin rash, constipation
Fosamprenavir (p. 516) (Lexiva)	**T:** 700 mg	**A:** 1,400–2,800 mg/day	Headaches, fatigue, rash, nausea, diarrhea, vomiting, abdominal pain
Indinavir (p. 612) (Crixivan)	**C:** 200 mg, 400 mg	**A:** 800 mg q8h	Nephrolithiasis, hyperbilirubinemia, abdominal pain, asthenia, fatigue, flank pain, nausea, vomiting, diarrhea, headaches, insomnia, dizziness, altered taste

Lopinavir/ritonavir (p. 704) **(Kaletra)**	**C:** 133/33 mg **OS:** 80/20 mg	**A:** 400/100 mg/day **C (4–12 yrs):** 10–13 mg/kg 2 times/day	Diarrhea, nausea, vomiting, abdominal pain, headaches, rash
Nelfinavir (p. 824) **(Viracept)**	**T:** 250 mg **Oral Powder:** 50 mg/g	**A:** 750 mg q8h **C:** 20–25 mg/kg q8h	Diarrhea, fatigue, asthenia, headaches, hypertension, impaired concentration
Ritonavir (p. 1035) **(Norvir)**	**C:** 100 mg **OS:** 80 mg/ml	**A:** Titrate up to 600 mg 2 times/day	Nausea, vomiting, diarrhea, altered taste, fatigue, elevated hepatic function tests and triglyceride levels
Saquinavir (p. 1048) **(Invirase)**	**C:** 200 mg	**A:** 600 mg 3 times/day	Diarrhea, elevated hepatic function tests, hypertriglycerides, cholesterol, abnormal fat accumulation, hyperglycemia
Tipranavir (p. 1149) **(Aptivus)**	**C:** 250 mg	**A:** 500 mg (with 200 mg ritonavir) 2 times/day	Diarrhea, nausea, fatigue, headaches, vomiting

Fusion Inhibitors

Enfuvirtide (p. 413) **(Fuzeon)**	**I:** 108 mg (90 mg when reconstituted)	**Subcutaneous:** 90 mg 2 times/day	Insomnia, depression, peripheral neuropathy, decreased appetite, constipation, asthenia, cough

A, Adults; ***C,*** capsules; ***C*** *(dosage),* children; ***I,*** injection; ***OS,*** oral solution; ***T,*** tablets.

Immunosuppressive Agents

USES

Improvement of both short- and long-term allograft survivals.

ACTION

Basiliximab: An interleukin-2 (IL-2) receptor antagonist inhibiting IL-2 binding. This prevents activation of lymphocytes and the response of the immune system to antigens is impaired.

Cyclosporine: Inhibits production and release of IL-2.

Daclizumab: An IL-2 receptor antagonist inhibiting IL-2 binding.

Mycophenolate: A prodrug that reversibly binds and inhibits inosine monophosphate dehydrogenase (IMPD), resulting in inhibition of purine nucleotide synthesis, inhibiting DNA and RNA synthesis and subsequent synthesis of T and B cells.

Sirolimus: Inhibits IL-2–stimulated T-lymphocyte activation and proliferation, which may occur through formation of a complex.

Tacrolimus: Inhibits IL-2–stimulated T-lymphocyte activation and proliferation, which may occur through formation of a complex.

IMMUNOSUPPRESSIVES

Name	Availability	Dosage	Side Effects
Basiliximab (p. 121) (Simulect)	**I:** 20 mg	20 mg for 2 doses	Abdominal pain, asthenia, cough, dizziness, dyspnea, dysuria, edema, hypertension, infection, tremors
Cyclosporine (p. 303) (Neoral, Sandimmune)	**C:** 25 mg, 50 mg, 100 mg **S:** 100 mg/ml **I:** 50 mg/ml	7–10 mg/kg/day	Hypertension, hyperkalemia, nephrotoxicity, coarsening of facial features, hirsutism, gingival hyperplasia, nausea, vomiting, diarrhea, hepatic toxicity, hyperuricemia, hypertriglyceridemia, hypercholesterolemia, tremors, paresthesia, seizures, risk of infection/malignancy
Daclizumab (p. 309) (Zenapax)	**I:** 25 mg/5 ml	1 mg/kg (**Maximum:** 100 mg)	Dyspnea, fever, hypertension, nausea, peripheral edema, tachycardia, tremors, vomiting, weakness, wound infection

Mycophenolate (p. 800) (CellCept)	**C**: 250 mg **I**: 500 mg **S**: 200 mg/ml **T**: 500 mg	1 g 2 times/day	Diarrhea, vomiting, leukopenia, neutropenia, infections
Sirolimus (p. 1065) (Rapamune)	**S**: 1 mg/ml **T**: 1 mg	2–10 mg/day	Dyspnea, leukopenia, thrombocytopenia, hyperlipidemia, abdominal pain, acne, arthralgia, fever, diarrhea, constipation, headaches, vomiting, weight gain
Tacrolimus (p. 1099) (Prograf)	**C**: 0.5 mg, 1 mg, 5 mg **I**: 5 mg/ml	0.1–0.15 mg/kg/day	Nephrotoxicity, neurotoxicity, hyperglycemia, nausea, vomiting, photophobia, infections, hypertension, hyperlipidemia

C, Capsules; ***I,*** injection; ***S,*** oral solution or suspension; ***T,*** tablets.

Laxatives

USES

Short-term treatment of constipation; colon evacuation before rectal/bowel examination; prevention of straining (e.g., after anorectal surgery, MI); to reduce painful elimination (e.g., episiotomy, hemorrhoids, anorectal lesions); modification of effluent from ileostomy, colostomy; prevention of fecal impaction; removal of ingested poisons.

ACTION

Laxatives ease or stimulate defecation. Mechanisms by which this is accomplished include (1) attracting, retaining fluid in colonic contents due to hydrophilic or osmotic properties; (2) acting directly or indirectly on mucosa to decrease absorption of water and NaCl; or (3) increasing intestinal motility, decreasing absorption of water and NaCl by virtue of decreased transit time.

Bulk-forming: Act primarily in small/large intestine. Retain water in stool, may bind water, ions in colonic lumen (soften feces, increase bulk); may increase colonic bacteria growth (increases fecal mass). Produce soft stool in 1–3 days.

Osmotic agents: Acts in colon. Similar to saline laxatives. Osmotic action may be enhanced in distal ileum/colon by bacterial metabolism to lactate, other organic acids. This decrease in pH increases motility, secretion. Produces soft stool in 1–3 days.

Saline: Acts in small/large intestine, colon (sodium phosphate). Poorly, slowly absorbed; causes hormone cholecystokinin release from duodenum (stimulates fluid secretion, motility); possesses osmotic properties; produces watery stool in 2–6 hrs (small doses produce semifluid stool in 6–12 hrs).

Stimulant: Acts in colon. Enhances accumulation of water/electrolytes in colonic lumen, enhances intestinal motility. May act directly on intestinal mucosa. Produces semifluid stool in 6–12 hrs.

◀ **ALERT** ▶ Bisacodyl suppository acts in 15–60 min.

Stool softener: Acts in small/large intestine. Hydrates and softens stools by its surfactant action, facilitating penetration of fat and water into stool. Produces soft stool in 1–3 days.

LAXATIVES

Name	Onset of Action	Uses	Side Effects/Precautions
Bulk-forming			
Methylcellulose (Citrucel) (p. 751)	12–24 hrs up to 3 days	Treatment of constipation for postpartum women, elderly, pts with diverticulosis, irritable bowel syndrome, hemorrhoids	Gas, bloating, esophageal obstruction, colonic obstruction, calcium and iron malabsorption
Psyllium (Metamucil) (p. 991)	Same as methylcellulose	Treatment of chronic constipation and constipation associated with rectal disorders; management of irritable bowel syndrome	Diarrhea, constipation, abdominal cramps, esophageal/colon obstruction, bronchospasm
Stool Softener			
Docusate (Colace, Surfak) (p. 381)	1–3 days	Treatment of constipation due to hard stools, in painful anorectal conditions, and for those who need to avoid straining during bowel movements	Stomach ache, mild nausea, cramping, diarrhea, irritated throat (with liquid and syrup dose forms)
Saline			
Magnesium hydroxide (p. 716)	30 min–3 hrs	Short-term treatment of occasional constipation	Electrolyte abnormalities can occur; Use caution in pts with renal or cardiac impairment; diarrhea, abdominal cramps, hypotension

(continued)

LAXATIVES *(continued)*

Name	Onset of Action	Uses	Side Effects/Precautions
Saline *(continued)*			
Magnesium citrate (Citrate of Magnesia, Citro-Mag) (p. 716)	30 min–3 hrs	Bowel evacuation prior to certain surgical and daignostic procedures	Hypotension, abdominal cramping diarrhea, gas formation, electrolyte abnormalities
Sodim phosphate (Fleets Phospho Soda)	2–15 min	Relief of occasional constipation; bowel evacuation prior to certain surgical and diagnostic procedures	Electrolyte abnormalities; do not use for pts with CHF, severe renal impairment, ascites, GI obstruction, active inflammatory bowel disease
Osmotic			
Lactulose (Kristalose) (p. 662)	24–48 hrs	Short-term relief of constipation	Nausea, vomiting, diarrhea, abdominal cramping, bloating, gas
Polyethylene glycol (Miralax) (p. 947)	24–48 hrs	Short-term relief of constipation	Bitter taste, diarrhea
Stimulant			
Bisacodyl (Dulcolax) (p. 140)	**PO:** 6–12 hrs **Rectal:** 15–60 min	Short-term relief of constipation	Elecrolyte imbalance, abdominal discomfort, gas, potential for overuse/abuse
Senna (Senokot) (p. 1056)	6–12 hrs	Short-term relief of constipation	Abdominal discomfort, cramps

Neuromuscular Blockers

USES

Adjuvant in surgical anesthesia to relax skeletal muscle (esp. abdominal wall) for surgery (allows lighter level of anesthesia; valuable in orthopedic procedures). Neuromuscular blocking agents of short duration often used to facilitate endotracheal intubation, laryngoscopy, bronchoscopy, and esophagoscopy in combination with general anesthetics. Provide muscle relaxation in pts undergoing mechanical ventilation, muscle relaxation in diagnosis of myasthenia gravis. Prevent convulsive movements during electroconvulsive therapy.

ACTION

Paralysis results from blocking of normal neuromuscular transmission. Succinylcholine, a depolarizing agent, attaches to the acetylcholine (ACh) receptor on the motor end plate, causing depolarization. It prevents the binding of ACh to the receptor. Nondepolarizing agents also bind to the receptor at the motor end plate but competitively block ACh from attaching to the receptor. These agents also block presynaptic channels that cause the release of ACh.

NEUROMUSCULAR BLOCKERS

Name	Class	Intubation Dose	ICU Dose	Side Effects
Atracurium (Tracrium)	Short	0.4–0.5 mg/kg	0.4–0.5 mg/kg bolus, then 4–12 mcg/kg/min	Flushed skin, urticaria
Cisatracurium (Nimbex)	Intermediate	0.15–2 mg/kg	0.10–0.2 mg/kg bolus, then 2.5–3 mcg/kg/min	Skin rash, flushing
Doxacurium (Nuromax)	Long	0.05 mg/kg	0.025–0.05 mg/kg bolus, then 0.3–0.5 mg/kg/min	Injection site reaction, urticaria

(continued)

NEUROMUSCULAR BLOCKERS *(continued)*

Name	Class	Intubation Dose	ICU Dose	Side Effects
Mivacurium (Mivacron)	Short	0.15–0.2 mg/kg	0.15–0.25 mg/kg bolus, then 9–10 mcg/kg/min	Flushing, hypotension, dizziness, muscle spasm
Pancuronium (Pavulon)	Long	0.06–0.1 mg/kg	0.05–0.1 mg/kg bolus, then 1–2 mcg/kg/hr	Increased B/P, increased salivation, pruritus
Rocuronium (Zemuron)	Intermediate	0.45–1.2 mg/kg	0.15–0.25 mg/kg bolus, then 10–12 mcg/kg/min	Pain at injection site, hypertension, hypotension
Succinylcholine (Anectine, Quelicin)	Ultrashort	1–2 mg/kg	NA	Increased intracranial pressure, increased intraocular pressure, postop muscle pain, weakness, increased salivation, bradycardia, cardiac arrhythmias
Tubocurarine	Intermediate	0.5–0.6 mg/kg	NA	Decreased B/P
Vecuronium (Norcuron)	Intermediate	0.08–0.1 mg/kg	0.08–0.1 mg/kg bolus, then 0.8–1.2 mcg/kg/min	Skeletal muscle weakness with prolonged use

Nitrates

USES

Sublingual: Acute relief of angina pectoris.

Oral, topical: Long-term prophylactic treatment of angina pectoris.

Intravenous: Adjunctive treatment in CHF associated with acute MI. Produce controlled hypotension during surgical procedures; control B/P in perioperative hypertension, angina unresponsive to organic nitrates or beta-blockers.

ACTION

Relax most smooth muscles, including arteries and veins. Effect is primarily on veins (decrease left/right ventricular end-diastolic pressure). In angina, nitrates decrease myocardial work and O_2 requirements (decrease preload by venodilation and after-load by arteriodilation). Nitrates also appear to redistribute blood flow to ischemic myocardial areas, improving perfusion without increase in coronary blood flow.

NITRATES

Name	Availability	Dosage Range	Side Effects
Isosorbide (p. 643) (Isordil)	**T:** 5 mg, 10 mg, 20 mg, 30 mg, 40 mg **T (ER):** 30 mg, 40 mg, 60 mg, 120 mg **SL:** 2.5 mg, 5 mg **T (chewable):** 5 mg, 10 mg **C (SR):** 40 mg	**SL:** 2.5–10 mg q2–3h **PO:** 10–40 mg q6h **PO (SR):** 40–80 mg q8–12h	Flushing, headaches, nausea, vomiting, orthostatic hypotension, restlessness, tachycardia

(continued)

NITRATES *(continued)*

Nitroglycerin (p. 844) (Minitran, Nitro-Bid, Nitro-Dur, Nitrostat)	**SL:** 0.4 mg **T (SR):** 2.6 mg, 6.5 mg, 9 mg **C (SR):** 2.5 mg, 6.5 mg, 9 mg, 13 mg **Topical:** 2% ointment **Trans:** 0.1 mg/hr, 0.2 mg/hr, 0.3 mg/hr, 0.4 mg/hr, 0.6 mg/hr, 0.8 mg/hr **I:** 0.5 mg/ml, 5 mg/ml **Infusion:** 100 mcg/ml, 200 mcg/ml	**SL:** 0.4 mg up to 3 times q15min **SR:** 2.5–26 mg 3–4 times/day **Trans:** 0.1–0.8 mg/hr **T:** 1–2 inches up to 4–5 inches q4h	Same as isosorbide

C, Capsules; ***ER,*** extended-release; ***I,*** injection; ***SL,*** sublingual; ***SR,*** sustained-release; ***T,*** tablets; ***Trans,*** transdermal.

Nonsteroidal Anti-Inflammatory Drugs (NSAIDs)

USES

Provide symptomatic relief from *pain/inflammation* in the treatment of musculoskeletal disorders (e.g., rheumatoid arthritis, osteoarthritis, ankylosing spondylitis), *analgesic* for low to moderate pain, *reduction in fever* (many agents not suited for routine/prolonged therapy due to toxicity). By virtue of its action on platelet function, aspirin is used in treatment or prophylaxis of diseases associated with hypercoagulability (reduces risk of stroke/heart attack).

ACTION

Exact mechanism for anti-inflammatory, analgesic, antipyretic effects unknown. Inhibition of enzyme cyclo-oxygenase, the enzyme responsible for prostaglandin synthesis, appears to be a major mechanism of action. May inhibit other mediators of inflammation (e.g., leukotrienes). Direct action on hypothalamus heat-regulating center may contribute to antipyretic effect.

NSAIDs

Name	Availability	Dosage Range	Side Effects
Aspirin (p. 96)	**T:** 81 mg, 160 mg, 325 mg **Supplement:** 300 mg, 600 mg	**P (A):** 325–650 mg q4h as needed **C:** Up to 60–80 mg/kg/day **Arthritis:** 3.2–6 g/day **JRA:** 60–110 mg/kg/day **RF (A):** 5–8 g/day **C:** 75–100 mg/kg/day **TIA:** 1,300 mg/day **MI:** 81–325 mg/day	GI discomfort, dizziness, headaches
Celecoxib (p. 227) (Celebrex)	**C:** 100 mg, 200 mg	**OA:** 200 mg/day **RA:** 100–200 mg 2 times/day **FAP:** 400 mg 2 times/day	Diarrhea, back pain, dizziness, heartburn, headaches, nausea, abdominal pain
Diclofenac (p. 353) (Voltaren)	**T:** 25 mg, 50 mg, 75 mg, 100 mg	**Arthritis:** 100–200 mg/day	Indigestion, constipation, diarrhea, nausea, headaches, fluid retention, abdominal cramps
Diflunisal (p. 359) (Dolobid)	**T:** 250 mg, 500 mg	**Arthritis:** 0.5–1 g/day **P:** 0.5 g q8–12h	Headaches, abdominal cramps, indigestion, diarrhea, nausea
Etodolac (p. 456) (Lodine)	**T:** 400 mg, 500 mg **T (ER):** 400 mg, 500 mg, 600 mg **C:** 200 mg, 300 mg	**Arthritis:** 600–800 mg/day **P:** 200–400 mg q6–8h	Indigestion, dizziness, headaches, bloated feeling, diarrhea, nausea, weakness, abdominal cramps
Fenoprofen (p. 473) (Nalfon)	**C:** 200 mg, 300 mg **T:** 600 mg	**Arthritis:** 300–600 mg 3–4 times/day **P:** 200 mg q4–6h as needed	Nausea, indigestion, anxiety, constipation, shortness of breath, heartburn

(continued)

NSAIDs ***(continued)***

Name	Availability	Dosage Range	Side Effects
Flurbiprofen (p. 503) (Ansaid)	**T**: 50 mg, 100 mg	**Arthritis:** 200–300 mg/day	Indigestion, nausea, fluid retention, headaches, abdominal cramps, diarrhea
Ibuprofen (p. 595) (Motrin, Advil)	**T**: 100 mg, 200 mg, 400 mg, 600 mg, 800 mg **T (chewable)**: 50 mg, 100 mg **C**: 200 mg **S**: 100 mg/5 ml, 100 mg/2.5 ml **Drops**: 40 mg/ml	**Arthritis:** 1.2–3.2 g/day **P**: 400 mg q4–6h as needed **Fever**: 200 mg q4–6h as needed **JA**: 30–40 mg/kg/day	Dizziness, abdominal cramps, abdominal pain, heartburn, nausea
Indomethacin (p. 614) evolve (Indocin)	**C**: 25 mg, 50 mg **C (SR)**: 75 mg **S**: 25 mg/5 ml **Supplement**: 50 mg	**Arthritis:** 50–200 mg/day **Bursitis/tendonitis:** 75–150 mg/day **GA**: 150 mg/day	Fluid retention, dizziness, headaches, abdominal pain, indigestion, nausea
Ketoprofen (p. 655) (Orudis KT)	**T**: 12.5 mg **C**: 25 mg, 50 mg, 75 mg **C (ER)**: 100 mg, 150 mg, 200 mg	**Arthritis:** 150–300 mg/day **P**: 25–50 mg q6–8h as needed	Headaches, anxiety, abdominal pain, bloated feeling, constipation, diarrhea, nausea
Ketorolac (p. 657) (Toradol)	**T**: 10 mg **I**: 15 mg/ml, 30 mg/ml	**P (PO)**: 10 mg q4–6h as needed; **(IM/IV)**: 60–120 mg/day	Fluid retention, abdominal pain, diarrhea, dizziness, headaches, nausea
Meloxicam (p. 728) (Mobic)	**C**: 7.5 mg	**Arthritis:** 7.5–15 mg/day	Heartburn, indigestion, nausea, diarrhea, headaches

Nabumetone (p. 804) (Relafen)	**T**: 500 mg, 750 mg	**Arthritis:** 1–2 g/day	Fluid retention, dizziness, headaches, abdominal pain, constipation, diarrhea, nausea
Naproxen (p. 816) (Anaprox, Naprosyn)	**T**: 200 mg, 250 mg, 375 mg, 500 mg **T (CR):** 375 mg **S:** 125 mg/5 ml	**Arthritis:** 250–550 mg/day **P:** 250 mg q6–8h **JA:** 10 mg/kg/day **GA:** 750 mg once, then 250 mg q8h	Tinnitus, fluid retention, shortness of breath, dizziness, drowsiness, headaches, abdominal pain, constipation, heartburn, nausea
Oxaprozin (p. 879) (Daypro)	**C:** 600 mg	**Arthritis:** 600–1,800 mg/day	Constipation, diarrhea, nausea, indigestion
Piroxicam (p. 944) evolve (Feldene)	**C:** 10 mg, 20 mg	**Arthritis:** 20 mg/day	Abdominal pain, stomach pain, nausea
Sulindac (p. 1092) (Clinoril)	**T**: 150 mg, 200 mg	**Arthritis:** 300 mg/day **GA:** 400 mg/day	Dizziness, abdominal pain, constipation, diarrhea, nausea
Tolmetin evolve (Tolectin)	**T**: 200 mg, 600 mg **C:** 400 mg	**Arthritis:** 600–1,800 mg/day **JA:** 15–30 mg/kg/day	Fluid retention, dizziness, headaches, weakness, abdominal pain, diarrhea, indigestion, nausea, vomiting

A, Adults; ***C,*** capsules; ***C*** *(dosage),* children; ***CR,*** controlled-release; ***ER,*** extended-release; ***FAP,*** familial adenomatous polyposis; ***GA,*** gouty arthritis; ***I,*** injection; ***JA,*** juvenile arthritis; ***JRA,*** juvenile rheumatoid arthritis; ***MI,*** myocardial infarction; ***OA,*** osteoarthritis; ***P,*** pain; ***RA,*** rheumatoid arthritis; ***RF,*** rheumatic fever; ***S,*** suspension; ***T,*** tablets; ***TIA,*** transient ischemic attack.

Nutrition: Enteral

	INDICATIONS	ROUTES OF ENTERAL NUTRITION DELIVERY
Enteral nutrition (EN), also known as *tube feedings,* provides food/nutrients via the GI tract using special formulas, delivery techniques, and equipment. All routes of EN consist of a tube through which liquid formula is infused.	Tube feedings are used in pts with major trauma, burns; those undergoing radiation and/or chemotherapy; pts with hepatic failure, severe renal impairment, physical or neurologic impairment; preop and postop to promote anabolism; prevention of cachexia, malnutrition.	**Nasogastric (NG):** **INDICATIONS:** Most common for short-term feeding in pts unable or unwilling to consume adequate nutrition by mouth. Requires at least a partially functioning GI tract. **ADVANTAGES:** Does not require surgical intervention and is fairly easily inserted. Allows full use of digestive tract. Decreases abdominal distention, nausea, vomiting that may be caused by hyperosmolar solutions. **DISADVANTAGES:** Temporary. May be easily pulled out during routine nursing care. Has potential for pulmonary aspiration of gastric contents, risk of refluxesophagitis, regurgitation. **Nasoduodenal (ND), Nasojejunal (NJ):** **INDICATIONS:** Pts unable or unwilling to consume adequate nutrition by mouth. Requires at least a partially functioning GI tract. **ADVANTAGES:** Does not require surgical intervention and is fairly easily inserted. Preferred for pts at risk for aspiration. Valuable for pts with gastroparesis.

ROUTES OF ENTERAL NUTRITION DELIVERY *(cont.)*

DISADVANTAGES: Temporary. May be pulled out during routine nursing care. May be dislodged by coughing, vomiting. Small lumen size increases risk of clogging when medication is administered via tube, more susceptible to rupturing when using infusion device. Must be radiographed for placement, frequently extubated.

Gastrostomy:

INDICATIONS: Pts with esophageal obstruction or impaired swallowing; pts in whom NG, ND, or NJ not feasible; when long-term feeding indicated.

ADVANTAGES: Permanent feeding access. Tubing has larger bore, allowing noncontinuous (bolus) feeding (300–400 ml over 30–60 min q3–6h). May be inserted endoscopically using local anesthetic (procedure called *percutaneous endoscopic gastrostomy* [PEG]).

DISADVANTAGES: Requires surgery; may be inserted in conjunction with other surgery or endoscopically (see **ADVANTAGES**). Stoma care required. Tube may be inadvertently dislodged. Risk of aspiration, peritonitis, cellulitis, leakage of gastric contents.

Jejunostomy:

INDICATIONS: Pts with stomach or duodenal obstruction, impaired gastric motility; pts in whom NG, ND, or NJ not feasible; when long-term feeding indicated.

ADVANTAGES: Allows early postop feeding (small bowel function is least affected by surgery). Risk of aspiration reduced. Rarely pulled out inadvertently.

DISADVANTAGES: Requires surgery (laparotomy). Stoma care required. Risk of intraperitoneal leakage. Can be dislodged easily.

INITIATING ENTERAL NUTRITION

With continuous feeding, initiation of isotonic (about 300 mOsm/L) or moderately hypertonic feeding (up to 495 mOsm/L) can be given full strength, usually at a slow rate (30–50 ml/hr) and gradually increased (25 ml/hr q6–24h). Formulas with osmolality greater than 500 mOsm/L are generally started at half strength and gradually increased in rate, then concentration. Tolerance is increased if the rate and concentration are not increased simultaneously.

Nutrition: Enteral *(continued)*

SELECTION OF FORMULAS

Protein: Has many important physiologic roles and is the primary source of nitrogen in the body. Provides 4 kcal/g protein. Sources of protein in enteral feedings: sodium caseinate, calcium caseinate, soy protein, dipeptides.

Carbohydrate (CHO): Provides energy for the body and heat to maintain body temperature. Provides 3.4 kcal/g carbohydrate. Sources of CHO in enteral feedings: corn syrup, cornstarch, maltodextrin, lactose, sucrose, glucose.

Fat: Provides concentrated source of energy. Referred to as *kilocalorie dense* or *protein sparing*. Provides 9 kcal/g fat. Sources of fat in enteral feedings: corn oil, safflower oil, medium-chain triglycerides.

Electrolytes, vitamins, trace elements: Contained in formulas (not found in specialized products for renal/hepatic insufficiency).

All products containing protein, fat, carbohydrate, vitamin, electrolytes, trace elements are nutritionally complete and designed to be used by pts for long periods.

COMPLICATIONS

MECHANICAL: Usually associated with some aspect of the feeding tube.

Aspiration pneumonia: Caused by delayed gastric emptying, gastroparesis, gastroesophageal reflux, or decreased gag reflex. May be prevented or treated by reducing infusion rate, using lower-fat formula, feeding beyond pylorus, checking residuals, using small-bore feeding tubes, elevating head of bed 30°–45° during and for 30–60 min after intermittent feeding, and regularly checking tube placement.

Esophageal, mucosal, pharyngeal irritation, otitis: Caused by using large-bore NG tube. Prevented by use of small bore whenever possible.

Irritation, leakage at ostomy site: Caused by drainage of digestive juices from site. Prevented by close attention to skin/stoma care.

Tube, lumen obstruction: Caused by thickened formula residue, formation of formula-medication complexes. Prevented by frequently irrigating tube with clear water (also before and after giving formulas/medication), avoiding instilling medication if possible.

GASTROINTESTINAL: Usually associated with formula, rate of delivery, unsanitary handling of solutions or delivery system.

Diarrhea: Caused by low-residue formulas, rapid delivery, use of hyperosmolar formula, hypoalbuminemia, malabsorption, microbial contamination, or rapid GI transit time. Prevented by using fiber supplemented formulas, decreasing rate of delivery, using dilute formula and gradually increasing strength.

Cramps, gas, abdominal distention: Caused by nutrient malabsorption, rapid delivery of refrigerated formula. Prevented by delivering formula by continuous methods, giving formulas at room temperature, decreasing rate of delivery.

Nausea, vomiting: Caused by rapid delivery of formula, gastric retention. Prevented by reducing rate of delivery, using dilute formulas, selecting low-fat formulas.

COMPLICATIONS *(cont.)*

Constipation: Caused by inadequate fluid intake, reduced bulk, inactivity. Prevented by supplementing fluid intake, using fiber-supplemented formula, encouraging ambulation.

METABOLIC: Fluid/serum electrolyte status should be monitored. Refer to monitoring section. In addition, the very young and very old are at greater risk in developing complications such as dehydration or overhydration.

MONITORING

Daily: Estimate nutrient intake, fluid intake/output, weight of pt, clinical observations.

Weekly: Serum electrolytes (potassium, sodium, magnesium, calcium, phosphorus), blood glucose, BUN, creatinine, hepatic function tests (e.g., AST, alkaline phosphatase), 24-hr urea and creatinine excretion, total iron-binding capacity (TIBC) or serum transferrin, triglycerides, cholesterol.

Monthly: Serum albumin.

Other: Urine glucose, acetone (when blood glucose is greater than 250), vital signs (temperature, respirations, pulse, B/P) q8h.

DRUG THERAPY: DOSAGE FOR SELECTION/ ADMINISTRATION:

Drug therapy should not have to be compromised in pts receiving enteral nutrition:

- Temporarily discontinue medications not immediately necessary
- Consider an alternate route for administering medications (e.g., transdermal, rectal, intravenous)
- Consider alternate medications when current medication is not available in alternate dosage forms

ENTERAL ADMINISTRATION OF MEDICATIONS: Medications may be given via feeding tube with several considerations:

- Tube type
- Tube location in the GI tract
- Site of drug action
- Site of drug absorption
- Effects of food on drug absorption
- Use of liquid dosage forms preferred whenever possible, many tablets may be crushed, contents of many capsules may be emptied and given through large-bore feeding tubes
- Many oral products should not be crushed (e.g., sustained-release, enteric coated)
- Some medications should not be given with enteral formulas because they form precipitates that may clog the feeding tube and reduce drug absorption
- Feeding tube should be flushed with water before and after administration of medications to clear any residual medication

Nutrition: Parenteral

Parenteral nutrition (PN), also known as *total parenteral nutrition* (TPN) or *hyperalimentation* (HAL), provides required nutrients to pts by IV route of administration. The goal of PN is to maintain or restore nutritional status caused by disease, injury, or inability to consume nutrients by other means.

INDICATIONS

Conditions when pt is unable to use alimentary tract via oral, gastrostomy, or jejunostomy route. Impaired absorption of protein caused by obstruction, inflammation, or antineoplastic therapy. Bowel rest necessary because of GI surgery or ileus, fistulas, or anastomotic leaks. Conditions with increased metabolic requirements (e.g., burns, infection, trauma). Preserve tissue reserves (e.g., acute renal failure). Inadequate nutrition from tube feeding methods.

COMPONENTS OF PN

To meet IV nutritional requirements, six essential categories in PN are needed for tissue synthesis and energy balance.

Protein: In the form of crystalline amino acids (CAA), primarily used for protein synthesis. Several products are designed to meet specific needs for pts with renal failure (e.g., NephrAmine), hepatic disease (e.g., HepatAmine), stress/trauma (e.g., Aminosyn HBC), use in neonates and pediatrics (e.g., Aminosyn PF, TrophAmine). Calories: 4 kcal/g protein.

Energy: In the form of dextrose, available in concentrations of 5%–70%. Dextrose less than 10% may be given peripherally; concentrations greater than 10% must be given centrally. Calories: 3.4 kcal/g dextrose.

IV fat emulsion: Available in 10% and 20% concentrations. Provides a concentrated source of energy/calories (9 kcal/g fat) and is a source of essential fatty acids. May be administered peripherally or centrally.

COMPONENTS OF PN (cont.)

Electrolytes: Major electrolytes (calcium, magnesium, potassium, sodium; also acetate, chloride, phosphate). Doses of electrolytes are individualized, based on many factors (e.g., renal/hepatic function, fluid status).

Vitamins: Essential components in maintaining metabolism and cellular function; widely used in PN.
Trace elements: Necessary in long-term PN administration. Trace elements include zinc, copper, chromium, manganese, selenium, molybdenum, iodine.

Miscellaneous: Additives include insulin, albumin, heparin, and histamine$_2$ blockers (e.g., cimetidine, ranitidine, famotidine). Other medication may be included, but compatibility for admixture should be checked on an individual basis.

ROUTE OF ADMINISTRATION

PN is administered via either peripheral or central vein.

Peripheral: Usually involves 2–3 L/day of 5%–10% dextrose with 3%–5% amino acid solution along with IV fat emulsion. Electrolytes, vitamins, trace elements are added according to pt needs. Peripheral solutions provide about 2,000 kcal/day and 60–90 g protein/day.
ADVANTAGES: Lower risks vs. central mode of administration.
DISADVANTAGES: Peripheral veins may not be suitable (esp. in pts with illness of long duration); more susceptible to phlebitis (due to osmolalities over 600 mOsm/L); veins may be viable only 1–2 wks; large volumes of fluid are needed to meet nutritional requirements, which may be contraindicated in many patients.

Central: Usually utilizes hypertonic dextrose (concentration range of 15%–35%) and amino acid solution of 3%–7% with IV fat emulsion. Electrolytes, vitamins, trace elements are added according to pt needs. Central solutions provide 2,000–4,000 kcal/day. Must be given through large central vein with high blood flow, allowing rapid dilution, avoiding phlebitis/thrombosis (usually through percutaneous insertion of catheter into subclavian vein then advancement of catheter to superior vena cava).
ADVANTAGES: Allows more alternatives/flexibility in establishing regimens; allows ability to provide full nutritional requirements without need of daily fat emulsion; useful in patients who are fluid restricted (increased concentration), those needing large nutritional requirements (e.g., trauma, malignancy), or those for whom PN indicated more than 7–10 days.

DISADVANTAGES: Risk with insertion, use, maintenance of central line; increased risk of infection, catheter-induced trauma, and metabolic changes.

Nutrition: Parenteral *(continued)*

MONITORING

May vary slightly from institution to institution.

Baseline: CBC, platelet count, prothrombin time, weight, body length/head circumference (in infants), serum electrolytes, glucose, BUN, creatinine, uric acid, total protein, cholesterol, triglycerides, bilirubin, alkaline phosphatase, LDH, AST, albumin, other tests as needed.

Daily: Weight, vital signs (TPR), nutritional intake (kcal, protein, fat), serum electrolytes (potassium, sodium chloride), glucose (serum, urine), acetone, BUN, osmolarity, other tests as needed.

2–3 times/wk: CBC, coagulation studies (PT, PTT), serum creatinine, calcium, magnesium, phosphorus, acid-base status, other tests as needed.

Weekly: Nitrogen balance, total protein, albumin, prealbumin, transferrin, hepatic function tests (AST, ALT), serum alkaline phosphatase, LDH, bilirubin, Hgb, uric acid, cholesterol, triglycerides, other tests as needed.

COMPLICATIONS

Mechanical: Malfunction in system for IV delivery (e.g., pump failure; problems with lines, tubing, administration sets, catheter). Pneumothorax, catheter misdirection, arterial puncture, bleeding, hematoma formation may occur with catheter placement.

Infectious: Infections (pts often more susceptible to infections), catheter sepsis (e.g., fever, shaking chills, glucose intolerance where no other site of infection is identified).

Metabolic: Includes hyperglycemia, elevated serum cholesterol and triglycerides, abnormal serum hepatic function tests.

Fluid, electrolyte, acid-base disturbances: May alter serum potassium, sodium, phosphate, magnesium levels.

Nutritional: Clinical effects seen may be due to lack of adequate vitamins, trace elements, essential fatty acids.

DRUG THERAPY/ADMINISTRATION METHODS: Compatibility of other intravenous medications pts may be administered while receiving parenteral nutrition is an important concern.

Intravenous medications usually are given as a separate admixture via piggyback to the parenteral nutrition line, but in some instances may be added directly to the parenteral nutrition solution. Because of the possibility of incompatibility when adding medication directly to the parenteral nutrition solution, specific criteria should be considered:

- Stability of the medication in the parenteral nutrition solution
- Properties of the medication, including pharmacokinetics that determine if the medication is appropriate for continuous infusion
- Documented chemical and physical compatibility with the parenteral nutrition solution

In addition, when medication is given via piggyback using the parenteral nutrition line, important criteria should include:

- Stability of the medication in the parenteral nutrition solution
- Documented chemical and physical compatibility with the parenteral nutrition solution

Obesity Management

USES

Adjunct to diet and physical activity in the treatment of chronic, relapsing obesity.

ACTIONS

Two categories of medications are used for weight control.

Appetite suppressants: Blocks neuronal uptake of norepinephrine, serotonin, dopamine causing a feeling of fullness or satiety.

Digestion inhibitors: Reversible lipase inhibitors that block the breakdown and absorption of fats, decreasing appetite and reducing calorie intake.

ANOREXIANTS

Name	Type	Availability	Dosage	Side Effects
Benzphetamine (Didrex)	AS	**T:** 50 mg	25–50 mg 1–3 times/day	Headaches, insomnia, nervousness, anxiety, irritability, dry mouth, constipation, euphoria, palpitations, hypertension
Diethylpropion (Tenuate)	AS	**T:** 25 mg, 75 mg	25 mg 3 times/day or 75 mg once/day	Headaches, insomnia, nervousness, anxiety, irritability, dry mouth, constipation, euphoria, palpitations, hypertension
Mazindol (Sanorex)	AS	**T:** 1 mg, 2 mg	1–3 mg/day with meals	Palpitations, restlessness, dizziness, headaches, depression, weakness, abdominal pain
Orlistat (p. 874) (Xenical)	DI	**C:** 120 mg	120 mg 3 times/day before meals	Flatulence, rectal incontinence, oily stools

(continued)

ANOREXIANTS *(continued)*

Name	Type	Availability	Dosage	Side Effects
Phendimetrazine (Bontril)	AS	**C:** 105 mg **T:** 35 mg	17.5–70 mg 2–3 times/day or 105 mg once/day	Headaches, insomnia, nervousness, anxiety, irritability, dry mouth, constipation, euphoria, palpitations, hypertension
Phenmetrazine (Preludin)	AS	**T:** 75 mg	75 mg once/day	Palpitations, hypertension, nervousness, headaches, dizziness, dry mouth, euphoria, constipation
Phenteramine (Ionamin)	AS	**C:** 15 mg, 30 mg, 37.5 mg	15–37.5 mg once/day	Headaches, insomnia, nervousness, anxiety, irritability, dry mouth, constipation, euphoria, palpitations, hypertension
Sibutramine (Meridia)	AS	**C:** 5 mg, 10 mg, 15 mg	Initially, 10 mg, then increase to 15 mg/day or decrease to 5 mg/day	Hypertension, tachycardia, headaches, dry mouth, loss of appetite, insomnia, constipation

AS, Appetite suppressant; ***C,*** capsules; ***DI,*** digestion inhibitor; ***T,*** tablets.

Opioid Analgesics

USES

Relief of moderate to severe pain associated with surgical procedures, MI, burns, cancer, or other conditions. May be used as an adjunct to anesthesia, either as a preop medication or intraoperatively as a supplement to anesthesia. Also used for obstetric analgesia. Codeine and hydrocodone have an antitussive effect. Opium tinctures, such as paregoric, are used for severe diarrhea. Methadone relieves severe pain but is used primarily as part of heroin detoxification.

ACTION

Opioids refer to all drugs having actions similar to morphine and to receptors combining with these agents. Major effects are on the CNS (produce analgesia, drowsiness, mood changes, impaired concentration, analgesia without loss of consciousness, nausea and vomiting) and GI tract (decrease HCl secretion; diminish biliary, pancreatic, and intestinal secretions; diminish propulsive peristalsis). Also affects respiration (depressed) and cardiovascular system (peripheral vasodilation, decrease peripheral resistance, inhibit baroreceptor reflexes).

OPIOID ANALGESICS

		Analgesic Effect			
Names	Equianalgesic Dose	Onset (min)	Peak (min)	Duration (hrs)	Dosage Range
Butorphanol (p. 170) **(Stadol)**	**IM:** 2 mg **IV:** —	**IM:** 10–30 **IV:** 2–3	**IM:** 30–60 **IV:** 30	**IM:** 3–4 **IV:** 2–4	**IM:** 1–4 mg q3–4h **IV:** 0.5–2 mg q3–4h
Codeine (p. 282)	**IM:** 15–30 mg **PO:** 15–30 mg	**IM:** 10–30 **PO:** 30–45	**IM:** 30–60 **PO:** 60–120	**IM/PO:** 4–6	**IM/PO (A):** 15–60 mg q4–6h; **(C):** 0.5 mg/kg q4–6h

(continued)

Opioid Analgesics *(continued)*

Names	Equianalgesic Dose	Onset (min)	Peak (min)	Duration (hrs)	Dosage Range
Fentanyl (p. 475) (Sublimaze)	**IM:** 0.1–0.2 mg **IV:** —	**IM:** 7–15 **IV:** 1–2	**IM:** 20–30 **IV:** 3–5	**IM:** 1–2 **IV:** 0.5–1	**IM:** 50–100 mcg q1–2h
Hydrocodone (p. 577)	**PO:** 5–10 mg	10–30	30–60	4–6	5–10 mg q4–6h
Hydromorphone (p. 582) (Dilaudid)	**PO:** 7.5 mg **IM:** 1.5 mg	**PO:** 30 **IM:** 15 **IV:** 10–15	**PO:** 90–120 **IM:** 30–60 **IV:** 15–30	**PO:** 4–5 **IM:** 4–5 **IV:** 4	**PO:** 1–4 mg q3–6h **IM:** 1–4 mg q3–6h **IV:** 0.5–1 mg q3h **R:** 3 mg q4–8h
Levorphanol (Levo-Dromoran)	**PO:** 4 mg **IM:** 2 mg	**PO:** 10–60 **IM:** —	**PO:** 90–120 **IM:** 60	4–5	**PO:** 2–4 mg q4h **IM:** 2–3 mg q4h
Meperidine (p. 732) (Demerol)	**PO:** 300 mg **IM:** 75 mg **IV:** —	**PO:** 15 **IM:** 10–15 **IV:** 1	**PO:** 60–90 **IM:** 30–60 **IV:** 5–7	2–4	**PO, IM (A):** 50–150 mg q3–4h; **(C):** 1–1.8 mg/kg q3–4h
Methadone (p. 745) (Dolophine)	**PO:** 10–20 mg **IM:** 10 mg	**PO:** 30–60 **IM:** 10–20 **IV:** —	**PO:** 90–120 **IM:** 60–120 **IV:** 15–30	**PO:** 4–6 **IM:** 4–5 **IV:** 3–4	**IM, PO:** 2.5–10 mg q3–4h
Morphine (p. 792) (Roxanol, MS Contin)	**PO:** 30 mg **IM:** 10 mg **IV:** —	**PO:** 30–60 **IM:** 10–30 **IV:** —	**PO:** 90 **IM:** 30–60 **IV:** 20	**PO:** 4 **IM/IV:** 4–5	**PO:** 10–30 mg q4h **IM:** 5–20 mg q4h **IV:** 0.05–0.1 mg/kg q4h
Nalbuphine (p. 810) (Nubain)	**IM:** 10 mg **IV:** —	**IM:** 2–15 **IV:** 2–3	**IM:** 60 **IV:** 30	**IM:** 3–6 **IV:** 3–4	**IM/IV:** 10–20 mg q3–6h
Oxycodone (p. 884) (Roxicodone)	**PO:** 20–30 mg	30	60	3–4	5–15 mg or 5 ml q4–6h **(ER):** q12h (dose titrated)
Oxymorphone (Opana, Opana ER) (p. 887)	N/A	N/A	N/A	N/A	**PO:** 10–20 mg q4–6h **ER:** Half PO total daily dose q12h
Propoxyphene (p. 982) (Darvon)	**PO:** 65 mg	15–60	60–120	4–6	**PO:** 100 mg q4–6h

A, Adults; ***C,*** children; ***ER,*** extended release.

Parkinson's Disease Treatment

USES	ACTION
To slow or stop clinical progression of Parkinson's disease and to improve pt function and quality of life in those with Parkinson's disease, a progressive neurodegenerative disorder.	Normal motor function is dependent on the synthesis and release of dopamine by neurons projecting from the substantia nigra to the corpus striatum. In Parkinson's disease, disruption of this pathway results in diminished levels of the neurotransmitter dopamine. Medication is aimed at providing improved function using the lowest effective dose.

TYPES OF MEDICATIONS FOR PARKINSON'S DISEASE

DOPAMINE PRECURSOR

Levodopa/carbidopa:

Levodopa: Dopamine precursor supplementation to enhance dopaminergic neurotransmission. A small amount of levodopa crosses the blood-brain barrier and is decarboxylated to dopamine, which is then available to stimulate dopaminergic receptors.

Carbidopa: Inhibits peripheral decarboxylation of levodopa, decreasing its conversion to dopamine in peripheral tissues, which results in an increased availability of levodopa for transport across the blood-brain barrier.

COMT INHIBITORS

Reversible inhibitor of catechol-O-methyltransferase (COMT). COMT is responsible for catalyzing levodopa. In the presence of a decarboxylase inhibitor (carbidopa), COMT becomes the major metabolizing enzyme for levodopa in the brain and periphery. By inhibiting COMT, higher plasma levels of levodopa are attained, resulting in more dopaminergic stimulation in the brain and lessening the symptoms of Parkinson's disease.

DOPAMINE RECEPTOR AGONISTS

Apomorphine: Stimulates dopamine receptors in the brain.

Bromocriptine: Stimulates postsynaptic dopamine type 2 receptors in the neostriatum of the CNS.

Pergolide: Directly stimulates post-synaptic dopamine receptors (at both D1 and D2 receptor sites) in the nigrostriatal system. Independent of presynaptic dopamine synthesis or stores.

Pramipexole: Stimulates dopamine receptors in the striatum of the CNS.

Ropinirole: Stimulates postsynaptic dopamine D2 type receptors within the caudate putamen in the brain.

MONOAMINE OXIDASE B INHIBITORS

Selegiline, rasagiline: Increases dopaminergic activity due to irreversible inhibition of monoamine oxidase type B (MAO B). MAO B is involved in the oxidative deamination of dopamine in the brain.

Parkinson's Disease Treatment

MEDICATIONS FOR TREATMENT OF PARKINSON'S DISEASE

Name	Type	Dosage	Side Effects
Apomorphine (p. 82) (Apokyn)	Dopamine agonist	2 mg, initially up to 2–6 mg given 3–5 times/day as needed	Drowsiness, increased salivation, headaches, vomiting, orthostatic hypotension
Bromocriptine (p. 156) (Parlodel)	Dopamine agonist	2.5 mg 3 times/day initially up to maximum of 90 mg/day divided into 2 or 3 doses/day	Hypotension, nausea, livedo reticularis, edema, confusion, hallucinations
Carbidopa/levodopa (p. 187) (Sinemet)	Dopamine precursor	25/100 mg 3 times/day initially up to 200/2,000 mg divided into 3–6 doses/day	Hypotension, nausea, confusion, dyskinesia
Entacapone (p. 416) (Comtan)	COMT inhibitor	200 mg with each dose of levodopa (maximum 8 tablets or 1,600 mg/day)	Urine discoloration (benign), diarrhea
Pergolide (p. 924) (Permax)	Dopamine agonist	0.05–0.25 mg 3 times/day initially up to 0.75–5 mg/day	Hypotension, nausea, livedo reticularis, edema, confusion, hallucinations
Pramipexole (p. 954) (Mirapex)	Dopamine agonist	0.125 mg 3 times/day initially up to 1.5–4.5 mg/day in divided doses	Nausea, hypotension, sedation, hallucinations
Rasagiline (p. 1014) (Azilect)	MAO B inhibitor	Initially, 0.5 mg once daily, up to 1 mg 2 times/day	Headache, depression, constipation, dry mouth, rash
Ropinirole (p. 1041) (Requip)	Dopamine agonist	0.25 mg 3 times/day up to 9–24 mg/day in 3 divided doses	Nausea, hypotension, sedation, hallucinations
Selegiline (p. 1054) (Eldepryl)	MAO B inhibitor	10 mg/day (5 mg at breakfast and lunch)	Nausea, dizziness, faintness, abdominal discomfort
Tolcapone (Tasmar)	COMT inhibitor	100 mg 3 times/day up to 200 mg 3 times/day	Urine discoloration (benign), diarrhea, hepatic toxicity (hepatic monitoring required)

Proton Pump Inhibitors

USES

Treatment of various gastric disorders, including gastric and duodenal ulcers, GERD, pathologic hypersecretory conditions.

ACTION

Suppress gastric acid secretion by specific inhibition of the hydrogen-potassium-adenosine triphosphatase (H^+/K^+ ATPase) enzyme system, which transports the acid at the gastric parietal cells. These agents do not have anticholinergic or histamine receptor antagonistic properties.

PROTON PUMP INHIBITORS

Name	Availability	Indications	Usual Dosage	Side Effects
Esomeprazole (p. 443) (Nexium)	**C:** 20 mg, 40 mg **I:** 20 mg	*H. pylori* eradication, GERD, erosive esophagitis	20–40 mg/day	Headaches, diarrhea, abdominal pain, nausea
Lansoprazole (p. 667) (Prevacid)	**C:** 15 mg, 30 mg **I:** 30 mg	Duodenal ulcer, gastric ulcer, NSAID-associated gastric ulcer, hypersecretory conditions, *H. pylori* eradication, GERD, erosive esophagitis	15–30 mg/day	Diarrhea, skin rash, pruritus, headaches
Omeprazole (p. 870) (Prilosec)	**C:** 10 mg, 20 mg, 40 mg	Duodenal ulcer, gastric ulcer, hypersecretory conditions, *H. pylori* eradication, GERD, erosive esophagitis	20–40 mg/day	Headaches, diarrhea, abdominal pain, nausea
Pantoprazole (p. 902) (Protonix)	**T:** 20 mg, 40 mg **I:** 40 mg	Erosive esophagitis, hypersecretory conditions	40 mg/day	Diarrhea, headaches
Rabeprazole (p. 1006) (Aciphex)	**T:** 20 mg	Duodenal ulcer, hypersecretory conditions, *H. pylori* eradication, GERD, erosive esophagitis	20 mg/day	Headaches

C, Capsules; ***GERD,*** gastroesophageal reflux disease; ***I,*** Injection; ***NSAID,*** nonsteroidal anti-inflammatory drug; ***T,*** tablets.

Sedative-Hypnotics

USES

Treatment of insomnia, e.g., difficulty falling asleep initially, frequent awakening, awakening too early.

ACTION

Benzodiazepines are the most widely used agents and largely replace barbiturates due to greater safety, lower incidence of drug dependence. Benzodiazepines nonselectively bind to at least three receptor subtypes accounting for sedative, anxiolytic, relaxant, and anticonvulsant properties. Benzodiazepines enhance the effect of the inhibitory neurotransmitter gamma-aminobutyric acid (GABA), which inhibits impulse transmission in the CNS reticular formation in brain. Benzodiazepines decrease sleep latency, number of nocturnal awakenings, and time spent in awake stage of sleep; increase total sleep time. The *nonbenzodiazepines* zaleplon and zolpidem preferentially bind with one receptor subtype, reducing sleep latency and nocturnal awakenings and increasing total sleep time.

SEDATIVE-HYPNOTICS

Name	Availability	Dosage Range	Side Effects
Benzodiazepines			
Estazolam evolve **(ProSom)**	**T:** 1 mg, 2 mg	**A:** 1–2 mg **E:** 0.5–1 mg	Daytime sedation, memory and psychomotor impairment, tolerance, withdrawal reactions, rebound insomnia, dependence
Flurazepam (p. 502) (Dalmane)	**C:** 15 mg, 30 mg	**A/E:** 15–30 mg	Headaches, unpleasant taste, dry mouth, dizziness, anxiety, nausea
Quazepam (Doral)	**T:** 7.5 mg, 15 mg	**A:** 7.5–15 mg **E:** 7.5 mg	Same as flurazepam
Temazepam (p. 1111) (Restoril)	**C:** 7.5 mg, 15 mg, 30 mg	**A:** 15–30 mg **E:** 7.5–15 mg	Same as flurazepam

Triazolam (p. 1182) (Halcion)	**T:** 0.125 mg, 0.25 mg	**A:** 0.125–0.25 mg **E:** 0.125 mg	Same as flurazepam
Nonbenzodiazepines			
Eszopiclone (p. 450) (Lunesta)	**T:** 1 mg, 2 mg, 3 mg	**A:** 2–3 mg **E:** 1–2 mg	Headaches, unpleasant taste, dry mouth, dizziness, anxiety, nausea
Ramelteon (p. 1008) (Rozerem)	**T:** 8 mg	**A, E:** 8 mg	Headaches, dizziness, fatigue, nausea
Zaleplon (p. 1235) (Sonata)	**C:** 5 mg, 10 mg	**A:** 5–10 mg **E:** 5 mg	Headaches, dizziness, myalgia, drowsiness, asthenia, abdominal pain
Zolpidem (p. 1246) (Ambien, Ambien CR)	**T:** 5 mg, 10 mg **CR:** 6.25 mg, 12.5 mg	**A:** 10 mg, 12.5 **E:** 5 mg, 6.25 mg	Dizziness, daytime drowsiness, headaches, confusion, depression, hangover, asthenia

A, Adults; ***C,*** capsules; ***CR,*** controlled-release; ***E,*** elderly; ***T,*** tablets.

Skeletal Muscle Relaxants

USES

Central acting muscle relaxants: Adjunct to rest, physical therapy for relief of discomfort associated with acute, painful musculoskeletal disorders, i.e., local spasms from muscle injury.

Baclofen, dantrolene, diazepam: Treatment of spasticity characterized by heightened muscle tone, spasm, loss of dexterity caused by multiple sclerosis, cerebral palsy, spinal cord lesions, CVA.

ACTION

Central acting muscle relaxants: Exact mechanism unknown. May act in CNS at various levels to depress polysynaptic reflexes; sedative effect may be responsible for relaxation of muscle spasm.

Baclofen, diazepam: May mimic actions of gamma-aminobutyric acid on spinal neurons; does not directly affect skeletal muscles.

Dantrolene: Acts directly on skeletal muscle, relieving spasticity.

SKELETAL MUSCLE RELAXANTS

Name	Indication	Dosage Range	Side Effects/Comments
Baclofen (Lioresal) (p. 120)	Spasticity associated with multiple sclerosis, spinal cord injury	Initially 5 mg 3 times/day. Increase by 5 mg 3 times/day q3days. **Maximum:** 20 mg 4 times/day	Drowsiness, dizziness, GI effects. Caution with renal impairment, seizure disorders. Withdrawal syndrome (e.g., hallucinations, psychosis, seizures)
Carisoprodol (Rela)	Discomfort due to acute, painful, musculoskeletal conditions	350 mg 4 times/day	Drowsiness, dizziness, GI effects. Hypomania at higher than recommended doses. Withdrawal syndrome. Hypersensitivity reaction (skin reaction, bronchospasm, weakness, burning eyes, fever) or idiosyncratic reaction (weakness, visual or motor disturbances, confusion) usually occurring within first 4 doses.
Chlorzoxazone (Parafon Forte)	Discomfort due to acute, painful, musculoskeletal conditions	Initially 250–500 mg 3–4 times/day. **Maximum:** 750 mg 3–4 times/day	Drowsiness, dizziness, GI effects. Rare hepatic toxicity. Hypersensitivity reaction (urticaria, itching). Urine discoloration to orange, red, or purple.
Cyclobenzaprine (Flexeril) (p. 299)	Muscle spasm, pain, tenderness, restricted movement due to acute, painful, musculoskeletal conditions	Initially 5–10 mg 3 times/day. **Maximum:** 20 mg 3 times/day.	Drowsiness, dizziness, GI effects. Anticholinergic effects (dry mouth, urinary retention). Quinidine-like effects on heart (QT prolongation). Long half-life.
Dantrolene (Dantrium) (p. 314)	Spasticity associated with multiple sclerosis, cerebral palsy, spinal cord injury	Initially 25 mg/day for 1 week, then 25 mg 3 times/day for 1 week, then 50 mg 3 times/day for 1 week, then 100 mg 3 times/day. **Maximum:** 100 mg 4 times/day	Drowsiness, dizziness, GI effects. Contraindicated with hepatic disease. Dose-dependent hepatic toxicity. Diarrhea that is dose dependent and may be severe, requiring discontinuation.

Diazepam (Valium) (p. 350)	Spasticity associated with cerebral palsy, spinal cord injury; reflex spasm due to muscle, joint trauma or inflammation	2–10 mg 3–4 times/day	Drowsiness, dizziness, GI effects. Abuse potential.
Metaxalone (Skelaxin)	Discomfort due to acute, painful, musculoskeletal conditions	800 mg 3–4 times/day	Drowsiness (low risk), dizziness, GI effects. Paradoxical muscle cramps. Mild withdrawal syndrome. Contraindicated in serious hepatic or renal disease.
Methocarbamol (Robaxin)	Discomfort due to acute, painful, musculoskeletal conditions	Initially 1,500 mg 4 times/day. **Maintenance:** 1,000 mg 4 times/day	Drowsiness, dizziness, GI effects. Urine discoloration to brown, brown-black, or green.
Orphenadrine (Norflex)	Discomfort due to acute, painful, musculoskeletal conditions	100 mg 2 times/day	Drowsiness, dizziness, GI effects. Long half-life. Anticholinergic effects (dry mouth, urinary retention). Rare aplastic anemia. Some products may contain sulfites.
Tizanidine (Zanaflex) (p. 1152)	Spasticity	Initially 4 mg q6–8 h (maximum 3 times/day), may increase by 2–4 mg as needed/tolerated. **Maximum:** 36 mg (limited information on doses greater than 24 mg)	Drowsiness, dizziness, GI effects. Hypotension (20% decrease in b/p). Hepatic toxicity (usually reversible). Withdrawal syndrome (hypertension, tachycardia, hypertonia). Effect is short lived (3–6 hrs) Dose cautiously with creatinine clearance less than 25 ml/min.

A, Adults; ***C,*** capsules; ***C** (dosage),* children; ***E,*** elderly; ***T,*** tablets.

Smoking Cessation Agents

Tobacco smoking is associated with the development of lung cancer and chronic obstructive pulmonary disease (COPD). Smoking is not just harmful to the smoker but also family members, coworkers and others breathing cigarette smoke.

Quitting smoking decreases the risk of developing lung cancer, other cancers, heart disease, stroke and respiratory illnesses. Several medications have proven useful as smoking cessation aids. Nausea and light-headedness are possible signs of overdose of nicotine warranting a reduction in dosage.

Smoking Cessation Agents

Name	Availability	Dose Duration	Cautions/Side Effects	Comments
Bupropion (Zyban) (p. 164)	**T:** 150 mg	150 mg every morning for 3 days, then 150 mg 2 times/day Start 1–2 wks before quit date. **Duration:** 7–12 wks up to 6 mos for maintenance	History of seizure, eating disorder, use of MAOI within previous 14 days, bipolar disorder. **Side effects:** Insomnia, dry mouth, tremor, rash	Stop smoking during second wk of treatment and use counseling support services along with medication.
Clonidine (Catapres, Catapres-TTS) (p. 273)	**T:** 0.1 mg, 0.2 mg. **Patch:** 0.1 mg/24 hrs, 0.2 mg/24 hrs, 0.3 mg/24 hrs	**Oral:** 0.15–0.75 mg/day **Patch:** 0.1–0.2 mg daily **Duration:** 3–10 weeks.	Rebound hypertension. **Side effects:** Dry mouth, drowsiness, dizziness, sedation, constipation	Abrupt discontinuation can result in anxiety, agitation, headaches, tremors accompanied or followed by rapid rise in B/P.
Nicotine gum (Nicorette) (p. 836)	**Squares:** 2 mg, 4 mg	1 gum q1–2h for 6 wks, then q2–4h for 3 wks **Maximum:** 24 pieces/day **Duration:** up to 12 wks	Recent MI (within 2 wks), serious arrhythmias, serious or worsening angina pectoris.	2 mg recommended for pts smoking less than 25 cigarettes/day, 4 mg for pts smoking 25 or more cigarettes/day Chew until a peppery or minty taste emerges

			Side effects: Dyspepsia, mouth soreness, hiccups	and then "park" between cheek and gums to facilitate nicotine absorption through oral mucosa. Chew slowly and intermittently to avoid jaw ache and achieve maximum benefit. Only water should be taken 15 min before and during chewing.
Nicotine inhaler (Nicotrol) (p. 836)	**Cartridge:** 10 mg (delivers 4 mg nicotine)	6–16 cartridges daily; taper frequency of use over the last 6–12 wks. **Duration:** up to 6 mos	Recent MI (within 2 wks), serious arrhythmias, serious or worsening angina pectoris. **Side effects:** Local irritation of mouth and throat, coughing, rhinitis	Use at or above room temperature (cold temperatures decrease amount of nicotine inhaled)
Nicotine lozenge (Commit) (p. 836)	**Lozenges:** 2 mg, 4 mg	One lozenge q1–2h for 6 wks, then q2–4h for 3 wks, then q4–8h for 3 wks **Duration:** 12 wks	Recent MI (within 2 wks), serious arrhythmias, serious or worsening angina pectoris. **Side effects:** Local skin reaction, insomnia, nausea, sore throat	First cigarette smoked within 30 min of waking, use 4 mg; after 30 min of waking, use 2 mg. Use at least 9 lozenges/day first 6 wks. Only 1 lozenge at a time, 5 per 6 hrs and 20 per 24 hrs Do not chew or swallow
Nicotine nasal spray (Nicotrol NS) (p. 836)	10 mg/ml (delivers 0.5 mg/spray)	8–40 doses/day A dose consists of one 0.5 mg delivery to each nostril; initial dose is 1–2 sprays/hr, increasing as needed. **Duration:** 3–6 mos	Recent MI (within 2 wks), serious arrhythmias, serious or worsening angina pectoris. **Side effects:** Nasal irritation	Do not sniff, swallow, or inhale through nose while administering nicotine doses (may increase irritation). Tilt head back slightly for best results

(continued)

Smoking Cessation Agents ***(continued)***

Name	Availability	Dose Duration	Cautions/Side Effects	Comments
Nicotine patch (Nicoderm CQ, Nicotrol) (p. 836)	**Nicoderm CQ:** 7 mg/24 hrs, 14 mg/24 hrs, 21 mg/24 hrs **Nicotrol:** 5 mg/16 hrs, 10 mg/16 hrs, 15 mg/16 hrs	Apply upon waking on quit date: **Nicoderm CQ:** 21 mg/24 hrs for 4 wks, then 14 mg/24 hrs for 2 wks, then 7 mg/24 hrs for 2 wks **Nicotrol:** 15 mg/16 hrs for 6 wks, then 10 mg/16 hrs for 2 wks, then 5 mg/16 hrs for 2 wks	Recent MI (within 2 wks), serious arrhythmias, serious or worsening angina pectoris. **Side effects:** Local skin reaction, insomnia	The 16- and 24-hr patches are of comparable efficacy Begin with a lower-dose patch in pts smoking 10 or fewer cigarettes/day. Place new patch on relatively hair-free location, usually between neck and waist, in the morning. If insomnia occurs, remove the 24-hr patch prior to bedtime or use the 16-hr patch. Rotate patch site to diminish skin irritation
Nortriptyline (Pamelor) (p. 854)	**T:** 25 mg, 50 mg, 75 mg, 100 mg	Initially 25 mg/day, increasing gradually to target dose of 75–100 mg/day. **Duration:** up to 12 wks	Risk of arrhythmias. **Side effects:** Sedation, dry mouth, blurred vision, urinary retention, light-headedness, shaky hands	Initiate therapy 10–28 days before the quit date to allow steady state of nortriptyline at target dose.
Varenicline (Chantix) (p. 1205)	**T:** 0.5 mg, 1 mg	Days 1–3: 0.5 mg; daily; days 4–7; 0.5 mg 2 times/day; day 8 to end of treatment: 1 mg 2 times/day **Duration:** begin 1 wk before set quit date continue for 12 wks. May use additional 12 wks if failed to quit after first 12 wks.	**Side effects:** Nausea, sleep disturbances, headaches	Use lower dosage if not able to tolerate nausea and vomiting. Use counseling support services along with medication

T, Tablets.

Sympathomimetics

USES

Stimulation of alpha$_1$-receptors: Induce vasoconstriction primarily in skin and mucous membranes, nasal decongestion; combine with local anesthetics to delay anesthetic absorption; increases B/P in certain hypotensive states; produce mydriasis, facilitating eye exams, ocular surgery.
Stimulation of beta$_1$-receptors: Treatment of cardiac arrest, heart failure, shock, AV block.
Stimulation of beta$_2$-receptors: Treatment of asthma.
Stimulation of dopamine receptors: Treatment of shock.

ACTION

The sympathetic nervous system (SNS) is involved in maintaining homeostasis (involved in regulation of heart rate, force of cardiac contractions, B/P, bronchial airway tone, carbohydrate, fatty acid meters (primarily norepinephrine, epinephrine, and dopamine), which act on adrenergic receptors. These receptors include beta$_1$, beta$_2$, alpha$_1$, alpha$_2$, and dopaminergic. Sympathomimetics differ widely in their actions based on their specificity to affect these receptors.

- *Alpha$_1$:* Causes mydriasis, constriction of arterioles, veins.
- *Alpha$_2$:* Inhibits transmitter release.
- *Beta$_1$:* Increases rate, force of contraction, conduction velocity of heart; releases renin from kidney.
- *Beta$_2$:* Dilates arterioles, bronchi, relaxes uterus.
- *Dopaminergic:* Dilates kidney vasculature.

SYMPATHOMIMETICS

Name	Availability	Receptor Specificity	Uses	Dosage Range
Dobutamine (p. 376) (Dobutrex)	**I:** 12.5 mg/ml, 500 mg/ 250 ml	Beta$_1$, beta$_2$, alpha$_1$	Inotropic support in cardiac decompensation	**IV infusion:** 2.5–10 mcg/kg/min
Dopamine (p. 385) (Intropin)	**I:** 40 mg, 80 mg, 160-ml vials, 800 mcg/ml, 1,600 mcg/ml	Beta$_1$, alpha$_1$, dopaminergic	Vasopressor, cardiac stimulant	**Dopaminergic:** 0.5–3 mcg/kg/min **Beta$_1$:** 2–10 mcg/ kg/min **Alpha$_1$:** more than 10 mcg/kg/min
Ephedrine	**I:** 50 mg/ml	Alpha, beta$_1$, beta$_2$	Acute hypotensive states, esp. with spinal anesthesia	**IV:** 5–25 mg

(continued)

SYMPATHOMIMETICS *(continued)*

Name	Availability	Receptor Specificity	Uses	Dosage Range
Epinephrine (p. 419) (Adrenalin)	**I:** 0.1 mg/ml, 1 mg/ml	$Beta_1$, $beta_2$, $alpha_1$	Cardiac arrest, anaphylactic shock	**Vasopressor:** 1–10 mcg/min **Cardiac arrest:** 1 mg q3–5min during resuscitation
Norepinephrine (p. 851) (Levophed)	**I:** 1 mg/ml	$Beta_1$, $alpha_1$	Vasopressor	**IV:** 0.5–1 mcg/min up to 2–12 mcg/min
Phenylephrine (p. 931) (Neo-Synephrine)	**I:** 10 mg/ml	$Alpha_1$	Vasopressor	**IV:** Initially, 10–180 mcg/min, then 40–60 mcg/min

I, Injection.

Thyroid

USES

Treatment of hypothyroidism, a common endocrine disorder in which the thyroid fails to release sufficient amounts of thyroid hormones.

ACTION

Thyroid hormones are necessary for proper metabolism, growth, and homeostasis. Thyroid hormone regulates energy and heat production; facilitates development of the central nervous system, growth, and puberty. Regulates the synthesis of proteins that are important in hepatic, cardiac, neurologic, and muscular functions.

THYROID

Name	Availability	Dosage Average	Side Effects
Levothyroxine (p. 687) (Levoxyl, Synthroid)	**T:** 25 mcg, 50 mcg, 75 mcg, 88 mcg, 100 mcg, 112 mcg, 125 mcg, 137 mcg, 150 mcg, 175 mcg, 200 mcg, 300 mcg	75–100 mcg/day	Side effects are due to excessive amounts of medication, including diarrhea, heat intolerance, palpitations, tremors, tachycardia, vomiting, weight loss, increased B/P.
Liothyronine (p. 693) evolve **(Cytomel)**	**T:** 5 mcg, 25 mcg, 50 mcg	25–50 mcg/day	Same as levothyroxine
Liotrix (Thyrolar)	**T:** ¼ grain, ½ grain, 1 grain, 2 grain, 3 grain	½–1 grain/day	Same as levothyroxine
Thyroid	**T:** 15 mg, 30 mg, 60 mg, 90 mg, 120 mg, 180 mg, 240 mg, 300 mg	60–120 mg/day	Same as levothyroxine

T, Tablets.

Vitamins

INTRODUCTION

Vitamins are organic substances required for growth, reproduction, and maintenance of health and are obtained from food or supplementation in small quantities (vitamins cannot be synthesized by the body or the rate of synthesis is too slow/inadequate to meet metabolic needs). Vitamins are essential for energy transformation and regulation of metabolic processes. They are catalysts for all reactions using proteins, fats, carbohydrates for energy, growth, and cell maintenance.

WATER SOLUBLE

Water-soluble vitamins include vitamin C (ascorbic acid), B_1 (thiamine), B_2 (riboflavin), B_3 (niacin), B_5 (pantothenic acid), B_6 (pyridoxine), folic acid, B_{12} (cyanocobalamin). Water-soluble vitamins act as coenzymes for almost every cellular reaction in the body. B-complex vitamins differ from one another in both structure and function but are grouped together because they first were isolated from the same source (yeast and liver).

FAT SOLUBLE

Fat-soluble vitamins include vitamins A, D, E, and K. They are soluble in lipids and are usually absorbed into the lymphatic system of the small intestine and then into the general circulation. Absorption is facilitated by bile. These vitamins are stored in the body tissue when excessive quantities are consumed. May be toxic when taken in large doses (see sections on individual vitamins).

Vitamins *(continued)*

VITAMINS

Name	Uses	RDA	Side Effects
Vitamin A (p. 1220) (Aquasol A)	Required for normal growth, bone development, vision, reproduction, maintenance of epithelial tissue	**M:** 1,000 mcg **F:** 800 mcg	**High dosages:** Hepatic toxicity, cheilitis, facial dermatitis, photosensitivity, mucosal dryness
Vitamin B_1 (p. 1129) (Thiamine)	Important in red blood cell formation, carbohydrate metabolism, neurologic function, myocardial contractility, growth, energy production	**M:** 1.5 mg **F:** 1.1 mg	**Large parenteral doses:** May cause pain on injection
Vitamin B_2 (Riboflavin)	Necessary for function of coenzymes in oxidation-reduction reactions, essential for normal cellular growth, assists in absorption of iron and pyridoxine	**M:** 1.7 mg **F:** 1.3 mg	Orange-yellow discoloration in urine
Vitamin B_3 (p. 832) (Niacin)	Coenzyme for many oxidation-reduction reactions	**M:** 19 mg **F:** 15 mg	**High dosage (over 500 mg):** Nausea, vomiting, diarrhea, gastritis, hepatic toxicity, skin rash, facial flushing, headaches
Vitamin B_5 (Pantothenic acid)	Precursor to coenzyme A, important in synthesis of cholesterol, hormones, fatty acids	**M:** 4–7 mg **F:** 4–7 mg	Occasional GI disturbances (e.g., diarrhea)
Vitamin B_6 (p. 995) (Pyridoxine)	Enzyme cofactor for amino acid metabolism, essential for erythrocyte production, Hgb synthesis	**M:** 2 mg **F:** 1.6 mg	**High dosages:** May cause sensory neuropathy

Vitamin B_{12} (p. 298) (Cyanocobalamin)	Coenzyme in cells, including bone marrow, CNS, and GI tract, necessary for lipid metabolism, formation of myelin	**M:** 2.4 mcg **F:** 2.4 mcg	Skin rash, diarrhea, pain at injection site
Vitamin C (p. 92) (Ascorbic acid)	Cofactor in various physiologic reactions, necessary for collagen formation, acts as antioxidant	**M:** 90 mg **F:** 75 mg (increased with smoking, pregnancy, lactation)	**High dosages:** May cause calcium oxalate crystalluria, esophagitis, diarrhea
Vitamin D (p. 1222) (Calciferol)	Necessary for proper formation of bone, calcium, mineral homeostasis, regulation of parathyroid hormone, calcitonin, phosphate	**M:** 200–400 units **F:** 200–400 units	Hypercalcemia, kidney stones, renal failure, hypertension, psychosis, diarrhea, nausea, vomiting, anorexia, fatigue, headaches, altered mental status
Vitamin E (p. 1224) (Aquasol E)	Antioxidant	**M:** 15 mg **F:** 15 mg	**High dosages:** GI disturbances, malaise, headaches

F, Females; ***M,*** males.

abacavir

ah-bah-**kay**-veer
(Ziagen)

FIXED-COMBINATION(S)

Epzicom: abacavir/lamivudine (antiretroviral): 600 mg/300 mg. **Trizivir:** abacavir/lamivudine (antiretroviral)/zidovudine (antiretroviral): 300 mg/150 mg/300 mg.

◆ CLASSIFICATION

PHARMACOTHERAPEUTIC: Antiretroviral agent. **CLINICAL:** Antiviral (see pp. 64C, 110C).

ACTION

Inhibits activity of HIV-1 reverse transcriptase by competing with natural substrate dGTP and by its incorporation into viral DNA. **Therapeutic Effect:** Inhibits viral DNA growth.

PHARMACOKINETICS

Rapidly and extensively absorbed after PO administration. Protein binding: 50%. Widely distributed, including to cerebrospinal fluid (CSF) and erythrocytes. Metabolized in the liver to inactive metabolites. Primarily excreted in urine. Unknown if removed by hemodialysis. **Half-life:** 1.5 hrs.

USES

Treatment of HIV infection, in combination with other agents.

PRECAUTIONS

CONTRAINDICATIONS: Moderate or severe hepatic impairment. **CAUTIONS:** Liver disease.

⌛ LIFESPAN CONSIDERATIONS:

Pregnancy/Lactation: Unknown if excreted in breast milk. Do not breast-feed while taking abacavir (may increase potential for HIV transmission, adverse effects). **Pregnancy Category C. Children:** No safety issues noted in those 3 mos–13 yrs. **Elderly:** No information available.

INTERACTIONS

DRUG: Alcohol may increase concentration and half-life. **HERBAL: St. John's wort** may decrease concentration, effect. **FOOD:** None known. **LAB VALUES:** May increase serum AST, ALT, GGT, blood glucose, triglycerides.

AVAILABILITY (Rx)

SOLUTION, ORAL: 20 mg/ml. **TABLETS:** 300 mg.

ADMINISTRATION/HANDLING

PO

- May give without regard to food.
- Oral solution may be refrigerated. Do not freeze.

INDICATIONS/ROUTES/DOSAGE

HIV INFECTION (IN COMBINATION WITH OTHER ANTIRETROVIRALS)

PO: ADULTS: 300 mg twice a day or 600 mg once daily. **CHILDREN 3 MOS–16 YRS:** 8 mg/kg twice a day. **Maximum:** 300 mg twice a day.

DOSAGE IN HEPATIC IMPAIRMENT

Mild impairment: 200 mg twice a day. **Moderate to severe impairment:** Not recommended.

SIDE EFFECTS

ADULT: **FREQUENT:** Nausea (47%), nausea with vomiting (16%), diarrhea (12%), decreased appetite (11%). **OCCASIONAL:** Insomnia (7%). CHILDREN: **FREQUENT:** Nausea with vomiting (39%), fever (19%), headache, diarrhea (16%), rash (11%). **OCCASIONAL:** Decreased appetite (9%).

ADVERSE EFFECTS/ TOXIC REACTIONS

Hypersensitivity reaction may be life-threatening. Signs and symptoms include fever, rash, fatigue, intractable nausea/

vomiting, severe diarrhea, abdominal pain, cough, pharyngitis, dyspnea. Life-threatening hypotension may occur. Lactic acidosis, severe hepatomegaly may occur.

NURSING CONSIDERATIONS

BASELINE ASSESSMENT

Question for possibility of pregnancy. Obtain baseline laboratory testing, esp. liver function tests, before beginning therapy and at periodic intervals during therapy. Offer emotional support.

INTERVENTION/EVALUATION

Assess for nausea, vomiting. Determine pattern of bowel activity and stool consistency. Assess eating pattern; monitor for weight loss. Monitor lab values carefully, particularly liver function.

PATIENT/FAMILY TEACHING

• Do not take any medications, including OTC drugs, without consulting physician. • Small, frequent meals may offset anorexia, nausea. • Abacavir is not a cure for HIV infection, nor does it reduce risk of transmission to others.

abarelix

ah-**bare**-eh-licks
(Plenaxis)

CLASSIFICATION

PHARMACOTHERAPEUTIC: Gonadotropin-releasing hormone antagonist. **CLINICAL:** Sex hormone.

ACTION

Inhibits gonadotropin and androgen production by blocking gonadotropin releasing-hormone (GnRH) receptors in the pituitary. **Therapeutic Effect:** Suppresses luteinizing hormone (LH) and follicle-stimulating hormone (FSH) secretion, reducing secretion of testosterone by testes.

PHARMACOKINETICS

Slowly absorbed following intramuscular administration. Distributed extensively. Protein binding: 96%–99%. **Half-life:** 13.2 days.

USES

Treatment of men with advanced symptomatic prostate cancer in whom luteinizing hormone releasing hormone (LHRH) agonist therapy is not appropriate, who refuse surgical castration, and have 1 or more of the following: 1) risk of neurologic compromise due to metastases, 2) ureteral or bladder outlet obstruction, or 3) severe bone pain from bone metastases.

PRECAUTIONS

CONTRAINDICATIONS: Female pts, children, pregnancy. **CAUTIONS:** Pts with prolonged QT interval, pts weighing more than 225 lb (103 kg).

LIFESPAN CONSIDERATIONS:

Pregnancy/Lactation: Embryolethal. Avoid breast-feeding. **Pregnancy Category X.** **Children:** Not indicated for use in pediatric pts. **Elderly:** No age-related precautions noted.

INTERACTIONS

DRUG: QT_c interval may be prolonged with **amiodarone, procainamide, guinidine, sotalol**. **HERBAL:** None significant. **FOOD:** None known. **LAB VALUES:** May increase serum transaminase, AST, ALT, triglycerides. May decrease bone mineral density.

AVAILABILITY (Rx)

INJECTION, POWDER FOR RECONSTITUTION: 113-mg kit containing 10 ml 0.9% NaCl, 18-gauge needle, 22-gauge needle (provides 100 mg/2 ml when reconstituted).

ADMINISTRATION/HANDLING

IM

Reconstitution • Before reconstitution, shake vial gently. Withdraw 2.2 ml 0.9% NaCl, and inject diluent quickly. • Shake immediately for approximately 15 sec. Let vial stand for 2 min. • Tap vial to reduce foaming and swirl vial occasionally. • Shake again for approximately 15 sec. • Allow vial to stand for 2 min.

Rate of administration • Following reconstitution, administer within 1 hr. • Administer at dorsogluteal or ventrogluteal region of buttock. • Following administration, monitor pt for 30 min (cumulative risk for allergic reaction increases with each injection).

Storage • Store at room temperature.

INDICATIONS/ROUTES/DOSAGE

PROSTATE CANCER

IM: ADULTS, ELDERLY: 100 mg on days 1, 15, 29 and q4wk thereafter. Treatment failure can be detected by obtaining serum testosterone concentration prior to abarelix administration, day 19 and q8wk thereafter.

SIDE EFFECTS

FREQUENT (79%–30%): Hot flashes, sleep disturbances, breast enlargement. **OCCASIONAL (20%–11%):** Breast pain, nipple tenderness, back pain, constipation, peripheral edema, dizziness, upper respiratory tract infection, diarrhea. **RARE (10%):** Fatigue, nausea, dysuria, micturition frequency, urinary retention, UTI.

ADVERSE EFFECTS/ TOXIC REACTIONS

◀ ALERT ▶ Immediate-onset systemic allergic reaction characterized by hypotension, urticaria, pruritus, periorbital and/or circumoral edema, shortness of breath, wheezing, syncope may occur. Prolongation of QT interval may occur.

NURSING CONSIDERATIONS

BASELINE ASSESSMENT

Inform pt of treatment duration and required monitoring procedures. Obtain serum transaminase levels before treatment and periodically thereafter.

INTERVENTION/EVALUATION

Monitor pt for at least 30 min each time abarelix is given. Assess for systemic allergic reaction. Measure serum testosterone concentration before administration beginning on day 29 and q8wk thereafter. Monitor periodic serum prostate-specific antigen (PSA) levels.

PATIENT/FAMILY TEACHING

• Notify physician or nurse immediately if rash, hives, itching, tingling, flushing occurs (skin reaction may occur immediately after injection or several days later).

abatacept

ah-**bah**-tah-cept
(Orencia)

CLASSIFICATION

PHARMACOTHERAPEUTIC: Selective T-cell co-stimulation modulator. **CLINICAL:** Rheumatoid arthritis agent.

ACTION

Inhibits T-lymphocyte activation, necessary in the inflammatory cascade leading to joint inflammation and destruction of rheumatoid arthritis. **Therapeutic Effect:** Induces major clinical response to adult pts with moderate to severely active rheumatoid arthritis.

PHARMACOKINETICS

Higher clearance with increasing body weight. Age, gender does not affect clearance. **Half-life:** 13–16 days.

USES

Reduces signs and symptoms, progression of structural damage in adults with moderate to severe rheumatoid arthritis unresponsive to other disease-modifying antirheumatic drugs.

PRECAUTIONS

CONTRAINDICATIONS: None known. **CAUTIONS:** Chronic, latent, or localized infection, chronic obstructive pulmonary disease (COPD), elderly.

LIFESPAN CONSIDERATIONS:

Pregnancy/Lactation: Crosses placenta; unknown if distributed in breast milk. **Pregnancy Category C. Children:** Safety and efficacy not established. **Elderly:** Cautious use due to increased risk of serious infection and malignancy.

INTERACTIONS

DRUG: May increase risk of infection, decrease efficacy of immune response associated with **live vaccines. Tumor necrosis factor (TNF) antagonists (adalimumab, etanercept, infliximab)** may increase risk of infection. **HERBAL:** None significant. **FOOD:** None known. **LAB VALUES:** None known.

AVAILABILITY (Rx)

INJECTION, POWDER FOR RECONSTITUTION: 250 mg in 15-ml vial.

ADMINISTRATION/HANDLING

IV

Reconstitution • Reconstitute powder in each vial with 10 ml Sterile Water for Injection using the silicone-free syringe provided with each vial and an 18–21 gauge needle. • Rotate solution gently to prevent foaming until powder is completely dissolved. • From a 100 ml 0.9% NaCl infusion bag, withdraw and discard an amount equal to the volume of the reconstituted vials (for 2 vials remove 20 ml, for 3 vials remove 30 ml, for 4 vials remove 40 ml). • Slowly add the reconstituted solution from each vial into the infusion bag using the same syringe provided with each vial. • Concentration in the infusion bag will be 5, 7.5, or 10 mg abatacept per ml of infusion, depending on the number of vials of abatacept used.

Rate of administration • Infuse over 30 min using a low-protein binding filter.

Storage • Any reconstitution that has been prepared by using siliconized syringes will develop translucent particles and must be discarded. • Solution should appear clear and colorless to pale yellow. Discard if solution is discolored or contains precipitate. • Solution is stable for up to 14 hrs after reconstitution. • Reconstituted solution may be stored at room temperature or refrigerated.

IV INCOMPATIBILITIES

Do not infuse concurrently in same IV line as other agents.

INDICATIONS/ROUTES/DOSAGE

RHEUMATOID ARTHRITIS

IV: BODY WEIGHT 101 KG OR MORE: 1 gram (4 vials) given as a 30-min infusion. Following initial therapy, give at 2 wks and 4 wks after first infusion, then q3wk thereafter. **BODY WEIGHT 60–100 KG:** 750 mg (3 vials) given as a 30-min infusion. Following initial therapy, give at 2 wks and 4 wks after first infusion, then q3wk thereafter. **BODY WEIGHT 59 KG OR LESS:** 500 mg (2 vials) given as a 30-min infusion. Following initial therapy, give at 2 wks and 4 wks after first infusion, then q3wk thereafter.

SIDE EFFECTS

FREQUENT (18%): Headache. **OCCASIONAL (9%–6%):** Dizziness, cough, back pain, hypertension, nausea.

ADVERSE EFFECTS/ TOXIC REACTIONS

Upper respiratory tract infection, nasopharyngitis, sinusitis, UTI, influenza, bronchitis occur in 5% of pts. Serious infections manifested as pneumonia, cellulitis, diverticulitis, acute pyelonephritis occur in 3% of pts. Hypersensitivity reaction (rash, uriticaria, hypotension, dyspnea) occurs rarely.

NURSING CONSIDERATIONS

BASELINE ASSESSMENT

Assess onset, type, location, duration of pain/inflammation. Inspect appearance of affected joint for immobility, deformities, skin condition.

INTERVENTION/EVALUATION

Assess for therapeutic response: relief of pain, stiffness, swelling, improved joint mobility, reduced joint tenderness, improved grip strength. Monitor COPD pts for worsening of respiratory symptoms; discontinuing drug therapy may be necessary.

PATIENT/FAMILY TEACHING

• Consult physician or nurse if infection occurs. • Do not receive live virus vaccine during treatment or within 3 mos of its discontinuation.

abciximab

ab-**six**-ih-mab
(c7E3 Fab, ReoPro)

CLASSIFICATION

PHARMACOTHERAPEUTIC: Glycoprotein IIb/IIIa receptor inhibitor. **CLINICAL:** Antiplatelet; antithrombotic (see p. 31C).

ACTION

Rapidly inhibits platelet aggregation by preventing the binding of fibrinogen to GP IIb/IIIa receptor sites on platelets. **Therapeutic Effect:** Prevents closure of treated coronary arteries. Prevents acute cardiac ischemic complications.

PHARMACOKINETICS

Rapidly cleared from plasma. Initial-phase half-life is less than 10 min; second-phase half-life is 30 min. Platelet function generally returns within 48 hrs.

USES

Adjunct to aspirin and heparin therapy to prevent cardiac ischemic complications in pts undergoing percutaneous coronary intervention (PCI) and those with unstable angina not responding to conventional medical therapy when PCI is planned within 24 hrs.

PRECAUTIONS

CONTRAINDICATIONS: Active internal bleeding, arteriovenous malformation or aneurysm, cerebrovascular accident (CVA) with residual neurologic defect, history of CVA (within the past 2 yrs) or oral anticoagulant use within the past 7 days unless PT is less than 1.2 × control, history of vasculitis, hypersensitivity to murine proteins, intracranial neoplasm, prior IV dextran use before or during percutaneous transluminal coronary angioplasty (PTCA), recent surgery or trauma (within the past 6 wks), recent (within the past 6 wks or less) GI or GU bleeding, thrombocytopenia (less than 100,000 cells/mcl), and severe uncontrolled hypertension. **CAUTIONS:** Pts who weigh less than 75 kg; those older than 65 yrs; those with history of GI disease; those receiving thrombolytics, heparin, aspirin, PTCA less than 12 hrs of onset

A

of symptoms for acute MI, prolonged PTCA (longer than 70 min), failed PTCA.

LIFESPAN CONSIDERATIONS:

Pregnancy/Lactation: Unknown if distributed in breast milk. **Pregnancy Category C. Children:** Safety and efficacy not established. **Elderly:** Increased risk of major bleeding.

INTERACTIONS

DRUG: **Heparin, other anticoagulants, thrombolytics**, or **antiplatelet medications** may increase risk of bleeding. **HERBAL:** None significant. **FOOD:** None known. **LAB VALUES:** Increases activated clotting time (ACT), prothrombin time (PT), activated partial thromboplastin time (aPTT); decreases platelet count.

AVAILABILITY (Rx)

INJECTION SOLUTION: 2 mg/ml (5-ml vial).

ADMINISTRATION/HANDLING

IV

Reconstitution • Use 0.2- to 0.22-micron filter; filtering may be done during preparation or at administration. • Bolus dose may be given undiluted. • Withdraw desired dose and further dilute in 250 ml of 0.9% NaCl or D_5W (e.g., 10 mg in 250 ml equals concentration of 40 mcg/ml).

Rate of administration • See Indications/Routes/Dosage.

Administration precautions • Give in separate IV line; do not add any other medication to infusion. • For bolus injection and continuous infusion, use sterile, nonpyrogenic, low protein-binding 0.2- or 0.22-micron filter. • While vascular sheath is in position, maintain pt on complete bed rest with head of bed elevated at 30°. • Maintain affected limb in straight position. • After sheath removal, apply femoral pressure for 30 min, either manually or mechanically, then apply pressure dressing.

Storage • Store vials in refrigerator. • Solution appears clear, colorless. Do not shake. Discard any unused portion left in vial or if preparation contains *any* opaque particles.

IV INCOMPATIBILITY

Administer in separate line; no other medication should be added to infusion solution.

INDICATIONS/ROUTES/DOSAGE

PERCUTANEOUS CORONARY INTERVENTION (PCI)

IV BOLUS: ADULTS: 0.25 mg/kg 10–60 min before angioplasty or atherectomy, then 12-hr IV infusion of 0.125 mcg/kg/min. **Maximum:** 10 mcg/min.

PCI (UNSTABLE ANGINA)

IV BOLUS: ADULTS: 0.25 mg/kg, followed by 18- to 24-hr infusion of 10 mcg/min, ending 1 hr after procedure.

SIDE EFFECTS

FREQUENT: Nausea (16%), hypotension (12%). **OCCASIONAL (9%):** Vomiting. **RARE (3%):** Bradycardia, confusion, dizziness, pain, peripheral edema, UTI.

ADVERSE EFFECTS/ TOXIC REACTIONS

Major bleeding complications may occur; stop infusion immediately. Hypersensitivity reaction may occur. Atrial fibrillation or flutter, pulmonary edema, and complete AV block occur occasionally.

NURSING CONSIDERATIONS

BASELINE ASSESSMENT

Heparin should be discontinued 4 hrs before arterial sheath removal. Maintain pt on bed rest for 6–8 hrs following sheath removal or drug discontinuation, whichever is later. Check platelet count, PT, aPTT before infusion (assess for preexisting blood abnormalities), 2–4 hrs following treatment, and at 24 hrs or before discharge, whichever is first. Check insertion site, distal pulse of affected limb while femoral artery sheath is in place, and then routinely for 6 hrs following femoral artery sheath removal. Minimize need for injections, blood draws, intubations, catheters.

INTERVENTION/EVALUATION

Stop abciximab and/or heparin infusion if any serious bleeding occurs that is uncontrolled by pressure. Assess skin for ecchymosis, petechiae, particularly femoral arterial access, also catheter insertion, arterial and venous puncture, cutdown, needle sites. Handle pt carefully and as infrequently as possible to prevent bleeding. Do not obtain B/P in lower extremities (possible deep vein thrombi). Assess for decrease in B/P, increase in pulse rate, complaint of abdominal or back pain, severe headache, evidence of GI hemorrhage. Monitor ACT, PT, aPTT, platelet counts. Question for increase in discharge during menses. Assess urinary output for hematuria. Monitor for hematoma. Use care in removing any dressing, tape.

Abelcet, *see amphotericin B*

Abilify, *see aripiprazole*

acamprosate

ah-**cam**-pro-sate
(Campral)

CLASSIFICATION

CLINICAL: Alcohol abuse deterrent.

ACTION

Appears to interact with glutamate and gamma-aminobutyric acid neurotransmitter systems centrally, restoring their balance. **Therapeutic Effect:** Reduces alcohol dependence.

PHARMACOKINETICS

Slowly absorbed from GI tract. Steady-state plasma concentrations are reached within 5 days. Does not undergo metabolism. Excreted in urine. **Half-life:** 20–33 hrs.

USES

Maintenance of alcohol abstinence in pts with alcohol dependence who are abstinent at treatment initiation.

PRECAUTIONS

CONTRAINDICATIONS: Severe renal impairment (creatinine clearance of 30 ml/min or less). **CAUTIONS:** Mental depression, renal impairment.

LIFESPAN CONSIDERATIONS:

Pregnancy/Lactation: Unknown if distributed in breast milk. **Pregnancy Category C. Children:** Safety and efficacy not established. **Elderly:** Age-related renal impairment may require dosage adjustment.

INTERACTIONS

DRUG: Naltrexone may increase concentration. **HERBAL:** None significant. **FOOD:** None known. **LAB VALUES:** None known.

AVAILABILITY (Rx)

TABLETS: 333 mg.

ADMINISTRATION/HANDLING

PO

• Do not crush, break enteric-coated tablets. • Give without regard to meals; however, giving with food may aid in compliance of pts who regularly eat three meals daily.

INDICATIONS/ROUTES/DOSAGE

ALCOHOL ABSTINENCE

PO: ADULTS, ELDERLY: Two tablets 3 times a day.

DOSAGE IN RENAL IMPAIRMENT

For pts with creatinine clearance of 30–49 ml/min, dosage is decreased to one tablet 3 times a day. Contraindicated in pts with severe renal impairment (creatinine clearance less than 30 ml/min).

SIDE EFFECTS

FREQUENT (17%): Diarrhea. **OCCASIONAL (6%–4%):** Insomnia, asthenia, fatigue, anxiety, flatulence, nausea, depression, pruritus. **RARE (3%–1%):** Dizziness, anorexia, paresthesia, diaphoresis, dry mouth.

ADVERSE EFFECTS/ TOXIC REACTIONS

Acute renal failure has been reported.

NURSING CONSIDERATIONS

BASELINE ASSESSMENT

Obtain BUN, serum creatinine before treatment. Assess motor responses (agitation, trembling, tension), autonomic responses (cold and clammy hands, diaphoresis).

INTERVENTION/EVALUATION

Monitor pattern of bowel activity and stool consistency. Assess sleep pattern and provide environment conducive to sleep (quiet environment, low lighting). Offer emotional support to anxious pt. Assist with ambulation if dizziness occurs.

PATIENT/FAMILY TEACHING

• Inform pt that medication does not eliminate or diminish withdrawal symptoms. • Avoid tasks that require alertness, motor skills until response to drug is established. • Advise pt that medication helps maintain abstinence only when used as a part of a treatment program that includes counseling and support.

acarbose

ah-**car**-bose

(Prandase ✱, Precose)

Do not confuse Precose with PreCare.

CLASSIFICATION

PHARMACOTHERAPEUTIC: Alpha glucosidase inhibitor. **CLINICAL:** Antidiabetic: Oral (see p. 41C).

ACTION

Delays glucose absorption and digestion of carbohydrates, resulting in a smaller rise in blood glucose concentration after meals. **Therapeutic Effect:** Lowers postprandial hyperglycemia.

USES

Adjunctive therapy to diet in treatment of pts with type 2 diabetes. May be used alone or in combination with other antidiabetic agents.

PRECAUTIONS

CONTRAINDICATIONS: Chronic intestinal diseases associated with marked disorders of digestion or absorption, cirrhosis, colonic ulceration, conditions that may deteriorate as a result of increased gas formation in intestine, diabetic ketoacidosis, hypersensitivity to acarbose, inflammatory bowel disease, partial intestinal obstruction or predisposition to intestinal obstruction, significant renal dysfunction (serum creatinine level greater than 2 mg/dl). **CAUTIONS:** Fever, infection, surgery, trauma (may cause loss of glycemic control). **Pregnancy Category B.**

INTERACTIONS

DRUG: **Digestive enzymes, intestinal absorbents (e.g., charcoal)** reduce acarbose effect. Do not use concurrently. **HERBAL:** None significant. **FOOD:** None known. **LAB VALUES:** May increase serum transaminase levels.

AVAILABILITY (Rx)

TABLETS: 25 mg, 50 mg, 100 mg.

ADMINISTRATION/HANDLING

PO

• Give with the first bite of each main meal.

INDICATIONS/ROUTES/DOSAGE

DIABETES MELLITUS

PO: **ADULTS, ELDERLY:** Initially, 25 mg 3 times a day with first bite of each main meal. May increase at 4- to 8-wk intervals. **Maximum:** For pts weighing more than 60 kg, 100 mg 3 times a day; for pts weighing 60 kg or less, 50 mg 3 times a day.

SIDE EFFECTS

Side effects diminish in frequency and intensity over time. **FREQUENT:** Transient GI disturbances: flatulence (77%), diarrhea (33%), abdominal pain (21%).

ADVERSE EFFECTS/ TOXIC REACTIONS

None known.

NURSING CONSIDERATIONS

BASELINE ASSESSMENT

Check blood glucose level. Discuss lifestyle to determine extent of learning, emotional needs.

INTERVENTION/EVALUATION

Monitor blood glucose, glycosylated hemoglobin, transaminase values, food intake. Assess for hypoglycemia (cool wet skin, tremors, dizziness, anxiety, headache, tachycardia, numbness in mouth, hunger, diplopia) or hyperglycemia (polyuria, polyphagia, polydipsia, nausea, vomiting, dim vision, fatigue, deep rapid breathing). Be alert to conditions that alter glucose requirements: fever, increased activity/stress, surgical procedure.

PATIENT/FAMILY TEACHING

• Do not skip or delay meals. • Check with physician when glucose demands are altered (e.g., fever, infection, trauma, stress, heavy physical activity). • Avoid alcoholic beverages. • Weight control, exercise, hygiene (including foot care), nonsmoking are essential parts of therapy.

Accupril, *see quinapril*

Accutane, *see isotretinoin*

acebutolol ⚑

ah-see-**beaut**-oh-lol

(Apo-acebutolol ♣, Monitan ♣, Novo-acebutolol ♣, Rhotral ♣, Sectral)

Do not confuse Sectral with Factrel or Septra.

◆ CLASSIFICATION

PHARMACOTHERAPEUTIC: Beta$_1$-adrenergic blocker. **CLINICAL:** Antihypertensive, antiarrhythmic (see pp. 15C, 64C).

ACTION

Competitively blocks beta$_1$-adrenergic receptors in cardiac tissue. Reduces rate of spontaneous firing of sinus pacemaker, delays AV conduction. **Therapeutic Effect:** Slows heart rate, decreases cardiac output, decreases B/P, exhibits antiarrhythmic activity.

PHARMACOKINETICS

Route	Onset	Peak	Duration
PO (hypotensive)	1–1.5 hrs	2–8 hrs	24 hrs
PO (antiarrhythmic)	1 hr	4–6 hrs	10 hrs

Well absorbed from GI tract. Protein binding: 26%. Undergoes extensive first-pass liver metabolism to active metabolite. Eliminated via bile, secreted into GI tract via intestine, excreted in urine. Removed by hemodialysis. **Half-life:** 3–4 hrs; metabolite, 8–13 hrs.

USES

Management of mild to moderate hypertension. Used alone or in combination with other antihypertensives. Management of cardiac arrhythmias (primarily premature ventricular contractions [PVCs]). **OFF-LABEL:** Treatment of anxiety, chronic angina pectoris, hypertrophic cardiomyopathy, MI, pheochromocytoma, syndrome of mitral valve prolapse, thyrotoxicosis, tremors.

PRECAUTIONS

CONTRAINDICATIONS: Cardiogenic shock, heart block greater than first degree, overt heart failure, severe bradycardia. **CAUTIONS:** Renal/hepatic impairment, peripheral vascular disease, hyperthyroidism, diabetes, inadequate cardiac function, bronchospastic disease.

⌛ LIFESPAN CONSIDERATIONS:

Pregnancy/Lactation: Readily crosses placenta; distributed in breast milk. May produce bradycardia, apnea, hypoglycemia, hypothermia during delivery, low birth-weight infants. **Pregnancy Category B (D if used in second or third trimester). Children:** No age-related precautions noted. Dosage not established. **Elderly:** Age-related peripheral vascular disease requires caution.

INTERACTIONS

DRUG: Diuretics, other hypertensives may increase hypotensive effect; **sympathomimetics, xanthines** may mutually inhibit effects; may mask symptoms of hypoglycemia; may prolong hypoglycemic effect of **insulin, oral hypoglycemics. HERBAL: Ginseng, yohimbe** may decrease antihypertensive effect. **FOOD:** None known. **LAB VALUES:** May increase serum ANA titer, AST, ALT, alkaline phosphatase, LDH, bilirubin, BUN, creatinine, potassium, uric acid, lipoproteins, triglycerides.

AVAILABILITY (Rx)

CAPSULES: 200 mg, 400 mg.

ADMINISTRATION/HANDLING

PO

- May be given without regard to meals.

INDICATIONS/ROUTES/DOSAGE

MILD TO MODERATE HYPERTENSION

PO: ADULTS: Initially, 400 mg/day in 12 divided doses. Range: Up to 1,200 mg/day in 2 divided doses. Maintenance: 400–800 mg/day.

VENTRICULAR ARRHYTHMIAS

PO: ADULTS: Initially, 200 mg q12h. Increase gradually to 600–1,200 mg/day in 2 divided doses. **ELDERLY:** Initially, 200–400 mg/day. **Maximum:** 800 mg/day.

ANGINA

PO: ADULTS: 600–1,600 mg in 2–3 divided doses.

DOSAGE IN RENAL IMPAIRMENT

Dosage is modified based on creatinine clearance.

Creatinine Clearance	% of Usual Dosage
Less than 50 ml/min	50
Less than 25 ml/min	25

SIDE EFFECTS

FREQUENT: Hypotension (manifested as dizziness, nausea, diaphoresis), headache, cold extremities, fatigue, constipation, diarrhea. **OCCASIONAL:** Insomnia, urinary frequency, impotence or decreased libido. **RARE:** Rash, arthralgia, myalgia, confusion (esp. the elderly), altered taste.

ADVERSE EFFECTS/ TOXIC REACTIONS

Abrupt withdrawal may result in diaphoresis, palpitations, headache, tremors. Administration may precipitate CHF or MI in pts with heart disease; thyroid storm in those with thyrotoxicosis; or peripheral ischemia in those with existing peripheral vascular disease. Overdose may produce profound bradycardia, hypotension. Hypoglycemia may occur in pts with previously controlled diabetes. Signs of thrombocytopenia, such as unusual bleeding or bruising, occur rarely.

NURSING CONSIDERATIONS

BASELINE ASSESSMENT

Assess B/P, apical pulse immediately before drug administration. If pulse is 60 beats/min or less or systolic B/P is less than 90 mm Hg, withhold medication, contact physician. **Antianginal:** Record onset, type (sharp, dull, squeezing), radiation, location, intensity and duration of anginal pain, precipitating factors (exertion, emotional stress).

INTERVENTION/EVALUATION

Monitor B/P for hypotension, respiration for shortness of breath. Assess pulse for quality, rate, rhythm. Monitor EKG for cardiac arrhythmias, shortening of QT interval, prolongation of PR interval. Assess frequency/consistency of stools. Assess for evidence of CHF: dyspnea (particularly on exertion or lying down), night cough, peripheral edema, distended neck veins, decreased urine output, weight gain. Assess for nausea, diaphoresis, headache, fatigue.

PATIENT/FAMILY TEACHING

• Do not abruptly discontinue medication. • Compliance with therapy regimen is essential to control hypertension, arrhythmias. • Report shortness of breath, excessive fatigue, weight gain, prolonged dizziness, headache. • Do not use nasal decongestants, OTC cold preparations (stimulants) without physician approval. • Restrict salt, alcohol intake.

acetaminophen

ah-see-tah-**min**-oh-fen

(Abenol ✤, Acephen, Apo-Acetaminophen ✤, Atasol ✤, Feverall, Genapap, Genapap Infant, Mapap, Tempra ✤, Tylenol, Tylenol Arthritis Pain, Tylenol Extra Strength)

Do not confuse Fioricet with Fiorinol, Hycet with Hycodan, Percocet with Percodan, or Tylenol with Tuinol.

FIXED-COMBINATION(S)

Anexsia: acetaminophen/hydrocodone: 500 mg/5 mg, 650 mg/7.5 mg, 660 mg/10 mg. **Balacet 325:** acetaminophen/propoxyphene napsylate: 325 mg/100 mg. **Capital with Codeine, Tylenol with Codeine:** acetaminophen/codeine: 120 mg/12 mg per 5 ml. **Darvocet-N:** acetaminophen/propoxyphene: 325 mg/50 mg, 650 mg/100 mg. **Fioricet:** acetaminophen/caffeine/butalbital: 325 mg/40 mg/50 mg. **Hycet:** acetaminophen/hydrocodone: 325 mg/7.5 mg per 15 ml. **Lortab:** acetaminophen/hydrocodone: 500 mg/2.5 mg; 500 mg/5 mg; 500 mg/7.5 mg. **Lortab Elixir:** acetaminophen/hydrocodone: 167 mg/2.5 mg per

5 ml. **Norco:** acetaminophen/hydrocodone: 325 mg/10 mg. **Percocet, Roxicet:** acetaminophen/oxycodone: 325 mg/5 mg. **Tylenol with Codeine:** acetaminophen/codeine: 300 mg/15 mg, 300 mg/30 mg, 300 mg/60 mg. **Tylox:** acetaminophen/oxycodone: 500 mg/5 mg. **Ultracet:** acetaminophen/tramadol: 325 mg/37.5 mg. **Vicodin:** acetaminophen/hydrocodone: 500 mg/5 mg. **Vicodin ES:** acetaminophen/hydrocodone: 750 mg/7.5 mg. **Vicodin HP:** acetaminophen/hydrocodone: 660 mg/10 mg. **Xodol:** acetaminophen/hydrocodone: 300 mg/5 mg. **Zydone:** acetaminophen/hydrocodone: 400 mg/5 mg; 400 mg/7.5 mg; 400 mg/10 mg.

CLASSIFICATION

PHARMACOTHERAPEUTIC: Central analgesic. **CLINICAL:** Non-narcotic analgesic, antipyretic.

ACTION

Appears to inhibit prostaglandin synthesis in the CNS and, to a lesser extent, block pain impulses through peripheral action. Acts centrally on hypothalamic heat-regulating center, producing peripheral vasodilation (heat loss, skin erythema, diaphoresis). **Therapeutic Effect:** Results in antipyresis. Produces analgesic effect.

PHARMACOKINETICS

Route	Onset	Peak	Duration
PO	15–30 min	1–1.5 hrs	4–6 hrs

Rapidly, completely absorbed from GI tract; rectal absorption variable. Protein binding: 20%–50%. Widely distributed to most body tissues. Metabolized in liver; excreted in urine. Removed by hemodialysis. **Half-life:** 1–4 hrs (half-life is increased in those with hepatic disease, elderly, neonates; decreased in children).

USES

Relief of mild to moderate pain, fever.

PRECAUTIONS

CONTRAINDICATIONS: Active alcoholism, liver disease, or viral hepatitis, all of which increase the risk of hepatotoxicity. **CAUTIONS:** Sensitivity to acetaminophen, severe renal impairment, phenylketonuria, G6PD deficiency.

LIFESPAN CONSIDERATIONS:

Pregnancy/Lactation: Crosses placenta; distributed in breast milk. Routinely used in all stages of pregnancy, appears safe for short-term use. **Pregnancy Category B. Children/Elderly:** No age-related precautions noted.

INTERACTIONS

DRUG: **Alcohol** (chronic use), **liver enzymes inducers (e.g., cimetidine), hepatotoxic medications (e.g., phenytoin)** may increase risk of hepatotoxicity with prolonged high dose or single toxic dose. May increase risk of bleeding with **warfarin** with regular use. **HERBAL:** **St. John's wort** may decrease blood levels. **FOOD:** None known. **LAB VALUES:** May increase serum AST, ALT, bilirubin, prothrombin levels (may indicate hepatotoxicity). Therapeutic serum level: 10–30 mcg/ml; toxic serum level: greater than 200 mcg/ml.

AVAILABILITY (OTC)

CAPLETS (GENAPAP, TYLENOL): 500 mg. **ELIXIR:** 160 mg/5 ml. **LIQUID (ORAL [TYLENOL EXTRA STRENGTH]):** 500 mg/15 ml. **SOLUTION (ORAL DROPS [GENAPAP INFANT]):** 80 mg/0.8 ml. **SUPPOSITORY:** (Acephen): 120 mg, 325 mg, 650 mg, (Feverall): 80 mg, 120 mg, 325 mg, 650 mg. **TABLETS (GENAPAP, MAPAP, TYLENOL):** 325 mg,

500 mg. **TABLETS (CHEWABLE [GENAPAP, MAPAP, TYLENOL]):** 80 mg. **CAPLETS: (EXTENDED-RELEASE [MAPAP, TYLENOL ARTHRITIS PAIN]):** 650 mg. **CAPSULES: (MAPAP):** 500 mg.

ADMINISTRATION/HANDLING

PO

- Give without regard to meals.
- Tablets may be crushed.

RECTAL

- Moisten suppository with cold water before inserting well up into rectum.

INDICATIONS/ROUTES/DOSAGE

ANALGESIA AND ANTIPYRESIS

PO: ADULTS, ELDERLY, CHILDREN 13 YRS AND OLDER: 325–650 mg q4–6h or 1 g 3–4 times/day. **Maximum:** 4 g/day. **CHILDREN 12 YRS AND YOUNGER:** 10–15 mg/kg/dose q4–6h as needed. **Maximum:** 5 doses/24 hrs. **NEONATES:** 10–15 mg/kg/dose q6–8h as needed. **RECTAL: ADULTS:** 650 mg q4–6h. **Maximum:** 6 doses/24 hrs. **CHILDREN:** 10–20 mg/kg/dose q4–6h as needed. **NEONATES:** 10–15 mg/kg/dose q6–8h as needed.

DOSAGE IN RENAL IMPAIRMENT

Creatinine Clearance	Frequency
10–50 ml/min	q6h
Less than 10 ml/min	q8h

SIDE EFFECTS

RARE: Hypersensitivity reaction.

ADVERSE EFFECTS/ TOXIC REACTIONS

EARLY SIGNS OF ACETAMINOPHEN TOXICITY: Anorexia, nausea, diaphoresis, fatigue within first 12–24 hrs. **LATER SIGNS OF TOXICITY:** Vomiting, right upper quadrant tenderness, elevated hepatic funtion tests within 48–72 hrs after ingestion. **ANTIDOTE:** Acetylcysteine.

NURSING CONSIDERATIONS

BASELINE ASSESSMENT

If given for analgesia, assess onset, type, location, duration of pain. Effect of medication is reduced if full pain response recurs prior to next dose. **Fixed-Combination:** Obtain vital signs before giving medication. If respirations are 12/min or less (20/min or less in children), withhold medication, contact physician.

INTERVENTION/EVALUATION

Assess for clinical improvement and relief of pain, fever. Therapeutic serum level: 10–30 mcg/ml; toxic serum level: greater than 200 mcg/ml.

PATIENT/FAMILY TEACHING

- Consult physician for use in children younger than 2 yrs; oral use longer than 5 days (children), longer than 10 days (adults), or fever longer than 3 days.
- Severe/recurrent pain or high/continuous fever may indicate serious illness.

*acetaZOLAMIDE

ah-seat-ah-**zole**-ah-myd

(Apo-Acetazolamide ✤, Diamox, Diamox Sequels)

Do not confuse acetazolamide with acetohexamide, or Diamox with Trimox.

CLASSIFICATION

PHARMACOTHERAPEUTIC: Carbonic anhydrase inhibitor. **CLINICAL:** Antiglaucoma, anticonvulsant, diuretic, urinary alkalinizer (see p. 50C).

ACTION

Reduces formation of hydrogen and bicarbonate ions by inhibiting the enzyme carbonic anhydrase. **Therapeutic Effect:** Increases excretion of sodium, potassium, bicarbonate, and water in kidney; decreases formation of aqueous humor in eye; retards abnormal discharge from CNS neurons.

USES

Treatment of glaucoma, control of intraocular pressure (IOP) before surgery, adjunct in management of seizures, edema, decreases incidence/severity of symptoms associated with acute altitude sickness. **OFF-LABEL:** Lowers IOP in treatment of malignant glaucoma, treatment of toxicity of weakly acidic medications, prevents uric acid/renal calculi by alkalinizing the urine.

PRECAUTIONS

CONTRAINDICATIONS: Hypersensitivity to sulfonamides, severe renal disease, adrenal insufficiency, hypochloremic acidosis. **CAUTIONS:** History of hypercalcemia, diabetes mellitus, gout, concurrent digoxin therapy, obstructive pulmonary disease. **Pregnancy Category C.**

INTERACTIONS

DRUG: May increase **digoxin** levels (due to hypokalemia). May increase effects/toxicity of **amphetamines;** may decrease effects of **methenamine**. **HERBAL:** None significant. **FOOD:** None known. **LAB VALUES:** May increase serum ammonia, bilirubin, glucose, chloride, uric acid, calcium; may decrease serum bicarbonate, potassium.

AVAILABILITY (Rx)

INJECTION, POWDER FOR RECONSTITUTION: 500 mg. **TABLETS (Diamox):** 125 mg, 250 mg.

CAPSULES (SUSTAINED-RELEASE [Diamox Sequels]): 500 mg.

IV INCOMPATIBILITY

Diltiazem.

IV COMPATIBILITIES

Cimetidine, ranitidine.

INDICATIONS/ROUTES/DOSAGE

GLAUCOMA

IV: ADULTS, ELDERLY: 250–500 mg; may repeat in 2–4 hrs, then continue with oral therapy. **CHILDREN:** 5–10 mg/kg q6h. **Maximum:** 1 g a day.

PO: ADULTS, ELDERLY: 250 mg 1–4 times a day. **CHILDREN:** 8–30 mg/kg/day in divided doses q8h.

PO (EXTENDED-RELEASE): ADULTS, ELDERLY: 500 mg twice a day.

EDEMA

PO, IV: ADULTS: 250–375 mg a day. **CHILDREN:** 5 mg/kg/dose once daily.

EPILEPSY

PO: ADULTS, ELDERLY, CHILDREN: 8–30 mg/kg/day in up to 4 divided doses. Sustained-release formulation not recommended for epilepsy.

ALTITUDE SICKNESS

PO: ADULTS: 250 mg q8–12h or 500 mg sustained-release capsule q12–24h. Begin 24–48 hrs before and continue during ascent and for at least 48 hrs following arrival at high altitude.

DOSAGE IN RENAL IMPAIRMENT

Creatinine Clearance	Dosage Interval
10–50 ml/min	q12h
Less than 10 ml/min	Not recommended

SIDE EFFECTS

FREQUENT: Fatigue, diarrhea, increased urination/frequency, decreased appetite/weight, altered taste (metallic), nausea, vomiting, paresthesia, circumoral numbness. **OCCASIONAL:** Depression, drowsiness. **RARE:** Headache, photosensitivity, confusion, tinnitus, severe muscle weakness, loss of taste.

ADVERSE EFFECTS/ TOXIC REACTIONS

Long-term therapy may result in acidotic state. Nephrotoxicity/hepatotoxicity occurs occasionally, manifested as dark urine/stools, pain in lower back, jaundice, dysuria, crystalluria, renal colic/calculi. Bone marrow depression may be manifested as aplastic anemia, thrombocytopenia, thrombocytopenic purpura, leukopenia, agranulocytosis, hemolytic anemia.

NURSING CONSIDERATIONS

BASELINE ASSESSMENT

Glaucoma: Assess affected pupil for dilation, response to light. **Epilepsy:** Obtain history of seizure disorder (length, intensity, duration of seizure, presence of aura, level of consciousness [LOC]).

INTERVENTION/EVALUATION

Monitor for acidosis (headache, lethargy progressing to drowsiness, CNS depression, Kussmaul's respiration).

PATIENT/FAMILY TEACHING

- Report tingling/tremor in hands or feet, unusual bleeding or bruising, unexplained fever, sore throat, flank pain.

*acetoHEXAMIDE

(Dymelor)

See Antidiabetics

acetylcysteine (*N*-acetylcysteine)

ah-sea-tyl-**sis**-teen

(Acetadote, Mucomyst, Parvolex ✤)

Do not confuse acetylcysteine with acetylcholine, or Mucomyst with Mucinex.

CLASSIFICATION

PHARMACOTHERAPEUTIC: Respiratory inhalant, intratracheal. **CLINICAL:** Mucolytic, antidote.

ACTION

Splits linkage of mucoproteins, reducing viscosity of pulmonary secretions. **Therapeutic Effect:** Facilitates removal of pulmonary secretions by coughing, postural drainage, mechanical means. Protects against acetaminophen overdose-induced hepatotoxicity.

USES

Inhalation: Adjunctive treatment for abnormally viscid mucous secretions present in acute and chronic bronchopulmonary disease and pulmonary complication of cystic fibrosis, tracheostomy care. **Injection, oral:** Antidote in acute acetaminophen toxicity. **OFF-LABEL:** Prevention of renal damage from dyes given during certain diagnostic tests (such as CT scans). Treatment *H. pylori* infection.

PRECAUTIONS

CONTRAINDICATIONS: None known. **CAUTIONS:** Bronchial asthma, elderly, debilitated with severe respiratory insufficiency. **Pregnancy Category B.**

INTERACTIONS

DRUG: None significant. **HERBAL:** None significant. **FOOD:** None known. **LAB VALUES:** None known.

AVAILABILITY (Rx)

INHALATION SOLUTION (MUCOMYST): 10% (100 mg/ml), 20% (200 mg/ml). **INJECTION SOLUTION (ACETADOTE):** 20% (200 mg/ml).

ADMINISTRATION/HANDLING

IV

- Give 3 infusions of different strengths: first dose (150 mg/kg) in 200 ml D_5W and infused over 60 min, second dose (50 mg/kg) in 500 ml D_5W and infused over 4 hrs, third dose (100 mg/kg) in 1,000 ml D_5W and infused over 16 hrs.

PO
• Give as a 5% solution. • Dilute 20% solution 1:3 with cola, orange juice, other soft drink. • Give within 1 hr of preparation.

INHALATION, NEBULIZATION
• May administer either undiluted or diluted with 0.9% NaCl.

INDICATIONS/ROUTES/DOSAGE

BRONCHOPULMONARY DISEASE

INHALATION, NEBULIZATION

◀ **ALERT** ▶ Bronchodilators should be given 10–15 min before acetylcysteine.
ADULTS, ELDERLY, CHILDREN: 3–5 ml (20% solution) 3–4 times a day or 6–10 ml (10% solution) 3–4 times a day. Range: 1–10 ml (20% solution) q2–6h or 2–20 ml (10% solution) q2–6h. **INFANTS:** 1–2 ml (20%) or 2–4 ml (10%) 3–4 times a day.
INTRATRACHEAL: ADULTS, CHILDREN: 1–2 ml of 10% or 20% solution instilled into tracheostomy q1–4h.

ACETAMINOPHEN OVERDOSE

PO (ORAL SOLUTION 5%): ADULTS, ELDERLY, CHILDREN: Loading dose of 140 mg/kg, followed in 4 hrs by maintenance dose of 70 mg/kg q4h for 17 additional doses (or until acetaminophen assay reveals nontoxic level). Repeat dose if emesis occurs within 1 hr of administration.

IV: ADULTS, ELDERLY, CHILDREN: 150 mg/kg infused over 60 min, then 50 mg/kg infused over 4 hrs, then 100 mg/kg infused over 16 hrs. See Administration/Handling.

PREVENTION OF RENAL DAMAGE

PO: ADULTS, ELDERLY: 600 mg twice a day for 4 doses starting the day before the procedure. Hydrate pt with 0.9% NaCl concurrently.

SIDE EFFECTS

FREQUENT: Inhalation: Stickiness on face, transient unpleasant odor. **OCCASIONAL: Inhalation:** Increased bronchial secretions, throat irritation, nausea, vomiting, rhinorrhea. **RARE: Inhalation:** Rash. **Oral:** Facial edema, bronchospasm, wheezing.

ADVERSE EFFECTS/ TOXIC REACTIONS

Large doses may produce severe nausea/vomiting.

NURSING CONSIDERATIONS

BASELINE ASSESSMENT

Mucolytic: Assess pretreatment respirations for rate, depth, rhythm.

INTERVENTION/EVALUATION

If bronchospasm occurs, discontinue treatment, notify physician; bronchodilator may be added to therapy. Monitor rate, depth, rhythm, type of respiration (abdominal, thoracic). Check sputum for color, consistency, amount.

PATIENT/FAMILY TEACHING

• Slight, disagreeable odor from solution may be noticed during initial administration but disappears quickly. • Explain importance of adequate hydration. • Teach proper coughing and deep breathing.

Aciphex, *see rabeprazole*

Actiq, *see fentanyl*

Activase, *see alteplase*

Actonel, *see risedronate*

Actos, *see pioglitazone*

acyclovir

aye-**sigh**-klo-veer
(Apo-Acyclovir ♣, Zovirax)
Do not confuse Zovirax with Zostrix, Zyvox.

♦CLASSIFICATION

PHARMACOTHERAPEUTIC: Synthetic nucleoside. **CLINICAL:** Antiviral (see p. 64C).

ACTION

Converts to acyclovir triphosphate, becoming part of DNA chain. **Therapeutic Effect:** Interferes with DNA synthesis and viral replication. Virustatic.

PHARMACOKINETICS

Poorly absorbed from GI tract; minimal absorption following topical application. Protein binding: 9%–36%. Widely distributed. Partially metabolized in liver. Excreted primarily in urine. Removed by hemodialysis. **Half-life:** 2.5 hrs (increased in renal impairment).

USES

Oral and/or parenteral: Treatment of herpes infections including genital (initial, recurrent), simplex (mucotaneous, neonatal, encephalitis), zoster (chickenpox, immunocompromised pts, shingles). **Topical:** Treatment of initial herpes simplex (genital, mucutaneous). **OFF-LABEL: Oral, parenteral:** Prophylaxis of herpes simplex and herpes zoster infections, infectious mononucleosis. **Topical:** Treatment adjunct for herpes zoster infections.

PRECAUTIONS

CONTRAINDICATIONS: Use in neonates when acyclovir is reconstituted with bacteriostatic water containing benzyl alcohol. **CAUTIONS:** Renal/hepatic impairment, dehydration, fluid/electrolyte imbalance, concurrent use of nephrotoxic agents, neurologic abnormalities.

LIFESPAN CONSIDERATIONS:

Pregnancy/Lactation: Crosses placenta; distributed in breast milk. **Pregnancy Category B. Children:** Safety and efficacy in children younger than 2 yrs not established (younger than 1 yr for IV use). **Elderly:** Age-related renal impairment may require decreased dosage.

INTERACTIONS

DRUG: Probenecid may increase half-life. **Nephrotoxic medications (e.g., aminoglycosides)** may increase nephrotoxicity. May decrease **varicella virus vaccine** effectiveness. **HERBAL:** None significant. **FOOD:** None known. **LAB VALUES:** May increase BUN, serum creatinine concentrations.

AVAILABILITY (Rx)

INJECTION, SOLUTION: 25 mg/ml. 50 mg/ml. **INJECTION, POWDER FOR RECONSTITUTION:** 500 mg, 1,000 mg. **OINTMENT:** 5%. **SUSPENSION, ORAL:** 200 mg/5 ml. **TABLETS:** 400 mg, 800 mg.

CAPSULES: 200 mg.

ADMINISTRATION/HANDLING

IV

Reconstitution • Add 10 ml Sterile Water for Injection to each 500-mg vial (50 mg/ml). Do not use Bacteriostatic Water for Injection containing benzyl alcohol or parabens (will cause precipitate). • Shake well until solution is clear. • Further dilute with at least 100 ml D_5W

or 0.9 NaCl. Final concentration should be 7 mg/ml or less.

Rate of administration • Infuse over at least 1 hr (renal tubular damage may occur with too rapid rate). • Maintain adequate hydration during infusion and for 2 hrs following IV administration.

Storage • Store vials at room temperature • Solutions of 50 mg/ml stable for 12 hrs at room temperature; may form precipitate if refrigerated. Potency not affected by precipitate and redissolution. • IV infusion (piggyback) stable for 24 hrs at room temperature. Yellow discoloration does not affect potency.

PO

• May give without regard to food. • Do not crush/break capsules. • Store capsules at room temperature.

TOPICAL

• Avoid eye contact. • Use finger cot/rubber glove to prevent autoinoculation.

IV INCOMPATIBILITIES

Aztreonam (Azactam), cefepime (Maxipime), diltiazem (Cardizem), dobutamine (Dobutrex), dopamine (Intropin), levofloxacin (Levaquin), lipids, meropenem (Merrem IV), ondansetron (Zofran), piperacillin and tazobactam (Zosyn), total parenteral nutrition (TPN).

IV COMPATIBILITIES

Allopurinol (Alloprim), amikacin (Amikin), ampicillin, cefazolin (Ancef), cefotaxime (Claforan), ceftazidime (Fortaz), ceftriaxone (Rocephin), cimetidine (Tagamet), clindamycin (Cleocin), famotidine (Pepcid), fluconazole (Diflucan), gentamicin, heparin, hydromorphone (Dilaudid), imipenem (Primaxin), lorazepam (Ativan), magnesium sulfate, methylprednisolone (SoluMedrol), metoclopramide (Reglan), metronidazole (Flagyl), morphine, multivitamins, potassium chloride, propofol (Diprivan), ranitidine (Zantac), vancomycin.

INDICATIONS/ROUTES/DOSAGE

GENITAL HERPES (INITIAL EPISODE)

IV: ADULTS, ELDERLY, CHILDREN 12 YRS AND OLDER: 5 mg/kg q8h for 5–7 days.

PO: ADULTS, ELDERLY, CHILDREN 12 YRS AND OLDER: 200 mg q4h 5 times a day for 10 days or 400 mg 3 times a day for 5–10 days.

GENITAL HERPES (RECURRENT)

Intermittent Therapy

PO: ADULTS, ELDERLY, CHILDREN 12 YRS AND OLDER: 200 mg q4h 5 times a day for 5 days or 400 mg 3 times a day for 5–10 days.

Chronic Supressive Therapy

PO: ADULTS, ELDERLY, CHILDREN 12 YRS AND OLDER: 400 mg 2 times a day or 200 mg 3–5 times a day for up to 12 mos. **CHILDREN**, 80 mg/kg/day in 3 divided doses. **Maximum:** 1 g/day.

HERPES SIMPLEX MUCOCUTANEOUS

PO: ADULTS, ELDERLY: 400 mg 5 times/day for 7–14 days.

IV: ADULTS, ELDERLY, CHILDREN 12 YRS AND OLDER: 5 mg/kg/dose q8h for 7–14 days. **CHILDREN YOUNGER THAN 12 YRS:** 10 mg/kg q8h for 7 days.

HERPES SIMPLEX NEONATAL

IV: CHILDREN YOUNGER THAN 4 MOS: 10 mg/kg q8h for 10 days.

HERPES SIMPLEX ENCEPHALITIS

IV: ADULTS, ELDERLY, CHILDREN 12 YRS AND OLDER: 10 mg/kg q8h for 10 days. **CHILDREN 3 MOS–YOUNGER THAN 12 YRS:** 20 mg/kg q8h for 10 days.

HERPES ZOSTER (CAUSED BY VARICELLA)

IV: ADULTS, ELDERLY, CHILDREN 12 YRS AND OLDER: 10 mg/kg q8h for 7 days. **CHILDREN YOUNGER THAN 12 YRS:** 20 mg/kg q8h for 7 days.

HERPES ZOSTER (SHINGLES)

PO: ADULTS, ELDERLY, CHILDREN 12 YRS AND OLDER: 800 mg q4h 5 times a day for 7–10 days.

HERPES SIMPLEX (COLD SORES)

TOPICAL: ADULTS, ELDERLY: Apply to affected area 3–6 times a day for 7 days.

VARICELLA (CHICKENPOX)

PO: ADULTS, ELDERLY, CHILDREN OLDER THAN 12 YRS OR CHILDREN 2–12 YRS, WEIGHING 40 KG OR MORE: 800 mg 4 times a day for 5 days. **CHILDREN 2–12 YRS, WEIGHING LESS THAN 40 KG:** 20 mg/kg 4 times a day for 5 days. **Maximum:** 800 mg/dose. **CHILDREN YOUNGER THAN 2 YRS:** 80 mg/kg/day.

DOSAGE IN RENAL IMPAIRMENT

Dosage and frequency are modified based on severity of infection and degree of renal impairment.

PO: Normal dose 200 mg q4h.

Creatinine clearance greater than 10 ml/min: Give usual dose and at normal interval, 200 mg q4h. **Creatinine clearance 10 ml/min and less:** 200 mg q12h.

PO: Normal dose 400 mg q12h.

Creatinine clearance greater than 10 ml/min: Give usual dose and at normal interval, 400 mg q12h. **Creatinine clearance 10 ml/min and less:** 200 mg q12h.

PO: Normal dose 800 mg q4h.

Creatinine clearance greater than 25 ml/min: Give usual dose and at normal interval, 800 mg q4h. **Creatinine clearance 10–25 ml/min:** 800 mg q8h. **Creatinine clearance less than 10 ml/min:** 800 mg q12h.

IV:

Creatinine Clearance	Dosage Percent	Dosage Interval
Greater than 50 ml/min	100	8 hrs
25–50 ml/min	100	12 hrs
10–24 ml/min	100	24 hrs
Less than 10 ml/min	50	24 hrs

SIDE EFFECTS

FREQUENT: Parenteral (9%–7%): Phlebitis or inflammation at IV site, nausea, vomiting. **Topical (28%):** Burning, stinging. **OCCASIONAL: Parenteral (3%):** Pruritus, rash, urticaria. **Oral (12%–6%):** Malaise, nausea. **Topical (4%):** Pruritus. **RARE: Oral (3%–1%):** Vomiting, rash, diarrhea, headache. **Parenteral (2%–1%):** Confusion, hallucinations, seizures, tremors. **Topical (less than 1%):** Rash.

ADVERSE EFFECTS/ TOXIC REACTIONS

Rapid parenteral administration, excessively high doses, or fluid and electrolyte imbalance may produce renal failure (abdominal pain, decreased urination, decreased appetite, increased thirst, nausea, vomiting). Toxicity not reported with oral or topical use.

NURSING CONSIDERATIONS

BASELINE ASSESSMENT

Question for history of allergies, particularly to acyclovir. Assess herpes simplex lesions before treatment to compare baseline with treatment effect.

INTERVENTION/EVALUATION

Assess IV site for phlebitis (heat, pain, red streaking over vein). Evaluate cutaneous lesions. Ensure adequate ventilation. Manage chickenpox and disseminated herpes zoster with strict isolation. Provide analgesics and comfort measures; esp. exhausting to elderly. Encourage fluids.

PATIENT/FAMILY TEACHING

• Drink adequate fluids. • Do not touch lesions with fingers to prevent spreading infection to new site. • **Genital Herpes:** Continue therapy for full length of treatment. • Space doses evenly. • Use finger cot/rubber glove to apply topical ointment. • Avoid sexual intercourse during duration of lesions to prevent infecting partner. • Acyclovir does not cure herpes infections. • Pap smear should be done at least annually due to increased risk of cervical cancer in women with genital herpes.

A

Adalat, *see nifedipine*

adalimumab

ah-dah-**lim**-you-mab
(Humira)

CLASSIFICATION

PHARMACOTHERAPEUTIC: Monoclonal antibody. **CLINICAL:** Rheumatoid arthritis agent.

ACTION

Binds specifically to tumor necrosis factor (TNF) alpha cell, blocking its interaction with cell surface TNF receptors. **Therapeutic Effect:** Reduces inflammation, tenderness, swelling of joints; slows or prevents progressive destruction of joints in rheumatoid arthritis.

PHARMACOKINETICS

Half-life: 10–20 days.

USES

Reduces signs, symptoms, progression of structural damage and improves physical function in adults with moderate to severe rheumatoid arthritis unresponsive to other disease-modifying antirheumatic drugs. First-line treatment of moderate to severe rheumatoid arthritis, treatment of psoriatic arthritis, treatment of ankylosing spondylitis.

PRECAUTIONS

CONTRAINDICATIONS: Active infections. **CAUTIONS:** History of sensitivity to monoclonal antibodies, cardiovascular disease, pregnancy, preexisting or recent-onset CNS demyelinating disorders, elderly.

LIFESPAN CONSIDERATIONS:

Pregnancy/Lactation: Unknown if excreted in breast milk. **Pregnancy Category B. Children:** Safety and efficacy not established. **Elderly:** Cautious use due to increased risk of serious infection and malignancy.

INTERACTIONS

DRUG: Anakinra may increase risk of infections. May decrease efficacy of immune response with **live vaccines. Methotrexate** reduces the absorption of adalimumab by 29%–40%, but dosage adjustment is unnecessary if given concurrently. **HERBAL:** None significant. **FOOD:** None known. **LAB VALUES:** May increase levels of serum cholesterol, other lipids, and alkaline phosphatase.

AVAILABILITY (Rx)

INJECTION SOLUTION: 40 mg/0.8 ml in prefilled syringes.

ADMINISTRATION/HANDLING

SUBCUTANEOUS

• Refrigerate; do not freeze. • Discard unused portion. • Rotate injection sites. Give new injection at least 1 inch from an old site and never into area where skin is tender, bruised, red, or hard.

INDICATIONS/ROUTES/DOSAGE

RHEUMATOID ARTHRITIS

SUBCUTANEOUS: ADULTS, ELDERLY: 40 mg every other week. Dose may be increased to 40 mg/wk in those not taking methotrexate.

ANKYLOSING SPONDYLITIS, PSORIATIC ARTHRITIS

SUBCUTANEOUS: ADULTS, ELDERLY: 40 mg every other week.

SIDE EFFECTS

FREQUENT(20%): Injection site erythema, pruritus, pain, and swelling. **OCCASIONAL (12%–9%):** Headache, rash, sinusitis, nausea. **RARE (7%–5%):** Abdominal or back pain, hypertension.

ADVERSE EFFECTS/ TOXIC REACTIONS

Hypersensitivity reactions, infections (primarily upper respiratory tract, bronchitis, urinary tract) occur rarely. More serious infections (pneumonia, tuberculosis, cellulitis, pyelonephritis, septic arthritis) also occur rarely.

NURSING CONSIDERATIONS

BASELINE ASSESSMENT

Assess onset, type, location, duration of pain or inflammation. Inspect appearance of affected joints for immobility, deformities, skin condition. If pt is to self-administer, instruct on subcutaneous injection technique, including areas of the body acceptable for injection sites.

INTERVENTION/EVALUATION

Monitor lab values, particularly alkaline phosphatase. Assess for therapeutic response: relief of pain, stiffness, swelling, increased joint mobility, reduced joint tenderness, improved grip strength.

PATIENT/FAMILY TEACHING

• Injection site reaction generally occurs in first month of treatment and decreases in frequency during continued therapy. • Do not receive live vaccines during treatment.

adefovir

add-eh-**foe**-vir
(Hepsera)

FIXED-COMBINATION(S)

Epzicom: abacavir/lamivudine (antiretroviral): 600 mg/300 mg. **Trizivir:** abacavir/lamivudine (antiretroviral)/zidovudine (antiretroviral): 300 mg/150 mg/300 mg.

CLASSIFICATION

PHARMACOTHERAPEUTIC: Antiviral. **CLINICAL:** Hepatitis B agent.

ACTION

Inhibits DNA polymerase, an enzyme, causing DNA chain termination after its incorporation into viral DNA. **Therapeutic Effect:** Prevents cell replication.

PHARMACOKINETICS

Binds to proteins after PO administration. Protein binding: less than 4%. Excreted in urine. **Half-life:** 7 hrs (increased in renal impairment).

USES

Treatment of chronic hepatitis B in adults with evidence of active viral replication and evidence of persistent elevations of serum AST or ALT or active disease.

PRECAUTIONS

CONTRAINDICATIONS: None known. **CAUTIONS:** Pts with known risk factors for hepatic disease, impaired renal function, elderly.

LIFESPAN CONSIDERATIONS:

Pregnancy/Lactation: Unknown if drug crosses placenta or is distributed in breast milk. **Pregnancy Category C.** **Children:** Safety and efficacy not established. **Elderly:** Age-related renal impairment, decreased cardiac function requires cautious use.

INTERACTIONS

DRUG: **Ibuprofen** increases adefovir plasma concentration. **Nephrotoxic agents (aminoglycosides, cyclosporin, NSAIDs, tacrolimus,**

vancomycin) may increase risk of nephrotoxicity. **HERBAL:** None significant. **FOOD:** None known. **LAB VALUES:** May increase serum ALT, AST, serum creatinine, amylase.

AVAILABILITY (Rx)

TABLETS: 10 mg.

ADMINISTRATION/HANDLING

PO

- Give without regard to food.

INDICATIONS/ROUTES/DOSAGE

CHRONIC HEPATITIS B (NORMAL RENAL FUCTION)

PO: ADULTS, ELDERLY: 10 mg once a day.

CHRONIC HEPATITIS B (IMPAIRED RENAL FUNCTION)

PO: ADULTS, ELDERLY WITH CREATININE CLEARANCE 20–49 ML/MIN: 10 mg q48h. **ADULTS, ELDERLY WITH CREATININE CLEARANCE 10–19 ML/MIN:** 10 mg q72h. **ADULTS, ELDERLY ON HEMODIALYSIS:** 10 mg every 7 days following dialysis.

SIDE EFFECTS

FREQUENT (13%): Asthenia. **OCCASIONAL (9%–4%):** Headache, abdominal pain, nausea, flatulence. **RARE (3%):** Diarrhea, dyspepsia.

ADVERSE EFFECTS/ TOXIC REACTIONS

Nephrotoxicity, characterized by increased serum creatinine and decreased serum phosphorus levels, is treatment-limiting toxicity of adefovir therapy. Lactic acidosis, severe hepatomegaly occur rarely, particularly in female pts.

NURSING CONSIDERATIONS

BASELINE ASSESSMENT

Obtain baseline renal function lab values before therapy begins and routinely thereafter. Those with preexisting renal insufficiency or during treatment may require dose adjustment. HIV antibody testing should be performed before therapy begins (unrecognized or untreated HIV infection may result in emergence of HIV resistance).

INTERVENTION/EVALUATION

Monitor I&O, serum creatinine; AST, ALT, alkaline phosphatase levels. Closely monitor for adverse reactions in those taking other medications that are excreted renally or with other drugs known to affect renal function.

Adenoscan, *see adenosine*

adenosine

ah-**den**-oh-seen

(Adenocard, Adenoscan)

CLASSIFICATION

PHARMACOTHERAPEUTIC: Cardiac agent, diagnostic aid. **CLINICAL:** Antiarrhythmic.

ACTION

Slows impulse formation in SA node and conduction time through AV node. Acts as a diagnostic aid in myocardial perfusion imaging or stress echocardiography. **Therapeutic Effect:** Depresses left ventricular function, restores normal sinus rhythm.

USES

Adenocard: Treatment of paroxysmal supraventricular tachycardia, including those associated with accessory bypass tracts (Wolff-Parkinson-White syndrome). **Adenoscan:** Adjunct in diagnosis in myocardial perfusion imaging or stress echocardiography.

PRECAUTIONS

CONTRAINDICATIONS: Atrial fibrillation or flutter, second- or third-degree AV block or sick sinus syndrome (with functioning pacemaker), ventricular tachycardia. **CAUTIONS:** Heart block, arrhythmias at time of conversion, asthma, hepatic/renal failure. **Pregnancy Category C.**

INTERACTIONS

DRUG: Methylxanthines (e.g., theophyline) may decrease effect. **Dipyridamole** may increase effect. **Carbamazepine** may increase degree of heart block caused by adenosine. **HERBAL:** None significant. **FOOD:** Avoid **Caffeine** (may decrease effect). **LAB VALUES:** None known.

AVAILABILITY (Rx)

INJECTION SOLUTION (ADENOCARD): 3 mg/ml in 2 ml, 4 ml syringes. **INJECTION SOLUTION (ADENOSCAN):** 3 mg/ml in 20 ml, 30 ml vials.

ADMINISTRATION/HANDLING

IV

Rate of administration • Administer very rapidly (over 1–2 sec) undiluted directly into vein, or if using IV line, use closest port to insertion site. If IV line is infusing any fluid other than 0.9% NaCl, flush line first. • After rapid bolus injection, follow with rapid 0.9% NaCl flush.

Storage • Store at room temperature. Solution appears clear. • Crystallization occurs if refrigerated; if crystallization occurs, dissolve crystals by warming to room temperature. Discard unused portion.

IV INCOMPATIBILITIES

Any drug or solution other than 0.9% NaCl or D_5W.

INDICATIONS/ROUTES/DOSAGE

PAROXYSMAL SUPRAVENTRICULAR TACHYCARDIA (PSVT)

RAPID IV BOLUS: ADULTS, ELDERLY, CHILDREN WEIGHING 50 KG AND MORE: Initially, 6 mg given over 1–2 sec. If first dose does not convert within 1–2 min, give 12 mg; may repeat 12-mg dose in 1–2 min if no response has occurred. **CHILDREN WEIGHING LESS THAN 50 KG:** Initially 0.05–01. mg/kg. If first dose does not convert within 1–2 min, may increase dose by 0.05–0.1 mg/kg. May repeat until sinus rhythm is established or up to a maximum single dose of 0.3 mg/kg or 12 mg.

DIAGNOSTIC TESTING

IV INFUSION: ADULTS: 140 mcg/kg/min for 6 min. **Total dose:** 0.84 mg/kg. Thallium is injected at midpoint (3 min) of infusion.

SIDE EFFECTS

FREQUENT (18%–12%): Facial flushing, dyspnea. **OCCASIONAL (7%–2%):** Headache, nausea, light-headedness, chest pressure. **RARE (1% or less):** Paresthesias, dizziness, diaphoresis, hypotension, palpitations; chest, jaw, or neck pain.

ADVERSE EFFECTS/ TOXIC REACTIONS

May produce short-lasting heart block.

NURSING CONSIDERATIONS

BASELINE ASSESSMENT

Identify arrhythmia per cardiac monitor and assess apical pulse.

INTERVENTION/EVALUATION

Assess cardiac performance per continuous EKG. Monitor B/P, apical pulse (rate, rhythm, quality). Auscultate pt breath sounds for clarity. Monitor respiratory rate. Monitor I&O; assess for fluid retention. Check electrolytes.

Advair, *see fluticasone*

Advair diskus, *see fluticasone and salmeterol*

Aggrenox, *see dipyridamole and aspirin*

albumin, human

al-**byew**-min

(Albuminar-5, Albuminar-25, Albutein, Buminate, Flexbumin, Plasbumin)

Do not confuse albumin with albuterol.

CLASSIFICATION

PHARMACOTHERAPEUTIC: Plasma protein fraction. **CLINICAL:** Blood derivative.

ACTION

Blood volume expander. **Therapeutic Effect:** Provides temporary increase in blood volume, reduces hemoconcentration and blood viscosity.

PHARMACOKINETICS

Route	Onset	Peak	Duration
IV	15 min (in well-hydrated pt)	N/A	N/A

Distributed throughout extracellular fluid. **Half-life:** 15–20 days.

USES

Treatment of hypovolemia, hypoproteinemia. Adjunct in treatment of severe burns, neonatal hyperbilirubinemia, adult respiratory distress syndrome (ARDS), cardiopulmonary bypass, ascites, acute nephrosis or nephrotic syndrome, hemodialysis, pancreatitis, intra-abdominal infections, acute hepatic failure. **OFF-LABEL:** Plasmapheresis (5% concentration).

PRECAUTIONS

CONTRAINDICATIONS: Heart failure, history of allergic reaction to albumin level, hypervolemia, normal serum albumin, pulmonary edema, severe anemia. **CAUTIONS:** Hypertension, normal serum albumin concentration, low cardiac reserve, pulmonary disease, hepatic/renal failure.

LIFESPAN CONSIDERATIONS:

Pregnancy/Lactation: Unknown if drug crosses placenta or is distributed in breast milk. **Pregnancy Category C.** **Children/Elderly:** No age-related precautions noted.

INTERACTIONS

DRUG: None significant. **HERBAL:** None significant. **FOOD:** None known. **LAB VALUES:** May increase serum alkaline phosphatase concentration.

AVAILABILITY (Rx)

INJECTION SOLUTION: (5%): 50 ml, 250 ml, 500 ml, 1,000 ml. **(25%):** 20 ml, 50 ml, 100 ml.

ADMINISTRATION/HANDLING

IV

Reconstitution • A 5% solution may be made from 25% solution by adding 1 volume 25% to 4 volumes 0.9% NaCl or D_5W (NaCl preferred). Do not use Sterile Water for Injection (life-threatening hemolysis, acute renal failure can result).

Rate of administration • Give by IV infusion. Rate is variable, depending on use, blood volume, concentration of solute. 5%: Do not exceed 2–4 ml/min in pts with normal plasma volume, 5–10 ml/min in pts with hypoproteinemia. 25%: Do not exceed 1 ml/min in pts with normal plasma volume, 2–3 ml/min in pts with hypoproteinemia. 5% administered undiluted; 25% may be administered undiluted or diluted with 0.9% NaCl or D_5W. NaCl preferred. • May give without regard to pt blood group or Rh factor.

Storage • Store at room temperature. Appears as clear, brownish, odorless, moderate viscous fluid. • Do not use if solution has been frozen, appears turbid, contains sediment, or if not used within 4 hrs of opening vial.

IV INCOMPATIBILITIES

Lipids, midazolam (Versed), vancomycin (Vancocin), verapamil (Isoptin).

IV COMPATIBILITIES

Diltiazem (Cardizem), lorazepam (Ativan).

INDICATIONS/ROUTES/DOSAGE

◀ **ALERT** ▶ 5% should be used in hypovolemic or intravascularly depleted pts. 25% should be used in pts in whom fluid and sodium intake must be minimized.

HYPOVOLEMIA

IV: ADULTS, ELDERLY: Initially, 25 g; may repeat in 15–30 min. **Maximum:** 250 g within 48 hrs. **CHILDREN:** 0.5–1 g/kg/dose (10–20 ml/kg/dose of 5% albumin) **Maximum:** 6 g/kg/day.

HYPOPROTEINEMIA

IV: ADULTS, ELDERLY, CHILDREN: 0.5–1 g/kg/dose (10–20 ml/kg/dose of 5% albumin). Repeat in 1–2 days.

BURNS

IV: ADULTS, ELDERLY, CHILDREN: Initially, give large volumes of crystalloid infusion to maintain plasma volume. After 24 hrs, give 25 g, then adjust dosage to maintain plasma albumin concentration of 2–2.5 g/100 ml.

CARDIOPULMONARY BYPASS

IV: ADULTS, ELDERLY: 5% or 25% albumin with crystalloid to maintain plasma albumin concentration of 2.5 g/100 ml.

ACUTE NEPHROSIS, NEPHROTIC SYNDROME

IV: ADULTS, ELDERLY: 25 g of 25% injection, with diuretic once a day for 7–10 days.

HEMODIALYSIS

IV: ADULTS, ELDERLY: 100 ml (25 g) of 25% albumin.

HYPERBILIRUBINEMIA, ERYTHROBLASTOSIS FETALIS

IV: INFANTS: 1 g/kg 1–2 hrs before transfusion.

SIDE EFFECTS

OCCASIONAL: Hypotension. **RARE:** High dose in repeated therapy: altered vital signs, chills, fever, increased salivation, nausea, vomiting, urticaria, tachycardia.

ADVERSE EFFECTS/ TOXIC REACTIONS

Fluid overload may occur, marked by increased B/P, distended neck veins. Neurological changes that may occur include headache, weakness, blurred vision, behavioral changes, incoordination, isolated muscle twitching. Pulmonary edema may also occur, evidenced by rapid respirations, rales, wheezing, coughing.

NURSING CONSIDERATIONS

BASELINE ASSESSMENT

Obtain B/P, pulse, respirations immediately before administration. Adequate hydration required before albumin is administered.

INTERVENTION/EVALUATION

Monitor B/P for hypotension/hypertension. Assess frequently for evidence of fluid overload, pulmonary edema (see Adverse Effects/Toxic Reactions). Check skin for flushing, urticaria. Monitor I&O ratio (watch for decreased output). Assess for therapeutic response (increased B/P, decreased edema).

Albuminar, *see albumin*

albuterol

ale-**beut**-er-all

(AccuNeb, Asmavent ✱, Novosalmol ✱, Proventil, Proventil HFA, Proventil Repetabs, Ventolin, Ventolin HFA, Volmax, Vospire ER)

Do not confuse albuterol with Albutein or atenolol, or Proventil with Prinivil.

FIXED-COMBINATION(S)

Combivent: albuterol/ipratropium (a bronchodilator): 103 mcg/18 mcg per actuation. **Duoneb:** albuterol/ipratropium 3 mg/0.5 mg.

CLASSIFICATION

PHARMACOTHERAPEUTIC: Sympathomimetic (adrenergic agonist). **CLINICAL:** Bronchodilator (see p. 70C).

ACTION

Stimulates beta$_2$-adrenergic receptors in lungs, resulting in relaxation of bronchial smooth muscle. **Therapeutic Effect:** Relieves bronchospasm and reduces airway resistance.

PHARMACOKINETICS

Route	Onset	Peak	Duration
PO	15–30 min	2–3 hrs	4–6 hrs
PO (extended-release)	30 min	2–4 hrs	12 hrs
Inhalation	5–15 min	0.5–2 hrs	2–5 hrs

Rapidly, well absorbed from GI tract; gradually absorbed from bronchi after inhalation. Metabolized in the liver. Primarily excreted in urine. **Half-life:** 2.7–5 hrs (PO); 3.8 hrs (inhalation).

USES

Relief of bronchospasm due to reversible obstructive airway disease, exercise-induced bronchospasm.

PRECAUTIONS

CONTRAINDICATIONS: History of hypersensitivity to sympathomimetics. **CAUTIONS:** Hypertension, cardiovascular disease, hyperthyroidism, diabetes mellitus.

LIFESPAN CONSIDERATIONS:

Pregnancy/Lactation: Appears to cross placenta; unknown if distributed in breast milk. May inhibit uterine contractility. **Pregnancy Category C. Children:** Safety and efficacy not established in children younger than 2 yrs (syrup) or younger than 6 yrs (tablets). **Elderly:** May be more sensitive to tremor or tachycardia due to age-related increased sympathetic sensitivity.

INTERACTIONS

DRUG: Beta-adrenergic blocking agents (beta-blockers) antagonize effects. May increase risk of arrhythmias with **digoxin. MAOIs, tricyclic antidepressants** may potentiate cardiovascular effects. **Thyroid hormones** may increase effect, enhance risk of coronary insufficiency in pts with coronary artery disease (CAD). **HERBAL: Ephedra, yohimbe** may cause CNS stimulation. **FOOD:** None known. **LAB VALUES:** May increase blood glucose level. May decrease serum potassium level.

AVAILABILITY (Rx)

INHALATION AEROSOL (PROVENTIL, VENTOLIN): 90 mcg/spray. **INHALATION**

SOLUTION (ACCUNEB): 0.75 mg/3 ml (0.63 mg/3 ml albuterol), 1.5 mg/3 ml (1.25 mg/3 ml albuterol). **INHALATION SOLUTION:** 0.083% (Proventil), 0.5% (Proventil, Ventolin). **SYRUP:** 2 mg/5 ml. **TABLETS (PROVENTIL, VENTOLIN):** 2 mg, 4 mg.

TABLETS (EXTENDED-RELEASE): 4 mg (Proventil Repetabs, Volmax, VoSpire ER), 8 mg (Volmax, VoSpire ER).

ADMINISTRATION/HANDLING

PO

• Do not crush/break extended-release tablets. • May give without regard to food.

INHALATION

• Shake container well before inhalation. • Wait 2 min before inhaling second dose (allows for deeper bronchial penetration). • Rinse mouth with water immediately after inhalation (prevents mouth/throat dryness).

NEBULIZATION

• Dilute 0.5 ml of 0.5% solution to final volume of 3 ml with 0.9% NaCl to provide 2.5 mg. • Administer over 5–15 min. • Nebulizer should be used with compressed air or O_2 at rate of 6–10 L/min.

INDICATIONS/ROUTES/DOSAGE

ACUTE BRONCHOSPASM

INHALATION: ADULTS, ELDERLY, CHILDREN OLDER THAN 12 YRS: 4–8 puffs q20min up to 4 hrs, then q1–4h as needed. **CHILDREN 12 YRS AND YOUNGER:** 4–8 puffs q20min for 3 doses, then q1–4h as needed.

NEBULIZATION: ADULTS, ELDERLY, CHILDREN OLDER THAN 12 YRS: 2.5–5 mg q20min for 3 doses, then 2.5–10 mg q1–4h or 10–15 mg/hr continuously. **CHILDREN 12 YRS AND YOUNGER:** 0.15 mg/kg q20min for 3 doses (minimum: 2.5 mg), then 0.15–0.3 mg/kg q1–4h as needed. **Maximum:** 10 mg or 0.5 mg/kg/hr by continuous infusion.

CHRONIC BRONCHOSPASM

PO: ADULTS, CHILDREN OLDER THAN 12 YRS: 2–4 mg 3–4 times a day. **Maximum:** 8 mg 4 times a day. **ELDERLY:** 2 mg 3–4 times a day. **Maximum:** 8 mg 4 times a day. **CHILDREN 6–12 YRS:** 2 mg 3–4 times a day. **Maximum:** 24 mg/day. **CHILDREN 2–5 YRS:** 0.1–0.2 mg/kg/dose 3 times a day. **Maximum:** 12 mg/day.

PO (EXTENDED-RELEASE): ADULTS, CHILDREN OLDER THAN 12 YRS: 4–8 mg q12h. **Maximum:** 32 mg/day.

NEBULIZATION: ADULTS, ELDERLY, CHILDREN OLDER THAN 12 YRS: 2.5 mg 3–4 times a day over 5–15 min. **CHILDREN 12 YRS AND YOUNGER:** 0.05 mg/kg q4–6h. **Minimum:** 1.25 mg/dose. **Maximum:** 2.5 mg/dose.

INHALATION: ADULTS, ELDERLY, CHILDREN 4 YRS AND OLDER: 1–2 puffs q4–6h. **Maximum:** 12 puffs per day.

EXERCISE-INDUCED BRONCHOSPASM

INHALATION: ADULTS, ELDERLY, CHILDREN OLDER THAN 12 YRS: 2 puffs 15–30 min before exercise. **CHILDREN 12 YRS AND YOUNGER:** 1–2 puffs 5 min before exercise.

SIDE EFFECTS

FREQUENT: Headache (27%); nausea (15%); restlessness, nervousness, tremors (20%); dizziness (less than 7%); throat dryness and irritation, pharyngitis (less than 6%); B/P changes, including hypertension (5%–3%); heartburn, transient wheezing (less than 5%). **OCCASIONAL (3%–2%):** Insomnia, asthenia, altered taste. **Inhalation:** Dry, irritated mouth or throat; cough; bronchial irritation. **RARE:** Somnolence, diarrhea, dry mouth, flushing, diaphoresis, anorexia.

ADVERSE EFFECTS/ TOXIC REACTIONS

Excessive sympathomimetic stimulation may produce palpitations, extrasystole, tachycardia, chest pain, slight increase in B/P followed by substantial decrease, chills, diaphoresis, blanching of skin. Too-frequent or excessive use may lead to decreased bronchodilating effectiveness and severe, paradoxical bronchoconstriction.

NURSING CONSIDERATIONS

BASELINE ASSESSMENT

Offer emotional support (high incidence of anxiety due to difficulty in breathing and sympathomimetic response to drug).

INTERVENTION/EVALUATION

Monitor rate, depth, rhythm, type of respiration; quality and rate of pulse; EKG; serum potassium, ABG determinations. Assess lung sounds for wheezing (bronchoconstriction), rales.

PATIENT/FAMILY TEACHING

• Instruct on proper use of inhaler. • Increase fluid intake (decreases lung secretion viscosity). • Do not take more than 2 inhalations at any one time (excessive use may produce paradoxical bronchoconstriction or decreased bronchodilating effect). • Rinsing mouth with water immediately after inhalation may prevent mouth/throat dryness. • Avoid excessive use of caffeine derivatives (chocolate, coffee, tea, cola, cocoa).

alclometasone

(Aclovate)

See Corticosteroids: topical (p. 94C)

aldesleukin

all-des-**lyew**-kin

(Interleukin-2, IL-2, Proleukin)

See Interleukin-2, pp. 75C, 631.

alefacept

ale-fah-cept

(Amevive)

CLASSIFICATION

PHARMACOTHERAPEUTIC: Immunologic agent. **CLINICAL:** Immunosuppressive.

ACTION

Interferes with activation of T-lymphocytes by binding to the lymphocyte antigen, inhibiting interaction of T-lymphocytes. **Therapeutic Effect:** Reduces number of circulating total lymphocytes, predominant in chronic plaque psoriasis.

PHARMACOKINETICS

Half-life: 270 hrs.

USES

Treatment of adults with moderate to severe chronic plaque psoriasis who are candidates for systemic therapy or phototherapy.

PRECAUTIONS

CONTRAINDICATIONS: History of systemic malignancy, concurrent use of immunosuppressive agents or phototherapy. Do not administer to pts infected with HIV (reduces $CD4^+$ T-lymphocyte count, which may accelerate disease progression or increase disease complications). **CAUTIONS:** Those at high risk for malignancy, chronic infections, history of recurrent infection, elderly.

LIFESPAN CONSIDERATIONS:

Pregnancy/Lactation: Unknown if drug crosses placenta or is distributed in breast milk. **Pregnancy Category B.** **Children:** Safety and efficacy not established. **Elderly:** Cautious use due to higher incidence of infections and certain malignancies.

INTERACTIONS

DRUG: **Immunosuppressive agents, methotrexate** may increase possibility of excessive immunosupression. **HERBAL:** None significant. **FOOD:** None known. **LAB VALUES:** Decreases serum T-lymphocyte levels. May increase serum AST, ALT levels.

AVAILABILITY (Rx)

INJECTION, POWDER FOR RECONSTITUTION: 7.5 mg for IV administration, 15 mg for IM administration.

ADMINISTRATION/HANDLING

◀ ALERT ▶ For both IM and IV administration, withdraw 0.6 ml of the supplied diluent and with the needle pointed at the side-wall of the vial, slowly inject the diluent into the vial of alefacept. Prevent excessive foaming by swirling gently to dissolve.

IV

Reconstitution • Reconstitute 7.5 mg with 0.6 ml of supplied diluent (Sterile Water for Injection); 0.5 ml of reconstituted solution contains 7.5 mg alefacept.

Rate of administration • Prepare 2 syringes with 3 ml 0.9% NaCl for pre- and post-administration flush. • Prime the winged infusion set with 3 ml 0.9% NaCl and insert the set into the vein. • Attach the medication-filled syringe to the infusion set and give over no more than 5 sec. • Flush with 3 ml 0.9% NaCl.

Storage • Store unopened vials at room temperature. • Following reconstitution, use immediately, or if refrigerated, within 4 hrs. • Discard unused portion within 4 hrs of reconstitution. • Reconstituted solution should be clear and colorless to slightly yellow. • Do not use if discolored or cloudy or if undissolved material remains.

IM

Reconstitution • Reconstitute 15 mg with 0.6 ml of supplied diluent (Sterile Water for Injection); 0.5 ml of reconstituted solution contains 15 mg alefacept. • Inject the full 0.5 ml of solution. • Use a different IM site for each new injection. Give new injections at least 1 inch from the old site. Avoid areas where the skin is tender, bruised, red, or hard.

Storage • Store unopened vials at room temperature. • Following reconstitution, use immediately, or if refrigerated, within 4 hrs. • Discard unused portion within 4 hrs of reconstitution. • Reconstituted solution should be clear and colorless to slightly yellow. • Do not use if discolored or cloudy or if undissolved material remains.

IV INCOMPATIBILITIES

Do not mix alefacept with any other medications. Do not reconstitute it with any diluent other than that supplied by the manufacturer.

INDICATIONS/ROUTES/DOSAGE

PLAQUE PSORIASIS

IV: ADULTS, ELDERLY: 7.5 mg once weekly for 12 wks.

IM: ADULTS, ELDERLY: 15 mg once weekly for 12 wks.

SIDE EFFECTS

FREQUENT (16%): Injection site pain and inflammation (with IM administration). **OCCASIONAL (5%):** Chills. **RARE (2% or less):** Pharyngitis, dizziness, cough, nausea, myalgia.

ADVERSE EFFECTS/ TOXIC REACTIONS

Hypersensitivity reaction, lymphopenia, malignancies, serious infections requiring hospitalization (abscess, pneumonia, postoperative wound infection) occur rarely. Coronary artery disease and MI occur in less than 1% of pts.

NURSING CONSIDERATIONS

BASELINE ASSESSMENT

Obtain baseline $CD4^+$ T-lymphocyte levels before treatment and weekly during the 12-wk dosing period.

INTERVENTION/EVALUATION

Closely monitor $CD4^+$ T-lymphocyte levels. Withhold dose if $CD4^+$ T-lymphocyte levels are below 250 cells/mcl. If levels remain below 250 cells/mcl for 1 mo, discontinue treatment.

PATIENT/FAMILY TEACHING

• Regular monitoring of WBC count during therapy is necessary. • Promptly report any signs of infection or evidence of malignancy.

alemtuzumab

ah-lem-**two**-zoo-mab
(Campath)

CLASSIFICATION

PHARMACOTHERAPEUTIC: Monoclonal antibody. **CLINICAL:** Antineoplastic (see p. 75C).

ACTION

Binds to CD52, cell surface glycoprotein, found on surface of all B- and T-lymphocytes, most monocytes, macrophages, natural killer cells, granulocytes. **Therapeutic Effect:** Produces cytotoxicity, reducing tumor size.

PHARMACOKINETICS

Half-life: About 12 days. Peak and trough levels rise during first few weeks of therapy and approach steady state by about week 6.

USES

Treatment of B-cell chronic lymphocytic leukemia (B-CLL) in pts who have been treated with alkylating agents and who have failed fludarabine (Fludara) therapy.

PRECAUTIONS

CONTRAINDICATIONS: Active systemic infections, history of hypersensitivity or anaphylactic reaction to alemtuzumab, other monoclonal antibodies, immunosuppression. **CAUTIONS:** None known.

LIFESPAN CONSIDERATIONS:

Pregnancy/Lactation: Has potential to cause fetal B- and T-lymphocyte depletion. Discontinue breast-feeding during treatment and for at least 3 mos after last dose. **Pregnancy Category C.** **Children:** Safety and efficacy not established. **Elderly:** No age-related precautions noted.

INTERACTIONS

DRUG: Concurrent use with **live virus vaccines** may potentiate virus replication, increase side effects, or decrease pt's antibody response. **Immunosuppressive agents** causing blood dyscrasias may have additive effects. **HERBAL:** None significant. **FOOD:** None known. **LAB VALUES:** May decrease Hgb level, platelet count, WBC count.

AVAILABILITY (Rx)

INJECTION SOLUTION: 30 mg/ml.

ADMINISTRATION/HANDLING

IV

◀ **ALERT** ▶ Do not give by IV push or bolus.

Reconstitution • Withdraw needed amount from ampule into a syringe. • Using a low-protein binding, non–fiber-releasing 5-micron filter, inject into 100 ml 0.9% NaCl or D_5W. • Invert bag to mix; do not shake.

Rate of administration • Give the 100 ml solution as a 2-hr IV infusion.

Storage • Refrigerate undiluted ampules; do not freeze. • Use within 8 hrs after dilution. Diluted solution may be stored at room temperature or refrigerated. • Discard if particulate matter is present or if solution is discolored.

IV INCOMPATIBILITIES

Do not mix with any other medications.

INDICATIONS/ROUTES/DOSAGE

◀ **ALERT** ▶ Pretreatment with acetaminophen 650 mg and diphenhydramine 50 mg before each infusion may prevent infusion-related side effects.

CHRONIC LYMPHOCYTIC LEUKEMIA

IV: ADULTS, ELDERLY: Initially, 3 mg/day as a 2-hr infusion. When the 3-mg daily dose is tolerated (with only low-grade or no infusion-related toxicities), increase daily dose to 10 mg. When the 10 mg/day dose is tolerated, maintenance dose may be initiated. Maintenance: 30 mg/day 3 times a wk on alternate days (such as Monday, Wednesday, and Friday or Tuesday, Thursday, and Saturday) for up to 12 wks. The increase to 30 mg/day is usually achieved in 3–7 days.

SIDE EFFECTS

FREQUENT: Rigors, tremors (86%), fever (85%), nausea (54%), vomiting (41%), rash (40%), fatigue (34%), hypotension (32%), urticaria (30%), pruritus, skeletal pain, headache (24%), diarrhea (22%), anorexia (20%). **OCCASIONAL (less than 10%):** Myalgia, dizziness, abdominal pain, throat irritation, vomiting, neutropenia, rhinitis, bronchospasm, urticaria.

ADVERSE EFFECTS/ TOXIC REACTIONS

Neutropenia occurs in 85% of pts, anemia occurs in 80% of pts, and thrombocytopenia occurs in 72% of pts. Rash occurs in 40% of pts. Respiratory toxicity, manifested as dyspnea, cough, bronchitis, pneumonitis, and pneumonia, occurs in 26%–16% of pts. Serious, sometimes fatal bacterial, viral, fungal, and protozoan infections have been reported.

NURSING CONSIDERATIONS

BASELINE ASSESSMENT

Pretreatment with acetaminophen and diphenhydramine before each infusion may prevent infusion-related side effects. CBC, platelet count should be obtained frequently during and after therapy to assess for neutropenia, anemia, thrombocytopenia.

INTERVENTION/EVALUATION

Monitor for infusion-related symptoms complex consisting mainly of rigors, fever, chills, hypotension, generally occurring within 30 min–2 hrs of beginning of first infusion. Slowing infusion rate resolves symptoms. Monitor for hematologic toxicity (fever, sore throat, signs of local infection, easy bruising, unusual bleeding from any site), symptoms of anemia (excessive fatigue, weakness).

PATIENT/FAMILY TEACHING

• Avoid crowds, those with known infection. • Avoid contact with those who recently received live virus vaccine; do not receive vaccinations.

alendronate

ah-**len**-drew-nate

(Apo-alendronate ✤, Fosamax, Novo-alendronate ✤)

Do not confuse Fosamax with Flomax.

FIXED-COMBINATION(S)

Fosamax Plus D: alendronate/cholecalciferol (vitamin D analog): 70 mg/2800 international units.

◆**CLASSIFICATION**

PHARMACOTHERAPEUTIC: Bisphosphonate. **CLINICAL:** Bone resorption inhibitor, calcium regulator.

ACTION

Inhibits normal and abnormal bone resorption, without retarding mineralization. **Therapeutic Effect:** Leads to significantly increased bone mineral density; reverses progression of osteoporosis.

PHARMACOKINETICS

Poorly absorbed after oral administration. Protein binding: 78%. After oral administration, rapidly taken into bone, with uptake greatest at sites of active bone turnover. Excreted in urine. **Terminal half-life:** Greater than 10 yrs (reflects release from skeleton as bone is resorbed).

USES

Treatment of osteoporosis in men. Treatment adjunct in glucocorticoid-induced osteoporosis, treatment and prevention of osteoporosis in postmenopausal women, treatment of Paget's disease. **OFF-LABEL:** Treatment of breast cancer.

PRECAUTIONS

CONTRAINDICATIONS: GI disease, including dysphagia, frequent heartburn, GI reflux disease, hiatal hernia, and ulcers, inability to stand or sit upright for at least 30 min; renal impairment; sensitivity to alendronate. **CAUTIONS:** Hypocalcemia, vitamin D deficiency.

⌛ **LIFESPAN CONSIDERATIONS:** **Pregnancy/Lactation:** Possible incomplete fetal ossification, decreased maternal weight gain, delay in delivery. Excretion in breast milk unknown. Do not give to breast-feeding women. **Pregnancy Category C. Children:** Safety and efficacy not established. **Elderly:** No age-related precautions noted.

INTERACTIONS

DRUG: IV ranitidine may double drug bioavailability. **Aspirin** may increase GI disturbances. **HERBAL:** None significant. **FOOD:** Concurrent **dietary supplements, food, beverages** may interfere with alendronate absorption. **Caffeine** may reduce efficacy. **LAB VALUES:** Reduces serum calcium, phosphate concentrations. Significant decrease in serum alkaline phosphatase noted in those with Paget's disease.

AVAILABILITY (Rx)

SOLUTION, ORAL: 70 mg/75 ml. **TABLETS:** 5 mg, 10 mg, 35 mg, 40 mg, 70 mg.

ADMINISTRATION/HANDLING

PO

• Give at least 30 min before first food, beverage, or medication of the day. • Give with 6–8 oz plain water only (mineral water, coffee, tea, juice will decrease absorption). • Instruct pt **not** to lie down or eat for at least 30 min after administering medication (allows medication to reach stomach quickly, minimizing esophageal irritation).

INDICATIONS/ROUTES/DOSAGE

OSTEOPOROSIS (IN MEN)

PO: ADULTS, ELDERLY: 10 mg once a day in the morning or 70 mg weekly.

GLUCOCORTICOID-INDUCED OSTEOPOROSIS

PO: ADULTS, ELDERLY: 5 mg once a day in the morning. **POST-MENOPAUSAL WOMEN NOT RECEIVING ESTROGEN:** 10 mg once a day in the morning.

POST-MENOPAUSAL OSTEOPOROSIS

PO (TREATMENT): ADULTS, ELDERLY: 10 mg once a day in the morning or 70 mg weekly.

PO (PREVENTION): ADULTS, ELDERLY: 5 mg once a day in the morning or 35 mg weekly.

PAGET'S DISEASE

PO: ADULTS, ELDERLY: 40 mg once a day in the morning for 6 mos.

SIDE EFFECTS

FREQUENT (8%–7%): Back pain, abdominal pain. **OCCASIONAL (3%–2%):** Nausea, abdominal distention, constipation, diarrhea, flatulence. **RARE (less than 2%):** Rash, severe bone, joint, muscle pain.

ADVERSE EFFECTS/ TOXIC REACTIONS

Overdose produces hypocalcemia, hypophosphatemia, significant GI disturbances. Esophageal irritation occurs if not given with 6–8 oz of plain water or if pt lies down within 30 min of administration.

NURSING CONSIDERATIONS

BASELINE ASSESSMENT

Hypocalcemia, vitamin D deficiency must be corrected before therapy. Check electrolytes (esp. calcium and alkaline phosphatase serum levels).

INTERVENTION/EVALUATION

Monitor electrolytes (esp. serum calcium and alkaline phosphatase levels).

PATIENT/FAMILY TEACHING

• Instruct pt that expected benefits occur only when medication is taken with full glass (6–8 oz) of plain water, first thing in the morning and at least 30 min before first food, beverage, or medication of the day is taken. Any other beverage (mineral water, orange juice, coffee) significantly reduces absorption of medication. • Do not lie down for at least 30 min after taking medication (potentiates delivery to stomach, reducing risk of esophageal irritation). • Consider weight-bearing exercises, modify behavioral factors (e.g., cigarette smoking, alcohol consumption).

alfentanil

(Alfenta)

See Opioid analgesics

alfuzosin

ale-few-**zoe**-sin

(Uroxatral, Xatral ✤)

CLASSIFICATION

PHARMACOTHERAPEUTIC: Alpha$_1$-adrenergic blocker. **CLINICAL:** Benign prostatic hyperplasia agent.

ACTION

Targets receptors around bladder neck and prostate capsule. **Therapeutic Effect:** Relaxes smooth muscle, improves urinary flow, symptoms of prostatic hyperplasia.

PHARMACOKINETICS

Rapidly absorbed and widely distributed. Protein binding: 90%. Extensively metabolized in the liver. Primarily excreted in urine. **Half-life:** 3–9 hrs.

USES

Treatment of signs and symptoms of benign prostatic hyperplasia.

PRECAUTIONS

CONTRAINDICATIONS: None known. **CAUTIONS:** Coronary artery disease, hepatic disease, orthostatic hypotension, general anesthesia.

⌛ LIFESPAN CONSIDERATIONS:

Pregnancy/Lactation: Not indicated for use in this pt population. **Pregnancy**

Category B. Children: Not indicated for use in this pt population. **Elderly:** No age-related precautions noted.

INTERACTIONS

DRUG: Atenolol, diltiazem blood levels may be increased with concomitant use. **Other alpha-blocking agents (prazosin, terazosin, doxazosin, tamsulosin)** may have additive effect. **Cimetidine** may increase alfuzosin concentration. **Itraconazole, ketoconazole, ritonavir** increase blood levels. **HERBAL:** None significant. **FOOD: Food** increases absorption. **LAB VALUES:** None known.

AVAILABILITY (Rx)

TABLETS (EXTENDED-RELEASE): 10 mg.

ADMINISTRATION/HANDLING

PO

- Give after the same meal each day.
- Do not chew or crush extended-release tablet.

INDICATIONS/ROUTES/DOSAGE

BENIGN PROSTATIC HYPERPLASIA

PO: ADULTS: 10 mg once a day, approximately 30 min after same meal each day.

SIDE EFFECTS

FREQUENT (7%–6%): Dizziness, headache, malaise. **OCCASIONAL (4%):** Dry mouth. **RARE (3%–2%):** Nausea, dyspepsia (heartburn, epigastric discomfort), diarrhea, orthostatic hypotension, tachycardia, drowsiness.

ADVERSE EFFECTS/ TOXIC REACTIONS

Ischemia-related chest pain may occur rarely (2%). Priapism has been reported.

NURSING CONSIDERATIONS

BASELINE ASSESSMENT

Question for sensitivity to alfuzosin, use of other alpha-blocking agents (prazosin, terazosin, doxazosin, tamsulosin). Obtain B/P.

INTERVENTION/EVALUATION

Assist with ambulation if dizziness occurs. Report headache. Monitor for hypotension.

PATIENT/FAMILY TEACHING

- Take after the same meal each day.
- Avoid tasks that require alertness, motor skills until response to drug is established.
- Do not chew/crush extended-release tablet.

Alimta, *see pemetrexed*

alitretinoin

ah-**lee**-tret-ih-nown

(Panretin)

Do not confuse Panretin with pancreatin.

CLASSIFICATION

PHARMACOTHERAPEUTIC: Second-generation retinoid. **CLINICAL:** Antineoplastic (see p. 76C).

ACTION

Binds to and activates all known retinoid receptors. Once activated, receptors act as transcription factors, regulating genes that control cellular differentiation and proliferation. **Therapeutic Effect:** Inhibits growth of Kaposi's sarcoma (KS) cells.

USES

Topical treatment of cutaneous lesions in those with AIDS-related KS. **OFF-LABEL:** Breast, cervical, ovarian, prostatic carcinomas; myelodysplastic syndrome; psoriasis.

PRECAUTIONS

CONTRAINDICATIONS: When systemic therapy is required (more than 10 new KS lesions in previous month), symptomatic pulmonary KS, symptomatic visceral involvement or symptomatic lymphedema in KS. **CAUTIONS:** None known. **Pregnancy Category D.**

INTERACTIONS

DRUG: Increased risk of toxicity to products containing **DEET** (component of insect repellent). **HERBAL:** None significant. **FOOD:** None known. **LAB VALUES:** None known.

AVAILABILITY (Rx)

GEL: 0.1%.

INDICATIONS/ROUTES/DOSAGE

KAPOSI'S SARCOMA

TOPICAL: ADULTS: Initially, apply twice a day to lesions. May increase to 3–4 times a day. Allow gel to dry 3–5 min before covering with clothing. Do not use occlusive dressings.

SIDE EFFECTS

FREQUENT (greater than 5%): Rash (erythema, scaling, irritation, redness, dermatitis), pruritus, exfoliative dermatitis (flaking, peeling, desquamation, exfoliation), stinging, tingling, edema, skin disorders (scabbing, crusting, drainage).

ADVERSE EFFECTS/ TOXIC REACTIONS

Severe local skin reaction (intense erythema, edema, vesiculation) may limit treatment.

NURSING CONSIDERATIONS

PATIENT/FAMILY TEACHING

• Do not apply dressings over medication gel. • Do not apply gel to healthy skin surrounding lesions or on or near mucosal surfaces. • If severe irritation occurs, frequency of application can be reduced or discontinued for a few days until symptoms subside.

Allegra, *see fexofenadine*

Allegra-D, *see fexofenadine and pseudoephedrine*

allopurinol

ah-low-**pure**-ih-nal

(Aloprim, Apo-Allopurinol ♣, Zyloprim)

Do not confuse Zyloprim with Zorprin.

CLASSIFICATION

PHARMACOTHERAPEUTIC: Xanthine oxidase inhibitor. **CLINICAL:** Antigout.

ACTION

Decreases uric acid production by inhibiting xanthine oxidase, an enzyme. **Therapeutic Effect:** Reduces uric acid concentrations in serum and urine.

PHARMACOKINETICS

Route	Onset	Peak	Duration
PO, IV	2–3 days	1–3 wks	1–2 wks

Well absorbed from GI tract. Widely distributed. Metabolized in the liver to active metabolite. Excreted primarily in urine. Removed by hemodialysis. **Half-life:** 1–3 hrs; metabolite, 12–30 hrs.

A

USES

Oral: Prevents attacks of gouty arthritis, nephropathy. Treatment of secondary hyperuricemia that may occur during cancer treatment. Prevents recurrent uric acid and calcium oxalate calculi. **Injection:** Management of elevated uric acid in cancer pts unable to tolerate oral therapy. **OFF-LABEL:** In mouthwash following fluorouracil therapy to prevent stomatitis.

PRECAUTIONS

CONTRAINDICATIONS: Asymptomatic hyperuricemia. **CAUTIONS:** Impaired renal/hepatic function, CHF, diabetes mellitus, hypertension.

LIFESPAN CONSIDERATIONS:

Pregnancy/Lactation: Unknown if drug crosses placenta or is distributed in breast milk. **Pregnancy Category C.** **Children/Elderly:** No age-related precautions noted.

INTERACTIONS

DRUG: **Thiazide diuretics** may decrease effect. May increase effect of **oral anticoagulants.** May increase effect, toxicity of **azathioprine, mercaptopurine. Ampicillin, amoxicillin** may increase incidence of rash. **HERBAL:** None significant. **FOOD:** None known. **LAB VALUES:** May increase serum phosphatase, AST, ALT, BUN, creatinine.

AVAILABILITY (Rx)

INJECTION, POWDER FOR RECONSTITUTION (ALOPRIM): 500 mg. **TABLETS (ZYLOPRIM):** 100 mg, 300 mg.

ADMINISTRATION/HANDLING

IV

Reconstitution • Reconstitute 500-mg vial with 25 ml Sterile Water for Injection, giving a clear, almost colorless solution (concentration of 20 mg/ml). • Further dilute with 0.9% NaCl or D_5W (19 ml of added diluent yields 1 mg/ml, 9 ml yields 2 mg/ml, 2.3 ml yields maximum concentration of 6 mg/ml).

Rate of administration • Infuse over 15–60 min.

Storage • Store unreconstituted vials at room temperature. • May store reconstituted solution at room temperature and give within 10 hrs. Do not use if precipitate forms or solution is discolored.

PO

• May give with or immediately after meals or milk. • Instruct pt to drink at least 10–12 eight-oz glasses of water/day. • Dosages greater than 300 mg/day to be administered in divided doses.

IV INCOMPATIBILITIES

Amikacin (Amikin), carmustine (BiCNU), cefotaxime (Claforan), chlorpromazine (Thorazine), cimetidine (Tagamet), clindamycin (Cleocin), cytarabine (Ara-C), dacarbazine (DTIC), diphenhydramine (Benadryl), doxorubicin (Adriamycin), doxycycline (Vibramycin), droperidol (Inapsine), fludarabine (Fludara), gentamicin (Garamycin), haloperidol (Haldol), hydroxyzine (Vistaril), idarubicin (Idamycin), imipenem-cilastatin (Primaxin), meperidine (Demerol), methylprednisolone (Solu-Medrol), metoclopramide (Reglan), ondansetron (Zofran), prochlorperazine (Compazine), promethazine (Phenergan), streptozocin (Zanosar), tobramycin (Nebcin), vinorelbine (Navelbine).

IV COMPATIBILITIES

Bumetanide (Bumex), calcium gluconate, furosemide (Lasix), heparin, hydromorphone (Dilaudid), lorazepam (Ativan), morphine, potassium chloride.

INDICATIONS/ROUTES/DOSAGE

GOUTY ARTHRITIS

PO: ADULTS, ELDERLY, CHILDREN OLDER THAN 10 YRS (Mild): 100–300 mg/day. **(Moderate to severe):** 400–600 mg/

day as single or 2–3 divided doses. **Maximum:** 800 mg/day.

TO PREVENT URIC ACID NEPHROPATHY DURING CHEMOTHERAPY

◀ **ALERT** ▶ Maintenance dosage is based on serum uric acid levels. Discontinue following period of tumor regression.

SECONDARY HYPERURICEMIA ASSOCIATED WITH CHEMOTHERAPY

PO: ADULTS, ELDERLY, CHILDREN OLDER THAN 10 YRS: 600–800 mg/day in 2–3 divided doses for 2–3 days starting 1–2 days before chemotherapy. **CHILDREN 6–10 YRS:** 300 mg/day 2–3 divided doses. **CHILDREN YOUNGER THAN 6 YRS:** 150 mg/day in 3 divided doses.

IV: ADULTS, ELDERLY, CHILDREN 10 YRS OR OLDER: 200–400 mg/m^2/day beginning 24–48 hrs before initiation of chemotherapy. **CHILDREN YOUNGER THAN 10 YRS:** 200 mg/m^2/day. **Maximum:** 600 mg/day.

PREVENTION OF URIC ACID CALCULI

PO: ADULTS: 100–200 mg 1–4 times a day or 300 mg once a day.

RECURRENT CALCIUM OXALATE CALCULI

PO: ADULTS: 200–300 mg/day. **ELDERLY:** Initially, 100 mg/day, gradually increase until optimal uric acid level is reached.

DOSAGE IN RENAL IMPAIRMENT

Dosage is modified based on creatinine clearance. **Oral:** Removed by hemodialysis, adult maintenance doses based on creatinine clearance. Administer dose post hemodialysis or administer 50% supplemental dose.

Creatinine Clearance	Dosage Adjustment
10–20 ml/min	200 mg/day
3–9 ml/min	100 mg/day
Less than 3 ml/min	100 mg at extended intervals

SIDE EFFECTS

OCCASIONAL: Oral: Somnolence, unusual hair loss. **IV:** Rash, nausea, vomiting. **RARE:** Diarrhea, headache.

ADVERSE EFFECTS/ TOXIC REACTIONS

Pruritic maculopapular rash possibly accompanied by malaise, fever, chills, joint pain, nausea, vomiting should be considered a toxic reaction. Severe hypersensitivity may follow appearance of rash. Bone marrow depression, hepatotoxicity, peripheral neuritis, acute renal failure occur rarely.

NURSING CONSIDERATIONS

BASELINE ASSESSMENT

Instruct pt to drink 10–12 glasses (8 oz) of fluid daily while taking medication.

INTERVENTION/EVALUATION

Discontinue medication immediately if rash or other evidence of allergic reaction appears. Monitor I&O (output should be at least 2,000 ml/day). Assess CBC, uric acid, hepatic function serum levels. Assess urinary for cloudiness, unusual color, odor. Assess for therapeutic response (reduced joint tenderness, swelling, redness, limited motion).

PATIENT/FAMILY TEACHING

• May take 1 wk or longer for full therapeutic effect. • Encourage drinking 10–12 glasses (8 oz) of fluid daily while taking medication. • Avoid tasks that require alertness, motor skills until response to drug is established.

almotriptan

al-moe-**trip**-tan
(Axert)

Do not confuse Axert with Antivert.

◆ **CLASSIFICATION**

PHARMACOTHERAPEUTIC: Serotonin receptor agonist. **CLINICAL:** Antimigraine (see p. 60C).

ACTION

Binds selectively to vascular receptors, producing a vasoconstrictive effect on cranial blood vessels. **Therapeutic Effect:** Produces relief of migraine headache.

PHARMACOKINETICS

Well absorbed after PO administration. Metabolized by the liver, excreted in urine. **Half-life:** 3–4 hrs.

USES

Acute treatment of migraine headache with or without aura.

PRECAUTIONS

CONTRAINDICATIONS: Arrhythmias associated with conduction disorders, hemiplegic or basilar migraine, ischemic heart disease (including angina pectoris, history of MI, silent ischemia, and Prinzmetal's angina), uncontrolled hypertension, use within 24 hrs of ergotamine-containing preparation or another serotonin receptor antagonist, use within 14 days of MAOIs, Wolff-Parkinson-White syndrome. **CAUTIONS:** Mild to moderate renal or hepatic impairment, pt profile suggesting cardiovascular risks, controlled hypertension, history of cerebrovascular accident (CVA).

⌛ LIFESPAN CONSIDERATIONS:

Pregnancy/Lactation: Unknown if distributed in breast milk. **Pregnancy Category C.** **Children:** Safety and efficacy not established in pts younger than 12 yrs. **Elderly:** No age-related precautions noted.

INTERACTIONS

DRUG: **Ergotamine-containing drugs** may produce vasospastic reaction. **MAOIs** may increase concentration. Combined use of **fluoxetine, fluvoxamine, paroxetine, sertraline** may produce weakness, hyperreflexia, incoordination. **Ketoconazole, itraconazole, ritonavir, erythromycin** may increase plasma concentration of almotriptan. **HERBAL:** None significant. **FOOD:** None known. **LAB VALUES:** None known.

AVAILABILITY (Rx)

TABLETS: 6.5 mg, 12.5 mg.

ADMINISTRATION/HANDLING

PO

• Swallow tablets whole. • Take with full glass of water.

INDICATIONS/ROUTES/DOSAGE

MIGRAINE HEADACHE

PO: ADULTS, ELDERLY: Initially, 6.25–12.5 mg as a single dose. If headache improves but then returns, dose may be repeated after 2 hrs. **Maximum:** 2 doses/24 hrs.

DOSAGE IN RENAL/HEPATIC IMPAIRMENT

For adult and elderly pts, recommended initial dose is 6.25 mg and maximum daily dose is 12.5 mg.

SIDE EFFECTS

FREQUENT: Nausea, dry mouth, paresthesia, flushing. **OCCASIONAL:** Changes in temperature sensation, asthenia, dizziness.

ADVERSE EFFECTS/ TOXIC REACTIONS

Excessive dosage may produce tremor, redness of extremities, decreased respirations, cyanosis, seizures, chest pain. Serious arrhythmias occur rarely but particularly in pts with hypertension, diabetes, obesity, smokers, and those with strong family history of coronary artery disease.

NURSING CONSIDERATIONS

BASELINE ASSESSMENT

Question for history of peripheral vascular disease. Question pt regarding onset, location, duration of migraine and possible precipitating symptoms.

INTERVENTION/EVALUATION

Evaluate for relief of migraine headache and resulting photophobia, phonophobia (sound sensitivity), nausea, vomiting.

PATIENT/FAMILY TEACHING

• Take a single dose as soon as symptoms of an actual migraine attack appear. • Medication is intended to relieve migraine, not to prevent or reduce number of attacks. • Lie down in quiet, dark room for additional benefit after taking medication. • Avoid tasks that require alertness, motor skills until response to drug is established. • If palpitations, pain or tightness in chest or throat, or pain or weakness of extremities occurs, contact physician immediately.

alprazolam

ale-**praz**-oh-lam

(Alprazolam Intensol, Apo-Alpraz ✤, Niravam, Novo-Alprazol ✤, Xanax, Xanax XR)

Do not confuse alprazolam with lorazepam, or Xanax with Tenex or Zantac.

CLASSIFICATION

PHARMACOTHERAPEUTIC: Benzodiazepine (**Schedule IV**). **CLINICAL:** Antianxiety (see p. 11C).

ACTION

Enhances the action of neurotransmitter, gamma-aminobutyric acid, in the brain. **Therapeutic Effect:** Produces anxiolytic effect due to CNS depressant action.

PHARMACOKINETICS

Well absorbed from GI tract. Protein binding: 80%. Metabolized in the liver. Primarily excreted in urinary. Minimal removal by hemodialysis. **Half-life:** 11–16 hrs.

USES

Management of anxiety disorders associated with depression, panic disorder. **OFF-LABEL:** Management of premenstrual syndrome symptoms (mood disturbances, insomnia, cramps), irritable bowel syndrome, treatment of agoraphobia, post-traumatic stress disorder, tremors, ethanol withdrawal, anxiety in children.

PRECAUTIONS

CONTRAINDICATIONS: Acute alcohol intoxication with depressed vital signs, acute angle-closure glaucoma, concurrent use of itraconazole or ketoconazole, myasthenia gravis, severe COPD. **CAUTIONS:** Renal/hepatic impairment.

LIFESPAN CONSIDERATIONS:

Pregnancy/Lactation: Crosses placenta; distributed in breast milk. Chronic ingestion during pregnancy may produce withdrawal symptoms, CNS depression in neonates. **Pregnancy Category D. Children:** Safety and efficacy not established. **Elderly:** Use small initial doses with gradual increase to avoid ataxia (muscular incoordination) or excessive sedation.

INTERACTIONS

DRUG: Potentiated effects when used with **other CNS depressants**

(including alcohol). Ketoconazole, nefazodone, fluvoxamine may inhibit hepatic metabolism, increase serum concentrations. **HERBAL: Kava kava, valerian** may increase CNS depressant effect. **St. John's wort** may decrease effectiveness. **FOOD: Grapefruit juice** may inhibit metabolism. **LAB VALUES:** None known.

AVAILABILITY (Rx)

SOLUTION, ORAL (ALPRAZOLAM INTENSOL): 1 mg/ml. **TABLETS (XANAX):** 0.25 mg, 0.5 mg, 1 mg, 2 mg. **TABLETS (ORALLY-DISINTEGRATING [NIRAVAM]):** 0.25 mg, 0.5 mg, 1 mg, 2 mg.

TABLETS (EXTENDED-RELEASE [XANAX XR]): 0.5 mg, 1 mg, 2 mg, 3 mg.

ADMINISTRATION/HANDLING

PO, IMMEDIATE-RELEASE

- May give without regard to meals.
- Tablets may be crushed.

PO, EXTENDED-RELEASE

- Administer once daily. • Do not crush, chew, break. Swallow whole.

PO, ORALLY-DISINTEGRATING

- Place tablet on tongue, allow to dissolve. • Swallow with saliva.

INDICATIONS/ROUTES/DOSAGE

ANXIETY DISORDERS

PO (IMMEDIATE-RELEASE): ADULTS: Initially, 0.25–0.5 mg 3 times a day. May titrate q3–4 days. **Maximum:** 4 mg/day in divided doses. **ELDERLY, DEBILITATED PTS, PTS WITH HEPATIC DISEASE OR LOW SERUM ALBUMIN:** Initially, 0.25 mg 2–3 times a day. Gradually increase to optimum therapeutic response.

PO (ORALLY-DISINTEGRATING): ADULTS: 0.25–0.5 mg 3 times a day. **Maximum:** 4 mg/day in divided doses.

ANXIETY WITH DEPRESSION

PO: ADULTS: 2.5–3 mg/day in divided doses.

PANIC DISORDER

PO (IMMEDIATE-RELEASE): ADULTS: Initially, 0.5 mg 3 times a day. May increase at 3- to 4-day intervals. Range: 5–6 mg/day. **Maximum:** 10 mg/day. **ELDERLY:** Initially, 0.125–0.25 mg twice a day. May increase in 0.125-mg increments until desired effect attained.

PO (EXTENDED-RELEASE):

◀ **ALERT** ▶ To switch from immediate-release to extended–release form, give total daily dose (immediate–release) as a single daily dose of extended–release form.

ADULTS: Initially, 0.5–1 mg once a day. May titrate at 3- to 4-day intervals. Range: 3–6 mg/day. **Maximum:** 10 mg/day. **ELDERLY:** Initially, 0.5 mg once daily.

PO (ORALLY-DISINTEGRATING): ADULTS: Initially, 0.5 mg 3 times a day. May increase at 3- to 4-day intervals. Range: 5–6 mg/day. **Maximum:** 10 mg/day.

PREMENSTRUAL SYNDROME

PO: ADULTS: 0.25 mg 3 times a day.

SIDE EFFECTS

FREQUENT: Ataxia; lightheadedness; transient, mild somnolence; slurred speech (particularly in elderly or debilitated pts). **OCCASIONAL:** Confusion, depression, blurred vision, constipation, diarrhea, dry mouth, headache, nausea. **RARE:** Behavioral problems such as anger, impaired memory; paradoxical reactions (insomnia, nervousness, irritability).

ADVERSE EFFECTS/ TOXIC REACTIONS

Abrupt or too rapid withdrawal may result in pronounced restlessness, irritability, insomnia, hand tremors, abdominal/muscle cramps, diaphoresis, vomiting, seizures. Overdose results in somnolence, confusion, diminished reflexes, coma. Blood dyscrasias noted rarely.

NURSING CONSIDERATIONS

BASELINE ASSESSMENT

Offer emotional support to anxious pt. Assess motor responses (agitation, trembling, tension), autonomic responses (cold/clammy hands, diaphoresis).

INTERVENTION/EVALUATION

For those on long-term therapy, perform hepatic/renal function tests, blood counts periodically. Assess for paradoxical reaction, particularly during early therapy. Evaluate for therapeutic response: calm facial expression, decreased restlessness, insomnia.

PATIENT/FAMILY TEACHING

• Drowsiness usually disappears during continued therapy. • If dizziness occurs, change positions slowly from recumbent to sitting position before standing. • Avoid tasks that require alertness, motor skills until response to drug is established. • Smoking reduces drug effectiveness. • Sour hard candy, gum, sips of tepid water may relieve dry mouth. • Do not abruptly withdraw medication after long-term therapy. • Avoid alcohol. • Do not take other medications without consulting physician.

alprostadil (prostaglandin E_1; PGE_1)

ale-**pros**-tah-dill

(Caverject, Edex, Edex Refill, Muse, Prostin VR Pediatric)

CLASSIFICATION

PHARMACOTHERAPEUTIC: Prostaglandin. **CLINICAL:** Patent ductus arteriosus agent, anti-impotence.

ACTION

Direct effect on vascular and ductus arteriosus smooth muscle; relaxes trabecular smooth muscle. **Therapeutic Effect:** Causes vasodilation; dilates cavernosal arteries, allowing blood flow to and entrapment in the lacunar spaces of the penis.

USES

Prostin VR Pediatric: Temporarily maintains patency of ductus arteriosus until surgery is performed in those with congenital heart defects and dependent on patent ductus for survival (e.g., pulmonary atresia or stenosis). **Caverject, Edex, Muse:** Treatment of erectile dysfunction due to neurogenic, vasculogenic, psychogenic causes. **Caverject:** Adjunct in diagnosis of erectile dysfunction. **OFF-LABEL:** Treatment of atherosclerosis, gangrene, pain due to severe peripheral arterial occlusive disease, treatment of pulmonary hypertension in infants, children.

PRECAUTIONS

CONTRAINDICATIONS: Conditions predisposing to anatomic deformation of penis, hyaline membrane disease, penile implants, priapism, respiratory distress syndrome. **CAUTIONS:** Severe hepatic disease, coagulation defects, leukemia, multiple myeloma, polycythemia, sickle cell disease, thrombocythemia. **Pregnancy Category X (Muse: C).**

INTERACTIONS

DRUG: **Anticoagulants, heparin, thrombolytics** may increase risk of bleeding. **Sympathomimetics** may decrease effect. **Antihypertensives** may increase risk of hypotension. **HERBAL:** None significant. **FOOD:** None known. **LAB VALUES:** May increase serum bilirubin. May decrease serum calcium glucose, potassium.

A

AVAILABILITY (Rx)

INJECTION, POWDER FOR RECONSTITUTION: (CAVERJECT, EDEX): 10 mcg, 20 mcg, 40 mcg. **INJECTION, SOLUTION (PROSTIN VR PEDIATRIC)** 500 mcg/ml. **URETHRAL PELLET (MUSE):** 125 mcg, 250 mcg, 500 mcg, 1,000 mcg.

ADMINISTRATION/HANDLING

URETHRAL PELLET

Storage: Refrigerate pellet unless used within 14 days.

IV

Reconstitution • Dilute 500-mcg ampule with D_5W or 0.9% NaCl to volume depending on infusion pump capabilities.

Rate of administration • Infuse for shortest time, lowest dose possible. • If significant decrease in arterial pressure is noted via umbilical artery catheter, auscultation, or Doppler transducer, decrease infusion rate immediately. • Discontinue infusion immediately if apnea or bradycardia occurs (overdosage).

Storage • Store parenteral form in refrigerator. • Must dilute before use. • Prepare fresh q24h. • Discard unused portions.

IV INCOMPATIBILITIES

No information available.

INDICATIONS/ROUTES/DOSAGE

MAINTAIN PATENCY OF DUCTUS ARTERIOSUS

IV INFUSION: NEONATES: Initially, 0.05–0.1 mcg/kg/min. Maintenance: 0.01–0.4 mcg/kg/min. **Maximum:** 0.4 mcg/kg/min.

IMPOTENCE

PELLET, INTRACAVERNOSAL: ADULTS: Dosage is individualized.

SIDE EFFECTS

FREQUENT: Intracavernosal (4%–1%): Penile pain (37%), prolonged erection, hypertension, localized pain, penile fibrosis, injection site hematoma or ecchymosis, headache, respiratory infection, flu-like symptoms. **Intraurethral (3%):** Penile pain (36%), urethral pain or burning, testicular pain, urethral bleeding, headache, dizziness, respiratory infection, flu-like symptoms. **Systemic (greater than 1%):** Fever, flushing, bradycardia, hypotension, tachycardia, diarrhea. **OCCASIONAL: Intracavernosal (less than 1%):** Hypotension, pelvic pain, back pain, dizziness, cough, nasal congestion. **Intraurethral (less than 3%):** Fainting, sinusitis, back and pelvic pain. **Systemic (less than 1%):** Anxiety, lethargy, myalgia, arrhythmias, respiratory depression, anemia, bleeding, hematuria.

ADVERSE EFFECTS/ TOXIC REACTIONS

◀ **ALERT** ▶ Apnea experienced by 10%–12% of neonates with congenital heart defects.

Overdose manifested as apnea, flushing of the face/arms, bradycardia. Cardiac arrest, sepsis occur rarely. Seizures, sepsis, thrombocytopenia occur rarely.

NURSING CONSIDERATIONS

INTERVENTION/EVALUATION

Patent Ductus Arteriosus: Monitor arterial pressure by umbilical artery catheter, auscultation, Doppler transducer. If significant decrease in arterial pressure occurs, decrease infusion rate immediately. Maintain continuous cardiac monitoring. Assess heart sounds, femoral pulse (circulation to lower extremities), respiratory status frequently. Monitor for symptoms of hypotension. Assess B/P, arterial blood gases, temperature. If apnea or bradycardia occurs, discontinue infusion and notify physician. In infants with restricted systemic blood flow, efficacy should be measured by monitoring improvement of systemic B/P and blood pH.

PATIENT/FAMILY TEACHING

• **Patent Ductus Arteriosus:** Explain purpose of this palliative therapy to parents. • **Impotence:** Erection is to occur within 2–5 min. • Do not use if female is pregnant (unless using condom barrier). • Inform physician if erection lasts longer than 4 hrs or becomes painful.

Altace, *see ramipril*

alteplase

all-teh-place

(Activase, Cathflo Activase)

Do not confuse alteplase or Activase with Altace.

CLASSIFICATION

PHARMACOTHERAPEUTIC: Tissue plasminogen activator (tPA). **CLINICAL:** Thrombolytic (see p. 32C).

ACTION

An enzyme binds to fibrin in a thrombus and converts entrapped plasminogen to plasmin, initiating fibrinolysis. **Therapeutic Effect:** Degrades fibrin clots, fibrinogen, other plasma proteins.

PHARMACOKINETICS

Rapidly metabolized in the liver. Primarily excreted in urine. **Half-life:** 35 min.

USES

Treatment of acute MI, acute ischemic stroke, acute massive pulmonary embolism. Treatment of occluded central venous catheters. **OFF-LABEL:** Acute peripheral occlusive disease, basilar artery occlusion, cerebral infarction, deep vein thrombosis, femoropopliteal artery occlusion, mesenteric or subclavian vein occlusion, pleural effusion (parapneumonic).

PRECAUTIONS

CONTRAINDICATIONS: Active internal bleeding, AV malformation or aneurysm, bleeding diathesis, intracranial neoplasm, intracranial or intraspinal surgery or trauma, recent (within past 2 mos) cerebrovascular accident, severe uncontrolled hypertension. **CAUTIONS:** Recent (within 10 days) major surgery or GI bleeding, OB delivery, organ biopsy, recent trauma or CPR, left heart thrombus, endocarditis, severe hepatic/renal disease, pregnancy, elderly, cerebrovascular disease, diabetic retinopathy, thrombophlebitis, occluded AV cannula at infected site.

LIFESPAN CONSIDERATIONS:

Pregnancy/Lactation: Use only when benefit outweighs potential risk to fetus. Unknown if drug crosses placenta or is distributed in breast milk. **Pregnancy Category C. Children:** Safety and efficacy not established. **Elderly:** Risk of bleeding with thrombolytic therapy increases; careful pt selection, monitoring recommended.

INTERACTIONS

DRUG: Oral anticoagulants, heparin, low molecular weight heparins, medications altering platelet function (e.g., NSAIDs, clopidogrel, thrombolytics) increase risk of hemorrhage. **HERBAL: Cat's claw, dong quai, evening primrose, feverfew, red clover, horse chestnut, garlic, green tea, ginseng, ginkgo** may increase risk of bleeding due to antiplatelet activity. **FOOD:** None known. **LAB VALUES:** Decreases plasminogen and fibrinogen levels during infusion, decreases clotting time (confirms the presence of lysis). Decreases Hgb, Hct.

AVAILABILITY (Rx)

INJECTION, POWDER FOR RECONSTITUTION: 2 mg (Cathflo Activase), 50 mg (Activase), 100 mg (Activase).

ADMINISTRATION/HANDLING

IV

Reconstitution • Reconstitute immediately before use with Sterile Water for Injection. • Reconstitute 100-mg vial with 100 ml Sterile Water for Injection (50-mg vial with 50 ml sterile water) without preservative to provide a concentration of 1 mg/ml. May be further diluted with equal volume D_5W or 0.9% NaCl to provide a concentration of 0.5 mg/ml. • Avoid excessive agitation; gently swirl or slowly invert vial to reconstitute.

Rate of administration • Give by IV infusion via infusion pump. See individual dosages. • If minor bleeding occurs at puncture sites, apply pressure for 30 sec; if unrelieved, apply pressure dressing. • If uncontrolled hemorrhage occurs, discontinue infusion immediately (slowing rate of infusion may produce worsening hemorrhage). • Avoid undue pressure when drug is injected into catheter (can rupture catheter or expel clot into circulation).

Storage • Store vials at room temperature. • After reconstitution, solutions appear colorless to pale yellow. • Solution is stable for 8 hrs after reconstitution. Discard unused portions.

IV INCOMPATIBILITIES

Dobutamine (Dobutrex), dopamine (Intropin), heparin, nitroglycerin.

IV COMPATIBILITIES

Lidocaine, metoprolol (Lopressor), morphine, nitroglycerin, propranolol (Inderal).

INDICATIONS/ROUTES/DOSAGE

ACUTE MI

IV INFUSION: ADULTS WEIGHING GREATER THAN 67 KG: Total dose: 100 mg over 90 min, starting with 15-mg bolus over 1–2 min, then 50 mg over 30 min, then 35 mg over 60 min. **ADULTS WEIGHING 67 KG OR LESS: Total dose:** 100 mg over 90 min, starting with 15-mg bolus, then 0.75 mg/kg over 30 min (**Maximum:** 50 mg), then 0.5 mg/kg over 60 min (**Maximum:** 35 mg).

ACUTE PULMONARY EMBOLI

IV INFUSION: ADULTS: 100 mg over 2 hrs. Institute or reinstitute heparin near end or immediately after infusion when aPTT or thrombin time (TT) returns to twice normal or less.

ACUTE ISCHEMIC STROKE

◀ **ALERT** ▶ Dose should be given within the first 3 hrs of the onset of symptoms.

IV INFUSION: ADULTS: 0.9 mg/kg over 60 min (load with 0.09 mg/kg [10% of 0.9 mg/kg dose] as IV bolus over 1 min).

CENTRAL VENOUS CATHETER CLEARANCE

IV: ADULTS, ELDERLY: Up to 2 mg; may repeat after 2 hrs.

SIDE EFFECTS

FREQUENT: Superficial bleeding at puncture sites, decreased B/P. **OCCASIONAL:** Allergic reaction (rash, wheezing, bruising).

ADVERSE EFFECTS/ TOXIC REACTIONS

Severe internal hemorrhage may occur. Lysis of coronary thrombi may produce atrial or ventricular arrhythmias or stroke.

NURSING CONSIDERATIONS

BASELINE ASSESSMENT

Obtain baseline B/P, apical pulse. Record weight. Evaluate 12-lead EKG, cardiac enzymes, electrolytes. Assess Hct, platelet count, thrombin (TT), prothrombin time (PT), activated partial thromboplastin time (aPTT), fibrinogen level before therapy is instituted. Type and crossmatch, hold blood.

INTERVENTION/EVALUATION

Perform continuous cardiac monitoring for arrhythmias. Check B/P, pulse, respirations q15min until stable, then hourly. Check peripheral pulses, heart and lung sounds. Monitor for chest pain relief and notify physician of continuation or recurrence (note location, type, intensity). Assess for bleeding: overt blood, blood in any body substance. Monitor aPTT per protocol. Maintain B/P; avoid any trauma that might increase risk of bleeding (e.g., injections, shaving). Assess neurologic status.

altretamine (hexamethylmelamine)

(Hexalen)

See Antineoplastics (p. 76C)

aluminum hydroxide

a-**loo**-mi-num hye-**drox**-ide

(Alternagel, Amphojel ✤, Basaljel ✤)

FIXED-COMBINATION(S)

With magnesium, an antacid (**Gaviscon, Maalox**); with magnesium and simethicone, an antiflatulent (**Gelusil, Maalox Plus, Mylanta, Silain-Gel**).

CLASSIFICATION

CLINICAL: Antacid (p. 9C).

ACTION

Reduces gastric acid. Binds with phosphate in intestine, then excreted as aluminum carbonate in feces. Resultant decreased serum phosphate level results in increased absorption of calcium. Astringent, adsorbent properties. **Therapeutic Effect:** Neutralizes or increases gastric pH; reduces phosphates in urine, preventing formation of phosphate urinary calculi; decreases fluidity of stools.

USES

Treatment of hyperacidity, hyperphosphatemia.

PRECAUTIONS

CONTRAINDICATIONS: Children age 6 yrs and younger, intestinal obstruction. **CAUTIONS:** Impaired renal function, gastric outlet obstruction, elderly, dehydration, fluid restriction, Alzheimer's disease, symptoms of appendicitis, GI/rectal bleeding, constipation, fecal impaction, chronic diarrhea. **Pregnancy Category C (considered safe except for chronic, high-dose usage)**.

INTERACTIONS

DRUG: May decrease excretion of **quinidine, anticholinergics.** May decrease effects of **methenamine.** May increase **salicylate** excretion. May decrease absorption of **quinolones, iron preparations, isoniazid, ketoconazole, tetracyclines.** **HERBAL:** None significant. **FOOD:** None known. **LAB VALUES:** May increase serum gastrin level, systemic and urinary pH. May decrease serum phosphate level.

AVAILABILITY (OTC)

SUSPENSION: 320 mg/5 ml, 600 mg/5 ml.

ADMINISTRATION/HANDLING

PO

• Usually administered 1–3 hrs after meals. • Individualize dose (based on neutralizing capacity of antacids). • Chewable tablets (fixed combinations): Thoroughly chew tablets before swallowing (follow with glass of water or milk). • If administering suspension, shake well before use.

INDICATIONS/ROUTES/DOSAGE

ANTACID

PO: ADULTS, ELDERLY: 600–1,200 mg between meals and at bedtime.

HYPERPHOSPHATEMIA

PO: ADULTS, ELDERLY: Initially, 300–600 mg 3 times a day with meals. **CHILDREN:** Initially, 50–150 mg/kg/day in divided doses q4–6h. Titrate to maintain serum phosphorus within normal range.

SIDE EFFECTS

FREQUENT: Chalky taste, mild constipation, abdominal cramps. **OCCASIONAL:** Nausea, vomiting, speckling or whitish discoloration of stools.

ADVERSE EFFECTS/ TOXIC REACTIONS

Prolonged constipation may result in intestinal obstruction. Excessive or chronic use may produce hypophosphatemia manifested as anorexia, malaise, muscle weakness, bone pain, resulting in osteomalacia, osteoporosis. Prolonged use may produce urinary calculi.

NURSING CONSIDERATIONS

BASELINE ASSESSMENT

Do not give other PO medication within 1–2 hrs of antacid administration.

INTERVENTION/EVALUATION

Assess daily pattern of bowel activity/ stool consistency. Monitor serum phosphate, calcium, uric acid, aluminum levels. Assess for relief of gastric distress.

PATIENT/FAMILY TEACHING

• **Chewable Tablets (fixed combinations):** Chew tablets thoroughly before swallowing (may be followed by water or milk). • Tablets may discolor stool. • Maintain adequate fluid intake.

amantadine

ah-**man**-tih-deen

(Endantadine ✱, PMS-Amantadine ✱, Symmetrel)

CLASSIFICATION

PHARMACOTHERAPEUTIC: Dopaminergic agonist. **CLINICAL:** Antiviral, antiparkinson agent (see p. 64C).

ACTION

Blocks uncoating of influenza A virus, preventing penetration into the host and inhibiting M2 protein in the assembly of progeny virions. Blocks reuptake of dopamine into presynaptic neurons and causes direct stimulation of postsynaptic receptors. **Therapeutic Effect:** Antiviral, antiparkinsonian activity.

PHARMACOKINETICS

Rapidly and completely absorbed from GI tract. Protein binding: 67%. Widely distributed. Primarily excreted in urine. Minimally removed by hemodialysis. **Half-life:** 11–15 hrs (increased in the elderly, decreased in renal impairment).

USES

Prevention, treatment of respiratory tract infections due to influenza virus, Parkinson's disease, drug-induced extrapyramidal reactions. **OFF-LABEL:** Treatment of ADHD, fatigue associated with multiple sclerosis.

PRECAUTIONS

CONTRAINDICATIONS: None known. **CAUTIONS:** History of seizures, ortho-static hypotension, CHF, peripheral edema, hepatic disease, recurrent eczematoid dermatitis, cerebrovascular disease, renal dysfunction, those receiving CNS stimulants.

LIFESPAN CONSIDERATIONS:

Pregnancy/Lactation: Unknown if drug crosses placenta; distributed in breast milk. **Pregnancy Category C.** **Children:** No age-related precautions noted in those older than 1 yr. **Elderly:** May exhibit increased sensitivity to anticholinergic effects. Age-related renal impairment may require dosage adjustment.

INTERACTIONS

DRUG: **Alcohol** may increase CNS effects. **Quinidine, quinine, trimethoprim/sulfamethoxazole (Bactrim, Septra)** may increase concentration. **Tricyclic antidepressants, antihistamines, phenothiazine, anticholinergics** may increase anticholinergic effects. **Hydrochlorothiazide, triamterene** may increase concentration, toxicity. **HERBAL:** None significant. **FOOD:** None known. **LAB VALUES:** None known.

AVAILABILITY (Rx)

CAPSULES: 100 mg. **SYRUP:** 50 mg/5 ml. **TABLETS:** 100 mg.

ADMINISTRATION/HANDLING

PO

- May give without regard to food.
- Administer nighttime dose several hours before bedtime (prevents insomnia).

INDICATIONS/ROUTES/DOSAGE

TREATMENT OF INFLUENZA A

PO: ADULTS, CHILDREN 13 YRS AND OLDER: 100 mg twice a day. Initiate within 24–48 hrs after onset of symptoms; discontinue as soon as possible based on clinical response. **ELDERLY:** 100 mg a day. **CHILDREN 10–12 YRS, WEIGHING 40 KG AND MORE:** 100 mg twice a day. **CHILDREN 10 YRS AND OLDER, WEIGHING LESS THAN 40 KG:** 5 mg/kg/day. **Maximum:** 150 mg/day. **CHILDREN 1–9 YRS:** 5 mg/kg/day. **Maximum:** 150 mg/day.

PREVENTION OF INFUENZA A

PO: ADULTS, CHILDREN 13 YRS AND OLDER: 100 mg twice a day.

PARKINSON'S DISEASE, EXTRAPYRAMIDAL SYMPTOMS

PO: ADULTS, ELDERLY: 100 mg twice a day. May increase up to 400 mg/day in divided doses.

DOSAGE IN RENAL IMPAIRMENT

Dose and frequency are modified based on creatinine clearance.

Creatinine Clearance	Dosage
30–50 ml/min	200 mg first day; 100 mg/day thereafter
15–29 ml/min	200 mg first day; 100 mg on alternate days
Less than 15 ml/min	200 mg every 7 days

SIDE EFFECTS

FREQUENT (10%–5%): Nausea, dizziness, poor concentration, insomnia, nervousness. **OCCASIONAL (5%–1%):** Orthostatic hypotension, anorexia, headache, livedo reticularis (reddish blue, netlike blotching of skin), blurred vision, urinary retention, dry mouth or nose. **RARE:** Vomiting, depression, irritation or swelling of eyes, rash.

ADVERSE EFFECTS/ TOXIC REACTIONS

CHF, leukopenia, neutropenia occur rarely. Hyperexcitability, seizures, ventricular arrhythmias may occur.

NURSING CONSIDERATIONS

BASELINE ASSESSMENT

When treating infections caused by influenza A virus, obtain specimens for viral diagnostic tests before giving first dose (therapy may begin before results are known).

INTERVENTION/EVALUATION

Monitor I&O, renal function tests if ordered; check for peripheral edema. Evaluate food tolerance, vomiting. Assess skin for mottling or rash. Assess for dizziness. **Parkinson's Disease:** Assess for clinical reversal of symptoms (improvement of tremor of head/hands at rest, mask-like facial expression, shuffling gait, muscular rigidity).

PATIENT/FAMILY TEACHING

• Continue therapy for full length of treatment. • Doses should be evenly spaced. • Do not take any other medications without consulting physician. • Avoid alcoholic beverages. • Do not drive, use machinery, or engage in other activities that require mental acuity if experiencing dizziness, blurred vision. • Get up slowly from a sitting or lying position. • Inform physician of new symptoms, esp. blotching, rash, dizziness, blurred vision, nausea/vomiting. • Take nighttime dose several hours before bedtime to prevent insomnia.

Amaryl, *see glimepiride*

Ambien, *see zolpidem*

AmBisome, *see amphotericin B*

amcinonide

(Cyclocort)

See Corticosteroids: topical (p. 94C)

amifostine

am-ih-**fos**-teen

(Ethyol)

Do not confuse Ethyol with ethanol.

CLASSIFICATION

PHARMACOTHERAPEUTIC: Antineoplastic adjunct. **CLINICAL:** Protective agent.

ACTION

Converted by alkaline phosphatase in tissues, allowing its ability to protect normal tissue relative to tumor tissue. **Therapeutic Effect:** Reduces toxic effect of chemotherapeutic agent cisplatin.

USES

Reduces cumulative renal toxicity associated with repeated administration of cisplatin in those with advanced ovarian cancer. Treatment of postop radiation-induced dry mouth in pts with head or neck cancer. **OFF-LABEL:** Prophylaxis of antineoplastic agent-induced bone marrow toxicity; cisplatin-induced neurotoxicity; protection of lung fibroblasts from damaging effects of chemotherapeutic agent paclitaxel; reduction of mucositis of radiation therapy or radiation therapy combined with chemotherapy; treatment of myelodysplastic syndrome.

PRECAUTIONS

CONTRAINDICATIONS: Sensitivity to aminothiol compounds or mannitol.

CAUTIONS: Uncorrected dehydration or hypotensive pts, those receiving antihypertensive therapy that cannot be interrupted prior to 24 hrs before amifostine treatment, preexisting cardiovascular or cerebrovascular conditions (i.e., ischemic heart disease, arrhythmias, CHF, history of stroke or transient ischemic attack [TIA]), pts receiving chemotherapy for malignancies that are potentially curable (e.g., certain malignancies of germ cell origin). **Pregnancy Category C.**

INTERACTIONS

DRUG: Antihypertensives, other **hypotensive agents** may increase risk of hypotension. **HERBAL:** None significant. **FOOD:** None known. **LAB VALUES:** May reduce serum calcium level, esp. in those with nephrotic syndrome.

AVAILABILITY (Rx)

INJECTION, POWDER FOR RECONSTITUTION: 500 mg in a 10-ml single-use vial.

ADMINISTRATION/HANDLING

IV

Reconstitution • Reconstitute with 9.7 ml 0.9% NaCl. • Further dilute with 0.9% NaCl for a concentration of 5–40 mg/ml.

Rate of administration • Administer over 15 min (30 min before chemotherapy). • If hypotension requires interruption of therapy, place pt in Trendelenburg position; give bolus infusion of normal saline using a separate IV line. • An antiemetic, dexamethasone 20 mg IV and serotonin 5-HT_3 (receptor antagonist) should be given before and concurrently with amifostine.

Storage • Reconstituted solution stable for 5 hrs at room temperature, 24 hrs if refrigerated. • Do not use if discolored or contains particulate matter.

IV INCOMPATIBILITIES

Do not mix amifostine in any solution other than 0.9% NaCl.

IV COMPATIBILITIES

Mannitol, potassium chloride.

INDICATIONS/ROUTES/DOSAGE

CYTOPROTECTIVE (CHEMOTHERAPY)

IV: ADULTS: 910 mg/m^2 once a day as 15-min infusion, beginning 30 min before chemotherapy. 15-min infusion is better tolerated than extended infusions. If full dose cannot be administered, dose for subsequent cycles should be 740 mg/m^2.

RADIATION-INDUCED XEROSTOMIA

IV: ADULTS: 200 mg/m^2 once a day as 3 min infusion, starting 15–30 min before radiation therapy.
SUBCUTANEOUS: ADULTS: 500 mg/day during radiation therapy.

SIDE EFFECTS

FREQUENT (62%): Transient reduction in B/P (usually starts 14 min into infusion, lasts about 6 min and returns to normal in 5–15 min); severe nausea, vomiting. **OCCASIONAL (20%–10%):** Flushing, feeling of warmth or chills, dizziness, hiccups, sneezing, somnolence. **RARE (less than 1%):** Clinically relevant hypocalcemia, mild rash.

ADVERSE EFFECTS/ TOXIC REACTIONS

Pronounced drop in B/P may require temporary cessation of amifostine and fluid resuscitation.

NURSING CONSIDERATIONS

BASELINE ASSESSMENT

Be sure pt is adequately hydrated before infusion. Pt should maintain supine position during the infusion. Interrupt infusion if systolic B/P decreases significantly from baseline (for baseline of less than 100, B/P drop by 20 mm Hg;

for baseline of 100–119, a drop by 25 mm Hg; for baseline of 120–139, a drop by 30 mm Hg; for baseline of 140–179, a drop by 40 mm Hg; for baseline of greater than 180, a drop by 50 mm Hg). If B/P returns to normal within 5 min and pt appears asymptomatic, begin infusion again so that full dose can be administered.

INTERVENTION/EVALUATION

Carefully monitor pt for fluid balance, adequate hydration. Monitor serum calcium levels in those at risk of hypocalcemia (nephrotic syndrome). Monitor B/P q5min during infusion.

amikacin

am-i-**kay**-sin

(Amikin, Amikin Pediatric)

Do not confuse amikacin or Amikin with Amicar.

CLASSIFICATION

PHARMACOTHERAPEUTIC: Aminoglycoside. **CLINICAL:** Antibiotic (see p. 19C).

ACTION

Irreversibly binds to protein on bacterial ribosomes. **Therapeutic Effect:** Interferes with protein synthesis of susceptible microorganisms.

PHARMACOKINETICS

Rapid, complete absorption after IM administration. Protein binding: 0%–10%. Widely distributed (does not cross blood-brain barrier, low concentrations in CSF). Excreted unchanged in urine. Removed by hemodialysis. **Half-life:** 2–4 hrs (increased in renal impairment, neonates; decreased in cystic fibrosis, burn pts, febrile pts).

USES

Treatment of susceptible infections due to Pseudomonas, other gram-negative organisms including biliary tract, bone and joint, CNS, intra-abdominal, skin and soft tissue and UTIs. Treatment of bacterial pneumonia, septicemia.

PRECAUTIONS

CONTRAINDICATIONS: Hypersensitivity to amikacin, other aminoglycosides (cross-sensitivity), or their components. **CAUTIONS:** Myasthenia gravis, parkinsonism, renal impairment, 8th cranial nerve impairment (vestibulocochlear nerve).

LIFESPAN CONSIDERATIONS:

Pregnancy/Lactation: Readily crosses placenta; small amounts distributed in breast milk. May produce fetal nephrotoxicity. **Pregnancy Category C.** **Children:** Neonates, premature infants may be more susceptible to toxicity due to immature renal function. **Elderly:** Higher risk of toxicity due to age-related renal impairment, increased risk of hearing loss.

INTERACTIONS

DRUG: **Nephrotoxic- and ototoxic-producing medications** may increase toxicity. May increase effects of **neuromuscular blocking agents.** **HERBAL:** None significant. **FOOD:** None known. **LAB VALUES:** May increase serum creatinine BUN, AST, ALT, bilirubin, LDH concentrations; may decrease serum calcium, magnesium, potassium, sodium concentrations. Therapeutic serum level: Peak: 20–30 mcg/ml; toxic serum level: greater than 30 mcg/ml; Trough: 1–9 mcg/ml; toxic trough serum level: greater than 10 mcg/ml.

AVAILABILITY (Rx)

INJECTION SOLUTION: 50 mg/ml (Amikin Pediatric), 62.5 mg/ml (Amikin), 250 mg/ml (Amikin).

ADMINISTRATION/HANDLING

IV

Reconstitution • Dilute each 500 mg with 100 ml 0.9% NaCl or D_5W.

Rate of administration • Infuse over 30–60 min for adults, older children; over 60–120 min for infants, young children.

Storage • Store vials at room temperature. • Solutions appear clear but may become pale yellow (does not affect potency). • Intermittent IV infusion (piggyback) is stable for 24 hrs at room temperature. • Discard if precipitate forms or dark discoloration occurs.

IM

• To minimize discomfort, give deep IM slowly. • Less painful if injected into gluteus maximus rather than in lateral aspect of thigh.

IV INCOMPATIBILITIES

Amphotericin, ampicillin, cefazolin (Ancef), heparin, propofol (Diprivan).

IV COMPATIBILITIES

Amiodarone (Cordarone), aztreonam (Azactam), calcium gluconate, cefepime (Maxipime), cimetidine (Tagamet), ciprofloxacin (Cipro), clindamycin (Cleocin), diltiazem (Cardizem), enalapril (Vasotec), esmolol (BreviBloc), fluconazole (Diflucan), furosemide (Lasix), levofloxacin (Levaquin), lorazepam (Ativan), lipids, magnesium sulfate, midazolam (Versed), morphine, ondansetron (Zofran), potassium chloride, ranitidine (Zantac), total parenteral nutrition (TPN), vancomycin.

INDICATIONS/ROUTES/DOSAGE

USUAL PARENTERAL DOSAGE

IV, IM: ADULTS, ELDERLY: 15 mg/kg/day in divided doses q8–12h. **Maximum:** 1.5 g/day. **CHILDREN, INFANTS:** 15–22.5 mg/kg/day in divided doses q8h. **NEONATES:** 7.5–10 mg/kg/dose q8–24h.

DOSAGE IN RENAL IMPAIRMENT

Dosage and frequency are modified based on degree of renal impairment and serum drug concentration. After a loading dose of 5–7.5 mg/kg, maintenance dose and frequency are based on serum creatinine levels and creatinine clearance.

SIDE EFFECTS

FREQUENT: Phlebitis, thrombophlebitis. **OCCASIONAL:** Hypersensitivity reactions (rash, fever, urticaria, pruritus). **RARE:** Neuromuscular blockade (difficulty breathing, drowsiness, weakness).

ADVERSE EFFECTS/ TOXIC REACTIONS

Serious reactions include nephrotoxicity (as evidenced by increased thirst, decreased appetite, nausea, vomiting, increased BUN and serum creatinine levels, decreased creatinine clearance); neurotoxicity (manifested as muscle twitching, visual disturbances, seizures, paresthesias); and ototoxicity (as evidenced by tinnitus, dizziness, loss of hearing).

NURSING CONSIDERATIONS

BASELINE ASSESSMENT

Dehydration must be treated prior to aminoglycoside therapy. Establish pt's baseline hearing acuity before beginning therapy. Question for history of allergies, esp. to aminoglycosides and sulfite. Obtain specimen for culture, sensitivity before giving the first dose (therapy may begin before results are known).

INTERVENTION/EVALUATION

Monitor I&O (maintain hydration), urinalysis (casts, RBC, WBC, decrease in specific gravity). Monitor results of serum peak/trough levels. Be alert to ototoxic, neurotoxic symptoms (see Adverse Effects/Toxic Reactions). Check IM injection site for pain, induration. Evaluate IV site for phlebitis (heat, pain, red streaking over vein). Assess for skin rash, superinfection (particularly genital/anal pruritus), changes of oral mucosa, diarrhea. When treating pts with neuromuscular disorders, assess respiratory response carefully. Therapeutic serum level: Peak: 20–30 mcg/ml; toxic serum level: greater than 30 mcg/ml; trough: 1–9 mcg/ml; toxic serum level: greater than 10 mcg/ml.

PATIENT/FAMILY TEACHING

• Continue antibiotic for full length of treatment. • Space doses evenly. • IM injection may cause discomfort. • Notify physician of any hearing, visual, balance, urinary problems even after therapy is completed. • Do not take other medications without consulting physician. • Lab tests are essential part of therapy.

amiloride

a-**mill**-oh-ride
(Midamor)

Do not confuse amiloride with amiodarone or amlodipine.

FIXED-COMBINATION(S)

Moduretic: amiloride/hydrothiazide (a diuretic): 5 mg/50 mg.

CLASSIFICATION

PHARMACOTHERAPEUTIC: Guanidine derivative. **CLINICAL:** Potassium-sparing diuretic, antihypertensive, antihypokalemic (see p. 97C).

ACTION

Directly interferes with sodium reabsorption in the distal tubule. **Therapeutic Effect:** Increases sodium and water excretion, decreases potassium excretion.

PHARMACOKINETICS

Route	Onset	Peak	Duration
PO	2 hrs	6–10 hrs	24 hrs

Incompletely absorbed from GI tract. Protein binding: Minimal. Primarily excreted in urine; partially eliminated in feces. **Half-life:** 6–9 hrs.

USES

Treatment of hypertension. Management of edema in CHF, hepatic cirrhosis, nephrotic syndrome. **OFF-LABEL:** Treatment of edema associated with CHF, liver cirrhosis, nephrotic syndrome; treatment of hypertension, reduces lithium-induced polyuria, slows pulmonary function reduction in cystic fibrosis.

PRECAUTIONS

CONTRAINDICATIONS: Acute or chronic renal insufficiency, anuria, diabetic nephropathy, pts on other potassium-sparing diuretics, serum potassium greater than 5.5 mEq/L. **CAUTIONS:** BUN greater than 30 mg/dl or serum creatinine greater than 1.5 mg/dl, elderly/debilitated pts, hepatic insufficiency, cardiopulmonary disease, diabetes mellitus.

LIFESPAN CONSIDERATIONS: **Pregnancy/Lactation:** Unknown if drug crosses placenta or is distributed in breast milk. **Pregnancy Category B (D if used in pregnancy-induced hypertension).** **Children:** No age-related precautions noted. **Elderly:** Increased risk of hyperkalemia, age-related renal impairment may require caution.

INTERACTIONS

DRUG: May decrease effect of **anticoagulants, heparin. NSAIDs** may decrease antihypertensive effect. **Cyclosporine, ACE inhibitors (e.g., captopril), potassium-sparing diuretics, potassium supplements** may increase potassium. May decrease **lithium** clearance, increase toxicity. **HERBAL:** None significant. **FOOD:** None known. **LAB VALUES:** May increase BUN, calcium excretion, serum creatinine, glucose, magnesium, potassium, uric acid. May decrease serum sodium.

AVAILABILITY (Rx)

TABLETS: 5 mg.

ADMINISTRATION/HANDLING

PO

- Give with food to prevent GI distress.

INDICATIONS/ROUTES/DOSAGE

HYPERTENSION, EDEMA

PO: ADULTS, CHILDREN WEIGHING MORE THAN 20 KG: 5–10 mg/day up to 20 mg. **ELDERLY:** Initially, 5 mg/day or every other day. **CHILDREN WEIGHING 6–20 KG:** 0.625 mg/kg/day. **Maximum:** 10 mg/day.

DOSAGE IN RENAL IMPAIRMENT

Creatinine Clearance	Dosage
10–50 ml/min	50% of normal
Less than 10 ml/min	Avoid use

SIDE EFFECTS

FREQUENT (8%–3%): Headache, nausea, diarrhea, vomiting, decreased appetite. **OCCASIONAL (3%–1%):** Dizziness, constipation, abdominal pain, weakness, fatigue, cough, impotence. **RARE (less than 1%):** Tremors, vertigo, confusion, nervousness, insomnia, thirst, dry mouth, heartburn, shortness of breath, increased urination, hypotension, rash.

ADVERSE EFFECTS/ TOXIC REACTIONS

Severe hyperkalemia may produce irritability, anxiety, sensation of heaviness of legs; paresthesia of hands/face/lips; hypotension, bradycardia, EKG changes (tented T waves, widening of QRS, ST depression).

NURSING CONSIDERATIONS

BASELINE ASSESSMENT

Assess baseline serum electrolytes, particularly for low potassium. Assess renal/hepatic functions. Assess edema (note location, extent), skin turgor, mucous membranes for hydration status. Assess muscle strength, mental status. Note skin temperature, moisture. Obtain baseline weight. Initiate strict I&O. Obtain baseline 12-lead EKG. Note pulse rate/rhythm.

INTERVENTION/EVALUATION

Monitor B/P, vital signs, electrolytes (particularly potassium), I&O, weight. Note extent of diuresis. Watch for changes from initial assessment; hyperkalemia may result in muscle strength changes, tremor, muscle cramps, change in mental status (orientation, alertness, confusion), cardiac arrhythmias. Monitor serum potassium level, particularly during initial therapy. Weigh daily. Assess lung sounds for rales, wheezing.

PATIENT/FAMILY TEACHING

• Expect increase in volume/frequency of urination. • Therapeutic effect takes several days to begin and can last for several days when drug is discontinued. • High-potassium diet/potassium supplements can be dangerous, esp. if pt has renal/hepatic problems. • Avoid foods high in potassium such as whole grains (cereals), legumes, meat, bananas, apricots, orange juice, potatoes (white, sweet), raisins. • Contact physician if confusion, irregular heartbeat, nervousness, numbness of hands, feet, lips, difficulty breathing, unusual fatigue, or weakness in legs occur (hyperkalemia).

aminocaproic acid

a-mee-noe-ka-**proe**-ik **ah**-sid

(Amicar)

Do not confuse Amicar with amikacin or Amikin.

CLASSIFICATION

PHARMACOTHERAPEUTIC: Systemic hemostatic. **CLINICAL:** Antifibrinolytic, antihemorrhagic.

ACTION

Inhibits activation of plasminogen activator substances. **Therapeutic Effect:** Prevents formation of fibrin clots.

USES

Treatment of excessive bleeding from hyperfibrinolysis or urinary fibrinolysis as noted in anemia, abruptio placentae, cirrhosis, carcinoma of prostate, lung, stomach, cervix. **OFF-LABEL:** Control of bleeding in thrombocytopenia, control of oral bleeding in congenital and acquired coagulation disorders, prevention of recurrence of subarachnoid hemorrhage, prevention of hemorrhage in hemophiliacs following dental surgery, treatment of traumatic hyphema.

PRECAUTIONS

CONTRAINDICATIONS: Active intravascular clotting process, disseminated intravascular coagulation without concurrent heparin therapy, hematuria of upper urinary tract origin (unless benefit outweighs risk); newborns (parenteral form). **CAUTIONS:** Cardiac, hepatic, renal impairment; those with hyperfibrinolysis, premature neonates. **Pregnancy Category C.**

INTERACTIONS

DRUG: **Oral contraceptives, estrogens** increase risk of hypercoagulability. **HERBAL:** None significant. **FOOD:** None known. **LAB VALUES:** May elevate serum potassium level.

AVAILABILITY (Rx)

INJECTION, SOLUTION: 250 mg/ml. **SYRUP:** 250 mg/ml. **TABLETS:** 500 mg.

ADMINISTRATION/HANDLING

IV

Reconstitution • Dilute each 1 g in up to 50 ml 0.9% NaCl, D_5W, Ringer's, or Sterile Water for Injection (do not use Sterile Water for Injection in pts with subarachnoid hemorrhage).

Rate of administration • Give only by IV infusion. • Infuse 5 g or less over first hr in 250 ml of solution; give each succeeding 1 g over 1 hr in 50–100 ml solution.

Administration precaution • Monitor for hypotension during infusion. • Rapid infusion may produce bradycardia, arrhythmias.

IV INCOMPATIBILITY

Sodium lactate.

INDICATIONS/ROUTES/DOSAGE

ACUTE BLEEDING

PO, IV INFUSION: ADULTS, ELDERLY: 4–5 g over first hr; then 1–1.25 g/hr. Continue for 8 hrs or until bleeding is controlled. **Maximum:** 30 g/24 hr. **CHILDREN:** 100–200 mg/kg over first hr then 33.3 mg/kg/hr or 100 mg/kg q6h. **Maximum:** 18 g/m^2/24 hrs.

DOSAGE IN RENAL IMPAIRMENT

Decrease dose to 25% of normal.

SIDE EFFECTS

OCCASIONAL: Nausea, diarrhea, cramps, decreased urination, decreased B/P, dizziness, headache, muscle fatigue and weakness, myopathy, bloodshot eyes.

ADVERSE EFFECTS/ TOXIC REACTIONS

Too-rapid IV administration produces tinnitus, rash, arrhythmias, unusual fatigue, weakness. Rarely, grand mal seizure occurs, generally preceded by weakness, dizziness, headache.

NURSING CONSIDERATIONS

INTERVENTION/EVALUATION

Question for any change in muscle strength as noted by pt. Monitor for increased serum creatine kinase (CK), AST serum levels (skeletal myopathy). Monitor heart rhythm. Assess for decrease in B/P, increase in pulse rate, abdominal/back pain, severe headache (may be evidence of hemorrhage). Assess peripheral pulses for quality, skin for ecchymoses, petechiae. Question for increased discharge during menses. Check for excessive bleeding from minor cuts, scratches. Assess gums for erythema, gingival bleeding. Observe urine for hematuria.

PATIENT/FAMILY TEACHING

- Report any sign of red/dark urine, black/red stool, coffee-ground vomitus, blood-tinged mucus from cough.

aminophylline evolve

am-in-**ah**-phil-lin

(Phyllocontin)

theophylline

(Elixophyllin, Quibron-T, Quibron-T/SR, Theo-24, Theolair, T-Phyl, Uniphyl)

Do not confuse aminophylline with amitriptyline or ampicillin, or Slo-Bid with Dolobid.

◆ CLASSIFICATION

PHARMACOTHERAPEUTIC: Xanthine derivative. **CLINICAL:** Bronchodilator (see p. 69C).

ACTION

Directly relaxes smooth muscle of bronchial airways and pulmonary blood vessels. **Therapeutic Effect:** Relieves bronchospasm, increases vital capacity.

USES

Symptomatic relief, prevention of bronchial asthma, reversible bronchospasm due to chronic bronchitis, emphysema, or chronic obstructive pumonary disease (COPD). **OFF-LABEL:** Treatment of apnea in neonates.

PRECAUTIONS

CONTRAINDICATIONS: History of hypersensitivity to caffeine or xanthine. **CAUTIONS:** Cardiac, renal, hepatic impairment; hypertension; hyperthyroidism; diabetes mellitus; peptic ulcer; glaucoma; severe hypoxemia; underlying seizure disorder. **Pregnancy Category C.**

INTERACTIONS

DRUG: **Phenytoin, primidone, rifampin** may increase metabolism. **Beta-blockers** may decrease effects. **Cimetidine, ciprofloxacin, clarithromycin, erythromycin, norfloxacin** may increase concentration, toxicity. **Smoking** may decrease concentration. **HERBAL:** None significant. **FOOD:** **Charcoal-broiled foods, high-protein/low-carbohydrate diet** may decrease serum level. **LAB VALUES:** None known.

AVAILABILITY (Rx)

ELIXIR (ELIXOPHYLLIN): 80 mg/15 ml. **INFUSION (THEOPHYLLINE):** 0.8 mg/ml, 1.6 mg/ml, 2 mg/ml, 3.2 mg/ml, 4 mg/ml. **INJECTION SOLUTION (AMINOPHYLLINE):** 25 mg/ml. **ORAL, SOLUTION:** 80 mg/15 ml.

CAPSULES (EXTENDED-RELEASE [THEO-24]): 100 mg, 200 mg, 300 mg, 400 mg.

TABLETS (CONTROLLED-RELEASE): 100 mg **(THEOCHRON)**, 200 mg **(THEOCHRON, T-PHYL)**, 300 mg **(QUIBRON-T/SR, THEOCHRON, THEOLAIR-SR)**, 400 mg **(UNIPHYL)**, 500 mg **(THEOLAIR-SR)**, 600 mg **(UNIPHYL)**.

ADMINISTRATION/HANDLING

IV

Dilution • Give loading dose diluted in 100–200 ml of D_5W or 0.9% NaCl. • Prepare maintenance dose in larger volume parenteral infusion.

Rate of administration • Do not exceed flow rate of 1 ml/min (25 mg/min) for either piggyback or infusion. • Administer loading dose over 20–30 min. • Use infusion pump or microdrip to regulate IV administration.

Storage • Store at room temperature. • Discard if solution contains precipitate.

PO

• Give with food to prevent GI distress.
• Do not crush/break extended-release forms.

IV INCOMPATIBILITIES

Amiodarone (Cordarone), ciprofloxacin (Cipro), dobutamine (Dobutrex), ondansetron (Zofran).

IV COMPATIBILITIES

Aztreonam (Azactam), ceftazidime (Fortaz), fluconazole (Diflucan), heparin, lipids, morphine, potassium chloride, total parenteral nutrition (TPN).

INDICATIONS/ROUTES/DOSAGE

ASTHMA

IV: ADULTS: Initially 5 mg/kg bolus over 20–30 min (to provide serum theophylline of 5–15 mg/ml), then 0.4 mg/kg/hr continuous infusion. **ELDERLY:** 5 mg/kg bolus, then 0.2 mg/kg/hr continuous infusion. **CHILDREN 9–16 YRS:** Initially 5 mg/kg bolus, then 0.7 mg/kg/hr. **CHILDREN 1–8 YRS:** Initially 5 mg/kg bolus, then 0.8 mg/kg/hr.

PO: ADULTS: Initially 5 mg/kg (use ideal body weight), then 300–600 mg/day in 3–4 divided doses. **ELDERLY:** Initially 5 mg/kg, then 2 mg/kg q8h.

PO (CONTROLLED-RELEASE 12-HR FORMULATIONS): ADULTS, CHILDREN WEIGHING 45 KG OR MORE: Initially 300 mg/day in 2 divided doses. May increase in 3 days to 400 mg/day in 2 divided doses. May increase in 3 days to 600 mg/day in 2 divided doses. **CHILDREN WEIGHING LESS THAN 45 KG:** Initially 12–24 mg/kg/day in divided doses. **Maximum:** 300 mg. May increase in 3 days to 16 mg/kg/day. **Maximum:** 400 mg. May increase in 3 days to 20 mg/kg/day. **Maximum:** 600 mg.

PO (EXTENDED-RELEASE 24-HR FORMULATIONS): ADULTS, CHILDREN WEIGHING 45 KG OR MORE: Initially 300–400 mg/day. May increase in 3 days to 400–600 mg/day, then titrate according to blood level. **CHILDREN WEIGHING LESS THAN 45 KG:** Initially 12–24 mg/kg/day. **Maximum:** 300 mg. May increase in 3 days to 16 mg/kg/day. **Maximum:** 400 mg. May increase in 3 days to 20 mg/kg/day. **Maximum:** 600 mg.

SIDE EFFECTS

FREQUENT: Altered smell (during IV administration), restlessness, tachycardia, tremor. **OCCASIONAL:** Heartburn, vomiting, headache, mild diuresis, insomnia, nausea.

ADVERSE EFFECTS/ TOXIC REACTIONS

Too-rapid IV administration may produce marked hypotension with accompanying syncope, light-headedness, palpitations, tachycardia, hyperventilation, nausea, vomiting, angina-like pain, seizures, ventricular fibrillation, cardiac standstill.

NURSING CONSIDERATIONS

BASELINE ASSESSMENT

Offer emotional support (high incidence of anxiety due to difficulty in breathing

A

and sympathomimetic response to drug). Peak serum concentration should be drawn 1 hr following IV dose, 1–2 hrs after immediate-release dose, 3–8 hrs after extended-release dose. Draw trough level just before next dose.

INTERVENTION/EVALUATION

Monitor rate, depth, rhythm, type of respiration; quality/rate of pulse. Assess lung sounds for rhonchi, wheezing, rales. Monitor ABGs. Observe lips, fingernails for cyanosis (blue or dusky color in light-skinned pts; gray in dark-skinned pts). Observe for clavicular retractions, hand tremor. Evaluate for clinical improvement (quieter, slower respirations, relaxed facial expression, cessation of clavicular retractions). Monitor serum theophylline levels (therapeutic serum level range: 10–20 mcg/ml).

PATIENT/FAMILY TEACHING

• Increase fluid intake (decreases lung secretion viscosity). • Avoid excessive caffeine derivatives (chocolate, coffee, tea, cola, cocoa). • Smoking, charcoal-broiled food, high-protein/low-carbohydrate diet may decrease serum theophylline level.

amiodarone

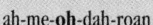

ah-me-**oh**-dah-roan

(Apo-Amiodarone ✦, Cordarone, Cordarone I.V., Novo-Amiodarone ✦, Pacerone)

Do not confuse amiodarone with amiloride or Cordarone with Cardura.

CLASSIFICATION

PHARMACOTHERAPEUTIC: Cardiac agent. **CLINICAL:** Antiarrhythmic (see p. 16C).

ACTION

Prolongs duration of myocardial cell action potential and refractory period by acting directly on all cardiac tissue. Decreases AV and sinus node function. **Therapeutic Effect:** Suppresses arrhythmias.

PHARMACOKINETICS

Route	Onset	Peak	Duration
PO	3 days–3 wks	1 wk–5 mos	7–50 days after discontinuation

Slowly, variably absorbed from GI tract. Protein binding: 96%. Extensively metabolized in the liver to active metabolite. Excreted via bile; not removed by hemodialysis. **Half-life:** 26–107 days; metabolite, 61 days.

USES

Oral: Management of life-threatening recurrent ventricular fibrillation, hemodynamically unstable ventricular tachycardia (VT). **IV:** Management/prophylaxis of frequently occurring ventricular fibrillation, unstable ventricular tachycardia (VT) unresponsive to other therapy. **OFF-LABEL:** Control of hemodynamically stable VT, control of rapid ventricular rate due to accessory pathway conduction in pre-excited atrial arrhythmias, conversion of atrial fibrillation to normal sinus rhythm, in cardiac arrest with persistent VT or ventricular fibrillation, paroxysmal supraventricular tachycardia, polymorphic VT or wide complex tachycardia of uncertain origin, prevention of postoperative atrial fibrillation.

PRECAUTIONS

CONTRAINDICATIONS: Bradycardia-induced syncope (except in the presence of a pacemaker), second- and third-degree AV block, severe hepatic disease, severe sinus node dysfunction. **CAUTIONS:** Thyroid disease, electrolyte imbalance, hepatic disease, hypotension, left ventricular dysfunction, photosensitivity, pulmonary disease.

LIFESPAN CONSIDERATIONS:

Pregnancy/Lactation: Crosses placenta; distributed in breast milk. May adversely affect fetal development. **Pregnancy Category D. Children:** Safety and efficacy not established. **Elderly:** May be more sensitive to effects on thyroid function. May experience increased incidence ataxia, other neurotoxic effects.

INTERACTIONS

DRUG: May increase cardiac effects with **other antiarrhythmics.** May increase effect of **beta-blockers, oral anticoagulants.** May increase concentration, toxicity of **digoxin, phenytoin. Simvastatin** may increase risk for myopathy, rhabdomyolysis. **HERBAL: St. John's wort** may decrease effect. **FOOD: Grapefruit, grapefruit juice** may decrease effect. **LAB VALUES:** May increase serum AST, ALT, alkaline phosphatase, ANA titer. May cause changes in EKG, thyroid function test results. Therapeutic serum level: 0.5–2.5 mcg/ml; toxic serum level not established.

AVAILABILITY (Rx)

INJECTION, SOLUTION (CORDARONE I.V.): 50 mg/ml. **TABLETS:** 100 mg (Pacerone), 200 mg (Cordarone, Pacerone) 300 mg (Pacerone), 400 mg (Pacerone).

ADMINISTRATION/HANDLING

IV

Reconstitution • Use glass or polyolefin containers for dilution. • Dilute loading dose (150 mg) in 100 ml D_5W (1.5 mg/ml). • Dilute maintenance dose (900 mg) in 500 ml D_5W (1.8 mg/ml). Concentrations greater than 3 mg/ml cause peripheral vein phlebitis.

Rate of administration • Does not need protection from light during administration. • Administer through central venous catheter (CVC) if possible, using in-line filter. • Bolus over 10 min (15 mg/min) not to exceed 30 mg/min; then 1 mg/min over 6 hrs; then 0.5 mg/min over 18 hrs. • Infusions longer than 1 hr, concentration not to exceed 2 mg/ml unless CVC used.

Storage • Store at room temperature. • Use in PVC containers within 2 hrs of dilution; within 24 hrs with glass or polyolefin containers.

PO

- Give with meals to reduce GI distress.
- Tablets may be crushed.

IV INCOMPATIBILITIES

Aminophylline (theophylline), cefazolin (Ancef), heparin, sodium bicarbonate.

IV COMPATIBILITIES

Dobutamine (Dobutrex), dopamine (Intropin), furosemide (Lasix), insulin (regular), labetalol (Normodyne), lidocaine, midazolam (Versed), morphine, nitroglycerin, norepinephrine (Levophed), phenylephrine (Neo-Synephrine), potassium chloride, vancomycin.

INDICATIONS/ROUTES/DOSAGE

VENTRICULAR ARRHYTHMIAS

PO: ADULTS, ELDERLY: Initially, 800–1,600 mg/day in 2–4 divided doses for 1–3 wks. After arrhythmia is controlled or side effects occur, reduce to 600–800 mg/day for about 4 wks. **Maintenance:** 200–600 mg/day. **CHILDREN:** Initially, 10–20 mg/kg/day for 4–14 days, then 5 mg/kg/day for several wks. **Maintenance:** 2.5 mg/kg/day or lowest effective maintenance dose for 5 of 7 days/wk.

IV INFUSION: ADULTS: Initially, 1,050 mg over 24 hrs; 150 mg over 10 min, then 360 mg over 6 hrs; then 540 mg over 18 hrs. May continue at 0.5 mg/min. After first 24 hrs, infuse

720 mg/24 hrs with a concentration of 1–6 mg/ml.

SIDE EFFECTS

EXPECTED: Corneal microdeposits noted in almost all pts treated for more than 6 mos (can lead to blurry vision). **FREQUENT (greater than 3%): Parenteral:** Hypotension, nausea, fever, bradycardia. **Oral:** Constipation, headache, decreased appetite, nausea, vomiting, paresthesias, photosensitivity, muscular incoordination. **OCCASIONAL (less than 3%): Oral:** Bitter or metallic taste; decreased libido; dizziness; facial flushing; blue-gray coloring of skin (face, arms, and neck); blurred vision; bradycardia; asymptomatic corneal deposits. **RARE (less than 1%): Oral:** Rash, vision loss, blindness.

ADVERSE EFFECTS/ TOXIC REACTIONS

Serious, potentially fatal pulmonary toxicity (alveolitis, pulmonary fibrosis, pneumonitis, acute respiratory distress syndrome) may begin with progressive dyspnea and cough with crackles, decreased breath sounds, pleurisy, CHF, or hepatotoxicity. May worsen existing arrhythmias or produce new arrhythmias.

NURSING CONSIDERATIONS

BASELINE ASSESSMENT

Obtain baseline pulmonary function tests, chest x-ray, hepatic enzyme tests, serum AST, ALT, alkaline phosphatase, 12-lead EKG. Assess B/P, apical pulse immediately before drug is administered (if pulse is 60/min or less or systolic B/P is less than 90 mm Hg, withhold medication, contact physician).

INTERVENTION/EVALUATION

Monitor for symptoms of pulmonary toxicity (progressively worsening dyspnea, cough). Dosage should be discontinued or reduced if toxicity occurs. Assess pulse for quality, rhythm, bradycardia. Monitor EKG for cardiac changes, (e.g., widening of QRS, prolongation of PR and QT intervals). Notify physician of any significant interval changes. Assess for nausea, fatigue, paresthesia, tremor. Monitor for signs of hypothyroidism (periorbital edema, lethargy, pudgy hands/feet, cool/pale skin, vertigo, night cramps) and hyperthyroidism (hot/dry skin, bulging eyes [exophthalmos], frequent urination, eyelid edema, weight loss, difficulty breathing). Monitor serum AST, ALT, alkaline phosphatase for evidence of hepatic toxicity. Assess skin, cornea for bluish discoloration in those who have been on drug therapy longer than 2 mos. Monitor hepatic function tests, thyroid test results. If elevated hepatic enzymes occur, dosage reduction or discontinuation is necessary. Monitor for therapeutic serum level (0.5–2.5 mcg/ml). Toxic serum level not established.

PATIENT/FAMILY TEACHING

• Protect against photosensitivity reaction on skin exposed to sunlight. • Bluish skin discoloration gradually disappears when drug is discontinued. • Report shortness of breath, cough. • Outpatients should monitor pulse before taking medication. • Do not abruptly discontinue medication. • Compliance with therapy regimen is essential to control arrhythmias. • Restrict salt, alcohol intake. • Recommend ophthalmic exams q6mo. • Report any vision changes.

amitriptyline

a-me-**trip**-tih-leen
(Apo-Amitriptyline ✤, Elavil, Levate ✤, Novo-Tryptyn ✤)

Do not confuse amitriptyline with aminophylline or nortriptyline, or Elavil with Equanil or Mellaril.

FIXED-COMBINATION(S)

Etrafon, Triavil: amitriptyline/perphenazine (an antipsychotic): 10 mg/2 mg; 25 mg/2 mg; 10 mg/4 mg; 25 mg/4 mg. **Limbitrol:** amitriptyline/chlordiaz epoxide (an antianxiety): 12.5 mg/5 mg; 25 mg/10 mg.

◆ CLASSIFICATION

PHARMACOTHERAPEUTIC: Tricyclic. **CLINICAL:** Antidepressant, antineuralgic, antibulimic (see p. 36C).

ACTION

Blocks reuptake of neurotransmitters, (norepinephrine, serotonin) at presynaptic membranes, increasing availability at postsynaptic receptor sites. Strong anticholinergic activity. **Therapeutic Effect:** Antidepressant effect.

PHARMACOKINETICS

Rapidly and well absorbed from the GI tract. Protein binding: 90%. Undergoes first-pass metabolism in the liver. Primarily excreted in urine. Minimal removal by hemodialysis. **Half-life:** 10–26 hrs.

USES

Treatment of various forms of depression, exhibited as persistent, prominent dysphoria (occurring nearly every day for at least 2 wks) manifested by 4 of 8 symptoms: appetite change, sleep pattern change, increased fatigue, impaired concentration, feelings of guilt or worthlessness, loss of interest in usual activities, psychomotor agitation or retardation, suicidal tendencies. **OFF-LABEL:** Relief of neuropathic pain, such as that experienced by pts with diabetic neuropathy or postherpetic neuralgia; treatment of anxiety, bulimia nervosa, migraine, nocturnal enuresis, panic disorder, peptic ulcer.

PRECAUTIONS

CONTRAINDICATIONS: Acute recovery period after MI, use within 14 days of MAOIs. **CAUTIONS:** Prostatic hypertrophy, history of urinary retention or obstruction, glaucoma, diabetes mellitus, history of seizures, hyperthyroidism, cardiac/hepatic/renal disease, schizophrenia, increased intraocular pressure (IOP), hiatal hernia.

⌛ LIFESPAN CONSIDERATIONS:

Pregnancy/Lactation: Crosses placenta; minimally distributed in breast milk. **Pregnancy Category C. Children:** More sensitive to increased dosage, toxicity, increased risk of suicidal ideation, worsening of depression. **Elderly:** Increased risk of toxicity. Increased sensitivity to anticholinergic effects. Cautions in those with cardiovascular disease.

INTERACTIONS

DRUG: CNS depressants (including alcohol, barbiturates, phenothiazines, sedative-hypnotics, anticonvulsants) may increase sedation, respiratory depression, hypotensive effects. **Antithyroid agents** may increase risk of agranulocytosis. **Phenothiazines** may increase sedative, anticholinergic effects. **Cimetidine, valproic acid** may increase concentration, toxicity. May decrease effects of **clonidine.** May increase cardiac effects with **sympathomimetics.** May increase risk of hypertensive crisis, hyperpyresis, seizures with **MAOIs. HERBAL: St. John's wort** may decrease levels. **Valerian, kava kava, gotu, kola, St. John's wort** may increase CNS depression. **FOOD:** None known. **LAB VALUES:** May alter EKG readings (flattened T wave), serum glucose. Therapeutic serum level: Peak: 120-250 ng/ml; toxic serum level: greater than 500 ng/ml.

AVAILABILITY (Rx)

INJECTION SOLUTION (ELAVIL): 10 mg/ml. **TABLETS (ELAVIL):** 10 mg, 25 mg, 50 mg, 75 mg, 100 mg, 150 mg.

ADMINISTRATION/HANDLING

IM

• Give by IM only if PO administration is not feasible. • Crystals may form in injectable solution. Redissolve by immersing ampule in hot water for 1 min. • Give deep IM slowly.

PO

• Give with food or milk if GI distress occurs.

INDICATIONS/ROUTES/DOSAGE

DEPRESSION

PO: ADULTS: 25–100 mg/day as a single dose at bedtime or in divided doses. May gradually increase up to 300 mg/day. Titrate to lowest effective dosage. **ELDERLY:** Initially, 10–25 mg at bedtime. May increase by 10–25 mg at weekly intervals. Range: 25–150 mg/day. **CHILDREN 6–12 YRS:** 1–5 mg/kg/day in 2 divided doses.

IM: ADULTS: 20–30 mg 4 times a day.

PAIN MANAGEMENT

PO: ADULTS, ELDERLY: 25–100 mg at bedtime.

SIDE EFFECTS

FREQUENT: Dizziness, somnolence, dry mouth, orthostatic hypotension, headache, increased appetite, weight gain, nausea, unusual fatigue, unpleasant taste. **OCCASIONAL:** Blurred vision, confusion, constipation, hallucinations, delayed micturition, eye pain, arrhythmias, fine muscle tremors, parkinsonian syndrome, anxiety, diarrhea, diaphoresis, heartburn, insomnia. **RARE:** Hypersensitivity, alopecia, tinnitus, breast enlargement, photosensitivity.

ADVERSE EFFECTS/ TOXIC REACTIONS

Overdose may produce confusion, seizures, severe somnolence, fast/slow/irregular heart rate, fever, hallucinations, agitation, dyspnea, vomiting, unusual fatigue, weakness. Abrupt withdrawal after prolonged therapy may produce headache, malaise, nausea, vomiting, vivid dreams. Blood dyscrasias, cholestatic jaundice occur rarely.

NURSING CONSIDERATIONS

BASELINE ASSESSMENT

Observe and record behavior. Assess psychological status, thought content, sleep patterns, appearance, interest in environment. For those on long-term therapy, hepatic/renal function tests, blood counts should be performed periodically.

INTERVENTION/EVALUATION

Supervise suicidal-risk pt closely during early therapy (as depression lessens, energy level improves, increasing suicide potential). Assess appearance, behavior, speech pattern, level of interest, mood. Monitor B/P, pulse for hypotension, arrhythmias. Therapeutic serum level: Peak: 120–250 ng/ml; toxic serum level: greater than 500 ng/ml.

PATIENT/FAMILY TEACHING

• Change positions slowly to avoid hypotensive effect. Tolerance to postural hypotension, sedative and anticholinergic effects usually develop during early therapy. • Maximum therapeutic effect may be noted in 2–4 wks. • Sensitivity to sun may occur. • Report visual disturbances. • Do not abruptly discontinue medication. • Avoid tasks that require alertness, motor skills until response to drug is established. • Sips of tepid water may relieve dry mouth.

amlodipine

am-**low**-dih-peen

(Norvasc)

Do not confuse amlodipine with amiloride, or Norvasc with Navane or Vascor.

FIXED-COMBINATIONS

Caduet: amlodipine/atorvastatin (hydroxamethylglutaryl-CoA [HMG-CoA] reductase inhibitor): 2.5 mg/10 mg; 2.5 mg/20 mg; 2.5 mg/40 mg; 5 mg/10 mg; 10 mg/10 mg; 5 mg/20 mg; 10 mg/20 mg; 5 mg/40 mg; 10 mg/40 mg; 5 mg/80 mg; 10 mg/80 mg. **Exforge:** amlodipine/valsartan (an angiotensin II receptor antagonist): 5 mg/160 mg; 10 mg/160 mg; 5 mg/320 mg; 10 mg/320 mg. **Lotrel:** amlodipine/benazepril (an angiotensin-converting enzyme [ACE] inhibitor): 2.5 mg/10 mg; 5 mg/10 mg; 5 mg/20 mg; 5 mg/40 mg; 10 mg/20 mg; 10 mg/40 mg.

CLASSIFICATION

PHARMACOTHERAPEUTIC: Calcium channel blocker. **CLINICAL:** Antihypertensive, antianginal (see p. 73C).

ACTION

Inhibits calcium movement across cardiac and vascular smooth muscle cell membranes. **Therapeutic Effect:** Dilates coronary arteries, peripheral arteries/arterioles. Decreases total peripheral vascular resistance and B/P by vasodilation.

PHARMACOKINETICS

Route	Onset	Peak	Duration
PO	0.5–1 hr	6–12 hrs	24 hrs

Slowly absorbed from GI tract. Protein binding: 93%. Undergoes first-pass metabolism in the liver. Excreted primarily in urine. Not removed by hemodialysis. **Half-life:** 30–50 hrs (increased in the elderly, those with hepatic cirrhosis).

USES

Management of hypertension, chronic stable angina, vasospastic (Prinzmetal's or variant) angina. May be used alone or with other antihypertensives or antianginals.

PRECAUTIONS

CONTRAINDICATIONS: Severe hypotension. **CAUTIONS:** Hepatic impairment, aortic stenosis, CHF.

LIFESPAN CONSIDERATIONS:

Pregnancy/Lactation: Unknown if drug crosses placenta or is distributed in breast milk. **Pregnancy Category C.** **Children:** Safety and efficacy not established. **Elderly:** Half-life may be increased, more sensitive to hypotensive effects.

INTERACTIONS

DRUG: None significant. **HERBAL:** **St. John's wort** may decrease concentration. **Ephedra, yohimbe** may worsen hypertension. **Garlic** may increase antihypertensive effect. **FOOD:** **Grapefruit, grapefruit juice** may increase concentration, hypotensive effects. **LAB VALUES:** None known.

AVAILABILITY (Rx)

TABLETS: 2.5 mg, 5 mg, 10 mg.

ADMINISTRATION/HANDLING

PO

- May give without regard to food.

INDICATIONS/ROUTES/DOSAGE

HYPERTENSION

PO: **ADULTS:** Initially, 5 mg/day as a single dose. May increase by 2.5 mg/day every 7–14 days. **Maximum:** 10 mg/day. **SMALL-FRAME, FRAGILE, ELDERLY:** Initially, 2.5 mg/day as a single dose. **CHILDREN 6–17 YRS:** 2.5–5 mg/day.

ANGINA (CHRONIC STABLE OR VASOSPASTIC)

PO: ADULTS: 5–10 mg/day as a single dose. **ELDERLY, PTS WITH HEPATIC INSUFFICIENCY:** 5 mg/day as a single dose.

DOSAGE IN RENAL IMPAIRMENT

ADULTS, ELDERLY: (Hypertension) 2.5 mg/day. (Angina) 5 mg/day.

SIDE EFFECTS

FREQUENT (greater than 5%): Peripheral edema, headache, flushing. **OCCASIONAL (5%–1%):** Dizziness, palpitations, nausea, unusual fatigue or weakness (asthenia). **RARE (less than 1%):** Chest pain, bradycardia, orthostatic hypotension.

ADVERSE EFFECTS/ TOXIC REACTIONS

Overdose may produce excessive peripheral vasodilation, marked hypotension with reflex tachycardia.

NURSING CONSIDERATIONS

BASELINE ASSESSMENT

Assess baseline renal/hepatic function tests, B/P, apical pulse.

INTERVENTION/EVALUATION

Assess B/P (if systolic B/P is less than 90 mm Hg, withhold medication, contact physician). Assess for peripheral edema behind medial malleolus (sacral area in bedridden pts). Assess skin for flushing. Question for headache, asthenia.

PATIENT/FAMILY TEACHING

• Do not abruptly discontinue medication. • Compliance with therapy regimen is essential to control hypertension. • Avoid tasks that require alertness, motor skills until response to drug is established. • Avoid concomitant ingestion of grapefruit juice.

amoxicillin

ah-mocks-ih-**sill**-in

(Amoxicot, Amoxil, Amoxil Pediatric Drops, Biomox, DisperMox, Moxilin, Novamoxin ✤, Polymox, Trimox, Wymox)

Do not confuse amoxicillin with amoxapine or DisperMox with Diamox or Trimox with Tylox.

CLASSIFICATION

PHARMACOTHERAPEUTIC: Penicillin. **CLINICAL:** Antibiotic (see p. 28C).

ACTION

Inhibits bacterial cell wall synthesis. **Therapeutic Effect:** Bactericidal in susceptible microorganisms.

PHARMACOKINETICS

Well absorbed from GI tract. Protein binding: 20%. Partially metabolized in the liver. Primarily excreted in urine. Removed by hemodialysis. **Half-life:** 1–1.3 hrs (increased in renal impairment).

USES

Treatment of susceptible infections due to *streptococci, E. coli, E. faecalis, P. mirabilis, H. influencae, N. gonorrhoeae* including ear, nose and throat, lower respiratory tract, skin and skin structure and UTIs, acute uncomplicated gonorrhea, *H. pylori*. **OFF-LABEL:** Treatment of Lyme disease and typhoid fever.

PRECAUTIONS

CONTRAINDICATIONS: Hypersensitivity to any penicillin, infectious mononucleosis. **CAUTIONS:** History of allergies (esp. cephalosporins), antibiotic-associated colitis.

LIFESPAN CONSIDERATIONS:

Pregnancy/Lactation: Crosses placenta, appears in cord blood, amniotic fluid. Distributed in breast milk in low concentrations. May lead to allergic sensitization, diarrhea, candidiasis, skin rash in infant. **Pregnancy Category B.** **Children:** Immature renal function in neonate/young infant may delay renal excretion. **Elderly:** Age-related renal impairment may require dosage adjustment.

INTERACTIONS

DRUG: **Allopurinol** may increase incidence of rash. **Probenecid** may increase concentration, toxicity risk. May decrease effects of **oral contraceptives.** **HERBAL:** None significant. **FOOD:** None known. **LAB VALUES:** May increase serum AST, ALT, LDH, bilirubin, creatinine, BUN. May cause positive Coomb's test.

AVAILABILITY (Rx)

CAPSULES: 250 mg, 500 mg. **POWDER FOR ORAL SUSPENSION:** 50 mg/ml, 125 mg/5 ml, 200 mg/5 ml, 250 mg/5 ml, 400 mg/5ml. **TABLETS** 500 mg, 875 mg. **TABLETS (CHEWABLE):** 125 mg, 200 mg, 250 mg, 400 mg. **TABLETS (FOR ORAL SUSPENSION):** 200 mg, 400 mg.

ADMINISTRATION/HANDLING

PO

• Store capsules, tablets at room temperature. • After reconstitution, oral solution is stable for 14 days at either room temperature or refrigerated. • Give without regard to meals. • Instruct pt to chew/crush chewable tablets thoroughly before swallowing. • **DisperMox:** Mix 1 tablet in 10 ml water. Do not chew or swallow tablets.

INDICATIONS/ROUTES/DOSAGE

SUSCEPTIBLE INFECTIONS

PO: ADULTS, ELDERLY: 250–500 mg q8h or 500–875 mg q12h. **CHILDREN OLDER THAN 3 MOS:** 25–50 mg/kg/day in 3 divided doses. **CHILDREN 3 MOS AND YOUNGER:** 30 mg/kg/day in 2 divided doses.

LOWER RESPIRATORY TRACT INFECTION

PO: ADULTS, ELDERLY: 500 mg q8h or 875 mg q12h.

***H. PYLORI* INFECTION**

PO: ADULTS, ELDERLY: 1 g twice a day in combination with clarithromycin and lansoprazole for 14 days.

OTITIS MEDIA

PO: CHILDREN: 80–90 mg/kg/day in 2 or 3 divided doses.

GONORRHEA

PO: ADULTS, ELDERLY: 3 g as a single dose.

ENDOCARDITIS PROPHYLAXIS

PO: ADULTS, ELDERLY: 2 g 1 hr before procedure. **CHILDREN:** 50 mg/kg 1 hr before procedure. **Maximum:** 2 g.

DOSAGE IN RENAL IMPAIRMENT

Dosage interval is modified based on creatinine clearance. **Creatinine Clearance 10–30 ml/min:** Usual dose q12h. **Creatinine Clearance less than 10 ml/min:** Usual dose q24h.

SIDE EFFECTS

FREQUENT: GI disturbances (mild diarrhea, nausea, vomiting), headache, oral/vaginal candidiasis. **OCCASIONAL:** Generalized rash, urticaria.

ADVERSE EFFECTS/ TOXIC REACTIONS

Antibiotic-associated colitis, other superinfections (abdominal cramps, severe watery diarrhea, fever) may result from altered bacterial balance. Severe hypersensitivity reactions, including anaphylaxis, acute interstitial nephritis occur rarely.

NURSING CONSIDERATIONS

BASELINE ASSESSMENT

Question for history of allergies, esp. penicillins, cephalosporins.

INTERVENTION/EVALUATION

Hold medication and promptly report rash, diarrhea (fever, abdominal pain, mucus and blood in stool may indicate antibiotic-associated colitis). Be alert for signs and symptoms of superinfection including increased fever, sore throat, vomiting, diarrhea, black/hairy tongue, stomatitis, anal/genital pruritus.

PATIENT/FAMILY TEACHING

• Continue antibiotic for full length of treatment. Space doses evenly. • Take with meals if GI upset occurs. • Thoroughly chew the chewable tablets before swallowing. • Notify physician if rash, diarrhea, other new symptoms occur.

amoxicillin/ clavulanate

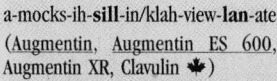

a-mocks-ih-**sill**-in/klah-view-**lan**-ate

(Augmentin, Augmentin ES 600, Augmentin XR, Clavulin ♣)

Do not confuse amoxicillin with amoxapine.

◆ CLASSIFICATION

PHARMACOTHERAPEUTIC: Penicillin. **CLINICAL:** Antibiotic (see p. 28C).

ACTION

Amoxicillin inhibits bacterial cell wall synthesis. Clavulanate inhibits bacterial beta-lactamase. **Therapeutic Effect:** Amoxicillin is bactericidal in susceptible microorganisms. Clavulanate protects amoxicillin from enzymatic degradation.

PHARMACOKINETICS

Well absorbed from GI tract. Protein binding: 20%. Partially metabolized in the liver. Primarily excreted in urine. Removed by hemodialysis. **Half-life:** 1–1.3 hrs (increased in renal impairment).

USES

Treatment of susceptible infections due to *streptococci, E. coli, E. faecalis, P. mirabilis,* beta-lactamase producing *H. influenzae, Klebsiella* species, *M. catarrhalis*, and *S. aureus* (not methicillin-resistant *Staphylococcus aureus* [MRSA]) including lower respiratory, skin and skin structure, UTIs, otitis media, sinusitis. **OFF-LABEL:** Treatment of bronchitis, chancroid.

PRECAUTIONS

CONTRAINDICATIONS: Hypersensitivity to any penicillins, infectious mononucleosis. **CAUTIONS:** History of allergies, esp. cephalosporins; antibiotic-associated colitis.

⌛ LIFESPAN CONSIDERATIONS:

Pregnancy/Lactation: Crosses placenta, appears in cord blood, amniotic fluid. Distributed in breast milk in low concentrations. May lead to allergic sensitization, diarrhea, candidiasis, skin rash in infant. **Pregnancy Category B. Children:** Immature renal function in neonate/young infant may delay renal excretion. **Elderly:** Age-related renal impairment may require dosage adjustment.

INTERACTIONS

DRUG: Allopurinol may increase incidence of rash. **Probenecid** may increase concentration, toxicity risk. May decrease effects of **oral contraceptives. HERBAL:** None significant. **FOOD:** None known. **LAB VALUES:** May increase serum AST, ALT. May cause positive Coomb's test.

AVAILABILITY (Rx)

POWDER FOR ORAL SUSPENSION (AUGMENTIN): 125 mg–31.25 mg/5 ml, 200 mg–28.5 mg/5 ml, 250 mg–62.5 mg/5 ml, 400 mg–57 mg/5 ml, 600 mg–42.9 mg/5 ml. **TABLETS (AUGMENTIN):** 250 mg–125 mg, 500 mg–125 mg, 875 mg–125 mg. **TABLETS (CHEWABLE [AUGMENTIN]):** 125 mg–31.25 mg, 200 mg–28.5 mg, 250 mg–62.5 mg, 400 mg–57 mg.

TABLETS (EXTENDED-RELEASE [AUGMENTIN XR]): 1,000 mg–62.5 mg.

ADMINISTRATION/HANDLING

PO

• Store tablets at room temperature. • After reconstitution, oral solution is stable for 14 days at room temperature or refrigerated. • Give without regard to meals. • Instruct pt to chew/crush chewable tablets thoroughly before swallowing.

INDICATIONS/ROUTES/DOSAGE

MILD TO MODERATE INFECTIONS

PO: ADULTS, ELDERLY: 500 mg q12h or 250 mg q8h.

SEVERE INFECTIONS, RESPIRATORY TRACT INFECTIONS

PO: ADULTS, ELDERLY: 875 mg q12h or 500 mg q8h.

COMMUNITY-ACQUIRED PNEUMONIA, SINUSITIS

PO: ADULTS, ELDERLY: 2 g (extended-release tablets) q12h for 7–10 days.

USUAL PEDIATRIC DOSAGE

PO: CHILDREN WEIGHING 40 KG AND LESS: 25–45 mg/kg/day (200 or 400 mg/5 ml powder or 200 mg–28.5 mg or 400 mg–57 mg chewable tablets) in 2 divided doses or 20–40 mg/kg/day (125 or 250 mg/5 ml powder or 125 mg–31.25 mg or 250 mg–62.5 mg chewable tablets) in 3 divided doses.

OTITIS MEDIA

PO: CHILDREN: 90 mg/kg/day (600 mg/5 ml suspension) in divided doses q12h for 10 days.

USUAL NEONATE DOSAGE

PO: NEONATES, CHILDREN YOUNGER THAN 3 MOS: 30 mg/kg/day (125 mg/5 ml suspension) in divided doses q12h.

DOSAGE IN RENAL IMPAIRMENT

Dosage and frequency are modified based on creatinine clearance.

Creatinine clearance 10–30 ml/min: 250–500 mg q12h.

Creatinine clearance less than 10 ml/min: 250–500 mg q24h.

SIDE EFFECTS

FREQUENT: GI disturbances (mild diarrhea, nausea, vomiting), headache, oral/vaginal candidiasis. **OCCASIONAL:** Generalized rash, urticaria.

ADVERSE EFFECTS/ TOXIC REACTIONS

Antibiotic-associated colitis, other superinfections (abdominal cramps, severe watery diarrhea, fever) may result from altered bacterial balance. Severe hypersensitivity reactions, including anaphylaxis, acute interstitial nephritis occur rarely.

NURSING CONSIDERATIONS

BASELINE ASSESSMENT

Question for history of allergies, esp. penicillins, cephalosporins.

INTERVENTION/EVALUATION

Hold medication and promptly report rash, diarrhea (with fever, abdominal pain, mucus and blood in stool may indicate antibiotic-associated colitis). Be alert for superinfection: increased fever, sore throat, vomiting, diarrhea, black/hairy tongue, ulceration or changes of oral mucosa, anal/genital pruritus.

PATIENT/FAMILY TEACHING

• Continue antibiotic for full length of treatment. • Space doses evenly. • Take with meals if GI upset occurs. • Thoroughly chew the chewable tablets before swallowing. • Notify physician if rash, diarrhea, other new symptoms occur.

Amoxil, *see amoxicillin*

amphotericin B

am-foe-**tear**-ih-sin

(Abelcet, AmBisome, Amphocin, Amphotec, Fungizone, Fungizone for Tissue Culture)

CLASSIFICATION

CLINICAL: Antifungal, antiprotozoal.

ACTION

Generally fungistatic but may become fungicidal with high dosages or very susceptible microorganisms. Binds to sterols in fungal cell membrane. **Therapeutic Effect:** Increases fungal cell-membrane permeability, allowing loss of potassium, other cellular components.

PHARMACOKINETICS

Protein binding: 90%. Widely distributed. Metabolic fate unknown. Cleared by nonrenal pathways. Minimal removal by hemodialysis. Amphotec and Abelcet are not dialyzable. **Half-life:** Fungizone, 24 hrs (increased in neonates and children); Abelcet, 7.2 days; AmBisome, 100–153 hrs; Amphotec, 26–28 hrs.

USES

Abelcet: Treatment of invasive fungal infections refractory or intolerant to Fungizone. **AmBisome:** Empiric treatment of fungal infection in febrile neutropenic pts. *Aspergillus,* candida, cryptococcus infections refractory to Fungizone or pt with renal impairment or toxicity with Fungizone. Treatment of visceral leishmaniasis. **Amphotec:** Treatment of invasive aspergillosis in pts with renal impairment or toxicity or prior treatment failure with Fungizone, Amphocin. **Fungizone:** Treatment of cryptococcosis, blastomycosis, systemic candidiasis, disseminated forms of moniliasis, coccidioidomycosis, and histoplasmosis, zygomycosis, sporotrichosis, aspergillosis. **Topical:** Treatment of cutaneous/mucocutaneous infections caused by *Candida albicans* (paronychia, oral thrush, perle'che, diaper rash, intertriginous candidiasis). **OFF-LABEL:** Febrile neutropenia, meningoencephalitis, paracoccidioidomycosis.

PRECAUTIONS

CONTRAINDICATIONS: Hypersensitivity to amphotericin B or sulfites. **CAUTIONS:** Renal impairment, in combination with antineoplastic therapy. Give only for progressive, potentially fatal fungal infection.

LIFESPAN CONSIDERATIONS:

Pregnancy/Lactation: Crosses placenta; unknown if distributed in breast milk. **Pregnancy Category B. Children:** Safety and efficacy not established, but use the least amount for therapeutic regimen. **Elderly:** No age-related precautions noted.

INTERACTIONS

DRUG: Antineoplastic agents may increase potential for bronchospasm, renal toxicity, hypotension. **Steroids** may cause severe hypokalemia. **Bone marrow depressants** may worsen anemia. May increase **digoxin** toxity (due to hypokalemia). **Nephrotoxic medications** may increase nephrotoxicity. **HERBAL:** None significant. **FOOD:** None known. **LAB VALUES:** May increase serum AST, ALT, alkaline phosphatase, BUN, serum creatinine. May decrease serum calcium, magnesium, potassium.

AVAILABILITY (Rx)

CREAM (FUNGIZONE): 3%. **INJECTION, POWDER FOR RECONSTITUTION:** 50 mg (AmBisome, Amphocin, Amphotec, Fungizone), 100 mg (Amphotec). **INJECTION, SUSPENSION (ABELCET):** 5 mg/ml.

ADMINISTRATION/HANDLING

IV

• Monitor B/P, temperature, pulse, respirations; assess for adverse reactions q15min twice, then q30min for 4 hrs after initial infusion. • Potential for thrombophlebitis may be less with use of pediatric scalp vein needles or (with physician order) adding dilute heparin solution. • Observe strict aseptic technique because no bacteriostatic agent or preservative is present in diluent.

Reconstitution

ABELCET

• Shake 20-ml (100-mg) vial gently until contents are dissolved. Withdraw required dose using 5-micron filter needle (supplied by manufacturer). • Inject dose into D_5W; 4 ml D_5W required for each 1 ml (5 mg) to final concentration of 1 mg/ml. Reduce dose by half for pediatric, fluid-restricted pts (2 mg/ml).

AMBISOME

• Reconstitute each 50-mg vial with 12 ml Sterile Water for Injection to provide concentration of 4 mg/ml. • Shake vial vigorously for 30 sec. Withdraw required dose and empty syringe contents through a 5-micron filter into an infusion of D_5W to provide final concentration of 1–2 mg/ml.

AMPHOTEC

• Add 10 ml Sterile Water for Injection to each 50-mg vial to provide concentration of 5 mg/ml. Shake gently. • Further dilute **only** with D_5W using specific amount recommended by manufacturer to provide concentration of 0.16–0.83 mg/ml.

FUNGIZONE

• Rapidly inject 10 ml Sterile Water for Injection to each 50-mg vial to provide concentration of 5 mg/ml. Immediately shake vial until solution is clear. • Further dilute each 1 mg in at least 10 ml D_5W to provide a concentration of 0.1 mg/ml.

Rate of administration

• Give by slow IV infusion. Infuse conventional amphotericin or Fungizone over 2–6 hrs; Abelcet over 2 hrs (shake contents if infusion longer than 2 hrs); Amphotec over 2–4 hrs; AmBisome over 1–2 hrs.

Storage

ABELCET

• Refrigerate unreconstituted solution. Reconstituted solution is stable for 48 hrs if refrigerated; 6 hrs at room temperature.

AMBISOME

• Refrigerate unreconstituted solution. Reconstituted solution of 4 mg/ml is stable for 24 hrs. Concentration of 1–2 mg/ml is stable for 6 hrs.

AMPHOTEC

• Store unreconstituted solution at room temperature. Reconstituted solution stable for 24 hrs.

FUNGIZONE

• Refrigerate unreconstituted solution. • Reconstituted solution is stable for 24 hrs at room temperature or 7 days if refrigerated. • Diluted solution 0.1 mg/ml or less to be used promptly. Do not use if cloudy or contains a precipitate.

IV INCOMPATIBILITIES

Abelcet, AmBisome, Amphotec: Do not mix with any other drug, diluent, or solution. Fungizone: Allopurinol (Aloprim), amifostine (Ethyol), aztreonam (Azactam), calcium gluconate, cefepime (Maxipime), cimetidine (Tagamet), ciprofloxacin (Cipro), docetaxel (Taxotere), dopamine (Intropin), doxorubicin (Adriamycin), enalapril (Vasotec), etoposide (VP-16), filgrastim (Neupogen), fluconazole (Diflucan), fludarabine (Fludara), foscarnet (Foscavir), gemcitabine (Gemzar), lipids, magnesium sulfate, meropenem (Merrem IV), ondansetron (Zofran), paclitaxel (Taxol), piperacillin and tazobactam (Zosyn), potassium chloride, propofol (Diprivan), total parenteral nutrition (TPN), vinorelbine (Navelbine).

IV COMPATIBILITIES

None known; do not mix with other medications or electrolytes.

INDICATIONS/ROUTES/DOSAGE

USUAL AMPHOCIN, FUNGIZONE DOSE

IV INFUSION (AMPHOCIN, FUNGIZONE): ADULTS, ELDERLY: Dosage based on pt tolerance and severity of infection. Initially, 1-mg test dose is given over 20–30 min. If test dose is tolerated, 5-mg dose may be given the same day. Subsequently, dosage is increased by 5 mg q12–24h until desired daily dose is reached. Alternatively, if test dose is tolerated, 0.25 mg/kg is given on same day and 0.5 mg/kg on second day; then dosage is increased until desired daily dose reached. Total daily dose: 1 mg/kg/day up to 1.5 mg/kg every other day. **Maximum:** 1.5 mg/kg/day. **CHILDREN:** Test dose of 0.1 mg/kg/dose (**Maximum:** 1 mg) is infused over 20–60 min. If test dose is tolerated, initial dose of 0.4 mg/kg may be given on same day; dosage is then increased in 0.25-mg/kg increments as needed. Maintenance dose: 0.25–1 mg/kg/day.

USUAL ABELCET DOSE

IV INFUSION (ABELCET): ADULTS, CHILDREN: 2.5–5 mg/kg at rate of 2.5 mg/kg/hr.

USUAL AMBISOME DOSE

IV INFUSION (AMBISOME): ADULTS, CHILDREN: 3–5 mg/kg over 1 hr.

USUAL AMPHOTEC DOSE

IV INFUSION (AMPHOTEC): ADULTS, CHILDREN: 3–4 mg/kg over 2–4 hrs. **Maximum:** 7.5 mg/kg/day.

USUAL TOPICAL DOSE

TOPICAL: ADULTS, ELDERLY, CHILDREN: Apply liberally to affected area and rub in 2–4 times a day.

SIDE EFFECTS

FREQUENT (greater than 10%): Abelcet: Chills, fever, increased serum creatinine, multiple organ failure. **Ambisome:** Hypokalemia, hypomagnesemia, hyperglycemia, hypocalcemia, edema, abdominal pain, back pain, chills, chest pain, hypotension, diarrhea, nausea, vomiting, headache, fever, rigors, insomnia, dyspnea, epistaxis, increased hepatic/renal function test results. **Amphotec:** Chills, fever, hypotension, tachycardia, increased serum creatinine, hypokalemia, bilirubinemia. **Fungizone:** Fever, chills, headache, anemia, hypokalemia, hypomagnesemia, anorexia, malaise, generalized pain, nephrotoxicity. **Topical:** Local irritation, dry skin. **RARE: Topical:** Rash.

ADVERSE EFFECTS/ TOXIC REACTIONS

Cardiovascular toxicity (hypotension, ventricular fibrillation), anaphylaxis occurs rarely. Altered vision/hearing, seizures, hepatic failure, coagulation defects, multiple organ failure, sepsis may be noted. Each alternative formulation is less nephrotoxic than conventional amphotericin (Fungizone).

NURSING CONSIDERATIONS

BASELINE ASSESSMENT

Question for history of allergies, esp. to amphotericin B, sulfite. Avoid, if possible, other nephrotoxic medications. Obtain premedication orders to reduce adverse reactions during IV therapy (antipyretics, antihistamines, antiemetics, corticosteroids).

INTERVENTION/EVALUATION

Monitor B/P, temperature, pulse, respirations; assess for adverse reactions (fever, tremors, chills, anorexia, nausea, vomiting, abdominal pain) q15min twice, then q30min for 4 hrs of initial infusion. If symptoms occur, slow infusion, administer medication for symptomatic relief. For severe reaction, stop infusion and notify physician. Evaluate IV site for phlebitis (heat, pain, red streaking over vein). Monitor I&O, renal function tests for nephrotoxicity. Check serum potassium and magnesium levels, hematologic and hepatic function test results. **Topical:** Assess for itching, irritation, burning.

PATIENT/FAMILY TEACHING

• Prolonged therapy (weeks or months) is usually necessary. • Fever reaction may decrease with continued therapy. • Muscle weakness may be noted during therapy (due to hypokalemia). **Topical:** Application may cause staining of skin or nails; soap and water or dry cleaning will remove fabric stains. • Do not use other preparations or occlusive coverings without consulting physician. • Keep areas clean, dry; wear light clothing. • Separate personal items with direct contact to area.

ampicillin

am-pi-**sill**-in

(Apo-Ampi ✱, Novo-Ampicillin ✱, Nu-Ampi ✱, Polycillin, Principen)

Do not confuse ampicillin with aminophylline, Imipenem, or Unipen.

CLASSIFICATION

PHARMACOTHERAPEUTIC: Penicillin.
CLINICAL: Antibiotic (see p. 28C).

ACTION

Inhibits cell wall synthesis in susceptible microorganisms. **Therapeutic Effect:** Bactericidal in susceptible microorganisms.

PHARMACOKINETICS

Moderately absorbed from GI tract. Protein binding: 28%. Widely distributed. Partially metabolized in the liver. Primarily excreted in urine. Removed by hemodialysis. **Half-life:** 1–1.5 hrs (increased in renal impairment).

USES

Treatment of susceptible infections due to *streptococci, S. pneumoniae, staphylococci* (non-penicillinase producing), *meningococci*, *Listeria*, some *Klebsiella*, *E. coli*, *H. influenzae*, *Salmonella*, *Shigella* including GI, GU, respiratory infections, meningitis, endocarditis prophylaxis.

PRECAUTIONS

CONTRAINDICATIONS: Hypersensitivity to any penicillin, infectious mononucleosis. **CAUTIONS:** History of allergies, particularly cephalosporins, antibiotic-associated colitis.

LIFESPAN CONSIDERATIONS:

Pregnancy/Lactation: Readily crosses placenta; appears in cord blood, amniotic fluid. Distributed in breast milk in low concentrations. May lead to allergic sensitization, diarrhea, candidiasis, skin rash in infant. **Pregnancy Category B.** **Children:** Immature renal function in neonates/young infants may delay renal excretion. **Elderly:** Age-related renal impairment may require dosage adjustment.

INTERACTIONS

DRUG: **Allopurinol** may increase incidence of rash. **Probenecid** may increase concentration, toxicity risk. May decrease effects of **oral contraceptives.** **HERBAL:** None significant. **FOOD:** None known. **LAB VALUES:** May increase serum AST, ALT. May cause positive Coomb's test.

AVAILABILITY (Rx)

CAPSULES: 250 mg, 500 mg. **INJECTION, POWDER FOR RECONSTITUTION:** 125 mg, 250 mg, 500 mg, 1 g, 2 g. **POWDER FOR ORAL SUSPENSION:** 125 mg/5 ml, 250 mg/5 ml.

ADMINISTRATION/HANDLING

IV

Reconstitution • For IV injection, dilute each vial with 5 ml Sterile Water for Injection (10 ml for 1- and 2-g vials). • For intermittent IV infusion (piggyback), further dilute with 50–100 ml 0.9% NaCl or D_5W.

Rate of administration • For IV injection, give over 3–5 min (10–15 min for 1- to 2-g dose). • For intermittent IV infusion (piggyback), infuse over 20–30 min. • Due to potential for hypersensitivity/anaphylaxis, start initial dose at few drops per min, increase slowly to ordered rate; stay with pt first 10–15 min, then check q10min. • Change to PO as soon as possible.

Storage • IV solution, diluted with 0.9% NaCl, is stable for 2–8 hrs at room temperature or 3 days if refrigerated. • If diluted with D_5W, is stable for 2 hrs at room temperature or 3 hrs if refrigerated. • Discard if precipitate forms.

IM

• Reconstitute each vial with Sterile Water for Injection or Bacteriostatic Water for Injection (consult individual vial for specific volume of diluent). • Stable for 1 hr. • Give deeply in large muscle mass.

PO

• Store capsules at room temperature. • Oral suspension, after reconstituted, is stable for 7 days at room temperature, 14 days if refrigerated. • Give orally 1 hr before or 2 hrs after meals for maximum absorption.

IV INCOMPATIBILITIES

Amikacin (Amikin), diltiazem (Cardizem), gentamicin, midazolam (Versed).

IV COMPATIBILITIES

Calcium gluconate, cefepime (Maxipime), dopamine (Intropin), famotidine (Pepcid), furosemide (Lasix), heparin, hydromorphone (Dilaudid), insulin (regular), levofloxacin (Levaquin), lipids, magnesium sulfate, morphine, multivitamins, potassium chloride, propofol (Diprivan), total parenteral nutrition (TPN) (if ampicillin sodium concentration is less than 40 mg/ml).

INDICATIONS/ROUTES/DOSAGE

USUAL DOSAGE

PO: ADULTS, ELDERLY: 250–500 mg q6h. **CHILDREN:** 50–100 mg/kg/day in divided doses q6h. **Maximum:** 3 g/day.
IV, IM: ADULTS, ELDERLY: 500 mg–3 g q4–6h. **Maximum:** 14 g/day. **CHILDREN:** 100–200 mg/kg/day in divided doses q6h. **NEONATES:** 50–100 mg/kg/day in divided doses q6–12h.

GI, GU INFECTIONS

IV, IM: ADULTS, ELDERLY: 500 mg q6h.
PO: ADULTS, ELDERLY: 500 mg q6h. **CHILDREN:** 100 mg/kg/day in 4 divided doses.

RESPIRATORY TRACT INFECTIONS

IV, IM: ADULTS, ELDERLY: 250–500 mg q6h.

PO: ADULTS, ELDERLY: 250 mg q6h.

ENDOCARDITIS PROPHYLAXIS

IV, IM: ADULTS, ELDERLY: 1–2 g (plus gentamicin) 30 min before procedure. **CHILDREN:** 50 mg/kg (plus gentamicin in high-risk pts), with follow-up dose of 25–50 mg/kg 6–8 hrs later.

MENINGITIS

IV: ADULTS, ELDERLY: 8–14 g/day in 4–6 divided doses. **CHILDREN:** 200–400 mg/kg/day in divided doses q6h. **Maximum:** 12 g/day. **NEONATES:** 100–200 mg/kg/day in divided doses q6–12h.

GONOCOCCAL INFECTIONS

PO: ADULTS: 3.5 g one time with 1 g probenecid.
IM: MALES: 500 mg for 2 doses.

PERIOPERATIVE PROPHYLAXIS

IV, IM: ADULTS, ELDERLY: 2 g 30 min before procedure. May repeat in 8 hrs. **CHILDREN:** 50 mg/kg 30 min before procedure. May repeat in 8 hrs.

DOSAGE IN RENAL IMPAIRMENT

Creatinine Clearance	% of Normal Dosage
10–30 ml/min	Give q6–12h
Less than 10 ml/min	Give q12h

SIDE EFFECTS

FREQUENT: Pain at IM injection site, GI disturbances (mild diarrhea, nausea, vomiting), oral or vaginal candidiasis. **OCCASIONAL:** Generalized rash, urticaria, phlebitis or thrombophlebitis (with IV administration), headache. **RARE:** Dizziness, seizures (esp. with IV therapy).

ADVERSE EFFECTS/ TOXIC REACTIONS

Antibiotic-associated colitis, other superinfections (abdominal cramps, severe watery diarrhea, fever) may result from altered bacterial balance. Severe hypersensitivity reactions, including anaphylaxis, acute interstitial nephritis occur rarely.

NURSING CONSIDERATIONS

BASELINE ASSESSMENT

Question for history of allergies, esp. penicillins, cephalosporins.

INTERVENTION/EVALUATION

Hold medication and promptly report rash (although common with ampicillin, may indicate hypersensitivity) or diarrhea (with fever, abdominal pain, mucus and blood in stool may indicate antibiotic-associated colitis). Evaluate IV site for phlebitis (heat, pain, red streaking over vein). Check IM injection site for pain, induration. Monitor I&O, urinalysis, renal function tests. Assess for signs of superinfection: increased fever, sore throat, vomiting, diarrhea, anal/genital pruritus, oral ulcerations or pain, black/hairy tongue.

PATIENT/FAMILY TEACHING

• Space doses evenly. • Take antibiotic for full length of treatment. • More effective if taken 1 hr before or 2 hrs after food/beverages. • Discomfort may occur with IM injection. • Notify physician of rash, diarrhea, or other new symptoms.

ampicillin/ sulbactam

amp-ih-**sill**-in/sull-**bak**-tam
(Unasyn)

◆ CLASSIFICATION

PHARMACOTHERAPEUTIC: Penicillin. **CLINICAL:** Antibiotic (see p. 28C).

ACTION

Ampicillin inhibits bacterial cell wall synthesis. Sulbactam inhibits bacterial beta-lactamase. **Therapeutic Effect:** Ampicillin is bactericidal in susceptible microorganisms. Sulbactam protects ampicillin from enzymatic degradation.

PHARMACOKINETICS

Protein binding: 28%–38%. Widely distributed. Partially metabolized in the liver. Primarily excreted in urine. Removed by hemodialysis. **Half-life:** 1 hr (increased in renal impairment).

USES

Treatment of susceptible infections due to beta-lactamase producing organisms including *H. influenzae, E. coli, Klebsiella, Acinetobacter, Enterobacter, S. aureus,* and *Bacteroides* species including intra-abdominal, skin/skin structure, gynecologic infections.

PRECAUTIONS

CONTRAINDICATIONS: Hypersensitivity to any penicillin or sulbactam, infectious mononucleosis. **CAUTIONS:** History of allergies, particularly to cephalosporins, antibiotic-associated colitis.

LIFESPAN CONSIDERATIONS:

Pregnancy/Lactation: Readily crosses placenta; appears in cord blood, amniotic fluid. Distributed in breast milk in low concentrations. May lead to allergic sensitization, diarrhea, candidiasis, skin rash in infant. **Pregnancy Category B. Children:** Safety and efficacy not established in children younger than 1 yr. **Elderly:** Age-related renal impairment may require dosage adjustment.

INTERACTIONS

DRUG: **Allopurinol** may increase incidence of rash. **Probenecid** may increase concentration, toxicity risk. May decrease effects of **oral contraceptives.** **HERBAL:** None significant. **FOOD:** None known. **LAB VALUES:** May increase serum AST, ALT, alkaline phosphatase, LDH, creatinine. May cause positive Coomb's test.

AVAILABILITY (Rx)

INJECTION, POWDER FOR RECONSTITUTION: 1.5 g (ampicillin 1 g/sulbactam 500 g), 3 g (ampicillin 2 g/sulbactam 1 g).

ADMINISTRATION/HANDLING

IV

Reconstitution • For IV injection, dilute with 10–20 ml Sterile Water for Injection. • For intermittent IV infusion (piggyback), further dilute with 50–100 ml D_5W or 0.9% NaCl.

Rate of administration • For IV injection, give slowly over minimum of 10–15 min. • For intermittent IV infusion (piggyback), infuse over 15–30 min. • Due to potential for hypersensitivity/anaphylaxis, start initial dose at few drops per min, increase slowly to ordered rate; stay with pt first 10–15 min, then check q10min. • Change to PO antibiotic as soon as possible.

Storage • When reconstituted with 0.9% NaCl, IV solution is stable for 8 hrs at room temperature, 48 hrs if refrigerated. Stability may be different with other diluents. • Discard if precipitate forms.

IM

• Reconstitute each 1.5-g vial with 3.2 ml Sterile Water for Injection to provide concentration of 250 mg ampicillin/ 125 mg sublactam/ml. • Give deeply into large muscle mass within 1 hr after preparation.

IV INCOMPATIBILITIES

Diltiazem (Cardizem), idarubicin (Idamycin), ondansetron (Zofran), sargramostim (Leukine), total parenteral nutrition (TPN).

IV COMPATIBILITIES

Famotidine (Pepcid), heparin, insulin (regular), lipids, morphine.

INDICATIONS/ROUTES/DOSAGE

SKIN AND SKIN-STRUCTURE, INTRA-ABDOMINAL, GYNECOLOGIC INFECTIONS

IV, IM: ADULTS, ELDERLY: 1.5 g (1 g ampicillin/500 mg sulbactam) to 3 g (2 g ampicillin/1 g sulbactam) q6h.

SKIN AND SKIN-STRUCTURE INFECTIONS

IV: CHILDREN 12 YRS AND YOUNGER: 150–400 mg/kg/day in divided doses q6h.

DOSAGE IN RENAL IMPAIRMENT

Dosage and frequency are modified based on creatinine clearance and severity of infection.

Creatinine Clearance	Dosage
Greater than 30 ml/min	0.5–3 g q6–8h
15–29 ml/min	1.5–3 g q12h
5–14 ml/min	1.5–3 g q24h
Less than 5 ml/min	Not recommended

SIDE EFFECTS

FREQUENT: Diarrhea, rash (most common), urticaria, pain at IM injection site, thrombophlebitis with IV administration, oral or vaginal candidiasis. **OCCASIONAL:** Nausea, vomiting, headache, malaise, urinary retention.

ADVERSE EFFECTS/ TOXIC REACTIONS

Antibiotic-associated colitis, other superinfections (abdominal cramps, severe watery diarrhea, fever) may result from altered bacterial balance. Severe hypersensitivity reactions, including anaphylaxis, acute interstitial nephritis, blood dyscrasias may occur. High dosage may produce seizures.

NURSING CONSIDERATIONS

BASELINE ASSESSMENT

Question for history of allergies, esp. penicillins, cephalosporins.

INTERVENTION/EVALUATION

Hold medication and promptly report rash (although common with ampicillin, may indicate hypersensitivity) or diarrhea (with fever, mucus and blood in stool, abdominal pain may indicate antibiotic-associated colitis). Evaluate IV site for phlebitis (heat, pain, red streaking over vein). Check IM injection site for pain, induration. Monitor I&O, urinalysis, renal function tests. Assess for initial signs of superinfection: increased fever, sore throat onset, vomiting, diarrhea, anal/genital pruritus, ulceration or changes of oral mucosa.

PATIENT/FAMILY TEACHING

• Space doses evenly. • Take antibiotic for full length of treatment. • Discomfort may occur with IM injection. • Notify physician of rash, diarrhea, or other new symptoms.

amprenavir

am-**pren**-eh-veer
(Agenerase)

Do not confuse Agenerase with asparaginase.

CLASSIFICATION

PHARMACOTHERAPEUTIC: Antiviral. **CLINICAL:** Protease inhibitor (see pp. 64C, 112C).

ACTION

Inhibits HIV-1 protease by binding to the enzyme's active site, thus preventing processing of viral precursors, resulting in formation of immature, noninfectious viral particles. **Therapeutic Effect:** Impairs HIV viral replication and proliferation.

PHARMACOKINETICS

Rapidly absorbed after PO administration. Protein binding: 90%. Metabolized in the liver. Primarily excreted in feces. **Half-life:** 7.1–10.6 hrs.

USES

Treatment of HIV-1 infection in combination with other antiretroviral agents.

PRECAUTIONS

CONTRAINDICATIONS: None known. **CAUTIONS:** Hepatic impairment, diabetes mellitus, hemophilia, hypersensitivity to sulfas, vitamin K deficiency due to anticoagulant/malabsorption.

LIFESPAN CONSIDERATIONS:

Pregnancy/Lactation: Unknown if drug crosses placenta or is distributed in breast milk. **Pregnancy Category C.** **Children:** Safety and efficacy of capsules not established in those younger than 4 yrs. **Elderly:** Age-related hepatic impairment may require decreased dosage.

INTERACTIONS

DRUG: May interfere with metabolism of **amiodarone, lidocaine, oral contraceptives, midazolam, triazolam, tricyclic antidepressants, quinidine, bepridil, ergotamine. Antacids, didanosine** may decrease absorption. **Carbamazepine, phenobarbital, phenytoin, rifampin** may decrease concentration. Amprenavir may increase concentration of **clozapine, HMG-CoA reductase inhibitors (statins), warfarin.** **HERBAL: St. John's wort** may decrease concentration. **FOOD: High-fat meals** may decrease absorption. **LAB VALUES:** May increase serum glucose, cholesterol, triglycerides.

AVAILABILITY (Rx)

CAPSULES: 50 mg. **SOLUTION, ORAL:** 15 mg/ml.

ADMINISTRATION/HANDLING

PO

- May give without regard to food.

INDICATIONS/ROUTES/DOSAGE

HIV-1 INFECTION (IN COMBINATION WITH OTHER ANTIRETROVIRALS)

PO: ADULTS, CHILDREN 17 YRS AND OLDER, CHILDREN 13–16 YRS WEIGHING 50 KG AND MORE: 1,200 mg twice a day. **CHILDREN 4–12 YRS, CHILDREN 13–16 YRS WEIGHING LESS THAN 50 KG:** 20 mg/kg twice a day or 15 mg/kg 3 times a day. **Maximum:** 2,400 mg/day.

ORAL SOLUTION: ADULTS, CHILDREN 17 YRS AND OLDER, CHILDREN 13–16 YRS WEIGHING 50 KG AND MORE: 1,400 mg twice a day. **CHILDREN 4–12 YRS, CHILDREN 13–16 YRS WEIGHING LESS THAN 50 KG:** 22.5 mg/kg/day (1.5 ml/kg) oral solution twice a day or 17 mg/kg/day (1.1 ml/kg) 3 times a day. **Maximum:** 2,800 mg/day.

DOSAGE IN HEPATIC IMPAIRMENT

Dosage and frequency are modified based on the Child-Pugh score.

Child-Pugh Score	Capsules	Oral Solution
5–8	450 mg bid	513 mg bid
9–12	300 mg bid	342 mg bid

SIDE EFFECTS

FREQUENT: Diarrhea, loose stools (56%), nausea (38%), oral paresthesia (30%), rash (25%), vomiting (20%). **OCCASIONAL:** Peripheral paresthesia (12%), depression (4%).

ADVERSE EFFECTS/ TOXIC REACTIONS

Severe hypersensitivity reactions, Stevens-Johnson syndrome as evidenced by blisters, peeling skin, loosening of skin/mucous membranes, fever may occur.

NURSING CONSIDERATIONS

BASELINE ASSESSMENT

Obtain baseline laboratory tests before beginning therapy and at periodic intervals during therapy. Offer emotional support.

INTERVENTION/EVALUATION

Assess for nausea, vomiting. Determine pattern of bowel activity and stool consistency. Assess eating pattern; monitor for weight loss. Assess for paresthesias. Assess skin for rash.

PATIENT/FAMILY TEACHING

• Avoid high-fat meals (decreases drug absorption). • Small, frequent meals may offset anorexia, nausea. • Amprenavir is not a cure for HIV infection, nor does it reduce risk of transmission to others.

anagrelide

ah-na-**greh**-lide
(Agrylin)

CLASSIFICATION

PHARMACOTHERAPEUTIC: Hematologic agent. **CLINICAL:** Antiplatelet.

ACTION

Reduces platelet production, prevents platelet shape changes caused by platelet aggregating agents. **Therapeutic Effect:** Inhibits platelet aggregation.

PHARMACOKINETICS

After oral administration, plasma concentration peaks within 1 hr. Extensively metabolized. Primarily excreted in urine. **Half-life:** About 3 days.

USES

Treatment of essential thrombocythemia, reducing elevated platelet count and risk of thrombosis. Treatment of thrombocythemia due to myeloproliferative disorders.

PRECAUTIONS

CONTRAINDICATIONS: Severe hepatic impairment. **CAUTIONS:** Cardiac disease; renal/hepatic impairment.

LIFESPAN CONSIDERATIONS:

Pregnancy/Lactation: Unknown if drug crosses placenta or is distributed in breast milk. May cause fetal harm. **Pregnancy Category C. Children:** Safety and efficacy in those younger than 16 yrs not established. **Elderly:** Age-related renal/hepatic impairment, cardiac disease requires caution.

INTERACTIONS

DRUG: None significant. **HERBAL: Ginkgo biloba** may increase the risk of bleeding. **FOOD:** None known. **LAB VALUES:** May increase serum hepatic enzyme levels (rare).

AVAILABILITY (Rx)

CAPSULES: 0.5 mg, 1 mg.

ADMINISTRATION/HANDLING

PO

• Give without regard to food.

INDICATIONS/ROUTES/DOSAGE

THROMBOCYTHEMIA

PO: ADULTS, ELDERLY: Initially, 0.5 mg 4 times a day or 1 mg twice a day. Adjust to lowest effective dosage, increasing by up to 0.5 mg/day or less in any 1 wk. **Maximum:** 10 mg/day or 2.5 mg/dose. **CHILDREN:** Initially, 0.5 mg/day. Range: 0.5 mg 1–4 times a day.

SIDE EFFECTS

FREQUENT (5% or more): Headache, palpitations, diarrhea, abdominal pain, nausea, flatulence, bloating, asthenia, pain, dizziness. **OCCASIONAL (less than**

5%): Tachycardia, chest pain, vomiting, paresthesia, peripheral edema, anorexia, dyspepsia, rash. **RARE:** Confusion, insomnia.

ADVERSE EFFECTS/ TOXIC REACTIONS

Angina, heart failure, arrhythmias occur rarely.

NURSING CONSIDERATIONS

BASELINE ASSESSMENT

Assess platelet count, Hgb, Hct, WBC before treatment, q2days during first wk of treatment, and weekly thereafter until therapeutic range is achieved. Ask if pt is breast-feeding, pregnant, or planning to become pregnant (may cause fetal harm).

INTERVENTION/EVALUATION

Monitor serum hepatic function, BUN, creatinine. Pts with suspected heart disease should be monitored closely. Assess skin for bruises, petechiae; catheter insertion site, needle site, GI sites for bleeding.

PATIENT/FAMILY TEACHING

• Platelet count responds within 7–14 days. • Not recommended in pregnancy. • Use contraceptives while taking anagrelide.

anakinra

an-a-**kin**-ra
(Kineret)

CLASSIFICATION

PHARMACOTHERAPEUTIC: Interleukin-1 receptor antagonist. **CLINICAL:** Anti-inflammatory.

ACTION

Blocks the binding of interleukin-1 (IL-1), a protein that is a major mediator of joint pathology and is present in excess amounts in pts with rheumatoid arthritis. **Therapeutic Effect:** Inhibits inflammatory response.

PHARMACOKINETICS

No accumulation of anakinra in tissues or organs was observed after daily subcutaneous doses. Excreted in urine. **Half-life:** 4–6 hrs.

USES

Treatment of signs and symptoms or to slow progression of structural damage of moderate to severely active rheumatoid arthritis in pts who have failed treatment with one or more disease-modifying antirheumatic drugs.

PRECAUTIONS

CONTRAINDICATIONS: Known hypersensitivity to *Escherichia coli*-derived proteins, serious infection. **CAUTIONS:** Renal impairment (risk of toxic reaction is increased), asthma (higher incidence of serious infection).

LIFESPAN CONSIDERATIONS:

Pregnancy/Lactation: Unknown if distributed in breast milk. **Pregnancy Category B. Children:** Safety and efficacy not established. **Elderly:** Age-related renal impairment may require caution.

INTERACTIONS

DRUG: Live/inactive virus vaccines may be ineffective. Increased risk of infection with **etanercept. HERBAL:** None significant. **FOOD:** None known. **LAB VALUES:** May decrease WBC count, platelet count, absolute neutrophil count (ANC). May increase eosinophil count.

AVAILABILITY (Rx)

INJECTION SOLUTION: 100-mg syringe.

ADMINISTRATION/HANDLING

SUBCUTANEOUS

• Store in refrigerator; do not freeze or shake. • Do not use if particulate or discoloration is noted. • Give by subcutaneous route.

INDICATIONS/ROUTES/DOSAGE

RHEUMATOID ARTHRITIS

SUBCUTANEOUS: ADULTS, ELDERLY: 100 mg/day, given at same time each day.

SIDE EFFECTS

OCCASIONAL: Injection site ecchymosis, erythema, inflammation. **RARE:** Headache, nausea, diarrhea, abdominal pain.

ADVERSE EFFECTS/ TOXIC REACTIONS

Infections, including upper respiratory tract infection, sinusitis, flu-like symptoms, and cellulitis, have been noted. Neutropenia may occur, particularly when anakinra is used in combination with tumor necrosis factor-blocking agents.

NURSING CONSIDERATIONS

BASELINE ASSESSMENT

Do not give live vaccines concurrently (vaccination may not be effective in those receiving anakinra).

INTERVENTION/EVALUATION

Monitor neutrophil count before therapy begins, monthly for 3 mos while receiving therapy, then quarterly for up to 1 yr. Assess for inflammatory reaction, esp. during first 4 wks of therapy (uncommon after first mo of therapy).

PATIENT/FAMILY TEACHING

• Instruct pt on proper dosage and administration, correct procedure to administer subcutaneous dosage. • Advise pt on importance of proper disposal of syringes and needles.

anastrozole

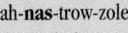

ah-**nas**-trow-zole

(Arimidex)

Do not confuse Arimidex with Imitrex.

CLASSIFICATION

PHARMACOTHERAPEUTIC: Aromatase inhibitor. **CLINICAL:** Antineoplastic hormone (see p. 76C).

ACTION

Decreases circulating estrogen level by inhibiting aromatase, the enzyme that catalyzes the final step in estrogen production. **Therapeutic Effect:** Inhibits growth of breast cancers that are stimulated by estrogens by lowering serum estradiol concentration.

PHARMACOKINETICS

Well absorbed into systemic circulation (absorption not affected by food). Protein binding: 40%. Extensively metabolized in the liver. Eliminated by biliary system and, to a lesser extent, kidneys. **Mean half-life:** 50 hrs in postmenopausal women. Steady-state plasma levels reached in about 7 days.

USES

Treatment of advanced breast cancer in postmenopausal women who have developed progressive disease while receiving tamoxifen therapy. First-line therapy in advanced or metastatic breast cancer. Adjuvant treatment in early breast cancer.

PRECAUTIONS

CONTRAINDICATIONS: None known. **CAUTIONS:** None known.

LIFESPAN CONSIDERATIONS:

Pregnancy/Lactation: Crosses placenta; may cause fetal harm. Unknown if excreted in breast milk. **Pregnancy Category D.** **Children:** Safety and efficacy not established. **Elderly:** No age-related precautions noted.

INTERACTIONS

DRUG: **Estrogen therapies** may reduce efficacy. **Tamoxifen** may reduce plasma concentration. **HERBAL:** Avoid **black cohosh, licorice, red clover, dong quai**. **FOOD:** None known. **LAB VALUES:** May elevate serum GGT level in pts with liver metastases. May increase serum AST, ALT, alkaline phosphate, total cholesterol, LDL cholesterol.

AVAILABILITY (Rx)

TABLETS: 1 mg.

ADMINISTRATION/HANDLING

PO

- Give without regard to food.

INDICATIONS/ROUTES/DOSAGE

BREAST CANCER

PO: ADULTS, ELDERLY: 1 mg once a day.

SIDE EFFECTS

FREQUENT (16%–8%): Asthenia, nausea, headache, hot flashes, back pain, vomiting, cough, diarrhea. **OCCASIONAL (6%–4%):** Constipation, abdominal pain, anorexia, bone pain, pharyngitis, dizziness, rash, dry mouth, peripheral edema, pelvic pain, depression, chest pain, paresthesia. **RARE (2%–1%):** Weight gain, diaphoresis.

ADVERSE EFFECTS/ TOXIC REACTIONS

Thrombophlebitis, anemia, leukopenia occur rarely. Vaginal hemorrhage occurs rarely (2%).

NURSING CONSIDERATIONS

INTERVENTION/EVALUATION

Monitor for asthenia and dizziness and assist with ambulation if needed. Assess for headache. Offer antiemetic for nausea and vomiting. Monitor for onset of diarrhea; offer antidiarrheal medication.

PATIENT/FAMILY TEACHING

- Notify physician if nausea, asthenia, hot flashes become unmanageable.

Ancef, *see cefazolin*

AndroGel, *see testosterone*

Angiomax, *see bivalirudin*

anidulafungin

a-nid-you-lah-**fun**-gin
(Eraxis)

CLASSIFICATION

PHARMACOTHERAPEUTIC: Echinocandin. **CLINICAL:** Antifungal.

ACTION

Inhibits synthesis of glucan, an enzyme, (vital component of fungal cell formation), preventing fungal cell wall formation. **Therapeutic Effect:** Fungistatic.

PHARMACOKINETICS

Distributed in tissue. Moderately bound to albumin. Protein binding: 84%. Slow chemical degradation; 30% excreted in feces over 9 days. Not removed by hemodialysis. **Half-life:** 40–50 hrs.

USES

Treatment of candidemia, other forms of *Candida* infections (intra-abdominal abscess, peritonitis), esophageal candidiasis.

PRECAUTIONS

CONTRAINDICATIONS: Hypersensitivity to anidulafungin, other echinocandin. **CAUTIONS:** Hepatic impairment, myelosuppression, renal insufficiency.

LIFESPAN CONSIDERATIONS:

Pregnancy/Lactation: May be embryotoxic. Crosses placental barrier. Unknown if distributed in breast milk. **Pregnancy Category C.** **Children:** Safety and efficacy not established. **Elderly:** No age-related precautions noted.

INTERACTIONS

DRUG: None significant. **HERBAL:** None significant. **FOOD:** None known. **LAB VALUES:** May increase serum ALT, AST, bilirubin, akaline phosphatase, LDH, transferase, amylase, lipase, CPK, creatinine, calcium. May decrease serum albumin, bicarbonate, magnesium, protein, potassium, Hgb, Hct, WBCs, neutrophils, platelet count.

AVAILABILITY (Rx)

INJECTION, POWDER FOR INJECTION: 50-mg vial.

ADMINISTRATION/HANDLING

IV

Reconstitution • Reconstitute each 50-mg vial with 15 ml of companion diluent (20% dehydrated alcohol in Sterile Water for Injection). • Further dilute with 85 ml D_5W or 0.9% NaCl only to provide a total infusion volume of 100 ml per each 50-mg vial for a concentration of 0.5 mg/ml.

Rate of administration • Do not exceed infusion rate of 1.1 mg/min.

Storage • May store unreconstituted vials or reconstituted vials with companion diluent at room temperature. • Final reconstituted infusion solution must be used within 24 hrs.

IV INCOMPATIBILITIES

Amphotericin B (Abelcet, AmBisome), ertapenem (Invanz), sodium bicarbonate.

IV COMPATIBILITIES

Dexamethasone, (Decadron) famotidine (Pepcid), furosemide (Lasix), hydromorphone (Dilaudid), lorazepam (Ativan), meperidine (Demerol), methylprednisolone (Solu-Medrol), morphine.

INDICATIONS/ROUTES/DOSAGE

◀ **ALERT** ▶ Duration of treatment based on pt's clinical response. In general, treatment is continued for at least 14 days after last positive culture.

CANDIDEMIA, OTHER CANDIDA INFECTIONS

IV: ADULTS, ELDERLY: Give single 200-mg loading dose on day 1, followed by 100 mg/day thereafter.

ESOPHAGEAL CANDIDIASIS

IV: ADULTS, ELDERLY: Give single 100-mg loading dose on day 1, followed by 50 mg/day thereafter for a minimum of 14 days and for at least 7 days following resolution of symptoms.

SIDE EFFECTS

RARE (3%–1%): Diarrhea, nausea, headache.

ADVERSE EFFECTS/ TOXIC REACTIONS

Hypokalemia occurs in 4% of pts. Hypersensitivity reaction characterized by facial flushing, hypotension, pruritus, urticaria, rash, occur rarely.

NURSING CONSIDERATIONS

BASELINE ASSESSMENT

Obtain specimens for fungal culture prior to therapy. Treatment may be instituted before results are known. Obtain baseline hepatic enzyme levels.

INTERVENTION/EVALUATION

Monitor serum chemistry results for evidence of hepatic dysfunction. Monitor daily pattern of bowel activity/stool consistency. Assess for rash, urticaria.

PATIENT/FAMILY TEACHING

• For esophageal candidiasis, maintain diligent oral hygiene.

antihemophilic factor (factor VIII, AHF)

an-tee-hee-moe-**fill**-ick **fak**-tor

(**Human:** Alphanate, Hemofil M, Humate-P, Koate-DVI, Monarc M, Monoclate-P. **Recombinant:** Advate, Hexilate FS, Kogenate FS, Recombinate, Refacto)

Do not confuse Alphanate with Alfenta.

CLASSIFICATION

PHARMACOTHERAPEUTIC: Antihemophilic agent. **CLINICAL:** Hemostatic.

ACTION

Assists in conversion of prothrombin to thrombin, essential for blood coagulation. Replaces missing clotting factor. **Therapeutic Effect:** Produces hemostasis; corrects or prevents bleeding episodes.

PHARMACOKINETICS

Half-Life: 12–17 hrs.

USES

Human: Management of hemophilia A. Humate P also indicated for treatment of spontaneous bleeding in pts with severe von Willebrand's disease and in mild von Willebrand's disease when desmopressin is known or suspected to be inadequate. **Recombinant:** Management of hemophilia A, prevention and control of bleeding episodes, perioperative management of hemophilia A. **OFF-LABEL:** Treatment of disseminated intravascular coagulation.

PRECAUTIONS

CONTRAINDICATIONS: None known. **CAUTIONS:** Hepatic disease, those with blood types A, B, AB.

LIFESPAN CONSIDERATIONS:

Pregnancy/Lactation: Unknown if drug crosses placenta or is distributed in breast milk. **Pregnancy Category C. Children:** Safety and efficacy not established. **Elderly:** No age-related precautions noted.

INTERACTIONS

DRUG: None significant. **HERBAL:** None significant. **FOOD:** None known. **LAB VALUES:** None known.

AVAILABILITY (Rx)

HUMAN INJECTION: Actual number of units listed on each vial. **RECOMBINANT: INJECTION POWDER FOR RECONSTITUTION: ADVATE:** 250 units, 500 units, 1000 units, 1500 units. **HEXILATE, KOGENATE, RECOMBINATE:** 250 units, 500 units, 1000 units. **REFACTO:** 250 units, 500 units, 1000 units, 2000 units.

ADMINISTRATION/HANDLING

IV

Reconstitution • Warm concentrate and diluent to room temperature. • Using needle supplied by the manufacturer, add diluent to powder to dissolve, gently agitate or rotate. Do not shake vigorously. Complete dissolution may take 5–10 min. • Use second filtered needle supplied by the manufacturer, and add to infusion bag.

Rate of administration • Administer IV at rate of approximately 2 ml/min. May give up to 10 ml/min.

Administration precautions • Check pulse rate prior to and following administration. If pulse rate increases, reduce or stop administration. • After administration, apply prolonged pressure on venipuncture site. • Monitor IV site for oozing q5–15min for 1–2 hrs following administration.

Storage • Refrigerate.

IV INCOMPATIBILITIES

Do not mix with other IV solutions or medications.

INDICATIONS/ROUTES/DOSAGE

HEMOPHILIA A, VON WILLEBRAND'S DISEASE

IV: ADULTS, ELDERLY, CHILDREN: Dosage is highly individualized and is based on pt's weight, severity of bleeding, coagulation studies.

SIDE EFFECTS

OCCASIONAL: Allergic reaction, including fever, chills, urticaria, wheezing, hypotension, nausea, feeling of chest tightness; stinging at injection site; dizziness; dry mouth; headache; altered taste.

ADVERSE EFFECTS/ TOXIC REACTIONS

Risk of transmitting viral hepatitis. Intravascular hemolysis may occur if large or frequent doses are used with blood group A, B, or AB.

NURSING CONSIDERATIONS

BASELINE ASSESSMENT

When monitoring B/P, avoid overinflation of cuff. Remove adhesive tape from any pressure dressing very carefully and slowly.

INTERVENTION/EVALUATION

Following IV administration, apply prolonged pressure on venipuncture site. Monitor IV site for oozing q5–15 min for 1–2 hrs following administration. Assess for allergic reaction. Report immediately any evidence of hematuria or change in vital signs. Assess for decreases in B/P, increased pulse rate, complaint of abdominal or back pain, severe headache (may be evidence of hemorrhage). Question for increased discharge during menses. Assess skin for bruises, petechiae. Check for excessive bleeding from minor cuts, scratches. Assess gums for erythema, gingival bleeding. Assess urine for hematuria. Evaluate for therapeutic relief of pain, reduction of swelling, restricted joint movement.

PATIENT/FAMILY TEACHING

• Use electric razor, soft toothbrush to prevent bleeding. • Report any sign of red or dark urine, black/red stool, coffee-ground vomitus, blood-tinged mucus from cough.

Anzemet, *see dolasetron*

Apokyn, *see apomorphine*

apomorphine

aye-poe-**more**-feen
(Apokyn)

CLASSIFICATION

PHARMACOTHERAPEUTIC: Dopaminergics. **CLINICAL:** Antiparkinson.

ACTION

Stimulates postsynaptic dopamine receptors in the brain. **Therapeutic Effect:** Relieves signs and symptoms of Parkinson's disease, improves motor function.

PHARMACOKINETICS

Rapidly absorbed after subcutaneous administration. Protein binding: 99.9%. Widely distributed. Rapidly eliminated from plasma. Not detected in urine or secretions. **Half-life:** 41–45 min.

USES

Acute, intermittent treatment of hypomobility, ("off" episodes) associated with advanced Parkinson's disease. **OFF-LABEL:** Induce emesis, treatment of acute poisoning.

PRECAUTIONS

CONTRAINDICATIONS: Concurrent use of 5-HT_3 antagonists (e.g., alosetron, dolasetron, granisetron, ondansetron, or palonosetron). **CAUTIONS:** Hepatic/renal impairment, cardiac decompensation.

LIFESPAN CONSIDERATIONS:

Pregnancy/Lactation: Unknown if drug is distributed in breast milk. **Pregnancy Category C.** **Children:** Safety and efficacy not established. **Elderly:** No age-related precautions noted, but hallucinations appear to occur more frequently.

INTERACTIONS

DRUG: Concurrent use of **ondansetron, dolasetron, granisetron, palonosetron, alosetron** may produce profound hypotension, loss of consciousness. **Phenothiazines, butyrophenones, thioxanthenes, metaclopramide** diminish effectiveness of apomorphine. Additive side effects with **CNS depressants.** **HERBAL:** None significant. **FOOD:** None known. **LAB VALUES:** May increase serum alkaline phosphatase.

AVAILABILITY (Rx)

INJECTION SOLUTION: 10 mg/ml.

ADMINISTRATION/HANDLING

SUBCUTANEOUS

Storage • Store at room temperature.

INDICATIONS/ROUTES/DOSAGE

PARKINSON'S DISEASE

SUBCUTANEOUS: ADULTS, ELDERLY: Initially, 0.2 ml (2 mg); may be increased in 0.1-ml (1-mg) increments every few days. **Maximum:** 0.6 ml (6 mg).

SIDE EFFECTS

OCCASIONAL (4%–3%): Injection site discomfort, arthralgia, somnolence, hypersalivation, pallor, yawning, headache, dizziness, diaphoresis, vomiting, orthostatic hypotension. **RARE (less than 2%):** Psychosis, stomatitis, altered taste, hallucinations.

ADVERSE EFFECTS/ TOXIC REACTIONS

Respiratory depression or CNS stimulation characterized by tachypnea, bradycardia, persistent vomiting may occur. May cause or exacerbate preexisting dyskinesia.

NURSING CONSIDERATIONS

INTERVENTION/EVALUATION

Instruct pt to change positions slowly to prevent risk of orthostatic hypotension. Assist with ambulation if dizziness occurs. Assess for clinical improvement, reversal of symptoms (improvement of tremor of head/hands at rest, mask-like facial expression, shuffling gait, muscular rigidity).

PATIENT/FAMILY TEACHING

• Drowsiness, dizziness may be an initial response to drug. • Avoid tasks that require alertness, motor skills until response to drug is established. • Inform pt and family that hallucinations may occur, esp. in the elderly.

apraclonidine

(Iopidine)

See Antiglaucoma agents (p. 49C)

aprepitant

ah-**prep**-ih-tant
(Emend, Emend 3-Day)

CLASSIFICATION

PHARMACOTHERAPEUTIC: Selective receptor antagonist. **CLINICAL:** Antinausea, antiemetic.

ACTION

Inhibits chemotherapy-induced nausea, vomiting centrally in the chemoreceptor trigger zone. **Therapeutic Effect:** Prevents the acute and delayed phases of chemotherapy-induced emesis, including vomiting caused by high-dose cisplatin.

PHARMACOKINETICS

Crosses blood-brain barrier. Extensively metabolized in the liver. Eliminated primarily by liver metabolism (not excreted renally). **Half-life:** 9–13 hrs.

USES

Prevention of acute and delayed nausea/vomiting associated with initial and repeat courses of emetogenic cancer chemotherapy, including high-dose cisplatin. Prevention of postoperative nausea, vomiting.

PRECAUTIONS

CONTRAINDICATIONS: Breast-feeding, concurrent use of astemizole, cisapride, pimozide, terfenadine. **CAUTIONS:** None known.

LIFESPAN CONSIDERATIONS:

Pregnancy/Lactation: Unknown if drug crosses placenta or is distributed in breast milk. **Pregnancy Category B.** **Children:** Safety and efficacy not established. **Elderly:** No age-related precautions noted.

INTERACTIONS

DRUG: **Carbamazepine, phenytoin, rifampin** reduce plasma concentration. **Antifungals, nefazodone, clarithromycin, ritonavir, nelfinavir, diltiazem** increase plasma concentration. Plasma concentrations of **docetaxel, paclitaxol, etoposide, irinotecan, ifosfamide, imatinib, vinorelbine, vinblastine, vincristine, midazolam, alprazolam, triazolam** may be elevated. May decrease effectiveness of **contraceptives.** Increases effects of **corticosteroids** (IV steroid dose should be reduced by 25%, oral dose by 50%). **Paroxetine** may decrease effectiveness of either drug. May decrease effectiveness of **warfarin.** **HERBAL:** **St. John's wort** may decrease plasma concentration. **FOOD:** **Grapefruit, grapefruit juice** may increase plasma concentration. **LAB VALUES:** May increase BUN, serum creatinine, AST, ALT. May produce proteinuria.

AVAILABILITY (Rx)

CAPSULES (EMEND): 40 mg, 80 mg, 125 mg. **KIT (EMEND 3-DAY):** 125 mg-80 mg.

ADMINISTRATION/HANDLING

PO

- Give without regard to food.

INDICATIONS/ROUTES/DOSAGE

PREVENTION OF CHEMOTHERAPY-INDUCED NAUSEA, VOMITING

PO: ADULTS, ELDERLY: 125 mg 1 hr before chemotherapy on day 1 and 80 mg once a day in the morning on days 2 and 3.

PREVENTION OF POSTOPERATIVE NAUSEA, VOMITTING

PO: ADULTS, ELDERLY: 40 mg once within 3 hrs prior to induction of anesthesia.

SIDE EFFECTS

FREQUENT (17%–10%): Fatigue, nausea, hiccups, diarrhea, constipation, anorexia. **OCCASIONAL (8%–4%):** Headache, vomiting, dizziness, dehydration, heartburn. **RARE (3% or less):** Abdominal pain, epigastric discomfort, gastritis, tinnitus, insomnia.

ADVERSE EFFECTS/ TOXIC REACTIONS

Neutropenia, mucous membrane disorders occur rarely.

NURSING CONSIDERATIONS

BASELINE ASSESSMENT

Assess for dehydration if excessive vomiting occurs (poor skin turgor, dry mucous membranes, longitudinal furrows in tongue). Provide emotional support.

INTERVENTION/EVALUATION

Monitor pt in environment. Assess bowel sounds for peristalsis. Assist with ambulation if dizziness occurs. Provide supportive measures. Monitor pattern of daily bowel activity and stool consistency. Record time of evacuation.

PATIENT/FAMILY TEACHING

- Relief from nausea/vomiting generally occurs shortly after drug administration.
- Report persistent vomiting, headache.

Aptivus, *see tipranavir*

Aranesp, *see darbepoetin alfa*

Arava, *see leflunomide*

arformoterol

are-four-**mow**-tear-ohl
(Brovana)

CLASSIFICATION

PHARMACOTHERAPEUTIC: Sympathomimetic (beta-$_2$ adrenergic agonist). **CLINICAL:** Bronchodilator (see p. 70C).

ACTION

Long-acting bronchodilator that stimulates beta-$_2$ adrenergic receptors in lungs, resulting in relaxation of bronchial smooth muscle. Inhibits release of mediators from various cells in lungs, including mast cells, with little effect on heart rate. **Therapeutic Effect:** Relieves bronchospasm, reduces airway resistance. Improves bronchodilation, nighttime asthma control, peak flow rates. Long-acting bronchodilating effects.

PHARMACOKINETICS

Absorbed from bronchi following nebulization. Metabolized in liver. Primarily excreted in urine. Unknown if removed by hemodialysis. **Half-life:** 26 hrs.

USES

Long-term, twice daily (morning and evening) maintenance treatment of bronchoconstriction in pts with chronic obstructive pulmonary disease (COPD), including chronic bronchitis and emphysema.

PRECAUTIONS

CONTRAINDICATIONS: History of sensitivity to formoterol. **CAUTIONS:** Hypertension, cardiovascular disease, convulsive disorder, thyrotoxicosis.

⌛ LIFESPAN CONSIDERATIONS:

Pregnancy/Lactation: Unknown if drug crosses placenta or is distributed in breast milk. **Pregnancy Category C. Children:** Safety and efficacy not established. **Elderly:** May be more sensitive to tremor or tachycardia due to age-related increased sympathetic sensitivity.

INTERACTIONS

DRUG: Beta-adrenergic blocking agents (beta blockers) can antagonize bronchodilating effects. May potentiate cardiovascular effects with **MAOIs, tricyclic antidepressants, drugs that can prolong QT interval (erythromycin, quinidine). Diuretics, theophylline, steroids** can increase risk of hypokalemia. **HERBAL:** None significant. **FOOD:** None known. **LAB VALUES:** May reduce serum potassium, increase blood glucose.

AVAILABILITY (Rx)

INHALATION, SOLUTION FOR NEBULIZATION: 15 mcg/2 ml.

ADMINISTRATION/HANDLING

NEBULIZATION

• Refrigerate, protect from light, excessive heat. • May store at room temperature for up to 6 wks. • Use only in standard jet nebulizer machine connected to an air compressor at adequate flow rates via facemask or mouthpiece. • Requires no dilution before administration by nebulization.

INDICATIONS/ROUTES/DOSAGE

BRONCHOCONSTRICTION

NEBULIZATION: ADULTS, ELDERLY: 15 mcg 2 times/day (morning and evening).

SIDE EFFECTS

OCCASIONAL: Pain, diarrhea, sinusitis, leg cramps, dyspnea, rash, flu syndrome, peripheral edema.

ADVERSE EFFECTS/ TOXIC REACTIONS

Excessive sympathomimetic stimulation may produce palpitations, extrasystoles, chest pain.

NURSING CONSIDERATIONS

BASELINE ASSESSMENT

Offer emotional support (high incidence of anxiety due to difficulty in breathing and sympathomimetic response to drug).

INTERVENTION/EVALUATION

Assess rate, depth, rhythm, type of respiration; quality and rate of pulse. Monitor EKG, serum potassium, ABG determinations. Assess lung sounds for wheezing (bronchoconstriction), rales.

PATIENT/FAMILY TEACHING

Instruct on proper use of nebulizer. Increase fluid intake (decreases lung secretion viscosity). Avoid excessive use of caffeine derivatives (e.g., coffee, cola). Call emergency medical care if breathing worsens quickly.

argatroban

our-ga-**trow**-ban
(Acova)

Do not confuse argatroban with Aggrestat or Orgaran.

◆ CLASSIFICATION

PHARMACOTHERAPEUTIC: Thrombin inhibitor. **CLINICAL:** Anticoagulant.

ACTION

Direct thrombin inhibitor that reversibly binds to thrombin-active sites. Inhibits thrombin-catalyzed or thrombin-induced reactions, including fibrin formation, activation of coagulant factors V, VIII, and XIII; inhibits protein C formation, platelet aggregation. **Therapeutic Effect:** Produces anticoagulation.

PHARMACOKINETICS

Following IV administration, distributed primarily in extracellular fluid. Protein binding: 54%. Metabolized in the liver. Primarily excreted in the feces, presumably through biliary secretion. **Half-life:** 39–51 min.

USES

Prophylaxis or treatment of thrombosis in heparin-induced thrombocytopenia (HIT). Prevention of HIT during percutaneous coronary procedures. **OFF-LABEL:** Cerebral thrombosis, MI.

PRECAUTIONS

CONTRAINDICATIONS: Overt major bleeding. **CAUTIONS:** Severe hypertension, immediately following lumbar puncture, spinal anesthesia, major surgery, pts with congenital or acquired bleeding disorders, ulcerations, hepatic impairment.

LIFESPAN CONSIDERATIONS:

Pregnancy/Lactation: Unknown if excreted in breast milk. **Pregnancy Category B.** **Children:** Safety and efficacy not established in those younger than 18 yrs. **Elderly:** No age-related precautions noted.

INTERACTIONS

DRUG: **Antiplatelet agents, thrombolytics, other anticoagulants** may increase the risk of bleeding. **HERBAL:** **Arnica, astragalus, bilberry, black currant, cat's claw, chaparral, dandelion, evening primrose, feverfew, garlic, ginger, ginkgo biloba, hawthorn, kava, licorice, tan-shen, vitamin A** may increase the risk of bleeding. **FOOD:** None known. **LAB VALUES:** Increases prothrombin time (PT), activated partial thromboplastin time (aPTT). International Normalized Ratio (INR). May increase Hgb, Hct.

AVAILABILITY (Rx)

INJECTION SOLUTION: 100 mg/ml.

ADMINISTRATION/HANDLING

IV

Reconstitution • Must be diluted 100-fold before infusion in 0.9% NaCl, D_5W, or lactated Ringer's solution to provide a final concentration of 1 mg/ml. • The solution must be mixed by repeated inversion of the diluent bag for 1 min. • After reconstitution, solution may show a brief haziness due to formation of microprecipitates that rapidly dissolve upon mixing.

Rate of administration • Rate of administration is based on body weight at 2 mcg/kg/min (e.g., 50-kg pt infuse at 6 ml/hr).

Storage • Discard if solution appears cloudy or an insoluble precipitate is noted. • Following reconstitution, stable for 24 hrs at room temperature, 48 hrs if refrigerated. • Avoid direct sunlight.

IV INCOMPATIBILITIES

Do not mix with other medications or solutions.

INDICATIONS/ROUTES/DOSAGE

HEPARIN-INDUCED THROMBOCYTOPENIA

IV INFUSION: ADULTS, ELDERLY: Initially, 2 mcg/kg/min administered as a continuous infusion. After initial infusion, dose may be adjusted until steady state aPTT is 1.5–3 times initial baseline value, not to exceed 100 sec.

PERCUTANEOUS CORONARY INTERVENTION

IV INFUSION: ADULTS, ELDERLY: Initially, 25 mcg/kg/min and administer bolus of 350 mcg/kg over 3–5 min. ACT (activated clotting time) checked in 5–10 min following bolus. If ACT is less than 300 sec, give additional bolus 150 mcg/kg, increase infusion to 30 mcg/kg/min. If ACT is greater than 450 sec, decrease infusion to 15 mcg/kg/min. Once ACT of 300–450 sec achieved, proceed with procedure.

DOSAGE IN HEPATIC IMPAIRMENT

ADULTS, ELDERLY: Initially, 0.5 mcg/kg/min.

SIDE EFFECTS

FREQUENT (8%–3%): Dyspnea, hypotension, fever, diarrhea, nausea, pain, vomiting, infection, cough.

ADVERSE EFFECTS/ TOXIC REACTIONS

Ventricular tachycardia, atrial fibrillation occur occasionally. Major bleeding, sepsis occur rarely.

NURSING CONSIDERATIONS

BASELINE ASSESSMENT

Check CBC, including platelet count, PT, PTT. Determine initial B/P. Minimize need for numerous injection sites, blood draws, catheters.

INTERVENTION/EVALUATION

Assess for any sign of bleeding: bleeding at surgical site, hematuria, blood in stool, bleeding from gums, petechiae, ecchymoses, bleeding from injection sites. Handle pt carefully and as infrequently as possible to prevent bleeding. Do not obtain B/P in lower extremities (possible deep vein thrombi). Assess for decreased B/P, increased pulse rate, complaint of abdominal/back pain, severe headache (indicates evidence of hemorrhage). Monitor ACT, PT, aPTT, platelet count. Question for increase in discharge during menses. Assess urinary output for hematuria. Observe skin for any occurring hematoma. Use care in removing any dressing, tape.

PATIENT/FAMILY TEACHING

• Use electric razor, soft toothbrush to prevent bleeding. • Report any sign of red/dark urine, black/red stool, coffee-ground vomitus, blood-tinged mucus from cough.

Aricept, *see donepezil*

Arimidex, *see anastrozole*

aripiprazole

air-ee-**pip**-rah-zole

(Abilify, Abilify Discmelt)

◆ CLASSIFICATION

PHARMACOTHERAPEUTIC: Dopamine agonist. **CLINICAL:** Antipsychotic agent.

ACTION

Provides partial agonist activity at dopamine and serotonin (5-HT_{1A}) receptors and antagonist activity at serotonin (5-HT_{2A}) receptors. **Therapeutic Effect:** Diminishes schizophrenic behavior.

PHARMACOKINETICS

Well absorbed through GI tract. Protein binding: 99% (primarily albumin). Reaches steady levels in 2 wks. Metabolized in the liver. Eliminated primarily in feces and, to a lesser extent, in urine. Not removed by hemodialysis. **Half-life:** 75 hrs.

USES

Treatment of schizophrenia. Maintains stability in pts with schizophrenia. Treatment of bipolar disorder. **IM:** Agitation associated with schizophrenia/bipolar disorder. **OFF-LABEL:** Schizoaffective disorder.

PRECAUTIONS

CONTRAINDICATIONS: None known. **CAUTIONS:** Concurrent use of CNS depressants (including alcohol), cardiovascular or cerebrovascular diseases (may induce hypotension), Parkinson's disease (potential for exacerbation), history of seizures or conditions that may lower seizure threshold (Alzheimer's disease), renal/hepatic impairment.

LIFESPAN CONSIDERATIONS:

Pregnancy/Lactation: Unknown if drug crosses placenta. May be distributed in breast milk; avoid breast-feeding. **Pregnancy Category C. Children:** Safety and efficacy not established. **Elderly:** No age-related precautions noted.

INTERACTIONS

DRUG: **Alcohol** may potentiate cognitive and motor effects. **Carbamazepine** may decrease concentration. **Ketoconazole, quinidine, fluoxetine, paroxetine** may increase concentrations. **HERBAL:** **St. John's wort** may decrease levels. **Kava kava, gotu kola, valerian, St. John's wort** may increase CNS depression. **FOOD:** None known. **LAB VALUES:** None known.

AVAILABILITY (Rx)

INJECTION, SOLUTION: 9.75 mg/1.3 ml. **SOLUTION ORAL:** 1 mg/ml. **TABLETS:** 2 mg, 5 mg, 10 mg, 15 mg, 20 mg, 30 mg. **TABLETS, ORAL DISINTEGRATION:** 10 mg, 15 mg.

ADMINISTRATION/HANDLING

IM

• For IM use only. Do not administer IV or subcutaneous.

PO

• Give without regard to food.

ODT

• Remove tablet, place entire tablet on tongue. • Do not break, split tablet. • May give without liquid.

INDICATIONS/ROUTES/DOSAGE

SCHIZOPHRENIA

PO: ADULTS, ELDERLY: Initially, 10–15 mg once a day. May increase up to 30 mg/day.

BIPOLAR DISORDER

PO: ADULTS, ELDERLY: 30 mg once a day. May decrease to 15 mg/day based on pt tolerance.

AGITATION WITH SCHIZOPHRENIA/ BIPOLAR DISORDER

IM: ADULTS, ELDERLY: 5.25–15 mg. May repeat after 2 hrs. **Maximum:** 30 mg/day.

SIDE EFFECTS

FREQUENT (11%–5%): Weight gain, headache, insomnia, vomiting. **OCCASIONAL (4%–3%):** Light-headedness, nausea, akathisia, somnolence. **RARE (2% or less):** Blurred vision, constipation, asthenia (loss of energy/strength), anxiety, fever, rash, cough, rhinitis, orthostatic hypotension.

ADVERSE EFFECTS/ TOXIC REACTIONS

Extrapyramidal symptoms, neuroleptic malignant syndrome occur rarely. Prolonged QT interval occurs rarely.

NURSING CONSIDERATIONS

BASELINE ASSESSMENT

Assess behavior, appearance, emotional status, response to environment, speech pattern, thought content. Correct dehydration, hypovolemia.

INTERVENTION/EVALUATION

Periodically monitor weight. Monitor for extrapyramidal symptoms (abnormal movement), tardive dyskinesia (protrusion of tongue, puffing of cheeks, chewing/puckering of the mouth). Periodically monitor B/P, pulse (particularly in those with preexisting cardiovascular disease). Assess for therapeutic response (greater interest in surroundings, improved self-care, increased ability to concentrate, relaxed facial expression).

PATIENT/FAMILY TEACHING

• Avoid alcohol. • Avoid tasks that require alertness, motor skills until response to drug is established.

Arixtra, *see fondaparinux*

Aromasin, *see exemestane*

Arranon, *see nelarbine*

arsenic trioxide

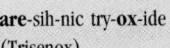

are-sih-nic try-**ox**-ide
(Trisenox)

Do not confuse Trisenox with Trimox.

CLASSIFICATION

CLINICAL: Antineoplastic (see p. 76C).

ACTION

Produces morphologic changes and DNA fragmentation in promyelocytic leukemia cells. **Therapeutic Effect:** Produces cell death.

PHARMACOKINETICS

Distributed in liver, kidneys, heart, lungs, hair, and nails. Metabolized in liver. Eliminated by kidneys. Does not have a half-life.

USES

Induction of remission and consolidations in pts with acute promyelocytic leukemia (APL) who are refractory to or have relapsed from retinoid and anthracycline chemotherapy.

PRECAUTIONS

CONTRAINDICATIONS: None known. **CAUTIONS:** Renal impairment, cardiac abnormalities.

LIFESPAN CONSIDERATIONS:

Pregnancy/Lactation: Distributed in breast milk. May cause fetal harm. **Pregnancy Category D. Children:** Safety and efficacy not established in children younger than 5 yrs. **Elderly:** Age-related renal impairment may require dosage adjustment.

INTERACTIONS

DRUG: May prolong QT interval in those taking **antiarrhythmics, moxifloxacin, thioridazine. Diuretics, amphotericin B, cyclosporine** may produce electrolyte abnormalities. **HERBAL:** None significant. **FOOD:** None known. **LAB VALUES:** May decrease WBC count, Hgb, platelet count, serum magnesium, calcium. May increase serum AST, ALT. Higher risk of hypokalemia than hyperkalemia, hyperglycemia than hypoglycemia.

AVAILABILITY (Rx)

INJECTION SOLUTION: 1 mg/ml.

ADMINISTRATION/HANDLING

IV

◄ **ALERT** ► Central venous line is not required for drug administration.

Reconstitution • After withdrawing drug from ampule, dilute with 100–250 ml D_5W or 0.9% NaCl.

Rate of administration • Infuse over 1–2 hrs. Duration of infusion may be extended up to 4 hrs.

Storage • Store at room temperature. • Diluted solution is stable for 24 hrs at room temperature, 48 hrs if refrigerated.

IV INCOMPATIBILITIES

Do not mix with any other medications.

INDICATIONS/ROUTES/DOSAGE

ACUTE PROMYELOCYTIC LEUKEMIA

IV: ADULTS, ELDERLY, CHILDREN OLDER THAN 5 YRS: Induction: 0.15 mg/kg/day until myelosuppression occurs. Do not exceed 60 induction doses. **Consolidation:** beginning 3–6 wks after completion of induction therapy, 0.15 mg/kg/day for maximum 25 doses over a period of up to 5 wks.

SIDE EFFECTS

EXPECTED (75%–50%): Nausea, cough, fatigue, fever, headache, vomiting, abdominal pain, tachycardia, diarrhea, dyspnea. **FREQUENT (43%–30%):** Dermatitis, insomnia, edema, rigors, prolonged QT interval, sore throat, pruritus, arthralgia, paresthesia, anxiety. **OCCASIONAL (28%–20%):** Constipation, myalgia, hypotension, epistaxis, anorexia, dizziness,sinusitis.**(15%–8%):** Ecchymosis, nonspecific pain, weight gain, herpes simplex, wheezing, flushing, diaphoresis, tremor, hypertension, palpitations, dyspepsia, eye irritation, blurred vision, asthenia, diminished breath sounds, crackles. **RARE:** Confusion, petechiae, dry mouth, oral candidiasis, incontinence, rhonchi.

ADVERSE EFFECTS/ TOXIC REACTIONS

Seizures, GI hemorrhage, renal impairment or failure, pleural or pericardial effusion, hemoptysis, sepsis occur rarely. Prolonged QT interval, complete AV block, unexplained fever, dyspnea, weight gain, effusion are evidence of arsenic toxicity. Treatment should be halted, steroid therapy instituted.

NURSING CONSIDERATIONS

BASELINE ASSESSMENT

Assess platelet count, Hgb, Hct, WBC before and frequently during treatment. Ask if pt is breast-feeding, pregnant, or planning to become pregnant (may cause fetal harm).

INTERVENTION/EVALUATION

Monitor hepatic function test results, CBC, serum values. Monitor for arsenic toxicity syndrome (fever, dyspnea, weight gain, confusion, muscle weakness, seizures).

PATIENT/FAMILY TEACHING

• Avoid crowds, those with known infection. • Avoid tasks that require alertness, motor skills, until response to drug is established. • Contact physician if high fever, vomiting, difficulty breathing, or rapid heart rate occur.

Arthrotec, *see diclofenac and misoprostil*

artificial tears

(Eye Tears, Hypotears, Isopto Tears, Refresh Aquasite, Tears Naturale, Tears Plus, Ultra Fresh Eyes, Visine Tears, Viva Drops)

CLASSIFICATION

PHARMACOTHERAPEUTIC: Ophthalmic lubricant.

ACTION

Stabilizes/thickens precorneal tear film, lengthening tear film breakup time. **Therapeutic Effect:** Protects, lubricates the eyes.

USES

Relief of dryness, irritation due to deficient tear production; ocular lubricant for artificial eyes; some products may be used with hard contact lenses. **OFF-LABEL:** Treatment of recurrent corneal erosions, decreased corneal sensitivity.

PRECAUTIONS

CONTRAINDICATIONS: Hypersensitivity to any component of preparation. **CAUTIONS:** None known. **Pregnancy Category A.**

INTERACTIONS

DRUG: None significant. **HERBAL:** None significant. **FOOD:** None known. **LAB VALUES:** None known.

INDICATIONS/ROUTES/DOSAGE

OPHTHALMIC LUBRICANT

ADULTS, ELDERLY: 1–2 drops 3–4 times a day as needed.

SIDE EFFECTS

OCCASIONAL: Eye irritation, blurred vision, stickiness of eyelashes.

ADVERSE EFFECTS/ TOXIC REACTIONS

None known.

NURSING CONSIDERATIONS

BASELINE ASSESSMENT

Determine extent of dryness, irritation.

INTERVENTION/EVALUATION

Monitor for increased irritation or discomfort. Assess therapeutic response.

PATIENT/FAMILY TEACHING

- Wash hands thoroughly before use.
- Do not touch tip of dropper or container to any surface.

Asacol, *see mesalamine*

ascorbic acid (vitamin C)

a-**skor**bic

(C-500-GR, Cecon, Cedvibid, C-Gram, Proflavanol C ✦, Revitalose C-1000 ✦, Vita-C)

CLASSIFICATION

CLINICAL: Vitamin (see p. 151C).

ACTION

Assists in collagen formation, tissue repair and is involved in oxidation reduction reactions, other metabolic reactions. **Therapeutic Effect:** Involved in carbohydrate utilization and metabolism, as well as synthesis of carnitine, lipids, proteins. Preserves blood vessel integrity.

PHARMACOKINETICS

Readily absorbed from GI tract. Protein binding: 25%. Metabolized in the liver. Excreted in urine. Removed by hemodialysis.

USES

Prevention and treatment of scurvy, acidification of urine, dietary supplement, prevention of and reduction in the severity of colds. **OFF-LABEL:** Chronic iron toxicity, control of idiopathic methemoglobinemia, macular degeneration, prevention of common cold, urinary acidifier.

PRECAUTIONS

CONTRAINDICATIONS: None known. **CAUTIONS:** Those on sodium restriction, daily salicylate treatment, warfarin therapy; diabetes mellitus; history of renal stones.

LIFESPAN CONSIDERATIONS:

Pregnancy/Lactation: Crosses placenta; excreted in breast milk. Large doses during pregnancy may produce scurvy in neonates. **Pregnancy Category A (C if used in doses above recommended daily allowance). Children/Elderly:** No age-related precautions noted.

INTERACTIONS

DRUG: Enhances **iron** absorption. May increase effect of **oral contraceptives.** May reduce effect of **oral contraceptives** with reduction in dosage of ascorbic acid. **HERBAL:** None significant. **FOOD:** None known. **LAB VALUES:** May decrease serum bilirubin, urinary pH. May increase serum uric acid, urinary oxalate.

AVAILABILITY

CAPSULES: 500 mg, 1000 mg. **CRYSTALS:** 4 g/tsp. **INJECTION, SOLUTION:** 250 mg/ml, 500 mg/ml. **SOLUTION, ORAL:** 90 mg/ml. **TABLETS:** 100 mg, 250 mg, 500 mg, 1,000 mg. **TABLETS (CHEWABLE):** 100 mg, 250 mg, 500 mg.

CAPSULES (TIMED RELEASE): 500 mg. **TABLETS (TIMED RELEASE):** 500 mg, 1,000 mg, 1,500 mg.

ADMINISTRATION/HANDLING

IV

Rate of administration • May give undiluted or dilute in D_5W, 0.9% NaCl, lactated Ringer's solution. • For IV push, dilute with equal volume D_5W or 0.9% NaCl and infuse over 10 min. For IV solution, infuse over 4–12 hrs.

Storage • Refrigerate. • Protect from freezing and light.

PO

• Give without regard to food.

IV INCOMPATIBILITIES

No information available for Y-site administration.

IV COMPATIBILITIES

Calcium gluconate, heparin.

INDICATIONS/ROUTES/DOSAGE

DIETARY SUPPLEMENT

PO: ADULTS, ELDERLY: 50–200 mg/day. **CHILDREN:** 35–100 mg/day.

ACIDIFICATION OF URINE

PO: ADULTS, ELDERLY: 4–12 g/day in 3–4 divided doses. **CHILDREN:** 500 mg q6–8h.

SCURVY

PO: ADULTS, ELDERLY: 100–250 mg 1–2 times a day. **CHILDREN:** 100–300 mg/day in divided doses.

PREVENTION AND REDUCTION OF SEVERITY OF COLDS

PO: ADULTS, ELDERLY: 1–3 g/day in divided doses.

SIDE EFFECTS

RARE: Abdominal cramps, nausea, vomiting, diarrhea, increased urination with doses exceeding 1 g. **Parenteral:** Flushing, headache, dizziness, sleepiness or insomnia, soreness at injection site.

ADVERSE EFFECTS/ TOXIC REACTIONS

May acidify urine, leading to crystalluria. Large doses of IV ascorbic acid may lead to deep vein thrombosis. Prolonged use of large doses may produce rebound ascorbic acid deficiency, when dosage is reduced to normal range.

NURSING CONSIDERATIONS

INTERVENTION/EVALUATION

Assess for clinical improvement (improved sense of well-being and sleep patterns). Observe for reversal of deficiency symptoms (gingivitis, bleeding gums, poor wound healing, digestive difficulties, joint pain).

PATIENT/FAMILY TEACHING

• Abrupt vitamin C withdrawal may produce rebound deficiency. Reduce dosage gradually. • Foods rich in vitamin C include rose hips, guava, black currant jelly, Brussels sprouts, green peppers, spinach, watercress, strawberries, citrus fruits.

asparaginase

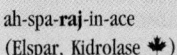

ah-spa-**raj**-in-ace

(Elspar, Kidrolase ♣)

Do not confuse asparaginase with pegaspargase.

CLASSIFICATION

PHARMACOTHERAPEUTIC: Enzyme. **CLINICAL:** Antineoplastic (see p. 76C).

ACTION

Inhibits DNA, RNA, protein synthesis by breaking down asparagine, thus depriving tumor cells of this essential amino acid. Cell cycle–specific for G_1 phase of cell division. **Therapeutic Effect:** Toxic to leukemic cells.

PHARMACOKINETICS

Metabolized by reticuloendothelial system through slow sequestration. **Half-life:** 39–49 hrs IM; 8–30 hrs IV.

USES

Treatment of acute lymphocytic leukemia (ALL), lymphoma in combination with other therapy. **OFF-LABEL:** Treatment of acute myelocytic leukemia, acute myelomonocytic leukemia, chronic lymphocytic leukemia, Hodgkin's disease, lymphosarcoma, melanosarcoma, reticulum cell sarcoma.

PRECAUTIONS

CONTRAINDICATIONS: History of hypersensitivity to asparaginase, pancreatitis. **CAUTIONS:** Existing or recent chickenpox, herpes zoster, diabetes mellitus, gout, infection, hepatic/renal impairment, recent cytotoxic/radiation therapy.

LIFESPAN CONSIDERATIONS:

Pregnancy/Lactation: If possible, avoid use during pregnancy, esp. first trimester. Breast-feeding not recommended. **Pregnancy Category C.** **Children/Elderly:** No age-related precautions noted.

INTERACTIONS

DRUG: Steroids, vincristine may increase hyperglycemia, risk of neuropathy, disturbances of erythropoiesis. May decrease effect of **antigout medications.** May block effects of **methotrexate. Live virus vaccines** may potentiate virus replication, increase vaccine side effects, decrease pt's antibody response to vaccine. **HERBAL:** None significant. **FOOD:** None known. **LAB VALUES:** May increase serum ammonia, BUN, uric acid, glucose, partial thromboplastin time (PTT), platelet count, prothrombin time (PT), thrombin time (TT), AST, ALT, alkaline phosphatase, bilirubin. May decrease blood clotting factors (plasma fibrinogen, antithrombin, plasminogen), serum albumin, calcium, cholesterol.

AVAILABILITY (Rx)

INJECTION, POWDER FOR RECONSTITUTION: 10,000 international units.

ADMINISTRATION/HANDLING

◀ **ALERT** ▶ May be carcinogenic, mutagenic, teratogenic. Handle with extreme care during preparation/administration. Handle voided urine as infectious waste. Powder, solution may irritate skin on contact. Wash area for 15 min if contact occurs.

IV

◀ **ALERT** ▶ Administer intradermal test dose (2 international units) before initiating therapy or when longer than 1 wk has elapsed between doses.

- Observe pt for 1 hr for appearance of wheal or erythema.

Test Solution • Reconstitute 10,000 international units vial with 5 ml Sterile Water for Injection or 0.9% NaCl. • Shake to dissolve.

Reconstitution • Withdraw 0.1 ml, inject into vial containing 9.9 ml same diluent for concentration of 20 international units/ml. • Reconstitute 10,000 international units vial with 5 ml Sterile Water for Injection or 0.9% NaCl to provide a concentration of 2,000 international units/ml. • Shake gently to ensure complete dissolution (vigorous shaking produces foam, some loss of potency).

Rate of administration • For IV injection, administer into tubing of freely running IV solution of D_5W or 0.9% NaCl over at least 30 min. • For IV infusion, further dilute with up to 1,000 ml D_5W or 0.9% NaCl.

Storage • Refrigerate powder for reconstitution. • Reconstituted solution stable for 8 hrs if refrigerated. • Gelatinous fiber-like particles may develop (remove via 5-micron filter during administration).

IM

- Add 2 ml 0.9% NaCl injection to 10,000 international units vial to provide a concentration of 5,000 international units/ml. • Administer no more than 2 ml at any one site.

IV INCOMPATIBILITIES

None known.

INDICATIONS/ROUTES/DOSAGE

ACUTE LYMPHOCYTIC LEUKEMIA

IV: ADULTS, ELDERLY: 200 units/kg/day for 28 days or 5,000–10,000 units/m^2/day for 7 days every 3 wks or 10,000–40,000 units every 2–3 wks. **CHILDREN:** 1,000 units/kg/day for 10 days.

IM: ADULTS, ELDERLY: 6,000–12,000 units/m^2. **CHILDREN:** 6,000 units/m^2 on days 4, 7, 10, 13, 16, 19, 22, 25, 28.

SIDE EFFECTS

FREQUENT: Allergic reaction (rash, urticaria, arthralgia, facial edema, hypotension, respiratory distress) pancreatitis (severe abdominal pain, nausea and vomiting). **OCCASIONAL:** CNS effects (confusion, drowsiness, depression, anxiety, fatigue), stomatitis, hypoalbuminemia or uric acid nephropathy, (manifested as pedal or lower extremity edema), hyperglycemia. **RARE:** Hyperthermia (including fever or chills), thrombosis, seizures.

ADVERSE EFFECTS/ TOXIC REACTIONS

Hepatotoxicity usually occurs within 2 wks of initial treatment. Risk of an allergic reaction, including anaphylaxis, increases after repeated therapy. Myelosuppression may be severe.

NURSING CONSIDERATIONS

BASELINE ASSESSMENT

Before giving medication, agents for adequate airway and allergic reaction (antihistamine, epinephrine, O_2, IV corticosteroid) should be readily available. Assess baseline CNS functions. CBC, comprehensive serum chemistry should be performed before therapy begins and when 1 or more wks have elapsed between doses.

INTERVENTION/EVALUATION

Assess serum amylase concentration frequently during therapy. Discontinue medication at first sign of renal failure (oliguria, anuria), pancreatitis (abdominal pain, nausea, vomiting). Monitor for hematologic toxicity (fever, sore throat, signs of local infection, unusual bruising/bleeding), symptoms of anemia (excessive fatigue, weakness).

PATIENT/FAMILY TEACHING

• Increase fluid intake (protects against renal impairment). • Nausea may decrease during therapy. • Do not have immunizations without physician's approval (drug lowers body's resistance). • Avoid contact with those who have recently taken a live virus vaccine.

aspirin (acetylsalicylic acid, ASA)

ass-purr-in

(Asaphen E.C. ♣, Bayer, Bufferin, Ecotrin, Entrophen ♣, Halfprin, Novasen ♣, ZORprin)

Do not confuse aspirin or Ascriptin with Aricept, Afrin, or Asendin, or Ecotrin with Edecrin.

FIXED-COMBINATION(S)

Aggrenox: aspirin/dipyridamole (an antiplatelet agent): 25 mg/200 mg. **Fiorinal:** aspirin/butalbital/caffeine (a barbiturate): 325 mg/50 mg/40 mg. **Lortab/ASA:** aspirin/hydrocodone (an analgesic): 325 mg/5 mg. **Percodan:** aspirin/oxycodone (an analgesic): 325 mg/4.5 mg; 325 mg/2.25 mg. **Pravigard:** aspirin/pravastatin (a cholesterol lowering agent): 81 mg/20 mg, 81 mg/40 mg, 81 mg/80 mg, 325 mg/20 mg, 325 mg/40 mg, 325 mg/80 mg.

CLASSIFICATION

PHARMACOTHERAPEUTIC: Nonsteroidal salicylate. **CLINICAL:** Anti-inflammatory, antipyretic, anticoagulant (see pp. 31C, 123C).

ACTION

Inhibits prostaglandin synthesis, acts on the hypothalamus heat-regulating center, interferes with production of thromboxane A, a substance that stimulates platelet aggregation. **Therapeutic Effect:** Reduces inflammatory response, intensity of pain; decreases fever; inhibits platelet aggregation.

PHARMACOKINETICS

Route	Onset	Peak	Duration
PO	1 hr	2–4 hrs	4–6 hrs

Rapidly and completely absorbed from GI tract; enteric-coated absorption delayed; rectal absorption delayed and incomplete. Protein binding: High. Widely distributed. Rapidly hydrolyzed to salicylate. **Half-life:** 15–20 min (aspirin); 2–3 hrs (salicylate at low dose); more than 20 hrs (salicylate at high dose).

USES

Treatment of mild to moderate pain, fever. Reduces inflammation including rheumatoid arthritis, juvenile arthritis, osteoarthritis, rheumatic fever. As platelet aggregation inhibitor in the prevention of transient ischemic attacks (TIAs), cerebral thromboembolism, MI or reinfarction. **OFF-LABEL:** Acute ischemic stroke, complications of pregnancy (prophylaxis), MI (prophylaxis), prevention of thromboembolism, rheumatic fever, treatment of Kawasaki's disease.

PRECAUTIONS

CONTRAINDICATIONS: Allergy to tartrazine dye, bleeding disorders, chickenpox or flu in children and teenagers, GI bleeding or ulceration, hepatic impairment, history of hypersensitivity to aspirin or NSAIDs. **CAUTIONS:** Vitamin K deficiency, chronic renal insufficiency, those with "aspirin triad" (rhinitis, nasal polyps, asthma).

LIFESPAN CONSIDERATIONS:

Pregnancy/Lactation: Readily crosses placenta; distributed in breast milk. May prolong gestation and labor; decrease fetal birth weight; increase incidence of stillbirths, neonatal mortality, hemorrhage. Avoid use during last trimester (may adversely affect fetal cardiovascular system: premature closure of ductus arteriosus). **Pregnancy Category C (D if full dose used in third trimester of pregnancy).** **Children:** Caution in children with acute febrile illness (Reye's syndrome). **Elderly:** May be more susceptible to toxicity; lower dosages recommended.

INTERACTIONS

DRUG: **Alcohol, NSAIDs** may increase risk of GI effects (e.g., ulceration). **Urinary alkalinizers, antacids** increase excretion. **Anticoagulants, heparin, thrombolytics** increase risk of bleeding. Large dose may increase effect of **insulin, oral hypoglycemics. Valproic acid, platelet aggregation inhibitors** may increase risk of bleeding. May increase toxicity of **methotrexate, zidovudine. Ototoxic medications, vancomycin** may increase ototoxicity. May decrease effect of **probenecid, sulfinpyrazone.** **HERBAL:** Avoid **cat's claw, dong quai, evening primrose, feverfew, garlic, ginger, ginkgo, red clover, horse chestnut, green tea, ginseng** (possess anti-platelet activity). **FOOD:** None known. **LAB VALUES:** May alter serum AST, ALT, alkaline phosphatase, uric acid; prolongs prothrombin time, bleeding time. May decrease serum cholesterol, potassium, T_3, T_4.

AVAILABILITY (OTC)

CAPLETS (BAYER): 81 mg, 325 mg, 500 mg. **GELCAPS (BAYER):** 325 mg, 500 mg. **SUPPOSITORIES:** 300 mg, 600 mg. **TABLETS:** 162 mg (Halfprin), 325 mg (Bayer), 500 mg (Bayer). **TABLETS (CHEWABLE [BAYER, ST. JOSEPH]):** 81 mg.

TABLETS (ENTERIC-COATED [BAYER, ECOTRIN, ST. JOSEPH]): 81 mg, 325 mg, 500 mg, 650 mg.

ADMINISTRATION/HANDLING

PO

• Do not crush or break enteric-coated tablet. • May give with water, milk, meals if GI distress occurs.

RECTAL

• Refrigerate suppositories. • If suppository is too soft, chill for 30 min in refrigerator or run cold water over foil wrapper. • Moisten suppository with cold water before inserting well into rectum.

INDICATIONS/ROUTES/DOSAGE

ANALGESIA, FEVER

PO, RECTAL: ADULTS, ELDERLY: 325–1,000 mg q4–6h. **CHILDREN:** 10–15 mg/kg/dose q4–6h. **Maximum:** 4 g/day.

ANTI-INFLAMMATORY

PO: ADULTS, ELDERLY: Initially, 2.4–3.6 g/day in divided doses; then 3.6–5.4 g/day. **CHILDREN:** Initially, 60–90 mg/kg/day in divided doses; then 80–100 mg/kg/day.

PLATELET AGGREGATION INHIBITOR

PO: ADULTS, ELDERLY: 80–325 mg/day.

KAWASAKI'S DISEASE

PO: CHILDREN: 80–100 mg/kg/day in divided doses, After fever resolves, 3–5 mg/kg once daily.

SIDE EFFECTS

OCCASIONAL: GI distress (including abdominal distention, cramping, heartburn, mild nausea); allergic reaction (including bronchospasm, pruritus, and urticaria).

ADVERSE EFFECTS/ TOXIC REACTIONS

High doses of aspirin may produce GI bleeding and/or gastric mucosal lesions. Dehydrated, febrile children may experience aspirin toxicity quickly. Reye's syndrome may occur in children with chickenpox or flu. Low-grade toxicity characterized by tinnitus, generalized pruritus (may be severe), headache, dizziness, flushing, tachycardia, hyperventilation, diaphoresis, thirst. Marked toxicity characterized by hyperthermia, restlessness, seizures, abnormal breathing patterns, respiratory failure, coma.

NURSING CONSIDERATIONS

BASELINE ASSESSMENT

Do not give to children or teenagers who have flu or chickenpox (increases risk of Reye's syndrome). Do not use if vinegar-like odor is noted (indicates chemical breakdown). Assess type, location, duration of pain, inflammation. Inspect appearance of affected joints for immobility, deformities, skin condition. Therapeutic serum level for anti-arthritic effect: 20–30 mg/dl (toxicity occurs if levels are greater than 30 mg/dl).

INTERVENTION/EVALUATION

Monitor urinary pH (sudden acidification, pH from 6.5 to 5.5, may result in toxicity). Assess skin for evidence of ecchymosis. If given as antipyretic, assess temperature directly before and 1 hr after giving medication. Evaluate for therapeutic response: relief of pain, stiffness, swelling; increase in joint mobility; reduced joint tenderness; improved grip strength.

PATIENT/FAMILY TEACHING

• Do not crush or chew enteric-coated tablets. • Report tinnitus or persistent abdominal GI pain. • Therapeutic anti-inflammatory effect noted in 1–3 wks. • Behavioral changes, vomiting may be early signs of Reye's syndrome. Contact physician.

Astelin, *see azelastine*

Atacand, *see candesartan*

atazanavir

ah-tah-**zan**-ah-veer

(Reyataz)

Do not confuse Reyataz with Retavase.

CLASSIFICATION

PHARMACOTHERAPEUTIC: Antiretroviral. **CLINICAL:** Protease inhibitor.

ACTION

Acts as an HIV-1 protease inhibitor, selectively preventing the processing of viral precursors found in cells infected with HIV-1. **Therapeutic Effect:** Prevents formation of mature HIV viral cells.

PHARMACOKINETICS

Rapidly absorbed after PO administration. Protein binding: 86%. Extensively metabolized in the liver. Excreted primarily in urine and, to a lesser extent, in feces. **Half-life:** 5–8 hrs.

USES

Treatment of HIV-1 infection in combination with other antiretroviral agents.

PRECAUTIONS

CONTRAINDICATIONS: Concurrent use with ergot derivatives, midazolam, pimozide, triazolam; severe hepatic insufficiency. **EXTREME CAUTION:** Hepatic impairment. **CAUTIONS:** Preexisting conduction system disease (first-degree AV block or second- or third-degree AV block), diabetes mellitus, elderly, renal impairment.

LIFESPAN CONSIDERATIONS:

Pregnancy/Lactation: Unknown if drug crosses placenta or distributed in breast milk. Lactic acidosis syndrome, hyperbilirubinemia, kernicterus have been reported. **Pregnancy Category B.** **Children:** Safety and efficacy not established in those younger than 3 mos. **Elderly:** Age-related hepatic impairment may require dose reduction.

INTERACTIONS

DRUG: May increase concentration, toxicity of **amiodarone, bepridil, lidocaine, atorvastatin, clarithromycin, cyclosporine, sirolimus, tacrolimus, diltiazem, felodipine, nicardipine, nifedfipine, verapamil, lovastatin, simvastatin, sildenafil, tadalafil, vardenafil, tricyclic antidepressants, warfarin.** **H_2-receptor antagonists, proton pump inhibitors, rifampin** decrease atazanavir concentration, effect. **Ritonavir, voriconazole** increase concentration. **HERBAL:** **St. John's wort** may decrease concentration. **FOOD:** **High-fat meals** may decrease absorption. **LAB VALUES:** May increase serum bilirubin, AST, ALT, amylase, lipase. May decrease Hgb, neutrophil count, platelets. May alter serum LDL cholesterol, triglycerides.

AVAILABILITY (Rx)

CAPSULES: 100 mg, 150 mg, 200 mg, 300 mg.

ADMINISTRATION/HANDLING

PO

- Give with food.

INDICATIONS/ROUTES/DOSAGE

HIV-1 INFECTION

PO: ADULTS, ELDERLY (ANTIRETROVIRAL-NAIVE): 400 mg (2 capsules) once a day with food. **ADULTS, ELDERLY (ANTIRETROVIRAL-EXPERIENCED):** 300 mg and ritonavir (Norvir) 100 mg once a day.

HIV-1 INFECTION (CONCURRENT THERAPY WITH EFAVIRENZ)

PO: ADULTS, ELDERLY: 300 mg atazanavir, 100 mg ritonavir, and 600 mg efavirenz as a single daily dose with food.

HIV-1 INFECTION (CONCURRENT THERAPY WITH DIDANOSINE)

PO: ADULTS, ELDERLY: Give atazanavir with food 2 hrs before or 1 hr after didanosine.

HIV-1 INFECTION (CONCURRENT THERAPY WITH TENOFOVIR)

PO: ADULTS, ELDERLY: 300 mg atazanavir and 100 mg ritonavir and 300 mg tenofovir given as a single daily dose with food.

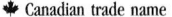

HIV-1 INFECTION IN PTS WITH MILD TO MODERATE HEPATIC IMPAIRMENT

◀ **ALERT** ▶ Avoid use in pts with severe hepatic impairment.

PO: ADULTS, ELDERLY: 300 mg once a day with food.

SIDE EFFECTS

FREQUENT (16%–14%): Nausea, headache. **OCCASIONAL (9%–4%):** Rash, vomiting, depression, diarrhea, abdominal pain, fever. **RARE (3% or less):** Dizziness, insomnia, cough, fatigue, back pain.

ADVERSE EFFECTS/ TOXIC REACTIONS

Severe hypersensitivity reaction (angioedema, chest pain), jaundice may occur.

NURSING CONSIDERATIONS

BASELINE ASSESSMENT

Obtain baseline laboratory tests, CBC, hepatic function tests, before beginning therapy and at periodic intervals during therapy. Offer emotional support.

INTERVENTION/EVALUATION

Assess for nausea, vomiting; assess eating pattern. Determine daily pattern of bowel activity/stool consistency. Assess skin for rash. Question for evidence of headache. Monitor for onset of depression.

PATIENT/FAMILY TEACHING

- Take with food.
- Small, frequent meals may offset nausea, vomiting.
- Atazanavir is not a cure for HIV infection, nor does it reduce risk of transmission to others.

atenolol

ay-**ten**-oh-lol
(Apo-Atenol ✱, Novo-Atenol ✱, Tenolin ✱, Tenormin)

Do not confuse atenolol with albuterol or timolol.

FIXED-COMBINATION(S)

Tenoretic: atenolol/chlorthalidone (a diuretic): 50 mg/25 mg; 100 mg/25 mg.

CLASSIFICATION

PHARMACOTHERAPEUTIC: $Beta_1$-adrenergic blocker. **CLINICAL:** Antihypertensive, antianginal, antiarrhythmic (see p. 67C).

ACTION

Blocks $beta_1$-adrenergic receptors in cardiac tissue. **Therapeutic Effect:** Slows sinus node heart rate, decreasing cardiac output, B/P. Decreases myocardial oxygen demand.

PHARMACOKINETICS

Route	Onset	Peak	Duration
PO	1 hr	2–4 hrs	24 hrs

Incompletely absorbed from GI tract. Protein binding: 6%–16%. Minimal liver metabolism. Primarily excreted unchanged in urine. Removed by hemodialysis. **Half-life:** 6–7 hrs (increased in renal impairment).

USES

Treatment of hypertension, alone or in combination with other agents; management of angina pectoris; reduces cardiovascular mortality in those with definite or suspected acute MI. **OFF-LABEL:** Acute alcohol withdrawal, arrhythmia (esp. supraventricular and ventricular tachycardia), improved survival in diabetics with heart disease, mild to moderately severe CHF (adjunct); prevention of migraine, thyrotoxicosis, tremors; treatment of hypertrophic cardiomyopathy, pheochromocytoma, syndrome of mitral valve prolapse.

PRECAUTIONS

CONTRAINDICATIONS: Cardiogenic shock, overt heart failure, second- or third-degree heart block, severe bradycardia. **CAUTIONS:** Renal/hepatic impairment, peripheral vascular disease, hyperthyroidism, diabetes, inadequate cardiac function, bronchospastic disease.

LIFESPAN CONSIDERATIONS:

Pregnancy/Lactation: Readily crosses placenta; distributed in breast milk. Avoid use during first trimester. May produce bradycardia, apnea, hypoglycemia, hypothermia during delivery; low birth-weight infants. **Pregnancy Category D.** **Children:** No age-related precautions noted. **Elderly:** Age-related peripheral vascular disease, renal impairment require caution.

INTERACTIONS

DRUG: **Diuretics, other hypotensives** may increase hypotensive effects. **Sympathomimetics, xanthines** may mutually inhibit effects. May mask symptoms of hypoglycemia, prolong hypoglycemic effect of **insulin, oral hypoglycemics. NSAIDs** may decrease antihypertensive effect. **Cimetidine** may increase concentration. **HERBAL:** **Ephedra, yohimbe, ginseng** may worsen hypertension. **Garlic** may increase antihypertensive effect. **FOOD:** None known. **LAB VALUES:** May increase serum ANA titer and BUN, serum creatinine, potassium, uric acid, lipoprotein, triglycerides.

AVAILABILITY (Rx)

INJECTION SOLUTION: 5 mg/10 ml. **TABLETS:** 25 mg, 50 mg, 100 mg.

ADMINISTRATION/HANDLING

IV

Reconstitution • May give undiluted or dilute in 10–50 ml 0.9% NaCl or D_5W.

Rate of administration • Give IV push over 5 min. • Give IV infusion over 15 min.

Storage • Store at room temperature. • After reconstitution, parenteral form is stable for 48 hrs at room temperature.

PO

• Give without regard to food. • Tablets may be crushed.

IV INCOMPATIBILITIES

Amphotericin complex (Abelcet, AmBisome, Amphotec).

INDICATIONS/ROUTES/DOSAGE

HYPERTENSION

PO: **ADULTS:** Initially, 25–50 mg once a day. May increase dose up to 100 mg once a day. **ELDERLY:** Usual initial dose, 25 mg/day. **CHILDREN:** Initially, 0.8–1 mg/kg/dose given once a day. Range: 0.8–1.5 mg/kg/day. **Maximum:** 2 mg/kg/day or 100 mg/day.

IV: **ADULTS, ELDERLY:** 1.25–5 mg of 6–12h.

ANGINA PECTORIS

PO: **ADULTS:** Initially, 50 mg once a day. May increase dose up to 200 mg once a day. **ELDERLY:** Usual initial dose, 25 mg/day.

ACUTE MI

IV: **ADULTS:** Give 5 mg over 5 min; may repeat in 10 min. In those who tolerate full 10-mg IV dose, begin 50-mg tablets 10 min after last IV dose followed by another 50-mg oral dose 12 hrs later. Thereafter, give 100 mg once a day or 50 mg twice a day for 6–9 days. Or, for those who do not tolerate full IV dose, give 50 mg orally twice a day or 100 mg once a day for at least 7 days.

DOSAGE IN RENAL IMPAIRMENT

Dosage interval is modified based on creatinine clearance.

Creatinine Clearance	Dosage Interval
15–35 ml/min	50 mg a day
Less than 15 ml/min	50 mg every other day

SIDE EFFECTS

Atenolol is generally well tolerated, with mild and transient side effects. **FREQUENT:** Hypotension manifested as cold extremities, constipation or diarrhea, diaphoresis, dizziness, fatigue, headache, nausea. **OCCASIONAL:** Insomnia, flatulence, urinary frequency, impotence or decreased libido, depression. **RARE:** Rash, arthralgia, myalgia, confusion (esp. in the elderly), altered taste.

ADVERSE EFFECTS/ TOXIC REACTIONS

Overdose may produce profound bradycardia, hypotension. Abrupt withdrawal may result in diaphoresis, palpitations, headache, tremors. May precipitate CHF, MI in pts with cardiac disease; thyroid storm in those with thyrotoxicosis; peripheral ischemia in those with existing peripheral vascular disease. Hypoglycemia may occur in previously controlled diabetes. Thrombocytopenia (unusual bruising, bleeding) occurs rarely.

NURSING CONSIDERATIONS

BASELINE ASSESSMENT

Assess B/P, apical pulse immediately before drug is administered (if pulse is 60/min or less, or systolic B/P is less than 90 mm Hg, withhold medication, contact physician). **Antianginal:** Record onset, quality (sharp, dull, squeezing), radiation, location, intensity, duration of anginal pain, precipitating factors (exertion, emotional stress). Assess baseline renal/hepatic function tests.

INTERVENTION/EVALUATION

Monitor B/P for hypotension, pulse for bradycardia, respiration for difficulty in breathing. Monitor daily pattern of bowel activity/stool consistency. Assess for evidence of CHF: dyspnea (particularly on exertion or lying down), night cough, peripheral edema, distended neck veins. Monitor I&O (increased weight, decreased urinary output may indicate CHF). Assess extremities for coldness. Assist with ambulation if dizziness occurs.

PATIENT/FAMILY TEACHING

• Do not abruptly discontinue medication. • Compliance with therapy essential to control hypertension, angina. • To reduce hypotensive effect, rise slowly from lying to sitting position and permit legs to dangle from bed momentarily before standing. • Avoid tasks that require alertness, motor skills until drug reaction is established. • Report dizziness, depression, confusion, rash, unusual bruising/bleeding. • Outpatients should monitor B/P, pulse before taking medication (teach correct technique). • Restrict salt, alcohol intake. • Therapeutic antihypertensive effect noted in 1–2 wks.

Ativan, *see lorazepam*

atomoxetine

ah-toe-**mocks**-eh-teen

(Strattera)

◆ CLASSIFICATION

PHARMACOTHERAPEUTIC: Norepinephrine reuptake inhibitor. **CLINICAL:** Psychotherapeutic agent.

ACTION

Enhances noradrenergic function by selective inhibition of the presynaptic norepinephrine transporter. **Therapeutic Effect:** Improves symptoms of attention-deficit hyperactivity disorder (ADHD).

PHARMACOKINETICS

Rapidly absorbed after PO administration. Protein binding: 98% (primarily to albumin). Eliminated primarily in urine and, to a lesser extent, in feces. Not removed by hemodialysis. **Half-life:** 4–5 hrs in general population, 22 hrs in 7% of Caucasians and 2% of African-Americans; (increased in moderate to severe hepatic insufficiency).

USES

Treatment of ADHD. **OFF-LABEL:** Treatment of depression.

PRECAUTIONS

CONTRAINDICATIONS: Angle-closure glaucoma, use within 14 days of MAOIs. **CAUTIONS:** Hypertension; tachycardia; cardiovascular disease; pts at risk for urinary retention, moderate or severe hepatic impairment.

⌛ LIFESPAN CONSIDERATIONS:

Pregnancy/Lactation: Unknown if excreted in breast milk. **Pregnancy Category C. Children:** Safety and efficacy in pts younger than 6 yrs have not been established. May produce suicidal thoughts in children and adolescents. **Elderly:** Age-related hepatic/renal impairment, cardiovascular or cerebrovascular disease may increase risk of effects.

INTERACTIONS

DRUG: MAOIs may increase toxic effects. **Paroxetine, fluoxetine, quinidine** may increase concentrations. Avoid concurrent use of **medications that can increase heart rate or B/P.** **HERBAL:** None significant. **FOOD:** None known. **LAB VALUES:** None known.

AVAILABILITY (Rx)

CAPSULES: 10 mg, 18 mg, 25 mg, 40 mg, 60 mg, 80 mg, 100 mg.

ADMINISTRATION/HANDLING

PO

- Give without regard to food.

INDICATIONS/ROUTES/DOSAGE

ADHD

PO: ADULTS, CHILDREN WEIGHING 70 KG AND MORE: 40 mg once a day. May increase after at least 3 days to 80 mg as a single daily dose or in divided doses. **Maximum:** 100 mg. **CHILDREN WEIGHING LESS THAN 70 KG:** Initially, 0.5 mg/kg/day. May increase after at least 3 days to 1.2 mg/kg/day. **Maximum:** 1.4 mg/kg/day or 100 mg.

DOSAGE IN HEPATIC IMPAIRMENT

Expect to administer 50% of normal atomoxetine dosage to pts with moderate hepatic impairment and 25% of normal dosage to those with severe hepatic impairment.

SIDE EFFECTS

FREQUENT: Headache, dyspepsia, nausea, vomiting, fatigue, decreased appetite, dizziness, altered mood. **OCCASIONAL:** Tachycardia, hypertension, weight loss, delayed growth in children, irritability. **RARE:** Insomnia, sexual dysfunction in adults, fever.

ADVERSE EFFECTS/ TOXIC REACTIONS

Urinary retention, urinary hesitancy may occur. In overdose, gastric lavage, activated charcoal may prevent systemic absorption. Severe hepatic injury occurs rarely.

NURSING CONSIDERATIONS

BASELINE ASSESSMENT

Assess pulse, B/P before therapy, following dose increases, and periodically while on therapy.

INTERVENTION/EVALUATION

Monitor urinary output; complaints of urinary retention/hesitancy may be a related adverse reaction. Assist with ambulation if dizziness occurs. Be alert to mood changes. Monitor fluid and electrolyte status in those with significant vomiting.

PATIENT/FAMILY TEACHING

• Avoid tasks that require alertness, motor skills until response to drug is established. • Take last dose early in evening to avoid insomnia. • Report palpitations, fever, vomiting, irritability.

atorvastatin

ah-tore-**vah**-stah-tin

(Lipitor)

Do not confuse Lipitor with Levatol.

FIXED-COMBINATION(S)

Caduet: atorvastatin/amlodipine (calcium channel blocker): 10 mg/2.5 mg, 10 mg/5 mg, 10 mg/10 mg, 20 mg/2.5 mg, 20 mg/5 mg, 20 mg/10 mg, 40 mg/2.5 mg, 40 mg/5 mg, 40 mg/10 mg, 80 mg/5 mg, 80 mg/10 mg.

CLASSIFICATION

PHARMACOTHERAPEUTIC: Hydroxymethylglutaryl CoA (HMG-CoA) reductase inhibitor. **CLINICAL:** Antihyperlipidemic (see p. 56C).

ACTION

Inhibits HMG-CoA reductase, the enzyme that catalyzes the early step in cholesterol synthesis. **Therapeutic Effect:** Decreases LDL and VLDL cholesterol, plasma triglyceride levels; increases HDL cholesterol concentration.

PHARMACOKINETICS

Poorly absorbed from GI tract. Protein binding: greater than 98%. Metabolized in the liver. Minimally eliminated in urine. Plasma levels markedly increased in chronic alcoholic hepatic disease but unaffected by renal disease. **Half-life:** 14 hrs.

USES

Primary prevention of cardiovascular disease in high-risk pts. Reduces risk of stroke and heart attack in pts with type 2 diabetes without evidence of heart disease but other risk factors. Reduces risk of stroke without evidence of heart disease but with multiple risk factors other than diabetes. Adjunct to diet therapy in management of hyperlipidemias (reduces elevations in total cholesterol, LDL-C, apolipoprotein B triglycerides in pts with primary hypercholesterolemia), homozygous familial hypercholesterolemia, heterozygous familial hypercholesterolemia in pts 10–17 yrs of age, females more than 1 yr postmenarche). **OFF-LABEL:** Secondary prevention of ischemia in pts with CHF.

PRECAUTIONS

CONTRAINDICATIONS: Active hepatic disease, lactation, pregnancy, unexplained elevated hepatic function test results. **CAUTIONS:** Anticoagulant therapy, history of hepatic disease, substantial alcohol consumption, major surgery, severe acute infection, trauma, hypotension, severe metabolic, endocrine, electrolyte disorders, uncontrolled seizures.

LIFESPAN CONSIDERATIONS:

Pregnancy/Lactation: Distributed in breast milk. Contraindicated during pregnancy. May produce skeletal malformation. **Pregnancy Category X. Children:** Safety and efficacy not established. **Elderly:** No age-related precautions noted.

INTERACTIONS

DRUG: **Antacids, colestipol, propranolol** decrease atorvastatin activity. **Warfarin, digoxin, oral contraceptives, itraconazole** may increase concentration, producing severe muscle pain, inflammation, weakness. Increased risk of rhabdomyolysis, acute renal failure with **cyclosporine, erythromycin, gemfibrozil, nicotinic acid**. **HERBAL:** **St. John's wort** may decrease levels. **FOOD:** May be given without regard to meals. **Grapefruit, grapefruit juice** may increase serum concentrations. **LAB VALUES:** May increase creatinine kinase, serum transaminase concentrations.

AVAILABILITY (Rx)

TABLETS: 10 mg, 20 mg, 40 mg, 80 mg.

ADMINISTRATION/HANDLING

PO

- Give without regard to food.
- Do not break film-coated tablets.

INDICATIONS/ROUTES/DOSAGE

PREVENTION OF CARDIOVASCULAR DISEASE (CVD)

PO: ADULTS, ELDERLY: 10 mg once daily.

HYPERLIPIDEMIAS

PO: ADULTS, ELDERLY: Initially, 10–20 mg/day (40 mg in pts requiring greater than 45% reduction in LDL-C). Range: 10–80 mg/day.

HETEROZYGOUS HYPERCHOLESTEROLEMIA

PO: CHILDREN 10–17 YRS: Initially, 10 mg/day. **Maximum:** 20 mg/day.

SIDE EFFECTS

COMMON: Atorvastatin is generally well tolerated. Side effects are usually mild and transient. **FREQUENT (16%):** Headache. **OCCASIONAL (5%–2%):** Myalgia, rash, pruritus, allergy. **RARE (less than 2%–1%):** Flatulence, dyspepsia.

ADVERSE EFFECTS/ TOXIC REACTIONS

Potential for cataracts, photosensitivity.

NURSING CONSIDERATIONS

BASELINE ASSESSMENT

Question for possibility of pregnancy before initiating therapy (Pregnancy Category X). Assess baseline lab results: cholesterol, triglycerides, hepatic function tests.

INTERVENTION/EVALUATION

Monitor for headache. Assess for rash, pruritus, malaise. Monitor cholesterol, triglyceride lab values for therapeutic response.

PATIENT/FAMILY TEACHING

• Follow special diet (important part of treatment). • Periodic lab tests are essential part of therapy. • Do not take other medications without consulting physician.

atovaquone

a-**toe**-va-kwone

(Mepron)

CLASSIFICATION

PHARMACOTHERAPEUTIC: Systemic anti-infective. **CLINICAL:** Antiprotozoal.

ACTION

Inhibits mitochondrial electron-transport system at the cytochrome bc1 complex (Complex III) interrupting nucleic acid, adenosine triphosphate synthesis. **Therapeutic Effect:** Antiprotozoal, antipneumocystic activity.

USES

Treatment or prevention of mild to moderate *Pneumocystis carinii* pneumonia (PCP) in those intolerant to trimethoprim-sulfamethoxazole (TMP-SMZ).

PRECAUTIONS

CONTRAINDICATIONS: Development or history of potentially life-threatening allergic reaction to the drug. **CAUTIONS:** Elderly, pts with severe PCP, chronic diarrhea, malabsorption syndromes. **Pregnancy Category C.**

INTERACTIONS

DRUG: **Rifampin, rifabutin, tetracycline** may decrease concentration. Atovaquone may increase **rifampin** concentration. **Metoclopramide** decreases bioavailability. **HERBAL:** None significant. **FOOD:** **High-fat meals** increase absorption. **LAB VALUES:** May elevate serum AST, ALT, alkaline phosphatase, amylase. May decrease serum sodium.

AVAILABILITY (Rx)

SUSPENSION, ORAL: 750 mg/5 ml.

INDICATIONS/ROUTES/DOSAGE

***PNEUMOCYSTIS CARINII* PNEUMONIA (PCP)**

PO: **ADULTS, CHILDREN OLDER THAN 12 YRS:** 750 mg twice a day with food for 21 days. **CHILDREN 12 YRS AND YOUNGER:** 40 mg/kg/day in 2 divided doses. **Maximum:** 1,500 mg/day.

PREVENTION OF PCP

PO: **ADULTS:** 1,500 mg once a day with food. **CHILDREN 4–24 MOS:** 45 mg/kg/day as single dose. **Maximum:** 1,500 mg/day. **CHILDREN 1–3 MOS AND OLDER THAN 24 MOS:** 30 mg/kg/day as single dose. **Maximum:** 1,500 mg/day.

SIDE EFFECTS

FREQUENT (greater than 10%): Rash, nausea, diarrhea, headache, vomiting, fever, insomnia, cough. **OCCASIONAL (less than 10%):** Abdominal discomfort, thrush, asthenia, anemia, neutropenia.

ADVERSE EFFECTS/ TOXIC REACTIONS

None known.

NURSING CONSIDERATIONS

INTERVENTION/EVALUATION

Assess for GI discomfort, nausea, vomiting. Check consistency and frequency of stools. Assess skin for rash. Monitor I&O, renal function tests, Hgb. Monitor elderly closely for decreased hepatic, renal, cardiac function.

PATIENT/FAMILY TEACHING

• Continue therapy for full length of treatment. • Do not take any other medications unless approved by physician. • Notify physician of rash, diarrhea, or other new symptoms.

atracurium

(Tracrium)

See Neuromuscular blockers (p. 119C)

atropine

ah-trow-peen

(AtroPen Auto Injector, Atropine-Care, Isopto Atropine, Sal-Tropine)

FIXED-COMBINATION(S)

Donnatal: atropine/hyoscyamine (anticholinergic)/phenobarbital (sedative)/scopolamine (anticholinergic): 0.0194 mg/0.1037 mg/16.2 mg/0.0065 mg. **Lomotil:** atropine/diphenoxylate: 0.025 mg/2.5 mg.

CLASSIFICATION

PHARMACOTHERAPEUTIC: Acetylcholine antagonist. **CLINICAL:** Antiarrhythmic, antispasmodic, antidote, cycloplegic, antisecretory, anticholinergic.

ACTION

Competes with acetylcholine for common binding sites on muscarinic receptors located on exocrine glands, cardiac, smooth-muscle ganglia, intramural neurons. **Therapeutic Effect:** Decreases GI motility and secretory activity, GU muscle tone (ureter, bladder); produces ophthalmic cycloplegia, mydriasis.

PHARMACOKINETICS

AtroPen auto injector: Rapidly and well absorbed after IM administration. Much of the drug is destroyed by enzymatic hydrolysis, particularly in the liver. Partially excreted unchanged in urine.

USES

Injection: Preoperative to inhibit salivation/secretions; treatment of symptomatic sinus bradycardia; AV block; ventricular asystole; antidote for organophosphate pesticide poisoning. **Ophthalmic:** Produce mydriasis and cycloplegia for examination of retina and optic disc; uveitis. **OFF-LABEL:** Malignant glaucoma.

PRECAUTIONS

CONTRAINDICATIONS: Bladder neck obstruction due to prostatic hypertrophy, cardiospasm, intestinal atony, myasthenia gravis in those not treated with neostigmine, narrow-angle glaucoma, obstructive disease of GI tract, paralytic ileus, severe ulcerative colitis, tachycardia secondary to cardiac insufficiency or thyrotoxicosis, toxic megacolon, unstable cardiovascular status in acute hemorrhage. **EXTREME CAUTION:** Autonomic neuropathy, known or suspected GI infections, diarrhea, mild to moderate ulcerative colitis. **CAUTIONS:** Hyperthyroidism, hepatic/renal disease, hypertension, tachyarrhythmias, CHF, coronary artery disease, gastric ulcer, esophageal reflux or hiatal hernia associated with reflux esophagitis, infants, elderly, systemic administration in those with chronic obstructive pulmonary disease (COPD). **Ophthalmic:** Spastic paralysis, brain damage, Down syndrome.

LIFESPAN CONSIDERATIONS:

Pregnancy/Lactation: Crosses placenta; distributed in breast milk. **Pregnancy Category C.** **Children/Elderly:** Increased susceptibility to atropine effects.

INTERACTIONS

DRUG: **Anticholinergics** may increase effects. **HERBAL:** None significant. **FOOD:** None known. **LAB VALUES:** None known.

AVAILABILITY (Rx)

INJECTION, SOLUTION: 0.05 mg/ml, 0.1 mg/ml, 0.4 mg/ml, 0.5 mg/ml. **INJECTION (ATROPEN):** 0.5 mg/0.7 ml, 1 mg/0.7 ml, 2 mg/0.7 ml. **OPHTHALMIC OINTMENT:** 1%. **OPHTHALMIC SOLUTION:** 1%.

ADMINISTRATION/HANDLING

IV

• Must be given rapidly (prevents paradoxical slowing of heart rate).

IM

• May be given subcutaneously or IM.

A

IM, Atro-Pen

• Store at room temperature. • Give as soon as symptoms of organophosphorous or carbamate poisoning appear. • Do not use more than three AtroPen auto injectors for each person at risk for nerve agent or organophosphate insecticide poisoning.

OPHTHALMIC

• Place gloved finger on lower eyelid and pull out until a pocket is formed between eye and lower lid. • Hold dropper above pocket and place prescribed number of drops or 1/4–1/2 inch of ointment into pocket. • Instruct pt to close eye gently (so medication will not be squeezed out of the sac). • For solution, apply digital pressure to lacrimal sac at inner canthus for 1 min to minimize systemic absorption. • For ointment, instruct pt to roll the eyeball to increase contact area of drug to the eye.

IV INCOMPATIBILITY

Pentothal (Thiopental).

IV COMPATIBILITIES

Diphenhydramine (Benadryl), droperidol (Inapsine), fentanyl (Sublimaze), glycopyrrolate (Robinul), heparin, hydromorphone (Dilaudid), midazolam (Versed), morphine, potassium chloride, propofol (Diprivan).

INDICATIONS/ROUTES/DOSAGE

ASYSTOLE, SLOW PULSELESS ELECTRICAL ACTIVITY

IV: ADULTS, ELDERLY: 1 mg; may repeat q3–5min up to total dose of 0.04 mg/kg.

PRE-ANESTHETIC

IV, IM, SUBCUTANEOUS: ADULTS, ELDERLY: 0.4–0.6 mg 30–60 min preop. **CHILDREN WEIGHING 5 KG AND MORE:** 0.01–0.02 mg/kg/dose to maximum of 0.4 mg/dose. **CHILDREN WEIGHING LESS THAN 5 KG:** 0.02 mg/kg/dose 30–60 min preop.

BRADYCARDIA

IV: ADULTS, ELDERLY: 0.5–1 mg q5min not to exceed 2 mg or 0.04 mg/kg. **CHILDREN:** 0.02 mg/kg with a minimum of 0.1 mg to a maximum of 0.5 mg in children and 1 mg in adolescents. May repeat in 5 min. **Maximum total dose:** 1 mg in children, 2 mg in adolescents.

CYCLOPLEGIC REFRACTION, POSTOPERATIVE MYDRIASIS, UVEITIS

OPHTHALMIC SOLUTION: ADULTS, ELDERLY: Instill 1 drop in affected eye(s) up to 4 times a day.

OPHTHALMIC OINTMENT: ADULTS, ELDERLY: Apply ointment several hours prior to examination when used for refraction.

POISONING BY SUSCEPTIBLE ORGANOPHOSPHOROUS NERVE AGENTS HAVING CHOLINESTERASE ACTIVITY, ORGANOPHOSPHOROUS OR CARBAMATE INSECTICIDES

IM: ADULTS, CHILDREN WEIGHING MORE THAN 90 LB: AtroPen 2 mg (green). **CHILDREN WEIGHING 40–90 LB:** AtroPen 1 mg (dark red). **CHILDREN WEIGHING 15–39 LB:** AtroPen 0.5 mg (blue). **INFANTS WEIGHING LESS THAN 15 LB:** AtroPen 0.25 mg (yellow).

SIDE EFFECTS

FREQUENT: Dry mouth, nose, throat that may be severe; decreased diaphoresis, constipation, irritation at subcutaneous or IM injection site. **OCCASIONAL:** Dyphagia, blurred vision, bloated feeling, impotence, urinary hesitancy. **Ophthalmic:** Mydriasis, blurred vision, photophobia, decreased visual acuity, tearing, dry eyes or dry conjunctiva, eye irritation, crusting of eyelid. **RARE:** Allergic reaction, including rash, urticaria; mental confusion or excitement, particularly in children; fatigue.

ADVERSE EFFECTS/ TOXIC REACTIONS

Overdose may produce tachycardia, palpitations, hot/dry/flushed skin, absence of bowel sounds, increased respiratory rate, nausea, vomiting, confusion, somnolence, slurred speech, dizziness, CNS stimulation. Overdose may also produce psychosis as evidenced by agitation, restlessness, rambling speech, visual hallucinations, paranoid behavior, delusions, followed by depression. Opthalmic form may rarely produce increased intraocular pressure.

NURSING CONSIDERATIONS

BASELINE ASSESSMENT

Before giving medication, instruct pt to void (reduces risk of urinary retention). Determine if pt is sensitive to atropine, homatropine, scopolamine. Treatment with AtroPen auto injector may be instituted without waiting for lab results.

INTERVENTION/EVALUATION

Monitor changes in B/P, pulse, temperature. Observe for tachycardia if pt has cardiac abnormalities. Assess skin turgor, mucous membranes to evaluate hydration status (encourage adequate fluid intake unless NPO for surgery) bowel sounds for peristalsis. Be alert for fever (increased risk of hyperthermia). Monitor I&O, palpate bladder for urinary retention. Assess stool frequency, consistency.

PATIENT/FAMILY TEACHING

- For preoperative use, explain that warm, dry, flushing feeling may occur.
- Remind pt to remain in bed and not eat or drink anything.

Atrovent, *see ipratropium*

Augmentin, *see amoxicillin/clavulanate potassium*

Augmentin ES-600, *see amoxicillin/clavulanate potassium*

Augmentin XR, *see amoxicillin/clavulanate potassium*

Avalide, *see hydrochlorothiazide and irbesartan*

Avandia, *see rosiglitazone*

Avapro, *see irbesartan*

Avastin, *see bevacizumab*

Avelox, *see moxifloxacin*

Avodart, *see dutasteride*

Avonex, *see interferon beta 1a*

Axid, *see nizatidine*

azacitidine

ay-zah-**sigh**-tih-deen
(Vidaza)

CLASSIFICATION

PHARMACOTHERAPEUTIC: Antineoplastic. **CLINICAL:** DNA demethylation agent.

ACTION

Exerts cytotoxic effect on rapidly dividing cells by causing demethylation of DNA in abnormal hematopoietic cells in bone marrow. **Therapeutic Effect:** Restores normal function to tumor-suppressor genes regulating cellular differentiation, proliferation.

PHARMACOKINETICS

Rapidly absorbed after subcutaneous administration. Metabolized by the liver. Eliminated in urine. **Half-life:** 4 hrs.

USES

Treatment of myelodysplastic syndromes, specifically refractory anemia, myelomonocytic leukemia. **OFF-LABEL:** Treatment of refractory acute lymophocytic and myelogenous leukemia.

PRECAUTIONS

CONTRAINDICATIONS: Advanced malignant hepatic tumors, hypersensitivity to mannitol. **CAUTIONS:** Hepatic disease, renal impairment.

LIFESPAN CONSIDERATIONS:

Pregnancy/Lactation: May be embryotoxic; may cause developmental abnormalities of the fetus. Mothers should avoid breast-feeding. **Pregnancy Category D. Children:** Safety and efficacy have not been established. **Elderly:** Age-related renal impairment may increase risk of renal toxicity.

INTERACTIONS

DRUG: Bone marrow suppressants may increase myelosuppression. **HERBAL:** None significant. **FOOD:** None known. **LAB VALUES:** May decrease Hgb, Hct, WBC, RBC, platelet counts. May increase serum creatinine, potassium.

AVAILABILITY (Rx)

INJECTION, POWDER FOR RECONSTITUTION: 100 mg.

ADMINISTRATION/HANDLING

SUBCUTANEOUS

Reconstitution • Reconstitute with 4 ml Sterile Water for Injection. • Reconstituted solution will appear cloudy. • Solution must be used within 1 hr after reconstitution.

Rate of administration • Doses greater than 4 ml should be divided equally into 2 syringes. • Contents of syringe must be resuspended by inverting the syringe 2–3 times and rolling the syringe between the palms for 30 sec immediately before administration. • Rotate site for each injection (thigh, upper arm, abdomen). New injections should be administered at least 1 inch from the old site.

Storage • Store vials at room temperature. • Reconstituted solution may be stored for up to 1 hr at room temperature or up to 8 hrs if refrigerated. • Solution may be allowed to return to room temperature and used within 30 min.

INDICATIONS/ROUTES/DOSAGE

REFRACTORY ANEMIA, CHRONIC MYELOMONOCYTIC LEUKEMIA

◀ **ALERT** ▶ Dosage adjustment based on hematology.

SUBCUTANEOUS: ADULTS, ELDERLY: 75 mg/m^2/day for 7 days every 4 wks.

Dosage may be increased to 100 mg/m² if initial dose is insufficient and toxicity is manageable. Treatment recommended for at least 4 cycles.

SIDE EFFECTS

FREQUENT (71%–29%): Nausea, vomiting, fever, diarrhea, fatigue, injection site erythema, constipation, ecchymosis, cough, dyspnea, weakness. **OCCASIONAL (26%–16%):** Rigors, petechiae, injection site pain, pharyngitis, arthralgia, headache, limb pain, dizziness, peripheral edema, back pain, erythema, epistaxis, weight loss, myalgia. **RARE (13%–8%):** Anxiety, abdominal pain, rash, depression, tachycardia, insomnia, night sweats, stomatitis.

ADVERSE EFFECTS/ TOXIC REACTIONS

Hematologic toxicity, manifested as anemia, leukopenia, neutropenia, thrombocytopenia occurs commonly.

NURSING CONSIDERATIONS

BASELINE ASSESSMENT

Give emotional support to pt and family. Use strict asepsis and protect pt from infection. Obtain blood counts as needed to monitor response and toxicity but particularly before each dosing cycle.

INTERVENTION/EVALUATION

Monitor for hematologic toxicity (fever, sore throat, signs of local infections, unusual bruising/bleeding), symptoms of anemia (excessive fatigue, weakness). Assess response to medication; monitor and report nausea, vomiting, diarrhea. Avoid rectal temperatures, other traumas that may induce bleeding.

PATIENT/FAMILY TEACHING

• Do not have immunizations without physician's approval (drug lowers body's resistance). • Avoid crowds, persons with known infections. • Report signs of infection (fever, flu-like symptoms) immediately. • Contact physician if nausea/vomiting continues at home. • Advise men to use barrier contraception while receiving treatment.

azathioprine

ay-za-**thye**-oh-preen

(Apo-Azathioprine ♣, Azasan, Azathioprine Sodium, Imuran, Novo-Azathioprine ♣)

Do not confuse azathioprine with Azulfidine or azatadine, or Imuran with Elmiron or Imferon.

CLASSIFICATION

PHARMACOTHERAPEUTIC: Immunologic agent. **CLINICAL:** Immunosuppressant.

ACTION

Antagonizes purine metabolism, inhibits DNA, protein, and RNA synthesis. **Therapeutic Effect:** Suppresses cell-mediated hypersensitivities; alters antibody production, immune response in transplant recipients. Reduces arthritis symptoms severity.

USES

Adjunct in prevention of rejection in kidney transplantation; treatment of rheumatoid arthritis in those unresponsive to conventional therapy. **OFF-LABEL:** Treatment of biliary cirrhosis, chronic active hepatitis, glomerulonephritis, inflammatory bowel disease, inflammatory myopathy, multiple sclerosis, myasthenia gravis, nephrotic syndrome, pemphigoid, pemphigus, polymyositis, systemic lupus erythematosus. Adjunct in preventing rejection of solid organ (nonrenal) transplants. Maintenance remission in Crohn's disease.

A

PRECAUTIONS

CONTRAINDICATIONS: Pregnant pts with rheumatoid arthritis. **CAUTIONS:** Immunosuppressed pts, those previously treated for rheumatoid arthritis with alkylating agents (cyclophosphamide, chlorambucil, melphalan), chickenpox (current or recent), herpes zoster, gout, hepatic/renal impairment, infection. **Pregnancy Category D.**

INTERACTIONS

DRUG: **Allopurinol** may increase activity, toxicity. **Bone marrow depressants** may increase myelosuppression. **Other immunosuppressants** may increase risk of infection or development of neoplasms. **Live virus vaccines** may potentiate virus replication, increase vaccine side effects, decrease pt's antibody response to vaccine. **HERBAL:** Avoid **cat's claw, echinacea** (immunostimulant properties). **FOOD:** None known. **LAB VALUES:** May decrease Hgb, albumin, uric acid. May increase AST, ALT, alkaline phosphatase, amylase, bilirubin.

AVAILABILITY (Rx)

INJECTION, POWDER FOR RECONSTITUTION (IMURAN): 100-mg vial. **TABLETS:** 25 mg (Azasan), 50 mg (Azasan, Imuran), 75 mg (Azasan), 100 mg (Azasan).

ADMINISTRATION/HANDLING

IV

Reconstitution • Reconstitute 100-mg vial with 10 ml Sterile Water for Injection to provide concentration of 10 mg/ml. • Swirl vial gently to mix and dissolve solution. • May further dilute in 50 ml D_5W or 0.9% NaCl.

Rate of administration • Infuse over 30–60 min. Range: 5 min–8 hrs.

Storage • Store parenteral form at room temperature. • After reconstitution, IV solution stable for 24 hrs.

PO

• Give during or after food to reduce potential for GI disturbances. • Store oral form at room temperature.

IV INCOMPATIBILITIES

Methyl and propyl parabens, phenol.

INDICATIONS/ROUTES/DOSAGE

PREVENTION OF RENAL ALLOGRAFT REJECTION

PO, IV: ADULTS, ELDERLY, CHILDREN: 3–5 mg/kg/day on day of transplant, then 1–3 mg/kg/day as maintenance dose.

RHEUMATOID ARTHRITIS

PO: ADULTS: Initially, 1 mg/kg/day as a single dose or in 2 divided doses for 6–8 wks. May increase by 0.5 mg/kg/day after 6–8 wks at 4-wk intervals up to maximum of 2.5 mg/kg/day. Maintenance: Lowest effective dosage. May decrease dose by 0.5 mg/kg or 25 mg/day q4wk (while other therapies, such as rest, physiotherapy, and salicylates, are maintained). **ELDERLY:** Initially, 1 mg/kg/day (50–100 mg); may increase by 25 mg/day until response or toxicity.

DOSAGE IN RENAL IMPAIRMENT

Dosage is modified based on creatinine clearance.

Creatinine Clearance	Dose
10–50 ml/min	75% of usual dose
Less than 10 ml/min	50% of usual dose

SIDE EFFECTS

FREQUENT: Nausea, vomiting, anorexia (particularly during early treatment and with large doses). **OCCASIONAL:** Rash. **RARE:** Severe nausea/vomiting with diarrhea, abdominal pain, hypersensitivity reaction.

ADVERSE EFFECTS/ TOXIC REACTIONS

Increases risk of neoplasia (new abnormal-growth tumors). Significant leukopenia and thrombocytopenia may occur, particularly in those undergoing renal transplant rejection. Hepatotoxicity occurs rarely.

NURSING CONSIDERATIONS

BASELINE ASSESSMENT

Arthritis: Assess onset, type, location, and duration of pain, fever, inflammation. Inspect appearance of affected joints for immobility, deformities, skin condition.

INTERVENTION/EVALUATION

CBC, platelet count, hepatic function studies should be performed weekly during first mo of therapy, twice monthly during second and third mos of treatment, then monthly thereafter. If WBC falls rapidly, dosage should be reduced or discontinued. Assess particularly for delayed myelosuppression. Routinely watch for any change from normal. **Arthritis:** Evaluate for therapeutic response: relief of pain, stiffness, swelling, increased joint mobility, reduced joint tenderness, improved grip strength.

PATIENT/FAMILY TEACHING

• Contact physician if unusual bleeding/bruising, sore throat, mouth sores, abdominal pain, fever occurs. • Therapeutic response in rheumatoid arthritis may take up to 12 wks. • Women of child-bearing age must avoid pregnancy.

azelastine

aye-zeh-**las**-teen

(Astelin, Optivar)

Do not confuse Optivar with Optiray.

CLASSIFICATION

PHARMACOTHERAPEUTIC: Antihistamine. **CLINICAL:** Antiallergy.

ACTION

Competes with histamine for histamine receptor sites on cells in blood vessels, GI tract, respiratory tract. **Therapeutic Effect:** Relieves symptoms associated with seasonal allergic rhinitis (increased mucus production, sneezing) and symptoms associated with allergic conjunctivitis, (redness, itching, excessive tearing).

PHARMACOKINETICS

Route	Onset	Peak	Duration
Nasal spray	0.5–1 hr	2–3 hrs	12 hrs
Ophthalmic	N/A	3 min	8 hrs

Well absorbed through nasal mucosa. Primarily excreted in feces. **Half-life:** 22 hrs.

USES

Nasal: Treatment of symptoms of seasonal and perennial allergic rhinitis. **Ophthalmic:** Treatment of itching associated with allergic conjunctivitis.

PRECAUTIONS

CONTRAINDICATIONS: Breast-feeding women; history of hypersensitivity to antihistamines; neonates or premature infants; third trimester of pregnancy. **CAUTIONS:** Renal impairment.

LIFESPAN CONSIDERATIONS:

Pregnancy/Lactation: Unknown if drug crosses placenta or is distributed in breast milk. Do not use during third trimester. **Pregnancy Category C.** **Children:** Safety and efficacy not established in those younger than 12 yrs. **Elderly:** No age-related precautions noted.

INTERACTIONS

DRUG: **Alcohol, CNS depressants** may increase CNS depression. **Cimetidine** may increase plasma concentration.

HERBAL: None significant. **FOOD:** None significant. **LAB VALUES:** May suppress wheal and flare reaction to antigen skin testing unless drug is discontinued 4 days before testing. May increase serum ALT.

AVAILABILITY (Rx)

NASAL SPRAY (ASTELIN): 137 mcg/spray. **OPHTHALMIC SOLUTION (OPTIVAR):** 0.05%.

ADMINISTRATION/HANDLING

NASAL

• Instruct pt to clear nasal passages as much as possible before use. • Tilt head slightly forward. • Insert spray tip into nostril, pointing toward nasal passage, away from nasal septum. • Spray into nostril while holding the other nostril closed and concurrently inhale through nose to permit medication as high into nasal passage as possible.

OPHTHALMIC

• Tilt pt's head back; place solution in conjunctival sac. • Have pt close eyes; press gently on lacrimal sac for 1 min.

INDICATIONS/ROUTES/DOSAGE

ALLERGIC RHINITIS

NASAL: ADULTS, ELDERLY, CHILDREN 12 YRS AND OLDER: 2 sprays in each nostril twice a day. **CHILDREN 5–11 YRS:** 1 spray in each nostril twice a day.

ALLERGIC CONJUNCTIVITIS

OPHTHALMIC: ADULTS, ELDERLY, CHILDREN 3 YRS OR OLDER: 1 drop into affected eye twice a day.

SIDE EFFECTS

NASAL: FREQUENT (20%–15%): Headache, bitter taste. **RARE:** Nasal burning, paroxysmal sneezing, somnolence. **Ophthalmic:** Transient eye burning or stinging, bitter taste, headache.

ADVERSE EFFECTS/ TOXIC REACTIONS

Epistaxis occurs rarely.

NURSING CONSIDERATIONS

BASELINE ASSESSMENT

Question for hypersensitivity to antihistamines.

INTERVENTION/EVALUATION

Assess therapeutic response to medication.

azithromycin

aye-zith-row-**my**-sin

(Apo-Azithromycin ✱, Novo-Azithromycin ✱, Zithromax, Zithromax TRI-PAK, Zithromax Z-PAK, Zmax)

Do not confuse azithromycin with erythromycin.

CLASSIFICATION

PHARMACOTHERAPEUTIC: Macrolide. **CLINICAL:** Antibiotic (see p. 25C).

ACTION

Binds to ribosomal receptor sites of susceptible organisms, inhibiting RNA-dependent protein synthesis. **Therapeutic Effect:** Bacteriostatic or bactericidal, depending on drug dosage.

PHARMACOKINETICS

Rapidly absorbed from GI tract. Protein binding: 7%–50%. Widely distributed. Eliminated primarily unchanged by biliary excretion. **Half-life:** 68 hrs.

USES

Treatment of susceptible infections due to *Chlamydia pneumoniae, C. trachomatis, H. influenza, Legionella, M. catarrhalis, Mycoplasma pneumoniae, N. gonorrhoeae, S. aureus. S. pneumoniae, S. pyogenes* including mild to moderate infections of upper respiratory tract (pharyngitis, tonsillitis), lower respiratory tract (acute bacterial exacerbations, chronic obstructive pulmonary disease [COPD], pneumonia), uncomplicated skin and skin-structure infections, sexually transmitted diseases (nongonococcal urethritis, cervicitis due to *Chlamydia trachomatis*), chancroid. Prevents disseminated *Mycobacterium avium* complex (MAC). Treatment of mycoplasma pneumonia. **Injection:** Community-acquired pneumonia, pelvic inflammatory disease (PID). **OFF-LABEL:** Treatment of chlamydial infections, gonococcal pharyngitis, uncomplicated gonococcal infections of cervix, urethra, rectum.

PRECAUTIONS

CONTRAINDICATIONS: Hypersensitivity to other macrolide antibiotics. **CAUTIONS:** Hepatic/renal dysfunction.

LIFESPAN CONSIDERATIONS:

Pregnancy/Lactation: Unknown if distributed in breast milk. **Pregnancy Category B. Children:** Safety and efficacy not established in those younger than 16 yrs for IV use and younger than 6 mos for oral use. **Elderly:** No age-related precautions in those with normal renal function.

INTERACTIONS

DRUG: May increase serum concentration of **carbamazepine, bromocriptine, cyclosporine, digoxin, ergot alkaloids, tacrolimus. Aluminum/magnesium-containing antacids** may decrease concentration (give 1 hr before or 2 hrs after antacid). **HERBAL:** None significant. **FOOD:** None known. **LAB VALUES:** May increase serum creatine phosphokinase (CPK), AST, ALT.

AVAILABILITY (Rx)

INJECTION, POWDER FOR RECONSTITUTION (ZITHROMAX): 500 mg. **SUSPENSION, ORAL (ZITHROMAX):** 100 mg/5 ml, 200 mg/5 ml. **SUSPENSION, ORAL (EXTENDED-RELEASE [ZMAX]):** 1 g single-dose packet, 2 g single-dose packet. **TABLETS:** 250 mg, 500 mg, 600 mg (Zithromax). Tri-Pak: 3 × 500 mg (Zithromax TRI-PAK). Z-Pak: 6 × 250 mg (Zithromax Z-PAK).

ADMINISTRATION/HANDLING

IV

Reconstitution • Reconstitute each 500-mg vial with 4.8 ml Sterile Water for Injection to provide concentration of 100 mg/ml. • Shake well to ensure dissolution. • Further dilute with 250 or 500 ml 0.9% NaCl or D_5W to provide final concentration of 2 mg with 250 ml diluent or 1 mg/ml with 500 ml diluent.

Rate of administration • Infuse over 60 min.

Storage • Store vials at room temperature. • Following reconstitution, suspension is stable for 24 hrs at room temperature or 7 days if refrigerated.

PO

• Give tablets without regard to food. • May store suspension at room temperature. Stable for 10 days after reconstitution. • Do not administer oral suspension with food. Give at least 1 hr before or 2 hrs after meals. Give Zmax within 12 hrs of reconstitution.

IV INCOMPATIBILITIES

Ceftriaxone (Rocephin), ciprofloxacin (Cipro), famotidine (Pepcid), furosemide (Lasix), ketorolac (Toradol), levofloxacin (Levaquin), morphine, piperacillin/tazobactam (Zosyn), potassium chloride.

IV COMPATIBILITY

Diphenhydramine (Benadryl).

INDICATIONS/ROUTES/DOSAGE

ACUTE EXACERBATIONS OF COPD

PO: ADULTS, ELDERLY, CHILDREN 16 YRS AND OLDER: 500 mg/day for 3 days or 500 mg on day 1, then 250 mg/day on days 2–5.

ACUTE BACTERIAL SINUSITIS

PO (ZMAX): ADULTS, ELDERLY: 2 g as a single dose.

PO: ADULTS, ELDERLY: 500 mg/day for 3 days. **CHILDREN 6 MOS AND OLDER:** 10 mg/kg for 3 days. **Maximum:** 500 mg/day.

CERVICITIS

PO: ADULTS, ELDERLY: 1–2 g as single dose.

CHANCROID

PO: ADULTS, ELDERLY: 1 g as single dose.

MAC PREVENTION

PO: ADULTS, ELDERLY: 1,200 mg once weekly. **CHILDREN:** 20 mg/kg once weekly. **Maximum:** 1,200 mg/dose.

MAC TREATMENT

PO: ADULTS, ELDERLY: 600 mg/day with ethambutol 15 mg/kg/day. **CHILDREN:** 5–20 mg/kg/day for 1 mo or longer.

OTITIS MEDIA

PO: CHILDREN 6 MOS AND OLDER: 30 mg/kg as single dose or 10 mg/kg/day for 3 days or 10 mg/kg on day 1, then 5 mg/kg on days 2–5.

PHARYNGITIS, TONSILLITIS

PO: ADULTS, ELDERLY, CHILDREN 16 YRS AND OLDER: 500 mg on day 1, then 250 mg on days 2–5. **CHILDREN 2–15 YRS:** 12 mg/kg daily for 5 days.

PNEUMONIA, COMMUNITY ACQUIRED

PO (ZMAX): ADULTS, ELDERLY: 2 g as a single dose.

PO: ADULTS, ELDERLY, CHILDREN 16 YRS AND OLDER: 500 mg on day 1, then 250 mg on days 2–5 or 500 mg/day IV for 2 days, then 500 mg/day PO to complete course of therapy. **CHILDREN 6 MOS–15 YRS:** 10 mg/kg on day 1, then 5 mg/kg on days 2–5.

SKIN AND SKIN-STRUCTURE INFECTIONS

PO: ADULTS, ELDERLY, CHILDREN 16 YRS AND OLDER: 500 mg on day 1, then 250 mg on days 2–5.

PELVIC INFLAMMATORY DISEASE (PID)

IV: ADULTS, ELDERLY: 500 mg/day for at least 2 days, then 250 mg/day to complete a 7-day course of therapy.

SIDE EFFECTS

OCCASIONAL: Nausea, vomiting, diarrhea, abdominal pain. **RARE:** Headache, dizziness, allergic reaction.

ADVERSE EFFECTS/ TOXIC REACTIONS

Antibiotic-associated colitis (abdominal cramps, severe watery diarrhea, fever), other superinfections may result from altered bacterial balance. Acute interstitial nephritis, hepatotoxicity occur rarely.

NURSING CONSIDERATIONS

BASELINE ASSESSMENT

Question for history of hepatitis, allergies to azithromycin, erythromycins.

INTERVENTION/EVALUATION

Check for GI discomfort, nausea, vomiting. Determine pattern of bowel activity and stool consistency. Monitor hepatic function tests, assess for hepatotoxicity: malaise, fever, abdominal pain, GI disturbances. Evaluate for superinfection: genital/anal pruritus, sore mouth or tongue, moderate to severe diarrhea.

PATIENT/FAMILY TEACHING

• Continue therapy for full length of treatment. • Doses should be evenly spaced. • Take oral medication with 8 oz of water at least 1 hr before or 2 hrs after food or beverage.

Azmacort, *see triamcinolone*

aztreonam

az-**tree**-oo-nam
(Azactam)

CLASSIFICATION

PHARMACOTHERAPEUTIC: Monobactam. **CLINICAL:** Antibiotic.

ACTION

Inhibits bacterial cell wall synthesis. **Therapeutic Effect:** Bactericidal.

PHARMACOKINETICS

Completely absorbed after IM administration. Protein binding: 56%–60%. Partially metabolized by hydrolysis. Primarily excreted unchanged in urine. Removed by hemodialysis. **Half-life:** 1.4–2.2 hrs (increased in renal hepatic impairment).

USES

Treatment of infections caused by susceptible gram-negative micro-organisms *P. aeruginose, E. coli, S. marcescens, K. pneumoniae, P. mirabilis, H. influenzae,* Enterobacter, Citrobacter species including lower respiratory tract, skin/skin structure, intra-abdominal, gynecologic, complicated/uncomplicated UTIs; septicemia, cystic fibrosis. **OFF-LABEL:** Treatment of bone and joint infections.

PRECAUTIONS

CONTRAINDICATIONS: None known. **CAUTIONS:** History of allergy, esp. antibiotics, hepatic/renal impairment.

LIFESPAN CONSIDERATIONS:

Pregnancy/Lactation: Crosses placenta, distributed in amniotic fluid; low concentration in breast milk. **Pregnancy Category B. Children:** Safety and efficacy not established in children younger than 9 mos. **Elderly:** Age-related renal impairment may require dosage adjustment.

INTERACTIONS

DRUG: None significant. **HERBAL:** None significant. **FOOD:** None known. **LAB VALUES:** May increase serum alkaline phosphatase, creatinine, LDH, AST, ALT levels. Produces a positive Coombs' test.

AVAILABILITY (Rx)

INJECTION, INFUSION SOLUTION: Premix 1 g/50 ml, 2 g/50 ml. **INJECTION, POWDER FOR RECONSTITUTION:** 500 mg, 1 g, 2 g.

ADMINISTRATION/HANDLING

IV

Reconstitution • For IV push, dilute each gram with 6–10 ml Sterile Water for Injection. • For intermittent IV infusion, further dilute with 50–100 ml D_5W or 0.9% NaCl.

Rate of administration • For IV push, give over 3–5 min. • For IV infusion, administer over 20–60 min.

Storage • Store vials at room temperature. • Solution appears colorless to light yellow. • Following reconstitution, solution is stable for 48 hrs at room temperature or 7 days if refrigerated. • Discard if precipitate forms. Discard unused portions.

IM

• Shake immediately, vigorously after adding diluent. • Inject deeply into large muscle mass. • Following reconstitution, solution is stable for 48 hrs at room temperature or 7 days if refrigerated.

IV INCOMPATIBILITIES

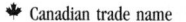

Acyclovir (Zovirax), amphotericin (Fungizone), daunorubicin (Cerubidine), ganciclovir (Cytovene), lorazepam (Ativan), metronidazole (Flagyl), vancomycin (Vancocin).

IV COMPATIBILITIES

Aminophylline, bumetanide (Bumex), calcium gluconate, cimetidine (Tagamet), diltiazem (Cardizem), dobutamine (Dobutrex), dopamine (Intropin), famotidine (Pepcid), furosemide (Lasix), heparin, hydromorphone (Dilaudid), insulin (regular), lipids, magnesium sulfate, morphine, potassium chloride, propofol (Diprivan), total parenteral nutrition (TPN).

INDICATIONS/ROUTES/DOSAGE

UTIs

IV, IM: **ADULTS, ELDERLY:** 500 mg–1 g q8–12h.

MODERATE TO SEVERE SYSTEMIC INFECTIONS

IV, IM: **ADULTS, ELDERLY:** 1–2 g q8–12h.

SEVERE OR LIFE-THREATENING INFECTIONS

IV: **ADULTS, ELDERLY:** 2 g q6–8h.

CYSTIC FIBROSIS

IV: **CHILDREN:** 50 mg/kg/dose q6–8h up to 200 mg/kg/day. **Maximum:** 8 g/day.

MILD TO SEVERE INFECTIONS IN CHILDREN

IV: **CHILDREN:** 30 mg/kg q6–8h. **Maximum:** 120 mg/kg/day. **NEONATES:** 60–120 mg/kg/day q6–12h.

DOSAGE IN RENAL IMPAIRMENT

Dosage and frequency are modified based on creatinine clearance and severity of infection:

Creatinine Clearance	Dosage
10–30 ml/min	1–2 g initially, then ½ usual dose at usual intervals
Less than 10 ml/min	1–2 g initially, then ¼ usual dose at usual intervals

SIDE EFFECTS

OCCASIONAL (less than 3%): Discomfort and swelling at IM injection site, nausea, vomiting, diarrhea, rash. **RARE (less than 1%):** Phlebitis or thrombophlebitis at IV injection site, abdominal cramps, headache, hypotension.

ADVERSE EFFECTS/ TOXIC REACTIONS

Antibiotic-associated colitis (abdominal cramps, severe watery diarrhea, fever), other superinfections may result from altered bacterial balance. Severe hypersensitivity reactions, including anaphylaxis, occur rarely.

NURSING CONSIDERATIONS

BASELINE ASSESSMENT

Question for history of allergies, esp. to aztreonam, other antibiotics.

INTERVENTION/EVALUATION

Evaluate for phlebitis (heat, pain, red streaking over vein), pain at IM injection site. Assess for GI discomfort, nausea, vomiting. Monitor stool frequency and consistency. Assess skin for rash. Be alert for superinfection: increased temperature, sore throat, vomiting, diarrhea, black/hairy tongue, ulceration or changes of oral mucosa, anal/genital pruritus.

PATIENT/FAMILY TEACHING

- Report nausea, vomiting, diarrhea, rash.

B

bacitracin

bah-cih-**tray**-sin

(AK-Tracin, Baciguent, Bacitracin)

Do not confuse bacitracin with Bactrim or Bactroban.

FIXED-COMBINATION(S)

With polymyxin B, an antibiotic **(Polysporin);** with polymyxin B and neomycin, antibiotics **(Mycitracin, Neosporin).**

CLASSIFICATION

PHARMACOTHERAPEUTIC: Anti-infective. **CLINICAL:** Antibiotic.

ACTION

Interferes with plasma membrane permeability, inhibits bacterial cell wall synthesis in susceptible microorganisms. **Therapeutic Effect:** Bacteriostatic.

USES

Ophthalmic: Superficial ocular infections (conjunctivitis, keratitis, corneal ulcers, blepharitis). **Topical:** Minor skin abrasions, superficial infections. **Irrigation:** Treatment, prophylaxis of surgical procedures.

PRECAUTIONS

CONTRAINDICATIONS: None known. **CAUTIONS:** None known. **Pregnancy Category C.**

INTERACTIONS

DRUG: None significant. **HERBAL:** None significant. **FOOD:** None known. **LAB VALUES:** None known.

AVAILABILITY (Rx)

OPHTHALMIC OINTMENT (AK-TRACIN): 500 units/g. **POWDER FOR IRRIGATION:** 50,000 units. **TOPICAL OINTMENT (BACIGUENT [OTC]):** 500 units/g.

ADMINISTRATION/HANDLING

OPHTHALMIC

• Place gloved finger on lower eyelid and pull out until a pocket is formed between eye and lower lid. Place ¼–½ inch ointment into pocket. • Instruct pt to close eye gently for 1–2 min, rolling eyeball (increases contact area of drug to eye).

TOPICAL

• Gently cleanse area prior to application. • Without touching application tip to skin, apply on area thoroughly.

INDICATIONS/ROUTES/DOSAGE

SUPERFICIAL OCULAR INFECTIONS

OPHTHALMIC: ADULTS: ½-inch ribbon in conjunctival sac q3–4h.

SKIN ABRASIONS, SUPERFICIAL SKIN INFECTIONS

TOPICAL: ADULTS, CHILDREN: Apply to affected area 1–5 times a day.

SURGICAL TREATMENT, PROPHYLAXIS

IRRIGATION: ADULTS, ELDERLY: 50,000–150,000 units, as needed.

SIDE EFFECTS

RARE: Ophthalmic: Burning, itching, redness, swelling, pain. **Topical:** Hypersensitivity reaction (allergic contact dermatitis, burning, inflammation, pruritus).

ADVERSE EFFECTS/ TOXIC REACTIONS

Severe hypersensitivity reaction (apnea, hypotension) occur rarely.

NURSING CONSIDERATIONS

INTERVENTION/EVALUATION

Topical: Evaluate for hypersensitivity reaction: itching, burning, inflammation. With preparations containing corticosteroids, consider masking effect on clinical signs. **Ophthalmic:** Assess eye for therapeutic response or increased

B

redness, swelling, burning, itching (hypersensitivity reaction).

PATIENT/FAMILY TEACHING

• Continue therapy for full length of treatment. • Doses should be evenly spaced. • Report burning, itching, rash, increased irritation.

baclofen

bak-loe-fen

(Apo-Baclofen ✤, Lioresal, Liotec ✤, Nu-Baclofen ✤)

Do not confuse baclofen with Bactroban or Beclovent.

CLASSIFICATION

PHARMACOTHERAPEUTIC: Skeletal muscle relaxant. **CLINICAL:** Antispastic, analgesic in trigeminal neuralgia (see p. 142C).

ACTION

Inhibits transmission of reflexes at spinal cord level. **Therapeutic Effect:** Relieves muscle spasticity.

PHARMACOKINETICS

Well absorbed from GI tract. Protein binding: 30%. Partially metabolized in the liver. Primarily excreted in urine. **Half-life:** 2.5–4 hrs; intrathecal: 1.5 hrs.

USES

Treatment of cerebral spasticity, reversible spasticity associated with multiple sclerosis, spinal cord lesions. **Intrathecal:** For those unresponsive to oral therapy or exhibiting intolerable side effects. **OFF-LABEL:** Treatment of bladder spasms, cerebral palsy, intractable hiccups or pain, Huntington's chorea, trigeminal neuralgia.

PRECAUTIONS

CONTRAINDICATIONS: Skeletal muscle spasm due to cerebral palsy, Parkinson's disease, rheumatic disorders, cerebrovascular accident (CVA), cough, intractable hiccups, neuropathic pain. **CAUTIONS:** Renal impairment, CVA, diabetes mellitus, epilepsy, preexisting psychiatric disorders.

LIFESPAN CONSIDERATIONS:

Pregnancy/Lactation: Unknown if drug crosses placenta or is distributed in breast milk. **Pregnancy Category C.** **Children:** Safety and efficacy not established in those younger than 12 yrs. **Elderly:** Increased risk of CNS toxicity (hallucinations, sedation, confusion, mental depression); age-related renal impairment may require decreased dosage.

INTERACTIONS

DRUG: Potentiated effects when used with other **CNS depressants (including alcohol). MAOI** may increase CNS depression, hypotensive effect. **HERBAL: St. John's wort, kava kava, gotu kola, valerian** may increase CNS sedation. **FOOD:** None known. **LAB VALUES:** May increase serum AST, ALT, alkaline phosphatase, blood glucose.

AVAILABILITY (Rx)

INTRATHECAL INJECTION: 50 mcg/ml, 500 mcg/ml, 2,000 mcg/ml. **TABLETS:** 10 mg, 20 mg.

ADMINISTRATION/HANDLING

PO

• Give without regard to food. • Tablets may be crushed.

INTRATHECAL

• For screening, a 50 mcg/ml concentration should be used for injection. • For maintenance therapy, solution should be diluted for pts who require concentrations other than 500 mcg/ml or 2,000 mcg/ml.

INDICATIONS/ROUTES/DOSAGE

SPASTICITY

PO: ADULTS: Initially, 5 mg 3 times a day. May increase by 15 mg/day at 3-day intervals. Range: 40–80 mg/day. **Maximum:** 80 mg/day. **ELDERLY:** Initially, 5 mg 2–3 times a day. May gradually increase dosage. **CHILDREN:** Initially, 10–15 mg/day in divided doses q8h. May increase by 5–15 mg/day at 3-day intervals. **Maximum:** 40 mg/day (children 2–7 yrs); 60 mg/day (children 8 yrs and older).

USUAL INTRATHECAL DOSAGE

ADULTS, ELDERLY, CHILDREN OLDER THAN 12 YRS: 300–800 mcg/day. **CHILDREN 12 YRS AND YOUNGER:** 100–300 mcg/day.

SIDE EFFECTS

FREQUENT (greater than 10%): Transient somnolence, asthenia, dizziness, lightheadedness, nausea, vomiting. **OCCASIONAL (10%–2%):** Headache, paresthesia, constipation, anorexia, hypotension, confusion, nasal congestion. **RARE (less than 1%):** Paradoxical CNS excitement or restlessness, slurred speech, tremor, dry mouth, diarrhea, nocturia, impotence.

ADVERSE EFFECTS/ TOXIC REACTIONS

Abrupt discontinuation may produce hallucinations, seizures. Overdose results in blurred vision, seizures, myosis, mydriasis, severe muscle weakness, strabismus, respiratory depression, vomiting.

NURSING CONSIDERATIONS

BASELINE ASSESSMENT

Record onset, type, location, duration of muscular spasm. Check for immobility, stiffness, swelling.

INTERVENTION/EVALUATION

Assess for paradoxical reaction. Assist with ambulation at all times. For those on long-term therapy, hepatic/renal function tests, blood counts should be performed periodically. Evaluate for therapeutic response: decreased intensity of skeletal muscle pain.

PATIENT/FAMILY TEACHING

• Drowsiness usually diminishes with continued therapy. • Avoid tasks that require alertness, motor skills until response to drug is established. • Do not abruptly withdraw medication after long-term therapy. • Avoid alcohol, CNS depressants.

Bactrim, *see co-trimoxazole*

Bactroban, *see mupirocin*

Baraclude, *see entecavir*

basiliximab

bay-zul-**ix**-ah-mab

(Simulect)

Do not confuse basiliximab with daclizumab.

CLASSIFICATION

PHARMACOTHERAPEUTIC: Monoclonal antibody. **CLINICAL:** Immunosuppressive (see p. 114C).

ACTION

Binds to and blocks receptor of interleukin-2, a protein that stimulates proliferation of T-lymphocytes, which play a

B

major role in organ transplant rejection. **Therapeutic Effect:** Prevents lymphocytic activity, impairs response of immune system to antigens, preventing acute renal transplant rejection.

PHARMACOKINETICS

Half-life: Adults, 4–10 days; children, 5–17 days.

USES

Adjunct with cyclosporine, corticosteroids in prevention of acute organ rejection in pts receiving renal transplant.

PRECAUTIONS

CONTRAINDICATIONS: None known. **CAUTIONS:** Infection, history of malignancy.

LIFESPAN CONSIDERATIONS:

Pregnancy/Lactation: Unknown if drug crosses placenta or is distributed in breast milk. **Pregnancy Category B.** **Children/Elderly:** No age-related precautions noted.

INTERACTIONS

DRUG: None significant. **HERBAL:** None significant. **FOOD:** None known. **LAB VALUES:** Alters serum calcium, glucose, potassium, Hgb, Hct. Increases serum cholesterol, BUN, creatinine, uric acid. Decreases serum magnesium, phosphate, platelet count.

AVAILABILITY (Rx)

INJECTION, POWDER FOR RECONSTITUTION: 10 mg, 20 mg.

ADMINISTRATION/HANDLING

IV

Reconstitution • Reconstitute with 5 ml Sterile Water for Injection. • Shake gently to dissolve. • Further dilute with 50 ml 0.9% NaCl or D_5W. • Gently invert to avoid foaming.

Rate of administration • Infuse over 20–30 min.

Storage • Refrigerate. • After reconstitution, use within 4 hrs (24 hrs if refrigerated). • Discard if precipitate forms.

IV INCOMPATIBILITIES

Specific information not available. Do not add other medications simultaneously, through same IV line.

INDICATIONS/ROUTES/DOSAGE

PROPHYLAXIS OF ORGAN REJECTION

IV: ADULTS, ELDERLY, CHILDREN WEIGHING 35 KG AND MORE: 20 mg within 2 hrs before transplant surgery and 20 mg 4 days after transplant. **CHILDREN WEIGHING LESS THAN 35 KG:** 10 mg within 2 hrs before transplant surgery and 10 mg 4 days after transplant.

SIDE EFFECTS

FREQUENT (greater than 10%): GI disturbances (constipation, diarrhea, dyspepsia), CNS effects (dizziness, headache, insomnia, tremor), respiratory tract infection, dysuria, acne, leg or back pain, peripheral edema, hypertension. **OCCASIONAL (10%–3%):** Angina, neuropathy, abdominal distention, tachycardia, rash, hypotension, urinary disturbances (urinary frequency, genital edema, hematuria), arthralgia, hirsutism, myalgia.

ADVERSE EFFECTS/ TOXIC REACTIONS

Severe acute hypersensitivity reactions including anaphylaxis characterized by hypotension, tachycardia, cardiac failure, dyspnea, wheezing, bronchospasm, pulmonary edema, respiratory failure, urticaria, rash, pruritus, and/or sneezing, as well as capillary leak syndrome and cytokine release syndrome, have been reported.

B

NURSING CONSIDERATIONS

BASELINE ASSESSMENT

Obtain baseline BUN, serum creatinine, potassium, uric acid, glucose, calcium, phosphatase levels and vital signs, particularly B/P, pulse rate. Breast-feeding not recommended.

INTERVENTION/EVALUATION

Diligently monitor CBC, all serum levels. Assess B/P for hypertension/hypotension; pulse for evidence of tachycardia. Question for GI disturbances, CNS effects, urinary changes. Monitor for presence of wound infection, signs of infection (fever, sore throat, unusual bleeding/bruising).

PATIENT/FAMILY TEACHING

• Report difficulty in breathing or swallowing, tachycardia, rash, itching, swelling of lower extremities, weakness. • Avoid pregnancy.

BCG, intravesical

(Immu Cyst ✦, Pacis, TheraCys, Tice BCG)

See Cancer Chemotherapeutic Agents (p. 76C)

becaplermin

beh-**cap**-lear-min
(Regranex)

Do not confuse Regranex with Repronex.

CLASSIFICATION

PHARMACOTHERAPEUTIC: Biologic response modifier. **CLINICAL:** Growth factor.

ACTION

Platelet-derived growth factor. **Therapeutic Effect:** Stimulates body to grow new tissue to heal open wounds.

USES

Treatment of lower extremity diabetic neuropathic ulcers extending into or beyond subcutaneous tissue.

PRECAUTIONS

CONTRAINDICATIONS: Skin neoplasms at site of application. **CAUTIONS:** Wounds showing exposed joints, tendons, ligaments, bones. **Pregnancy Category C.**

INTERACTIONS

DRUG: None significant. **HERBAL:** None significant. **FOOD:** None known. **LAB VALUES:** None known.

AVAILABILITY (Rx)

GEL: 0.01%.

ADMINISTRATION/HANDLING

• Refrigerate gel. • Measure gel on a clean, nonabsorbable surface. • Transfer to ulcer and spread as a thin, continuous layer onto the ulcer. • With a gauze pad moistened with 0.9% NaCl, cover ulcer for 12 hrs; remove and wash any residual gel from ulcer and replace with new gauze pad moistened with 0.9% NaCl until time of next application.

INDICATIONS/ROUTES/DOSAGE

ULCERS

TOPICAL: ADULTS, ELDERLY: Apply once a day (spread evenly; cover with saline-moistened gauze dressing). After 12 hrs, rinse ulcer, recover with saline moistened gauze.

SIDE EFFECTS

OCCASIONAL (2%): Local rash near ulcer.

B

ADVERSE EFFECTS/ TOXIC REACTIONS

None known.

NURSING CONSIDERATIONS

INTERVENTION/EVALUATION

Do not allow tip of tube to come in contact with ulcer.

PATIENT/FAMILY TEACHING

• Dosage requires recalculation weekly or biweekly, depending on rate of change in width and length of ulcer.

beclomethasone

be-kloe-**meth**-a-sone

(Apo-Beclomethasone ✤, Beconase AQ, Propaderm ✤, Qvar, Rivanuse AQ ✤)

Do not confuse Beconase with baclofen.

CLASSIFICATION

PHARMACOTHERAPEUTIC: Adrenocorticosteroid. **CLINICAL:** Anti-inflammatory, immunosuppressant (see pp. 71C, 92C).

ACTION

Controls or prevents inflammation by altering rate of protein synthesis; migration of polymorphonuclear leukocytes, fibroblasts; reverses capillary permeability. **Therapeutic Effect: Inhalation:** Inhibits bronchoconstriction, produces smooth muscle relaxation, decreases mucus secretion. **Intranasal:** Decreases response to seasonal and perennial rhinitis.

PHARMACOKINETICS

Rapidly absorbed from pulmonary, nasal, GI tissue. Undergoes extensive first-pass metabolism in the liver. Protein binding: 87%. Primarily eliminated in feces. **Half-life:** 15 hrs.

USES

Inhalation: Long-term control of bronchial asthma. Reduces need for oral corticosteroid therapy for asthma. **Intranasal:** Relief of seasonal/perennial rhinitis; prevention of nasal polyp recurrence after surgical removal; treatment of nonallergic rhinitis. **OFF-LABEL:** Prevention of seasonal rhinitis (nasal form).

PRECAUTIONS

CONTRAINDICATIONS: Hypersensitivity to beclomethasone, acute exacerbation of asthma, status asthmaticus. **CAUTIONS:** Cirrhosis, glaucoma, hypothyroidism, untreated systemic infections, osteoporosis, tuberculosis.

⌛ LIFESPAN CONSIDERATIONS:

Pregnancy/Lactation: Unknown if drug crosses placenta or is distributed in breast milk. **Pregnancy Category C.** **Children:** Prolonged treatment/high dosages may decrease short-term growth rate, cortisol secretion. **Elderly:** No age-related precautions noted.

INTERACTIONS

DRUG: None significant. **HERBAL:** None significant. **FOOD:** None known. **LAB VALUES:** None known.

AVAILABILITY (Rx)

INHALATION, ORAL (QVAR): 40 mcg/inhalation, 80 mcg/inhalation. **NASAL INHALATION (BECONASE AQ):** 42 mcg/inhalation.

ADMINISTRATION/HANDLING

INHALATION

• Shake container well, exhale completely, place mouthpiece between lips, inhale, hold breath as long as possible before exhaling. • Allow at least 1 min between inhalations. • Rinse mouth after each use to decrease dry mouth, hoarseness.

INTRANASAL

• Clear nasal passages as much as possible. • Insert spray tip into nostril, pointing toward nasal passages, away from nasal septum. • Spray into nostril while holding other nostril closed, concurrently inspire through nose to permit medication as high into nasal passages as possible.

INDICATIONS/ROUTES/DOSAGE

LONG-TERM CONTROL OF BRONCHIAL ASTHMA, REDUCES NEED FOR ORAL CORTICOSTEROID THERAPY FOR ASTHMA

ORAL INHALATION: **ADULTS, ELDERLY, CHILDREN 12 YRS AND OLDER:** 40–160 mcg twice a day. **Maximum:** 320 mcg twice a day. **CHILDREN 5–11 YRS:** 40 mcg twice a day. **Maximum:** 80 mcg twice a day.

RHINITIS, PREVENTION OF RECURRENCE OF NASAL POLYPS

NASAL INHALATION: **ADULTS, ELDERLY, CHILDREN 12 YRS AND OLDER:** 1 spray in each nostril 2–4 times a day or 2 sprays twice a day. Maintenance: 1 spray 3 times a day. **CHILDREN 6–12 YRS:** 1 spray 3 times a day.

SIDE EFFECTS

FREQUENT: Inhalation (14%–4%): Throat irritation, dry mouth, hoarseness, cough. **Intranasal:** Nasal burning, mucosal dryness. **OCCASIONAL: Inhalation (3%–2%):** Localized fungal infection (thrush). **Intranasal:** Nasal-crusting epistaxis, sore throat, ulceration of nasal mucosa. **RARE: Inhalation:** Transient bronchospasm, esophageal candidiasis. **Intranasal:** Nasal and pharyngeal candidiasis, eye pain.

ADVERSE EFFECTS/ TOXIC REACTIONS

Acute hypersensitivity reaction, (urticaria, angioedema, severe bronchospasm) occurs rarely. Transfer from systemic to local steroid therapy may unmask previously suppressed bronchial asthma condition.

NURSING CONSIDERATIONS

BASELINE ASSESSMENT

Question for hypersensitivity to any corticosteroids.

INTERVENTION/EVALUATION

In those receiving bronchodilators by inhalation concomitantly with inhalation of steroid therapy, advise to use bronchodilator several minutes before corticosteroid aerosol (enhances penetration of steroid into bronchial tree).

PATIENT/FAMILY TEACHING

• Do not change dose schedule or stop taking drug; must taper off gradually under medical supervision. • **Inhalation:** Maintain careful oral hygiene. • Rinse mouth with water immediately after inhalation (prevents mouth/throat dryness, fungal infection of mouth). • Contact physician/nurse if sore throat or mouth occurs. • **Intranasal:** Contact physician if symptoms do not improve or sneezing, nasal irritation occurs. • Clear nasal passages prior to use. • Improvement noted after several days.

Benadryl, *see diphenhydramine*

benazepril

ben-**ayz**-ah-prill

(Lotensin)

Do not confuse benazepril with Benadryl, or Lotensin with Loniten or lovastatin.

B

FIXED-COMBINATION(S)

Lotensin HCT: benazepril/hydrochlorothiazide (a diuretic): 5 mg/625 mg; 10 mg/12.5 mg; 20 mg/12.5 mg; 20 mg/25 mg. **Lotrel:** benazepril/amlodipine (a calcium blocker): 2.5 mg/10 mg; 5 mg/10 mg; 5 mg/20 mg; 5 mg/40 mg; 10 mg/20 mg; 10 mg/40 mg.

◆CLASSIFICATION

PHARMACOTHERAPEUTIC: Angiotensin-converting enzyme (ACE) inhibitor. **CLINICAL:** Antihypertensive (see p. 7C).

ACTION

Decreases rate of conversion of angiotensin I to angiotensin II, a potent vasoconstrictor. Reduces peripheral arterial resistance. **Therapeutic Effect:** Lowers B/P.

PHARMACOKINETICS

Route	Onset	Peak	Duration
PO	1 hr	2–4 hrs	24 hrs

Partially absorbed from GI tract. Protein binding: 97%. Metabolized in the liver to active metabolite. Primarily excreted in urine. Minimal removal by hemodialysis. **Half-life:** 35 min; metabolite 10–11 hrs.

USES

Treatment of hypertension. Used alone or in combination with other antihypertensives. **OFF-LABEL:** Treatment of CHF.

PRECAUTIONS

CONTRAINDICATIONS: History of angioedema from previous treatment with ACE inhibitors, pregnancy. **CAUTIONS:** Renal impairment, sodium depletion, diuretic therapy, dialysis, hypovolemia, coronary or cerebrovascular insufficiency, hepatic impairment, diabetes mellitus.

⌛ LIFESPAN CONSIDERATIONS:

Pregnancy/Lactation: Crosses placenta. Unknown if distributed in breast milk. May cause fetal, neonatal mortality or morbidity. **Pregnancy Category C (D if used in second or third trimester).** **Children:** Safety and efficacy not established. **Elderly:** May be more sensitive to hypotensive effects.

INTERACTIONS

DRUG: **Alcohol, diuretics, hypotensive agents** may increase effects. **NSAIDs** may decrease effect. **Potassium-sparing diuretics, potassium supplements** may cause hyperkalemia. May increase **lithium** concentration, toxicity. **HERBAL:** **Ephedra, ginseng, yohimbe** may worsen hypertension. **Garlic** may have increased antihypertensive effect. **FOOD:** None known. **LAB VALUES:** May increase serum potassium, AST, ALT, alkaline phosphatase, bilirubin, BUN, creatinine. May decrease serum sodium. May cause positive ANA titer.

AVAILABILITY (Rx)

TABLETS: 5 mg, 10 mg, 20 mg, 40 mg.

ADMINISTRATION/HANDLING

- Give without regard to food.

INDICATIONS/ROUTES/DOSAGE

HYPERTENSION (MONOTHERAPY)

PO: **ADULTS:** Initially, 10 mg/day. Maintenance: 20–40 mg/day as single or in 2 divided doses. **Maximum:** 80 mg/day. **ELDERLY:** Initially, 5–10 mg/day. Range: 20–40 mg/day.

HYPERTENSION (COMBINATION THERAPY)

PO: **ADULTS:** Discontinue diuretic 2–3 days prior to initiating benazepril, then dose as noted above. If unable to discontinue diuretic, begin benazepril at 5 mg/day.

USUAL PEDIATRIC DOSAGE

PO: CHILDREN 6 YRS AND OLDER: Initially, 0.2 mg/kg/day. Range: 0.1–0.6 mg/kg/day. **Maximum:** 40 mg/day.

DOSAGE IN RENAL IMPAIRMENT

For adult pts with creatinine clearance less than 30 ml/min, initially, 5 mg/day titrated up to maximum of 40 mg/day.

SIDE EFFECTS

FREQUENT (6%–3%): Cough, headache, dizziness. **OCCASIONAL (2%):** Fatigue, somnolence or drowsiness, nausea. **RARE (less than 1%):** Rash, fever, myalgia, diarrhea, loss of taste.

ADVERSE EFFECTS/ TOXIC REACTIONS

Excessive hypotension ("first-dose syncope") may occur in those with CHF, severe salt or volume depletion. Angioedema (swelling of face, lips), hyperkalemia occur rarely. Agranulocytosis, neutropenia may be noted in those with renal impairment, collagen vascular disease (scleroderma, systemic lupus erythematosus). Nephrotic syndrome may be noted in pts with history of renal disease.

NURSING CONSIDERATIONS

BASELINE ASSESSMENT

Obtain B/P immediately before each dose, in addition to regular monitoring (be alert to fluctuations). If excessive reduction in B/P occurs, place pt in supine position with legs elevated. In pts with renal impairment, autoimmune disease, or taking drugs that affect leukocytes or immune response, CBC should be performed before therapy begins and q2wk for 3 mos, then periodically thereafter.

INTERVENTION/EVALUATION

Assist with ambulation if dizziness occurs. Monitor B/P, renal function, urinary protein, leukocyte count.

PATIENT/FAMILY TEACHING

• To reduce hypotensive effect, rise slowly from lying to sitting position, permit legs to dangle from bed momentarily before standing. • Full therapeutic effect may take 2–4 wks. • Skipping doses or noncompliance with drug therapy may produce severe, rebound hypertension.

Benicar, *see olmesartan*

benzocaine

(Americaine, Anbesol, Cetacaine, Chloraseptic Lozenges, Dermoplast, Hurricane, Orajel)

See Anesthetics: local

benzonatate

evolve

ben-**zoe**-na-tate

(Tessalon, Tessalon Perles)

CLASSIFICATION

PHARMACOTHERAPEUTIC: Nonnarcotic antitussive. **CLINICAL:** Anticough.

ACTION

Anesthetizes stretch receptors in respiratory passages, lungs, pleura. **Therapeutic Effect:** Reduces cough production.

B

USES

Relief of nonproductive cough, including acute cough of minor throat/bronchial irritation.

PRECAUTIONS

CONTRAINDICATIONS: None known. **CAUTIONS:** Productive cough. **Pregnancy Category C.**

INTERACTIONS

DRUG: **CNS depressants** may increase effect. **HERBAL:** None significant. **FOOD:** None known. **LAB VALUES:** None known.

AVAILABILITY (Rx)

CAPSULES (TESSALON): 100 mg, 200 mg.

ADMINISTRATION/HANDLING

PO

- Give without regard to food.
- Swallow whole, do not chew/dissolve in mouth (may produce temporary local anesthesia/choking).

INDICATIONS/ROUTES/DOSAGE

ANTITUSSIVE

PO: ADULTS, ELDERLY, CHILDREN OLDER THAN 10 YRS: 100 mg 3 times a day or q4h up to 600 mg/day.

SIDE EFFECTS

OCCASIONAL: Mild somnolence, mild dizziness, constipation, GI upset, skin eruptions, nasal congestion.

ADVERSE EFFECTS/ TOXIC REACTIONS

Paradoxical reaction (restlessness, insomnia, euphoria, nervousness, tremor) has been noted.

NURSING CONSIDERATIONS

BASELINE ASSESSMENT

Assess type, severity, frequency of cough; monitor amount, color, consistency of sputum.

INTERVENTION/EVALUATION

Initiate deep breathing/coughing exercises, particularly in pts with impaired pulmonary function. Monitor for paradoxical reaction. Increase fluid intake, environmental humidity to lower viscosity of lung secretions. Assess for clinical improvement and record onset of relief of cough.

PATIENT/FAMILY TEACHING

- Avoid tasks that require alertness, motor skills until response to drug is established.
- Dry mouth, drowsiness, dizziness may be an expected response to drug.

benztropine

benz-**trow**-peen

(Apo-Benthropine ✱, Cogentin)

Do not confuse benztropine with bromocriptine.

CLASSIFICATION

PHARMACOTHERAPEUTIC: Anticholinergic. **CLINICAL:** Antiparkinson agent.

ACTION

Selectively blocks central cholinergic receptors, assists in balancing cholinergic/dopaminergic activity. **Therapeutic Effect:** Reduces incidence/severity of akinesia, rigidity, tremor.

PHARMACOKINETICS

Well absorbed following oral and IM administration. Oral onset of action: 1–2 hrs, IM onset of action: minutes. Pharmacologic effects may not be apparent until 2–3 days after initiation of therapy and may persist for up to 24 hrs after discontinuation of drug. **Half-life:** Extended.

USES

Treatment of Parkinson's disease, drug-induced extrapyramidal reactions (except tardive dyskinesia).

PRECAUTIONS

CONTRAINDICATIONS: Angle-closure glaucoma, benign prostatic hyperplasia, children younger than 3 yrs, GI obstruction, intestinal atony, megacolon, myasthenia gravis, paralytic ileus, severe ulcerative colitis. **CAUTIONS:** Treated open-angle glaucoma, heart disease, hypertension; pts with tachycardia, arrhythmias, prostatic hypertrophy, hepatic/renal impairment, obstructive diseases of GI/GU tract, urinary retention.

LIFESPAN CONSIDERATIONS:

Pregnancy/Lactation: Unknown if drug crosses placenta or is distributed in breast milk. **Pregnancy Category C. Children:** Safety and efficacy not established. **Elderly:** No age-related precautions noted, but there is a higher risk for adverse effects.

INTERACTIONS

DRUG: **Alcohol, CNS depressants** may increase sedation. **Amantadine, anticholinergics, MAOIs** may increase effects. **Antacids, antidiarrheals** may decrease absorption, effects. **HERBAL:** None significant. **FOOD:** None known. **LAB VALUES:** None known.

AVAILABILITY (Rx)

INJECTION, SOLUTION: 1 mg/ml. **TABLETS:** 0.5 mg, 1 mg, 2 mg.

ADMINISTRATION/HANDLING

IM

- Inject slow, deep IM.

PO

- Give without regard to food.

INDICATIONS/ROUTES/DOSAGE

PARKINSONISM

PO: ADULTS: 0.5–6 mg/day as a single dose or in 2 divided doses. Titrate by 0.5 mg at 5–6 day intervals. **ELDERLY:** Initially, 0.5 mg once or twice a day. Titrate by 0.5 mg at 5–6 day intervals. **Maximum:** 4 mg/day.

DRUG-INDUCED EXTRAPYRAMIDAL SYMPTOMS

PO, IM, IV: ADULTS: 1–4 mg once or twice a day. **CHILDREN OLDER THAN 3 YRS:** 0.02–0.05 mg/kg/dose once or twice a day.

ACUTE DYSTONIC REACTIONS

IV, IM: ADULTS: Initially, 1–2 mg; then 1–2 mg PO twice a day to prevent recurrence.

SIDE EFFECTS

FREQUENT: Somnolence, dry mouth, blurred vision, constipation, decreased diaphoresis or urination, GI upset, photosensitivity. **OCCASIONAL:** Headache, memory loss, muscle cramps, anxiety, peripheral paresthesia, orthostatic hypotension, abdominal cramps. **RARE:** Rash, confusion, eye pain.

ADVERSE EFFECTS/ TOXIC REACTIONS

Overdose may produce severe anticholinergic effects (unsteadiness, somnolence, tachycardia, dyspnea, skin flushing, dryness of mouth/nose/throat). Severe paradoxical reactions (hallucinations, tremor, seizures, toxic psychosis) may occur.

NURSING CONSIDERATIONS

BASELINE ASSESSMENT

Assess mental status for confusion, disorientation, agitation, psychotic-like symptoms (medication frequently produces such side effects in those older than 60 yrs).

INTERVENTION/EVALUATION

Be alert to neurologic effects: headache, drowsiness, mental confusion, agitation. Assess for clinical reversal of symptoms (improvement of tremor of head and hands at rest, mask-like facial

B

expression, shuffling gait, muscular rigidity).

PATIENT/FAMILY TEACHING

• Avoid tasks that require alertness, motor skills until response to drug is established. • Dry mouth, drowsiness, dizziness may be an expected response to drug. • Avoid alcoholic beverages during therapy. • Drowsiness tends to diminish or disappear with continued therapy.

beractant

burr-**act**-ant
(Survanta Intratracheal)

Do not confuse Survanta with Sufenta.

CLASSIFICATION

PHARMACOTHERAPEUTIC: Natural bovine lung extract. **CLINICAL:** Pulmonary surfactant.

ACTION

Lowers alveolar surface tension during respiration, stabilizing alveoli. **Therapeutic Effect:** Improves lung compliance, respiratory gas exchange.

PHARMACOKINETICS

Not absorbed systemically.

USES

Prevention and treatment (rescue) of respiratory distress syndrome (RDS—hyaline membrane disease) in premature infants. **Prevention:** Body weight less than 1,250 g in infants at risk for developing or with evidence of surfactant deficiency (give within 15 min of birth). **Rescue Therapy:** Treatment of infants with RDS confirmed by X-ray and requiring mechanical ventilation (give within 8 hrs of birth).

PRECAUTIONS

CONTRAINDICATIONS: None known. **CAUTIONS:** Those at risk for circulatory overload. This drug is for use only in neonates. **Pregnancy Category:** Not indicated for use in pregnant women.

INTERACTIONS

DRUG: None significant. **HERBAL:** None significant. **FOOD:** None known. **LAB VALUES:** None known.

AVAILABILITY (Rx)

SUSPENSION FOR INHALATION: 25 mg/ml (4 ml, 8 ml).

ADMINISTRATION/HANDLING

INTRATRACHEAL

Administration • Instill through catheter inserted into infant's endotracheal tube. Do not instill into main stem bronchus. • Monitor for bradycardia, decreased O_2 saturation during administration. Stop dosing procedure if these effects occur; begin appropriate measures before reinstituting therapy.

Storage • Refrigerate vials. • Warm by standing vial at room temperature for 20 min or warm in hand 8 min. • If settling occurs, gently swirl vial (do not shake) to redisperse. • After warming, may return to refrigerator within 8 hrs one time only. • Each vial should be injected with a needle only one time; discard unused portions. • Color appears off-white to light brown.

INDICATIONS/ROUTES/DOSAGE

PREVENTION AND RESCUE TREATMENT OF RDS OR HYALINE MEMBRANE DISEASE IN PREMATURE INFANTS

INTRATRACHEAL: INFANTS: 100 mg of phospholipids/kg birth weight (4 ml/kg). Give within 15 min of birth if infant weighs less than 1,250 g and has evidence of surfactant deficiency; give within 8 hrs when RDS is confirmed by X-ray and requires mechanical ventilation. May repeat 6 hrs or longer after preceding dose. **Maximum:** 4 doses in the first 48 hrs of life.

SIDE EFFECTS

FREQUENT: Transient bradycardia, oxygen (O_2) desaturation, increased carbon dioxide (CO_2) retention. **OCCASIONAL:** Endotracheal tube reflux. **RARE:** Apnea, endotracheal tube blockage, hypotension or hypertension, pallor, vasoconstriction.

ADVERSE EFFECTS/ TOXIC REACTIONS

Life-threatening nosocomial sepsis may occur.

NURSING CONSIDERATIONS

BASELINE ASSESSMENT

Drug must be administered in highly supervised setting. Clinicians caring for neonate must be experienced with intubation, ventilator management. Offer emotional support to parents.

INTERVENTION/EVALUATION

Monitor infant with arterial or transcutaneous measurement of systemic O_2, CO_2. Assess lung sounds for rales, moist breath sounds.

betamethasone

bay-ta-**meth**-a-sone

(Beta-Val, Betaderm ♣, Betaject ♣, Betnesol ♣, Betnovate ♣, Celestone, Celestone Soluspan, Diprolene, Diprolene AF, Ectosone ♣, Luxiq, Maxivate)

FIXED-COMBINATION(S)

Lotrisone: betamethasone/clotrimazole (an antifungal): 0.05%/1%. **Taclonex:** betamethasone/calcipotriene (an anti-psoriatic): 0.064%/0.005%

CLASSIFICATION

PHARMACOTHERAPEUTIC: Adrenocorticosteroid. **CLINICAL:** Anti-inflammatory, immunosuppressant (see pp. 92C, 94C).

ACTION

Controls rate of protein synthesis, depresses migration of polymorphonuclear leukocytes/fibroblasts, reverses capillary permeability, prevents or controls inflammation. **Therapeutic Effect:** Decreases tissue response to inflammatory process.

PHARMACOKINETICS

Rapidly and almost completely absorbed following PO administration. After topical application, limited absorption systemically. Metabolized in liver. Excreted in urine. **Half-life:** 36–54 hrs.

USES

Systemic: Anti-inflammatory, immunosuppressant, corticosteroid replacement therapy. **Topical:** Relief of inflammatory and pruritic dermatoses. **Foam:** Relief of inflammation, itching associated with dermatosis.

PRECAUTIONS

CONTRAINDICATIONS: Hypersensitivity to systemic fungal infections. **CAUTIONS:** Hypothyroidism, cirrhosis, nonspecific ulcerative colitis, pts at increased risk for peptic ulcer.

LIFESPAN CONSIDERATIONS:

Pregnancy/Lactation: Crosses placenta, distributed in breast milk. **Pregnancy Category C (D if used in first trimester).** **Children:** Prolonged treatment, high-dose therapy may decrease short-term growth rate, cortisol secretion. **Elderly:** Higher risk for developing hypertension, osteoporosis.

B

INTERACTIONS

DRUG: **Amphotericin** may increase hypokalemia. May decrease effect of **oral hypoglycemics, insulin, diuretics, potassium supplements.** May increase **digoxin** toxicity (due to hypokalemia). **Hepatic enzyme inducers** may decrease effect. **Live virus vaccines** may potentiate virus replication, increase vaccine side effects, decrease pt's antibody response to vaccine. **HERBAL:** **Cat's claw, echinacea** possess immunostimulant effects. **FOOD:** None known. **LAB VALUES:** May decrease serum calcium, potassium, thyroxine. May increase serum cholesterol, lipids, glucose, sodium, amylase.

AVAILABILITY (Rx)

CREAM: 0.05% **(DIPROLENE AF, MAXIVATE),** 0.1% **(BETAVAL). FOAM: (LUXIQ):** 0.12%. **GEL:** 0.05%. **INJECTION, SUSPENSION (CELESTONE SOLUSPAN):** 3 mg/ml. **LOTION:** 0.05% **(DIPROLENE, MAXIVATE),** 0.1% **(BETA-VAL). OINTMENT:** 0.05%, 0.1%. **SYRUP (CELESTONE):** 0.6 mg/5 ml.

ADMINISTRATION/HANDLING

IM

- Inject slowly, deep IM into large muscle mass.

PO

- Protect syrup from light and tablets from excessive moisture. • Give with milk or food (decreases GI upset). • Give single doses before 9 AM; give multiple doses at evenly spaced intervals.

TOPICAL

- Gently cleanse area before application. • Apply sparingly and rub into area thoroughly. • When using aerosol, spray area 3 sec from 15-cm (approximately 12 in) distance; avoid inhalation.

STORAGE

- Store all forms at room temperature.
- Protect parenteral form from light.

INDICATIONS/ROUTES/DOSAGE

ANTI-INFLAMMATION, IMMUNOSUPPRESSION, CORTICOSTEROID REPLACEMENT THERAPY

PO: ADULTS, ELDERLY: 0.6–7.2 mg/day. **CHILDREN:** 0.0175–0.25 mg/kg/day in 3–4 divided doses.

IM: ADULTS, ELDERLY: 0.5–9 mg/day in 2 divided doses. **CHILDREN:** 0.0175–0.125 mg/kg/day in 3–4 divided doses.

RELIEF OF INFLAMMED AND PRURITIC DERMATOSES

TOPICAL: ADULTS, ELDERLY: 1–3 times a day. **Foam:** Apply twice a day.

SIDE EFFECTS

FREQUENT: Systemic: Increased appetite, abdominal distention, nervousness, insomnia, false sense of well-being. **Topical:** Burning, stinging, pruritus. **OCCASIONAL: Systemic:** Dizziness, facial flushing, diaphoresis, decreased or blurred vision, mood swings. **Topical:** Allergic contact dermatitis, purpura or blood-containing blisters, thinning of skin with easy bruising, telangiectases or raised dark red spots on skin.

ADVERSE EFFECTS/ TOXIC REACTIONS

Overdose may cause systemic hypercorticism, adrenal suppression.

NURSING CONSIDERATIONS

BASELINE ASSESSMENT

Question for hypersensitivity to any of the corticosteroids, sulfite. Obtain baselines for height, weight, B/P, glucose, electrolytes. Check results of initial tests (tuberculosis [TB] skin test, X-rays, EKG).

INTERVENTION/EVALUATION

Monitor B/P, blood glucose, electrolytes. Apply topical preparation sparingly. Not for use on broken skin or in areas of infection. Do not apply to wet skin, face, inguinal areas.

B

PATIENT/FAMILY TEACHING

• Take with food, milk. • Take single daily dose in the morning. • Do not stop abruptly. • Apply topical preparations in a thin layer. • Do not receive smallpox vaccination during or immediately after therapy.

Betaseron, *see interferon beta 1b*

betaxolol

bay-**tax**-oh-lol
(Betoptic, Betoptic-S, Kerlone)

Do not confuse betaxolol with bethanechol.

CLASSIFICATION

PHARMACOTHERAPEUTIC: Beta-adrenergic blocker. **CLINICAL:** Antihypertensive; antiglaucoma (see pp. 49C, 67C).

ACTION

Blocks $beta_1$-adrenergic receptors in cardiac tissue. Reduces aqueous humor production. **Therapeutic Effect:** Slows sinus heart rate, decreases B/P, reduces intraocular pressure (IOP).

USES

Ophthalmic: Treatment of chronic open-angle glaucoma, ocular hypertension. **Systemic:** Management of hypertension. **OFF-LABEL:** Treatment of angle-closure glaucoma during or after iridectomy, malignant glaucoma, secondary glaucoma; with miotics, to decrease IOP in acute and chronic angle-closure glaucoma.

PRECAUTIONS

CONTRAINDICATIONS: Cardiogenic shock, overt cardiac failure, second- or third-degree heart block, sinus bradycardia. **CAUTIONS:** Renal/hepatic impairment, peripheral vascular disease, hyperthyroidism, diabetes mellitus, inadequate cardiac function. **Pregnancy Category C (D if used in second or third trimester).**

INTERACTIONS

DRUG: **Diuretics, other antihypertensives** may increase hypotensive effect. **Sympathomimetics, xanthines** may mutually inhibit effect. May mask symptoms of hypoglycemia, prolong hypoglycemic effect of **insulin, oral hypoglycemics. NSAIDs** may decrease antihypertensive effect. **Cimetidine** may increase concentration. **HERBAL:** **Ephedra, ginseng, yohimbe** may worsen hypertension. **Garlic** may have increased antihypertensive effect. **FOOD:** None known. **LAB VALUES:** May increase ANA titer, BUN, serum creatinine, potassium, uric acid, lipoproteins, triglycerides.

AVAILABILITY (Rx)

OPHTHALMIC SOLUTION (BETOPTIC): 0.5%. **OPHTHALMIC SUSPENSION (BETOPTIC-S):** 0.25%. **TABLETS (KERLONE):** 10 mg, 20 mg.

ADMINISTRATION/HANDLING

PO

• Give without regard to meals. • Obtain standing systolic B/P 1 hr after drug administration.

OPHTHALMIC

• Place gloved finger on lower eyelid and pull out until a pocket is formed between eye and lower lid. • Hold dropper above pocket and place prescribed number of drops into pocket. • Instruct pt to close eye gently (so medication will not be squeezed out of the sac). • Apply digital pressure to the lacrimal sac for 1 min to minimize systemic absorption.

INDICATIONS/ROUTES/DOSAGE

HYPERTENSION

PO: ADULTS: Initially, 5–10 mg/day. May increase to 20 mg/day after 7–14 days. **ELDERLY:** Initially, 5 mg/day.

CHRONIC OPEN-ANGLE GLAUCOMA AND OCULAR HYPERTENSION

OPHTHALMIC (SOLUTION): ADULTS, ELDERLY: 1 drop twice a day.

OPHTHALMIC (SUSPENSION): ADULTS, ELDERLY: 1–2 drops twice a day.

DOSAGE IN RENAL IMPAIRMENT

For adult and elderly pts who are on dialysis, initially give 5 mg/day; increase by 5 mg/day q2wk. **Maximum:** 20 mg/day.

SIDE EFFECTS

Betaxolol is generally well tolerated, with mild and transient side effects. **FREQUENT: Systemic:** Hypotension manifested as dizziness, nausea, diaphoresis, headache, fatigue, constipation or diarrhea, dyspnea. **Ophthalmic:** Eye irritation, visual disturbances. **OCCASIONAL: Systemic:** Insomnia, flatulence, urinary frequency, impotence or decreased libido. **Ophthalmic:** Increased light sensitivity, watering of eye. **RARE: Systemic:** Rash, arrhythmias, arthralgia, myalgia, confusion, altered taste, increased urination. **Ophthalmic:** Dry eye, conjunctivitis, eye pain.

ADVERSE EFFECTS/ TOXIC REACTIONS

Overdose may produce profound bradycardia, hypotension, bronchospasm. Abrupt withdrawal may result in diaphoresis, palpitations, headache, tremors. May precipitate CHF, MI in pts with cardiac disease; thyroid storm in those with thyrotoxicosis, peripheral ischemia in those with existing peripheral vascular disease. Hypoglycemia may occur in previously controlled diabetes. Ophthalmic overdose may produce bradycardia, hypotension, bronchospasm, acute cardiac failure.

NURSING CONSIDERATIONS

BASELINE ASSESSMENT

PO: Assess baseline renal and hepatic function tests. Assess B/P, apical pulse immediately before drug is administered (if pulse is 60/min or less or systolic B/P is less than 90 mm Hg, withhold medication, contact physician).

INTERVENTION/EVALUATION

Monitor B/P for hypotension. Assess pulse for quality, irregular rate, bradycardia. Monitor daily pattern of bowel activity/stool consistency. Assist with ambulation if dizziness occurs. Assess for evidence of CHF: dyspnea (particularly on exertion or lying down), night cough, peripheral edema, distended neck veins, increase in weight, decrease in urine output. Assess for nausea, diaphoresis, headache, fatigue.

PATIENT/FAMILY TEACHING

• Do not abruptly discontinue medication. • Compliance with therapy regimen is essential to control glaucoma, hypertension. • To avoid hypotensive effect, rise slowly from lying to sitting position, wait momentarily before standing. • Avoid tasks that require alertness, motor skills until response to drug is established. • Report shortness of breath, excessive fatigue, prolonged dizziness, headache. • Do not use nasal decongestants, OTC cold preparations (stimulants) without physician approval. • Restrict salt, alcohol intake.

bethanechol

be-**than**-e-kole
(Duvoid, Myotonachol ✤, Urecholine)

Do not confuse bethanechol with betaxolol.

CLASSIFICATION

PHARMACOTHERAPEUTIC: Cholinergic (see p. 85C).

ACTION

Acts directly at cholinergic receptors in smooth muscle of urinary bladder, GI tract. Increases detrusor muscle tone. **Therapeutic Effect:** May initiate micturition, bladder emptying. Stimulates gastric, intestinal motility.

PHARMACOKINETICS

Poorly absorbed following PO administration. Does not cross blood-brain barrier. **Half-life:** Unknown.

USES

Treatment of nonobstructive urinary retention, retention due to neurogenic bladder. **OFF-LABEL:** Treatment of congenital megacolon, gastroesophageal reflux, postoperative gastric atony.

PRECAUTIONS

CONTRAINDICATIONS: Active or latent bronchial asthma, acute inflammatory GI tract conditions, anastomosis, bladder wall instability, cardiac or coronary artery disease, epilepsy, hypertension, hyperthyroidism, hypotension, mechanical GI or urinary tract obstruction or recent GI resection, parkinsonism, peptic ulcer, pronounced bradycardia, vasomotor instability. **CAUTIONS:** Presence of bacteremia, urinary retention.

LIFESPAN CONSIDERATIONS:

Pregnancy/Lactation: Unknown if drug crosses placenta or is distributed in breast milk. **Pregnancy Category C.** **Children/Elderly:** No age-related precautions noted.

INTERACTIONS

DRUG: **Cholinesterase inhibitors** may increase effects/toxicity. **Procainamide, quinidine** may decrease effect. **HERBAL:** None significant. **FOOD:** None known. **LAB VALUES:** May increase serum amylase, lipase, AST.

AVAILABILITY (Rx)

INJECTION, SOLUTION: 5 mg/ml (Urecholine). **TABLETS:** 5 mg (Urecholine), 10 mg (Duvoid, Urecholine), 25 mg (Duvoid, Urecholine), 50 mg (Duvoid, Urecholine).

INDICATIONS/ROUTES/DOSAGE

POSTOPERATIVE AND POSTPARTUM URINE RETENTION, ATONY OF BLADDER

PO: ADULTS, ELDERLY: 10–50 mg 3–4 times a day. Minimum effective dose determined by giving 5–10 mg initially, repeating same amount at 1-hr intervals until desired response is achieved. **CHILDREN:** 0.6 mg/kg/day in 3–4 divided doses.

SUBCUTANEOUS: ADULTS, ELDERLY: Initially, 2.5–5 mg. Minimum effective dose determined by giving 2.5 mg (0.5 ml), repeating same amount at 15- to 30-min intervals up to a maximum of 4 doses. Minimum dose repeated 3–4 times a day. **CHILDREN:** 0.2 mg/kg/day in 3–4 divided doses.

SIDE EFFECTS

OCCASIONAL: Belching, changes in vision, blurred vision, diarrhea, frequent urinary urgency. **RARE:** **Subcutaneous:** Shortness of breath, chest tightness, bronchospasm.

ADVERSE EFFECTS/ TOXIC REACTIONS

Overdose produces CNS stimulation (insomnia, anxiety, orthostatic hypotension), cholinergic stimulation, (headache, increased salivation/diaphoresis, nausea, vomiting, flushed skin, abdominal pain, seizures).

NURSING CONSIDERATIONS

BASELINE ASSESSMENT

Violent cholinergic reaction if given IM or IV (circulatory collapse, severe hypotension, bloody diarrhea, shock, cardiac arrest). **Antidote:** 0.6–1.2 mg atropine sulfate.

INTERVENTION/EVALUATION

Assess for cholinergic reaction: GI discomfort or cramping, feeling of facial warmth, excessive salivation/diaphoresis, lacrimation, pallor, urinary urgency, blurred vision. Question for complaints of difficulty chewing, swallowing, progressive muscle weakness.

PATIENT/FAMILY TEACHING

- Report nausea, vomiting, diarrhea, diaphoresis, increased salivary secretions, irregular heartbeat, muscle weakness, severe abdominal pain, difficulty breathing.

bevacizumab

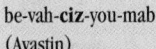

be-vah-**ciz**-you-mab
(Avastin)

CLASSIFICATION

PHARMACOTHERAPEUTIC: Monoclonal antibody. **CLINICAL:** Antineoplastic.

ACTION

Binds to and inhibits vascular endothelial growth factor, a protein that plays a major role in formation of new blood vessels to tumors. **Therapeutic Effect:** Inhibits metastatic disease progression.

PHARMACOKINETICS

Clearance varies by body weight, gender, tumor burden. **Half-life:** 20 days (range, 11–50 days).

USES

Combination chemotherapy with 5-fluorouracil (5-FU) for first-line treatment of pts with colorectal cancer. First-line treatment on nonsquamous, non-small cell lung cancer (NSCLC). **OFF-LABEL:** Adjunctive therapy in breast cancer, malignant mesothelioma, ovarian cancer, prostate cancer, renal cell carcinoma.

PRECAUTIONS

CONTRAINDICATIONS: GI perforation, hypertensive crisis, nephrotic syndrome, recent hemoptysis, serious bleeding, wound dehiscence requiring medical intervention. **CAUTIONS:** Hypertension, proteinuria, CHF, epistaxis, renal insufficiency.

LIFESPAN CONSIDERATIONS:

Pregnancy/Lactation: Teratogenic. Potential for fertility impairment. May decrease maternal and fetal body weight; increase risk of skeletal fetal abnormalities. Do not breast-feed. **Pregnancy Category C.** **Children:** Safety and efficacy not established. **Elderly:** Higher incidence of severe adverse reactions in pts older than 65 yrs.

INTERACTIONS

DRUG: None significant. **HERBAL:** None significant. **FOOD:** None known. **LAB VALUES:** May decrease serum potassium, sodium, WBC count, Hgb, Hct, platelet count.

AVAILABILITY (Rx)

INJECTION, SOLUTION: 25-mg/ml vial.

ADMINISTRATION/HANDLING

IV

◄ **ALERT** ► Do not give by IV push or bolus.

Reconstitution • Withdraw amount of bevacizumab for a dose of 5 mg/kg and dilute in 100 ml 0.9% NaCl. • Discard any unused portion.

Rate of administration • Infuse IV over 90 min following chemotherapy. • If first infusion is well tolerated, second infusion may be administered over 60 min. • If 60-min infusion is well tolerated, all subsequent infusions may be administered over 30 min.

Storage • Refrigerate vials. • Diluted solution may be stored for up to 8 hrs if refrigerated.

IV INCOMPATIBILITIES

Do not mix with dextrose solutions.

INDICATIONS/ROUTES/DOSAGE

COLORECTAL CANCER

IV: ADULTS, ELDERLY: 5 mg/kg once every 14 days.

NSCLC

IV: ADULTS, ELDERLY: 15 mg/kg every 3 wks.

DOSE ADJUSTMENT FOR TOXICITY

Temporary Suspension: Mild to moderate proteinuria, severe hypertension not controlled with medical management. **Permanent Discontinuation:** Wound dehiscence requiring intervention, GI perforation, hypertensive crises, serious bleeding, nephrotic syndrome.

SIDE EFFECTS

FREQUENT (73%–25%): Asthenia, vomiting, anorexia, hypertension, epistaxis, stomatitis, constipation, headache, dyspnea. **OCCASIONAL (21%–15%):** Altered taste, dry skin, exfoliative dermatitis, dizziness, flatulence, excessive lacrimation, skin discoloration, weight loss, myalgia. **RARE (8%–6%):** Nail disorder, skin ulcer, alopecia, confusion, abnormal gait, dry mouth.

ADVERSE EFFECTS/ TOXIC REACTIONS

UTI, manifested as urinary frequency/ urgency and proteinuria, occurs frequently. Most serious adverse effects include CHF, deep vein thrombosis, GI perforation, wound dehiscence, hypertensive crisis, nephrotic syndrome, severe hemorrhage. Anemia, neutropenia, thrombocytopenia occur occasionally. Hypersensitivity reactions occur rarely.

NURSING CONSIDERATIONS

BASELINE ASSESSMENT

Monitor B/P regularly during treatment. Assess for proteinuria with urinalysis. For those with 2+ or greater urine dipstick reading, a 24-hr urine collection is advisable. Monitor CBC, serum potassium, sodium levels at regular intervals during therapy.

INTERVENTION/EVALUATION

Assess for asthenia (loss of strength, energy). Assist with ambulation if asthenia occurs. Monitor for fever, chills, abdominal pain. Offer antiemetic if nausea, vomiting occurs. Monitor daily pattern of bowel activity/stool consistency.

PATIENT/FAMILY TEACHING

• Do not have immunizations without physician's approval (lowers body's resistance). • Avoid contact with anyone who recently received a live virus vaccine. • Avoid crowds, those with infection. • Warn female pt of childbearing age of potential fetal risk if pregnancy occurs.

bexarotene (High Alert)

becks-**aye**-row-teen
(Targretin, Targretin Topical)

CLASSIFICATION

PHARMACOTHERAPEUTIC: Retinoid. **CLINICAL:** Antineoplastic (see p. 76C).

B

ACTION

Binds to and activates retinoid X receptor subtypes that regulate the genes that control cellular differentiation and proliferation. **Therapeutic Effect:** Inhibits growth of tumor cell lines of hematopoietic and squamous cell origin, induces tumor regression.

PHARMACOKINETICS

Moderately absorbed from GI tract. Protein binding: greater than 99%. Metabolized in the liver. Primarily eliminated through the hepatobiliary system. **Half-life:** 7 hrs.

USES

Oral: Treatment of cutaneous T-cell lymphoma (CTCL) in those refractory to at least one prior systemic therapy. **Topical:** Treatment of cutaneous lesions in those with refractory CTCL (stage 1A and 1B) or not tolerant of other therapies. **OFF-LABEL:** Treatment of diabetes mellitus; head, neck, lung, renal cell carcinomas; Kaposi's sarcoma.

PRECAUTIONS

CONTRAINDICATIONS: None known. **CAUTIONS:** Hepatic impairment, diabetes mellitus, lipid abnormalities.

LIFESPAN CONSIDERATIONS:

Pregnancy/Lactation: May cause fetal harm. Unknown if distributed in breast milk. **Pregnancy Category X. Children:** Safety and efficacy not established. **Elderly:** No age-related precautions noted.

INTERACTIONS

DRUG: Bone marrow depressants, medications causing blood dyscrasias may have adverse additive effects. **Phenobarbital, phenytoin, rifampin** may decrease plasma concentrations. **Erythromycin, gemfibrozil, itraconazole, ketoconazole** may increase plasma concentrations. Bexarotene may reduce **tamoxifen** concentrations, may enhance hypoglycemic effect of **insulin, oral hypoglycemics. Live virus vaccines** may potentiate virus replication, increase vaccine side effects, decrease pt's antibody response to vaccine. **HERBAL: Dong quai, St. John's wort** may cause photosensitization. **St. John's wort** may decrease plasma concentrations. **FOOD: Grapefruit, grapefruit juice** may increase concentration/toxicity. **LAB VALUES:** CA-125 in ovarian cancer may be increased. May produce abnormal hepatic function tests; increase serum cholesterol, triglycerides, total and LDL cholesterol; decrease HDL cholesterol.

AVAILABILITY (Rx)

CAPSULES (SOFT GELATIN [TARGRETIN]): 75 mg. **TOPICAL GEL (TARGRETIN TOPICAL):** 1%.

ADMINISTRATION/HANDLING

PO

- Give with food.

TOPICAL

- Generously coat lesions with gel.
- Allow to dry before covering.
- Avoid applying gel to normal skin surrounding lesions or near mucosal surfaces.

INDICATIONS/ROUTES/DOSAGE

CUTANEOUS T-CELL LYMPHOMA REFRACTORY TO AT LEAST ONE PRIOR SYSTEMIC THERAPY

PO: ADULTS: 300 mg/m^2/day. If no tumor response after 8 wks and initial dose is well tolerated, may be increased to 400 mg/m^2/day. If not tolerated, may decrease to 200 mg/m^2/day, then to 100 mg/m^2/day, or temporarily suspended to manage toxicity. **TOPICAL: ADULTS:** Initially, apply once every other day for first wk. May increase at weekly intervals to once daily, then twice a day, then 3 times a day up to 4 times a day.

SIDE EFFECTS

FREQUENT: Hyperlipidemia (79%), headache (30%), hypothyroidism (29%), asthenia (20%). **OCCASIONAL:** Rash (17%); nausea (15%); peripheral edema (13%); dry skin, abdominal pain (11%); chills, exfoliative dermatitis (10%); diarrhea (7%).

ADVERSE EFFECTS/ TOXIC REACTIONS

Pancreatitis, hepatic failure, pneumonia occur rarely.

NURSING CONSIDERATIONS

BASELINE ASSESSMENT

Assess baseline lipid profile, WBC, hepatic function, thyroid function. Question about possibility of pregnancy (Pregnancy Category X). Warn women of childbearing age about potential fetal risk if pregnancy occurs. Instruct on need for use of 2 reliable forms of contraceptives concurrently during therapy and for 1 mo after discontinuation of therapy, even in infertile, premenopausal woman.

INTERVENTION/EVALUATION

Monitor serum cholesterol, triglycerides, CBC, hepatic and thyroid function tests.

PATIENT/FAMILY TEACHING

• Do not use medicated, drying, abrasive soaps; wash with gentle, bland soap. • Inform physician if pregnant or planning to become pregnant (Pregnancy Category X).

Biaxin, *see clarithromycin*

Biaxin XL, *see clarithromycin*

bicalutamide

by-kale-**yew**-tah-myd
(Casodex)

CLASSIFICATION

PHARMACOTHERAPEUTIC: Antiandrogen hormone. **CLINICAL:** Antineoplastic (see p. 76C).

ACTION

Competitively inhibits androgen action by binding to androgen receptors in target tissue. **Therapeutic Effect:** Decreases growth of prostatic carcinoma.

PHARMACOKINETICS

Well absorbed from GI tract. Protein binding: 96%. Metabolized in the liver to inactive metabolite. Excreted in urine and feces. Not removed by hemodialysis. **Half-life:** 5.8 days.

USES

Treatment of advanced metastatic prostatic carcinoma (in combination with luteinizing hormone-releasing hormone [LHRH] agonistic analogues—i.e., leuprolide). Treatment with both drugs must be started at same time.

PRECAUTIONS

CONTRAINDICATIONS: Women, esp. those who may become pregnant. **CAUTIONS:** Moderate to severe hepatic impairment.

LIFESPAN CONSIDERATIONS:

Pregnancy/Lactation: May inhibit spermatogenesis, not used in women. **Pregnancy Category X.** **Children:** Safety and efficacy not established. **Elderly:** No age-related precautions noted.

INTERACTIONS

DRUG: May increase **warfarin** effect. **HERBAL:** None significant. **FOOD:** None known. **LAB VALUES:** May increase

B

serum AST, ALT, alkaline phosphatase, creatinine, bilirubin, BUN. May decrease WBC, Hgb.

AVAILABILITY (Rx)

TABLETS: 50 mg.

ADMINISTRATION/HANDLING

PO

• Give without regard to food. • Take at same time each day.

INDICATIONS/ROUTES/DOSAGE

PROSTATIC CARCINOMA

PO: ADULTS, ELDERLY: 50–150 mg once a day in morning or evening, given concurrently with an LHRH analogue or after surgical castration.

SIDE EFFECTS

FREQUENT: Hot flashes (49%), breast pain (38%), muscle pain (27%), constipation (17%), asthenia (15%), diarrhea (10%), nausea (11%). **OCCASIONAL (9%–8%):** Nocturia, abdominal pain, peripheral edema. **RARE (7%–3%):** Vomiting, weight loss, dizziness, insomnia, rash, impotence, gynecomastia.

ADVERSE EFFECTS/ TOXIC REACTIONS

Sepsis, CHF, hypertension, iron deficiency anemia, interstitial pneumonitis, pulmonary fibrosis may occur. Severe hepatotoxicity occurs rarely within the first 3–4 mos after treatment initiation.

NURSING CONSIDERATIONS

INTERVENTION/EVALUATION

Perform periodic hepatic function tests. If transaminases increase over 2 times the upper limit of normal, discontinue treatment. Monitor for diarrhea, nausea, vomiting.

PATIENT/FAMILY TEACHING

• Do not stop taking medication (both drugs must be continued). • Take medications at same time each day. • Explain possible expectancy of frequent side effects. • Contact physician if persistent nausea, vomiting occur.

bimatoprost

(Lumigan)

See Antiglaucoma agents (p. 49C)

bisacodyl

bise-ah-**co**-dahl

(Alophen, Apo-Bisacodyl ✤, Dulcolax, Fleet, Gentlax, Modane, Veracolate)

Do not confuse Veracolate with Accolate or Modane with Mudrane.

CLASSIFICATION

PHARMACOTHERAPEUTIC: GI stimulant. **CLINICAL:** Laxative (see p. 118C).

ACTION

Direct effect on colonic smooth musculature by stimulating intramural nerve plexi. **Therapeutic Effect:** Promotes fluid and ion accumulation in colon increasing peristalsis, producing laxative effect.

PHARMACOKINETICS

Route	Onset	Peak	Duration
PO	6–12 hrs	N/A	N/A
Rectal	15–60 min	N/A	N/A

Minimal absorption following oral and rectal administration. Absorbed drug is excreted in urine; remainder is eliminated in feces.

USES

Treatment of constipation, colonic evacuation before examinations or procedures.

PRECAUTIONS

CONTRAINDICATIONS: Abdominal pain, appendicitis, intestinal obstruction, nausea, undiagnosed rectal bleeding, vomiting. **CAUTIONS:** Excessive use may lead to fluid, electrolyte imbalance.

LIFESPAN CONSIDERATIONS:

Pregnancy/Lactation: Unknown if drug crosses placenta or is distributed in breast milk. **Pregnancy Category C.** **Children:** Avoid in children younger than 6 yrs (usually unable to describe symptoms or more severe side effects). **Elderly:** Repeated use may cause weakness, orthostatic hypotension due to electrolyte loss.

INTERACTIONS

DRUG: **Antacids, cimetidine, famotidine, ranitidine** may cause rapid dissolution of bisacodyl, producing abdominal cramping, vomiting. May decrease transit time of concurrently administered **oral medications,** decreasing absorption. **HERBAL:** None significant. **FOOD:** **Milk** may cause rapid dissolution of bisacodyl. **LAB VALUES:** May increase blood glucose concentration. May decrease serum potassium.

AVAILABILITY (OTC)

RECTAL ENEMA (FLEET): 10 mg/30 ml. **SUPPOSITORIES (DULCOLAX, FLEET):** 10 mg.

TABLETS (ENTERIC-COATED [DULCOLAX, FLEET]): 5 mg.

ADMINISTRATION/HANDLING

PO

• Give on empty stomach (faster action). • Offer 6–8 glasses of water a day (aids stool softening). • Administer tablets whole; do not chew or crush. • Avoid giving within 1 hr of antacids, milk, other oral medication.

RECTAL, ENEMA

• Shake bottle, and remove orange protective shield from tip. • Position pt on left side with left knee slightly bent and right leg drawn up, or in knee-chest position. • Insert tip into rectum, aiming at pt's umbilicus.

RECTAL, SUPPOSITORY

• If suppository is too soft, chill for 30 min in refrigerator or run cold water over foil wrapper. • Moisten suppository with cold water before inserting well into rectum.

STORAGE

• Store rectal enema, suppositories at room temperature.

INDICATIONS/ROUTES/DOSAGE

TREATMENT OF CONSTIPATION

PO: **ADULTS, CHILDREN OLDER THAN 12 YRS:** 5–15 mg as needed. **Maximum:** 30 mg. **CHILDREN 3–12 YRS:** 5–10 mg or 0.3 mg/kg at bedtime or after breakfast. **ELDERLY:** Initially, 5 mg/day.

RECTAL, ENEMA: **ADULTS, CHILDREN OLDER THAN 12 YRS:** One 1.25-oz bottle in a single daily dose.

RECTAL, SUPPOSITORY: **ADULTS, CHILDREN OLDER THAN 12 YRS:** 10 mg to induce bowel movement. **CHILDREN 2–12 YRS:** 5–10 mg as a single dose. **CHILDREN YOUNGER THAN 2 YRS:** 5 mg. **ELDERLY:** 5–10 mg/day.

SIDE EFFECTS

FREQUENT: Some degree of abdominal discomfort, nausea, mild cramps, faintness. **OCCASIONAL:** Rectal administration: burning of rectal mucosa, mild proctitis.

ADVERSE EFFECTS/ TOXIC REACTIONS

Long-term use may result in laxative dependence, chronic constipation, loss of normal bowel function. Chronic use or

B

overdose may result in electrolyte or metabolic disturbances (hypokalemia, hypocalcemia, metabolic acidosis, alkalosis), persistent diarrhea, vomiting, muscle weakness, malabsorption, weight loss.

NURSING CONSIDERATIONS

INTERVENTION/EVALUATION

Encourage adequate fluid intake. Assess bowel sounds for peristalsis. Monitor daily pattern of bowel activity/stool consistency; record time of evacuation. Assess for abdominal disturbances. Monitor serum electrolytes in those exposed to prolonged, frequent, or excessive use of medication.

PATIENT/FAMILY TEACHING

• Institute measures to promote defecation: increase fluid intake, exercise, high-fiber diet. • Do not take antacids, milk, or other medication within 1 hr of taking medication (decreased effectiveness). • Report unrelieved constipation, rectal bleeding, muscle pain or cramps, dizziness, weakness.

bismuth

bis-muth

(Bismed 🍁, Diotame, Kaopectate, Maalox Total Stomach Relief, Pepto-Bismol)

FIXED-COMBINATION(S)

Helidac: bismuth/metronidazole/tetracycline: 262 mg/250 mg/500 mg.

CLASSIFICATION

PHARMACOTHERAPEUTIC: Antisecretory, antimicrobial. **CLINICAL:** Antidiarrheal, antinauseant, antiulcer (see p. 43C).

ACTION

Absorbs water, toxins in large intestine, forms a protective coating in intestinal mucosa. Possesses antisecretory and antimicrobial effects. **Therapeutic Effect:** Prevents diarrhea.

USES

Treatment of diarrhea, indigestion, nausea. Adjunct in treatment of *H. pylori*–associated peptic ulcer disease. **OFF-LABEL:** Prevention of traveler's diarrhea.

PRECAUTIONS

CONTRAINDICATIONS: Bleeding ulcers, gout, hemophilia, hemorrhagic states, renal impairment. **CAUTIONS:** Elderly, diabetic pts. **Pregnancy Category C.**

INTERACTIONS

DRUG: **Anticoagulants, heparin, thrombolytics** may increase the risk of bleeding. **Aspirin, other salicylates** may increase risk of salicylate toxicity. Large dose may increase the effects of **insulin, oral antidiabetics.** May decrease absorption of **tetracyclines**. **HERBAL:** None significant. **FOOD:** None known. **LAB VALUES:** May alter serum alkaline phosphatase, AST, ALT, uric acid levels. May decrease serum potassium. May prolong PT.

AVAILABILITY (OTC)

CAPLET: **(PEPTO-BISMOL):** 262 mg. **LIQUID:** 262 mg/15 ml **(DIOTAME, KAOPECTATE, PEPTO-BISMOL)**, 525 mg/15 ml **(KAOPECTATE EXTRA STRENGTH, MAALOX TOTAL STOMACH RELIEF, PEPTO-BISMOL MAXIMUM STRENGTH)**. **SUSPENSION:** 262 mg/15 ml. **TABLETS, CHEWABLE:** **(DIOTAME, PEPTO-BISMOL):** 262 mg.

ADMINISTRATION/HANDLING

• Shake suspension well. • Chew or dissolve chewable tablet before swallowing.

INDICATIONS/ROUTES/DOSAGE

DIARRHEA, GASTRIC DISTRESS

PO: ADULTS, ELDERLY: 2 tablets (30 ml) q30–60min. **Maximum:** 8 doses in 24 hrs. **CHILDREN 9–12 YRS:** 1 tablet or 15 ml q30–60min. **Maximum:** 8 doses in 24 hrs. **CHILDREN 6–8 YRS:** ⅔ tablet or 10 ml q30–60min. **Maximum:** 8 doses in 24 hrs. **CHILDREN 3–5 YRS:** ⅓ tablet or 5 ml q30–60min. **Maximum:** 8 doses in 24 hrs.

***H. PYLORI*–ASSOCIATED DUODENAL ULCER, GASTRITIS**

PO: ADULTS, ELDERLY: 525 mg 4 times a day, with 500 mg amoxicillin and 500 mg metronidazole, 3 times a day after meals, for 7–14 days.

CHRONIC INFANT DIARRHEA

PO: CHILDREN 2–24 MOS: 2.5 ml q4h.

SIDE EFFECTS

FREQUENT: Grayish black stools. **RARE:** Constipation.

ADVERSE EFFECTS/ TOXIC REACTIONS

Debilitated pts and infants may develop impaction.

NURSING CONSIDERATIONS

INTERVENTION/EVALUATION

Encourage adequate fluid intake. Assess bowel sounds for peristaltic activity. Monitor daily pattern of bowel activity/stool consistency.

PATIENT/FAMILY TEACHING

• Stool may appear gray/black. • Chew the chewable tablets thoroughly before swallowing.

bisoprolol ⚑

bye-**sew**-pro-lol

(Monocor ✤, Zebeta)

Do not confuse Zebeta with DiaBeta.

FIXED-COMBINATION(S)

Ziac: bisoprolol/hydrochlorothiazide (a diuretic): 2.5 mg/6.25 mg; 5 mg/6.25 mg; 10 mg/6.25 mg.

CLASSIFICATION

PHARMACOTHERAPEUTIC: Beta-adrenergic blocker. **CLINICAL:** Antihypertensive (see p. 68C).

ACTION

Blocks $beta_1$-adrenergic receptors in cardiac tissue. **Therapeutic Effect:** Slows sinus heart rate, decreases B/P.

PHARMACOKINETICS

Well absorbed from GI tract. Protein binding: 26%–33%. Metabolized in the liver. Primarily excreted in urine. Not removed by hemodialysis. **Half-life:** 9–12 hrs (increased in renal impairment).

USES

Management of hypertension, alone or in combination with diuretics, other medications. **OFF-LABEL:** Angina pectoris, premature ventricular contractions, supraventricular arrhythmias, CHF.

PRECAUTIONS

CONTRAINDICATIONS: Cardiogenic shock, marked sinus bradycardia, overt cardiac failure, second- or third-degree heart block. **CAUTIONS:** Renal/hepatic impairment, peripheral vascular disease, hyperthyroidism, diabetes, inadequate cardiac function, bronchospastic disease.

LIFESPAN CONSIDERATIONS:

Pregnancy/Lactation: Readily crosses placenta; distributed in breast milk. Avoid use during first trimester. May produce bradycardia, apnea, hypoglycemia, hypothermia during delivery, low birth-weight infants. **Pregnancy Category C (D if used in second or third trimester).** **Children:** Safety and efficacy not established. **Elderly:** Age-related peripheral vascular disease may increase risk of decreased peripheral circulation.

INTERACTIONS

DRUG: **Diuretics, other antihypertensives** may increase hypotensive effect. **Sympathomimetics, xanthines** may mutually inhibit effects. May mask symptoms of hypoglycemia, prolong hypoglycemic effect of **insulin, oral hypoglycemics. NSAIDs** may decrease antihypertensive effect. **Cimetidine** may increase concentration. **HERBAL:** **Ephedra, yohimbe, ginseng** may worsen hypertension. **Garlic** may have increased antihypertensive effect. **FOOD:** None known. **LAB VALUES:** May increase ANA titer, BUN, serum creatinine, potassium, uric acid, lipoproteins, triglycerides.

AVAILABILITY (Rx)

TABLETS: 5 mg, 10 mg.

ADMINISTRATION/HANDLING

PO

• Give without regard to food. • Scored tablet may be crushed.

INDICATIONS/ROUTES/DOSAGE

HYPERTENSION

PO: ADULTS: Initially, 2.5–5 mg/day. May increase up to 20 mg/day. **ELDERLY:** Initially, 2.5 mg/day. May increase by 2.5–5 mg/day. **Maximum:** 20 mg/day.

DOSAGE IN HEPATIC/RENAL IMPAIRMENT

For adults and elderly pts with cirrhosis or hepatitis whose creatinine clearance is less than 40 ml/min, initially give 2.5 mg.

SIDE EFFECTS

FREQUENT: Hypotension manifested as dizziness, nausea, diaphoresis, headache, cold extremities, fatigue, constipation, diarrhea. **OCCASIONAL:** Insomnia, flatulence, urinary frequency, impotence or decreased libido. **RARE:** Rash, arthralgia, myalgia, confusion (esp. in the elderly), altered taste.

ADVERSE EFFECTS/ TOXIC REACTIONS

Overdose may produce profound bradycardia, hypotension. Abrupt withdrawal may result in diaphoresis, palpitations, headache, tremors. May precipitate CHF, MI in pts with cardiac disease, thyroid storm in those with thyrotoxicosis, peripheral ischemia in those with existing peripheral vascular disease. Hypoglycemia may occur in previously controlled diabetes. Thrombocytopenia, unusual bruising, bleeding, occur rarely.

NURSING CONSIDERATIONS

BASELINE ASSESSMENT

Assess baseline renal/hepatic function tests. Assess B/P, apical pulse immediately before drug is administered (if pulse is 60/min or less or systolic B/P is less than 90 mm Hg, withhold medications, contact physician).

INTERVENTION/EVALUATION

Assess pulse for quality, irregular rate, bradycardia. Assist with ambulation if dizziness occurs. Assess for peripheral edema (usually, first area of lower extremity swelling is behind medial malleolus in ambulatory, sacral area in bedridden). Monitor daily pattern of bowel activity/stool consistency.

PATIENT/FAMILY TEACHING

• Do not abruptly discontinue medication. • Compliance with therapy regimen is essential to control hypertension. • If dizziness occurs, sit or lie down immediately. • Avoid tasks that require alertness, motor skills until response to drug is established. • Teach pts how to take pulse properly before each dose and to report excessively slow pulse rate (less than 60 beats/min), peripheral numbness, dizziness. • Do not use nasal decongestants, OTC cold preparations (stimulants) without physician approval. • Restrict salt, alcohol intake.

bivalirudin

bye-**vail**-ih-rhu-din
(Angiomax)

CLASSIFICATION

PHARMACOTHERAPEUTIC: Thrombin inhibitor. **CLINICAL:** Anticoagulant.

ACTION

Specifically and reversibly inhibits thrombin by binding to its receptor sites. **Therapeutic Effect:** Decreases acute ischemic complications in pts with unstable angina pectoris.

PHARMACOKINETICS

Route	Onset	Peak	Duration
IV	Immediate	N/A	1 hr

Primarily eliminated by kidneys. Twenty-five percent removed by hemodialysis. **Half-life:** 25 min (increased in moderate to severe renal impairment).

USES

Anticoagulant in pts with unstable angina undergoing percutaneous transluminal coronary angioplasty (PTCA) in conjunction with aspirin. Pts with heparin induced thrombocytopenia (HIT) and thrombosis syndrome (HITTS) while undergoing percutaneous coronary intervention.

PRECAUTIONS

CONTRAINDICATIONS: Active major bleeding. **CAUTIONS:** Conditions associated with increased risk of bleeding (e.g., bacterial endocarditis, recent major bleeding, cerebrovascular accident [CVA], stroke, intracerebral surgery, hemorrhagic diathesis, severe hypertension, severe renal/hepatic impairment, recent major surgery).

LIFESPAN CONSIDERATIONS:

Pregnancy/Lactation: Unknown if drug is distributed in breast milk or crosses placenta. **Pregnancy Category B.** **Children:** Safety and efficacy not established. **Elderly:** Age-related renal impairment may require dosage adjustment.

INTERACTIONS

DRUG: Warfarin, platelet aggregation inhibitors other than aspirin, thrombolytics may increase risk of bleeding complication. **HERBAL: Ginkgo biloba** may increase risk of bleeding **FOOD:** None known. **LAB VALUES:** Prolongs aPTT, PT.

AVAILABILITY (Rx)

INJECTION, POWDER FOR RECONSTITUTION: 250 mg.

ADMINISTRATION/HANDLING

IV

Reconstitution • To each 250-mg vial add 5 ml Sterile Water for Injection. • Gently swirl until all material is dissolved. • Further dilute each vial in 50 ml D_5W or 0.9% NaCl to yield final concentration of 5 mg/ml (1 vial in 50 ml, 2 vials in 100 ml, 5 vials in 250 ml). • If low-rate infusion is used after initial infusion, reconstitute the 250-mg vial with added 5 ml Sterile

B

Water for Injection. • Gently swirl until all material is dissolved. • Further dilute each vial in 500 ml D_5W or 0.9% NaCl to yield final concentration of 0.5 mg/ml. • Produces a clear, colorless solution (do not use if cloudy or contains a precipitate).

Rate of administration • Adjust IV infusion based on aPTT or pt's body weight.

Storage • Store unreconstituted vials at room temperature. • Reconstituted solution may be refrigerated for 24 hrs or less. • Diluted drug with a concentration of 0.5–5 mg/ml is stable at room temperature for up to 24 hrs.

IV INCOMPATIBILITIES

Alteplase (Activase), amiodarone (Cordarone), amphotericin B (AmBisome, Abelcet), chlorpromazine (Thorazine), diazepam (Valium), dobutamine (incompatible at 12.5 mg/ml, compatible at 4 mg/ml) (Dobutrex), prochlorperazine (Compazine), reteplase (Retavase), streptokinase (Streptase), vancomycin (Vancocin).

INDICATIONS/ROUTES/DOSAGE

ANTICOAGULANT IN PTS WITH UNSTABLE ANGINA, HITS, OR HITTS WHO ARE UNDERGOING PTCA IN CONJUNCTION WITH ASPIRIN

IV: ADULTS, ELDERLY: 0.75 mg/kg as IV bolus, followed by IV infusion at rate of 1.75 mg/kg/hr for duration of procedure and up to 4 hrs postprocedure. IV infusion may be continued beyond initial 4 hrs at rate of 0.2 mg/kg/hr for up to 20 hrs.

DOSAGE IN RENAL IMPAIRMENT

◄ **ALERT** ► Initial bolus dose remains unchanged.

Creatinine Clearance	IV Infusion Rate
30 ml/min or greater	20% to 1.75 mg/kg/hr
10–29 ml/min	60% to 1 mg/kg/hr
Dialysis	90% to 0.25 mg/kg/hr

SIDE EFFECTS

FREQUENT (42%): Back pain. **OCCASIONAL (15%–12%):** Nausea, headache, hypotension, generalized pain. **RARE (8%–4%):** Injection site pain, insomnia, hypertension, anxiety, vomiting, pelvic or abdominal pain, bradycardia, nervousness, dyspepsia, fever, urinary retention.

ADVERSE EFFECTS/ TOXIC REACTIONS

Hemorrhagic event occurs rarely, characterized by a fall in B/P or Hct.

NURSING CONSIDERATIONS

BASELINE ASSESSMENT

Assess CBC, bleeding time, renal function. Determine initial B/P.

INTERVENTION/EVALUATION

Monitor aPTT, Hct, urine and stool culture for occult blood, renal function studies. Assess for decrease in B/P, increase in pulse rate. Question for increase in amount of discharge during menses. Assess urine for hematuria.

black cohosh

(Black Cohosh Softgel, Remifemin)

Also known as baneberry, bugbane, bugwort, fairy candles.

CLASSIFICATION

HERBAL: See Appendix G.

ACTION

May target serotonin receptors to help regulate body temperature. **Effect:** Reduces symptoms of menopause (e.g., hot flashes).

USES

Treatment of symptoms of menopause, induction of labor in pregnant women. May reduce lipids and/or B/P (esp. when combined with prescription medications). Mild sedative action.

PRECAUTIONS

CONTRAINDICATIONS: Preterm pregnancy (has menstrual and uterine stimulant effects that may increase risk of miscarriage). Not to be taken for longer than 6 mos. **CAUTIONS:** Pts with breast, uterine, ovarian cancer; endometriosis; uterine fibroids.

LIFESPAN CONSIDERATIONS:

Pregnancy/Lactation: Contraindicated. **Children:** Safety and efficacy not established. **Elderly:** No age-related precautions noted.

INTERACTIONS

DRUG: May have additive antiproliferative effect with **tamoxifen**. May increase action of **antihypertensives. HERBAL:** None significant. **FOOD:** None known. **LAB VALUES:** May decrease serum luteinizing hormone (LH) concentration.

AVAILABILITY

CAPSULES (SOFT GELATIN): 40 mg. **TABLETS:** 20 mg.

INDICATIONS/ROUTES/DOSAGE

MENOPAUSE, LABOR INDUCTION, REDUCES LIPIDS AND/OR B/P, SEDATIVE

PO: ADULTS, ELDERLY: 20–80 mg twice a day.

SIDE EFFECTS

Nausea, headache, dizziness, weight gain, visual changes, migraines.

ADVERSE EFFECTS/ TOXIC REACTIONS

Overdose may cause nausea/vomiting, decreased heart rate, diaphoresis. May produce hepatotoxicity.

NURSING CONSIDERATIONS

BASELINE ASSESSMENT

Assess if pt is pregnant or breast-feeding (contraindicated).

INTERVENTION/EVALUATION

Monitor B/P, lipid levels.

PATIENT/FAMILY TEACHING

• Inform physician if pregnancy occurs or planning to become pregnant, breast-feeding. • Do not take for longer than 6 mos.

bleomycin

blee-oh-**my**-sin

(Blenoxane)

CLASSIFICATION

PHARMACOTHERAPEUTIC: Glycopeptide antibiotic. **CLINICAL:** Antineoplastic, sclerosing agent (see p. 77C).

ACTION

Binds to portions of DNA, producing DNA single-strand breaks. Most effective in G_2 phase of cell division. **Therapeutic Effect:** Inhibits cell replication.

PHARMACOKINETICS

Protein binding: Low (1%). Metabolism varies. Excreted in urine as unchanged drug. **Half-life:** 115 min.

USES

Treatment of Hodgkin's and non-Hodgkin's lymphoma, malignant pleural effusions, squamous cell carcinoma (e.g., head, neck, penis, cervix, vulva), testicular carcinoma. **OFF-LABEL:** Sclerosing agent for malignant pleural effusion, treatment of mycosis fungoides, osteosarcoma, ovarian tumors, renal carcinoma, soft-tissue sarcoma.

B

PRECAUTIONS

CONTRAINDICATIONS: Previous allergic reaction. **CAUTIONS:** Severe renal or pulmonary impairment.

LIFESPAN CONSIDERATIONS:

Pregnancy/Lactation: May cause fetal harm. Avoid breast-feeding. **Pregnancy Category D. Children:** Safety and efficacy not established. **Elderly:** Increased risk of pulmonary toxicity.

INTERACTIONS

DRUG: Cisplatin may decrease bleomycin clearance and increase the risk of bleomycin toxicity (from cisplatin-induced renal impairment). **Live virus vaccines** may potentiate virus replication, increase vaccine side effects, and decrease pt's antibody response to the vaccine. **Other antineoplastics** may increase risk of bleomycin toxicity. **HERBAL:** None significant. **FOOD:** None known. **LAB VALUES:** None known.

AVAILABILITY (Rx)

INJECTION, POWDER FOR RECONSTITUTION, (BLENOXANE): 15 units, 30 units.

ADMINISTRATION/HANDLING

◀ ALERT ▶ May be carcinogenic, mutagenic, teratogenic. Handle with extreme care during preparation/administration.

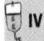

IV

Reconstitution • Reconstitute 15-unit vial with at least 5 ml (30-unit vial with at least 10 ml) 0.9% NaCl to provide a concentration not greater than 3 units/ml.

Rate of administration • Administer over at least 10 min for IV injection.

Storage • Refrigerate powder. • After reconstitution with 0.9% NaCl, solution is stable for 24 hrs at room temperature.

IM, SUBCUTANEOUS

Rate of administration • Reconstitute 15-unit vial with 1–5 ml (30-unit vial with 2–10 ml) Sterile Water for Injection, 0.9% NaCl, or Bacteriostatic Water for Injection to provide concentration of 3–15 units/ml. Do not use D_5W.

Storage • Refrigerate powder • After reconstitution, solution is stable for 24 hrs at room temperature.

IV INCOMPATIBILITIES

Hydrocortisone sodium succinate (Solo-Cortef).

IV COMPATIBILITIES

Cefepime (Maxipime), dacarbazine (DTIC), dexamethasone (Decadron), diphenhydramine (Benadryl), fludarabine (Fludara), gemcitabine (Gemzar), ondansetron (Zofran), paclitaxel (Taxol), piperacillin and tazobactam (Zosyn), vinblastine (Velban), vinorelbine (Navelbine).

INDICATIONS/ROUTES/DOSAGE

USUAL DOSAGE (refer to individual protocols)

IV, IM, SUBCUTANEOUS: ADULTS, ELDERLY: 10–20 units/m^2 (0.25–0.5 units/kg) 1–2 times a wk.

IV (CONTINUOUS): ADULTS, ELDERLY: 15 units/m^2 over 24 hrs for 4 days.

SCLEROSING AGENT

ADULTS, ELDERLY: 60 units as a single infusion. May repeat at intervals of several days if fluid continues to accumulate (may add lidocaine 100–200 mg to reduce local discomfort).

DOSAGE IN RENAL IMPAIRMENT

Creatinine Clearance	Dosage
10–50 ml/min	75% of normal dosage
Less than 10 ml/min	50% of normal dosage

B

SIDE EFFECTS

FREQUENT: Anorexia, weight loss, erythematous skin swelling, urticaria, rash, striae, vesiculation, hyperpigmentation (particularly at areas of pressure, skin folds, cuticles, IM injection sites, scars), stomatitis (usually evident 1–3 wks after initial therapy); may be accompanied by decreased skin sensitivity followed by skin hypersensitivity, nausea, vomiting, alopecia, and with parenteral form-fever or chills (typically occurring a few hrs after large single dose and lasting 4–12 hrs).

ADVERSE EFFECTS/ TOXIC REACTIONS

Interstitial pneumonitis occurs in 10% of pts, occasionally progresses to pulmonary fibrosis. Appears to be dose-, age-related (older than 70 yrs, those receiving total dose greater than 400 units). Nephrotoxicity, hepatotoxicity occur infrequently.

NURSING CONSIDERATIONS

BASELINE ASSESSMENT

Obtain chest x-rays q1–2wk.

INTERVENTION/EVALUATION

Monitor breath sounds for pulmonary toxicity (rales, rhonchi). Observe for dyspnea. Monitor hematologic, pulmonary function, hepatic, renal function tests. Assess skin daily for cutaneous toxicity. Monitor for stomatitis (burning or erythema of oral mucosa at inner margin of lips), hematologic toxicity (fever, sore throat, signs of local infection, unusual bruising/bleeding), symptoms of anemia (excessive fatigue, weakness).

PATIENT/FAMILY TEACHING

• Fever or chills reaction occurs less frequently with continued therapy. • Improvement of Hodgkin's disease, testicular tumors noted within 2 wks, squamous cell carcinoma within 3 wks. • Do not have immunizations without doctor's approval (drug lowers body's resistance). • Avoid contact with those who have recently taken live virus vaccine or have a cold.

bortezomib

bor-**teh**-zoe-mib
(Velcade)

CLASSIFICATION

PHARMACOTHERAPEUTIC: Proteasome inhibitor. **CLINICAL:** Antineoplastic.

ACTION

Degrades conjugated proteins required for cell-cycle progression and mitosis, disrupting cell proliferation. **Therapeutic Effect:** Produces antitumor and chemosensitizing activity, cell death.

PHARMACOKINETICS

Distributed to tissues and organs, with highest level in GI tract and liver. Protein binding: 83%. Primarily metabolized by enzymatic action. Rapidly cleared from the circulation. Significant biliary excretion, with lesser amount excreted in the urine. **Half-life:** 9–15 hrs.

USES

Treatment of multiple myeloma, mantle cell lymphoma in pts who have had one prior treatment and disease progression during that therapy.

PRECAUTIONS

CONTRAINDICATIONS: Hypersensitivity to boron or mannitol. **CAUTIONS:** History

B

of syncope, pts receiving medication known to be associated with hypotension, dehydrated pts, renal/hepatic impairment.

LIFESPAN CONSIDERATIONS:

Pregnancy/Lactation: May induce degenerative effects in ovary, degenerative changes in testes. May affect male and female fertility. Breast-feeding not recommended. **Pregnancy Category D.** **Children:** Safety and efficacy not established. **Elderly:** Increased incidence of grades 3 and 4 thrombocytopenia.

INTERACTIONS

DRUG: **Amiodarone, antivirals, isoniazid, nitrofurantoin, statins** may increase risk of peripheral neuropathy. May affect **antihypertensives, medications associated with hypotension.** May alter **oral hypoglycemic** response. **HERBAL:** None significant. **FOOD:** None known. **LAB VALUES:** May significantly decrease WBC, Hgb, Hct, platelet count, neutrophils.

AVAILABILITY (Rx)

INJECTION, POWDER FOR RECONSTITUTION: 3.5 mg.

ADMINISTRATION/HANDLING

IV

Reconstitution • Reconstitute vial with 3.5 ml 0.9% NaCl.

Rate of administration • Give as bolus IV injection over 3–5 sec.

Storage • Store unopened vials at room temperature. • Once reconstituted, solution may be stored at room temperature up to 8 hrs after preparation.

INDICATIONS/ROUTES/DOSAGE

MULTIPLE MYELOMA, MANTLE CELL LYMPHOMA

IV: ADULTS, ELDERLY: Treatment cycle consists of 1.3 mg/m^2 twice weekly on days 1, 4, 8, and 11 for 2 wks followed by a 10-day rest period on days 12 to 21. Consecutive doses separated by at least 72 hrs.

DOSAGE ADJUSTMENT GUIDELINES

Therapy is withheld at onset of grade 3 nonhematologic or grade 4 hematologic toxicities, excluding neuropathy. When symptoms resolve, therapy is restarted at a 25% reduced dosage.

NEUROPATHIC PAIN, PERIPHERAL SENSORY NEUROPATHY

IV: ADULTS, ELDERLY: For grade 1 with pain or grade 2 (interfering with function but not activities of daily living [ADL]), 1 mg/m^2. For grade 2 with pain or grade 3 (interfering with ADL), withhold drug until toxicity is resolved, then reinitiate with 0.7 mg/m^2. For grade 4 (permanent sensory loss that interferes with function), discontinue bortezomib.

SIDE EFFECTS

EXPECTED (65%–36%): Fatigue, malaise, asthenia, nausea, diarrhea, anorexia, constipation, fever, vomiting. **FREQUENT (28%–21%):** Headache, insomnia, arthralgia, limb pain, edema, paresthesia, dizziness, rash. **OCCASIONAL (18%–11%):** Dehydration, cough, anxiety, bone pain, muscle cramps, myalgia, back pain, abdominal pain, taste alteration, dyspepsia, pruritus, hypotension (including orthostatic hypotension), rigors, blurred vision.

ADVERSE EFFECTS/ TOXIC REACTIONS

Thrombocytopenia occurs in 40% of pts. Platelet count peaks at day 11, returns to baseline by day 21. GI, intracerebral hemorrhage are associated with drug-induced thrombocytopenia. Anemia occurs in 32% of pts. New onset or worsening of existing neuropathy occurs in 37% of pts. Symptoms may improve in some pts upon drug discontinuation. Pneumonia occurs occasionally.

NURSING CONSIDERATIONS

BASELINE ASSESSMENT

Obtain baseline CBC; monitor CBC, esp. platelet count, throughout treatment. Antiemetics, antidiarrheals may be effective in preventing, treating nausea, vomiting, diarrhea.

INTERVENTION/EVALUATION

Routinely assess B/P; monitor pt for orthostatic hypotension. Maintain strict I&O. Encourage adequate fluid intake to prevent dehydration. Monitor temperature and be alert to high potential for fever. Monitor for peripheral neuropathy (burning sensation, neuropathic pain, paresthesia, hyperesthesia). Avoid IM injections, rectal temperatures, other traumas that may induce bleeding.

PATIENT/FAMILY TEACHING

• Discuss importance of pregnancy testing, avoidance of pregnancy, measures to prevent pregnancy. • Increase fluid intake. • Avoid tasks requiring mental alertness, motor skills until response to drug is established.

bosentan

bo-sen-tan

(Tracleer)

Do not confuse Tracleer with Tricor.

CLASSIFICATION

PHARMACOTHERAPEUTIC: Endothelin receptor antagonist. **CLINICAL:** Vasodilator, neurohormonal blocker.

ACTION

Blocks the neurohormone that constricts pulmonary arteries. **Therapeutic Effect:** Improves exercise ability, slows clinical worsening of pulmonary arterial hypertension (PAH).

PHARMACOKINETICS

Highly bound to plasma proteins, mainly albumin. Metabolized in the liver. Eliminated by biliary excretion. **Half-life:** Approximately 5 hrs.

USES

Treatment of PAH in those with class III or IV symptoms (World Health Organization). **OFF-LABEL:** CHF, pulmonary hypertension secondary to scleroderma.

PRECAUTIONS

CONTRAINDICATIONS: Administration with cyclosporine or glyburide, pregnancy. **EXTREME CAUTION:** Moderate to severe hepatic impairment. **CAUTIONS:** Mild hepatic impairment.

⌛ LIFESPAN CONSIDERATIONS:

Pregnancy/Lactation: May induce male infertility, atrophy of seminiferous tubules of testes; reduce sperm count. Expected to cause fetal harm, teratogenic effects, including malformations of head, mouth, face, large vessels. Breastfeeding not recommended. **Pregnancy Category X.** **Children:** Safety and efficacy not established. **Elderly:** Use caution in dosage due to higher frequency of decreased hepatic, renal, cardiac function.

INTERACTIONS

DRUG: May decrease concentration of **atorvastatin, glyburide, hormonal contraceptives (including oral, injectable, and implantable), lovastatin, simvastatin, warfarin. Cyclosporine, ketoconazole** may increase plasma concentration of bosentan.

B

HERBAL: None significant. **FOOD:** None known. **LAB VALUES:** May increase serum bilirubin, AST, ALT levels. May decrease blood Hgb, Hct levels.

AVAILABILITY (Rx)

TABLETS: 62.5 mg, 125 mg.

ADMINISTRATION/HANDLING

• Give in morning and evening, with or without food. • Do not chew film-coated tablets.

INDICATIONS/ROUTES/DOSAGE

PULMONARY ARTERIAL HYPERTENSION

PO: ADULTS, ELDERLY: 62.5 mg twice a day for 4 wks; then increase to maintenance dosage of 125 mg twice a day. **CHILDREN WEIGHING LESS THAN 40 KG:** 62.5 mg twice a day.

◀ **ALERT** ▶ When discontinuing adult/elderly dosage, reduce dosage to 62.5 mg twice a day for 3–7 days to avoid clinical deterioration.

DOSAGE BASED ON TRANSAMINASE ELEVATIONS

Any elevation accompanied by symptoms of hepatic injury or serum bilirubin 2 or more times upper limit of normal, stop treatment. **AST/ALT greater than 3 or less than 6 times upper limit of normal,** reduce dose or interrupt treatment. **AST/ALT greater than 5 and up to 8 times upper limit of normal,** confirm with additional test and, if confirmed, stop treatment. **AST/ALT greater than 8 times upper limit of normal,** stop treatment.

SIDE EFFECTS

OCCASIONAL: Headache, nasopharyngitis, flushing. **RARE:** Dyspepsia (heartburn, epigastric distress), fatigue, pruritus, hypotension.

ADVERSE EFFECTS/ TOXIC REACTIONS

Abnormal hepatic function, lower extremity edema, palpitations occur rarely.

NURSING CONSIDERATIONS

BASELINE ASSESSMENT

Pregnancy must be excluded before starting treatment and prevented thereafter. A negative result from a urine or serum pregnancy test performed during the first 5 days of a normal menstrual period and at least 11 days after the last act of sexual intercourse must be obtained. Monthly follow-up pregnancy tests must be maintained.

INTERVENTION/EVALUATION

Assess hepatic enzyme levels (aminotransferase) before initiating therapy and then monthly thereafter. If elevation in hepatic enzymes is noted, changes in monitoring and treatment must be initiated. If clinical symptoms of hepatic injury (nausea, vomiting, fever, abdominal pain, fatigue, jaundice) occur or if serum bilirubin level increases, stop treatment. Monitor Hgb levels at 1 mo and 3 mos of treatment, then q3mo. Monitor Hgb, Hct levels for decrease.

PATIENT/FAMILY TEACHING

• Discuss importance of pregnancy testing, avoidance of pregnancy, measures to prevent pregnancy.

botulinum toxin type A

botch-you-lin-em **tocks**-in **tipe A**
(Botox, Botox Cosmetic)

CLASSIFICATION

PHARMACOTHERAPEUTIC: Neurotoxin. **CLINICAL:** Neuromuscular conduction blocker.

ACTION

Blocks neuromuscular conduction by binding to receptor sites on motor nerve endings, inhibiting release of acetylcholine, resulting in muscle denervation. **Therapeutic Effect:** Reduces muscle activity.

PHARMACOKINETICS

In treatment of blepharospasm, each treatment lasts approximately 3 mos. In treatment of strabismus, paralysis lasts for 2–6 wks and gradually resolves over an additional 2–6 wks. In treatment of hemifacial spasm, treatment may last 6 mos.

USES

Treatment of strabismus, blepharospasm associated with dystonia; cervical dystonia. Temporary improvement of brow furrow lines in those 65 yrs and younger. **OFF-LABEL:** Treatment of dynamic muscle contracture in children with cerebral palsy, focal task-specific dystonia, head and neck tremor unresponsive to drug therapy, hemifacial spasms, laryngeal dystonia, oromandibular dystonia, spasmoditic torticollis, writer's cramp.

PRECAUTIONS

CONTRAINDICATIONS: Infection at proposed injection sites. **CAUTIONS:** Pts with neuromuscular junctional disorders (amyotrophic lateral sclerosis, motor neuropathy, myasthenia gravis, Lambert-Eaton syndrome) may experience significant systemic effects (severe dysphagia, respiratory compromise).

LIFESPAN CONSIDERATIONS:

Pregnancy/Lactation: Unknown if drug crosses placenta or is distributed is breast milk. **Pregnancy Category C. Children:** Safety and efficacy not established. **Elderly:** No age-related precautions noted.

INTERACTIONS

DRUG: **Aminoglycoside antibiotics, neuromuscular blocking agents** may potentiate effects. **HERBAL:** None significant. **FOOD:** None known. **LAB VALUES:** None known.

AVAILABILITY (Rx)

INJECTION, POWDER FOR RECONSTITUTION: 100 units/vial.

ADMINISTRATION/HANDLING

IM

Reconstitution • 0.9% NaCl is recommended diluent. • For resulting dose of units/0.1 ml, draw up 1 ml diluent to provide 10 units, 2 ml to provide 5 units, 4 ml to provide 2.5 units, 8 ml to provide 1.25 units. • Slowly, gently inject diluent into the vial, avoid bubbles, rotate vial gently to mix.

Rate of administration • Administer within 4 hrs after reconstitution. • Inject into affected muscle using 25-, 27-, or 30-gauge needle for superficial muscles and 22-gauge needle for deeper musculature.

Storage • Store in freezer. • Administer within 4 hrs after removal from freezer and reconstituted. • May store reconstituted solution in refrigerator for up to 4 hrs. • Appears as a clear, colorless solution (discard if particulates form).

INDICATIONS/ROUTES/DOSAGE

CERVICAL DYSTONIA IN PTS WHO HAVE PREVIOUSLY TOLERATED BOTULINUM TOXIN TYPE A

IM: ADULTS, ELDERLY: Mean dose of

B

236 units (range: 198–300 units) divided among the affected muscles, based on pt's head and neck position, localization of pain, muscle hypertrophy, pt response, adverse reaction history.

CERVICAL DYSTONIA IN PTS WHO HAVE NOT PREVIOUSLY BEEN TREATED WITH BOTULINUM TOXIN TYPE A

IM: ADULTS, ELDERLY: Administer at lower dosage than for pts who have previously tolerated the drug.

STRABISMUS

IM: ADULTS, CHILDREN OLDER THAN 12 YRS: 1.25–2.5 units into any one muscle. **CHILDREN 2 MOS–12 YRS:** 1–2.5 units into any one muscle.

BLEPHAROSPASM

IM: ADULTS, CHILDREN 12 YRS AND OLDER: Initially, 1.25–2.5 units. May increase up to 2.5–5.0 units at repeat treatments. **Maximum:** 5 units per injection or cumulative dose of 200 units over a 30-day period.

CEREBRAL PALSY SPASTICITY

IM: CHILDREN OLDER THAN 18 MOS: 1–6 units/kg. **Maximum:** 50 units per injection site. No more than 400 units per visit or during a 3-mo period.

IMPROVEMENT OF BROW FURROW

IM: ADULTS 65 YRS AND YOUNGER: Individualized.

SIDE EFFECTS

◄ **ALERT** ► Side effects usually occur within the first week after injection. **FREQUENT (15%–11%):** Localized pain, tenderness, bruising at injection site; localized weakness in injected muscle; upper respiratory tract infection; neck pain; headache. **OCCASIONAL (10%–2%):** Increased cough, flu-like symptoms, back pain, rhinitis, dizziness, hypertonia, soreness at injection site, asthenia, dry mouth, nausea, somnolence. **RARE:** Stiffness, numbness, diplopia, ptosis.

ADVERSE EFFECTS/ TOXIC REACTIONS

Mild to moderate dysphagia occurs in approximately 20% of pts. Arrhythmias and severe dysphagia (manifested as aspiration, pneumonia, dyspnea) occur rarely. Overdose produces systemic weakness, muscle paralysis.

NURSING CONSIDERATIONS

BASELINE ASSESSMENT

Assess onset, type, location, duration of dystonia.

INTERVENTION/EVALUATION

Clinical improvement begins within first 2 wks after injection. Maximum benefit appears at approximately 6 wks after injection.

PATIENT/FAMILY TEACHING

- Resume activity slowly and carefully.
- Seek medical attention immediately if swallowing, speech, respiratory difficulties occur.

botulinum toxin type B

botch-you-lin-em **tocks**-in **tipe B** (Myobloc)

CLASSIFICATION

PHARMACOTHERAPEUTIC: Neurotoxin. **CLINICAL:** Neuromuscular conduction blocker.

ACTION

Inhibits acetylcholine release at neuromuscular junction by binding to the protein complex responsible for fusion to the presynaptic membrane, a necessary step to neurotransmitter release. **Therapeutic Effect:** Produces flaccid paralysis.

PHARMACOKINETICS

Duration of effect is 12–16 wks at doses of 5,000 or 10,000 units.

USES

Treatment of cervical dystonia (CD) to reduce severity of abnormal head position, neck pain associated with CD. **OFF-LABEL:** Treatment of cervical dystonia in pts resistant to botulinum toxin type A.

PRECAUTIONS

CONTRAINDICATIONS: None known. **CAUTIONS:** Pts with neuromuscular junctional disorders (amyotrophic lateral sclerosis, motor neuropathy, myasthenia gravis, Lambert-Eaton syndrome) may experience significant systemic effects (severe dysphagia, respiratory compromise).

⌛ LIFESPAN CONSIDERATIONS:

Pregnancy/Lactation: Unknown if drug crosses placenta or is distributed in breast milk. **Pregnancy Category C.** **Children:** Safety and efficacy not established. **Elderly:** No age-related precautions noted.

INTERACTIONS

DRUG: **Aminoglycoside antibiotics, neuromuscular blocking agents** may potentiate effects. **HERBAL:** None significant. **FOOD:** None known. **LAB VALUES:** None known.

AVAILABILITY (Rx)

INJECTION SOLUTION: 5,000 units/ml.

ADMINISTRATION/HANDLING

IM

Reconstitution • 0.9% NaCl is recommended diluent. • Slowly, gently inject diluent into the vial; avoid bubbles, rotate vial gently to mix.

Rate of administration • Administer within 4 hrs after reconstitution. • Inject into affected muscle using 25-, 27-, or 30-gauge needle for superficial muscles and 22-gauge needle for deeper musculature.

Storage • May be refrigerated for up to 21 mos. Do not freeze. • Administer within 4 hrs after removal from refrigerator and reconstitution. • May store reconstituted solution in refrigerator for up to 4 hrs. • Appears as a clear, colorless solution (discard if particulate forms).

INDICATIONS/ROUTES/DOSAGE

TO REDUCE SEVERITY OF SYMPTOMS IN PTS WITH CERVICAL DYSTONIA WHO HAVE PREVIOUSLY TOLERATED BOTULINUM TOXIN TYPE B

IM: ADULTS, ELDERLY: 2,500–5,000 units divided among the affected muscles.

TO REDUCE SEVERITY OF SYMPTOMS IN PTS WITH CERVICAL DYSTONIA WHO HAVE NOT PREVIOUSLY BEEN TREATED WITH BOTULINUM TOXIN TYPE B

IM: ADULTS, ELDERLY: Administer at lower dosage than for pts who have previously tolerated the drug.

SIDE EFFECTS

◀ ALERT ▶ Side effects usually occur within the first week after the injection. **FREQUENT (19%–12%):** Infection, neck pain, headache, injection site pain, dry mouth. **OCCASIONAL (10%–4%):** Flu-like symptoms, generalized pain, increased cough, back pain, myasthenia. **RARE:** Dizziness, nausea, rhinitis, headache, vomiting, edema, allergic reaction.

ADVERSE EFFECTS/ TOXIC REACTIONS

Mild to moderate dysphagia occurs in approximately 10% of pts. Arrhythmias

B

and severe dysphagia (manifested as aspiration, pneumonia, dyspnea) occur rarely. Overdose produces systemic weakness, muscle paralysis.

NURSING CONSIDERATIONS

BASELINE ASSESSMENT

Assess onset, type, location, duration of dystonia.

INTERVENTION/EVALUATION

Duration of effect lasts between 12–16 wks at doses of 5,000 units or 10,000 units.

PATIENT/FAMILY TEACHING

- Resume activity slowly and carefully.
- Seek medical attention immediately if swallowing, speech, respiratory difficulties appear.

Brethine, *see terbutaline*

bretylium tosylate

bre-**till**-ee-um

(Bretylate ♣, Bretylol)

See Antiarrhythmics

Brevibloc, *see esmolol*

brimonidine

(Alphagan)

See Antiglaucoma agents (p. 49C)

brinzolamide

(Azopt)

See Antiglaucoma agents (p. 50C)

bromocriptine

broe-moe-**krip**-teen

(Apo-Bromocriptine ♣, Parlodel)

Do not confuse bromocriptine with benztropine, or Parlodel with pindolol.

CLASSIFICATION

PHARMACOTHERAPEUTIC: Dopamine agonist. **CLINICAL:** Infertility therapy adjunct, antihyperprolactinemic, lactation inhibitor, antidyskinetic, growth hormone suppressant.

ACTION

Directly stimulates dopamine receptors in corpus striatum, inhibits prolactin secretion. Suppresses secretion of growth hormone. **Therapeutic Effect:** Improves symptoms of parkinsonism, suppresses galactorrhea, reduces serum growth hormone concentrations in acromegaly.

PHARMACOKINETICS

Indication	Onset	Peak	Duration
Prolactin lowering	2 hrs	8 hrs	24 hrs
Antiparkinson	0.5–1.5 hrs	2 hrs	N/A
Growth hormone suppressant	1–2 hrs	4–8 wks	4–8 hrs

Minimally absorbed from GI tract. Protein binding: 90%–96%. Metabolized in the liver. Excreted in feces by biliary secretion. **Half-life:** 15 hrs.

USES

Treatment of pituitary prolactinomas, conditions associated with hyperprolactinemia (amenorrhea, galactorrhea, hypogonadism, infertility), parkinsonism. **OFF-LABEL:** Treatment of cocaine addiction, hyperprolactinemia associated with pituitary adenomas, neuroleptic malignant syndrome.

PRECAUTIONS

CONTRAINDICATIONS: Hypersensitivity to ergot alkaloids, peripheral vascular disease, pregnancy, severe ischemic heart disease, uncontrolled hypertension. **CAUTIONS:** Impaired hepatic or cardiac function, hypertension, psychiatric disorders.

⌛ LIFESPAN CONSIDERATIONS:

Pregnancy/Lactation: Not recommended during pregnancy or while breast-feeding. **Pregnancy Category B.** **Children:** Safety and efficacy not established. **Elderly:** CNS effects may occur more frequently.

INTERACTIONS

DRUG: Disulfram-like reactions (chest pain, confusion, flushed face, nausea, vomiting) may occur with **alcohol. Estrogens, progestins** may decrease effects. **Phenothiazines, haloperidol, MAOIs** may decrease prolactin effect. **Antihypertensive agents** may increase hypotension. **Levodopa** may increase effects. **Erythromycin, ritonavir** may increase concentration, toxicity. **Risperidone** may increase serum prolactin concentrations, interfere with bromocriptine effects. **HERBAL:** None significant. **FOOD:** None known. **LAB VALUES:** May increase plasma concentration of growth hormone.

AVAILABILITY (Rx)

CAPSULES: 5 mg. **TABLETS:** 2.5 mg.

ADMINISTRATION/HANDLING

PO

• Pt should be lying down before administering first dose. • Give after food intake (decreases incidence of nausea).

INDICATIONS/ROUTES/DOSAGE

HYPERPROLACTINEMIA

PO: ADULTS, ELDERLY: Initially, 1.25–2.5 mg at bedtime. May increase by 2.5 mg q3–7 days up to 5–7.5 mg/day in divided doses. Maintenance: 2.5 mg 2–3 times a day.

PITUITARY PROLACTINOMAS

PO: ADULTS, ELDERLY: Initially, 1.25 mg 2–3 times a day. May gradually increase over several weeks to 10–20 mg/day in divided doses. Maintenance: 2.5–20 mg/day in divided doses.

PARKINSONISM

PO: ADULTS, ELDERLY: Initially, 1.25 mg 1–2 times a day. May take single doses at bedtime. May increase by 2.5 mg/day at 14–28 day intervals. Maintenance: 2.5–40 mg/day in divided doses. **Range:** 30–90 mg/day in 3 divided doses. **Maximum:** 100 mg/day.

ACROMEGALY

PO: ADULTS, ELDERLY: Initially, 1.25–2.5 mg at bedtime. May increase by 1.25–2.5 mg q3–7days up to 30 mg/day in divided doses. Maintenance: 10–30 mg/day in divided doses. **Maximum:** 100 mg/day.

SIDE EFFECTS

FREQUENT: Nausea (49%), headache (19%), dizziness (17%). **OCCASIONAL (7%–3%):** Fatigue, light-headedness, vomiting, abdominal cramps, diarrhea, constipation, nasal congestion, somnolence, dry mouth. **RARE:** Muscle cramps, urinary hesitancy.

ADVERSE EFFECTS/ TOXIC REACTIONS

Visual or auditory hallucinations noted in pts with Parkinson's disease. Long-term,

B

high-dose therapy may produce continuing rhinorrhea, syncope, GI hemorrhage, peptic ulcer, severe abdominal pain.

NURSING CONSIDERATIONS

BASELINE ASSESSMENT

Evaluation of pituitary (rule out tumor) should be done before treatment for hyperprolactinemia with amenorrhea or galactorrhea, infertility. Obtain pregnancy test.

INTERVENTION/EVALUATION

Assist with ambulation if dizziness is noted after administration. Assess for therapeutic response (decrease in engorgement, parkinsonism symptoms). Monitor for constipation.

PATIENT/FAMILY TEACHING

• To reduce lightheadedness, rise slowly from lying to sitting position, permit legs to dangle momentarily before standing. Avoid sudden posture changes. • Avoid tasks that require alertness, motor skills until response to drug is established. • Must use contraceptive measures (other than oral) during treatment. • Report any watery nasal discharge to physician.

brompheniramine

(Brovex, Brovex CT)

See Antihistamines (p. 51C)

budesonide

byew-**des**-oh-nyd

(Entocort EC, Pulmicort Respules, Pulmicort Turbuhaler, Rhinocort, Rhinocort Aqua)

FIXED-COMBINATION(S)

Symbicort: budesonide/formoterol (bronchodilator): 80 mcg/4.5 mcg, 160 mcg/4.5 mcg.

◆CLASSIFICATION

PHARMACOTHERAPEUTIC: Glucocorticosteroid. **CLINICAL:** Anti-inflammatory, antiallergy (see pp. 71C, 92C).

ACTION

Inhibits accumulation of inflammatory cells, decreases and prevents tissues from responding to inflammatory process. **Therapeutic Effect:** Relieves symptoms of allergic rhinitis, Crohn's disease.

PHARMACOKINETICS

Minimally absorbed from nasal tissue; moderately absorbed from inhalation. Protein binding: 88%. Primarily metabolized in the liver. **Half-life:** 2–3 hrs.

USES

Nasal: Management of seasonal or perennial allergic rhinitis, nonallergic rhinitis. **Inhalation:** Maintenance or prophylaxis therapy for bronchial asthma. **Oral:** Treatment of mild to moderate active Crohn's disease. Maintenance of clinical remission of mild to moderate Crohn's disease. **OFF-LABEL:** Treatment of vasomotor rhinitis.

PRECAUTIONS

CONTRAINDICATIONS: Hypersensitivity to any corticosteroid or its components, persistently positive sputum cultures for *Candida albicans,* primary treatment of status asthmaticus, systemic fungal infections, untreated localized infection involving nasal mucosa. **CAUTIONS:** Adrenal insufficiency, cirrhosis, glaucoma, hypothyroidism, untreated infection, osteoporosis, tuberculosis.

LIFESPAN CONSIDERATIONS:

Pregnancy/Lactation: Unknown if drug crosses placenta or is distributed in breast milk. **Pregnancy Category B (Inhalation); C (Oral). Children:** Prolonged treatment or high dosages may decrease short-term growth rate, cortisol secretion. **Elderly:** No age-related precautions noted.

INTERACTIONS

DRUG: Bupropion may lower seizure threshold. **Itraconazole, ketoconazole** may increase plasma concentration. **HERBAL:** None significant. **FOOD: Grapefruit, grapefruit juice** may increase systemic exposure of budesonide. **LAB VALUES:** None known.

AVAILABILITY (Rx)

CAPSULES (ENTOCORT EC): 3 mg. **INHALATION POWDER (PULMICORT TURBUHALER):** 200 mcg per inhalation. **INHALATION SUSPENSION (PULMICORT RESPULES):** 0.25 mg/2 ml; 0.5 mg/2 mg. **NASAL SPRAY (RHINOCORT AQUA):** 32 mcg/spray.

ADMINISTRATION/HANDLING

INHALATION

• Shake container well. Instruct pt to exhale completely, place mouthpiece between lips, inhale, hold breath as long as possible before exhaling. • Allow at least 1 min between inhalations. • Rinse mouth after each use to decrease dry mouth, hoarseness.

INTRANASAL

• Instruct pt to clear nasal passages before use. • Tilt head slightly forward. • Insert spray tip into nostril, pointing toward nasal passages, away from nasal septum. • Spray into one nostril while holding other nostril closed and concurrently inspire through nostril to allow medication as high into nasal passages as possible.

INDICATIONS/ROUTES/DOSAGE

RHINITIS

INTRANASAL: ADULTS, ELDERLY, CHILDREN 6 YRS AND OLDER: 1 spray in each nostril once a day. **Maximum:** 8 sprays/day for adults and children 12 yrs and older; 4 sprays/day for children younger than 12 yrs.

BRONCHIAL ASTHMA

NEBULIZATION: CHILDREN 6 MOS–8 YRS: 0.25–1 mg/day titrated to lowest effective dosage.

INHALATION: ADULTS, ELDERLY, CHILDREN 6 YRS AND OLDER: Initially, 200–400 mcg twice a day. **Maximum:** *Adults:* 800 mcg twice a day. *Children:* 400 mcg twice a day.

CROHN'S DISEASE

PO: ADULTS, ELDERLY: 9 mg once a day for up to 8 wks. Recurring episodes may be treated with a repeat 8-wk course of treatment.

SIDE EFFECTS

FREQUENT (greater than 3%): Nasal: Mild nasopharyngeal irritation, burning, stinging, dryness; headache, cough. **Inhalation:** Flu-like symptoms, headache, pharyngitis. **OCCASIONAL (3%–1%): Nasal:** Dry mouth, dyspepsia, rebound congestion, rhinorrhea, loss of taste. **Inhalation:** Back pain, vomiting, altered taste, voice changes, abdominal pain, nausea, dyspepsia.

ADVERSE EFFECTS/ TOXIC REACTIONS

Acute hypersensitivity reaction (urticaria, angioedema, severe bronchospasm) occurs rarely.

NURSING CONSIDERATIONS

BASELINE ASSESSMENT

Question for hypersensitivity to any corticosteroids, components.

B

INTERVENTION/EVALUATION

Monitor for relief of symptoms.

PATIENT/FAMILY TEACHING

• Improvement noted in 24 hrs, but full effect may take 3–7 days. • Contact physician if no improvement in symptoms, sneezing, nasal irritation occurs.

bumetanide

byew-**met**-ah-nide
(Bumex, Burinex ✱)

CLASSIFICATION

PHARMACOTHERAPEUTIC: Loop. **CLINICAL:** Diuretic (see p. 97C).

ACTION

Enhances excretion of sodium, chloride, and to lesser degree, potassium, by direct action at ascending limb of loop of Henle and in proximal tubule. **Therapeutic Effect:** Produces diuresis.

PHARMACOKINETICS

Route	Onset	Peak	Duration
PO	30–60 min	60–120 min	4–6 hrs
IV	Rapid	15–30 min	2–3 hrs
IM	40 min	60–120 min	4–6 hrs

Completely absorbed from GI tract (absorption decreased in CHF, nephrotic syndrome). Protein binding: 94%–96%. Partially metabolized in the liver. Primarily excreted in urine. Not removed by hemodialysis. **Half-life:** 1–1.5 hrs.

USES

Treatment of edema associated with CHF, chronic renal failure (including nephrotic syndrome), hepatic cirrhosis with ascites, acute pulmonary edema. **OFF-LABEL:** Treatment of hypercalcemia, hypertension.

PRECAUTIONS

CONTRAINDICATIONS: Anuria, hepatic coma, severe electrolyte depletion. **CAUTIONS:** Hypersensitivity to sulfonamides, renal/hepatic impairment, diabetes mellitus, elderly/debilitated.

LIFESPAN CONSIDERATIONS:

Pregnancy/Lactation: Unknown if drug is distributed in breast milk. **Pregnancy Category C (D if used in pregnancy-induced hypertension). Children:** Safety and efficacy not established. **Elderly:** May be more sensitive to hypotension/electrolyte effects. Increased risk for circulatory collapse or thrombolytic episode. Age-related renal impairment may require reduced or extended dosage interval.

INTERACTIONS

DRUG: Amphotericin B, ototoxic, nephrotoxic agents may increase risk of toxicity. May decrease effect of **anticoagulants, heparin. Agents inducing hypokalemia** may have increased hypokalemic effect. May increase risk of **lithium** toxicity. **HERBAL: Ephedra, ginseng, yohimbe** may worsen hypertension. **Garlic** may have increased antihypertensive effect. **FOOD:** None known. **LAB VALUES:** May increase serum glucose, BUN, uric acid, urinary phosphate. May decrease serum calcium, chloride, magnesium, potassium, sodium.

AVAILABILITY (Rx)

INJECTION SOLUTION: 0.25 mg/ml. **TABLETS:** 0.5 mg, 1 mg, 2 mg.

ADMINISTRATION/HANDLING

IV

Rate of administration • May give undiluted but is compatible with D_5W,

0.9% NaCl, or Lactated Ringer's solution. • Administer IV push over 1–2 min. • May give through Y tube or 3-way stopcock. • May give as continuous infusion.

Storage • Store at room temperature. • Stable for 24 hrs if diluted.

PO

• Give with food to avoid GI upset, preferably with breakfast (may prevent nocturia).

IV INCOMPATIBILITY

Midazolam (Versed).

IV COMPATIBILITIES

Aztreonam (Azactam), cefepime (Maxipime), diltiazem (Cardizem), dobutamine (Dobutrex), furosemide (Lasix), lipids, lorazepam (Ativan), milrinone (Primacor), morphine, piperacillin and tazobactam (Zosyn), propofol (Diprivan).

INDICATIONS/ROUTES/DOSAGE

EDEMA

PO: ADULTS, CHILDREN OLDER THAN 18 YRS: 0.5–2 mg as a single dose in the morning. May repeat at q4–5h. **ELDERLY:** 0.5 mg/day, increased as needed.

IV, IM: ADULTS, ELDERLY: 0.5–2 mg/dose; may repeat in 2–3 hrs or 0.5–1 mg/hr by continuous IV infusion.

HYPERTENSION

PO: ADULTS, ELDERLY: Initially, 0.5 mg/day. Range: 1–4 mg/day. **Maximum:** 5 mg/day. Larger doses may be given 2–3 doses/day.

USUAL PEDIATRIC DOSAGE

IV, IM, PO: CHILDREN: 0.015–0.1 mg/kg/dose q6–24h. **Maximum:** 10 mg/day.

SIDE EFFECTS

EXPECTED: Increased urinary frequency and urine volume. **FREQUENT:** Orthostatic hypotension, dizziness. **OCCASIONAL:** Blurred vision, diarrhea, headache, anorexia, premature ejaculation, impotence, dyspepsia. **RARE:** Rash, urticaria, pruritus, asthenia, muscle cramps, nipple tenderness.

ADVERSE EFFECTS/ TOXIC REACTIONS

Vigorous diuresis may lead to profound water and electrolyte depletion, resulting in hypokalemia, hyponatremia, dehydration, coma, circulatory collapse. Ototoxicity manifested as deafness, vertigo, tinnitus may occur, esp. in pts with severe renal impairment or those taking other ototoxic drugs. Blood dyscrasias, acute hypotensive episodes have been reported.

NURSING CONSIDERATIONS

BASELINE ASSESSMENT

Check vital signs, esp. B/P for hypotension, before administration. Assess baseline electrolytes; particularly check for low serum potassium. Assess for edema. Observe skin turgor, mucous membranes for hydration status. Initiate I&O.

INTERVENTION/EVALUATION

Continue to monitor B/P, vital signs, electrolytes, I&O, weight. Note extent of diuresis. Watch for changes from initial assessment (hypokalemia may result in muscle strength changes, tremor, muscle cramps, altered mental status, cardiac arrhythmias; hyponatremia may result in confusion, thirst, cold/clammy skin).

PATIENT/FAMILY TEACHING

• Expect increased urinary frequency/volume. • Report hearing abnormalities (e.g., sense of fullness in ears, tinnitus) to physician. • Eat foods high in potassium such as whole grains (cereals), legumes, meat, bananas,

B

apricots, orange juice, potatoes (white, sweet), raisins. • Get up slowly from sitting/lying position.

Bumex, *see bumetanide*

Buminate, *see albumin*

bupivacaine

(Marcaine, Sensorcaine)

See Anesthetics: local (p. 4C)

buprenorphine

byew-**pren**-or-phen

(Buprenex, Suboxone, Subutex)

Do not confuse buprenorphine with bupropion.

FIXED-COMBINATION(S)

Suboxone: buprenorphine/naloxone (narcotic antagonist): 2 mg/0.5 mg, 8 mg/2 mg.

CLASSIFICATION

PHARMACOTHERAPEUTIC: Opioid agonist, antagonist injection **(Schedule V)**; tablet **(Schedule III)**. **CLINICAL:** Opioid dependence adjunct, analgesic.

ACTION

Binds to opioid receptors within CNS. **Therapeutic Effect:** Suppresses opioid withdrawal symptoms, cravings. Alters pain perception, emotional response to pain.

PHARMACOKINETICS

Route	Onset	Peak	Duration
Sublingual	15 min	1 hr	6 hrs
IV	Less than 15 min	Less than 1 hr	6 hrs
IM	15 min	1 hr	6 hrs

Excreted primarily in feces with lesser amount eliminated in urine. **Half-life:** (Parenteral): 2–3 hrs, (Sublingual): 37 hrs (increased in pts with hepatic impairment).

USES

Treatment of opioid dependence. Relief of moderate to severe pain.

PRECAUTIONS

CONTRAINDICATIONS: Hypersensitivity to naloxone. **CAUTIONS:** Hepatic/renal impairment, elderly, debilitated, head injury/increased intracranial pressure, respiratory impairment, hypothyroidism, myxedema, adrenal cortical insufficiency (e.g., Addison's disease), urethral stricture, CNS depression, toxic psychosis, prostatic hypertrophy, delirium tremens, kyphoscoliosis, biliary tract dysfunction, acute abdominal conditions, acute alcoholism.

LIFESPAN CONSIDERATIONS:

Pregnancy/Lactation: Crosses placenta. Distributed in breast milk (breastfeeding not recommended). Neonatal withdrawal noted in infant if mother was treated with buprenorphine during pregnancy with onset of withdrawal symptoms generally noted on day 1, manifested as hypertonia, tremor, agitation, myoclonus. Apnea, bradycardia, seizures occur rarely. **Pregnancy Category C. Children:** Safety and efficacy of injection form not established in children 2–12 yrs. Safety and efficacy of tablet, fixed-combination form not established in children 16 yrs or younger. **Elderly:** Age-related hepatic impairment may require dosage adjustment.

INTERACTIONS

DRUG: **CNS depressants, MAOIs** may increase CNS or respiratory depression, hypotension. **Azole antifungals, macrolide antibiotics, protease inhibitors** may increase plasma concentration. **Phenobarbital, carbamazepine, phenytoin, rifampin** may cause increased clearance of buprenorphine. May decrease effects of **other opioid analgesics.** **HERBAL:** None significant. **FOOD:** None known. **LAB VALUES:** May increase serum amylase, lipase.

AVAILABILITY (Rx)

INJECTION SOLUTION (BUPRENEX): 0.3 mg/1 ml. **TABLETS, SUBLINGUAL (SUBUTEX):** 2 mg, 8 mg. **TABLETS, SUBLINGUAL (FIXED-COMBINATION [SUBOXONE]):** 2 mg/0.5 mg, 8 mg/2 mg.

ADMINISTRATION/HANDLING

IV

Reconstitution • May be diluted with isotonic saline, lactated Ringer's solution, D_5W, 0.9% NaCl.

Rate of administration • If given as IV push, administer over at least 2 min.

IM

Give deep IM into large muscle mass.

SUBLINGUAL

Dissolve tablet(s) under tongue; do not swallow (reduces drug bioavailability). For doses more than 2 tablets, either place all tablets at once or 2 tablets at a time under the tongue.

Storage • Store parenteral form at room temperature. • Protect from prolonged exposure to light. • Store tablets at room temperature.

IV INCOMPATIBILITIES

Amphotericin B (Abelcet, AmBisome), diazepam (Valium), lansoprazole (Prevacid), lorazepam (Ativan).

IV COMPATIBILITIES

Allopurinol (Aloprim, Zyloprim), aztreonam (Azactam), cefepime (Maxipime), granisetron (Kytril), haloperidol (Haldol), heparin, linezolid (Zyvox), lipids, midazolam (Versed), piperacillin/tazobactam (Zosyn), propofol (Diprivan).

INDICATIONS/ROUTES/DOSAGE

OPIOID DEPENDENCE, ANALGESIA

SUBLINGUAL: ADULTS, CHILDREN 13 YRS AND OLDER: 12–16 mg/day of Subutex used as induction with switch to Suboxone for maintenance.

IM/IV: ADULTS, CHILDREN 13 YRS AND OLDER: 0.3 mg (1 ml) q6h prn; may repeat 30–60 min after initial dose. May increase to 0.6 mg and/or reduce dosing interval to q4h if necessary. **CHILDREN 2–12 YRS:** 2–6 mcg/kg q4–6h prn.

USUAL ELDERLY DOSAGE

IM/IV: 0.15 mg q6h prn.
SUBLINGUAL: ADULTS, ELDERLY: 12–16 mg/day. For pts taking heroin/other short-acting opioids, give at least 4 hrs after pt last used opioids or when early signs of withdrawal appear.

SIDE EFFECTS

FREQUENT: Sedation (67%), dizziness, nausea (10%). **OCCASIONAL (5%–1%):** Headache, hypotension, vomiting, miosis, diaphoresis. **RARE (Less than 1%):** Dry mouth, pallor, visual abnormalities, injection site reaction.

ADVERSE EFFECTS/ TOXIC REACTIONS

Overdosage results in cold, clammy skin, weakness, confusion, severe respiratory depression, cyanosis, pinpoint pupils, extreme somnolence progressing to seizures, stupor, coma.

B

NURSING CONSIDERATIONS

BASELINE ASSESSMENT

Obtain baseline B/P, pulse rate. Assess mental status, alertness. Obtain history of when pt last used opioids. Assess for early signs of withdrawal symptoms before initiating therapy.

INTERVENTION/EVALUATION

Monitor for change in respirations, B/P, rate/quality of pulse. Initiate deep breathing, coughing exercises, particularly in those with pulmonary impairment. Assess for clinical improvement, record onset of relief of pain.

PATIENT/FAMILY TEACHING

Change positions slowly to avoid dizziness, orthostatic hypotension. Avoid tasks that require alertness, motor skills until response to drug is established. Overdose may occur if alcohol, sedatives, antidepressants, tranquilizers are taken concurrently with buprenorphine.

*buPROPion

byew-**pro**-peon

(Wellbutrin, Wellbutrin SR, Wellbutrin XL, Zyban)

Do not confuse bupropion with buspirone, Wellbutrin with Wellcovorin or Wellferon, or Zyban with Zagam.

CLASSIFICATION

PHARMACOTHERAPEUTIC: Aminoketone. **CLINICAL:** Antidepressant, smoking cessation aid (see pp. 38C, 144C).

ACTION

Blocks reuptake of neurotransmitters, (serotonin, norepinephrine) at CNS presynaptic membranes, increasing availability at postsynaptic receptor sites. Reduces firing rate of noradrenergic neurons. **Therapeutic Effect:** Relieves depression. Eliminates nicotine withdrawal symptoms.

PHARMACOKINETICS

Rapidly absorbed from GI tract. Protein binding: 84%. Crosses the blood-brain barrier. Undergoes extensive first-pass metabolism in the liver to active metabolite. Primarily excreted in urine. **Half-life:** 14 hrs.

USES

Treatment of depression, particularly endogenous depression, exhibited as persistent and prominent dysphoria (occurring nearly every day for at least 2 wks) manifested by 4 of 8 symptoms: change in appetite, change in sleep pattern, increased fatigue, impaired concentration, feelings of guilt or worthlessness, loss of interest in usual activities, psychomotor agitation or retardation, or suicidal tendencies. Assists in smoking cessation. Prevents depression in pts with seasonal affective disorder (SAD). **OFF-LABEL:** Treatment of attention deficit hyperactivity disorder in adults, children.

PRECAUTIONS

CONTRAINDICATIONS: Current or prior diagnosis of anorexia nervosa or bulimia, seizure disorder, use within 14 days of MAOIs, concomitant use of other bupropion products. **CAUTIONS:** History of seizure, cranial trauma; those currently taking antipsychotics, antidepressants; renal/hepatic impairment.

LIFESPAN CONSIDERATIONS:

Pregnancy/Lactation: Unknown if drug crosses placenta or is distributed in breast milk. **Pregnancy Category B.**

Children: More sensitive to increased dosage, toxicity, increased risk of suicidal ideation, worsening of depression. Safety and efficacy not established in those younger than 18 yrs. **Elderly:** More sensitive to anticholinergic, sedative, cardiovascular effects. Age-related renal impairment may require dosage adjustment.

INTERACTIONS

DRUG: **Alcohol, lithium, ritonavir, steroids, trazodone, tricyclic antidepressants** may increase risk of seizures. **Fosphenytoin, phenytoin, phenobarbital** may decrease the effectiveness of bupropion. May increase plasma levels of **haloperidol. Levodopa** may increase risk of adverse effects (nausea, vomiting, excitation, restlessness, postural tremor). **MAOIs** may increase risk of neuroleptic malignant syndrome, acute bupropion toxicity. **HERBAL:** **St. John's wort, gotu kola, kava kava, valerian** may increase CNS depression. **FOOD:** None known. **LAB VALUES:** May decrease WBC.

AVAILABILITY (Rx)

TABLETS (SUSTAINED-RELEASE [WELLBUTRIN SR]): 100 mg, 150 mg, 200 mg. **TABLETS (SUSTAINED-RELEASE [ZYBAN]):** 150 mg. **TABLETS (WELLBUTRIN):** 75 mg, 100 mg.

TABLETS (EXTENDED-RELEASE [WELLBUTRIN XL]): 150 mg, 300 mg.

ADMINISTRATION/HANDLING

PO

• Give without regard to food (give with food if GI irritation occurs). • Give at least 4-hr interval for immediate onset and 8-hr interval for sustained-release tablet to avoid seizures. • Avoid bedtime dosage (decreases risk of insomnia). • Do not crush sustained-release preparations.

INDICATIONS/ROUTES/DOSAGE

DEPRESSION

PO (IMMEDIATE-RELEASE): ADULTS: Initially, 100 mg twice a day. May increase to 100 mg 3 times a day no sooner than 3 days after beginning therapy. **Maximum:** 450 mg/day. **ELDERLY:** 37.5 mg twice a day. May increase by 37.5 mg q3–4 days. Maintenance: Lowest effective dosage.

PO (SUSTAINED-RELEASE): ADULTS: Initially, 150 mg/day as a single dose in the morning. May increase to 150 mg twice a day as early as day 4 after beginning therapy. **Maximum:** 400 mg/day. **ELDERLY:** Initially, 50–100 mg/day. May increase by 50–100 mg/day q3–4 days. Maintenance: Lowest effective dosage.

PO (EXTENDED-RELEASE): ADULTS: 150 mg once a day. May increase to 300 mg once a day. **Maximum:** 450 mg a day.

SMOKING CESSATION

PO: ADULTS: Initially, 150 mg a day for 3 days; then 150 mg twice a day for 7–12 wks.

PREVENTION SAD

PO: ADULTS, ELDERLY: (WELLBUTRIN XL): 150 mg/day for 1 wk, then 300 mg/day. Begin in autumn (Sept–Nov). End of treatment begins in spring (Mar–Apr) by decreasing dose to 150 mg/day for 2 wks before discontinuation.

DOSAGE IN HEPATIC IMPAIRMENT

Mild–moderate: Use caution, reduce dosage. **Severe:** Use extreme caution, maximum dose. Wellbutrin: 75 mg/day. Wellbutrin SR: 100 mg/day or 150 mg every other day. Wellbutrin XL: 150 mg every other day. Zyban: 150 mg every other day.

SIDE EFFECTS

FREQUENT (32%–18%): Constipation, weight gain or loss, nausea, vomiting, anorexia, dry mouth, headache, diaphoresis, tremor, sedation, insomnia,

B

dizziness, agitation. **OCCASIONAL (10%–5%):** Diarrhea, akinesia, blurred vision, tachycardia, confusion, hostility, fatigue.

ADVERSE EFFECTS/ TOXIC REACTIONS

Risk of seizures increases in pts taking more than 150 mg/dose, history of bulimia, seizure disorders, discontinuing drugs that may lower seizure threshold.

NURSING CONSIDERATIONS

BASELINE ASSESSMENT

For those on long-term therapy, hepatic/renal function tests should be performed periodically.

INTERVENTION/EVALUATION

Closely supervise suicidal-risk pt during early therapy (as depression lessens, energy level improves, increasing suicide potential). Assess appearance, behavior, speech pattern, level of interest, mood.

PATIENT/FAMILY TEACHING

• Full therapeutic effect may be noted in 4 wks. • Avoid tasks that require alertness, motor skills until response to drug is established.

*busPIRone hydrochloride

byew-spear-own

(Apo-Buspirone ✤, BuSpar, BuSpar Dividose, Buspirex ✤, Bustab ✤, Novo-Buspirone✤)

Do not confuse buspirone with bupropion.

◆ CLASSIFICATION

PHARMACOTHERAPEUTIC: Nonbarbiturate. **CLINICAL:** Antianxiety (see p. 12C).

ACTION

Binds to serotonin, dopamine at presynaptic neurotransmitter receptors in CNS. **Therapeutic Effect:** Produces anxiolytic effect.

PHARMACOKINETICS

Rapidly and completely absorbed from GI tract. Protein binding: 95%. Undergoes extensive first-pass metabolism. Metabolized in the liver to active metabolite. Primarily excreted in urine. Not removed by hemodialysis. **Half-life:** 2–3 hrs.

USES

Short-term management (up to 4 wks) of anxiety disorders. **OFF-LABEL:** Augmenting medication for antidepressants; management of aggression in mental retardation, secondary mental disorders, major depression, panic attack; premenstrual syndrome (aches, pain, fatigue, irritability).

PRECAUTIONS

CONTRAINDICATIONS: Concurrent use of MAOIs, severe hepatic/renal impairment. **CAUTIONS:** Renal/hepatic impairment.

⌛ LIFESPAN CONSIDERATIONS:

Pregnancy/Lactation: Unknown if drug crosses placenta or is distributed in breast milk. **Pregnancy Category B.** **Children:** Safety and efficacy not established. **Elderly:** No age-related precautions noted.

INTERACTIONS

DRUG: **Alcohol, other CNS depressants** potentiate effects, may increase sedation. **Erythromycin, itraconazole** may increase concentration, risk of toxicity. **MAOIs** may increase B/P. **HERBAL:** **St. John's wort, kava kava, gotu kola, valerian** may increase CNS depression. **FOOD:** **Grapefruit,**

grapefruit juice may increase concentration, risk of toxicity. **LAB VALUES:** None known.

AVAILABILITY (Rx)

TABLETS: 5 mg (BuSpar), 7.5 mg, 10 mg (BuSpar), 15 mg (BuSpar, BuSpar Dividose), 30 mg (BuSpar Dividose).

ADMINISTRATION/HANDLING

PO

• Give without regard to food. • Tablets may be crushed.

INDICATIONS/ROUTES/DOSAGE

SHORT-TERM MANAGEMENT (UP TO 4 WKS) OF ANXIETY DISORDERS

PO: ADULTS: 5 mg 2–3 times a day or 7.5 mg twice a day. May increase by 5 mg/day every 2–4 days. Maintenance: 15–30 mg/day in 2–3 divided doses. **Maximum:** 60 mg/day. **ELDERLY:** Initially, 5 mg twice a day. May increase by 5 mg/day every 2–3 days. **Maximum:** 60 mg/day. **CHILDREN:** Initially, 5 mg/day. May increase by 5 mg/day at weekly intervals. **Maximum:** 60 mg/day.

SIDE EFFECTS

FREQUENT (12%–6%): Dizziness, somnolence, nausea, headache. **OCCASIONAL (5%–2%):** Nervousness, fatigue, insomnia, dry mouth, light-headedness, mood swings, blurred vision, poor concentration, diarrhea, paraesthesia. **RARE:** Muscle pain/stiffness, nightmares, chest pain, involuntary movements.

ADVERSE EFFECTS/ TOXIC REACTIONS

No evidence of drug tolerance, psychological or physical dependence, withdrawal syndrome. Overdose may produce severe nausea, vomiting, dizziness, drowsiness, abdominal distention, excessive pupil contraction.

NURSING CONSIDERATIONS

BASELINE ASSESSMENT

Offer emotional support to anxious pt. Assess motor responses (agitation, trembling, tension), autonomic responses (cold, clammy hands; diaphoresis).

INTERVENTION/EVALUATION

For those on long-term therapy, hepatic/renal function tests, blood counts should be performed periodically. Assist with ambulation if drowsiness, light-headedness occur. Evaluate for therapeutic response: calm, facial expression, decreased restlessness, insomnia.

PATIENT/FAMILY TEACHING

• Improvement may be noted in 7–10 days, but optimum therapeutic effect generally takes 3–4 wks. • Drowsiness usually disappears during continued therapy. • If dizziness occurs, change position slowly from recumbent to sitting position before standing. • Avoid tasks that require alertness, motor skills until response to drug is established.

busulfan

bew-**sull**-fan

(Busulfex, Myleran)

Do not confuse Myleran with Alkeran, Leukeran, or Mylicon.

◆CLASSIFICATION

PHARMACOTHERAPEUTIC: Alkylating agent. **CLINICAL:** Antineoplastic (see p. 77C).

B

ACTION

Interferes with DNA replication, RNA synthesis. Cell cycle-phase nonspecific. **Therapeutic Effect:** Disrupts nucleic acid function. Myelosuppressant.

PHARMACOKINETICS

Completely absorbed from GI tract. Protein binding: 33%. Metabolized in the liver. Primarily excreted in urine. Minimally removed by hemodialysis. **Half-life:** 2.5 hrs.

USES

Treatment of chronic myelogenous leukemia (CML). **OFF-LABEL:** Treatment of acute myelocytic leukemia.

PRECAUTIONS

CONTRAINDICATIONS: Disease resistance to previous therapy with this drug. **EXTREME CAUTION:** Compromised bone marrow reserve. **CAUTIONS:** Chickenpox, herpes zoster, infection, history of gout.

LIFESPAN CONSIDERATIONS:

Pregnancy/Lactation: If possible, avoid use during pregnancy, esp. first trimester. May cause fetal harm. Unknown if distributed in breast milk. Breast-feeding not recommended. **Pregnancy Category D. Children/Elderly:** No age-related precautions noted.

INTERACTIONS

DRUG: May decrease effect of **antigout medications. Cytotoxic agents** may increase cytotoxicity. **Bone marrow depressants** may increase risk of myelosuppression. **Live virus vaccines** may potentiate virus replication, increase vaccine side effects, decrease antibody response to vaccine. **HERBAL: St. John's wort** may decrease concentration. **FOOD:** None known. **LAB VALUES:** May decrease serum magnesium, potassium, phosphate, sodium. May increase serum glucose, calcium, bilirubin, ALT, creatinine, alkaline phosphatase, BUN.

AVAILABILITY (Rx)

INJECTION SOLUTION (BUSULFAN): 60-mg ampule. **TABLETS (MYLERAN):** 2 mg.

ADMINISTRATION/HANDLING

◀ ALERT ▶ May be carcinogenic, mutagenic, teratogenic. Handle with extreme care during administration. Use of gloves recommended. If contact occurs with skin/mucosa, wash thoroughly with water.

IV

Reconstitution • Dilute with 0.9% NaCl or D_5W only. Diluent quantity must be 10 times the volume of busulfan (e.g., 9.3 ml busulfan must be diluted with 93 ml diluent). • Use filter to withdraw busulfan from ampule. • Add busulfan to calculated diluent. • Use infusion pump to administer busulfan.

Rate of administration • Infuse over 2 hrs. • Before and after infusion, flush catheter line with 5 ml 0.9% NaCl or D_5W.

Storage • Refrigerate ampules. • Following dilution, stable for 8 hrs at room temperature, 12 hrs if refrigerated when diluted with 0.9% NaCl.

PO

• Give at same time each day. • Give on empty stomach if nausea/vomiting occur.

IV INCOMPATIBILITIES

Do not mix busulfan with any other medications.

INDICATIONS/ROUTES/DOSAGE

REMISSION INDUCTION IN CML

PO: ADULTS, ELDERLY: 4–8 mg/day up to 12 mg/day. Maintenance: 1–4

B

mg/day to 2 mg/wk. Continue until WBC count is 10,000–20,000/mm^3, resume when WBC count reaches 50,000/mm^3. **CHILDREN:** 0.06–0.12 mg/kg/day. Maintenance: Titrate to maintain leukocyte count above 40,000/mm^3, reduce dose by 50% if count is 30,000–40,000/mm^3, and discontinue if the count is 20,000/mm^3 or less.

MARROW ABLATIVE CONDITIONING AND BONE MARROW TRANSPLANTATION

IV: ADULTS, ELDERLY, CHILDREN WEIGHING MORE THAN 12 KG: 0.8 mg/kg/dose q6h for total of 16 doses. (Use IBW or ABW, whichever is lower). **CHILDREN WEIGHING 12 KG OR LESS:** 1.1 mg/kg/dose (IBW) q6h for 16 doses.

PO: ADULTS, ELDERLY, CHILDREN: 1 mg/kg/dose (IBW) q6h for 16 doses.

SIDE EFFECTS

EXPECTED (98%–72%): Nausea, stomatitis, vomiting, anorexia, insomnia, diarrhea, fever, abdominal pain, anxiety. **FREQUENT (69%–44%):** Headache, rash, asthenia, infection, chills, tachycardia, dyspepsia. **OCCASIONAL (38%–16%):** Constipation, dizziness, edema, pruritus, cough, dry mouth, depression, abdominal enlargement, pharyngitis, hiccups, back pain, alopecia, myalgia. **RARE (13%–5%):** Injection site pain, arthralgia, confusion, hypotension, lethargy.

ADVERSE EFFECTS/ TOXIC REACTIONS

Major adverse effect is myelosuppression resulting in hematologic toxicity (anemia, severe leukopenia, severe thrombocytopenia). Very high dosages may produce blurred vision, muscle twitching, tonic-clonic seizures. Long-term therapy (more than 4 yrs) may produce pulmonary syndrome ("busulfan lung"), characterized by persistent cough, congestion, crackles, dyspnea. Hyperuricemia may produce uric acid nephropathy, renal calculi, acute renal failure.

NURSING CONSIDERATIONS

BASELINE ASSESSMENT

CBC with differential, hepatic/renal function studies should be performed weekly (dosage based on hematologic values).

INTERVENTION/EVALUATION

Monitor lab values diligently for evidence of bone marrow depression. Assess mouth for onset of stomatitis (redness/ulceration of oral mucous membranes, gum inflammation, difficulty swallowing). Initiate antiemetics to prevent nausea/vomiting. Monitor daily pattern of bowel activity/stool consistency.

PATIENT/FAMILY TEACHING

Educate pt/family regarding expected effects of therapy. • Maintain adequate daily fluid intake (may protect against renal impairment). • Report consistent cough, congestion, difficulty breathing. • Promptly report fever, sore throat, signs of local infection, unusual bruising/bleeding from any site. • Do not have immunizations without physician's approval (drug lowers body's resistance). • Avoid contact with those who have recently taken live virus vaccine. • Take at same time each day. • Contraception is recommended during therapy.

butenafine

(Mentax)

See Antifungals: topical (p. 46C)

B

butorphanol

byew-**tore**-phen-awl
(Stadol, Stadol NS)

Do not confuse butorphanol with butabarbital or Stadol with Haldol.

CLASSIFICATION

PHARMACOTHERAPEUTIC: Opioid (**Schedule IV**). **CLINICAL:** Analgesic, anesthesia adjunct (see p. 135C).

ACTION

Binds to opiate receptor sites in CNS. Reduces intensity of pain stimuli incoming from sensory nerve endings. **Therapeutic Effect:** Alters pain perception, emotional response to pain.

PHARMACOKINETICS

Route	Onset	Peak	Duration
IM	10–30 min	30–60 min	3–4 hrs
IV	Less than 1 min	30 min	2–4 hrs
Nasal	15 min	1–2 hrs	4–5 hrs

Rapidly absorbed after IM injection. Protein binding: 80%. Extensively metabolized in the liver. Primarily excreted in urine. **Half-life:** 2.5–4 hrs.

USES

Management of pain (including postoperative pain). **Nasal:** Migraine headache pain. **Parenteral:** Preoperative, preanesthetic medication, supplement balanced anesthesia, relief of pain during labor.

PRECAUTIONS

CONTRAINDICATIONS: CNS disease that affects respirations, hypersensitivity to the preservative benzethonium chloride, physical dependence on other opioid analgesics, preexisting respiratory depression, pulmonary disease. **CAUTIONS:** Hepatic/renal impairment, elderly, debilitated, head injury, hypertension, use before biliary tract surgery (produces spasm of sphincter of Oddi), MI, narcotic dependence.

LIFESPAN CONSIDERATIONS:

Pregnancy/Lactation: Readily crosses placenta. Distributed in breast milk. Breast-feeding not recommended. **Pregnancy Category C, D if used for prolonged time, high dose at term. Children:** Safety and efficacy not known in those younger than 18 yrs. **Elderly:** May be more sensitive to effects; adjust dose and interval.

INTERACTIONS

DRUG: **Alcohol, CNS depressants** may increase CNS or respiratory depression, hypotension. Effects may be decreased with **buprenorphine. MAOIs** may produce severe, fatal reaction unless dose is reduced by ¼. **HERBAL:** **St. John's wort, kava kava, gotu kola, valerian** may increase CNS depression. **FOOD:** None known. **LAB VALUES:** None known.

AVAILABILITY (Rx)

INJECTION SOLUTION (STADOL): 1 mg/ml, 2 mg/ml. **NASAL SPRAY (STADOL NS):** 10 mg/ml.

ADMINISTRATION/HANDLING

INTRANASAL

• Instruct pt to blow nose to clear nasal passages as much as possible. • Tilt head slightly forward, insert spray tip into nostril, pointing toward nasal passages, away from nasal septum. • Spray into nostril while holding other nostril closed, concurrently inspire through nose to permit medication as high into nasal passages as possible.

IV INCOMPATIBILITIES

Amphotericin B complex (Abelcet, AmBisome, Amphotec).

B

IV COMPATIBILITIES

Atropine, diphenhydramine (Benadryl), droperidol (Inapsine), hydroxyzine (Vistaril), lipids, morphine, promethazine (Phenergan), propofol (Diprivan).

INDICATIONS/ROUTES/DOSAGE

ANALGESIA

IV: ADULTS: Initially 1 mg, then 0.5–2 mg q3–4h as needed. **ELDERLY:** 1 mg q4–6h as needed.

IM: ADULTS: Initially 2 mg, then 1–4 mg q3–4h as needed. **ELDERLY:** 1 mg q4–6h as needed.

MIGRAINE

NASAL: ADULTS: 1 mg or 1 spray in one nostril. May repeat in 60–90 min. May repeat 2-dose sequence q3–4h as needed. Alternatively, 2 mg or 1 spray in each nostril if pt remains recumbent, may repeat in 3–4 hrs.

SIDE EFFECTS

FREQUENT: Parenteral: Somnolence (43%), dizziness (19%). **Nasal:** Nasal congestion (13%), insomnia (11%). **OCCASIONAL: Parenteral (9%–3%):** Confusion, diaphoresis, clammy skin, lethargy, headache, nausea, vomiting, dry mouth. **Nasal (9%–3%):** Vasodilation, constipation, unpleasant taste, dyspnea, epistaxis, nasal irritation, upper respiratory tract infection, tinnitus. **RARE: Parenteral:** Hypotension, pruritus, blurred vision, sensation of heat, CNS stimulation, insomnia. **Nasal:** Hypertension, tremor, ear pain, paresthesia, depression, sinusitis.

ADVERSE EFFECTS/ TOXIC REACTIONS

Abrupt withdrawal after prolonged use may produce symptoms of narcotic withdrawal (abdominal cramping, rhinorrhea, lacrimation, anxiety, increased temperature, piloerection [goose bumps]). Overdose results in severe respiratory depression, skeletal muscle flaccidity, cyanosis, extreme somnolence progressing to seizures, stupor, coma. Tolerance to analgesic effect, physical dependence may occur with chronic use.

NURSING CONSIDERATIONS

BASELINE ASSESSMENT

Obtain vital signs before giving medication. If respirations are 12/min or less (20/min or less in children), withhold medication, contact physician. Assess onset, type, location, duration of pain. Effect of medication is reduced if full pain recurs before next dose. Protect from falls. During labor, assess fetal heart tones, uterine contractions.

INTERVENTION/EVALUATION

Monitor for change in respirations, B/P, rate/quality of pulse. Initiate deep breathing, coughing exercises, particularly in those with pulmonary impairment. Change pt's position q2–4h. Assess for clinical improvement, record onset of relief of pain.

PATIENT/FAMILY TEACHING

• Change positions slowly to avoid dizziness. • Avoid tasks that require alertness, motor skills until response to drug is established. • Instruct pt on proper use of nasal spray. • Avoid use of alcohol, CNS depressants.

Byetta, *see exenatide*

cabergoline

cab-**err**-go-leen
(Dostinex)

CLASSIFICATION

CLINICAL: Antihyperprolactinemic.

ACTION

Agonist at dopamine D_2 receptors suppressing prolactin secretion. **Therapeutic Effect:** Shrinks prolactinomas, restores gonadal function.

PHARMACOKINETICS

Extensive tissue distribution. Protein binding: 40%–42%. Hydrolyzed to inactive metabolite. Excreted primarily in feces. **Half-life:** 63–69 hrs.

USES

Treatment of hyperprolactinemic disorders, either idiopathic or due to pituitary adenomas.

PRECAUTIONS

CONTRAINDICATIONS: Uncontrolled hypertension, hypersensitivity to ergot alkaloids.
CAUTIONS: Hepatic impairment.

LIFESPAN CONSIDERATIONS:

Pregnancy/Lactation: Adequate studies not done. Unknown if distributed in breast milk. Not recommended during pregnancy. **Pregnancy Category B. Children/Elderly:** Safety and efficacy not established.

INTERACTIONS

DRUG: **Other antihypertensives** may increase hypotensive effect if given concurrently. May decrease effects of **metoclopramide, haloperidol, phenothiazines**. **HERBAL:** None significant. **FOOD:** None known. **LAB VALUES:** None known.

AVAILABILITY (Rx)

TABLETS: 0.5 mg.

INDICATIONS/ROUTES/DOSAGE

HYPERPROLACTINEMIA

PO: ADULTS, ELDERLY: Initially, 0.25 mg twice a wk. May increase by 0.25 mg a wk at 4-wk intervals up to a maximum of 1 mg twice a wk according to pt's serum prolactin level.

SIDE EFFECTS

FREQUENT (29%): Nausea. **OCCASIONAL (20%–5%):** Headache, vertigo, dizziness, dyspepsia, postural hypotension, constipation. **RARE (4%–2%):** Vomiting, dry mouth, diarrhea, flatulence.

ADVERSE EFFECTS/ TOXIC REACTIONS

Overdosage may produce nasal congestion, syncope, hallucinations.

NURSING CONSIDERATIONS

BASELINE ASSESSMENT

Obtain baseline hepatic function tests.

INTERVENTION/EVALUATION

Monitor prolactin monthly until levels equalize.

PATIENT/FAMILY TEACHING

- Rise slowly from lying to sitting position, permit legs to dangle momentarily before rising to reduce hypotensive effect.

caffeine citrate

(Cafcit)

ACTION

Stimulates medullary respiratory center. Appears to increase sensitivity of respiratory center to stimulatory effects of CO_2.

Therapeutic Effect: Increases alveolar ventilation, reducing severity, frequency of apneic episodes.

USES

Short-term treatment of apnea in premature infants from 28 wks to younger than 33 wks gestational age.

PRECAUTIONS

Pregnancy Category C.

INTERACTIONS

DRUG: None significant. **HERBAL:** None signifcant. **FOOD:** None known. **LAB VALUES:** None known.

AVAILABILITY (Rx)

INJECTION SOLUTION: 20 mg/ml. **ORAL SOLUTION:** 20 mg/ml.

INDICATIONS/ROUTES/DOSAGE

APNEA

PO, IV: Loading dose: 10–20 mg/kg as caffeine citrate (5–10 mg/kg as caffeine base). If theophylline given within previous 72 hrs, a modified dose (50%–75%) may be given. Maintenance: 5 mg/kg/day as caffeine citrate (2.5 mg/kg/day as caffeine base). Dosage adjusted based on pt response.

SIDE EFFECTS

FREQUENT (10%–5%): Feeding intolerance, rash.

ADVERSE EFFECTS/ TOXIC REACTIONS

Sepsis, necrotizing enterocolitis may occur.

NURSING CONSIDERATIONS

INTERVENTION/EVALUATION

Monitor respirations diligently. Assess skin for rash.

calcitonin

kal-sih-**toe**-nin

(Apo-Calcitonin ✤, Calcimar ✤, Caltine ✤, Cibacalcin, Fortical, Miacalcin, Miacalcin Nasal)

Do not confuse calcitonin with calcitriol, Miacalcin with Micatin.

CLASSIFICATION

PHARMACOTHERAPEUTIC: Synthetic hormone. **CLINICAL:** Calcium regulator, bone resorption inhibitor, osteoporosis therapy.

ACTION

Decreases osteoclast activity in bones, decreases tubular reabsorption of sodium and calcium in kidneys, increases absorption of calcium in GI tract. **Therapeutic Effect:** Regulates serum calcium concentrations.

PHARMACOKINETICS

Injection form rapidly metabolized (primarily in kidneys); primarily excreted in urine. Nasal form rapidly absorbed. **Half-life:** 70–90 min (injection); 43 min (nasal).

USES

Parenteral: Treatment of Paget's disease, hypercalcemia, postmenopausal osteoporosis, osteogenesis imperfecta. **Intranasal:** Postmenopausal osteoporosis. **OFF-LABEL:** Treatment of secondary osteoporosis due to drug therapy or hormone disturbance.

PRECAUTIONS

CONTRAINDICATIONS: Hypersensitivity to gelatin desserts or salmon protein. **CAUTIONS:** History of allergy, renal dysfunction.

LIFESPAN CONSIDERATIONS:

Pregnancy/Lactation: Drug does not cross placenta; unknown if distributed in breast milk. Safe usage during lactation not established (inhibits lactation in animals). **Pregnancy Category C. Children:** Safety and efficacy not established. **Elderly:** No age-related precautions noted.

INTERACTIONS

DRUG: Preparations containing calcium, vitamin D may antagonize effects. **HERBAL:** None significant. **FOOD:** None known. **LAB VALUES:** None known.

AVAILABILITY (Rx)

INJECTION SOLUTION (MIACALCIN): 200 international units/ml (calcitonin-salmon), 500 mg (calcitonin-human). **NASAL SPRAY (FORTICAL, MIACALCIN NASAL):** 200 international units/activation (calcitonin-salmon).

ADMINISTRATION/HANDLING

IM, SUBCUTANEOUS

No more than 2-ml dose should be given IM. • Skin test should be performed before therapy in pts suspected of sensitivity to calcitonin. • Bedtime administration may reduce nausea, flushing.

INTRANASAL

• Refrigerate unopened nasal spray. Store at room temperature after initial use. • Instruct pt to clear nasal passages as much as possible. • Tilt head slightly forward, insert spray tip into nostril, pointing toward nasal passages, away from nasal septum. • Spray into nostril while pt holds other nostril closed and concurrently inspires through nose to permit medication as high into nasal passage as possible.

INDICATIONS/ROUTES/DOSAGE

SKIN TESTING BEFORE TREATMENT IN PTS WITH SUSPECTED SENSITIVITY TO CALCITONIN-SALMON

INTRACUTANEOUS: ADULTS, ELDERLY: Prepare a 10-international units/ml dilution; withdraw 0.05 ml from a 200-international units/ml vial in a tuberculin syringe; fill up to 1 ml with 0.9% NaCl. Take 0.1 ml and inject intracutaneously on inner aspect of forearm. Observe after 15 min; a positive response is the appearance of more than mild erythema or wheal.

PAGET'S DISEASE

IM, SUBCUTANEOUS: ADULTS, ELDERLY: Initially, 100 international units/day. Maintenance: 50 international units/day or 50–100 international units every 1–3 days.

OSTEOPOROSIS IMPERFECTA

IM, SUBCUTANEOUS: ADULTS: 2 international units/kg 3 times a week.

POSTMENOPAUSAL OSTEOPOROSIS

IM, SUBCUTANEOUS: ADULTS, ELDERLY: 100 international units every other day with adequate calcium and vitamin D intake. **INTRANASAL: ADULTS, ELDERLY:** 200 international units/day as a single spray, alternating nostrils daily.

HYPERCALCEMIA

IM, SUBCUTANEOUS: ADULTS, ELDERLY: Initially, 4 international units/kg q12h; may increase to 8 international units/kg q12h if no response in 2 days; may further increase to 8 international units/kg q6h if no response in another 2 days.

SIDE EFFECTS

FREQUENT: IM, Subcutaneous (10%): Nausea (may occur 30 min after injection, usually diminishes with continued therapy), inflammation at injection site. **Nasal (12%–10%):** Rhinitis, nasal irritation, redness, sores. **OCCASIONAL: IM, Subcutaneous (5%–2%):** Flushing of face, hands. **Nasal (5%–3%):** Back pain, arthralgia, epistaxis, headache. **RARE: IM, Subcutaneous:** Epigastric discomfort, dry mouth, diarrhea, flatulence. **Nasal:** Itching of earlobes, pedal edema, rash, diaphoresis.

ADVERSE EFFECTS/ TOXIC REACTIONS

Pts with a protein allergy may develop a hypersensitivity reaction.

NURSING CONSIDERATIONS

BASELINE ASSESSMENT

Establish baseline electrolytes.

INTERVENTION/EVALUATION

Ensure rotation of injection sites; check for inflammation. Assess vertebral bone mass (document stabilization/improvement). Assess for allergic response: rash, urticaria, swelling, shortness of breath, tachycardia, hypotension.

PATIENT/FAMILY TEACHING

• Instruct pt and family on aseptic technique, proper injection of medication, including rotation of sites. • Nausea is transient and usually decreases with continued therapy. • Notify physician immediately if rash, itching, shortness of breath, significant nasal irritation occur. • Explain to pt and family that improvement in biochemical abnormalities and bone pain usually occurs in the first few months of treatment. • Explain to pts with neurologic lesions, improvement may take more than a year.

calcium acetate

(PhosLo)

calcium carbonate

(Apo-Cal ✤, Caltrate, Caltrate 600 ✤, OsCal ✤, Os-Cal 500, Titralac, Tums)

calcium chloride

calcium citrate

(Citracal, Cal-Citrate, Osteocit ✤)

calcium glubionate

calcium gluconate

kal-see-um

Do not confuse OsCal with Asacol, Citracal with Citrucel, PhosLo with PhosChol.

CLASSIFICATION

PHARMACOTHERAPEUTIC: Electrolyte replenisher. **CLINICAL:** Antacid, antihypocalcemic, antihyperkalemic, antihypermagnesemic, antihyperphosphatemic (see p. 10C).

ACTION

Essential for function, integrity of nervous, muscular, skeletal systems. Plays an important role in normal cardiac/renal function, respiration, blood coagulation, cell membrane and capillary permeability. Assists in regulating release/storage of neurotransmitters/hormones. Neutralizes/reduces gastric acid (increases pH). **Calcium acetate:** Combines with dietary phosphate, forming insoluble calcium phosphate. **Therapeutic Effect:** Replaces calcium in deficiency states; controls hyperphosphatemia in end-stage renal disease.

PHARMACOKINETICS

Moderately absorbed from small intestine (absorption depends on presence of vitamin D metabolites and pt's pH). Primarily eliminated in feces.

USES

Parenteral: Acute hypocalcemia (e.g., neonatal hypocalcemic tetany, alkalosis), electrolyte depletion, cardiac arrest (strengthens myocardial contractions), hyperkalemia (reverses cardiac depression), hypermagnesemia (aids in reversing CNS depression). **Calcium carbonate:** Antacid, treatment/prevention of calcium deficiency, hyperphosphatemia. **Calcium citrate:** Antacid, treatment/prevention of calcium deficiency, hyperphosphatemia. **Calcium acetate:** Controls hyperphosphatemia in end-stage renal disease.

C

PRECAUTIONS

CONTRAINDICATIONS: Calcium renal calculi, digoxin toxicity, hypercalcemia, hypercalciuria, sarcoidosis, ventricular fibrillation. **Calcium acetate:** Renal impairment, hypoparathyroidism. **CAUTIONS:** Dehydration, history of renal calculi, chronic renal impairment, decreased cardiac function, ventricular fibrillation during cardiac resuscitation.

LIFESPAN CONSIDERATIONS:

Pregnancy/Lactation: Distributed in breast milk. Unknown whether calcium chloride or gluconate is distributed in breast milk. **Pregnancy Category C.** **Children:** Extreme irritation, possible tissue necrosis or sloughing with IV. Restrict IV use due to small vasculature. **Elderly:** Oral absorption may be decreased.

INTERACTIONS

DRUG: **Digoxin** may increase risk of arrhythmias. May antagonize effects of **etidronate, gallium.** May decrease absorption of **ketoconazole, phenytion, tetracyclines.** May decrease effects of **methenamine, parenteral magnesium.** **HERBAL:** None significant. **FOOD:** Food may increase calcium absorption. **LAB VALUES:** May increase serum pH, calcium, gastrin. May decrease serum phosphate, potassium.

AVAILABILITY

CALCIUM ACETATE

GELCAP (PHOSLO): 667 mg (equivalent to 169 mg elemental calcium). **TABLETS (PHOSLO):** 667 mg (equivalent to 169 mg elemental calcium).

CALCIUM CARBONATE

TABLETS: equivalent to 500 mg elemental calcium (Os-Cal 500), equivalent to 600 mg elemental calcium (Caltrate 600). **TABLETS (CHEWABLE):** equivalent to 200 mg elemental calcium (Tums), equivalent to 500 mg elemental calcium (Os-Cal 500).

CALCIUM CHLORIDE

INJECTION SOLUTION: 10% (100 mg/ml) equivalent to 27.2 mg elemental calcium per ml.

CALCIUM CITRATE

TABLETS: 125 mg (Citracal Prenatal Rx), 250 mg (equivalent to 53 mg elemental calcium) (Cal-Citrate), 950 mg (equivalent to 200 mg elemental calcium) (Citracal).

CALCIUM GLUBIONATE

SYRUP: 1.8 g/5 ml (equivalent to 115 mg of elemental calcium per 5 ml).

CALCIUM GLUCONATE

INJECTION SOLUTION: 10% (equivalent to 9 mg elemental calcium per ml).

ADMINISTRATION/HANDLING

IV

DILUTION

Calcium chloride • May give undiluted or may dilute with equal amount 0.9% NaCl or Sterile Water for Injection.

Calcium gluconate • May give undiluted or may dilute in up to 1,000 ml NaCl.

Rate of administration

Calcium chloride • Give by slow IV push: 0.5–1 ml/min (rapid administration may produce bradycardia, metallic/chalky taste, drop in B/P, sensation of heat, peripheral vasodilation).

Calcium gluconate • Give by IV push: 0.5–1 ml/min (rapid administration may produce vasodilation, drop in B/P, arrhythmias, syncope, cardiac arrest). • Maximum rate for intermittent IV infusion is 200 mg/min (e.g., 10 ml/min when 1 g diluted with 50 ml diluent).

Storage • Store at room temperature.

PO

• Take tablets with full glass of water 0.5–1 hr after meals. Give syrup before meals (increases absorption), diluted in juice, water. • Chew chewable tablets well before swallowing.

IV INCOMPATIBILITIES

Calcium chloride: Amphotericin B complex (Abelcet, AmBisone, Amphotec), propofol (Diprivan), sodium bicarbonate. **Calcium gluconate:** Amphotericin B complex (Abelcet, AmBisome, Amphotec), fluconazole (Diflucan).

IV COMPATIBILITIES

Calcium chloride: Amikacin (Amikin), dobutamine (Dobutrex), lidocaine, milrinone (Primacor), morphine, norepinephrine (Levophed). **Calcium gluconate:** Ampicillin, aztreonam (Azactam), cefazolin (Ancef), cefepime (Maxipime), ciprofloxacin (Cipro), dobutamine (Dobutrex), enalapril (Vasotec), famotidine (Pepcid), furosemide (Lasix), heparin, lidocaine, lipids, magnesium sulfate, meropenem (Merrem IV), midazolam (Versed), milrinone (Primacor), norepinephrine (Levophed), piperacillin and tazobactam (Zosyn), potassium chloride, propofol (Diprivan).

INDICATIONS/ROUTES/DOSAGE

HYPERPHOSPHATEMIA

PO (CALCIUM ACETATE): ADULTS, ELDERLY: 2 tablets 3 times a day with meals. May increase gradually to bring serum phosphate level to less than 6 mg/dl as long as hypercalcemia does not develop.

HYPOCALCEMIA

PO (CALCIUM CARBONATE): ADULTS, ELDERLY: 1–2 g/day in 3–4 divided doses. **CHILDREN:** 45–65 mg/kg/day in 3–4 divided doses.

PO (CALCIUM GLUBIONATE): ADULTS, ELDERLY: 6–18 g/day in 4–6 divided doses. **CHILDREN, INFANTS:** 0.6–2 g/kg/day in 4 divided doses. **NEONATES:** 1.2 g/kg/day in 4–6 divided doses.

IV (CALCIUM CHLORIDE): ADULTS, ELDERLY: 0.5–1 g repeated q4–6h as needed. **CHILDREN:** 2.5–5 mg/kg/dose in q4–6h.

IV (CALCIUM GLUCONATE): ADULTS, ELDERLY: 2–15 g/24 hr. **CHILDREN:** 200–500 mg/kg/day.

ANTACID

PO (CALCIUM CARBONATE): ADULTS, ELDERLY: 1–2 tabs (5–10 ml) in q2h as needed.

OSTEOPOROSIS

PO (CALCIUM CARBONATE): ADULTS, ELDERLY: 1,200 mg/day.

CARDIAC ARREST

IV (CALCIUM CHLORIDE): ADULTS, ELDERLY: 2–4 mg/kg. May repeat q10 min. **CHILDREN:** 20 mg/kg. May repeat in 10 min.

HYPOCALCEMIA TETANY

IV (CALCIUM CHLORIDE): ADULTS, ELDERLY: 1 g may repeat in 6 hrs. **CHILDREN:** 10 mg/kg over 5–10 min. May repeat in q6–8h.

IV (CALCIUM GLUCONATE): ADULTS, ELDERLY: 1–3 g until therapeutic response achieved. **CHILDREN:** 100–200 mg/kg/dose in 6–8 hrs.

SUPPLEMENT

PO (CALCIUM CITRATE): ADULTS, ELDERLY: 0.5–2 g 2–4 times a day.

SIDE EFFECTS

FREQUENT: PO: Chalky taste. **Parenteral:** Pain, rash, redness, burning at injection site, flushing, feeling of warmth, nausea, vomiting, diaphoresis, hypotension. **OCCASIONAL: PO:** Mild constipation, fecal impaction, peripheral edema, metabolic alkalosis (muscle pain, restlessness, slow respirations, altered taste). **Calcium carbonate:** Milk-alkali syndrome (headache, decreased appetite, nausea, vomiting, unusual fatigue). **RARE:** Urinary urgency, painful urination.

ADVERSE EFFECTS/ TOXIC REACTIONS

Hypercalcemia: Early signs: Constipation, headache, dry mouth, increased thirst, irritability, decreased appetite, metallic taste, fatigue, weakness, depression. **Later signs:** Confusion, somnolence, hypertension, photosensitivity, arrhythmias, nausea, vomiting, painful urination.

NURSING CONSIDERATIONS

BASELINE ASSESSMENT

Assess B/P, EKG and cardiac rhythm, renal function, serum magnesium, phosphate, potassium concentrations.

INTERVENTION/EVALUATION

Monitor B/P, EKG, cardiac rhythm, serum magnesium, phosphate, potassium, renal function. Monitor serum, urine calcium concentrations. Monitor for signs of hypercalcemia.

PATIENT/FAMILY TEACHING

• Stress importance of diet. • Take tablets with full glass of water, ½–1 hr after meals. • Give liquid before meals. • Do not take within 1–2 hrs of other oral medications, fiber-containing foods. • Avoid excessive alcohol, tobacco, caffeine.

calfactant

cal-**fac**-tant
(Infasurf)

CLASSIFICATION

PHARMACOTHERAPEUTIC: Natural lung extract. **CLINICAL:** Pulmonary surfactant.

ACTION

Reduces alveolar surface tension, stabilizing the alveoli. **Therapeutic Effect:** Restores surface activity to infant lungs, improves lung compliance, respiratory gas exchange.

PHARMACOKINETICS

No studies have been performed.

USES

Prevention of respiratory distress syndrome (RDS) in premature infants younger than 29 wks of gestational age; treatment of premature infants younger than 72 hrs of age who develop RDS and require endotracheal intubation.

PRECAUTIONS

CONTRAINDICATIONS: None known. **CAUTIONS:** Hypersensitivity to calfactant.

LIFESPAN CONSIDERATIONS:

Pregnancy/Lactation: Not indicated in this pt population. **Pregnancy Category:** Not indicated for use in pregnant women. **Children:** Used only in neonates. No age-related precautions noted. **Elderly:** Not indicated in this pt population.

INTERACTIONS

DRUG: None significant. **HERBAL:** None significant. **FOOD:** None known. **LAB VALUES:** None known.

AVAILABILITY (Rx)

INTRATRACHEAL SUSPENSION: 35-mg/ml vials.

ADMINISTRATION/HANDLING

INTRATRACHEAL

• Refrigerate. • Unopened, unused vials may be returned to refrigerator only once after having been warmed to room temperature. • Do not shake. • Enter vial only once, discard unused suspension.

INDICATIONS/ROUTES/DOSAGE

RESPIRATORY DISTRESS SYNDROME (RDS)

INTRATRACHEAL: NEONATES: 3 ml/kg of birth weight administered as soon as possible after birth in 2 doses of 1.5 ml/kg. Repeat 3-ml/kg doses, up to a total of 3 doses given 12 hrs apart.

SIDE EFFECTS

FREQUENT: Cyanosis (65%), airway obstruction (39%), bradycardia (34%), reflux of surfactant into endotracheal tube (21%), need for manual ventilation (16%). **OCCASIONAL:** Need for reintubation (3%).

ADVERSE EFFECTS/ TOXIC REACTIONS

None known.

NURSING CONSIDERATIONS

BASELINE ASSESSMENT

Drug must be administered in highly supervised setting. Clinicians in charge of care of neonate must be experienced with intubation, ventilator management. Offer emotional support to parents.

INTERVENTION/EVALUATION

Monitor infant with arterial or transcutaneous measurement of systemic O_2, CO_2. Assess lung sounds for rales, moist breath sounds.

Camptosar, *see irinotecan*

Cancidas, *see caspofungin*

candesartan

kan-de-**sar**-tan

(Atacand)

FIXED-COMBINATION(S)

Atacand HCT: candesartan/hydrochlorothiazide (a diuretic): 16 mg/ 12.5 mg; 32 mg/12.5 mg.

◆ CLASSIFICATION

PHARMACOTHERAPEUTIC: Angiotensin II receptor antagonist. **CLINICAL:** Antihypertensive (see p. 8C).

ACTION

Blocks vasoconstrictor, aldosterone-secreting effects of angiotensin II, inhibiting binding of angiotensin II to AT_1 receptors. **Therapeutic Effect:** Produces vasodilation, decreases peripheral resistance, B/P.

PHARMACOKINETICS

Route	Onset	Peak	Duration
PO	2–3 hrs	6–8 hrs	Greater than 24 hrs

Rapidly, completely absorbed. Protein binding: greater than 99%. Undergoes minor hepatic metabolism to inactive metabolite. Excreted unchanged in urine and in feces through biliary system. Not removed by hemodialysis. **Half-life:** 9 hrs.

USES

Treatment of hypertension alone or in combination with other antihypertensives, heart failure (reduces risk of death from cardiovascular causes, reduces hospitalization for heart failure).

PRECAUTIONS

CONTRAINDICATIONS: Hypersensitivity to candesartan. **CAUTIONS:** Severe CHF, dehydration (increased risk for hypotension), renal/hepatic impairment, renal artery stenosis.

C

LIFESPAN CONSIDERATIONS:

Pregnancy/Lactation: Unknown if distributed in breast milk. May cause fetal/neonatal morbidity/mortality. **Pregnancy Category C (D if used in second or third trimester). Children:** Safety and efficacy not established. **Elderly:** No age-related precautions noted.

INTERACTIONS

DRUG: May increase risk of **lithium** toxicity. **HERBAL: Ephedra, ginseng, yohimbe** may worsen hypertension. **Garlic** may increase antihypertensive effect. **FOOD:** None known. **LAB VALUES:** May increase BUN, serum alkaline phosphatase, bilirubin, creatinine, AST, ALT. May decrease Hgb, Hct.

AVAILABILITY (Rx)

TABLETS: 4 mg, 8 mg, 16 mg, 32 mg.

ADMINISTRATION/HANDLING

PO

- Give without regard to food.

INDICATIONS/ROUTES/DOSAGE

HYPERTENSION

PO: ADULTS, ELDERLY, PTS WITH MILDLY IMPAIRED LIVER OR KIDNEY FUNCTION: Initially, 16 mg once a day in those who are not volume depleted. Can be given once or twice a day with total daily doses of 8–32 mg. Give lower dosage in those treated with diuretics or with severely renal impairment.

HEART FAILURE

PO: ADULTS, ELDERLY: Initially, 4 mg once daily. May double dose at approximately 2-wk intervals up to a target dose of 32 mg/day.

SIDE EFFECTS

OCCASIONAL (6%–3%): Upper respiratory tract infection, dizziness, back/leg pain. **RARE (2%–1%):** Pharyngitis, rhinitis, headache, fatigue, diarrhea, nausea, dry cough, peripheral edema.

ADVERSE EFFECTS/ TOXIC REACTIONS

Overdosage may manifest as hypotension, tachycardia. Bradycardia occurs less often. Institute supportive measures.

NURSING CONSIDERATIONS

BASELINE ASSESSMENT

Obtain B/P, apical pulse immediately before each dose, in addition to regular monitoring (be alert to fluctuations). If excessive reduction in B/P occurs, place pt in supine position, feet slightly elevated. Question for possibility of pregnancy (see Pregnancy Category). Assess medication history (esp. diuretic). Question for history of hepatic/renal impairment, renal artery stenosis. Obtain BUN, serum creatinine, AST, ALT, alkaline phosphatase, bilirubin, Hgb, Hct.

INTERVENTION/EVALUATION

Maintain hydration (offer fluids frequently). Assess for evidence of upper respiratory infection. Assist with ambulation if dizziness occurs. Monitor all serum levels. Assess B/P for hypertension/hypotension.

PATIENT/FAMILY TEACHING

• Inform female pt regarding consequences of second- and third-trimester exposure to candesartan. • Report pregnancy to physician as soon as possible. • Avoid tasks that require alertness, motor skills until response to drug is established. • Report any sign of infection (sore throat, fever). • Do not stop taking medication. • Explain need for lifelong control. • Caution against exercising during hot weather (risk of dehydration, hypotension).

capecitabine

cap-eh-**site**-ah-bean

(Xeloda)

Do not confuse Xeloda with Xenical.

CLASSIFICATION

PHARMACOTHERAPEUTIC: Antimetabolite. **CLINICAL:** Antineoplastic (see p. 77C).

ACTION

Enzymatically converted to 5-fluorouracil (5-FU). Inhibits enzymes necessary for synthesis of essential cellular components. **Therapeutic Effect:** Interferes with DNA synthesis, RNA processing, protein synthesis.

PHARMACOKINETICS

Readily absorbed from GI tract. Protein binding: less than 60%. Metabolized in the liver. Primarily excreted in urine. **Half-life:** 45 min.

USES

Treatment of metastatic breast cancer resistant to other therapy, colon cancer. Adjuvant (postsurgical) treatment of Dukes' C colon cancer.

PRECAUTIONS

CONTRAINDICATIONS: Severe renal impairment, dihydropyrimidine dehydrogenase (DPD) deficiency, hypersensitivity to 5-FU. **CAUTIONS:** Existing bone marrow depression, chickenpox, herpes zoster, hepatic impairment, moderate renal impairment, previous cytotoxic therapy/radiation therapy.

LIFESPAN CONSIDERATIONS:

Pregnancy/Lactation: May be harmful to fetus. Unknown if distributed in breast milk. **Pregnancy Category D.** **Children:** Safety and efficacy in those younger than 18 yrs not established. **Elderly:** May be more sensitive to GI side effects.

INTERACTIONS

DRUG: **Warfarin** may increase risk of bleeding. Myelosuppression may be enhanced when given concurrently with **bone marrow depressants. Live virus vaccines** may potentiate virus replication, increase vaccine side effects, decrease pt's antibody response to vaccine. **HERBAL:** None significant. **FOOD:** None known. **LAB VALUES:** May increase serum alkaline phosphatase, bilirubin, AST, ALT. May decrease Hgb, Hct, WBC count.

AVAILABILITY (Rx)

TABLETS: 150 mg, 500 mg.

ADMINISTRATION/HANDLING

- Give after meals with water.

INDICATIONS/ROUTES/DOSAGE

METASTATIC BREAST CANCER, COLON CANCER, ADJUVANT (POST SURGERY) TREATMENT OF DUKES' C COLON CANCER

PO: ADULTS, ELDERLY: Initially, 2,500 mg/m^2/day in 2 equally divided doses approximately q12h for 2 wks. Follow with a 1-wk rest period; given in 3-wk cycles.

DOSAGE IN RENAL IMPAIRMENT

Creatinine clearance 50–80 ml/min: No adjustment. **Creatinine clearance 30–49 ml/min:** 75% of normal dose. **Creatinine clearance less than 30 ml/min:** Not recommended.

SIDE EFFECTS

FREQUENT (greater than 5%): Diarrhea (sometimes severe), nausea, vomiting, stomatitis, hand-and-foot syndrome (painful palmar-plantar swelling with paresthesia, erythema, blistering), fatigue, anorexia, dermatitis. **OCCASIONAL**

(less than 5%): Constipation, dyspepsia, nail disorder, headache, dizziness, insomnia, edema, myalgia.

ADVERSE EFFECTS/ TOXIC REACTIONS

Serious reactions include myelosuppression (neutropenia, thrombocytopenia, anemia), cardiovascular toxicity (angina, cardiomyopathy, deep vein thrombosis), respiratory toxicity (dyspnea, epistaxis, pneumonia), lymphedema.

NURSING CONSIDERATIONS

BASELINE ASSESSMENT

Assess sensitivity to capecitabine or 5-fluorouracil. Obtain baseline Hgb, Hct, serum chemistries.

INTERVENTION/EVALUATION

Monitor for severe diarrhea; if dehydration occurs, fluid and electrolyte replacement therapy should be ordered. Assess hands/feet for erythema (chemotherapy induced). Monitor CBC for evidence of bone marrow depression. Monitor for blood dyscrasias (fever, sore throat, signs of local infection, unusual bruising/bleeding from any site), symptoms of anemia (excessive fatigue, weakness).

PATIENT/FAMILY TEACHING

• Inform pt of potential for, and need to notify physician if nausea, vomiting, possibly severe diarrhea, hand-and-foot syndrome, stomatitis occur. • Do not have immunizations without physician's approval (drug lowers body's resistance). • Avoid contact with those who have recently received live virus vaccine. • Promptly report fever higher than 100.5°F, sore throat, signs of local infection, unusual bruising/bleeding from any site.

Capoten, *see captopril*

capsaicin

cap-**say**-sin

(ArthriCare, Axsain, Capzasin-P, Zostrix)

Do not confuse Zostrix with Zestril or Zovirax.

CLASSIFICATION

PHARMACOTHERAPEUTIC: Counter-irritant. **CLINICAL:** Topical analgesic.

ACTION

Depletes/prevents reaccumulation of the chemomediator of pain impulses (substance P) from peripheral sensory neurons to CNS. **Therapeutic Effect:** Relieves pain.

USES

Treatment of neuralgia (e.g., pain with herpes zoster, painful diabetic neuropathy), osteoarthritis, rheumatoid arthritis. **OFF-LABEL:** Treatment of neurogenic pain, pruritis associated with hemodialysis and exposure to water.

PRECAUTIONS

CONTRAINDICATIONS: None known. **CAUTIONS:** For external use only. **Pregnancy Category C.**

INTERACTIONS

DRUG: None significant. **HERBAL:** None significant. **FOOD:** None known. **LAB VALUES:** None known.

AVAILABILITY (Rx)

CREAM (ARTHRICARE, AXSAIN, CAPZASIN-P, ZOSTRIX): 0.025%; **(CAPZASIN-HP, ZOSTRIX HP):** 0.075%. **LOTION (ARTHRICARE):** 0.025%. **STICK (ZOSTRIX):** 0.025%; **(ZOSTRIX HP):** 0.075%.

INDICATIONS/ROUTES/DOSAGE

USUAL TOPICAL DOSAGE

TOPICAL: ADULTS, ELDERLY, CHILDREN 2 YRS AND OLDER: Apply directly to affected area 3–4 times a day. Continue for 14–28 days for optimal clinical response.

SIDE EFFECTS

FREQUENT (greater than 30%): Burning, stinging, erythema at application site.

ADVERSE EFFECTS/ TOXIC REACTIONS

None known.

NURSING CONSIDERATIONS

PATIENT/FAMILY TEACHING

• Avoid contact with eyes, broken/ irritated skin. • Transient burning may occur on application; usually disappears after 72 hrs. • Wash hands immediately after application. • If there is no improvement or condition deteriorates after 28 days, discontinue use and consult physician.

captopril

cap-toe-pril

(Apo-Capto ♣, Capoten, Novo-Captoril ♣)

Do not confuse captopril with Capitrol.

FIXED-COMBINATION(S)

Capozide: captopril/hydrochlorothiazide (a diuretic): 25 mg/15 mg; 25 mg/25 mg; 50 mg/15 mg; 50 mg/25 mg.

♦CLASSIFICATION

PHARMACOTHERAPEUTIC: Angiotensin-converting enzyme (ACE) inhibitor. **CLINICAL:** Antihypertensive, vasodilator (see p. 7C).

ACTION

Suppresses renin-angiotensin-aldosterone system (prevents conversion of angiotensin I to angiotensin II, a potent vasoconstrictor; may inhibit angiotensin II at local vascular and renal sites). Decreases plasma angiotensin II, increases plasma renin activity, decreases aldosterone secretion. **Therapeutic Effect:** Reduces peripheral arterial resistance, pulmonary capillary wedge pressure; improves cardiac output, exercise tolerance.

PHARMACOKINETICS

Route	Onset	Peak	Duration
PO	0.25 hr	0.5–1.5 hrs	Dose-related

Rapidly, well absorbed from GI tract (absorption decreased in presence of food). Protein binding: 25%–30%. Metabolized in the liver. Primarily excreted in urine. Removed by hemodialysis. **Half-life:** less than 3 hrs (increased in those with renal impairment).

USES

Treatment of hypertension, CHF, diabetic nephropathy, post-MI for prevention of ventricular failure. **OFF-LABEL:** Treatment of hypertensive crisis, rheumatoid arthritis, diagnosis of renal artery stenosis, hypertension secondary to sclerodema renal crisis, diagnosis of aldosteronism, idiopathic edema, Bartter's syndrome to increase circulation in Raynaud's phenomenon.

PRECAUTIONS

CONTRAINDICATIONS: History of angioedema from previous treatment with ACE inhibitors. **CAUTIONS:** Renal impairment, those with sodium depletion or on diuretic therapy, dialysis, hypovolemia, coronary/cerebrovascular insufficiency.

C

LIFESPAN CONSIDERATIONS:

Pregnancy/Lactation: Crosses placenta; distributed in breast milk. May cause fetal/neonatal mortality/morbidity. **Pregnancy Category C (D if used in second or third trimester). Children:** Safety and efficacy not established. **Elderly:** May be more sensitive to hypotensive effects; caution recommended.

INTERACTIONS

DRUG: Alcohol, antihypertensives, diuretics may increase effects. May increase **lithium** concentration, toxicity. **NSAIDs** may decrease effect. **Potassium-sparing diuretics, potassium supplements** may cause hyperkalemia. **HERBAL: Ephedra, ginseng, yohimbe** may worsen hypertension. **Garlic** may increase antihypertensive effect. **FOOD: All foods** significantly reduce absorption. **LAB VALUES:** May increase BUN, serum alkaline phosphatase, bilirubin, creatinine, potassium, AST, ALT. May decrease serum sodium. May cause positive ANA titer.

AVAILABILITY (Rx)

TABLETS: 12.5 mg, 25 mg, 50 mg, 100 mg.

ADMINISTRATION/HANDLING

PO

• Best taken 1 hr before meals for maximum absorption (food significantly decreases drug absorption). • Tablets may be crushed.

INDICATIONS/ROUTES/DOSAGE

HYPERTENSION

PO: ADULTS, ELDERLY: Initially, 12.5–25 mg 2–3 times a day. After 1–2 wks, may increase to 50 mg 2–3 times a day. Diuretic may be added if no response in additional 1–2 wks. If taken in combination with diuretic, may increase to 100–150 mg 2–3 times a day after 1–2 wks. Maintenance: 25–150 mg 2–3 times a day. **Maximum:** 450 mg/day. **CHILDREN:** 0.05–0.5 mg three times/day. **Maximum:** 2 mg/kg/dose 2–3 times/day. **INFANTS:** 0.01–0.25 mg/kg q12h. **Maximum:** 2 mg/kg/dose 2–3 times/day.

CHF

PO: ADULTS, ELDERLY: Initially, 6.25–25 mg 3 times a day. Increase to 50 mg 3 times a day. After at least 2 wks, may increase to 50–100 mg 3 times a day. **Maximum:** 450 mg/day.

POST-MI, HEPATIC IMPAIRMENT

PO: ADULTS, ELDERLY: Initially, 6.25 mg, then 12.5 mg 3 times a day. Increase to 25 mg 3 times a day over several days up to 50 mg 3 times a day over several wks.

DIABETIC NEPHROPATHY, PREVENTION OF RENAL FAILURE

PO: ADULTS, ELDERLY: 25 mg 3 times a day.

DOSAGE IN RENAL IMPAIRMENT

Creatinine clearance 10–50 ml/min: 75% of normal dosage. **Creatinine clearance less than 10 ml/min:** 50% of normal dosage.

SIDE EFFECTS

FREQUENT (7%–4%): Rash. **OCCASIONAL (4%–2%):** Pruritus, dysgeusia (altered taste). **RARE (less than 2%–0.5%):** Headache, cough, insomnia, dizziness, fatigue, parasthesia, malaise, nausea, diarrhea or constipation, dry mouth, tachycardia.

ADVERSE EFFECTS/ TOXIC REACTIONS

Excessive hypotension ("first-dose syncope") may occur in pts with CHF and in those who are severely salt and volume depleted. Angioedema (swelling of face/lips), hyperkalemia occur rarely. Agranulocytosis, neutropenia may be noted in those with collagen vascular disease (scleroderma, systemic lupus erythematosus), renal impairment.

Nephrotic syndrome may be noted in those with history of renal disease.

NURSING CONSIDERATIONS

BASELINE ASSESSMENT

Obtain B/P immediately before each dose, in addition to regular monitoring (be alert to fluctuations). If excessive reduction in B/P occurs, place pt in supine position with legs elevated. In pts with prior renal disease or receiving dosages greater than 150 mg/day, urine test for protein by dipstick method should be made with first urine of day before therapy begins and periodically thereafter. In pts with renal impairment, autoimmune disease, or taking drugs that affect leukocytes or immune response, CBC should be performed before beginning therapy, q2wk for 3 mos, then periodically thereafter.

INTERVENTION/EVALUATION

Assess skin for rash, pruritus. Assist with ambulation if dizziness occurs. Monitor urinalysis for proteinuria. Assess for anorexia secondary to altered taste perception. Monitor serum potassium levels in those on concurrent diuretic therapy.

PATIENT/FAMILY TEACHING

• Several wks may be needed for full therapeutic effect of B/P reduction. • Skipping doses or voluntarily discontinuing drug may produce severe, rebound hypertension. • Avoid alcohol.

carbachol

(Isopto-Carbachol)

See Antiglaucoma agents (p. 48C)

carbamazepine

car-bah-**may**-zeh-peon

(Apo-Carbamazepine ✤, Carbatrol, Equetro, Novo-Carbamax ✤, Tegretol, Tegretol XR)

Do not confuse Tegretol with Cartrol, Topamax, Toprol XL, Toradol, or Trental.

◆CLASSIFICATION

PHARMACOTHERAPEUTIC: Iminostilbene derivative. **CLINICAL:** Anticonvulsant, antineuralgic, antimanic, antipsychotic (see p. 33C).

ACTION

Decreases sodium, calcium ion influx into neuronal membranes, reducing post-tetanic potentiation at synapses. **Therapeutic Effect:** Produces anticonvulsant effect.

PHARMACOKINETICS

Slowly, completely absorbed from GI tract. Protein binding: 75%. Metabolized in the liver to active metabolite. Primarily excreted in urine. Not removed by hemodialysis. **Half-life:** 25–65 hrs (decreased with chronic use).

USES

Carbatrol, Tegretol, Tegretol XR: Treatment of partial seizures with complex symptomatology, generalized tonic-clonic seizures, mixed seizure patterns, pain relief of trigeminal neuralgia, diabetic neuropathy. **Equetro:** Acute manic and mixed episodes associated with bipolar disorder. **OFF-LABEL:** Treatment of alcohol withdrawal, diabetes insipidus, neurogenic pain, psychotic disorders.

PRECAUTIONS

CONTRAINDICATIONS: Concomitant use of MAOIs, history of myelosuppression,

C

hypersensitivity to tricyclic antidepressants. **CAUTIONS:** Mental illness, increased intraocular pressure (IOP), history of atypical absence seizures, cardiac, hepatic, renal impairment.

LIFESPAN CONSIDERATIONS:

Pregnancy/Lactation: Crosses placenta; distributed in breast milk. Accumulates in fetal tissue. **Pregnancy Category D. Children:** Behavioral changes more likely to occur. **Elderly:** More susceptible to confusion, agitation, AV block, bradycardia, syndrome of inappropriate antidiuretic hormone (SIADH).

INTERACTIONS

DRUG: May decrease effects of **anticoagulants, clarithromycin, diltiazem, erythromycin, estrogens, propoxyphene, quinidine, steroids.** May increase CNS depressant effects of **antipsychotic medications, haloperidol, tricyclic antidepressants.** May increase metabolism of **other anticonvulsant medications, barbiturates, benzodiazepines, valproic acid. Cimetidine, itraconazole, ketoconazole** may increase concentration, toxicity. **Isoniazid** may increase concentration, toxicity. May increase metabolism of **isoniazid. MAOIs** may cause seizures, hypertensive crisis. **HERBAL: Evening primrose** may decrease seizure threshold. **Gotu kola, kava kava, St. John's wort, valerian** may increase CNS depression. **FOOD: Grapefruit, grapefruit juice** may increase absorption, concentration. **LAB VALUES:** May increase BUN, serum glucose, alkaline phosphatase, bilirubin, AST, ALT, protein, cholesterol, HDL, triglycerides. May decrease serum calcium, thyroid hormone (T_3, T_4 index) levels. Therapeutic serum level: 4–12 mcg/ml; toxic serum level: greater than 12 mcg/ml.

AVAILABILITY (Rx)

SUSPENSION (TEGRETOL): 100 mg/5 ml. **TABLETS (EPITOL, TEGRETOL):** 200 mg. **TABLETS (CHEWABLE [TEGRETOL]):** 100 mg.

CAPSULES (EXTENDED-RELEASE): Carbatrol, Equetro: 100 mg, 200 mg, 300 mg. **TABLETS (EXTENDED-RELEASE [TEGRETOL XR]):** 100 mg, 200 mg, 400 mg.

ADMINISTRATION/HANDLING

PO

• Store oral suspension, tablets at room temperature. • Give with meals to reduce risk of GI distress. • Shake oral suspension well. Do not administer simultaneously with other liquid medicine. • Do not crush extended-release capsules or tablets.

INDICATIONS/ROUTES/DOSAGE

SEIZURE CONTROL

PO: ADULTS, CHILDREN OLDER THAN 12 YRS: Initially, 200 mg twice a day. May increase dosage by 200 mg/day at weekly intervals. Range: 400–1,200 mg/day in 2–4 divided doses. **Maximum:** 1.6–2.4 g/day. **CHILDREN 6–12 YRS:** Initially, 100 mg twice a day. May increase by 100 mg/day at weekly intervals. Range: 400–800 mg/day. **Maximum:** 1,000 mg/day. **CHILDREN YOUNGER THAN 6 YRS:** Initially 10–20 mg/kg/day in 2–3 divided doses. May increase at weekly intervals until optimal response and therapeutic levels are achieved. **Maximum:** 35 mg/kg/day. **ELDERLY:** Initially 100 mg 1–2 times a day. May increase by 100 mg/day at weekly intervals. Usual dose 400–1,000 mg/day.

TRIGEMINAL NEURALGIA, DIABETIC NEUROPATHY

PO: ADULTS: Initially, 100 mg twice a day. May increase by 100 mg twice a day up to 400–800 mg/day. **Maximum:** 1200 mg/day. **ELDERLY:** Initially 100 mg 1–2 times a day. May increase by 100 mg/day at weekly intervals. Usual dose 400–1,000 mg/day.

C

BIPOLAR DISORDER

PO: ADULTS, ELDERLY (Equetro): Initially, 400 mg/day in 2 divided doses. May adjust dose in 200 mg increments. **Maximum:** 1,600 mg/day in divided doses.

SIDE EFFECTS

FREQUENT: Drowsiness, dizziness, nausea, vomiting. **OCCASIONAL:** Visual abnormalities (spots before eyes, difficulty focusing, blurred vision), dry mouth/pharynx, tongue irritation, headache, fluid retention, diaphoresis, constipation, diarrhea, behavioral changes in children.

ADVERSE EFFECTS/ TOXIC REACTIONS

Toxic reactions appear as blood dyscrasias (aplastic anemia, agranulocytosis, thrombocytopenia, leukopenia, leukocytosis, eosinophilia), cardiovascular disturbances (CHF, hypotension/hypertension, thrombophlebitis, arrhythmias), dermatologic effects (rash, urticaria, pruritus, photosensitivity). Abrupt withdrawal may precipitate status epilepticus.

NURSING CONSIDERATIONS

BASELINE ASSESSMENT

Seizures: Review history of seizure disorder (intensity, frequency, duration, level of consciousness [LOC]). Provide safety precautions, quiet/dark environment. CBC, serum iron determination, urinalysis, BUN should be performed before therapy begins and periodically during therapy.

INTERVENTION/EVALUATION

Seizures: Observe frequently for recurrence of seizure activity. Monitor for therapeutic serum levels. Assess for clinical improvement (decrease in intensity, frequency of seizures). Assess for clinical evidence of early toxic signs (fever, sore throat, mouth ulcerations, unusual bruising/bleeding, joint pain). **Neuralgia:** Avoid triggering tic douloureux (draft, talking, washing face, jarring bed, hot/warm/cold food or liquids). Therapeutic serum level: 4–12 mcg/ml; toxic serum level: greater than 12 mcg/ml.

PATIENT/FAMILY TEACHING

• Do not abruptly withdraw medication after long-term use (may precipitate seizures). • Strict maintenance of drug therapy is essential for seizure control. • Drowsiness usually disappears during continued therapy. • Avoid tasks that require alertness, motor skills until response to drug is established. • Report visual disturbances. • Blood tests should be repeated frequently during first 3 mos of therapy and at monthly intervals thereafter for 2–3 yrs. • Do not take oral suspension simultaneously with other liquid medicine. • Do not take with grapefruit juice.

carbenicillin

(Geocillin)

See Antibiotic: penicillins (p. 28C)

carbidopa/levodopa

car-bih-dope-ah/**lev**-oh-dope-ah

(Apo-Levocarb ♣, Novo-Levocarbidopa ♣, Parcopa, Sinemet, Sinemet CR)

FIXED-COMBINATION(S)

Stalevo: carbidopa/levodopa/entacapone (antiparkinson agent): 12.5 mg/50 mg/200 mg, 25 mg/100 mg/200 mg, 37.5 mg/150 mg/200 mg.

C

♦ CLASSIFICATION

PHARMACOTHERAPEUTIC: Dopamine precursor. **CLINICAL:** Antiparkinson agent.

ACTION

Converted to dopamine in basal ganglia, increasing dopamine concentration in brain, inhibiting hyperactive cholinergic activity. Carbidopa prevents peripheral breakdown of levodopa, making more levodopa available for transport into brain. **Therapeutic Effect:** Reduces tremor.

PHARMACOKINETICS

Carbidopa is rapidly and completely absorbed from GI tract. Widely distributed. Excreted primarily in urine. Levodopa is converted to dopamine. Excreted primarily in urine. **Half-life:** 1–2 hrs (carbidopa); 1–3 hrs (levodopa).

USES

Treatment of idiopathic Parkinson's disease (paralysis agitans), postencephalitic parkinsonism, symptomatic parkinsonism following CNS injury by CO_2 poisoning, manganese intoxication.

PRECAUTIONS

CONTRAINDICATIONS: Angle-closure glaucoma, use within 14 days of MAOIs, skin lesions (Sinemet CR), history of melanoma (Sinemet CR). **CAUTIONS:** History of MI, bronchial asthma (tartrazine sensitivity), emphysema; severe cardiac, pulmonary, renal, hepatic, endocrine disease; active peptic ulcer; treated open-angle glaucoma.

LIFESPAN CONSIDERATIONS:

Pregnancy/Lactation: Unknown if drug crosses placenta or is distributed in breast milk. May inhibit lactation. Do not breast-feed. **Pregnancy Category C.** **Children:** Safety and efficacy not established in those younger than 18 yrs. **Elderly:** More sensitive to effects of levodopa. Anxiety, confusion, nervousness more common when receiving anticholinergics.

INTERACTIONS

DRUG: Anticonvulsants, benzodiazepines, haloperidol, phenothiazines may decrease effects of carbidopa and levodopa. **MAOIs** may increase risk of hypertensive crisis. **Selegiline** may increase levodopa-induced dyskinesias, nausea, orthostatic hypotension, confusion, hallucinations. **HERBAL: Kava kava** may decrease effect. **FOOD: High-protein** diets may cause decreased or erratic response to levodopa. **LAB VALUES:** May increase BUN, serum LDH, alkaline phosphatase, bilirubin, AST, ALT.

AVAILABILITY (Rx)

TABLETS (SINEMET): 10 mg carbidopa/100 mg levodopa, 25 mg carbidopa/100 mg levodopa, 25 mg carbidopa/250 mg levodopa. **TABLETS (ORAL-DISINTEGRATING [PARCOPA]):** 10 mg carbidopa/100 mg levodopa, 25 mg carbidopa/100 mg levodopa, 25 mg carbidopa/250 mg levodopa.

TABLETS (EXTENDED-RELEASE [SINEMET CR]): 25 mg carbidopa/100 mg levdopa, 50 mg carbidopa/200 mg levodopa.

ADMINISTRATION/HANDLING

PO

• Scored tablets may be crushed. • Give without regard to food. • Do not crush extended-release tablet; may cut in half.

PO (PARCOPA)

• Place oral disintegrating tablet on top of tongue. Tablet will dissolve in seconds, pt to swallow with saliva. Not necessary to administer with liquid.

INDICATIONS/ROUTES/DOSAGE

PARKINSONISM

PO: ADULTS (IMMEDIATE RELEASE): Initially, 25/100 mg 2–4 times a day.

May increase up to 200/2,000 mg daily. **ELDERLY:** Initially, 25/100 mg twice a day. May increase as necessary. When converting a pt from Sinemet to Sinemet CR (50 mg/200 mg), dosage is based on total daily dose of levodopa, as follows:

Sinemet	Sinemet CR
300–400 mg	1 tablet twice a day
500–600 mg	1.5 tablet twice a day or 1 tab 3 times a day
700–800 mg	4 tablets in 3 or more divided doses
900–1,000 mg	5 tablets in 3 or more divided doses

Intervals between doses of Sinemet CR should be 4–8 hrs while awake, with smaller doses at end of day if doses are not equal.

SIDE EFFECTS

FREQUENT: Uncontrolled movements of face, tongue, arms, upper body; nausea/vomiting (80%); anorexia (50%). **OCCASIONAL:** Depression, anxiety, confusion, nervousness, urinary retention, palpitations, dizziness, light-headedness, decreased appetite, blurred vision, constipation, dry mouth, flushed skin, headache, insomnia, diarrhea, unusual fatigue, darkening of urine and sweat. **RARE:** Hypertension, ulcer, hemolytic anemia (marked by fatigue).

ADVERSE EFFECTS/ TOXIC REACTIONS

High incidence of involuntary choreiform, dystonic, dyskinetic movements in those on long-term therapy. Numerous mild to severe CNS and psychiatric disturbances may occur, (reduced attention span, anxiety, nightmares, daytime somnolence, euphoria, fatigue, paranoia, psychotic episodes, depression, hallucinations).

NURSING CONSIDERATIONS

BASELINE ASSESSMENT

Instruct pt to void before giving medication (reduces risk of urinary retention).

INTERVENTION/EVALUATION

Be alert to neurologic effects (headache, lethargy, mental confusion, agitation). Monitor for evidence of dyskinesia (difficulty with movement). Assess for clinical reversal of symptoms (improvement of tremor of head and hands at rest, mask-like facial expression, shuffling gait, muscular rigidity).

PATIENT/FAMILY TEACHING

• Avoid tasks that require alertness, motor skills until response to drug is established. • Avoid alcoholic beverages during therapy. • Sugarless gum, sips of tepid water may relieve dry mouth. • Take with food to minimize GI upset. • Effects may be delayed from several wks to mos. • May cause darkening of urine or sweat (not harmful). • Instruct pt taking oral disintegrating tablet to report any uncontrolled movement of face, eyelids, mouth, tongue, arms, hands, legs; mental changes; palpitations; severe or persistent nausea/vomiting; difficulty urinating.

carboplatin

car-bow-**play**-tin

(Paraplatin, Paraplatin-AQ ✤)

Do not confuse carboplatin with Cisplatin or Platinol.

CLASSIFICATION

PHARMACOTHERAPEUTIC: Platinum coordination complex. **CLINICAL:** Antineoplastic (see p. 77C).

C

ACTION

Inhibits DNA synthesis by cross-linking with DNA strands, preventing cell division. Cell cycle-phase nonspecific. **Therapeutic Effect:** Interferes with DNA function.

PHARMACOKINETICS

Protein binding: Low. Hydrolyzed in solution to active form. Primarily excreted in urine. **Half-life:** 2.6–5.9 hrs.

USES

Treatment of ovarian carcinoma. **OFF-LABEL:** Brain tumors, Hodgkin's and non-Hodgkin's lymphomas, malignant melanoma, retinoblastoma, treatment of breast, bladder, endometrial, esophageal, small cell lung, non-small cell lung, head and neck, testicular carcinomas.

PRECAUTIONS

CONTRAINDICATIONS: History of severe allergic reaction to cisplatin, platinum compounds, mannitol; severe bleeding, severe myelosuppression. **CAUTIONS:** Chickenpox, herpes zoster, renal impairment.

LIFESPAN CONSIDERATIONS:

Pregnancy/Lactation: If possible, avoid use during pregnancy, esp. first trimester. May cause fetal harm. Unknown if distributed in breast milk. Breast-feeding not recommended. **Pregnancy Category D. Children:** Safety and efficacy not established. **Elderly:** Peripheral neurotoxicity increased, myelotoxicity may be more severe. Age-related renal impairment may require decreased dosage, more careful monitoring of blood counts.

INTERACTIONS

DRUG: **Bone marrow depressants** may increase myelosuppression. **Live virus vaccines** may potentiate virus replication, increase vaccine side effects, decrease pt's antibody response to vaccine. **Nephrotoxic, ototoxic medications** may increase risk of toxicity. **HERBAL:** Avoid **black cohosh, dong quai** in estrogen-dependent tumors. **FOOD:** None known. **LAB VALUES:** May decrease serum calcium, magnesium, potassium, sodium. High dosages (more than 4 times the recommended dosage) may elevate BUN, serum alkaline phosphatase, bilirubin, creatinine, AST.

AVAILABILITY (Rx)

INJECTION, POWDER FOR RECONSTITUTION: 50 mg, 150 mg, 450 mg. **INJECTION SOLUTION:** 10 mg/ml.

ADMINISTRATION/HANDLING

◄ **ALERT** ► May be carcinogenic, mutagenic, teratogenic. Handle with extreme care during preparation/administration.

IV

Reconstitution • Reconstitute immediately before use. • Do not use aluminum needles or administration sets that come in contact with drug (may produce black precipitate, loss of potency). • Reconstitute each 50 mg with 5 ml Sterile Water for Injection, D_5W, or 0.9% NaCl to provide concentration of 10 mg/ml. • May be further diluted with D_5W or 0.9% NaCl to provide concentration as low as 0.5 mg/ml.

Rate of administration • Infuse over 15–60 min. • Rarely, anaphylactic reaction occurs minutes after administration. Use of epinephrine, corticosteroids alleviates symptoms.

Storage • Store vials at room temperature. • After reconstitution, solution is stable for 8 hrs. Discard unused portion after 8 hrs.

IV INCOMPATIBILITIES

Amphotericin B complex (Abelcet, AmBisome, Amphotec).

IV COMPATIBILITIES

Etoposide (VePesid), granisetron (Kytril), lipids, ondansetron (Zofran), paclitaxel (Taxol).

INDICATIONS/ROUTES/DOSAGE

OVARIAN CARCINOMA (MONOTHERAPY)

IV: ADULTS: 360 mg/m^2 on day 1, every 4 wks. Do not repeat dose until neutrophil and platelet counts are within acceptable levels. Adjust drug dosage in previously treated pts based on lowest post-treatment platelet or neutrophil count. Increase dosage only once to no more than 125% of starting dose.

OVARIAN CARCINOMA (COMBINATION THERAPY)

IV: ADULTS: 300 mg/m^2 (with cyclophosphamide) on day 1, every 4 wks. Do not repeat dose until neutrophil and platelet counts are within acceptable levels.

USUAL DOSE FOR CHILDREN

300–600 mg/m^2 every 4 wks for solid tumor, or 175 mg/m^2 every 4 wks for brain tumor.

DOSAGE IN RENAL IMPAIRMENT

Initial dosage is based on creatinine clearance; subsequent dosages are based on pt's tolerance, degree of myelosuppression.

Creatinine Clearance	Dosage Day 1
60 ml/min or greater	360 mg/m^2
41–59 ml/min	250 mg/m^2
16–40 ml/min	200 mg/m^2

SIDE EFFECTS

FREQUENT: Nausea (75%–80%), vomiting (65%). **OCCASIONAL:** Generalized pain (17%), diarrhea/constipation (6%), peripheral neuropathy (4%). **RARE (3%–2%):** Alopecia, asthenia, hypersensitivity reaction (erythema, pruritus, rash, urticaria).

ADVERSE EFFECTS/ TOXIC REACTIONS

Myelosuppression may be severe, resulting in anemia, infection, (sepsis, pneumonia), bleeding. Prolonged treatment may result in peripheral neurotoxicity.

NURSING CONSIDERATIONS

BASELINE ASSESSMENT

Offer emotional support. Do not repeat treatment until WBC recovers from previous therapy. Transfusions may be needed in those receiving prolonged therapy (myelosuppression increased in those with previous therapy, renal impairment).

INTERVENTION/EVALUATION

Monitor hematologic status, pulmonary function studies, hepatic/renal function tests. Monitor for fever, sore throat, signs of local infection, unusual bruising/bleeding from any site, symptoms of anemia (excessive fatigue, weakness).

PATIENT/FAMILY TEACHING

• Nausea, vomiting generally abate in less than 24 hrs. • Do not have immunizations without physician's approval (drug lowers body's resistance). • Avoid contact with those who have recently received live virus vaccine.

Cardizem, *see diltiazem*

carisoprodol

(Soma)

See Skeletal muscle relaxants

C

carmustine

car-**muss**-teen
(BiCNU, Gliadel Wafer)

CLASSIFICATION

PHARMACOTHERAPEUTIC: Alkylating agent, nitrosourea. **CLINICAL:** Antineoplastic (see p. 77C).

ACTION

Inhibits DNA, RNA synthesis by cross-linking with DNA, RNA strands, preventing cell division. Cell cycle-phase nonspecific. **Therapeutic Effect:** Interferes with DNA, RNA function.

PHARMACOKINETICS

Crosses blood-brain barrier. Metabolized in liver. Excreted in urine. **Half-life:** 1.4 min (first phase); 17.8 min (second phase).

USES

Treatment of brain tumors, Hodgkin's lymphomas, non-Hodgkin's lymphomas, multiple myeloma. **Gliadel Wafer:** Adjunct to surgery to prolong survival in recurrent glioblastoma multiforme. **OFF-LABEL:** Treatment of colorectal, hepatic, GI carcinoma, malignant melanoma, mycosis fungoides.

PRECAUTIONS

CONTRAINDICATIONS: None known. **CAUTIONS:** Pts with decreased platelet, leukocyte, erythrocyte counts.

LIFESPAN CONSIDERATIONS:

Pregnancy/Lactation: Avoid during pregnancy, particularly first trimester; may cause fetal harm. Unknown if distributed in breast milk; do not breastfeed. **Pregnancy Category D. Children:** Safety and efficacy not established in children. **Elderly:** No age-related precautions noted.

INTERACTIONS

DRUG: Bone marrow depressants, cimetidine may enhance myelosuppressive effect. **Hepatotoxic, nephrotoxic medications** may increase risk of hepatotoxicity, nephrotoxicity. **Live-virus vaccines** may potentiate virus replication, increase vaccine side effects, decrease pt's antibody response to vaccine. **HERBAL:** None significant. **FOOD:** None known. **LAB VALUES:** May increase BUN, serum alkaline phosphatase, bilirubin, AST, ALT.

AVAILABILITY (Rx)

INJECTION, POWDER FOR RECONSTITUTION (BICNU): 100 mg. **IMPLANT DEVICE (GLIADEL WAFER):** 7.7 mg.

ADMINISTRATION/HANDLING

◄ ALERT ► May be carcinogenic, mutagenic, teratogenic. Wear protective gloves during preparation of drug; may cause transient burning, brown staining of skin.

IV

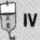

Reconstitution • Reconstitute 100-mg vial with 3 ml sterile dehydrated (absolute) alcohol, followed by 27 ml Sterile Water for Injection to provide concentration of 3.3 mg/ml. • Further dilute with 50–250 ml D_5W or 0.9% NaCl.

Rate of administration • Infuse over 1–2 hrs (shorter duration may produce intense burning pain at injection site, intense flushing of skin, conjunctiva). • Flush IV line with 5–10 ml 0.9% NaCl or D_5W before and after administration to prevent irritation at injection site.

Storage • Refrigerate unopened vials of dry powder. • Reconstituted vials are stable for 8 hrs at room temperature or 24 hrs if refrigerated. • Solutions further diluted to 0.2 mg/ml with D_5W or 0.9% NaCl are stable for 48 hrs if refrigerated or an additional 8 hrs at room temperature. • Solutions appear clear, colorless to yellow. • Discard if precipitate forms, color change occurs, or oily film develops on bottom of vial.

IV INCOMPATIBILITY

Allopurinol (Aloprim).

INDICATIONS/ROUTES/DOSAGE

USUAL DOSAGE

IV (BiCNU): ADULTS, ELDERLY: 150–200 mg/m^2 as a single dose q6–8wk or 75–100 mg/m^{2}on 2 successive days q6–8wk. **CHILDREN:** 200–250 mg/m^2 q4–6wk as a single dose.

◄ ALERT ► Next dosage is based on clinical and hematologic response to previous dose (platelets greater than 100,000/mm^3 and leukocytes greater than 4,000/mm^3).

IMPLANTATION: (GLIADEL WAFER): ADULTS, ELDERLY, CHILDREN: Up to 8 wafers (62.6 mg) may be placed in resection cavity.

SIDE EFFECTS

FREQUENT: Nausea/vomiting within minutes to 2 hrs after administration (may last up to 6 hrs). **OCCASIONAL:** Diarrhea, esophagitis, anorexia, dysphagia. **RARE:** Thrombophlebitis.

ADVERSE EFFECTS/ TOXIC REACTIONS

Hematologic toxicity due to myelosuppression occurs frequently. Thrombocytopenia occurs about 4 wks after carmustine treatment begins and lasts 1–2 wks. Leukopenia is evident 5–6 wks after treatment begins and lasts 1–2 wks. Anemia occurs less frequently, is less severe. Mild reversible hepatotoxicity occurs frequently. Prolonged high-dose carmustine therapy may produce impaired renal function, pulmonary toxicity (pulmonary infiltrate/fibrosis).

NURSING CONSIDERATIONS

BASELINE ASSESSMENT

Perform CBC, renal/hepatic function studies before beginning therapy and periodically thereafter. Perform blood counts weekly during and for at least 6 wks after therapy ends.

INTERVENTION/EVALUATION

Monitor CBC, BUN, serum transaminase, alkaline phosphatase, bilirubin; pulmonary, renal/hepatic function tests. Monitor for hematologic toxicity (fever, sore throat, signs of local infection, unusual bruising/bleeding from any site), symptoms of anemia (excessive fatigue, weakness). Monitor lung sounds for pulmonary toxicity (dyspnea, fine lung rales).

PATIENT/FAMILY TEACHING

• Maintain adequate daily fluid intake (may protect against renal impairment). • Do not have immunizations without physician's approval (drug lowers body's resistance). • Avoid contact with those who have recently received live virus vaccine. • Contact physician if nausea/vomiting continues at home.

carteolol

(Cartrol, Ocupress)

See Beta-adrenergic blockers (pp. 49C, 68C)

carvedilol ⚑

car-**veh**-dih-lol

(Apo-Carvedilol ✤, Coreg, Coreg CR, Novo-Carvedilol ✤)

C

Do not confuse carvedilol with carteolol.

CLASSIFICATION

PHARMACOTHERAPEUTIC: Beta-adrenergic blocker. **CLINICAL:** Antihypertensive (see p. 68C).

ACTION

Possesses non-selective beta-blocking and alpha-adrenergic blocking activity. Causes vasodilation. **Therapeutic Effect:** Reduces cardiac output, exercise-induced tachycardia, reflex orthostatic tachycardia; reduces peripheral vascular resistance.

PHARMACOKINETICS

Route	Onset	Peak	Duration
PO	30 min	1–2 hrs	24 hrs

Rapidly, extensively absorbed from GI tract. Protein binding: 98%. Metabolized in the liver. Excreted primarily via bile into feces. Minimally removed by hemodialysis. **Half-life:** 7–10 hrs. Food delays rate of absorption.

USES

Treatment of mild to severe heart failure, left ventricular dysfunction following MI, hypertension. Reduces risk of second MI in pts with damaged heart or heart failure. **OFF-LABEL:** Treatment of angina pectoris, idiopathic cardiomyopathy.

PRECAUTIONS

CONTRAINDICATIONS: Bronchial asthma or related bronchospastic conditions, cardiogenic shock, pulmonary edema, second- or third-degree AV block, severe bradycardia. **CAUTIONS:** CHF controlled with digitalis, diuretics, angiotensin-converting enzyme (ACE) inhibitor; peripheral vascular disease; anesthesia; diabetes mellitus; hypoglycemia; thyrotoxicosis; hepatic impairment.

LIFESPAN CONSIDERATIONS:

Pregnancy/Lactation: Unknown if drug crosses placenta or is distributed in breast milk. May produce bradycardia, apnea, hypoglycemia, hypothermia during delivery, low birth-weight infants. **Pregnancy Category C (D if used in the second or third trimester). Children:** Safety and efficacy not established. **Elderly:** Incidence of dizziness may be increased.

INTERACTIONS

DRUG: Calcium channel blockers increase risk of cardiac conduction disturbances. **Diuretics, other antihypertensives** may potentiate hypotensive effects. **Cimetidine** may increase concentration. May increase concentration of **cyclosporine, digoxin.** May decrease effect of **insulin, oral hypoglycemics. Rifampin** decreases concentration. **HERBAL: Ephedra, ginseng, yohimbe** may worsen hypertension. **Garlic** may increase antihypertensive effect. **FOOD:** None known. **LAB VALUE:** None known.

AVAILABILITY (Rx)

TABLETS: 3.125 mg, 6.25 mg, 12.5 mg, 25 mg.

CAPSULES, EXTENDED-RELEASE (Coreg CR): 10 mg, 20 mg, 40 mg, 80 mg.

ADMINISTRATION/HANDLING

PO

- Give with food (slows rate of absorption, reduces risk of orthostatic effects).
- Take standing systolic B/P 1 hr after dosing as guide for tolerance.

INDICATIONS/ROUTES/DOSAGE

HYPERTENSION

PO: ADULTS, ELDERLY: Initially, 6.25 mg twice a day. May double at 7- to 14-day intervals to highest tolerated dosage. **Maximum:** 50 mg/day.

CHF

PO: ADULTS, ELDERLY: Initially, 3.125 mg twice a day. May double at 2-wk intervals to highest tolerated dosage. **Maximum:** For pts weighing more than 85 kg, give 50 mg twice a day, for those weighing 85 kg or less, give 25 mg twice a day.

LEFT VENTRICULAR DYSFUNCTION

PO: ADULTS, ELDERLY: Initially, 3.125–6.25 mg twice a day. May increase at intervals of 3–10 days up to 25 mg twice a day.

USUAL DOSAGE FOR EXTENDED-RELEASE CAPSULES

PO: ADULTS, ELDERLY: 10–80 mg once daily.

SIDE EFFECTS

Carvedilol is generally well tolerated, with mild transient side effects. **FREQUENT (6%–4%):** Fatigue, dizziness. **OCCASIONAL (2%):** Diarrhea, bradycardia, rhinitis, back pain. **RARE (less than 2%):** Orthostatic hypotension, somnolence, UTI, viral infection.

ADVERSE EFFECTS/ TOXIC REACTIONS

Overdose may produce profound bradycardia, hypotension, bronchospasm, cardiac insufficiency, cardiogenic shock, cardiac arrest. Abrupt withdrawal may result in diaphoresis, palpitations, headache, tremors. May precipitate CHF, MI in pts with cardiac disease; thyroid storm in those with thyrotoxicosis, peripheral ischemia in those with existing peripheral vascular disease. Hypoglycemia may occur in pts with previously controlled diabetes.

NURSING CONSIDERATIONS

BASELINE ASSESSMENT

Assess B/P, apical pulse immediately before drug is administered (if pulse is 60/min or less or systolic B/P is less than 90 mm Hg, withhold medication, contact physician).

INTERVENTION/EVALUATION

Monitor B/P for hypotension, respiration for dyspnea. Assess pulse for quality, irregular rate, bradycardia. Monitor EKG for cardiac arrhythmias. Assist with ambulation if dizziness occurs. Assess for evidence of CHF: dyspnea (particularly on exertion or lying down), night cough, peripheral edema, distended neck veins. Monitor I&O (increase in weight, decrease in urine output may indicate CHF).

PATIENT/FAMILY TEACHING

• Full antihypertensive effect noted in 1–2 wks. • Contact lens wearers may experience decreased lacrimation. • Take with food. • Do not abruptly discontinue medication. Compliance with therapy regimen is essential to control hypertension. • Avoid tasks that require alertness, motor skills until response to drug is established. • Report excessive fatigue, prolonged dizziness. • Do not use nasal decongestants, OTC cold preparations (stimulants) without physician approval. • Monitor B/P, pulse before taking medication. • Restrict salt, alcohol intake.

cascara sagrada

cass-**care**-ah sah-**graud**-ah
(Cascara Sagrada)

FIXED-COMBINATION(S)

With milk of magnesia, a saline laxative.

◆CLASSIFICATION

PHARMACOTHERAPEUTIC: GI stimulant. **CLINICAL:** Laxative.

ACTION

Increases peristalsis of colonic smooth musculature by stimulating intramural

C

nerve plexi. **Therapeutic Effect:** Promotes fluid, ion accumulation in colon, promoting a laxative effect.

PHARMACOKINETICS

Poorly absorbed following PO administration. Metabolized in intestinal wall. Excreted in urine and bile. **Half life:** Unknown.

USES

Temporary relief of constipation, sometimes used with milk of magnesia.

PRECAUTIONS

CONTRAINDICATIONS: Abdominal pain, appendicitis, intestinal obstruction, nausea, vomiting. **CAUTIONS:** None known.

LIFESPAN CONSIDERATIONS:

Pregnancy/Lactation: May be distributed in breast milk. **Pregnancy Category C.** **Children:** Safety and efficacy not established in children younger than 6 yrs. **Elderly:** No age-related precautions noted.

INTERACTIONS

DRUG: **Oral medications** may decrease transit time of concurrently administered oral medications, decreasing absorption. **HERBAL:** None significant. **FOOD:** None known. **LAB VALUES:** May increase serum glucose. May decrease serum calcium, potassium.

AVAILABILITY (Rx)

LIQUID: (18% alcohol) 1 g/ml. **TABLETS:** 150 mg, 325 mg.

INDICATIONS/ROUTES/DOSAGE

TREATMENT OF CONSTIPATION

PO: ADULTS, ELDERLY: 5 ml or 1–2 tablets at bedtime. **CHILDREN 2–11 YRS:** 2.5 ml, 1–3 ml as a single dose. **INFANT:** 1.25 ml, 0.5–2 ml as a single dose.

SIDE EFFECTS

FREQUENT: Pink-red, red-violet, red-brown, or yellow-brown discoloration of urine. **OCCASIONAL:** Abdominal discomfort, nausea, mild cramps, faintness.

ADVERSE EFFECTS/ TOXIC REACTIONS

Long-term use may result in laxative dependence, chronic constipation, loss of normal bowel function. Prolonged use or overdose may result in electrolyte or metabolic disturbances (hypokalemia, hypocalcemia, metabolic acidosis, alkalosis), persistent diarrhea, vomiting, muscle weakness, malabsorption, weight loss.

NURSING CONSIDERATIONS

INTERVENTION/EVALUATION

Encourage adequate fluid intake. Assess bowel sounds for peristalsis. Monitor daily pattern of bowel activity/stool consistency; record time of evacuation. Assess for abdominal disturbances. Monitor serum electrolytes in those exposed to prolonged/frequent/excessive use of medication.

PATIENT/FAMILY TEACHING

• Urine may turn pink-red, red-violet, red-brown, yellow-brown (only temporary, not harmful). • Institute measures to promote defecation: increase fluid intake, exercise, high-fiber diet. • Laxative effect generally occurs in 6–12 hrs but may take 24 hrs. • Do not use in presence of nausea, vomiting, abdominal pain longer than 1 wk. • Do not take other oral medication within 1 hr of taking this medicine (decreased effectiveness due to increased peristalsis).

Casodex, *see bicalutamide*

caspofungin

cas-poe-**fun**-gin
(Cancidas)

CLASSIFICATION

CLINICAL: Antifungal.

ACTION

Inhibits synthesis of glucan, a vital component of fungal cell formation, damaging fungal cell membrane. **Therapeutic Effect:** Fungistatic.

PHARMACOKINETICS

Distributed in tissue. Extensively bound to albumin. Protein binding: 97%. Slowly metabolized in liver to active metabolite. Excreted primarily in urine and to a lesser extent in feces. Not removed by hemodialysis. **Half-life:** 40–50 hrs.

USES

Treatment of invasive aspergillosis, candidemia, intra-abdominal abscess, peritonitis, esophageal candidiasis. Empiric therapy for presumed fungal infections in febrile neutropenia.

PRECAUTIONS

CONTRAINDICATIONS: None known. **CAUTIONS:** Myelosuppression, renal insufficiency, hepatic impairment.

LIFESPAN CONSIDERATIONS:

Pregnancy/Lactation: May be embryotoxic. Crosses placental barrier. Distributed in breast milk. **Pregnancy Category C. Children:** Safety and efficacy not established. **Elderly:** Age-related moderate renal impairment may require dosage adjustment.

INTERACTIONS

DRUG: Carbamazepine, cyclosporine, dexamethasone, efavirenz, nelfinavir, nevirapine, phenytoin, rifampin may increase concentration. Concurrent use with **cyclosporine** may increase ALT, AST levels. May decrease concentration, effect of **tacrolimus. HERBAL:** None significant. **FOOD:** None known. **LAB VALUES:** May increase PT, serum alkaline phosphatase, bilirubin, creatinine, LDH, AST, ALT, uric acid. May increase urine pH, protein, RBCs, WBCs. May decrease serum albumin, bicarbonate, protein, potassium, Hgb, Hct, platelet count.

AVAILABILITY (Rx)

INJECTION, POWDER FOR RECONSTITUTION: 50-mg, 70-mg vials.

ADMINISTRATION/HANDLING

IV

Reconstitution • For a 70-mg dose, add 10.5 ml of 0.9% NaCl to the 70-mg vial. Transfer 10 ml of reconstituted solution to 250 ml 0.9% NaCl. • For a 50-mg dose, add 10.5 ml of 0.9% NaCl to the 50-mg vial. Transfer 10 ml of the reconstituted solution to 100 ml or 250 ml 0.9% NaCl. • For a 35-mg dose, add 10.5 ml of 0.9% NaCl to the 50-mg vial. Transfer 7 ml of the reconstituted solution to 100 ml or 250 ml 0.9% NaCl.

Rate of administration • Infuse over 60 min.

Storage • Refrigerate but warm to room temperature before preparing with diluent. • Reconstituted solution, prior to preparation of pt infusion solution, may be stored at room temperature for 1 hr before infusion. • Final infusion solution can be stored at room temperature for 24 hrs. • Discard if solution contains particulate or is discolored.

IV INCOMPATIBILITIES

Do not mix caspofungin with any other medication or use dextrose as a diluent.

C

INDICATIONS/ROUTES/DOSAGE

ASPERGILLOSIS

IV: ADULTS, ELDERLY, CHILDREN OLDER THAN 12 YRS: Give single 70-mg loading dose on day 1, followed by 50 mg/day thereafter. For pts with moderate hepatic insufficiency, reduce daily dose to 35 mg.

INVASIVE CANDIDIASIS

IV: ADULTS, ELDERLY: Initially, 70 mg followed by 50 mg daily.

ESOPHAGEAL CANDIDIASIS

IV: ADULTS, ELDERLY: 50 mg a day.

EMPIRIC THERAPY

IV: ADULTS, ELDERLY: Initially, 70 mg then 50 mg/day. May increase to 70 mg/day.

SIDE EFFECTS

FREQUENT (26%): Fever. **OCCASIONAL (11%–4%):** Headache, nausea, phlebitis. **RARE (3% or less):** Paresthesia, vomiting, diarrhea, abdominal pain, myalgia, chills, tremor, insomnia.

ADVERSE EFFECTS/ TOXIC REACTIONS

Hypersensitivity reaction (rash, facial edema, pruritus, sensation of warmth) may occur.

NURSING CONSIDERATIONS

BASELINE ASSESSMENT

Determine baseline temperature, hepatic function tests. Assess allergies.

INTERVENTION/EVALUATION

Assess for signs/symptoms of hepatic dysfunction. Monitor hepatic enzyme tests in pts with preexisting hepatic dysfunction.

Catapres, *see clonidine*

Catapres TTS, *see clonidine*

cefaclor

sef-a-klor

(Apo-Cefaclor ✦, Ceclor, Ceclor CD, Ceclor Pulvules, Novo-Cefaclor ✦, Ramiclor)

CLASSIFICATION

PHARMACOTHERAPEUTIC: Second-generation cephalosporin. **CLINICAL:** Antibiotic (see p. 21C).

ACTION

Binds to bacterial cell membranes, inhibits cell wall synthesis. **Therapeutic Effect:** Bactericidal.

PHARMACOKINETICS

Well absorbed from GI tract. Protein binding: 25%. Widely distributed. Primarily excreted unchanged in urine. Moderately removed by hemodialysis. **Half-life:** 0.6–0.9 hr (increased in renal impairment).

USES

Treatment of susceptible infections due to *S. pneumoniae*, *S. pyogenes*, *S. aureus*, *H. influenzae*, *E. coli*, *M. catarrhalis*, *Klebsiella* species, *P. mirabilis*, including acute otitis media, bronchitis, pharyngitis/tonsillitis, respiratory tract, skin/skin structure and UTIs.

PRECAUTIONS

CONTRAINDICATIONS: History of anaphylactic reaction to penicillins, hypersensitivity to cephalosporins. **CAUTIONS:** Renal impairment, history of GI disease (esp. ulcerative colitis, antibiotic-associated colitis), concurrent use of nephrotoxic medications.

LIFESPAN CONSIDERATIONS:

Pregnancy/Lactation: Readily crosses placenta. Distributed in breast milk. **Pregnancy Category B. Children:** No age-related precautions noted in those older than 1 mo. **Elderly:** Age-related renal impairment may require dosage adjustment.

INTERACTIONS

DRUG: Aminoglycosides, furosemide may increase risk of nephrotoxicity. **Probenecid** may increase concentration. Bleeding may occur with concomitant use of **warfarin. HERBAL:** None significant. **FOOD:** None known. **LAB VALUES:** May increase BUN, serum alkaline phosphatase, bilirubin, creatinine, LDH, AST, ALT. May cause positive direct/indirect Coombs' test.

AVAILABILITY (Rx)

CAPSULES (CECLOR PULVULES): 250 mg, 500 mg. **POWDER FOR ORAL SUSPENSION (CECLOR):** 125 mg/5 ml, 187 mg/5 ml, 250 mg/5 ml, 375 mg/5 ml. **TABLETS (CHEWABLE [RANICLOR]):** 125 mg, 187 mg, 250 mg, 375 mg.

TABLETS (EXTENDED-RELEASE [CECLOR CD]): 375 mg, 500 mg.

ADMINISTRATION/HANDLING

PO

- After reconstitution, oral solution is stable for 14 days if refrigerated.
- Shake oral suspension well before using.
- Give without regard to food; if GI upset occurs, give with food, milk.
- Do not cut, crush, chew extended-release tablets.

INDICATIONS/ROUTES/DOSAGE

BRONCHITIS

PO (EXTENDED-RELEASE): ADULTS, ELDERLY: 500 mg q12h for 7 days.

LOWER RESPIRATORY TRACT INFECTIONS

PO: ADULTS, ELDERLY: 250–500 mg q8h.

OTITIS MEDIA

PO: CHILDREN: 20–40 mg/kg/day in 2–3 divided doses. **Maximum:** 1 g/day.

PHARYNGITIS, SKIN/SKIN STRUCTURE INFECTIONS, TONSILLITIS

PO (EXTENDED-RELEASE): ADULTS, ELDERLY: 375 mg q12h.

PO (REGULAR-RELEASE): ADULTS, ELDERLY: 250–500 mg q8h. **CHILDREN:** 20–40 mg/kg/day in 2–3 divided doses. **Maximum:** 1 g/day.

UTI

PO: ADULTS, ELDERLY: 250–500 mg q8h. **CHILDREN:** 20–40 mg/kg/day in 2–3 divided doses q8h. **Maximum:** 1 g/day.

PO (EXTENDED-RELEASE): ADULTS, CHILDREN OLDER THAN 16 YRS: 375–500 mg q12h.

DOSAGE IN RENAL IMPAIRMENT

Decreased dosage may be necessary in pts with creatinine clearance less than 40 ml/min.

SIDE EFFECTS

FREQUENT: Oral candidiasis, mild diarrhea, mild abdominal cramping, vaginal candidiasis. **OCCASIONAL:** Nausea, serum sickness-like reaction (fever, joint pain; usually occurs after second course of therapy and resolves after drug is discontinued). **RARE:** Allergic reaction (pruritus, rash, urticaria).

ADVERSE EFFECTS/ TOXIC REACTIONS

Antibiotic-associated colitis (severe abdominal pain, tenderness, fever, severe watery diarrhea), other superinfections may result from altered bacterial balance. Nephrotoxicity may occur, esp. in pts with preexisting renal disease. Pts with a history of allergies, esp. to penicillin, are at increased risk for developing a severe hypersensitivity reaction, (severe pruritus, angioedema, bronchospasm, anaphylaxis).

NURSING CONSIDERATIONS

BASELINE ASSESSMENT

Question for history of allergies, particularly cephalosporins, penicillins.

C

INTERVENTION/EVALUATION

Assess oral cavity for white patches on mucous membranes, tongue (thrush). Monitor daily pattern of bowel activity/stool consistency carefully; mild GI effects may be tolerable (increasing severity may indicate onset of antibiotic-associated colitis). Monitor I&O, renal function tests for nephrotoxicity. Be alert for superinfection (severe genital/anal pruritus, abdominal pain, severe mouth soreness, moderate to severe diarrhea).

PATIENT/FAMILY TEACHING

• Continue therapy for full length of treatment. • Doses should be evenly spaced. • May cause GI upset (may take with food, milk). • Refrigerate oral suspension.

cefadroxil

sef-a-**drox**-ill

(Apo-Cefadroxil ♣, Duricef, Novo-Cefadroxil ♣)

CLASSIFICATION

PHARMACOTHERAPEUTIC: First-generation cephalosporin. **CLINICAL:** Antibiotic (see p. 21C).

ACTION

Binds to bacterial cell membranes, inhibits cell wall synthesis. **Therapeutic Effect:** Bactericidal.

PHARMACOKINETICS

Well absorbed from GI tract. Protein binding: 15%–20%. Widely distributed. Primarily excreted unchanged in urine. Removed by hemodialysis. **Half-life:** 1.2–1.5 hrs (increased in renal impairment).

USES

Treatment of susceptible infections due to group A *streptococci, staphylococci, S. pneumoniae, H. influenzae, Klebsiella* species, *E. coli, P. mirabilis,* including impetigo, pharyngitis/tonsillitis, skin/skin structure and UTIs.

PRECAUTIONS

CONTRAINDICATIONS: History of anaphylactic reaction to penicillins, hypersensitivity to cephalosporins. **CAUTIONS:** Renal impairment, history of GI disease (esp. ulcerative colitis, antibiotic-associated colitis), concurrent use of nephrotoxic medications.

LIFESPAN CONSIDERATIONS:

Pregnancy/Lactation: Readily crosses placenta. Distributed in breast milk. **Pregnancy Category B. Children:** No age-related precautions noted. **Elderly:** Age-related renal impairment may require dosage adjustment.

INTERACTIONS

DRUG: Probenecid may increase concentration. Bleeding may occur with concomitant use of **warfarin. HERBAL:** None significant. **FOOD:** None known. **LAB VALUES:** May increase BUN, serum alkaline phosphatase, bilirubin, creatinine, LDH, AST, ALT. May cause positive direct/indirect Coombs' test.

AVAILABILITY (Rx)

CAPSULES: 500 mg. **POWDER FOR ORAL SUSPENSION:** 250 mg/5 ml, 500 mg/5 ml. **TABLETS:** 1 g.

ADMINISTRATION/HANDLING

PO

• After reconstitution, oral solution is stable for 14 days if refrigerated. • Shake oral suspension well before using. • Give without regard to meals; if GI upset occurs, give with food, milk.

INDICATIONS/ROUTES/DOSAGE

UTI

PO: ADULTS, ELDERLY: 1–2 g/day as a single dose or in 2 divided doses.

CHILDREN: 30 mg/kg/day in 2 divided doses. **Maximum:** 2 g/day.

SKIN/SKIN STRUCTURE INFECTIONS, GROUP A BETA-HEMOLYTIC STREPTOCOCCAL PHARYNGITIS, TONSILLITIS

PO: ADULTS, ELDERLY: 1–2 g/day in 2 divided doses. **CHILDREN:** 30 mg/kg/day in 2 divided doses. **Maximum:** 2 g/day.

IMPETIGO

PO: CHILDREN: 30 mg/kg/day as a single or in 2 divided doses. **Maximum:** 2 g/day.

DOSAGE IN RENAL IMPAIRMENT

After initial 1-g dose, dosage and frequency are modified based on creatinine clearance and severity of infection.

Creatinine Clearance	Dosage Interval
25–50 ml/min	500 mg q12h
10–25 ml/min	500 mg q24h
0–10 ml/min	500 mg q36h

SIDE EFFECTS

FREQUENT: Oral candidiasis, mild diarrhea, mild abdominal cramping, vaginal candidiasis. **OCCASIONAL:** Nausea, unusual bruising/bleeding, serum sickness-like reaction (fever, joint pain; usually occurs after second course of therapy and resolves after drug is discontinued). **RARE:** Allergic reaction (rash, pruritus, urticaria), thrombophlebitis (pain, redness, swelling at injection site).

ADVERSE EFFECTS/ TOXIC REACTIONS

Antibiotic-associated colitis (severe abdominal pain, tenderness, fever, severe watery diarrhea), other superinfections may result from altered bacterial balance. Nephrotoxicity may occur, esp. in pts with preexisting renal disease. Pts with a history of allergies, esp. to penicillin, are at increased risk for developing a severe hypersensitivity reaction (severe pruritus, angioedema, bronchospasm, anaphylaxis).

NURSING CONSIDERATIONS

BASELINE ASSESSMENT

Question for history of allergies, particularly cephalosporins, penicillins.

INTERVENTION/EVALUATION

Assess oral cavity for white patches on mucous membranes, tongue (thrush). Monitor daily pattern of bowel activity/stool consistency carefully; mild GI effects may be tolerable (increasing severity may indicate onset of antibiotic-associated colitis). Monitor I&O, renal function tests for nephrotoxicity. Be alert for superinfection (genital/anal pruritus, moniliasis, abdominal pain, sore mouth/tongue, moderate to severe diarrhea).

PATIENT/FAMILY TEACHING

• Continue therapy for full length of treatment. • Doses should be evenly spaced. • May cause GI upset (may take with food, milk). • Refrigerate oral suspension.

cefazolin

cef-ah-**zoe**-lin

(Ancef, Kefzol)

Do not confuse cefazolin with cefprozil or Cefzil.

CLASSIFICATION

PHARMACOTHERAPEUTIC: First-generation cephalosporin. **CLINICAL:** Antibiotic (see p. 21C).

ACTION

Binds to bacterial cell membranes, inhibits cell wall synthesis. **Therapeutic Effect:** Bactericidal.

PHARMACOKINETICS

Widely distributed. Protein binding: 85%. Primarily excreted unchanged in urine. Moderately removed by hemodialysis.

C

Half-life: 1.4–1.8 hrs (increased in renal impairment).

USES

Treatment of susceptible infections due to *S. aureus, S. epidermidis,* Group A *beta-hemolytic streptococci, S. pneumoniae, E. coli, P. mirabilis, Klebsiella* species, *H. influenzae* including biliary tract, bone and joint, genital, respiratory tract, skin/skin structure and UTIs, endocarditis, perioperative prophylaxis, septicemia.

PRECAUTIONS

CONTRAINDICATIONS: History of anaphylactic reaction to penicillins, hypersensitivity to cephalosporins. **CAUTIONS:** Renal impairment, history of GI disease (esp. ulcerative colitis, antibiotic-associated colitis), concurrent use of nephrotoxic medications.

LIFESPAN CONSIDERATIONS:

Pregnancy/Lactation: Readily crosses placenta; distributed in breast milk. **Pregnancy Category B. Children:** No age-related precautions noted. **Elderly:** Age-related renal impairment may require reduced dosage.

INTERACTIONS

DRUG: Aminoglycosides, furosemide may increase risk of nephrotoxicity. **Probenecid** may increase concentration. Bleeding may occur with concomitant use of **warfarin. HERBAL:** None significant. **FOOD:** None known. **LAB VALUES:** May increase BUN, serum alkaline phosphatase, bilirubin, creatinine, LDH, AST, ALT. May cause positive direct/indirect Coombs' test.

AVAILABILITY (Rx)

INJECTION, POWDER FOR RECONSTITUTION (ANCEF, KEFZOL): 500 mg, 1 g. **READY-TO-HANG INFUSION (ANCEF):** 500 mg/50 ml, 1 g/50 ml, 2 g/100 ml.

ADMINISTRATION/HANDLING

IV

Reconstitution • Reconstitute each 1 g with at least 10 ml Sterile Water for Injection. • May further dilute in 50–100 ml D_5W or 0.9% NaCl (decreases incidence of thrombophlebitis).

Rate of administration • For IV push, administer over 3–5 min. • For intermittent IV infusion (piggyback), infuse over 20–30 min.

Storage • Solution appears light yellow to yellow. • IV infusion (piggyback) stable for 24 hrs at room temperature, 96 hrs if refrigerated. • Discard if precipitate forms.

IM

• To minimize discomfort, inject deep IM slowly. • Less painful if injected into gluteus maximus rather than lateral aspect of thigh.

IV INCOMPATIBILITIES

Amikacin (Amikin), amiodarone (Cordarone), hydromorphone (Dilaudid).

IV COMPATIBILITIES

Calcium gluconate, diltiazem (Cardizem), famotidine (Pepcid), heparin, insulin (regular), lidocaine, lipids, magnesium sulfate, midazolam (Versed), morphine, multivitamins, potassium chloride, propofol (Diprivan), total parenteral nutrition (TPN), vecuronium (Norcuron).

INDICATIONS/ROUTES/DOSAGE

UNCOMPLICATED UTIs

IV, IM: ADULTS, ELDERLY: 1 g q12h.

MILD TO MODERATE INFECTIONS

IV, IM: ADULTS, ELDERLY: 500 mg–1 g q6–8h.

SEVERE INFECTIONS

IV, IM: ADULTS, ELDERLY: 1–2 g q6–8h.

LIFE-THREATENING INFECTIONS

IV, IM: ADULTS, ELDERLY: 1–2 g q4–6h. **Maximum:** 12 g/day.

PERIOPERATIVE PROPHYLAXIS

IV, IM: ADULTS, ELDERLY: 1 g 30–60 min before surgery, 0.5–1 g during surgery, and q6–8h for up to 24 hrs postoperatively.

USUAL PEDIATRIC DOSAGE

CHILDREN: 50–100 mg/kg/day in divided doses q8h. **Maximum:** 6 g/day. **NEONATES OLDER THAN 7 DAYS:** 40–60 mg/kg/day in divided doses q8–12h. **NEONATES 7 DAYS AND YOUNGER:** 40 mg/kg/day in divided doses q12h.

DOSAGE IN RENAL IMPAIRMENT

Dosing frequency is modified based on creatinine clearance.

Creatinine Clearance	Dosage Interval
10–30 ml/min	Usual dose q12h
Less than 10 ml/min	Usual dose q24h

SIDE EFFECTS

FREQUENT: Discomfort with IM administration, oral candidiasis, mild diarrhea, mild abdominal cramping, vaginal candidiasis. **OCCASIONAL:** Nausea, serum sickness-like reaction (fever, joint pain; usually occurs after second course of therapy and resolves after drug is discontinued). **RARE:** Allergic reaction (rash, pruritus, urticaria), thrombophlebitis (pain, redness, swelling at injection site).

ADVERSE EFFECTS/ TOXIC REACTIONS

Antibiotic-associated colitis (severe abdominal pain, tenderness, fever, severe watery diarrhea), other superinfections may result from altered bacterial balance. Nephrotoxicity may occur, esp. in pts with preexisting renal disease. Pts with a history of allergies, esp. to penicillin, are at increased risk for developing a severe hypersensitivity reaction (severe pruritus, angioedema, bronchospasm, anaphylaxis).

NURSING CONSIDERATIONS

BASELINE ASSESSMENT

Question for history of allergies, particularly cephalosporins, penicillins.

INTERVENTION/EVALUATION

Evaluate IM site for induration and tenderness. Assess oral cavity for white patches on mucous membranes, tongue (thrush). Monitor daily pattern of bowel activity/stool consistency carefully; mild GI effects may be tolerable (increasing severity may indicate onset of antibiotic-associated colitis). Monitor I&O, renal function tests for nephrotoxicity. Be alert for superinfection (severe genital/anal pruritus, abdominal pain, severe mouth soreness, moderate to severe diarrhea).

PATIENT/FAMILY TEACHING

- Discomfort may occur with IM injection.

cefdinir

sef-di-neer

(Omnicef)

CLASSIFICATION

PHARMACOTHERAPEUTIC: Third-generation cephalosporin. **CLINICAL:** Antibiotic (see p. 22C).

ACTION

Binds to bacterial cell membranes, inhibits cell wall synthesis. **Therapeutic Effect:** Bactericidal.

PHARMACOKINETICS

Moderately absorbed from GI tract. Protein binding: 60%–70%. Widely distributed. Not appreciably metabolized. Primarily excreted unchanged in urine. Minimally removed by hemodialysis. **Half-life:** 1–2 hrs (increased in renal impairment).

C

USES

Treatment of susceptible infections due to *S. pyogenes, S. pneumoniae, H. influenzae, H. parainfluenzae, M. catarrhalis* including community-acquired pneumonia, acute exacerbation of chronic bronchitis, acute maxillary sinusitis, pharyngitis, tonsillitis, uncomplicated skin/skin structure infections, otitis media.

PRECAUTIONS

CONTRAINDICATIONS: History of anaphylactic reaction to penicillins, hypersensitivity to cephalosporins. **CAUTIONS:** Hypersensitivity to penicillins, other drugs; history of GI disease (e.g., colitis); renal impairment, hepatic impairment.

⌛ LIFESPAN CONSIDERATIONS:

Pregnancy/Lactation: Crosses placenta. Not detected in breast milk. **Pregnancy Category B. Children:** Newborns, infants may have lower renal clearance. **Elderly:** Age-related renal impairment may require decreased dosage or increased dosing interval.

INTERACTIONS

DRUG: **Aminoglycosides** may increase risk of nephrotoxicity. **Antacids, iron preparations** may interfere with absorption. **Probenecid** increases concentration. **HERBAL:** None significant. **FOOD:** None known. **LAB VALUES:** May produce false-positive reaction for urine ketones. May increase serum alkaline phosphatase, bilirubin, LDH, AST, ALT.

AVAILABILITY (Rx)

CAPSULES: 300 mg. **POWDER FOR ORAL SUSPENSION:** 125 mg/5 ml, 250 mg/5 ml.

ADMINISTRATION/HANDLING

PO

• Give without regard to food. • To reconstitute oral suspension, for the 60-ml bottle, add 39 ml water; for the 120-ml bottle, add 65 ml water. • Shake oral suspension well before administering. • Store mixed suspension at room temperature. Discard unused portion after 10 days.

INDICATIONS/ROUTES/DOSAGE

COMMUNITY-ACQUIRED PNEUMONIA

PO: ADULTS, ELDERLY, CHILDREN 13 YRS AND OLDER: 300 mg q12h for 10 days.

ACUTE EXACERBATION OF CHRONIC BRONCHITIS

PO: ADULTS, ELDERLY: 300 mg q12h for 5–10 days or 600 mg once daily for 10 days.

ACUTE MAXILLARY SINUSITIS

PO: ADULTS, ELDERLY, CHILDREN 13 YRS AND OLDER: 300 mg q12h or 600 mg q24h for 10 days. **CHILDREN 6 MOS–12 YRS:** 7 mg/kg q12h or 14 mg/kg q24h for 10 days. **Maximum:** 600 mg/day.

PHARYNGITIS, TONSILLITIS

PO: ADULTS, ELDERLY, CHILDREN 13 YRS AND OLDER: 300 mg q12h for 5–10 days or 600 mg q24h for 10 days. **CHILDREN 6 MOS–12 YRS:** 7 mg/kg q12h for 5–10 days or 14 mg/kg q24h for 10 days. **Maximum:** 600 mg/day.

UNCOMPLICATED SKIN/SKIN STRUCTURE INFECTIONS

PO: ADULTS, ELDERLY, CHILDREN 13 YRS AND OLDER: 300 mg q12h for 10 days. **CHILDREN 6 MOS–12 YRS:** 7 mg/kg q12h for 10 days. **Maximum:** 600 mg/day.

ACUTE BACTERIAL OTITIS MEDIA

PO (CAPSULES): CHILDREN: 6 MOS–12 YRS: 7 mg/kg q12h or 14 mg/kg q24h for 10 days. **Maximum:** 600 mg/day.

USUAL PEDIATRIC DOSAGE FOR ORAL SUSPENSION

CHILDREN WEIGHING 81–95 LB (37–43 KG): 12.5 ml (2.5 tsp) q12h or 25 ml (5 tsp) q24h. **CHILDREN WEIGHING 61–80 LB (28–36 KG):** 10 ml (2 tsp) q12h or 20 ml (4 tsp) q24h. **CHILDREN WEIGHING 41–60 LB (19–27 KG):** 7.5 ml (1 tsp) q12h or 15 ml (3 tsp) q24h. **CHILDREN WEIGHING 20–40 LB (9–18 KG):** 5 ml (1 tsp) q12h or 10 ml (2 tsp) q24h. **INFANTS WEIGHING LESS THAN 20 LB**

(LESS THAN 9 KG): 2.5 ml (½ tsp) q12h or 5 ml (1 tsp) q24h.

DOSAGE IN RENAL IMPAIRMENT

For pts with creatinine clearance less than 30 ml/min, dosage is 300 mg/day as single daily dose. For hemodialysis pts, dosage is 300 mg or 7 mg/kg/dose every other day.

SIDE EFFECTS

FREQUENT: Oral candidiasis, mild diarrhea, mild abdominal cramping, vaginal candidiasis. **OCCASIONAL:** Nausea, serum sickness-like reaction (fever, joint pain; usually occurs after second course of therapy and resolves after drug is discontinued). **RARE:** Allergic reaction (rash, pruritus, urticaria).

ADVERSE EFFECTS/ TOXIC REACTIONS

Antibiotic-associated colitis (severe abdominal pain, tenderness, fever, severe watery diarrhea), other superinfections may result from altered bacterial balance. Nephrotoxicity may occur, esp. in pts with preexisting renal disease. Pts with a history of allergies, esp. to penicillin, are at increased risk for developing a severe hypersensitivity reaction (severe pruritus, angioedema, bronchospasm, anaphylaxis).

NURSING CONSIDERATIONS

BASELINE ASSESSMENT

Question for hypersensitivity to cefdinir or other cephalosporins, penicillins.

INTERVENTION/EVALUATION

Monitor daily pattern of bowel activity/stool consistency carefully; mild GI effects may be tolerable, (increasing severity may indicate onset of antibiotic-associated colitis). Be alert for superinfection (e.g., genital/anal pruritus, ulceration or changes in oral mucosa, moderate to severe diarrhea, new/increased fever). Monitor hematology reports.

PATIENT/FAMILY TEACHING

• Take antacids 2 hrs before or following medication. • Continue medication for full length of treatment; do not skip doses. • Doses should be evenly spaced. • Report persistent diarrhea to nurse/physician.

cefditoren

sef-dih-**toe**-rin
(Spectracef)

◆ CLASSIFICATION

PHARMACOTHERAPEUTIC: Third-generation cephalosporin. **CLINICAL:** Antibiotic.

ACTION

Binds to bacterial cell membranes, inhibits cell wall synthesis. **Therapeutic Effect:** Bactericidal.

PHARMACOKINETICS

Moderately absorbed from GI tract. Protein binding: 88%. Not metabolized. Excreted in urine. Minimally removed by hemodialysis. **Half-life:** 1.6 hrs (half-life increased with renal impairment).

USES

Treatment of susceptible infections due to *S. pneumoniae, S. pyogenes, S. aureus, H. influenzae, M. catarrhalis* including acute bacterial exacerbations of chronic bronchitis, pharyngitis or tonsillitis, uncomplicated skin/skin structure infections, community-acquired pneumonia.

PRECAUTIONS

CONTRAINDICATIONS: Carnitine deficiency, inborn errors of metabolism, known allergy to cephalosporins, hypersensitivity to milk protein. **CAUTIONS:** Hypersensitivity to penicillins or other drugs; allergies; history of GI disease (e.g., colitis); renal impairment.

C

LIFESPAN CONSIDERATIONS:

Pregnancy/Lactation: Unknown if distributed in breast milk. **Pregnancy Category B. Children:** Safety and efficacy not established in those younger than 12 yrs. **Elderly:** Age-related renal impairment may require reduced dosage adjustment.

INTERACTIONS

DRUG: Antacids containing aluminum, magnesium, H_2 antagonists may decrease absorption. **Probenecid** may increase absorption. Bleeding may occur with concomitant use of **warfarin. HERBAL:** None significant. **FOOD: High-fat meals** increase concentration. **LAB VALUES:** May cause positive direct/indirect Coombs' test. May cause false-positive reaction for urine glucose.

AVAILABILITY (Rx)

TABLETS: 200 mg.

ADMINISTRATION/HANDLING

PO

- Give with food (enhances absorption).

INDICATIONS/ROUTES/DOSAGE

PHARYNGITIS, TONSILLITIS, SKIN INFECTIONS

PO: ADULTS, ELDERLY, CHILDREN OLDER THAN 12 YRS: 200 mg twice a day for 10 days.

ACUTE EXACERBATION OF CHRONIC BRONCHITIS

PO: ADULTS, ELDERLY, CHILDREN OLDER THAN 12 YRS: 400 mg twice a day for 10 days.

COMMUNITY-ACQUIRED PNEUMONIA

PO: ADULTS, ELDERLY, CHILDREN OLDER THAN 12 YRS: 400 mg 2 twice a day for 14 days.

DOSAGE IN RENAL IMPAIRMENT

Dosage and frequency are modified based on creatinine clearance.

Creatinine Clearance	Dosage
50–80 ml/min	No adjustment necessary.
30–49 ml/min	200 mg twice a day
Less than 30 ml/min	200 mg once a day

SIDE EFFECTS

OCCASIONAL (11%): Diarrhea. **RARE (4%–1%):** Nausea, headache, abdominal pain, vaginal candidiasis, dyspepsia, vomiting.

ADVERSE EFFECTS/ TOXIC REACTIONS

Antibiotic-associated colitis (severe abdominal pain, tenderness, fever, severe watery diarrhea), other superinfections may occur. Pts with a history of allergies, esp. to penicillin, are at increased risk for developing a severe hypersensitivity reaction (severe pruritus, angioedema, bronchospasm, anaphylaxis).

NURSING CONSIDERATIONS

BASELINE ASSESSMENT

Question for history of allergies, particularly cephalosporins, penicillins.

INTERVENTION/EVALUATION

Monitor daily pattern of bowel activity/ stool consistency; mild GI effects may be tolerable, (increasing severity may indicate onset of antibiotic-associated colitis). Be alert for superinfection (severe genital or anal pruritus, abdominal pain, stomatitis, moderate to severe diarrhea). Monitor carnitine deficiency (muscle damage, hypoglycemia, fatigue, confusion).

PATIENT/FAMILY TEACHING

• Continue medication for full length of treatment; do not skip doses. • Doses should be evenly spaced. • May cause GI upset (may take with food).

C

cefepime

sef-eh-**peem**
(Maxipime)

Do not confuse cefepime with ceftidine.

✦CLASSIFICATION

PHARMACOTHERAPEUTIC: Fourth-generation cephalosporin. **CLINICAL:** Antibiotic (see p. 23C).

ACTION

Binds to bacterial cell membranes, inhibits cell wall synthesis. **Therapeutic Effect:** Bactericidal.

PHARMACOKINETICS

Well absorbed after IM administration. Protein binding: 20%. Widely distributed. Primarily excreted unchanged in urine. Removed by hemodialysis. **Half-life:** 2–2.3 hrs (increased in renal impairment, elderly pts).

USES

Susceptible infections due to aerobic gram-negative organisms including *P. aeruginosa,* gram-positive organisms including *S. aureus.* Treatment of empiric febrile neutropenia, intra-abdominal, skin/skin structure, UTIs, pneumonia.

PRECAUTIONS

CONTRAINDICATIONS: History of anaphylactic reaction to penicillins, hypersensitivity to cephalosporins. **CAUTIONS:** Renal impairment.

LIFESPAN CONSIDERATIONS:

Pregnancy/Lactation: Unknown if distributed in breast milk. **Pregnancy Category B. Children:** No age-related precautions noted in those older than 2 mos. **Elderly:** Age-related renal impairment may require reduced dosage or increased dosing interval.

INTERACTIONS

DRUG: Aminoglycosides, furosemide may increase risk of nephrotoxicity. **Probenecid** may increase concentration. **HERBAL:** None significant. **FOOD:** None known. **LAB VALUES:** May increase BUN, serum alkaline phosphatase, bilirubin, LDH, AST, ALT. May cause positive direct/indirect Coombs' test.

AVAILABILITY (Rx)

INJECTION, POWDER FOR RECONSTITUTION: 500 mg, 1 g, 2 g.

ADMINISTRATION/HANDLING

IV

Reconstitution • Add 5 ml to 500-mg vial (10 ml for 1-g and 2-g vials). • Further dilute with 50–100 ml 0.9% NaCl, or D_5W.

Rate of administration • For IV push, administer over 3–5 min. • For intermittent IV infusion (piggyback), infuse over 30 min.

Storage • Solution is stable for 24 hrs at room temperature, 7 days if refrigerated.

IM

• Add 1.3 ml Sterile Water for Injection, 0.9% NaCl, or D_5W to 500-mg vial (2.4 ml for 1-g and 2-g vials). • Inject into a large muscle mass (e.g., upper gluteus maximus).

IV INCOMPATIBILITIES

Acyclovir (Zovirax), amphotericin (Fungizone), cimetidine (Tagamet), ciprofloxacin (Cipro), cisplatin (Platinol), dacarbazine (DTIC), daunorubicin (Cerubidine), diazepam (Valium), diphenhydramine (Benadryl), dobutamine (Dobutrex), dopamine (Intropin), doxorubicin (Adriamycin), droperidol (Inapsine), famotidine (Pepcid), ganciclovir (Cytovene), haloperidol (Haldol), magnesium, magnesium sulfate, mannitol, meperidine (Demerol), metoclopramide (Reglan), morphine, ofloxacin

(Floxin), ondansetron (Zofran), vancomycin (Vancocin).

C

IV COMPATIBILITIES

Bumetanide (Bumex), calcium gluconate, furosemide (Lasix), hydromorphone (Dilaudid), lorazepam (Ativan), propofol (Diprivan).

INDICATIONS/ROUTES/DOSAGE

PNEUMONIA

IV: ADULTS, ELDERLY: 1–2 g q12h for 7–10 days. **CHILDREN 2 MOS AND OLDER:** 50 mg/kg q12h. **Maximum:** 2 g/dose.

INTRA-ABDOMINAL INFECTIONS

IV: ADULTS, ELDERLY: 2 g q12h for 10 days.

SKIN/SKIN STRUCTURE INFECTIONS

IV: ADULTS, ELDERLY: 2 g q12h for 10 days. **CHILDREN 2 MOS AND OLDER:** 50 mg/kg q12h. **Maximum:** 2 g/dose.

UTIs

IV: ADULTS, ELDERLY: 0.5–2 g q12h for 7–10 days. **CHILDREN 2 MOS AND OLDER:** 50 mg/kg q12h. **Maximum:** 2 g/dose.

FEBRILE NEUTROPENIA

IV: ADULTS, ELDERLY: 2 g q8h. **CHILDREN 2 MOS AND OLDER:** 50 mg/kg q8h. **Maximum:** 2 g/dose.

DOSAGE IN RENAL IMPAIRMENT

Dosage and frequency are modified based on creatinine clearance and severity of infection.

Creatinine Clearance	Dose Range
30–60 ml/min	0.5 g q24h–2 g q12h
11–29 ml/min	0.5–2 g q24h
10 ml/min or less	0.25–1 g q24h

SIDE EFFECTS

FREQUENT: Discomfort with IM administration, oral candidiasis, mild diarrhea, mild abdominal cramping, vaginal candidiasis. **OCCASIONAL:** Nausea, serum sickness-like reaction (fever, joint pain; usually occurs after second course of therapy and resolves after drug is discontinued). **RARE:** Allergic reaction (rash, pruritus, urticaria), thrombophlebitis (pain, redness, swelling at injection site).

ADVERSE EFFECTS/ TOXIC REACTIONS

Antibiotic-associated colitis (severe abdominal pain, tenderness, fever, severe watery diarrhea), other superinfections may result from altered bacterial balance. Nephrotoxicity may occur, esp. in pts with preexisting renal disease. Pts with a history of allergies, esp. to penicillin, are at increased risk for developing a severe hypersensitivity reaction (severe pruritus, angioedema, bronchospasm, anaphylaxis).

NURSING CONSIDERATIONS

BASELINE ASSESSMENT

Question for history of allergies, particularly cephalosporins, penicillins.

INTERVENTION/EVALUATION

Evaluate IM site for induration and tenderness. Assess oral cavity for white patches on mucous membranes, tongue (thrush). Monitor daily pattern of bowel activity/stool consistency carefully; mild GI effects may be tolerable (increasing severity may indicate onset of antibiotic-associated colitis). Monitor I&O, renal function tests for nephrotoxicity. Be alert for superinfection (severe genital/anal pruritus, abdominal pain, severe mouth soreness, moderate to severe diarrhea).

PATIENT/FAMILY TEACHING

• Discomfort may occur with IM injection. • Continue therapy for full length of treatment. • Doses should be evenly spaced.

C

cefixime

sef-ih-zeem

(Suprax)

Do not confuse Suprax with Sporanox, Surbex, or Surfak.

CLASSIFICATION

PHARMACOTHERAPEUTIC: Third-generation cephalosporin. **CLINICAL:** Antibiotic.

ACTION

Binds to bacterial cell membranes, inhibits cell wall synthesis. **Therapeutic Effect:** Bactericidal.

PHARMACOKINETICS

Moderately absorbed from GI tract. Protein binding: 65%–70%. Widely distributed. Primarily excreted unchanged in urine. Minimally removed by hemodialysis. **Half-life:** 3–4 hrs (increased in renal impairment).

USES

Treatment of susceptible infections due to *S. pneumoniae, S. pyogenes, M. catarrhalis, H. influenzae, N. gonorrhoeae, E. coli, P. mirabilis* including otitis media, acute bronchitis, acute exacerbations of chronic bronchitis, pharyngitis, tonsillitis, uncomplicated UTI, uncomplicated gonorrhea.

PRECAUTIONS

CONTRAINDICATIONS: History of anaphylactic reaction to penicillins, hypersensitivity to cephalosporins. **CAUTIONS:** Hypersensitivity to penicillins, other drugs; allergies; history of GI disease (e.g., colitis); renal impairment.

LIFESPAN CONSIDERATIONS:

Pregnancy/Lactation: Not recommended during labor and delivery. Unknown if distributed in breast milk. **Pregnancy Category B. Children:** Safety and efficacy not established in those younger than 6 mos. **Elderly:** Age-related renal impairment may require dosage adjustment.

INTERACTIONS

DRUG: Aminoglycosides, furosemide may increase risk of nephrotoxicity. **Probenecid** may increase concentration. Bleeding may occur with concomitant use of **warfarin. HERBAL:** None significant. **FOOD:** None known. **LAB VALUES:** May increase BUN, serum alkaline phosphatase, bilirubin, creatinine, LDH, AST, ALT. May cause a positive direct/indirect Coombs' test.

AVAILABILITY (Rx)

ORAL SUSPENSION: 100 mg/5 ml. **TABLETS:** 200 mg, 400 mg.

ADMINISTRATION/HANDLING

PO

• Give without regard to food. • After reconstitution, oral suspension is stable for 14 days at room temperature. • Do not refrigerate. • Shake oral suspension well before administering.

INDICATIONS/ROUTES/DOSAGE

USUAL DOSAGE

PO: ADULTS, ELDERLY, CHILDREN WEIGHING MORE THAN 50 KG: 400 mg/day as a single dose or in 2 divided doses. **CHILDREN 6 MOS–12 YRS WEIGHING LESS THAN 50 KG:** 8 mg/kg/day as a single dose or in 2 divided doses. **Maximum:** 400 mg.

UNCOMPLICATED GONORRHEA

PO: ADULTS: 400 mg as a single dose.

DOSAGE IN RENAL IMPAIRMENT

Dosage is modified based on creatinine clearance.

Creatinine Clearance	% of Usual Dose
21–60 ml/min	75%
20 ml/min or less	50%

SIDE EFFECTS

FREQUENT: Oral candidiasis, mild diarrhea, mild abdominal cramping, vaginal candidiasis. **OCCASIONAL:** Nausea, serum sickness-like reaction (arthralgia, fever; usually occurs after second course of therapy and resolves after drug is discontinued). **RARE:** Allergic reaction (rash, pruritus, urticaria).

ADVERSE EFFECTS/ TOXIC REACTIONS

Antibiotic-associated colitis (severe abdominal pain, tenderness, fever, severe watery diarrhea), other superinfections may result from altered bacterial balance. Nephrotoxicity may occur, esp. in pts with preexisting renal disease. Pts with a history of allergies, esp. to penicillin, are at increased risk for developing a severe hypersensitivity reaction (severe pruritus, angioedema, bronchospasm, anaphylaxis).

NURSING CONSIDERATIONS

BASELINE ASSESSMENT

Question for hypersensitivity to cefixime or other cephalosporins, penicillins, other drugs.

INTERVENTION/EVALUATION

Assess oral cavity for white patches on mucous membranes, tongue (thrush). Monitor daily pattern of bowel activity/stool consistency; mild GI effects may be tolerable, (increasing severity may indicate onset of antibiotic-associated colitis). Monitor renal function tests for evidence of nephrotoxicity. Be alert for superinfection (severe genital/anal pruritus, abdominal pain, stomatitis, moderate to severe diarrhea).

PATIENT/FAMILY TEACHING

• Continue medication for full length of treatment; do not skip doses. • Doses should be evenly spaced. • May cause GI upset (may take with food or milk).

cefotaxime

sef-oh-**taks**-eem

(Claforan)

Do not confuse cefotaxime with cefoxitin, ceftizoxime, or cefuroxime, or Claforan with Claritin.

CLASSIFICATION

PHARMACOTHERAPEUTIC: Third-generation cephalosporin. **CLINICAL:** Antibiotic (see p. 22C).

ACTION

Binds to bacterial cell membranes, inhibits cell wall synthesis. **Therapeutic Effect:** Bactericidal.

PHARMACOKINETICS

Widely distributed (including to cerebrospinal fluid [CSF]). Protein binding: 30%–50%. Partially metabolized in the liver to active metabolite. Primarily excreted in urine. Moderately removed by hemodialysis. **Half-life:** 1 hr (increased in renal impairment).

USES

Treatment of susceptible infections due to gram-negative organisms including bone, joint, GU, gynecologic, intra-abdominal, lower respiratory tract, skin/skin structure infections, septicemia, meningitis, preoperative prophylaxis. **OFF-LABEL:** Treatment of Lyme disease.

PRECAUTIONS

CONTRAINDICATIONS: History of anaphylactic reaction to penicillins, hypersensitivity to cephalosporins. **CAUTIONS:** Concurrent use of nephrotoxic medications, history of GI disease (esp. ulcerative colitis, antibiotic-associated colitis), renal impairment with creatinine clearance less than 20 ml/min.

LIFESPAN CONSIDERATIONS:

Pregnancy/Lactation: Readily crosses placenta. Distributed in breast milk. **Pregnancy Category B. Children:** No age-related precautions noted. **Elderly:** Age-related renal impairment may require dosage adjustment.

INTERACTIONS

DRUG: Aminoglycosides, furosemide may increase risk of nephrotoxicity. **Probenecid** may increase concentration. **HERBAL:** None significant. **FOOD:** None known. **LAB VALUES:** May cause positive direct/indirect Coombs' test. May increase hepatic enzyme levels, AST, ALT.

AVAILABILITY (Rx)

INJECTION, POWDER FOR RECONSTITUTION: 500 mg, 1 g, 2 g. **INTRAVENOUS SOLUTION:** 1 g/50 ml, 2 g/50 ml.

ADMINISTRATION/HANDLING

IV

Reconstitution • Reconstitute with 10 ml Sterile Water for Injection to provide a concentration of 50 mg, 95 mg, or 180 mg/ml for 500-mg, 1-g, or 2-g vials, respectively. • May further dilute with 50–100 ml 0.9% NaCl or D_5W.

Rate of administration • For IV push, administer over 3–5 min. • For intermittent IV infusion (piggyback), infuse over 20–30 min.

Storage • Solution appears light yellow to amber. IV infusion (piggyback) may darken in color (does not indicate loss of potency). • IV infusion (piggyback) is stable for 24 hrs at room temperature, 5 days if refrigerated. • Discard if precipitate forms.

IM

• Reconstitute with Sterile Water for Injection or Bacteriostatic Water for Injection. • Add 2, 3, or 5 ml to 500-mg, 1-g, or 2-g vial, respectively, providing a concentration of 230 mg, 300 mg, or 330 mg/ml, respectively. • To minimize discomfort, inject deep IM slowly. Less painful if injected into gluteus maximus than lateral aspect of thigh. For 2-g IM dose, give at 2 separate sites.

IV INCOMPATIBILITIES

Allopurinol (Aloprim), filgrastim (Neupogen), fluconazole (Diflucan), hetastarch (Hespan), lipids, pentamidine (Pentam IV), vancomycin (Vancocin).

IV COMPATIBILITIES

Diltiazem (Cardizem), famotidine (Pepcid), hydromorphone (Dilaudid), lorazepam (Ativan), magnesium sulfate, midazolam (Versed), morphine, propofol (Diprivan), total parenteral nutrition (TPN).

INDICATIONS/ROUTES/DOSAGE

UNCOMPLICATED INFECTIONS

IV, IM: ADULTS, ELDERLY: 1 g q12h.

MILD TO MODERATE INFECTIONS

IV, IM: ADULTS, ELDERLY: 1–2 g q8h.

SEVERE INFECTIONS

IV, IM: ADULTS, ELDERLY: 2 g q6–8h.

LIFE-THREATENING INFECTIONS

IV, IM: ADULTS, ELDERLY: 2 g q4h. **CHILDREN:** 2 g q4h. **Maximum:** 12 g/day.

GONORRHEA

IM: ADULTS: (Male): 1 g as a single dose. **(Female):** 0.5 g as a single dose.

PERIOPERATIVE PROPHYLAXIS

IV, IM: ADULTS, ELDERLY: 1 g 30–90 min before surgery.

CESAREAN SECTION

IV: ADULTS: 1 g as soon as umbilical cord is clamped, then 1 g 6 and 12 hrs after first dose.

USUAL PEDIATRIC DOSAGE

CHILDREN WEIGHING 50 KG OR MORE: 1–2 g q6–8h. **CHILDREN 1 MOS–12 YRS WEIGHING LESS THAN 50 KG:** 100–200 mg/kg/day in divided doses q6–8h.

C

DOSAGE IN RENAL IMPAIRMENT

For pts with creatinine clearance less than 20 ml/min, give half of dose at usual dosing intervals.

SIDE EFFECTS

FREQUENT: Discomfort with IM administration, oral candidiasis, mild diarrhea, mild abdominal cramping, vaginal candidiasis. **OCCASIONAL:** Nausea, serum sickness-like reaction (fever, joint pain; usually occurs after second course of therapy and resolves after drug is discontinued). **RARE:** Allergic reaction (rash, pruritus, urticaria), thrombophlebitis (pain, redness, swelling at injection site).

ADVERSE EFFECTS/ TOXIC REACTIONS

Antibiotic-associated colitis (severe abdominal pain, tenderness, fever, severe watery diarrhea), other superinfections may result from altered bacterial balance. Nephrotoxicity may occur, esp. in pts with preexisting renal disease. Pts with a history of allergies, esp. to penicillin, are at increased risk for developing a severe hypersensitivity reaction (severe pruritus, angioedema, bronchospasm, anaphylaxis).

NURSING CONSIDERATIONS

BASELINE ASSESSMENT

Question for history of allergies, particularly cephalosporins, penicillins.

INTERVENTION/EVALUATION

Check IM injection sites for induration, tenderness. Assess oral cavity for white patches on mucous membranes, tongue (thrush). Monitor daily pattern of bowel activity/stool consistency carefully; mild GI effects may be tolerable (increasing severity may indicate onset of antibiotic-associated colitis). Monitor I&O, renal function tests for nephrotoxicity. Be alert for superinfection (severe genital/ anal pruritus, abdominal pain, severe mouth soreness, moderate to severe diarrhea).

PATIENT/FAMILY TEACHING

- Discomfort may occur with IM injection.
- Doses should be evenly spaced.
- Continue antibiotic therapy for full length of treatment.

cefoxitin

se-**fox**-i-tin

(Mefoxin)

Do not confuse cefoxitin with cefotaxime, cefotetan, or Cytoxan.

CLASSIFICATION

PHARMACOTHERAPEUTIC: Second-generation cephalosporin. **CLINICAL:** Antibiotic (see p. 21C).

ACTION

Binds to bacterial cell membranes, inhibits cell wall synthesis. **Therapeutic Effect:** Bactericidal.

PHARMACOKINETICS

Well distributed. Protein binding: 41%–75%. Primarily excreted in urine. Removed by hemodialysis. **Half-life:** 0.8–1 hr.

USES

Treatment of susceptible infections due to *S. pneumoniae, S. aureus,* gram-negative enteric bacilli, anaerobes (e.g., bacteroides species) including bone, joint, gynecologic, intra-abdominal, lower respiratory, skin/skin structure, UTIs, perioperative prophylaxis.

PRECAUTIONS

CONTRAINDICATIONS: History of anaphylactic reaction to penicillins, hypersensitivity to cephalosporins. **CAUTIONS:** Renal impairment, history of GI disease (esp. ulcerative colitis, antibiotic-associated colitis), concurrent use of nephrotoxic medications.

LIFESPAN CONSIDERATIONS:

Pregnancy/Lactation: Readily crosses placenta; distributed in breast milk. **Preg-nancy Category B. Children:** No age-related precautions noted. **Elderly:** Age-related renal impairment may require dosage adjustment.

INTERACTIONS

DRUG: Aminoglycosides, furosemide may increase risk of nephrotoxicity. **Probenecid** may increase concentration. **HERBAL:** None significant. **FOOD:** None known. **LAB VALUES:** May increase BUN, serum alkaline phosphatase, creatinine, AST, ALT. May cause positive direct/indirect Coombs' test; may interfere with blood crossmatching and hematologic tests.

AVAILABILITY (Rx)

INJECTION, POWDER FOR RECONSTITUTION: 1 g, 2 g. **INTRAVENOUS SOLUTION:** 1 g/50 ml, 2 g/50 ml.

ADMINISTRATION/HANDLING

◄ **ALERT** ► Give IM, IV push, intermittent IV infusion (piggyback).

IV

Reconstitution • Reconstitute each 1 g with 10 ml Sterile Water for Injection to provide concentration of 95 mg/ml. • May further dilute with 50–100 ml 0.9% Sterile Water for Injection, NaCl, or D_5W.

Rate of administration • For IV push, administer over 3–5 min. • For intermittent IV infusion (piggyback), infuse over 15–30 min.

Storage • Solution appears colorless to light amber but may darken (does not indicate loss of potency). • IV infusion (piggyback) is stable for 24 hrs at room temperature, 48 hrs if refrigerated. • Discard if precipitate forms.

IM

• Reconstitute each 1 g with 2 ml Sterile Water for Injection or lidocaine to provide concentration of 400 mg/ml. • To minimize discomfort, inject deep IM slowly. Less painful if injected into gluteus maximus than lateral aspect of thigh.

IV INCOMPATIBILITIES

Filgrastim (Neupogen), pentamidine (Pentam IV), vancomycin (Vancocin).

IV COMPATIBILITIES

Diltiazem (Cardizem), famotidine (Pepcid), heparin, hydromorphone (Dilaudid), lipids, magnesium sulfate, morphine, multivitamins, propofol (Diprivan).

INDICATIONS/ROUTES/DOSAGE

MILD TO MODERATE INFECTIONS

IV, IM: ADULTS, ELDERLY: 1–2 g q6–8h.

SEVERE INFECTIONS

IV, IM: ADULTS, ELDERLY: 1 g q4h or 2 g q6–8h up to 2 g q4h.

PERIOPERATIVE PROPHYLAXIS

IV, IM: ADULTS, ELDERLY: 1–2 g 30–60 min before surgery, then q6h for up to 24 hrs after surgery. **CHILDREN OLDER THAN 3 MOS:** 30–40 mg/kg 30–60 min before surgery, then q6h for up to 24 hrs after surgery.

CESAREAN SECTION

IV: ADULTS: 2 g as soon as umbilical cord is clamped, then 2 g 4 and 8 hrs after first dose, then q6h for up to 24 hrs.

USUAL PEDIATRIC DOSAGE

CHILDREN OLDER THAN 3 MOS: 80–160 mg/kg/day in 4–6 divided doses. **Maximum:** 12 g/day. **NEONATES:** 90–100 mg/kg/day in divided doses q8h.

DOSAGE IN RENAL IMPAIRMENT

After a loading dose of 1–2 g, dosage and frequency are modified based on creatinine clearance and severity of infection.

C

Creatinine Clearance	Dosage
30–50 ml/min	1–2 g q8–12h
10–29 ml/min	1–2 g q12–24h
5–9 ml/min	500 mg–1 g q12–24h
Less than 5 ml/min	500 mg–1 g q24–48h

SIDE EFFECTS

FREQUENT: Discomfort with IM administration, oral candidiasis, mild diarrhea, mild abdominal cramping, vaginal candidiasis. **OCCASIONAL:** Nausea, serum sickness-like reaction (fever, joint pain; usually occurs after second course of therapy and resolves after drug is discontinued). **RARE:** Allergic reaction (pruritus, rash, urticaria), thrombophlebitis (pain, redness, swelling at injection site).

ADVERSE EFFECTS/ TOXIC REACTIONS

Antibiotic-associated colitis (severe abdominal pain, tenderness, fever, severe watery diarrhea), other superinfections may result from altered bacterial balance. Nephrotoxicity may occur, esp. in pts with preexisting renal disease. Pts with a history of allergies, esp. to penicillin, are at increased risk for developing a severe hypersensitivity reaction (severe pruritus, angioedema, bronchospasm, anaphylaxis).

NURSING CONSIDERATIONS

BASELINE ASSESSMENT

Question for history of allergies, particularly cephalosporins, penicillins.

INTERVENTION/EVALUATION

Evaluate IV site for phlebitis (heat, pain, red streaking over vein). Assess IM injection sites for induration, tenderness. Assess oral cavity for white patches on mucous membranes, tongue (thrush). Monitor daily pattern of bowel activity/ stool consistency carefully; mild GI effects may be tolerable, (increasing severity may indicate onset of antibiotic-associated colitis). Monitor I&O, renal function tests for nephrotoxicity. Be alert for superinfection (severe genital or anal pruritus, abdominal pain, severe mouth soreness, moderate to severe diarrhea).

PATIENT/FAMILY TEACHING

• Discomfort may occur with IM injection. • Doses should be evenly spaced. • Continue antibiotic therapy for full length of treatment.

cefpodoxime

sef-poe-**docks**-em
(Vantin)

Do not confuse Vantin with Ventolin.

CLASSIFICATION

PHARMACOTHERAPEUTIC: Third-generation cephalosporin. **CLINICAL:** Antibiotic (see p. 21C).

ACTION

Binds to bacterial cell membranes, inhibits cell wall synthesis. **Therapeutic Effect:** Bactericidal.

PHARMACOKINETICS

Well absorbed from GI tract (food increases absorption). Protein binding: 21%–40%. Widely distributed. Primarily excreted unchanged in urine. Partially removed by hemodialysis. **Half-life:** 2.3 hrs (increased in renal impairment and elderly pts).

USES

Treatment of susceptible infections due to *S. pneumoniae, S pyogenes, S. aureus, H. influenzae, M. catarrhalis, E. coli, Proteus, Klebsiella* including acute maxillary sinusitis, chronic bronchitis, community-acquired pneumonia, gonorrhea, otitis media, pharyngitis, tonsillitis, skin/skin structure, UTIs.

PRECAUTIONS

CONTRAINDICATIONS: History of anaphylactic reaction to penicillins, hypersensitivity to cephalosporins. **CAUTIONS:** Renal impairment, history of allergies or GI disease (esp. ulcerative colitis, antibiotic-associated colitis), concurrent use of nephrotoxic medications.

LIFESPAN CONSIDERATIONS:

Pregnancy/Lactation: Readily crosses placenta. Distributed in breast milk. **Pregnancy Category B. Children:** Safety and efficacy not established in those younger than 6 mos. **Elderly:** Age-related renal impairment may require dosage adjustment.

INTERACTIONS

DRUG: **Antacids containing aluminum, magnesium, H_2 antagonists** may decrease absorption. **Aminoglycosides, furosemide** may increase risk of nephrotoxicity. **Probenecid** may increase concentration. **HERBAL:** None significant. **FOOD:** None known. **LAB VALUES:** May increase BUN, serum alkaline phosphatase, bilirubin, creatinine, LDH, AST, ALT. May cause positive direct/indirect Coombs' test.

AVAILABILITY (Rx)

ORAL SUSPENSION: 50 mg/5 ml, 100 mg/5 ml. **TABLETS:** 100 mg, 200 mg.

ADMINISTRATION/HANDLING

PO

• Administer with food (enhances absorption). • After reconstitution, oral suspension is stable for 14 days if refrigerated.

INDICATIONS/ROUTES/DOSAGE

CHRONIC BRONCHITIS, PNEUMONIA

PO: ADULTS, ELDERLY, CHILDREN OLDER THAN 13 YRS: 200 mg q12h for 10–14 days.

GONORRHEA, RECTAL GONOCOCCAL INFECTION (FEMALE PTS ONLY)

PO: ADULTS, CHILDREN OLDER THAN 13 YRS: 200 mg as a single dose.

SKIN/SKIN STRUCTURE INFECTIONS

PO: ADULTS, ELDERLY, CHILDREN OLDER THAN 13 YRS: 400 mg q12h for 7–14 days.

PHARYNGITIS, TONSILLITIS

PO: ADULTS, ELDERLY, CHILDREN OLDER THAN 13 YRS: 100 mg q12h for 5–10 days. **CHILDREN 6 MOS–13 YRS:** 5 mg/kg q12h for 5–10 days. **Maximum:** 100 mg/dose.

ACUTE MAXILLARY SINUSITIS

PO: ADULTS, CHILDREN OLDER THAN 13 YRS: 200 mg twice a day for 10 days. **CHILDREN 2 MOS–13 YRS:** 5 mg/kg q12h for 10 days. **Maximum:** 200 mg/dose.

UTIs

PO: ADULTS, ELDERLY, CHILDREN OLDER THAN 13 YRS: 100 mg q12h for 7 days.

ACUTE OTITIS MEDIA

PO: CHILDREN 6 MOS–13 YRS: 5 mg/kg q12h for 5 days. **Maximum:** 400 mg/dose.

DOSAGE IN RENAL IMPAIRMENT

For pts with creatinine clearance less than 30 ml/min, usual dose is given q24h. For pts on hemodialysis, usual dose is given 3 times/wk after dialysis.

SIDE EFFECTS

FREQUENT: Oral candidiasis, mild diarrhea, mild abdominal cramping, vaginal candidiasis. **OCCASIONAL:** Nausea, serum sickness-like reaction (fever, joint pain; usually occurs after second course of therapy and resolves after drug is discontinued). **RARE:** Allergic reaction (pruritus, rash, urticaria).

ADVERSE EFFECTS/ TOXIC REACTIONS

Antibiotic-associated colitis (severe abdominal pain, tenderness, fever, severe watery diarrhea), other superinfections may result from altered bacterial balance. Nephrotoxicity may occur, esp.

in pts with preexisting renal disease. Pts with a history of allergies, esp. to penicillin, are at increased risk for developing a severe hypersensitivity reaction (severe pruritus, angioedema, bronchospasm anaphylaxis).

NURSING CONSIDERATIONS

BASELINE ASSESSMENT

Question for history of allergies, particularly cephalosporins, penicillins.

INTERVENTION/EVALUATION

Assess oral cavity for white patches on mucous membranes, tongue (thrush). Monitor daily pattern of bowel activity/stool consistency carefully; mild GI effects may be tolerable, (increasing severity may indicate onset of antibiotic-associated colitis). Monitor I&O, renal function tests for nephrotoxicity. Be alert for superinfection (severe genital/anal pruritus, abdominal pain, severe mouth soreness, moderate to severe diarrhea).

PATIENT/FAMILY TEACHING

• Doses should be evenly spaced. • Shake oral suspension well before using. • Continue antibiotic therapy for full length of treatment. • Take with food. • Refrigerate oral suspension.

cefprozil

sef-**proz**-ill

(Cefzil)

Do not confuse cefprozil with Cefazolin or Cefzil with Cefol, Ceftin, or Kefzol.

CLASSIFICATION

PHARMACOTHERAPEUTIC: Second-generation cephalosporin. **CLINICAL:** Antibiotic (see p. 21C).

ACTION

Binds to bacterial cell membranes, inhibits cell wall synthesis. **Therapeutic Effect:** Bactericidal.

PHARMACOKINETICS

Well absorbed from GI tract. Protein binding: 36%–45%. Widely distributed. Primarily excreted unchanged in urine. Moderately removed by hemodialysis. **Half-life:** 1.3 hrs (increased in renal impairment).

USES

Treatment of susceptible infections due to *S. pneumoniae, S pyogenes, S. aureus, H. influenzae, M. catarrhalis* including pharyngitis, tonsillitis, otitis media, secondary bacterial infection of acute bronchitis, acute bacterial exacerbation of chronic bronchitis, uncomplicated skin/skin structure infections, acute sinusitis.

PRECAUTIONS

CONTRAINDICATIONS: History of anaphylactic reaction to penicillins, hypersensitivity to cephalosporins. **CAUTIONS:** Renal impairment, history of GI disease (esp. ulcerative colitis, antibiotic-associated colitis), concurrent use of nephrotoxic medications.

LIFESPAN CONSIDERATIONS:

Pregnancy/Lactation: Readily crosses placenta. Distributed in breast milk. **Pregnancy Category B. Children:** Safety and efficacy not established in those younger than 6 mos. **Elderly:** Age-related renal impairment may require dosage adjustment.

INTERACTIONS

DRUG: **Aminoglycosides, furosemide** may increase risk of nephrotoxicity. **Probenecid** may increase concentration. **HERBAL:** None significant. **FOOD:** None known. **LAB VALUES:** May cause positive direct/indirect Coombs' test; may interfere with blood crossmatching and hematologic tests. May increase hepatic enzyme levels, AST, ALT.

AVAILABILITY (Rx)

ORAL SUSPENSION: 125 mg/5 ml, 250 mg/5 ml. **TABLETS:** 250 mg, 500 mg.

ADMINISTRATION/HANDLING

PO

• After reconstitution, oral suspension is stable for 14 days if refrigerated. • Shake oral suspension well before using. • Give without regard to food; if GI upset occurs, give with food, milk.

INDICATIONS/ROUTES/DOSAGE

PHARYNGITIS, TONSILLITIS

PO: ADULTS, ELDERLY: 500 mg q24h for 10 days. **CHILDREN 2–12 YRS:** 7.5 mg/kg q12h for 10 days. **Maximum:** 1 g/day.

ACUTE BACTERIAL EXACERBATION OF CHRONIC BRONCHITIS, SECONDARY BACTERIAL INFECTION OF ACUTE BRONCHITIS

PO: ADULTS, ELDERLY: 500 mg q12h for 10 days.

SKIN/SKIN STRUCTURE INFECTIONS

PO: ADULTS, ELDERLY, CHILDREN OLDER THAN 12 YRS: 250–500 mg q12h for 10 days. **CHILDREN 2–12 YRS:** 20 mg/kg q24h for 10 days. **Maximum:** 1 g/day.

ACUTE SINUSITIS

PO: ADULTS, ELDERLY: 250–500 mg q12h for 10 days. **CHILDREN 6 MOS–12 YRS:** 7.5–15 mg/kg q12h for 10 days.

OTITIS MEDIA

PO: CHILDREN 6 MOS–12 YRS: 15 mg/kg q12h for 10 days. **Maximum:** 1 g/day.

DOSAGE IN RENAL IMPAIRMENT

Pts with creatinine clearance less than 30 ml/min receive 50% of usual dose at usual interval.

SIDE EFFECTS

FREQUENT: Oral candidiasis, mild diarrhea, mild abdominal cramping, vaginal candidiasis. **OCCASIONAL:** Nausea, serum sickness reaction (fever, joint pain; usually occurs after second course of therapy and resolves after drug is discontinued). **RARE:** Allergic reaction (pruritus, rash, urticaria).

ADVERSE EFFECTS/ TOXIC REACTIONS

Antibiotic-associated colitis (severe abdominal pain, tenderness, fever, severe watery diarrhea), other superinfections may result from altered bacterial balance. Nephrotoxicity may occur, esp. in pts with preexisting renal disease. Pts with a history of allergies, esp. to penicillin, are at increased risk for developing a severe hypersensitivity reaction (severe pruritus, angioedema, bronchospasm, anaphylaxis).

NURSING CONSIDERATIONS

BASELINE ASSESSMENT

Question for history of allergies, particularly cephalosporins, penicillins.

INTERVENTION/EVALUATION

Assess oral cavity for evidence of stomatitis. Monitor daily pattern of bowel activity/stool consistency carefully; mild GI effects may be tolerable, (but increasing severity may indicate onset of antibiotic-associated colitis). Monitor I&O, renal function tests for nephrotoxicity. Be alert for superinfection (severe genital/anal pruritus, abdominal pain, severe mouth soreness, moderate to severe diarrhea).

PATIENT/FAMILY TEACHING

• Doses should be evenly spaced. • Continue antibiotic therapy for full length of treatment. • May cause GI upset (may take with food or milk).

C

ceftazidime

sef-**taz**-ih-deem

(Ceptaz, Fortaz, Tazicef, Tazidime)

Do not confuse ceftazidime with ceftizoxime or Ceptaz with Septra.

CLASSIFICATION

PHARMACOTHERAPEUTIC: Third-generation cephalosporin. **CLINICAL:** Antibiotic (see p. 22C).

ACTION

Binds to bacterial cell membranes, inhibits cell wall synthesis. **Therapeutic Effect:** Bactericidal.

PHARMACOKINETICS

Widely distributed (including to cerebrospinal fluid [CSF]). Protein binding: 5%–17%. Primarily excreted unchanged in urine. Removed by hemodialysis. **Half-life:** 2 hrs (increased in renal impairment).

USES

Treatment of susceptible infections due to gram-negative organisms including *Pseudomonas* and *Enterobactereaceae* including bone, joint, CNS (including meningitis), gynecologic, intra-abdominal, lower respiratory tract, skin/skin structure, UTIs, septicemia.

PRECAUTIONS

CONTRAINDICATIONS: History of anaphylactic reaction to penicillins, hypersensitivity to cephalosporins. **CAUTIONS:** Renal impairment, history of GI disease (esp. ulcerative colitis, antibiotic-associated colitis), concurrent use of nephrotoxic medications.

LIFESPAN CONSIDERATIONS:

Pregnancy/Lactation: Readily crosses placenta. Distributed in breast milk. **Pregnancy Category B. Children:** No age-related precautions noted. **Elderly:** Age-related renal impairment may require dosage adjustment.

INTERACTIONS

DRUG: **Aminoglycosides, furosemide** may increase risk of nephrotoxicity. **HERBAL:** None significant. **FOOD:** None known. **LAB VALUES:** May increase BUN, serum alkaline phosphatase, creatinine, LDH, AST, ALT. May cause positive direct/indirect Coombs' test; may interfere with blood crossmatching and hematologic tests.

AVAILABILITY (Rx)

INJECTION, POWDER FOR RECONSTITUTION (FORTAZ, TAZICEF, TAZIDIME): 500 mg, 1 g, 2 g.

ADMINISTRATION/HANDLING

◀ **ALERT** ▶ Give by IM injection, direct IV injection (IV push), or intermittent IV infusion (piggyback).

IV

Reconstitution • Add 10 ml Sterile Water for Injection to each 1 g to provide concentration of 90 mg/ml. • May further dilute with 50–100 ml 0.9% NaCl, D_5W or other compatible diluent.

Rate of administration • For IV push, administer over 3–5 min. • For intermittent IV infusion (piggyback), infuse over 15–30 min.

Storage • Solution appears light yellow to amber, tends to darken (color change does not indicate loss of potency). • IV infusion (piggyback) stable for 18 hrs at room temperature, 7 days if refrigerated. • Discard if precipitate forms.

IM

• For reconstitution, add 1.5 ml Sterile Water for Injection or lidocaine 1% to 500 mg or 3 ml to 1-g vial to provide a concentration of 280 mg/ml.

• To minimize discomfort, inject deep IM slowly. Less painful if injected into gluteus maximus than lateral aspect of thigh.

IV INCOMPATIBILITIES

Amphotericin B complex (Abelcet, AmBisome, Amphotec), doxorubicin liposomal (Doxil), fluconazole (Diflucan), idarubicin (Idamycin), midazolam (Versed), pentamidine (Pentam IV), vancomycin (Vancocin), total parenteral nutrition (TPN).

IV COMPATIBILITIES

Diltiazem (Cardizem), famotidine (Pepcid), heparin, hydromorphone (Dilaudid), lipids, morphine, propofol (Diprivan).

INDICATIONS/ROUTES/DOSAGE

UTIs

IV, IM: ADULTS: 250–500 mg q8–12h.

MILD TO MODERATE INFECTIONS

IV, IM: ADULTS: 1 g q8–12h.

UNCOMPLICATED PNEUMONIA, SKIN/SKIN STRUCTURE INFECTIONS

IV, IM: ADULTS: 0.5–1 g q8h.

BONE, JOINT INFECTIONS

IV, IM: ADULTS: 2 g q12h.

MENINGITIS, SERIOUS GYNECOLOGIC AND INTRA-ABDOMINAL INFECTIONS

IV, IM: ADULTS: 2 g q8h.

PSEUDOMONAL PULMONARY INFECTIONS IN PTS WITH CYSTIC FIBROSIS

IV: ADULTS: 30–50 mg/kg q8h. **Maximum:** 6 g/day.

USUAL ELDERLY DOSAGE

ELDERLY (NORMAL RENAL FUNCTION): 500 mg–1 g q12h.

USUAL PEDIATRIC DOSAGE

CHILDREN 1 MO–12 YRS: 100–150 mg/kg/day in divided doses q8h. **Maximum:** 6 g/day. **NEONATES 0–4 WKS:** 100–150 mg/kg/day in divided doses q8–12h.

DOSAGE IN RENAL IMPAIRMENT

After an initial 1-g dose, dosage and frequency are modified based on creatinine clearance and severity of infection.

Creatinine Clearance	Dosage Interval
31–50 ml/min	q12h
10–30 ml/min	q24h
Less than 10 ml/min	q48–72h

SIDE EFFECTS

FREQUENT: Discomfort with IM administration, oral candidiasis, mild diarrhea, mild abdominal cramping, vaginal candidiasis. **OCCASIONAL:** Nausea, serum sickness-like reaction (fever, joint pain; usually occurs after second course of therapy and resolves after drug is discontinued). **RARE:** Allergic reaction (pruritus, rash, urticaria), thrombophlebitis (pain, redness, swelling at injection site).

ADVERSE EFFECTS/TOXIC REACTIONS

Antibiotic-associated colitis (severe abdominal pain, tenderness, fever, severe watery diarrhea), other superinfections may result from altered bacterial balance. Nephrotoxicity may occur, esp. in pts with preexisting renal disease. Pts with a history of allergies, esp. to penicillin, are at increased risk for developing a severe hypersensitivity reaction (severe pruritus, angioedema, bronchospasm, anaphylaxis).

NURSING CONSIDERATIONS

BASELINE ASSESSMENT

Question for history of allergies, particularly cephalosporins, penicillins.

INTERVENTION/EVALUATION

Evaluate IV site for phlebitis (heat, pain, red streaking over vein). Assess IM injection sites for induration, tenderness. Check oral cavity for white patches on mucous membranes, tongue (thrush). Monitor daily pattern of bowel activity/stool consistency carefully; mild GI effects may be tolerable (increasing severity may indicate onset of antibiotic-associated colitis). Monitor I&O, renal function tests for nephrotoxicity. Be alert for superinfection (severe genital/anal pruritus, abdominal pain, severe mouth soreness, moderate to severe diarrhea).

PATIENT/FAMILY TEACHING

• Discomfort may occur with IM injection. • Doses should be evenly spaced. • Continue antibiotic therapy for full length of treatment.

ceftibuten

sef-tih-**byew**-ten
(Cedax)

CLASSIFICATION

PHARMACOTHERAPEUTIC: Third-generation cephalosporin. **CLINICAL:** Antibiotic (see p. 23C).

ACTION

Binds to bacterial cell membranes, inhibits cell wall synthesis. **Therapeutic Effect:** Bactericidal.

PHARMACOKINETICS

Rapidly absorbed from GI tract. Protein binding: 65%–77%. Excreted primarily in urine. **Half-life:** 2–3 hrs.

USES

Treatment of susceptible infections due to *S. pneumoniae, S pyogenes, H. influenzae, M. catarrhalis* including chronic bronchitis, acute bacterial otitis media, pharyngitis, tonsillitis.

PRECAUTIONS

CONTRAINDICATIONS: History of anaphylactic reaction to penicillins, hypersensitivity to cephalosporins. **CAUTIONS:** Hypersensitivity to penicillins, other drugs, history of GI disease (e.g., colitis), renal impairment.

LIFESPAN CONSIDERATIONS:

Pregnancy/Lactation: Unknown if drug crosses placenta or is distributed in breast milk. **Pregnancy Category B.** **Children:** Safety and efficacy not established in children younger than 6 mos. **Elderly:** Age-related renal impairment may require dosage adjustment.

INTERACTIONS

DRUG: **Aminoglycosides** may increase risk of nephrotoxicity. **Probenecid** may increase concentration. **HERBAL:** None significant. **FOOD:** None known. **LAB VALUES:** May increase BUN, serum alkaline phosphatase, bilirubin, creatinine, LDH, AST, ALT. May cause positive direct/indirect Coombs' test.

AVAILABILITY (Rx)

CAPSULES: 400 mg. **ORAL SUSPENSION:** 90 mg/5 ml.

INDICATIONS/ROUTES/DOSAGE

CHRONIC BRONCHITIS

PO: ADULTS, ELDERLY: 400 mg/day once a day for 10 days.

PHARYNGITIS, TONSILLITIS

PO: ADULTS, ELDERLY: 400 mg once a day for 10 days. **CHILDREN OLDER THAN 6 MOS:** 9 mg/kg once a day for 10 days. **Maximum:** 400 mg/day.

OTITIS MEDIA

PO: CHILDREN OLDER THAN 6 MOS: 9 mg/kg once a day for 10 days. **Maximum:** 400 mg/day.

DOSAGE IN RENAL IMPAIRMENT

Dosage is modified based on creatinine clearance.

Creatinine Clearance	Dosage
50 ml/min and higher	400 mg or 9 mg/kg q24h
30–49 ml/min	200 mg or 4.5 mg/kg q24h
Less than 30 ml/min	100 mg or 2.25 mg/kg q24h

SIDE EFFECTS

FREQUENT: Oral candidiasis, mild diarrhea (discharge, itching). **OCCASIONAL:** Nausea, serum sickness-like reaction (fever, joint pain; usually occurs after second course of therapy and resolves after drug is discontinued). **RARE:** Allergic reaction (rash, pruritus, urticaria).

ADVERSE EFFECTS/ TOXIC REACTIONS

Antibiotic-associated colitis (severe abdominal pain, tenderness, fever, severe watery diarrhea), other superinfections may result from altered bacterial balance. Nephrotoxicity may occur, esp. in pts with preexisting renal disease. Pts with a history of allergies, esp. to penicillin, are at increased risk for developing a severe hypersensitivity reaction (severe pruritus, angioedema, bronchospasm, anaphylaxis).

NURSING CONSIDERATIONS

BASELINE ASSESSMENT

Question for history of allergies, particularly cephalosporins, penicillins.

INTERVENTION/EVALUATION

Assess oral cavity for white patches on mucous membranes, tongue (thrush). Monitor daily pattern of bowel activity/stool consistency carefully; mild GI effects may be tolerable (increasing severity may indicate onset of antibiotic-associated colitis). Monitor I&O, serum renal function tests for nephrotoxicity. Be alert for superinfection (severe genital/anal pruritus, abdominal pain, severe mouth soreness, moderate to severe diarrhea).

PATIENT/FAMILY TEACHING

• Continue medication for full length of treatment; do not skip doses. • Doses should be evenly spaced. • May cause GI upset (may take with food or milk).

Ceftin, *see cefuroxime*

ceftizoxime

sef-ti-**zox**-eem

(Cefizox)

Do not confuse ceftizoxime with cefotaxime or ceftazidime.

CLASSIFICATION

PHARMACOTHERAPEUTIC: Third-generation cephalosporin. **CLINICAL:** Antibiotic (see p. 23C).

ACTION

Binds to bacterial cell membranes, inhibits cell wall synthesis. **Therapeutic Effect:** Bactericidal.

PHARMACOKINETICS

Widely distributed (including to cerebrospinal fluid [CSF]). Protein binding: 30%. Primarily excreted unchanged in urine. Moderately removed by hemodialysis. **Half-life:** 1.7 hrs (increased in renal impairment).

USES

Treatment of intra-abdominal, biliary tract, respiratory tract, GU tract, skin, bone infections; gonorrhea; meningitis; septicemia; pelvic inflammatory disease (PID).

PRECAUTIONS

CONTRAINDICATIONS: History of anaphylactic reaction to penicillins, hypersensitivity to cephalosporins. **CAUTIONS:** History of GI disease (esp. ulcerative colitis, antibiotic-associated colitis), hepatic/renal impairment.

LIFESPAN CONSIDERATIONS:

Pregnancy/Lactation: Readily crosses placenta. Distributed in breast milk.

C

Pregnancy Category B. Children: Associated with transient elevations of eosinophils, serum AST, ALT, creatine kinase. **Elderly:** Age-related renal impairment may require dosage adjustment.

INTERACTIONS

DRUG: Aminoglycosides, furosemide may increase risk of nephrotoxicity. **Probenecid** may increase concentration. **HERBAL:** None significant. **FOOD:** None known. **LAB VALUES:** May increase BUN, serum alkaline phosphatase, bilirubin, creatinine, LDH, AST, ALT. May cause positive direct/indirect Coombs' test.

AVAILABILITY (Rx)

INJECTION, POWDER FOR RECONSTITUTION: 500 mg, 1 g, 2 g. **INTRAVENOUS SOLUTION:** 1 g/50 ml, 2 g/50 ml.

ADMINISTRATION/HANDLING

IV

Reconstitution • Add 5 ml Sterile Water for Injection to each 0.5 g to provide concentration of 95 mg/ml. • May further dilute with 50–100 ml 0.9% NaCl, D_5W, or other compatible fluid.

Rate of administration • For IV push, administer over 3–5 min. • For intermittent IV infusion (piggyback), infuse over 15–30 min.

Storage • Solution appears clear to pale yellow. Color change from yellow to amber does not indicate loss of potency. • IV infusion (piggyback) is stable for 24 hrs at room temperature, 96 hrs if refrigerated. • Discard if precipitate forms.

IM

• Add 1.5 ml Sterile Water for Injection to each 0.5 g to provide concentration of 270 mg/ml. • Inject deep IM slowly to minimize discomfort. • When giving 2-g dose, divide dose and give in different large muscle masses.

IV INCOMPATIBILITY

Filgrastim (Neupogen).

IV COMPATIBILITIES

Hydromorphone (Dilaudid), lipids, morphine, propofol (Diprivan).

INDICATIONS/ROUTES/DOSAGE

UNCOMPLICATED UTIs

IV, IM: ADULTS, ELDERLY: 500 mg q12h.

MILD, MODERATE, OR SEVERE INFECTIONS

IV, IM: ADULTS, ELDERLY: 1–2 g q8–12h.

LIFE-THREATENING INFECTIONS

IV: ADULTS, ELDERLY: 3–4 g q8h, up to 2 g q4h.

PID

IV: ADULTS: 2 g q4–8h.

UNCOMPLICATED GONORRHEA

IM: ADULTS: 1 g one time.

USUAL PEDIATRIC DOSAGE

IV, IM: CHILDREN: OLDER THAN 6 MOS: 50 mg/kg q6–8h. **Maximum:** 12 g/day.

DOSAGE IN RENAL IMPAIRMENT

After a loading dose of 0.5–1 g, dosage and frequency are modified based creatinine clearance and severity of infection.

Creatinine Clearance	Dosage
50–79 ml/min	0.5 g–1.5 g q8h
5–49 ml/min	0.25 g–1 g q12h
Less than 5 ml/min	0.25–0.5 g q24h or 0.5 g–1 g q48h

SIDE EFFECTS

FREQUENT: Discomfort with IM administration, oral candidiasis, mild diarrhea, mild abdominal cramping, vaginal candidiasis. **OCCASIONAL:** Nausea, serum sickness-like reaction (fever, joint pain; usually occurs after second course of therapy and resolves after drug is discontinued). **RARE:** Allergic reaction (rash, pruritus, urticaria), thrombophlebitis (pain, redness, swelling at injection site).

C

ADVERSE EFFECTS/ TOXIC REACTIONS

Antibiotic-associated colitis (severe abdominal pain, tenderness, fever, severe watery diarrhea), other superinfections may result from altered bacterial balance. Nephrotoxicity may occur, esp. in pts with preexisting renal disease. Pts with a history of allergies, esp. to penicillin, are at increased risk for developing a severe hypersensitivity reaction (severe pruritus, angioedema, bronchospasm, anaphylaxis).

NURSING CONSIDERATIONS

BASELINE ASSESSMENT

Question for history of allergies, particularly cephalosporins, penicillins.

INTERVENTION/EVALUATION

Assess oral cavity for white patches on mucous membranes, tongue (thrush). Monitor daily pattern of bowel activity/ stool consistency carefully; mild GI effects may be tolerable, but increasing severity may indicate onset of antibiotic-associated colitis. Monitor I&O, renal function reports for nephrotoxicity. Be alert for superinfection: severe genital or anal pruritus, abdominal pain, severe mouth soreness, moderate to severe diarrhea.

PATIENT/FAMILY TEACHING

• Doses should be evenly spaced. • Continue therapy for full length of treatment. • Discomfort may occur with IM injection.

ceftriaxone

sef-try-**ax**-zone

(Rocephin, Rocephin IM Convenience Kit)

CLASSIFICATION

PHARMACOTHERAPEUTIC: Third-generation cephalosporin. **CLINICAL:** Antibiotic (see p. 23C).

ACTION

Binds to bacterial cell membranes, inhibits cell wall synthesis. **Therapeutic Effect:** Bactericidal.

PHARMACOKINETICS

Widely distributed (including to cerebrospinal fluid [CSF]). Protein binding: 83%–96%. Primarily excreted unchanged in urine. Not removed by hemodialysis. **Half-life:** 4.3–4.6 hrs IV; 5.8–8.7 hrs IM (increased in renal impairment).

USES

Treatment of susceptible infections due to gram-negative aerobic organisms, some gram-positive organisms including respiratory tract, GU tract, skin, bone, intra-abdominal, biliary tract infections; septicemia; meningitis; gonorrhea; Lyme disease; acute bacterial otitis media.

PRECAUTIONS

CONTRAINDICATIONS: History of anaphylactic reaction to penicillins, hypersensitivity to cephalosporins. **CAUTIONS:** Renal/hepatic impairment, history of GI disease (esp. ulcerative colitis, antibiotic-associated colitis), concurrent administration of nephrotoxic medications.

LIFESPAN CONSIDERATIONS:

Pregnancy/Lactation: Readily crosses placenta. Distributed in breast milk. **Pregnancy Category B. Children:** May displace bilirubin from serum albumin. Caution in hyperbilirubinemic neonates. **Elderly:** Age-related renal impairment may require dosage adjustment.

C

INTERACTIONS

DRUG: Probenecid may increase excretion. **HERBAL:** None significant. **FOOD:** None known. **LAB VALUES:** May increase BUN, serum alkaline phosphatase, bilirubin, creatinine, LDH, AST, ALT. May cause positive direct/indirect Coombs' test; may interfere with blood crossmatching and hematologic tests.

AVAILABILITY (Rx)

INJECTION, POWDER FOR RECONSTITUTION (ROCEPHIN): 250 mg, 500 mg, 1 g, 2 g. **INTRAVENOUS SOLUTION (ROCEPHIN):** 1 g/50 ml, 2 g/50 ml. **KIT (INTRAMUSCULAR [ROCEPHIN IM CONVENIENCE KIT]):** 500 mg, 1 g.

ADMINISTRATION/HANDLING

IV

Reconstitution • Add 2.4 ml Sterile Water for Injection to each 250 mg to provide concentration of 100 mg/ml. • May further dilute with 50–100 ml 0.9% NaCl, D_5W.

Rate of administration • For intermittent IV infusion (piggyback), infuse over 15–30 min for adults, 10–30 min in children, neonates. • Alternating IV sites, use large veins to reduce potential for phlebitis.

Storage • Solution appears light yellow to amber. • IV infusion (piggyback) is stable for 3 days at room temperature, 10 days if refrigerated. • Discard if precipitate forms.

IM

• Add 0.9 ml Sterile Water for Injection, 0.9% NaCl, D_5W, or lidocaine to each 250 mg to provide concentration of 250 mg/ml. (ml/min) • To minimize discomfort, inject deep IM slowly. Less painful if injected into gluteus maximus than lateral aspect of thigh.

IV INCOMPATIBILITIES

Aminophylline, amphotericin B complex (Abelcet, AmBisome, Amphotec), filgrastim (Neupogen), fluconazole (Diflucan), labetalol (Normodyne), pentamidine (Pentam IV), vancomycin (Vancocin).

IV COMPATIBILITIES

Diltiazem (Cardizem), heparin, lidocaine, lipids, morphine, propofol (Diprivan), total parenteral nutrition (TPN).

INDICATIONS/ROUTES/DOSAGE

MILD TO MODERATE INFECTIONS

IV, IM: ADULTS, ELDERLY: 1–2 g as a single dose or in 2 divided doses. **CHILDREN:** 50–75 mg/kg/day in 1–2 divided doses q12–24h. **Maximum:** 2 g/day.

SERIOUS INFECTIONS

IV, IM: ADULTS, ELDERLY: Up to 4 g/day in 2 divided doses. **CHILDREN:** 80–100 mg/kg/day in divided doses q12h. **Maximum:** 4 g/day.

MENINGITIS

IV: CHILDREN: Initially, 75–100 mg/kg, then 100 mg/kg/day as a single dose or in divided doses q12h. **Maximum:** 4 g/day.

LYME DISEASE

IV: ADULTS, ELDERLY: 2–4 g a day for 10–14 days.

ACUTE BACTERIAL OTITIS MEDIA

IM: CHILDREN: 50 mg/kg once. **Maximum:** 1 g/day.

PERIOPERATIVE PROPHYLAXIS

IV, IM: ADULTS, ELDERLY: 1 g 0.5–2 hrs before surgery.

UNCOMPLICATED GONORRHEA

IM: ADULTS: 125–250 mg plus doxycycline one time.

DOSAGE IN RENAL IMPAIRMENT

Dosage modification is usually unnecessary but hepatic/renal function test results should be monitored in those with renal and liver impairment or severe renal impairment.

SIDE EFFECTS

FREQUENT: Discomfort with IM administration, oral candidiasis, mild diarrhea, mild abdominal cramping, vaginal candidiasis. **OCCASIONAL:** Nausea, serum sickness-like reaction (fever, joint pain; usually occurs after second course of therapy and resolves after drug is discontinued). **RARE:** Allergic reaction (rash, pruritus, urticaria), thrombophlebitis (pain, redness, swelling at injection site).

ADVERSE EFFECTS/ TOXIC REACTIONS

Antibiotic-associated colitis (severe abdominal pain, tenderness, fever, severe watery diarrhea), other superinfections may result from altered bacterial balance. Nephrotoxicity may occur, esp. in pts with preexisting renal disease. Pts with a history of allergies, esp. to penicillin, are at increased risk for developing a severe hypersensitivity reaction (severe pruritus, angioedema, bronchospasm, anaphylaxis).

NURSING CONSIDERATIONS

BASELINE ASSESSMENT

Question for history of allergies, particularly cephalosporins, penicillins.

INTERVENTION/EVALUATION

Assess oral cavity for white patches on mucous membranes, tongue (thrush). Monitor daily pattern of bowel activity/ stool consistency carefully; mild GI effects may be tolerable, (increasing severity may indicate onset of antibiotic-associated colitis). Monitor I&O, renal function tests for nephrotoxicity. Be alert for superinfection (severe genital/anal pruritus, abdominal pain, severe mouth soreness, moderate to severe diarrhea).

PATIENT/FAMILY TEACHING

• Discomfort may occur with IM injection. • Doses should be evenly spaced. • Continue antibiotic therapy for full length of treatment.

cefuroxime axetil

sef-yur-**ox**-ime

(Ceftin)

Do not confuse cefuroxime with cefotaxime or deferoxamine; Ceftin with Cefzil or Cipro; or Zinacef with Zithromax.

cefuroxime sodium

(Kefurox, Zinacef)

CLASSIFICATION

PHARMACOTHERAPEUTIC: Second-generation cephalosporin. **CLINICAL:** Antibiotic (see p. 22C).

ACTION

Binds to bacterial cell membranes, inhibits cell wall synthesis. **Therapeutic Effect:** Bactericidal.

PHARMACOKINETICS

Rapidly absorbed from GI tract. Protein binding: 33%–50%. Widely distributed (including to cerebrospinal fluid [CSF]). Primarily excreted unchanged in urine. Moderately removed by hemodialysis. **Half-life:** 1.3 hrs (increased in renal impairment).

USES

Treatment of susceptible infections due to group B *streptococci*, pneumococci, staphylococci, *H. influenzae, E. coli, Enterobacter, Klebsiella* including acute/chronic bronchitis, gonorrhea, impetigo, early Lyme disease, otitis media, pharyngitis/tonsillitis, sinusitis, skin/skin structure, UTIs.

PRECAUTIONS

CONTRAINDICATIONS: History of anaphylactic reaction to penicillins, hypersensitivity to cephalosporins. **CAUTIONS:** Renal impairment, history of GI disease (esp. ulcerative colitis, antibiotic-associated colitis), concurrent use of nephrotoxic medications.

LIFESPAN CONSIDERATIONS:

Pregnancy/Lactation: Readily crosses placenta. Distributed in breast milk. **Pregnancy Category B. Children:** No age-related precautions noted. **Elderly:** Age-related renal impairment may require dosage adjustment.

INTERACTIONS

DRUG: Aminoglycosides, furosemide may increase risk of nephrotoxicity. **Probenecid** may increase concentration. **HERBAL:** None significant. **FOOD:** None known. **LAB VALUES:** May increase serum alkaline phosphatase, bilirubin, LDH, AST, ALT. May cause positive direct/indirect Coombs' test; may interfere with blood crossmatching and hematologic tests.

AVAILABILITY (Rx)

INJECTION, POWDER FOR RECONSTITUTION: 750 mg, 1.5 g. **INJECTION, SOLUTION:** 750 mg/50 ml, 1.5 g/50 ml. **ORAL SUSPENSION (CEFTIN):** 125 mg/5 ml, 250 mg/5 ml. **TABLETS (CEFTIN):** 125 mg, 250 mg, 500 mg.

ADMINISTRATION/HANDLING

IV

Reconstitution • Reconstitute 750 mg in 8 ml (1.5 g in 14 ml) Sterile Water for Injection to provide a concentration of 100 mg/ml. • For intermittent IV infusion (piggyback), further dilute with 50–100 ml 0.9% NaCl or D_5W.

Rate of administration • For IV push, administer over 3–5 min. • For intermittent IV infusion (piggyback), infuse over 15–60 min.

Storage • Solution appears light yellow to amber (may darken, but color change does not indicate loss of potency). • IV infusion (piggyback) is stable for 24 hrs at room temperature, 7 days if refrigerated. • Discard if precipitate forms.

IM

• To minimize discomfort, inject deep IM slowly. Less painful if injected into gluteus maximus than lateral aspect of thigh.

PO

• Give tablets without regard to food. If GI upset occurs, give with food, milk. • Avoid crushing tablets due to bitter taste. • Suspension must be given with food.

IV INCOMPATIBILITIES

Filgrastim (Neupogen), fluconazole (Diflucan), midazolam (Versed), vancomycin (Vancocin).

IV COMPATIBILITIES

Diltiazem (Cardizem), hydromorphone (Dilaudid), lipids, morphine, propofol (Diprivan), total parenteral nutrition (TPN).

INDICATIONS/ROUTES/DOSAGE

USUAL DOSAGE

IV, IM: ADULTS, ELDERLY: 750 mg–1.5 g q8h. **CHILDREN:** 75–150 mg/kg/day divided q8h. **Maximum:** 6 g/day. **NEONATES:** 50–100 mg/kg/day divided q12h.

PO: ADULTS, ELDERLY: 250–500 mg twice a day, depending on the infection.

PHARYNGITIS, TONSILLITIS

PO: CHILDREN 3 MOS–12 YRS: 125 mg (tablets) q12h or 20 mg/kg/day (suspension) in 2 divided doses for 10 days.

ACUTE OTITIS MEDIA, ACUTE BACTERIAL MAXILLARY SINUSITIS, IMPETIGO

PO: CHILDREN 3 MOS–12 YRS: 250 mg (tablets) q12h or 30 mg/kg/day (suspension) in 2 divided doses for 10 days.

BACTERIAL MENINGITIS

IV: CHILDREN 3 MOS–12 YRS: 200–240 mg/kg/day in divided doses q6–8h.

GONORRHEA

PO: ADULTS, ELDERLY: 1 g as single dose.

URINARY TRACT INFECTION

PO: ADULTS, ELDERLY: 125–250 mg q12h for 7–10 days.

PERIOPERATIVE PROPHYLAXIS

IV: ADULTS, ELDERLY: 1.5 g 30–60 min before surgery and 750 mg q8h after surgery.

USUAL NEONATAL DOSAGE

IV, IM: NEONATES: 20–100 mg/kg/day in divided doses q12h.

DOSAGE IN RENAL IMPAIRMENT

Adult dosage and frequency are modified based on creatinine clearance and severity of infection.

Creatinine Clearance	Dosage Interval
Greater than 20 ml/min	q8h
10–20 ml/min	q12h
Less than 10 ml/min	q24h

SIDE EFFECTS

FREQUENT: Discomfort with IM administration, oral candidiasis, mild diarrhea, mild abdominal cramping, vaginal candidiasis. **OCCASIONAL:** Nausea, serum sickness-like reaction (fever, joint pain; usually occurs after second course of therapy and resolves after drug is discontinued). **RARE:** Allergic reaction (rash, pruritus, urticaria), thrombophlebitis (pain, redness, swelling at injection site).

ADVERSE EFFECTS/ TOXIC REACTIONS

Antibiotic-associated colitis (severe abdominal pain, tenderness, fever, severe watery diarrhea), other superinfections may result from altered bacterial balance. Nephrotoxicity may occur, esp. in pts with preexisting renal disease. Pts with a history of allergies, esp. to penicillin, are at increased risk for developing a severe hypersensitivity reaction (severe pruritus, angioedema, bronchospasm anaphylaxis).

NURSING CONSIDERATIONS

BASELINE ASSESSMENT

Question for history of allergies, particularly cephalosporins, penicillins.

INTERVENTION/EVALUATION

Assess oral cavity for white patches on mucous membranes, tongue (thrush). Monitor daily pattern of bowel activity/stool consistency carefully; mild GI effects may be tolerable, (increasing severity may indicate onset of antibiotic-associated colitis). Monitor I&O, renal function tests for nephrotoxicity. Be alert for superinfection (severe genital/anal pruritus, abdominal pain, severe mouth soreness, moderate to severe diarrhea).

PATIENT/FAMILY TEACHING

• Discomfort may occur with IM injection. • Doses should be evenly spaced. • Continue antibiotic therapy for full length of treatment. • May cause GI upset (may take with food, milk).

Cefzil, *see cefprozil*

Celebrex, *see celecoxib*

celecoxib

sell-eh-**cox**-ib

(Celebrex)

Do not confuse Celebrex with Cerebyx or Celexa.

CLASSIFICATION

PHARMACOTHERAPEUTIC: Nonsteroidal anti-inflammatory. **CLINICAL:** Anti-inflammatory (see p. 123C).

C

ACTION

Inhibits cyclo-oxygenase-2, the enzyme responsible for prostaglandin synthesis. **Therapeutic Effect:** Reduces inflammation, relieves pain.

PHARMACOKINETICS

Widely distributed. Protein binding: 97%. Metabolized in the liver. Primarily eliminated in feces. **Half-life:** 11.2 hrs.

USES

Relief of signs/symptoms of osteoarthritis, rheumatoid arthritis in adults. Treatment of acute pain, menstrual pain. Used to reduce number of adenomatous colorectal polyps in familial adenomatous polyposis (FAP). Relief of signs/symptoms associated with ankylosing spondylitis.

PRECAUTIONS

◀ **ALERT** ▶ May increase cardiovascular risk when high doses given to prevent colon cancer.

CONTRAINDICATIONS: Hypersensitivity to aspirin, NSAIDs, sulfonamides. **CAUTIONS:** History of peptic ulcer, older than 60 yrs, those receiving anticoagulant therapy, steroids, alcohol consumption, smoking.

LIFESPAN CONSIDERATIONS:

Pregnancy/Lactation: Unknown if drug crosses placenta or is distributed in breast milk. Avoid use during third trimester (may adversely affect fetal cardiovascular system: premature closure of ductus arteriosus). **Pregnancy Category C (D if used in third trimester or near delivery).** **Children:** Safety and efficacy not established in those younger than 18 yrs. **Elderly:** No age-related precautions noted.

INTERACTIONS

DRUG: Fluconazole may significantly increase concentration. May significantly increase **lithium** concentration. **Warfarin** may increase risk of bleeding. **HERBAL:** None significant. **FOOD:** None known. **LAB VALUES:** May increase serum AST, ALT.

AVAILABILITY (Rx)

CAPSULES: 100 mg, 200 mg, 400 mg.

ADMINISTRATION/HANDLING

PO

• Give without regard to food. • Do not break capsules.

INDICATIONS/ROUTES/DOSAGE

◀ **ALERT** ▶ Decrease dose by 50% in pts with moderate hepatic impairment.

OSTEOARTHRITIS

PO: ADULTS, ELDERLY: 200 mg/day as a single dose or 100 mg twice a day.

RHEUMATOID ARTHRITIS

PO: ADULTS, ELDERLY: 100–200 mg twice a day.

ACUTE PAIN

PO: ADULTS, ELDERLY: Initially, 400 mg with additional 200 mg on day 1, if needed. Maintenance: 200 mg twice a day as needed.

FAMILIAL ADENOMATOUS POLYPOSIS

PO: ADULTS, ELDERLY: 400 mg twice a day (with food).

PRIMARY DYSMENORRHEA

PO: ADULTS: 200 mg twice a day as needed (with food).

ANKYLOSING SPONDYLITIS

PO: ADULTS, ELDERLY: 200 mg/day as a single dose or in 2 divided doses. May increase to 400 mg/day if no effect is seen after 6 wks.

SIDE EFFECTS

FREQUENT (greater than 5%): Diarrhea, dyspepsia, headache, upper respiratory tract infection. **OCCASIONAL (5%–1%):** Abdominal pain, flatulence, nausea, back pain, peripheral edema, dizziness, rash.

ADVERSE EFFECTS/ TOXIC REACTIONS

Increased risk of cardiovascular events, (MI, cerebrovascular accident), serious, potentially life-threatening, GI bleeding.

NURSING CONSIDERATIONS

BASELINE ASSESSMENT

Assess onset, type, location, duration of pain/inflammation. Inspect appearance of affected joints for immobility, deformity, skin condition.

INTERVENTION/EVALUATION

Evaluate for therapeutic response: pain relief, decreased stiffness, swelling, increased joint mobility, decreased tenderness, improved grip strength.

PATIENT/FAMILY TEACHING

- If GI upset occurs, take with food.
- Avoid aspirin, alcohol (increases risk of GI bleeding).

Celexa, *see citalopram*

CellCept, *see mycophenolate*

Cenestin, *see conjugated estrogens*

cephalexin

cef-ah-**lex**-in

(Apo-Cephalex ✤, Biocef, Keflex, Keftab, Novolexin ✤, Panixine DisperDose)

CLASSIFICATION

PHARMACOTHERAPEUTIC: First-generation cephalosporin. **CLINICAL:** Antibiotic (see p. 21C).

ACTION

Binds to bacterial cell membranes, inhibits cell wall synthesis. **Therapeutic Effect:** Bactericidal.

PHARMACOKINETICS

Rapidly absorbed from GI tract. Protein binding: 10%–15%. Widely distributed. Primarily excreted unchanged in urine. Moderately removed by hemodialysis. **Half-life:** 0.9–1.2 hrs (increased in renal impairment).

USES

Treatment of susceptible infections due to Staphylococci, group A *Streptococcus, K. pneumoniae, E. coli, P. mirabilis, H. influenzae, M. catarrhalis* including respiratory tract, GU tract, skin, soft tissue, bone infections; otitis media; rheumatic fever prophylaxis; follow-up to parenteral therapy.

PRECAUTIONS

CONTRAINDICATIONS: History of anaphylactic reaction to penicillins, hypersensitivity to cephalosporins. **CAUTIONS:** Renal impairment, history of GI disease (esp. ulcerative colitis, antibiotic-associated colitis), concurrent use of nephrotoxic medications.

LIFESPAN CONSIDERATIONS:

Pregnancy/Lactation: Readily crosses placenta. Distributed in breast milk. **Pregnancy Category B. Children:** No age-related precautions noted. **Elderly:** Age-related renal impairment may require dosage adjustment.

INTERACTIONS

DRUG: Aminoglycosides, furosemide may increase risk of nephrotoxicity. **Probenecid** increases concentration.

C

HERBAL: None significant. **FOOD:** None known. **LAB VALUES:** May increase serum alkaline phosphatase, bilirubin, LDH, AST, ALT. May cause positive direct/indirect Coombs' test; may interfere with blood crossmatching and hematologic tests.

AVAILABILITY (Rx)

CAPSULES (BIOCEF, KEFLEX) 250 mg, 500 mg, 750 mg. **POWDER FOR ORAL SUSPENSION (BIOCEF, KEFLEX):** 125 mg/5 ml, 250 mg/5 ml. **TABLETS:** 250 mg, 500 mg. **TABLETS FOR ORAL SUSPENSION (PANIXINE):** 125 mg, 250 mg.

ADMINISTRATION/HANDLING

PO

• After reconstitution, oral suspension is stable for 14 days if refrigerated. • Shake oral suspension well before using. • Give without regard to food. If GI upset occurs, give with food, milk.

INDICATIONS/ROUTES/DOSAGE

USUAL DOSAGE RANGE

PO: ADULTS, ELDERLY: 250–1,000 mg q6h. **Maximum:** 4 g/day. **CHILDREN:** 25–100 mg/kg/day in 3–4 divided doses.

STREPTOCOCCAL PHARYNGITIS, SKIN/SKIN STRUCTURE INFECTIONS

PO: ADULTS, ELDERLY: 500 mg q12h. **CHILDREN:** 25–50 mg/kg/day in 2 divided doses.

UNCOMPLICATED CYSTITIS

PO: ADULTS, ELDERLY, CHILDREN OLDER THAN 15 YRS: 500 mg q12h for 7–14 days.

OTITIS MEDIA

PO: CHILDREN: 75–100 mg/kg/day in 4 divided doses.

DOSAGE IN RENAL IMPAIRMENT

After usual initial dose, dosing frequency is modified based on creatinine clearance and severity of infection.

Creatinine Clearance	Dosage Interval
10–40 ml/min	Usual dose q8–12h
Less than 10 ml/min	Usual dose q12–24h

SIDE EFFECTS

FREQUENT: Oral candidiasis, mild diarrhea, mild abdominal cramping, vaginal candidiasis. **OCCASIONAL:** Nausea, serum sickness-like reaction (fever, joint pain; usually occurs after second course of therapy and resolves after drug is discontinued). **RARE:** Allergic reaction (rash, pruritus, urticaria).

ADVERSE EFFECTS/TOXIC REACTIONS

Antibiotic-associated colitis (severe abdominal pain, tenderness, fever, severe watery diarrhea), other superinfections may result from altered bacterial balance. Nephrotoxicity may occur, esp. in pts with preexisting renal disease. Pts with a history of allergies, esp. to penicillin, are at increased risk for developing a severe hypersensitivity reaction (severe pruritus, angioedema, bronchospasm, anaphylaxis).

NURSING CONSIDERATIONS

BASELINE ASSESSMENT

Question for history of allergies, particularly cephalosporins, penicillins.

INTERVENTION/EVALUATION

Assess oral cavity for white patches on mucous membranes, tongue (thrush). Monitor daily pattern of bowel activity/stool consistency carefully; mild GI effects may be tolerable (increasing severity may indicate onset of antibiotic-associated colitis). Monitor I&O, renal function tests for nephrotoxicity. Be alert for superinfection (severe genital/anal pruritus, abdominal pain, severe mouth soreness, moderate to severe diarrhea).

PATIENT/FAMILY TEACHING

• Doses should be evenly spaced. • Continue therapy for full length of treatment. • May cause GI upset (may take with food, milk). • Refrigerate oral suspension.

Cerebyx, *see fosphenytoin*

Cervidil, *see dinoprostone*

cetirizine

sih-**tier**-eh-zeen

(Apo-Cetirizine ✤, Reactine ✤, Zyrtec)

Do not confuse Zyrtec with Zantac or Zyprexa.

FIXED-COMBINATION(S)

Zyrtec D 12 Hour Tablets: cetirizine/pseudoephedrine: 5 mg/120 mg.

CLASSIFICATION

PHARMACOTHERAPEUTIC: Second-generation piperazine. **CLINICAL:** Antihistamine (see p. 51C).

ACTION

Competes with histamine for H_1-receptor sites on effector cells in GI tract, blood vessels, respiratory tract. **Therapeutic Effect:** Prevents allergic response, produces mild bronchodilation, blocks histamine-induced bronchitis.

PHARMACOKINETICS

Route	Onset	Peak	Duration
PO	Less than 1 hr	4–8 hrs	Less than 24 hrs

Rapidly, almost completely absorbed from GI tract (absorption not affected by food). Protein binding: 93%. Undergoes low first-pass metabolism; not extensively metabolized. Primarily excreted in urine (more than 80% as unchanged drug). **Half-life:** 6.5–10 hrs.

USES

Relief of symptoms (sneezing, rhinorrhea, postnasal discharge, nasal pruritus, ocular pruritus, tearing) of seasonal and perennial allergic rhinitis (hay fever). Treatment of chronic urticaria (hives). **OFF-LABEL:** Treatment of bronchial asthma.

PRECAUTIONS

CONTRAINDICATIONS: Hypersensitivity to cetirizine, hydroxyzine. **CAUTIONS:** Hepatic/renal impairment. May cause drowsiness at dosage greater than 10 mg/day.

LIFESPAN CONSIDERATIONS:

Pregnancy/Lactation: Not recommended during early months of pregnancy. Unknown if excreted in breast milk. Breast-feeding not recommended. **Pregnancy Category B. Children:** Less likely to cause anticholinergic effects. **Elderly:** More sensitive to anticholinergic effects (e.g., dry mouth, urinary retention). Dizziness, sedation, confusion more likely to occur.

INTERACTIONS

DRUG: Alcohol, other CNS depressants may increase CNS depression. **Anticholinergics** may increase anticholinergic effects. **MAOIs** may prolong or increase anticholinergic, CNS depressant effects. **HERBAL:** None significant. **FOOD:** None known. **LAB VALUES:** May suppress wheal and flare reactions to antigen skin testing unless drug is discontinued 4 days before testing.

AVAILABILITY (Rx)

SYRUP: 5 mg/5 ml. **TABLETS:** 5 mg, 10 mg. **TABLETS (CHEWABLE):** 5 mg, 10 mg.

ADMINISTRATION/HANDLING

PO

- Give without regard to food.

C

INDICATIONS/ROUTES/DOSAGE

ALLERGIC RHINITIS, URTICARIA

PO: ADULTS, ELDERLY, CHILDREN OLDER THAN 5 YRS: Initially, 5–10 mg/day as a single or in 2 divided doses. **CHILDREN 2–5 YRS:** 2.5 mg/day. May increase up to 5 mg/day as a single or in 2 divided doses. **CHILDREN 12–23 MOS:** Initially, 2.5 mg/day. May increase up to 5 mg/day in 2 divided doses. **CHILDREN 6–11 MOS:** 2.5 mg once a day.

DOSAGE IN RENAL/HEPATIC IMPAIRMENT

For adult/elderly pts with renal impairment (creatinine clearance 11–31 ml/min), those receiving hemodialysis (creatinine clearance less than 7 ml/min), those with hepatic impairment, dosage is decreased to 5 mg once a day. **CHILDREN 6–11 YRS:** Less than 2.5 mg once daily.

SIDE EFFECTS

OCCASIONAL (10%–2%): Pharyngitis; dry mucous membranes, nose, throat; nausea/vomiting; abdominal pain; headache; dizziness; fatigue; thickening of mucus; somnolence; photosensitivity; urinary retention.

ADVERSE EFFECTS/ TOXIC REACTIONS

Children may experience paradoxical reaction (restlessness, insomnia, euphoria, nervousness, tremor). Dizziness, sedation, confusion more likely to occur in elderly.

NURSING CONSIDERATIONS

BASELINE ASSESSMENT

Assess lung sounds. Assess severity of rhinitis, urticaria, other symptoms. Obtain baseline hepatic function tests.

INTERVENTION/EVALUATION

For upper respiratory allergies, increase fluids to maintain thin secretions and offset thirst. Monitor symptoms for therapeutic response.

PATIENT/FAMILY TEACHING

• Avoid tasks that require alertness, motor skills until response to drug is established (may cause drowsiness). • Avoid alcohol during antihistamine therapy. • Avoid prolonged exposure to sunlight.

cetrorelix

(Cetrotide)

See Fertility agents (p. 99C)

cetuximab

ceh-**tux**-ih-mab
(Erbitux)

CLASSIFICATION

PHARMACOTHERAPEUTIC: Monoclonal antibody. **CLINICAL:** Antineoplastic.

ACTION

Binds to the epidermal growth factor receptor (EGFR), a glycoprotein on normal and tumor cells. **Therapeutic Effect:** Inhibits tumor cell growth, inducing apoptosis.

PHARMACOKINETICS

Reaches steady-state levels by the third weekly infusion. Clearance decreases as dose increases. **Half-life:** 114 hrs (Range: 75–188 hrs).

USES

As a single agent or in combination with irinotecan for treatment of EGFR-expressing, metastatic colorectal carcinoma in pts who are refractory or intolerant to irinotecan-based chemotherapy.

Treatment of advanced squamous cell cancer of head/neck (with radiation). Treatment of head/neck cancer that metastasized (as monotherapy). **OFF-LABEL:** Breast cancer, tumors overexpressing EGFR.

PRECAUTIONS

CONTRAINDICATIONS: None known. **CAUTIONS:** Hypersensitivity to murine proteins.

LIFESPAN CONSIDERATIONS:

Pregnancy/Lactation: Crosses placental barrier; has potential to cause fetal harm, abortifactant. Do not breast-feed. **Pregnancy Category C. Children:** Safety and efficacy not established. **Elderly:** No age-related precautions noted.

INTERACTIONS

DRUG: None significant. **HERBAL:** None significant. **FOOD:** None known. **LAB VALUES:** May decrease WBCs, Hgb, Hct.

AVAILABILITY (Rx)

INJECTION SOLUTION: 2 mg/ml.

ADMINISTRATION/HANDLING

IV

◄ ALERT ► Do not give by IV push or bolus.

Reconstitution • Solution should appear clear, colorless; may contain a small amount of visible, white particulates. • Do not shake or dilute. • Infuse with a low protein-binding 0.22 micron in-line filter.

Rate of administration • First dose should be given as a 120-min IV infusion. • Maintenance infusion should be infused over 60 min. • Maximum infusion rate should not exceed 5 ml/min.

Storage • Refrigerate vials. • Preparations in infusion containers are stable for up to 12 hrs if refrigerated, up to 8 hrs at room temperature. • Discard any unused portion.

IV COMPATIBILITY

Irinotecan (Camptosar).

INDICATIONS/ROUTES/DOSAGE

HEAD/NECK CANCER, METASTATIC COLORECTAL CARCINOMA

IV: ADULTS, ELDERLY: Initially, 400 mg/m^2 as a loading dose. Maintenance: 250 mg/m^2 infused over 60 min weekly.

SIDE EFFECTS

FREQUENT (90%–25%): Acneiform rash, malaise, fever, nausea, diarrhea, constipation, headache, abdominal pain, anorexia, vomiting. **OCCASIONAL (16%–10%):** Nail disorder, back pain, stomatitis, peripheral edema, pruritus, cough, insomnia. **RARE (9%–5%):** Weight loss, depression, dyspepsia, conjunctivitis, alopecia.

ADVERSE EFFECTS/ TOXIC REACTIONS

Anemia occurs in 10% of pts. Severe infusion reaction (rapid onset of airway obstruction, precipitous drop in B/P, severe urticaria), occurs rarely. Dermatologic toxicity, pulmonary embolus, leukopenia, renal failure occur rarely.

NURSING CONSIDERATIONS

BASELINE ASSESSMENT

Monitor Hgb, Hct. Assess signs/symptoms for evidence of anemia. Question pt regarding possibility of pregnancy. Advise pt to avoid pregnancy due to potential to cause fetal harm.

INTERVENTION/EVALUATION

Diligently monitor pt for evidence of infusion reaction (rapid onset of bronchospasm, stridor, hoarseness, urticaria, hypotension). Be aware that pt may

C

experience first severe infusion reaction during later infusions. Assess skin for evidence of dermatologic toxicity (development of inflammatory sequelae, dry skin, exfoliative dermatitis, rash).

PATIENT/FAMILY TEACHING

• Do not have immunizations without physician's approval (drug lowers resistance). • Avoid contact with anyone who recently received a live virus vaccine. • Avoid crowds, those with infection. • Instruct pt to wear sunscreen, limit sun exposure during therapy (sunlight can exacerbate skin reactions).

chamomile

ka-mow-meal

Also known as German chamomile, pinheads (Blossom 120/jar, 45/jar, 30/jar).

CLASSIFICATION

HERBAL: See Appendix G.

ACTION

Antiallergic, anti-inflammatory action due to inhibiting release of histamine. Possesses antiallergic, antiflatulent, antispasmodic, mild sedative, anti-inflammatory action. **Effect:** Reduces GI symptoms, produces mild CNS depression.

USES

Treatment of symptoms of flatulence, travel sickness, diarrhea, insomnia, GI spasms.

PRECAUTIONS

CONTRAINDICATIONS: Pregnancy. **CAUTIONS:** Pts with asthma (may exacerbate condition), those allergic to ragweed, aster, daisies, chrysanthemums.

LIFESPAN CONSIDERATIONS:

Pregnancy/Lactation: Contraindicated. A teratogen, affects menstrual cycle, has uterine stimulant effects. **Children:** Safety and efficacy not established. **Elderly:** No age-related precautions noted.

INTERACTIONS

DRUG: May increase anticoagulation, risk of bleeding with **aspirin, clopidogrel, dalteparin, enoxaparin, heparin, warfarin.** May have additive effects with **benzodiazepines. HERBAL:** Sedative effects may increase with **ginseng, kava kava, St. John's wort, valerian.** May increase risk of bleeding with **feverfew, garlic, ginger, ginkgo, licorice. FOOD:** None known. **LAB VALUES:** None known.

AVAILABILITY

WHOLE FLOWERS: 30 g/jar, 45 g/jar, 120 g/jar.

INDICATIONS/ROUTES/DOSAGE

FLATULENCE, TRAVEL SICKNESS, DIARRHEA, INSOMNIA, GI SPASMS

PO: ADULTS, ELDERLY: 2–8 g of dried flower heads 3 times a day or 1 cup of tea 3–4 times a day.

SIDE EFFECTS

Allergic reaction (contact dermatitis, severe hypersensitivity reaction, anaphylactic reaction), eye irritation.

ADVERSE EFFECTS/ TOXIC REACTIONS

Anaphylactic reaction (bronchospasm, severe pruritus, angioedema) occurs rarely.

NURSING CONSIDERATIONS

BASELINE ASSESSMENT

Assess if pt is pregnant, breast-feeding, or asthmatic. Assess if pt is taking other medications, esp. those that increase risk of bleeding or have sedative properties. Assess for allergies to ragweed, aster, daisies, chrysanthemums.

INTERVENTION/EVALUATION

Monitor for signs of allergic reaction.

PATIENT/FAMILY TEACHING

• Inform physician if pregnancy occurs or if planning to become pregnant or breast-feed. • May cause mild sedation. • Avoid tasks that require alertness, motor skills until response to herbal is established. • Avoid use with other sedatives, alcohol, anticoagulants.

chloral hydrate

klor-al **hye**-drate

(Aquachloral Supprettes, PMS-Chloral Hydrate ✤, Somnote)

CLASSIFICATION

PHARMACOTHERAPEUTIC: Nonbarbiturate chloral derivative. **CLINICAL:** Sedative, hypnotic.

ACTION

Nonbarbiturate that produces CNS depression. **Therapeutic Effect:** Induces quiet, deep sleep, with only slight decrease in respiratory rate, B/P.

PHARMACOKINETICS

Readily absorbed from GI tract following PO administration. Well absorbed following rectal administration. Protein binding: 70%–80%. Metabolized in liver, erythrocytes to active metabolite, trichloroethanol, which may be further metabolized to inactive metabolites. Excreted in urine. **Half-life:** 7–10 hrs (trichloroethanol).

USES

Sedative/hypnotic for dental or diagnostic procedures, sedative before EEG evaluations.

PRECAUTIONS

CONTRAINDICATIONS: Gastritis, marked hepatic/renal impairment, severe cardiac disease. **CAUTIONS:** History of drug abuse, clinical depression.

LIFESPAN CONSIDERATIONS:

Pregnancy/Lactation: Crosses placenta; distributed in breast milk. **Pregnancy Category C. Children:** Safety and efficacy not established. **Elderly:** No age-related precautions noted.

INTERACTIONS

DRUG: Alcohol, other CNS depressants may increase effects of chloral hydrate. **Furosemide (IV)** may alter B/P and cause diaphoresis if given within 24 hrs. May increase effect of **warfarin. HERBAL:** None significant. **FOOD:** None known. **LAB VALUES:** May interfere with copper sulfate test for glycosuria, fluorometric tests for urine catecholamines, urinary 17-hydroxycorticosteroid determinations.

AVAILABILITY (Rx)

CAPSULES (SOMNOTE): 500 mg. **SUPPOSITORIES (AQUACHLORAL SUPPRETTES):** 324 mg, 648 mg. **SYRUP:** 500 mg/5 ml.

ADMINISTRATION/HANDLING

PO

• Give capsules with full glass of water or fruit juice. Swallow capsules whole; do not chew. • Dilute syrup in water to minimize gastric irritation.

RECTAL

• Store suppositories at room temperature.

INDICATIONS/ROUTES/DOSAGE

PREMEDICATION FOR DENTAL OR MEDICAL PROCEDURES

PO, RECTAL: ADULTS: 0.5–1 g. **CHILDREN:** 75 mg/kg up to 1 g total.

PREMEDICATION FOR EEG

PO, RECTAL: ADULTS: 0.5–1.5 g. **CHILDREN:** 25–50 mg/kg/dose 30–60 min prior to EEG. May repeat in 30 min. **Maximum:** 1 g for infants, 2 g for children.

SIDE EFFECTS

OCCASIONAL: Gastric irritation (nausea, vomiting, flatulence, diarrhea), rash, sleepwalking. **RARE:** Headache, paradoxical CNS hyperactivity or nervousness in children, excitement or restlessness in the elderly (particularly in pts with pain).

ADVERSE EFFECTS/ TOXIC REACTIONS

Overdose may produce somnolence, confusion, slurred speech, severe incoordination, respiratory depression, coma. Allergic-type reaction may occur in those with tartrazine sensitivity.

NURSING CONSIDERATIONS

BASELINE ASSESSMENT

Assess B/P, pulse, respirations immediately before administration. Provide safety measures, e.g., raise bedrails. Provide environment conducive to sleep (back rub, quiet environment, low lighting).

INTERVENTION/EVALUATION

Monitor mental status, vital signs. Gastric irritation decreased by diluting dose in water. Assess sleep pattern. Assess elderly and children for paradoxical reaction. Evaluate for therapeutic response to insomnia: decrease in number of nocturnal awakenings, increase in length of sleep.

PATIENT/FAMILY TEACHING

• Take capsule with full glass of water or fruit juice. • Swallow capsules whole; do not chew. • If taking at home before procedure, do not drive. • Do not abruptly withdraw medication after long-term use. • Tolerance, dependence may occur with prolonged use.

chlorambucil

klor-**am**-bew-sill

(Leukeran)

Do not confuse Leukeran with Alkeran, Chloromycetin, Leukine, or Myleran.

CLASSIFICATION

PHARMACOTHERAPEUTIC: Alkylating agent, nitrogen mustard. **CLINICAL:** Antineoplastic (see p. 77C).

ACTION

Inhibits DNA, RNA synthesis by cross-linking with DNA, RNA strands. Cell cycle–phase nonspecific. **Therapeutic Effect:** Interferes with nucleic acid function.

PHARMACOKINETICS

Rapidly, completely absorbed from GI tract. Protein binding: 99%. Rapidly metabolized in the liver to active metabolite. Not removed by hemodialysis. **Half-life:** 1.5 hrs; metabolite 2.5 hrs.

USES

Treatment of chronic lymphocytic leukemia, Hodgkin's and non-Hodgkin's lymphomas. **OFF-LABEL:** Treatment of cutaneous T-cell lymphomas, epithelial carcinoma, hairy cell leukemia, nephrotic syndrome, ovarian or testicular carcinoma, breast cancer, polycythemia vera, trophoblastic gestational tumors.

PRECAUTIONS

CONTRAINDICATIONS: Previous allergic reaction, disease resistance to drug. **EXTREME CAUTIONS:** Within 4 wks after full-course radiation therapy or myelosuppressive drug regimen.

LIFESPAN CONSIDERATIONS:

Pregnancy/Lactation: If possible, avoid use during pregnancy, esp. first trimester. Breast-feeding not recommended. **Pregnancy Category D.** **Children:** No age-related precautions noted. When taken for nephritic syndrome, may increase seizures. **Elderly:** No age-related precautions noted.

INTERACTIONS

DRUG: May decrease effect of **antigout medications. Bone marrow depressants** may increase myelosuppression. **Other immunosuppressants (e.g., steroids)** may increase risk of infection or development of neoplasms. **Live virus vaccines** may potentiate virus replication, increase vaccine side effects, decrease antibody response to vaccine. **HERBAL:** None significant. **FOOD:** None known. **LAB VALUES:** May increase serum AST, alkaline phosphatase, uric acid.

AVAILABILITY (Rx)

TABLETS: 2 mg.

ADMINISTRATION/HANDLING

PO

- Give without regard to food.

INDICATIONS/ROUTES/DOSAGE

USUAL DOSAGE

PO: ADULTS, ELDERLY, CHILDREN: For initial or short-course therapy, 0.1–0.2 mg/kg/day as a single or in divided doses for 3–6 wks (average dose, 4–10 mg/day). Alternatively, 0.4 mg/kg initially as a single daily dose every 2 wks and increased by 0.1 mg/kg every 2 wks until response and myelosuppression occur. **Maintenance:** 0.03–0.1 mg/kg/day (average dose, 2–4 mg/day).

SIDE EFFECTS

EXPECTED: GI effects (nausea, vomiting, anorexia, diarrhea, abdominal distress) generally mild, last less than 24 hrs, occur only if single dose exceeds 20 mg. **OCCASIONAL:** Rash, dermatitis, pruritus, cold sores. **RARE:** Alopecia, urticaria, erythema, hyperuricemia.

ADVERSE EFFECTS/ TOXIC REACTIONS

Hematologic toxicity due to severe myelosuppression occurs frequently, manifested as neutropenia, anemia, thrombocytopenia. After discontinuation of therapy, thrombocytopenia, neutropenia usually last for 1–2 wks but may persist for 3–4 wks. Neutrophil count may continue to decrease for up to 10 days after last dose. Toxicity appears to be less severe with intermittent rather than continuous drug administration. Overdosage may produce seizures in children. Excessive uric acid level, hepatotoxicity occur rarely.

NURSING CONSIDERATIONS

BASELINE ASSESSMENT

CBC should be performed before therapy and each week during therapy, WBC count performed 3–4 days following each weekly CBC during first 3–6 wks of therapy (4–6 wks if pt on intermittent dosing schedule).

INTERVENTION/EVALUATION

Monitor for hematologic toxicity (fever, sore throat, signs of local infection, unusual bruising/bleeding from any site), symptoms of anemia (excessive fatigue, weakness). Assess skin for rash, pruritus, urticaria.

C

PATIENT/FAMILY TEACHING

• Increase fluid intake (may protect against hyperuricemia). • Do not have immunizations without physician's approval (drug lowers resistance). • Avoid contact with those who have recently received live virus vaccine. • Promptly report fever, sore throat, signs of local infection, unusual bruising/bleeding from any site.

chlordiazepoxide

evolve

klor-dye-az-e-**pox**-ide

(Apo-Chlordiazepoxide ✦, Librium)

Do not confuse Librium with Librax.

FIXED-COMBINATION(S)

Limbitrol: amitriptyline/chlordiazepoxide: 5 mg/12.5 mg; 10 mg/25 mg. **Librax:** chlordiazepoxide-clidinium: 5 mg/2.5 mg.

CLASSIFICATION

PHARMACOTHERAPEUTIC: Benzodiazepine. **CLINICAL:** Antianxiety (see p. 11C).

ACTION

Enhances action of inhibitory neurotransmitter gamma-aminobutyric acid in CNS. **Therapeutic Effect:** Produces anxiolytic effect.

PHARMACOKINETICS

Widely distributed. Protein binding: 90–98%. Metabolized in liver. Primarily excreted in urine. **Half-life:** 6.6–25 hrs.

USES

Management of anxiety disorders, acute alcohol withdrawal symptoms; short-term relief of symptoms of anxiety, preop anxiety, tension. **OFF-LABEL:** Treatment of panic disorder, tension headache, tremors.

PRECAUTIONS

CONTRAINDICATIONS: Acute alcohol intoxication, acute angle-closure glaucoma. **CAUTIONS:** Renal/hepatic impairment.

LIFESPAN CONSIDERATIONS:

Pregnancy/Lactation: Crosses placenta; distributed in breast milk. **Pregnancy Category D. Children/Elderly:** Reduce initial dose, increase dosage gradually (prevents excessive sedation).

INTERACTIONS

DRUG: **Alcohol, other CNS depressants** may increase CNS depression. **Azole antifungals** may increase serum concentration, increase risk of toxicity. **HERBAL:** **Kava kava, valerian** may increase CNS depression. **St. John's wort** may decrease effectiveness. **FOOD:** None known. **LAB VALUES:** Therapeutic serum level: 1–3 mcg/ml; toxic serum level: greater than 5 mcg/ml.

AVAILABILITY (Rx)

CAPSULES (LIBRIUM): 5 mg, 10 mg, 25 mg. **INJECTION, POWDER FOR RECONSTITUTION (LIBRIUM):** 100 mg.

ADMINISTRATION/HANDLING

◄ **ALERT** ► Keep pt recumbent for up to 3 hrs after parenteral administration (reduces drug's hypotensive effect).

INDICATIONS/ROUTES/DOSAGE

ALCOHOL WITHDRAWAL SYMPTOMS

PO, IV: ADULTS, ELDERLY: 50–100 mg. May repeat q2–4h. **Maximum:** 300 mg/24 hrs.

C

ANXIETY

PO: ADULTS: 15–100 mg/day in 3–4 divided doses. **ELDERLY:** 5 mg 2–4 times a day.

IV, IM: ADULTS: Initially, 50–100 mg, then 25–50 mg 3–4 times a day as needed.

PREOPERATIVE ANXIETY

IM: ADULTS, ELDERLY: 50–100 mg once.

SIDE EFFECTS

FREQUENT: Pain at IM injection site; somnolence, ataxia, dizziness, confusion with oral dose (particularly in elderly or debilitated pts). **OCCASIONAL:** Rash, peripheral edema, GI disturbances. **RARE:** Paradoxical CNS reactions (hyperactivity, nervousness in children; excitement, restlessness in the elderly, generally noted during first 2 wks of therapy, particularly in presence of uncontrolled pain).

ADVERSE EFFECTS/ TOXIC REACTIONS

IV administration may produce pain, swelling, thrombophlebitis, carpal tunnel syndrome. Abrupt or too-rapid withdrawal may result in pronounced restlessness, irritability, insomnia, hand tremors, abdominal/muscle cramps, diaphoresis, vomiting, seizures. Overdose results in somnolence, confusion, diminished reflexes, coma.

NURSING CONSIDERATIONS

BASELINE ASSESSMENT

Assess B/P, pulse, respirations immediately before administration. Pt must remain recumbent for up to 3 hrs (individualized) after parenteral administration to reduce hypotensive effect.

INTERVENTION/EVALUATION

Assess motor responses (agitation, tremors, tension), autonomic responses (cold/clammy hands, diaphoresis). Assess children, elderly for paradoxical reaction, particularly during early therapy. Assist with ambulation if drowsiness, ataxia occur. Therapeutic serum level: 1–3 mcg/ml; toxic serum level: greater than 5 mcg/ml.

PATIENT/FAMILY TEACHING

• Discomfort may occur with IM injection. • Drowsiness usually disappears during continued therapy. • If dizziness occurs, change positions slowly from recumbent to sitting before standing. • Smoking reduces drug effectiveness. • Do not abruptly withdraw medication after long-term therapy.

chloroprocaine

(Nesacaine)

See Anesthetics: local (p. 4C)

chloroquine

klor-oh-kwin

(Aralen, Novo-Chloroquin ✱)

CLASSIFICATION

PHARMACOTHERAPEUTIC: Amebicide. **CLINICAL:** Antimalarial.

ACTION

Concentrates in parasite acid vesicles. May interfere with parasite protein synthesis. **Therapeutic Effect:** Increases pH (inhibits parasite growth).

PHARMACOKINETICS

Rapidly absorbed from GI tract. Widely distributed. Metabolized in liver, excreted in urine. **Half-life:** 3–5 days.

USES

Suppression/chemoprophylaxis of malaria in chloroquine-sensitive areas. Treatment of uncomplicated or mild to moderate malaria, extraintestinal amebiasis. **OFF-LABEL:** Treatment of sarcoid-associated hypercalcemia, juvenile

C

arthritis, rheumatoid arthritis, systemic lupus erythematosus, solar urticaria, chronic cutaneous vasculitis.

PRECAUTIONS

CONTRAINDICATIONS: Hypersensitivity to 4-aminoquinolones, retinal/visual field changes, psoriasis, porphyria. **CAUTIONS:** Alcoholism, severe hematologic disorders, hepatic disease, neurologic disorders, G6PD deficiency. Children are esp. susceptible to chloroquine fatalities. **Pregnancy Category C.**

INTERACTIONS

DRUG: May increase concentration of **penicillamine,** increase risk of hematologic/renal or severe skin reaction. **HERBAL:** None significant. **FOOD:** None known. **LAB VALUES:** Acute decrease in Hct, Hgb, RBC count may occur.

AVAILABILITY (Rx)

TABLETS: 250 mg, 500 mg.

INDICATIONS/ROUTES/DOSAGE

◀ ALERT ▶ Chloroquine PO_4 500 mg = 300 mg base; chloroquine HCl 50 mg = 40 mg base.

CHLOROQUINE PHOSPHATE

TREATMENT OF MALARIA (acute attack): Dose (mg base)

Dose	Time	Adults	Children
Initial	Day 1	600 mg	10 mg/kg
Second	6 hrs later	300 mg	5 mg/kg
Third	Day 2	300 mg	5 mg/kg
Fourth	Day 3	300 mg	5 mg/kg

SUPPRESSION OF MALARIA

PO: ADULTS: 500 mg (300 mg base)/wk on same day each week beginning 2 wks before exposure; continue for 6–8 wks after leaving endemic area. **CHILDREN:** 5 mg base/kg/wk. If therapy is not begun before exposure, then double initial loading dose to 10 mg base/kg in 2 divided doses 6 hrs apart. Follow with usual dosage regimen. **PO: ADULTS:** 600 mg base initially given in 2 divided doses 6 hrs apart. **CHILDREN:** 10 mg base/kg.

AMEBIASIS

PO: ADULTS: 1 g (600 mg base) a day for 2 days; then 500 mg (300 mg base) a day for at least 2–3 wks. **CHILDREN:** 10 mg base/kg once daily for 2–3 wks. **Maximum:** 300 mg base a day.

SIDE EFFECTS

FREQUENT: Mild transient headache, anorexia, nausea/vomiting. **OCCASIONAL:** Visual disturbances (blurring, difficulty focusing), anxiety, fatigue, pruritus (esp. of palms, soles, scalp), bleaching of hair, irritability, personality changes, diarrhea, skin eruptions. **RARE:** Stomatitis (redness/burning of oral mucosa, gingivitis, glossitis), exfoliative dermatitis.

ADVERSE EFFECTS/ TOXIC REACTIONS

Ocular toxicity (tinnitus), ototoxicity (reduced hearing) has been noted. Prolonged therapy may produce peripheral neuritis and neuromyopathy, hypotension, EKG changes, agranulocytosis, aplastic anemia, thrombocytopenia, seizures, psychosis. Overdosage results in headache, vomiting, visual disturbance, drowsiness, seizures, hypokalemia followed by cardiovascular collapse, death.

NURSING CONSIDERATIONS

INTERVENTION/EVALUATION

Check for, promptly report any visual disturbances. Evaluate for GI distress. Monitor hepatic function tests; assess for fatigue, jaundice, other signs of hepatic effects. Assess skin/buccal mucosa, inquire about pruritus. Check vital signs; be alert to signs/symptoms of overdosage (esp. with parenteral administration, children). Notify physician of tinnitus, reduced hearing. With prolonged therapy, test for muscle weakness.

C

PATIENT/FAMILY TEACHING

• IM administration may cause local discomfort. • Continue drug for full length of treatment. • Notify physician immediately of **any** new symptom, visual difficulties, decreased hearing, tinnitus. • Periodic lab, visual tests are important part of therapy.

chlorothiazide

(Diuril)

See Diuretics (p. 96C)

chlorpheniramine

(Chlor-Trimeton, Teldrin)

See Antihistamines (p. 52C)

*chlorproMAZINE

evolve

klor-**proe**-ma-zeen

(Apo-Chlorpromazine ♣, Chlorpromanyl ♣, Largactil ♣, Novo-Chlorpromazine ♣, Thorazine)

Do not confuse chlorpromazine with chlorpropamide, clomipramine, or prochlorperazine, or Thorazine with thiamine or thioridazine.

CLASSIFICATION

PHARMACOTHERAPEUTIC: Phenothiazine. **CLINICAL:** Antipsychotic, antiemetic, antianxiety, antineuralgia adjunct (see p. 62C).

ACTION

Blocks dopamine neurotransmission at postsynaptic dopamine receptor sites. Possesses strong anticholinergic, sedative, antiemetic effects; moderate extrapyramidal effects; slight antihistamine action. **Therapeutic Effect:** Improves psychotic conditions; relieves nausea/vomiting; controls intractable hiccups, porphyria.

PHARMACOKINETICS

Rapidly absorbed from GI tract. Protein binding: 92–97%. Metabolized in liver, excreted in urine. **Half-life:** Initial 2 hrs; **Terminal:** 30 hrs.

USES

Management of psychotic disorders, manic phase of manic-depressive illness, severe nausea/vomiting, severe behavioral disturbances in children. Relief of intractable hiccups, acute intermittent porphyria. **OFF-LABEL:** Treatment of choreiform movement of Huntington's disease.

PRECAUTIONS

CONTRAINDICATIONS: Comatose states, myelosuppression, severe cardiovascular disease, severe CNS depression, subcortical brain damage. **CAUTIONS:** Impaired respiratory/hepatic/renal/cardiac function, alcohol withdrawal, history of seizures, urinary retention, glaucoma, prostatic hypertrophy, hypocalcemia (increases susceptibility to dystonias).

LIFESPAN CONSIDERATIONS: **Pregnancy/Lactation:** Crosses placenta; distributed in breast milk. **Pregnancy Category C. Children:** Those with acute illnesses (chickenpox, measles, gastroenteritis, CNS infection) are at risk of developing neuromuscular, extrapyramidal symptoms (EPS), particularly dystonias. **Elderly:** Susceptible to anticholinergic, neuromuscular, EPS.

INTERACTIONS

DRUG: **Alcohol, CNS depressants** may increase respiratory depression, hypotensive effects. **Tricyclic antidepressants, MAOIs** may increase sedative, anticholinergic effects. **Antithyroid agents** may increase risk of agranulocytosis. Increased risk of EPS with **EPS-producing medications. Antihypertensives** may increase hypotension. May decrease **levodopa** effects. **Lithium** may decrease absorption, produce adverse neurologic effects. **HERBAL: St. John's wort** may decrease concentration, increase photosensitization, sedative effect. **Dong quai** may increase photosensitization. **Kava kava, gotu kola, valerian** may increase sedative effect. **FOOD:** None known. **LAB VALUES:** May produce false-positive pregnancy test, phenylketonuria (PKU) test. EKG changes may occur, including Q- and T-wave disturbances. Therapeutic serum level: 50-300 mcg/ml; toxic serum level: greater than 750 mcg/ml.

AVAILABILITY (Rx)

CAPSULES (SUSTAINED-RELEASE): 30 mg, 75 mg, 150 mg. **INJECTION SOLUTION:** 25 mg/ml. **ORAL CONCENTRATE:** 30 mg/ml, 100 mg/ml. **SUPPOSITORIES:** 25 mg, 100 mg. **SYRUP:** 10 mg/5 ml. **TABLETS:** 10 mg, 25 mg, 50 mg, 100 mg, 200 mg.

ADMINISTRATION/HANDLING

IM

◀ ALERT ▶ Do not give chlorpromazine by subcutaneous route (risk for severe tissue necrosis).

• Dilute the injection solution as prescribed, with Sodium Chloride for Injection or 2% procaine to reduce injection site irritation. • Slowly inject drug deep into large muscle, such as gluteus maximus rather than lateral aspect of the thigh, to minimize discomfort.

PO

• Avoid skin contact with oral concentrate and syrup to prevent contact dermatitis. • Slight yellow color in oral concentrate or syrup will not affect drug's potency; discard if markedly discolored or it contains precipitate. • Dilute each dose of oral concentrate immediately before administration with 60 ml or more of water, coffee, tea, milk, carbonated beverage, tomato or fruit juice, simple syrup, orange syrup, soup, pudding. Use immediately; discard any remaining mixture.

RECTAL

• Wash hands with soap, water before using suppository. • Remove foil or wrapper from suppository before inserting it. • Lie pt on left side with left leg straight or slightly bent, and right knee bent upward. Gently push pointed end of suppository into rectum about 1 inch. • Have pt remain lying down for about 15 min to allow suppository to melt. • Wash hands after inserting suppository.

INDICATIONS/ROUTES/DOSAGE

SEVERE NAUSEA/VOMITING

PO: ADULTS, ELDERLY: 10–25 mg q4–6h. **CHILDREN:** 0.5–1 mg/kg q4–6h.
IV, IM: ADULTS, ELDERLY: 25–50 mg q4–6h. **CHILDREN:** 0.5–1 mg/kg q6–8h.
RECTAL: ADULTS, ELDERLY: 50–100 mg q6–8h. **CHILDREN:** 1 mg/kg q6–8h.

PSYCHOTIC DISORDERS

PO: ADULTS, ELDERLY: 30–800 mg/day in 1–4 divided doses. **CHILDREN OLDER THAN 6 MOS:** 0.5–1 mg/kg q4–6h.
IV, IM: ADULTS, ELDERLY: Initially, 25 mg; may repeat in 1–4 hrs. May gradually increase to 400 mg q4–6h. Usual dose: 300–800 mg/day. **CHILDREN OLDER THAN 6 MOS:** 0.5–1 mg/kg q6–8h. **Maximum:** 75 mg/day for children 5–12 yrs; 40 mg/day for children younger than 5 yrs.

INTRACTABLE HICCUPS

PO, IV, IM: ADULTS: 25–50 mg 3–4 times a day.

PORPHYRIA

PO: ADULTS: 25–50 mg 3–4 times a day.
IM: ADULTS, ELDERLY: 25 mg 3–4 times a day.

SIDE EFFECTS

FREQUENT: Somnolence, blurred vision, hypotension, color vision or night vision disturbances, dizziness, decreased diaphoresis, constipation, dry mouth, nasal congestion. **OCCASIONAL:** Urinary retention, photosensitivity, rash, decreased sexual function, swelling/pain in breasts, weight gain, nausea, vomiting, abdominal pain, tremors.

ADVERSE EFFECTS/ TOXIC REACTIONS

EPS appear to be dose related (particularly high dosage) and are divided into three categories: akathisia (inability to sit still, tapping of feet), parkinsonian symptoms (mask-like face, tremors, shuffling gait, hypersalivation), acute dystonias (torticollis [neck muscle spasm] opisthotonos [rigidity of back muscles] and oculogyric crisis [rolling back of eyes]). Dystonic reaction may produce diaphoresis, pallor. Tardive dyskinesia (tongue protrusion, puffing of cheeks, puckering of the mouth) occurs rarely (may be irreversible). Abrupt discontinuation after long-term therapy may precipitate nausea, vomiting, gastritis, dizziness, tremors. Blood dyscrasias, particularly agranulocytosis mild leukopenia, may occur. May lower seizure threshold.

NURSING CONSIDERATIONS

BASELINE ASSESSMENT

Avoid skin contact with solution (contact dermatitis). **Antiemetic:** Assess for dehydration (poor skin turgor, dry mucous membranes, longitudinal furrows in tongue). **Antipsychotic:** Assess behavior, appearance, emotional status, response to environment, speech pattern, thought content.

INTERVENTION/EVALUATION

Monitor B/P for hypotension. Assess for EPS. Monitor WBC, differential count for blood dyscrasias, fine tongue movement (may be early sign of tardive dyskinesia). Supervise suicidal-risk pt closely during early therapy (as depression lessens, energy level improves, increasing suicide potential). Assess for therapeutic response (interest in surroundings, improvement in self-care, increased ability to concentrate, relaxed facial expression). Therapeutic serum level: 50–300 mcg/ml; toxic serum level: greater than 750 mcg/ml.

PATIENT/FAMILY TEACHING

• Full therapeutic response may take up to 6 wks. • Urine may darken. • Do not abruptly withdraw from long-term drug therapy. • Report visual disturbances. • Drowsiness generally subsides with continued therapy. • Avoid tasks that require alertness, motor skills until response to drug is established. • Avoid alcohol, exposure to sunlight.

*chlorproPAMIDE

(Diabinese)

See Antidiabetics (p. 41C)

chlorzoxazone

(Paraflex, Parafon Forte DSC)

See Skeletal muscle relaxants (p. 142C)

cholestyramine

coal-es-**tie**-rah-meen

(Novo-Cholamine ♣, Prevalite, Questran, Questran Lite)

CLASSIFICATION

PHARMACOTHERAPEUTIC: Bile acid sequestrant. **CLINICAL:** Antihyperlipoproteinemic (see p. 54C).

C

ACTION

Binds with bile acids in intestine, forming insoluble complex. Binding results in partial removal of bile acid from enterohepatic circulation. **Therapeutic Effect:** Removes LDL cholesterol from plasma.

PHARMACOKINETICS

Not absorbed from GI tract. Decreases in serum LDL apparent in 5–7 days and in serum cholesterol in 1 mo. Serum cholesterol returns to baseline levels about 1 mo after drug is discontinued.

USES

Adjunct to dietary therapy to decrease elevated serum cholesterol levels in pts with primary hypercholesterolemia. Relief of pruritus associated with elevated levels of bile acids. **OFF-LABEL:** Treatment of diarrhea (due to bile acids), hyperoxaluria.

PRECAUTIONS

CONTRAINDICATIONS: Complete biliary obstruction, hypersensitivity to cholestyramine, tartrazine (frequently seen in aspirin hypersensitivity). **CAUTIONS:** GI dysfunction (esp. constipation), hemorrhoids, hematologic disorders, osteoporosis.

LIFESPAN CONSIDERATIONS:

Pregnancy/Lactation: Not systemically absorbed. May interfere with maternal absorption of fat-soluble vitamins. **Pregnancy Category B. Children:** No age-related precautions noted. Limited experience in those younger than 10 yrs. **Elderly:** Increased risk of GI side effects, adverse nutritional effects.

INTERACTIONS

DRUG: May increase effects of **anticoagulants** by decreasing vitamin K level. May decrease **warfarin** absorption. May bind with, decrease absorption of **digoxin, folic acid, pencillins, propranolol, tetracyclines, thiazides, thyroid hormones, other medications.** May bind with, decrease effects of **oral vancomycin. HERBAL:** None significant. **FOOD:** None known. **LAB VALUES:** May increase serum alkaline phosphatase, magnesium, AST, ALT. May decrease serum calcium, potassium, sodium. May prolong PT.

AVAILABILITY (Rx)

POWDER FOR ORAL SUSPENSION: 4 g/5.7 g powder (Questran Light), 4 g/9 g powder (Prevalite, Questran).

ADMINISTRATION/HANDLING

PO

• Give other drugs at least 1 hr before or 4–6 hrs following cholestyramine (capable of binding drugs in GI tract). • Do not give in dry form (highly irritating). Mix with 3–6 oz water, milk, fruit juice, soup. • Place powder on surface for 1–2 min (prevents lumping), then mix thoroughly. • Excessive foaming with carbonated beverages; use extra large glass, stir slowly. • Administer before meals.

INDICATIONS/ROUTES/DOSAGE

HYPERCHOLESTEROLEMIA

PO: ADULTS, ELDERLY: Initially, 4 g 1–2 times a day. Maintenance: 8–16 g/day in divided doses. **Maximum:** 24 g/day. **CHILDREN:** 80 mg/kg 3 times a day.

PRURITIS

PO: ADULTS, ELDERLY: Initially, 4 g 1–2 times a day. Maintenance: 8–16 g/day in divided doses. **Maximum:** 24 g/day.

SIDE EFFECTS

FREQUENT: Constipation (may lead to fecal impaction), nausea, vomiting, abdominal pain, indigestion. **OCCASIONAL:** Diarrhea, belching, bloating, headache, dizziness. **RARE:** Gallstones, peptic ulcer disease, malabsorption syndrome.

ADVERSE EFFECTS/ TOXIC REACTIONS

GI tract obstruction, hyperchloremic acidosis, osteoporosis secondary to calcium excretion may occur. High dosage may interfere with fat absorption, resulting in steatorrhea.

NURSING CONSIDERATIONS

BASELINE ASSESSMENT

Question for history of hypersensitivity to cholestyramine, tartrazine, aspirin. Obtain baseline serum cholesterol, triglycerides, electrolytes, hepatic enzyme levels.

INTERVENTION/EVALUATION

Monitor daily pattern of bowel activity/stool consistency. Evaluate food tolerance, abdominal discomfort, flatulence. Monitor serum electrolytes. Encourage several glasses of water between meals.

PATIENT/FAMILY TEACHING

• Complete full course of therapy; do not omit or change doses. • Take other drugs at least 1 hr before or 4–6 hrs after cholestyramine. • Never take in dry form; mix with 3–6 oz water, milk, fruit juice, soup (place powder on surface for 1–2 min to prevent lumping, then mix well). • Use extra large glass, stir slowly when mixing with carbonated beverages due to foaming. • Take before meals, drink several glasses of water between meals. • Eat high-fiber foods (whole grain cereals, fruits, vegetables) to reduce potential for constipation.

chorionic gonadotropin, hCG

kore-ee-**on**-ik goe-**nad**-oh-troe-pin

(APL, Humegon ✤, Novarel, Pregnyl, Profasi HP ✤)

CLASSIFICATION

PHARMACOTHERAPEUTIC: Gonadotropin. **CLINICAL:** Infertility therapy adjunct, diagnostic aid (hypogonadism).

ACTION

Stimulates production of gonadal steroid hormones by stimulating interstitial cells (Leydig cells) of testes to produce androgen and corpus luteum of the ovary to produce progesterone. **Therapeutic Effect:** Androgen stimulation in male causes production of secondary sex characteristics, may stimulate descent of testes when no anatomic impediment exists. In women of childbearing age with normally functioning ovaries, causes maturation of corpus luteum, triggers ovulation.

PHARMACOKINETICS

Excreted in urine. **Half-life:** 23–29 hrs.

USES

Treatment of hypogonadotropic hypogonadism, prepubertal cryptorchidism. Induces ovulation. **OFF-LABEL:** Diagnosis of male hypogonadism, treatment of corpus luteum dysfunction.

PRECAUTIONS

CONTRAINDICATIONS: Precocious puberty, carcinoma of prostate, other androgen-dependent neoplasia. Undiagnosed abnormal vaginal bleeding, fibroid tumors of uterus, ovarian cyst or enlargement not associated with polycystic ovarian disease. Active thrombophlebitis. **CAUTIONS:** Prepubertal males, conditions aggravated by fluid retention (cardiac/renal disease, epilepsy, migraine, asthma), polycystic ovarian disease. **Pregnancy Category C.**

C

INTERACTIONS

DRUG: None significant. **HERBAL:** None significant. **FOOD:** None known. **LAB VALUES:** None known.

AVAILABILITY (Rx)

INJECTION, POWDER FOR RECONSTITUTION: 10,000 units.

ADMINISTRATION/HANDLING

IM

• Reconstituted drug is stable for 30–90 days when refrigerated.

INDICATIONS/ROUTES/DOSAGE

PREPUBERTAL CRYPTORCHIDISM, HYPOGONADOTROPIC HYPOGONADISM

IM: CHILDREN: Dosage is individualized based on indication, age, weight of pt, and physician preference.

INDUCTION OF OVULATION

IM: ADULTS (AFTER PRETREATMENT WITH MENOTROPINS): 5,000–10,000 international units 1 day after last dose of menotropins.

SIDE EFFECTS

FREQUENT: Pain at injection site. **Induction of ovulation:** Ovarian cysts, uncomplicated ovarian enlargement. **OCCASIONAL:** Enlarged breasts, headache, irritability, fatigue, depression. **Induction of ovulation:** Severe ovarian hyperstimulation, peripheral edema. **Cryptorchidism:** Precocious puberty (acne, deepening voice, penile growth, pubic/axillary hair).

ADVERSE EFFECTS/ TOXIC REACTIONS

When used with menotropins: increased risk of arterial thromboembolism, ovarian hyperstimulation with high incidence (20%) of multiple births (premature deliveries and neonatal prematurity), ruptured ovarian cysts.

NURSING CONSIDERATIONS

BASELINE ASSESSMENT

Obtain baseline weight, B/P.

INTERVENTION/EVALUATION

Assess for edema: weigh every 2–3 days, report weight gain greater than 5 lb/wk; monitor B/P periodically during treatment; check for decreased urinary output, peripheral edema.

PATIENT/FAMILY TEACHING

• Promptly report abdominal pain, vaginal bleeding, signs of precocious puberty in males (deepening of voice; axillary, facial, pubic hair; acne; penile growth), signs of edema. • In anovulation treatment, begin recording daily basal temperature; initiate intercourse daily beginning the day preceding human chorionic gonadotropin (hCG) treatment. • Possibility of multiple births.

ciclopirox

(Loprox, Penlac)

See Antifungals: topical (p. 46C)

cidofovir

ci-**dah**-fo-veer

(Vistide)

CLASSIFICATION

PHARMACOTHERAPEUTIC: Anti-infective. **CLINICAL:** Antiviral (see p. 64C).

ACTION

Inhibits viral DNA synthesis by incorporating itself into growing viral DNA chain.

Therapeutic Effect: Suppresses replication of cytomegalovirus (CMV).

PHARMACOKINETICS

Protein binding: less than 6%. Excreted primarily unchanged in urine. Effect of hemodialysis unknown. **Elimination half-life:** 1.4–3.8 hrs.

USES

Treatment of CMV retinitis in those with acquired immunodeficiency syndrome (AIDS). Should be given with Probenecid. **OFF-LABEL:** Treatment of acyclovir-resistant herpes simplex virus, adenovirus, foscarnet-resistant CMV, ganciclovir-resistant CMV, varicella-zoster virus.

PRECAUTIONS

CONTRAINDICATIONS: Direct intraocular injection, history of clinically severe hypersensitivity to probenecid or other sulfa-containing drugs, renal impairment (serum creatinine level greater than 1.5 mg/dl, creatinine clearance 55 ml/min or less, or urine protein level greater than 100 mg/dl). **CAUTION:** Preexisting diabetes.

LIFESPAN CONSIDERATIONS:

Pregnancy/Lactation: Embryotoxic (reduced fetal body weight) in animals. Unknown if excreted in breast milk. Do not administer to breast-feeding women. HIV-infected women should not breast-feed. **Pregnancy Category C. Children:** Safety and efficacy not established. **Elderly:** Age-related renal impairment may require dosage adjustment.

INTERACTIONS

DRUG: **Nephrotoxic medications (e.g., aminoglycosides, amphotericin B, foscarnet, IV pentamidine)** increase risk of nephrotoxicity. **HERBAL:** None significant. **FOOD:** None known. **LAB VALUES:** May decrease neutrophil count serum bicarbonate, phosphate, uric acid. May elevate serum creatinine.

AVAILABILITY (Rx)

INJECTION SOLUTION: 75 mg/ml (5-ml ampule).

ADMINISTRATION/HANDLING

◄ ALERT ► Do not exceed recommended dosage, frequency, infusion rate.

IV

Reconstitution • Dilute in 100 ml 0.9% NaCl.

Rate of administration • Infuse over 1 hr. • IV hydration with 0.9% NaCl and probenecid therapy **must** be used with each cidofovir infusion (minimizes risk of nephrotoxicity). • Ingestion of food before each dose of probenecid may reduce nausea/vomiting. Antiemetic may reduce potential for nausea.

Storage • Store at controlled room temperature (68°–77°F). • Admixtures may be refrigerated for no more than 24 hrs. • Allow refrigerated admixtures to warm to room temperature before use.

IV INCOMPATIBILITIES

No information available for Y-site administration.

INDICATIONS/ROUTES/DOSAGE

CMV RETINITIS IN PTS WITH AIDS (IN COMBINATION WITH PROBENECID)

IV INFUSION: ADULTS, CHILDREN: Induction: Usual dosage, 5 mg/kg at constant rate over 1 hr once weekly for 2 consecutive wks. Give 2 g of PO probenecid 3 hrs before cidofovir dose, then give 1 g 2 hrs and 8 hrs after completion of the 1-hr cidofovir infusion (total of 4 g). In addition, give 1 L of 0.9% NaCl over 1–2 hrs immediately before cidofovir infusion. If tolerated, a second liter may be infused over 1–3 hrs at start of infusion or immediately afterward. **Maintenance: ADULTS, ELDERLY:** 5 mg/kg once every 2 wks. **CHILDREN:** 3 mg/kg once every 2 wks.

C

DOSAGE IN RENAL IMPAIRMENT

Changes During Therapy: If creatinine increases by 0.3–0.4 mg/dl, reduce dose to 3 mg/kg; if creatinine increases by 0.5 mg/dl or greater or development of 3+ or greater proteinuria, discontinue therapy.

Preexisting Renal Impairment: Do not use with serum creatinine greater than 1.5 mg/dl, creatinine clearance less than 55 ml/min, or urine protein 100 mg/dl or greater (2+ or greater proteinuria).

SIDE EFFECTS

FREQUENT: Nausea, vomiting (65%), fever (57%), asthenia (46%), rash (30%), diarrhea (27%), headache (27%), alopecia (25%), chills (24%), anorexia (22%), dyspnea (22%), abdominal pain (17%).

ADVERSE EFFECTS/ TOXIC REACTIONS

Serious adverse effects include proteinuria (80%), nephrotoxicity (53%), neutropenia (31%), elevated serum creatinine (29%), infection (24%), anemia (20%), decrease in intraocular pressure (12%), pneumonia (9%). Concurrent use of probenecid may produce a hypersensitivity reaction characterized by rash, fever, chills, anaphylaxis. Acute renal failure occurs rarely.

NURSING CONSIDERATIONS

BASELINE ASSESSMENT

For those taking zidovudine, temporarily discontinue zidovudine administration or decrease zidovudine dose by 50% on days of infusion (probenecid reduces metabolic clearance of zidovudine). Closely monitor renal function (urinalysis, serum creatinine) during therapy.

INTERVENTION/EVALUATION

Monitor serum creatinine, WBC count, urine protein before each dose. Monitor for proteinuria (may be early indicator of dose-dependent nephrotoxicity). Periodically monitor visual acuity, ocular symptoms.

PATIENT/FAMILY TEACHING

• Obtain regular follow-up ophthalmologic exams. • Those of childbearing age should use effective contraception during and for 1 mo after treatment. • Men should practice barrier contraceptive methods during and for 3 mos after treatment. • Do not breast-feed. • Must complete full course of probenecid with each cidofovir dose.

cilostazol

sill-oh-**stay**-zole

(Pletal)

Do not confuse Pletal with Plendil.

CLASSIFICATION

PHARMACOTHERAPEUTIC: Phosphodiesterase III inhibitor. **CLINICAL:** Antiplatelet.

ACTION

Inhibits platelet aggregation. Dilates vascular beds with greatest dilation in femoral beds. **Therapeutic Effect:** Improves walking distance in those with intermittent claudication; usually noted in 2–4 wks but may take as long as 12 wks.

PHARMACOKINETICS

Moderately absorbed from GI tract. Protein binding: 95%–98%. Extensively metabolized in the liver. Excreted primarily in the urine and, to a lesser extent, in the feces. Not removed by hemodialysis. **Half-life:** 11–13 hrs.

USES

Management of peripheral vascular disease, primarily intermittent claudication.

OFF-LABEL: Treatment of acute coronary syndrome, graft patency improvement in percutaneous coronary intervention with/without stenting.

PRECAUTIONS

CONTRAINDICATIONS: CHF of any severity; hemostatic disorders or active pathologic bleeding (bleeding peptic ulcer, intracranial bleeding). **CAUTIONS:** None known.

⌛ LIFESPAN CONSIDERATIONS:

Pregnancy/Lactation: Unknown if drug crosses placenta or is distributed in breast milk. **Pregnancy Category C.** **Children:** Safety and efficacy not established. **Elderly:** No age-related precautions noted.

INTERACTIONS

DRUG: **Aspirin** may potentiate inhibition of platelet aggregation. **Clarithromycin, diltiazem, erythromycin, fluconazole, fluoxetine, omeprazole, sertraline** may increase concentration. **HERBAL:** None significant. **FOOD:** **Grapefruit, grapefruit juice** may increase blood concentration, toxicity. **LAB VALUES:** May increase BUN, serum creatinine. May decrease Hgb, Hct.

AVAILABILITY (Rx)

TABLETS: 50 mg, 100 mg.

ADMINISTRATION/HANDLING

PO

• Give at least 30 min before or 2 hrs after meals. • Do not take with grapefruit juice.

INDICATIONS/ROUTES/DOSAGE

PERIPHERAL VASCULAR DISEASE

PO: ADULTS, ELDERLY: 100 mg twice a day at least 30 min before or 2 hrs after meals. 50 mg twice a day during concurrent therapy with CYP3A4 or CYP2C19 (e.g., clarithromycin, diltiazem, erythromycin, fluconazole, fluoxetine, omeprazole, sertraline).

SIDE EFFECTS

FREQUENT (34%–10%): Headache, diarrhea, palpitations, dizziness, pharyngitis. **OCCASIONAL (7%–3%):** Nausea, rhinitis, back pain, peripheral edema, dyspepsia, abdominal pain, tachycardia, cough, flatulence, myalgia. **RARE (2%–1%):** Leg cramps, paresthesia, rash, vomiting.

ADVERSE EFFECTS/ TOXIC REACTIONS

Overdose noted as severe headache, diarrhea, hypotension, cardiac arrhythmias.

NURSING CONSIDERATIONS

BASELINE ASSESSMENT

Assess platelet count, Hgb, Hct before treatment and periodically during treatment.

PATIENT/FAMILY TEACHING

• Take on an empty stomach (at least 30 min before or 2 hrs after meals). • Do not take with grapefruit juice.

Ciloxan, *see ciprofloxacin*

cimetidine

sih-**met**-ih-deen

(Apo-Cimetidine ♣, Tagamet, Tagamet HB 200)

Do not confuse cimetidine with simethicone.

CLASSIFICATION

PHARMACOTHERAPEUTIC: H_2 receptor antagonist. **CLINICAL:** Antiulcer, gastric acid secretion inhibitor (see p. 103C).

C

ACTION

Inhibits histamine action at histamine 2 (H_2) receptor sites of parietal cells. **Therapeutic Effect:** Inhibits gastric acid secretion during fasting, at night, or when stimulated by food, caffeine, insulin.

PHARMACOKINETICS

Well absorbed from GI tract. Protein binding: 15%–20%. Widely distributed. Metabolized in the liver. Primarily excreted in urine. Not removed by hemodialysis. **Half-life:** 2 hrs; increased with renal impairment.

USES

Short-term treatment of active duodenal ulcer. Prevention of duodenal ulcer recurrence, upper GI bleeding in critically ill pts. Treatment of benign gastric ulcer, pathologic GI hypersecretory conditions, gastroesophageal reflux disease (GERD). **OTC use:** Heartburn, acid indigestion, sour stomach. **OFF-LABEL:** Prevention of aspiration pneumonia; treatment of acute urticaria, chronic warts, upper GI bleeding; *H. pylori* eradication.

PRECAUTIONS

CONTRAINDICATIONS: Hypersensitivity to other H_2-antagonists. **CAUTIONS:** Renal/hepatic impairment, elderly. Cimetidine may interfere with skin tests.

LIFESPAN CONSIDERATIONS:

Pregnancy/Lactation: Crosses placenta. Distributed in breast milk. In infants, may suppress gastric acidity, inhibit drug metabolism, produce CNS stimulation. **Pregnancy Category B. Children:** Long-term use may induce cerebral toxicity, affect hormonal system. **Elderly:** More likely to experience confusion, esp. in pts with renal impairment.

INTERACTIONS

DRUG: Antacids may decrease absorption. May increase concentration, decrease metabolism of **calcium channel blockers, cyclosporine, lidocaine, metoprolol, metronidazole, oral anticoagulants, oral hypoglycemics, phenytoin, propranolol, theophylline, tricyclic antidepressants.** May decrease absorption of **ketoconazole. HERBAL: St. John's wort** may decrease concentration. **FOOD:** None known. **LAB VALUES:** Interferes with skin tests using allergen extracts. May increase serum prolactin, creatinine, transaminase. May decrease parathyroid hormone concentration.

AVAILABILITY (Rx)

INJECTION, SOLUTION: 150 mg/ml. **LIQUID, ORAL:** 300 mg/5 mL. **TABLETS:** 200 mg (OTC), 300 mg, 400 mg, 800 mg.

ADMINISTRATION/HANDLING

IV

Reconstitution • Dilute each 300 mg (2 ml) with 18 ml 0.9% NaCl, 0.45% NaCl, 0.2% NaCl, D_5W, $D_{10}W$, Ringer's solution, or lactated Ringer's to a total volume of 20 ml.

Rate of administration • For IV push, administer over not less than 2 min (prevents arrhythmias, hypotension). • For intermittent IV (piggyback), infuse over 15–20 min. • For IV infusion, dilute with 100–1,000 ml 0.9% NaCl, D_5W, or other compatible solution (see Reconstitution) and infuse over 24 hrs.

Storage • Store at room temperature. • Reconstituted drug is stable for 48 hrs at room temperature.

IM

• Administer undiluted. • Inject deep into large muscle mass.

PO

• Give without regard to food. Best given with meals and at bedtime. • Do not administer within 1 hr of antacids.

IV INCOMPATIBILITIES

Allopurinol (Aloprim), amphotericin B complex (Abelcet, AmBisome, Amphotec), cefepime (Maxipime).

IV COMPATIBILITIES

Aminophylline, diltiazem (Cardizem), furosemide (Lasix), heparin, hydromorphone (Dilaudid), insulin (regular), lidocaine, lipids, lorazepam (Ativan), midazolam (Versed), morphine, potassium chloride, propofol (Diprivan).

INDICATIONS/ROUTES/DOSAGE

ACTIVE DUODENAL ULCER

PO: ADULTS, ELDERLY: 300 mg 4 times a day or 400 mg twice a day or 800 mg at bedtime for up to 8 wks.

IV, IM: ADULTS, ELDERLY: 300 mg q6h or 150 mg as single dose followed by 37.5 mg/hr continuous infusion.

PREVENTION OF DUODENAL ULCER

PO: ADULTS, ELDERLY: 400–800 mg at bedtime.

GASTRIC HYPERSECRETORY SECRETIONS

PO, IV, IM: ADULTS, ELDERLY: 300–600 mg q6h. **Maximum:** 2,400 mg/day.

GASTROESOPHAGEAL REFLUX DISEASE

PO: ADULTS, ELDERLY: 800 mg twice a day or 400 mg 4 times a day for 12 wks.

OTC USE

PO: ADULTS, ELDERLY: 100 mg up to 30 min before meals. **Maximum:** 2 doses/day.

PREVENTION OF UPPER GI BLEEDING

IV INFUSION: ADULTS, ELDERLY: 50 mg/hr.

USUAL PEDIATRIC DOSE

CHILDREN: 20–40 mg/kg/day in divided doses q6h. **INFANTS:** 10–20 mg/kg/day in divided doses q6–12h. **NEONATES:** 5–10 mg/kg/day in divided doses q8–12h.

DOSAGE IN RENAL IMPAIRMENT

Dosage is based on a 300-mg dose in adults. Dosage interval is modified based on creatinine clearance.

Creatinine Clearance	Dosage Interval
Greater than 40 ml/min	q6h
20–40 ml/min	q8h or decrease dose by 25%
Less than 20 ml/min	q12h or decrease dose by 50%

Give after hemodialysis and q12h between dialysis sessions.

SIDE EFFECTS

OCCASIONAL (4%–2%): Headache. **Elderly, severely ill pts, pts with renal impairment:** Confusion, agitation, psychosis, depression, anxiety, disorientation, hallucinations. Effects reverse 3–4 days after discontinuance. **RARE (less than 2%):** Diarrhea, dizziness, somnolence, nausea, vomiting, gynecomastia, rash, impotence.

ADVERSE EFFECTS/ TOXIC REACTIONS

Rapid IV administration may produce cardiac arrhythmias, hypotension.

NURSING CONSIDERATIONS

BASELINE ASSESSMENT

Do not administer antacids concurrently (separate by 1 hr).

INTERVENTION/EVALUATION

Monitor B/P for hypotension during IV infusion. Assess for GI bleeding: hematemesis, blood in stool. Check mental status in elderly, severely ill, those with renal impairment.

PATIENT/FAMILY TEACHING

• May produce transient discomfort at IM injection site. • Do not take antacids within 1 hr of cimetidine administration. • Avoid tasks that require alertness,

C

motor skills until drug response is established. • Avoid smoking. • Report any blood in vomitus/stool, or dark, tarry stool.

cinacalcet

sin-ah-**kal**-set
(Sensipar)

CLASSIFICATION

PHARMACOTHERAPEUTIC: Calcium receptor agonist. **CLINICAL:** Calcimimetic.

ACTION

Increases sensitivity of calcium-sensing receptor on parathyroid gland to activation by extracellular calcium, thus lowering parathyroid hormone (PTH) levels. **Therapeutic Effect:** Decreases serum calcium, PTH levels.

PHARMACOKINETICS

Extensively distributed after PO administration. Protein binding: 93%–97%. Rapidly, extensively metabolized by multiple enzymes. Primarily eliminated in urine with a lesser amount excreted in feces. **Half-life:** 30–40 hrs.

USES

Treatment of hypercalcemia in pts with parathyroid carcinoma. Treatment of secondary hyperparathyroidism in pts on dialysis with chronic renal disease. **OFF-LABEL:** Primary hyperthyroidism.

PRECAUTIONS

CONTRAINDICATIONS: None known. **CAUTIONS:** Hepatic impairment.

LIFESPAN CONSIDERATIONS:

Pregnancy/Lactation: May cross placental barrier; unknown if distributed in breast milk. Safe usage during lactation not established (potential adverse reaction in infants). **Pregnancy Category C. Children:** Safety and efficacy not established. **Elderly:** No age-related precautions noted.

INTERACTIONS

DRUG: Increases **amitriptyline** plasma concentration. **Erythromycin, itraconazole, ketoconazole** increase plasma concentration. Concurrent administration of **flecainide, thioridazine, tricyclic antidepressants, vinblastine** may require dosage adjustment. **HERBAL:** None significant. **FOOD: High-fat meals** increase plasma concentration. **LAB VALUES:** Reduces serum calcium level.

AVAILABILITY (Rx)

TABLETS: 30 mg, 60 mg, 90 mg.

ADMINISTRATION/HANDLING

PO

• Store at room temperature. • Do not break/crush film-coated tablets. • Administer with food or shortly after a meal.

INDICATIONS/ROUTES/DOSAGE

HYPERCALCEMIA IN PARATHYROID CARCINOMA

PO: ADULTS, ELDERLY: Initially, 30 mg twice a day. Titrate dosage sequentially (60 mg twice a day, 90 mg twice a day, and 90 mg 3–4 times a day) every 2–4 wks as needed to normalize serum calcium level.

SECONDARY HYPERPARATHYROIDISM IN PTS ON DIALYSIS

PO: ADULTS, ELDERLY: Initially, 30 mg once a day. Titrate dosage sequentially (60, 90, 120, and 180 mg once a day) every 2–4 wks.

SIDE EFFECTS

FREQUENT (31%–21%): Nausea, vomiting, diarrhea. **OCCASIONAL (15%–10%):** Myalgia, dizziness. **RARE (7%–5%):** Asthenia, hypertension, anorexia, non-cardiac chest pain.

ADVERSE EFFECTS/ TOXIC REACTIONS

Overdose may lead to hypocalcemia.

NURSING CONSIDERATIONS

BASELINE ASSESSMENT

Establish baseline serum electrolyte levels.

INTERVENTION/EVALUATION

Monitor serum calcium. Monitor daily pattern of bowel activity/stool consistency. Obtain order for antidiarrhea, antiemetic medication to prevent serum electrolyte imbalance. Assess for evidence of dizziness, institute fall risk precautions.

PATIENT/FAMILY TEACHING

• Instruct pt to take cinacalcet with food or shortly after a meal. • Notify physician or nurse immediately if vomiting, diarrhea occur.

Cipro, *see ciprofloxacin*

Cipro IV, *see ciprofloxacin*

ciprofloxacin

sip-row-**flocks**-ah-sin

(Ciloxan, Cipro, Cipro I.V., Cipro XR, Proquin XR)

Do not confuse ciprofloxacin with cephalexin, Ciloxan with Cytoxan, Cipro with Ceftin.

FIXED-COMBINATION(S)

Cipro HC Otic: ciprofloxacin/ hydrocortisone (a steroid): 0.2%/ 1%. **CiproDex Otic:** ciprofloxacin/ dexamethasone (a corticosteroid): 0.3%/0.1%.

CLASSIFICATION

PHARMACOTHERAPEUTIC: Fluoroquinolone. **CLINICAL:** Anti-infective (see p. 24C).

ACTION

Inhibits enzyme, DNA gyrase, in susceptible bacteria, interfering with bacterial cell replication. **Therapeutic Effect:** Bactericidal.

PHARMACOKINETICS

Well absorbed from GI tract (food delays absorption). Protein binding: 20%–40%. Widely distributed (including to cerebrospinal fluid [CSF]). Metabolized in the liver to active metabolite. Primarily excreted in urine. Minimal removal by hemodialysis. **Half-life:** 4–6 hrs (increased in renal impairment, elderly).

USES

Treatment of susceptible infections due to *E. coli, K. pneumoniae, E. cloacae, P. mirabilis, P. vulgaris, P. aeruginosa, H. influenzae, M. catarrhalis, S. pneumoniae, S. aureus* (methicillin susceptible), *S. epidermidis, S. pyogenes, C. jejuni,* Shigella species, *S. typhi* including intra-abdominal, bone, joint, lower respiratory tract, skin/skin structure, UTIs, infectious diarrhea, prostatitis, sinusitis, typhoid fever, febrile neutropenia. **OFF-LABEL:** Treatment of chancroid. Acute pulmonary exacerbations in cystic fibrosis, disseminated gonococcal infections, prophylaxis to *Neisseria meninigitidis* following close contact with infected person.

PRECAUTIONS

CONTRAINDICATIONS: Hypersensitivity to ciprofloxacin, other quinolones; for ophthalmic administration: vaccinia, varicella, epithelial herpes simplex, keratitis, mycobacterial infection, fungal disease of ocular structure, use after uncomplicated removal of foreign body. **CAUTIONS:** Renal impairment, CNS disorders, seizures, those taking theophylline, caffeine. Suspension not for use in NG tube.

LIFESPAN CONSIDERATIONS:

Pregnancy/Lactation: Unknown if distributed in breast milk. If possible, do not use during pregnancy/lactation (risk of arthropathy to fetus/infant). **Pregnancy Category C. Children:** Safety and efficacy not established in those younger than 18 yrs. Arthropathy may occur if given to children younger than 18 yrs. **Elderly:** Age-related renal impairment may require dosage adjustment.

INTERACTIONS

DRUG: **Antacids, iron preparations, sucralfate** may decrease absorption. May increase effects of **caffeine, oral anticoagulants.** May decrease concentration of **phenytoin, fosphenytoin.** May increase concentration, toxicity of **theophylline.** Decreases **theophylline** clearance. **HERBAL:** **Dong quai, St. John's wort** may increase photosensitization. **FOOD:** None known. **LAB VALUES:** May increase serum alkaline phosphatase, bilirubin, BUN, creatinine, LDH, AST, ALT.

AVAILABILITY (Rx)

INJECTION, SOLUTION (CIPRO): 100 mg/ml. **OPHTHALMIC OINTMENT (CILOXAN):** 0.3%. **OPHTHALMIC SOLUTION (CILOXAN):** 0.3%. **ORAL SUSPENSION (CIPRO):** 250 mg/5 ml, 500 mg/5 ml. **TABLET (CIPRO):** 100 mg, 250 mg, 500 mg, 750 mg.

TABLET (EXTENDED-RELEASE) (CIPRO XR, PROQUIN XR): 500 mg.

ADMINISTRATION/HANDLING

IV

Reconstitution • Available prediluted in infusion container ready for use.

Rate of administration • Infuse over 60 min.

Storage • Store at room temperature. • Solution appears clear, colorless to slightly yellow.

PO

• May be given without regard to food (preferred dosing time: 2 hrs after meals). • Do not administer antacids (aluminum, magnesium) within 2 hrs of ciprofloxacin. • Encourage cranberry juice, citrus fruits (acidifies urine). • Suspension may be stored for 14 days at room temperature.

OPHTHALMIC

• Tilt pt's head back; place solution in conjunctival sac. • Instruct pt to close eyes and press gently on lacrimal sac at inner canthus for 1 min (reduces systemic absorption). • Do not use ophthalmic solution for injection.

IV INCOMPATIBILITIES

Aminophylline, ampicillin and sulbactam (Unasyn), cefepime (Maxipime), dexamethasone (Decadron), furosemide (Lasix), heparin, hydrocortisone (Solu-Cortef), methylprednisolone (Solu-Medrol), phenytoin (Dilantin), sodium bicarbonate, total parenteral nutrition (TPN).

IV COMPATIBILITIES

Calcium gluconate, diltiazem (Cardizem), dobutamine (Dobutrex), dopamine (Intropin), lidocaine, lipids, lorazepam (Ativan), magnesium, midazolam (Versed), potassium chloride.

INDICATIONS/ROUTES/DOSAGE

BONE, JOINT INFECTIONS

IV: ADULTS, ELDERLY: 400 mg q8–12h for 4–6 wks.

PO: ADULTS, ELDERLY: 500 mg q12h for 4–6 wks.

CONJUNCTIVITIS

OPHTHALMIC: ADULTS, ELDERLY: 1–2 drops q2h for 2 days, then 2 drops q4h for next 5 days.

C

CORNEAL ULCER
OPHTHALMIC: ADULTS, ELDERLY: 2 drops q15min for 6 hrs, then 2 drops q30min for the remainder of first day, 2 drops q1h on second day, and 2 drops q4h on days 3–14.

CYSTIC FIBROSIS
IV: CHILDREN: 40 mg/kg/day in 2–3 divided doses. **Maximum:** 1.2 g/day.
PO: CHILDREN: 40 mg/kg/day. **Maximum:** 2 g/day.

FEBRILE NEUTROPENIA
IV: ADULTS, ELDERLY: 400 mg q8h for 7–14 days (in combination).

GONORRHEA
PO: ADULTS, ELDERLY: 250–500 mg as a single dose.

INFECTIOUS DIARRHEA
PO: ADULTS, ELDERLY: 500 mg q12h for 5–7 days.

INTRA-ABDOMINAL INFECTIONS (WITH METRONIDAZOLE)
IV: ADULTS, ELDERLY: 400 mg q12h for 7–14 days.
PO: ADULTS, ELDERLY: 500 mg q12h for 7–14 days.

LOWER RESPIRATORY TRACT INFECTIONS
IV: ADULTS, ELDERLY: 400 mg q12h for 7–14 days.
PO: ADULTS, ELDERLY: 500–750 mg q12h for 7–14 days.

NOSOCOMIAL PNEUMONIA
IV: ADULTS, ELDERLY: 400 mg q8h for 10–14 days.

PROSTATITIS
IV: ADULTS, ELDERLY: 400 mg q12h for 28 days.
PO: ADULTS, ELDERLY: 500 mg q12h for 28 days.

SINUSITIS
IV: ADULTS, ELDERLY: 400 mg q12h for 10 days.
PO: ADULTS, ELDERLY: 500 mg q12h for 10 days.

SKIN/SKIN STRUCTURE INFECTIONS
IV: ADULTS, ELDERLY: 400 mg q12h for 7–14 days.
PO: ADULTS, ELDERLY: 500–750 mg q12h for 7–14 days.

SUSCEPTIBLE INFECTIONS
IV: ADULTS, ELDERLY: 400 mg q8–12h.
PO: ADULTS, ELDERLY: 500–750 mg q12h.

TYPHOID FEVER
PO: ADULTS, ELDERLY: 500 mg q12h for 10 days.

UTIs
IV: ADULTS, ELDERLY: 200–400 mg q12h for 7–14 days.
PO: ADULTS, ELDERLY: Immediate Release: 100–250 mg q12h for 3 days for acute uncomplicated infections; 250 mg q12h for 7–14 days for mild to moderate infections; 500 mg q12h for 7–14 days for severe or complicated infections. **Extended Release:** 1,000 mg q24h for 7–14 days.

DOSAGE IN RENAL IMPAIRMENT
Dosage and frequency are modified based on creatinine clearance and the severity of the infection.

Creatinine Clearance	Dosage Interval
Less than 30 ml/min	Usual dose q18–24h

HEMODIALYSIS
ADULTS, ELDERLY: 250–500 mg q24h (after dialysis).

PERITONEAL DIALYSIS
ADULTS, ELDERLY: 250–500 mg q24h (after dialysis).

SIDE EFFECTS

FREQUENT (5%–2%): Nausea, diarrhea, dyspepsia, vomiting, constipation, flatulence, confusion, crystalluria. **Ophthalmic:** Burning, crusting in corner of eye.
OCCASIONAL (less than 2%): Abdominal pain/discomfort, headache, rash.

C

Ophthalmic: Bad taste, sensation of foreign body in eye, eyelid redness, itching. **RARE (less than 1%):** Dizziness, confusion, tremors, hallucinations, hypersensitivity reaction, insomnia, dry mouth, paresthesia.

ADVERSE EFFECTS/ TOXIC REACTIONS

Superinfection (esp. enterococcal, fungal), nephropathy, cardiopulmonary arrest, cerebral thrombosis may occur. Hypersensitivity reaction, (rash, pruritus, blisters, edema, burning skin), photosensitivity have occurred. Sensitization to ophthalmic form may contraindicate later systemic use of ciprofloxacin.

NURSING CONSIDERATIONS

BASELINE ASSESSMENT

Question for history of hypersensitivity to ciprofloxacin, quinolones.

INTERVENTION/EVALUATION

Evaluate food tolerance. Monitor daily pattern of bowel activity/stool consistency. Monitor for dizziness, headache, visual changes, tremors. Assess for chest, joint pain. **Ophthalmic:** Observe therapeutic response.

PATIENT/FAMILY TEACHING

• Do not skip doses; take full course of therapy. • Take with 8 oz water; drink several glasses of water between meals. • Eat, drink high sources of ascorbic acid (cranberry juice, citrus fruits) to prevent crystalluria. • Do not take antacids (reduces/destroys effectiveness). • Shake suspension well before using; do not chew microcapsules in suspension. • Sugarless gum, hard candy may relieve bad taste. • **Ophthalmic:** Explain possibility of crystal precipitate forming, usual resolution in 1–7 days.

cisatracurium

(Nimbex)

See Neuromuscular blockers (p. 119C)

cisplatin

sis-**plah**-tin

(Platinol-AQ)

Do not confuse cisplatin with carboplatin, or Platinol with Paraplatin or Patanol.

CLASSIFICATION

PHARMACOTHERAPEUTIC: Platinum coordination complex. **CLINICAL:** Antineoplastic (see p. 77C).

ACTION

Inhibits DNA and, to a lesser extent, RNA protein synthesis by cross-linking with DNA strands. Cell cycle–phase nonspecific. **Therapeutic Effect:** Prevents cellular division.

PHARMACOKINETICS

Widely distributed. Protein binding: greater than 90%. Undergoes rapid nonenzymatic conversion to inactive metabolite. Excreted in urine. Removed by hemodialysis. **Half-life:** 58–73 hrs (increased with renal impairment).

USES

Treatment of metastatic testicular tumors, metastatic ovarian tumors, advanced bladder carcinoma. **OFF-LABEL:** Adrenocortical, anal, biliary tract, breast, cervical, endometrial, esophageal, gastric, head and neck, lung (small cell, non–small cell), primary hepatocellular, prostatic skin, thyroid, vulvar carcinomas; germ cell, gestational trophoblastic, ovarian germ cell tumors; Hodgkin's and non-Hodgkin's lymphomas; Kaposi's sarcoma, malignant melanoma, neuroblastoma, osteosarcoma, soft tissue sarcoma, Wilm's tumor.

PRECAUTIONS

CONTRAINDICATIONS: Hearing impairment, myelosuppression, preexisting renal impairment. **CAUTIONS:** Previous therapy with other antineoplastic agents, radiation.

LIFESPAN CONSIDERATIONS:

Pregnancy/Lactation: If possible, avoid use during pregnancy, esp. first trimester. Breast-feeding not recommended. **Pregnancy Category D. Children:** Ototoxic effects may be more severe. **Elderly:** Age-related renal impairment may require dosage adjustment.

INTERACTIONS

DRUG: May decrease effects of **antigout medications. Bone marrow depressants** may increase myelosuppression. **Live virus vaccines** may potentiate virus replication, increase vaccine side effects, decrease pt's antibody response to vaccine. **Nephrotoxic, ototoxic agents** may increase risk of toxicity. **HERBAL:** Avoid **black cohosh, dong quai** with estrogen-dependent tumors. **FOOD:** None known. **LAB VALUES:** May increase BUN, serum creatinine, uric acid, AST. May decrease creatinine clearance, serum calcium, magnesium, phosphate, potassium, sodium. May cause positive Coombs' test.

AVAILABILITY (Rx)

INJECTION SOLUTION: 1 mg/ml.

ADMINISTRATION/HANDLING

◄ ALERT ► Wear protective gloves during handling of cisplatin. May be carcinogenic, mutagenic, teratogenic. Handle with extreme care during preparation/administration.

IV

Reconstitution • For IV infusion, dilute desired dose in up to 1,000 ml D_5W, 0.33% or 0.45% NaCl containing 12.5–50 g mannitol/L.

Rate of administration • Infuse over 2–24 hrs. • Avoid rapid infusion (increases risk of nephrotoxicity, ototoxicity). • Monitor for anaphylactic reaction during first few minutes of IV infusion.

Storage • Protect from sunlight; do not refrigerate (may precipitate). Discard if precipitate forms. Stable for 20 hrs at room temperature.

IV INCOMPATIBILITIES

Amifostine (Ethyol), amphotericin B complex (Abelcet, AmBisome, Amphotec), cefepime (Maxipime), piperacillin and tazobactam (Zosyn), sodium bicarbonate, thiotepa.

IV COMPATIBILITIES

Etoposide (VePesid), granisetron (Kytril), heparin, hydromorphone (Dilaudid), lipids, lorazepam (Ativan), magnesium sulfate, mannitol, morphine, ondansetron (Zofran).

INDICATIONS/ROUTES/DOSAGE

BLADDER CARCINOMA

IV: ADULTS, ELDERLY: (Single agent): 50–70 mg/m^2 q3–4wks.

OVARIAN TUMORS

IV: ADULTS, ELDERLY: 75–100 mg/m^2 q3–4wks.

TESTICULAR TUMORS

IV: ADULTS, ELDERLY: 10–20 mg/m^2 daily for 5 days repeated q3–4wks.

DOSAGE IN RENAL IMPAIRMENT

Dosage is modified based on creatinine clearance.

C

Creatinine Clearance	% of Dose
10–50 ml/min	75%
Less than 10 ml/min	50%

SIDE EFFECTS

FREQUENT: Nausea, vomiting (generally beginning 1–4 hrs after administration and lasting up to 24 hrs); myelosuppression (affecting 25%–30% of pts, with recovery generally occurring in 18–23 days). **OCCASIONAL:** Peripheral neuropathy (with prolonged therapy [4–7 mos]). Pain/redness at injection site, loss of taste, appetite. **RARE:** Hemolytic anemia, blurred vision, stomatitis.

ADVERSE EFFECTS/ TOXIC REACTIONS

Anaphylactic reaction (angioedema, wheezing, tachycardia, hypotension) may occur in first few minutes of IV administration in those previously exposed to cisplatin. Nephrotoxicity occurs in 28%–36% of pts treated with single dose of cisplatin, usually during second week of therapy. Ototoxicity, (tinnitus, hearing loss) occurs in 31% of pts treated with single dose of cisplatin (more severe in children). May become more frequent, severe with repeated doses.

NURSING CONSIDERATIONS

BASELINE ASSESSMENT

Pts should be well hydrated before and 24 hrs after medication to ensure good urinary output, decrease risk of nephrotoxicity.

INTERVENTION/EVALUATION

Measure all vomitus (general guideline requiring immediate notification of physician: 750 ml/8 hrs, urinary output less than 100 ml/hr). Monitor I&O q1–2h beginning with pretreatment hydration, continue for 48 hrs after cisplatin therapy. Assess vital signs q1–2h during infusion. Monitor urinalysis, renal function tests for nephrotoxicity.

PATIENT/FAMILY TEACHING

• Report signs of ototoxicity (tinnitus, hearing loss). • Do not have immunizations without physician's approval (lowers body's resistance). • Avoid contact with those who have recently taken oral polio vaccine. • Contact physician if nausea/vomiting continues at home. • Teach signs of peripheral neuropathy.

citalopram

sigh-**tail**-oh-pram

(Apo-Citalopram ✱, Celexa, Novo-Citalopram ✱)

Do not confuse Celexa with Celebrex, Zyprexa, or Cerebyx.

CLASSIFICATION

PHARMACOTHERAPEUTIC: Serotonin reuptake inhibitor. **CLINICAL:** Antidepressant (see p. 37C).

ACTION

Blocks uptake of the neurotransmitter serotonin at CNS presynaptic neuronal membranes, increasing its availability at postsynaptic receptor sites. **Therapeutic Effect:** Relieves depression.

PHARMACOKINETICS

Well absorbed after PO administration. Protein binding: 80%. Primarily metabolized in the liver. Primarily excreted in feces with a lesser amount eliminated in urine. **Half-life:** 35 hrs.

USES

Treatment of depression. **OFF-LABEL:** Treatment of alcohol abuse, dementia, diabetic neuropathy, obsessive-compulsive disorder, panic disorder, smoking cessation.

C

PRECAUTIONS

CONTRAINDICATIONS: Sensitivity to citalopram, use within 14 days of MAOIs. **CAUTIONS:** Hepatic/renal impairment, history of seizures, mania, hypomania.

LIFESPAN CONSIDERATIONS:

Pregnancy/Lactation: Distributed in breast milk. **Pregnancy Category C.** **Children:** May cause increased anticholinergic effects, hyperexcitability. **Elderly:** More sensitive to anticholinergic effects (e.g., dry mouth), more likely to experience dizziness, sedation, confusion, hypotension, hyperexcitability.

INTERACTIONS

DRUG: **Antifungals, cimetidine, macrolide antibiotics** may increase plasma level. **Carbamazepine** may decrease plasma level. **MAOIs** may cause serotonin syndrome (excitement, diaphoresis, rigidity, hyperthermia, autonomic hyperactivity, coma). Increases plasma level of **metoprolol.** **HERBAL:** **Gotu kola, kava kava, SAMe, St. John's wort, valerian** may increase CNS depression. **FOOD:** None known. **LAB VALUES:** May reduce serum sodium.

AVAILABILITY (Rx)

ORAL SOLUTION: 10 mg/5 ml. **TABLETS:** 10 mg, 20 mg, 40 mg. **TABLETS (ORALLY DISINTEGRATING):** 10 mg, 20 mg, 40 mg.

ADMINISTRATION/HANDLING

PO

• Give without regard to food. • Scored tablets may be crushed.

PO (ORALLY DISINTEGRATING)

• Place tablet on tongue, allow to dissolve. • Swallow with saliva.

INDICATIONS/ROUTES/DOSAGE

DEPRESSION

PO: ADULTS: Initially, 20 mg once a day in the morning or evening. May increase in 20-mg increments at intervals of no less than 1 wk. **Maximum:** 60 mg/day. **ELDERLY, PTS WITH HEPATIC IMPAIRMENT:** 20 mg/day. May titrate to 40 mg/day only for nonresponding pts.

SIDE EFFECTS

FREQUENT (21%–11%): Nausea, dry mouth, somnolence, insomnia, diaphoresis. **OCCASIONAL (8%–4%):** Tremor, diarrhea, abnormal ejaculation, dyspepsia, fatigue, anxiety, vomiting, anorexia. **RARE (3%–2%):** Sinusitis, sexual dysfunction, menstrual disorder, abdominal pain, agitation, decreased libido.

ADVERSE EFFECTS/ TOXIC REACTIONS

Overdose manifested as dizziness, drowsiness, tachycardia, somnolence, confusion, seizures.

NURSING CONSIDERATIONS

BASELINE ASSESSMENT

Hepatic/renal function tests, blood counts should be performed periodically for pts on long-term therapy. Observe, record behavior. Assess psychological status, thought content, sleep pattern, appearance, interest in environment.

INTERVENTION/EVALUATION

Closely supervise suicidal-risk pt during early therapy (as energy level improves, suicide potential increases). Assess appearance, behavior, speech pattern, level of interest, mood.

PATIENT/FAMILY TEACHING

• Do not stop taking medication or increase dosage. • Avoid alcohol. • Avoid tasks that require alertness, motor skills until response to drug is established.

citrates

sih-traits

(Bicitra, Citrolith, Oracit, Polycitra, Polycitra-K, Polycitra-LC, Urocit-K)

C

CLASSIFICATION

CLINICAL: Alkalinizer.

ACTION

Increases urinary pH, urinary citrate level, decreasing calcium ion activity, saturation of calcium oxalate. Increases plasma bicarbonate, buffers excess hydrogen ion concentration. **Therapeutic Effect:** Increases blood and urinary pH, reverses metabolic acidosis.

USES

Treatment of metabolic acidosis. **Potassium citrate:** Prevents uric acid nephrolithiasis, calcium renal stones, urinary alkalizer when sodium citrate is contraindicated.

PRECAUTIONS

CONTRAINDICATIONS: Acute dehydration, anuria, azotemia, heat cramps, hypersensitivity to citrates, severe myocardial damage, severe renal impairment, sodium-restricted diet, untreated Addison's disease. **Urocit-K:** Concurrent use of anticholinergics, delayed gastric emptying, intestinal obstruction or stricture, severe peptic ulcer disease. **CAUTIONS:** Those with CHF, hypertension, pulmonary edema. May increase risk of urolithiasis.

LIFESPAN CONSIDERATIONS:

Pregnancy/Lactation: Unknown if drug crosses placenta or is distributed in breast milk. **Pregnancy Category C (potassium citrate); other forms not expected to cause fetal harm. Children:** Safety and efficacy not established. **Elderly:** No age-related precautions noted.

INTERACTIONS

DRUG: **Angiotensin-converting enzyme (ACE) inhibitors, NSAIDs, potassium-containing medications, potassium-sparing diuretics** may increase risk of hyperkalemia. **Antacids** may increase risk of systemic alkalosis. May decrease the effects of **methenamine.** May increase the excretion of **quinidine.** **HERBAL:** None significant. **FOOD:** None known. **LAB VALUES:** None known.

AVAILABILITY (Rx)

ORAL SOLUTION: 490 mg sodium citrate and 640 mg citric acid per 5 ml (Oracit), 500 mg sodium citrate and 334 mg citric acid per 5 ml (Bicitra), 550 mg potassium citrate, 500 mg sodium citrate, and 334 mg citric acid per 5 ml (Polycitra-LC), 1,100 mg potassium citrate and 334 mg citric acid per 5 ml (Polycitra-K). **SYRUP (POLYCITRA):** 550 mg potassium citrate, plus 500 mg sodium citrate, plus 334 mg citric acid per 5 ml. **TABLETS:** 5 mEq, 10 mEq. **TABLETS (CITROLITH):** 50 mg potassium citrate and 950 mg sodium citrate.

ADMINISTRATION/HANDLING

- Give after meals and at bedtime.

INDICATIONS/ROUTES/DOSAGE

METABOLIC ACIDOSIS

PO: ADULTS, ELDERLY: 15–30 ml after meals and at bedtime or 30–60 mEq/day in 3–4 divided doses. **CHILDREN:** 5–15 ml after meals and at bedtime or 2–3 mEq/kg/day in 3–4 divided doses.

SIDE EFFECTS

OCCASIONAL: Diarrhea, mild abdominal pain, nausea, vomiting.

ADVERSE EFFECTS/ TOXIC REACTIONS

Metabolic alkalosis, bowel obstruction/perforation, hyperkalemia, hypernatremia occur rarely.

NURSING CONSIDERATIONS

INTERVENTION/EVALUATION

Assess urinary pH, EKG in pts with cardiac disease, serum acid-base balance, CBC, Hgb, Hct, serum creatinine.

PATIENT/FAMILY TEACHING

• Take after meals. • Mix in water or juice; follow with additional liquid if desired.

cladribine

clad-rih-bean

(Leustatin)

Do not confuse Leustatin with lovastatin.

CLASSIFICATION

PHARMACOTHERAPEUTIC: Antimetabolite. **CLINICAL:** Antineoplastic (see p. 77C).

ACTION

Disrupts cellular metabolism by incorporating into DNA of dividing cells. Cytotoxic to both actively dividing and quiescent lymphocytes, monocytes. **Therapeutic Effect:** Prevents DNA synthesis.

PHARMACOKINETICS

Protein binding: 20%. Metabolized in liver. Primarily excreted in urine. **Half-life:** 5.4 hrs.

USES

Treatment of active hairy cell leukemia defined by clinically significant anemia, neutropenia, thrombocytopenia. **OFF-LABEL:** Treatment of chronic lymphocytic leukemia, non-Hodgkin's lymphoma, acute myeloid leukemia, autoimmune hemolytic anemia.

PRECAUTIONS

CONTRAINDICATIONS: None known. **CAUTIONS:** Renal/hepatic impairment, bone marrow suppression.

LIFESPAN CONSIDERATIONS:

Pregnancy/Lactation: May produce fetal harm; may be embryotoxic, fetotoxic; potential for serious reactions in breast-fed infants. **Pregnancy Category D. Children:** Safety and efficacy not established. **Elderly:** No age-related precautions noted.

INTERACTIONS

DRUG: Bone marrow depressants may increase myelosuppression. Concurrent administration of **cyclophosphamide,** total body irradiation may cause severe, irreversible neurologic toxicity, acute renal dysfunction. **Nephrotoxic, neurotoxic medications** may increase toxicity. **Live virus vaccines** may potentiate virus replication, increase vaccine side effects, decrease pt's antibody response to vaccine. **HERBAL:** None significant. **FOOD:** None known. **LAB VALUES:** None known.

AVAILABILITY (Rx)

INJECTION SOLUTION: 1 mg/ml.

ADMINISTRATION/HANDLING

IV

Reconstitution • Must dilute before administration. • Wear gloves, protective clothing during handling; if contact with skin, rinse with copious amounts of water. • Add calculated dose (0.09 mg/kg) to 500 ml 0.9% NaCl. Avoid D_5W (increases degradation of medication).

Rate of administration • Monitor vital signs during infusion, esp. during first hour. Observe for hypotension, bradycardia (usually both do not occur during same course). • Immediately discontinue administration if severe hypersensitivity reaction occurs.

Storage • Refrigerate unopened vials. • May refrigerate dilution solution for no more than 8 hrs before

C

administration. • Solution is stable for at least 24 hrs at room temperature. • Discard unused portion.

IV INCOMPATIBILITIES

Do not mix with other IV drugs/additives or infuse concurrently via a common IV line.

INDICATIONS/ROUTES/DOSAGE

HAIRY CELL LEUKEMIA

IV INFUSION: ADULTS, CHILDREN: 0.09–0.1 mg/kg/day as continuous infusion for 7 days. May repeat in 4–5 wks.

CHRONIC LYMPHOCYTIC LEUKEMIA

IV INFUSION: ADULTS, ELDERLY: 0.1 mg/kg/day days 1–7.

CHRONIC MYELOGENOUS LEUKEMIA

IV INFUSION: ADULTS, ELDERLY: 15 mg/m^2/day days 1–5. Give as a 1-hr infusion. If no response, increase to 20 mg/m^2/day with second course.

ACUTE LEUKEMIAS

IV INFUSION: 6.2–7.5 mg/m^2/day for days 1–5.

SIDE EFFECTS

FREQUENT: Fever (69%), fatigue (45%), nausea (28%), rash (27%), headache (22%), injection site reactions (19%), anorexia (17%), vomiting (13%). **OCCASIONAL (10%–5%):** Diarrhea, cough, purpura, chills, diaphoresis, constipation, dizziness, petechiae, myalgia, shortness of breath, malaise, pruritus, erythema, insomnia, edema, tachycardia, abdominal/trunk pain, epistaxis, arthralgia.

ADVERSE EFFECTS/ TOXIC REACTIONS

Myelosuppression characterized as severe neutropenia (less than 500 cells/mm^3); severe anemia (Hgb less than 8.5 g/dl), thrombocytopenia occur commonly. High-dose treatment may produce acute nephrotoxicity (increased BUN, creatinine levels), neurotoxicity (irreversible motor weakness of upper/lower extremities).

NURSING CONSIDERATIONS

BASELINE ASSESSMENT

Offer emotional support to pt, family. Perform neurologic function tests before chemotherapy. Use strict asepsis; protect pt from infection.

INTERVENTION/EVALUATION

Monitor temperature, report fever promptly. Assess for signs of infection. Assess skin for evidence of rash, purpura, petechiae. Monitor Hgb, Hct, BUN, platelet count, WBC, serum creatinine, potassium, sodium.

PATIENT/FAMILY TEACHING

• Narrow margin between therapeutic and toxic response. • Avoid crowds, persons with known infections; report signs of infection at once (fever, flu-like symptoms). • Do not have immunizations without physician's approval (drug lowers resistance). • Avoid contact with those who have recently received live virus vaccine. • Women of childbearing potential should not become pregnant during treatment.

Clarinex, *see desloratadine*

clarithromycin

clair-**rith**-row-my-sin

(Biaxin, Biaxin XL, Biaxin XL-Pak)

CLASSIFICATION

PHARMACOTHERAPEUTIC: Macrolide. **CLINICAL:** Antibiotic (see p. 25C).

C

ACTION

Binds to ribosomal receptor sites of susceptible organisms, inhibiting protein synthesis of bacterial cell wall. **Therapeutic Effect:** Bacteriostatic; may be bactericidal with high dosages or very susceptible microorganisms.

PHARMACOKINETICS

Well absorbed from GI tract. Protein binding: 65%–75%. Widely distributed. Metabolized in the liver to active metabolite. Primarily excreted in urine. Not removed by hemodialysis. **Half-life:** 3–7 hrs; metabolite 5–7 hrs (increased in renal impairment).

USES

Treatment of susceptible infections due to *C. pneumoniae, H. influenzae, H. parainfluenzae, H. pylori, M. catarrhalis, M. avium, M. pneumoniae, S. aureus, S. pneumoniae, S. pyogenes,* including bacterial exacerbation of bronchitis, otitis media, acute maxillary sinusitis, *Mycobacterium avium* complex (MAC), pharyngitis, tonsillitis, *H. pylori* duodenal ulcer, bacterial pneumonia, skin and soft tissue infections. Prevention of MAC disease. **Biaxin XL:** Treatment of community-acquired pneumonia.

PRECAUTIONS

CONTRAINDICATIONS: Hypersensitivity to other macrolide antibiotics. **CAUTIONS:** Hepatic/renal dysfunction, elderly with severe renal impairment.

⌛ LIFESPAN CONSIDERATIONS:

Pregnancy/Lactation: Unknown if distributed in breast milk. **Pregnancy Category C.** **Children:** Safety and efficacy not established in those younger than 6 mos. **Elderly:** Age-related renal impairment may require dosage adjustment.

INTERACTIONS

DRUG: May increase concentration, toxicity of **carbamazepine, digoxin, theophylline. Rifampin** may decrease plasma concentration. May increase **warfarin** effects. May decrease concentration of **zidovudine.** **HERBAL: St. John's wort** may decrease plasma concentration. **FOOD:** None known. **LAB VALUES:** May rarely increase BUN, serum AST, ALT.

AVAILABILITY (Rx)

ORAL SUSPENSION (BIAXIN): 125 mg/5 ml, 250 mg/5 ml. **TABLETS (BIAXIN):** 250 mg, 500 mg.

TABLETS (EXTENDED-RELEASE [BIAXIN XL, BIAXIN XL PAK]): 500 mg.

ADMINISTRATION/HANDLING

PO

• Give without regard to food. • Do not crush/break tablets.

INDICATIONS/ROUTES/DOSAGE

BRONCHITIS

PO: ADULTS, ELDERLY: 250–500 mg q12h for 7–14 days.

PO (EXTENDED-RELEASE): ADULTS, ELDERLY: 1 g once daily for 7 days.

SKIN, SOFT TISSUE INFECTIONS

PO: ADULTS, ELDERLY: 250 mg q12h for 7–14 days. **CHILDREN:** 7.5 mg/kg q12h for 10 days. **Maximum:** 1 g/day.

MAC PROPHYLAXIS

PO: ADULTS, ELDERLY: 500 mg twice a day. **CHILDREN:** 7.5 mg/kg q12h. **Maximum:** 500 mg twice a day.

MAC TREATMENT

PO: ADULTS, ELDERLY: 500 mg twice a day in combination. **CHILDREN:** 7.5 mg/kg q12h in combination. **Maximum:** 500 mg twice a day.

PHARYNGITIS, TONSILLITIS

PO: ADULTS, ELDERLY: 250 mg q12h for 10 days. **CHILDREN:** 7.5 mg/kg q12h for 10 days. **Maximum:** 1 g/day.

PNEUMONIA

PO: ADULTS, ELDERLY: 250 mg q12h for 7–14 days. **CHILDREN:** 7.5 mg/kg q12h.

PO (EXTENDED-RELEASE): ADULTS, ELDERLY: 1 g/day.

C

MAXILLARY SINUSITIS

PO: ADULTS, ELDERLY: 500 mg q12h or 1,000 mg (2×500 mg extended-release) once daily for 14 days. **CHILDREN:** 7.5 mg/kg q12h. **Maximum:** 500 mg twice a day.

H. PYLORI

PO: ADULTS, ELDERLY: 500 mg q8–12h for 10–14 days in combination.

ACUTE OTITIS MEDIA

PO: CHILDREN: 7.5 mg/kg q12h for 10 days. **Maximum:** 500 mg q12h.

DOSAGE IN RENAL IMPAIRMENT

For pts with creatinine clearance less than 30 ml/min, reduce dose by 50% and administer once or twice a day.

SIDE EFFECTS

OCCASIONAL (6%–3%): Diarrhea, nausea, altered taste, abdominal pain. **RARE (2%–1%):** Headache, dyspepsia.

ADVERSE EFFECTS/ TOXIC REACTIONS

Antibiotic-associated colitis (severe abdominal pain, tenderness, fever, severe watery diarrhea), other superinfections may result from altered bacterial balance. Hepatotoxicity, thrombocytopenia occur rarely.

NURSING CONSIDERATIONS

BASELINE ASSESSMENT

Question pt for history of hepatitis, allergies to clarithromycin, erythromycins.

INTERVENTION/EVALUATION

Monitor daily pattern of bowel activity/ stool consistency carefully; mild GI effects may be tolerable, but increasing severity may indicate onset of antibiotic-associated colitis. Be alert for superinfection (genital/anal pruritus, abdominal pain, mouth soreness, moderate to severe diarrhea).

PATIENT/FAMILY TEACHING

• Continue therapy for full length of treatment. • Doses should be evenly spaced. • Take medication with 8 oz water without regard to food.

Claritin, *see loratadine*

clemastine

kleh-**mass**-teen

(Contac 12 Hour Allergy, Dayhist Allergy, Tavist Allergy)

CLASSIFICATION

PHARMACOTHERAPEUTIC: Ethanolamine. **CLINICAL:** Antihistamine (see p. 52C).

ACTION

Competes with histamine on effector cells in GI tract, blood vessels, respiratory tract. **Therapeutic Effect:** Relieves allergic symptoms (urticaria, rhinitis, pruritus). Anticholinergic effects cause drying of nasal mucosa.

PHARMACOKINETICS

Route	Onset	Peak	Duration
PO	15–60 min	5–7 hrs	10–12 hrs

Well absorbed from GI tract. Metabolized in the liver. Excreted primarily in urine. **Half-life:** 21 hrs.

USES

Perennial and seasonal allergic rhinitis, other allergic symptoms (e.g., urticaria, pruritus).

PRECAUTIONS

CONTRAINDICATIONS: Angle-closure glaucoma, hypersensitivity to clemastine, use within 14 days of MAOIs. **CAUTIONS:** Peptic ulcer, GI/GU obstruction, asthma, prostatic hypertrophy.

LIFESPAN CONSIDERATIONS:

Pregnancy/Lactation: Excreted in breast milk. **Pregnancy Category B.** **Children:** Safety and efficacy not established in those younger than 6 yrs. **Elderly:** Age-related renal impairment may require dosage adjustment.

INTERACTIONS

DRUG: **Alcohol, other CNS depressants** may increase CNS depression. **MAOIs** may increase anticholinergic, CNS depressant effects. **HERBAL:** None significant. **FOOD:** None known. **LAB VALUES:** May suppress wheal, flare reactions to antigen skin testing unless drug is discontinued 4 days before testing.

AVAILABILITY (Rx)

SYRUP (TAVIST): 0.67 mg/5 ml. **TABLETS:** 1.34 mg (Contac 12 Hour Allergy), 2.68 mg (Tavist).

ADMINISTRATION/HANDLING

PO

• Give without regard to food. • Scored tablets may be crushed.

INDICATIONS/ROUTES/DOSAGE

ALLERGIC RHINITIS, ALLERGIC SYMPTOMS

PO: ADULTS, CHILDREN OLDER THAN 11 YRS: 1.34 mg twice a day up to 2.68 mg 3 times a day. **Maximum:** 8.04 mg/day. **CHILDREN 6–11 YRS:** 0.67–1.34 mg twice a day. **Maximum:** 4.02 mg/day. **CHILDREN YOUNGER THAN 6 YRS:** 0.05 mg/kg/day or 2.5–5 ml daily divided into 2–3 doses per day. **Maximum:** 1.34 mg/day. **ELDERLY:** 1.34 mg 1–2 times a day.

SIDE EFFECTS

FREQUENT: Somnolence, dizziness, urinary retention, thickening of bronchial secretions, dry mouth, nose, throat; in elderly, sedation, dizziness, hypotension. **OCCASIONAL:** Epigastric distress, flushing, blurred vision, tinnitus, paresthesia, diaphoresis, chills.

ADVERSE EFFECTS/ TOXIC REACTIONS

Children may experience paradoxical reactions (restlessness, insomnia, euphoria, anxiety, tremors). Overdose in children may result in hallucinations, seizures, death. Hypersensitivity reaction (eczema, pruritus, rash, cardiac disturbances, angioedema, photosensitivity) may occur. Overdose symptoms may vary from paradoxical reaction (hallucinations, tremors, seizure) to CNS depression (sedation, apnea, cardiovascular collapse).

NURSING CONSIDERATIONS

BASELINE ASSESSMENT

If pt is experiencing allergic reaction, obtain history of recently ingested foods, drugs, environmental exposure, recent emotional stress. Monitor rate, depth, rhythm, type of respiration; quality and rate of pulse. Assess lung sounds for rhonchi, wheezing, rales.

INTERVENTION/EVALUATION

Monitor B/P, esp. in elderly (increased risk of hypotension). Monitor children closely for paradoxical reaction.

PATIENT/FAMILY TEACHING

• Tolerance to antihistaminic effect generally does not occur; tolerance to sedative effect may occur. • Avoid tasks that require alertness, motor skills until response to drug is established. • Dry mouth, drowsiness, dizziness may be an expected response of drug. • Avoid alcoholic beverages during antihistamine therapy. • Coffee, tea may help reduce drowsiness.

Climara, *see estradiol*

C

clindamycin

klin-da-**mye**-sin
(Cleocin, Cleocin Pediatric, Cleocin T, Cleocin Vaginal, Clinda-Derm, Clindagel, Clindamax, Clindesse, Clindets Pledget, Dalacin ✤, Dalacin C ✤)

CLASSIFICATION

PHARMACOTHERAPEUTIC: Lincosamide. **CLINICAL:** Antibiotic.

ACTION

Inhibits protein synthesis of bacterial cell wall by binding to bacterial ribosomal receptor sites. Topically, decreases fatty acid concentration on skin. **Therapeutic Effect:** Bacteriostatic. Prevents outbreaks of acne vulgaris.

PHARMACOKINETICS

Rapidly absorbed from GI tract. Protein binding: 92%–94%. Widely distributed. Metabolized in the liver to some active metabolites. Primarily excreted in urine. Not removed by hemodialysis. **Half-life:** 2.4–3 hrs (increased in renal impairment, premature infants).

USES

Systemic: Treatment of aerobic gram-positive staphylococci and streptococci (not enterococci), *Fusobacgterium, Bacteroides* species and *Actinomyces* for treatment of respiratory tract infections. Skin/soft tissue infections, sepsis, intra-abdominal infections, infections of female pelvis and genital tract, bacterial endocarditis prophylaxis for dental and upper respiratory procedures in penicillin-allergic pts, perioperative prophylaxis. **Topical:** Treatment of acne vulgaris. **Intravaginal:** Treatment of bacterial vaginosis. **OFF-LABEL:** Treatment of actinomycosis, babesiosis, erysipelas, malaria, otitis media, *Pneumocystis carinii* pneumonia, sinusitis, toxoplasmosis.

PRECAUTIONS

CONTRAINDICATIONS: History of antibiotic-associated colitis, regional enteritis, ulcerative colitis; hypersensitivity to clindamycin, lincomycin; known allergy to tartrazine dye. **CAUTIONS:** Severe renal/hepatic dysfunction, concomitant use of neuromuscular blocking agents, neonates. Topical preparations should not be applied to abraded areas of skin or near eyes.

⌛ LIFESPAN CONSIDERATIONS:

Pregnancy/Lactation: Readily crosses placenta. Distributed in breast milk. **Topical/vaginal:** Unknown if distributed in breast milk. **Pregnancy Category B. Children:** Caution in those younger than 1 mo. **Elderly:** No age-related precautions noted.

INTERACTIONS

DRUG: Adsorbent antidiarrheals may delay absorption. **Chloramphenicol, erythromycin** may antagonize effects. May increase the effects of **neuromuscular blockers. HERBAL: St. John's wort** may decrease plasma concentration. **FOOD:** None known. **LAB VALUES:** May increase serum alkaline phosphatase, AST, ALT levels.

AVAILABILITY (Rx)

CAPSULES: 75 mg, 150 mg, 300 mg. **CREAM, VAGINAL (CLEOCIN, CLINDESSE):** 2%. **GEL, TOPICAL: (CLEOCIN T, CLINDAGEL, CLINDAMAX):** 1%. **INFUSION, PRE-MIX: (CLEOCIN):** 300 mg/50 ml, 600 mg/50 ml, 900 mg/50 ml. **INJECTION, SOLUTION: (CLEOCIN):** 150 mg/ml. **LOTION: (CLEOCIN T, CLINDAMAX):** 1%. **ORAL SOLUTION: (CLEOCIN PEDIATRIC):** 75 mg/5 ml. **SUPPOSITORIES, VAGINAL: (CLEOCIN):** 100 mg. **SWABS, TOPICAL: (CLINDETS, CLEOCIN T):** 1%.

C

ADMINISTRATION/HANDLING

IV

Reconstitution • Dilute 300–600 mg with 50 ml D_5W or 0.9% NaCl (900–1,200 mg with 100 ml). • Never exceed concentration of 18 mg/ml.

Rate of administration • 50 ml (300–600 mg) piggyback is infused over 10–20 min; 100 ml (900 mg–1.2 g) piggyback is infused over 30–40 min. Severe hypotension, cardiac arrest can occur with too-rapid administration. • No more than 1.2 g should be given in a single infusion.

Storage • IV infusion (piggyback) is stable for 16 days at room temperature.

IM

• Do not exceed 600 mg/dose. • Administer deep IM.

PO

• Store capsules at room temperature. • After reconstitution, oral solution is stable for 2 wks at room temperature. • Do not refrigerate oral solution (avoids thickening). • Give with 8 oz water. Give without regard to food.

TOPICAL

• Wash skin, allow to dry completely before application. • Shake topical lotion well before each use. • Apply liquid, solution, or gel in thin film to affected area. • Avoid contact with eyes or abraded areas.

VAGINAL, CREAM OR SUPPOSITORY

• Use one applicatorful or suppository at bedtime. • Fill applicator that comes with cream or suppository to indicated level. • Instruct pt to lie on back with knees drawn upward and spread apart. • Insert applicator into vagina and push plunger to release medication. • Withdraw, wash applicator with soap and warm water. • Wash hands promptly to avoid spreading infection.

IV INCOMPATIBILITIES

Allopurinol (Aloprim), filgrastim (Neupogen), fluconazole (Diflucan), idarubicin (Idamycin).

IV COMPATIBILITIES

Amiodarone (Cordarone), diltiazem (Cardizem), heparin, hydromorphone (Dilaudid), lipids, magnesium sulfate, midazolam (Versed), morphine, multivitamins, propofol (Diprivan), total parenteral nutrition (TPN).

INDICATIONS/ROUTES/DOSAGE

SUSCEPTIBLE INFECTIONS

IV, IM: ADULTS, ELDERLY: 1.2–1.8 g/day in 2–4 divided doses. **Maximum:** 4.8 g/day. **CHILDREN 1 MOS–16 YRS:** 25–40 mg/kg/day in 2–4 divided doses. **Maximum:** 4.8 g/day. **CHILDREN YOUNGER THAN 1 MO:** 15–20 mg/kg/day in 2–3 divided doses.
PO: ADULTS, ELDERLY: 150–450 mg q6h. **CHILDREN:** 8–25 mg/kg/day in 3–4 divided doses.

BACTERIAL VAGINOSIS

PO: ADULTS, ELDERLY: 300 mg twice a day for 7 days.
INTRAVAGINAL: ADULTS: One applicatorful at bedtime for 3–7 days or 1 suppository at bedtime for 3 days.
INTRAVAGINAL (CLINDESSE CREAM): ADULTS: One applicatorful once at any time of the day.

ACNE VULGARIS

TOPICAL: ADULTS: Apply thin layer to affected area twice a day.

SIDE EFFECTS

FREQUENT: Systemic: Abdominal pain, nausea, vomiting, diarrhea. **Topical:** Dry scaly skin. **Vaginal:** Vaginitis, pruritus. **OCCASIONAL: Systemic:** Phlebitis, thrombophlebitis with IV administration, pain, induration at IM injection site, allergic reaction, urticaria, pruritus. **Topical:** Contact dermatitis, abdominal pain, mild diarrhea, burning, stinging.

C

Vaginal: Headache, dizziness, nausea, vomiting, abdominal pain. **RARE: Vaginal:** Hypersensitivity reaction.

ADVERSE EFFECTS/ TOXIC REACTIONS

Antibiotic-associated colitis, other superinfections may occur during and several weeks after clindamycin therapy (including topical form). Blood dyscrasias (leukopenia, thrombocytopenia), nephrotoxicity (proteinuria, azotemia, oliguria) occur rarely.

NURSING CONSIDERATIONS

BASELINE ASSESSMENT

Question pt for history of allergies, particularly to clindamycin, lincomycin, aspirin. Avoid, if possible, concurrent use of neuromuscular blocking agents.

INTERVENTION/EVALUATION

Monitor daily pattern of bowel activity/ stool consistency; report diarrhea promptly due to potential for serious colitis (even with topical or vaginal administration). Assess skin for rash (dryness, irritation) with topical application. With all routes of administration, assess for superinfection (severe diarrhea, genital/anal pruritus, elevated temperature, change of oral mucosa).

PATIENT/FAMILY TEACHING

• Continue therapy for full length of treatment. • Doses should be evenly spaced. • Take oral doses with 8 oz water. • Caution should be used when applying topical clindamycin concurrently with peeling or abrasive acne agents, soaps, alcohol-containing cosmetics to avoid cumulative effect. • Do not apply topical preparations near eyes, abraded areas. • Notify physician if severe persistent diarrhea, cramps, bloody stool occur. • **Vaginal:** In event of accidental contact with eyes, rinse with copious amounts of cool tap water. • Do not engage in sexual intercourse during treatment. • Advise pt to wear sanitary napkin to protect clothes against stains. Tampons should not be used.

clobetasol

(Temovate)

See Corticosteroids: topical (p. 94C)

clofarabine

klo-**fare**-ah-been

(Clolar)

CLASSIFICATION

PHARMACOTHERAPEUTIC: Antimetabolite. **CLINICAL:** Antineoplastic.

ACTION

Metabolized intracellularly to ribonucleotide reductase. Alters mitochondrial membrane necessary in DNA synthesis. **Therapeutic Effect:** Decreases cell replication, affects cell repair. Produces cell death.

PHARMACOKINETICS

Protein binding: 47%, primarily to albumin. Metabolized intracellularly. Partially excreted unchanged in urine. **Half-life:** 5.2 hrs.

USES

Treatment of relapsed or refractory acute lymphoblastic leukemia (ALL) in pediatric pts (1–21 yrs) whose disease relapsed after or was refractory to at least 2 prior regimens. **OFF-LABEL:** Relapsed or refractory acute myeloid leukemia (AML), chronic myeloid leukemia (CML) in blast phase, acute lymphocytic leukemia (ALL), myelodysplastic syndrome.

PRECAUTIONS

CONTRAINDICATIONS: None known. **CAUTIONS:** Renal/hepatic impairment, dehydration, hypotension.

LIFESPAN CONSIDERATIONS:

Pregnancy/Lactation: May cause fetal harm. Breast-feeding not recommended. **Pregnancy Category D.** **Children:** Safety and efficacy not established. **Elderly:** No age-related precautions noted.

INTERACTIONS

DRUG: **Hepatotoxic, nephrotoxic medications** may increase risk of hepatic/renal toxicity. **HERBAL:** None significant. **FOOD:** None known. **LAB VALUES:** May increase serum creatinine, uric acid, AST, ALT, bilirubin. May decrease WBCs, Hgb, Hct, thrombocytes.

AVAILABILITY (Rx)

INJECTION, SOLUTION: 1 mg/ml.

ADMINISTRATION/HANDLING

IV

Reconstitution • Filter clofarabine through sterile, 0.2-micrometer syringe filter prior to further dilution with D_5W or 0.9% NaCl.

Rate of administration • Administer over 2 hrs. • Continuously infuse IV fluids to decrease risk of tumor lysis syndrome, other adverse events.

Storage • Store undiluted or diluted solution at room temperature. • Use diluted solution within 24 hrs.

IV INCOMPATIBILITIES

Do not administer any other medication through same IV line.

INDICATIONS/ROUTES/DOSAGE

ALL

IV: CHILDREN 1–21 YRS: 52 mg/m^2 over 2 hrs once daily for 5 consecutive days; repeat q2–6wk following recovery or return to baseline organ function.

SIDE EFFECTS

FREQUENT: Vomiting (83%); nausea (75%); diarrhea (53%); pruritus (47%); headache (46%); fever, dermatitis (41%); rigors (38%); abdominal pain, fatigue (36%); tachycardia (34%); epistaxis (31%); anorexia (30%); petechiae, limb pain, hypotension (29%); anxiety (22%); constipation (21%); edema (20%). **OCCASIONAL:** Cough (19%); mucosal inflammation, erythema, flushing (18%); hematuria (17%); dizziness (16%); gingival bleeding (15%); injection site pain, respiratory distress, pharyngitis (14%); back pain, palmar-plantar erythrodysesthesia syndrome, myalgia, oral candidiasis (13%); hypertension, depression, irritability, arthralgia, anorexia (11%). **RARE (10%):** Tremor, weight gain, somnolence.

ADVERSE EFFECTS/ TOXIC REACTIONS

Neutropenia occurs in 57% of pts; pericardial effusion in 35%; left ventricular systolic dysfunction in 27%; hepatomegaly, jaundice in 15%; pleural effusion, pneumonia, bacteremia in 10%; capillary leak syndrome in less than 10%.

NURSING CONSIDERATIONS

BASELINE ASSESSMENT

Monitor Hgb, Hct; assess for signs/symptoms of anemia. Question pt regarding possibility of pregnancy. Assess AST, ALT, bilirubin, creatinine clearance, BUN, creatinine levels prior to therapy.

INTERVENTION/EVALUATION

Monitor B/P, hepatic/renal function tests. Monitor daily pattern of bowel activity/stool consistency. Assess for GI disturbances. Assess skin for pruritus, dermatitis, petechiae, erythema on palms of hands and soles of feet. Assess for fever, sore throat; obtain blood cultures to detect evidence of infection.

PATIENT/FAMILY TEACHING

• Do not have immunizations without physician's approval (drug lowers resistance). • Avoid contact with anyone who recently received a live virus vaccine. • Avoid crowds, those with infection. • Avoid pregnancy due to risk of fetal harm; advise pts of childbearing potential to use effective contraception. • Maintain fastidious oral hygiene and frequent handwashing. • Notify physician if fever, respiratory distress, prolonged nausea, vomiting, diarrhea occur.

*clomiPRAMINE

klow-**mih**-prah-meen

(Anafranil, Apo-Clomipramine ✱)

Do not confuse clomipramine with chlorpromazine, clomiphene, or imipramine, or Anafranil with alfentanil, enalapril, or nafarelin.

♦CLASSIFICATION

PHARMACOTHERAPEUTIC: Tricyclic. **CLINICAL:** Antidepressant (see p. 36C).

ACTION

Blocks reuptake of neurotransmitters (norepinephrine, serotonin) at CNS presynaptic membranes, increasing availability at postsynaptic receptor sites. **Therapeutic Effect:** Reduces obsessive-compulsive behavior.

PHARMACOKINETICS

Rapidly absorbed. Metabolized in liver. **Half-life:** 20–30 hrs.

USES

Treatment of obsessive-compulsive disorder manifested as repetitive tasks producing marked distress, time-consuming, or significant interference with social or occupational behavior. **OFF-LABEL:** Treatment of bulimia nervosa, cataplexy associated with narcolepsy, mental depression, neurogenic pain, chronic pain, panic disorder, ejaculatory disorders, pervasive developmental disorder.

PRECAUTIONS

CONTRAINDICATIONS: Acute recovery period after MI, use within 14 days of MAOIs. **CAUTIONS:** Prostatic hypertrophy, history of urinary retention/obstruction, glaucoma, diabetes mellitus, seizures, hyperthyroidism, cardiac/hepatic/renal disease, schizophrenia, increased intraocular pressure, hiatal hernia. **Pregnancy Category C.**

INTERACTIONS

DRUG: **Alcohol, other CNS depressants** may increase CNS, respiratory depression, hypotensive effects. **Antithyroid agents** may increase the risk of agranulocytosis. **Cimetidine** may increase plasma concentration, risk of toxicity. May decrease the effects of **clonidine. MAOIs** may increase risk of neuroleptic malignant syndrome, seizures, hyperpyresis, hypertensive crisis. **Phenothiazines** may increase anticholinergic, sedative effects. **Sympathomimetics** may increase the risk of cardiac effects. **HERBAL:** **St. John's wort** may increase the risk of serotonin syndrome. **Gota kola, kava kava, SAMe, St. John's wort, valerian** may increase CNS depression. **FOOD:** **Grapefruit, grapefruit juice** may increase serum concentration, toxicity. **LAB VALUES:** May alter serum glucose, EKG readings.

AVAILABILITY (Rx)

CAPSULES: 25 mg, 50 mg, 75 mg.

INDICATIONS/ROUTES/DOSAGE

OBSESSIVE-COMPULSIVE DISORDER

PO: **ADULTS, ELDERLY:** Initially, 25 mg/day. May gradually increase to 100 mg/

day in the first 2 wks. **Maximum:** 250 mg/day. **CHILDREN 10 YRS AND OLDER:** Initially, 25 mg/day. May gradually increase up to maximum of 3 mg/kg/day or 200 mg, whichever is smaller.

SIDE EFFECTS

FREQUENT: Somnolence, fatigue, dry mouth, blurred vision, constipation, sexual dysfunction (42%), ejaculatory failure (20%), impotence, weight gain (18%), delayed micturition, orthostatic hypotension, diaphoresis, impaired concentration, increased appetite, urinary retention. **OCCASIONAL:** GI disturbances (nausea, GI distress, metallic taste), asthenia, aggressiveness, muscle weakness. **RARE:** Paradoxical reactions (agitation, restlessness, nightmares, insomnia), extrapyramidal symptoms (particularly fine hand tremor), laryngitis, seizures.

ADVERSE EFFECTS/ TOXIC REACTIONS

Overdose may produce seizures; cardiovascular effects (severe orthostatic hypotension, dizziness, tachycardia, palpitations, arrhythmias), altered temperature regulation (hyperpyrexia, hypothermia). Abrupt discontinuation after prolonged therapy may produce headache, malaise, nausea, vomiting, vivid dreams. Anemia, agranulocytosis have been noted.

NURSING CONSIDERATIONS

INTERVENTION/EVALUATION

Closely supervise suicidal-risk pt during early therapy (as depression lessens, energy level improves, increasing suicide potential). Assess appearance, behavior, speech pattern, level of interest, mood.

PATIENT/FAMILY TEACHING

• May cause dry mouth, constipation, blurred vision. • Tolerance to postural hypotension, sedative, anticholinergic effects usually develop during early therapy. • Maximum therapeutic effect may be noted in 2–4 wks. • Do not abruptly discontinue medication. • Avoid tasks that require alertness, motor skills until response to drug is established. • Avoid alcohol.

clonazepam

klon-**nah**-zih-pam

(Apo-Clonazepam ♣, Clonapam ♣, Klonopin, Klonopin Wafer, Novo-Clonazepam ♣, Rivotril ♣)

Do not confuse clonazepam with clonidine or lorazepam.

◆CLASSIFICATION

PHARMACOTHERAPEUTIC: Benzodiazepine **(Schedule IV). CLINICAL:** Anticonvulsant, antianxiety (see p. 33C).

ACTION

Depresses all levels of CNS; depresses nerve impulse transmission in motor cortex. Suppresses abnormal discharge in petit mal seizures. **Therapeutic Effect:** Produces anxiolytic, anticonvulsant effects.

PHARMACOKINETICS

Well absorbed from GI tract. Protein binding: 85%. Metabolized in the liver. Excreted in urine. Not removed by hemodialysis. **Half-life:** 18–50 hrs.

USES

Adjunct in treatment of Lennox-Gastaut syndrome (petit mal variant epilepsy); akinetic, myoclonic seizures; absence seizures (petit mal). Treatment of panic disorder. **OFF-LABEL:** Restless leg syndrome, neuralgia, multifocal tic disorder, parkinsonian dysarthria, bipolar disorder, adjunct therapy for schizophrenia.

C

PRECAUTIONS

CONTRAINDICATIONS: Narrow-angle glaucoma, significant hepatic disease. **CAUTIONS:** Renal/hepatic impairment chronic respiratory disease.

LIFESPAN CONSIDERATIONS:

Pregnancy/Lactation: Crosses placenta. May be distributed in breast milk. Chronic ingestion during pregnancy may produce withdrawal symptoms, CNS depression in neonates. **Pregnancy Category D. Children:** Long-term use may adversely affect physical/mental development. **Elderly:** Usually more sensitive to CNS effects (e.g., ataxia, dizziness, oversedation). Use low dosage, increase gradually.

INTERACTIONS

DRUG: Alcohol, other CNS depressants may increase CNS depressant effect. **Azole antifungals** may increase serum concentration, toxicity. **HERBAL: Gotu kola, kava kava, SAMe, St. John's wort, valerian** may increase CNS depression. **FOOD:** None known. **LAB VALUES:** None known.

AVAILABILITY (Rx)

TABLETS (KLONOPIN): 0.5 mg, 1 mg, 2 mg. **TABLETS (DISINTEGRATING [KLONOPIN WAFER]):** 0.125 mg, 0.25 mg, 0.5 mg, 1 mg, 2 mg.

ADMINISTRATION/HANDLING

PO

• Give without regard to food. • Tablets may be crushed.

ORAL DISINTEGRATING TABLET

• Open pouch, peel back foil; do not push tablet through foil. • Remove tablet with dry hands, place in mouth. • Swallow with or without water. • Use immediately after removing from package.

INDICATIONS/ROUTES/DOSAGE

SEIZURES

PO: ADULTS, ELDERLY, CHILDREN 10 YRS AND OLDER: 1.5 mg/day in 3 divided doses; may be increased in 0.5- to 1-mg increments every 3 days until seizures are controlled or adverse effects occur. **Maintenance:** 0.05–0.2 mg/kg. **Maximum:** 20 mg/day. **INFANTS, CHILDREN YOUNGER THAN 10 YRS OR WEIGHING LESS THAN 30 KG:** 0.01–0.03 mg/kg/day in 2–3 divided doses; may be increased by no more than 0.5 mg every 3 days until seizures are controlled or adverse effects occur. Do not exceed maintenance dosage of 0.2 mg/kg/day.

PANIC DISORDER

PO: ADULTS, ELDERLY: Initially, 0.25 mg twice a day; increased in increments of 0.125–0.25 mg twice a day every 3 days. **Maximum:** 4 mg/day.

SIDE EFFECTS

FREQUENT: Mild, transient drowsiness; ataxia; behavioral disturbances (aggression, irritability, agitation), esp. in children. **OCCASIONAL:** Rash, ankle or facial edema, nocturia, dysuria, change in appetite or weight, dry mouth, sore gums, nausea, blurred vision. **RARE:** Paradoxical CNS reactions (hyperactivity/nervousness in children; excitement, restlessness in elderly, particularly in the presence of uncontrolled pain).

ADVERSE EFFECTS/ TOXIC REACTIONS

Abrupt withdrawal may result in pronounced restlessness, irritability, insomnia, hand tremors, abdominal/muscle cramps, diaphoresis, vomiting, status epilepticus. Overdose results in somnolence, confusion, diminished reflexes, coma.

NURSING CONSIDERATIONS

BASELINE ASSESSMENT

Review history of seizure disorder (frequency, duration, intensity, level of consciousness [LOC]). For panic attack, assess motor responses (agitation, trembling, tension), autonomic responses (cold/clammy hands, diaphoresis).

INTERVENTION/EVALUATION

Assess children, elderly for paradoxical reaction, particularly during early therapy. Implement safety measures, observe frequently for recurrence of seizure activity. Assist with ambulation if drowsiness, ataxia occur. For those on long-term therapy, liver/renal function tests, blood counts should be performed periodically. Evaluate for therapeutic response: decreased intensity and frequency of seizures or, if used in panic attack, calm facial expression, decreased restlessness.

PATIENT/FAMILY TEACHING

• Drowsiness usually diminishes with continued therapy. • Avoid tasks that require alertness, motor skills until response to drug is established. • Smoking reduces drug effectiveness. • Do not abruptly withdraw medication after long-term therapy. • Strict maintenance of drug therapy is essential for seizure control. • Avoid alcohol.

clonidine

klon-ih-deen

(Apo-Clonidine ✦, Catapres, Catapres-TTS-1, Catapres-TTS-2, Catapres-TTS-3, Clonidine TTS-1, Clonidine TTS-2, Clonidine TTS-3, Dixarit ✦, Duraclon, Novo-Clonidine ✦)

Do not confuse clonidine with clomiphene, Klonopin, Loniten, or quinidine, or Catapres with Cetapred, Cataflam, Combipres.

FIXED-COMBINATION(S)

Combipres: clonidine/chlorthalidone (a diuretic): 0.1 mg/15 mg, 0.2 mg/15 mg, 0.3 mg/15 mg.

CLASSIFICATION

PHARMACOTHERAPEUTIC: Antiadrenergic, sympatholytic. **CLINICAL:** Antihypertensive (see pp. 58C, 144C).

ACTION

Prevents pain signal transmission to brain and produces analgesia at pre- and post-alpha-adrenergic receptors in spinal cord. **Therapeutic Effect:** Reduces peripheral resistance; decreases B/P, heart rate.

PHARMACOKINETICS

Route	Onset	Peak	Duration
PO	0.5–1 hr	2–4 hrs	Up to 8 hrs

Well absorbed from GI tract. Transdermal best absorbed from chest and upper arm; least absorbed from thigh. Protein binding: 20%–40%. Metabolized in the liver. Primarily excreted in urine. Minimally removed by hemodialysis. **Half-life:** 12–16 hrs (increased with renal impairment).

USES

Treatment of hypertension alone or in combination with other antihypertensive agents. **Epidural:** Combined with opiates for relief of severe pain. **OFF-LABEL:** ADHD, diagnosis of pheochromocytoma, opioid withdrawal, prevention of migraine headaches, treatment of diarrhea in diabetes mellitus, treatment of dysmenorrhea, menopausal flushing.

PRECAUTIONS

CONTRAINDICATIONS: Epidural contraindicated in pts with bleeding diathesis or infection at the injection site, those receiving anticoagulation therapy. **CAUTIONS:** Severe coronary insufficiency, recent MI, cerebrovascular disease, chronic renal failure, Raynaud's disease, thromboangiitis obliterans.

LIFESPAN CONSIDERATIONS:

Pregnancy/Lactation: Crosses placenta. Distributed in breast milk. **Pregnancy Category C.** **Children:** More sensitive to effects, use caution. **Elderly:** May be more sensitive to hypotensive effect. Age-related renal impairment may require dosage adjustment.

INTERACTIONS

DRUG: Discontinuation of concurrent **beta-blocker** therapy may increase risk of clonidine-withdrawal hypertensive crisis. **Tricyclic antidepressants** may decrease effect. **HERBAL:** **Gotu kola, kava kava, SAMe, St. John's wort, valerian** may increase CNS depression. **Ephedra, ginseng, yohimbe** may decrease antihypertensive effects. **FOOD:** None known. **LAB VALUES:** None known.

AVAILABILITY (Rx)

INJECTION SOLUTION (DURACLON): 100 mcg/ml, 500 mcg/ml. **TABLETS (CATAPRES):** 0.1 mg, 0.2 mg, 0.3 mg. **TRANSDERMAL PATCH:** 2.5 mg (release at 0.1 mg/24 hrs) (Catapres-TTS-1, Clonidine TTS-1), 5 mg (release at 0.2 mg/24 hrs) (Catapres-TTS-2, Clonidine TTS-2), 7.5 mg (release at 0.3 mg/24 hrs) (Catapres-TTS-3, Clonidine TTS-3).

ADMINISTRATION/HANDLING

PO

• Give without regard to food. • Tablets may be crushed. • Give last oral dose just before bedtime.

TRANSDERMAL • Apply transdermal system to dry, hairless area of intact skin on upper arm or chest. • Rotate sites (prevents skin irritation). • Do not trim patch to adjust dose.

IV INCOMPATIBILITIES

None known.

IV COMPATIBILITIES

Bupivacaine (Marcaine, Sensorcaine), fentanyl (Sublimaze), heparin, ketamine (Ketalar), lidocaine, lorazepam (Ativan).

INDICATIONS/ROUTES/DOSAGE

HYPERTENSION

PO: ADULTS: Initially, 0.1 mg twice a day. Increase by 0.1–0.2 mg q2–4days. Maintenance: 0.2–1.2 mg/day in 2–4 divided doses up to maximum of 2.4 mg/day. **ELDERLY:** Initially, 0.1 mg at bedtime. May increase gradually. **CHILDREN:** Initially, 5–10 mcg/kg/day in divided doses q8–12h. Increase at 5- to 7-day intervals up to 25 mcg/kg/day in divided doses q6h. **Maximum:** 0.9 mg/day.

TRANSDERMAL: ADULTS, ELDERLY: System delivering 0.1 mg/24 hrs up to 0.6 mg/24 hrs q7days.

ATTENTION DEFICIT HYPERACTIVITY DISORDER (ADHD)

PO: CHILDREN: Initially 0.05 mg/day. May increase by 0.05 mg/day q3–7days up to 3–5 mcg/kg/day in divided doses 3–4 times a day. **Maximum:** 0.3–0.4 mg/day.

SEVERE PAIN

EPIDURAL: ADULTS, ELDERLY: 30–40 mcg/hr. **CHILDREN:** **Range:** 0.5–2 mcg/kg/hr, not to exceed adult dose.

SIDE EFFECTS

FREQUENT: Dry mouth (40%), somnolence (33%), dizziness (16%), sedation, constipation (10%). **OCCASIONAL (5%–1%):** **Tablets, Injection:** Depression, pedal edema, loss of appetite, decreased sexual function, itching eyes, dizziness, nausea, vomiting, nervousness. **Transdermal:** Pruritus, redness or darkening of skin. **RARE (less than 1%):** Nightmares, vivid dreams, feeling of coldness in distal extremities (esp. the digits).

ADVERSE EFFECTS/ TOXIC REACTIONS

Overdose produces profound hypotension, irritability, bradycardia, respiratory depression, hypothermia, miosis (pupillary constriction), arrhythmias, apnea. Abrupt withdrawal may result in rebound hypertension associated with nervousness, agitation, anxiety, insomnia, paresthesia, tremor, flushing, diaphoresis.

NURSING CONSIDERATIONS

BASELINE ASSESSMENT

Obtain B/P immediately before each dose is administered, in addition to regular monitoring (be alert to B/P fluctuations).

INTERVENTION/EVALUATION

Monitor daily pattern of bowel activity/stool consistency. If clonidine is to be withdrawn, discontinue concurrent beta-blocker therapy several days before discontinuing clonidine (prevents clonidine withdrawal hypertensive crisis). Slowly reduce clonidine dosage over 2–4 days.

PATIENT/FAMILY TEACHING

• Sugarless gum, sips of tepid water may relieve dry mouth. • To reduce hypotensive effect, rise slowly from lying to sitting position, permit legs to dangle momentarily before standing. • Skipping doses or voluntarily discontinuing drug may produce severe, rebound hypertension. • Side effects tend to diminish during therapy.

clopidogrel

klow-**pih**-duh-grel

(Plavix)

Do not confuse Plavix with Paxil.

CLASSIFICATION

PHARMACOTHERAPEUTIC: Thienopyridine derivative. **CLINICAL:** Antiplatelet (see p. 31C).

ACTION

Inhibits binding of enzyme adenosine phosphate (ADP) to its platelet receptor and subsequent ADP-mediated activation of a glycoprotein complex. **Therapeutic Effect:** Inhibits platelet aggregation.

PHARMACOKINETICS

Route	Onset	Peak	Duration
PO	1 hr	2 hrs	N/A

Rapidly absorbed. Protein binding: 98%. Extensively metabolized by the liver. Eliminated equally in the urine and feces. **Half-life:** 8 hrs.

USES

Reduction of atherosclerotic event (e.g., MI, stroke, vascular death) in pts with documented atherosclerosis. Treatment of acute coronary syndrome (reduces MI, stroke, refractory ischemia, cardiovascular death). **OFF-LABEL:** Graft patency (saphenous vein), mitral regurgitation, mitral stenosis, noncardioembolic stroke, percutaneous coronary intervention.

PRECAUTIONS

CONTRAINDICATIONS: Active bleeding, coagulation disorders, severe hepatic disease. **CAUTIONS:** Hypertension, hepatic/renal impairment, history of bleeding, hematologic disorders, preoperative pts.

LIFESPAN CONSIDERATIONS:

Pregnancy/Lactation: Unknown if drug crosses placenta or is distributed in breast milk. **Pregnancy Category B.** **Children:** Safety and efficacy not established. **Elderly:** No age-related precautions noted.

INTERACTIONS

DRUG: Aspirin, NSAIDS may increase risk of bleeding. May interfere with metabolism of **fluvastatin, NSAIDs, phenytoin, tamoxifen, tolbutamide, torsemide, warfarin.** HERBAL: **Cat's claw, dong quai, evening primrose, feverfew, garlic, ginger, ginkgo, red clover, horse chestnut, green tea, ginseng** may have additive antiplatelet effects. **FOOD:** None known. **LAB VALUES:** Prolongs clotting time, ACT.

AVAILABILITY (Rx)

TABLETS: 75 mg.

ADMINISTRATION/HANDLING

PO

- Give without regard to food.

INDICATIONS/ROUTES/DOSAGE

REDUCTION OF ATHEROSCLEROTIC EVENTS

PO: ADULTS, ELDERLY: 75 mg once a day.

ACUTE CORONARY SYNDROME

PO: ADULTS, ELDERLY: Initially, 300 mg loading dose, then 75 mg once a day (in combination with aspirin).

SIDE EFFECTS

FREQUENT (15%): Skin disorders. **OCCASIONAL (8%–6%):** Upper respiratory tract infection, chest pain, flu-like symptoms, headache, dizziness, arthralgia. **RARE (5%–3%):** Fatigue, edema, hypertension, abdominal pain, dyspepsia, diarrhea, nausea, epistaxis, dyspnea, rhinitis.

ADVERSE EFFECTS/ TOXIC REACTIONS

Agranulocytosis, aplastic anemia/pancytopenia, thrombotic thrombocytopenic purpura (TTP) occur rarely. Hepatitis, hypersensitivity reaction, anaphylactoid reaction have been reported.

NURSING CONSIDERATIONS

BASELINE ASSESSMENT

Perform platelet counts before drug therapy, q2days during first week of treatment, and weekly thereafter until therapeutic maintenance dose is reached. Abrupt discontinuation of drug therapy produces elevated platelet count within 5 days.

INTERVENTION/EVALUATION

Monitor platelet count for evidence of thrombocytopenia. Assess BUN, serum creatinine, bilirubin, AST, ALT, WBC, Hgb, signs/symptoms of hepatic insufficiency during therapy.

PATIENT/FAMILY TEACHING

- Inform pt that it may take longer to stop bleeding during drug therapy.
- Report any unusual bleeding.
- Inform physicians, dentists if clopidogrel is being taken, esp. before surgery is scheduled or before taking any new drug.

clorazepate

klor-**az**-e-pate

(Apo-Clorazepate ✱, Novo-Clopate ✱, Tranxene, Tranxene SD, Tranxene SD Half-Strength, Tranxene T-Tab)

Do not confuse clorazepate with clofibrate, clonazepam.

CLASSIFICATION

PHARMACOTHERAPEUTIC: Benzodiazepine. **CLINICAL:** Antianxiety, anticonvulsant (see p. 11C).

ACTION

Depresses all levels of CNS, including limbic and reticular formation, by binding to benzodiazepine receptor sites on gamma-aminobutyric acid (GABA) receptor complex. Modulates GABA, a major inhibitory neurotransmitter in the brain. **Therapeutic Effect:** Produces

C

anxiolytic effect, suppresses seizure activity.

PHARMACOKINETICS

Readily absorbed from GI tract. Metabolized in liver. Excreted primarily in urine.

USES

Management of anxiety disorders; short-term relief of anxiety symptoms, partial seizures, acute alcohol withdrawal symptoms.

PRECAUTIONS

CONTRAINDICATIONS: Acute narrow-angle glaucoma. **CAUTIONS:** Renal/hepatic impairment, acute alcohol intoxication.

⌛ LIFESPAN CONSIDERATIONS:

Pregnancy/Lactation: Crosses placenta; distributed in breast milk. **Pregnancy Category D. Children:** May experience paradoxical excitement. **Elderly:** Increased risk of dizziness, sedation, confusion, hypotension, hyperexcitability.

INTERACTIONS

DRUG: Alcohol, other CNS depressants may increase CNS depressant effects. **Azole antifungals** may increase plasma concentration, toxicity. **HERBAL: Gotu kola, kava kava, SAMe, St. John's wort, valerian** may increase CNS depression. **FOOD:** None known. **LAB VALUES:** Therapeutic serum level is 0.12–1.5 mcg/ml; toxic serum level is greater than 5 mcg/ml.

AVAILABILITY (Rx)

TABLETS (TRANXENE, TRANXENE T-TAB): 3.75 mg, 7.5 mg, 15 mg.

TABLETS (SUSTAINED-RELEASE): 11.25 mg (Tranxene SD Half-Strength), 22.5 mg (Tranxene SD).

ADMINISTRATION/HANDLING

◄ ALERT ► If the pt requires change to another anticonvulsant, decrease clorazepate dosage gradually as low-dose therapy begins with replacement drug.

INDICATIONS/ROUTES/DOSAGE

ANXIETY

PO (REGULAR-RELEASE): ADULTS, ELDERLY: 7.5–15 mg 2–4 times a day.
PO (SUSTAINED-RELEASE): ADULTS, ELDERLY: 11.25 mg or 22.5 mg once a day at bedtime.

PARTIAL SEIZURES

PO: ADULTS, ELDERLY, CHILDREN OLDER THAN 12 YRS: Initially, 7.5 mg 2–3 times a day. May increase by 7.5 mg at weekly intervals. Maintenance: 0.5–1 mg/kg/day. **Maximum:** 90 mg/day. **CHILDREN 9–12 YRS:** Initially, 3.75–7.5 mg twice a day. May increase by 3.75 mg at weekly intervals. **Maximum:** 60 mg/day in 2–3 divided doses.

ALCOHOL WITHDRAWAL

PO: ADULTS, ELDERLY: Initially, 30 mg, then 15 mg 2–4 times a day on first day. Gradually decrease dosage over subsequent days. **Maximum:** 90 mg/day.

SIDE EFFECTS

FREQUENT: Somnolence. **OCCASIONAL:** Dizziness, GI disturbances, anxiety, blurred vision, dry mouth, headache, confusion, ataxia, rash, irritability, slurred speech. **RARE:** Paradoxical CNS reactions (hyperactivity, nervousness in children, excitement, restlessness in elderly, debilitated, generally noted during first 2 wks of therapy, particularly in presence of uncontrolled pain).

ADVERSE EFFECTS/TOXIC REACTIONS

Abrupt or too-rapid withdrawal may result in pronounced restlessness, irritability, insomnia, hand tremors, abdominal/muscle cramps, diaphoresis, vomiting, seizures. Overdose results in somnolence, confusion, diminished reflexes, coma.

NURSING CONSIDERATIONS

BASELINE ASSESSMENT

Anxiety: Assess autonomic response (cold/clammy hands, diaphoresis), motor response (agitation, trembling, tension). Offer emotional support to anxious pt. **Seizures:** Review history of seizure disorder (intensity, frequency, duration, level of consciousness [LOC]). Observe frequently for recurrence of seizure activity. Initiate seizure precautions.

INTERVENTION/EVALUATION

Assess for paradoxical reaction, particularly during early therapy. Assist with ambulation if drowsiness, dizziness occur. Evaluate for therapeutic response: **Anxiety:** Calm facial expression; decreased restlessness. **Seizures:** Decrease in intensity/frequency of seizures. Therapeutic serum level: Peak: 0.12–1.5 mcg/ml; toxic serum level: greater than 5 mcg/ml.

PATIENT/FAMILY TEACHING

• Do not abruptly withdraw medication after long-term use (may precipitate seizures). • Strict maintenance of drug therapy is essential for seizure control. • Drowsiness usually disappears during continued therapy. • Avoid tasks that require alertness, motor skills until response to drug is established. • If dizziness occurs, change positions slowly from recumbent to sitting position before standing. • Smoking reduces drug effectiveness. • Avoid alcohol.

clotrimazole

kloe-**try**-mah-zole
(Canesten ♣, Clotrimaderm ♣, Cruex, Gyne-Lotrimin, Lotrimin, Mycelex)

Do not confuse clotrimazole with cotrimoxazole, or Lotrimin with Lotrisone, or Mycelex, Mycelex-G with Myoflex.

FIXED-COMBINATION(S)

Lotrisone: clotrimazole/betamethasone (a corticosteroid): 1%/0.05%.

CLASSIFICATION

PHARMACOTHERAPEUTIC: Anti-infective. **CLINICAL:** Antifungal (see p. 46C).

ACTION

Binds with phospholipids in fungal cell membrane. **Therapeutic Effect:** Alters cell membrane permeability, inhibits yeast growth.

USES

Oral Lozenges: Treatment/prophylaxis of oropharyngeal candidiasis due to *Candida* sp. **Topical:** Treatment of tinea pedis, tinea cruris, tinea corporis, tinea versicolor, cutaneous candidiasis (moniliasis) due to *Candida albicans.* **Intravaginal:** Treatment of vulvovaginal candidiasis (moniliasis) due to *Candida* sp. **OFF-LABEL: Topical:** Treatment of paronychia, tinea barbae, tinea capitis.

PRECAUTIONS

CONTRAINDICATIONS: Hypersensitivity to clotrimazole or any ingredient in preparation, children younger than 3 yrs. **CAUTIONS:** Hepatic disorder with oral therapy.

LIFESPAN CONSIDERATIONS:

Pregnancy/Lactation: Oral: Unknown if distributed in breast milk. **Pregnancy Category C. Topical:** Unknown if distributed in breast milk. No adverse effects noted in fetus when given in 2nd or 3rd trimesters. **Pregnancy Category B. Vaginal:** Unknown if distributed in breast milk. **Pregnancy Category B. Children: Oral:** No specific problems

C

noted in children 3 yrs and older. Not recommended in children younger than 3 yrs. **Topical:** No age-related precautions noted. **Vaginal:** Safety and efficacy not established in children up to 12 yrs of age. **Elderly: Oral/Topical/Vaginal:** No age-related precautions noted.

INTERACTIONS

DRUG: None significant. **HERBAL:** None significant. **FOOD:** None known. **LAB VALUES:** May increase serum AST.

AVAILABILITY (Rx)

TOPICAL CREAM (CRUEX, LOTRIMIN): 1%. **TOPICAL SOLUTION (LOTRIMIN):** 1%. **TROCHE (MYCELEX):** 10 mg. **VAGINAL CREAM (MYCELEX):** 1%, 2%. **VAGINAL TABLET (GYNE-LOTRIMIN):** 200 mg.

ADMINISTRATION/HANDLING

PO

• Lozenges must be dissolved in mouth longer than 15–30 min for oropharyngeal therapy. • Swallow saliva.

TOPICAL

• Rub well into affected, surrounding areas. • Do not apply occlusive covering or other preparations to affected area.

VAGINAL

• Use vaginal applicator; insert high into vagina.

INDICATIONS/ROUTES/DOSAGE

ORAL-LOCAL/OROPHARYNGEAL

PO: ADULTS, ELDERLY, CHILDREN 3 YRS AND OLDER: 10 mg 5 times a day for 14 days.

PROPHYLAXIS VS. OROPHARYNGEAL CANDIDIASIS

PO: ADULTS, ELDERLY: 10 mg 3 times a day.

USUAL TOPICAL DOSAGE

TOPICAL: ADULTS, ELDERLY, CHILDREN 3 YRS AND OLDER: Twice a day. Therapeutic effect may take up to 8 wks.

VULVOVAGINAL CANDIDIASIS

VAGINAL (TABLETS): ADULTS, ELDERLY, CHILDREN 12 YRS AND OLDER: 1 tablet (100 mg) at bedtime for 7 days; 2 tablets (200 mg) at bedtime for 3 days; or 500-mg tablet one time.

VAGINAL (CREAM): ADULTS, ELDERLY, CHILDREN 12 YRS AND OLDER: (1%): One applicator at bedtime for 7 days. (2%): One applicator at bedtime for 3 days.

SIDE EFFECTS

FREQUENT: PO: Nausea, vomiting, diarrhea, abdominal pain. **OCCASIONAL: Topical:** Pruritis, burning, stinging, erythema, urticaria. **Vaginal:** Mild burning (tablets/cream); irritation, cystitis (cream). **RARE: Vaginal:** Pruritis, rash, lower abdominal cramping, headache.

ADVERSE EFFECTS/ TOXIC REACTIONS

None known.

NURSING CONSIDERATIONS

BASELINE ASSESSMENT

Assess pt's ability to understand, follow directions regarding use of oral lozenges.

INTERVENTION/EVALUATION

With oral therapy, assess for nausea, vomiting. With topical therapy, check skin for erythema, urticaria, blistering; inquire about pruritis, burning, stinging. With vaginal therapy, evaluate for vulvovaginal irritation, abdominal cramping, urinary frequency, discomfort.

PATIENT/FAMILY TEACHING

• Continue for full length of therapy. • Inform physician of increased irritation. • Avoid contact with eyes. • **Topical:** Keep areas clean, dry; wear light clothing to promote ventilation. • Separate personal items, linens. • **Vaginal:** Continue use during menses. • Refrain from sexual intercourse or advise partner to use condom during therapy.

C

cloxacillin

(Tegopen)

See Antibiotic: penicillins (p. 27C)

clozapine

evolve

klo-za-peen

(Apo-Clozapine ✦, Clozaril, FazaClo)

Do not confuse clozapine with Cloxapen or clofazimine, or Clozaril with Clinoril or Colazal.

◆CLASSIFICATION

PHARMACOTHERAPEUTIC: Dibenzodiazepine derivative. **CLINICAL:** Antipsychotic (see p. 62C).

ACTION

Interferes with binding of dopamine at dopamine receptor sites; binds primarily at nondopamine receptor sites. **Therapeutic Effect:** Diminishes schizophrenic behavior.

PHARMACOKINETICS

Readily absorbed from GI tract. Protein binding: 97%. Metabolized in liver. Excreted in urine. **Half-life:** 12 hrs.

USES

Management of severely ill schizophrenic pts who fail to respond to other antipsychotic therapy. Treatment of recurrent suicidal behavior.

PRECAUTIONS

CONTRAINDICATIONS: Coma, concurrent use of other drugs that may suppress bone marrow function, history of clozapine-induced agranulocytosis or severe granulocytopenia, myeloproliferative disorders, paralytic ileus, severe CNS depression. **CAUTIONS:** History of seizures, cardiovascular disease, myocarditis; respiratory, hepatic, renal impairment; alcohol withdrawal; urinary retention; glaucoma; prostatic hypertrophy. **Pregnancy Category B.**

INTERACTIONS

DRUG: Antihypertensive medications may increase risk of hypotension. **Alcohol, other CNS depressants** may increase CNS depressant effects. **Bone marrow depressants** may increase myelosuppression. **SSRIs (e.g., paroxetine)** may increase concentration. **Lithium** may increase the risk of confusion, dyskinesia, seizures. **HERBAL:** None significant. **FOOD:** None known. **LAB VALUES:** May increase serum glucose, cholesterol, triglycerides.

AVAILABILITY (Rx)

TABLETS (CLOZARIL): 12.5 mg, 25 mg, 100 mg, 200 mg. **TABLETS (ORALLY-DISINTEGRATING [FAZACLO]):** 25 mg, 100 mg.

ADMINISTRATION/HANDLING

PO

• Give without regard to food.

ORALLY DISINTEGRATING TABLETS

• Remove from foil blister; do not push tablet through foil. • Remove tablet with dry hands, place in mouth. • Allow to dissolve in mouth, swallow with saliva.• If dose requires splitting tablet, discard unused portion.

INDICATIONS/ROUTES/DOSAGE

SCHIZOPHRENIC DISORDERS, REDUCE SUICIDAL BEHAVIOR

◄ **ALERT** ► For initiation of therapy, must have WBC equal to or greater than 3,500 mm^3 and ANC equal to or greater than 2,000 mm^3.

PO: ADULTS: Initially, 25 mg once or twice a day. May increase by 25–50 mg/day over 2 wks until dosage of 300–450 mg/day is achieved. May further increase by 50–100 mg/day no more than once or twice a week. **Range:** 200–600 mg/

day. **Maximum:** 900 mg/day. **ELDERLY:** Initially, 25 mg/day. May increase by 25 mg/day. **Maximum:** 450 mg/day.

SIDE EFFECTS

FREQUENT: Somnolence (39%), salivation (31%), tachycardia (25%), dizziness (19%), constipation (14%). **OCCASIONAL:** Hypotension (9%); headache (7%); tremor, syncope, diaphoresis, dry mouth (6%); nausea, visual disturbances (5%); nightmares, restlessness, akinesia, agitation, hypertension, abdominal discomfort, heartburn, weight gain (4%). **RARE:** Rigidity, confusion, fatigue, insomnia, diarrhea, rash.

ADVERSE EFFECTS/ TOXIC REACTIONS

Seizures occur occasionally (3%). Overdose produces CNS depression (sedation, delirium, coma) respiratory depression, hypersalivation. Blood dyscrasias, particularly agranulocytosis, mild leukopenia, may occur.

NURSING CONSIDERATIONS

BASELINE ASSESSMENT

Obtain baseline WBC, absolute neutrophil count (ANC) before initiating treatment. Monitor WBC, ANC count every week for first 6 mos of continuous therapy, then biweekly for 6 mos. If CBC and ANC are normal after 12 mos, then monthly monitoring of CBC and ANC is recommended. Assess behavior, appearance, emotional status, response to environment, speech pattern, thought content.

INTERVENTION/EVALUATION

Monitor B/P for hypertension/hypotension. Assess pulse for tachycardia (common side effect). Monitor CBC for blood dyscrasias. Supervise suicidal-risk pt closely during early therapy (as depression lessens, energy level improves, increasing suicide potential). Assess for therapeutic response (interest in surroundings, improvement in self-care, increased ability to concentrate, relaxed facial expression).

PATIENT/FAMILY TEACHING

• Do not abruptly withdraw from long-term drug therapy. • Drowsiness generally subsides during continued therapy. • Avoid tasks that require alertness, motor skills until response to drug is established. • Avoid alcohol.

cocaine

evolve

koe-**kane**

FIXED-COMBINATION(S)

AC Gel: cocaine/epinephrine (a sympathomimetic): 11.8%/1:1,000. **TAC:** tetracaine/epinephrine/cocaine: 0.5%/1:2,000/11.8%.

CLASSIFICATION

PHARMACOTHERAPEUTIC: Amide. **CLINICAL:** Topical anesthetic.

ACTION

Decreases membrane permeability; increases norepinephrine at postsynaptic receptor sites, producing intense vasoconstriction. **Therapeutic Effect:** Blocks conduction of nerve impulses.

USES

Topical anesthesia for mucous membranes of orolaryngeal, nasal areas; minor, uncomplicated facial lacerations.

PRECAUTIONS

CONTRAINDICATIONS: Hypersensitivity to cocaine, local anesthetics; systemic or ophthalmic use. **CAUTIONS:** Hypertension, severe cardiovascular disease, thyrotoxicosis, infants, those with severely traumatized mucosa in area of intended application. **Pregnancy Category C (X if nonmedical use).**

C

INTERACTIONS

DRUG: Effects of **beta-blockers** may be decreased. **Cholinesterase inhibitor** may increase effects, risk of toxicity. **CNS agonist agents** may increase CNS effects. **Sympathomimetics** increase CNS stimulation, risk of cardiovascular effects. **Tricyclic antidepressants, digoxin, methyldopa** may increase arrhythmias. **HERBAL:** None significant. **FOOD:** None known. **LAB VALUES:** None known.

AVAILABILITY (Rx)

TOPICAL SOLUTION: 4%, 10%.

INDICATIONS/ROUTES/DOSAGE

USUAL TOPICAL DOSAGE

TOPICAL: ADULTS, ELDERLY: 1%–10% solution. **Maximum single dose:** 1 mg/kg.

SIDE EFFECTS

FREQUENT: Loss of sense of smell/taste.

ADVERSE EFFECTS/ TOXIC REACTIONS

Repeated nasal application may produce stuffy nose, chronic rhinitis. Early signs of overdosage include increased B/P, increased pulse, palpitations, chills/fever, agitation, anxiety, confusion, restlessness, nausea, vomiting, abdominal pain, diaphoresis, tachypnea, dilated pupils. Advanced signs of overdosage include arrhythmias, CNS hemorrhage, CHF, seizures, delirium, hyperreflexia, loss of bladder/bowel control, respiratory depression. Late signs of overdosage include loss of reflexes, muscle paralysis, dilated pupils, diminished level of consciousness (LOC), cyanosis, pulmonary edema, cardiac/respiratory failure.

NURSING CONSIDERATIONS

INTERVENTION/EVALUATION

Monitor for anesthetic response. Be alert to CNS stimulation. Assess for euphoria; restlessness; increased B/P, pulse, respirations. Be prepared to provide ventilatory support and emergency medications in event of progression of CNS response.

PATIENT/FAMILY TEACHING

- Do not eat, chew gum until sensation returns when used for throat anesthesia.
- One time or infrequent use for procedures will not cause dependence.
- Report feelings of euphoria, restlessness, tachycardia if these develop during procedure.

codeine phosphate

koe-deen

(Codeine Phosphate Injection)

codeine sulfate

(Codeine Contin ✱)

Do not confuse codeine with Cardene or Lodine.

FIXED-COMBINATION(S)

Capital with Codeine, Tylenol with Codeine: acetaminophen/codeine: 120 mg/12 mg per 5 ml. **Tylenol with Codeine:** acetaminophen/codeine: 300 mg/15 mg, 300 mg/30 mg, 300 mg/60 mg.

CLASSIFICATION

PHARMACOTHERAPEUTIC: Opioid agonist. **CLINICAL:** Analgesic: **Schedule II;** fixed-combination form: **Schedule III** (see p. 135C).

ACTION

Binds to opioid receptors in CNS, particularly in medulla. Inhibits ascending pain pathways. **Therapeutic Effect:** Alters perception of and emotional response to pain, suppresses cough reflex.

C

PHARMACOKINETICS

Well absorbed following PO administration. Protein binding: Very low. Metabolized in liver. Excreted in urine. **Half-life:** 2.5–3.5 hrs.

USES

Relief of mild to moderate pain and/or nonproductive cough. **OFF-LABEL:** Treatment of diarrhea.

PRECAUTIONS

CONTRAINDICATIONS: Premature infants. **EXTREME CAUTION:** CNS depression, anoxia, hypercapnia, respiratory depression, seizures, acute alcoholism, shock, untreated myxedema, respiratory dysfunction. **CAUTIONS:** Increased intracranial pressure (ICP), hepatic impairment, acute abdominal conditions, hypothyroidism, prostatic hypertrophy, Addison's disease, urethral stricture, chronic obstructive pulmoney disease (COPD). **Pregnancy Category C (D if used for prolonged periods or at high dosages at term).**

INTERACTIONS

DRUG: Alcohol, other CNS depressants may increase CNS, respiratory depression, hypotension. **MAOIs** may produce a severe, sometimes fatal reaction (reduce dosage to ¼ usual dose). **HERBAL: St. John's wort** may decrease plasma concentration. **Gotu kola, kava kava, SAMe, St. John's wort, valerian** may increase CNS depression. **FOOD:** None known. **LAB VALUES:** May increase serum amylase, lipase.

AVAILABILITY (Rx)

INJECTION SOLUTION: 15 mg/ml, 30 mg/ml, 60 mg/ml. **ORAL SOLUTION:** 15 mg/5 ml. **TABLETS (PHOSPHATE):** 30 mg, 60 mg. **TABLETS (SULFATE):** 15 mg, 30 mg, 60 mg.

ADMINISTRATION/HANDLING

PO

- Give with food or milk (minimizes adverse GI effects).

INDICATIONS/ROUTES/DOSAGE

◄ ALERT ► Reduce initial dosage in those with hypothyroidism, Addison's disease, renal insufficiency; those using other CNS depressants concurrently.

ANALGESIA

PO, IM, SUBCUTANEOUS: ADULTS, ELDERLY: 30 mg q4–6h. Range: 15–60 mg. **CHILDREN:** 0.5–1 mg/kg q4–6h. **Maximum:** 60 mg/dose.

COUGH

PO: ADULTS, ELDERLY, CHILDREN 12 YR AND OLDER: 10–20 mg q4–6yrs. **Maximum:** 120 mg/day. **CHILDREN 6–11 YRS:** 5–10 mg q4–6h. **Maximum:** 60 mg/day. **CHILDREN 2–5 YRS:** 2.5–5 mg q4–6h. **Maximum:** 30 mg/day.

DOSAGE IN RENAL IMPAIRMENT

Dosage is modified based on creatinine clearance.

Creatinine Clearance	Dosage
10–50 ml/min	75% of usual dose
Less than 10 ml/min	50% of usual dose

SIDE EFFECTS

◄ ALERT ► Ambulatory pts, those not in severe pain may experience dizziness, nausea, vomiting, hypotension more frequently than those in supine position or with severe pain. **FREQUENT:** Constipation, somnolence, nausea, vomiting. **OCCASIONAL:** Paradoxical excitement, confusion, palpitations, facial flushing, decreased urination, blurred vision, dizziness, dry mouth, headache, hypotension (including orthostatic hypotension), decreased appetite, injection site redness, burning, or pain. **RARE:** Hallucinations, depression, abdominal pain, insomnia.

ADVERSE EFFECTS/ TOXIC REACTIONS

Too-frequent use may result in paralytic ileus. Overdose may produce cold/clammy skin, confusion, seizures, decreased B/P, restlessness, pinpoint pupils, bradycardia, respiratory depression, decreased LOC, severe weakness. Tolerance to drug's analgesic effect, physical dependence may occur with repeated dosage.

C

NURSING CONSIDERATIONS

BASELINE ASSESSMENT

Analgesic: Assess onset, type, location, duration of pain. Effect of medication is reduced if full pain response recurs before next dose. **Antitussive:** Assess type, severity, frequency of cough, sputum production.

INTERVENTION/EVALUATION

Monitor daily pattern of bowel activity/stool consistency. Increase fluid intake, environmental humidity to improve viscosity of lung secretions. Initiate deep breathing, coughing exercises. Assess for clinical improvement; record onset of relief of pain, cough.

PATIENT/FAMILY TEACHING

• Change positions slowly to avoid orthostatic hypotension. • Avoid tasks that require alertness, motor skills until response to drug is established. • Tolerance, dependence may occur with prolonged use of high dosages. • Avoid alcohol.

colchicine

kol-chi-seen
(Colchicine)

CLASSIFICATION

PHARMACOTHERAPEUTIC: Alkaloid. **CLINICAL:** Antigout.

ACTION

Decreases leukocyte motility, phagocytosis, lactic acid production. **Therapeutic Effect:** Decreases urate crystal deposits, reduces inflammatory process.

PHARMACOKINETICS

Rapidly absorbed from GI tract. Highest concentration is in liver, spleen, and kidney. Protein binding: 30%–50%. Reenters intestinal tract by biliary secretion and is reabsorbed from intestines. Partially metabolized in liver. Eliminated primarily in feces.

USES

Treatment of acute gouty arthritis, prophylaxis of recurrent gouty arthritis. **OFF-LABEL:** To reduce frequency of recurrence of familial Mediterranean fever; treatment of acute calcium pyrophosphate deposition, amyloidosis, biliary cirrhosis, recurrent pericarditis, sarcoid arthritis.

PRECAUTIONS

CONTRAINDICATIONS: Blood dyscrasias; severe cardiac, GI, hepatic, renal disorders. **CAUTIONS:** Hepatic impairment, elderly, debilitated.

LIFESPAN CONSIDERATIONS:

Pregnancy/Lactation: Unknown if drug crosses placenta or is distributed in breast milk. **Pregnancy Category D (Parenteral), C (Oral). Children:** Safety and efficacy not established. **Elderly:** May be more susceptible to cumulative toxicity. Age-related renal impairment may increase risk of myopathy.

INTERACTIONS

DRUG: Bone marrow depressants may increase risk of blood dyscrasias. **Clarithromycin, erythromycin** may increase plasma levels, toxicity. **NSAIDs** may increase the risk of myelosuppression, neutropenia, thrombocytopenia. **HERBAL:** None significant. **FOOD:** None known. **LAB VALUES:** May increase serum alkaline phosphatase, AST. May decrease platelet count.

AVAILABILITY (Rx)

INJECTION SOLUTION: 0.5 mg/ml. **TABLETS:** 0.6 mg.

ADMINISTRATION/HANDLING

IV

◀ **ALERT** ▶ Subcutaneous, IM administration produces severe local reaction. Use via IV route only. Avoid concurrent IV and oral administration.

Reconstitution • May dilute with 0.9% NaCl or Sterile Water for Injection. • Do not dilute with D_5W.

Rate of administration • Administer over 2–5 min.

Storage • Store at room temperature.

PO
• Give without regard to food.

IV INCOMPATIBILITIES

No information available on Y-site administration.

INDICATIONS/ROUTES/DOSAGE

ACUTE GOUTY ARTHRITIS

PO: ADULTS, ELDERLY: Initially, 0.6–1.2 mg; then 0.6 mg q1–2h until pain is relieved or nausea, vomiting, diarrhea occurs. Total dose: 6 mg.

IV: ADULTS, ELDERLY: Initially 1–2 mg, then 0.5 mg q6h until satisfactory response. **Maximum:** 4 mg/wk or 4 mg/one course of treatment. If pain recurs, may give 1–2 mg/day for several days but no sooner than 7 days after a full course of IV therapy (total of 4 mg).

CHRONIC GOUTY ARTHRITIS

PO: ADULTS, ELDERLY: 0.6 mg every other day up to 3 times a day.

SIDE EFFECTS

FREQUENT: PO: Nausea, vomiting, abdominal discomfort. **OCCASIONAL: PO:** Anorexia. **RARE:** Hypersensitivity reaction, including angioedema. **Parenteral:** Nausea, vomiting, diarrhea, abdominal discomfort, pain/redness at injection site, neuritis in injected arm.

ADVERSE EFFECTS/ TOXIC REACTIONS

Bone marrow depression (aplastic anemia, agranulocytosis, thrombocytopenia) may occur with long-term therapy. Overdose initially causes burning feeling in skin/throat, severe diarrhea, abdominal pain. Second stage manifests as fever, seizures, delirium, renal impairment (hematuria, oliguria). Third stage causes hair loss, leukocytosis, stomatitis.

NURSING CONSIDERATIONS

BASELINE ASSESSMENT

Instruct pt to drink 8–10 glasses (8 oz) of fluid daily while taking medication. Discontinue medication if GI symptoms occur.

INTERVENTION/EVALUATION

Discontinue medication immediately if GI symptoms occur. Encourage high fluid intake (3,000 ml a day). Monitor I&O (output should be at least 2,000 ml a day). Assess serum uric acid. Assess for therapeutic response (reduced joint tenderness, swelling, redness, limitation of motion).

PATIENT/FAMILY TEACHING

• Encourage low-purine food intake, drink 8–10 glasses (8 oz) of fluid daily while taking medication. • Report skin rash, sore throat, fever, unusual bruising/bleeding, weakness, fatigue, numbness. • Stop medication as soon as gout pain is relieved or at first sign of nausea, vomiting, diarrhea.

colesevelam

koh-le-**sev**-e-lam
(Welchol)

C

CLASSIFICATION

PHARMACOTHERAPEUTIC: Bile acid sequestrant. **CLINICAL:** Antihyperlipidemic agent (see p. 54C).

ACTION

Binds with bile acids in intestine, preventing their reabsorption and removing them from the body. **Therapeutic Effect:** Decreases LDL cholesterol.

USES

Adjunctive therapy to diet, exercise used either alone or in combination with hydroxamethylglutaryl CoA reductase inhibitor (e.g., simvastatin) to decrease elevated LDL cholesterol in pts with primary hypercholesterolemia (Fredrickson type IIa).

PRECAUTIONS

CONTRAINDICATIONS: Complete biliary obstruction. **CAUTIONS:** Dysphagia, swallowing disorders, severe GI motility disorders, major GI tract surgery, those susceptible to fat-soluble vitamin deficiency. **Pregnancy Category B.**

INTERACTIONS

DRUG: None significant. **HERBAL:** None significant. **FOOD:** None known. **LAB VALUES:** None known.

AVAILABILITY (Rx)

TABLETS: 625 mg.

INDICATIONS/ROUTES/DOSAGE

CHOLESTEROL REDUCTION (INCLUDING PRIMARY HYPERCHOLESTEROLEMIA [FREDRICKSON TYPE IIA]).

PO: ADULTS, ELDERLY: 3 tablets with meals twice a day or 6 tablets once a day with a meal. May increase daily dose to 7 tablets a day.

SIDE EFFECTS

FREQUENT: (12%–8%) Flatulence, constipation, infection, dyspepsia (heartburn, epigastric distress).

ADVERSE EFFECTS/ TOXIC REACTIONS

GI tract obstruction may occur.

NURSING CONSIDERATIONS

BASELINE ASSESSMENT

Assess baseline lab results: cholesterol, triglycerides, hepatic function tests.

INTERVENTION/EVALUATION

Monitor cholesterol, triglyceride lab results for therapeutic response. Monitor daily pattern of bowel activity/ stool consistency.

PATIENT/FAMILY TEACHING

• Follow special, low-cholesterol diet (important part of treatment). • Periodic lab tests are essential part of therapy. • Do not take other medications without physician's knowledge.

colestipol

(Colestid)

See Antihyperlipidemics

Combivent, *see albuterol and ipratropium*

Combivir, *see lamivudine and zidovudine*

Concerta, *see methylphenidate*

conivaptan

kon-ih-**vap**-tan
(Vaprisol)

CLASSIFICATION

PHARMACOTHERAPEUTIC: Vasopressin antagonist. **CLINICAL:** Hyponatremia adjunct.

ACTION

Promotes excretion of free water (without loss of serum electrolytes) resulting in net fluid loss, increased urine output, decreased urine osmolarlity. **Therapeutic Effect:** Restores normal serum sodium level.

PHARMACOKINETICS

Metabolized in liver to active metabolites. Protein binding: 99%. Mainly eliminated in feces with lesser amount excreted in urine. **Half-life:** 5 hrs.

USES

Treatment of euvolemic hyponatremia (syndrome of inappropriate secretion of antidiuretic hormone, in setting of hypothyroidism, adrenal insufficiency, pulmonary disorders) in hospitalized pts.

PRECAUTIONS

CONTRAINDICATIONS: Hypovolemic hyponatremia; concurrent use with strong CYP3A4 inhibitors (ketoconazole, ritonavir, clarithromycin). **CAUTIONS:** Hepatic/renal impairment, underlying congestive heart failure.

LIFESPAN CONSIDERATIONS:

Pregnancy/Lactation: Accumulates in placenta; systemic exposure to fetus likely. Potential for decreased neonatal viability, delayed growth/development at doses lower than those required for therapeutic efficacy. Unknown if distributed in breast milk. **Pregnancy Category C.** **Children:** Safety and efficacy not established. **Elderly:** No age-related precautions noted.

INTERACTIONS

DRUG: **Aminoglutethimide, carbamazepine, nafcillin, nevirapine, phenobarbital, phenytoin, rifamycins** may decrease levels/effects. **Azole antifungals, clarithromycin, diclofenac, doxcycline, erythromycin, imatinib, isoniazid, ketoconazole, nefazodone, nicardipine, propofol, protease inhibitors, quinidine, telithromycin, verapamil** may increase levels/effects. May increase levels/effects of **benzodiazepines, calcium channel blockers, cyclosporine, mirtazapine, nateglinide, nefazodone, sildenafil, tacrolimus, venlafaxine.** May increase levels/toxicity of **digoxin.** **HERBAL:** None significant. **FOOD:** None known. **LAB VALUES:** May decrease Hgb, Hct, serum potassium, magnesium. May alter serum glucose.

AVAILABILITY (Rx)

INJECTION SOLUTION (VAPRISOL): 5 mg/ml (4-ml single-use ampule).

ADMINISTRATION/HANDLING

◀ **ALERT** ▶ Administer through large veins; change peripheral IV site every 24 hrs (minimizes risk of vascular irritation).

IV

Reconstitution • For intermittent infusion (piggyback), withdraw 4 ml (20 mg) conivaptan and dilute with 100 ml D_5W. Invert bag several times to ensure mixing solution. • For continuous infusion, withdraw 4 ml (20 mg) conivaptan and dilute with 250 ml D_5W. Invert bag serveral times to ensure mixing solution.

Rate of administration • For 100-ml infusion, infuse over 30 min. For 250-ml infusion, infuse over 24 hrs.

C

Storage • Store ampules at room temperature. • Protect from prolonged exposure to light. • Diluted solution must be used within 24 hrs of mixing.

IV INCOMPATIBILITIES

Ringer's lactate, 0.9% NaCl.

IV COMPATIBILITIES

Do not infuse concurrently with any other medication or solution.

INDICATIONS/ROUTES/DOSAGE

EUVOLEMIC HYPONATREMIA

IV: ADULTS, ELDERLY: Loading dose: 20 mg given over 30 min. Follow with 20 mg in a continuous IV infusion over 24 hrs. Administer for an additional 1–3 days as a continuous infusion of 20 mg/day. May be titrated upward to 40 mg/day as a continuous infusion if serum sodium is not rising at desired rate. Duration of infusion after loading dose should not exceed 4 days.

SIDE EFFECTS

FREQUENT: Peripheral injection site reactions (pain, erythema, phlebitis, swelling) (53%); headache (12%). **OCCASIONAL (10%–4%):** Thirst, vomiting, hypertension, polyuria, orthostatic hypotension, diarrhea, constipation, fever, confusion, dry mouth, nausea. **RARE (3%–2%):** Atrial fibrillation, hypotension, insomnia, dehydration, oral candidiasis.

ADVERSE EFFECTS/ TOXIC REACTIONS

Overly rapid increase in serum sodium may produce temporary neurologic symptoms. Urinary tract infection, anemia, hematuria, pneumonia occur occasionally.

NURSING CONSIDERATIONS

BASELINE ASSESSMENT

Obtain baseline serum sodium, hepatic enzyme levels, BUN, creatinine, CBC. Start peripheral IV in large vein. Assess for increased pulse rate, poor skin turgor, nausea, diarrhea (signs of hyponatremia).

INTERVENTION/EVALUATION

Obtain, monitor frequent serum sodium levels. Assess peripheral IV site for pain, erythema, phlebitis, swelling; if vein irritation occurs, change IV site. New IV site should be obtained every 24 hrs (minimizes vein irritation). Monitor for improvement in signs/symptoms of hyponatremia, impending signs/symptoms of hypernatremia (flushing, edema, restlessness, dry mucous membranes, fever).

PATIENT/FAMILY TEACHING

Change positions slowly to avoid orthostatic hypotension.

conjugated estrogens

ess-troe-jenz

(Cenestin, C.E.S. ♣, Congest ♣, Enjuvia, Premarin, Premarin Intravenous, Premarin Vaginal)

Do not confuse Premarin with Primaxin or Remeron.

FIXED-COMBINATION(S)

Premphase, Prempro: estrogen/ methyltestosterone (an androgen): 0.3 mg/1.5 mg; 0.45 mg/1.5 mg; 0.625 mg/2.5 mg; 0.625 mg/5 mg.

CLASSIFICATION

PHARMACOTHERAPEUTIC: Estrogen. **CLINICAL:** Hormone.

ACTION

Increases synthesis of DNA, RNA, various proteins in target tissues; reduces release of gonadotropin-releasing hormone, reduces follicle-stimulating hormone

(FSH), leuteinizing hormone (LH) release. **Therapeutic Effect:** Promotes normal growth, development of female sex organs, maintains GU function, vasomotor stability. Prevents accelerated bone loss by inhibiting bone resorption, restoring balance of bone resorption/formation. Inhibits LH, decreases serum concentration of testosterone.

PHARMACOKINETICS

Well absorbed from GI tract. Widely distributed. Protein binding: 50%–80%. Metabolized in the liver. Primarily excreted in urine.

USES

Premarin: Management of moderate to severe vasomotor symptoms associated with menopause. Treatment of atrophic vaginitis, kraurosis vulvae, female hypogonadism and castration, primary ovarian failure. Retardation of osteoporosis in postmenopausal women. Palliative treatment of inoperable, progressive cancer of the prostate in men and of the breast in postmenopausal women. **Cenestin:** Treatment of moderate to severe vasomotor symptoms of menopause, treatment of vulvar/vaginal atrophy. **OFF-LABEL:** Prevention of estrogen deficiency–induced premenopausal osteoporosis. **Cream:** Prevention of nosebleeds.

PRECAUTIONS

CONTRAINDICATIONS: Breast cancer (with some exceptions), hepatic disease, thrombophlebitis, undiagnosed vaginal bleeding. **CAUTIONS:** Asthma, epilepsy, migraine headaches, diabetes, cardiac/renal dysfunction.

LIFESPAN CONSIDERATIONS:

Pregnancy/Lactation: Distributed in breast milk. May be harmful to fetus. Not for use during lactation. **Pregnancy Category X. Children:** Safety and efficacy not established. **Elderly:** No age-related precautions noted.

INTERACTIONS

DRUG: May increase serum concentration, enhance hepatotoxic effect of **cyclosporine**. **Hepatotoxic medications** may increase the risk of hepatotoxicity. **HERBAL: Black cohosh, dong quai** may increase estrogenic activity. **Ginseng, red clover, saw palmetto** may increase hormonal effects. **St. John's wort** may decrease plasma concentration. **FOOD:** None known. **LAB VALUES:** May increase blood glucose, HDL, serum calcium, triglycerides. May decrease serum cholesterol, LDH. May affect serum metapyrone testing, thyroid function tests.

AVAILABILITY (Rx)

CREAM, VAGINAL: (PREMARIN): 0.625 mg/g. **INJECTION, POWDER FOR RECONSTITUTION:** 25 mg. **TABLET (CENESTIN, PREMARIN):** 0.3 mg, 0.45 mg, 0.625 mg, 0.9 mg, 1.25 mg, 2.5 mg. **(ENJUVIA):** 0.3 mg, 0.45 mg, 0.625 mg, 1.25 mg.

ADMINISTRATION/HANDLING

IV

Reconstitution • Reconstitute with 5 ml Sterile Water for Injection containing benzyl alcohol (diluent provided). • Slowly add diluent, shaking gently. Avoid vigorous shaking.

Rate of administration • Give slowly to prevent flushing reaction.

Storage • Refrigerate vials for IV use. • Reconstituted solution stable for 60 days if refrigerated. • Do not use if solution darkens or precipitate forms.

PO

- Administer at same time each day.
- Give with milk, food if nausea occurs.

IV INCOMPATIBILITIES

No information available on Y-site administration.

C

INDICATIONS/ROUTES/DOSAGE

VASOMOTOR SYMPTOMS ASSOCIATED WITH MENOPAUSE, ATROPHIC VAGINITIS, KRAUROSIS VULVAE

PO: ADULTS, ELDERLY: 0.3–0.625 mg/day cyclically (21 days on, 7 days off) or continuously.

INTRAVAGINAL: ADULTS, ELDERLY: 0.5–2 g/day cyclically, such as 21 days on and 7 days off.

FEMALE HYPOGONADISM

PO: ADULTS: 0.3–0.625 mg/day in divided doses for 20 days; then a rest period of 10 days.

FEMALE CASTRATION, PRIMARY OVARIAN FAILURE

PO: ADULTS: Initially, 1.25 mg/day cyclically. Adjust dosage, upward or downward, according to severity of symptoms and pt response. For maintenance, adjust dosage to lowest level that will provide effective control.

OSTEOPOROSIS PREVENTION

PO: ADULTS, ELDERLY: 0.3–0.625 mg/day, cyclically, such as 25 days on and 5 days off.

BREAST CANCER

PO: ADULTS, ELDERLY: 10 mg 3 times a day for at least 3 mos.

PROSTATE CANCER

PO: ADULTS, ELDERLY: 1.25–2.5 mg 3 times a day.

ABNORMAL UTERINE BLEEDING

PO: ADULTS: 1.25 mg q4h for 24 hrs, then 1.25 mg/day for 7–10 days.

IV, IM: ADULTS: 25 mg; may repeat once in 6–12 hrs.

SIDE EFFECTS

FREQUENT: Vaginal bleeding (spotting, breakthrough bleeding); breast pain/tenderness; gynecomastia. **OCCASIONAL:** Headache, hypertension, intolerance to contact lenses. **High-doses:** Anorexia, nausea. **RARE:** Loss of scalp hair, depression.

ADVERSE EFFECTS/ TOXIC REACTIONS

Prolonged administration may increase risk of breast, cervical, endometrial, hepatic, vaginal carcinoma; cerebrovascular disease, coronary heart disease, gallbladder disease, hypercalcemia.

NURSING CONSIDERATIONS

BASELINE ASSESSMENT

Question for hypersensitivity to estrogen, previous jaundice, thromboembolic disorders associated with pregnancy, estrogen therapy.

INTERVENTION/EVALUATION

Assess B/P periodically. Check for edema; weigh daily. Promptly report signs/symptoms of thromboembolic, thrombotic disorders: sudden severe headache, shortness of breath, vision/speech disturbance, weakness/numbness of an extremity, loss of coordination, pain in chest, groin, leg.

PATIENT/FAMILY TEACHING

• Avoid smoking due to increased risk of heart attack, blood clots. • Explain importance of diet, exercise when taken to retard osteoporosis. • Teach how to perform Homans' test, signs/symptoms of blood clots (report these to physician immediately). • Notify physician of abnormal vaginal bleeding, depression. • Teach female pts to perform breast self-exam. • Report weight gain of more than 5 lb a wk. • Stop taking medication, contact physician if pregnancy is suspected.

Copaxone, *see glatiramer*

Cordarone, *see amiodarone*

Coreg, *see carvedilol*

Corlopam, *see fenoldopam*

cortisone

kor-ti-sone
(Cortone)

Do not confuse cortisone with Cort-Dome.

CLASSIFICATION

PHARMACOTHERAPEUTIC: Adrenocortical steroid. **CLINICAL:** Glucocorticoid (see p. 92C).

ACTION

Inhibits accumulation of inflammatory cells at inflammation sites, phagocytosis, lysosomal enzyme release, synthesis, release of mediators of inflammation. **Therapeutic Effect:** Prevents/suppresses cell-mediated immune reactions. Decreases/prevents tissue response to inflammatory process.

PHARMACOKINETICS

Slowly absorbed from GI tract. Widely distributed. Metabolized in liver. Excreted in urine/feces. **Half-life:** 0.5–2 hrs.

USES

Treatment of adrenocortical insufficiency, conditions treated by immunosuppression, inflammatory conditions.

PRECAUTIONS

CONTRAINDICATIONS: Hypersensitivity to corticosteroids, administration of live virus vaccine, peptic ulcers (except in life-threatening situations), systemic fungal infection. **CAUTIONS:** Thromboembolic disorders, history of tuberculosis (may reactivate disease), hypothyroidism, cirrhosis, nonspecific ulcerative colitis, CHF, hypertension, psychosis, renal insufficiency, seizure disorders. Prolonged therapy should be discontinued slowly.

LIFESPAN CONSIDERATIONS:

Pregnancy/Lactation: Crosses placenta; distributed in breast milk. **Pregnancy Category C (D if used in the first trimester). Children:** Monitor growth, development of children, infants on prolonged steroid therapy. **Elderly:** Higher risk for hypertension, osteoporosis.

INTERACTIONS

DRUG: Amphotericin may increase hypokalemia. **Bupropion** may lower the seizure threshold. May increase **digoxin** toxicity caused by hypokalemia. May decrease the effects of **diuretics, insulin, oral hypoglycemics, potassium supplements. Hepatic enzyme inducers** may decrease effects. **Live-virus vaccines** may decrease pt's antibody response to vaccine, increase vaccine side effects, potentiate virus replication. **HERBAL: Echinacea, Ma huang** may decrease corticosteroid effectiveness. **FOOD:** None known. **LAB VALUES:** May increase blood glucose, serum cholesterol, amylase, sodium. May decrease serum calcium, potassium, thyroxine.

AVAILABILITY (Rx)

TABLETS: 5 mg, 10 mg, 25 mg.

INDICATIONS/ROUTES/DOSAGE

Dosage is dependent on condition being treated and pt response.

PHYSIOLOGIC REPLACEMENT

PO: ADULTS, ELDERLY: 25–35 mg/day. **CHILDREN:** 0.5–0.75 mg/kg/day in 3 divided doses.

IM: CHILDREN: 0.25–0.35 mg/kg/day.

INFLAMMATORY CONDITIONS

PO: ADULTS, ELDERLY: 25–300 mg/day. **CHILDREN:** 2.5–10 mg/kg/day in 3–4 divided doses.

IM: ADULTS, ELDERLY: 25–300 mg/day. **CHILDREN:** 1–5 mg/kg/day in 1–2 doses/day.

SIDE EFFECTS

FREQUENT: Insomnia, heartburn, anxiety, abdominal distention, increased diaphoresis, acne, mood swings, increased appetite, facial flushing, delayed wound healing, increased susceptibility to infection, diarrhea, constipation. **OCCASIONAL:** Headache, edema, change in skin color, frequent urination. **RARE:** Tachycardia, allergic reaction (rash, urticaria), psychological changes, hallucinations, depression.

ADVERSE EFFECTS/ TOXIC REACTIONS

Long-term therapy: Hypocalcemia, hypokalemia, muscle wasting (esp. arms, legs) osteoporosis, spontaneous fractures, amenorrhea, cataracts, glaucoma, peptic ulcer, CHF. **Abrupt withdrawal following long-term therapy:** Anorexia, nausea, fever, headache, joint pain, rebound inflammation, fatigue, weakness, lethargy, dizziness, orthostatic hypotension.

NURSING CONSIDERATIONS

BASELINE ASSESSMENT

Question for hypersensitivity to any of the corticosteroids. Obtain baseline values for weight, B/P, serum glucose, cholesterol, electrolytes.

INTERVENTION/EVALUATION

Be alert to infection (reduced immune response): sore throat, fever, vague symptoms. For pts on long-term therapy, monitor for hypocalcemia (muscle twitching, cramps, positive Trousseau's or Chvostek's signs), hypokalemia (weakness, muscle cramps, numbness/tingling [esp. lower extremities], nausea/vomiting, irritability, EKG changes). Assess emotional status, ability to sleep.

PATIENT/FAMILY TEACHING

• Do not change dose or schedule or stop taking drug; **must** taper off under medical supervision. • Notify physician of fever, sore throat, muscle aches, sudden weight gain/swelling. • Inform dentist, other physicians of cortisone therapy now or within past 12 mos.

cosyntropin

koe-syn-**troe**-pin

(Cortrosyn)

Do not confuse Cortrosyn with Cotazym.

◆CLASSIFICATION

PHARMACOTHERAPEUTIC: Adrenocortical steroid. **CLINICAL:** Glucocorticoid.

ACTION

Stimulates initial reaction in synthesis of adrenal steroids from cholesterol. **Therapeutic Effect:** Increases endogenous corticoid synthesis.

USES

Diagnostic testing of adrenocortical function.

PRECAUTIONS

CONTRAINDICATIONS: Hypersensitivity to cosyntropin, corticotropin. **CAUTIONS:** None known. **Pregnancy Category C.**

INTERACTIONS

DRUG: None significant. **HERBAL:** None significant. **FOOD:** None known. **LAB VALUES:** None known.

AVAILABILITY (Rx)

POWDER FOR INJECTION: 0.25 mg.

INDICATIONS/ROUTES/DOSAGE

ADRENOCORTICAL INSUFFICIENCY

IM, IV: ADULTS, ELDERLY, CHILDREN OLDER THAN 2 YRS: 0.25–0.75 mg.

CHILDREN 2 YRS AND YOUNGER: 0.125 mg. **NEONATES:** 0.015 mg/kg/dose.
IV INFUSION: ADULTS, ELDERLY, CHILDREN OLDER THAN 2 YRS: 0.25 mg over 4–8 hrs at 0.04 mg/hr.

SIDE EFFECTS

OCCASIONAL: Nausea, vomiting. **RARE:** Hypersensitivity reaction (fever, pruritus).

ADVERSE EFFECTS/ TOXIC REACTIONS

None known.

NURSING CONSIDERATIONS

BASELINE ASSESSMENT

Hold cortisone, hydrocortisone, spironolactone on test day. Ensure that baseline plasma cortisol concentration has been drawn before start of test or 24-hr urine for 17-KS or 17-OHCS is initiated.

INTERVENTION/EVALUATION

Adhere to time frame for blood draws; monitor urine collection if indicated.

PATIENT/FAMILY TEACHING

- Explain procedure, purpose of test.

co-trimoxazole (sulfamethoxazole-trimethoprim)

koe-try-**mox**-oh-zole

(Apo-Sulfatrim ♣, Bactrim, Bactrim DS, Bactrim Pediatric, Novotrimel ♣, Septra, Septra DS)

Do not confuse Bactrim with bacitracin, co-trimoxazole with clotrimazole, or Septra with Sectral or Septa.

FIXED-COMBINATION(S)

Zotrim: co-trimoxazole/phenazopyridine. **Bactrim, Septra** (sulfamethoxazole/trimethoprim): 5:1 ratio remains constant in all dosage forms (e.g., 400 mg/80 mg).

CLASSIFICATION

PHARMACOTHERAPEUTIC: Sulfonamide/folate antagonist. **CLINICAL:** Antibiotic.

ACTION

Blocks bacterial synthesis of essential nucleic acids. **Therapeutic Effect:** Bactericidal in susceptible microorganisms.

PHARMACOKINETICS

Rapidly, well absorbed from GI tract. Protein binding: 45%–60%. Widely distributed. Metabolized in the liver. Excreted in urine. Minimally removed by hemodialysis. **Half-life:** sulfamethoxazole 6–12 hrs, trimethoprim 8–10 hrs (increased in renal impairment).

USES

Treatment of susceptible infecitons due to *S. pneumoniae, H. influenzae, E. coli,* Klebsiella sp, Enterobacter sp, *M. morganii, P. mirabilis, P. vulgaris, S. flexneri, Pneumocystis carinii* including acute or complicated and recurrent or chronic UTI, *Pneumocystis carinii* pneumonia (PCP), shigellosis, enteritis, otitis media, chronic bronchitis, traveler's diarrhea. Prophylaxis of PCP. **OFF-LABEL:** Treatment of bacterial endocarditis; gonorrhea; meningitis; septicemia; sinusitis; biliary tract, bone, joint, chancroid, chlamydial, intra-abdominal, skin, soft-tissue infections.

PRECAUTIONS

CONTRAINDICATIONS: Hypersensitivity to trimethoprim or any sulfonamides, infants younger than 2 mos, megaloblastic anemia due to folate deficiency. **CAUTIONS:** Those with G6PD deficiency, renal/hepatic impairment.

LIFESPAN CONSIDERATIONS:

Pregnancy/Lactation: Contraindicated during pregnancy at term and during lactation. Readily crosses placenta. Distributed in breast milk. May produce kernicterus in newborn. **Pregnancy Category C (D at term).** **Children:** Contraindicated in those younger than 2 mos, may increase risk of kernicterus in newborn. **Elderly:** Increased risk for severe skin reaction, myelosuppression, decreased platelet count.

INTERACTIONS

DRUG: **Hemolytics** may increase risk of toxicity. **Hepatotoxic medications** may increase risk of hepatotoxicity. May increase, prolong effects, increase toxicity of **hydantoin anticonvulsants, oral hypoglyemics, warfarin.** **Methenamine** may form a precipitate. May increase effects of **methotrexate.** **HERBAL:** **Dong quai, St. John's wort** may increase photosensitization reaction. **FOOD:** None known. **LAB VALUES:** May increase BUN, serum alkaline phosphatase, creatinine, potassium, AST, ALT.

AVAILABILITY (Rx)

◀ ALERT ▶ All dosage forms have same 5:1 ratio of sulfamethoxazole (SMX) to trimethoprim (TMP).

INJECTION SOLUTION: SMX 80 mg and TMP 16 mg per ml. **ORAL SUSPENSION (BACTRIM PEDIATRIC):** SMX 200 mg and TMP 40 mg per 5 ml. **TABLETS (BACTRIM, SEPTRA):** SMX 400 mg and TMP 80 mg. **TABLETS (DOUBLE STRENGTH [BACTRIM DS, SEPTRA DS]):** SMX 800 mg and TMP 160 mg.

ADMINISTRATION/HANDLING

IV

Reconstitution • For IV infusion (piggyback), dilute each 5 ml with 75–125 l D_5W. • Do not mix with other drugs or solutions.

Rate of administration • Infuse over 60–90 min. Must avoid bolus or rapid infusion. • Do not give IM. • Ensure adequate hydration.

Storage • IV infusion (piggyback) stable for 2–6 hrs (use immediately). • Discard if cloudy or precipitate forms.

PO

• Store tablets, suspension at room temperature. • Administer on empty stomach with 8 oz water. • Give several extra glasses of water/day.

IV INCOMPATIBILITIES

Fluconazole (Diflucan), foscarnet (Foscavir), midazolam (Versed), vinorelbine (Navelbine), total parenteral nutrition (TPN).

IV COMPATIBILITIES

Diltiazem (Cardizem), heparin, hydromorphone (Dilaudid), lorazepam (Ativan), magnesium sulfate, morphine.

INDICATIONS/ROUTES/DOSAGE

CHRONIC BRONCHITIS

PO: ADULTS, ELDERLY: 1 double-strength or 2 single-strength tablets or 20 ml suspension q12h for 10–14 days.

PCP

PO: ADULTS, ELDERLY: 1 double-strength tablet daily or 3 times a wk or 1 single-strength tablet daily. **CHILDREN 1 MO AND OLDER:** 150 mg/m^2 as trimethoprim each day in 2 divided doses 3 times a wk on consecutive days.

PCP TREATMENT

PO, IV: ADULTS, ELDERLY, CHILDREN 2 MOS AND OLDER: 15–20 mg/kg as trimethoprim a day in 4 divided doses for 14–21 days.

SHIGELLOSIS

PO: ADULTS, ELDERLY: 1 double-strength tablet or 2 single-strength tablets or 20 ml suspension q12h for 5 days.

IV: ADULTS, CHILDREN: 8–10 mg/kg as trimethoprim a day in 2–4 divided doses for up to 5 days.

OTITIS MEDIA

PO: CHILDREN 2 MOS AND OLDER: 8 mg/kg trimethoprim a day q12h for 10 days.

UTI

PO: ADULTS, ELDERLY: 1 double-strength or 2 single-strength tablets or 20 ml suspension q12h for 3–14 days depending on severity. **CHILDREN 2 MOS AND OLDER:** 8 mg/kg as trimethoprim a day in 2 divided doses for 10 days.

TRAVELERS' DIARRHEA

PO: ADULTS, ELDERLY: 1 double-strength or 2 single-strength tablets or 20 ml suspension q12h for 5 days.

DOSAGE IN RENAL IMPAIRMENT

Creatinine Clearance	Dosage
15–30 ml/min	50% of usual dosage
Less than 15 ml/min	Not recommended

SIDE EFFECTS

FREQUENT: Anorexia, nausea, vomiting, rash (generally 7–14 days after therapy begins), urticaria. **OCCASIONAL:** Diarrhea, abdominal pain, pain/irritation at IV infusion site. **RARE:** Headache, vertigo, insomnia, seizures, hallucinations, depression.

ADVERSE EFFECTS/ TOXIC REACTIONS

Rash, fever, sore throat, pallor, purpura, cough, shortness of breath may be early signs of serious adverse effects. Fatalities are rare but have occurred in sulfonamide therapy following Stevens-Johnson syndrome, toxic epidermal necrolysis, fulminant hepatic necrosis, agranulocytosis, aplastic anemia, other blood dyscrasias. Myelosuppression, decreased platelet count, severe dermatologic reactions may occur, esp. in the elderly.

NURSING CONSIDERATIONS

BASELINE ASSESSMENT

Obtain history for hypersensitivity to trimethoprim or any sulfonamide, sulfite sensitivity, bronchial asthma. Determine renal, hepatic, hematologic baselines.

INTERVENTION/EVALUATION

Monitor daily pattern of bowel activity/stool consistency. Assess skin for rash, pallor, purpura. Check IV site, flow rate. Monitor renal, hepatic, hematology reports. Assess I&O. Check for CNS symptoms (headache, vertigo, insomnia, hallucinations). Monitor vital signs at least twice a day. Monitor for cough, shortness of breath. Assess for overt bleeding, ecchymosis, edema.

PATIENT/FAMILY TEACHING

• Continue medication for full length of therapy. • Space doses evenly around the clock. • Take oral doses with 8 oz water and drink several extra glasses of water daily. • Notify physician immediately of new symptoms, esp. rash, other skin changes, bleeding/bruising, fever, sore throat.

Coumadin, *see warfarin*

Cozaar, *see losartan*

Crestor, *see rosuvastatin*

Crixivan, *see indinavir*

C

cromolyn

kroe-moe-lin

(Apo-Cromolyn ✦, Crolom, Gastrocom, Intal, Nasalcrom, Opticon)

Do not confuse Nasalcrom with Nasacort, Nasalide.

CLASSIFICATION

PHARMACOTHERAPEUTIC: Mast cell stabilizer. **CLINICAL:** Antiasthmatic, antiallergic (see p. 71C).

ACTION

Prevents mast cell release of histamine, leukotrienes, slow-reacting substances of anaphylaxis by inhibiting degranulation after contact with antigens. **Therapeutic Effect:** Assists in preventing symptoms of asthma, allergic rhinitis, mastocytosis, exercise-induced bronchospasm.

PHARMACOKINETICS

Minimal absorption after PO, inhalation, or nasal administration. Absorbed portion excreted in urine or by biliary system. **Half-life:** 80–90 min.

USES

Oral inhalation, nebulization: Prophylactic management of allergic disorders including bronchial asthma, prevention of exercise-induced bronchospasm. **Intranasal:** Prevention/treatment of perennial or seasonal allergic rhinitis. **Systemic:** Symptomatic treatment of systemic mastocytosis. **Ophthalmic:** Conjunctivitis. **OFF-LABEL:** Food allergy, treatment of inflammatory bowel disease (IBD).

PRECAUTIONS

CONTRAINDICATIONS: Status asthmaticus. **CAUTIONS:** Coronary artery disease, arrhythmias, tapering dose or discontinuing therapy (symptoms may recur).

LIFESPAN CONSIDERATIONS:

Pregnancy/Lactation: Unknown if drug crosses placenta or is distributed in breast milk. **Pregnancy Category B.** **Children:** No age-related precautions noted. **Elderly:** Age-related renal/hepatic impairment may require dosage adjustment.

INTERACTIONS

DRUG: None significant. **HERBAL:** None significant. **FOOD:** None known. **LAB VALUES:** None known.

AVAILABILITY (Rx)

CAPSULES (GASTROCROM): 100 mg. **INHALATION SOLUTION (INTAL):** 800 mcg/inhalation. **NASAL SPRAY (NASALCROM):** 40 mg/ml. **NEBULIZATION SOLUTION (INTAL):** 10 mg/ml. **OPHTHALMIC SOLUTION (CROLOM, OPTICROM):** 4%. **ORAL SOLUTION (GASTROCROM):** 100 mg/5 ml.

ADMINISTRATION/HANDLING

PO

• Give at least 30 min before meals. • Pour contents of capsule in hot water, stir until completely dissolved; add equal amount cold water while stirring. • Do not mix with fruit juice, milk, food.

INHALATION

• Shake container well; exhale completely; place mouthpiece fully into mouth, inhale deeply/slowly while depressing the canister; hold breath as long as possible before exhaling. • Wait 1–10 min before inhaling second dose (allows for deeper bronchial penetration). • Rinse mouth with water immediately after inhalation (prevents mouth/throat dryness). **Nebulization, inhalation capsules:** Do not swallow inhalation capsules; instruct pt on use of Spinhaler.

NASAL

• Nasal passages should be clear (may require nasal decongestant). • Inhale through nose.

OPHTHALMIC

• Place finger on lower eyelid; pull down until pocket is formed between eye and lower lid. • Hold dropper above pocket; place prescribed number of drops in pocket. • Instruct pt to close eyes gently so that medication will not be squeezed out of sac. • Apply gentle finger pressure to lacrimal sac at inner canthus for 1 min after installation (reduces risk of systemic absorption).

INDICATIONS/ROUTES/DOSAGE

ASTHMA

INHALATION (NEBULIZATION): **ADULTS, ELDERLY, CHILDREN OLDER THAN 2 YRS:** 20 mg 3–4 times a day.

AEROSOL SPRAY: **ADULTS, ELDERLY, CHILDREN 12 YRS AND OLDER:** Initially, 2 sprays 4 times a day. Maintenance: 2–4 sprays 3–4 times a day. **CHILDREN 5–11 YRS:** Initially, 2 sprays 4 times a day, then 1–2 sprays 3–4 times a day.

PREVENTION OF BRONCHOSPASM

INHALATION (NEBULIZATION): **ADULTS, ELDERLY, CHILDREN OLDER THAN 2 YRS:** 20 mg within 1 hr before exercise or exposure to allergens.

AEROSOL SPRAY: **ADULTS, ELDERLY, CHILDREN OLDER THAN 5 YRS:** 2 sprays within 1 hr before exercise or exposure to allergens.

FOOD ALLERGY, INFLAMMATORY BOWEL DISEASE

PO: **ADULTS, ELDERLY, CHILDREN OLDER THAN 12 YRS:** 200–400 mg 4 times a day. **CHILDREN 2–12 YRS:** 100–200 mg 4 times a day. **Maximum:** 40 mg/kg/day.

ALLERGIC RHINITIS

INTRANASAL: **ADULTS, ELDERLY, CHILDREN OLDER THAN 6 YRS:** 1 spray each nostril 3–4 times a day. May increase up to 6 times a day.

SYSTEMIC MASTOCYTOSIS

PO: **ADULTS, ELDERLY, CHILDREN OLDER THAN 12 YRS:** 200 mg 4 times a day. **CHILDREN 2–12 YRS:** 100 mg 4 times a day. **Maximum:** 40 mg/kg/day. **CHILDREN YOUNGER THAN 2 YRS:** 20 mg/kg/day in 4 divided doses. **Maximum:** 30 mg/kg/day (children 6 mos–2 yrs).

CONJUNCTIVITIS

OPHTHALMIC: **ADULTS, ELDERLY, CHILDREN OLDER THAN 4 YRS:** 1–2 drops in both eyes 4–6 times a day.

SIDE EFFECTS

FREQUENT: PO: Headache, diarrhea. **Inhalation:** Cough, dry mouth/throat, nasal congestion, throat irritation, unpleasant taste. **Nasal:** Nasal burning, stinging, irritation; increased sneezing. **Ophthalmic:** Eye burning/stinging. **OCCASIONAL: PO:** Rash, abdominal pain, arthralgia, nausea, insomnia. **Inhalation:** Bronchospasm, hoarseness, lacrimation. **Nasal:** Cough, headache, unpleasant taste, postnasal drip. **Ophthalmic:** Lacrimation, itching of eye. **RARE: Inhalation:** Dizziness, painful urination, arthralgia, myalgia, rash. **Nasal:** Epistaxis, rash. **Ophthalmic:** Chemosis or edema of conjunctiva, eye irritation.

ADVERSE EFFECTS/ TOXIC REACTIONS

Anaphylaxis occurs rarely when given by inhalation, nasal, oral route.

NURSING CONSIDERATIONS

INTERVENTION/EVALUATION

Monitor rate, depth, rhythm, type of respiration; quality/rate of pulse. Assess lung sounds for rhonchi, wheezing, rales. Observe for cyanosis (lips, fingernails for blue or dusky color in light-skinned pts; gray in dark-skinned pts).

PATIENT/FAMILY TEACHING

• Increase fluid intake (decreases lung secretion viscosity). • Rinsing mouth with water immediately after inhalation may prevent mouth/throat dryness. • Effect of therapy dependent on administration at regular intervals.

C

cyanocobalamin (vitamin B_{12})

sye-an-oh-koe-**bal**-a-min
(Bedoz ✦, Nascobal)

CLASSIFICATION

PHARMACOTHERAPEUTIC: Coenzyme. **CLINICAL:** Vitamin, antianemic (see p. 151C).

ACTION

Coenzyme for metabolic functions (fat, carbohydrate metabolism, protein synthesis). **Therapeutic Effect:** Necessary for cell growth and replication, hematopoiesis, myelin synthesis.

PHARMACOKINETICS

In presence of calcium, absorbed systemically in lower half of ileum. Initially, bound to intrinsic factor; this complex passes down intestine, binding to receptor sites on ileal mucosa. Protein binding: High. Metabolized in the liver. Primarily eliminated unchanged in urine. **Half-life:** 6 days.

USES

Treatment of pernicious anemia, vitamin B_{12} deficiency due to malabsorption diseases, increased B_{12} requirement due to pregnancy, thyrotoxicosis, hemorrhage, malignancy, hepatic/renal disease.

PRECAUTIONS

CONTRAINDICATIONS: Folic acid deficiency anemia, hereditary optic nerve atrophy, history of allergy to cobalamins. **CAUTIONS:** None known.

LIFESPAN CONSIDERATIONS:

Pregnancy/Lactation: Crosses placenta. Excreted in breast milk. **Pregnancy Category A (C if used in doses above recommended daily allowance) C (intranasal). Children/Elderly:** No age-related precautions noted.

INTERACTIONS

DRUG: Alcohol, colchicine may decrease absorption. **Ascorbic acid** may destroy cyanocobalamin. **Folic acid (large doses)** may decrease serum concentration. **HERBAL:** None significant. **FOOD:** None known. **LAB VALUES:** None known.

AVAILABILITY (Rx)

INJECTION SOLUTION: 1,000 mcg/ml. **NASAL GEL (NASCOBAL):** 500 mcg/0.1 ml. **TABLETS:** 50 mcg, 100 mcg, 250 mcg, 500 mcg, 1,000 mcg, 5,000 mcg. **TABLETS (EXTENDED-RELEASE):** 1,500 mcg.

ADMINISTRATION/HANDLING

IM, SUBCUTANEOUS

- Avoid IV route.

PO

- Give with food (increases absorption).

INTRANASAL

- Clear both nostrils. • Pull clear cover off top of pump. • Press down firmly and quickly on pump's finger grips until a droplet of gel appears at top of the pump. Then press down on finger grips two more times. • Place the tip of pump halfway into nostril, pointing tip toward back of nose. • Press down firmly and quickly on finger grips to release medication into one nostril while pressing other nostril closed. • Massage medicated nostril for a few seconds.
- Administer nasal preparation at least 1 hr before or 1 hr after hot foods or liquids are consumed.

INDICATIONS/ROUTES/DOSAGE

PERNICIOUS ANEMIA

IM, SUBCUTANEOUS: ADULTS, ELDERLY: 100 mcg/day for 7 days, then every other day for 7 days, then every 3–4 days for 2–3 wks. Maintenance: 100 mcg/mo (oral 1,000–2,000 mcg/day). **CHILDREN:** 30–50 mcg/day for 2 or more wks. Maintenance: 100 mcg/mo. **NEONATES:** 1,000 mcg/day for 2 or more wks. Maintenance: 50 mcg/mo.

VITAMIN DEFICIENCY

IM, SUBCUTANEOUS: ADULTS, ELDERLY: 30 mcg/day for 5–10 days, then 100–200 mcg/mo.
PO: ADULTS, ELDERLY: 250 mcg/day.
INTRANASAL: ADULTS, ELDERLY: 500 mcg in one nostril once weekly.

HEMATOLOGIC REMISSION

IM, SUBCUTANEOUS: ADULTS, ELDERLY: 100–1000 mcg/mo.
PO: ADULTS, ELDERLY: 1000–2000 mcg/day.
INTRANASAL: ADULTS, ELDERLY: 500 mcg in one nostril once weekly.

SIDE EFFECTS

OCCASIONAL: Diarrhea, pruritus.

ADVERSE EFFECTS/ TOXIC REACTIONS

Impurities in preparation may cause rare allergic reaction. Peripheral vascular thrombosis, pulmonary edema, hypokalemia, CHF occur rarely.

NURSING CONSIDERATIONS

BASELINE ASSESSMENT

Before and during therapy, assess for signs, symptoms of vitamin B_{12} deficiency (anorexia, ataxia, fatigue, hyporeflexia, insomnia, irritability, loss of positional sense, pallor, palpitations on exertion).

INTERVENTION/EVALUATION

Assess for CHF, pulmonary edema, hypokalemia in cardiac pts receiving subcutaneous/IM therapy. Monitor serum potassium (3.5–5 mEq/L), serum B_{12} (200–800 mcg/ml), rise in reticulocyte count (peaks in 5–8 days). Assess for reversal of deficiency symptoms (hyporeflexia, loss of positional sense, ataxia, fatigue, irritability, insomnia, anorexia, pallor, palpitations on exertion). Therapeutic response to treatment usually dramatic within 48 hrs.

PATIENT/FAMILY TEACHING

• Lifetime treatment may be necessary with pernicious anemia. • Report symptoms of infection. • Foods rich in vitamin B_{12} include organ meats, clams, oysters, herring, red snapper, muscle meats, fermented cheese, dairy products, egg yolks. • Use nasal preparation at least 1 hr before or 1 hr after consuming hot foods, liquids.

cyclobenzaprine

sye-kloe-**ben**-za-preen
(Apo-cyclobenzaprine ✤, Flexeril, Flexitec ✤, Novo-Cycloprine ✤)

Do not confuse cyclobenzaprine with cycloserine or cyproheptadine, or Flexeril with Floxin.

CLASSIFICATION

CLINICAL: Skeletal muscle relaxant.

ACTION

Centrally acting skeletal muscle relaxant that reduces tonic somatic muscle activity at level of brainstem. **Therapeutic Effect:** Relieves local skeletal muscle spasm.

PHARMACOKINETICS

Route	Onset	Peak	Duration
PO	1 hr	3–4 hrs	12–24 hrs

Well but slowly absorbed from GI tract. Protein binding: 93%. Metabolized in GI tract and liver. Primarily excreted in urine. **Half-life:** 1–3 days.

USES

Treatment of muscle spasm associated with acute, painful musculoskeletal conditions. **OFF-LABEL:** Treatment of fibromyalgia.

PRECAUTIONS

CONTRAINDICATIONS: Acute recovery phase of MI, arrhythmias, CHF, heart block, conduction disturbances,

C

hyperthyroidism, use within 14 days of MAOIs. **CAUTIONS:** Renal/hepatic impairment, history of urinary retention, angle-closure glaucoma, increased intraocular pressure (IOP).

LIFESPAN CONSIDERATIONS:

Pregnancy/Lactation: Unknown if drug crosses placenta or is distributed in breast milk. **Pregnancy Category B.** **Children:** Safety and efficacy not established. **Elderly:** Increased sensitivity to anticholinergic effects (e.g., confusion, urinary retention).

INTERACTIONS

DRUG: **Alcohol, other CNS depressant medications (e.g., tricyclic antidepressants)** may increase CNS depression. **MAOIs** may increase risk of hypertensive crisis, seizures. **Tramadol** may increase risk of seizures. **HERBAL:** **Gotu kola, kava kava, SAMe, St. John's wort, valerian** may increase CNS depression. **FOOD:** None known. **LAB VALUES:** None known.

AVAILABILITY (Rx)

TABLETS: 5 mg, 10 mg.

ADMINISTRATION/HANDLING

PO

- Give without regard to food.

INDICATIONS/ROUTES/DOSAGE

ACUTE, PAINFUL MUSCULOSKELETAL CONDITIONS

PO: ADULTS: Initially, 5 mg 3 times a day. May increase to 10 mg 3 times a day. **ELDERLY:** 5 mg 3 times a day.

DOSAGE IN HEPATIC IMPAIRMENT

MILD: 5 mg 3 times a day. **MODERATE AND SEVERE:** Not recommended.

SIDE EFFECTS

FREQUENT: Somnolence (39%), dry mouth (27%), dizziness (11%). **RARE (3%–1%):** Fatigue, asthenia, blurred vision, headache, anxiety, confusion, nausea, constipation, dyspepsia, unpleasant taste.

ADVERSE EFFECTS/ TOXIC REACTIONS

Overdose may result in visual hallucinations, hyperactive reflexes, muscle rigidity, vomiting, hyperpyrexia.

NURSING CONSIDERATIONS

BASELINE ASSESSMENT

Record onset, type, location, duration of muscular spasm. Check for immobility, stiffness, swelling.

INTERVENTION/EVALUATION

Assist with ambulation at all times. Evaluate for therapeutic response (decreased intensity of skeletal muscle pain/tenderness, improved mobility, decrease in stiffness).

PATIENT/FAMILY TEACHING

• Drowsiness usually diminishes with continued therapy. • Avoid tasks that require alertness, motor skills until response to drug is established. • Avoid alcohol, other depressants while taking medication. • Avoid sudden changes in posture. • Sugarless gum, sips of water may relieve dry mouth.

cyclophosphamide

sye-kloe-**foss**-fa-mide

(Cytoxan, Cytoxan Lyophilized, Neosar, Procytox ✤)

Do not confuse Cytoxan with cefoxitin, Ciloxan, Cytotec, or Cytosar, or cyclophosphamide with cyclosporine.

◆CLASSIFICATION

PHARMACOTHERAPEUTIC: Alkylating agent. **CLINICAL:** Antineoplastic (see p. 77C).

ACTION

Inhibits DNA, RNA protein synthesis by cross-linking with DNA, RNA strands. Cell cycle–phase nonspecific. **Therapeutic Effect:** Prevent cell growth. Potent immunosuppressant.

PHARMACOKINETICS

Well absorbed from GI tract. Protein binding: Low. Crosses blood-brain barrier. Metabolized in the liver to active metabolites. Primarily excreted in urine. Removed by hemodialysis. **Half-life:** 3–12 hrs.

USES

Treatment of acute lymphocytic, acute nonlymphocytic, chronic myelocytic, chronic lymphocytic leukemias; ovarian, breast carcinomas; neuroblastoma, retinobalstoma, Hodgkin's, non-Hodgkin's lymphomas; multiple myeloma, mycosis fungoides, nephrotic syndrome. **OFF-LABEL:** Adrenocortical, bladder, cervical, endometrial, prostatic, testicular carcinomas; Ewing's sarcoma; multiple sclerosis: non–small cell, small cell lung cancer; organ transplant rejection; osteosarcoma; ovarian germ cell, primary brain, trophoblastic tumors; rheumatoid arthritis; soft-tissue sarcomas, systemic dermatomyositis, systemic lupus erythematosus, Wilms' tumor.

PRECAUTIONS

CONTRAINDICATIONS: Severe myelosuppression. **CAUTIONS:** Severe leukopenia, thrombocytopenia, tumor infiltration of bone marrow, previous therapy with other antineoplastic agents, radiation.

LIFESPAN CONSIDERATIONS:

Pregnancy/Lactation: If possible, avoid use during pregnancy. May cause fetal malformations (limb abnormalities, cardiac anomalies, hernias). Distributed in breast milk. Breast-feeding not recommended. **Pregnancy Category D.** **Children:** No age-related precautions noted. **Elderly:** Age-related renal impairment may require dosage adjustment.

INTERACTIONS

DRUG: Allopurinol, bone marrow depressants may increase myelosuppression. May decrease effects of **anti-gout medications. Cytarabine** may increase risk of cardiomyopathy. **Immunosuppressants** may increase risk of infection, development of neoplasms. **Live virus vaccines** may potentiate virus replication, increase vaccine side effects, decrease pt's antibody response to vaccine. **HERBAL:** None significant. **FOOD:** None known. **LAB VALUES:** May increase serum uric acid.

AVAILABILITY (Rx)

INJECTION, POWDER FOR RECONSTITUTION (CYTOXAN, NEOSAR): 100 mg, 200 mg, 500 mg, 1 g, 2 g. **TABLETS (CYTOXAN):** 25 mg, 50 mg.

ADMINISTRATION/HANDLING

◀ **ALERT** ▶ May be carcinogenic, mutagenic, teratogenic. Handle with extreme care during preparation/administration.

IV

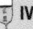

Reconstitution • For IV push, reconstitute each 100 mg with 5 ml Sterile Water for Injection or Bacteriostatic Water for Injection to provide concentration of 20 mg/ml. • Shake to dissolve. Allow to stand until clear.

Rate of administration • May give by IV push or further dilute with 250 ml D_5W, 0.9% NaCl, 0.45% NaCl, lactated

C

Ringer's (LR) solution or D_5W/LR. • Infuse each 100 mg or fraction thereof over 15 min or longer. • IV route may produce faintness, facial flushing, diaphoresis, oropharyngeal sensation.

Storage • Reconstituted solution is stable for 24 hrs at room temperature or up to 6 days if refrigerated.

PO

• Give on an empty stomach. If GI upset occurs, give with food.

IV INCOMPATIBILITIES

Amphotericin B complex (Abelcet, AmBisome, Amphotec).

IV COMPATIBILITIES

Granisetron (Kytril), heparin, hydromorphone (Dilaudid), lipids, lorazepam (Ativan), morphine, ondansetron (Zofran), propofol (Diprivan).

INDICATIONS/ROUTES/DOSAGE

USUAL DOSAGE (REFER TO INDIVIDUAL PROTOCOLS)

IV: ADULTS, ELDERLY, CHILDREN: (Single Dose): 400–1,800 mg/m^2 (30–50 mg/kg) per treatment course (1–5 days), which may be repeated q2–4wk.

PO: ADULTS, ELDERLY, CHILDREN: 50–100 mg/m^2 day as continuous therapy or 400–1,000 mg/m^2 in divided doses over 4–5 days as intermittent therapy.

BIOPSY-PROVEN MINIMAL-CHANGE NEPHROTIC SYNDROME

PO: ADULTS, CHILDREN: 2.5–3 mg/kg/day for 60–90 days.

SIDE EFFECTS

EXPECTED: Marked leukopenia 8–15 days after initial therapy. **FREQUENT:** Nausea, vomiting (beginning about 6 hrs after administration and lasting about 4 hrs); alopecia (33%). **OCCASIONAL:** Diarrhea, darkening of skin/fingernails, stomatitis, headache, diaphoresis. **RARE:** Pain/redness at injection site.

ADVERSE EFFECTS/ TOXIC REACTIONS

Major toxic effect is myelosuppression resulting in blood dyscrasias (leukopenia, anemia, thrombocytopenia, hypoprothrombinemia). Expect leukopenia to resolve in 17–28 days. Anemia generally occurs after large doses or prolonged therapy. Thrombocytopenia may occur 10–15 days after drug initiation. Hemorrhagic cystitis occurs commonly in long-term therapy (esp. in children). Pulmonary fibrosis, cardiotoxicity noted with high doses. Amenorrhea, azoospermia, hyperkalemia may occur.

NURSING CONSIDERATIONS

BASELINE ASSESSMENT

Obtain WBC count weekly during therapy or until maintenance dose is established, then at 2- to 3-wk intervals.

INTERVENTION/EVALUATION

Monitor CBC, serum uric acid, electrolytes. Monitor WBC closely during initial therapy. Monitor for hematologic toxicity (fever, sore throat, signs of local infection, unusual bruising/bleeding from any site), symptoms of anemia (excessive fatigue, weakness). Recovery from marked leukopenia due to myelosuppression can be expected in 17–28 days.

PATIENT/FAMILY TEACHING

• Encourage copious fluid intake, frequent voiding (assists in preventing cystitis) at least 24 hrs before, during, after therapy. • Do not have immunizations without physician's approval (drug lowers resistance). • Avoid contact with those who have recently received live virus vaccine. • Promptly report fever, sore throat, signs of local infection, unusual bruising/bleeding from any site. • Alopecia is reversible, but new hair growth may have different color, texture.

*cycloSPORINE

sye-kloe-**spor**-in
(Apo-Cyclosporine ✤, Gengraf, Neoral, Restasis, Sandimmune)

Do not confuse cyclosporine with cycloserine or cyclophosphamide.

◆CLASSIFICATION

PHARMACOTHERAPEUTIC: Cyclic polypeptide. **CLINICAL:** Immunosuppressant (see p. 114C).

ACTION

Inhibits cellular, humoral immune responses by inhibiting interleukin-2, a proliferative factor needed for T-cell activity. **Therapeutic Effect:** Prevents organ rejection, relieves symptoms of psoriasis, arthritis.

PHARMACOKINETICS

Variably absorbed from GI tract. Protein binding: 90%. Widely distributed. Metabolized in the liver. Eliminated primarily by biliary or fecal excretion. Not removed by hemodialysis. **Half-life:** Adults, 10–27 hrs; children, 7–19 hrs.

USES

Prevents organ rejection of kidney, liver, heart in combination with steroid therapy. Treatment of chronic allograft rejection in those previously treated with other immunosuppressives. **Capsules/Solution:** Treatment of severe, active rheumatoid arthritis, psoriasis. **Ophthalmic:** Chronic dry eyes. **OFF-LABEL:** Treatment of alopecia areata, aplastic anemia, atopic dermatitis, Behçet's disease, biliary cirrhosis, prevention of corneal transplant rejection, ulcerative colitis.

PRECAUTIONS

CONTRAINDICATIONS: History of hypersensitivity to cyclosporine, polyoxyethylated castor oil. **CAUTIONS:** Hepatic, renal, cardiac impairment; malabsorption syndrome; pregnancy; chickenpox; herpes zoster infection; hypokalemia. **Ophthalmic:** Active eye infection.

⌛ LIFESPAN CONSIDERATIONS:

Pregnancy/Lactation: Readily crosses placenta. Distributed in breast milk. Avoid breast-feeding. **Pregnancy Category C. Children:** No age-related precautions noted in transplant pts. **Elderly:** Increased risk of hypertension, increased serum creatinine.

INTERACTIONS

DRUG: Allopurinol, bromocriptine, cimetidine, clarithromycin, danazol, diltiazem, estrogens, erythromycin, fluconazole, itraconazole, ketoconazole may increase plasma concentration, risk of hepatic/renal toxicity. **ACE inhibitors, potassium-sparing diuretics, potassium supplements** may cause hyperkalemia. **Immunosuppressants** may increase risk of infection, lymphoproliferative disorders. **Lovastatin** may increase risk of rhabdomyolysis, acute renal failure. **Live virus vaccines** may potentiate virus replication, increase vaccine side effects, decrease pt's response to vaccine. **HERBAL:** Avoid **cat's claw, echinacea** (possess immunostimulant properties). **St. John's wort** may decrease plasma concentration. **FOOD: Grapefruit, grapefruit juice** may increase absorption, risk of toxicity. **LAB VALUES:** May increase BUN, serum alkaline phosphatase, amylase, bilirubin, creatinine, potassium, uric acid, AST, ALT. May decrease serum magnesium. Therapeutic peak serum level is 50–300 ng/ml; toxic serum level is greater than 400 ng/ml.

C

AVAILABILITY (Rx)

CAPSULES (GENGRAF, NEORAL [MODIFIED] SANDIMMUNE [NONMODIFIED]): 25 mg, 100 mg. **INJECTION, SOLUTION (SANDIMMUNE):** 50 mg/ml. **OPHTHALMIC EMULSION (RESTASIS):** 0.05%. **ORAL SOLUTION (GENGRAF, NEORAL [MODIFIED] SANDIMMUNE [NONMODIFIED]):** 100 mg/ml.

ADMINISTRATION/HANDLING

◀ **ALERT** ▶ Oral solution available in bottle form with calibrated liquid measuring device. Oral form should replace IV administration as soon as possible.

IV

Reconstitution • Dilute each ml concentrate with 20–100 ml 0.9% NaCl or D_5W.

Rate of administration • Infuse over 2–6 hrs. • Monitor pt continuously for first 30 min after instituting infusion and frequently thereafter for hypersensitivity reaction (facial flushing, dyspnea).

Storage • Store parenteral form at room temperature. • Protect IV solution from light. • After diluted, stable for 24 hrs.

PO

• Oral solution may be mixed in glass container with milk, chocolate milk, orange juice (preferably at room temperature). Stir well. Drink immediately. • Add more diluent to glass container. Mix with remaining solution to ensure total amount is given. • Dry outside of calibrated liquid measuring device before replacing in cover. Do not rinse with water. • Avoid refrigeration of oral solution (solution may separate). Discard oral solution after 2 mos once bottle is opened.

OPHTHALMIC

• Invert vial several times to obtain uniform suspension. • Instruct pt to remove contacts before administration (may reinsert 15 min after administration). • May use with artificial tears.

IV INCOMPATIBILITIES

Amphotericin B complex (Abelcet, AmBisome, Amphotec), magnesium.

IV COMPATIBILITY

Lipids, propofol (Diprivan).

INDICATIONS/ROUTES/DOSAGE

TRANSPLANTATION, PREVENTION OF ORGAN REJECTION

PO: ADULTS, ELDERLY, CHILDREN: NOT MODIFIED: 10–18 mg/kg/dose given 4–12 hrs prior to organ transplantation. Maintenance: 5–15 mg/kg/day in divided doses then tapered to 3–10 mg/kg/day. Modified (dose dependent upon type of transplant): Renal: 6–12 mg/kg/day in 2 divided doses. Hepatic: 4–12 mg/kg/day in 2 divided doses. Heart: 4–10 mg/kg/day in 2 divided doses.

IV: ADULTS, ELDERLY, CHILDREN: Initially, 5–6 mg/kg/dose given 4–12 hrs prior to organ transplantation. Maintenance: 2–10 mg/kg/day in divided doses.

RHEUMATOID ARTHRITIS

PO: ADULTS, ELDERLY: Initially, 2.5 mg/kg a day in 2 divided doses. May increase by 0.5–0.75 mg/kg/day. **Maximum:** 4 mg/kg/day.

PSORIASIS

PO: ADULTS, ELDERLY: Initially, 2.5 mg/kg/day in 2 divided doses. May increase by 0.5 mg/kg/day. **Maximum:** 4 mg/kg/day.

DRY EYE

OPHTHALMIC: ADULTS, ELDERLY: Instill 1 drop in each affected eye q12h.

SIDE EFFECTS

FREQUENT: Mild to moderate hypertension (26%), hirsutism (21%), tremor (12%). **OCCASIONAL (4%–2%):** Acne, leg cramps, gingival hyperplasia (red, bleeding, tender gums), paresthesia, diarrhea, nausea, vomiting, headache. **RARE (less than 1%):** Hypersensitivity reaction, abdominal discomfort, gynecomastia, sinusitis.

ADVERSE EFFECTS/ TOXIC REACTIONS

Mild nephrotoxicity occurs in 25% of renal transplants, 38% of cardiac transplants, 37% of liver transplants, generally 2–3 mos after transplantation (more severe toxicity may occur soon after transplantation). Hepatotoxicity occurs in 4% of renal, 7% of cardiac, and 4% of liver transplants, generally within first mo after transplantation. Both toxicities usually respond to dosage reduction. Severe hyperkalemia, hyperuricemia occur occasionally.

NURSING CONSIDERATIONS

BASELINE ASSESSMENT

If nephrotoxicity occurs, mild toxicity is generally noted 2–3 mos after transplantation; more severe toxicity noted early after transplantation; hepatotoxicity may be noted during first month after transplantation.

INTERVENTION/EVALUATION

Diligently monitor BUN, serum creatinine, bilirubin, AST, ALT, LDH levels for evidence of hepatotoxicity, nephrotoxicity (mild toxicity noted by slow rise in serum levels; more overt toxicity noted by rapid rise in levels; hematuria also noted in nephrotoxicity). Monitor serum potassium for evidence of hyperkalemia. Encourage diligent oral hygiene (gingival hyperplasia). Monitor B/P for evidence of hypertension. Therapeutic serum level: Peak: 50–300 ng/ml; toxic serum level: greater than 400 ng/ml.

PATIENT/FAMILY TEACHING

• Essential to repeat blood testing on a routine basis while receiving medication. • Headache, tremor may occur as a response to medication. • Avoid grapefruit, grapefruit juice (increases concentration, side effects).

cytarabine

sigh-**tar**-ah-bean

(Ara-C, Cytosar ♣, Cytosar-U, Depo-Cyt)

Do not confuse cytarabine with Cytoxan, vidarabine or Cytosar with Cytoxan, Neosar.

CLASSIFICATION

PHARMACOTHERAPEUTIC: Antimetabolite. **CLINICAL:** Antineoplastic (see p. 78C).

ACTION

Converted intracellularly to nucleotide. Cell cycle–specific for S phase of cell division. **Therapeutic Effect:** Appears to inhibit DNA synthesis. Potent immunosuppressive activity.

PHARMACOKINETICS

Widely distributed; moderate amount crosses blood-brain barrier. Protein binding: 15%. Primarily excreted in urine. **Half-life:** 1–3 hrs.

USES

Treatment of acute lymphocytic, acute nonlymphocytic, chronic myelocytic, meningeal leukemias. **Depo-Cyt:** Treatment of neoplastic meningitis.

C

OFF-LABEL: Carcinomatous meningitis, Hodgkin's and non-Hodgkin's lymphomas, myelodysplastic syndrome.

PRECAUTIONS

CONTRAINDICATIONS: None known. **CAUTIONS:** Hepatic impairment.

LIFESPAN CONSIDERATIONS:

Pregnancy/Lactation: If possible, avoid use during pregnancy. May cause fetal malformations. Unknown if distributed in breast milk. Breast-feeding not recommended. **Pregnancy Category D.** **Children:** No age-related precautions noted. **Elderly:** Age-related renal impairment may require dosage adjustment.

INTERACTIONS

DRUG: May decrease effects of **antigout medications**. **Bone marrow depressants** may increase myelosuppression. **Cyclophosphamide** may increase risk of cardiomyopathy. **Live virus vaccines** may potentiate virus replication, increase vaccine side effects, and decrease pt's antibody response to vaccine. **HERBAL:** None significant. **FOOD:** None known. **LAB VALUES:** May increase serum alkaline phosphatase, bilirubin, uric acid, AST.

AVAILABILITY (Rx)

INJECTION, POWDER FOR RECONSTITUTION: (ARA-C, CYTOSAR U): 100 mg, 500 mg, 1 g, 2 g. **INJECTION SOLUTION (ARA-C, CYTOSAR U):** 20 mg/ml, 100 mg/ml. **INJECTION, SUSPENSION (DEPO-CYT):** 10 mg/ml.

ADMINISTRATION/HANDLING

◄ **ALERT** ► May give by subcutaneous, IV push, IV infusion, intrathecal routes. May be carcinogenic, mutagenic, teratogenic (embryonic deformity). Handle with extreme care during preparation/administration. Depo-Cyt for intrathecal use only.

IV, SUBCUTANEOUS, INTRATHECAL

IV

Reconstitution • Reconstitute 100-mg vial with 5 ml Bacteriostatic Water for Injection with benzyl alcohol (10 ml for 500–mg vial) to provide concentration of 20 mg/ml and 50 mg/ml, respectively. • Dose may be further diluted with up to 1,000 ml D_5W or 0.9% NaCl for IV infusion. • For intrathecal use, reconstitute vial with preservative-free 0.9% NaCl or pt's spinal fluid. Dose usually administered in 5–15 ml of solution, after equivalent volume of cerebrospinal fluid (CSF) removed.

Rate of administration • For IV push, give over 1–3 min. • For IV infusion, give over 30 min–24 hrs.

Storage • Reconstituted solution is stable for 48 hrs at room temperature. • IV infusion solution at concentration up to 0.5 mg/ml is stable for 7 days at room temperature. • Discard if slight haze develops.

IV INCOMPATIBILITIES

Amphotericin B complex (Abelcet, AmBisome, Amphotec), ganciclovir (Cytovene), heparin, insulin (regular).

IV COMPATIBILITIES

Dexamethasone (Decadron), diphenhydramine (Benadryl), filgrastim (Neupogen), granisetron (Kytril), hydromorphone (Dilaudid), lipids, lorazepam (Ativan), morphine, ondansetron (Zofran), potassium chloride, propofol (Diprivan), total parenteral nutrition (TPN).

INDICATIONS/ROUTES/DOSAGE

USUAL DOSAGE FOR INDUCTION

IV: ADULTS, ELDERLY, CHILDREN: (Induction): 200 mg/m^2/day for 5 days q2wk as monotherapy or 100–200 mg/m^2/day

for 5- to 10-day course of therapy every q2–4wk in combination therapy. Maintenance: 70–200 mg/m^2/day for 2–5 days at monthly intervals.
INTRATHECAL: ADULTS, ELDERLY, CHILDREN: 5–7.5 mg/m^2 every 2–7 days.

USUAL MAINTENANCE DOSAGE
IV: ADULTS, ELDERLY, CHILDREN: 70–200 mg/m^2/day for 2–5 days every mo.
IM, SUBCUTANEOUS: ADULTS, ELDERLY, CHILDREN: 1–1.5 mg/m^2 as single dose q1–4wk.
INTRATHECAL: ADULTS, ELDERLY, CHILDREN: 5–7.5 mg/m^2 every 2–7 days.

USUAL DOSAGE FOR DEPOCYT
INTRATHECALY: ADULTS, ELDERLY: **(Induction):** 50 mg q14days for 2 doses (wks 1, 3). **(Consolidation):** 50 mg q14days for 3 doses (wks 5, 7, 9) followed by additional dose at wk 13. **(Maintenance):** 50 mg q28 days for 4 doses (wks 17, 21, 25, 29).

SIDE EFFECTS

FREQUENT: IV, Subcutaneous (33%–16%): Asthenia, fever, pain, altered taste/smell, nausea, vomiting (risk greater with IV push than with continuous IV infusion). **Intrathecal (28%–11%):** Headache, asthenia, altered taste/smell, confusion, somnolence, nausea, vomiting. **OCCASIONAL: IV, Subcutaneous (11%–7%):** Abnormal gait, somnolence, constipation, back pain, urinary incontinence, peripheral edema, headache, confusion. **Intrathecal (7%–3%):** Peripheral edema, back pain, constipation, abnormal gait, urinary incontinence.

ADVERSE EFFECTS/ TOXIC REACTIONS

Major toxic reaction is myelosuppression resulting in blood dyscrasias (leukopenia, anemia, thrombocytopenia, megaloblastosis, reticulocytopenia) occurring minimally after single IV dose. Leukopenia, anemia, thrombocytopenia should be expected with daily or continuous IV therapy. Cytarabine syndrome, (fever, myalgia, rash, conjunctivitis, malaise, chest pain), hyperuricemia may occur. High-dose therapy may produce severe CNS, GI, pulmonary toxicity.

NURSING CONSIDERATIONS

BASELINE ASSESSMENT

Leukocyte count decreases within 24 hrs after initial dose, continues to decrease for 7–9 days followed by brief rise at 12 days, decreases again at 15–24 days, then rises rapidly for next 10 days. Platelet count decreases 5 days after drug initiation to its lowest count at 12–15 days, then rises rapidly for next 10 days.

INTERVENTION/EVALUATION

Monitor CBC for evidence of myelosuppression. Monitor for blood dyscrasias (fever, sore throat, signs of local infection, unusual bruising/bleeding from any site), symptoms of anemia (excessive fatigue, weakness). Monitor for signs of neuropathy (gait disturbances, handwriting difficulties, paresthesias).

PATIENT/FAMILY TEACHING

• Increase fluid intake (may protect against hyperuricemia). • Do not have immunizations without physician's approval (drug lowers resistance). • Avoid contact with those who have recently received live virus vaccine. • Promptly report fever, sore throat, signs of local infection, unusual bruising/bleeding from any site.

D

dacarbazine

day-**car**-bah-zeen
(DTIC ✱, DTIC-Dome)

Do not confuse dacarbazine with Dicarbosil or procarbazine.

CLASSIFICATION

PHARMACOTHERAPEUTIC: Alkylating agent. **CLINICAL:** Antineoplastic (see p. 78C).

ACTION

Forms methyldiazonium ions, which attack nucleophilic groups in DNA. Cross-links DNA strands. **Therapeutic Effect:** Inhibits DNA, RNA, protein synthesis.

PHARMACOKINETICS

Minimally crosses blood-brain barrier. Protein binding: 5%. Metabolized in liver. Excreted in urine. **Half-life:** 5 hrs (increased in renal impairment).

USES

Treatment of metastatic malignant melanoma, second-line therapy of Hodgkin's disease. **OFF-LABEL:** Treatment of islet cell carcinoma, neuroblastoma, soft-tissue sarcoma.

PRECAUTIONS

CONTRAINDICATIONS: Demonstrated hypersensitivity to dacarbazine. **CAUTIONS:** Hepatic impairment.

LIFESPAN CONSIDERATIONS:

Pregnancy/Lactation: If possible, avoid use during pregnancy, esp. first trimester. Breast-feeding not recommended. **Pregnancy Category C. Children:** Safety and efficacy not established. **Elderly:** Age-related renal impairment may require dosage adjustment.

INTERACTIONS

DRUG: Bone marrow depressants may enhance myelosuppression. **Live virus vaccines** may potentiate virus replication, increase vaccine side effects, decrease pt's antibody response to the vaccine. **HERBAL: Dong quai, St. John's wort** may increase photosensitization. **FOOD:** None known. **LAB VALUES:** May increase BUN, serum alkaline phosphatase, AST, ALT.

AVAILABILITY (Rx)

INJECTION, POWDER FOR RECONSTITUTION: 100-mg vials, 200-mg vials, 500-mg vials.

ADMINISTRATION/HANDLING

◀ **ALERT** ▶ Give by IV push or IV infusion. May be carcinogenic, mutagenic, teratogenic. Handle with extreme care during preparation/administration.

IV

Reconstitution • Reconstitute 100-mg vial with 9.9 ml Sterile Water for Injection (19.7 ml for 200-mg vial) to provide concentration of 10 mg/ml.

Rate of administration • Give IV push over 2–3 min. • For IV infusion, further dilute with up to 250 ml D_5W or 0.9% NaCl. Infuse over 15–30 min. • Apply hot packs if local pain, burning sensation, irritation at injection site occurs. • Avoid extravasation (stinging, swelling, coolness, slight or no blood return at injection site).

Storage • Protect from light; refrigerate vials. • Color change from ivory to pink indicates decomposition; discard. • Solution containing 10 mg/ml is stable for 8 hrs at room temperature or 72 hrs if refrigerated. • Solution diluted with up to 500 ml D_5W or 0.9% NaCl is stable for at least 8 hrs at room temperature or 24 hrs if refrigerated.

IV INCOMPATIBILITIES

Allopurinol (Aloprim), cefepime (Maxipime), heparin, piperacillin and tazobactam (Zosyn).

IV COMPATIBILITIES

Etoposide (VePesid), granisetron (Kytril), ondansetron (Zofran), paclitaxel (Taxol).

INDICATIONS/ROUTES/DOSAGE

MALIGNANT MELANOMA

IV: ADULTS, ELDERLY: 2–4.5 mg/kg/day for 10 days, repeated q4wk; or 150–250 mg/m^2 a day for 5 days, repeated q3–4wk.

HODGKIN'S DISEASE

IV: ADULTS, ELDERLY: 100 mg/m^2/day for 5 days, repeated q4wk; or 375 mg/m^2 once, repeated every 15 days (as combination therapy). **CHILDREN:** 375 mg/m^2 on days 1 and 15; repeated every 28 days (as combination therapy).

SOLID TUMORS

IV: CHILDREN: 200–470 mg/m^2/day over 5 days every 21–28 days.

NEUROBLASTOMA

IV: CHILDREN: 800–900 mg/m^2 as single dose on day 1 of therapy, repeated q3–4wk (as combination therapy).

SIDE EFFECTS

FREQUENT (90%): Nausea, vomiting, anorexia (occurs within 1 hr of initial dose, may last up to 12 hrs). **OCCASIONAL:** Facial flushing, paresthesia, alopecia, flu-like symptoms (fever, myalgia, malaise), dermatologic reactions, confusion, blurred vision, headache, lethargy. **RARE:** Diarrhea, stomatitis, photosensitivity.

ADVERSE EFFECTS/ TOXIC REACTIONS

Myelosuppression resulting in blood dyscrasias (leukopenia, thrombocytopenia) generally appears 2–4 wks after last dacarbazine dose. Hepatotoxicity occurs rarely.

NURSING CONSIDERATIONS

BASELINE ASSESSMENT

Some clinicians recommend food, fluid restriction 4–6 hrs before treatment; other clinicians believe good hydration to within 1 hr of treatment will prevent dehydration due to vomiting. Conflicting reports of effectiveness of administering antiemetics for nausea, vomiting.

INTERVENTION/EVALUATION

Monitor leukocyte, erythrocyte, platelet counts for evidence of myelosuppression. Monitor for hematologic toxicity (fever, sore throat, signs of local infection, unusual bleeding/bruising from any site).

PATIENT/FAMILY TEACHING

• Tolerance to GI effects occurs rapidly (generally after 1–2 days of treatment). • Do not have immunizations without physician's approval (drug lowers resistance). • Avoid contact with those who have recently received live virus vaccine. • Promptly report fever, sore throat, signs of local infection, unusual bleeding/bruising from any site. • Notify physician of persistent nausea, vomiting.

daclizumab

day-**cly**-zu-mab
(Zenapax)

CLASSIFICATION

PHARMACOTHERAPEUTIC: Monoclonal antibody. **CLINICAL:** Immunosuppressive (see p. 114C).

ACTION

Binds to interleukin-2 (IL-2) receptor complex, inhibiting IL-2–mediated activation of T lymphocytes, a critical pathway in cellular immune response involved in allograft rejection. **Therapeutic Effect:** Prevents organ rejection.

PHARMACOKINETICS

Half-life: Adults: 20 days. **Children:** 13 days.

D

USES

Prophylaxis of acute organ rejection in pts receiving renal transplants (in combination with an immunosuppressive regimen). **OFF-LABEL:** Treatment of aplastic anemia, graft vs. host disease.

PRECAUTIONS

CONTRAINDICATIONS: None known. **CAUTIONS:** Infection, history of malignancy.

LIFESPAN CONSIDERATIONS:

Pregnancy/Lactation: Unknown if drug crosses placenta or is distributed in breast milk. **Pregnancy Category C.** **Children/Elderly:** No age-related precautions noted.

INTERACTIONS

DRUG: None significant. **HERBAL:** None significant. **FOOD:** None known. **LAB VALUES:** None known.

AVAILABILITY (Rx)

INJECTION SOLUTION: 5 mg/ml.

ADMINISTRATION/HANDLING

IV

Reconstitution • Dilute in 50 ml 0.9% NaCl. • Invert gently. • Avoid shaking.

Rate of administration • Infuse over 15 min.

Storage • Protect from light; refrigerate vials. • Once reconstituted, stable for 4 hrs at room temperature, 24 hrs if refrigerated.

IV INCOMPATIBILITIES

Do not mix daclizumab with any other drugs.

INDICATIONS/ROUTES/DOSAGE

PREVENTION OF ACUTE RENAL TRANSPLANT REJECTION (IN COMBINATION WITH AN IMMUNOSUPPRESSIVE)

IV: ADULTS, CHILDREN: 1 mg/kg over 15 min q14days for 5 doses, beginning no more than 24 hrs before transplantation. **Maximum:** 100 mg.

SIDE EFFECTS

OCCASIONAL (greater than 2%): Constipation, nausea, diarrhea, vomiting, abdominal pain, edema, headache, dizziness, fever, pain, fatigue, insomnia, weakness, arthralgia, myalgia, diaphoresis.

ADVERSE EFFECTS/ TOXIC REACTIONS

Hypersensitivity reaction (dyspnea, tachycardia, dysphagia, peripheral edema, rash, pruritus) occurs rarely.

NURSING CONSIDERATIONS

BASELINE ASSESSMENT

Obtain baseline laboratory studies, vital signs, particularly B/P, pulse.

INTERVENTION/EVALUATION

Diligently monitor all serum levels, CBC. Assess B/P for hypertension/hypotension; pulse for evidence of tachycardia. Question for GI disturbances, urinary changes. Monitor for presence of wound infection, signs of systemic infection (fever, sore throat), unusual bleeding/bruising.

PATIENT/FAMILY TEACHING

• Report difficulty in breathing or swallowing, tachycardia, rash, pruritus, swelling of lower extremities, weakness. • Avoid pregnancy.

Dalmane, *see flurazepam*

dalteparin

dawl-teh-pear-in
(Fragmin)

CLASSIFICATION

PHARMACOTHERAPEUTIC: Low-molecular-weight-heparin. **CLINICAL:** Anticoagulant (see p. 29C).

ACTION

Antithrombin in presence of low-molecular-weight heparin inhibits factor Xa, thrombin. Only slightly influences platelet aggregation, PT, aPTT. **Therapeutic Effect:** Produces anticoagulation.

PHARMACOKINETICS

Route	Onset	Peak	Duration
Subcutaneous	N/A	4 hrs	N/A

Protein binding: less than 10%. **Half-life:** 3–5 hrs.

USES

Treatment of unstable angina and non–Q-wave MI to prevent ischemic events. Prevention of deep vein thrombosis (DVT) in pts undergoing hip replacement or abdominal surgery who are at risk for thromboembolic complications. Those at risk are 40 yrs and older, obese, undergoing surgery under general anesthesia lasting longer than 30 min, malignancy, history of DVT or pulmonary embolism. Prevention of DVT or pulmonary embolism in acutely ill pts with severely restricted mobility.

PRECAUTIONS

CONTRAINDICATIONS: Active major bleeding; concurrent heparin therapy; hypersensitivity to dalteparin, heparin, pork products; thrombocytopenia associated with positive in vitro test for antiplatelet antibody. **CAUTIONS:** Conditions with increased risk for hemorrhage, bacterial endocarditis, history of heparin-induced thrombocytopenia, renal/hepatic impairment, uncontrolled hypertension, history of recent GI ulceration/hemorrhage, hypertensive/diabetic retinopathy.

LIFESPAN CONSIDERATIONS:

Pregnancy/Lactation: Use with caution, particularly during last trimester, immediate postpartum period (increased risk of maternal hemorrhage). Unknown if distributed in breast milk. **Pregnancy Category B. Children:** Safety and efficacy not established. **Elderly:** No age-related precautions noted.

INTERACTIONS

DRUG: Anticoagulants, platelet inhibitors may increase risk of bleeding. **HERBAL: Cat's claw, dong quai, evening primrose, garlic, ginseng** may increase antiplatelet activity. **FOOD:** None known. **LAB VALUES:** Increases (reversible) LDH, serum alkaline phosphatase, AST, ALT.

AVAILABILITY (Rx)

INJECTION, SOLUTION (SYRINGE): 2,500 international units/0.2 ml, 5,000 international units/0.2 ml, 7,500 international units/0.3 ml, 10,000 international units/ml. **(VIAL):** 10,000 international units/ml, 25,000 international units/ml.

ADMINISTRATION/HANDLING

SUBCUTANEOUS

• Store at room temperature. • Instruct pt to sit/lie down before administering by deep subcutaneous injection. • Inject in U-shaped area around the navel, upper outer side of thigh, upper outer quadrangle of buttock. • Use fine needle (25–26 gauge) to minimize tissue trauma. • Introduce entire length of needle (½ inch) into skin fold held between thumb and forefinger, holding needle during injection at 45°–90° angle. • Do not rub injection site after administration (prevents bruising).

• Alternate administration site with each injection.

INDICATIONS/ROUTES/DOSAGE

LOW- TO MODERATE-RISK ABDOMINAL SURGERY

SUBCUTANEOUS: ADULTS, ELDERLY: 2,500 international units 1–2 hrs before surgery, then daily for 5–10 days.

HIGH-RISK ABDOMINAL SURGERY

SUBCUTANEOUS: ADULTS, ELDERLY: 5,000 international units 1–2 hrs before surgery, then daily for 5–10 days.

TOTAL HIP SURGERY

SUBCUTANEOUS: ADULTS, ELDERLY: 2,500 international units 1–2 hrs before surgery, then 2,500 units 6 hrs after surgery, then 5,000 units/day for 7–10 days.

UNSTABLE ANGINA, NON–Q-WAVE MI

SUBCUTANEOUS: ADULTS, ELDERLY: 120 international units/kg q12h (**Maximum:** 10,000 international units/dose) given with aspirin until clinically stable.

PREVENTION OF DVT, PULMONARY EDEMA IN ACUTELY ILL PT

SUBCUTANEOUS: ADULTS, ELDERLY: 5,000 international units once a day.

SIDE EFFECTS

OCCASIONAL (7%–3%): Hematoma at injection site. **RARE (less than 1%):** Hypersensitivity reaction (chills, fever, pruritus, urticaria, asthma, rhinitis, lacrimation, headache); mild, local skin irritation.

ADVERSE EFFECTS/ TOXIC REACTIONS

Overdose may lead to bleeding complications ranging from local ecchymoses to major hemorrhage. Thrombocytopenia occurs rarely.

NURSING CONSIDERATIONS

BASELINE ASSESSMENT

Assess CBC, esp. platelet count. Determine initial B/P.

INTERVENTION/EVALUATION

Periodically monitor CBC, platelet count, stool for occult blood (no need for daily monitoring in pts with normal presurgical coagulation parameters). Assess for any sign of bleeding: (bleeding at surgical site, hematuria, blood in stool, bleeding from gums, petechiae, bruising/bleeding at injection sites).

PATIENT/FAMILY TEACHING

• Usual length of therapy is 5–10 days. • Do not take any OTC medication (esp. aspirin) without consulting physician. • Report bleeding, bruising, dizziness, lightheadedness, rash, itching, fever, swelling, breathing difficulty. • Rotate injection sites daily. • Teach proper injection technique. • Excessive bruising at injection site may be lessened by ice massage before injection.

danazol

evolve

dan-ah-zole

(Cyclomen ✤, Danocrine)

Do not confuse Danocrine with Dantrium.

CLASSIFICATION

PHARMACOTHERAPEUTIC: Testosterone derivative. **CLINICAL:** Androgen, hormone.

ACTION

Suppresses pituitary-ovarian axis by inhibiting output of pituitary gonadotropins. In endometriosis, causes atrophy of both normal and ectopic endometrial tissue. For fibrocystic breast disease, follicle-stimulating hormone (FSH), luteinizing hormone (LH) are depressed. Inhibits steroid synthesis, binding of steroids to their receptors in breast tissue. Increases serum esterase inhibitor. **Therapeutic**

Effect: Produces anovulation, amenorrhea. Reduces estrogen production. Corrects biochemical deficiency as seen in hereditary angioedema.

PHARMACOKINETICS

Metabolized in liver. Excreted in urine. **Half-life:** 4.5 hrs.

USES

Palliative treatment of endometriosis, fibrocystic breast disease; prophylactic treatment of hereditary angioedema. **OFF-LABEL:** Treatment of gynecomastia, menorrhagia, precocious puberty.

PRECAUTIONS

CONTRAINDICATIONS: Severe cardiac/hepatic/renal impairment. Active or history of thromboembolic disease, androgen tumor, abnormal vaginal bleeding. **CAUTIONS:** Renal impairment, cardiac impairment, epilepsy, migraine headaches, diabetes. **Pregnancy Category X.**

INTERACTIONS

DRUG: May enhance effects of **anticoagulants**. May increase nephrotoxicity with **cyclosporine, tacrolimus** **HERBAL:** None significant. **FOOD: High-fat meals** increase concentration. **LAB VALUES:** May increase hepatic function values.

AVAILABILITY (Rx)

CAPSULES: 50 mg, 100 mg, 200 mg.

ADMINISTRATION/HANDLING

PO

- High-fat meals increase concentration.

INDICATIONS/ROUTES/DOSAGE

◄ ALERT ► Initiate therapy during menstruation or when pt is not pregnant.

ENDOMETRIOSIS

PO: ADULTS: 200–800 mg a day in 2 divided doses for 3–9 mos.

FIBROCYSTIC BREAST DISEASE

PO: ADULTS: 100–400 mg a day in 2 divided doses.

HEREDITARY ANGIOEDEMA

PO: ADULTS: Initially, 200 mg 2–3 times a day. Decrease dosage by 50% or less at 1- to 3-mo intervals. If attack occurs, increase dosage by up to 200 mg a day.

SIDE EFFECTS

FREQUENT: Females: Amenorrhea, breakthrough bleeding/spotting, decreased breast size, weight gain, irregular menstrual period. **OCCASIONAL: Males/Females:** Edema, rhabdomyolysis (abnormal urine color [dark, red, cola colored], muscle cramps, unusual fatigue), virilism (acne, oily skin), flushed skin, altered moods. **RARE: Males/Females:** Hematuria, gingivitis, carpal tunnel syndrome, cataracts, severe headache, vomiting, rash, photosensitivity. **Females:** Enlarged clitoris, hoarseness, deepening voice, hair growth, monilial vaginitis. **Males:** Decreased testicle size.

ADVERSE EFFECTS/ TOXIC REACTIONS

Jaundice may occur in those receiving 400 mg or more per day. Hepatic dysfunction, eosinophilia, thrombocytopenia, pancreatitis occur rarely.

NURSING CONSIDERATIONS

BASELINE ASSESSMENT

Inquire about menstrual cycle. Therapy should begin during menstruation. Establish baseline weight, B/P.

INTERVENTION/EVALUATION

Weigh 2–3 times/wk; report 5 lb or more/wk gain or swelling of fingers/feet. Monitor B/P periodically. Check for jaundice (yellow sclera/skin, dark urine, clay-colored stools).

PATIENT/FAMILY TEACHING

• Pt should use nonhormonal contraceptive during therapy. • Do not take drug, notify physician if pregnancy suspected (risk to fetus). • Stress importance of full length of therapy, regular visits to physician's office (hepatic function tests, CBC, serum amylase, lipase). • Notify physician promptly of masculinizing effects (may not be reversible), weight gain, muscle cramps, fatigue. • Spotting/bleeding may occur in first mos of therapy for endometriosis (does not mean lack of efficacy). • In fibrocystic breast disease, irregular menstrual periods, amenorrhea may occur with or without ovulation.

dantrolene

dan-troe-leen

(Dantrium, Dantrium Intravenous)

Do not confuse Dantrium with Daraprim.

CLASSIFICATION

CLINICAL: Skeletal muscle relaxant.

ACTION

Reduces muscle contraction by interfering with release of calcium ion. Reduces calcium ion concentration. **Therapeutic Effect:** Dissociates excitation-contraction coupling. Interferes with catabolic process associated with malignant hyperthermic crisis.

PHARMACOKINETICS

Poorly absorbed from GI tract. Protein binding: High. Metabolized in the liver. Primarily excreted in urine. **Half-life: IV:** 4–8 hrs; **PO:** 8.7 hrs.

USES

PO: Relief of symptoms of spasticity due to spinal cord injuries, stroke, cerebral palsy, multiple sclerosis, esp. flexor spasms, concomitant pain, clonus, muscular rigidity. **Parenteral:** Management of fulminant hypermetabolism of skeletal muscle due to malignant hyperthermia crisis. **OFF-LABEL:** Relief of exercise-induced pain in pts with muscular dystrophy; treatment of flexor spasms, neuroleptic malignant syndrome.

PRECAUTIONS

CONTRAINDICATIONS: Active hepatic disease. **CAUTIONS:** Cardiac/pulmonary impairment, history of previous hepatic disease.

LIFESPAN CONSIDERATIONS:

Pregnancy/Lactation: Readily crosses placenta. Do not use in breast-feeding mothers. **Pregnancy Category C.** **Children:** No age-related precautions noted in those 5 yrs and older. **Elderly:** No information available.

INTERACTIONS

DRUG: **Central nervous system (CNS) depressants** may increase CNS depression with short-term use. **Hepatotoxic medications** may increase risk of hepatic toxicity with chronic use. **HERBAL:** **Gotu kola, kava kava, St. John's wort, valerian** may increase CNS depression. **FOOD:** None known. **LAB VALUES:** May alter hepatic function test results.

AVAILABILITY (Rx)

CAPSULES (DANTRIUM): 25 mg, 50 mg, 100 mg. **INJECTION, POWDER FOR RECONSTITUTION (DANTRIUM INTRAVENOUS):** 20-mg vial.

ADMINISTRATION/HANDLING

IV

Reconstitution • Reconstitute 20-mg vial with 60 ml Sterile Water for Injection to provide concentration of 0.33 mg/ml.

Rate of administration • For IV infusion, administer over 1 hr. • Diligently monitor for extravasation (high pH of

IV preparation). May produce severe complications.

Storage • Store at room temperature. • Use within 6 hrs after reconstitution. Solution is clear, colorless. Discard if cloudy, precipitate forms.

PO

- Give without regard to food.

IV INCOMPATIBILITY

None known.

INDICATIONS/ROUTES/DOSAGE

SPASTICITY

PO: ADULTS, ELDERLY: Initially, 25 mg/day. Increase to 25 mg 2–4 times a day, then by 25-mg increments up to 100 mg 2–4 times a day. **CHILDREN:** Initially, 0.5 mg/kg twice a day. Increase to 0.5 mg/kg 3–4 times a day, then in increments of 0.5 mg/kg/day up to 3 mg/kg 2–4 times a day. **Maximum:** 400 mg/day.

PREVENTION OF MALIGNANT HYPERTHERMIC CRISIS

PO: ADULTS, ELDERLY, CHILDREN: 4–8 mg/kg/day in 3–4 divided doses 1–2 days before surgery; give last dose 3–4 hrs before surgery.

IV: ADULTS, ELDERLY, CHILDREN: 2.5 mg/kg about 1.25 hrs before surgery.

MANAGEMENT OF MALIGNANT HYPERTHERMIC CRISIS

IV: ADULTS, ELDERLY, CHILDREN: Initially a minimum of 1 mg/kg rapid IV; may repeat up to total cumulative dose of 10 mg/kg. May follow with 4–8 mg/kg/day PO in 4 divided doses up to 3 days after crisis.

SIDE EFFECTS

FREQUENT: Drowsiness, dizziness, weakness, general malaise, diarrhea (mild). **OCCASIONAL:** Confusion, diarrhea (severe), headache, insomnia, constipation, urinary frequency. **RARE:** Paradoxical CNS excitement or restlessness, paresthesia, tinnitus, slurred speech, tremor, blurred vision, dry mouth, nocturia, impotence, rash, pruritus.

ADVERSE EFFECTS/ TOXIC REACTIONS

Risk of hepatotoxicity, most notably in females, those 35 yrs and older, those taking other medications concurrently. Overt hepatitis noted most frequently between 3rd and 12th mo of therapy. Overdosage results in vomiting, muscular hypotonia, muscle twitching, respiratory depression, seizures.

NURSING CONSIDERATIONS

BASELINE ASSESSMENT

Obtain baseline hepatic function tests (AST, ALT, alkaline phosphatase, total bilirubin). Record onset, type, location, duration of muscular spasm. Check for immobility, stiffness, swelling.

INTERVENTION/EVALUATION

Assist with ambulation. For those on long-term therapy, hepatic/renal function tests, CBC should be performed periodically. Evaluate for therapeutic response (decreased intensity of skeletal muscle pain, spasm).

PATIENT/FAMILY TEACHING

• Drowsiness usually diminishes with continued therapy. • Avoid tasks that require alertness, motor skills until response to drug is established. • Avoid alcohol/other depressants while taking medication. • Report continued weakness, fatigue, nausea, diarrhea, skin rash, itching, bloody/tarry stools.

daptomycin

dap-toe-my-sin

(Cubicin)

Do not confuse daptomycin with dactinomycin.

CLASSIFICATION

PHARMACOTHERAPEUTIC: Lipopeptide antibacterial agent. **CLINICAL:** Antibiotic.

D

ACTION

Binds to bacterial membranes and causes rapid depolarization of membrane potential. Inhibits protein, DNA, RNA synthesis. **Therapeutic Effect:** Bactericidal.

PHARMACOKINETICS

Widely distributed. Protein binding: 90%. Primarily excreted unchanged in urine. Moderately removed by hemodialysis. **Half-life:** 7–8 hrs (increased in renal impairment).

USES

Treatment of complicated skin/skin structure infections caused by susceptible strains of gram-positive pathogens, including penicillin-resistant *Streptococcus pneumoniae*, methicillin-resistant *Staphyloccus aureus*, vancomycin-resistant enterococci. Treatment of *S. aureus* systemic infections caused by methicillin susceptible and resistant *S. aureus*.

PRECAUTIONS

CONTRAINDICATIONS: None known. **CAUTIONS:** Renal impairment, history of or current musculoskeletal disorders (risk of exacerbation), pregnancy.

LIFESPAN CONSIDERATIONS:

Pregnancy/Lactation: Unknown if drug is distributed in breast milk. **Pregnancy Category B. Children:** Safety and efficacy not established in those younger than 18 yrs. **Elderly:** No age-related precautions noted.

INTERACTIONS

DRUG: Concurrent use with hydroxamethylglutaryl-CoA (HMG-CoA) reductase inhibitors (statins) may cause myopathy (discontinue use). **Tobramycin** increases serum concentration. **HERBAL:** None significant. **FOOD:** None known. **LAB VALUES:** May increase serum CPK levels. May alter hepatic function test results.

AVAILABILITY (Rx)

INJECTION, POWDER FOR RECONSTITUTION: 250 mg/vial, 500 mg/vial.

ADMINISTRATION/HANDLING

IV

Reconstitution • Reconstitute 250-mg vial with 5 ml 0.9% NaCl; reconstitute 500-mg vial with 10 ml 0.9% NaCl. Further dilute in 50 ml 0.9% NaCl.

Rate of administration • For intermittent IV infusion (piggyback), infuse over 30 min.

Storage • Refrigerate. • Appears as pale yellow to light brown lyophilized cake. • Reconstituted solution is stable for 12 hrs at room temperature or up to 48 hrs if refrigerated. • Discard if particulate forms.

IV INCOMPATIBILITIES

Diluents containing dextrose. If same IV line is used to administer different drugs, flush line with 0.9% NaCl.

INDICATIONS/ROUTES/DOSAGE

COMPLICATED SKIN/ SKIN STRUCTURE INFECTIONS

IV: ADULTS, ELDERLY: 4 mg/kg every 24 hrs for 7–14 days.

SYSTEMIC INFECTIONS

IV: ADULTS, ELDERLY: 6 mg/kg once daily.

DOSAGE IN RENAL IMPAIRMENT

For pts with creatinine clearance of less than 30 ml/min, dosage is 4 mg/kg q48h for 7–14 days.

SIDE EFFECTS

FREQUENT (6%–5%): Constipation, nausea, peripheral injection site reactions, headache, diarrhea. **OCCASIONAL (4%–3%):** Insomnia, rash, vomiting. **RARE (less than 3%):** Pruritus, dizziness, hypotension.

ADVERSE EFFECTS/ TOXIC REACTIONS

Skeletal muscle myopathy (muscle pain/weakness, particularly of distal extremities) occurs rarely. Antibiotic-associated colitis (severe abdominal pain, tenderness, fever, severe watery diarrhea) may result from altered bacterial balance.

NURSING CONSIDERATIONS

BASELINE ASSESSMENT

Obtain culture, sensitivity test before first dose (therapy may begin before results are known).

INTERVENTION/EVALUATION

Assess oral cavity for white patches on mucous membranes, tongue (thrush). Monitor daily pattern of bowel activity/stool consistency carefully; mild GI effects may be tolerable, but increasing severity may indicate onset of antibiotic-associated colitis. Be alert for superinfection (severe genital/anal pruritus, abdominal pain, severe mouth soreness, moderate to severe diarrhea). Monitor for dizziness, institute appropriate measures.

PATIENT/FAMILY TEACHING

- Report rash, headache, nausea, any new symptom.

darbepoetin alfa

dar-bee-eh-poe-**ee**-tin

(Aranesp)

Do not confuse Aranesp with Aricept.

CLASSIFICATION

PHARMACOTHERAPEUTIC: Glycoprotein. **CLINICAL:** Hematopoietic.

ACTION

Stimulates formation of RBCs in bone marrow; increases serum half-life of epoetin. **Therapeutic Effect:** Induces erythropoiesis, release of reticulocytes from bone marrow.

PHARMACOKINETICS

Well absorbed after subcutaneous administration. **Half-life:** 48.5 hrs.

USES

Treatment of anemia associated with chronic renal failure, chemotherapy-induced anemia.

PRECAUTIONS

CONTRAINDICATIONS: History of sensitivity to mammalian cell-derived products or human albumin, uncontrolled hypertension. **CAUTIONS:** Pts with known porphyria (impairment of erythrocyte formation in bone marrow or responsible for hepatic impairment), hemolytic anemia, sickle cell anemia, thalassemia, history of seizures.

LIFESPAN CONSIDERATIONS:

Pregnancy/Lactation: Unknown if drug crosses placenta or is distributed in breast milk. **Pregnancy Category C.** **Children:** Safety and efficacy not established. **Elderly:** Age-related renal impairment may require dosage adjustment.

INTERACTIONS

DRUG: None significant. **HERBAL:** None significant. **FOOD:** None known. **LAB VALUES:** May increase BUN, serum creatinine, phosphorus, potassium, uric acid, sodium. May decrease bleeding time, serum iron concentration, ferritin.

AVAILABILITY (Rx)

INJECTION SOLUTION: 25 mcg/ml, 40 mcg/ml, 60 mcg/ml, 100 mcg/ml, 150 mcg/ml, 200 mcg/ml, 300 mcg/ml. **PREFILLED SYRINGE:** 25 mcg/0.42 ml, 40 mcg/0.4 ml, 60 mcg/0.3 ml, 100 mcg/0.5 ml, 200 mcg/0.4 ml, 300 mcg/0.6 ml, 500 mcg/ml.

ADMINISTRATION/HANDLING

◄ **ALERT** ► Avoid excessive agitation of vial; do not shake (will cause foaming).

D

IV

Reconstitution • No reconstitution necessary.

Rate of administration • May be given as IV bolus.

Storage • Refrigerate vials. Vigorous shaking may denature medication, rendering it inactive.

SUBCUTANEOUS

• Use 1 dose per vial; do not reenter vial. Discard unused portion. May be mixed in a syringe with Bacteriostatic 0.9% NaCl with Benzyl Alcohol 0.9% (Bacteriostatic Saline) at a 1:1 ratio (benzyl alcohol acts as a local anesthetic; may reduce injection site discomfort).

IV INCOMPATIBILITIES

Do not mix with other medications.

INDICATIONS/ROUTES/DOSAGE

ANEMIA IN CHRONIC RENAL FAILURE

IV BOLUS, SUBCUTANEOUS: ADULTS, ELDERLY: Initially, 0.45 mcg/kg once weekly. Adjust dosage to achieve and maintain target Hgb not to exceed 12 g/dl. Do not increase dosage more frequently than once monthly. Limit increases in Hgb to less than 1 g/dl over any 2-wk period.

ANEMIA ASSOCIATED WITH CHEMOTHERAPY

IV, SUBCUTANEOUS: ADULTS, ELDERLY: 2.25 mcg/kg/dose once a wk or 500 mcg every 3 wks. May increase up to 4.5 mcg/kg/dose once a wk.

SIDE EFFECTS

FREQUENT: Myalgia, hypertension/hypotension, headache, diarrhea. **OCCASIONAL:** Fatigue, edema, vomiting, reaction at injection site, asthenia, dizziness.

ADVERSE EFFECTS/ TOXIC REACTIONS

Vascular access thrombosis, CHF, sepsis, arrhythmias, anaphylactic reaction occur rarely.

NURSING CONSIDERATIONS

BASELINE ASSESSMENT

Assess B/P before drug administration (80% of pts with chronic renal failure have history of hypertension). B/P often rises during early therapy in those with history of hypertension. Assess serum iron (transferrin saturation should be greater than 20%), serum ferritin (greater than 100 ng/ml) before and during therapy. Consider that all pts will eventually need supplemental iron therapy. Establish baseline CBC (esp. note Hct).

INTERVENTION/EVALUATION

Monitor Hct level diligently (if level increases greater than 4 points in 2 wks, dosage should be reduced). Monitor Hgb, serum ferritin, CBC with differential, serum creatinine, BUN, potassium, phosphorus, reticulocyte count. Monitor B/P aggressively for increase (25% of pts taking medication require antihypertension therapy, dietary restrictions).

PATIENT/FAMILY TEACHING

• Frequent blood tests needed to determine correct dose. • Inform physician if severe headache develops. • Avoid tasks requiring alertness, motor skills until response to drug is established.

darifenacin

dare-ih-**fen**-ah-sin
(Enablex)

CLASSIFICATION

PHARMACOTHERAPEUTIC: Muscarinic receptor antagonist. **CLINICAL:** Urinary antispasmodic.

D

ACTION

Acts as a direct antagonist at muscarinic receptor sites in cholinergically innervated organs. Blockade of the receptor limits bladder contractions. **Therapeutic Effect:** Reduces symptoms of bladder irritability/overactivity (urge incontinence, urinary urgency/frequency), improves bladder capacity.

PHARMACOKINETICS

Well absorbed following PO administration. Protein binding: 98%. Extensively metabolized in liver. Primarily excreted in urine with a lesser amount eliminated in feces. **Half-life:** 13–19 hrs.

USES

Management of symptoms of bladder overactivity (urge incontinence, urinary urgency/frequency).

PRECAUTIONS

CONTRAINDICATIONS: Uncontrolled narrow-angle glaucoma, paralytic ileus, GI/GU obstruction, urine retention, severe hepatic impairment. **CAUTIONS:** Bladder outflow obstruction, nonobstructive prostatic hyperplasia, urine retention, GI obstructive disorders, decreased GI motility, constipation, hiatal hernia, reflux esophagitis, ulcerative colitis, controlled narrow-angle glaucoma, myasthenia gravis.

LIFESPAN CONSIDERATIONS:

Pregnancy/Lactation: Unknown if drug crosses placenta or is distributed in breast milk. **Pregnancy Category C.** **Children:** Safety and efficacy not established. **Elderly:** No age-related precautions noted.

INTERACTIONS

DRUG: May increase adverse anticholinergic effects of **anticholinergic drugs. Azole antifungals, (e.g., itraconazole, ketoconazole), clarithromycin, erythromycin, protease inhibitors, verapamil** may increase serum concentration. May increase serum level of **digoxin**. May increase concentration/effects of **beta-blockers, fluoxetine, lidocaine, mirtazapine, paroxetine, risperidone, ritonavir, thioridazine, tricyclic antidepressants, venlafaxine**. **HERBAL:** None significant. **FOOD:** None known. **LAB VALUES:** None known.

AVAILABILITY (Rx)

TABLETS (EXTENDED-RELEASE): 7.5 mg, 15 mg.

ADMINISTRATION/HANDLING

PO

• Give without regard to food. • Swallow extended-release tablets whole; do not crush.

INDICATIONS/ROUTES/DOSAGE

OVERACTIVE BLADDER

PO: ADULTS, ELDERLY: Initially, 7.5 mg once daily. If response is not adequate after at least 2 wks, may increase to 15 mg once daily. Do not exceed 7.5 mg once daily in moderate hepatic impairment.

SIDE EFFECTS

FREQUENT (35%–21%): Dry mouth, constipation. **OCCASIONAL (8%–4%):** Dyspepsia, headache, nausea, abdominal pain. **RARE (3%–2%):** Asthenia, diarrhea, dizziness, ocular dryness.

ADVERSE EFFECTS/ TOXIC REACTIONS

UTI occurs occasionally.

NURSING CONSIDERATIONS

BASELINE ASSESSMENT

Monitor voiding pattern, assess signs/symptoms of overactive bladder prior to therapy as baseline.

INTERVENTION/EVALUATION

Monitor I&O. Palpate bladder for urine retention. Monitor daily bowel activity/

stool consistency for evidence of constipation. Dry mouth may be relieved with sips of tepid water. Assess for relief of symptoms of overactive bladder (urge incontinence, urinary frequency/urgency).

PATIENT/FAMILY TEACHING

• Swallow tablet whole; do not crush, divide, chew. • Increase fluid intake to reduce risk of constipation. • Avoid tasks that require alertness, motor skills until response to drug is established.

darunavir

dah-**run**-ah-vir
(Prezista)

CLASSIFICATION

PHARMACOTHERAPEUTIC: Antiretroviral. **CLINICAL:** Protease inhibitor.

ACTION

Prevents virus-specifc processing of polyproteins, HIV-1 protease infected cells. **Therapeutic Effect:** Prevents formation of mature viral cells.

PHARMACOKINETICS

Readily absorbed following PO administration. Protein binding: 95%. Metabolized in liver. Eliminated mainly in feces with a lesser amount eliminated in urine. Not significantly removed by hemodialysis. **Half-life:** 15 hrs.

USES

Treatment of HIV infection in combination with ritonavir and other antiretroviral agents.

PRECAUTIONS

CONTRAINDICATIONS: Concurrent therapy with phenobarbital, phenytoin, carbamazepine, astemizole, terfenadine, pimozide, rifampin, dihydroergotamine, ergonovine, ergotamine, methylergonovine, St. John's wort, lovastatin, simvastatin, midazolam, triamzolam, cisapride, pimozide. **CAUTIONS:** Diabetes mellitus, hemophilia, known sulfonamide allergy, hepatic impairment.

LIFESPAN CONSIDERATIONS:

Pregnancy/Lactation: Unknown if drug crosses placenta or is distributed in breast milk. Do not breast-feed. **Pregnancy Category C. Children:** Safety and efficacy not established. **Elderly:** No age-related precautions noted.

INTERACTIONS

DRUG: May interfere with metabolism of **amiodarone, bepredil, lidocaine, quinidine, oral contraceptives, midazolam, triazolam, paroxetine, sertraline. Dexamethasone, lopinavir, rifabutin, rifampin** may decrease darunavir concentration. May increase concentration of **atorvastatin, clarithromycin, cyclosporine, inhaled fluticasone, lovastatin, pravastatin, simvastatin, sirolimus, tacrolimus, trazodone, felodipine, nifedipine, nicardipine.** May alter **warfarin, methadone, sildenafil, tadalafil, vardenafil** concentration. **Efavirenz, itraconazole, ketoconazole, voriconazole** may increase darunavir concentration. **Ergot derivatives** may cause peripheral vasospasm/ischemia. **HERBAL: St. John's wort** may lead to loss of virologic response, potential resistance to darunavir. **FOOD: Food** increases plasma concentration of darunavir. **LAB VALUES:** May increase aPTT, PT, serum alkaline phosphatase, bilirubin, amylase, lipase, cholesterol, triglycerides, uric acid. May decrease lymphocytes/neutrophil count, platelets, WBC count, serum bicarbonate, albumin, calcium. May alter glucose, sodium.

AVAILABILITY (Rx)

TABLETS (PREZISTA): 300 mg.

ADMINISTRATION/HANDLING

PO

• Give with food (increases plasma concentration). • Do not crush, chew film-coated tablets.

INDICATIONS/ROUTES/DOSAGE

HIV INFECTION, CONCURRENT THERAPY WITH RITONAVIR

PO: ADULTS, ELDERLY: 600 mg (2 300-mg tablets) administered with 100 mg ritonavir and with food twice daily.

SIDE EFFECTS

FREQUENT (19%–13%): Diarrhea, nausea, headache, nasopharyngitis. **OCCASIONAL (3%–2%):** Constipation, abdominal pain, vomiting. **RARE (Less than 2%):** Allergic dermatitis, dyspepsia, flatulence, abdominal distension, anorexia, arthralgia, myalgia, paresthesia, memory impairment.

ADVERSE EFFECTS/ TOXIC REACTIONS

Hypertension, MI, TIA occur in less than 2% of pts. Stevens-Johnson syndrome, acute renal failure, diabetes mellitus, dyspnea, worsening of hepatic impairment occur rarely.

NURSING CONSIDERATIONS

BASELINE ASSESSMENT

Obtain baseline laboratory testing, esp. hepatic function tests, before beginning therapy and at periodic intervals during therapy. Offer emotional support. Obtain medication history.

INTERVENTION/EVALUATION

Closely monitor for evidence of GI discomfort. Monitor daily pattern of bowel activity/stool consistency. Assess skin for evidence of rash. Monitor serum chemistry tests for marked laboratory abnormalities, particularly hepatic profile. Assess for opportunistic infections (onset of fever, oral mucosa changes, cough, other respiratory symptoms).

PATIENT/FAMILY TEACHING

Take medication with food. Continue therapy for full length of treatment. Doses should be evenly spaced. Medication is not a cure for HIV infection, nor does it reduce risk of transmission to others. Pt may continue to experience illnesses, including opportunistic infections. Diarrhea can be controlled with OTC medication.

D

Darvocet-N, *see propoxyphene*

dasatinib

dah-**sah**-tin-ib

(Sprycel)

CLASSIFICATION

PHARMACOTHERAPEUTIC: Protein-tyrosine kinase inhibitor. **CLINICAL:** Antineoplastic.

ACTION

Reduces activity of proteins responsible for uncontrolled growth of leukemia cells by binding to most imatinib-resistant BCR-ABL mutations of pts with chronic myelogenous leukemia (CML) or acute lymphoblastic leukemia (ALL). **Therapeutic Effect:** Inhibits proliferation, tumor growth of CML and ALL cancer cell lines.

PHARMACOKINETICS

Extensively distributed in extravascular space. Protein binding: 96%. Extensively metabolized. Eliminated primarily in feces. **Half-life:** 3–5 hrs.

D

USES

Treatment of adults with chronic, accelerated, myeloid or lymphoid blast phase of CML with resistance, intolerance to prior therapy, including imatinib. Treatment of adults with Philadelphia chromosome-positive (Ph+) ALL.

PRECAUTIONS

CONTRAINDICATIONS: None known. **CAUTIONS:** Hepatic/renal impairment, myelosuppression, particularly thrombocytopenia, pts prone to fluid retention, those with prolonged QT interval.

LIFESPAN CONSIDERATIONS:

Pregnancy/Lactation: Has potential for severe teratogenic effects, fertility impairment. Avoid breast-feeding. **Pregnancy Category C. Children:** Safety and efficacy not established in children younger than 18 yrs. **Elderly:** No age-related precautions noted.

INTERACTIONS

DRUG: Ketoconazole, itraconazole, erythromycin, clarithromycin, ritonavir, atazanavir, indinavir, nefazodone, nelfinavir, saquinavir, telethromycin may increase dasatinib concentrations. **Dexamethasone, phenytoin, carbamazepine, rifampicin, phenobarbital** may decrease dasatinib concentrations. **Antacids** alter pH-dependent solubility of dasatinib. **Famotidine, omeprazole** reduce dasatinib exposure. May alter **alfentanil, astemizole, terfenadine, cisapride, cyclosporine, fentanyl, pimozide, quinidine, sirolimus, tacrolimus, ergot alkaloids** plasma concentrations. **HERBAL: St. John's wort** may decrease dasatinib concentration. **FOOD:** None known. **LAB VALUES:** May decrease WBC, platelets, Hgb, Hct, RBC, serum calcium, phosphates. May increase serum bilirubin, ALT, AST, creatinine.

AVAILABILITY (Rx)

TABLETS (FILM-COATED): 20 mg, 50 mg, 70 mg.

ADMINISTRATION/HANDLING

PO

• Give without regard to food. • Do not crush/cut film-coated tablets. • Store at room temperature. • Do not give antacids either 2 hrs prior to or within 2 hrs after dasatinib administration.

INDICATIONS/ROUTES/DOSAGE

CML, ALL

PO: ADULTS 18 YRS AND OLDER, ELDERLY: 140 mg/day given in 2 divided doses (70 mg twice daily), 1 in the morning and 1 in the evening. Dose increase or reduction in 20-mg increments per dose is recommended based on pt safety, tolerability.

SIDE EFFECTS

FREQUENT (50%–32%): Fluid retention, diarrhea, headache, fatigue, musculoskeletal pain, fever, rash, nausea, dyspnea. **OCCASIONAL (28%–12%):** Cough, abdominal pain, vomiting anorexia, asthenia (loss of strength, energy), arthralgia, stomatitis, dizziness, constipation, peripheral neuropathy, myalgia. **RARE (less than 12%):** Abdominal distention, chills, weight increase, pruritus.

ADVERSE EFFECTS/ TOXIC REACTIONS

Pleural effusion occurs in 8% of pts, febrile neutropenia in 7%, GI bleeding, pneumonia in 6%, thrombocytopenia in 5%, dyspnea in 4%, anemia, cardiac failure in 3%.

NURSING CONSIDERATIONS

BASELINE ASSESSMENT

Obtain CBC weekly for first mo, biweekly for second mo, and periodically thereafter. Monitor hepatic function tests (bilirubin, alkaline phosphatase, AST,

ALT) before treatment begins and monthly thereafter.

INTERVENTION/EVALUATION

Assess lower extremities for pedal edema for early evidence of fluid retention. Weigh, monitor for unexpected rapid weight gain. Offer antiemetics to control nausea, vomiting. Monitor daily pattern of bowel activity/stool consistency. Assess oral mucous membranes for evidence of stomatitis. Monitor CBC for neutropenia, thrombocytopenia; monitor hepatic function tests for hepatotoxicity.

PATIENT/FAMILY TEACHING

Avoid crowds, those with known infection. Avoid contact with anyone who recently received live virus vaccine; do not receive vaccinations. Antacids may be taken up to 2 hrs before or 2 hrs after taking dasatinib.

*DAUNOrubicin

dawn-oh-**rue**-bih-sin

(Cerubidine, DaunoXome)

Do not confuse daunorubicin with dactinomycin or doxorubicin.

CLASSIFICATION

PHARMACOTHERAPEUTIC: Anthracycline antibiotic. **CLINICAL:** Antineoplastic (see p. 78C).

ACTION

Inhibits DNA, DNA-dependent RNA synthesis by binding with DNA strands. Liposomal encapsulation increases uptake by tumors, prolongs drug action, may decrease toxicity. Cell cycle-phase nonspecific. **Therapeutic Effect:** Prevents cell division.

PHARMACOKINETICS

Widely distributed. Protein binding: High. Does not cross blood-brain barrier. Metabolized in the liver to active metabolite. Excreted in urine; eliminated by biliary excretion. **Half-life:** 18.5 hrs; metabolite: 26.7 hrs.

USES

Cerubidine: Treatment of leukemias (acute lymphocytic [ALL], acute nonlymphocytic [ANLL]) in combination with other agents. **DaunoXome:** Advanced HIV-related Kaposi's sarcoma. **OFF-LABEL:** Treatment of chronic myelocytic leukemia, Ewing's sarcoma, neuroblastoma, non-Hodgkin's lymphoma, Wilms' tumor.

PRECAUTIONS

CONTRAINDICATIONS: Arrhythmias, CHF, left ventricular ejection fraction less than 40%, preexisting myelosuppression. **CAUTIONS:** Hepatic, biliary, renal impairment.

LIFESPAN CONSIDERATIONS:

Pregnancy/Lactation: If possible, avoid use during pregnancy, esp. first trimester. May cause fetal harm. Breastfeeding not recommended. **Pregnancy Category D. Children:** Safety and efficacy not established. **Elderly:** Cardiotoxicity may be more frequent; reduced bone marrow reserves requires caution. Age-related renal impairment may require dosage adjustment.

INTERACTIONS

DRUG: May decrease effects of **antigout medications. Bone marrow depressants** may enhance myelosuppression. **Live virus vaccines** may potentiate virus replication, increase vaccine side effects, decrease pt's antibody response to the vaccine. **HERBAL:** None significant. **FOOD:** None known. **LAB VALUES:** May increase serum alkaline phosphatase, bilirubin, uric acid, AST.

AVAILABILITY (Rx)

INJECTION, POWDER FOR RECONSTITUTION (CERUBIDINE): 20 mg.

INJECTION SOLUTION (CERUBIDINE): 5 mg/ml. **INJECTION SOLUTION (DAUNOXOME):** 2 mg/ml.

ADMINISTRATION/HANDLING

IV

◀ **ALERT** ▶ Give by IV push or IV infusion. Peripheral IV infusion not recommended due to vein irritation, risk of thrombophlebitis. Avoid small veins, swollen/edematous extremities, areas overlying joints/tendons. May be carcinogenic, mutagenic, teratogenic. Handle with extreme care during preparation/administration.

Reconstitution

Cerubidine • Reconstitute each 20-mg vial with 4 ml Sterile Water for Injection to provide concentration of 5 mg/ml. • Gently agitate vial until completely dissolved.

DaunoXome • Must dilute with equal part D_5W to provide concentration of 1 mg/ml. • Do not use any other diluent.

Rate of administration

Cerubidine • For IV push, withdraw desired dose into syringe containing 10–15 ml 0.9% NaCl. Inject over 2–3 min into tubing of running IV solution of D_5W or 0.9% NaCl. • For IV infusion, further dilute with 100 ml D_5W or 0.9% NaCl. Infuse over 30–45 min. • Extravasation produces immediate pain, severe local tissue damage. Aspirate as much infiltrated drug as possible, then infiltrate area with hydrocortisone sodium succinate injection (50–100 mg hydrocortisone) and/or isotonic sodium thiosulfate injection or ascorbic acid injection (1 ml of 5% injection). Apply cold compresses.

DaunoXome • Infuse over 60 min.

Storage

Cerubidine • Reconstituted solution is stable for 24 hrs at room temperature or 48 hrs if refrigerated. • Color change from red to blue-purple indicates decomposition; discard.

DaunoXome • Refrigerate unopened vials • Reconstituted solution is stable for 6 hrs if refrigerated. • Do not use if opaque.

IV INCOMPATIBILITIES

Allopurinol (Aloprim), aztreonam (Azactam), cefepime (Maxipime), fludarabine (Fludara), piperacillin and tazobactam (Zosyn). **DaunoXome:** Do not mix with any other solution, esp. NaCl or bacteriostatic agents (e.g., benzyl alcohol).

IV COMPATIBILITIES

Cytarabine (Cytosar), etoposide (VePesid), filgrastim (Neupogen), granisetron (Kytril), ondansetron (Zofran).

INDICATIONS/ROUTES/DOSAGE

ALL

IV (CERUBIDINE): ADULTS, ELDERLY: 45 mg/m^2 on days 1, 2, and 3 of induction course. **CHILDREN 2 YRS AND OLDER:** 25 mg/m^2 on day 1 of every wk. **CHILDREN YOUNGER THAN 2 YRS, BODY SURFACE AREA LESS THAN 0.5:** 1 mg/kg/dose.

ANLL

IV (CERUBIDINE): ADULTS YOUNGER THAN 60 YRS: 45 mg/m^2 on days 1, 2, and 3 of induction course then on days 1 and 2 of subsequent courses. **ADULTS 60 YRS AND OLDER:** 30 mg/m^2 on days 1, 2, and 3 of induction course, then on days 1 and 2 of subsequent courses.

KAPOSI'S SARCOMA

IV (DAUNOXOME): ADULTS: 20–40 mg/m^2 over 1 hr repeated q2wk; or 100 mg/m^2 q3wk.

DOSAGE IN RENAL IMPAIRMENT

CERUBIDINE: CREATININE CLEARANCE LESS THAN 10 ML/MIN: 75% of normal dose. **SERUM CREATININE GREATER THAN 3 MG/DL:** 50% of normal dose. **DAUNOXOME: SERUM CREATININE GREATER THAN 3 MG/DL:** 50% of normal dose.

DOSAGE IN HEPATIC IMPAIRMENT
CERUBIDINE: **BILIRUBIN 1.2–3 MG/DL:** 75% of normal dose. **BILIRUBIN 3.1–5 MG/DL:** 50% of normal dose. **BILIRUBIN GREATER THAN 5 MG/DL:** Daunorubicin is not recommended for use in this pt population.
DAUNOXOME: **BILIRUBIN 1.2–3 MG/DL:** 75% of normal dose. **BILIRUBIN GREATER THAN 3 MG/DL:** 50% of normal dose.

SIDE EFFECTS

FREQUENT: Complete alopecia (scalp, axillary, pubic), nausea, vomiting (beginning a few hrs after administration and lasting 24–48 hrs). **DAUNOXOME:** Mild to moderate nausea, fatigue, fever. **OCCASIONAL:** Diarrhea, abdominal pain, esophagitis, stomatitis, transverse pigmentation of fingernails, toenails. **RARE:** Transient fever, chills.

ADVERSE EFFECTS/ TOXIC REACTIONS

Myelosuppression manifested as hematologic toxicity (severe leukopenia, anemia, thrombocytopenia). Decrease in platelet count, WBC count occurs in 10–14 days, returns to normal level by third week. Cardiotoxicity noted as either acute, transient, abnormal. EKG findings and/or cardiomyopathy manifested as CHF (risk increases when cumulative dose exceeds 550 mg/m^2 in adults, 300 mg/m^2 in children 2 yrs and older, or total dosage greater than 10 mg/kg in children younger than 2 yrs).

NURSING CONSIDERATIONS

BASELINE ASSESSMENT

Obtain WBC, platelet, erythrocyte counts before and at frequent intervals during therapy. EKG should be obtained before therapy. Antiemetics may be effective in preventing, treating nausea.

INTERVENTION/EVALUATION

Monitor for stomatitis (burning, erythema of oral mucosa). May lead to ulceration within 2–3 days. Assess skin, nailbeds for hyperpigmentation. Monitor hematologic status, renal/hepatic function studies, serum uric acid. Monitor daily pattern of bowel activity/stool consistency. Monitor for hematologic toxicity (fever, sore throat, signs of local infection, unusual bruising/bleeding from any site), symptoms of anemia (excessive fatigue, weakness).

PATIENT/FAMILY TEACHING

• Urine may turn reddish color for 1–2 days after beginning therapy. • Alopecia is reversible, but new hair growth may have different color, texture. • New hair growth resumes about 5 wks after last therapy dose. • Maintain fastidious oral hygiene. • Do not have immunizations without physician's approval (drug lowers resistance). • Avoid contact with those who have recently received live virus vaccine. • Promptly report fever, sore throat, signs of local infection, unusual bruising/bleeding from any site. • Increase fluid intake (may protect against hyperuricemia). • Contact physician for persistent nausea, vomiting.

DDAVP, *see desmopressin*

Decadron, *see dexamethasone*

decitabine

deh-**sit**-tah-bean
(Dacogen)

CLASSIFICATION

PHARMACOTHERAPEUTIC: Antineoplastic. **CLINICAL:** DNA demethylation agent.

D

D

ACTION

Exerts cytotoxic effect on rapidly dividing cells by causing demethylation of DNA in abnormal hematopoietic cells in bone marrow. **Therapeutic Effect:** Restores normal function to tumor suppressor-genes regulating cellular differentiation, proliferation.

PHARMACOKINETICS

Protein binding: Less than 1%. Elimination appears to occur by removal of an amino group from the enzyme cytidine deaminase, found principally in liver, but also in granulocytes, intestinal epithelium, whole blood. **Half-life:** 30 min.

USES

Treatment of myelodysplastic syndromes, specifically refractory anemia, myelomonocytic leukemia.

PRECAUTIONS

CONTRAINDICATIONS: None known. **CAUTIONS:** Hepatic/renal impairment.

LIFESPAN CONSIDERATIONS:

Pregnancy/Lactation: May be embryotoxic; may cause developmental abnormalities of fetus. Nursing mothers should avoid breast-feeding. Men should not father a child while receiving treatment and for 2 mos after treatment. **Pregnancy Category D. Children:** Safety and efficacy not established. **Elderly:** No age-related precautions noted.

INTERACTIONS

DRUG: None significant. **HERBAL:** None significant. **FOOD:** None known. **LAB VALUES:** May decrease Hgb, Hct, WBC, RBC, platelets. May increase serum creatinine, potassium, AST, alkaline phosphatase, bicarbonate, lactate dehydrogenase, BUN, bilirubin, glucose, albumin, magnesium, sodium. May alter serum potassium.

AVAILABILITY (Rx)

POWDER FOR INJECTION: 50 mg.

ADMINISTRATION/HANDLING

IV

Reconstitution Reconstitute with 10 ml Sterile Water for Injection. Further dilute with 0.9% NaCl, D_5W, or Ringer's lactate.

Rate of administration Give by continuous IV infusion over 3 hrs.

Storage • Store vials at room temperature. • Unless used within 15 min of reconstitution, diluted solution must be prepared using cold infusion fluids and stored in refrigerator up to maximum of 7 hrs until administration.

INDICATIONS/ROUTES/DOSAGE

◀ **ALERT** ▶ Premedicate with antiemetics prior to therapy.

REFRACTORY ANEMIA, MYELOMONOCYTIC LEUKEMIA

IV Infusion: ADULTS, ELEDERLY: 15 mg/m^2 given over 3 hrs for 3 days. Subsequent treatment cycles should be repeated every 6 wks for a minimum of 4 cycles.

SIDE EFFECTS

FREQUENT (53%–20%): Pyrexia, nausea, cough, petechiae, constipation, diarrhea, insomnia, headache, vomiting, peripheral edema, pallor, ecchymosis, rigors, arthralgia. **OCCASIONAL (19%–11%):** Rash, limb pain, dizziness, back pain, anorexia, pharyngitis, abdominal pain, erythema, oral mucosal petechiae, stomatitis, confusion, lethargy, dyspepsia, anxiety, pruritus, hypoesthesia. **RARE (10%–5%):** Candidiasis, ascites, alopecia, chest wall pain, rales, catheter site infection, facial edema, hypotension, urticaria, dehydration, blurred vision, musculoskeletal discomfort, malaise, sinusitis, gastroesophageal reflux.

ADVERSE EFFECTS/ TOXIC REACTIONS

Pneumonia occurs in 22% of pts, cellulitus in 12%. Hematologic toxicity manifested most commonly as neutropenia (90%; recovery 28–50 days), thrombocytopenia (89%), anemia (82%), febrile neutropenia (29%), leukopenia (28%), lymphadenopathy (12%). UTI occurs in 7%.

NURSING CONSIDERATIONS

BASELINE ASSESSMENT

Give emotional support to pt, family. Use strict asepsis, protect pt from infection. Perform blood counts as needed to monitor response, toxicity but esp. prior to each dosing cycle.

INTERVENTION/EVALUATION

Monitor for hematologic toxicity (fever, sore throat, signs of local infections, unusual bleeding/bruising), symptoms of anemia (excessive fatigue, weakness). Assess response to medication; monitor, report nausea, vomiting, diarrhea. Avoid rectal temperatures, other traumas that may induce bleeding. If serum creatinine increases to 2 mg/dL, ALT, total bilirubin at least 2 times upper limit of normal, and pt has active or uncontrolled infection, treatment should be stopped and not restarted until toxicity is resolved.

PATIENT/FAMILY TEACHING

Do not have immunizations without physician's approval (drug lowers resistance). Avoid crowds, persons with known infections. Report signs of infection (fever, flu-like symptoms) immediately. Contact physician if nausea/vomiting continues at home. Advise men to use barrier contraception while receiving treatment.

deferasirox

daeh-fur-**ah**-sir-ox
(Exjade)

CLASSIFICATION

PHARMACOTHERAPEUTIC: Iron chelating agent. **CLINICAL:** Iron reduction.

ACTION

Selective for iron. Binds iron with high affinity in a 2:1 ratio. **Therapeutic Effect:** Induces iron excretion.

PHARMACOKINETICS

Well absorbed following PO administration. Protein binding: 99%. Minimally metabolized. Primarily excreted in feces with a lesser amount eliminated in urine. **Half-life:** 8–16 hrs.

USES

Treatment of chronic iron overload due to blood transfusions (transfusional hemosiderosis).

PRECAUTIONS

CONTRAINDICATIONS: None known. **CAUTIONS:** Renal/hepatic impairment, preexisting hearing loss, vision disturbances.

LIFESPAN CONSIDERATIONS:

Pregnancy/Lactation: Unknown if drug crosses placenta or is distributed in breast milk. **Pregnancy Category B.** **Children:** Not recommended for children younger than 2 yrs. **Elderly:** No age-related precautions noted.

INTERACTIONS

DRUG: **Antacids containing aluminium** decrease effects. **Iron-chelating agents** may increase risk of toxic effects. **HERBAL:** None significant. **FOOD:** Bioavailability is variably increased when given with **food**. **LAB VALUES:** Decreases serum ferritin. May increase serum creatinine, transaminase, AST, ALT, urine protein.

AVAILABILITY (Rx)

TABLETS (EXJADE): 125 mg, 250 mg, 500 mg.

ADMINISTRATION/HANDLING

PO

• Give on empty stomach 30 min before food. • Tablets should not be chewed or swallowed whole. • Disperse tablet by stirring in water, apple juice, orange juice until fine suspension is achieved. • Dosage less than 1 gram should be dispersed in 2.5 oz of liquid, dosage more than 1 gram should be dispersed in 7 oz of liquid. If any residue remains in glass, re-suspend with a small amount of liquid.

INDICATIONS/ROUTES/DOSAGE

IRON OVERLOAD

PO: ADULTS, ELDERLY, CHILDREN 2 YRS AND OLDER: Initially, 20 mg/kg once daily. Adjust dosage of 5 or 10 mg/kg every 3–6 mos based on serum ferritin levels. **Maximum:** 30 mg/kg once daily.

SIDE EFFECTS

FREQUENT (19%–10%): Fever, headache, abdominal pain, cough, nasopharyngitis, diarrhea, nausea, vomiting. **OCCASIONAL (9%–4%):** Rash, arthralgia, fatigue, back pain, urticaria. **RARE (1%):** Edema, sleep disorder, dizziness, anxiety.

ADVERSE EFFECTS/ TOXIC REACTIONS

Bronchitis, pharyngitis, acute tonsillitis, ear infection occur occasionally. Hepatitis, auditory disturbances, ocular abnormalities occur rarely.

NURSING CONSIDERATIONS

BASELINE ASSESSMENT

Obtain baseline serum creatinine, ALT, AST, transaminase, then monthly thereafter. Auditory, ophthalmic testing should be obtained before therapy and annually therafter. Monitor serum ferritin monthly.

INTERVENTION/EVALUATION

Treatment should be interrupted if serum ferritin levels are consistently less than 500 mcg/L. Suspend treatment if severe rash occurs.

PATIENT/FAMILY TEACHING

• Take on empty stomach 30 min before food. • Do not chew; swallow tablet whole; disperse tablet completely in water, apple juice, orange juice; drink resulting suspension immediately. • Do not take aluminum-containing antacids concurrently.

deferoxamine

deaf-er-**ox**-ah-meen

(Desferal)

Do not confuse deferoxamine with cefuroxime, or Desferal with Desyrel or Disophrol.

CLASSIFICATION

CLINICAL: Antidote.

ACTION

Binds with iron to form complex. **Therapeutic Effect:** Promotes urinary excretion of iron.

PHARMACOKINETICS

Erratic absorption following IM administration. Widely distributed. Rapidly metabolized in tissues, plasma. Excreted in urine, eliminated in feces via biliary excretion. Removed by hemodialysis. **Half-life:** 6 hrs.

USES

Treatment of acute iron toxicity, chronic iron toxicity secondary to multiple transfusions associated with some chronic anemias (e.g., thalassemia). **OFF-LABEL:** Treatment/diagnosis of aluminum toxicity.

PRECAUTIONS

CONTRAINDICATIONS: Severe renal disease, anuria, primary hemochromatosis.

CAUTIONS: Renal impairment. **Pregnancy Category C.**

INTERACTIONS

DRUG: **Vitamin C** may increase effect. **HERBAL:** None significant. **FOOD:** None known. **LAB VALUES:** May cause falsely elevated total iron-binding capacity (TIBC).

AVAILABILITY (Rx)

INJECTION, POWER FOR RECONSTITUTION: 500 mg, 2 g.

ADMINISTRATION/HANDLING

◀ **ALERT** ▶ Reconstitute each 500-mg vial with 2 ml Sterile Water for Injection to provide a concentration of 250 mg/ml.

IV

• For IV infusion, further dilute with 0.9% NaCl, D_5W, and administer at no more than 15 mg/kg/hr. • Too-rapid IV administration may produce skin flushing, urticaria, hypotension, shock.

IM

• Inject deeply into upper outer quadrant of buttock; may give undiluted.

SUBCUTANEOUS

• Administer subcutaneous very slowly; may give undiluted.

IV INCOMPATIBILITY

Do not mix with any other IV medications.

INDICATIONS/ROUTES/DOSAGE

ACUTE IRON INTOXICATION

IM: ADULTS: Initially, 1 g, then 0.5 g q4h for 2 doses; may give additional doses of 0.5 g q4–12h. **CHILDREN:** 50 mg/kg/dose q6h. **Maximum:** 6 g/day.

IV: ADULTS: 15 mg/kg/hr. **CHILDREN:** 15 mg/kg/hr. **Maximum:** 6 g/day.

CHRONIC IRON OVERLOAD

SUBCUTANEOUS: ADULTS: 1–2 g/day over 8–24 hrs. **CHILDREN:** 20–50 mg/kg/day over 8–12 hrs. **Maximum:** 2 g/day.

IM: ADULTS: 0.5–1 g/day. Also, 2 g with each unit blood.

IV: ADULTS, CHILDREN: 2 g after each unit blood at 15 mg/kg/hr. **Maximum:** 12 g/day.

SIDE EFFECTS

FREQUENT: Pain, induration at injection site, urine color change (to orange-rose). **OCCASIONAL:** Abdominal discomfort, diarrhea, leg cramps, impaired vision.

ADVERSE EFFECTS/ TOXIC REACTIONS

High-frequency hearing loss, tinnitus have been noted.

NURSING CONSIDERATIONS

BASELINE ASSESSMENT

Assess serum iron levels, total iron-binding capacity before and during therapy.

INTERVENTION/EVALUATION

Question for evidence of hearing loss (neurotoxicity). Periodic slit-lamp ophthalmic exams should be obtained in those treated for chronic iron overload. For IV administration, monitor serum ferritin, iron, TIBC, body weight, growth, B/P. If using subcutaneous technique, monitor for pruritus, erythema, skin irritation, edema.

PATIENT/FAMILY TEACHING

• Inform pt medication may produce discomfort at IM or subcutaneous injection site. • Urine will appear reddish.

delavirdine

deh-la-**ver**-deen

(Rescriptor)

Do not confuse Rescriptor with Retrovir or Ritonavir.

CLASSIFICATION

PHARMACOTHERAPEUTIC: Nonnucleoside reverse transcriptase inhibitor. **CLINICAL:** Antiretroviral (see pp. 64C, 112C).

D

ACTION
Binds directly to HIV-1 reverse transcriptase, blocks RNA- and DNA-dependent DNA polymerase activities. **Therapeutic Effect:** Interrupts HIV replication, slowing progression of HIV infection.

PHARMACOKINETICS
Rapidly absorbed after PO administration. Protein binding: 98%. Primarily distributed in plasma. Metabolized in the liver. Eliminated in feces and urinary. **Half-life:** 2–11 hrs.

USES
Treatment of HIV infection (in combination with other antivirals).

PRECAUTIONS
CONTRAINDICATIONS: None known. **CAUTIONS:** Hepatic impairment.

LIFESPAN CONSIDERATIONS:
Pregnancy/Lactation: Unknown if drug crosses placenta or is distributed in breast milk. **Pregnancy Category C.** **Children:** Safety and efficacy not established in those younger than 16 yrs. **Elderly:** Safety and efficacy not established.

INTERACTIONS
DRUG: Concurrent administration of **alprazolam, carbamazepine, ergotamine, lovastatin, midazolam, phenobarbital, phenytoin, rifabutin, rifampin, simvastatin** may cause serious adverse effects. **H_2 blockers, proton pump inhibitors** may decrease absorption. May increase concentration/effect of **amprenavir, antiarrhythmic agents (e.g., amiodarone, lidocaine), bepridil, clarithromycin, calcium channel blockers (e.g., amlodipine, diltiazem), atorvastatin, fluvastatin, immunosuppressants (e.g., cyclosporine, tacrolimus), indinavir, methadone, ritonavir, saquinavir, warfarin. HERBAL: St. John's wort** may increase concentration. **FOOD:** None known. **LAB VALUES:** May increase serum AST, ALT. May decrease neutrophil count.

AVAILABILITY (Rx)
TABLETS: 100 mg, 200 mg.

ADMINISTRATION/HANDLING
PO
• May disperse in water before consumption. • Give without regard to food. • Pts with achlorhydria should take with orange juice, cranberry juice.

INDICATIONS/ROUTES/DOSAGE
HIV INFECTION (IN COMBINATION WITH OTHER ANTIRETROVIRALS)
PO: ADULTS: 400 mg 3 times a day.

SIDE EFFECTS
FREQUENT (18%): Rash, pruritus. **OCCASIONAL (greater than 2%):** Headache, nausea, diarrhea, fatigue, anorexia.

ADVERSE EFFECTS/ TOXIC REACTIONS
Hepatic failure, severe rash, hemolytic anemia, rhabdomyolysis, erythema multiforme, Stevens-Johnson syndrome, acute renal failure have been reported.

NURSING CONSIDERATIONS
BASELINE ASSESSMENT
Obtain baseline lab tests, esp. hepatic function tests, before initiation of therapy and at periodic intervals during therapy. Offer emotional support.

INTERVENTION/EVALUATION
Assess skin for rash. Question if nausea is noted. Monitor daily pattern of bowel activity/stool consistency. Assess eating pattern; monitor for weight loss. Monitor lab values carefully, particularly hepatic function.

PATIENT/FAMILY TEACHING
• Do not take any medications, including OTC drugs, without consulting physician. • Small, frequent meals may

offset anorexia, nausea. • Delavirdine is not a cure for HIV infection, nor does it reduce risk of transmission to others.

demecarium

(Humorsol)

See Antiglaucoma agents

demeclocycline

deh-meh-clo-**sigh**-clean

(Declomycin)

CLASSIFICATION

PHARMACOTHERAPEUTIC: Tetracycline. **CLINICAL:** Antibiotic.

ACTION

Inhibits bacterial protein synthesis by binding to ribosomal receptor sites; inhibits ADH-induced water reabsorption. **Therapeutic Effect:** Bacteriostatic. Produces water diuresis.

PHARMACOKINETICS

Food, dairy products interfere with absorption. Protein binding: 41%–91%. Metabolized in liver. Excreted in urine. Removed by hemodialysis. **Half-life:** 10–15 hrs.

USES

Treatment of acne, gonorrhea, pertussis, chronic bronchitis, UTI, syndrome of inappropriate ADH secretion (SIADH).

PRECAUTIONS

CONTRAINDICATIONS: Children 8 yrs and younger, last half of pregnancy. **CAUTIONS:** Renal impairment, sun/ultraviolet exposure (severe photosensitivity reaction).

LIFESPAN CONSIDERATIONS:

Pregnancy/Lactation: Crosses placenta; distributed in breast milk. May inhibit skeletal growth of fetus; avoid use in last half of pregnancy. **Pregnancy Category D. Children:** Not recommended in those 8 yrs and younger; may cause permanent discoloration of teeth, enamel hypoplasia; may inhibit skeletal growth. **Elderly:** No age-related precautions noted.

INTERACTIONS

DRUG: Antacids containing aluminum, calcium, or magnesium, **laxatives** containing magnesium, **oral iron preparations** impair absorption. **Cholestyramine, colestipol** may decrease absorption. May decrease effects of **oral contraceptives. HERBAL: Dong quai, St. John's wort** may increase photosensitization. **FOOD: Dairy products** may decrease absorption. **LAB VALUES:** May increase BUN, serum alkaline phosphatase, amylase, bilirubin, AST, ALT.

AVAILABILITY (Rx)

TABLETS: 150 mg, 300 mg.

ADMINISTRATION/HANDLING

PO

• Give antacids containing aluminum, calcium, magnesium, laxatives containing magnesium, oral iron preparations 1–2 hrs before or after demeclocycline (impair drug's absorption).

INDICATIONS/ROUTES/DOSAGE

MILD TO MODERATE INFECTION, INCLUDING ACNE, PERTUSSIS, CHRONIC BRONCHITIS, UTI

PO: ADULTS, ELDERLY: 150 mg 4 times a day or 300 mg 2 times a day. **CHILDREN OLDER THAN 8 YRS:** 8–12 mg/kg/day in 2–4 divided doses.

UNCOMPLICATED GONORRHEA

PO: ADULTS: Initially, 600 mg, then 300 mg q12h for 4 days for total of 3 g.

D

SIADH

PO: ADULTS, ELDERLY: Initially, 900–1,200 mg/day in 3–4 divided doses, then decrease dose to 600–900 mg/day in divided doses.

SIDE EFFECTS

FREQUENT: Anorexia, nausea, vomiting, diarrhea, dysphagia, possibly severe photosensitivity, (with moderate to high demeclocycline dosage). **OCCASIONAL:** Urticaria, rash. Long-term therapy may result in diabetes insipidus syndrome (polydipsia, polyuria, weakness).

ADVERSE EFFECTS/ TOXIC REACTIONS

Superinfection (esp. fungal), anaphylaxis, benign intracranial hypertension occur rarely. Bulging fontanelles occur rarely in infants.

NURSING CONSIDERATIONS

BASELINE ASSESSMENT

Question for history of allergies, esp. to tetracyclines.

INTERVENTION/EVALUATION

Monitor daily pattern of bowel activity/stool consistency. Assess food intake, tolerance. Monitor I&O, renal function test results. Assess for rash. Be alert to superinfection (diarrhea, ulceration/changes of oral mucosa, tongue, anal/genital pruritus). Monitor B/P, level of consciousness (LOC) (potential for increased intracranial pressure [ICP]).

PATIENT/FAMILY TEACHING

• Continue antibiotic for full length of treatment. • Space doses evenly. • Take oral doses on empty stomach with full glass of water. • Avoid sun/ultraviolet light exposure.

Demedex, *see torsemide*

Demerol, *see meperidine*

denileukin

den-ee-**lew**-kin

(Ontak)

CLASSIFICATION

PHARMACOTHERAPEUTIC: Biologic response modifier. **CLINICAL:** Antineoplastic (see p. 78C).

ACTION

Cytotoxic fusion protein that targets cells expressing interleukin-2 (IL-2) receptors. After binding to IL-2 receptor, directs cytocidal action to malignant cutaneous T-cell lymphoma (CTCL) cells. **Therapeutic Effect:** Causes inhibition of protein synthesis, cell death.

PHARMACOKINETICS

Metabolized in liver. **Half-life:** 70–80 mins.

USES

Treatment of persistent/recurrent T-cell lymphoma whose malignant cells express CD25 component of IL-2 receptor.

PRECAUTIONS

CONTRAINDICATIONS: None known. **CAUTIONS:** Preexisting cardiovascular disease, hypoalbuminemia. **Pregnancy Category C.**

INTERACTIONS

DRUG: None significant. **HERBAL:** None significant. **FOOD:** None known. **LAB VALUES:** May decrease serum albumin, calcium, potassium, WBC, Hgb, Hct. Increases serum transaminase.

AVAILABILITY (Rx)

INJECTION SOLUTION: 150 mcg/ml.

ADMINISTRATION/HANDLING

IV

Reconstitution • Thaw in refrigerator for up to 24 hrs or at room temperature for 1–2 hrs. • Inject calculated dose into empty infusion bag. Add no more than 9 ml 0.9% NaCl to each ml denileukin.

Rate of administration • Infuse over 15 min.

Storage • Store frozen. • Solutions for IV infusion stable for 6 hrs.

IV INCOMPATIBILITIES

Do not mix with any other IV medications.

INDICATIONS/ROUTES/DOSAGE

CTCL

IV INFUSION: ADULTS: 9 or 18 mcg/kg/day for 5 consecutive days q21days. Infuse over at least 15 min.

SIDE EFFECTS

FREQUENT: Two distinct syndromes occur commonly: a hypersensitivity reaction (69%), consisting of 2 or more of the following: hypotension, back pain, dyspnea, vasodilation, vascular leak syndrome characterized by hypotension, edema, hypoalbuminemia, rash, chest tightness, tachycardia, dysphagia, syncope; and a flu-like symptom complex (91%), consisting of 2 or more of the following: fever, chills, nausea, vomiting, diarrhea, myalgia, arthralgia. **OCCASIONAL (25%–10%):** Dizziness, chest pain, weight loss, rhinitis, pruritus.

ADVERSE EFFECTS/ TOXIC REACTIONS

Pancreatitis, acute renal insufficiency, hematuria, hypothyroidism/hyperthyroidism occur rarely.

NURSING CONSIDERATIONS

BASELINE ASSESSMENT

CBC, blood chemistries (including renal/hepatic function tests), chest x-ray should be performed before therapy and weekly thereafter. Assess serum albumin level before initiation of each treatment (should be equal to or greater than 3 g/dl).

INTERVENTION/EVALUATION

Monitor serum albumin for hypoalbuminemia (generally occurs 1–2 wks after administration). Monitor for evidence of infection (lowered immune response: sore throat, fever, other vague symptoms).

PATIENT/FAMILY TEACHING

• At home, increase fluid intake (protects against renal impairment). • Do not have immunizations without physician's approval (drug lowers resistance); avoid contact with those who have recently taken live virus vaccine.

Depacon, *see valproic acid*

Depakene, *see valproic acid*

Depakote, *see valproic acid*

Depakote ER, *see valproic acid*

Depo-Medrol, *see methylprednisolone*

Depo-Provera, *see medroxyprogesterone*

D

desipramine

deh-**sip**-rah-meen

(Apo-Desipramine ✱, Norpramin)

Do not confuse desipramine with clomipramine, disopyramide, imipramine, or nortriptyline.

CLASSIFICATION

PHARMACOTHERAPEUTIC: Tricyclic. **CLINICAL:** Antidepressant (see p. 36C).

ACTION

Blocks reuptake of neurotransmitters, (norepinephrine, serotonin) at presynaptic membranes, increasing their availability at postsynaptic receptor sites. Strong anticholinergic activity. **Therapeutic Effect:** Relieves depression.

PHARMACOKINETICS

Rapidly, well absorbed from GI tract. Protein binding: 90%. Metabolized in the liver. Primarily excreted in urine. Minimally removed by hemodialysis. **Half-life:** 12–27 hrs.

USES

Treatment of various forms of depression, often in conjunction with psychotherapy. **OFF-LABEL:** Treatment of attention deficit hyperactivity disorder, bulimia nervosa, cataplexy associated with narcolepsy, cocaine withdrawal, neurogenic pain, panic disorder.

PRECAUTIONS

CONTRAINDICATIONS: Angle-closure glaucoma, within 14 days of MAOIs. **CAUTIONS:** Cardiovascular disease, cardiac conduction disturbances, urinary retention, seizure disorders, hyperthyroidism, those taking thyroid replacement therapy.

LIFESPAN CONSIDERATIONS:

Pregnancy/Lactation: Crosses placenta. Minimally distributed in breast milk. **Pregnancy Category C. Children:** Not recommended in those 6 yrs and younger. Children and adolescents with major depressive disorder (MDD), other psychiatric disorders are at increased risk for suicidal thinking, behavior while taking desipramine, esp. during first few months of treatment. **Elderly:** Use lower dosages (higher dosages not tolerated, increases risk of toxicity).

INTERACTIONS

DRUG: Alcohol, other CNS depressants may increase CNS, respiratory depression; hypotensive effects. **Antithyroid agents** may increase risk of agranulocytosis. **Cimetidine** may increase desipramine blood concentration, risk of toxicity. **Clonidine** may decrease effects. **MAOIs** may increase risk of neuroleptic malignant syndrome, hyperpyrexia, hypertensive crisis, seizures. **Phenothiazines** may increase anticholinergic, sedative effects. **Phenytoin** may decrease concentration. **Sympathomimetics** may increase risk of cardiac effects. **HERBAL: Kava kava, SAMe, St. John's wort, valerian** may increase sedation, risk of serotonin syndrome. **FOOD: Grapefruit, grapefruit juice** may increase concentration/toxicity. **LAB VALUES:** May alter serum glucose, EKG readings. Therapeutic serum level is 115–300 ng/ml; toxic serum level is greater than 400 ng/ml.

AVAILABILITY (Rx)

TABLETS: 10 mg, 25 mg, 50 mg, 75 mg, 100 mg, 150 mg.

ADMINISTRATION/HANDLING

PO

◀ **ALERT** ▶ Fourteen days must elapse between use of MAOIs and despiramine. • Give with food, milk if GI distress occurs.

INDICATIONS/ROUTES/DOSAGE

DEPRESSION

PO: ADULTS: 75 mg/day. May gradually increase to 150–200 mg/day. **Maximum:** 300 mg/day. **ELDERLY:** Initially, 10–25 mg/day. May gradually increase to 75–100 mg/day. **Maximum:** 300 mg/day. **CHILDREN OLDER THAN 12 YRS:** Initially, 25–50 mg/day. May gradually increase to 100 mg/day. **Maximum:** 150 mg/day. **CHILDREN 6–12 YRS:** 1–3 mg/kg/day. **Maximum:** 5 mg/kg/day.

SIDE EFFECTS

FREQUENT: Somnolence, fatigue, dry mouth, blurred vision, constipation, delayed micturition, orthostatic hypotension, diaphoresis, impaired concentration, increased appetite, urinary retention. **OCCASIONAL:** GI disturbances (nausea, GI distress, metallic taste). **RARE:** Paradoxical reactions (agitation, restlessness, nightmares, insomnia), extrapyramidal symptoms (particularly fine hand tremor).

ADVERSE EFFECTS/ TOXIC REACTIONS

Overdose may produce confusion, seizures, somnolence, arrhythmias, fever, hallucinations, dyspnea, vomiting, unusual fatigue, weakness. Abrupt discontinuation after prolonged therapy may produce severe headache, malaise, nausea, vomiting, vivid dreams.

NURSING CONSIDERATIONS

BASELINE ASSESSMENT

For those on long-term therapy, hepatic/renal function tests, blood counts should be performed periodically. For those at risk for arrhythmias, perform baseline EKG.

INTERVENTION/EVALUATION

Supervise suicidal-risk pt closely during early therapy (as depression lessens, energy level improves, increasing suicide potential). Assess appearance, behavior, speech pattern, level of interest, mood. Therapeutic serum level: 115–300 ng/ml; toxic serum level: greater than 400 ng/ml. Monitor EKG if pt has history of arrhythmias.

PATIENT/FAMILY TEACHING

• Change positions slowly to avoid hypotensive effect. • Tolerance to postural hypotension, sedative, anticholinergic effects usually develops during early therapy. • Maximum therapeutic effect may be noted in 2–4 wks. • Do not abruptly discontinue medication.

desloratadine

des-low-**rah**-tah-deen

(Aerius ✤, Clarinex, Clarinex Redi-Tabs)

Do not confuse Clarinex with Claritin.

FIXED-COMBINATION(S)

Clarinex-D 24 Hour: desloratadine/pseudoephedrine, (a sympathomimetic): 5 mg/240 mg. **Clarinex-D 12 Hour:** desloratadine/pseudoephedrine: 2.5 mg/120 mg.

CLASSIFICATION

PHARMACOTHERAPEUTIC: H_1 antagonist. **CLINICAL:** Nonsedating antihistamine.

ACTION

Exhibits selective peripheral histamine H_1 receptor blocking action. Competes

D

with histamine at receptor sites. **Therapeutic Effect:** Prevents allergic response mediated by histamine (rhinitis, urticaria).

PHARMACOKINETICS

Rapidly, almost completely absorbed from GI tract. Distributed mainly in liver, lungs, GI tract, bile. Metabolized in the liver to active metabolite and undergoes extensive first-pass metabolism. Eliminated in urine, feces. **Half-life:** 27 hrs (increased in elderly, renal/hepatic impairment).

USES

Relief of nasal/non-nasal symptoms of rhinitis (sneezing, rhinorrhea, itching/tearing of eyes, stuffiness), chronic idiopathic urticaria (hives).

PRECAUTIONS

CONTRAINDICATIONS: None known. **CAUTIONS:** Hepatic impairment. Safety in children younger than 6 yrs unknown.

LIFESPAN CONSIDERATIONS:

Pregnancy/Lactation: Excreted in breast milk. **Pregnancy Category C.** **Children/Elderly:** More sensitive to anticholinergic effects (e.g., dry mouth, nose, throat). Safety in children younger than 6 yrs unknown.

INTERACTIONS

DRUG: **Erythromycin, ketoconazole** may increase concentration. **HERBAL:** None significant. **FOOD:** None known. **LAB VALUES:** May suppress wheal, flare reactions to antigen skin testing unless antihistamines are discontinued 4 days before testing.

AVAILABILITY (Rx)

SYRUP (CLARINEX): 2.5 mg/5 ml. **TABLETS (CLARINEX):** 5 mg. **TABLETS (ORALLY DISINTEGRATING [CLARINEX REDITABS]):** 2.5 mg, 5 mg.

ADMINISTRATION/HANDLING

PO

- May give with or without food.

ORAL DISINTEGRATING TABLET

- Place on tongue. • May give with or without water.

INDICATIONS/ROUTES/DOSAGE

ALLERGIC RHINITIS, URTICARIA

PO: ADULTS, ELDERLY, CHILDREN OLDER THAN 12 YRS: 5 mg once a day. **CHILDREN 6–12 YRS:** 2.5 mg once a day. **CHILDREN 1–5 YRS:** 1.25 mg once a day. **CHILDREN 6–11 MOS:** 1 mg once a day.

DOSAGE IN HEPATIC/RENAL IMPAIRMENT

Dosage is decreased to 5 mg every other day.

SIDE EFFECTS

FREQUENT (12%): Headache. **OCCASIONAL (3%):** Dry mouth, somnolence. **RARE (less than 3%):** Fatigue, dizziness, diarrhea, nausea.

ADVERSE EFFECTS/ TOXIC REACTIONS

None known.

NURSING CONSIDERATIONS

BASELINE ASSESSMENT

Assess lung sounds for wheezing; skin for urticaria, hives.

INTERVENTION/EVALUATION

For upper respiratory allergies, increase fluids to decrease viscosity of secretions, offset thirst, replace loss of fluids from diaphoresis. Monitor symptoms for therapeutic response.

PATIENT/FAMILY TEACHING

- Does not cause drowsiness; however, if blurred vision or eye pain occurs, do not drive, perform activities requiring visual acuity. • Avoid alcohol.

desmopressin

des-moe-**press**-in

(Apo-Desmopressin ✦, DDAVP, DDAVP Nasal, DDAVP Rhinal Tube, Minirin, Octostim ✦, Stimate)

CLASSIFICATION

PHARMACOTHERAPEUTIC: Synthetic pituitary hormone. **CLINICAL:** Antidiuretic.

ACTION

Increases reabsorption of water by increasing permeability of collecting ducts of kidneys. Plasminogen activator. **Therapeutic Effect:** Increases plasma factor VIII (antihemophilic factor). Decreases urinary output.

PHARMACOKINETICS

Route	Onset	Peak	Duration
PO	1 hr	2–7 hrs	6–8 hrs
IV	15–30 min	1.5–3 hrs	N/A
Intranasal	15 min–1 hr	1–5 hrs	5–21 hrs

Poorly absorbed after oral, nasal administration. Metabolism: Unknown. **Half-life: Oral:** 1.5–2.5 hrs. **Intranasal:** 3.3–3.5 hrs. **IV:** 0.4–4 hrs.

USES

DDAVP Intranasal: Primary nocturnal enuresis, central cranial diabetes insipidus. **Parenteral:** Central cranial diabetes insipidus, hemophilia A, von Willebrand's disease (type I). **Stimate intranasal:** Hemophilia A, von Willebrand's disease (type I). **PO:** Central cranial diabetes insipidus. **OFF-LABEL:** Prophylaxis, treatment of central diabetes insipidus, treatment of hemophilia A, primary nocturnal enuresis, von Willebrand's disease.

PRECAUTIONS

CONTRAINDICATIONS: Hemophilia A with factor VIII levels less than 5%; hemophilia B; severe type I, type IIB, platelet-type von Willebrand's disease. **CAUTIONS:** Predisposition to thrombus formation, conditions with fluid, electrolyte imbalance, coronary artery disease, hypertensive cardiovascular disease.

LIFESPAN CONSIDERATIONS:

Pregnancy/Lactation: Pregnancy Category B. Children: Caution in neonates, those younger than 3 mos (increased risk of fluid balance problems). Careful fluid restrictions recommended in infants. **Elderly:** Increased risk of hyponatremia, water intoxication.

INTERACTIONS

DRUG: Carbamazepine, chlorpropamide, clofibrate may increase effects. **Demeclocycline, lithium, norepinephrine** may decrease effects. **HERBAL:** None significant. **FOOD:** None known. **LAB VALUES:** None known.

AVAILABILITY (Rx)

INJECTION SOLUTION (DDAVP): 4 mcg/ml. **NASAL SOLUTION (DDAVP):** 100 mcg/ml. **NASAL SPRAY:** 1.5 mg/ml (150 mcg/spray) (Stimate), 100 mcg/ml (10 mcg/spray) (DDAVP). **TABLETS (DDAVP):** 0.1 mg, 0.2 mg.

ADMINISTRATION/HANDLING

IV

Reconstitution • For IV infusion, dilute in 10–50 ml 0.9% NaCl.

Rate of administration • Infuse over 15–30 min. • For preop use, administer 30 min before procedure. • Monitor B/P, pulse during IV infusion. • IV dose = $\frac{1}{10}$ intranasal dose.

Storage • Refrigerate. Stable for 2 wks at room temperature.

SUBCUTANEOUS

• Estimate response by adequate sleep duration. • Morning, evening doses should be adjusted separately.

INTRANASAL
• Refrigerate DDAVP nasal solution, Stimate nasal spray. Nasal solution, Stimate nasal spray are stable for 3 wks at room temperature if unopened. • DDAVP nasal spray is stable at room temperature. • Calibrated catheter (rhinyle) is used to draw up measured quantity of desmopressin; with one end inserted in nose, pt blows on other end to deposit solution deep in nasal cavity. • For infants, young children, obtunded pts, air-filled syringe may be attached to catheter to deposit solution.

INDICATIONS/ROUTES/DOSAGE

PRIMARY NOCTURNAL ENURESIS
PO: CHILDREN 6 YRS AND OLDER: 0.2–0.6 mg once before bedtime.
INTRANASAL: CHILDREN 6 YRS AND OLDER: Initially, 20 mcg (0.2 ml) at bedtime; use ½ dose in each nostril. Adjust to maximum of 40 mcg/day. Range: 10–40 mcg.

CENTRAL CRANIAL DIABETES INSIPIDUS
PO: ADULTS, ELDERLY, CHILDREN 12 YRS AND OLDER: Initially, 0.05 mg twice a day. Range: 0.1–1.2 mg/day in 2–3 divided doses. **CHILDREN YOUNGER THAN 12 YRS:** Initially, 0.05 mg; then twice a day. Range: 0.1–0.8 mg daily.
IV, SUBCUTANEOUS: ADULTS, ELDERLY, CHILDREN 12 YRS AND OLDER: 2–4 mcg/day in 2 divided doses or $\frac{1}{10}$ of maintenance intranasal dose.
INTRANASAL (USE 100 MCG/ML CONCENTRATION): ADULTS, ELDERLY, CHILDREN OLDER THAN 12 YRS: 5–40 mcg (0.05–0.4 ml) in 1–3 doses/day. **CHILDREN 3 MOS–12 YRS:** Initially, 5 mcg (0.05 ml)/day. Range: 5–30 mcg (0.05–0.3 ml)/day.

HEMOPHILIA A, VON WILLEBRAND'S DISEASE (TYPE I)
IV INFUSION: ADULTS, ELDERLY, CHILDREN WEIGHING MORE THAN 10 KGS.: 0.3 mcg/kg diluted in 50 ml 0.9% NaCl. **CHILDREN WEIGHING 10 KG AND LESS:** 0.3 mcg/kg diluted in 10 ml 0.9% NaCl.
INTRANASAL (USE 1.5 MG/ML CONCENTRATION PROVIDING 150 MCG/SPRAY): ADULTS, ELDERLY, CHILDREN 12 YRS AND OLDER WEIGHING MORE THAN 50 KG: 300 mcg; use 1 spray in each nostril. **ADULTS, ELDERLY, CHILDREN 12 YRS AND OLDER WEIGHING 50 KG OR LESS:** 150 mcg as a single spray.

SIDE EFFECTS

OCCASIONAL: IV: Pain, redness, swelling at injection site; headache; abdominal cramps; vulvular pain; flushed skin; mild B/P elevation; nausea with high dosages. **Nasal:** Rhinorrhea, nasal congestion, slight B/P elevation.

ADVERSE EFFECTS/ TOXIC REACTIONS

Water intoxication, hyponatremia (headache, somnolence, confusion, decreased urination, rapid weight gain, seizures, coma) may occur in overhydration. Children, elderly pts, infants are esp. at risk.

NURSING CONSIDERATIONS

BASELINE ASSESSMENT
Establish baselines for B/P, pulse, weight, serum electrolytes, urine specific gravity. Check lab values for factor VIII coagulant concentration for hemophilia A, von Willebrand's disease; bleeding times.

INTERVENTION/EVALUATION
Check B/P, pulse with IV infusion. Monitor pt weight, fluid intake, urine volume, urine specific gravity, osmolality, serum electrolytes for diabetes insipidus. Assess factor VIII antigen levels, partial thromboplastin time (aPTT), factor VIII activity level for hemophilia.

PATIENT/FAMILY TEACHING
• Avoid overhydration. • Teach proper technique for intranasal administration. • Inform physician if headache,

shortness of breath, heartburn, nausea, abdominal cramps occur.

desonide

(Otic Tridesilon, Tridesilon)

See Corticosteroids: topical (p. 94C)

desoximetasone

(Topicort)

See Corticosteroids: topical (p. 94C)

Desyrel, *see trazodone*

Detrol, *see tolterodine*

Detrol LA, *see tolterodine*

dexamethasone

dex-a-**meth**-a-sone

(Apo-Dexamethasone ✤, Decadron, Dexamethasone Intensol, Dexpak Taperpak, Diodex ✤, Maxidex)

Do not confuse dexamethasone with desoximetasone or dextramethophan, or Maxidex with Maxzide.

FIXED-COMBINATION(S)

Ciprodex Otic: dextramethasone/ciprofloxacin (antibiotic): 0.1%/0.3%. **Dexacidin, Maxitrol:** dexamethasone/neomycin/polymyxin (anti-infectives): 0.1%/3.5 mg/10,000 units per g or ml.

CLASSIFICATION

PHARMACOTHERAPEUTIC: Long-acting glucocorticoid. **CLINICAL:** Corticosteroid (see pp. 92C, 94C).

ACTION

Inhibits accumulation of inflammatory cells at inflammation sites, phagocytosis, lysosomal enzyme release and synthesis, and/or release of mediators of inflammation. **Therapeutic Effect:** Prevents/suppresses cell/tissue immune reactions, inflammatory process.

PHARMACOKINETICS

Rapidly, completely absorbed from GI tract after PO administration. Widely distributed. Protein binding: High. Metabolized in the liver. Primarily excreted in urine. Minimally removed by hemodialysis. **Half-life:** 3–4.5 hrs.

USES

Acute exacerbations of chronic allergic disorders, cerebral edema, conditions treated by immunosupression, inflammatory conditions, otitis externa, ophthalmic conditions (corneal injury, inflammatory conditions, infective conjunctivitis). **OFF-LABEL:** Antiemetic, treatment of croup.

PRECAUTIONS

CONTRAINDICATIONS: Active untreated infections, fungal, tuberculosis, viral diseases of the eye. **CAUTIONS:** Respiratory tuberculosis, untreated systemic infections, ocular herpes simplex, hyperthyroidism, cirrhosis, ulcerative colitis, hypertension, osteoporosis pts at high thromboembolic risk, CHF, seizure disorders, peptic ulcer, diabetes. Prolonged use may result in cataracts, glaucoma.

LIFESPAN CONSIDERATIONS:

Pregnancy/Lactation: Crosses placenta. Distributed in breast milk. **Pregnancy Category C (D if used in the first trimester). Children:** Prolonged treatment with high-dose therapy may decrease short-term growth rate, cortisol secretion. **Elderly:** Higher risk for developing hypertension, osteoporosis.

INTERACTIONS

DRUG: Amphotericin may increase hypokalemia. May increase **digoxin** toxicity caused by hypokalemia. May decrease effects of **diuretics, insulin, oral hypoglycemics, potassium supplements. Hepatic enzyme inducers** may decrease effects. **Live virus vaccines** may decrease pt's antibody response to vaccine, increase vaccine side effects, potentiate virus replication. **HERBAL: Cat's claw, echinacea** may increase immunosuppresant effect. **FOOD:** Interferes with **calcium** absorption. **LAB VALUES:** May increase serum glucose lipids, amylase, sodium levels. May decrease serum calcium, potassium, thyroxine.

AVAILABILITY (Rx)

ELIXIR: 0.5 mg/5 ml. **INJECTION, SOLUTION:** 4 mg/ml, 10 mg/ml. **OPHTHALMIC OINTMENT:** 0.05%. **OPHTHALMIC SOLUTION:** 0.1%. **OPHTHALMIC SUSPENSION (MAXIDEX):** 0.1%. **SOLUTION, ORAL:** 0.5 mg/5ml. **SOLUTION, ORAL CONCENTRATE (DEXAMETHASONE INTENSOL):** 1 mg/ml. **TABLET:** 0.5 mg. 0.75 mg, 1 mg, 1.5 mg, 2 mg, 4 mg, 6 mg. **TABLET (TAPER PAK [DEX PAK]):** 1.5 mg (51 tablets on taper dose card).

ADMINISTRATION/HANDLING

IV

◄ **ALERT** ► Dexamethasone sodium phosphate may be given by IV push or IV infusion.

• For IV push, give over 1–4 min. • For IV infusion, mix with 0.9% NaCl or D_5W and infuse over 15–30 min. • For neonates, solution must be preservative free. • IV solution must be used within 24 hrs.

IM

• Give deep IM, preferably in gluteus maximus.

PO

• Give with milk, food.

OPHTHALMIC • Place finger on lower eyelid and pull out until a pocket is formed between eye and lower lid. • Hold dropper above pocket and place correct number of drops (¼–½ inch ointment) into pocket. • Close eye gently.
Solution: Apply digital pressure to lacrimal sac for 1–2 min (minimizes drainage into nose/throat, reducing risk of systemic effects).
Ointment: Close eye for 1–2 min. Instruct pt to roll eyeball (increases contact area of drug to eye). Remove excess solution or ointment around eye with tissue. • Ointment may be used at night to reduce frequency of solution administration. • As with other corticosteroids, taper dosage slowly when discontinuing.

TOPICAL • Gently cleanse area before application. • Use occlusive dressings only as ordered. • Apply sparingly, rub into area thoroughly.

IV INCOMPATIBILITIES

Ciprofloxacin (Cipro), daunorubicin (Cerubidine), idarubicin (Idamycin), midazolam (Versed).

IV COMPATIBILITIES

Aminophylline, cimetidine (Tagamet), cisplatin (Platinol), cyclophosphamide (Cytoxan), cytarabine (Cytosar), docetaxel (Taxotere), doxorubicin (Adriamycin), etoposide (VePesid), granisetron (Kytril), heparin, hydromorphone (Dilaudid), lipids, lorazepam (Ativan), morphine, ondansetron (Zofran), paclitaxel (Taxol), potassium chloride, propofol (Diprivan), total parenteral nutrition (TPN).

INDICATIONS/ROUTES/DOSAGE

ANTI-INFLAMMATORY

PO, IV, IM: ADULTS, ELDERLY: 0.75–9 mg/day in divided doses q6–12h. **CHILDREN:** 0.08–0.3 mg/kg/day in divided doses q6–12h.

CEREBRAL EDEMA

IV: ADULTS, ELDERLY: Initially, 10 mg, then 4 mg (IV or IM) q6h.

PO, IV, IM: CHILDREN: Loading dose of 1–2 mg/kg, then 1–1.5 mg/kg/day in divided doses q4–6h.

NAUSEA/VOMITING IN CHEMOTHERAPY PTS

IV: ADULTS, ELDERLY: 8–20 mg once, then 4 mg (PO) q4–6h or 8 mg q8h. **CHILDREN:** 10 mg/m^2/dose (**Maximum:** 20 mg), then 5 mg/m^2/dose q6h.

USUAL TOPICAL DOSAGE

TOPICAL: ADULTS, ELDERLY, CHILDREN: Apply to affected area 3–4 times a day.

PHYSIOLOGIC REPLACEMENT

PO, IV, IM: CHILDREN: 0.03–0.15 mg/kg/day in divided doses q6–12h.

USUAL OPHTHALMIC DOSAGE, OCULAR INFLAMMATORY CONDITIONS

OINTMENT: ADULTS, ELDERLY, CHILDREN: Thin coating 3–4 times/day.

SUSPENSION: ADULTS, ELDERLY, CHILDREN: Initially, 2 drops q1h while awake and q2h at night for 1 day, then reduce to 3–4 times/day.

SIDE EFFECTS

FREQUENT: Inhalation: Cough, dry mouth, hoarseness, throat irritation. **Intranasal:** Burning, mucosal dryness. **Ophthalmic:** Blurred vision. **Systemic:** Insomnia, facial edema (cushingoid appearance ["moon face"]), moderate abdominal distention, indigestion, increased appetite, nervousness, facial flushing, diaphoresis. **OCCASIONAL: Inhalation:** Localized fungal infection (thrush). **Intranasal:** Crusting inside nose, epistaxis, sore throat, ulceration of nasal mucosa. **Ophthalmic:** Decreased vision; watering of eyes; eye pain; burning, stinging, redness of eyes; nausea; vomiting. **Systemic:** Dizziness, decreased/blurred vision. **Topical:** Allergic contact dermatitis, purpura, thinning of skin with easy bruising, telangiectasis (raised dark red spots on skin). **RARE: Inhalation:** Increased bronchospasm, esophageal candidiasis. **Intranasal:** Nasal/pharyngeal candidiasis, eye pain. **Systemic:** Generalized allergic reaction (rash, urticaria); pain, redness, swelling at injection site; psychological changes; false sense of well-being; hallucinations; depression.

ADVERSE EFFECTS/ TOXIC REACTIONS

Long-term therapy. Muscle wasting (esp. arms, legs), osteoporosis, spontaneous fractures, amenorrhea, cataracts, glaucoma, peptic ulcer disease, CHF. **Ophthalmic:** Glaucoma, ocular hypertension, cataracts. **Abrupt withdrawal following long-term therapy:** Severe joint pain, severe headache, anorexia, nausea, fever, rebound inflammation, fatigue, weakness, lethargy, dizziness, orthostatic hypotension.

NURSING CONSIDERATIONS

BASELINE ASSESSMENT

Question for hypersensitivity to any corticosteroids. Obtain baselines for height, weight, B/P, serum glucose, electrolytes.

INTERVENTION/EVALUATION

Monitor I&O, daily weight. Assess for edema. Evaluate food tolerance, bowel activity/stool consistency. Report hyperacidity promptly. Check vital signs at least twice a day. Be alert to infection (sore throat, fever, vague symptoms). Monitor serum electrolytes, esp. for hypercalcemia (muscle twitching, cramps), hypokalemia (weakness, muscle cramps, paresthesia, [esp. lower extremities], nausea/vomiting, irritability). Assess emotional status, ability to sleep.

PATIENT/FAMILY TEACHING

• Do not change dose/schedule or stop taking drug. • **Must** taper off gradually under medical supervision. • Notify physician of fever, sore throat, muscle aches, sudden weight gain, edema. • Severe stress (serious infection, surgery, trauma) may require increased dosage. • Inform dentist, other physicians of dexamethasone therapy now or within past 12 mos. • **Topical:** Apply after shower/bath for best absorption.

dexmedetomidine

decks-meh-deh-**tome**-ih-deen

(Precedex)

Do not confuse Precedex with Peridex or Percocet.

CLASSIFICATION

PHARMACOTHERAPEUTIC: Alpha$_2$-agonist. **CLINICAL:** Nonbarbiturate sedative, hypnotic.

ACTION

Selective alpha$_2$-adrenergic agonist. **Therapeutic Effect:** Produces analgesic, hypnotic, sedative effects.

PHARMACOKINETICS

Protein binding: 94%. Metabolized in liver. Excreted in urine. **Half-life:** 2 hrs.

USES

Sedation of initially intubated, mechanically ventilated adults during treatment in intensive care setting. **OFF-LABEL:** Pain relief, treatment of shivering.

PRECAUTIONS

CONTRAINDICATIONS: None known. **CAUTIONS:** Advanced heart block, severe CHF, hepatic/renal impairment, hypovolemia. **Pregnancy Category C.**

INTERACTIONS

DRUG: **Isoniazid, miconazole** may increase concentration/effects. May increase concentration/effects of **beta-blockers, fluoxetine, lidocaine, mirtazapine, paroxetine, risperidone, ritonavir, thioridazine, tricyclic antidepressants, venlafaxine. Vasodilators** may increase hypotensive effect. May decrease concentration of **codeine, hydrocodone, oxycodone, tramadol.** **HERBAL:** None significant. **FOOD:** None known. **LAB VALUES:** May increase serum alkaline phosphatase, potassium, AST, ALT.

AVAILABILITY (Rx)

INJECTION SOLUTION: 100 mcg/ml.

ADMINISTRATION/HANDLING

IV

Reconstitution • Dilute 2 ml of dexmedetomidine with 48 ml 0.9 NaCl.

Rate of administration • Give as maintenance infusion.

Storage • Store at room temperature.

IV INCOMPATIBILITIES

Do not mix dexmedetomidine with any other medications.

INDICATIONS/ROUTES/DOSAGE

SEDATION FOR INTUBATION/MECHANICAL VENTILATION

IV: ADULTS: Loading dose of 1 mcg/kg over 10 min followed by maintenance infusion of 0.2–0.7 mcg/kg/hr. **ELDERLY:** May require decreased dosage. No guidelines available.

SIDE EFFECTS

FREQUENT: Hypotension (30%), nausea (11%). **OCCASIONAL (3%–2%):** Pain, fever, oliguria, thirst.

ADVERSE EFFECTS/ TOXIC REACTIONS

Bradycardia, atrial fibrillation, hypoxia, anemia, pain, pleural effusion may occur with too-rapid IV infusion.

NURSING CONSIDERATIONS

INTERVENTION/EVALUATION

Monitor EKG for atrial fibrillation, pulse for bradycardia, B/P for hypotension, level of sedation. Assess respiratory rate, rhythm. Monitor ventilator settings.

dexmethylphenidate

dex-meth-ill-**fen**-i-date
(Focalin, Focalin XR)

◆CLASSIFICATION

CLINICAL: CNS stimulant (**Schedule II**).

ACTION

Blocks reuptake of norepinephrine, dopamine into presynaptic neurons, increasing release of these neurotransmitters into synaptic cleft. **Therapeutic Effect:** Decreases motor restlessness, fatigue; increases motor activity, mental alertness, attention span; elevates mood.

PHARMACOKINETICS

Route	Onset	Peak	Duration
PO	N/A	N/A	4–5 hrs

Readily absorbed from GI tract. Plasma concentrations increase rapidly. Metabolized in the liver. Excreted unchanged in urine. **Half-life:** 2.2 hrs.

USES

Adjunct in treatment of attention deficit hyperactivity disorder (ADHD) with moderate to severe distractability, short attention spans, hyperactivity, emotional impulsivity in children 6 yrs and older.

PRECAUTIONS

CONTRAINDICATIONS: Diagnosis or family history of Tourette syndrome; glaucoma; history of marked agitation, anxiety, tension; motor tics; use of MAOIs within 14 days. **CAUTIONS:** Cardiovascular disease, seizure disorder, psychosis. Avoid use in those with history of substance abuse.

⌛ LIFESPAN CONSIDERATIONS:

Pregnancy/Lactation: Unknown if excreted in breast milk. **Pregnancy Category C.** **Children:** May be more susceptible to developing anorexia, insomnia, abdominal pain, weight loss. Chronic use may inhibit growth. In psychotic children, may exacerbate symptoms of behavior disturbance, thought disorder. **Elderly:** No age-related precautions noted.

INTERACTIONS

DRUG: **Antacids, acid suppressants** may alter absorption. Other **CNS stimulants** may have additive effects. **MAOIs** may increase effects. Decreased dosages for **phenobarbital, phenytoin, primidone, tricyclic antidepressants** may be necessary. May inhibit effects of **warfarin.** **HERBAL:** **Ephedra** may cause hypertension, arrhythmias. **Yohimbe** may increase CNS stimulation. **FOOD:** None known. **LAB VALUES:** None known.

AVAILABILITY (Rx)

TABLETS (FOCALIN): 2.5 mg.

CAPSULES (EXTENDED-RELEASE [FOCALIN XR]): 5 mg, 10 mg, 20 mg.

ADMINISTRATION/HANDLING

PO

• Do not give drug in afternoon or evening (causes insomnia). • Tablets may be crushed. • Give without regard

D

to food. • Swallow extended-release capsules whole; do not chew, crush, divide. • May sprinkle contents of extended-release capsules on small amount of applesauce. • Give extended-release capsules once each day in the morning, before breakfast.

INDICATIONS/ROUTES/DOSAGE

ADHD

Pts not currently taking methylphenidate:

Capsules

PO: ADULTS, ELDERLY: Initially, 10 mg/day. May increase in increments of 10 mg/day at weekly intervals. **Maximum:** 20 mg/day. **CHILDREN 6 YRS AND OLDER:** Initially, 5 mg/day. May increase in increments of 5 mg/day at weekly intervals. **Maximum:** 20 mg/day

Tablets

PO: ADULTS, ELDERLY, CHILDREN 6 YRS AND OLDER: Initially, 2.5 mg 2 times/day. May increase in increments of 2.5–5 mg at weekly intervals. **Conversion from methylphenidate:** Initially, half the dose of methyphenidate. **Conversion from dexmethylphenidate immediate-release to extended-release:** Switch to same dose using extended-release formulation.

SIDE EFFECTS

FREQUENT: Abdominal pain, nausea, anorexia, fever. **OCCASIONAL:** Tachycardia, arrhythmias, palpitations, insomnia, twitching. **RARE:** Blurred vision, rash, arthralgia.

ADVERSE EFFECTS/ TOXIC REACTIONS

Withdrawal after prolonged therapy may unmask symptoms of underlying disorder. May lower seizure threshold in those with history of seizures. Overdose produces excessive sympathomimetic effects (vomiting, tremor, hyperreflexia, seizures, confusion, hallucinations, diaphoresis). Prolonged administration to children may delay growth. Neuroleptic malignant syndrome occurs rarely.

NURSING CONSIDERATIONS

INTERVENTION/EVALUATION

CBC, differential, platelet count should be performed routinely during therapy. If paradoxical return of attention deficit occurs, dosage should be reduced or discontinued. Weigh pediatric pt regularly to detect delayed growth.

PATIENT/FAMILY TEACHING

• Avoid tasks that require alertness, motor skills until response to drug is established. • Report any increase in seizures. • Last dose should be given several hours before bedtime to prevent insomnia. • Report anxiety, fever.

dexrazoxane

dex-ray-**zoks**-ane
(Zinecard)

CLASSIFICATION

PHARMACOTHERAPEUTIC: Antineoplastic. **CLINICAL:** Cytoprotective agent.

ACTION

Rapidly penetrates myocardial cell membrane. Binds intracellular iron, prevents generation of free radicals by anthracyclines. **Therapeutic Effect:** Protects against anthracycline-induced cardiomyopathy.

PHARMACOKINETICS

Rapidly distributed after IV administration. Not bound to plasma proteins. Primarily excreted in urine. Removed by peritoneal dialysis. **Half-life:** 2.1–2.5 hrs.

USES

Reduction of incidence, severity of cardiomyopathy associated with doxorubicin therapy in women with metastatic breast cancer. Not recommended with initiation of doxorubicin therapy.

PRECAUTIONS

CONTRAINDICATIONS: Hypersensitivity to nonanthracycline chemotherapy regimens. **CAUTIONS:** Chemotherapeutic agents that are additive to myelosuppression, concurrent fluorouracil, adriamycin, cyclophosphamide (FAC) therapy.

LIFESPAN CONSIDERATIONS:

Pregnancy/Lactation: May be embryotoxic, teratogenic. Unknown if distributed in breast milk. Breast-feeding not recommended. **Pregnancy Category C.** **Children:** Safety and efficacy not established. **Elderly:** Information not available.

INTERACTIONS

DRUG: **Bone marrow depressants** may increase myelosuppression. **Concurrent FAC (5-fluorouracil, adriamycin, cyclophosphamide) therapy** may produce severe blood dyscrasias. **HERBAL:** None significant. **FOOD:** None known. **LAB VALUES:** Concurrent FAC therapy may produce abnormal hepatic/renal function test results.

AVAILABILITY (Rx)

INJECTION, POWDER FOR RECONSTITUTION: 250 mg (10 mg/ml reconstituted in 25-ml single-use vial), 500 mg (10 mg/ml reconstituted in 50-ml single-use vial).

ADMINISTRATION/HANDLING

◄ ALERT ► Do not mix with other drugs. Use caution in handling/preparation of reconstituted solution (glove use recommended).

IV

Reconstitution • Reconstitute with 0.167 molar (M/6) sodium lactate injection to give concentration of 10 mg dexrazoxane for each ml of sodium lactate. • May further dilute with 0.9% NaCl or D_5W. Concentration should range from 1.3–5 mg/ml.

Rate of administration • Give reconstituted solution by slow IV push or IV infusion over 15–30 min. • After infusion is completed and before total elapsed time of 30 min from beginning of dexrazoxane infusion, give IV injection of doxorubicin.

Storage • Store vials at room temperature. • Reconstituted solution is stable for 6 hrs at room temperature or if refrigerated. Discard unused solution.

IV INCOMPATIBILITIES

Do not mix dexrazoxane with other medications.

INDICATIONS/ROUTES/DOSAGE

CARDIOPROTECTIVE

IV: ADULTS, CHILDREN: Recommended dosage ratio is 10 parts dexrazoxane to 1 part doxorubicin (e.g., 500 mg/m^2 dexrazoxane for every 50 mg/m^2 doxorubicin).

DOSAGE IN RENAL IMPAIRMENT:

IV, ADULTS, ELDERLY: Moderate to severe (creatinine clearance less than 40 ml/min): use 5:1 ratio of dexrazoxane to doxorubicin.

SIDE EFFECTS

FREQUENT: Alopecia, nausea, vomiting, fatigue, malaise, anorexia, stomatitis, fever, infection, diarrhea. **OCCASIONAL:** Pain at injection site, neurotoxicity, phlebitis, dysphagia, streaking/erythema at injection site. **RARE:** Urticaria, skin reaction.

D

ADVERSE EFFECTS/ TOXIC REACTIONS

FAC (fluorouracil, adriamycin, cyclophosphamide) therapy with dexrazoxane increases risk for severe leukopenia, granulocytopenia, thrombocytopenia than in those receiving FAC without dextrazoxane. Overdose can be removed with peritoneal dialysis or hemodialysis.

NURSING CONSIDERATIONS

BASELINE ASSESSMENT

Use gloves when preparing solution. If powder/solution comes in contact with skin, wash immediately with soap and water. Antiemetics may be effective in preventing, treating nausea.

INTERVENTION/EVALUATION

Frequently monitor CBC with differential for evidence of blood dyscrasias. Assess for stomatitis (burning/erythema of oral mucosa at inner margin of lips, sore throat, difficulty swallowing). Monitor hematologic status, renal/hepatic function studies, cardiac function. Monitor daily pattern of bowel activity/stool consistency. Monitor for hematologic toxicity (fever, signs of local infection, unusual bruising/bleeding from any site).

PATIENT/FAMILY TEACHING

• Alopecia is reversible, but new hair growth may have different color/texture. • New hair growth resumes 2–3 mos after last therapy dose. • Maintain fastidious oral hygiene. • Promptly report fever, sore throat, signs of local infection. • Contact physician if persistent nausea/vomiting continues at home.

dextran, low molecular weight (dextran 40)

dex-tran
(Gentran LMD, Rheomacrodex ✤)

dextran, high molecular weight (dextran 70)

(Gentran, Macrodex)

◆CLASSIFICATION

PHARMACOTHERAPEUTIC: Branched polysaccharide. **CLINICAL:** Plasma volume expander.

ACTION

Produces plasma volume expansion due to high colloidal osmotic effect. Draws interstitial fluid into intravascular space. May increase blood flow in microcirculation. **Therapeutic Effect:** Increases central venous pressure (CVP), cardiac output, stroke volume, B/P, urine output, capillary perfusion, pulse pressure. Decreases heart rate, peripheral resistance, blood viscosity. Corrects hypovolemia.

USES

Fluid replacement, blood volume expander in treatment of hypovolemia, shock, impending shock.

PRECAUTIONS

CONTRAINDICATIONS: Hypervolemia, renal failure, severe bleeding disorders, severe CHF, severe thrombocytopenia. **CAUTIONS:** Those with extreme dehydration, chronic hepatic disease.

⌛ LIFESPAN CONSIDERATIONS:

Pregnancy/Lactation: Crosses placenta; unknown if distributed in breast milk. **Pregnancy Category C. Children:** No age-related precautions noted. **Elderly:** No age-related precautions noted.

INTERACTIONS

DRUG: None significant. **HERBAL:** None significant. **FOOD:** None known. **LAB VALUES:** Prolongs bleeding time, depresses platelet count. Decreases clotting factors V, VIII, IX.

AVAILABILITY (Rx)

INJECTION (HIGH MOLECULAR WEIGHT [GENTRAN]): 6% dextran 70 in 500 ml 0.9% NaCl. **INJECTION (LOW MOLECULAR WEIGHT [GENTRAN LMD]):** 10% dextran 40 in 500 ml D_5W, 10% dextran 40 in 500 ml 0.9% NaCl.

ADMINISTRATION/HANDLING

IV

Rate of administration • Give by IV infusion only. • Monitor pt closely during first 15 min of infusion for anaphylactoid reaction. Monitor vital signs q5min. • Monitor urinary flow rates during administration (if oliguria/anuria occurs, dextran 40 should be discontinued and osmotic diuretic given [minimizes vascular overloading]). • Monitor CVP when given by rapid infusion. If CVP rises precipitously, immediately discontinue drug (overexpansion of blood volume). • Monitor B/P diligently during infusion; if marked hypotension occurs, stop infusion immediately (imminent anaphylactic reaction). • If evidence of blood volume overexpansion occurs, discontinue drug until blood volume adjusts via diuresis.

Storage • Store at room temperature. • Use only clear solutions. • Discard partially used containers.

IV INCOMPATIBILITIES

Do not add medications to dextran solution.

INDICATIONS/ROUTES/DOSAGE

VOLUME EXPANSION, SHOCK

IV: ADULTS, ELDERLY: 500–1,000 ml at rate of 20–40 ml/min. **Maximum:** 20 ml/kg for first 24 hrs, and 10 ml/kg thereafter. **CHILDREN:** Total dose not to exceed 20 ml/kg on day 1 and 10 ml/kg/day thereafter.

SIDE EFFECTS

OCCASIONAL: Mild hypersensitivity reaction (urticaria, nasal congestion, wheezing).

ADVERSE EFFECTS/ TOXIC REACTIONS

Severe or fatal anaphylaxis (marked hypotension, cardiac/respiratory arrest) may occur early during IV infusion, generally in those not previously exposed to IV dextran.

NURSING CONSIDERATIONS

INTERVENTION/EVALUATION

Monitor urinary output closely (increased output generally occurs in oliguric pts after dextran administration). If no increase is observed after 500 ml dextran is infused, discontinue drug until diuresis occurs. Monitor for fluid overload (peripheral and/or pulmonary edema, impending CHF symptoms). Assess lung sounds for rales. Monitor CVP (detects overexpansion of blood volume). Monitor vital signs, observe closely for allergic reaction. Assess for bleeding, esp. following surgery or in those on anticoagulant therapy (overt bleeding, esp. at surgical site; bruising; development of petechiae).

D

dextroamphetamine

dex-troe-am-**fet**-a-meen

(Dexedrine, Dexedrine Spansule, Dextrostat)

Do not confuse dextroamphetamine with dextromethorphan, or Dexedrine with Dextran or Excedrin.

◆ CLASSIFICATION

PHARMACOTHERAPEUTIC: Amphetamine (**Schedule II**). **CLINICAL:** CNS stimulant.

ACTION

Enhances action of dopamine, norepinephrine by blocking reuptake from synapses. Inhibits monoamine oxidase, facilitates release of catecholamines. **Therapeutic Effect:** Increases motor activity, mental alertness; decreases drowsiness, fatigue; suppresses appetite.

PHARMACOKINETICS

Well absorbed following PO administration. Metabolized in liver. Excreted in urine. Removed by hemodialysis. **Half-life:** 7–34 hrs.

USES

Treatment of narcolepsy; treatment of attention deficit disorder (ADD) in hyperactive children; short-term treatment to assist caloric restriction in exogenous obesity.

PRECAUTIONS

CONTRAINDICATIONS: Advanced arteriosclerosis, agitated mental states, glaucoma, history of drug abuse, hypersensitivity to sympathomimetic amines, hyperthyroidism, moderate to severe hypertension, symptomatic cardiovascular disease, use of MAOIs within 14 days. **CAUTIONS:** Elderly, debilitated pts; tartrazine-sensitive pts.

LIFESPAN CONSIDERATIONS:

Pregnancy/Lactation: Distributed in breast milk. **Pregnancy Category C.** **Children:** Safety and efficacy not established in children younger than 3 yrs. **Elderly:** Age-related cardiovascular, cerebrovascular disease, hepatic/renal impairment may increase risk of side effects.

INTERACTIONS

DRUG: **Beta-blockers** may increase risk of bradycardia, heart block, hypertension. **Digoxin** may increase risk of arrhythmias. **MAOIs** may prolong, intensify effects. **Meperidine** may increase risk of hypotension, respiratory depression, seizures, vascular collapse. **Other CNS stimulants** may increase effects. **Thyroid hormones** may increase effects. **Tricyclic antidepressants** may increase cardiovascular effects. **HERBAL:** None significant. **FOOD:** None known. **LAB VALUES:** May increase plasma corticosteroid.

AVAILABILITY (Rx)

TABLETS (DEXTROSTAT): 5 mg, 10 mg.

CAPSULES (SUSTAINED-RELEASE [DEXEDRINE SPANSULE]): 5 mg, 10 mg, 15 mg.

INDICATIONS/ROUTES/DOSAGE

NARCOLEPSY

PO: ADULTS, CHILDREN OLDER THAN 12 YRS: Initially, 10 mg/day. Increase by 10 mg/day at weekly intervals until therapeutic response is achieved. **Maximum:** 60 mg/day. **CHILDREN 6–12 YRS:** Initially, 5 mg/day. Increase by 5 mg/day at weekly intervals until therapeutic response is achieved. **Maximum:** 60 mg/day.

ATTENTION DEFICIT HYPERACTIVITY DISORDER (ADHD)

PO: CHILDREN 6 YRS AND OLDER: Initially, 5 mg once or twice a day. Increase by 5 mg/day at weekly intervals until therapeutic response is achieved.

Range: 5–20 mg/day. **Maximum:** 40 mg/day. **CHILDREN 3–5 YRS:** Initially, 2.5 mg/day. Increase by 2.5 mg/day at weekly intervals until therapeutic response is achieved. Range: 0.1–0.5 mg/kg/dose. **Maximum:** 40 mg/day.

APPETITE SUPPRESSANT

PO: ADULTS: 5–30 mg daily in divided doses of 5–10 mg each, given 30–60 min before meals; or 1 extended-release capsule in the morning.

SIDE EFFECTS

FREQUENT: Increased motor activity, talkativeness, nervousness, mild euphoria, insomnia. **OCCASIONAL:** Headache, chills, dry mouth, GI distress, worsening depression in pts who are clinically depressed, tachycardia, palpitations, chest pain, dizziness, decreased appetite.

ADVERSE EFFECTS/ TOXIC REACTIONS

Overdose may produce skin pallor/flushing, arrhythmias, psychosis. Abrupt withdrawal after prolonged use of high doses may produce lethargy (may last for wks). Prolonged administration to children with ADHD may temporarily suppress normal weight/height pattern.

NURSING CONSIDERATIONS

INTERVENTION/EVALUATION

Monitor for CNS overstimulation, increase in B/P, weight loss.

PATIENT/FAMILY TEACHING

• Normal dosage levels may produce tolerance to drug's anorexic mood-elevating effects within a few wks. • Avoid tasks that require alertness, motor skills until response to drug is established. • Dry mouth may be relieved with sugarless gum, sips of tepid water. • Take early in day. • May mask extreme fatigue. • Report pronounced anxiety, dizziness, decreased appetite, dry mouth.

DHEA

Also known as prasterone.

CLASSIFICATION

HERBAL: See Appendix G.

ACTION

Produced in adrenal glands, liver; metabolized to androstenedione, major precursor to androgens and estrogens. Also produced in CNS, concentrated in limbic regions; may function as excitatory neuroregulator. **Effect:** Androgen, estrogen-like hormonal effects may be responsible for DHEA benefits.

USES

Increases strength, energy, muscle mass; stimulates immune system; improves cognitive function and memory; improves depressed mood/fatigue in HIV pts. Treatment of atherosclerosis, hyperglycemia, cancer; prevention of osteoporosis; increase bone mineral density.

PRECAUTIONS

CONTRAINDICATIONS: None known. **CAUTIONS:** May increase risk of prostate, breast, hormone-sensitive cancers. Avoid use in those with breast, uterine, ovarian cancer; endometriosis; uterine fibroids; diabetes (can increase insulin resistance/sensitivity); depression (may increase risk of adverse psychiatric effects).

LIFESPAN CONSIDERATIONS:

Pregnancy/Lactation: May adversely affect pregnancy by increasing androgen levels; avoid use. **Children:** Safety and efficacy not established. **Elderly:** Age-related hepatic impairment may require dosage adjustment.

INTERACTIONS

DRUG: May interfere with **estrogen/androgen therapy**. May increase

triazolam concentration. **HERBAL:** None significant. **FOOD:** None known. **LAB VALUES:** None known.

D

AVAILABILITY (OTC)

CAPSULES: 25 mg. **TABLETS:** 25 mg.

INDICATIONS/ROUTES/DOSAGE

DEPRESSION

PO: ADULTS, ELDERLY: 30–90 mg/day.

USUAL ADULT DOSAGE

PO: ADULTS, ELDERLY: 25–50 mg/day.

SIDE EFFECTS

Acne, hair loss, hirsutism, voice deepening, insulin resistance, altered menstrual cycle, hypertension, abdominal pain, fatigue, headache, nasal congestion.

ADVERSE EFFECTS/ TOXIC REACTIONS

None known.

NURSING CONSIDERATIONS

BASELINE ASSESSMENT

Assess for hormone-sensitive tumors (may stimulate growth). Avoid use of hormone replacement therapy.

INTERVENTION/EVALUATION

Assess changes in mood, sleep pattern. Monitor changes in aggressiveness, irritability, restlessness.

PATIENT/FAMILY TEACHING

- Avoid use in pregnancy/lactation; concurrent hormone replacement therapy.
- Lower dosage if acne develops.

Diabeta, *see glyburide*

diazepam

dye-**az**-e-pam

(Apo-Diazepam ✤, Diastat, Diazepam Intensol, Novo-Dipam ✤, Diazemuls ✤, Valium)

Do not confuse diazepam with diazoxide or Ditropan, or Valium with Valcyte.

◆ CLASSIFICATION

PHARMACOTHERAPEUTIC: Benzodiazepine (**Schedule IV**). **CLINICAL:** Antianxiety, skeletal muscle relaxant, anticonvulsant (see pp. 11C, 34C, 143C).

ACTION

Depresses all levels of CNS by enhancing action of gamma-aminobutyric acid, a major inhibitory neurotransmitter in the brain. **Therapeutic Effect:** Produces anxiolytic effect, elevates seizure threshold, produces skeletal muscle relaxation.

PHARMACOKINETICS

Route	Onset	Peak	Duration
PO	30 min	1–2 hrs	2–3 hrs
IV	1–5 min	15 min	15–60 min
IM	15 min	30–90 min	30–90 min

Well absorbed from GI tract. Widely distributed. Protein binding: 98%. Metabolized in the liver to active metabolite. Excreted in urine. Minimally removed by hemodialysis. **Half-life:** 20–70 hrs (increased in hepatic dysfunction, elderly).

USES

Short-term relief of anxiety symptoms, preanesthetic medication, relief of acute alcohol withdrawal. Adjunct for relief of acute musculoskeletal conditions, treatment of seizures (IV route used for termination of status epilepticus). **Gel:** Control of increased seizure activity in refractory epilepsy in those on stable regimens. **OFF-LABEL:** Treatment of panic disorder, tension headache, tremors.

PRECAUTIONS

CONTRAINDICATIONS: Angle-closure glaucoma, coma, preexisting CNS depression, respiratory depression, severe, uncontrolled pain. **CAUTIONS:** Those receiving other CNS depressants, renal/hepatic impairment, hypoalbuminemia.

LIFESPAN CONSIDERATIONS:

Pregnancy/Lactation: Crosses placenta. Distributed in breast milk. May increase risk of fetal abnormalities if administered during first trimester of pregnancy. Chronic ingestion during pregnancy may produce withdrawal symptoms, CNS depression in neonates. **Pregnancy Category D. Children/Elderly:** Use small initial doses with gradual increases to avoid ataxia, excessive sedation.

INTERACTIONS

DRUG: **Alcohol, CNS depressants** may increase CNS depression. **Fluvoxamine, itraconazole, ketoconazole** may increase concentration/toxicity. **HERBAL:** **Gotu kola, kava kava, St. John's wort, valerian** may increase CNS depression. **FOOD:** None known. **LAB VALUES:** May elevate serum alkaline phosphatase, bilirubin, LDH, AST, ALT. May produce abnormal renal function test results. Therapeutic serum level is 0.5–2 mcg/ml; toxic serum level is greater than 3 mcg/ml.

AVAILABILITY (Rx)

INJECTION, SOLUTION: 5 mg/ml. **ORAL SOLUTION:** 5 mg/5 ml. **ORAL CONCENTRATE (DIAZEPAM INTENSOL):** 5 mg/ml. **RECTAL GEL (DIASTAT):** 5 mg/ml. **TABLET (VALIUM):** 2 mg, 5 mg, 10 mg.

ADMINISTRATION/HANDLING

IV

Rate of administration • Give by IV push into tubing of flowing IV solution as close as possible to vein insertion point. • Administer directly into large vein (reduces risk of thrombosis/phlebitis). Do not use small veins (e.g., wrist/dorsum of hand). • Administer IV at rate not exceeding 5 mg/min. For children, give over a 3-min period (too-rapid IV may result in hypotension, respiratory depression). • Monitor respirations q5–15min for 2 hrs.

Storage • Store at room temperature.

IM

• Injection may be painful. Inject deeply into deltoid muscle.

PO

• Give without regard to meals. • Dilute oral concentrate with water, juice, carbonated beverages; may be mixed in semisolid food (applesauce, pudding). • Tablets may be crushed.

IV INCOMPATIBILITIES

Amphotericin B complex (Abelcet, AmBisome, Amphotec), cefepime (Maxipime), diltiazem (Cardizem), fluconazole (Diflucan), foscarnet (Foscavir), heparin, hydrocortisone (Solu-Cortef), hydromorphone (Dilaudid), meropenem (Merrem IV), potassium chloride, propofol (Diprivan), vitamins.

IV COMPATIBILITIES

Dobutamine (Dobutrex), fentanyl, morphine.

INDICATIONS/ROUTES/DOSAGE

ANXIETY, SKELETAL MUSCLE RELAXATION

PO: ADULTS: 2–10 mg 2–4 times a day. **ELDERLY:** 2–5 mg 2–4 times a day. **CHILDREN:** 0.12–0.8 mg/kg/day in divided doses q6–8h.

IV, IM: ADULTS: 2–10 mg repeated in 3–4 hrs. **CHILDREN:** 0.04–0.3 mg/kg/dose q2–4h. **Maximum:** 0.6 mg/kg in an 8-hr period.

PREANESTHESIA

IV: ADULTS, ELDERLY: 5–15 mg 5–10 min before procedure. **CHILDREN:** 0.2–0.3 mg/kg. **Maximum:** 10 mg.

ALCOHOL WITHDRAWAL

PO: ADULTS, ELDERLY: 10 mg 3–4 times during first 24 hrs, then reduced to 5–10 mg 3–4 times a day as needed.

IV, IM: ADULTS, ELDERLY: Initially, 10 mg, followed by 5–10 mg q3–4h.

STATUS EPILEPTICUS

IV: ADULTS, ELDERLY: 5–10 mg q10–15min up to 30 mg/8 hr. **CHILDREN 5 YRS AND OLDER:** 0.05–0.3 mg/kg/dose q15–30min. **Maximum:** 10 mg/dose. **CHILDREN 1 MO TO 5 YRS:** 0.05–0.3 mg/kg/dose q15–30min. **Maximum:** 5 mg/dose.

CONTROL OF INCREASED SEIZURE ACTIVITY (BREAKTHROUGH SEIZURES) IN PTS WITH REFRACTORY EPILEPSY WHO ARE ON STABLE REGIMENS OF ANTICONVULSANTS

RECTAL GEL: ADULTS, CHILDREN 12 YRS AND OLDER: 0.2 mg/kg; may be repeated in 4–12 hrs. **CHILDREN 6–11 YRS:** 0.3 mg/kg; may be repeated in 4–12 hrs. **CHILDREN 2–5 YRS:** 0.5 mg/kg; may be repeated in 4–12 hrs.

SIDE EFFECTS

FREQUENT: Pain with IM injection, somnolence, fatigue, ataxia. **OCCASIONAL:** Slurred speech, orthostatic hypotension, headache, hypoactivity, constipation, nausea, blurred vision. **RARE:** Paradoxical CNS reactions (hyperactivity/nervousness in children, excitement/restlessness in elderly/debilitated) generally noted during first 2 wks of therapy, particularly in presence of uncontrolled pain.

ADVERSE EFFECTS/ TOXIC REACTIONS

IV route may produce pain, swelling, thrombophlebitis, carpal tunnel syndrome. Abrupt or too-rapid withdrawal may result in pronounced restlessness, irritability, insomnia, hand tremor, abdominal/muscle cramps, diaphoresis, vomiting, seizures. Abrupt withdrawal in pts with epilepsy may produce increase in frequency/severity of seizures. Overdose results in somnolence, confusion, diminished reflexes, CNS depression, coma.

NURSING CONSIDERATIONS

BASELINE ASSESSMENT

Assess B/P, pulse, respirations immediately before administration. Pt must remain recumbent for up to 3 hrs (individualized) after parenteral administration to reduce hypotensive effect. **Anxiety:** Assess autonomic response (cold, clammy hands, diaphoresis), motor response (agitation, trembling, tension). **Musculoskeletal spasm:** Record onset, type, location, duration of pain. Check for immobility, stiffness, swelling. **Seizures:** Review history of seizure disorder (length, intensity, frequency, duration, level of consciousness [LOC]). Observe frequently for recurrence of seizure activity. Initiate seizure precautions.

INTERVENTION/EVALUATION

Monitor heart rate, respiratory rate, B/P. Assess children, elderly for paradoxical reaction, particularly during early therapy. Evaluate for therapeutic response (decrease in intensity/frequency of seizures; calm, facial expression, decreased restlessness; decreased intensity of skeletal muscle pain). Therapeutic serum level: 0.5–2 mcg/ml; toxic serum level: greater than 3 mcg/ml.

PATIENT/FAMILY TEACHING

• Avoid alcohol. • Limit caffeine. • May cause drowsiness, impair ability to perform activities requiring mental alertness (e.g., driving). • May be habit forming. • Avoid abrupt discontinuation after prolonged use.

dibucaine

(Nupercainal)

See Anesthetics: local

diclofenac

dye-**klo**-feh-nak

(Apo-Diclo ♣, Cataflam, Diclotec ♣, Novo-Difenac ♣, Solaraze, Voltaren, Voltaren Ophthalmic, Voltaren XR)

Do not confuse diclofenac with Diflucan or Duphalac, or Voltaren with Verelan.

FIXED-COMBINATION(S)

Arthrotec: diclofenac/misoprostol (an antisecretory gastric protectant): 50 mg/200 mcg; 75 mg/200 mcg.

◆ CLASSIFICATION

PHARMACOTHERAPEUTIC: Nonsteroidal anti-inflammatory. **CLINICAL:** Analgesic, anti-inflammatory (see p. 123C).

ACTION

Inhibits prostaglandin synthesis, intensity of pain stimulus reaching sensory nerve endings. Constricts iris sphincter. **Therapeutic Effect:** Produces analgesic, anti-inflammatory effects. Prevents miosis during cataract surgery.

PHARMACOKINETICS

Route	Onset	Peak	Duration
PO	30 min	2–3 hrs	Up to 8 hrs

Completely absorbed from GI tract; penetrates cornea after ophthalmic administration (may be systemically absorbed). Protein binding: greater than 99%. Widely distributed. Metabolized in the liver. Primarily excreted in urine. Minimally removed by hemodialysis. **Half-life:** 1.2–2 hrs.

USES

Oral: (Immediate-release): Treatment of rheumatoid arthritis, oesteoarthritis, ankylosing spondylitis, primary dysmenorrhea. (Delayed-release): Treatment of rheumatoid arthritis, oesteoarthritis, ankylosing spondylitis. (Extended-release): Treatment of rheumatoid arthritis, oesteoarthritis. **Ophthalmic:** Treatment of photophobia, pain in pts undergoing corneal refractive surgery. **Topical:** Treatment of actinic keratoses. **OFF-LABEL:** Treatment of vascular headaches (oral); to reduce the occurrence/severity of cystoid macular edema after cataract surgery (ophthalmic form).

PRECAUTIONS

CONTRAINDICATIONS: Hypersensitivity to aspirin, diclofenac, other NSAIDs; porphyria. **CAUTIONS:** CHF, hypertension, renal/hepatic impairment, history of GI disease. Avoid topical gel to open skin wounds, infections, exfoliative dermatitis, eyes, neonates, infants, children.

⌛ LIFESPAN CONSIDERATIONS:

Pregnancy/Lactation: Crosses placenta. Unknown if distributed in breast milk. Avoid use during last trimester (may adversely affect fetal cardiovascular system: premature closure of ductus arteriosus). **Pregnancy Category B (D if used in third trimester or near delivery; C for ophthalmic solution).** **Children:** Safety and efficacy not established. **Elderly:** GI bleeding, ulceration more likely to cause serious adverse effects. Age-related renal impairment may increase risk of hepatic/renal toxicity; reduced dosage recommended.

D

INTERACTIONS

DRUG: May decrease effects of **antihypertensives, diuretics. Aspirin, other salicylates** may increase risk of GI side effects/bleeding. **Bone marrow depressants** may increase risk of hematologic reactions. May increase effects of **heparin, oral anticoagulants, thrombolytics.** May increase serum **lithium** concentration/toxicity. May increase risk of **methotrexate** toxicity. **Probenecid** may increase concentration. **Ophthalmic:** May decrease antiglaucoma effects of **epinephrine, antiglaucoma agents.** May decrease effects of **acetylcholine, carbachol. HERBAL: Cat's claw, dong quai, evening primrose, garlic, ginseng** may increase antiplatelet activity. **FOOD:** None known. **LAB VALUES:** May increase urine protein, BUN, serum alkaline phosphatase, creatinine, LDH, potassium, AST, ALT. May decrease serum uric acid.

AVAILABILITY (Rx)

OPHTHALMIC SOLUTION (VOLTAREN OPHTHALMIC): 0.1%. **TABLETS [CATAFLAM]):** 50 mg. **TOPICAL GEL (SOLARAZE):** 3%.

TABLETS (DELAYED-RELEASE [VOLTAREN]): 25 mg, 50 mg, 75 mg. **TABLETS (EXTENDED-RELEASE [VOLTAREN XR]):** 100 mg.

ADMINISTRATION/HANDLING

PO

• Do not crush, break enteric-coated form. • May give with food, milk, antacids if GI distress occurs.

OPHTHALMIC • Place finger on lower eyelid and pull out until pocket is formed between eye and lower lid. Hold dropper above pocket and place prescribed number of drops in pocket. • Close eye gently. Apply digital pressure to lacrimal sac for 1–2 min (minimized drainage into nose and throat, reducing risk of systemic effects). • Remove excess solution with tissue.

INDICATIONS/ROUTES/DOSAGE

OSTEOARTHRITIS

PO (CATAFLAM, VOLTAREN): ADULTS, ELDERLY: 50 mg 2–3 times a day.

PO (VOLTAREN XR): ADULTS, ELDERLY: 100–200 mg/day as a single dose.

RHEUMATOID ARTHRITIS

PO (CATAFLAM, VOLTAREN): ADULTS, ELDERLY: 50 mg 2–4 times a day. **Maximum:** 225 mg/day.

PO (VOLTAREN XR): ADULTS, ELDERLY: 100 mg once a day. **Maximum:** 100 mg twice a day.

ANKYLOSING SPONDYLITIS

PO (VOLTAREN): ADULTS, ELDERLY: 100–125 mg/day in 4–5 divided doses.

ANALGESIA, PRIMARY DYSMENORRHEA

PO (CATAFLAM): ADULTS, ELDERLY: 50 mg 3 times a day.

USUAL PEDIATRIC DOSAGE

CHILDREN: 2–3 mg/kg/day in 2–4 divided doses.

ACTINIC KERATOSES

TOPICAL: ADULTS, ADOLESCENTS: Apply twice a day to lesion for 60–90 days.

CATARACT SURGERY

OPHTHALMIC: ADULTS, ELDERLY: Apply 1 drop to eye 4 times a day commencing 24 hrs after cataract surgery. Continue for 2 wks afterward.

PAIN, RELIEF OF PHOTOPHOBIA IN PTS UNDERGOING CORNEAL REFRACTIVE SURGERY

OPHTHALMIC: ADULTS, ELDERLY: Apply 1–2 drops to affected eye 1 hr before surgery, within 15 min after surgery, then 4 times a day for up to 3 days.

SIDE EFFECTS

FREQUENT (9%–4%): PO: Headache, abdominal cramps, constipation, diarrhea, nausea, dyspepsia. **Ophthalmic:** Burning, stinging on instillation, ocular discomfort. **OCCASIONAL (3%–1%): PO:** Flatulence, dizziness, epigastric pain.

Ophthalmic: Ocular itching, tearing. **RARE (less than 1%): PO:** Rash, peripheral edema, fluid retention, visual disturbances, vomiting, drowsiness.

ADVERSE EFFECTS/ TOXIC REACTIONS

Overdose may result in acute renal failure. In those treated chronically, peptic ulcer, GI bleeding, gastritis, severe hepatic reaction (jaundice), nephrotoxicity (hematuria, dysuria, proteinuria), severe hypersensitivity reaction (bronchospasm, angioedema) occur rarely.

NURSING CONSIDERATIONS

BASELINE ASSESSMENT

Anti-inflammatory: Assess onset, type, location, duration of pain, inflammation. Inspect appearance of affected joints for immobility, deformities, skin condition.

INTERVENTION/EVALUATION

Monitor for headache, dyspepsia. Monitor daily pattern of bowel activity/ stool consistency. Evaluate for therapeutic response (relief of pain, stiffness, swelling; increase in joint mobility; reduced joint tenderness; improved grip strength).

PATIENT/FAMILY TEACHING

• Swallow tablet whole; do not crush, chew. • Avoid aspirin, alcohol during therapy (increases risk of GI bleeding). • If GI upset occurs, take with food, milk. • Report skin rash, itching, weight gain, changes in vision, black stools, persistent headache. • **Ophthalmic:** Do not use hydrogel soft contact lenses. • **Topical:** Avoid exposure to sunlight, sun lamps. • Inform physician if rash occurs.

dicloxacillin

(Dycill, Dynapen, Pathocil)

See Antibiotic: penicillins (p. 27C)

dicyclomine

dye-**sye**-kloe-meen

(Bentyl, Bentylol ✤, Dicyclocot, Formulex ✤, Lomine ✤)

Do not confuse dicyclomine with doxycycline or dyclonime, or Bentyl with Aventyl or Benadryl.

CLASSIFICATION

CLINICAL: GI antispasmodic, anticholinergic.

ACTION

Directly acts as smooth muscle relaxant. **Therapeutic Effect:** Reduces tone, motility of GI tract.

PHARMACOKINETICS

Route	Onset	Peak	Duration
PO	1–2 hrs	N/A	4 hrs

Readily absorbed from GI tract. Widely distributed. Metabolized in the liver. **Half-life:** 9–10 hrs.

USES

Treatment of functional disturbances of GI motility (e.g., irritable bowel syndrome).

PRECAUTIONS

CONTRAINDICATIONS: Bladder neck obstruction due to prostatic hyperplasia, coronary vasospasm, intestinal atony, myasthenia gravis in pts not treated with neostigmine, narrow-angle glaucoma, obstructive disease of GI tract, paralytic ileus, severe ulcerative colitis, tachycardia secondary to cardiac insufficiency/

thyrotoxicosis, toxic megacolon, unstable cardiovascular status in acute hemorrhage. **EXTREME CAUTION:** Autonomic neuropathy, known/suspected GI infections, diarrhea, mild to moderate ulcerative colitis. **CAUTIONS:** Hyperthyroidism, hepatic/renal disease, hypertension, tachyarrhythmias, CHF, coronary artery disease, gastric ulcer, esophageal reflux/hiatal hernia associated with reflux esophagitis, infants, elderly, chronic obstructive pulmonary disease (COPD).

LIFESPAN CONSIDERATIONS:

Pregnancy/Lactation: Unknown if drug crosses placenta or is distributed in breast milk. **Pregnancy Category B.** **Children:** Infants, young children more susceptible to toxic effects. **Elderly:** May cause excitement, agitation, drowsiness, confusion.

INTERACTIONS

DRUG: **Antacids, antidiarrheals** may decrease absorption. May decrease absorption of **ketoconazole. Other anticholinergics** may increase effects. **Potassium chloride** may increase severity of GI lesions with wax matrix formulation. **HERBAL:** None significant. **FOOD:** None known. **LAB VALUES:** None known.

AVAILABILITY (Rx)

CAPSULES (BENTYL): 10 mg. **INJECTION SOLUTION (BENTYL, DICYCLOCOT):** 10 mg/ml. **SYRUP (BENTYL):** 10 mg/5 ml. **TABLETS (BENTYL):** 20 mg.

ADMINISTRATION/HANDLING

• Store capsules, tablets, syrup, parenteral form at room temperature.

IM

• Injection should appear colorless. • Do not administer IV or subcutaneous. • Inject deep into large muscle mass. • Do not give for longer than 2 days.

PO

• Dilute oral solution with equal volume of water just before administration. • May give without regard to meals (food may slightly decrease absorption).

INDICATIONS/ROUTES/DOSAGE

FUNCTIONAL DISTURBANCES OF GI MOTILITY

PO: ADULTS: 10–20 mg 3–4 times a day up to 40 mg 4 times/day. **CHILDREN OLDER THAN 2 YRS:** 10 mg 3–4 times a day. **CHILDREN 6 MOS–2 YRS:** 5 mg 3–4 times a day. **ELDERLY:** 10–20 mg 4 times a day. May increase up to 160 mg/day.
IM: ADULTS: 20 mg q4–6h.

SIDE EFFECTS

FREQUENT: Dry mouth (sometimes severe), constipation, diminished sweating ability. **OCCASIONAL:** Blurred vision; photophobia; urinary hesitancy; somnolence (with high dosage); agitation, excitement, confusion, somnolence noted in elderly (even with low dosages); transient light-headedness (with IM route), irritation at injection site (with IM route). **RARE:** Confusion, hypersensitivity reaction, increased intraocular pressure, nausea, vomiting, unusual fatigue.

ADVERSE EFFECTS/ TOXIC REACTIONS

Overdose may produce temporary paralysis of ciliary muscle; pupillary dilation; tachycardia; palpitations; hot/dry/flushed skin; absence of bowel sounds; hyperthermia; increased respiratory rate; EKG abnormalities; nausea; vomiting; rash over face/upper trunk; CNS stimulation, psychosis (agitation, restlessness, rambling speech, visual hallucinations, paranoid behavior, delusions) followed by depression.

NURSING CONSIDERATIONS

BASELINE ASSESSMENT

Before giving medication, instruct pt to void (reduces risk of urinary retention).

INTERVENTION/EVALUATION

Monitor daily pattern of bowel activity/stool consistency. Assess for urinary retention. Monitor changes in B/P, temperature. Be alert for fever (increased risk of hyperthermia). Assess skin turgor, mucous membranes to evaluate hydration status (encourage adequate fluid intake), bowel sounds for peristalsis.

PATIENT/FAMILY TEACHING

• Do not become overheated during exercise in hot weather (may result in heat stroke). • Avoid hot baths, saunas. • Avoid tasks that require alertness, motor skills until response to drug is established. • Do not take antacids or antidiarrheals within 1 hr of taking this medication (decreased effectiveness).

didanosine

dye-**dan**-o-seen
(Videx, Videx-EC)

CLASSIFICATION

PHARMACOTHERAPEUTIC: Purine nucleoside analogue. **CLINICAL:** Antiviral (see pp. 64C, 110C).

ACTION

Intracellularly converted into triphosphate, which interferes with RNA-directed DNA polymerase (reverse transcriptase). **Therapeutic Effect:** Inhibits replication of retroviruses, including HIV.

PHARMACOKINETICS

Variably absorbed from GI tract. Protein binding: less than 5%. Rapidly metabolized intracellularly to active form. Primarily excreted in urine. Partially (20%) removed by hemodialysis. **Half-life:** 1.5 hrs; metabolite: 8–24 hrs.

USES

Treatment of HIV infection in combination with other antiretroviral agents.

PRECAUTIONS

CONTRAINDICATIONS: Hypersensitivity to didanosine or any of its components. **CAUTIONS:** Renal/hepatic impairment, alcoholism, elevated triglycerides, T-cell counts less than 100 cells/mm^3; extreme caution with history of pancreatitis. Phenylketonuria, sodium-restricted diets due to phenylalanine, sodium content of preparations.

LIFESPAN CONSIDERATIONS:

Pregnancy/Lactation: Use during pregnancy only if clearly needed. Discontinue breast-feeding during didanosine therapy. **Pregnancy Category B. Children:** Well tolerated in children older than 3 mos. **Elderly:** Age-related renal impairment may require dosage adjustment.

INTERACTIONS

DRUG: May decrease absorption of **dapsone, flouroquinolones, itraconazole, ketoconazole, tetracyclines. Medications producing pancreatitis or peripheral neuropathy** may increase risk of pancreatitis, peripheral neuropathy. **Stavudine** may increase risk of fatal lactic acidosis in pregnancy. **HERBAL:** None significant. **FOOD: All foods** decrease absorption. **LAB VALUES:** May increase serum alkaline phosphatase, amylase, bilirubin, lipase, triglycerides, AST, ALT, uric acid. May decrease serum potassium.

AVAILABILITY (Rx)

PEDIATRIC POWDER FOR ORAL SOLUTION (VIDEX): 10 mg/ml. **POWDER FOR ORAL SOLUTION (VIDEX):** 100 mg, 167 mg, 250 mg. **TABLETS (CHEWABLE [VIDEX]):** 25 mg, 50 mg, 100 mg, 150 mg, 200 mg.

CAPSULES (DELAYED-RELEASE): (VIDEX EC): 125 mg, 200 mg, 250 mg, 400 mg.

ADMINISTRATION/HANDLING

PO

• Store at room temperature. • Tablets dispersed in water are stable for 1 hr at room temperature; after reconstitution of buffered powder, oral solution is stable for 4 hrs at room temperature. • Pediatric powder for oral solution following reconstitution as directed, stable for 30 days refrigerated. • Give 1 hr before or 2 hrs after meals (food decreases rate/extent of absorption). • **Chewable tablets:** Thoroughly crush, disperse in at least 30 ml water before swallowing. Mixture should be stirred well (2–3 min), swallowed immediately. • **Buffered powder for oral solution:** Reconstitute before administration by pouring contents of packet into 4 oz water; stir until completely dissolved (up to 2–3 min). Do not mix with fruit juice, other acidic liquid (didanosine is unstable at acidic pH). • **Unbuffered pediatric powder:** Add 100–200 ml water to 2 or 4 g, respectively, to provide concentration of 20 mg/ml. Immediately mix with equal amount of antacid to provide concentration of 10 mg/ml. Shake thoroughly before removing each dose. • **Enteric-coated capsules:** Swallow whole, take on empty stomach.

INDICATIONS/ROUTES/DOSAGE

HIV INFECTION

PO (CHEWABLE TABLETS): ADULTS, CHILDREN 13 YRS AND OLDER, WEIGHING 60 KG AND MORE: 200 mg q12h or 400 mg once a day. **ADULTS, CHILDREN 13 YRS AND OLDER, WEIGHING LESS THAN 60 KG:** 125 mg q12h or 250 mg once a day. **CHILDREN 8 MOS–12 YRS:** 180–300 mg/m²/day in divided doses q12h. **CHILDREN YOUNGER THAN 8 MOS:** 50 mg/m²/day in divided doses q12h.

PO (DELAYED-RELEASE CAPSULES): ADULTS, CHILDREN 13 YRS AND OLDER, WEIGHING 60 KG AND MORE: 400 mg once a day. **ADULTS, CHILDREN 13 YRS AND OLDER, WEIGHING LESS THAN 60 KG:** 250 mg once a day.

PO (ORAL SOLUTION): ADULTS, CHILDREN 13 YRS AND OLDER WEIGHING 60 KG AND MORE: 200 mg q12h or 400 mg once a day. **ADULTS, CHILDREN 13 YRS AND OLDER WEIGHING LESS THAN 60 KG:** 125 mg q12h or 250 mg once a day.

PO (PEDIATRIC POWDER FOR ORAL SOLUTION): CHILDREN 8 MOS–12 YRS: 180–300 mg/m²/day in divided doses q12h. **CHILDREN YOUNGER THAN 8 MOS:** 50 mg/m²/day in divided doses q12h.

DOSAGE IN RENAL IMPAIRMENT

Pts weighing less than 60 kg:

CrCl	Tablets	Oral Solution	Delayed-Release Capsules
30–59 ml/min	75 mg twice a day	100 mg twice a day	125 mg once a day
10–29 ml/min	100 mg once a day	100 mg once a day	125 mg once a day
Less than 10 ml/min	75 mg once a day	100 mg once a day	N/A

CrCl = creatinine clearance

Pts weighing 60 kg or more:

CrCl	Tablets	Oral Solution	Delayed-Release Capsules
30–59 ml/min	100 mg twice a day	100 mg twice a day	200 mg once a day
10–29 ml/min	150 mg once a day	167 mg once a day	125 mg once a day
Less than 10 ml/min	100 mg once a day	100 mg once a day	125 mg once a day

CrCl = creatinine clearance

SIDE EFFECTS

FREQUENT: Adults (greater than 10%): Diarrhea, neuropathy, chills, fever. **Children (greater than 25%):** Chills, fever, decreased appetite, pain, malaise, nausea, vomiting, diarrhea, abdominal pain, headache, nervousness, cough, rhinitis, dyspnea, asthenia, rash, pruritus. **OCCASIONAL: Adults (9%–2%):** Rash, pruritus, headache, abdominal pain, nausea, vomiting, pneumonia, myopathy, decreased appetite, dry mouth, dyspnea. **Children (25%–10%):** Failure to thrive, weight loss, stomatitis, oral thrush, ecchymosis, arthritis, myalgia, insomnia, epistaxis, pharyngitis.

ADVERSE EFFECTS/ TOXIC REACTIONS

Pneumonia, opportunistic infections occur occasionally. Peripheral neuropathy, potentially fatal pancreatitis are major toxic effects.

NURSING CONSIDERATIONS

BASELINE ASSESSMENT

Obtain baseline values for CBC, serum renal/hepatic function tests, vital signs, weight.

INTERVENTION/EVALUATION

In event of abdominal pain, nausea, vomiting, elevated serum amylase, triglycerides, contact physician before administering medication (potential for pancreatitis). Be alert to sensation of burning feet, "restless leg syndrome" (unable to find comfortable position for legs or feet), lack of coordination, other signs of peripheral neuropathy. Monitor daily pattern of bowel activity/stool consistency. Check skin for rash, eruptions. Monitor serum electrolytes, CBC. Assess for opportunistic infections (onset of fever, oral mucosa changes, cough, other respiratory symptoms). Check weight at least twice per wk. Assess for visual, auditory difficulty; provide protection from light if photophobia develops.

PATIENT/FAMILY TEACHING

• Avoid alcohol. • Inform physician if numbness, tingling, persistent severe abdominal pain, nausea, vomiting occur. • Shake oral suspension well before use, keep refrigerated. • Discard solution after 30 days, obtain new supply.

Diflucan, *see fluconazole*

diflunisal

dye-**flew**-neh-sol

(Apo-Diflunisal ✤, Dolobid, Novo-Diflunisal ✤)

Do not confuse diflunisal with Dicarbosil or Dolobid with Slo-bid.

CLASSIFICATION

PHARMACOTHERAPEUTIC: Nonsteroidal anti-inflammatory. **CLINICAL:** Antirheumatic, analgesic, vascular headache suppressant (see p. 123C).

ACTION

Inhibits prostaglandin synthesis, reducing inflammatory response/intensity of pain stimulus reaching sensory nerve endings. **Therapeutic Effect:** Produces analgesic and anti-inflammatory effect.

PHARMACOKINETICS

Route	Onset	Peak	Duration
PO	1 hr	2–3 hrs	8–12 hrs

Completely absorbed from GI tract. Widely distributed. Protein binding: greater than 99%. Metabolized in liver. Primarily excreted in urine. Not removed by hemodialysis. **Half-life:** 8–12 hrs.

USES

Treatment of mild to moderate pain, rheumatoid arthritis, osteoarthritis.

D

OFF-LABEL: Treatment of psoriatic arthritis, vascular headache.

PRECAUTIONS

CONTRAINDICATIONS: Active GI bleeding, factor VII/factor IX deficiencies, hypersensitivity to aspirin, NSAIDs. **CAUTIONS:** Renal/hepatic impairment, edema, elevated hepatic function tests, platelet/bleeding disorders, peptic ulcer disease, erosive gastritis, vitamin K deficiency.

LIFESPAN CONSIDERATIONS:

Pregnancy/Lactation: Crosses placenta. Distributed in breast milk. Avoid use during last trimester (may adversely affect fetal cardiovascular system: premature closure of ductus arteriosus). **Pregnancy Category C (D if used in third trimester or near delivery). Children:** Safety and efficacy not established. **Elderly:** GI bleeding/ulceration more likely to cause serious adverse effects. Age-related renal impairment may increase risk of hepatic/renal toxicity; decreased dosage recommended.

INTERACTIONS

DRUG: May decrease effects of **antihypertensives, diuretics. Aspirin, salicylates** may increase risk of GI bleeding, side effects. **Bone marrow depressants** may increase risk of hematologic reactions. May increase effects of **heparin, oral anticoagulants, thrombolytics.** May increase concentration, risk of toxicity of **lithium.** May increase risk of toxicity of **methotrexate. Probenecid** may increase concentration. **HERBAL: Cat's claw, dong quai, evening primrose, garlic, ginseng** may increase antiplatelet activity. **FOOD:** None known. **LAB VALUES:** May increase serum AST, ALT. May decrease serum uric acid.

AVAILABILITY (Rx)

TABLETS: 250 mg, 500 mg.

ADMINISTRATION/HANDLING

PO

- May give with water, milk, meals.
- Do not crush, break film-coated tablets.

INDICATIONS/ROUTES/DOSAGE

MILD TO MODERATE PAIN

PO: ADULTS, ELDERLY: Initially, 0.5–1 g, then 250–500 mg q8–12h. **Maximum:** 1.5 g/day.

OSTEOARTHRITIS

PO: ADULTS, ELDERLY: 500–750 mg/day in divided doses.

RHEUMATOID ARTHRITIS

PO: ADULTS, ELDERLY: 0.5–1 g/day in 2 divided doses. **Maximum:** 1.5 g/day.

SIDE EFFECTS

Side effects are less common with short-term treatment.

OCCASIONAL (9%–3%): Nausea, dyspepsia (heartburn, indigestion, epigastric pain), diarrhea, headache, rash. **RARE (3%–1%):** Vomiting, constipation, flatulence, dizziness, somnolence, insomnia, fatigue, tinnitus.

ADVERSE EFFECTS/ TOXIC REACTIONS

Overdosage may produce drowsiness, vomiting, nausea, diarrhea, hyperventilation, tachycardia, diaphoresis, stupor, coma. Peptic ulcer, GI bleeding, gastritis, severe hepatic reaction (cholestasis, jaundice) occur rarely. Nephrotoxicity (dysuria, hematuria, proteinuria, nephrotic syndrome), severe hypersensitivity reaction (bronchospasm, angioedema) occur rarely.

NURSING CONSIDERATIONS

BASELINE ASSESSMENT

Assess onset, type, location, duration of pain, inflammation. Inspect affected joints for immobility, deformities, skin condition.

INTERVENTION/EVALUATION

Monitor for nausea, dyspepsia. Assess skin for evidence of rash. Monitor daily pattern of bowel activity/stool consistency. Evaluate for therapeutic response (relief of pain, stiffness, swelling; increase in joint mobility; reduced joint tenderness; improved grip strength).

PATIENT/FAMILY TEACHING

• Swallow tablet whole; do not crush, chew. • If GI upset occurs, take with food, milk. • Report GI distress, headache, rash.

Digitek, *see digoxin*

digoxin

di-**jox**-in

(Digitek, Lanoxicaps, Lanoxin)

Do not confuse digoxin with Desoxyn or doxepin, or Lanoxin with Levsinex or Lonox.

CLASSIFICATION

PHARMACOTHERAPEUTIC: Cardiac glycoside. **CLINICAL:** Antiarrhythmic, cardiotonic (see p. 74C).

ACTION

Increases influx of calcium from extracellular to intracellular cytoplasm. **Therapeutic Effect:** Potentiates activity of contractile cardiac muscle fibers, increases force of myocardial contraction. Slows the heart rate by decreasing conduction through SA, AV nodes.

PHARMACOKINETICS

Route	Onset	Peak	Duration
PO	0.5–2 hrs	28 hrs	3–4 days
IV	5–30 min	1–4 hrs	3–4 days

Readily absorbed from GI tract. Widely distributed. Protein binding: 30%. Partially metabolized in the liver. Primarily excreted in urine. Minimally removed by hemodialysis. **Half-life:** 36–48 hrs (increased with renal impairment, elderly).

USES

Prophylactic management/treatment of CHF, control of ventricular rate in pts with atrial fibrillation. Treatment/prevention of recurrent paroxysmal atrial tachycardia.

PRECAUTIONS

CONTRAINDICATIONS: Ventricular fibrillation, ventricular tachycardia unrelated to CHF. **CAUTIONS:** Renal/hepatic impairment, hypokalemia, advanced cardiac disease, acute MI, incomplete AV block, cor pulmonale, hyperthyroidism, hypothyroidism, pulmonary disease, severe bradycardia, sick sinus syndrome, Wolff-Parkinson-White syndrome.

LIFESPAN CONSIDERATIONS: Pregnancy/Lactation: Crosses placenta. Distributed in breast milk. **Pregnancy Category C. Children:** Premature infants more susceptible to toxicity. **Elderly:** Age-related hepatic/renal impairment may require dosage adjustment. Increased risk of loss of appetite.

INTERACTIONS

DRUG: Amiodarone may increase concentration/toxicity. **Beta-blockers, calcium channel blockers** may have additive effect on slowing AV nodal conduction. **Potassium-depleting diuretics** may increase toxicity due to hypokalemia. **Sympathomimetics** may increase risk of arrhythmias. **HERBAL: Ephedra** may increase risk of arrhythmias. **Licorice** may cause sodium and water retention, loss of potassium. **FOOD: Meals with increased fiber (bran) or high in pectin** may decrease absorption. **LAB VALUES:** None known.

D

AVAILABILITY (Rx)

CAPSULES (LANOXICAPS): 50 mcg, 100 mcg, 200 mcg. **ELIXIR (LANOXIN):** 50 mcg/ml. **INJECTION SOLUTION (LANOXIN):** 100 mcg/ml, 250 mcg/ml. **TABLETS (DIGITEK, LANOXIN):** 125 mcg, 250 mcg.

ADMINISTRATION/HANDLING

◀ **ALERT** ▶ IM rarely used (produces severe local irritation, erratic absorption). If no other route possible, give deep into muscle followed by massage. Give no more than 2 ml at any one site.

IV

- May give undiluted or dilute with at least a 4-fold volume of Sterile Water for Injection, or D_5W (less may cause precipitate). Use immediately. • Give IV slowly over at least 5 min.

PO

- May give without regard to meals.
- Tablets may be crushed.

IV INCOMPATIBILITIES

Amphotericin B complex (Abelcet, AmBisome, Amphotec), fluconazole (Diflucan), foscarnet (Foscavir), propofol (Diprivan).

IV COMPATIBILITIES

Cimetidine (Tagamet), diltiazem (Cardizem), furosemide (Lasix), heparin, insulin regular (physically compatible for 3 hrs in 0.9% NaCl. In D_5W, a slight haze develops within 1 hr.), lidocaine, lipids, midazolam (Versed), milrinone (Primacor), morphine, potassium chloride.

INDICATIONS/ROUTES/DOSAGE

LOADING DOSE

PO: ADULTS, ELDERLY: Initially, 0.5–0.75 mg, additional doses of 0.125–0.375 mg at 6- to 8-hr intervals. Range: 0.75–1.25 mg. **CHILDREN 10 YRS AND OLDER:** 10–15 mcg/kg. **CHILDREN 5–9 YRS:** 20–35 mcg/kg. **CHILDREN 2–4 YRS:** 30–40 mcg/kg. **CHILDREN 1–23 MOS:** 35–60 mcg/kg. **NEONATE, FULL-TERM:** 25–35 mcg/kg. **NEONATE, PREMATURE:** 20–30 mcg/kg.

IV: ADULTS, ELDERLY: 0.6–1 mg. **CHILDREN 10 YRS AND OLDER:** 8–12 mcg/kg. **CHILDREN 5–9 YRS:** 15–30 mcg/kg. **CHILDREN 2–4 YRS:** 25–35 mcg/kg. **CHILDREN 1–23 MOS:** 30–50 mcg/kg. **NEONATES, FULL-TERM:** 20–30 mcg/kg. **NEONATES, PREMATURE:** 15–25 mcg/kg.

MAINTENANCE DOSAGE

PO, IV: ADULTS, ELDERLY: 0.125–0.375 mg/day. **CHILDREN:** 25%–35% loading dose (20%–30% for premature neonates).

DOSAGE IN RENAL IMPAIRMENT

Dosage adjustment is based on creatinine clearance. Total digitalizing dose: decrease by 50% in end-stage renal disease.

Creatinine Clearance	Dosage
10–50 ml/min	25%–75% usual
Less than 10 ml/min	10%–25% usual

SIDE EFFECTS

None known. However, there is a very narrow margin of safety between therapeutic and toxic results. Long-term therapy may produce mammary gland enlargement in women but is reversible when drug is withdrawn.

ADVERSE EFFECTS/ TOXIC REACTIONS

Most common early manifestations of digoxin toxicity are GI disturbances (anorexia, nausea, vomiting), neurologic abnormalities (fatigue, headache, depression, weakness, drowsiness, confusion, nightmares). Facial pain, personality change, ocular disturbances (photophobia, light flashes, halos around bright objects, yellow or green color perception) may occur.

NURSING CONSIDERATIONS

BASELINE ASSESSMENT

Assess apical pulse for 60 sec (30 sec if on maintenance therapy). If pulse is 60 or less/min (70 or less/min for children), withhold drug, contact physician. Blood samples are best taken 6–8 hrs after dose or just before next dose.

INTERVENTION/EVALUATION

Monitor pulse for bradycardia, EKG for arrhythmias for 1–2 hrs after administration (excessive slowing of pulse may be first clinical sign of toxicity). Assess for GI disturbances, neurologic abnormalities (signs of toxicity) q2–4h during loading dose (daily during maintenance). Monitor serum potassium, magnesium. Therapeutic serum level: 0.8–2 ng/ml; toxic serum level: greater than 2 ng/ml.

PATIENT/FAMILY TEACHING

• Stress importance of follow-up visits, blood tests. • Teach pt to take apical pulse correctly and to report pulse 60 or less/min (or as indicated by physician). • Ensure pt understands signs of toxicity and need to notify physician if any occur. • Wear/carry identification of digoxin therapy and inform dentist, other physician of taking digoxin. • Do not increase or skip doses. • Do not take OTC medications without consulting physician. • Inform physician of decreased appetite, nausea/vomiting, diarrhea, visual changes.

digoxin immune FAB

di-**jox**-in

(Digibind, DigiFab)

Do not confuse digoxin immune FAB with Desoxyn or doxepin.

CLASSIFICATION

CLINICAL: Antidote.

ACTION

Binds molecularly to digoxin in extracellular space. **Therapeutic Effect:** Makes digoxin unavailable for binding at its site of action on cells in the body.

PHARMACOKINETICS

Route	Onset	Peak	Duration
IV	30 min	N/A	3–4 days

Widely distributed into extracellular space. Excreted in urine. **Half-life:** 15–20 hrs.

USES

Treatment of potentially life-threatening digoxin toxicity.

PRECAUTIONS

CONTRAINDICATIONS: None known. **CAUTIONS:** Cardiac, renal impairment.

LIFESPAN CONSIDERATIONS:

Pregnancy/Lactation: Unknown if drug crosses placenta or is distributed in breast milk. **Pregnancy Category C.** **Children:** No age-related precautions noted. **Elderly:** Age-related renal impairment may require dosage adjustment.

INTERACTIONS

DRUG: None significant. **HERBAL:** None significant. **FOOD:** None known. **LAB VALUES:** May alter serum potassium. Serum digoxin may increase precipitously and persist for up to 1 wk until FAB/digoxin complex is eliminated from body.

AVAILABILITY (Rx)

INJECTION, POWDER FOR RECONSTITUTION: 38-mg vial (Digibind), 40-mg vial (DigiFab).

D

ADMINISTRATION/HANDLING

IV

Reconstitution • Reconstitute each 38-mg vial with 4 ml Sterile Water for Injection to provide concentration of 9.5 mg/ml. • Further dilute with 50 ml 0.9% NaCl.

Rate of administration • Infuse over 30 min (recommended that solution be infused through a 0.22-micron filter). • If cardiac arrest is imminent, may give IV push.

Storage • Refrigerate vials. • After reconstitution, stable for 4 hrs if refrigerated. • Use immediately after reconstitution.

IV INCOMPATIBILITY

None known.

INDICATIONS/ROUTES/DOSAGE

POTENTIALLY LIFE-THREATENING DIGOXIN OVERDOSE

IV: ADULTS, ELDERLY, CHILDREN: Dosage varies according to amount of digoxin to be neutralized. Refer to manufacturer's dosing guidelines.

SIDE EFFECTS

RARE: Allergic reaction.

ADVERSE EFFECTS/ TOXIC REACTIONS

Digoxin toxicity may result in hyperkalemia (diarrhea, paresthesias, heaviness of legs, decreased B/P, cold skin, grayish pallor, hypotension, mental confusion, irritability, flaccid paralysis, tented T waves, widening QRS, ST depression). When effect of digitalis is reversed, hypokalemia may develop rapidly (muscle cramping, nausea, vomiting, hypoactive bowel sounds, abdominal distention, difficulty breathing, postural hypotension). Low cardiac output conditions, CHF occur rarely.

NURSING CONSIDERATIONS

BASELINE ASSESSMENT

Obtain serum digoxin level before administering drug. If drawn less than 6 hrs before last digoxin dose, test result may be unreliable. Those with renal impairment may require more than 1 wk before serum digoxin assay is reliable. Assess muscle strength, mental status.

INTERVENTION/EVALUATION

Closely monitor temperature, B/P, EKG, serum potassium during and after drug is administered. Watch for changes from initial assessment (hypokalemia may result in muscle strength changes, tremor, muscle cramps, altered mental status, cardiac arrhythmias; hyponatremia may result in confusion, thirst, cold/clammy skin).

dihydroergotamine

See ergotamine

dihydrotachysterol

See vitamin D

Dilacor XR, *see diltiazem*

Dilantin, *see phenytoin*

Dilaudid, *see hydromorphone*

diltiazem

dil-**tye**-a-zem

(Apo-Diltiaz ♣, Cardizem, Cardizem CD, Cardizem LA, Cardizem SR, Cartia XT, Dilacor XR, Diltia XT, Novo-Diltiazem ♣, Taztia XT, Tiazac)

Do not confuse Cardizem with Cardene or Cardene SR, or Tiazac with Ziac.

FIXED-COMBINATION(S)

Teczem: diltiazem/enalapril (angiotensin-converting enzyme [ACE] inhibitor): 180 mg/5 mg.

CLASSIFICATION

PHARMACOTHERAPEUTIC: Calcium channel blocker. **CLINICAL:** Antianginal, antihypertensive, antiarrhythmic (see pp. 16C, 73C).

ACTION

Inhibits calcium movement across cardiac, vascular smooth-muscle cell membranes (causes dilation of coronary arteries, peripheral arteries, arterioles). **Therapeutic Effect:** Decreases heart rate, myocardial contractility; slows SA, AV conduction; decreases total peripheral vascular resistance by vasodilation.

PHARMACOKINETICS

Route	Onset	Peak	Duration
PO	0.5–1 hr	N/A	N/A
PO (extended-release)	2–3 hrs	N/A	N/A
IV	3 min	N/A	N/A

Well absorbed from GI tract. Protein binding: 70%–80%. Undergoes first-pass metabolism in the liver to active metabolite. Primarily excreted in urine. Not removed by hemodialysis. **Half-life:** 3–8 hrs.

USES

PO: Treatment of angina due to coronary artery spasm (Prinzmetal's variant angina), chronic stable angina (effort-associated angina). **Extended-release:** Treatment of essential hypertension, angina. **Cardizem LA:** Treatment of chronic stable angina. **Parenteral:** Temporary control of rapid ventricular rate in atrial fibrillation/flutter. Rapid conversion of paroxysmal supraventricular tachycardia (PSVT) to normal sinus rhythm. **OFF-LABEL:** Therapy for Duchenne muscular dystrophy.

PRECAUTIONS

CONTRAINDICATIONS: Acute MI, pulmonary congestion, hypersensitivity to diltiazem or other calcium channel blockers, second- or third-degree AV block (except in presence of pacemaker), severe hypotension (less than 90 mm Hg, systolic), sick sinus syndrome. **CAUTIONS:** Renal/hepatic impairment, CHF.

LIFESPAN CONSIDERATIONS:

Pregnancy/Lactation: Distributed in breast milk. **Pregnancy Category C. Children:** No age-related precautions noted. **Elderly:** Age-related renal impairment may require dosage adjustment.

INTERACTIONS

DRUG: **Beta-blockers** may have additive effect. **Carbamazepine, quinidine, theophylline** may increase concentration, risk of toxicity. May increase serum **digoxin** concentration. **Procainamide, quinidine** may increase risk of QT-interval prolongation. **HERBAL: Ephedra** may worsen arrhythmias, hypertension. **Ginseng, yohimbe** may worsen hypertension. **Garlic** may increase antihypertensive effect. **FOOD:** None known. **LAB VALUES:** May increase PR interval.

D

AVAILABILITY (Rx)

INJECTION, SOLUTION: 5 mg/ml (5 ml, 10 ml, 25 ml). **INJECTION, INFUSION (READY TO HANG):** 1 mg./ml. **TABLETS:** 30 mg, 60 mg, 90 mg, 120 mg

CAPSULES, EXTENDED-RELEASE: (CARDIZEM CD): 120 mg, 180 mg, 240 mg, 300 mg, 360 mg. **(CARTIA XT):** 120 mg, 180 mg, 240 mg, 300 mg. **(DILACOR XR, DILTIA XT):** 120 mg, 180 mg, 240 mg. **(TAZTIA, XT):** 120 mg, 180 mg, 240 mg, 300 mg, 360 mg. **(TIAZAC):** 120 mg, 180 mg, 240 mg, 300 mg, 360 mg, 420 mg. **CAPSULES, SUSTAINED-RELEASE: (CARDIZEM SR):** 60 mg, 90 mg, 120 mg. **TABLETS, EXTENDED-RELEASE: (CARDIZEM LA):** 120 mg, 180 mg, 240 mg, 300 mg, 360 mg, 420 mg.

ADMINISTRATION/HANDLING

IV

Reconstitution • Add 125 mg to 100 ml D_5W, 0.9% NaCl to provide concentration of 1 mg/ml. Add 250 mg to 250 or 500 ml diluent to provide concentration of 0.83 mg/ml or 0.45 mg/ml, respectively. Maximum concentration: 1.25 g/250 ml (5 mg/ml).

Rate of administration • Infuse per dilution/rate chart provided by manufacturer.

Storage • Refrigerate vials. • After dilution, stable for 24 hrs.

PO

• Give before meals and at bedtime. • Tablets may be crushed. • Do not crush sustained-release capsules or extended-release capsules or tablets.

IV INCOMPATIBILITIES

Acetazolamide (Diamox), acyclovir (Zovirax), aminophylline, ampicillin, ampicillin/sulbactam (Unasyn), cefoperazone (Cefobid), diazepam (Valium), furosemide (Lasix), heparin, insulin, nafcillin, phenytoin (Dilantin), rifampin (Rifadin), sodium bicarbonate.

IV COMPATIBILITIES

Albumin, aztreonam (Azactam), bumetanide (Bumex), cefazolin (Ancef), cefotaxime (Claforan), ceftazidime (Fortaz), ceftriaxone (Rocephin), cefuroxime (Zinacef), cimetidine (Tagamet), ciprofloxacin (Cipro), clindamycin (Cleocin), digoxin (Lanoxin), dobutamine (Dobutrex), dopamine (Intropin), gentamicin (Garamycin), hydromorphone (Dilaudid), lidocaine, lorazepam (Ativan), metoclopramide (Reglan), metronidazole (Flagyl), midazolam (Versed), morphine, multivitamins, nitroglycerin, norepinephrine (Levophed), potassium chloride, potassium phosphate, tobramycin (Nebcin), vancomycin (Vancocin).

INDICATIONS/ROUTES/DOSAGE

ANGINA

PO (CARDIZEM): ADULTS, ELDERLY: Initially, 30 mg 4 times a day. Range: 180–360 mg/day.

PO (CARDIZEM CD, CARTIA XT, DILACOR XR, DILTIA XT, TIAZAC): ADULTS, ELDERLY: Initially, 120–180 mg/day. **Maximum:** 480 mg/day.

PO (CARDIZEM LA): ADULTS, ELDERLY: Initially, 180 mg/day. May increase at 7- to 14-day intervals. **Maximum:** 360 mg/day.

HYPERTENSION

PO (CARDIZEM CD, CARTIA XT, DILACOR XR, DILTIA XT, TIAZAC): ADULTS, ELDERLY: Initially, 180–240 mg/day. Range: 180–420 mg/day, **Tiazac:** 120–540 mg/day.

PO (CARDIZEM SR): ADULTS, ELDERLY: Initially, 60–120 mg twice a day. May increase at 14-day intervals. Maintenance: 240–360 mg/day.

PO (CARDIZEM LA): ADULTS, ELDERLY: Initially, 180–240 mg/day. May increase at 14-day intervals. Range: 120–540 mg/day.

TEMPORARY CONTROL OF RAPID VENTRICULAR RATE IN ATRIAL

FIBRILLATION/FLUTTER; RAPID CONVERSION OF PAROXYSMAL SUPRAVENTRICULAR TACHYCARDIA TO NORMAL SINUS RHYTHM

IV PUSH: ADULTS, ELDERLY: Initially, 0.25 mg/kg actual body weight over 2 min. May repeat in 15 min at dose of 0.35 mg/kg actual body weight. Subsequent doses individualized.

IV INFUSION: ADULTS, ELDERLY: After initial bolus injection, may begin infusion at 5–10 mg/hr; may increase by 5 mg/hr up to a maximum of 15 mg/hr. Infusion duration should not exceed 24 hrs.

SIDE EFFECTS

FREQUENT (10%–5%): Peripheral edema, dizziness, light-headedness, headache, bradycardia, asthenia (loss of strength, weakness). **OCCASIONAL (5%–2%):** Nausea, constipation, flushing, EKG changes. **RARE (less than 2%):** Rash, micturition disorder (polyuria, nocturia, dysuria, frequency of urination), abdominal discomfort, somnolence.

ADVERSE EFFECTS/ TOXIC REACTIONS

Abrupt withdrawal may increase frequency, duration of angina, CHF, second- and third-degree AV block occur rarely. Overdose produces nausea, somnolence, confusion, slurred speech, profound bradycardia.

NURSING CONSIDERATIONS

BASELINE ASSESSMENT

Concurrent therapy with sublingual nitroglycerin may be used for relief of anginal pain. Record onset, type (sharp, dull, squeezing), radiation, location, intensity, duration of anginal pain, precipitating factors (exertion, emotional stress). Assess baseline renal/hepatic function tests. Assess B/P, apical pulse immediately before drug is administered.

INTERVENTION/EVALUATION

Assist with ambulation if dizziness occurs. Assess for peripheral edema behind medial malleolus (sacral area in bedridden pts). Monitor pulse rate for bradycardia. With IV therapy, assess B/P, renal/hepatic function tests, EKG. Question for asthenia, headache.

PATIENT/FAMILY TEACHING

• Do not abruptly discontinue medication. • Compliance with therapy regimen is essential to control anginal pain. • To avoid hypotensive effect, rise slowly from lying to sitting position, wait momentarily before standing. • Avoid tasks that require alertness, motor skills until response to drug is established. • Contact physician if palpitations, shortness of breath, pronounced dizziness, nausea, constipation occurs.

*dimenhyDRINATE

(Dramamine)

See Antihistamines (p. 52C)

dinoprostone

dye-noe-**pros**-tone

(Cervidil, Prepidil, Prostin E_2)

Do not confuse Cervidil or Prepidil with bepridil or Prostin with Prostigmin.

♦CLASSIFICATION

PHARMACOTHERAPEUTIC: Prostaglandin. **CLINICAL:** Oxytocic, abortifacient, antihemorrhagic.

ACTION

Directly acts on myometrium, causing softening, dilation effect of cervix.

Therapeutic Effect: Stimulates myometrial contractions in gravid uterus.

PHARMACOKINETICS

Undergoes rapid enzymatic deactivation primarily in maternal lungs. Protein binding: 73%. Primarily excreted in urine. **Half-life:** Less than 5 min.

USES

Suppository: To induce abortion from wk 12 of pregnancy through the second trimester, to evacuate uterine contents in missed abortion or intrauterine fetal death up to 28 wks gestational age (as calculated from first day of last normal menstrual period), benign hydatidiform mole. Treatment of postpartum/postabortion hemorrhage, induction of labor at or near term. **Gel:** Ripening unfavorable cervix in pregnant women at or near term with medical/obstetric need for labor induction. Induction of labor at or near term. **Vaginal insert:** Initiation and/or cervical ripening in pts with medical indication for induction of labor.

PRECAUTIONS

CONTRAINDICATIONS: Gel: Active cardiac, hepatic, pulmonary, renal disease; acute pelvic inflammatory disease (PID); fetal malpresentation; grand multiparae with 6 or more previous term pregnancy cases with nonvertex presentation; history of cesarean section, major uterine surgery; history of difficult labor, traumatic delivery; hypersensitivity to other prostaglandins; placenta previa, unexplained vaginal bleeding during this pregnancy; pts for whom vaginal delivery is not indicated (vasa previa, active herpes genitalia); significant cephalopelvic disproportion. **Vaginal suppository:** Active cardiac, hepatic, pulmonary, renal disease; acute PID. **CAUTIONS:** Cervicitis, infected endocervical lesions, acute vaginitis, history of asthma, hypotension/hypertension, anemia, jaundice, diabetes, epilepsy, uterine fibroids, compromised (scarred) uterus, history of cardiovascular, renal, hepatic disease.

LIFESPAN CONSIDERATIONS:

Pregnancy/Lactation: Suppository: Teratogenic, therefore abortion must be complete. **Gel:** Sustained uterine hyperstimulation may affect fetus (e.g., abnormal heart rate). **Pregnancy Category C.** **Children/Elderly:** Not used in these pt populations.

INTERACTIONS

DRUG: Oxytocics may cause uterine hypertonus, possibly resulting in uterine rupture, cervical laceration. **HERBAL:** None significant. **FOOD:** None known. **LAB VALUES:** None known.

AVAILABILITY (Rx)

VAGINAL GEL (PREPIDIL): 0.5 mg. **VAGINAL INSERTS (CERVIDIL):** 10 mg. **VAGINAL SUPPOSITORIES (PROSTIN E_2 VAGINAL CREAM):** 20 mg.

ADMINISTRATION/HANDLING

GEL • Refrigerate. • Use caution in handling, prevent skin contact. Wash hands thoroughly with soap and water following administration. • Bring to room temperature just before use (avoid forcing the warming process). • Assemble dosing apparatus as described in manufacturer insert. • Place pt in dorsal position with cervix visualized using a speculum. • Introduce gel into cervical canal just below level of internal os. • Have pt remain in supine position at least 15–30 min (minimizes leakage from cervical canal).

SUPPOSITORY

• Keep frozen (less than 4°F); bring to room temperature just before use. • Administer only in hospital setting with emergency equipment available. • Warm suppository to room temperature before removing foil wrapper. • Avoid skin contact (risk of absorption). • Insert high into vagina.

• Pt should remain supine for 10 min after administration.

INDICATIONS/ROUTES/DOSAGE

ABORTIFACIENT

INTRAVAGINAL: ADULTS: 20 mg (or one suppository) high into vagina. May repeat at 3- to 5-hr intervals until abortion occurs. Do not administer for longer than 2 days. **Maximum:** 240 mg.

RIPENING OF UNFAVORABLE CERVIX

INTRACERVICAL (PREPIDIL): ADULTS: Initially, 0.5 mg (2.5 ml); if no cervical or uterine response, may repeat 0.5-mg dose in 6 hrs. **Maximum:** 1.5 mg (7.5 ml) for a 24-hr period.

INTRACERVICAL (CERVIDIL): ADULTS: 10 mg over 12-hr period; remove upon onset of active labor or 12 hrs after insertion.

SIDE EFFECTS

FREQUENT: Vomiting (66%), diarrhea (40%), nausea (33%). **OCCASIONAL:** Headache (10%), chills/shivering (10%), urticaria, bradycardia, increased uterine pain accompanying abortion, peripheral vasoconstriction. **RARE:** Flushing of skin, vulvar edema.

ADVERSE EFFECTS/ TOXIC REACTIONS

Overdose may cause uterine hypertonicity with spasm and tetanic contraction, leading to cervical laceration/perforation, uterine rupture/hemorrhage.

NURSING CONSIDERATIONS

BASELINE ASSESSMENT

Offer emotional support. **Suppository:** Obtain orders for antiemetics, antidiarrheals, meperidine, other pain medication for abdominal cramps. Assess any uterine activity, vaginal bleeding. **Gel:** Assess Bishop score. Assess degree of effacement (determines size of shielded endocervical catheter).

INTERVENTION/EVALUATION

Suppository: Check strength, duration, frequency of contractions. Monitor vital signs q15min until stable, then hourly until abortion complete. Check resting uterine tone. Administer medications for relief of GI effects if indicated or for abdominal cramps. **Gel:** Monitor uterine activity (onset of uterine contractions), fetal status (heart rate), character of cervix (dilation, effacement). Have pt remain recumbent 12 hrs after application with continuous electronic monitoring of fetal heart rate, uterine activity. Record maternal vital signs at least hourly in presence of uterine activity. Reassess Bishop score.

PATIENT/ FAMILY TEACHING

• **Suppository:** Report promptly fever, chills, foul-smelling/increased vaginal discharge, uterine cramps, pain.

Diovan, *see valsartan*

Diovan HCT, *see hydrochlorothiazide and valsartan*

*diphenhydrAMINE

dye-fen-**hye**-dra-meen

(Allerdry ♣, Banophen, Benadryl, Diphen, Diphenhist, Genahist, Nytol ♣)

Do not confuse diphenhydramine with dimenhydrinate, or Benadryl with benazepril, Bentyl, or Benylin, or Banophen with baclofen.

D

FIXED-COMBINATION(S)

Advil PM: diphenhydramine/ibuprofen (NSAID): 38 mg/200 mg. With calamine, an astringent, and camphor, a counterirritant **(Caladryl).**

CLASSIFICATION

PHARMACOTHERAPEUTIC: Ethanolamine. **CLINICAL:** Antihistamine, anticholinergic, antipruritic, antitussive, antiemetic, antidyskinetic (see p. 52C).

ACTION

Competitively blocks effects of histamine at peripheral H_1 receptor sites. **Therapeutic Effect:** Produces anticholinergic, antipruritic, antitussive, antiemetic, antidyskinetic, sedative effects.

PHARMACOKINETICS

Route	Onset	Peak	Duration
PO	15–30 min	1–4 hrs	4–6 hrs
IV, IM	Less than 15 min	1–4 hrs	4–6 hrs

Well absorbed after PO, parenteral administration. Protein binding: 98%–99%. Widely distributed. Metabolized in the liver. Primarily excreted in urine. **Half-life:** 1–4 hrs.

USES

Treatment of allergic reactions, parkinsonism; prevention/treatment of nausea, vomiting, vertigo due to motion sickness; antitussive; short-term management of insomnia. Topical form used for relief of pruritus, insect bites, skin irritations. **OFF-LABEL:** Treatment of nausea/vomiting, antitussive.

PRECAUTIONS

CONTRAINDICATIONS: Acute exacerbation of asthma, use of MAOIs within 14 days. **CAUTIONS:** Narrow-angle glaucoma, peptic ulcer, prostatic hypertrophy, pyloroduodenal/bladder neck obstruction, asthma, chronic obstructive pulmonary disease (COPD), increased intraocular pressure (IOP), cardiovascular disease, hyperthyroidism, hypertension, seizure disorders.

LIFESPAN CONSIDERATIONS:

Pregnancy/Lactation: Crosses placenta. Detected in breast milk (may produce irritability in breast-fed infants). Increased risk of seizures in neonates, premature infants if used during third trimester of pregnancy. May prohibit lactation. **Pregnancy Category B.** **Children:** Not recommended in newborns, premature infants (increased risk of paradoxical reaction, seizures). **Elderly:** Increased risk for dizziness, sedation, confusion, hypotension, hyperexcitability.

INTERACTIONS

DRUG: **Alcohol, other CNS depressants** may increase CNS depressant effects. **Anticholinergics** may increase anticholinergic effects. **MAOIs** may increase anticholinergic, CNS depressant effects. **HERBAL:** **Gotu kola, kava kava, St John's wort, valerian** may increase CNS depression. **FOOD:** None known. **LAB VALUES:** May suppress wheal/flare reactions to antigen skin testing unless drug is discontinued 4 days before testing.

AVAILABILITY (OTC)

CAPSULES: 25 mg (Banophen, Diphen, DNC Genahist), 50 mg (Nytol). **CREAM (BENADRYL):** 1%, 2%. **INJECTION SOLUTION (BENADRYL):** 50 mg/ml. **SPRAY (BENADRYL):** 1%, 2%. **SYRUP (DIPHEN, DIPHENHIST):** 12.5 mg/5 ml. **TABLETS (BANOPHEN, BENADRYL, GENAHIST, NYTOL):** 25 mg, 50 mg.

ADMINISTRATION/HANDLING

IV

• May be given undiluted. • Give IV injection over at least 1 min.

IM
- Give deep IM into large muscle mass.

PO
- Give without regard to meals.
- Scored tablets may be crushed.

IV INCOMPATIBILITIES

Allopurinol (Aloprim), amphotericin B complex (Abelcet, AmBisome, Amphotec), cefepime (Maxipime), dexamethasone (Decadron), foscarnet (Foscavir).

IV COMPATIBILITIES

Atropine, cisplatin (Platinol), cyclophosphamide (Cytoxan), cytarabine (Ara-C), droperidol (Inapsine), fentanyl, glycopyrrolate (Robinul), heparin, hydrocortisone (Solu-Cortef), hydromorphone (Dilaudid), hydroxyzine (Vistaril), lidocaine, lipids, metoclopramide (Reglan), ondansetron (Zofran), promethazine (Phenergan), potassium chloride, propofol (Diprivan).

INDICATIONS/ROUTES/DOSAGE

MODERATE TO SEVERE ALLERGIC REACTION

PO, IV, IM: ADULTS, ELDERLY: 25–50 mg q4h. **Maximum:** 400 mg/day. **CHILDREN:** 5 mg/kg/day in divided doses q6–8h. **Maximum:** 300 mg/day.

MOTION SICKNESS

PO: ADULTS, ELDERLY, CHILDREN 12 YRS AND OLDER: 25–50 mg q4–6h. **Maximum:** 300 mg/day. **CHILDREN 6–11 YRS:** 12.5–25 mg q4–6h. **Maximum:** 150 mg/day. **CHILDREN 2–5 YRS:** 6.25 mg q4–6h. **Maximum:** 37.5 mg/day.

PARKINSON'S DISEASE

PO: ADULTS, ELDERLY: 25–50 mg 3–4 times a day.

ANTITUSSIVE

PO: ADULTS, ELDERLY, CHILDREN 12 YRS AND OLDER: 25 mg q4h. **Maximum:** 150 mg/day. **CHILDREN 6–11 YRS:** 12.5 mg q4h. **Maximum:** 75 mg/day. **CHILDREN 2–5 YRS:** 6.25 mg q4h. **Maximum:** 37.5 mg/day.

NIGHTTIME SLEEP AID

PO: ADULTS, ELDERLY, CHILDREN 12 YRS AND OLDER: 50 mg at bedtime. **CHILDREN 2–11 YRS:** 1 mg/kg/dose. **Maximum:** 50 mg.

PRURITUS

TOPICAL: ADULTS, ELDERLY, CHILDREN 12 YRS AND OLDER: Apply 1% or 2% cream or spray 3–4 times a day. **CHILDREN 2–11 YRS:** Apply 1% cream or spray 3–4 times a day.

D

SIDE EFFECTS

FREQUENT: Drowsiness, dizziness, muscle weakness, hypotension, urinary retention, thickening of bronchial secretions, dry mouth, nose, throat, lips; in elderly: sedation, dizziness, hypotension. **OCCASIONAL:** Epigastric distress, flushing, visual/hearing disturbances, paresthesia, diaphoresis, chills.

ADVERSE EFFECTS/ TOXIC REACTIONS

Hypersensitivity reactions (eczema, pruritus, rash, cardiac disturbances, photosensitivity) may occur. Overdose symptoms may vary from CNS depression (sedation, apnea, hypotension, cardiovascular collapse, death) to severe paradoxical reactions (hallucinations, tremor, seizures). Children, infants, neonates may experience paradoxical reactions (restlessness, insomnia, euphoria, nervousness, tremors). Overdosage in children may result in hallucinations, seizures, death.

NURSING CONSIDERATIONS

BASELINE ASSESSMENT

If pt is having acute allergic reaction, obtain history of recently ingested foods, drugs, environmental exposure, emotional stress. Monitor B/P, rate, depth, rhythm, type of respiration; quality, rate of pulse. Assess lung sounds for rhonchi, wheezing, rales.

D

INTERVENTION/EVALUATION

Monitor B/P, esp. in elderly (increased risk of hypotension). Monitor children closely for paradoxical reaction.

PATIENT/FAMILY TEACHING

• Tolerance to antihistaminic effect generally does not occur; tolerance to sedative effect may occur. • Avoid tasks that require alertness, motor skills until response to drug is established. • Dry mouth, drowsiness, dizziness may be an expected response of drug. • Avoid alcohol.

diphenoxylate with atropine

dye-fen-**ox**-i-late
(Lomotil, Lonox)

Do not confuse Lomotil with Lamictal or Lonox with Lanoxin, Loprox, or Lovenox.

FIXED-COMBINATION(S)

Lomotil: diphenoxylate/atropine (anticholinergic, antispasmodic): 2.5 mg/0.025 mg.

CLASSIFICATION

PHARMACOTHERAPEUTIC: Meperidine derivative. **CLINICAL:** Antidiarrheal (see p. 43C).

ACTION

Acts locally and centrally on gastric mucosa. **Therapeutic Effect:** Reduces intestinal motility.

PHARMACOKINETICS

Well absorbed from GI tract. Metabolized in the liver to active metabolite. Primarily eliminated in feces. **Half-life:** 2.5 hrs; metabolite, 12–24 hrs.

USES

Adjunctive treatment of acute, chronic diarrhea.

PRECAUTIONS

CONTRAINDICATIONS: Children younger than 2 yrs, dehydration, jaundice, narrow-angle glaucoma, severe hepatic disease. **CAUTIONS:** Cirrhosis, renal/hepatic disease, renal impairment, acute ulcerative colitis.

LIFESPAN CONSIDERATIONS:

Pregnancy/Lactation: Unknown if drug crosses placenta or is distributed in breast milk. **Pregnancy Category C.** **Children:** Not recommended (increased susceptibility to toxicity, including respiratory depression). **Elderly:** More susceptible to anticholinergic effects, confusion, respiratory depression.

INTERACTIONS

DRUG: **Alcohol, other CNS depressants** may increase CNS depressant effects. **Anticholinergics** may increase the effects of atropine. May increase serum **digoxin** levels. **MAOIs** may precipitate hypertensive crisis. **HERBAL:** None significant. **FOOD:** None known. **LAB VALUES:** May increase serum amylase.

AVAILABILITY (Rx)

LIQUID (LOMOTIL): 2.5 mg/5 ml. **TABLETS (LOMOTIL, LONOX):** 2.5 mg diphenoxylate/0.025 mg atropine.

ADMINISTRATION/HANDLING

PO

• Give without regard to meals. If GI irritation occurs, give with food. • Use liquid for children 2–12 yrs (use graduated dropper for administration of liquid medication).

INDICATIONS/ROUTES/DOSAGE

DIARRHEA

PO: ADULTS, ELDERLY: Initially, 15–20 mg/day in 3–4 divided doses; then 5–15 mg/day in 2–3 divided doses. **CHILDREN 9–12 YRS:** 2 mg 5 times a day. **CHILDREN 6–8 YRS:** 2 mg 4 times a day. **CHILDREN 2–5 YRS:** 2 mg 3 times a day.

SIDE EFFECTS

FREQUENT: Drowsiness, light-headedness, dizziness, nausea. **OCCASIONAL:** Headache, dry mouth. **RARE:** Flushing, tachycardia, urinary retention, constipation, paradoxical reaction (marked by restlessness, agitation), blurred vision.

ADVERSE EFFECTS/ TOXIC REACTIONS

Dehydration may predispose pt to diphenoxylate toxicity. Paralytic ileus, toxic megacolon (constipation, decreased appetite, abdominal pain with nausea/vomiting) occur rarely. Severe anticholinergic reaction (severe lethargy, hypotonic reflexes, hyperthermia) may result in severe respiratory depression, coma.

NURSING CONSIDERATIONS

BASELINE ASSESSMENT

Check baseline hydration status: skin turgor, mucous membranes for dryness, urinary status.

INTERVENTION/EVALUATION

Encourage adequate fluid intake. Assess bowel sounds for peristalsis. Monitor daily pattern of bowel activity/stool consistency; record time of evacuation. Assess for abdominal disturbances. Discontinue medication if abdominal distention occurs.

PATIENT/FAMILY TEACHING

• Avoid tasks that require alertness, motor skills until response to drug is established. • Avoid alcohol, barbiturates. • Contact physician if fever, palpitations occur or diarrhea persists. • Report abdominal distention.

dipivefrin

(Propine)

See Antiglaucoma agents (p. 49C)

Diprivan, *see propofol*

dipyridamole

dye-pie-**rid**-ah-mole

(Apo-Dipyridamole FC ✤, Persantine)

Do not confuse Aggrenox with Aggrastat, or dipyridamole with disopyramide, or Persantine with Periactin.

FIXED-COMBINATION(S)

Aggrenox: dipyridamole/aspirin (antiplatelet): 200 mg/25 mg.

CLASSIFICATION

PHARMACOTHERAPEUTIC: Blood modifier, platelet aggregation inhibitor. **CLINICAL:** Antiplatelet, antianginal, diagnostic agent (see p. 31C).

ACTION

Inhibits activity of adenosine deaminase and phosphodiesterase, enzymes causing accumulation of adenosine, cyclic adenosine monophosphate (AMP). **Therapeutic Effect:** Inhibits platelet aggregation; may cause coronary vasodilation.

PHARMACOKINETICS

Slowly, variably absorbed from the GI tract. Widely distributed. Protein binding: 91%–99%. Metabolized in the liver.

D

Primarily eliminated via biliary excretion. **Half-life:** 10–15 hrs.

USES

Adjunct to warfarin (Coumadin) anticoagulant therapy in prevention of postop thromboembolic complications of cardiac valve replacement. **IV:** Alternative to exercise in thallium myocardial perfusion imaging for evaluation of coronary artery disease. **OFF-LABEL:** Reduces risk of reinfarction in pts recovering from MI, treatment of transient ischemic attacks (TIAs).

PRECAUTIONS

CONTRAINDICATIONS: None known. **CAUTIONS:** Hypotension.

LIFESPAN CONSIDERATIONS:

Pregnancy/Lactation: Distributed in breast milk. **Pregnancy Category B. Children:** Safety and efficacy not established. **Elderly:** No age-related precautions noted.

INTERACTIONS

DRUG: Anticoagulants, aspirin, heparin, salicylates, thrombolytics may increase risk of bleeding. **HERBAL: Cat's claw, dong quai, evening primrose, garlic, ginseng** may increase antiplatelet activity. **FOOD:** None known. **LAB VALUES:** None known.

AVAILABILITY (Rx)

INJECTION: 5 mg/ml. **TABLETS:** 25 mg, 50 mg, 75 mg.

ADMINISTRATION/HANDLING

IV

• Dilute to at least 1:2 ratio with 0.9% NaCl or D_5W for total volume of 20–50 ml (undiluted may cause irritation). • Infuse over 4 min. • Inject thallium within 5 min after dipyridamole infusion.

PO

• Best taken on empty stomach with full glass of water.

IV INCOMPATIBILITIES

No information available on Y-site administration.

INDICATIONS/ROUTES/DOSAGE

PREVENTION OF THROMBOEMBOLIC DISORDERS

PO: ADULTS, ELDERLY: 75–100 mg 4 times a day in combination with other medications. **CHILDREN:** 3–6 mg/kg/day in 3 divided doses.

DIAGNOSTIC AID

IV: ADULTS, ELDERLY (BASED ON WEIGHT): 0.142 mg/kg/min infused over 4 min; doses greater than 60 mg have been determined to be unnecessary for any pt.

SIDE EFFECTS

FREQUENT (14%): Dizziness. **OCCASIONAL (6%–2%):** Abdominal distress, headache, rash. **RARE (less than 2%):** Diarrhea, vomiting, flushing, pruritus.

ADVERSE EFFECTS/ TOXIC REACTIONS

Overdose produces peripheral vasodilation, resulting in hypotension.

NURSING CONSIDERATIONS

BASELINE ASSESSMENT

Assess for presence of chest pain. Obtain baseline B/P, pulse. When used as antiplatelet, check hematologic status.

INTERVENTION/EVALUATION

Assist with ambulation if dizziness occurs. Assess B/P for hypotension. Assess skin for flushing, rash.

PATIENT/FAMILY TEACHING

• Avoid alcohol. • If nausea occurs, cola, unsalted crackers, dry toast may relieve effect. • Therapeutic response may not be achieved before 2–3 mos of continuous therapy. • Use caution when rising suddenly from lying or sitting position.

disopyramide

dye-soe-**peer**-a-mide

(Norpace, Norpace CR, Rythmodan ✦, Rythmodan LA ✦)

Do not confuse disopyramide with desipramine, dipyridamole, or Rythmol.

CLASSIFICATION

CLINICAL: Antiarrhythmic (see p. 13C).

ACTION

Prolongs refractory period of cardiac cell by direct effect, decreasing myocardial excitability, conduction velocity. **Therapeutic Effect:** Depresses myocardial contractility. Has anticholinergic, negative inotropic effects.

PHARMACOKINETICS

Rapidly, almost completely absorbed from GI tract. Protein binding: 50%–65%. Metabolized in liver. Excreted in urine. Removed by hemodialysis. **Half-life:** 4–10 hrs.

USES

Suppression/prevention of ventricular ectopy (premature ventricular contractions, ventricular tachycardia). **OFF-LABEL:** Prophylaxis/treatment of supraventricular tachycardia.

PRECAUTIONS

CONTRAINDICATIONS: Cardiogenic shock, congenital QT-interval prolongation, narrow-angle glaucoma (unless pt is undergoing cholinergic therapy), preexisting second- or third-degree AV block, preexisting urinary retention. **CAUTIONS:** CHF, myasthenia gravis, prostatic hypertrophy, sick sinus syndrome (bradycardia/tachycardia), Wolff-Parkinson-White syndrome, bundle-branch block, renal/hepatic impairment.

LIFESPAN CONSIDERATIONS:

Pregnancy/Lactation: Distributed in breast milk. **Pregnancy Category C. Children:** Safety and efficacy not established in children. **Elderly:** Increased sensitivity to anticholinergic effects.

INTERACTIONS

DRUG: **Other antiarrhythmics (e.g., diltiazem, propranolol, verapamil)** may prolong cardiac conduction, decrease cardiac output. **Erythomycin** may increase concentration. **Medications prolonging QT-interval (e.g., clarithromycin, tricyclic antidepressants)** may have additive effects. **HERBAL: Ephedra** may worsen arrhythmias. **St. John's wort** may decrease concentration. **FOOD:** None known. **LAB VALUES:** May decrease serum glucose. May cause EKG changes. May increase serum cholesterol, triglycerides. Therapeutic serum level is 2–8 mcg/ml; toxic serum level is greater than; 8 mcg/ml.

AVAILABILITY (Rx)

CAPSULES (NORPACE): 100 mg, 150 mg.

CAPSULES (EXTENDED-RELEASE [NORPACE CR]): 100 mg, 150 mg.

ADMINISTRATION/HANDLING

PO

• Administer immediate-release capsules in divided doses. • Swallow extended-release capsules whole.

INDICATIONS/ROUTES/DOSAGE

SUPPRESSION/PREVENTION OF VENTRICULAR ECTOPY

PO: ADULTS, ELDERLY WEIGHING 50 KG AND MORE: 150 mg q6h (300 mg q12h with extended-release). **ADULTS, ELDERLY WEIGHING LESS THAN 50 KG:** 100 mg q6h (200 mg q12h with extended-release).

USUAL PEDIATRIC DOSAGE

PO (IMMEDIATE-RELEASE CAPSULES): CHILDREN 12–18 YRS: 6–15 mg/

kg/day in divided doses q6h. **CHILDREN 5–11 YRS:** 10–15 mg/kg/day in divided doses q6h. **CHILDREN 1–4 YRS:** 10–20 mg/kg/day in divided doses q6h. **CHILDREN YOUNGER THAN 1 YR:** 10–30 mg/kg/day in divided doses q6h.

DOSAGE IN RENAL IMPAIRMENT
With or without loading dose of 150 mg:

Creatinine Clearance	Dosage
40 ml/min and higher	100 mg q6h (extended-release 200 mg q12h)
30–39 ml/min	100 mg q8h
15–29 ml/min	100 mg q12h
Less than 15 ml/min	100 mg q24h

DOSAGE IN HEPATIC IMPAIRMENT
ADULTS, ELDERLY WEIGHING 50 KG AND MORE: 100 mg q6h (200 mg q12h with extended-release).

DOSAGE IN CARDIOMYOPATHY, CARDIAC DECOMPENSATION
ADULTS, ELDERLY WEIGHING 50 KG AND MORE: No loading dose; 100 mg q6–8h with gradual dosage adjustments.

SIDE EFFECTS

FREQUENT (greater than 9%): Dry mouth (32%), urinary hesitancy, constipation. **OCCASIONAL (9%–3%):** Blurred vision, dry eyes, nose, throat, urinary retention, headache, dizziness, fatigue, nausea. **RARE (less than 1%):** Impotence, hypotension, edema, weight gain, shortness of breath, syncope, chest pain, nervousness, diarrhea, vomiting, decreased appetite, rash, pruritus.

ADVERSE EFFECTS/ TOXIC REACTIONS

May produce/aggravate CHF. May produce severe hypotension, shortness of breath, chest pain, syncope (esp. in pts with primary cardiomyopathy, CHF). Hepatotoxicity occurs rarely.

NURSING CONSIDERATIONS

BASELINE ASSESSMENT
Before giving medication, instruct pt to void (reduces risk of urinary retention).

INTERVENTION/EVALUATION
Monitor EKG for cardiac changes, particularly widening of QRS complex, prolongation of PR, QT intervals. Monitor B/P, EKG, serum potassium, glucose, hepatic enzymes. Monitor I&O (be alert to urinary retention). Assess for evidence of CHF (cough, dyspnea [particularly on exertion], rales at base of lungs, fatigue). Assist with ambulation if dizziness occurs. Therapeutic serum level: 2–8 mcg/ml; toxic serum level: greater than 8 mcg/ml.

PATIENT/FAMILY TEACHING
• Report shortness of breath, productive cough. • Do not use nasal decongestants, OTC cold preparations (stimulants) without physician approval. • Restrict salt, alcohol intake.

Ditropan, *see oxybutynin*

Ditropan XL, *see oxybutynin*

**DOBUTamine*

doe-**byoo**-ta-meen
(Dobutrex)

Do not confuse dobutamine with dopamine.

CLASSIFICATION

PHARMACOTHERAPEUTIC: Sympathomimetic. **CLINICAL:** Cardiac stimulant (see p. 147C).

D

ACTION

Direct-action inotropic agent acting primarily on $beta_1$-adrenergic receptors, decreasing preload, afterload. **Therapeutic Effect:** Enhances myocardial contractility, stroke volume, cardiac output. Improves renal blood flow, urinary output.

PHARMACOKINETICS

Route	Onset	Peak	Duration
IV	1–2 min	10 min	Length of infusion

Metabolized in liver. Primarily excreted in urine. Not removed by hemodialysis. **Half-life:** 2 min.

USES

Short-term management of cardiac decompensation.

PRECAUTIONS

CONTRAINDICATIONS: Hypovolemia, idiopathic hypertrophic subaortic stenosis, sulfite sensitivity. **CAUTIONS:** Atrial fibrillation, hypertension, severe coronary artery disease, MI.

LIFESPAN CONSIDERATIONS:

Pregnancy/Lactation: Unknown if drug crosses placenta or is distributed in breast milk. Has not been administered to pregnant women. **Pregnancy Category B. Children/Elderly:** No age-related precautions noted.

INTERACTIONS

DRUG: Beta-blockers may antagonize effects. **Digoxin** may increase risk of arrhythmias, enhance inotropic effect. **Entacapone** may increase risk of arrhythmias, hypertension, tachycardia. **MAOIs, oxytocics, tricyclic antidepressants** may increase adverse effects (e.g., arrhythmias, hypertension). **HERBAL:** None significant. **FOOD:** None known. **LAB VALUES:** Decreases serum potassium.

AVAILABILITY (Rx)

INFUSION (READY-TO-USE): 1 mg/ml, 2 mg/ml, 4 mg/ml. **INJECTION SOLUTION:** 12.5-mg/ml vial.

ADMINISTRATION/HANDLING

◀ **ALERT** ▶ Correct hypovolemia with volume expanders before dobutamine infusion. Those with atrial fibrillation should be digitalized before infusion. Administer by IV infusion only.

IV

Reconstitution • Dilute 250-mg ampule with 10 ml Sterile Water for Injection or D_5W for Injection. Resulting solution: 25 mg/ml. Add additional 10 ml of diluent if not completely dissolved (resulting solution: 12.5 mg/ml). • Further dilute 250-mg vial with D_5W or 0.9% NaCl. Maximum concentration: 3.125 g/250 ml (12.5 mg/ml).

Rate of administration • Use infusion pump to control flow rate. • Titrate dosage to individual response. • Infiltration causes local inflammatory changes. • Extravasation may cause dermal necrosis.

Storage • Store at room temperature (Freezing produces crystallization). • Pink discoloration of solution (due to oxidation) does not indicate loss of potency if used within recommended time period. • Further diluted solution for infusion must be used within 24 hrs.

IV INCOMPATIBILITIES

Acyclovir (Zovirax), alteplase (Activase), amphotericin B complex (Abelcet, AmBisome, Amphotec), bumetanide (Bumex), cefepime (Maxipime), foscarnet (Foscavir), furosemide (Lasix), heparin, piperacillin/tazobactam (Zosyn).

IV COMPATIBILITIES

Amiodarone (Cordarone), calcium chloride, calcium gluconate, diltiazem (Cardizem), dopamine (Intropin), enalapril (Vasotec), famotidine (Pepcid), hydromorphone (Dilaudid), insulin (regular), lidocaine, lipids, lorazepam (Ativan), magnesium sulfate, midazolam (Versed), milrinone (Primacor), morphine, nitroglycerin, norepinephrine (Levophed), potassium chloride, propofol (Diprivan), total parenteral nutrition (TPN).

INDICATIONS/ROUTES/DOSAGE

◀ **ALERT** ▶ Dosage determined by pt response to drug.

MANAGEMENT OF CARDIAC DECOMPENSATION

IV INFUSION: ADULTS, ELDERLY, CHILDREN: 2.5–20 mcg/kg/min. May be infused at a rate of up to 40 mcg/kg/min to increase cardiac output. **NEONATES:** 2–15 mcg/kg/min.

SIDE EFFECTS

FREQUENT (greater than 5%): Increased heart rate, B/P. **OCCASIONAL (5%–3%):** Pain at injection site. **RARE (3%–1%):** Nausea, headache, anginal pain, shortness of breath, fever.

ADVERSE EFFECTS/ TOXIC REACTIONS

Overdose may produce marked increase in heart rate (30 beats/min or higher), marked increase in B/P (50 mm Hg or higher), anginal pain, premature ventricular contractions (PVCs).

NURSING CONSIDERATIONS

BASELINE ASSESSMENT

Pt must be on continuous cardiac monitoring. Determine weight (for dosage calculation). Obtain initial B/P, heart rate, respirations. Correct hypovolemia before drug therapy.

INTERVENTION/EVALUATION

Continuously monitor for cardiac rate, arrhythmias. With physician, establish parameters for adjusting rate, stopping infusion. Maintain accurate I&O; measure urinary output frequently. Assess serum potassium, plasma dobutamine (therapeutic range: 40–190 ng/ml). Monitor B/P continuously (hypertension risk greater in pts with preexisting hypertension). Check cardiac output, pulmonary wedge pressure/central venous pressure (CVP) frequently. Immediately notify physician of decreased urinary output, cardiac arrhythmias, significant increase in B/P, heart rate, or less commonly hypotension.

Dobutrex, *see dobutamine*

docetaxel

dox-eh-**tax**-el

(Taxotere)

Do not confuse docetaxel with Taxol.

CLASSIFICATION

PHARMACOTHERAPEUTIC: Antimitotic agent, taxoid. **CLINICAL:** Antineoplastic (see p. 78C).

ACTION

Disrupts microtubular cell network, essential for cellular function. **Therapeutic Effect:** Inhibits cellular mitosis.

PHARMACOKINETICS

Distributed into peripheral compartments. Protein binding: 94%. Extensively metabolized. Excreted primarily in feces, with lesser amount in urine. **Half-life:** 11.1 hrs.

USES

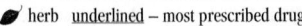

Treatment of locally advanced or metastatic breast carcinoma after failure of prior chemotherapy. Treatment of metastatic non–small cell lung cancer. Treatment of metastatic prostate cancer, head and neck cancer (with prednisone). Treatment of stomach cancer. **OFF-LABEL:** Bladder, esophageal, gastric, ovarian, small cell lung carcinoma.

PRECAUTIONS

CONTRAINDICATIONS: History of severe hypersensitivity to drugs formulated with polysorbate 80, neutrophil count less than 1,500 cells/mm^3. **CAUTIONS:** Hepatic impairment; myelosuppression; herpes zoster (shingles); varicella zoster (chickenpox); preexisting pleural effusion, infection, chemotherapy, radiation.

LIFESPAN CONSIDERATIONS:

Pregnancy/Lactation: May cause fetal harm. Unknown if distributed in breast milk; do not breast-feed. **Pregnancy Category D. Children:** Safety and efficacy not established in those younger than 16 yrs. **Elderly:** No age-related precautions noted.

INTERACTIONS

DRUG: Cyclosporine, erythromycin, ketoconazole may significantly inhibit docetaxel metabolism. **Hepatic enzyme inhibitors (e.g., erythromycin, ketoconazole)** may increase concentration/toxicity. **Immunosuppresants (e.g., cyclophosphamide, cyclosporine)** may increase risk of infection. **Live virus vaccines** may potentiate replication, increase vaccine side effects, decrease pt's antibody response to vaccine. **HERBAL: St. John's wort** may decrease concentration. **FOOD:** None known. **LAB VALUES:** May significantly increase BUN, serum alkaline phosphatase, bilirubin, creatinine, AST, ALT. Reduces neutrophil, thrombocyte, WBC counts.

AVAILABILITY (Rx)

INJECTION SOLUTION: 20 mg/0.5 ml with diluent, 80 mg/2 ml with diluent.

ADMINISTRATION/HANDLING

◀ ALERT ▶ Pt should be premedicated with oral corticosteroids (e.g., dexamethasone 16 mg/day for 5 days beginning day 1 before docetaxel therapy); reduces severity of fluid retention, hypersensitivity reaction.

IV

Reconstitution • Withdraw contents of diluent (provided by manufacturer) and add to vial of docetaxel. • Gently rotate to ensure thorough mixing to provide a solution of 10 mg/ml. • Withdraw dose and add to 250 ml 0.9% NaCl or D_5W in glass or polyolefin container to provide a final concentration of 0.3–0.9 mg/ml.

Rate of administration • Administer as a 1-hr infusion. • Monitor closely for hypersensitivity reaction (flushing, localized skin reaction, bronchospasm [may occur within a few min after beginning infusion]).

Storage • Refrigerate vial. Freezing does not adversely affect drug. • Protect from bright light. • Stand vial at room temperature for 5 min before administering (do not store in PVC bags). • Remixed solution is stable for 8 hrs either at room temperature or if refrigerated.

IV INCOMPATIBILITIES

Amphotericin B (Fungizone), doxorubicin liposomal (DaunoXome), methylprednisolone (Solu-Medrol), nalbuphine (Nubain).

IV COMPATIBILITIES

Bumetanide (Bumex), calcium gluconate, dexamethasone (Decadron), diphenhydramine (Benadryl), dobutamine (Dobutrex), dopamine (Inotropin), furosemide (Lasix), granisetron (Kytril), heparin, hydromorphone (Dilaudid), lorazepam (Ativan), magnesium sulfate, mannitol, morphine, ondansetron (Zofran), potassium chloride.

INDICATIONS/ROUTES/DOSAGE

BREAST CARCINOMA

IV: ADULTS: 60–100 mg/m^2 given over 1 hr q3wk. If pt develops febrile neutropenia, neutrophil count less than 500 cells/mm^3 for longer than 1 wk, severe or cumulative cutaneous reactions, severe peripheral neuropathy with initial dose of 100 mg/m^2, dosage should be decreased to 75 mg/m^2. If reaction continues, dosage should be further reduced to 55 mg/m^2 or therapy should be discontinued. Pts who do not experience these symptoms at a dose of 60 mg/m^2 may tolerate an increased docetaxel dose.

NON–SMALL CELL LUNG CARCINOMA

IV: ADULTS: 75 mg/m^2 q3wk. Adjust dosage if toxicity occurs.

PROSTATE CANCER

IV: ADULTS, ELDERLY: 75 mg/m^2 q3wk with concurrent administration of prednisone 5 mg twice a day.

STOMACH CANCER, HEAD/NECK CANCER

IV: ADULTS, ELDERLY: 75 mg/m^2 followed by cisplatin 75 mg/m^2 on day 1 only, then followed by 5-fluorouracil 750 mg/m^2 as 24 hr infusion for 5 days. Repeat q3wk.

SIDE EFFECTS

FREQUENT: Alopecia (80%), asthenia (62%), hypersensitivity reaction e.g., dermatitis (59%), decreases to 16% in those pretreated with oral corticosteroids), fluid retention (49%), stomatitis (43%), nausea, diarrhea (40%), fever (30%), nail changes (28%), vomiting (24%), myalgia (19%). **OCCASIONAL:** Hypotension, edema, anorexia, headache, weight gain, infection (urinary tract, injection site, indwelling catheter tip), dizziness. **RARE:** Dry skin, sensory disorders (vision, speech, taste), arthralgia, weight loss, conjunctivitis, hematuria, proteinuria.

ADVERSE EFFECTS/ TOXIC REACTIONS

In pts with normal hepatic function tests, neutropenia (neutrophil count less than 2,000 cells/mm^3), leukopenia (WBC count less than 4,000 cells/mm^3) occur in 96% of pts; anemia (hemoglobin level less than 11 g/dl) occurs in 90% of pts; thrombocytopenia (platelet count less than 100,000 cells/mm^3) occurs in 8% of pts; infection occurs in 28% of pts. Neurosensory, neuromotor disturbances (distal paresthesias, weakness) occur in 54% and 13% of pts, respectively.

NURSING CONSIDERATIONS

BASELINE ASSESSMENT

Offer emotional support to pt, family. Antiemetics may be effective in preventing, treating nausea/vomiting. Pt should be pretreated with corticosteroids before therapy to reduce fluid retention, hypersensitivity reaction.

INTERVENTION/ EVALUATION

Frequent monitoring of blood counts is essential, particularly neutrophil count (less than 1,500 cells/mm^3 requires discontinuation of therapy). Monitor renal/hepatic function tests; serum uric acid levels. Observe for cutaneous reactions (rash with eruptions, mainly on hands, feet). Assess for extravascular fluid accumulation: rales in lungs, dependent edema, dyspnea at rest, pronounced abdominal distention (due to ascites).

PATIENT/FAMILY TEACHING

• Alopecia is reversible, but new hair growth may have different color or texture. • New hair growth resumes 2–3 mos after last therapy dose. • Maintain fastidious oral hygiene. • Do not have immunizations without physician approval (drug lowers resistance). • Avoid those who have recently taken any live virus vaccine.

docusate

dok-yoo-sate

(Apo-Docusate ✤, Colace ✤, Diocto, Docusoft-S, Novo-Ducosate ✤, PMS-Docusate ✤, Pro-Cal-Sof, Regulex ✤, Selax ✤, Soflax ✤, Surfak)

CLASSIFICATION

PHARMACOTHERAPEUTIC: Bulk-producing laxative. **CLINICAL:** Stool softener (see p. 117C).

ACTION

Decreases surface film tension by mixing liquid with bowel contents. **Therapeutic Effect:** Increases infiltration of liquid to form a softer stool.

PHARMACOKINETICS

Minimal absorption from GI tract. Acts in small and large intestines. Results usually occur 1–2 days after first dose but may take 3–5 days.

USES

Stool softener for those who need to avoid straining during defecation; constipation associated with hard, dry stools.

PRECAUTIONS

CONTRAINDICATIONS: Acute abdominal pain, concomitant use of mineral oil, intestinal obstruction, nausea, vomiting. **CAUTIONS:** Do not use for longer than 1 wk.

LIFESPAN CONSIDERATIONS:

Pregnancy/Lactation: Unknown if drug is distributed in breast milk. **Pregnancy Category C. Children:** Not recommended in children younger than 6 yrs. **Elderly:** No age-related precautions noted.

INTERACTIONS

DRUG: May increase absorption of **danthron** or **mineral oil. HERBAL:** None significant. **FOOD:** None known. **LAB VALUES:** None known.

AVAILABILITY (OTC)

CAPSULES: 50 mg (Colace), 100 mg (Colace, Ducosoft-S), 240 mg (Surfak). **LIQUID (COLACE, DIOCTO):** 50 mg/5 ml (sodium). **SYRUP (COLACE, DIOCTO):** 60 mg/15 ml.

ADMINISTRATION/HANDLING

• Drink 6–8 glasses of water a day (aids stool softening). • Give each dose with full glass of water, fruit juice. • Administer docusate liquid with milk, fruit juice, infant formula (masks bitter taste).

INDICATIONS/ROUTES/DOSAGE

STOOL SOFTENER

PO: ADULTS, ELDERLY, CHILDREN 12 YRS AND OLDER: 50–500 mg/day in 1–4 divided doses. **CHILDREN 6–11 YRS:** 40–150 mg/day in 1–4 divided doses. **CHILDREN 3–5 YRS:** 20–60 mg/day in 1–4 divided doses. **CHILDREN YOUNGER THAN 3 YRS:** 10–40 mg in 1–4 divided doses.

SIDE EFFECTS

OCCASIONAL: Mild GI cramping, throat irritation (with liquid preparation). **RARE:** Rash.

ADVERSE EFFECTS/ TOXIC REACTIONS

None known.

NURSING CONSIDERATIONS

INTERVENTION/EVALUATION

Encourage adequate fluid intake. Assess bowel sounds for peristalsis. Monitor daily pattern of bowel activity/stool consistency; record time of evacuation.

PATIENT/FAMILY TEACHING

• Institute measures to promote defecation: increase fluid intake, exercise, high-fiber diet. • Do not use for longer than 1 wk.

D

dolasetron

dole-**ah**-seh-tron
(Anzemet)

Do not confuse Anzemet with Aldomet.

CLASSIFICATION

PHARMACOTHERAPEUTIC: Selective receptor antagonist. **CLINICAL:** Antiemetic.

ACTION

Acts centrally in chemoreceptor trigger zone, peripherally at the vagal nerve terminals to antagonize 5-HT_3 receptors. **Therapeutic Effect:** Prevents nausea/vomiting.

PHARMACOKINETICS

Readily absorbed from GI tract after PO administration. Protein binding: 69%–77%. Metabolized in the liver. Primarily excreted in urine. Unknown if removed by hemodialysis. **Half-life:** 5–10 hrs.

USES

Oral: Prevention of nausea/vomiting associated with cancer chemotherapy, including high-dose cisplatin; prevention of postop nausea/vomiting. **Injection:** Treatment of postop nausea/vomiting. **OFF-LABEL:** Radiation therapy-induced nausea/vomiting.

PRECAUTIONS

CONTRAINDICATIONS: None known. **CAUTIONS:** Those who have or may have prolongation of cardiac conduction intervals, hypokalemia, hypomagnesemia, those taking diuretics with potential for inducing electrolyte disturbances, congenital prolonged QT interval syndrome, those taking antiarrhythmics that may lead to QT prolongation, cumulative high-dose anthracycline therapy.

LIFESPAN CONSIDERATIONS:

Pregnancy/Lactation: Unknown if drug is distributed in breast milk. **Pregnancy Category B. Children:** Safety and efficacy not established in those younger than 2 yrs. **Elderly:** No age-related precautions noted.

INTERACTIONS

DRUG: Medications prolonging QT interval (e.g., clarithromycin, tricyclic antidepressants) may have additive effects. **HERBAL: St. John's wort** may decrease concentration. **FOOD:** None known. **LAB VALUES:** May transiently increase AST, ALT.

AVAILABILITY (Rx)

INJECTION, SOLUTION: 20 mg/ml in single use 0.625 ml amps, 0.625 ml fill in 2 ml Carpuject and 5 ml vials.

TABLETS: 50 mg, 100 mg.

ADMINISTRATION/HANDLING

IV

Reconstitution • May dilute in 0.9% NaCl, D_5W, D_5W with 0.45% NaCl, D_5W with lactated Ringer's, lactated Ringer's, or 10% mannitol injection to 50 ml.

Rate of administration • Can be given as IV push as rapidly as 100 mg/30 sec. • Intermittent IV infusion (piggyback) may be infused over 15 min.

Storage • Store vials at room temperature. • After dilution, solution is stable for 24 hrs at room temperature or 48 hrs if refrigerated.

PO

• Do not cut, break, chew film-coated tablets. • For children 2–16 yrs, injection form may be mixed in juice for oral dosing at 1.8 mg/kg up to a maximum of 100 mg.

IV INCOMPATIBILITIES

No information available on Y-site administration.

INDICATIONS/ROUTES/DOSAGE

TREATMENT/PREVENTION OF CHEMOTHERAPY-INDUCED NAUSEA/VOMITING

PO: ADULTS: 100 mg within 1 hr of chemotherapy. **CHILDREN 2–16 YRS:** 1.8 mg/kg within 1 hr of chemotherapy. **Maximum:** 100 mg.

IV: ADULTS, CHILDREN 1–16 YRS: 1.8 mg/kg as a single dose 30 min before chemotherapy. **Maximum:** 100 mg.

TREATMENT/PREVENTION OF POSTOPERATIVE NAUSEA/VOMITING

PO: ADULTS: 100 mg within 2 hrs of surgery. **CHILDREN 2–16 YRS:** 1.2 mg/kg within 2 hrs of surgery. **Maximum:** 100 mg.

IV: ADULTS: 12.5 mg 15 min before cessation of anesthesia or as soon as nausea occurs. **CHILDREN 2–16 YRS:** 0.35 mg/kg 15 min before cessation of anesthesia or as soon as nausea occurs. **Maximum:** 12.5 mg.

SIDE EFFECTS

FREQUENT (10%–5%): Headache, diarrhea, fatigue. **OCCASIONAL (5%–1%):** Fever, dizziness, tachycardia, dyspepsia.

ADVERSE EFFECTS/ TOXIC REACTIONS

Overdose may produce a combination of CNS stimulant, depressant effects.

NURSING CONSIDERATIONS

BASELINE ASSESSMENT

Assess for dehydration if excessive vomiting occurs (poor skin turgor, dry mucous membranes, longitudinal furrows in tongue). Provide emotional support.

INTERVENTION/EVALUATION

Monitor for therapeutic relief from nausea/vomiting, EKG in high-risk pts. Maintain quiet, supportive atmosphere.

Dolobid, *see diflunisal*

Dolophine, *see methadone*

donepezil

doh-**neh**-peh-zil

(Aricept, Aricept ODT)

Do not confuse Aricept with Aciphex or Ascriptin.

CLASSIFICATION

PHARMACOTHERAPEUTIC: Cholinesterase inhibitor. **CLINICAL:** Cholinergic.

ACTION

Inhibits enzyme acetylcholinesterase, increasing concentration of acetylcholine at cholinergic synapses, enhancing cholinergic function in CNS. **Therapeutic Effect:** Slows progression of Alzheimer's disease.

PHARMACOKINETICS

Well absorbed after PO administration. Protein binding: 96%. Extensively metabolized. Eliminated in urine, feces. **Half-life:** 70 hrs.

USES

Treatment of mild to moderate to severe dementia of Alzheimer's disease. **OFF-LABEL:** Treatment of attention deficit hyperactivity disorder, autism, behavioral syndromes in dementia.

PRECAUTIONS

CONTRAINDICATIONS: History of hypersensitivity to piperidine derivatives. **CAUTIONS:** Asthma, chronic obstructive pulmonary disease (COPD), bladder outflow obstruction, history of ulcer disease, those taking concurrent NSAIDs, supraventricular cardiac conduction disturbances (e.g., "sick sinus syndrome," Wolff-Parkinson-White syndrome), seizures.

D

LIFESPAN CONSIDERATIONS:

Pregnancy/Lactation: Unknown if drug is distributed in breast milk. **Pregnancy Category C.** **Children:** Safety and efficacy not established. **Elderly:** No age-related precautions noted.

INTERACTIONS

DRUG: May decrease effect of **anticholinergic medications.** May increase synergistic effects of **cholinergic agonists, neuromuscular blockers, succinylcholine. Ketoconazole, quinidine** may inhibit metabolism of donepezil. May increase gastric acid secretion with **NSAIDs. Paroxetine** may decrease metabolism, increase concentration of donepezil. **HERBAL: St. John's wort** may decrease concentration. **FOOD:** None known. **LAB VALUES:** May increase serum glucose, creatine kinase, LDH. May decrease serum potassium.

AVAILABILITY (Rx)

TABLETS (ARICEPT): 5 mg, 10 mg. **TABLETS (ORALLY DISINTEGRATING [ARICEPT ODT]):** 5 mg, 10 mg.

ADMINISTRATION/HANDLING

PO

• May be given without regard to meals or time of administration, although it is suggested dose be given in the evening, just before bedtime.

ODT

• Allow to dissolve completely on tongue. • Follow dose with water.

INDICATIONS/ROUTES/DOSAGE

ALZHEIMER'S DISEASE

PO: ADULTS, ELDERLY: Initially 5–10 mg/day at bedtime. May increase at 4–6 wk intervals to maximum 10 mg/day at bedtime.

SIDE EFFECTS

FREQUENT (11%–8%): Nausea, diarrhea, headache, insomnia, nonspecific pain, dizziness. **OCCASIONAL (6%–3%):** Mild muscle cramps, fatigue, vomiting, anorexia, ecchymosis. **RARE (3%–2%):** Depression, abnormal dreams, weight loss, arthritis, somnolence, syncope, frequent urination.

ADVERSE EFFECTS/ TOXIC REACTIONS

Overdose may result in cholinergic crisis (severe nausea, increased salivation, diaphoresis, bradycardia, hypotension, flushed skin, abdominal pain, respiratory depression, seizures, cardiorespiratory collapse). Increasing muscle weakness may occur, resulting in death if muscles of respiration become involved. **ANTIDOTE:** Atropine sulfate 1–2 mg IV with subsequent doses based on therapeutic response.

NURSING CONSIDERATIONS

BASELINE ASSESSMENT

Obtain baseline vital signs. Assess history for peptic ulcer, urinary obstruction, asthma, COPD, seizure disorder, cardiac conduction disturbances.

INTERVENTION/EVALUATION

Monitor for cholinergic reaction (GI discomfort/cramping, feeling of facial warmth, excessive salivation/diaphoresis), lacrimation, pallor, urinary urgency, dizziness. Monitor for nausea, diarrhea, headache, insomnia.

PATIENT/FAMILY TEACHING

• Report nausea, vomiting, diarrhea, diaphoresis, increased salivary secretions, severe abdominal pain, dizziness. • May take without regard to food. • Not a cure for Alzheimer's disease but may slow progression of symptoms.

D

dong quai

Also known as Chinese angelica, dang gui, tang kuei, toki.

CLASSIFICATION

HERBAL: See Appendix G.

ACTION

Competitively inhibits estradiol binding to estrogen receptors. Has vasodilatory, antispasmodic, CNS stimulant activity. **Effect:** Reduces symptoms of menopause.

USES

Gynecologic ailments, including menstrual cramps, menopause symptoms; uterine stimulant. Used as antihypertensive, anti-inflammatory, vasodilator, immunosuppressant, analgesic, antipyretic.

PRECAUTIONS

CONTRAINDICATIONS: Pregnancy due to uterine stimulant effect, bleeding disorders, excessive menstrual flow. **CAUTIONS:** Lactation; breast, ovarian, uterine cancer.

LIFESPAN CONSIDERATIONS:

Pregnancy/Lactation: Contraindicated. **Children:** Safety and efficacy not established. **Elderly:** No age-related precautions noted.

INTERACTIONS

DRUG: Anticoagulant effect risk of bleeding increased with **warfarin.** **HERBAL:** **Feverfew, garlic, ginger, ginkgo, ginseng** may increase risk of bleeding. **FOOD:** None known. **LAB VALUES:** May increase prothrombin time (PT), INR.

AVAILABILITY (Rx)

DONG QUAI SOFTGEL: 200 mg, 530 mg, 565 mg.

INDICATIONS/ROUTES/DOSAGE

GYNECOLOGIC AILMENTS, OTHER USES

PO: ADULTS, ELDERLY: 3–4 g a day in divided doses with meals.

SIDE EFFECTS

Diarrhea, photosensitivity, nausea, vomiting, anorexia, increased menstrual flow.

ADVERSE EFFECTS/ TOXIC REACTIONS

None known.

NURSING CONSIDERATIONS

BASELINE ASSESSMENT

Assess if pt is pregnant or breastfeeding, taking other medications, esp. those that increase risk of bleeding.

INTERVENTION/EVALUATION

Assess for hypersensitivity reaction.

PATIENT/FAMILY TEACHING

• Inform physician if pregnant or planning to become pregnant. • Do not breast-feed. • May cause photosensitivity reaction; sunscreen, protective clothing should be worn.

*DOPamine

dope-a-meen

(Intropin)

Do not confuse dopamine with dobutamine or Dopram, or Intropin with Isoptin.

CLASSIFICATION

PHARMACOTHERAPEUTIC: Sympathomimetic (adrenergic agonist). **CLINICAL:** Cardiac stimulant, vasopressor (see p. 147C).

ACTION

Stimulates adrenergic receptors. Effects are dose dependent. **Low dosage (less than 5 mcg/kg/min):** Stimulates dopaminergic receptors, causing renal vasodilation. **Low to moderate dosages (10 mcg/kg/min or less):** Has a positive inotropic effect by direct action, release of norepinephrine. **High dosage (greater than 10 mcg/kg/min):** Stimulates alpha-receptors. **Therapeutic Effect: Low dosage:** Increases renal blood flow, urinary flow, sodium excretion. **Low to moderate dosages:** Increases myocardial contractility, stroke volume, cardiac output. **High dosage:** Increases peripheral resistance, renal vasoconstriction, B/P.

PHARMACOKINETICS

Route	Onset	Peak	Duration
IV	1–2 min	N/A	Less than 10 min

Widely distributed. Does not cross blood-brain barrier. Metabolized in liver, kidney, plasma. Primarily excreted in urine. Not removed by hemodialysis. **Half-life:** 2 min.

USES

Prophylaxis/treatment of acute hypotension, shock (associated with MI, trauma, renal failure, cardiac decompensation, open heart surgery), treatment of low cardiac output, congestive heart failure (CHF).

PRECAUTIONS

CONTRAINDICATIONS: Pheochromocytoma, sulfite sensitivity, uncorrected tachyarrhythmias, ventricular fibrillation. **CAUTIONS:** Ischemic heart disease, occlusive vascular disease, hypovolemia, recent use of MAOIs, ventricular arrhythmias.

LIFESPAN CONSIDERATIONS:

Pregnancy/Lactation: Unknown if drug crosses placenta or is distributed in breast milk. **Pregnancy Category C. Children:** Recommended close hemodynamic monitoring (gangrene due to extravasation reported). **Elderly:** No age-related precautions noted.

INTERACTIONS

DRUG: Beta-blockers may decrease effects of dopamine. **Digoxin** may increase risk of arrhythmias. **Ergot alkaloids** may increase vasoconstriction. **MAOIs** may increase cardiac stimulation, vasopressor effects. **Tricyclic antidepressants** may increase cardiovascular effects. **HERBAL:** None significant. **FOOD:** None known. **LAB VALUES:** None known.

AVAILABILITY (Rx)

INJECTION SOLUTION: 40 mg/ml, 80 mg/ml, 160 mg/ml. **INJECTION (PREMIX WITH DEXTROSE):** 80 mg/100 ml, 160 mg/100 ml, 320 mg/100 ml.

ADMINISTRATION/HANDLING

◀ **ALERT** ▶ Blood volume depletion must be corrected before administering dopamine (may be used concurrently with fluid replacement).

IV

Reconstitution • Available prediluted in 250 or 500 ml D_5W or dilute each 5-ml (200-mg) ampule in 250–500 ml 0.9% NaCl, D_5W/0.45 NaCl, D_5W/0.45 NaCl, D_5W/lactated Ringer's, or lactated Ringer's (concentration is dependent on dosage and fluid requirement of pt); 250 ml solution yields 800 mcg/ml; 500 ml solution yields 400 mcg/ml. Maximum concentration: 3.2 g/250 ml (12.8 mg/ml).

Rate of administration • Administer into large vein (antecubital fossa, central line preferred) to prevent extravasation.

• Use infusion pump to control flow rate. • Titrate drug to desired hemodynamic, renal response (optimum urinary flow determines dosage).

Storage • Do not use solutions darker than slightly yellow or discolored to yellow, brown, pink to purple (indicates decomposition of drug). • Stable for 24 hrs after dilution.

IV INCOMPATIBILITIES

Acyclovir (Zovirax), amphotericin B complex (Abelcet, AmBisome, Amphotec), cefepime (Maxipime), furosemide (Lasix), insulin, sodium bicarbonate.

IV COMPATIBILITIES

Amiodarone (Cordarone), calcium chloride, diltiazem (Cardizem), dobutamine (Dobutrex), enalapril (Vasotec), heparin, hydromorphone (Dilaudid), labetalol (Trandate), levofloxacin (Levaquin), lidocaine, lipids, lorazepam (Ativan), methylprednisolone (Solu-Medrol), midazolam (Versed), milrinone (Primacor), morphine, nicardipine (Cardene), nitroglycerin, norepinephrine (Levophed), piperacillin/tazobactam (Zosyn), potassium chloride, propofol (Diprivan), total parenteral nutrition (TPN).

INDICATIONS/ROUTES/DOSAGE

ACUTE HYPOTENSION, SHOCK

IV INFUSION: ADULTS, ELDERLY: Initially, 2–5 mcg/kg/min. Increase in 5–10 mcg/kg/min increments. **Maximum:** 50 mcg/kg/min. **CHILDREN:** Initally, 2–5 mcg/kg/min. Increase in 5–10 mcg/kg/min increments. **Maximum:** 30 mcg/kg/min.

CHF

IV INFUSION: ADULTS, ELDERLY: Initially, 2–5 mcg/kg/min. Increase in 5–10 mcg/kg/min increments. **Maximum:** 50 mcg/kg/min. **CHILDREN:** Initally, 2–5 mcg/kg/min. Increase in 5–10 mcg/kg/min increments. **Maximum:** 20–30 mcg/kg/min.

SIDE EFFECTS

FREQUENT: Headache, arrhythmias, tachycardia, anginal pain, palpitations, vasoconstriction, hypotension, nausea, vomiting, dyspnea. **OCCASIONAL:** Piloerection (goose bumps), bradycardia, widening of QRS complex.

ADVERSE EFFECTS/ TOXIC REACTIONS

High doses may produce ventricular arrhythmias. Pts with occlusive vascular disease are at high risk for further compromise of circulation to extremities, which may result in gangrene. Tissue necrosis with sloughing may occur with extravasation of IV solution.

NURSING CONSIDERATIONS

BASELINE ASSESSMENT

Check for MAOI therapy within last 2–3 wks (requires dosage reduction). Pt must be on continuous cardiac monitoring. Determine weight (for dosage calculation). Obtain initial B/P, heart rate, respirations.

INTERVENTION/EVALUATION

Continuously monitor for cardiac arrhythmias. Measure urinary output frequently. If extravasation occurs, immediately infiltrate affected tissue with 10–15 ml 0.9% NaCl solution containing 5–10 mg phentolamine mesylate. Monitor B/P, heart rate, respirations q15min during administration (more often if indicated). Assess cardiac output, pulmonary wedge pressure, or central venous pressure (CVP) frequently. Assess peripheral circulation (palpate pulses, note color/temperature of extremities). Immediately notify physician of decreased urinary output, cardiac arrhythmias, significant changes in B/P, heart rate, or failure to respond to increase or decrease in infusion rate, decreased peripheral circulation (cold, pale, mottled extremities). Taper dosage before discontinuing (abrupt cessation of therapy may result in marked hypotension). Be alert to excessive vasoconstriction (decreased urine output, increased heart rate, arrhythmias, disproportionate increase in diastolic B/P, decrease in pulse pressure); slow or temporarily stop infusion, notify physician.

D

dorzolamide

(Trusopt)

See Antiglaucoma agents (p. 50C)

doxacurium

(Nuromax)

See Neuromuscular blockers (p. 119C)

doxazosin

dox-ay-**zoe**-sin

(Apo-Doxazosin ✱, Cardura)

Do not confuse doxazosin with doxapram, doxepin, or doxorubicin, or Cardura with Cardene, Cordarone, Coumadin, K-Dur, or Ridaura.

◆ CLASSIFICATION

PHARMACOTHERAPEUTIC: Alpha-adrenergic blocker. **CLINICAL:** Antihypertensive (see p. 59C).

ACTION

Selectively blocks alpha$_1$-adrenergic receptors, decreasing peripheral vascular resistance. **Therapeutic Effect:** Causes peripheral vasodilation, lowering B/P. Relaxes smooth muscle of bladder, prostate.

PHARMACOKINETICS

Route	Onset	Peak	Duration
PO	N/A	2–6 hrs	24 hrs

Well absorbed from GI tract. Protein binding: 98%–99%. Metabolized in liver. Primarily eliminated in feces. Not removed by hemodialysis. **Half-life:** 19–22 hrs.

USES

Treatment of mild to moderate hypertension. Used alone or in combination with other antihypertensives. Treatment of benign prostatic hyperplasia alone or in combination with finasteride (Proscar).

PRECAUTIONS

CONTRAINDICATIONS: Hypersensitivity to other quinazolines. **CAUTIONS:** Carcinoma of the prostate, chronic renal failure, hepatic impairment, recent cerebrovascular accident (CVA).

⌛ LIFESPAN CONSIDERATIONS:

Pregnancy/Lactation: Unknown if drug crosses placenta or is distributed in breast milk. **Pregnancy Category C. Children:** Safety and efficacy not established. **Elderly:** May be more sensitive to hypotensive effects.

INTERACTIONS

DRUG: NSAIDS may decrease effect. **Hypotension-producing medications (e.g., antihypertensives, diuretics)** may increase effect. **Sildenafil, tadalafil, vardenafil** may potentiate hypotensive effects. **Sympathomimetics** may decrease antihypertensive effect. **HERBAL: Ephedra, ginseng, yohimbe** may worsen hypertension. **Garlic** may increase antihypertensive effect. Avoid **saw palmetto** (limited experience with this combination). **FOOD:** None known. **LAB VALUES:** None known.

AVAILABILITY (Rx)

TABLETS: 1 mg, 2 mg, 4 mg, 8 mg.

ADMINISTRATION/HANDLING

PO

- Give without regard to food.

INDICATIONS/ROUTES/DOSAGE

HYPERTENSION

PO: ADULTS: Initially, 1 mg once a day. May increase to a maximum of 16 mg/day. **ELDERLY:** Initially, 0.5 mg once a day.

BENIGN PROSTATIC HYPERPLASIA

PO: ADULTS, ELDERLY: Initially, 1 mg/day. May increase q1–2wk. **Maximum:** 8 mg/day.

SIDE EFFECTS

FREQUENT (20%–10%): Dizziness, asthenia, headache, edema. **OCCASIONAL (9%–3%):** Nausea, pharyngitis, rhinitis, pain in extremities, somnolence. **RARE (3%–1%):** Palpitations, diarrhea, constipation, dyspnea, myalgia, altered vision, anxiety.

ADVERSE EFFECTS/ TOXIC REACTIONS

First-dose syncope (hypotension with sudden loss of consciousness) may occur 30–90 min following initial dose of 2 mg or greater, too-rapid increase in dosage, addition of another antihypertensive agent to therapy. First-dose syncope may be preceded by tachycardia (pulse rate 120–160 beats/min).

NURSING CONSIDERATIONS

BASELINE ASSESSMENT

Give first dose at bedtime. If initial dose is given during daytime, pt must remain recumbent for 3–4 hrs. Assess B/P, pulse immediately before each dose, and q15–30min until B/P is stabilized (be alert to fluctuations).

INTERVENTION/EVALUATION

Monitor pulse diligently (first-dose syncope may be preceded by tachycardia). Assess for edema, headache. Assist with ambulation if dizziness, light-headedness occurs.

PATIENT/FAMILY TEACHING

• Full therapeutic effect may not occur for 3–4 wks. • May cause syncope (fainting). • Avoid tasks that require alertness, motor skills until response to drug is established.

doxepin

dox-eh-pin

(Apo-Doxepin ✤, Novo-Doxepin ✤, Prudoxin, Sinequan, Zonalon)

Do not confuse doxepin with doxapram, doxazosin, or Doxidan, or Sinequan with saquinavir.

CLASSIFICATION

PHARMACOTHERAPEUTIC: Tricyclic. **CLINICAL:** Antidepressant, antianxiety, antineuralgic, antiulcer, antipruritic (see p. 37C).

ACTION

Increases synaptic concentrations of norepinephrine, serotonin. **Therapeutic Effect:** Produces antidepressant, anxiolytic effects.

PHARMACOKINETICS

Rapidly, well absorbed from GI tract. Protein binding: 80%–85%. Metabolized in liver to active metabolite. Primarily excreted in urine. Not removed by hemodialysis. **Half-life:** 6–8 hrs. **Topical:** Absorbed through skin. Distributed to body tissues. Metabolized to active metabolite. Excreted in urine.

D

USES

Treatment of various forms of depression, often in conjunction with psychotherapy. Treatment of anxiety. **Topical:** Treatment of pruritus associated with eczema. **OFF-LABEL:** Treatment of neurogenic pain, panic disorder; prophylaxis for vascular headache, pruritus in idiopathic urticaria.

PRECAUTIONS

CONTRAINDICATIONS: Angle-closure glaucoma, hypersensitivity to other tricyclic antidepressants, urinary retention. **CAUTIONS:** Schizophrenia, cardiac/hepatic/renal disease, diabetes mellitus, increased intraocular pressure, glaucoma, history of seizures, history of urinary retention/obstruction, hyperthyroidism, prostatic hypertrophy, hiatal hernia.

LIFESPAN CONSIDERATIONS:

Pregnancy/Lactation: Crosses placenta. Distributed in breast milk. **Pregnancy Category C (B for topical form). Children:** Safety and efficacy not established in children younger than 12 yrs. **Elderly:** Increased risk of toxicity (lower dosages recommended).

INTERACTIONS

DRUG: Alcohol, other CNS depressants may increase CNS, respiratory depression, hypotensive effects. **Antithyroid agents** may increase risk of agranulocytosis. **Cimetidine** may increase concentration, risk of toxicity. May decrease effects of **clonidine. MAOIs** may increase risk of seizures, hyperpyrexia, hypertensive crisis. **Phenothiazines** may increase anticholinergic, sedative effects. **Sympathomimetics** may increase cardiac effects. **HERBAL: Kava kava, SAMe, St. John's wort, valerian** may increase sedation, risk of serotonin syndrome. **FOOD: Grapefruit, grapefruit juice** may increase concentration/toxicity. **LAB VALUES:** May alter serum glucose, EKG readings. Therapeutic serum level: 110–250 ng/ml; toxic serum level: greater than 300 ng/ml.

AVAILABILITY (Rx)

CAPSULES (SINEQUAN): 10 mg, 25 mg, 50 mg, 75 mg, 100 mg, 150 mg. **CREAM (PRUDOXIN, ZONALON):** 5%. **ORAL CONCENTRATE (SINEQUAN):** 10 mg/ml.

ADMINISTRATION/HANDLING

PO

• Give with food, milk if GI distress occurs. • Dilute concentrate in 4-oz glass of water, milk, orange, tomato, prune, pineapple juice. Incompatible with carbonated drinks. • Give larger portion of daily dose at bedtime.

TOPICAL

• Apply thin film of cream on affected areas of skin. • Do not use for more than 8 days. • Do not use occlusive dressing.

INDICATIONS/ROUTES/DOSAGE

DEPRESSION, ANXIETY

PO: ADULTS: 25–150 mg/day at bedtime or in 2–3 divided doses. May increase gradually to 300 mg/day. **ELDERLY:** Initially, 10–25 mg at bedtime. May increase by 10–25 mg/day every 3–7 days. **Maximum:** 75 mg/day. **ADOLESCENTS:** Initially, 25–50 mg/day as a single dose or in divided doses. May increase to 100 mg/day. **CHILDREN 12 YRS AND YOUNGER:** 1–3 mg/kg/day.

PRURITUS ASSOCIATED WITH ECZEMA

TOPICAL: ADULTS, ELDERLY: Apply thin film 4 times a day at 3–4 hr intervals. Not recommended for more than 8 days.

SIDE EFFECTS

FREQUENT: Oral: Orthostatic hypotension, somnolence, dry mouth, headache, increased appetite, weight gain, nausea, unusual fatigue, unpleasant taste. **Topical:** Edema; increased pruritus, eczema; burning, tingling, stinging at application site; altered taste; dizziness; drowsiness; dry skin; dry mouth; fatigue;

headache; thirst. **OCCASIONAL: Oral:** Blurred vision, confusion, constipation, hallucinations, difficult urination, eye pain, irregular heartbeat, fine muscle tremors, nervousness, impaired sexual function, diarrhea, diaphoresis, heartburn, insomnia. **Topical:** Anxiety, skin irritation/cracking, nausea. **RARE: Oral:** Allergic reaction, alopecia, tinnitus, breast enlargement. **Topical:** Fever, photosensitivity.

ADVERSE EFFECTS/ TOXIC REACTIONS

Abrupt or too-rapid withdrawal may result in headache, malaise, nausea, vomiting, vivid dreams. Overdose may produce confusion, severe drowsiness, agitation, tachycardia, arrhythmias, shortness of breath, vomiting.

NURSING CONSIDERATIONS

BASELINE ASSESSMENT

Assess B/P, pulse, EKG (those with history of cardiovascular disease). Peform CBC, serum electrolyte tests before long-term therapy. Assess pt's appearance, behavior, level of interest, mood, sleep pattern.

INTERVENTION/EVALUATION

Monitor B/P, pulse, weight. Perform CBC, serum electrolyte tests periodically to assess renal/hepatic function. Supervise suicidal-risk pt closely during early therapy (as depression lessens, energy level improves, increasing suicide potential). Assess appearance, behavior, speech pattern, level of interest, mood. Therapeutic serum level: 110–250 ng/ml; toxic serum level: greater than 300 ng/ml.

PATIENT/FAMILY TEACHING

• Do not discontinue abruptly. • Change positions slowly to avoid dizziness. • Avoid tasks that require alertness, motor skills until response to drug is established. • Do not cover affected area with occlusive dressing after applying cream. • May cause dry mouth. • Avoid alcohol, limit caffeine. • May increase appetite. • Avoid exposure to sunlight/artificial light source. • Therapeutic effect may be noted within 2–5 days, maximum effect within 2–3 wks.

D

doxercalciferol

(Hectorol)

See vitamin D

Doxil, *see doxorubicin*

**DOXOrubicin*

dox-o-**roo**-bi-sin

(Adriamycin, Adriamycin PFS, Adriamycin RDF, Caelyx ✤, Doxil, Rubex)

Do not confuse doxorubicin with daunorubicin, or Adriamycin with idamycin or idarubicin.

✦CLASSIFICATION

PHARMACOTHERAPEUTIC: Anthracycline antibiotic. **CLINICAL:** Antineoplastic (see p. 78C).

ACTION

Inhibits DNA, DNA-dependent RNA synthesis by binding with DNA strands. Liposomal encapsulation increases uptake by tumors, prolongs drug action, may decrease toxicity. **Therapeutic Effect:** Prevents cell division.

PHARMACOKINETICS

Widely distributed. Protein binding: 74%–76%. Does not cross blood-brain barrier. Metabolized rapidly in liver to active metabolite. Primarily eliminated by biliary system. Not removed by hemodialysis. **Half-life:** 16 hrs; metabolite, 32 hrs.

USES

Adriamycin, Rubex: Treatment of acute lymphocytic, nonlymphocytic leukemia, breast, gastric, small cell lung, ovarian, epithelial, thyroid, bladder carcinomas, neuroblastoma, Wilms' tumor, Hodgkin's/non-Hodgkin's lymphoma, osteosarcoma, soft tissue sarcoma. **Doxil:** Treatment of AIDS-related Kaposi's sarcoma, metastatic ovarian cancer. **OFF-LABEL:** Ewing's sarcoma; germ cell, gestational trophoblastic, prostatic tumors; multiple myeloma; retinoblastoma; treatment of cervical, endometrial, esophageal, head/neck, non–small cell lung, pancreatic carcinoma.

PRECAUTIONS

CONTRAINDICATIONS: Cardiomyopathy; preexisting myelosuppression; previous or concomitant treatment with cyclophosphamide, idarubicin, mitoxantrone, or irradiation of cardiac region; severe CHF. **CAUTIONS:** Hepatic impairment.

LIFESPAN CONSIDERATIONS:

Pregnancy/Lactation: If possible, avoid use during pregnancy, esp. first trimester. Breast-feeding not recommended. **Pregnancy Category D.** **Children/Elderly:** Cardiotoxicity may be more frequent in those younger than 2 yrs or older than 70 yrs.

INTERACTIONS

DRUG: May decrease effects of **antigout medications. Bone marrow depressants** may increase myelosuppression. **Daunorubicin** may increase risk of cardiotoxicity. **Live virus vaccines** may potentiate virus replication, increase vaccine side effects, decrease pt's antibody response vaccine. **HERBAL:** **St. John's wort** may decrease concentration. Avoid **black cohosh, dong quai** in estrogen-dependent tumors. **FOOD:** None known. **LAB VALUES:** May cause EKG changes, increase serum uric acid. May reduce neutrophil, RBC counts.

AVAILABILITY (Rx)

INJECTION, POWDER FOR RECONSTITUTION: 10 mg (Adriamycin RDF), 20 mg (Adriamycin RDF), 50 mg (Adriamycin RDF, Rubex), 100 mg (Rubex), 150 mg (Adriamycin RDF). **INJECTION SOLUTION (ADRIAMYCIN PFS):** 2 mg/ml. **LIPID COMPLEX (DOXIL):** 2 mg/ml.

ADMINISTRATION/HANDLING

◄ **ALERT** ► Wear gloves. If powder or solution comes in contact with skin, wash thoroughly. Avoid small veins; swollen/edematous extremities; areas overlying joints, tendons. **Doxil:** Do not use with in-line filter or mix with any diluent except D_5W. May be carcinogenic, mutagenic, teratogenic. Handle with extreme care during preparation/administration.

IV

Reconstitution • Reconstitute each 10-mg vial with 5 ml preservative-free 0.9% NaCl (10 ml for 20 mg; 25 ml for 50 mg) to provide concentration of 2 mg/ml. • Shake vial; allow contents to dissolve. • Withdraw appropriate volume of air from vial during reconstitution (avoids excessive pressure buildup). • May be further diluted with 50 ml D_5W or 0.9% NaCl and given as continuous infusion through a central venous line. **Doxil:** Dilute each dose in 250 ml D_5W.

Rate of administration • For IV push, administer into tubing of freely running IV infusion of D_5W or 0.9% NaCl, preferably via butterfly needle over 3–5 min (avoids local erythematous streaking along vein and facial flushing). • Must test for flashback q30sec to be certain needle remains in vein during injection. • Extravasation produces immediate pain, severe local tissue damage. Terminate administration immediately; withdraw as much medication as possible, obtain extravasation kit, follow protocol. **Doxil:** Give as infusion over 30 min. Do not use in-line filter.

Storage • Store at room temperature. • Reconstituted solution is stable for 24 hrs at room temperature or 48 hrs if refrigerated. • Protect from prolonged exposure to sunlight; discard unused solution. **Doxil:** Refrigerate unopened vials. After solution is diluted, use within 24 hrs.

IV INCOMPATIBILITIES

Doxorubicin: Allopurinol (Aloprim), amphotericin B complex (Abelcet, AmBisome, Amphotec), cefepime (Maxipime), furosemide (Lasix), ganciclovir (Cytovene), heparin, lipids, piperacillin/tazobactam (Zosyn), propofol (Diprivan). **Doxil:** Do not mix with any other medications.

IV COMPATIBILITIES

Dexamethasone (Decadron), diphenhydramine (Benadryl), etoposide (VePesid), granisetron (Kytril), hydromorphone (Dilaudid), lorazepam (Ativan), morphine, ondansetron (Zofran), paclitaxel (Taxol).

INDICATIONS/ROUTES/DOSAGE

USUAL DOSAGE

IV: ADULTS: 60–75 mg/m^2 as a single dose every 21 days, 20 mg/m^2 once weekly, or 25–30 mg/m^2/day on 2–3 successive days q4wk. Because of risk of cardiotoxicity, do not exceed cumulative dose of 550 mg/m^2 (400–450 mg/m^2 for those previously treated with related compounds or irradiation of cardiac region). **CHILDREN:** 35–75 mg/m^2 as a single dose q3wk or 20–30 mg/m^2 weekly, or 60–90 mg/m^2 as continuous infusion over 96 hrs q3–4wk.

KAPOSI'S SARCOMA

IV (DOXIL): ADULTS: 20 mg/m^2 q3wk infused over 30 min.

OVARIAN CANCER

IV (DOXIL): ADULTS: 50 mg/m^2 q4wk.

DOSAGE IN RENAL IMPAIRMENT

Creatinine Clearance	Dosage
Less than 10 ml/min	75% of normal

DOSAGE IN HEPATIC IMPAIRMENT

Hepatic Function	Dosage
ALT/AST 2–3 times ULN	75% of dose
ALT/AST greater than 3 times ULN or Bilirubin 1.2–3 mg/dl	50% of dose
Bilirubin 3.1–5 mg/dl	25% of dose
Bilirubin greater than 5 mg/dl	Not recommended

UNL = upper limit of normal.

SIDE EFFECTS

FREQUENT: Complete alopecia (scalp, axillary, pubic hair), nausea, vomiting, stomatitis, esophagitis (esp. if drug is given on several successive days), reddish urine. **Doxil:** Nausea. **OCCASIONAL:** Anorexia, diarrhea; hyperpigmentation of nailbeds, phalangeal, dermal creases. **RARE:** Fever, chills, conjunctivitis, lacrimation.

ADVERSE EFFECTS/ TOXIC REACTIONS

Myelosuppression manifested as hematologic toxicity (principally leukopenia and, to lesser extent, anemia, thrombocytopenia) generally occurs within 10–15 days, returns to normal levels by third week. Cardiotoxicity (either acute, manifested as transient EKG abnormalities, or chronic, manifested as CHF) may occur.

D

NURSING CONSIDERATIONS

BASELINE ASSESSMENT

Obtain WBC, platelet, erythrocyte counts before and at frequent intervals during therapy. Obtain EKG before therapy, hepatic function studies before each dose. Antiemetics may be effective in preventing, treating nausea.

INTERVENTION/EVALUATION

Monitor for stomatitis (burning or erythema of oral mucosa at inner margin of lips, difficulty swallowing). May lead to ulceration of mucous membranes within 2–3 days. Assess dermal creases, nailbeds for hyperpigmentation. Monitor hematologic status, renal/hepatic function studies, serum uric acid levels. Monitor daily pattern of bowel activity/stool consistency. Monitor for hematologic toxicity (fever, sore throat, signs of local infection, unusual bruising/bleeding from any site), symptoms of anemia (excessive fatigue, weakness).

PATIENT/ FAMILY TEACHING

• Alopecia is reversible, but new hair growth may have different color, texture. New hair growth resumes 2–3 mos after last therapy dose. • Maintain fastidious oral hygiene. • Do not have immunizations without physician's approval (drug lowers resistance). • Avoid contact with those who have recently received live virus vaccine. • Promptly report fever, sore throat, signs of local infection, unusual bruising/bleeding from any site. • Contact physician for persistent nausea/vomiting. • Avoid alcohol (may cause GI irritation, a common side effect with liposomal doxorubicin).

doxycycline

dox-i-**sye**-kleen

(Adoxa, Apo-Doxy ♣, Doryx, Doxy-100, Doxycin ♣, Monodox, Oracea, Periostat, Vibramycin, Vibra-Tabs).

Do not confuse doxycycline with Dicyclomine or doxylamine, or Monodox with Monopril.

CLASSIFICATION

PHARMACOTHERAPEUTIC: Tetracycline. **CLINICAL:** Antibiotic.

ACTION

Inhibits bacterial protein synthesis by binding to ribosomes. **Therapeutic Effect:** Bacteriostatic.

PHARMACOKINETICS

Rapidly, almost completely absorbed after PO administration. Protein binding: greater than 90%. Metabolized in liver. Partially excreted in urine; partially eliminated in bile. **Half-life:** 15–24 hrs.

USES

Treatment of susceptible infections due to *H. ducreyi, Pasteurella pestis, tularnsis,* Bacteroides species, *V. cholerae,* Brucella species, *Rickettsiae, Y. pestis, Francisella tularesis, M. pneumoniae* including brucellosis, chlamydia, cholera, granuloma inguinale, lymphogranuloma venereum, malaria prophylaxis, nongonococcal urethritis, pelvic inflammatory disease, plague, psittacosis, relapsing fever, rickettsia infections, primary and secondary syphilis, tularemia. Treatment of inflammatory lesions in adults with rosacea. **OFF-LABEL:** Treatment of atypical mycobacterial infections, gonorrhea, malaria, rheumatoid arthritis, prevention of Lyme disease; prevention, treatment of traveler's diarrhea.

PRECAUTIONS

CONTRAINDICATIONS: Children 8 yrs and younger, hypersensitivity to tetracyclines or sulfites, last half of pregnancy, severe hepatic dysfunction. **CAUTIONS:** Sun, ultraviolet light exposure (severe photosensitivity reaction).

LIFESPAN CONSIDERATIONS:

Pregnancy/Lactation: Crosses placenta; distributed in breast milk. **Pregnancy Category D. Children:** May cause permanent discoloration of teeth, enamel hypoplasia. **Elderly:** No age-related precautions noted.

INTERACTIONS

DRUG: **Antacids containing aluminum, calcium, magnesium; laxatives containing magnesium** decrease absorption. **Barbiturates, carbamazepine, phenytoin** may decrease concentration. **Cholestyramine, colestipol** may decrease absorption. May decrease effects of **oral contraceptives**. **Oral iron preparations** impair absorption. **HERBAL:** **St. John's wort, dong quai** may increase photosensitization. **FOOD:** None known. **LAB VALUES:** May increase serum alkaline phosphatase, amylase, bilirubin, AST, ALT. May alter CBC.

AVAILABILITY (Rx)

CAPSULES: 40 mg (Oracea), 50 mg (Monodox), 75 mg (Doryx), 100 mg (Doryx, Monodox, Vibramycin). **INJECTION, POWDER FOR RECONSTITUTION (DOXY-100):** 100 mg. **ORAL SUSPENSION (VIBRAMYCIN):** 25 mg/5 ml. **SYRUP (VIBRAMYCIN):** 50 mg/5 ml. **TABLETS:** 20 mg (Periostat), 50 mg (Adoxa), 75 mg (Adoxa), 100 mg (Adoxa, Vibra-Tabs).

ADMINISTRATION/HANDLING

◄ **ALERT** ► Do not administer IM or subcutaneous. Space doses evenly around clock.

IV

Reconstitution • Reconstitute each 100-mg vial with 10 ml Sterile Water for Injection for concentration of 10 mg/ml. • Further dilute each 100 mg with at least 100 ml D_5W, 0.9% NaCl, lactated Ringer's.

Rate of administration • Give by intermittent IV infusion (piggyback). • Infuse over 1–4 hrs.

Storage • After reconstitution, IV infusion (piggyback) is stable for 12 hrs at room temperature or 72 hrs if refrigerated. • Protect from direct sunlight. Discard if precipitate forms.

PO

• Store capsules, tablets at room temperature. • Oral suspension is stable for 2 wks at room temperature. • Give with full glass of fluid. • May take with food, milk.

IV INCOMPATIBILITIES

Allopurinol (Aloprim), heparin, lipids, piperacillin/tazobactam (Zosyn).

IV COMPATIBILITIES

Amiodarone (Cordarone), diltiazem (Cardizem), hydromorphone (Dilaudid), magnesium sulfate, morphine, propofol (Diprivan), total parenteral nutrition (TPN).

INDICATIONS/ROUTES/DOSAGE

USUAL DOSAGE

IV/PO: ADULTS, ELDERLY, CHILDREN 8 YRS AND OLDER: 2–5 mg/kg/day (maximum: 200 mg/day) in 1–2 divided doses or 100–200 mg/day in 1–2 divided doses.

ACUTE GONOCOCCAL INFECTIONS

PO: ADULTS: Initially, 200 mg, then 100 mg at bedtime on first day; then 100 mg twice a day for 14 days.

SYPHILIS

PO, IV: ADULTS: 200 mg/day in divided doses for 14–28 days.

D

TRAVELER'S DIARRHEA

PO: ADULTS, ELDERLY: 100 mg/day during a period of risk (up to 14 days) and for 2 days after returning home.

ROSACEA

PO: ADULTS, ELDERLY: 40 mg once daily.

PERIODONTITIS

PO: ADULTS: 20 mg twice a day.

SIDE EFFECTS

FREQUENT: Anorexia, nausea, vomiting, diarrhea, dysphagia, photosensitivity (may be severe). **OCCASIONAL:** Rash, urticaria.

ADVERSE EFFECTS/ TOXIC REACTIONS

Superinfection (esp. fungal), benign intracranial hypertension (headache, visual changes) may occur. Hepatoxicity, fatty degeneration of liver, pancreatitis occur rarely.

NURSING CONSIDERATIONS

BASELINE ASSESSMENT

Question for history of allergies, esp. to tetracyclines, sulfites.

INTERVENTION/EVALUATION

Monitor daily pattern of bowel activity/stool consistency. Assess skin for rash. Monitor level of consciousness (LOC) due to potential for increased intracranial pressure (ICP). Be alert for superinfection (diarrhea, ulceration/changes of oral mucosa, anal/genital pruritus).

PATIENT/FAMILY TEACHING

• Avoid unnecessary exposure to sunlight. • Do not take with antacids, iron products, dairy products. • Complete full course of therapy. • After application of dental gel, avoid brushing teeth, flossing the treated areas for 7 days.

dronabinol

droe-**nab**-i-nol

(Marinol)

Do not confuse dronabinol with droperidol.

CLASSIFICATION

PHARMACOTHERAPEUTIC: Controlled substance (**Schedule III**). **CLINICAL:** Antinausea, antiemetic, appetite stimulant.

ACTION

Inhibits vomiting control mechanisms in medulla oblongata. **Therapeutic Effect:** Inhibits nausea/vomiting, stimulates appetite.

PHARMACOKINETICS

Well absorbed after PO administration. Protein binding: 97%. Undergoes first-pass metabolism. Highly lipid soluble. Primarily excreted in feces. **Half-life:** 4 hrs.

USES

Prevention, treatment of nausea/vomiting due to cancer chemotherapy; appetite stimulant in AIDS, cancer pts. **OFF-LABEL:** Postoperative nausea/vomiting.

PRECAUTIONS

CONTRAINDICATIONS: Treatment of nausea/vomiting not caused by chemotherapy, hypersensitivity to sesame oil, tetrahydrocannabinol products. **CAUTIONS:** Cardiac disorders, history of psychiatric illness, history of substance abuse, hypertension.

LIFESPAN CONSIDERATIONS:

Pregnancy/Lactation: Unknown if drug crosses placenta. Distributed in breast milk. **Pregnancy Category C.** **Children:** Not recommended. **Elderly:** Monitor carefully during therapy.

INTERACTIONS

DRUG: **Alcohol, other CNS suppressants** may increase CNS depression. **HERBAL:** **St. John's wort** may decrease concentration. **FOOD:** None known. **LAB VALUES:** None known.

AVAILABILITY (Rx)

CAPSULES (GELATIN [MARINOL]): 2.5 mg, 5 mg, 10 mg.

ADMINISTRATION/HANDLING

PO

• Refrigerate capsules. • Give before meals.

INDICATIONS/ROUTES/DOSAGE

PREVENTION OF CHEMOTHERAPY INDUCED NAUSEA AND VOMITING

PO: ADULTS, CHILDREN: Initially, 5 mg/m^2 1–3 hrs before chemotherapy, then q2–4h after chemotherapy for total of 4–6 doses a day. May increase by 2.5 mg/m^2 up to 15 mg/m^2 per dose.

APPETITE STIMULANT

PO: ADULTS: Initially, 2.5 mg twice a day (before lunch and dinner). Range: 2.5–20 mg/day.

SIDE EFFECTS

FREQUENT (24%–3%): Euphoria, dizziness, paranoid reaction, somnolence. **OCCASIONAL (less than 3%–1%):** Asthenia, ataxia, confusion, abnormal thinking, depersonalization. **RARE (less than 1%):** Diarrhea, depression, nightmares, speech difficulties, headache, anxiety, tinnitus, flushed skin.

ADVERSE EFFECTS/ TOXIC REACTIONS

Mild intoxication may produce increased sensory awareness (taste, smell, sound), altered time perception, reddened conjunctiva, dry mouth, tachycardia. Moderate intoxication may produce memory impairment, urine retention. Severe intoxication may produce lethargy, decreased motor coordination, slurred speech, orthostatic hypotension.

NURSING CONSIDERATIONS

BASELINE ASSESSMENT

Assess dehydration status if excessive vomiting occurs (skin turgor, mucous membranes, urinary output).

INTERVENTION/EVALUATION

Supervise closely for serious mood, behavior responses, esp. in pts with history of psychiatric illness. Monitor B/P, heart rate.

PATIENT/FAMILY TEACHING

• Change positions slowly to avoid dizziness. • Relief from nausea/vomiting generally occurs within 15 min of drug administration. • Do not take any other medications, including OTC, without physician approval. • Avoid alcohol, barbiturates. • Avoid tasks that require alertness, motor skills until response to drug is established. • For appetite stimulation, take before lunch and dinner.

droperidol

droe-**pear**-ih-dall
(Inapsine)

CLASSIFICATION

PHARMACOTHERAPEUTIC: General anesthetic. **CLINICAL:** Anesthesia adjunct, antiemetic.

ACTION

Antagonizes dopamine neurotransmission at synapses by blocking postsynaptic dopamine receptor sites; partially blocks adrenergic receptor binding sites.

D

Therapeutic Effect: Produces tranquilization, antiemetic effect.

PHARMACOKINETICS

Onset	Peak	Duration
IM		
3–10 min	30 min	2–4 hrs
IV		
3–10 min	30 min	2–4 hrs

Well absorbed after IM administration. Crosses blood-brain barrier. Metabolized in liver. Primarily excreted in urine. **Half-life:** 2.3 hrs.

USES

Treatment of nausea/vomiting associated with surgical and diagnostic procedures. **OFF-LABEL:** Adjunct in induction and maintenance of general and regional anesthesia, produces sedation for diagnostic procedures, treatment of acute psychotic episodes.

PRECAUTIONS

CONTRAINDICATIONS: Known or suspected QT interval prolongation, congenital long QT syndrome. **CAUTIONS:** Hepatic/renal/cardiac impairment (may cause cardiac arrhythmias during administration).

LIFESPAN CONSIDERATIONS:

Pregnancy/Lactation: Crosses placenta. Unknown if drug is distributed in breast milk. **Pregnancy Category C. Children:** Dystonias more likely. **Elderly:** May be more sensitive to sedative, hypotensive effects.

INTERACTIONS

DRUG: **Antihypertensives** may increase hypotension. **CNS depressants** may increase CNS depressant effect. **Volatile anesthetics, benzodiazepines, diuretics, IV opioids** may have additive effect on prolongation of QT interval. **HERBAL:** None significant. **FOOD:** None known. **LAB VALUES:** None known.

AVAILABILITY (Rx)

INJECTION SOLUTION: 2.5 mg/ml.

ADMINISTRATION/HANDLING

◀ **ALERT** ▶ Pt must remain recumbent for 30–60 min in head-low position with legs raised, to minimize hypotensive effect.

Storage • Store parenteral form at room temperature.

IV

• May give undiluted as IV push over 2–5 min. • Dose for high-risk pts should be added to D_5W or lactated Ringer's injection to a concentration of 1 mg/50 ml and given as an IV infusion.

IM

• Inject slowly, deep IM into upper outer quadrant of gluteus maximus.

IV INCOMPATIBILITIES

Allopurinol (Aloprim), amphotericin B complex (Abelcet, AmBisome, Amphotic), cefepime (Maxipime), foscarnet (Foscavir), heparin, lipids, methotrexate, piperacillin/tazobactam (Zosyn).

IV COMPATIBILITIES

Atropine, diphenhydramine (Benadryl), glycopyrrolate (Robinul), metoclopramide (Reglan), midazolam (Versed), morphine, potassium chloride, promethazine (Phenergan).

INDICATIONS/ROUTES/DOSAGE

NAUSEA, VOMITING

IM, IV: ADULTS, ELDERLY: Initially, 2.5 mg. Additional doses of 1.25 mg may be given to achieve desired effect. **CHILDREN 2–12 YRS:** 0.05–0.06 mg/kg (maximum initial dose of 0.1 mg/kg). Additional dose may be given to achieve desired effect.

D

SIDE EFFECTS

FREQUENT: Mild to moderate hypotension. **OCCASIONAL:** Tachycardia, postop drowsiness, dizziness, chills, shivering. **RARE:** Postop nightmares, facial diaphoresis, bronchospasm.

ADVERSE EFFECTS/ TOXIC REACTIONS

May produce cardiac arrhythmias. Extrapyramidal symptoms (EPS) may appear as akathisia (motor restlessness), dystonias: torticollis (neck muscle spasm), opisthotonos (rigidity of back muscles), oculogyric crisis (rolling back of eyes).

NURSING CONSIDERATIONS

BASELINE ASSESSMENT

Assess vital signs. Have pt void. Raise side rails. Instruct pt to remain recumbent.

INTERVENTION/EVALUATION

Monitor B/P, pulse diligently for hypotensive reaction during and after procedure. Assess pulse for tachycardia. Monitor for EPS. Evaluate for therapeutic response from anxiety (calm facial expression, decreased restlessness). Monitor for decreased nausea, vomiting.

drotrecogin alfa

dro-trae-**coe**-gin **al**-fa

(Xigris)

CLASSIFICATION

PHARMACOTHERAPEUTIC: Activated protein C. **CLINICAL:** Antisepsis agent.

ACTION

Recombinant form of human-activated protein C that exerts antithrombotic effect. Also exerts anti-inflammatory effect by inhibiting tumor necrosis factor (TNF) production. **Therapeutic Effect:** Produces anti-inflammatory, antithrombotic, profibrinolytic effects.

PHARMACOKINETICS

Inactivated by endogenous plasma protease inhibitors. Clearance occurs within 2 hrs of initiating infusion. **Half-life:** 1.6 hrs.

USES

Treatment of severe sepsis, septic shock with evidence of organ dysfunction in pts at high risk for death.

PRECAUTIONS

CONTRAINDICATIONS: Active internal bleeding, evidence of cerebral herniation, intracranial neoplasm/mass lesion, presence of epidural catheter, recent (within the past 3 mos) hemorrhagic stroke, recent (within the past 2 mos) intracranial or intraspinal surgery or severe head trauma, trauma with increased risk of life-threatening bleeding. **CAUTIONS:** Concurrent use of heparin, platelet count less than 30,000/mm^3, prolonged prothrombin time (PT), recent (6 wks or less) GI bleeding, recent (3 days or less) thrombolytic therapy, recent (7 days or less) anticoagulant or aspirin therapy, intracranial aneurysm, chronic severe hepatic disease.

⌛ LIFESPAN CONSIDERATIONS:

Pregnancy/Lactation: Unknown if the drug can cause fetal harm. Unknown if excreted in breast milk. **Pregnancy Category C. Children/Elderly:** Safety and efficacy not established.

INTERACTIONS

DRUG: **Aspirin, platelet inhibitors, heparin, thrombolytic agents, warfarin** may increase risk of bleeding.

D

HERBAL: **Cat's claw, dong quai, evening primrose, garlic, ginseng** may increase antiplatelet activity. **FOOD:** None known. **LAB VALUES:** May prolong activated partial thromboplastin time (aPTT).

AVAILABILITY (Rx)

INJECTION, POWDER FOR RECONSTITUTION: 5 mg, 20 mg.

ADMINISTRATION/HANDLING

IV

Reconstitution • Reconstitute 5-mg vials with 2.5 ml Sterile Water for Injection and 20-mg vials with 10 ml Sterile Water for Injection. Resulting concentration is 2 mg/ml. • Slowly add Sterile Water for Injection by swirling; do not shake, invert vial. • Further dilute with 0.9% NaCl. • Withdraw amount from vial and add to infusion bag containing 0.9% NaCl for final concentration between 100 and 200 mcg/ml; direct stream to side of bag (minimizes agitation). • Invert infusion bag to mix solution.

Rate of administration • Administer via dedicated IV line or dedicated lumen of multilumen central venous line (CVL). • Administer infusion rate of 24 mcg/kg/hr for 96 hrs. • If infusion is interrupted, restart drug at 24 mcg/kg/hr.

Storage • Store unreconstituted vials at room temperature. • Start infusion within 3 hrs after reconstitution.

IV INCOMPATIBILITIES

Amiodarone (Cordarone), ciprofloxacin (Ciloxan), cyclosporine (Sandimmune), furosemide (Lasix), levofloxacin (Levoquin).

IV COMPATIBILITIES

Lactated Ringer's solution, 0.9% NaCl, dextrose are only solutions that can be administered through same line.

INDICATIONS/ROUTES/DOSAGE

SEVERE SEPSIS

IV INFUSION: ADULTS, ELDERLY: 24 mcg/kg/hr for 96 hrs. Immediately stop infusion if clinically significant bleeding is identified.

SIDE EFFECTS

None known.

ADVERSE EFFECTS/TOXIC REACTIONS

Bleeding (intrathoracic, retroperitoneal, GI, GU, intra-abdominal, intracranial) occurs in 2% of pts.

NURSING CONSIDERATIONS

BASELINE ASSESSMENT

Criteria that must be met before initiating drug therapy: age older than 18 yrs, no pregnancy or breastfeeding, actual body weight less than 135 kg, 3 or more systemic inflammatory response criteria (fever, heart rate over 90 beats/min, respiratory rate over 20 breaths/min, increased WBC count), and at least one sepsis-induced organ or system failure (cardiovascular, renal, respiratory, hematologic, unexplained metabolic acidosis).

INTERVENTION/EVALUATION

Monitor closely for hemorrhagic complication.

Dulcolax, *see bisacodyl*

duloxetine

dew-**lox**-ah-teen
(Cymbalta)

CLASSIFICATION

CLINICAL: Antidepressant.

ACTION

Appears to inhibit serotonin and norepinephrine reuptake at CNS neuronal presynaptic membranes; is a less potent inhibitor of dopamine reuptake. **Therapeutic Effect:** Produces antidepressant effect.

PHARMACOKINETICS

Well absorbed from GI tract. Protein binding: greater than 90%. Extensively metabolized to active metabolites. Excreted primarily in urine and, to a lesser extent, in feces. **Half-life:** 8–17 hrs.

USES

Treatment of major depression exhibited as persistent, prominent dysphoria (occurring nearly every day for at least 2 wks) manifested by 4 of 8 symptoms: change in appetite, change in sleep pattern, increased fatigue, impaired concentration, feelings of guilt or worthlessness, loss of interest in usual activities, psychomotor agitation or retardation, or suicidal tendencies. **OFF-LABEL:** Treatment of chronic pain syndromes, fibromyalgia, stress incontinence, urinary incontinence.

PRECAUTIONS

CONTRAINDICATIONS: End-stage renal disease (creatinine clearance less than 30 ml/min), severe hepatic impairment, uncontrolled angle-closure glaucoma, use within 14 days of MAOIs. **CAUTIONS:** Renal impairment, history of alcoholism, chronic liver disease, hepatic insufficiency, history of seizures, history of mania, conditions that may slow gastric emptying, those with suicidal ideation and behavior.

LIFESPAN CONSIDERATIONS:

Pregnancy/Lactation: May produce neonatal adverse reactions (constant crying, feeding difficulty, hyperreflexia, irritability). Unknown if distributed in breast milk; do not breast-feed. **Pregnancy Category C. Children:** Safety and efficacy not established. **Elderly:** Caution required when increasing dosage.

INTERACTIONS

DRUG: Alcohol increases risk of hepatic injury. **Fluoxetine, fluvoxamine, paroxetine, quinidine, quinolone antimicrobials** may increase plasma concentration. **MAOIs** may cause serotonin syndrome (autonomic hyperactivity, coma, diaphoresis, excitement, hyperthermia, rigidity). May increase concentration, potential toxicity of **tricyclic antidepressants, propafenone, phenothiazines. Thioridazine** may produce ventricular arrhythmias. May increase **warfarin** plasma concentration. **HERBAL: Gotu kola, kava kava, St. John's wort, valerian** may increase CNS depression. **FOOD:** None known. **LAB VALUES:** May increase serum bilirubin, AST, ALT.

AVAILABILITY (Rx)

CAPSULES: 20 mg, 30 mg, 60 mg.

ADMINISTRATION/HANDLING

◀ **ALERT** ▶ Allow at least 14 days to elapse between use of MAOIs and duloxetine.

PO

• Give without regard to meals. Give with food, milk if GI distress occur. • Do not crush, chew enteric-coated capsules. • Do not sprinkle capsule contents on food or mix with liquids.

INDICATIONS/ROUTES/DOSAGE

MAJOR DEPRESSIVE DISORDER

PO: ADULTS: 20 mg twice a day, increased up to 60 mg/day as a single dose or in 2 divided doses.

DIABETIC NEUROPATHY PAIN

PO: ADULTS: 60 mg once a day.

SIDE EFFECTS

FREQUENT (20%–11%): Nausea, dry mouth, constipation, insomnia. **OCCASIONAL (9%–5%):** Dizziness, fatigue, diarrhea, somnolence, anorexia, diaphoresis, vomiting. **RARE (4%–2%):** Blurred vision, erectile dysfunction, delayed or failed ejaculation, anorgasmia, anxiety, decreased libido, hot flashes.

ADVERSE EFFECTS/ TOXIC REACTIONS

May slightly increase heart rate. Colitis, dysphagia, gastritis, irritable bowel syndrome occur rarely.

NURSING CONSIDERATIONS

BASELINE ASSESSMENT

Assess appearance, behavior, speech pattern, level of interest, mood, sleep pattern.

INTERVENTION/EVALUATION

For those on long-term therapy, serum chemistry profile to assess hepatic function should be performed periodically. Supervise suicidal risk pt closely during early therapy (as depression lessens, energy level improves, increasing suicide potential).

PATIENT/FAMILY TEACHING

• Therapeutic effect may be noted within 1–4 wks. • Do not abruptly discontinue medication. • Avoid tasks that require alertness, motor skills until response to drug is established. • Inform physician if intention of pregnancy or if pregnancy occurs. • Inform physician if anxiety, agitation, panic attacks, worsening of depression occurs. • Avoid heavy alcohol intake (associated with severe hepatic injury).

DuoNeb, *see albuterol and ipratropium*

Duragesic, *see fentanyl*

Duramorph, *see morphine*

dutasteride

do-tah-**stir**-eyed
(Avodart)

CLASSIFICATION

PHARMACOTHERAPEUTIC: Androgen hormone inhibitor. **CLINICAL:** Benign prostatic hyperplasia agent.

ACTION

Inhibits 5-alpha reductase, an intracellular enzyme that converts testosterone into dihydrotestosterone (DHT) in the prostate gland, reducing serum DHT level. **Therapeutic Effect:** Reduces enlarged prostate gland.

PHARMACOKINETICS

Route	Onset	Peak	Duration
PO	24 hrs	N/A	3–8 wks

Moderately absorbed after PO administration. Widely distributed. Protein binding: 99%. Metabolized in liver. Primarily excreted in feces. **Half-life:** Up to 5 wks.

USES

Treatment of benign prostatic hyperplasia (BPH). **OFF-LABEL:** Treatment of hair loss.

PRECAUTIONS

CONTRAINDICATIONS: Females, physical handling of tablets by those who are or may be pregnant. **CAUTIONS:** Hepatic disease/impairment, obstructive uropathy, preexisting sexual dysfunction (reduced male libido, impotence). **Pregnancy Category X.**

INTERACTIONS

DRUG: **Cimetidine, ciprofloxacin, diltiazem, ketoconazole, ritonavir, verapamil** may increase concentration. **HERBAL:** Avoid **saw plametto** (limited experience with this combination). **St. John's wort** may decrease concentration. **FOOD:** None known. **LAB VALUES:** Decreases serum prostate-specific antigen (PSA) level.

AVAILABILITY (Rx)

CAPSULE: 0.5 mg.

ADMINISTRATION/HANDLING

PO

• Do not open/break capsules. • Give without regard to meals.

INDICATIONS/ROUTES/DOSAGE

BENIGN PROSTATIC HYPERPLASIA (BPH)

PO: ADULTS, ELDERLY (MEN ONLY): 0.5 mg once a day.

SIDE EFFECTS

OCCASIONAL: Gynecomastia, sexual dysfunction (decreased libido, impotence, decreased volume of ejaculate).

ADVERSE EFFECTS/ TOXIC REACTIONS

Toxicity manifested as rash, diarrhea, abdominal pain.

NURSING CONSIDERATIONS

BASELINE ASSESSMENT

Serum PSA determination should be performed in pts with BPH before beginning therapy and periodically thereafter.

INTERVENTION/EVALUATION

Diligently monitor I&O. Assess for signs/symptoms of BPH (hesitancy, reduced force of urinary stream, postvoid dribbling, sensation of incomplete bladder emptying).

PATIENT/FAMILY TEACHING

• Discuss potential for impotence; volume of ejaculate may be decreased during treatment. • May not notice improved urinary flow for up to 6 mos after treatment. • Women who may be or are pregnant should not handle capsules (risk of fetal anomaly to male fetus).

Dyazide, *see hydrochlorothiazide and triamterene*

DynaCirc, *see isradipine*

echinacea

Also known as black susans, comb flower, red sunflower, scurvy root.

CLASSIFICATION

HERBAL: See Appendix G.

ACTION

Stimulates immune system. Possesses antiviral/immune stimulatory effects. Increases phagocytosis, lymphocyte activity (possibly by releasing tumor necrosis factor [TNF], interleukin-1, interferon). **Effect:** Prevents/reduces symptoms associated with upper respiratory infection.

USES

Immune system stimulant used for treatment/prevention of the common cold, other upper respiratory infections. Also used for UTI, vaginal candidiasis.

PRECAUTIONS

CONTRAINDICATIONS: Pregnancy/lactation, children 2 yrs and younger, those with autoimmune disease (e.g., multiple sclerosis, systemic lupus erythematosus [SLE], HIV/AIDS), tuberculosis, history of allergic conditions. **CAUTIONS:** Diabetes (may alter control of blood sugar). Do not use for more than 8 wks (may decrease effectiveness).

LIFESPAN CONSIDERATIONS:

Pregnancy/Lactation: Contraindicated. **Pregnancy Category C. Children:** Safety and efficacy not established in those younger than 2 yrs. **Elderly:** No age-related precautions noted.

INTERACTIONS

DRUG: May interfere with **immunosuppressant therapy (corticosteroids, cyclosporine, mycophenolate). Topical econazole** may reduce recurring vaginal candida infections. **HERBAL:** None significant. **FOOD:** None known. **LAB VALUES:** None known.

AVAILABILITY (OTC)

CAPSULES: 200 mg, 380 mg, 400 mg, 500 mg. **POWDER:** 25 g, 100 g, 500 g. **TINCTURE:** 475 mg/ml.

INDICATIONS/ROUTES/DOSAGE

USUAL ADULT DOSAGE

PO: ADULTS, ELDERLY: 6–9 ml herbal juice for maximum of 8 wks.

◄ **ALERT** ► A variety of doses have been used depending on the preparation.

SIDE EFFECTS

Well tolerated. May cause allergic reaction (urticaria, acute asthma/dyspnea, angioedema), fever, nausea, vomiting, diarrhea, unpleasant taste, abdominal pain, dizziness.

ADVERSE EFFECTS/ TOXIC REACTIONS

None known.

NURSING CONSIDERATIONS

BASELINE ASSESSMENT

Assess if pt is pregnant or breastfeeding, history of autoimmune disease, receiving immunosuppressant therapy.

INTERVENTION/EVALUATION

Assess for hypersensitivity reaction, improvement in infection.

PATIENT/FAMILY TEACHING

- Do not use during pregnancy or lactation, children younger than 2 yrs.
- Do not use for more than 8 wks without at least 1-wk break in therapy.

echothiophate

(Phospholine Iodide)

See Antiglaucoma agents (p. 48C)

Ecotrin, *see aspirin*

edetate calcium

See Appendix M

EES, *see erythromycin*

efalizumab

ef-ah-**liz**-ewe-mab
(Raptiva)

CLASSIFICATION

PHARMACOTHERAPEUTIC: Monoclonal antibody. **CLINICAL:** Immunosuppressive.

ACTION

Interferes with lymphocyte activation by binding to lymphocyte antigen, inhibiting adhesion of leukocytes to other cell types. **Therapeutic Effect:** Prevents release of cytokines, growth/migration of circulating total lymphocytes, predominant in psoriatic lesions.

PHARMACOKINETICS

Clearance is affected by body weight, not by gender or race, after subcutaneous injection. Serum concentration reaches steady state at 4 wks. Mean time to elimination: 25 days.

USES

Treatment of adults 18 yrs and older with chronic moderate to severe plaque psoriasis who are candidates for systemic therapy or phototherapy.

PRECAUTIONS

CONTRAINDICATIONS: Concurrent use of immunosuppressive agents, hypersensitivity to any murine or humanized monoclonal antibody preparation. **CAUTIONS:** History of malignancy, chronic infection, history of recurrent infection, asthma, history of allergic reaction.

LIFESPAN CONSIDERATIONS:

Pregnancy/Lactation: Unknown if drug is distributed in breast milk. **Pregnancy Category C. Children:** Not indicated for use in pediatric pts. **Elderly:** Age-related increased incidence of infection requires cautious use in the elderly.

INTERACTIONS

DRUG: Immunosuppressive agents increase risk of infection. **Live virus vaccines** decrease immune response. **HERBAL:** None significant. **FOOD:** None known. **LAB VALUES:** May increase lymphocyte count.

AVAILABILITY (Rx)

INJECTION, POWDER FOR RECONSTITUTION: 150 mg, designed to deliver 125 mg/1.25 ml.

ADMINISTRATION/HANDLING

SUBCUTANEOUS

Reconstitution • Slowly inject 1.3 ml Sterile Water for Injection provided into efalizumab vial, using provided prefilled diluent syringe. • Swirl vial gently to dissolve; do not shake (causes foaming). • Dissolution takes less than 5 min.

Rate of administration • Administer into thigh, abdomen, buttocks, upper arm.

Storage • Refrigerate unopened vial. • Reconstituted solution may be stored at room temperature for up to 8 hrs.

INDICATIONS/ROUTES/DOSAGE

PSORIASIS

SUBCUTANEOUS: ADULTS, ELDERLY: Initially, 0.7 mg/kg followed by weekly doses of 1 mg/kg. **Maximum:** 200 mg (single dose).

E

SIDE EFFECTS

FREQUENT (32%–10%): Headache, chills, nausea, injection site pain. **OCCASIONAL (8%–7%):** Myalgia, flu-like symptoms, fever. **RARE (4%):** Back pain, acne.

ADVERSE EFFECTS/ TOXIC REACTIONS

Worsening of psoriasis, serious infections (abscess, cellulitis, postoperative wound infection, pneumonia), thrombocytopenia, malignancies occur rarely.

NURSING CONSIDERATIONS

BASELINE ASSESSMENT

Inform pt of treatment duration and required monitoring procedures. Obtain CBC to assess platelet count, lymphocyte before therapy and periodically thereafter. Inform pt of increased risk of developing infection while undergoing treatment. Assess skin before therapy and document extent, location of psoriasis lesions.

INTERVENTION/EVALUATION

Assess skin throughout therapy for evidence of improvement of psoriasis lesions. Monitor for worsening of lesions. Offer pt teaching to assure accurate and sterile preparation and self-injection of medication.

PATIENT/FAMILY TEACHING

• If appropriate, pts may self-inject after proper training in preparation and injection technique. • Inform physician if bleeding from gums, bruising/petechiae of skin, or onset of signs of infection occurs. • If new diagnosis of malignancy occurs, inform physician of current treatment with efalizumab. • Advise pts not to undergo phototherapy treatments.

efavirenz

eh-fah-**vir**-enz

(Sustiva)

Do not confuse Sustiva with Survanta.

FIXED COMBINATION(S)

Atripla: efavirenz/emtricitabine (an antiretroviral)/tenofovir (an antiretroviral) 600 mg/200 mg/300 mg.

◆CLASSIFICATION

PHARMACOTHERAPEUTIC: Nonnucleoside reverse transcriptase inhibitor. **CLINICAL:** Antiretroviral (see pp. 65C, 112C).

ACTION

Inhibits activity of HIV-1 reverse transcriptase. **Therapeutic Effect:** Interrupts HIV replication, slowing progression of HIV infection.

PHARMACOKINETICS

Rapidly absorbed after PO administration. Protein binding: 99%. Metabolized to major isoenzymes in liver. Eliminated in urine, feces. **Half-life:** 40–55 hrs.

USES

Treatment of HIV infection in combination with other appropriate antiretroviral agents.

PRECAUTIONS

CONTRAINDICATIONS: Concurrent use with ergot derivatives, midazolam, triazolam; efavirenz as monotherapy. **CAUTIONS:** History of mental illness, substance abuse, hepatic impairment.

LIFESPAN CONSIDERATIONS:

Pregnancy/Lactation: Breast-feeding not recommended. **Pregnancy Category C.** **Children:** Safety and efficacy not established in those younger than 3 yrs; may have increased incidence of rash. **Elderly:** No age-related precautions noted.

INTERACTIONS

DRUG: **Alcohol, psychoactive drugs** may produce additive CNS effects. Decreases **clarithromycin, voriconazole** plasma levels. **Ergot derivatives, midazolam, triazolam** may cause serious or life-threatening reactions (cardiac arrhythmias, prolonged sedation, respiratory depression). Decreases plasma concentrations of **amprenavir, indinavir, saquinavir.** Increases plasma concentrations of **nelfinavir, ritonavir. Phenobarbital, rifabutin, rifampin** decrease concentration. Alters **warfarin** plasma concentration. **HERBAL:** **St. John's wort** may decrease concentration. **FOOD:** **High-fat meals** may increase drug absorption. **LAB VALUES:** May produce false-positive urine test results for cannabinoid; increases total serum cholesterol, AST, ALT, triglycerides.

AVAILABILITY (Rx)

CAPSULES: 50 mg, 100 mg, 200 mg. **TABLETS:** 600 mg.

ADMINISTRATION/HANDLING

PO

• Give without regard to meals. • Avoid high-fat meals (may increase absorption).

INDICATIONS/ROUTES/DOSAGE

HIV INFECTION (IN COMBINATION WITH OTHER ANTIRETROVIRALS)

PO: ADULTS, ELDERLY, CHILDREN 3 YRS AND OLDER WEIGHING 40 KG OR MORE: 600 mg once a day at bedtime. **CHILDREN 3 YRS AND OLDER WEIGHING 32.5 KG–LESS THAN 40 KG:** 400 mg once a day. **CHILDREN 3 YRS AND OLDER WEIGHING 25 KG–LESS THAN 32.5 KG:** 350 mg once a day. **CHILDREN 3 YRS AND OLDER WEIGHING 20 KG–LESS THAN 25 KG:** 300 mg once a day. **CHILDREN 3 YRS AND OLDER WEIGHING 15 KG–LESS THAN 20 KG:** 250 mg once a day. **CHILDREN 3 YRS AND OLDER WEIGHING 10 KG–LESS THAN 15 KG:** 200 mg once a day.

E

SIDE EFFECTS

FREQUENT (52%): **Mild to severe:** Dizziness, vivid dreams, insomnia, confusion, impaired concentration, amnesia, agitation, depersonalization, hallucinations, euphoria. **OCCASIONAL:** **Mild to moderate:** Maculopapular rash (27%); nausea, fatigue, headache, diarrhea, fever, cough (less than 26%).

ADVERSE EFFECTS/ TOXIC REACTIONS

Serious psychiatric adverse experiences (aggressive reactions, agitation, delusions, emotional lability, mania, neurosis, paranoia, psychosis, suicide) have been reported.

NURSING CONSIDERATIONS

BASELINE ASSESSMENT

Offer emotional support to pt/family. Obtain baseline AST, ALT in pts with history of hepatitis B or C; serum cholesterol or triglycerides before initiating therapy and at intervals during therapy. Obtain history of all prescription and OTC medications (high level of drug interaction).

INTERVENTION/EVALUATION

Monitor for CNS, psychological symptoms: severe acute depression, including suicidal ideation or attempts, dizziness, impaired concentration, somnolence, abnormal dreams, insomnia (begins during first or second day of therapy, generally resolves in 2–4 wks). Assess for evidence of rash (common side effect). Monitor hepatic enzyme studies for abnormalities. Assess for headache, nausea, diarrhea.

PATIENT/FAMILY TEACHING

• Avoid high-fat meals during therapy. • If rash appears, contact physician immediately. • CNS, psychological symptoms occur in more than half the pts (dizziness, impaired concentration, delusions, depression). • Take medication every day as prescribed. • Do not alter dose or discontinue medication without informing physician. • Avoid tasks that require alertness, motor skills until response to drug is established. • Drug is not a cure for HIV infection, nor does it reduce risk of transmission to others.

Effexor, *see venlafaxine*

Effexor CR, *see venlafaxine*

Effexor XR, *see venlafaxine*

Efudex, *see fluorouracil*

Elavil, *see amitriptyline*

eletriptan

el-eh-**trip**-tan
(Relpax)

CLASSIFICATION

PHARMACOTHERAPEUTIC: Serotonin receptor agonist. **CLINICAL:** Antimigraine.

ACTION

Binds selectively to vascular receptors, producing vasoconstrictive effect on cranial blood vessels. **Therapeutic Effect:** Relieves migraine headache.

PHARMACOKINETICS

Well absorbed after PO administration. Metabolized by liver to inactive metabolite. Eliminated in urine. **Half-life:** 4.4 hrs (increased in hepatic impairment, elderly [older than 65 yrs]).

USES

Treatment of acute migraine headache with or without aura.

PRECAUTIONS

CONTRAINDICATIONS: Arrhythmias associated with conduction disorders, cerebrovascular syndrome including strokes and transient ischemic attacks (TIAs), coronary artery disease, hemiplegic or basilar migraine, ischemic heart disease, peripheral vascular disease including ischemic bowel disease, severe hepatic impairment, uncontrolled hypertension, use within 24 hrs of treatment with another 5-HT1 agonist, an ergotamine-containing or ergot-type medication such as dihydroergotamine (DHE) or methysergide. **CAUTIONS:** Mild to moderate renal/hepatic impairment, controlled hypertension, history of cerebrovascular accident (CVA).

LIFESPAN CONSIDERATIONS:

Pregnancy/Lactation: May decrease possibility of ovulation. Distributed in breast milk. **Pregnancy Category C. Children:** Safety and efficacy not established in pts younger than 18 yrs. **Elderly:** Increased risk of hypertension in pts older than 65 yrs.

INTERACTIONS

DRUG: **Clarithromycin, itraconazole, ketoconazole, nefazodone, nelfinavir, ritonavir** may decrease metabolism. **Ergotamine-containing medications** may produce vasospastic reaction. **HERBAL:** None significant. **FOOD:** None known. **LAB VALUES:** None known.

AVAILABILITY (Rx)

TABLETS: 20 mg, 40 mg.

ADMINISTRATION/HANDLING

PO

• Do not crush, break film-coated tablets.

INDICATIONS/ROUTES/DOSAGE

ACUTE MIGRAINE HEADACHE

PO: ADULTS, ELDERLY: 20–40 mg. If headache improves but then returns, dose may be repeated after 2 hrs. **Maximum:** 80 mg/day.

SIDE EFFECTS

OCCASIONAL (6%–5%): Dizziness, somnolence, asthenia, nausea. **RARE (3%–2%):** Paresthesia, headache, dry mouth, warm or hot sensation, dyspepsia, dysphagia.

ADVERSE EFFECTS/ TOXIC REACTIONS

Cardiac reactions (ischemia, coronary artery vasospasm, MI), noncardiac vasospasm-related reactions (hemorrhage, CVA) occur rarely, particularly in pts with hypertension, obesity, diabetes, strong family history of coronary artery disease; smokers; males older than 40 yrs; postmenopausal women.

NURSING CONSIDERATIONS

BASELINE ASSESSMENT

Question pt regarding onset, location, duration of migraine, possible precipitating symptoms. Obtain baseline B/P for evidence of uncontrolled hypertension (contraindication).

INTERVENTION/EVALUATION

Assess for relief of migraine headache, potential for photophobia, phonophobia (sound sensitivity), nausea, vomiting.

PATIENT/FAMILY TEACHING

• Take a single dose as soon as symptoms of an actual migraine attack appear. • Medication is intended to relieve migraine headaches, not to prevent or reduce number of attacks. • Avoid tasks that require alertness, motor skills until response to drug is established. • Contact physician immediately if palpitations, pain/tightness in chest/throat, sudden or severe abdominal pain, pain/weakness of extremities occur.

Elidel, *see pimecrolimus*

Eloxatin, *see oxaliplatin*

emtricitabine

em-trih-**sit**-ah-bean

(Emtriva)

FIXED-COMBINATION(S)

Atripla: emtricitabine/efavirenz (an antiretroviral)/tenofovir (an antiretroviral): 200 mg/600 mg/300 mg. **Truvada:** emtricitabine/tenofovir (an antiretroviral): 200 mg/300 mg.

CLASSIFICATION

PHARMACOTHERAPEUTIC: Nucleoside reverse transcriptase inhibitor. **CLINICAL:** Antiretroviral agent.

E

ACTION

Inhibits HIV-1 reverse transcriptase by incorporating itself into viral DNA, resulting in chain termination. **Therapeutic Effect:** Impairs HIV replication, slowing progression of HIV infection.

PHARMACOKINETICS

Rapidly, extensively absorbed from GI tract. Excreted primarily in urine (86%) and, to a lesser extent, in feces (14%); 30% removed by hemodialysis. Unknown if removed by peritoneal dialysis. **Half-life:** 10 hrs.

USES

Used in combination with other antiretroviral agents for treatment of HIV-1 infection in adults.

PRECAUTIONS

CONTRAINDICATIONS: None known. **CAUTIONS:** Hepatic/renal impairment.

LIFESPAN CONSIDERATIONS:

Pregnancy/Lactation: Breast-feeding not recommended. **Pregnancy Category B. Children:** Safety and effectiveness not established. **Elderly:** Age-related renal impairment may require dosage adjustment.

INTERACTIONS

DRUG: None significant. **HERBAL:** None significant. **FOOD:** None known. **LAB VALUES:** May increase serum amylase, lipase, ALT, AST, triglycerides. May alter serum glucose.

AVAILABILITY (Rx)

CAPSULES: 200 mg. **ORAL SOLUTION:** 10 mg/ml.

ADMINISTRATION/HANDLING

PO

- Give without regard to food.

INDICATIONS/ROUTES/DOSAGE

HIV

Capsules

PO: ADULTS, ELDERLY, CHILDREN 3 MOS–17 YRS, WEIGHT GREATER THAN 33 KG: 200 mg once daily.

Oral Solution

PO: ADULTS, ELDERLY: 240 mg once daily. **CHILDREN 3 MOS–17 YRS:** 6 mg/kg once daily. **Maximum:** 240 mg once daily.

DOSAGE IN RENAL IMPAIRMENT

Creatinine Clearance	Capsule	Oral Solution
30–49 ml/min	200 mg q48h	120 mg q24h
15–29 ml/min	200 mg q72h	80 mg q24h
Less than 15 ml/min; hemodialysis pts	200 mg q96h	60 mg q24h

Administer after dialysis on dialysis days.

SIDE EFFECTS

FREQUENT (23%–13%): Headache, rhinitis, rash, diarrhea, nausea. **OCCASIONAL (14%–4%):** Cough, vomiting, abdominal pain, insomnia, depression, paresthesia, dizziness, peripheral neuropathy, dyspepsia, myalgia. **RARE (3%–2%):** Arthralgia, abnormal dreams.

ADVERSE EFFECTS/ TOXIC REACTIONS

Lactic acidosis, hepatomegaly with steatosis (excess fat in liver) occur rarely; may be severe.

NURSING CONSIDERATIONS

BASELINE ASSESSMENT

Obtain baseline laboratory tests, esp. serum hepatic function, triglycerides before beginning and at periodic intervals during emtricitabine therapy. Offer emotional support.

INTERVENTION/EVALUATION

Monitor daily pattern of bowel activity/stool consistency. Question for evidence of nausea, pruritus (itching). Assess skin for rash, urticaria (hives). Monitor serum chemistry tests for marked abnormalities.

PATIENT/FAMILY TEACHING

• May cause redistribution of body fat. • Continue therapy for full length of treatment. • Emtricitabine is not a cure for HIV infection, nor does it reduce risk of transmission to others. • Pts may continue to acquire illnesses associated with advanced HIV infection.

enalapril

en-**al**-ah-pril
(Vasotec)

Do not confuse enalapril with Anafranil, Eldepryl, or ramipril.

FIXED-COMBINATION(S)

Lexxel: enalapril/felodipine (calcium channel blocker): 5 mg/2.5 mg; 5 mg/5 mg. **Teczem:** enalapril/diltiazem (calcium channel blocker): 5 mg/180 mg. **Vaseretic:** enalapril/hydrochlorothiazide (diuretic): 5 mg/12.5 mg; 10 mg/25 mg.

CLASSIFICATION

PHARMACOTHERAPEUTIC: Angiotensin-converting enzyme (ACE) inhibitor. **CLINICAL:** Antihypertensive, vasodilator (see p. 7C).

ACTION

Suppresses renin-angiotensin-aldosterone system (prevents conversion of angiotensin I to angiotensin II, a potent vasoconstrictor; may inhibit angiotensin II at local vascular, renal sites). Decreases plasma angiotensin II, increases plasma renin activity, decreases aldosterone secretion. **Therapeutic Effect:** In hypertension, reduces peripheral arterial resistance. In congestive heart failure (CHF), increases cardiac output; decreases peripheral vascular resistance, B/P, pulmonary capillary wedge pressure, heart size.

PHARMACOKINETICS

Route	Onset	Peak	Duration
PO	1 hr	4–6 hrs	24 hrs
IV	15 min	1–4 hrs	6 hrs

Readily absorbed from GI tract (not affected by food). Protein binding: 50%–60%. Converted to active metabolite. Primarily excreted in urine. Removed by hemodialysis. **Half-life:** 11 hrs (half-life is increased in renal impairment).

USES

Treatment of hypertension alone or in combination with other antihypertensives. Adjunctive therapy for CHF. **OFF-LABEL:** Diabetic nephropathy, hypertension due to scleroderma, renal crisis, hypertensive crisis, idiopathic edema, renal artery stenosis, rheumatoid arthritis, post MI for prevention of ventricular failure.

PRECAUTIONS

CONTRAINDICATIONS: History of angioedema from previous treatment with ACE inhibitors. **CAUTIONS:** Renal impairment, those with sodium depletion or on diuretic therapy, dialysis, hypovolemia, coronary/cerebrovascular insufficiency.

LIFESPAN CONSIDERATIONS:

Pregnancy/Lactation: Crosses placenta. Distributed in breast milk. May cause fetal/neonatal mortality, morbidity. **Pregnancy Category D (C if used in first trimester). Children:** Safety and efficacy not established. **Elderly:** May be more susceptible to hypotensive effects.

E

INTERACTIONS

DRUG: Alcohol, diuretics, antihypertensive agents may increase effect. **NSAIDs** may decrease effect. **Potassium-sparing diuretics, potassium supplements** may cause hyperkalemia. May increase **lithium** concentration/toxicity. **HERBAL: Ephedra, ginseng, yohimbe** may worsen hypertension. **Garlic** may increase antihypertensive effect. **Licorice** may cause sodium/water retention, loss of potassium. **FOOD:** None known. **LAB VALUES:** May increase BUN, serum alkaline phosphatase, bilirubin, creatinine, potassium, AST, ALT. May decrease serum sodium. May cause positive ANA titer.

AVAILABILITY (Rx)

INJECTION SOLUTION: 1.25 mg/ml. **TABLETS:** 2.5 mg, 5 mg, 10 mg, 20 mg.

ADMINISTRATION/HANDLING

IV

Reconstitution • May give undiluted or dilute with D_5W or 0.9% NaCl.

Rate of administration • For IV push, give undiluted over 5 min. • For IV piggyback, infuse over 10–15 min.

Storage • Store parenteral form at room temperature. • Use only clear, colorless solution. • Diluted IV solution is stable for 24 hrs at room temperature.

PO

• Give without regard to food. • Tablets may be crushed.

IV INCOMPATIBILITIES

Amphotericin B (Fungizone), amphotericin B complex (Abelcet, AmBisome, Amphotec), cefepime (Maxipime), phenytoin (Dilantin).

IV COMPATIBILITIES

Calcium gluconate, dobutamine (Dobutrex), dopamine (Inotropin), fentanyl (Sublimaze), heparin, lidocaine, lipids, magnesium sulfate, morphine, nitroglycerin, potassium chloride, potassium phosphate, propofol (Diprivan).

INDICATIONS/ROUTES/DOSAGE

HYPERTENSION

PO: ADULTS, ELDERLY: Initially, 2.5–5 mg/day. May increase at 1–2 wk intervals. Range: 10–40 mg/day in 1–2 divided doses. **CHILDREN 1 MO–16 YRS:** 0.1 mg/kg/day in 1–2 divided doses. **Maximum:** 0.5 mg/kg/day. **NEONATES:** 0.1 mg/kg/day q24h.

IV: ADULTS, ELDERLY: 0.625–1.25 mg q6h up to 5 mg q6h. **CHILDREN, NEONATES:** 5–10 mcg/kg/dose q8–24h.

ADJUNCTIVE THERAPY FOR CHF

PO: ADULTS, ELDERLY: Initially, 2.5–5 mg/day. Range: 5–20 mg/day in 2 divided doses.

DOSAGE IN RENAL IMPAIRMENT

Creatinine Clearance	Oral	IV
30 ml/min or greater	5 mg/day; titrate to maximum 40 mg/day	1.25 mg q6h; titrate to desired response
Less than 30 ml/min	2.5 mg/day; titrate to control B/P	0.626 mg q6h; titrate to desired response

SIDE EFFECTS

FREQUENT (7%–5%): Headache, dizziness. **OCCASIONAL (3%–2%):** Orthostatic hypotension, fatigue, diarrhea, cough, syncope. **RARE (less than 2%):** Angina, abdominal pain, vomiting, nausea, rash, asthenia (loss of strength, energy).

ADVERSE EFFECTS/ TOXIC REACTIONS

Excessive hypotension ("first-dose syncope") may occur in pts with CHF, severe salt or volume depleted. Angioedema (facial, lip swelling), hyperkalemia occur rarely. Agranulocytosis, neutropenia may be noted in pts with renal impairment, collagen vascular diseases (scleroderma, systemic lupus erythematosus). Nephrotic syndrome may be noted in those with history of renal disease.

NURSING CONSIDERATIONS

BASELINE ASSESSMENT

Obtain B/P immediately before each dose (be alert to fluctuations). In pts with renal impairment, autoimmune disease, or taking drugs that affect leukocytes/immune response, CBC should be performed before beginning therapy, q2wks for 3 mos, then periodically thereafter.

INTERVENTION/EVALUATION

Assist with ambulation if dizziness occurs. Monitor serum potassium, BUN, serum creatinine, B/P. Monitor daily pattern of bowel activity/stool consistency.

PATIENT/FAMILY TEACHING

• To reduce hypotensive effect, rise slowly from lying to sitting position, permit legs to dangle from bed momentarily before standing. • Several wks may be needed for full therapeutic effect of B/P reduction. • Skipping doses or voluntarily discontinuing drug may produce severe, rebound hypertension. • Limit alcohol intake. • Inform physician if vomiting, diarrhea, diaphoresis, swelling of face, lips, tongue, difficulty in breathing occurs.

Enbrel, *see etanercept*

enfuvirtide

en-**few**-vir-tide

(Fuzeon)

Do not confuse Fuzeon with Furoxone.

CLASSIFICATION

PHARMACOTHERAPEUTIC: Fusion inhibitor. **CLINICAL:** Antiretroviral agent.

ACTION

Interferes with entry of HIV-1 into CD4+ cells by inhibiting fusion of viral, cellular membranes. **Therapeutic Effect:** Impairs HIV replication, slowing progression of HIV infection.

PHARMACOKINETICS

Comparable absorption when injected into subcutaneous tissue of abdomen, arm, thigh. Protein binding: 92%. Undergoes catabolism to amino acids. **Half-life:** 3.8 hrs.

USES

Used in combination with other antiretroviral agents for treatment of HIV-1 infection in treatment-experienced pts with evidence of HIV-1 replication.

PRECAUTIONS

CONTRAINDICATIONS: None known. **CAUTIONS:** None known.

LIFESPAN CONSIDERATIONS:

Pregnancy/Lactation: Breast-feeding not recommended. **Pregnancy Category B. Children:** Safety and effectiveness not established in children 6 yrs and younger. **Elderly:** No age-related precautions noted.

INTERACTIONS

DRUG: None significant. **HERBAL:** None significant. **FOOD:** None known. **LAB VALUES:** May elevate serum glucose, amylase, creatine kinase (CK), lipase, triglycerides, AST, ALT. May decrease hemoglobin (Hgb), WBC count.

AVAILABILITY (Rx)

INJECTION, POWDER FOR RECONSTITUTION: 108 mg (approximately 90 mg/ml when reconstituted) vials.

E

E

ADMINISTRATION/HANDLING

SUBCUTANEOUS

Reconstitution • Reconstitute with 1.1 ml Sterile Water for Injection. • Visually inspect vial for particulate matter. Solution should appear clear, colorless. • Discard unused portion.

Rate of administration • Administer into upper arm, anterior thigh, abdomen. Rotate injection sites.

Storage • Store at room temperature. • Refrigerate reconstituted solution; use within 24 hrs. • Bring reconstituted solution to room temperature before injection.

INDICATIONS/ROUTES/DOSAGE

HIV INFECTION

SUBCUTANEOUS: ADULTS, ELDERLY: 90 mg (1 ml) twice a day. **CHILDREN 6–16 YRS:** 2 mg/kg twice a day. **Maximum:** 90 mg twice a day.

PEDIATRIC DOSING GUIDELINES

Weight: kg (lb)	Dose: mg (ml)
11–15.5 (24–34)	27 (0.3)
15.6–20 (35–44)	36 (0.4)
20.1–24.5 (45–54)	45 (0.5)
24.6–29 (55–64)	54 (0.6)
29.1–33.5 (65–74)	63 (0.7)
33.6–38 (75–84)	72 (0.8)
38.1–42.5 (85–94)	81 (0.9)
Greater than 42.5 (greater than 94)	90 (1)

SIDE EFFECTS

EXPECTED (98%): Local injection site reactions (pain, discomfort, induration, erythema, nodules, cysts, pruritus, ecchymosis). **FREQUENT (26%–16%):** Diarrhea, nausea, fatigue. **OCCASIONAL (11%–4%):** Insomnia, peripheral neuropathy, depression, cough, decreased appetite or weight loss, sinusitis, anxiety, asthenia (loss of strength, energy), myalgia, cold sores. **RARE (3%–2%):** Constipation, influenza, upper abdominal pain, anorexia, conjunctivitis.

ADVERSE EFFECTS/ TOXIC REACTIONS

May potentiate bacterial pneumonia. Hypersensitivity (rash, fever, chills, rigors, hypotension), thrombocytopenia, neutropenia, renal insufficiency/failure occur rarely.

NURSING CONSIDERATIONS

BASELINE ASSESSMENT

Obtain baseline laboratory tests, esp. serum hepatic function, triglycerides before beginning enfuvirtide therapy and at periodic intervals during therapy. Offer emotional support.

INTERVENTION/EVALUATION

Assess skin for local injection site hypersensitivity reaction. Question for evidence of nausea, fatigue. Assess sleep pattern. Monitor for insomnia, signs/symptoms of depression. Monitor serum chemistry tests for marked abnormalities.

PATIENT/FAMILY TEACHING

• Advise pt that increased rate of bacterial pneumonia has occurred with enfuvirtide therapy and to seek medical attention if cough with fever, difficult breathing occurs. • Continue therapy for full length of treatment. • Enfuvirtide is not a cure for HIV infection, nor does it reduce risk of transmission to others; pt must continue practices to prevent HIV transmission.

enoxacin

(Penetrex)

See Antibiotic: fluoroquinolones

enoxaparin

en-**ox**-ah-pear-in
(Lovenox)

Do not confuse Lovenox with Lotronex.

CLASSIFICATION

PHARMACOTHERAPEUTIC: Low-molecular-weight heparin. **CLINICAL:** Anticoagulant (see p. 30C).

ACTION

Potentiates action of antithrombin III, inactivates coagulation factor Xa. **Therapeutic Effect:** Produces anticoagulation. Does not significantly influence bleeding time, PT, aPTT.

PHARMACOKINETICS

Route	Onset	Peak	Duration
Subcutaneous	N/A	3–5 hrs	12 hrs

Well absorbed after subcutaneous administration. Eliminated primarily in urine. Not removed by hemodialysis. **Half-life:** 4.5 hrs.

USES

Prevention of postop deep vein thrombosis (DVT) following hip or knee replacement surgery, abdominal surgery. Long-term DVT prevention following hip replacement surgery, nonsurgical acute illness. Treatment of unstable angina, non–Q-wave MI, acute DVT (with warfarin). **OFF-LABEL:** Prevention of DVT following general surgical procedures.

PRECAUTIONS

CONTRAINDICATIONS: Active major bleeding, concurrent heparin therapy, hypersensitivity to heparin, pork products, thrombocytopenia associated with positive in vitro test for antiplatelet antibodies. **CAUTIONS:** Conditions with increased risk of hemorrhage, history of heparin-induced thrombocytopenia, renal impairment, elderly, uncontrolled arterial hypertension, history of recent GI ulceration or hemorrhage. When neuraxial anesthesia (epidural or spinal anesthesia) or spinal puncture is used, pts anticoagulated or scheduled to be anticoagulated with enoxaparin for prevention of thromboembolic complications are at risk for developing an epidural or spinal hematoma that can result in long-term or permanent paralysis.

LIFESPAN CONSIDERATIONS: **Pregnancy/Lactation:** Use with caution, particularly during last trimester, immediate postpartum period (increased risk of maternal hemorrhage). Unknown if excreted in breast milk. **Pregnancy Category B. Children:** Safety and efficacy not established. **Elderly:** May be more susceptible to bleeding.

INTERACTIONS

DRUG: NSAIDs, aspirin, antiplatelet agents, thrombolytics may increase risk of bleeding. **HERBAL: Cat's claw, dong quai, evening primrose, feverfew, garlic, ginger, ginkgo, ginseng** may increase antiplatelet action. **FOOD:** None known. **LAB VALUES:** Increases (reversible) LDH, serum alkaline phosphatase, AST, ALT.

AVAILABILITY (Rx)

INJECTION SOLUTION: 30 mg/0.3 ml, 40 mg/0.4 ml, 60 mg/0.6 ml, 80 mg/0.8 ml, 100 mg/ml, 120 mg/0.8 ml, 150 mg/ml in prefilled syringes.

ADMINISTRATION/HANDLING

◄ **ALERT** ► Do not mix with other injections, infusions. Do not give IM.

SUBCUTANEOUS

• Parenteral form appears clear, colorless to pale yellow. • Store at room temperature. • Instruct pt to lie down before administering by deep subcutaneous injection. • Inject between left and right anterolateral and left and right posterolateral abdominal wall. • Introduce entire length of needle (½ inch) into skin fold held between thumb and forefinger, holding skin fold during injection.

E

INDICATIONS/ROUTES/DOSAGE

PREVENTION OF DVT AFTER HIP AND KNEE SURGERY

SUBCUTANEOUS: ADULTS, ELDERLY: 30 mg twice a day, generally for 7–10 days.

PREVENTION OF DVT AFTER ABDOMINAL SURGERY

SUBCUTANEOUS: ADULTS, ELDERLY: 40 mg a day for 7–10 days.

PREVENTION OF LONG-TERM DVT IN NONSURGICAL ACUTE ILLNESS

SUBCUTANEOUS: ADULTS, ELDERLY: 40 mg once a day for 3 wks.

PREVENTION OF ISCHEMIC COMPLICATIONS OF UNSTABLE ANGINA, NON–Q-WAVE MI (WITH ORAL ASPIRIN THERAPY)

SUBCUTANEOUS: ADULTS, ELDERLY: 1 mg/kg q12h.

ACUTE DVT

SUBCUTANEOUS: ADULTS, ELDERLY: 1 mg/kg q12h or 1.5 mg/kg once daily.

USUAL PEDIATRIC DOSAGE

SUBCUTANEOUS: CHILDREN: 0.5 mg/kg q12h (prophylaxis); 1 mg/kg q12h (treatment).

DOSAGE IN RENAL IMPAIRMENT

Clearance is decreased when creatinine clearance is less than 30 ml/min. Monitor and adjust dosage as necessary.

Use	Dosage
Abdominal surgery, pts with acute illness	30 mg once/day
Hip, knee surgery	30 mg once/day
DVT, angina, MI	1 mg/kg once/day

SIDE EFFECTS

OCCASIONAL (4%–1%): Injection site hematoma, nausea, peripheral edema.

ADVERSE EFFECTS/ TOXIC REACTIONS

Overdose may lead to bleeding complications ranging from local ecchymoses to major hemorrhage. **Antidote** IV injection of protamine sulfate (1% solution) equal to dose of enoxaparin injected. One mg protamine sulfate neutralizes 1 mg enoxaparin. A second dose of 0.5 mg protamine sulfate per 1 mg enoxaparin may be given if aPTT tested 2–4 hrs after first injection remains prolonged.

NURSING CONSIDERATIONS

BASELINE ASSESSMENT

Assess CBC, including platelet count.

INTERVENTION/EVALUATION

Periodically monitor CBC, platelet count, stool for occult blood (no need for daily monitoring in pts with normal presurgical coagulation parameters). Assess for any sign of bleeding (bleeding at surgical site, hematuria, blood in stool, bleeding from gums, petechiae, bruising, bleeding from injection sites).

PATIENT/FAMILY TEACHING

• Usual length of therapy is 7–10 days.
• Do not take any OTC medication (esp. aspirin) without consulting physician.

entacapone

en-**tah**-cah-pone
(Comtan)

FIXED-COMBINATION(S)

Stalevo: entacapone/carbidopa-levodopa (an antiparkinson agent) 200 mg/12.5 mg/50 mg; 200 mg/25 mg/100 mg; 200 mg/37.5 mg/150 mg.

◆ **CLASSIFICATION**

PHARMACOTHERAPEUTIC: Enzyme inhibitor. **CLINICAL:** Antiparkinson agent.

ACTION

Inhibits the enzyme, catechol-*O*-methyltransferase (COMT), potentiating dopamine activity, increasing duration of action of levodopa. **Therapeutic Effect:** Decreases signs, symptoms of Parkinson's disease.

PHARMACOKINETICS

Rapidly absorbed after PO administration. Protein binding: 98%. Metabolized in liver. Primarily eliminated by biliary excretion. Not removed by hemodialysis. **Half-life:** 2.4 hrs.

USES

In conjunction with levodopa/carbidopa, improves quality of life in pts with Parkinson's disease.

PRECAUTIONS

CONTRAINDICATIONS: Hypersensitivity, use within 14 days of MAOIs. **CAUTIONS:** Renal/hepatic impairment. May increase risk of orthostatic hypotension and syncope, exacerbate dyskinesias.

⌛ LIFESPAN CONSIDERATIONS:

Pregnancy/Lactation: Unknown if distributed in breast milk. **Pregnancy Category C. Children:** Not used in children. **Elderly:** No age-related precautions noted.

INTERACTIONS

DRUG: Ampicillin, cholestyramine, erythromycin, probenecid may decrease excretion of entacapone. **Bitolterol, dobutamine, dopamine, epinephrine, isoetharine, isoproterenol, epinephrine, methyldopa, norepinephrine** may increase risk of arrhythmias, alter B/P. **Nonselective MAOIs (including phenelzine)** may inhibit catecholamine metabolism. **Other CNS depressants** may increase CNS depression. **HERBAL:** None significant. **FOOD:** None known. **LAB VALUES:** None known.

AVAILABILITY (Rx)

TABLETS: 200 mg.

ADMINISTRATION/HANDLING

PO

- Give without regard to food.

INDICATIONS/ROUTES/DOSAGE

◀ **ALERT** ▶ Always administer with levodopa/carbidopa.

ADJUNCTIVE TREATMENT OF PARKINSON'S DISEASE

PO: ADULTS, ELDERLY: 200 mg concomitantly with each dose of carbidopa and levodopa up to a maximum of 8 times a day (1,600 mg).

SIDE EFFECTS

FREQUENT (greater than 10%): Dyskinesia (uncontrolled body movements), nausea, dark yellow or orange urine and sweat, diarrhea. **OCCASIONAL (9%–3%):** Abdominal pain, vomiting, constipation, dry mouth, fatigue, back pain. **RARE (less than 2%):** Anxiety, somnolence, agitation, dyspepsia, flatulence, diaphoresis, asthenia, dyspnea.

ADVERSE EFFECTS/ TOXIC REACTIONS

Hallucinations may be noted.

NURSING CONSIDERATIONS

INTERVENTION/EVALUATION

Monitor for evidence of dyskinesia (difficulty with movement). Assess for clinical reversal of symptoms (improvement of tremor of head and hands at rest, mask-like facial expression, shuffling gait, muscular rigidity). Monitor B/P. Assess for orthostatic hypotension, diarrhea.

PATIENT/FAMILY TEACHING

• Avoid tasks that require alertness, motor skills until response to drug is established. • May cause color change in urine or sweat (dark yellow, orange). • Report any uncontrolled movement of face, eyelids, mouth, tongue, arms, hands, legs.

E

entecavir

en-**tech**-ah-veer

(Baraclude)

CLASSIFICATION

PHARMACOTHERAPEUTIC: Reverse transcriptase inhibitor. **CLINICAL:** Antiretroviral.

ACTION

Inhibits hepatitis B viral polymerase, an enzyme blocking reverse transcriptase activity. **Therapeutic Effect:** Interferes with viral DNA synthesis.

PHARMACOKINETICS

Poorly absorbed from GI tract. Protein binding: 13%. Extensively distributed into tissues. Partially metabolized in liver. Eliminated mainly in urine. **Half-life:** 5–6 days (half-life increased in renal impairment).

USES

Treatment of chronic hepatitis B infection with evidence of active viral replication and either evidence of persistent transaminase elevations or histologically-active disease.

PRECAUTIONS

CONTRAINDICATIONS: None known. **CAUTIONS:** Renal impairment, pts receiving concurrent therapy that may reduce renal function, hepatic transplant pts receiving concurrent therapy of cyclosporine or tacrolimus.

LIFESPAN CONSIDERATIONS:

Pregnancy/Lactation: Unknown if drug crosses placenta or is distributed in breast milk. **Pregnancy Category C. Children:** Safety and efficacy not established in children younger than 16 yrs. **Elderly:** Age-related renal impairment may require dosage adjustment.

INTERACTIONS

DRUG: Drugs that reduce renal function may increase serum concentrations of entecavir or coadministered drug. **HERBAL:** None significant. **FOOD: Food** delays absorption, decreases concentration. **LAB VALUES:** May increase serum amylase, lipase, bilirubin, ALT, AST, creatinine, glucose. May decrease serum albumin, platelets.

AVAILABILITY (Rx)

ORAL SOLUTION: 0.05 mg/ml. **TABLETS:** 0.5 mg, 1 mg.

ADMINISTRATION/HANDLING

PO

• Administer tablets on an empty stomach (at least 2 hrs after a meal and 2 hrs before the next meal). • Do not dilute, mix oral solution with water or any other liquid. • Each bottle of oral solution is accompanied by a dosing spoon. Before administering, hold spoon in vertical position, fill it gradually to mark corresponding to prescribed dose.

Storage • Store tablets oral solution at room temperature.

INDICATIONS/ROUTES/DOSAGE

CHRONIC HEPATITIS B (NO PREVIOUS NUCLEOSIDE TREATMENT)

PO: ADULTS, ELDERLY, CHILDREN 16 YRS AND OLDER: 0.5 mg once daily.

CHRONIC HEPATITIS B (RECEIVING LAMIVUDINE, KNOWN LAMIVUDINE RESISTANCE)

PO: ADULTS, ELDERLY, CHILDREN 16 YRS AND OLDER: 1 mg once daily.

DOSAGE IN RENAL IMPAIRMENT

Creatinine Clearance	Dosage
50 ml/min and greater	0.5 mg once daily
30–49 ml/min	0.25 mg once daily
10–29 ml/min	0.15 mg once daily
9 ml/min and less	0.05 mg once daily

SIDE EFFECTS

OCCASIONAL (4%–3%): Headache, fatigue. **RARE (less than 1%):** Diarrhea, dyspepsia, nausea, vomiting, dizziness, insomnia.

ADVERSE EFFECTS/ TOXIC REACTIONS

Lactic acidosis, severe hepatomegaly with steatosis have been reported. Severe, acute exacerbations of hepatitis B have been reported in pts who have discontinued therapy; reinitiation of antihepatitis B therapy may be required. Hematuria occurs occasionally.

NURSING CONSIDERATIONS

BASELINE ASSESSMENT

Obtain baseline laboratory tests, esp. hepatic function, before beginning therapy and at periodic intervals during therapy. Offer emotional support. Obtain medication history.

INTERVENTION/EVALUATION

Hepatic function should be monitored closely with both clinical and laboratory follow-up for at least several mos in pts who discontinue antihepatitis B therapy. For pts on therapy, closely monitor amylase, lipase, bilirubin, ALT, AST, creatinine, glucose, albumin, platelet count. Assess for evidence of GI discomfort.

PATIENT/FAMILY TEACHING

• Take medication at least 2 hrs after a meal and 2 hrs before the next meal. • Avoid transmission of hepatitis B infection to others through sexual contact, blood contamination. • Notify physician immediately if unusual muscle pain, abdominal pain with nausea/vomiting, cold feeling in extremities, dizziness occur (signs and symptoms signaling onset of lactic acidosis).

epinephrine

eh-pih-**nef**-rin

(Adrenalin, EpiPen, EpiPen 2-Pak, EpiPen Auto Injector, EpiPen Jr. Auto-Injector, Primatene, Sus-Phrine Injection, Vaponephrin ✤)

Do not confuse epinephrine with ephedrine.

FIXED-COMBINATION(S)

LidoSite: epinephrine/lidocaine (anesthetic): 0.1%/10%.

CLASSIFICATION

PHARMACOTHERAPEUTIC: Sympathomimetic (adrenergic agonist). **CLINICAL:** Antiglaucoma, bronchodilator, cardiac stimulant, antiallergic, antihemorrhagic, priapism reversal agent (see pp. 49C, 148C).

ACTION

Stimulates alpha-adrenergic receptors (vasoconstriction, pressor effects), beta$_1$-adrenergic receptors (cardiac stimulation), beta$_2$-adrenergic receptors, (bronchial dilation, vasodilation). **Ophthalmic:** Increases outflow of aqueous humor from anterior eye chamber. **Therapeutic Effect:** Relaxes smooth muscle of bronchial tree, produces cardiac stimulation, dilates skeletal muscle vasculature. **Ophthalmic:** Dilates pupils, constricts conjunctival blood vessels.

PHARMACOKINETICS

Route	Onset	Peak	Duration
IM	5–10 min	20 min	1–4 hrs
Subcutaneous	5–10 min	20 min	1–4 hrs
Inhalation	3–5 min	20 min	1–3 hrs
Ophthalmic	1 hr	4–8 hrs	12–24 hrs

Well absorbed after parenteral administration; minimally absorbed after inhalation. Metabolized in liver, other tissues, sympathetic nerve endings. Excreted in urine. Ophthalmic form may be systemically absorbed as a result of drainage into nasal pharyngeal passages. Mydriasis occurs within several min and persists several hrs; vasoconstriction occurs within 5 min, and lasts less than 1 hr.

E

USES

Systemic: Treatment of asthma (acute exacerbation, reversible bronchospasm), anaphylaxis, hypersensitivity reaction, cardiac arrest. **Ophthalmic:** Management of chronic open-angle glaucoma. **OFF-LABEL:** **Systemic:** Treatment of gingival, pulpal hemorrhage; priapism. **Ophthalmic:** Treatment of conjunctival congestion during surgery, secondary glaucoma.

PRECAUTIONS

CONTRAINDICATIONS: Cardiac arrhythmias, cerebrovascular insufficiency, hypertension, hyperthyroidism, ischemic heart disease, narrow-angle glaucoma, shock-type states. **CAUTIONS:** Elderly, diabetes mellitus, angina pectoris, tachycardia, MI, severe renal/hepatic impairment, psychoneurotic disorders, hypoxia.

LIFESPAN CONSIDERATIONS:

Pregnancy/Lactation: Crosses placenta. Distributed in breast milk. **Pregnancy Category C.** **Children/Elderly:** No age-related precautions noted.

INTERACTIONS

DRUG: May decrease effects of **beta blockers. Digoxin, sympathomimetics** may increase risk of arrhythmias. **Ergonovine, methergine, oxytocin** may increase vasoconstriction. **MAOIs, tricyclic antidepressants** may increase cardiovascular effects. **HERBAL:** **Ephedra, yohimbe** may increase CNS stimulation. **FOOD:** None known. **LAB VALUES:** May decrease serum potassium.

AVAILABILITY (Rx)

AEROSOL FOR ORAL INHALATION: (Primatene Mist): 0.22 mg/inhalation. **INJECTION, SOLUTION (PREFILLED SYRINGES): (Epi-Pen):** 0.3 mg/0.3 ml **(Epi-Pen Jr):** 0.15 mg/0.3 ml **(Twinject):** 0.15 mg/0.15 ml. **INJECTION, SOLUTION:** 0.1 mg/ml (1:10,000), 1 mg/ml (1:1,000). **SOLUTION FOR ORAL INHALATION: (Adrenalin):** 1%(1:100) 10 mg/ml.

ADMINISTRATION/HANDLING

IV

Reconstitution • For injection, dilute each 1 mg of 1:1,000 solution with 10 ml 0.9 NaCl to provide 1:10,000 solution and inject each 1 mg or fraction thereof over 1 min or more (except in cardiac arrest). • For infusion, further dilute with 250–500 D_5W. Maximum concentration: 64 mg/250 ml.

Rate of administration • For IV infusion, give at 1–10 mcg/min (titrate to desired response).

Storage • Store parenteral forms at room temperature. • Do not use if solution appears discolored or contains a precipitate.

SUBCUTANEOUS

• Shake ampule thoroughly. • Use tuberculin syringe for injection into lateral deltoid region. • Massage injection site (minimizes vasoconstriction effect).

INHALATION

• Shake container well. • Instruct pt to exhale as completely as possible then place mouthpiece fully into mouth, and while holding inhaler upright, inhale deeply and slowly while pressuring top of canister. • Hold breath as long as possible, then exhale slowly. • Wait 1 min between inhalations when multiple inhalations are ordered (allows for deeper bronchial penetration). • Rinse mouth with water immediately after inhalation (prevents mouth, throat dryness).

NEBULIZER

• No more than 10 drops Adrenalin Chloride solution 1:100 should be placed in reservoir of nebulizer, nozzle placed just inside partially opened mouth. • As bulb is squeezed once or twice, instruct pt to inhale deeply, drawing vaporized solution into lungs. • Rinse mouth with water immediately after inhalation (prevents mouth/throat dryness). • When nebulizer is not in use, replace stopper, keep in upright position.

OPHTHALMIC

• Place finger on lower eyelid, pull out until pocket is formed between eye and lower lid. • Hold dropper above pocket and place prescribed number of drops into pocket. • Close eye gently so medication will not be squeezed out of sac. • Apply gentle digital pressure to lacrimal sac at inner canthus for 1 min after installation to lessen risk of systemic absorption.

IV INCOMPATIBILITY

Aminophylline, ampicillin (Omnipen, Polycillin), sodium bicarbonate.

IV COMPATIBILITIES

Calcium chloride, calcium gluconate, diltiazem (Cardizem), dobutamine (Dobutrex), dopamine (Intropin), fentanyl (Sublimaze), heparin, hydromorphone (Dilaudid), lorazepam (Ativan), midazolam (Versed), milrinone (Primacor), morphine, nitroglycerin, norepinephrine (Levophed), potassium chloride, propofol (Diprivan).

INDICATIONS/ROUTES/DOSAGE

ANAPHYLAXIS

IM: **ADULTS, ELDERLY:** 0.3 mg (0.3 ml of 1:1,000 solution). May repeat if anaphylaxis persists. **CHILDREN:** 0.15–0.3 mg or 0.01 mg/kg for pts weighing less than 30 kg. May repeat if anaphylaxis persists.

ASTHMA

SUBCUTANEOUS: **ADULTS, ELDERLY:** 0.2–0.5 mg (0.2–0.5 ml of 1:1,000 solution) q2h as needed. In severe attacks, may repeat q20min times 3 doses. **CHILDREN:** 0.01 ml/kg/dose (1:1,000 solution). **Maximum:** 0.4–0.5 ml/dose. May repeat q15–20min for 3–4 doses or q4h as needed.

INHALATION: **ADULTS, ELDERLY, CHILDREN 4 YRS AND OLDER:** 1 inhalation, wait at least 1 min. May repeat once. Do not use again for at least 3 hrs.

CARDIAC ARREST

IV: **ADULTS, ELDERLY:** Initially, 1 mg. May repeat q3–5min as needed. **CHILDREN:** Initially, 0.01 mg/kg (0.1 ml/kg of a 1:10,000 solution). May repeat q3–5min as needed.

ENDOTRACHEAL: **CHILDREN:** 0.1 mg/kg (0.1 ml/kg of a 1:1,000 solution). May repeat q3–5min as needed.

HYPERSENSITIVITY REACTION

IM, SUBCUTANEOUS: **ADULTS, ELDERLY:** 0.3–0.5 mg q15–20min.

SUBCUTANEOUS: **CHILDREN:** 0.01 mg/kg q15min for 2 doses, then q4h. **Maximum single dose:** 0.5 mg.

GLAUCOMA

OPHTHALMIC: **ADULTS, ELDERLY:** 1–2 drops 1–2 times a day.

SIDE EFFECTS

FREQUENT: Systemic: Tachycardia, palpitations, anxiety. **Ophthalmic:** Headache, eye irritation, watering of eyes. **OCCASIONAL: Systemic:** Dizziness, lightheadedness, facial flushing, headache, diaphoresis, increased B/P, nausea, trembling, insomnia, vomiting, fatigue. **Ophthalmic:** Blurred/decreased vision, eye pain. **RARE: Systemic:** Chest discomfort/pain, arrhythmias, bronchospasm, dry mouth/throat.

ADVERSE EFFECTS/ TOXIC REACTIONS

Excessive doses may cause acute hypertension, arrhythmias. Prolonged/excessive use may result in metabolic acidosis due to increased serum lactic acid. Metabolic acidosis may cause disorientation, fatigue, hyperventilation, headache, nausea, vomiting, diarrhea.

NURSING CONSIDERATIONS

INTERVENTION/EVALUATION

Monitor for vital sign changes. Assess lung sounds for rhonchi, wheezing, rales. Monitor ABGs. In cardiac arrest, monitor EKG, pt condition.

PATIENT/FAMILY TEACHING

• Avoid excessive use of caffeine derivatives (chocolate, coffee, tea, cola, cocoa). • **Ophthalmic:** Slight burning, stinging may occur on initial instillation. • Report any new symptoms (tachycardia, shortness of breath, dizziness) immediately: may be systemic effects.

epirubicin

eh-pea-**rew**-bih-sin

(Ellence, Pharmorubicin ♣, Pharmorubicin PFS ♣, Pharmorubicin RDS ♣)

CLASSIFICATION

PHARMACOTHERAPEUTIC: Anthracycline antibiotic. **CLINICAL:** Antineoplastic (see p. 78C).

ACTION

May include formation of complex with DNA, subsequent inhibition of DNA, RNA, protein synthesis. Inhibits DNA helicase activity, preventing enzymatic separation of double-stranded DNA, interfering with replication, transcription. **Therapeutic Effect:** Produces antiproliferative, cytotoxic activity.

PHARMACOKINETICS

Widely distributed into tissues. Protein binding: 77%. Metabolized in liver and RBCs. Primarily eliminated through biliary excretion. Not removed by hemodialysis. **Half-life:** 33 hrs.

USES

Component of adjuvant therapy in pts with evidence of axillary node tumor involvement following resection of primary breast cancer. **OFF-LABEL:** Esophageal, gastric, small cell lung, non–small cell lung, ovarian carcinomas; Hodgkin's, non-Hodgkin's lymphomas; soft tissue sarcoma; neoplasms of bladder.

PRECAUTIONS

CONTRAINDICATIONS: Baseline neutrophil count less than 1,500/mm^3, hypersensitivity to epirubicin, previous treatment with anthracyclines up to maximum cumulative dose, recent MI, severe hepatic impairment, severe myocardial insufficiency. **CAUTIONS:** Renal or hepatic impairment.

LIFESPAN CONSIDERATIONS:

Pregnancy/Lactation: May cause fetal harm. Unknown if distributed in breast milk. **Pregnancy Category D. Children:** Safety and efficacy not established. **Elderly:** No age-related precautions noted but monitor for toxicity.

INTERACTIONS

DRUG: Medications causing blood dyscrasias may increase risk of developing leukopenia, thrombocytopenia. **Bone marrow depressants** may cause additive myelosuppression. **Calcium channel blockers** may increase risk of developing heart failure. **Cimetidine** may increase serum concentration, toxicity. **Daunorubicin, doxorubicin, idarubicin, mitoxantrone** may increase risk of GI, hematologic, hepatic effects; cardiotoxicity. **Hepatotoxic medications** may increase risk of hepatotoxicity. **Live virus vaccines** may potentiate virus replication, increase vaccine side effects, decrease pt's antibody response to vaccine. **HERBAL: St. John's wort** may decrease concentration. Avoid **black cohosh, dong quai** in estrogen-dependent tumors. **FOOD:** None known. **LAB VALUES:** None known.

AVAILABILITY (Rx)

INJECTION SOLUTION: 2-mg/ml single-use vials.

ADMINISTRATION/HANDLING

◀ **ALERT** ▶ Exclude pregnant staff from working with epirubicin; wear protective clothing. If accidental contact with skin or eyes occurs, flush area immediately with copious amounts of water.

IV

Reconstitution • Ready-to-use vials require no reconstitution.

Rate of administration • Infuse medication into tubing of free-flowing IV of 0.9% NaCl or D_5W over 3–5 min.

Storage • Refrigerate vial. • Protect from light. • Use within 24 hrs of first penetration of rubber stopper. • Discard unused portion.

IV INCOMPATIBILITIES

Heparin, fluorouracil (5-FU). Do not mix epirubicin in same syringe with other medications.

INDICATIONS/ROUTES/DOSAGE

BREAST CANCER

IV: ADULTS: Initially, 100–120 mg/m^2 in repeated cycles of 3–4 wks, in combination with 5-FU and Cytoxan. Total dose may be given on day 1 of each cycle or in equally divided doses on days 1 and 8 of each cycle.

SIDE EFFECTS

FREQUENT (83%–70%): Nausea, vomiting alopecia, amenorrhea. **OCCASIONAL (9%–5%):** Stomatitis, diarrhea, hot flashes. **RARE (2%–1%):** Rash, pruritus, fever, lethargy, conjunctivitis.

ADVERSE EFFECTS/ TOXIC REACTIONS

Risk of cardiotoxicity (either acute, manifested as transient EKG abnormalities, or chronic, manifested as CHF) increases when total cumulative dose exceeds 900 mg/m^2. Extravasation during administration may result in severe local tissue necrosis. Myelosuppression may produce hematologic toxicity, manifested principally as leukopenia and, to lesser extent, anemia, thrombocytopenia.

NURSING CONSIDERATIONS

BASELINE ASSESSMENT

Obtain WBC, platelet, erythrocyte counts before and at frequent intervals during therapy. Obtain EKG before therapy, serum hepatic function studies before each dose. Antiemetics may be effective in preventing, treating nausea.

INTERVENTION/EVALUATION

Monitor for stomatitis (may lead to ulceration of mucous membranes within 2–3 days). Monitor blood counts for evidence of myelosuppression, renal/hepatic function studies, cardiac function. Monitor daily pattern of bowel activity/stool consistency. Monitor for hematologic toxicity (fever, sore throat, signs of local infection, unusual bruising/bleeding from any site), symptoms of anemia (excessive fatigue, weakness).

PATIENT/FAMILY TEACHING

• Alopecia is reversible, but new hair growth may have different color, texture. New hair growth resumes 2–3 mos after last therapy dose. • Maintain fastidious oral hygiene. • Do not have immunizations without physician's approval (drug lowers resistance). • Avoid contact with those who have recently received live virus vaccine. • Promptly report fever, sore throat, signs of local infection, easy unusual bruising/bleeding from any site.

E

Epivir, *see lamivudine*

eplerenone

eh-**pleh**-reh-known
(Inspra)

CLASSIFICATION

PHARMACOTHERAPEUTIC: Aldosterone receptor antagonist. **CLINICAL:** Antihypertensive.

ACTION

Binds to mineralocorticoid receptors in kidney, heart, blood vessels, brain, blocking binding of aldosterone. **Therapeutic Effect:** Reduces B/P.

PHARMACOKINETICS

Absorption unaffected by food. Protein binding: 50%. No active metabolites. Excreted in urine with lesser amount eliminated in feces. Not removed by hemodialysis. **Half-life:** 4–6 hrs.

USES

Treatment of hypertension alone or in combination with other antihypertensive agents. Treatment of CHF following acute myocardial infarction (AMI).

PRECAUTIONS

CONTRAINDICATIONS: Concurrent use of potassium supplements, potassium-sparing diuretics (e.g., amiloride, spironolactone, triamterene), strong inhibitors of cytochrome P450 3A4 enzyme system (e.g., ketoconazole, itraconazole), creatinine clearance less than 50 ml/min, serum creatinine level greater than 2 mg/dl in males or 1.8 mg/dl in females, serum potassium level greater than 5.5 mEq/L, type 2 diabetes mellitus with microalbuminuria. **CAUTIONS:** Hepatic insufficiency, hyperkalemia.

LIFESPAN CONSIDERATIONS:

Pregnancy/Lactation: Unknown if drug crosses placenta or is distributed in breast milk. **Pregnancy Category B.** **Children:** Safety and efficacy not established. **Elderly:** No age-related precautions noted.

INTERACTIONS

DRUG: **Angiotensin-converting enzyme (ACE) inhibitors, angiotensin II antagonists, erythromycin, fluconazole, saquinavir, verapamil** increase risk of hyperkalemia. **Potassium-sparing diuretics (e.g., spironolactone), potassium supplements** increase risk of hyperkalemia. **Itraconazole, ketoconazole** increase concentration fivefold (use is contraindicated). **HERBAL:** **St. John's wort** decreases effectiveness. **FOOD:** **Grapefruit, grapefruit juice** produces slight increase in serum potassium. **LAB VALUES:** May increase serum potassium. May decrease serum sodium.

AVAILABILITY (Rx)

TABLETS: 25 mg, 50 mg.

ADMINISTRATION/HANDLING

• Do not break, crush, chew film-coated tablets.

INDICATIONS/ROUTES/DOSAGE

HYPERTENSION

PO: ADULTS, ELDERLY: 50 mg once a day. If 50 mg once a day produces an inadequate B/P response, may increase dosage to 50 mg twice a day. If pt is concurrently receiving erythromycin, saquinavir, verapamil, or fluconazole, reduce initial dose to 25 mg once a day.

CHF FOLLOWING MI

PO: ADULTS, ELDERLY: Initially, 25 mg once a day. If tolerated, titrate up to 50 mg once a day within 4 wks.

DOSAGE ADJUSTMENT FOR SERUM POTASSIUM CONCENTRATIONS IN CHF

5 mEq/L or less: Increase from 25 mg daily to 50 mg daily. Increase from 25 mg every other day to 25 mg daily.
5–5.4 mEq/L: No adjustment needed.
5.5–5.9 mEq/L: Decrease dose from 50 mg daily to 25 mg daily. Decrease dose from 25 mg daily to 25 mg every other day. Decrease dose from 25 mg every other day to withhold medication.
6 mEq/L or greater: Withhold medication until potassium is less than 5.5 mEq/L.

DOSAGE IN RENAL IMPAIRMENT

Use is contraindicated in pts with hypertension with creatinine clearance less than 50 mL/min or serum creatinine greater than 2 mg/dL in males or greater than 1.8 mg/dL in females.

SIDE EFFECTS

RARE (3%–1%): Dizziness, diarrhea, cough, fatigue, flu-like symptoms, abdominal pain.

ADVERSE EFFECTS/ TOXIC REACTIONS

Hyperkalemia may occur, particularly in pts with type 2 diabetes mellitus and microalbuminuria.

NURSING CONSIDERATIONS

BASELINE ASSESSMENT

Obtain B/P, apical pulse immediately before each dose, in addition to regular monitoring (be alert to fluctuations). If excessive reduction in B/P occurs, place pt in supine position, feet slightly elevated.

INTERVENTION/EVALUATION

Assist with ambulation if dizziness occurs. Monitor serum potassium levels. Assess B/P for hypertension and hypotension. Monitor daily pattern of bowel activity/stool consistency. Assess for evidence of flu-like symptoms.

PATIENT/FAMILY TEACHING

• Avoid tasks that require alertness, motor skills until response to drug is established (possible dizziness effect). • Discuss need for lifelong control. • Caution against exercising during hot weather (risk of dehydration, hypotension).

epoetin alfa

eh-po-**ee**-tin-**al**-fa
(Epogen, Eprex ✤, Procrit)
Do not confuse Epogen with Neupogen.

CLASSIFICATION

PHARMACOTHERAPEUTIC: Glycoprotein. **CLINICAL:** Erythropoietin.

ACTION

Stimulates division, differentiation of erythroid progenitor cells in bone marrow. **Therapeutic Effect:** Induces erythropoiesis, releases reticulocytes from bone marrow.

PHARMACOKINETICS

Well absorbed after subcutaneous administration. Following administration, an increase in reticulocyte count occurs within 10 days, and increases in Hgb, Hct, and RBC count are seen within 2–6 wks. **Half-life:** 4–13 hrs.

USES

Treatment of anemia in pts receiving or who have received chemotherapy, those with chronic renal failure, HIV-infected pts on zidovudine (AZT) therapy, those scheduled for elective non-cardiac, nonvascular surgery, reducing need for allogenic blood transfusions. **OFF-LABEL:** Anemia associated with frequent blood donations, anemia in critically ill pts, malignancy, management of hepatitis C, myelodysplastic syndromes.

E

PRECAUTIONS

CONTRAINDICATIONS: History of sensitivity to mammalian cell-derived products or human albumin, uncontrolled hypertension. **CAUTIONS:** Pts with known porphyria (impairment of erythrocyte formation in bone marrow); history of seizures.

LIFESPAN CONSIDERATIONS:

Pregnancy/Lactation: Unknown if drug crosses placenta or is distributed in breast milk. **Pregnancy Category C.** **Children:** Safety and efficacy not established in those 12 yrs and younger. **Elderly:** No age-related precautions noted.

INTERACTIONS

DRUG: Increase in RBC volume may enhance blood clotting. **Heparin** dosage may need to be increased. **HERBAL:** None significant. **FOOD:** None known. **LAB VALUES:** May increase BUN, serum phosphorus, potassium, creatinine, uric acid, sodium. May decrease bleeding time, iron concentration, serum ferritin.

AVAILABILITY (Rx)

INJECTION SOLUTION (EPOGEN, PROCRIT): 2,000 units/ml, 3,000 units/ml, 4,000 units/ml, 10,000 units/ml, 20,000 units/ml, 40,000 units/ml.

ADMINISTRATION/HANDLING

◄ ALERT ► Avoid excessive agitation of vial; do not shake (foaming).

IV

Reconstitution • No reconstitution necessary.

Rate of administration • May be given as an IV bolus.

Storage • Refrigerate. • Vigorous shaking may denature medication, rendering it inactive.

SUBCUTANEOUS

Mix in syringe with bacteriostatic 0.9% NaCl with benzyl alcohol 0.9% (bacteriostatic saline) at a 1:1 ratio (benzyl alcohol acts as a local anesthetic; may reduce injection site discomfort). • Use 1 dose per vial; do not reenter vial. Discard unused portion.

IV INCOMPATIBILITIES

Do not mix injection form with other medications.

INDICATIONS/ROUTES/DOSAGE

TREATMENT OF ANEMIA IN CHEMOTHERAPY PTS

IV, SUBCUTANEOUS: ADULTS, ELDERLY: 150 units/kg/dose 3 times a wk or 40,000 units/wk. Doses range from 10,000 units 3 times a wk to 40,000 units once weekly. **CHILDREN:** Initially, 150 units/kg. **Range:** 25–300 units/kg 3–7 times/wk.

REDUCTION OF ALLOGENIC BLOOD TRANSFUSIONS IN ELECTIVE SURGERY

SUBCUTANEOUS: ADULTS, ELDERLY: 300 units/kg/day 10 days before and 4 days after surgery.

CHRONIC RENAL FAILURE

IV BOLUS, SUBCUTANEOUS: ADULTS, ELDERLY: Initially, 50–100 units/kg 3 times a wk. **CHILDREN:** Initially, 50 units/kg 3 times a wk. Target hematocrit (Hct) range: 30%–36%. Adjust dosage no earlier than 1-mo intervals unless prescribed. Decrease dosage if Hct is increasing and approaching 36%. Plan to temporarily withhold doses if Hct continues to rise and to reinstate lower dosage when Hct begins to decrease. If Hct increases by more than 4 points in 2 wks, monitor Hct twice a wk for 2–6 wks. Increase dose if Hct does not increase 5–6 points after 8 wks (with adequate iron stores) and if Hct is below target range. Maintenance (Adults): *Pts on dialysis:* 75 units/kg 3 times a wk. Range: 12.5–525 units/kg. *Pts not on dialysis:* 75–150 units/kg/wk. Maintenance (Children): *Pts on dialysis:* 167 units/kg/wk or 76 units/kg 2–3 times/wk. *Pts not on dialysis:* 50–250 units 1–3 times/wk.

HIV INFECTION IN PTS TREATED WITH AZT

IV, SUBCUTANEOUS: ADULTS: Initially, 100 units/kg 3 times a wk for 8 wks; may increase by 50–100 units/kg 3 times a wk. Evaluate response q4–8wk thereafter. Adjust dosage by 50–100 units/kg 3 times a wk. If dosages larger than 300 units/kg 3 times a wk are not eliciting response, it is unlikely pt will respond. Maintenance: Titrate to maintain desired Hct.

SIDE EFFECTS

PTS RECEIVING CHEMOTHERAPY

FREQUENT (20%–17%): Fever, diarrhea, nausea, vomiting, edema. **OCCASIONAL (13%–11%):** Asthenia, shortness of breath, paresthesia. **RARE (5%–3%):** Dizziness, trunk pain.

PTS WITH CHRONIC RENAL FAILURE

FREQUENT (24%–11%): Hypertension, headache, nausea, arthralgia. **OCCASIONAL (9%–7%):** Fatigue, edema, diarrhea, vomiting, chest pain, skin reactions at administration site, asthenia, dizziness.

PTS WITH HIV INFECTION TREATED WITH AZT

FREQUENT (38%–15%): Fever, fatigue, headache, cough, diarrhea, rash, nausea. **OCCASIONAL (14%–9%):** Shortness of breath, asthenia, skin reaction at injection site, dizziness.

ADVERSE EFFECTS/ TOXIC REACTIONS

Hypertensive encephalopathy, thrombosis, cerebrovascular accident, MI, seizures occur rarely. Hyperkalemia occurs occasionally in pts with chronic renal failure, usually in those who do not comply with medication regimen, dietary guidelines, frequency of dialysis regimen.

NURSING CONSIDERATIONS

BASELINE ASSESSMENT

Assess B/P before drug initiation (80% of pts with chronic renal failure have history of hypertension). B/P often rises during early therapy in pts with history of hypertension. Consider that all pts eventually need supplemental iron therapy. Assess serum iron (should be greater than 20%), serum ferritin (should be greater than 100 ng/ml) before and during therapy. Establish baseline CBC (esp. note Hct). Monitor aggressively for increased B/P (25% of pts on medication require antihypertensive therapy, dietary restrictions).

INTERVENTION/EVALUATION

Monitor Hct level diligently (if level increases greater than 4 points in 2 wks, dosage should be reduced); assess CBC routinely. Monitor temperature, esp. in cancer pts on chemotherapy and zidovudine-treated HIV pts. Monitor BUN, serum uric acid, creatinine, phosphorus, potassium, esp. in chronic renal failure pts.

PATIENT/FAMILY TEACHING

• Frequent blood tests needed to determine correct dosage. • Inform physician if severe headache develops. • Avoid potentially hazardous activity during first 90 days of therapy (increased risk of seizures in pts with chronic renal failure during first 90 days).

Epogen, *see epoetin alfa*

E

epoprostenol sodium, PG_2, PGX, prostacyclin

e-poe-**pros**-ten-ol
(Flolan)

CLASSIFICATION

PHARMACOTHERAPEUTIC: Vasodilator. **CLINICAL:** Antihypertensive.

ACTION

Directly dilates pulmonary, systemic arterial vascular beds; inhibits platelet aggregation. **Therapeutic Effect:** Reduces right and left ventricular afterload; increases cardiac output, stroke volume.

PHARMACOKINETICS

Rapidly hydrolyzed. Excreted in urine. **Half-life:** 6 min.

USES

Long-term treatment of primary pulmonary hypertension in class III and IV pts (New York Heart Association). **OFF-LABEL:** Cardiopulmonary bypass surgery, hemodialysis, pulmonary hypertension associated with acute respiratory distress syndrome (ARDS), systemic lupus erythematosus, congenital heart disease, neonatal pulmonary hypertension, refractory CHF, severe community-acquired pneumonia.

PRECAUTIONS

CONTRAINDICATIONS: Long-term use in pts with CHF (severe ventricular systolic dysfunction). **CAUTIONS:** Elderly.

LIFESPAN CONSIDERATIONS:

Pregnancy/Lactation: Unknown if drug crosses placenta or is distributed in breast milk. **Pregnancy Category B.** **Children:** Safety and efficacy not established. **Elderly:** No age-related precautions noted.

INTERACTIONS

DRUG: **Acetate in dialysis fluids, other vasodilators** may increase hypotensive effect. **Anticoagulants, antiplatelet agents** may increase risk of bleeding. **Vasoconstrictors** may decrease effects. **HERBAL:** None significant. **FOOD:** None known. **LAB VALUES:** None known.

AVAILABILITY (Rx)

INJECTION, POWDER FOR RECONSTITUTION: 0.5 mg, 1.5 mg.

ADMINISTRATION/HANDLING

IV

Reconstitution • Must use diluent provided by manufacturer. • Follow instructions of manufacturer for dilution to specific concentrations.

Rate of administration
◄ **ALERT** ► Infused continuously through permanent indwelling central venous catheter using an infusion pump. May give through peripheral vein only on temporary basis.

Storage • Store unopened vial at room temperature. • Do not freeze. • Reconstituted solutions may be refrigerated for up to 48 hrs.

IV INCOMPATIBILITIES

Do not mix epoprostenol with other medications.

INDICATIONS/ROUTES/DOSAGE

TREATMENT OF PRIMARY PULMONARY HYPERTENSION

IV INFUSION: ADULTS, ELDERLY: Procedure to determine dose range: Initially, 2 ng/kg/min, increased in increments of 2 ng/kg/min q15min until dose-limiting adverse effects occur. Chronic infusion: Start at 4 ng/kg/min less than the maximum dose rate tolerated during acute dose ranging (or ½ of the maximum rate if rate was less than 5 ng/kg/min).

SIDE EFFECTS

ACUTE PHASE: **FREQUENT:** Flushing (58%), headache (49%), nausea (32%), vomiting (32%), hypotension (16%), anxiety (11%), chest pain (11%), dizziness (8%). **OCCASIONAL (5%–2%):** Bradycardia, abdominal pain, muscle pain, dyspnea, back pain. **RARE (less than 2%):** Diaphoresis, dyspepsia, paresthesia, tachycardia.

CHRONIC PHASE: **FREQUENT (greater than 20%):** Dyspnea, asthenia, dizziness, headache, chest pain, nausea, vomiting, palpitations, edema, jaw pain, tachycardia, flushing, myalgia, nonspecific muscle pain, paresthesia, diarrhea, anxiety, chills/fever/flu-like symptoms. **OCCASIONAL (20%–10%):** Rash, depression, hypotension, pallor, syncope, bradycardia, ascites.

ADVERSE EFFECTS/ TOXIC REACTIONS

Overdose may cause hyperglycemia, ketoacidosis (polyuria, polydipsea, fruit-like breath odor). Angina, MI, thrombocytopenia occur rarely. Abrupt withdrawal, including large reduction in dosage or interruption in drug delivery, may produce rebound pulmonary hypertension (dyspnea, dizziness, asthenia).

NURSING CONSIDERATIONS

INTERVENTION/EVALUATION

Monitor orthostatic B/P measurements for several hrs after any dosage adjustment. Assess for therapeutic response (improvement in pulmonary function, decreased dyspnea on exertion, fatigue, syncope, chest pain, pulmonary vascular resistance, pulmonary arterial pressure).

PATIENT/FAMILY TEACHING

• Instruct pt about drug reconstitution, drug administration, care of permanent central venous catheter. • Brief interruptions in drug delivery may result in rapid, deteriorating symptoms. • Drug therapy will be necessary for a prolonged period, possibly years.

eprosartan

eh-pro-**sar**-tan
(Teveten)

FIXED COMBINATION(S)

Teveten HCT: eprosartan/hydrochlorothiazide (a diuretic) 400 mg/12.5 mg.

CLASSIFICATION

PHARMACOTHERAPEUTIC: Angiotensin II receptor antagonist. **CLINICAL:** Antihypertensive (see p. 8C).

ACTION

Potent vasolidator. Blocks vasoconstrictor, aldosterone-secreting effects of angiotensin II, inhibiting binding of angiotensin II to AT_1 receptors. **Therapeutic Effect:** Causes vasodilation, decreases peripheral resistance, decreases B/P.

PHARMACOKINETICS

Rapidly absorbed after PO administration. Protein binding: 98%. Undergoes first-pass metabolism in liver to active metabolites. Excreted in urine, biliary system. Minimally removed by hemodialysis. **Half-life:** 5–9 hrs.

USES

Treatment of hypertension.

PRECAUTIONS

CONTRAINDICATIONS: Bilateral renal artery stenosis, hyperaldosteronism. **CAUTIONS:** Unilateral renal artery stenosis, preexisting renal insufficiency, significant aortic/mitral stenosis.

LIFESPAN CONSIDERATIONS:

Pregnancy/Lactation: Has caused fetal and neonatal morbidity and mortality.

Potential for adverse effects on breast-feeding infant. Do not breast-feed. **Pregnancy Category C (D if used in second or third trimester). Children:** Safety and efficacy not established. **Elderly:** No age-related precautions noted.

INTERACTIONS

DRUG: Potassium-sparing diuretics, potassium supplements may increase risk of hyperkalemia. May produce additive effect with **antihypertensive agents. HERBAL: Ephedra, ginseng, yohimbe** may worsen hypertension. **Garlic** may increase antihypertensive effect. **FOOD:** None known. **LAB VALUES:** May increase BUN, serum alkaline phosphatase, bilirubin, creatinine, AST, ALT. May decrease Hgb, Hct.

AVAILABILITY (Rx)

TABLETS: 400 mg, 600 mg.

ADMINISTRATION/HANDLING

PO

• Give without regard to food.

INDICATIONS/ROUTES/DOSAGE

HYPERTENSION

PO: ADULTS, ELDERLY: Initially, 600 mg/day. Range: 400–800 mg/day as single or 2 divided doses.

SIDE EFFECTS

OCCASIONAL (5%–2%): Headache, cough, dizziness. **RARE (less than 2%):** Muscle pain, fatigue, diarrhea, upper respiratory tract infection, dyspepsia.

ADVERSE EFFECTS/ TOXIC REACTIONS

Overdosage may manifest as hypotension, tachycardia. Bradycardia occurs less often.

NURSING CONSIDERATIONS

BASELINE ASSESSMENT

Obtain B/P, apical pulse immediately before each dose, in addition to regular monitoring (be alert to fluctuations). Question for possibility of pregnancy (see Pregnancy Category), history of hepatic/renal impairment, renal artery stenosis. Assess medication history (esp. diuretics).

INTERVENTION/EVALUATION

Monitor B/P, electrolytes, serum creatinine, BUN, urinalysis, pulse for tachycardia.

PATIENT/FAMILY TEACHING

• Inform female pt regarding consequences of second and third trimester exposure to medication. • Avoid tasks that require alertness, motor skills until response to drug is established (possible dizziness effect). • Restrict sodium, alcohol intake. • Follow diet, control weight. • Do not stop taking medication. Discuss need for lifelong control. • Caution against exercising during hot weather (risk of dehydration, hypotension). • Check B/P regularly.

eptifibatide

ep-tih-**fye**-bah-tide
(Integrilin)

CLASSIFICATION

PHARMACOTHERAPEUTIC: Glycoprotein IIb/IIIa inhibitor. **CLINICAL:** Antiplatelet, antithrombotic (see p. 31C).

ACTION

Produces rapid inhibition of platelet aggregation by preventing binding of fibrinogen to receptor sites on platelets. **Therapeutic Effect:** Prevents thrombus formation within coronary arteries. Prevents acute cardiac ischemic complications.

PHARMACOKINETICS

Protein binding: 25%. Excreted in urine. **Half-life:** 2.5 hrs.

USES

Treatment of pts with acute coronary syndrome (ACS), including those managed medically and those undergoing percutaneous coronary intervention (PCI).

PRECAUTIONS

CONTRAINDICATIONS: Active internal bleeding, AV malformation or aneurysm, history of cerebrovascular accident (CVA) within 2 yrs or CVA with residual neurologic defect, history of vasculitis, intracranial neoplasm, oral anticoagulant use within last 7 days unless prothrombin time (PT) is less than 1.22 times the control, recent (6 wks or less) GI/GU bleeding, recent (6 wks or less) surgery or trauma, prior IV dextran use prior to or during percutaneous transluminal coronary angioplasty (PTCA), severe uncontrolled hypertension, thrombocytopenia (less than 100,000 cells/mcL). **CAUTIONS:** Pts who weigh less than 75 kg; those 65 yrs and older; history of GI disease; pts receiving thrombolytics, heparin, aspirin; PTCA less than 12 hrs of onset of symptoms for acute MI; prolonged PTCA (greater than 70 min); failed PTCA. **Pregnancy Category B.**

INTERACTIONS

DRUG: Anticoagulants, heparin may increase risk of hemorrhage. **Dextran, other platelet aggregation inhibitors (e.g., aspirin, dextran, thrombolytics), thrombolytic agents** may increase risk of bleeding. **HERBAL: Cat's claw, dong quai, evening primrose, feverfew, garlic, ginger, ginkgo, ginseng** may increase antiplatelet effects. **FOOD:** None known. **LAB VALUES:** Increases PT, activated partial thromboplastin time (aPTT), clotting time. Decreases platelet count.

AVAILABILITY (Rx)

INJECTION SOLUTION: 0.75 mg/ml, 2 mg/ml.

ADMINISTRATION/HANDLING

IV

Reconstitution • Withdraw bolus dose from 10-ml vial (2 mg/ml); for IV infusion, withdraw from 100-ml vial (0.75 mg/ml). IV push and infusion administration may be given undiluted.

Rate of administration • Give bolus dose IV push over 1–2 min.

Storage • Store vials in refrigerator. Solution appears clear, colorless. Do not shake. Discard any unused portion left in vial or if preparation contains *any* opaque particles.

IV INCOMPATIBILITIES

Administer in separate line; do not add other medications to infusion solution.

INDICATIONS/ROUTES/DOSAGE

ADJUNCT TO PERCUTANEOUS CORONARY INTERVENTION (PCI)

IV BOLUS, IV INFUSION: ADULTS, ELDERLY: 180 mcg/kg (Maximum: 22.6 mg) before PCI initiation; then continuous drip of 2 mcg/kg/min and a second 180 mcg/kg (Maximum: 22.6 mg) bolus 10 min after the first. **Maximum:** 15 mg/hr. Continue until hospital discharge or for up to 18–24 hrs. Minimum 12 hrs is recommended. Concurrent aspirin and heparin therapy is recommended.

ACUTE CORONARY SYNDROME

IV BOLUS, IV INFUSION: ADULTS, ELDERLY: 180 mcg/kg (Maximum: 22.6 mg) bolus then 2 mcg/kg/min until discharge or coronary artery bypass graft, up to 72 hrs. **Maximum:** 15 mg/hr. Concurrent aspirin and heparin therapy is recommended.

DOSAGE IN RENAL IMPAIRMENT

Creatinine clearance less than 50 ml/min: Use 180 mcg/kg bolus

(**Maximum:** 22.6 mg) and 1 mcg/kg/min infusion (**Maximum:** 7.5 mg/hr).

SIDE EFFECTS

OCCASIONAL (7%): Hypotension.

ADVERSE EFFECTS/ TOXIC REACTIONS

Minor to major bleeding complications may occur, most commonly at arterial access site for cardiac catheterization.

NURSING CONSIDERATIONS

BASELINE ASSESSMENT

Assess platelet count, Hgb, Hct before treatment. If platelet count less than 90,000/mm^3, additional platelet counts should be obtained routinely to avoid thrombocytopenia.

INTERVENTION/EVALUATION

Diligently monitor for potential bleeding, particularly at other arterial, venous puncture sites. If possible, urinary catheters, nasogastric tubes should be avoided.

Erbitux, *see cetuximab*

ergoloid mesylates

ur-go-loyd mess-**ah**-lates

CLASSIFICATION

PHARMACOTHERAPEUTIC: Ergot alkaloid. **CLINICAL:** Psychotherapeutic.

ACTION

Central action decreases vascular tone, slows heart rate. Peripheral action blocks alpha-adrenergic receptors. **Therapeutic Effect:** Improves O_2 uptake, improves cerebral metabolism.

USES

Treatment of age-related (those older than 60 yrs) decline in mental capacity (cognitive/interpersonal skills, mood, self-care, apparent motivation).

PRECAUTIONS

CONTRAINDICATIONS: Acute or chronic psychosis, regardless of etiology. **CAUTIONS:** Bradycardia, hypotension. **Pregnancy Category C.**

INTERACTIONS

DRUG: None significant. **HERBAL:** None significant. **FOOD:** None known. **LAB VALUES:** None known.

AVAILABILITY (Rx)

TABLETS (ORAL): 1 mg. **TABLETS (SUBLINGUAL):** 1 mg.

INDICATIONS/ROUTES/DOSAGE

AGE-RELATED DECLINE IN MENTAL CAPACITY

PO, SUBLINGUAL: ADULTS, ELDERLY: Initially, 1 mg 3 times a day. Range: 1.5–12 mg a day.

SIDE EFFECTS

OCCASIONAL: GI distress, transient nausea, sublingual irritation.

ADVERSE EFFECTS/ TOXIC REACTIONS

Overdose may produce blurred vision, dizziness, syncope, headache, facial flushing, nausea, vomiting, anorexia, abdominal cramps, stuffy nose.

NURSING CONSIDERATIONS

BASELINE ASSESSMENT

Exclude possibility that pt's signs/symptoms arise from possibly reversible, treatable condition secondary to systemic disease, neurologic disease, primary disturbance of mood prior to administering medication.

INTERVENTION/EVALUATION

Monitor B/P, pulse, peripheral circulation. Assess for relief of symptoms.

PATIENT/FAMILY TEACHING

• Elimination of symptoms appears gradually: results may not be noted for 3–4 wks. • May cause nausea, GI upset. • Allow sublingual tablets to dissolve completely under tongue.

ergotamine

er-**got**-a-meen
(Cafergot ✤, Ergomar, Ergostat, Gynergen, Medihaler Ergotamine ✤)

dihydroergotamine

(D.H.E. 45, Dihydroergotamine Sandoz ✤, Migranal)

FIXED-COMBINATION(S)

Bellergal-S: ergotamine/belladonna (anticholinergic)/phenobarbital (sedative-hypnotic): 0.6 mg/0.2 mg/ 40 mg. **Cafergot, Wigraine:** ergotamine/caffeine (stimulant): 1 mg/ 100 mg; 2 mg/100 mg.

CLASSIFICATION

PHARMACOTHERAPEUTIC: Ergotamine derivative. **CLINICAL:** Antimigraine.

ACTION

Directly stimulates vascular smooth muscle, resulting in peripheral and cerebral vasoconstriction. May have antagonist effects on serotonin. **Therapeutic Effect:** Suppresses vascular headaches, migraine headaches.

PHARMACOKINETICS

Slowly, incompletely absorbed from GI tract; rapidly and extensively absorbed after rectal administration. Protein binding: greater than 90%. Undergoes extensive first-pass metabolism in liver to active metabolite. Eliminated in feces by the biliary system. **Half-life:** 21 hrs.

USES

Ergotamine: Prevents or aborts vascular headaches (e.g., migraine, cluster headaches). **Dihydroergotamine:** Treatment of migraine headache with or without aura. Injection used to treat cluster headache. **OFF-LABEL:** Prevention of deep venous thrombosis, prevention and treatment of orthostatic hypotension, pulmonary thromboembolism.

PRECAUTIONS

CONTRAINDICATIONS: Coronary artery disease, hypertension, hepatic/renal impairment, malnutrition, peripheral vascular diseases (e.g., thromboangitis obliterans, syphilitic arteritis, severe arteriosclerosis, thrombophlebitis, Raynaud's disease), sepsis, severe pruritus. **CAUTIONS:** None known.

LIFESPAN CONSIDERATIONS:

Pregnancy/Lactation: Contraindicated in pregnancy (produces uterine stimulant action, resulting in possible fetal death or retarded fetal growth); increases vasoconstriction of placental vascular bed. Drug distributed in breast milk. May produce diarrhea, vomiting in neonate. May prohibit lactation. **Pregnancy Category X. Children:** No precautions in those 6 yrs and older, but use only when unresponsive to other medication. **Elderly:** Age-related occlusive peripheral vascular disease increases risk of peripheral vasoconstriction. Age-related renal impairment may require dosage adjustment.

INTERACTIONS

DRUG: Beta blockers, erythromycin may increase risk of vasospasm.

Ergot alkaloids, systemic vasoconstrictors may increase pressor effect. May decrease effects of **nitroglycerin**. **HERBAL:** None significant. **FOOD: Tea, cola, coffee** may increase absorption. **Grapefruit, grapefruit juice** may increase concentration/toxicity. **LAB VALUES:** None known.

E

AVAILABILITY (Rx)

ERGOTAMINE

TABLETS, SUBLINGUAL (ERGOMAR): 2 mg.

DIHYDROERGOTAMINE

INJECTION, SOLUTION: 1 mg/ml. **INTRANASAL SPRAY, SOLUTION (MIGRANAL):** 4 mg/ml (0.5 mg/spray).

ADMINISTRATION/HANDLING

SUBLINGUAL

- Place under tongue; do not swallow.

INDICATIONS/ROUTES/DOSAGE

VASCULAR HEADACHES

ERGOTAMINE

PO: ADULTS, ELDERLY: *(Cafergot):* 2 mg at onset of headache, then 1–2 mg q30min. **Maximum:** 6 mg/episode; 10 mg/wk.

Sublingual: ADULTS, ELDERLY: *(Ergomar):* 1 tablet at onset of headache, then 1 tablet q30min. **Maximum:** 3 tablets/24 hrs; 5 tabs/wk.

Rectal: ADULTS, ELDERLY: 1 suppository at onset of headache, then second dose in 1 hr. **Maximum:** 2/episode; 5/wk.

DIHYDROERGOTAMINE

IM/Subcutaneous: ADULTS, ELDERLY: 1 mg at onset of headache; repeat hourly. **Maximum:** 3 mg/day; 6 mg/wk.

IV: ADULTS, ELDERLY: 1 mg at onset of headache; repeat hourly. **Maximum:** 2 mg/day; 6 mg/wk.

Intranasal: ADULTS, ELDERLY: 1 spray (0.5 mg) into each nostril; repeat in 15 min. **Maximum:** 4 sprays/day; 8 sprays/wk.

SIDE EFFECTS

OCCASIONAL (5%–2%): Cough, dizziness. **RARE (less than 2%):** Myalgia, fatigue, diarrhea, upper respiratory tract infection, dyspepsia.

ADVERSE EFFECTS/ TOXIC REACTIONS

Prolonged administration, excessive dosage may produce ergotamine poisoning, manifested as nausea, vomiting; paresthesia of fingers/toes, muscle pain/weakness; precordial pain; tachycardia/bradycardia; hypertension/hypotension. Vasoconstriction of peripheral arteries/arterioles may result in localized edema, pruritus. Feet, hands will become cold, pale. Muscle pain will occur when walking and later, even at rest. Other rare effects include confusion, depression, drowsiness, seizures, gangrene.

NURSING CONSIDERATIONS

BASELINE ASSESSMENT

Question for history of peripheral vascular disease, renal/hepatic impairment, possibility of pregnancy. Question regarding onset, location, duration of migraine, possible precipitating symptoms.

INTERVENTION/EVALUATION

Monitor closely for evidence of ergotamine overdosage as result of prolonged administration or excessive dosage.

PATIENT/FAMILY TEACHING

• Initiate therapy at first sign of migraine headache. • Report if there is need to progressively increase dose to relieve vascular headaches or if palpitations, nausea, vomiting, paresthesias, pain or weakness of extremities is noted. • Discuss contraception with physician; report suspected pregnancy immediately (Pregnancy Category X).

erlotinib

er-**low**-tih-nib

(Tarceva)

◆ CLASSIFICATION

PHARMACOTHERAPEUTIC: Human epidermal growth factor. **CLINICAL:** Antineoplastic.

ACTION

Inhibits tyrosine kinases (TK) associated with transmembrane cell surface receptors found on both normal and cancer cells. One such receptor is epidermal growth factor receptor (EGFR). **Therapeutic Effect:** TK activity appears to be vitally important to cell proliferation and survival.

PHARMACOKINETICS

About 60% is absorbed after PO administration; bioavailability is increased by food to almost 100%. Protein binding: 93%. Extensively metabolized in liver. Primarily eliminated in feces; minimal excretion in urine. **Half-life:** 36 hrs.

USES

Treatment of locally advanced or metastatic non–small cell lung cancer after failure of at least one prior chemotherapy regimen. Treatment of locally advanced, unresectable, or metastatic pancreatic cancer (in combination with gemcitabine). **OFF-LABEL:** Salvage therapy of advanced or metastatic breast, colorectal, and head and neck tumors.

PRECAUTIONS

CONTRAINDICATIONS: Pregnancy. **CAUTIONS:** Severe hepatic/renal impairment.

⌛ LIFESPAN CONSIDERATIONS:

Pregnancy/Lactation: Unknown if drug crosses the placenta or is distributed in breast milk. **Pregnancy Category D. Children:** Safety and efficacy not established. **Elderly:** No age-related precautions noted.

INTERACTIONS

DRUG: Atanzavir, clarithromycin, indinavir, itraconazole, ketoconazole, nefazodone, nelfinavir, ritonavir, saquinavir, telithromycin may increase concentration, effects. **Carbamazepine, phenobarbital, phenytoin, rifampin** may decrease concentration, effects. **Warfarin** may increase risk of bleeding. **HERBAL: St. John's wort** may decrease concentration, effects. **FOOD:** None known. **LAB VALUES:** May increase ALT, AST, serum bilirubin.

AVAILABILITY (Rx)

TABLETS: 25 mg, 100 mg, 150 mg.

ADMINISTRATION/HANDLING

PO

• Give at least 1 hr before or 2 hrs after ingestion of food.

INDICATIONS/ROUTES/DOSAGE

LUNG CANCER

PO: ADULTS, ELDERLY: 150 mg/day until disease progression or unacceptable toxicity occurs.

PANCREATIC CANCER

PO: ADULTS, ELDERLY: 100 mg/day in combination with gemcitabine until disease progression or unacceptable toxicity occurs.

SIDE EFFECTS

FREQUENT (greater than 10%): Fatigue, anxiety, headache, depression, insomnia, rash, pruritus, dry skin, erythema, diarrhea, anorexia, nausea, vomiting, mucositis, constipation, dyspepsia, weight loss, dysphagia, abdominal pain, arthralgia, dyspnea, cough. **OCCASIONAL (10%–1%):** Keratitis. **RARE (less than 1%):** Corneal ulceration.

ADVERSE EFFECTS/ TOXIC REACTIONS

Urinary tract infection occurs occasionally. Pneumonitis, GI bleeding occur rarely.

NURSING CONSIDERATIONS

BASELINE ASSESSMENT

Obtain hepatic enzyme levels, CBC before beginning therapy.

INTERVENTION/EVALUATION

Assess hepatic enzyme levels, CBC periodically.

PATIENT/FAMILY TEACHING

• Take drug on empty stomach. • Notify physician if rash, blood in stool, diarrhea, irritated eyes, fever occur.

E

ertapenem

er-tah-**pen**-em
(Invanz)

CLASSIFICATION

PHARMACOTHERAPEUTIC: Carbapenem. **CLINICAL:** Antibiotic.

ACTION

Penetrates bacterial cell wall of microorganisms, binds to penicillin-binding proteins, inhibiting cell wall synthesis. **Therapeutic Effect:** Produces bacterial cell death.

PHARMACOKINETICS

Almost completely absorbed after IM administration. Protein binding: 85%–95%. Widely distributed. Primarily excreted in urine with smaller amount eliminated in feces. Removed by hemodialysis. **Half-life:** 4 hrs.

USES

Treatment of susceptible infections due to *S. aureus* (methicillin susceptible only), *S. agalactiae, S. pneumoniae* (penicillin susceptible only), *S. pyogenes, E. coli, H. influenzae* (beta-lactamase negative strains only), *K. pneumoniae, M. catarrhalis, Bacteroides* species, *C. clostridioforme, Peptostreptococcus* species, including moderate to severe intra-abdominal, skin/skin-structure infections; community-acquired pneumonia; complicated UTI; acute pelvic infection; adult diabetic foot infections without osteomyelitis. Prevention of surgical site infection.

PRECAUTIONS

CONTRAINDICATIONS: History of hypersensitivity to beta-lactams (imipenem and cilastin, meropenem), hypersensitivity to amide-type local anesthetics (IM). **CAUTIONS:** Hypersensitivity to penicillins, cephalosporins, other allergens; renal impairment; CNS disorders, esp. brain lesions or history of seizures.

LIFESPAN CONSIDERATIONS:

Pregnancy/Lactation: Distributed in breast milk. **Pregnancy Category B. Children:** Safety and efficacy not established in those younger than 18 yrs. **Elderly:** Advanced or end-stage renal insufficiency may require dosage adjustment.

INTERACTIONS

DRUG: Probenecid reduces renal excretion of ertapenem (do not use concurrently). **HERBAL:** None significant. **FOOD:** None known. **LAB VALUES:** May increase serum alkaline phosphatase, AST, ALT. May decrease platelet count, Hgb, Hct, serum potassium.

AVAILABILITY (Rx)

INJECTION POWDER FOR RECONSTITUTION: 1 g.

ADMINISTRATION/HANDLING

IV

Reconstitution • Dilute 1-g vial with 10 ml 0.9% NaCl or Bacteriostatic Water for Injection. • Shake well to dissolve. • Further dilute with 50 ml 0.9% NaCl.

Rate of administration • Give by intermittent IV infusion (piggyback).

Do not give IV push. • Infuse over 20–30 min.

Storage • Solution appears colorless to yellow (variation in color does not affect potency). • Discard if solution contains precipitate. • Reconstituted solution is stable for 6 hrs at room temperature or 24 hrs if refrigerated.

IM

• Reconstitute with 3.2 ml 1% lidocaine HCl injection (without epinephrine). • Shake vial thoroughly. • Inject deep in large muscle mass (gluteal or lateral part of thigh). • Administer suspension within 1 hr after preparation.

IV INCOMPATIBILITIES

Do not mix or infuse with any other medications. Do not use diluents or IV solutions containing dextrose.

IV COMPATIBILITIES

Sterile Water for Injection, 0.9% NaCl.

INDICATIONS/ROUTES/DOSAGE

INTRA-ABDOMINAL INFECTION

IV, IM: ADULTS, ELDERLY: 1 g/day for 5–14 days.

SKIN/SKIN STRUCTURE INFECTION

IV, IM: ADULTS, ELDERLY: 1 g/day for 7–14 days.

PNEUMONIA, UTI

IV, IM: ADULTS, ELDERLY: 1 g/day for 10–14 days.

PELVIC INFECTION

IV, IM: ADULTS, ELDERLY: 1 g/day for 3–10 days.

DIABETIC FOOT INFECTION

IV, IM: ADULTS, ELDERLY: 1 g/day for 7–14 days.

DOSAGE IN RENAL IMPAIRMENT

For adults and elderly pts with creatinine clearance less than 30 ml/min: dosage is 500 mg once a day.

SIDE EFFECTS

FREQUENT (10%–6%): Diarrhea, nausea, headache. **OCCASIONAL (5%–2%):** Altered mental status, insomnia, rash, abdominal pain, constipation, vomiting, edema, fever. **RARE (less than 2%):** Dizziness, cough, oral candidiasis, anxiety, tachycardia, phlebitis at IV site.

ADVERSE EFFECTS/ TOXIC REACTIONS

Antibiotic-associated colitis, other superinfections may occur. Anaphylactic reactions have been reported. Seizures may occur in those with CNS disorders (brain lesions, history of seizures), bacterial meningitis, severe renal impairment.

NURSING CONSIDERATIONS

BASELINE ASSESSMENT

Question for history of allergies, particularly to beta-lactams, penicillins, cephalosporins. Inquire about history of seizures.

INTERVENTION/EVALUATION

Monitor daily pattern of bowel activity/ stool consistency. Monitor for nausea, vomiting. Evaluate hydration status. Evaluate for inflammation at IV injection site. Assess skin for rash. Observe mental status; be alert to tremors, possible seizures. Assess sleep pattern for evidence of insomnia.

PATIENT/FAMILY TEACHING

• Notify physician in event of tremors, seizures, rash, diarrhea, other new symptoms.

Eryc, *see erythromycin*

Erythrocin, *see erythromycin*

erythromycin

er-rith-row-**my**-sin

(A/T/S, Akne-Mycin, Apo-Erythro Base ♣, EES, E-Mycin, Erybid ♣, Eryc, Eryc-125 ♣, Eryc-250 ♣, EryDerm, EryPed, Ery-Tab, Erythra-Derm, Erythrocin, PCE Dispertab, Romycin, Staticin, Theramycin Z, T-Stat)

Do not confuse erythromycin with azithromycin or Ethmozine, or Eryc with Emct.

FIXED-COMBINATION(S)

Eryzole, Pediazole: erythromycin/sulfisoxazole (sulfonamide): 200 mg/600 mg per 5 ml.

CLASSIFICATION

PHARMACOTHERAPEUTIC: Macrolide. **CLINICAL:** Antibiotic, antiacne (see p. 26C).

ACTION

Penetrates bacterial cell membranes, reversibly binds to bacterial ribosomes, inhibiting protein synthesis. **Therapeutic Effect:** Bacteriostatic.

PHARMACOKINETICS

Variably absorbed from GI tract (depending on dosage form used). Protein binding: 70%–90%. Widely distributed. Metabolized in liver. Primarily eliminated in feces by bile. Not removed by hemodialysis. **Half-life:** 1.4–2 hrs (increased in renal impairment).

USES

Treatment of susceptible infections due to *S. pyogenes, S. pneumoniae, S. aureus, M. pneumoniae, Legionella,* diphtheria, pertussis, chancroid, *Chlamydia, N. gonorrheae, E, histolytica,* syphilis, nongonococcal urethritis, *Campylobacter* gastroenteritis. **Topical:** Treatment of acne vulgaris. **Ophthalmic:** Prevention of gonococcal ophthalmia neonatorum. **OFF-LABEL: Systemic:** Treatment of acne vulgaris, chancroid, *Campylobacter* enteritis, gastroparesis, Lyme disease. **Topical:** Treatment of minor bacterial skin infections. **Ophthalmic:** Treatment of blepharitis, conjunctivitis, keratitis, chlamydial trachoma.

PRECAUTIONS

CONTRAINDICATIONS: Administration of fixed-combination product, Pediazole, to infants younger than 2 mos; history of hepatitis due to macrolides; hypersensitivity to macrolides; preexisting hepatic disease. **CAUTIONS:** Hepatic dysfunction. If combination therapy is used (Pediazole), consider precautions of sulfonamides. IV route may cause tachycardia, prolonged QT interval.

⌛ LIFESPAN CONSIDERATIONS:

Pregnancy/Lactation: Crosses placenta. Distributed in breast milk. Erythromycin estolate may increase hepatic enzymes in pregnant women. **Pregnancy Category B. Children/Elderly:** No age-related precautions noted. High dosage in those with decreased hepatic/renal function increases risk of hearing loss.

INTERACTIONS

DRUG: May increase concentration, toxicity of **buspirone, cyclosporine, felodipine, lovastatin, simvastatin, valproic acid.** May inhibit metabolism of **carbamazepine.** May decrease effects of **clindamycin. Hepatotoxic medications** may increase risk of hepatotoxicity. **Theophylline** may increase risk of theophylline toxicity. May increase effects of **warfarin. HERBAL: St. John's wort** may decrease concentration. **FOOD:** None known. **LAB VALUES:** May increase serum alkaline phosphatase, bilirubin, AST, ALT.

AVAILABILITY (Rx)

GEL, TOPICAL: (A/T/S, ERYGEL): 2%. **OINTMENT, OPHTHALMIC: (ROMYCIN):** 0.5%. **OINTMENT, TOPICAL: (AKNE-MYCIN):** 2%. **ORAL SUSPENSION: (EES, ERYPED):** 200 mg/5 ml, 400 mg/5ml. **ORAL SUSPENSION, DROPS: (ERYPED):** 100 mg/2.5 ml. **TABLET AS BASE:** 250 mg, 333 mg, 500 mg. **TABLET AS ETHYL-SUCCINATE (EES):** 400 mg. **TABLET AS STEARATE (ERYTHROCIN):** 250 mg, 500 mg. **TABLETS, CHEWABLE (ERYPED):** 200 mg.

CAPSULES, DELAYED-RELEASE: (ERYC): 250 mg. **TABLETS, DELAYED-RELEASE: (ERY-TAB):** 250 mg, 333 mg, 500 mg.

ADMINISTRATION/HANDLING

IV

Reconstitution • Reconstitute each 500 mg with 10 ml Sterile Water for Injection without preservative to provide a concentration of 50 mg/ml. • Further dilute with 100–250 ml D_5W or 0.9% NaCl.

Rate of administration • For intermittent IV infusion (piggyback), infuse over 20–60 min. • For continuous infusion, infuse over 6–24 hrs.

Storage • Store parenteral form at room temperature. • Initial reconstituted solution in vial is stable for 2 wks refrigerated or 24 hrs at room temperature. • Diluted IV solution stable for 8 hrs at room temperature or 24 hrs if refrigerated. • Discard if precipitate forms.

PO

• Store capsules, tablets at room temperature. • Oral suspension is stable for 14 days at room temperature. • Administer erythromycin base, stearate 1 hr before or 2 hrs following ingestion of food. Erythromycin estolate, ethylsuccinate may be given without regard to meals, but optimal absorption occurs when given on empty stomach. • Give with 8 oz water. • If swallowing difficulties occur, sprinkle capsule contents on teaspoon of applesauce, follow with water. • Do not swallow chewable tablets whole.

OPHTHALMIC

• Place finger on lower eyelid, pull out until a pocket is formed between eye and lower lid. Place ¼–½ inch layer of ointment into pocket. • Have pt close eye gently for 1–2 min, rolling eyeball (increases contact area of drug to eye). • Remove excess ointment around eye with tissue.

IV INCOMPATIBILITY

Fluconazole (Diflucan), furosemide (Lasix), metoclopramide (Reglan).

IV COMPATIBILITIES

Aminophylline, amiodarone (Cordarone), diltiazem (Cardizem), heparin, hydromorphone (Dilaudid), lidocaine, lipids, lorazepam (Ativan), magnesium sulfate, midazolam (Versed), morphine, multivitamins, potassium chloride, total parenteral nutrition (TPN).

INDICATIONS/ROUTES/DOSAGE

MILD TO MODERATE INFECTIONS OF UPPER AND LOWER RESPIRATORY TRACT, PHARYNGITIS, SKIN INFECTIONS

PO: ADULTS, ELDERLY: 250 mg q6h, 500 mg q12h, or 333 mg q8h. **Maximum:** 4 g/day. **CHILDREN:** 30–50 mg/kg/day in divided doses up to 60–100 mg/kg/day for severe infections. **NEONATES:** 20–40 mg/kg/day in divided doses q6–12h.

IV: ADULTS, ELDERLY, CHILDREN: 15–20 mg/kg/day in divided doses. **Maximum:** 4 g/day.

PREOPERATIVE INTESTINAL ANTISEPSIS

PO: ADULTS, ELDERLY: 1 g at 1 PM, 2 PM, and 11 PM on day before surgery (with neomycin). **CHILDREN:** 20 mg/kg at 1 PM, 2 PM, and 11 PM on day before surgery (with neomycin).

ACNE VULGARIS

TOPICAL: ADULTS: Apply thin layer to affected area twice a day.

GONOCOCCAL OPHTHALMIA NEONATORUM

OPHTHALMIC: NEONATES: 0.5–2 cm no later than 1 hr after delivery.

SIDE EFFECTS

FREQUENT: IV: Abdominal cramping/discomfort, phlebitis/thrombophlebitis. **Topical:** Dry skin (50%). **OCCASIONAL:** Nausea, vomiting, diarrhea, rash, urticaria. **RARE: Ophthalmic:** Sensitivity reaction with increased irritation, burning, itching, inflammation. **Topical:** Urticaria.

ADVERSE EFFECTS/ TOXIC REACTIONS

Superinfections, esp. antibiotic-associated colitis (genital/anal pruritus, sore mouth/tongue, moderate to severe diarrhea), reversible cholestatic hepatitis may occur. High dosage in pts with renal impairment may lead to reversible hearing loss. Anaphylaxis occurs rarely. Ventricular arrhythmias, prolonged QT interval occur rarely with IV form.

NURSING CONSIDERATIONS

BASELINE ASSESSMENT

Question for history of allergies (particularly erythromycins), hepatitis.

INTERVENTION/EVALUATION

Monitor daily pattern of bowel activity/stool consistency. Assess skin for rash. Assess for hepatotoxicity (malaise, fever, abdominal pain, GI disturbances). Evaluate for superinfection. Check for phlebitis (heat, pain, red streaking over vein). Monitor for high-dose hearing loss.

PATIENT/FAMILY TEACHING

• Continue therapy for full length of treatment. • Doses should be evenly spaced. • Do *not* swallow chewable tablets whole. • Take medication with 8 oz water 1 hr before or 2 hrs following food or beverage. • **Ophthalmic:** Report burning, itching, inflammation. • **Topical:** Report excessive skin dryness, itching, burning. • Improvement of acne may not occur for 1–2 mos; maximum benefit may take 3 mos; therapy may last mos or yrs. • Use caution if using other topical acne preparations containing peeling or abrasive agents, medicated or abrasive soaps, cosmetics containing alcohol (e.g., astringents, aftershave lotion).

escitalopram

es-sih-**tail**-oh-pram

(Cipralex ✤, Lexapro)

CLASSIFICATION

PHARMACOTHERAPEUTIC: Serotonin reuptake inhibitor. **CLINICAL:** Antidepressant (see p. 37C).

ACTION

Blocks uptake of neurotransmitter serotonin at neuronal presynaptic membranes, increasing its availability at postsynaptic receptor sites. **Therapeutic Effect:** Antidepressant effect.

PHARMACOKINETICS

Well absorbed after PO administration. Primarily metabolized in liver. Primarily excreted in feces with a lesser amount eliminated in urine. **Half-life:** 35 hrs.

USES

Treatment of major depressive disorder exhibited as persistent, prominent dysphoria (occurring nearly every day for at least 2 wks) manifested by 4 of 8 symptoms: appetite change, sleep pattern change, increased fatigue, impaired concentration, feelings of guilt or worthlessness, loss of interest in usual activities, psychomotor agitation or retardation, suicidal tendencies. Treatment of generalized anxiety disorder (GAD). **OFF-LABEL:** Mixed anxiety and depressive disorder.

PRECAUTIONS

CONTRAINDICATIONS: Breast-feeding, use within 14 days of MAOIs. **CAUTIONS:** Hepatic/renal impairment; history of seizures, mania, hypomania; concurrent use of CNS depressants.

LIFESPAN CONSIDERATIONS:

Pregnancy/Lactation: Distributed in breast milk. **Pregnancy Category C.** **Children:** May cause increased anticholinergic effects or hyperexcitability. **Elderly:** More sensitive to anticholinergic effects (e.g., dry mouth), more likely to experience dizziness, sedation, confusion, hypotension, hyperexcitability.

INTERACTIONS

DRUG: **Alcohol, other CNS suppressants** may increase CNS depression. **Antifungals, cimetidine, macrolide antibiotics** may increase plasma concentration. **Carbamazepine** may decrease plasma concentration. May increase **lithium** concentration, risk of serotonin syndrome. **Linezolid, MAOIs** may cause serotonin syndrome (autonomic hyperactivity, diaphoresis, excitement, hyperthermia, rigidity, neuroleptic malignant syndrome, coma). Increases plasma level of **metoprolol.** **HERBAL:** **Gotu kola, kava kava, St. John's wort, SAMe, valerian** may increase CNS depression. **Ginkgo biloba, St. John's wort** may increase risk of serotonin syndrome. **FOOD:** None known. **LAB VALUES:** May reduce serum sodium.

AVAILABILITY (Rx)

ORAL SOLUTION: 5 mg/5 ml.

TABLETS: 5 mg, 10 mg, 20 mg.

ADMINISTRATION/HANDLING

PO

- Give without regard to food.

INDICATIONS/ROUTES/DOSAGE

DEPRESSION, GENERAL ANXIETY DISORDER (GAD)

PO: ADULTS: Initially, 10 mg once a day in the morning or evening. May increase to 20 mg after a minimum of 1 wk. **ELDERLY:** 10 mg/day.

DOSAGE IN RENAL IMPAIRMENT

Use caution in pts with creatinine clearance less than 20 ml/min.

DOSAGE IN HEPATIC IMPAIRMENT

10 mg/day.

SIDE EFFECTS

FREQUENT (21%–11%): Nausea, dry mouth, somnolence, insomnia, diaphoresis. **OCCASIONAL (8%–4%):** Tremor, diarrhea, abnormal ejaculation, dyspepsia, fatigue, anxiety, vomiting, anorexia. **RARE (3%–2%):** Sinusitis, sexual dysfunction, menstrual disorder, abdominal pain, agitation, decreased libido.

ADVERSE EFFECTS/ TOXIC REACTIONS

Overdose manifested as dizziness, drowsiness, tachycardia, somnolence, confusion, seizures.

NURSING CONSIDERATIONS

BASELINE ASSESSMENT

For pts on long-term therapy, hepatic/renal function tests, blood counts should be performed periodically. Observe, record behavior. Assess psychological status, thought content, sleep pattern, appearance, interest in environment.

INTERVENTION/EVALUATION

Supervise suicidal-risk pt closely during early therapy (as energy level improves, suicide potential increases). Assess appearance, behavior, speech pattern, level of interest, mood.

PATIENT/FAMILY TEACHING

• Do not stop taking medication or increase dosage. • Avoid use of alcohol. • Avoid tasks that require alertness, motor skills until response to drug is established.

E

Eskalith, *see lithium carbonate*

esmolol

ess-moe-lol
(Brevibloc)

CLASSIFICATION

PHARMACOTHERAPEUTIC: Beta$_1$-adrenergic blocker. **CLINICAL:** Antiarrhythmic (see pp. 15C, 68C).

ACTION

Selectively blocks beta$_1$-adrenergic receptors. **Therapeutic Effect:** Slows sinus heart rate, decreases cardiac output, reducing B/P.

PHARMACOKINETICS

Rapidly metabolized primarily by esterase in cytosol of red blood cells. Protein binding: 55%. Less than 1%–2% excreted in urine. **Half-life:** 9 min.

USES

Rapid, short-term control of ventricular rate in supraventricular tachycardia, atrial fibrillation or flutter; treatment of tachycardia and/or hypertension (esp. intraoperative or postop).

PRECAUTIONS

CONTRAINDICATIONS: Cardiogenic shock, overt cardiac failure, second- and third-degree heart block, sinus bradycardia. **CAUTIONS:** History of allergy, bronchial asthma, emphysema, bronchitis, CHF, diabetes, renal impairment.

LIFESPAN CONSIDERATIONS:

Pregnancy/Lactation: Crosses placenta; distributed in breast milk. **Pregnancy Category C. Children:** Safety and efficacy not established. **Elderly:** No age-related precautions noted.

INTERACTIONS

DRUG: May mask symptoms of hypoglycemia, prolong hypoglycemic effect of **insulin, oral hypoglycemics. MAOIs** may cause significant hypertension. **Sympathomimetics, xanthines** may mutually inhibit effects. **HERBAL:** None significant. **FOOD:** None known. **LAB VALUES:** None known.

AVAILABILITY (Rx)

INJECTION SOLUTION: 10 mg/ml, 20 mg/ml, 250 mg/ml.

ADMINISTRATION/HANDLING

◀ **ALERT** ▶ Give by IV infusion. Avoid butterfly needles, very small veins.

IV

Reconstitution • The 250 mg/ml ampule is not for direct IV injection but must be diluted to a final concentration not to exceed 10 mg/ml (prevents vein irritation). • For IV infusion, remove 20 ml from 500-ml container of D_5W, Ringer's, D_5W/Ringer's, D_5W/lactated D_5W/0.9% NaCl, D_5W/0.45% NaCl, 0.9% NaCl, lactated Ringer's or 0.45% NaCl and dilute 250 mg/ml concentration esmolol to remaining 480 ml of solution to provide concentration of 10 mg/ml. Maximum concentration: 10 g/250 ml (40 mg/ml).

Rate of administration • Administer by controlled infusion device; titrate to tolerance and response. • Infuse IV loading dose over 1–2 min.

• Hypotension (systolic B/P less than 90 mm Hg) is greatest during first 30 min of IV infusion.

Storage • Use only clear and colorless to light yellow solution. • After dilution, solution is stable for 24 hrs. • Discard solution if discolored or precipitate forms.

IV INCOMPATIBILITIES

Amphotericin B complex (Abelcet, AmBisome, Amphotec), furosemide (Lasix).

IV COMPATIBILITIES

Amiodarone (Cordarone), diltiazem (Cardizem), dopamine (Intropin), heparin, magnesium, midazolam (Versed), potassium chloride, propofol (Diprivan).

INDICATIONS/ROUTES/DOSAGE

RATE CONTROL IN SUPRAVENTRICULAR ARRHYTHMIAS

IV: ADULTS, ELDERLY: Initially, loading dose of 500 mcg/kg/min for 1 min, followed by 50 mcg/kg/min for 4 min. If optimum response is not attained in 5 min, give second loading dose of 500 mcg/kg/min for 1 min, followed by infusion of 100 mcg/kg/min for 4 min. Additional loading doses can be given and infusion increased by 50 mcg/kg/min, up to 200 mcg/kg/min, for 4 min. Once desired response is attained, cease loading dose and increase infusion by no more than 25 mcg/kg/min. Interval between doses may be increased to 10 min. Infusion usually administered over 24–48 hrs in most pts. Range: 50–200 mcg/kg/min, with average dose of 100 mcg/kg/min.

INTRA/POSTOPERATIVE TACHYCARDIA HYPERTENSION (IMMEDIATE CONTROL)

IV: ADULTS, ELDERLY: Initially, 80 mg over 30 sec, then 150 mcg/kg/min infusion up to 300 mcg/kg/min.

SIDE EFFECTS

Generally well tolerated, with transient, mild side effects. **FREQUENT:** Hypotension (systolic B/P less than 90 mm Hg) manifested as dizziness, nausea, diaphoresis, headache, cold extremities, fatigue. **OCCASIONAL:** Anxiety, drowsiness, flushed skin, vomiting, confusion, inflammation at injection site, fever.

ADVERSE EFFECTS/ TOXIC REACTIONS

Overdose may produce profound hypotension, bradycardia, dizziness, syncope, drowsiness, breathing difficulty, bluish fingernails or palms of hands, seizures. May potentiate insulin-induced hypoglycemia in diabetic pts.

NURSING CONSIDERATIONS

BASELINE ASSESSMENT

Assess B/P, apical pulse immediately before drug is administered (if pulse is 60 or less/min or systolic B/P is 90 mm Hg or less, withhold medication, contact physician).

INTERVENTION/EVALUATION

Monitor B/P for hypotension, EKG, heart rate, respiratory rate, development of diaphoresis, dizziness (usually first sign of impending hypotension). Assess pulse for quality, irregular rate, bradycardia, extremities for coldness. Assist with ambulation if dizziness occurs. Assess for nausea, diaphoresis, headache, fatigue.

esomeprazole

es-oh-**mep**-rah-zole
(Nexium, Nexium IV)

CLASSIFICATION

PHARMACOTHERAPEUTIC: Proton pump inhibitor. **CLINICAL:** Gastric acid inhibitor (see p. 139C).

ACTION

Converted to active metabolites that irreversibly bind to, inhibit hydrogen-potassium adenosine triphosphates, enzymes on surface of gastric parietal cells. Inhibits hydrogen ion transport into gastric lumen. **Therapeutic Effect:** Increases gastric pH, reducing gastric acid production.

E

PHARMACOKINETICS

Well absorbed after PO administration. Protein binding: 97%. Extensively metabolized by the liver. Primarily excreted in urine. **Half-life:** 1–1.5 hrs.

USES

Oral: Short-term treatment (4–8 wks) of erosive esophagitis (diagnosed by endoscopy); symptomatic gastroesophageal reflux disease (GERD). Treatment of Zollinger-Ellison syndrome. Used in triple therapy with amoxicillin and clarithromycin for treatment of *H. pylori* infection in pts with duodenal ulcer. Reduce risk of NSAID gastric ulcer. **IV:** Short-term treatment of GERD when oral therapy is not appropriate.

PRECAUTIONS

CONTRAINDICATIONS: Hypersensitivity to benzimidazoles. **CAUTIONS:** None known.

LIFESPAN CONSIDERATIONS:

Pregnancy/Lactation: Unknown if drug crosses placenta or is distributed in breast milk. **Pregnancy Category B. Children:** Safety and efficacy not established. **Elderly:** No age-related precautions noted.

INTERACTIONS

DRUG: May decrease concentration of **digoxin, iron, ketoconazole.** May increase effect of **warfarin. HERBAL:** None significant. **FOOD:** None known. **LAB VALUES:** None known.

AVAILABILITY (Rx)

INJECTION, POWDER FOR RECONSTITUTION (SODIUM [NEXIUM IV]): 20 mg, 40 mg. **ORAL SUSPENSION, DELAYED-RELEASE:** 20 mg, 40 mg.

CAPSULES (DELAYED-RELEASE, [NEXIUM]): 20 mg, 40 mg.

ADMINISTRATION/HANDLING

IV

Reconstitution • For IV push, add 5 mL of 0.9% NaCl to esomeprazole vial. • Use only half reconstituted solution when administering a 20 mg dose. • Discard unused solution.

Infusion • For IV infusion, dissolve content of one vial in up to 100 ml 0.9% NaCl.

Rate of administration • For IV push, administer over not less than 3 min. For intermittent infusion (piggyback) infuse over 15–30 min. • Flush line with 0.9% NaCl, lactated Ringer's, or D_5W, both before and after administration.

Storage • Use only clear and colorless to very slightly yellow solution. • Discard solution if particulate forms.

PO

• Give 1 hr or more before eating. • Do not crush, chew capsule; swallow whole. For those with difficulty swallowing capsules, open capsule and mix pellets with 1 tbsp applesauce. Swallow spoonful without chewing.

IV INCOMPATIBILITIES

Do not mix esomeprazole with any other medications through the same IV line or tubing.

INDICATIONS/ROUTES/DOSAGE

EROSIVE ESOPHAGITIS

PO: ADULTS, ELDERLY: 20–40 mg once daily for 4–8 wks.

MAINTENANCE THERAPY FOR EROSIVE ESOPHAGITIS

PO: ADULTS, ELDERLY: 20 mg/day.

TO REDUCE THE RISK OF NSAID-INDUCED GASTRIC ULCER
PO: ADULTS, ELDERLY: 20 mg once a day for 4 wks.

GERD
IV: ADULTS, ELDERLY: 20 or 40 mg once daily.
PO: ADULTS, ELDERLY, CHILDREN, 12–17 YRS: 20 mg once daily.

ZOLLINGER-ELLISON
PO: ADULTS, ELDERLY: 40 mg 2 times/day. Doses up to 240 mg/day have been used.

DUODENAL ULCER CAUSED BY *HELICOBACTER PYLORI*
PO: ADULTS, ELDERLY: 40 mg (esomeprazole) once a day, with amoxicillin 1,000 mg and clarithromycin 500 mg twice a day for 10 days.

SIDE EFFECTS

FREQUENT (7%): Headache. **OCCASIONAL (3%–2%):** Diarrhea, abdominal pain, nausea. **RARE (less than 2%):** Dizziness, asthenia (loss of strength), vomiting, constipation, rash, cough.

ADVERSE EFFECTS/ TOXIC REACTIONS

None known.

NURSING CONSIDERATIONS

INTERVENTION/EVALUATION

Evaluate for therapeutic response (relief of GI symptoms). Question if GI discomfort, nausea, diarrhea occur.

PATIENT/FAMILY TEACHING

• Report headache. • Take more than 1 hr before eating. • For pts with difficulty swallowing capsules, open capsule and mix pellets with 1 tbsp applesauce. Swallow spoonful without chewing.

Estrace, *see estradiol*

Estraderm, *see estradiol*

estradiol

ess-tra-**dye**-ole

(Alora, Climara, Delestrogen, Depo-Estradiol, Elestrin, Esclim, Estrace, Estraderm, Estradot ✤, Estrasorb, Estrogel, Estring, Femring, Menostar, Oesclim ✤, Vagifem, Vivelle, Vivelle Dot)

Do not confuse Estraderm with Testoderm.

FIXED-COMBINATION(S)

Activella: estradiol/norethindrone (hormone): 1 mg/0.5 mg. **Climara PRO:** estradiol/levonorgestrel (progestin): 0.045 mg/24 hr; 0.015 mg/24 hr. **Combi-patch:** estradiol/norethindrone (hormone): 0.05 mg/0.14 mg; 0.05 mg/0.25 mg. **Femhrt:** estradiol/norethindrone (hormone): 5 mcg/1 mg. **Lunelle:** estradiol/medroxy-progesterone(progestin): 5 mg/25 mg per 0.5 ml.

◆ CLASSIFICATION

PHARMACOTHERAPEUTIC: Estrogen. **CLINICAL:** Estrogen, antineoplastic.

ACTION

Increases synthesis of DNA, RNA, proteins in target tissues; reduces release of gonadotropin-releasing hormone from hypothalamus; reduces follicle-stimulating hormone (FSH), luteinizing hormone (LH) release from pituitary. **Therapeutic Effect:** Promotes normal growth/development of female sex organs, maintains GU function, vasomotor stability. Prevents accelerated bone loss by inhibiting bone resorption, restoring balance of bone resorption, formation. Inhibits

LH, decreases serum testosterone concentration.

PHARMACOKINETICS

Well absorbed from GI tract. Widely distributed. Protein binding: 50%–80%. Metabolized in liver. Primarily excreted in urine. **Half-life:** Unknown.

E

USES

Treatment of moderate to severe vasomotor symptoms associated with menopause, hypoestrogenism (due to hypogonadism, primary ovarian failure), breast cancer, prostate cancer, prevention of osteoporosis, vaginal atrophy, atrophic vaginitis, abnormal uterine bleeding due to hormone imbalance, postmenopausal urogenital symptoms of lower urinary tract. **OFF-LABEL:** Treatment of Turner's syndrome.

PRECAUTIONS

CONTRAINDICATIONS: Undiagnosed abnormal vaginal bleeding, active arterial thrombosis, blood dyscrasias, estrogen-dependent cancer, known or suspected breast cancer, pregnancy, thrombophlebitis or thromboembolic disorders, thyroid dysfunction. **CAUTIONS:** Renal/hepatic insufficiency, diseases that may be exacerbated by fluid retention, diabetes mellitus, endometriosis, hypercalcemia, hyperlipidemias, hypertension, hypocalcemia, hypothyroidism, history of jaundice during pregnancy, vaginal infection, children in whom bone growth is not complete.

LIFESPAN CONSIDERATIONS:

Pregnancy/Lactation: Distributed in breast milk. May be harmful to infant. Not for use during breast-feeding. **Pregnancy Category X. Children:** Caution in those whom bone growth is not complete (may accelerate epiphyseal closure). **Elderly:** No age-related precautions noted.

INTERACTIONS

DRUG: May interfere with effects of **bromocriptine.** May increase **cyclosporine** concentration, risk of hepatotoxicity, nephrotoxicity. **Hepatotoxic medications** may increase risk of hepatotoxicity. **HERBAL:** Avoid **black cohosh, dong quai, saw palmetto. St. John's wort** may decrease plasma concentration, effectiveness of estrogens. **FOOD:** None known. **LAB VALUES:** May increase serum glucose, calcium, HDL, triglycerides. May decrease serum cholesterol level, LDH. May affect metapyrone testing, thyroid function tests.

AVAILABILITY (Rx)

EMULSION (TOPICAL [ESTRASORB]): 2.5 mg/g. **GEL: ELESTRIN. INJECTION (CYPIONATE [DEPO-ESTRADIOL]):** 5 mg/ml. **INJECTION (VALERATE [DELESTROGEN]):** 10 mg/ml. **TABLETS (ESTRACE):** 0.5 mg, 1 mg, 2 mg. **TOPICAL GEL (ESTROGEL):** 1.25 g. **TRANSDERMAL SYSTEM (ALORA):** twice weekly: 0.025 mg, 0.05 mg, 0.075 mg, 0.1 mg. **TRANSDERMAL SYSTEM (CLI-MARA):** once weekly: 0.025 mg, 0.0375 mg, 0.05 mg, 0.06 mg, 0.075 mg, 0.1 mg. **TRANSDERMAL SYSTEM (ESCLIM):** twice weekly: 0.025 mg, 0.0375 mg, 0.05 mg, 0.075 mg, 0.1 mg. **TRANSDERMAL SYSTEM (ESTRADERM):** twice weekly: 0.05 mg, 0.1 mg. **TRANSDERMAL SYS-TEM (MENOSTAR):** once weekly: 1 mg. **TRANSDERMAL SYSTEM (VIVELLE):** twice weekly: 0.025 mg, 0.0375 mg, 0.05 mg, 0.075 mg, 0.1 mg. **TRANSDERAMAL SYSTEM (VIVELLE DOT):** twice weekly: 0.0375 mg, 0.05 mg, 0.075 mg, 0.1 mg. **VAGINAL CREAM (ESTRACE):** 0.1 mg/g. **VAGINAL RING (ESTRING):** 2 mg. **VAGINAL RING (FEMRING):** 0.05 mg. **VAGINAL TABLET (VAGIFEM):** 25 mcg.

ADMINISTRATION/HANDLING

IM

- Rotate vial to disperse drug in solution.
- Inject deep IM in large muscle mass.

PO
• Administer at same time each day.

TRANSDERMAL
• Remove old patch; select new site (buttocks are alternative application site). • Peel off protective strip to expose adhesive surface. • Apply to clean, dry, intact skin on trunk of body (area with as little hair as possible). • Press in place for at least 10 sec (do not apply to breasts or waistline).

VAGINAL
• Apply at bedtime for best absorption. • Insert end of filled applicator into vagina, directed slightly toward sacrum; push plunger down completely. • Avoid skin contact with cream (prevents skin absorption).

INDICATIONS/ROUTES/DOSAGE

PROSTATE CANCER
IM (ESTRADIOL VALERATE): ADULTS, ELDERLY: 30 mg or more q1–2wk.
PO: ADULTS, ELDERLY: 10 mg 3 times a day for at least 3 mos.

BREAST CANCER
PO: ADULTS, ELDERLY: 10 mg 3 times a day for at least 3 mos.

OSTEOPOROSIS PROPHYLAXIS IN POSTMENOPAUSAL FEMALES
PO: ADULTS, ELDERLY: 0.5 mg/day cyclically (3 wks on, 1 wk off).
TRANSDERMAL (CLIMARA): ADULTS, ELDERLY: Initially, 0.025 mg weekly, adjust dose as needed.
TRANSDERMAL (ALORA, VIVELLE, VIVELLE-DOT): ADULTS, ELDERLY: Initially, 0.025 mg patch twice weekly, adjust dose as needed.
TRANSDERMAL (ESTRADERM): ADULTS, ELDERLY: 0.05 mg twice weekly.
TRANSDERMAL (MENOSTAR): ADULTS, ELDERLY: 1 mg weekly.

FEMALE HYPOESTROGENISM
PO: ADULTS, ELDERLY: 1–2 mg/day, adjust dose as needed.
IM (CYPIONATE): ADULTS, ELDERLY: 1.5–2 mg monthly.
IM (ESTRADIOL VALERATE): ADULTS, ELDERLY: 10–20 mg q4wk.

VASOMOTOR SYMPTOMS ASSOCIATED WITH MENOPAUSE
PO: ADULTS, ELDERLY: 1–2 mg/day cyclically (3 wks on, 1 wk off), adjust dose as needed.
IM (ESTRADIOL CYPIONATE): ADULTS, ELDERLY: 1–5 mg q3–4wk.
IM (ESTRADIOL VALERATE): ADULTS, ELDERLY: 10–20 mg q4wk.
TOPICAL EMULSION (ESTRASORB): ADULTS, ELDERLY: 3.84 g once a day in the morning.
TOPICAL GEL (ESTROGEL): ADULTS, ELDERLY: 1.25 g/day.
TRANSDERMAL (CLIMARA): ADULTS, ELDERLY: 0.025 mg weekly. Adjust dose as needed.
TRANSDERMAL (ALORA, ESCLIM, ESTRADER, VIVELLE-DOT): ADULTS, ELDERLY: 0.05 mg twice a wk.
TRANSDERMAL (VIVELLE): ADULTS, ELDERLY: 0.0375 mg twice a wk.
VAGINAL RING (FEMRING): ADULTS, ELDERLY: 0.05 mg. May increase to 0.1 mg if needed.

VAGINAL ATROPHY
VAGINAL RING (ESTRING): ADULTS, ELDERLY: 2 mg.
VAGINAL CREAM (ESTRACE): Insert 2–4 g/day intravaginally for 2 wks, then reduce dose by ½ initial dose for 2 wks, then maintenance dose of 1 g 1–3 times/wk.

ATROPHIC VAGINITIS
VAGINAL TABLET (VAGIFEM): ADULTS, ELDERLY: Initially, 1 tablet/day for 2 wks. Maintenance: 1 tablet twice a week.

SIDE EFFECTS

FREQUENT: Anorexia, nausea, swelling of breasts, peripheral edema marked by swollen ankles and feet. **Transdermal:** Skin irritation, redness. **OCCASIONAL:** Vomiting (esp. with high doses), headache (may be severe), intolerance to contact lenses, hypertension, glucose intolerance, brown spots on exposed skin. **Vaginal:** Local irritation, vaginal discharge, changes in vaginal bleeding (spotting, breakthrough, prolonged bleeding). **RARE:** Chorea/involuntary movements, hirsutism/abnormal hairiness, loss of scalp hair, depression.

E

ADVERSE EFFECTS/ TOXIC REACTIONS

Prolonged administration increases risk of gallbladder disease, thromboembolic disease, breast, cervical, vaginal, endometrial, hepatic carcinoma. Cholestatic jaundice occurs rarely.

NURSING CONSIDERATIONS

BASELINE ASSESSMENT

Question for hypersensitivity to estrogen, previous jaundice, thromboembolic disorders associated with pregnancy, estrogen therapy. Question for possibility of pregnancy (Pregnancy Category X).

INTERVENTION/EVALUATION

Monitor B/P, weight, serum calcium, glucose, hepatic enzymes.

PATIENT/FAMILY TEACHING

• Limit alcohol, caffeine. • Inform physician if sudden headache, vomiting, disturbance of vision/speech, numbness/weakness of extremities, chest pain, calf pain, shortness of breath, severe abdominal pain, mental depression, unusual bleeding occurs.

estramustine

es-trah-**mew**-steen

(Emcyt)

Do not confuse Emcyt with Eryc.

CLASSIFICATION

PHARMACOTHERAPEUTIC: Alkylating agent, estrogen/nitrogen mustard. **CLINICAL:** Antineoplastic (see p. 79C).

ACTION

Binds to microtubule-associated proteins, causing their disassembly. **Therapeutic Effect:** Reduces serum testosterone concentration.

PHARMACOKINETICS

Well absorbed from GI tract. Highly localized in prostatic tissue. Rapidly dephosphorylated during absorption into peripheral circulation. Metabolized in the liver. Primarily eliminated in feces by biliary system. **Half-life:** 20 hrs.

USES

Treatment of metastatic or progressive carcinoma of prostate gland.

PRECAUTIONS

CONTRAINDICATIONS: Active thrombophlebitis or thromboembolic disorders (unless tumor is cause of thromboembolic disorder and benefits outweigh risk), hypersensitivity to estradiol nitrogen mustard. **CAUTIONS:** History of thrombophlebitis, thrombosis, thromboembolic disorders; cerebrovascular, coronary artery disease; hepatic impairment; metabolic bone disease in those with hypercalcemia, renal insufficiency.

LIFESPAN CONSIDERATIONS:

Pregnancy/Lactation: **Pregnancy Category C.** **Children:** Not used in this population. **Elderly:** Age-related renal impairment and/or peripheral vascular disease may require dosage adjustment.

INTERACTIONS

DRUG: **Calcium-containing antacids** may impair absorption. **Hepatotoxic medications** may increase risk of hepatotoxicity. **HERBAL:** None significant. **FOOD:** **Milk, dairy products, other calcium-rich foods** may impair absorption. **LAB VALUES:** May increase serum glucose, bilirubin, cortisol, LDH, phospholipid, prolactin, AST, sodium, triglyceride. May decrease urine pregnanediol, serum antithrombin III, folate, phosphate. May alter thyroid function test results.

AVAILABILITY (Rx)

CAPSULES: 140 mg.

ADMINISTRATION/HANDLING

PO

• Refrigerate capsules (may remain at room temperature for 24–48 hrs without loss of potency). • Give with water 1 hr before or 2 hrs after meals.

INDICATIONS/ROUTES/DOSAGE

PROSTATIC CARCINOMA

PO: ADULTS, ELDERLY: 10–16 mg/kg/day (most common: 14 mg/kg/day) or 140 mg 4 times a day.

SIDE EFFECTS

FREQUENT: Peripheral edema (esp. lower extremities), breast tenderness/enlargement, diarrhea, flatulence, nausea. **OCCASIONAL:** Increase in B/P, thirst, dry skin, ecchymosis, flushing, alopecia, night sweats. **RARE:** Headache, rash, fatigue, insomnia, vomiting.

ADVERSE EFFECTS/ TOXIC REACTIONS

May exacerbate CHF; increased risk of pulmonary emboli, thrombophlebitis, cerebrovascular accident.

NURSING CONSIDERATIONS

INTERVENTION/EVALUATION

Monitor B/P periodically.

PATIENT/FAMILY TEACHING

• Do not take with milk, milk products, calcium-rich food, calcium-containing antacids. • Use contraceptive measures during therapy. • If headache (migraine or severe), vomiting, disturbed speech/vision, dizziness, numbness, shortness of breath, calf pain, chest pain/pressure, unexplained cough occurs, contact physician.

estropipate

ess-troe-**pie**-pate
(Ogen, Ortho-Est)

CLASSIFICATION

PHARMACOTHERAPEUTIC: Estrogen.
CLINICAL: Hormone.

ACTION

Increases synthesis of DNA, RNA, proteins in target tissues; reduces release of gonadotropin-releasing hormone from hypothalamus; reduces follicle-stimulating hormone (FSH), luteinizing hormone (LH) from pituitary. **Therapeutic Effect:** Promotes normal growth, development of female sex organs, maintains GU function, vasomotor stability. Prevents accelerated bone loss by inhibiting bone resorption, restoring balance of bone resorption, formation. Inhibits LH, decreases serum testosterone.

PHARMACOKINETICS

Well absorbed from GI tract. Metabolized in liver.

USES

Treatment of vasomotor symptoms associated with menopause, vulvar/vaginal atrophy, hypoestrogenism, osteoporosis prophylaxis.

PRECAUTIONS

CONTRAINDICATIONS: Abnormal vaginal bleeding, active arterial thrombosis, blood dyscrasias, estrogen-dependent cancer, known or suspected breast cancer, pregnancy, thrombophlebitis, thromboembolic disorders, thyroid dysfunction. **CAUTIONS:** Renal/hepatic insufficiency, diseases that may be exacerbated by fluid retention. **Pregnancy Category X.**

INTERACTIONS

DRUG: May interfere with effects of **bromocriptine.** May increase **cyclosporine** concentration, risk of hepatotoxicity, nephrotoxicity. **Hepatotoxic medications** may increase risk of hepatotoxicity. **HERBAL:** **St. John's wort** may decrease concentration. Avoid **black cohosh, dong quai, saw palmetto.** **FOOD:** None known. **LAB VALUES:** May increase serum glucose, calcium, HDL, triglycerides. May decrease serum cholesterol, LDH. May affect metapyrone testing, thyroid function tests.

E

AVAILABILITY (Rx)

TABLETS (OGEN, ORTHO-EST): 0.625 mg (0.75 mg estropipate), 1.25 mg (1.5 mg estropipate), 2.5 mg (3 mg estropipate).

ADMINISTRATION/HANDLING

- Administer at same time each day.

INDICATIONS/ROUTES/DOSAGE

VASOMOTOR SYMPTOMS, ATROPHIC VAGINITIS, KRAUROSIS VULVAE

PO: ADULTS, ELDERLY: 0.625–5 mg/day cyclically.

FEMALE HYPOGONADISM, CASTRATION, PRIMARY OVARIAN FAILURE

PO: ADULTS, ELDERLY: 1.25–7.5 mg/day for 21 days; then off for 8–10 days. Repeat if bleeding does not occur by end of off cycle.

PREVENTION OF OSTEOPOROSIS

PO: ADULTS, ELDERLY: 0.625 mg/day (25 days of 31-day cycle/mo).

SIDE EFFECTS

FREQUENT: Anorexia, nausea, swelling of breasts, peripheral edema marked by swollen ankles and feet. **OCCASIONAL:** Vomiting (esp. with high doses), headache (may be severe), intolerance to contact lenses, hypertension, glucose intolerance, brown spots on exposed skin. **Vaginal:** Local irritation, vaginal discharge, changes in vaginal bleeding (spotting, breakthrough, prolonged bleeding). **RARE:** Chorea (involuntary movements), hirsutism (abnormal hairiness), loss of scalp hair, depression.

ADVERSE EFFECTS/ TOXIC REACTIONS

Prolonged administration increases risk of cerebrovascular disease, coronary artery disease, gallbladder disease, hypercalcemia; breast, cervical, vaginal, endometrial, hepatic carcinoma. Cholestatic jaundice occurs rarely.

NURSING CONSIDERATIONS

BASELINE ASSESSMENT

Question for hypersensitivity to estrogen, previous jaundice, thromboembolic disorders associated with pregnancy, estrogen therapy. Question for possibility of pregnancy (Pregnancy Category X).

INTERVENTION/EVALUATION

Promptly report signs/symptoms of thromboembolic/thrombotic disorders (sudden severe headache, shortness of breath, vision/speech disturbance, numbness of an extremity).

PATIENT/FAMILY TEACHING

• Avoid smoking due to increased risk of heart attack and blood clots. • Notify physician of abnormal vaginal bleeding, depression. • With vaginal application, remain recumbent at least 30 min after application; do not use tampons. • Stop taking medication and contact physician at once if pregnancy is suspected.

eszopiclone

es-zoe-**pick**-lone
(Lunesta)

CLASSIFICATION

PHARMACOTHERAPEUTIC: Nonbenzodiazepine. **CLINICAL:** Hypnotic (**Schedule IV**).

ACTION

May interact with GABA-receptor complexes at binding domains located close to or allosterically coupled to benzodiazepine receptors. **Therapeutic Effect:** Prevents insomnia, difficulty maintaining normal sleep.

PHARMACOKINETICS

Rapidly absorbed following PO administration. Weakly bound to plasma proteins. Metabolized in liver. Excreted in urine. **Half-life:** 5–6 hrs.

USES

Long-term treatment of insomnia in pts who experience difficulty falling asleep, or are unable to sleep through the night (sleep maintenance difficulty).

PRECAUTIONS

CONTRAINDICATIONS: None known. **CAUTIONS:** Hepatic impairment, compromised respiratory function, clinical depression.

LIFESPAN CONSIDERATIONS:

Pregnancy/Lactation: Unknown if drug crosses placenta or is distributed in breast milk. **Pregnancy Category C.** **Children:** Safety and efficacy not established. **Elderly:** Those with impaired motor or cognitive performance may require dosage adjustment.

INTERACTIONS

DRUG: **Alcohol, anticonvulsants, antihistamines, other CNS depressants** may increase CNS depression. **Clarithromycin, itraconazole, ketoconazole, nelfinavir, ritonavir, (CYP3A4 inhibitors)** may increase concentration/toxicity. **HERBAL: Gotu kola, kava kava, St. John's wort, valerian** may increase CNS depression. **FOOD:** Onset of action may be reduced if taken with or immediately after a **high-fat meal**. **LAB VALUES:** None known.

AVAILABILITY (Rx)

TABLETS, FILM-COATED: 1 mg, 2 mg, 3 mg (Lunesta).

ADMINISTRATION/HANDLING

PO

- Should be administered immediately before bedtime.
- Do not give with or immediately following a high-fat meal.
- Do not crush, break tablet.

INDICATIONS/ROUTES/DOSAGE

INSOMNIA

PO: ADULTS: 2 mg before bedtime. **Maximum:** 3 mg. **Concurrent use with CYP3A4 inhibitors** (e.g., clarithromycin, erythromycin, azole antifungals) 1 mg before bedtime; if needed, dose may be increased to 2 mg. **ELDERLY:** Initially, 1 mg before bedtime. **Maximum:** 2 mg.

SLEEP MAINTENANCE DIFFICULTY

PO: ADULTS: 2 mg before bedtime.

SIDE EFFECTS

FREQUENT (34%–21%): Unpleasant taste, headache. **OCCASIONAL (10%–4%):** Somnolence, dry mouth, dyspepsia, dizziness, nervousness, nausea, rash, pruritus, depression, diarrhea. **RARE (3%–2%):** Hallucinations, anxiety, confusion, abnormal dreams, decreased libido, neuralgia.

ADVERSE EFFECTS/ TOXIC REACTIONS

Chest pain, peripheral edema occur occasionally.

NURSING CONSIDERATIONS

BASELINE ASSESSMENT

Assess B/P, pulse, respirations. Raise bed rails, provide call light. Provide environment conducive to sleep (quiet environment, low or no lighting, TV off).

INTERVENTION/EVALUATION

Assess sleep pattern of pt. Evaluate for therapeutic response (decrease in number of nocturnal awakenings, increase in length of sleep).

PATIENT/FAMILY TEACHING

• Do not abruptly withdraw medication following long-term use. • Avoid alcohol. • At least 8 hrs must be devoted for sleep time before daily activity begins. • Advise pt to take eszopiclone immediately before bedtime.

etanercept

ee-**tan**-er-cept
(Enbrel)

CLASSIFICATION

PHARMACOTHERAPEUTIC: Protein. **CLINICAL:** Antiarthritic.

ACTION

Binds to tumor necrosis factor (TNF), blocking its interaction with cell surface receptors. Elevated levels of TNF, involved in inflammatory and immune responses, are found in synovial fluid of rheumatoid arthritis pts. **Therapeutic Effect:** Relieves symptoms of rheumatoid arthritis.

PHARMACOKINETICS

Well absorbed after subcutaneous administration. **Half-life:** 115 hrs.

USES

Reduces signs/symptoms of moderate to severely active rheumatoid arthritis (RA). Treatment of active juvenile RA, ankylosing spondylitis, psoriatic arthritis. Treatment of chronic, moderate to severe plaque psoriasis. Improvement of physical function in pts with psoriatic arthritis. **OFF-LABEL:** Treatment of Crohn's disease, reactive arthritis.

PRECAUTIONS

CONTRAINDICATIONS: Serious active infection or sepsis. **CAUTIONS:** History of recurrent infections, illnesses that predispose to infection (e.g., diabetes).

LIFESPAN CONSIDERATIONS:

Pregnancy/Lactation: Unknown if drug is excreted in breast milk. **Pregnancy Category B. Children:** No age-related precautions noted in those 4 yrs and older. **Elderly:** No age-related precautions noted.

INTERACTIONS

DRUG: **Anakinra** may increase risk of infection. Use of **live virus vaccines** may potentiate virus replication, increase vaccine side effects, decrease pt's antibody response to vaccine. **HERBAL:** None significant. **FOOD:** None known. **LAB VALUES:** None known.

AVAILABILITY (Rx)

INJECTION, POWDER FOR RECONSTITUTION: 25 mg. **INJECTION, SOLUTION PREFILLED SYRINGE:** 50 mg/ml. **INJECTION, SOLUTION (AUTO INJECTOR):** 50 mg/ml.

ADMINISTRATION/HANDLING

◀ **ALERT** ▶ Do not add other medications to solution. Do not use filter during reconstitution or administration.

SUBCUTANEOUS

• Reconstitute with 1 ml of Bacteriostatic Water for Injection (0.9% benzyl alcohol). Do not reconstitute with other diluents. • Slowly inject diluent into vial. Some foaming will occur. To avoid excessive foaming, slowly swirl contents until powder is dissolved (less than 5 min). • Visually inspect solution for particles, discoloration. Reconstituted solution should appear clear, colorless.

If discolored, cloudy, or particles remain, discard solution; do not use. • Withdraw all the solution into syringe. Final volume should be approximately 1 ml. • Inject into thigh, abdomen, upper arm. Rotate injection sites. • Give new injection at least 1 inch from an old site and never into area where skin is tender, bruised, red, hard. • Refrigerate. • Once reconstituted, may be stored up to 6 hrs if refrigerated.

INDICATIONS/ROUTES/DOSAGE

RHEUMATOID ARTHRITIS, PSORIATIC ARTHRITIS, ANKYLOSING SPONDYLITIS

SUBCUTANEOUS: ADULTS, ELDERLY: 25 mg twice weekly given 72–96 hrs apart or 50 mg once weekly. **Maximum:** 50 mg/wk.

JUVENILE RHEUMATOID ARTHRITIS

SUBCUTANEOUS: CHILDREN 4–17 YRS: 0.4 mg/kg (**Maximum:** 25 mg dose) twice weekly given 72–96 hrs apart or 50 mg once weekly. **Maximum:** 25 mg/dose.

PLAQUE PSORIASIS

SUBCUTANEOUS: ADULTS, ELDERLY: 50 mg twice a wk (give 3–4 days apart) for 3 mos. Maintenance: 50 mg once a wk.

SIDE EFFECTS

FREQUENT (37%): Injection site erythema, pruritus, pain, swelling; abdominal pain, vomiting (more common in children than adults). **OCCASIONAL (16%–4%):** Headache, rhinitis, dizziness, pharyngitis, cough, asthenia, abdominal pain, dyspepsia. **RARE (less than 3%):** Sinusitis, allergic reaction.

ADVERSE EFFECTS/ TOXIC REACTIONS

Infection (pyelonephritis, cellulitis, osteomyelitis, wound infection, leg ulcer, septic arthritis, diarrhea, bronchitis, pneumonia) occur in 38%–29% of pts. Rare adverse effects include heart failure, hypertension, hypotension, pancreatitis, GI hemorrhage.

NURSING CONSIDERATIONS

BASELINE ASSESSMENT

Assess onset, type, location, duration of pain, inflammation. If significant exposure to varicella virus has occurred during treatment, therapy should be temporarily discontinued and treatment with varicella-zoster immune globulin considered.

INTERVENTION/EVALUATION

Assess for joint swelling, pain, tenderness. Monitor erythrocyte sedimentation rate (ESR), C-reactive protein level, CBC with differential, platelet count.

PATIENT/FAMILY TEACHING

• Instruct in subcutaneous injection technique, including areas of body acceptable as injection sites. • Injection site reaction generally occurs in first mo of treatment and decreases in frequency during continued therapy. • Do not receive live vaccines during treatment. • Inform physician if persistent fever, bruising, bleeding, pallor occurs.

ethambutol

eth-**am**-bew-tol

(Etibi ✤, Myambutol)

Do not confuse ethambutol or Myambutol with Nembutal.

CLASSIFICATION

PHARMACOTHERAPEUTIC: Isonicotinic acid derivative. **CLINICAL:** Antitubercular.

ACTION

Interferes with RNA synthesis. **Therapeutic Effect:** Suppresses multiplication of mycobacteria.

PHARMACOKINETICS

Rapidly, well absorbed from GI tract. Protein binding: 20%–30%. Widely distributed. Metabolized in liver. Primarily excreted in urine. Removed by hemodialysis. **Half-life:** 3–4 hrs (increased in renal impairment).

USES

In conjunction with at least one other antitubercular agent for initial treatment and retreatment of clinical tuberculosis. **OFF-LABEL:** Treatment of atypical mycobacterial infections (e.g., *Mycobacterium avium* complex [MAC]).

PRECAUTIONS

CONTRAINDICATIONS: Optic neuritis. **CAUTIONS:** Renal dysfunction, gout, ocular defects: diabetic retinopathy, cataracts, recurrent ocular inflammatory conditions. Not recommended for children 13 yrs and younger.

LIFESPAN CONSIDERATIONS:

Pregnancy/Lactation: Crosses placenta. Excreted in breast milk. **Pregnancy Category B. Children:** Safety and efficacy not established in those younger than 13 yrs. **Elderly:** Age-related renal impairment may require dosage adjustment.

INTERACTIONS

DRUG: **Neurotoxic medications** may increase risk of neurotoxicity. **HERBAL:** None significant. **FOOD:** None known. **LAB VALUES:** May increase serum uric acid.

AVAILABILITY (Rx)

TABLETS: 100 mg, 400 mg.

ADMINISTRATION/HANDLING

PO

- Give with food (decreases GI upset).

INDICATIONS/ROUTES/DOSAGE

TUBERCULOSIS, OTHER MYOBACTERIAL DISEASES

PO: ADULTS, ELDERLY: 15–25 mg/kg/day. **Maximum:** 1.6 g/dose **or** 50 mg/kg twice weekly. **Maximum:** 4 g regardless of weight. **CHILDREN:** 15–20 mg/kg/day. **Maximum:** 1 g/day **or** 50 mg/kg twice weekly. **Maximum:** 4 g regardless of weight.

DOSAGE IN RENAL IMPAIRMENT

Dosage interval is modified based on creatinine clearance.

Creatinine Clearance	Dosage Interval
10–50 ml/min	q24–36h
Less than 10 ml/min	q48h

SIDE EFFECTS

OCCASIONAL: Acute gouty arthritis (chills, pain, swelling of joints with hot skin), confusion, abdominal pain, nausea, vomiting, anorexia, headache. **RARE:** Rash, fever, blurred vision, red-green color blindness.

ADVERSE EFFECTS/ TOXIC REACTIONS

Optic neuritis (more common with high-dosage, long-term therapy), peripheral neuritis, thrombocytopenia, anaphylactoid reaction occur rarely.

NURSING CONSIDERATIONS

BASELINE ASSESSMENT

Evaluate initial CBC, renal/hepatic fuction test results.

INTERVENTION/EVALUATION

Assess for vision changes (altered color perception, decreased visual acuity may be first signs): discontinue drug and notify physician immediately. Give with food if GI distress occurs. Monitor serum uric acid. Assess for hot, painful, swollen joints, esp. great toe, ankle, knee (gout). Report numbness, tingling, burning of extremities (peripheral neuritis).

PATIENT/FAMILY TEACHING

• Do not skip doses; take for full length of therapy (may take mos or yrs). • Notify physician immediately of any visual problem (visual effects generally reversible with discontinuation of ethambutol but in rare cases may take up to 1 yr to disappear or may be permanent); promptly report swelling or pain of joints, numbness or tingling/burning of extremities.

ethosuximide

(Zarontin)

See Anticonvulsants

etidronate

eh-**tye**-droe-nate

(Didronel, Didronel I.V.)

Do not confuse etidronate with etidocaine or etomidate.

CLASSIFICATION

PHARMACOTHERAPEUTIC: Bisphosphonate. **CLINICAL:** Calcium regulator.

ACTION

Decreases mineral release, matrix in bone, inhibits osteocytic osteolysis. **Therapeutic Effect:** Decreases bone reabsorption.

PHARMACOKINETICS

Variable absorption following PO administration. Not metabolized. Approximately 50% of drug is excreted in urine. Unabsorbed drug is excreted intact in feces. **Half-life:** 1–6 hrs (oral); 6 hrs (IV).

USES

PO: Treatment of symptomatic Paget's disease of bone, prevention/treatment of heterotopic ossification following hip replacement or due to spinal injury. **IV:** Treatment of hypercalcemia associated with malignant neoplasms inadequately managed by dietary modification, oral hydration; treatment of hypercalcemia of malignancy persisting after adequate hydration has been restored.

PRECAUTIONS

CONTRAINDICATIONS: Clinically overt osteomalacia. **CAUTIONS:** Those with restricted calcium/vitamin D intake, renal impairment, hyperphosphatemia.

LIFESPAN CONSIDERATIONS:

Pregnancy/Lactation: Unknown if drug is distributed in breast milk. **Pregnancy Category C (parenteral), B (oral). Children:** Safety and efficacy not established. **Elderly:** Prone to overhydration when treated with parenteral etidronate in conjunction with hydration therapy.

INTERACTIONS

DRUG: Mineral supplements; antacids containing aluminum, calcium, magnesium may decrease absorption. **HERBAL:** None significant. **FOOD: Foods high in calcium** may decrease absorption. **LAB VALUES:** None known.

AVAILABILITY (Rx)

INJECTION SOLUTION (DIDRONEL I.V.): 300-mg ampule (50 mg/ml). **TABLETS (DIDRONEL):** 200 mg, 400 mg.

ADMINISTRATION/HANDLING

IV

Reconstitution • Must dilute with at least 250 ml 0.9% NaCl or D_5W.

Rate of administration • Infuse over at least 2 hrs.

Storage • Store at room temperature.

IV INCOMPATIBILITIES

Do not mix with other medications.

INDICATIONS/ROUTES/DOSAGE

PAGET'S DISEASE

PO: ADULTS, ELDERLY: Initially, 5–10 mg/kg/day not to exceed 6 mos, or 11–20 mg/kg/day not to exceed 3 mos. Repeat only after drug-free period of at least 90 days.

HETEROTOPIC OSSIFICATION CAUSED BY SPINAL CORD INJURY

PO: ADULT, ELDERLY: 20 mg/kg/day for 2 wks; then 10 mg/kg/day for 10 wks.

HETEROTOPIC OSSIFICATION COMPLICATING TOTAL HIP REPLACEMENT

PO: ADULTS, ELDERLY: 20 mg/kg/day for 1 mo before surgery; then 20 mg/kg/day for 3 mos after surgery.

HYPERCALCEMIA ASSOCIATED WITH MALIGNANCY

IV: ADULTS, ELDERLY: 7.5 mg/kg/day for 3 days. For retreatment, allow 7 days between treatment courses. Follow with oral therapy on day after last infusion. Begin with 20 mg/kg/day for 30 days; may extend up to 90 days.

SIDE EFFECTS

FREQUENT: Nausea; diarrhea; continuing or more frequent bone pain in pts with Paget's disease. **OCCASIONAL:** Bone fractures (esp. femur). **Parenteral:** Metallic, altered taste. **RARE:** Hypersensitivity reaction.

ADVERSE EFFECTS/ TOXIC REACTIONS

Nephrotoxicity (hematuria, dysuria, proteinuria) noted with parenteral route.

NURSING CONSIDERATIONS

BASELINE ASSESSMENT

Obtain baseline laboratory tests, esp. serum electrolytes, renal function.

INTERVENTION/EVALUATION

Assess for diarrhea. Monitor electrolytes. Monitor I&O, BUN, serum creatinine in pts with renal impairment. Evaluate pain in pts with Paget's disease.

PATIENT/FAMILY TEACHING

- May take up to 3 mos for therapeutic response.
- Ensure milk, dairy products in diet for calcium, vitamin D.
- Take medication on empty stomach, 2 hrs after food, vitamins, antacids.

etodolac

eh-**toe**-doe-lack

(Apo-Etodolac ✱, Lodine, Lodine XL, Ultradol ✱)

Do not confuse Lodine with codeine or iodine.

CLASSIFICATION

PHARMACOTHERAPEUTIC: NSAID. **CLINICAL:** Nonsteroidal anti-inflammatory, analgesic (see p. 123C).

ACTION

Produces analgesic, anti-inflammatory effects by inhibiting prostaglandin synthesis. **Therapeutic Effect:** Reduces inflammatory response, intensity of pain.

PHARMACOKINETICS

Route	Onset	Peak	Duration
PO (analgesic)	30 min	N/A	4–12 hrs

Completely absorbed from GI tract. Protein binding: greater than 99%. Widely distributed. Metabolized in liver. Primarily excreted in urine. Not removed by hemodialysis. **Half-life:** 6–7 hrs.

USES

Acute and long-term treatment of osteoarthritis, management of pain, treatment of rheumatoid arthritis (RA), juvenile rheumatoid arthritis (JRA). **OFF-LABEL:** Treatment of acute gouty arthritis, vascular headache.

PRECAUTIONS

CONTRAINDICATIONS: Active peptic ulcer disease, chronic inflammation of GI tract, GI bleeding/ulceration, history of hypersensitivity to aspirin, NSAIDs. **CAUTIONS:** Renal/hepatic impairment, history of GI tract disease, predisposition to fluid retention.

LIFESPAN CONSIDERATIONS:

Pregnancy/Lactation: Unknown if drug crosses placenta or is distributed in breast milk. Avoid use during last trimester (may adversely affect fetal cardiovascular system: premature closure of ductus arteriosus). **Pregnancy Category C (D if used in third trimester or near delivery). Children:** Safety and efficacy not established. **Elderly:** GI bleeding, ulceration more likely to cause serious adverse effects. Age-related renal impairment may increase risk of hepatic/renal toxicity; decreased dosage recommended.

INTERACTIONS

DRUG: May decrease effects of **antihypertensives, diuretics. Aspirin, other salicylates** may increase risk of GI side effects, bleeding. May increase concentration/toxicity of **cyclosporine. Bone marrow depressants** may increase risk of hematologic reactions. May increase effects of **heparin, oral anticoagulants, thrombolytics.** May increase concentration, risk of toxicity of **lithium.** May increase risk of **methotrexate** toxicity. **Probenecid** may increase concentration. **HERBAL: Cat's claw, dong quai, evening primrose, feverfew, garlic, ginger, ginkgo, ginseng** may increase antiplatelet action, risk of bleeding. **FOOD:** None known. **LAB VALUES:** May increase bleeding time, hepatic function test results, serum creatinine. May decrease serum uric acid.

AVAILABILITY (Rx)

TABLETS (LODINE): 400 mg, 500 mg.

CAPSULES (LODINE): 200 mg, 300 mg. **TABLETS (EXTENDED-RELEASE [LODINE XL]):** 400 mg, 500 mg, 600 mg.

ADMINISTRATION/HANDLING

PO

• Do not crush, break capsules, extended-release tablets. • May give with food, milk, antacids if GI distress occurs.

INDICATIONS/ROUTES/DOSAGE

OSTEOARTHRITIS, RHEUMATOID ARTHRITIS

PO (IMMEDIATE-RELEASE): ADULTS, ELDERLY: Initially, 300 mg 2–3 times a day or 400–500 mg twice a day. Maintenance: 600–1,000 mg/day in 2–4 divided doses.

PO (EXTENDED-RELEASE): ADULTS, ELDERLY: 400–1,000 mg once daily. **Maximum:** 1,200 mg/day.

JUVENILE RHEUMATOID ARTHRITIS

PO (EXTENDED-RELEASE): CHILDREN 6–16 YRS: 1,000 mg in children weighing more than 60 kg, 800 mg once daily in children weighing 46–60 kg, 600 mg once daily in children weighing 31–45 kg, 400 mg once daily in children weighing 20–30 kg.

ANALGESIA

PO: ADULTS, ELDERLY: 200–400 mg q6–8h as needed. **Maximum:** 1,200 mg/day.

SIDE EFFECTS

OCCASIONAL (9%–4%): Dizziness, headache, abdominal pain/cramping, bloated feeling, diarrhea, nausea, indigestion. **RARE (3%–1%):** Constipation, rash, pruritus, visual disturbances, tinnitus.

ADVERSE EFFECTS/ TOXIC REACTIONS

Overdose may result in acute renal failure. Increased risk of cardiovascular events (MI, CVA) and serious, potentially life-threatening GI bleeding. Rare reactions with long-term use include peptic ulcer, gastritis, jaundice, nephrotoxicity (hematuria, dysuria, proteinuria), severe hypersensitivity reaction (bronchospasm, angioedema).

NURSING CONSIDERATIONS

BASELINE ASSESSMENT

Assess onset, type, location, duration of pain/inflammation. Inspect appearance of affected joints for immobility, deformities, skin condition.

INTERVENTION/EVALUATION

Monitor CBC, hepatic/renal function tests. Observe for bleeding/ecchymosis. Evaluate for therapeutic response (relief of pain, stiffness, swelling; increase in joint mobility; reduced joint tenderness; improved grip strength).

PATIENT/FAMILY TEACHING

• Swallow capsule whole; do not crush, chew. • Avoid aspirin, alcohol during therapy (increases risk of GI bleeding). • Report GI distress, visual disturbances, rash, edema, headache. • Report any signs of bleeding. • Take with food, milk, antacid if GI distress occurs. • Avoid tasks that require alertness, motor skills until response to drug is established (possibility of dizziness).

etoposide, VP-16

eh-**toe**-poe-side

(Etopophos, Toposar, VePesid)

Do not confuse VePesid with Pepcid or Versed.

CLASSIFICATION

PHARMACOTHERAPEUTIC: Epipodophyllotoxin. **CLINICAL:** Antineoplastic (see p. 79C).

ACTION

Induces single- and double-stranded breaks in DNA. Cell cycle-dependent and phase-specific; most effective in S and G_2 phases of cell division. **Therapeutic Effect:** Inhibits, alters DNA synthesis.

PHARMACOKINETICS

Variably absorbed from GI tract. Rapidly distributed, low concentrations in cerebrospinal fluid (CSF). Protein binding: 97%. Metabolized in liver. Primarily excreted in urine. Not removed by hemodialysis. **Half-life:** 3–12 hrs.

USES

Treatment of refractory testicular tumors, small cell lung carcinoma. **OFF-LABEL:** Acute lymphocytic, acute nonlymphocytic leukemias; Ewing's and Kaposi's sarcoma; Hodgkin's and non-Hodgkin's lymphomas; endometrial, gastric, non–small cell lung carcinomas; multiple myeloma; myelodysplastic syndromes; neuroblastoma; osteosarcoma; ovarian germ cell tumors; primary brain, gestational trophoblastic tumors; soft tissue sarcomas; Wilms' tumor.

PRECAUTIONS

CONTRAINDICATIONS: Pregnancy. **CAUTIONS:** Hepatic/renal impairment, myelosuppression.

LIFESPAN CONSIDERATIONS:

Pregnancy/Lactation: If possible, avoid use during pregnancy, esp. first trimester. May cause fetal harm. Breastfeeding not recommended. **Pregnancy Category D.** **Children:** Safety and efficacy not established. **Elderly:** Age-related renal impairment may require dosage adjustment.

INTERACTIONS

DRUG: **Bone marrow depressants** may increase myelosuppression. **Live-virus vaccines** may potentiate virus replication, increase vaccine side effects, decrease pt's antibody response to vaccine. **HERBAL:** **St. John's wort** may decrease concentration. **FOOD:** None known. **LAB VALUES:** None known

AVAILABILITY (Rx)

CAPSULES (VEPESID): 50 mg. **INJECTION, POWDER FOR RECONSTITUTION (WATER-SOLUBLE [ETOPOPHOS]):** 100 mg. **INJECTION SOLUTION (TOPOSAR, VEPESID):** 20 mg/ml.

ADMINISTRATION/HANDLING

◄ ALERT ► Administer by slow IV infusion. Wear gloves when preparing solution. If powder or solution comes in contact with skin, wash immediately and thoroughly with soap, water. May be carcinogenic, mutagenic, teratogenic. Handle with extreme care during preparation, administration.

IV

Reconstitution

VEPESID • Dilute each 100 mg (5 ml) with at least 250 ml D_5W or 0.9% NaCl to provide concentration of 0.4 mg/ml (500 ml for concentration of 0.2 mg/ml).

ETOPOPHOS • Reconstitute each 100 mg with 5–10 ml Sterile Water for Injection, D_5W, or 0.9% NaCl to provide concentration of 20 mg/ml or 10 mg/ml, respectively. • May give without further dilution or further dilute to concentration as low as 0.1 mg/ml with 0.9% NaCl or D_5W.

Rate of administration

VEPESID • Infuse slowly, over 30–60 min (rapid IV may produce marked hypotension). • Monitor for anaphylactic reaction during infusion (chills, fever, dyspnea, diaphoresis, lacrimation, sneezing, throat, back, chest pain).

ETOPOPHOS • May give over as little as 5 min up to 210 min.

Storage

VEPESID • Store injection at room temperature before dilution. • Concentrate for injection is clear, yellow. • Diluted solution is stable at room temperature for 96 hrs at 0.2 mg/ml, 48 hrs at 0.4 mg/ml. • Discard if crystallization occurs.

ETOPOPHOS • Refrigerate vials. • Stable for 24 hrs after reconstitution.

PO

Storage • Refrigerate gelatin capsules.

IV INCOMPATIBILITIES

VePesid: Cefepime (Maxipime), filgrastim (Neupogen), idarubicin (Idamycin). **Etopophos:** Amphotericin B (Fungizone), cefepime (Maxipime), chlorpromazine (Thorazine), methylprednisolone (Solu-Medrol), prochlorperazine (Compazine).

IV COMPATIBILITIES

VePesid: Carboplatin (Paraplatin), cisplatin (Platinol), cytarabine (Cytosar), daunorubicin (Cerubidine), doxorubicin (Adriamycin), granisetron (Kytril), mitoxantrone (Novantrone), ondansetron (Zofran). **Etopophos:** Carboplatin (Paraplatin), cisplatin (Platinol), cytarabine (Cytosar), dacarbazine (DTIC-Dome), daunorubicin (Cerubidine), dexamethasone (Decadron), diphenhydramine (Benadryl), doxorubicin (Adriamycin), granisetron (Kytril), magnesium sulfate, mannitol, mitoxantrone (Novantrone), ondansetron (Zofran), potassium chloride.

INDICATIONS/ROUTES/DOSAGE

◄ ALERT ► Dosage individualized based on clinical response, tolerance to

E

adverse effects. Treatment repeated at 3- to 4-wk intervals.

REFRACTORY TESTICULAR TUMORS

IV: ADULTS: 50–100 mg/m²/day on days 1–5, or 100 mg/m²/day on days 1, 3, 5 (as combination therapy). Given q3–4 wk for 3–4 courses.

ACUTE MYELOCYTIC LEUKEMIA

IV: CHILDREN: 150 mg/m²/day for 2–3 days and 2–3 cycles.

BRAIN TUMOR

IV: CHILDREN: 150 mg/m²/day on days 2 and 3 of treatment course.

NEUROBLASTOMA

IV: CHILDREN: 100 mg/m²/day on days 1–5 of treatment course; repeated q4wk.

SMALL-CELL LUNG CARCINOMA

PO: ADULTS: Twice the IV dose rounded to nearest 50 mg. Give once a day for doses 400 mg or less, in divided doses for dosages greater than 400 mg.

IV: ADULTS: 35 mg/m²/day for 4 consecutive days up to 50 mg/m²/day for 5 consecutive days (as combination therapy).

LEUKEMIA, RHABDOMYOSARCOMA

IV: CHILDREN: 60–150 mg/m²/day for 2–5 days q3–6wk.

DOSAGE IN RENAL IMPAIRMENT

Creatinine Clearance	Dosage
10–50 ml/min	75% normal dose
Less than 10 ml/min	50% normal dose

SIDE EFFECTS

FREQUENT (66%–43%): Mild to moderate nausea/vomiting, alopecia. **OCCASIONAL (13%–6%):** Diarrhea, anorexia, stomatitis. **RARE (2% or less):** Hypotension, peripheral neuropathy.

ADVERSE EFFECTS/ TOXIC REACTIONS

Myelosuppression manifested as hematologic toxicity, principally anemia, leukopenia (occurring 7–14 days after drug administration), thrombocytopenia (occurring 9–16 days after administration) and, to lesser extent, pancytopenia. Bone marrow recovery occurs by day 20. Hepatotoxicity occurs occasionally.

NURSING CONSIDERATIONS

BASELINE ASSESSMENT

Obtain hematologic tests before and at frequent intervals during therapy. Antiemetics readily control nausea, vomiting.

INTERVENTION/EVALUATION

Monitor Hgb, Hct, WBC, platelet count. Monitor daily pattern of bowel activity/ stool consistency. Monitor for hematologic toxicity (fever, sore throat, signs of local infection, unusual ecchymosis or bleeding from any site), symptoms of anemia (excessive fatigue, weakness). Assess for paresthesias (peripheral neuropathy). Monitor for stomatitis.

PATIENT/FAMILY TEACHING

• Alopecia is reversible, but new hair growth may have different color, texture. • Do not have immunizations without physician's approval (drug lowers resistance). • Avoid contact with those who have recently received live virus vaccine. • Promptly report fever, sore throat, signs of local infection, unusual bruising or bleeding from any site.

Eulexin, *see flutamide*

Evista, *see raloxifene*

Exelon, *see rivastigmine*

exemestane

x-eh-**mess**-tane
(Aromasin)

CLASSIFICATION

PHARMACOTHERAPEUTIC: Hormone. **CLINICAL:** Antineoplastic (see p. 79C).

ACTION

Inactivates aromatase, the principal enzyme that converts androgens to estrogens in both premenopausal and postmenopausal women, lowering circulating estrogen level. **Therapeutic Effect:** Inhibits growth of breast cancers stimulated by estrogens.

PHARMACOKINETICS

Rapidly absorbed after PO administration. Protein binding: 90%. Distributed extensively into tissues. Metabolized in liver; eliminated in urine and feces. **Half-life:** 24 hrs.

USES

Treatment of advanced breast cancer in postmenopausal women whose disease has progressed following tamoxifen therapy. Adjuvant treatment of postmenopausal women with estrogen-receptor positive early breast cancer after 2–3 yrs of tamoxifen therapy for completion of 5 consecutive yrs of adjuvant hormonal therapy. **OFF-LABEL:** Prevention of prostate cancer.

PRECAUTIONS

CONTRAINDICATIONS: Pregnancy. **CAUTIONS:** Do not give to premenopausal women.

LIFESPAN CONSIDERATIONS:

Pregnancy/Lactation: Indicated for postmenopausal women. **Pregnancy Category D. Children:** Not indicated in children. **Elderly:** No age-related precautions noted.

INTERACTIONS

DRUG: Estrogens may interfere with action. **HERBAL: St. John's wort** may decrease concentration. Avoid **black cohosh, dong quai** in estrogen-dependent tumors. **FOOD:** None known. **LAB VALUES:** May increase serum alkaline phosphatase, AST, ALT.

AVAILABILITY (Rx)

TABLETS: 25 mg.

ADMINISTRATION/HANDLING

PO

- Give after meals.

INDICATIONS/ROUTES/DOSAGE

BREAST CANCER

PO: ADULTS, ELDERLY: 25 mg once a day after a meal. 50 mg/day when used concurrently with potent CYP3A4 inducers (e.g., rifampin, phenytoin).

SIDE EFFECTS

FREQUENT (22%–10%): Fatigue, nausea, depression, hot flashes, pain, insomnia, anxiety, dyspnea. **OCCASIONAL (8%–5%):** Headache, dizziness, vomiting, peripheral edema, abdominal pain, anorexia, flu-like symptoms, diaphoresis, constipation, hypertension. **RARE (4%):** Diarrhea.

ADVERSE EFFECTS/ TOXIC REACTIONS

Myocardial infarction (MI) has been noted.

NURSING CONSIDERATIONS

INTERVENTION/EVALUATION

Monitor for onset of depression. Assess sleep pattern. Monitor for and assist with ambulation if dizziness occurs. Assess for headache. Offer antiemetic for nausea/vomiting.

PATIENT/FAMILY TEACHING

- Notify physician if nausea, hot flashes become unmanageable. • Avoid tasks that require alertness, motor skills until response to drug is established. • Best taken after meals and at same time each day.

E

exenatide

ex-**nah**-tide
(Byetta)

CLASSIFICATION

PHARMACOTHERAPEUTIC: Antihyperglycemic. **CLINICAL:** Antidiabetic.

ACTION

Stimulates release of insulin from beta cells of pancreas, mimics enhancement of glucose-dependent insulin secretion, suppresses elevated glucagon secretion, slows gastric emptying. **Therapeutic Effect:** Improves glycemic control by reducing fasting and postprandial glucose concentrations in pts with type 2 diabetes mellitus.

PHARMACOKINETICS

Minimal systemic metabolism. Eliminated by glomerular filtration with subsequent proteolytic degradation. **Half-life:** 2.4 hrs.

USES

Adjunct to diet, exercise to improve glycemic control in pts with type 2 diabetes mellitus who are taking metformin (Glucophage) and a sulfonylurea or metformin and a thiazolidinedione.

PRECAUTIONS

CONTRAINDICATIONS: Diabetic ketoacidosis, type 1 diabetes mellitus. Not recommended in severe renal impairment, severe GI disease. **CAUTIONS:** Mild-to-moderate renal impairment.

LIFESPAN CONSIDERATIONS:

Pregnancy/Lactation: Unknown if distributed in breast milk. **Pregnancy Category C. Children:** Safety and efficacy not established. **Elderly:** No age-related precautions noted.

INTERACTIONS

DRUG: Reduces, delays optimal absorption, peak levels of **antibiotics, acetaminophen, digoxin, lisinopril, lovastatin, oral contraceptives** if administered within 1 hr of exenatide dose. **Ethanol** increases risk of hypoglycemia. May reduce rate, extent of absorption of **oral medications**. **HERBAL:** None significant. **FOOD:** None known. **LAB VALUES:** Decreases serum glucose.

AVAILABILITY (Rx)

INJECTION, SOLUTION: (PREFILLED PEN): 250 mcg/ml (1.2 ml provides 5 mcg/dose; 2.4 ml provides 10 mcg/dose).

ADMINISTRATION/HANDLING

SUBCUTANEOUS

• May be given in thigh, abdomen, upper arm. • Rotation of injection sites is essential; maintain careful injection site record. • Give within 60 min before morning and evening meals.

Storage • Refrigerate prefilled pens. • Discard if freezing occurs. • Discard pen 30 days after initial use.

INDICATIONS/ROUTE/DOSAGE

DIABETES MELLITUS

SUBCUTANEOUS: ADULTS, ELDERLY: 5 mcg per dose given twice a day at any time with the 60-min period before the morning and evening meals. Dose may be increased to 10 mcg twice a day after 1 mo of therapy.

◀ **ALERT** ▶ Not recommeded in pts with creatinine clearance less than 30 ml/min.

SIDE EFFECTS

FREQUENT (44%): Nausea. **OCCASIONAL (13%–6%):** Diarrhea, vomiting, dizziness, anxiety, dyspepsia. **RARE (less than 6%):** Weakness, decreased appetite.

ADVERSE EFFECTS/ TOXIC REACTIONS

With concurrent sulfonylurea, hypoglycemia occurs in 36% when given a 10 mcg dose exenatide, 16% when given a 5 mcg dose.

NURSING CONSIDERATIONS

BASELINE ASSESSMENT

Check serum glucose before administration. Discuss lifestyle to determine extent of learning, emotional needs. Assure follow-up instruction if pt or family does not thoroughly understand diabetes management, glucose-testing technique. At least 1 mo should elapse to assess response to drug before new dose adjustment is made.

INTERVENTION/EVALUATION

Monitor serum glucose, food intake. Assess for hypoglycemia (cool wet skin, tremors, dizziness, anxiety, headache, tachycardia, numbness in mouth, hunger, diplopia), hyperglycemia (polyuria, polyphagia, polydipsia, nausea, vomiting, dim vision, fatigue, deep rapid breathing). Be alert to conditions that alter glucose requirements (fever, increased activity or stress, surgical procedure).

PATIENT/FAMILY TEACHING

• Diabetes mellitus requires lifelong control. • Prescribed diet and exercise is principal part of treatment; do not skip, delay meals. • Continue to adhere to dietary instructions, regular exercise program, regular testing of serum glucose. • When taking combination therapy with a sulfonylurea, have source of glucose available to treat symptoms of hypoglycemia.

Exjade, *see deferasirox*

ezetimibe

eh-**zeh**-tih-myb

(Ezetrol ✤, Zetia)

Do not confuse Zetia with Zestril.

FIXED-COMBINATION(S)

Vytorin: ezetimibe/simvastatin (Hydroxamethyglutaryl CoA [HMG-CoA] reductase inhibitor): 10 mg/10 mg, 10 mg/20 mg, 10 mg/40 mg, 10 mg/80 mg.

CLASSIFICATION

PHARMACOTHERAPEUTIC: Antihyperlipidemic. **CLINICAL:** Anticholesterol agent.

ACTION

Inhibits cholesterol absorption in small intestine, leading to decrease in delivery of intestinal cholesterol to liver. **Therapeutic Effect:** Reduces total serum cholesterol, LDL cholesterol, triglyceride; increases HDL cholesterol.

PHARMACOKINETICS

Well absorbed following PO administration. Protein binding: greater than 90%. Metabolized in small intestine and liver. Excreted by kidneys and bile. **Half-life:** 22 hrs.

USES

Adjunct to diet for treatment of primary hypercholesterolemia (monotherapy or in combination with HMG-CoA reductase inhibitors or fenofibrate) homozygous sitosterolemia, homozygous familial hypercholesterolemia (combined with atrovastatin or simvastatin).

E

PRECAUTIONS

CONTRAINDICATIONS: Concurrent use of an hydroxamethylglutaryl-CoA (HMG-CoA) reductase inhibitor (atorvastatin, fluvastatin, lovastatin, pravastatin, simvastatin) in pts with active hepatic disease or unexplained persistent elevations in serum transaminase; moderate or severe hepatic insufficiency. **CAUTIONS:** Diabetes, hypothyroidism, obstructive hepatic disease, chronic renal failure, hepatic impairment.

LIFESPAN CONSIDERATIONS:

Pregnancy/Lactation: Unknown if drug crosses placenta or is distributed in breast milk. **Pregnancy Category C.** **Children:** Safety and efficacy not established in pts 10 yrs and younger. **Elderly:** Age-related mild hepatic impairment may require dosage adjustment. Not recommended in pts with moderate or severe hepatic impairment.

INTERACTIONS

DRUG: **Antacids containing aluminum or magnesium, cyclosporine, fenofibrate, gemfibrozil** increase plasma concentration. **Cholestyramine resin** decreases drug effectiveness. **HERBAL:** None significant. **FOOD:** None known. **LAB VALUES:** May increase serum alkaline phosphatase, bilirubin, AST, ALT.

AVAILABILITY (Rx)

TABLETS: 10 mg.

ADMINISTRATION/HANDLING

- Give without regard to food.

INDICATIONS/ROUTES/DOSAGE

HYPERCHOLESTEROLEMIA

PO: ADULTS, ELDERLY, CHILDREN, 10 YRS AND OLDER: Initially, 10 mg once a day, given with or without food. If pt is also receiving a bile acid sequestrant, give ezetimibe at least 2 hrs before or at least 4 hrs after bile acid sequestrant.

SITOSTEROLEMIA

PO: ADULTS, ELDERLY: 10 mg/day.

SIDE EFFECTS

OCCASIONAL (4%–3%): Back pain, diarrhea, arthralgia, sinusitis, abdominal pain. **RARE (2%):** Cough, pharyngitis, fatigue.

ADVERSE EFFECTS/ TOXIC REACTIONS

Hepatitis, hypersensitivity reaction, myopathy, rhabdomyolysis occur rarely.

NURSING CONSIDERATIONS

BASELINE ASSESSMENT

Obtain serum cholesterol, triglycerides, hepatic function tests, blood counts during initial therapy and periodically during treatment. Treatment should be discontinued if hepatic enzyme levels persist more than 3 times normal limit.

INTERVENTION/EVALUATION

Monitor daily pattern of bowel activity/ stool consistency. Question pt for signs/ symptoms of back pain, abdominal disturbances. Monitor serum cholesterol, triglyceride for therapeutic response.

PATIENT/FAMILY TEACHING

• Periodic laboratory tests are essential part of therapy. • Do not stop medication without consulting physician.

famciclovir

fam-**sigh**-klo-veer

(Famvir)

Do not confuse Famvir with Femhrt.

CLASSIFICATION

PHARMACOTHERAPEUTIC: Synthetic nucleoside. **CLINICAL:** Antiviral (see p. 65C).

ACTION

Inhibits viral DNA synthesis. **Therapeutic Effect:** Suppresses replication of herpes simplex virus, varicella-zoster virus.

PHARMACOKINETICS

Rapidly, extensively absorbed after PO administration. Protein binding: 20%–25%. Rapidly metabolized to penciclovir by enzymes in GI wall, liver, plasma. Eliminated unchanged in urine. Removed by hemodialysis. **Half-life:** 2 hrs.

USES

Management of acute herpes zoster (shingles), treatment and suppression of recurrent genital herpes, treatment of recurrent mucocutaneous herpes simplex in immunocompromised pts. Treatment of recurrent herpes labialis (cold sores).

PRECAUTIONS

CONTRAINDICATIONS: Hypersensitivity to penciclovir cream. **CAUTIONS:** Renal/hepatic impairment.

LIFESPAN CONSIDERATIONS:

Pregnancy/Lactation: Increased mammary adenocarcinoma in animals. Unknown if excreted in breast milk. **Pregnancy Category B. Children:** Safety and efficacy not established. **Elderly:** Age-related renal impairment may require dosage adjustment.

INTERACTIONS

DRUG: Probenecid may increase concentration. **HERBAL:** None significant. **FOOD:** None known. **LAB VALUES:** None known.

AVAILABILITY (Rx)

TABLETS: 125 mg, 250 mg, 500 mg.

ADMINISTRATION/HANDLING

PO

- Give without regard to meals.

INDICATIONS/ROUTES/DOSAGE

HERPES ZOSTER

PO: ADULTS: 500 mg q8h for 7 days.

GENITAL HERPES, INITIAL EPISODE

PO: ADULTS, ELDERLY: 250 mg 3 times a day for 7–10 days.

RECURRENT GENITAL HERPES

PO: ADULTS: 125 mg twice a day for 5 days or 1,000 mg twice a day for one day.

SUPPRESSION OF RECURRENT GENITAL HERPES

PO: ADULTS: 250 mg twice a day for up to 1 yr.

RECURRENT HERPES SIMPLEX

PO: ADULTS: 500 mg twice a day for 7 days.

HERPES LABIALIS (COLD SORES)

PO: ADULTS, ELDERLY: 1,500 mg as a single dose.

DOSAGE IN RENAL IMPAIRMENT

Dosage and frequency are modified based on creatinine clearance.

F

Creatinine Clearance	Herpes Zoster	Recurrent Genital Herpes	Suppression of Recurrent Genital Herpes	Recurrent Orolabial or Genital Herpes in Immuno-compromised Pts
60 ml/min or greater	500 mg q8h			
40–59 ml/min	500 mg q12h			
40 ml/min or greater		125 mg q12h	250 mg q12h	500 mg q12h
20–39 ml/min	500 mg q24h	125 mg q24h	125 mg q12h	500 mg q24h
Less than 20 ml/min	250 mg q24h	125 mg q48h	125 mg q24h	250 mg q24h

DOSAGE IN HEMODIALYSIS PTS

For adults with herpes zoster, give 250 mg after each dialysis treatment; for adults with genital herpes, give 125 mg after each dialysis treatment.

SIDE EFFECTS

FREQUENT: Headache (23%), nausea (12%). **OCCASIONAL (10%–2%):** Dizziness, somnolence, paresthesia (esp. feet), diarrhea, vomiting, constipation, decreased appetite, fatigue, fever, pharyngitis, sinusitis, pruritus. **RARE (less than 2%):** Insomnia, abdominal pain, dyspepsia, flatulence, back pain, arthralgia.

ADVERSE EFFECTS/ TOXIC REACTIONS

Urticaria, hallucinations, confusion, (delirium, disorientation, occurs predominantly in elderly) have been reported.

NURSING CONSIDERATIONS

INTERVENTION/EVALUATION

Evaluate cutaneous lesions. Be alert to neurologic effects: headache, dizziness. Provide analgesics, comfort measures; esp. exhausting in elderly.

PATIENT/FAMILY TEACHING

• Drink adequate fluids. • Fingernails should be kept short, hands clean. • Do not touch lesions with fingers to avoid spreading infection to new site. • **Genital herpes:** Continue therapy for full length of treatment. • Space doses evenly. • Avoid contact with lesions during duration of outbreak to prevent cross-contamination. • Notify physician if lesions recur or do not improve.

famotidine

fah-**mow**-tih-deen

(Apo-Famotidine ✤, Fluxid, Novo-Famotidine ✤, Pepcid, Pepcid AC, Ulcidine ✤)

FIXED-COMBINATION(S)

Pepcid Complete: famotidine/calcium chloride/magnesium hydroxide (antacids): 10 mg/800 mg/165 mg.

CLASSIFICATION

PHARMACOTHERAPEUTIC: H_2 receptor antagonist. **CLINICAL:** Antiulcer, gastric acid secretion inhibitor (see p. 104C).

ACTION

Inhibits histamine action H_2 receptors of parietal cells. **Therapeutic Effect:** Inhibits gastric acid secretion (fasting, nocturnal, or stimulated by food, caffeine, insulin).

PHARMACOKINETICS

Route	Onset	Peak	Duration
PO	1 hr	1–4 hrs	10–12 hrs
IV	1 hr	0.5–3 hrs	10–12 hrs

Rapidly, incompletely absorbed from GI tract. Protein binding: 15%–20%. Partially metabolized in liver. Primarily excreted in urine. Not removed by hemodialysis. **Half-life:** 2.5–3.5 hrs (increased with renal impairment).

USES

Short-term treatment of active duodenal ulcer. Prevention, maintenance of duodenal ulcer recurrence. Treatment of active benign gastric ulcer, pathologic GI hypersecretory conditions. Short-term treatment of gastroesophageal reflux disease (GERD), including erosive esophagitis. OTC formulation for relief of heartburn, acid indigestion, sour stomach. **OFF-LABEL:** Autism, prophylaxis of aspiration pneumonitis, *H. pylori* eradication.

PRECAUTIONS

CONTRAINDICATIONS: None known. **CAUTIONS:** Renal/hepatic impairment.

LIFESPAN CONSIDERATIONS:

Pregnancy/Lactation: Unknown if drug crosses placenta or is distributed in breast milk. **Pregnancy Category B. Children:** No age-related precautions noted. **Elderly:** Confusion more likely to occur, esp. in those with renal/hepatic impairment.

INTERACTIONS

DRUG: Antacids may decrease absorption. May decrease absorption of **itraconazole, ketoconazole**. **HERBAL:** None significant. **FOOD:** None known. **LAB VALUES:** Interferes with skin tests using allergen extracts. May increase hepatic enzymes.

AVAILABILITY (Rx)

GELCAP: (PEPCID AC): 10 mg. **INJECTION, SOLUTION: (PEPCID):** 10 mg/ml. **POWDER FOR ORAL SUSPENSION: (PEPCID):** 40 mg/5 ml. **TABLETS: (PEPCID AC):** 10 mg. **(PEPCID):** 20 mg, 40 mg. **TABLETS, CHEWABLE: (PEPCID AC):** 10 mg.

TABLETS, ORALLY DISINTEGRATING: (FLUXID): 20 mg, 40 mg.

ADMINISTRATION/HANDLING

IV

Reconstitution • For IV push, dilute 20 mg with 5–10 ml 0.9% NaCl, D_5W, $D_{10}W$, lactated Ringer's, or 5% sodium bicarbonate. • For intermittent IV infusion (piggyback), dilute with 50–100 ml D_5W, or 0.9% NaCl.

Rate of administration • Give IV push over at least 2 min. • Infuse piggyback over 15–30 min.

Storage • Refrigerate unreconstituted vials. • IV solution appears clear, colorless. • After dilution, IV solution is stable for 48 hrs at room temperature.

PO

• Store tablets, suspension at room temperature. • Following reconstitution, oral suspension is stable for 30 days at room temperature. • Give without regard to meals. Best given after meals, at bedtime. • Shake suspension well before use.

ORAL DISINTEGRATING TABLETS

• Place tablet on tongue with dry hands. • Tablet dissolves rapidly in saliva. • Do not break, crush tablets.

IV INCOMPATIBILITIES

Amphotericin B complex (Abelcet, AmBisome, Amphotec), cefepime (Maxipime), furosemide (Lasix), piperacillin/tazobactam (Zosyn).

IV COMPATIBILITIES

Calcium gluconate, dobutamine (Dobutrex), dopamine (Intropin), heparin, hydromorphone (Dilaudid), insulin

F

(regular), lidocaine, lipids, lorazepam (Ativan), magnesium sulfate, midazolam (Versed), morphine, nitroglycerin, norepinephrine (Levophed), potassium chloride, potassium phosphate, propofol (Diprivan), total parenteral nutrition (TPN).

INDICATIONS/ROUTES/DOSAGE

F

DUODENAL, GASTRIC ULCERS

PO: ADULTS, ELDERLY, CHILDREN 12 YRS AND OLDER: 40 mg/day at bedtime. **CHILDREN 1–11 YRS:** 0.5 mg/kg/day at bedtime. **Maximum:** 40 mg/day.

DUODENAL ULCER MAINTENANCE

PO: ADULTS, ELDERLY: 20 mg/day at bedtime.

GASTROESOPHAGEAL REFLUX DISEASE

PO: ADULTS, ELDERLY, CHILDREN 12 YRS AND OLDER: 20 mg twice a day. **CHILDREN 1–11 YRS:** 1 mg/kg/day in 2 divided doses. **CHILDREN 3 MOS–11 MOS:** 0.5 mg/kg/dose twice a day. **CHILDREN YOUNGER THAN 3 MOS:** 0.5 mg/kg/dose once a day.

ESOPHAGITIS

PO: ADULTS, ELDERLY, CHILDREN 12 YRS AND OLDER: 20–40 mg twice a day.

HYPERSECRETORY CONDITIONS

PO: ADULTS, ELDERLY, CHILDREN 12 YRS AND OLDER: Initially, 20 mg q6h. May increase up to 160 mg q6h.

ACID INDIGESTION, HEARTBURN (OTC USE)

PO: ADULTS, ELDERLY, CHILDREN 12 YRS AND OLDER: 10–20 mg 15–60 min before eating. **Maximum:** 2 doses per day.

USUAL PARENTERAL DOSAGE

IV: ADULTS, ELDERLY, CHILDREN 16 YRS AND OLDER: 20 mg q12h. **CHILDREN 1–16 YRS:** 0.25–0.5 mg/kg q12h. **Maximum:** 40 mg/day.

DOSAGE IN RENAL IMPAIRMENT

Dosing frequency is modified based on creatinine clearance.

Creatinine Clearance	Dosing Frequency
10–50 ml/min	q24h
Less than 10 ml/min	q36–48h

SIDE EFFECTS

OCCASIONAL (5%): Headache. **RARE (2% or less):** Constipation, diarrhea, dizziness.

ADVERSE EFFECTS/ TOXIC REACTIONS

None known.

NURSING CONSIDERATIONS

INTERVENTION/EVALUATION

Monitor daily pattern of bowel activity/stool consistency. Monitor for diarrhea, constipation, headache.

PATIENT/FAMILY TEACHING

• May take without regard to meals, antacids. • Report headache. • Avoid excessive amounts of coffee, aspirin. • If symptoms of heartburn, acid indigestion, sour stomach persist with medication, consult physician.

Famvir, *see famciclovir*

Faslodex, *see fulvestrant*

felodipine

feh-**low**-dih-peen

(Plendil, Renedil ✦)

Do not confuse Plendil with Pletal, or Renedil with Prinivil.

FIXED-COMBINATION(S)

Lexxel: felodipine/enalapril (angiotensin-converting enzyme [ACE] inhibitor): 2.5 mg/5 mg; 5 mg/5 mg.

◆ **CLASSIFICATION**

PHARMACOTHERAPEUTIC: Calcium channel blocker. **CLINICAL:** Antihypertensive, antianginal (see p. 73C).

ACTION

Inhibits calcium movement across cardiac, vascular smooth muscle cell membranes. Potent peripheral vasodilator (does not depress SA, AV nodes). **Therapeutic Effect:** Increases myocardial contractility, heart rate, cardiac output; decreases peripheral vascular resistance, B/P.

PHARMACOKINETICS

Route	Onset	Peak	Duration
PO	2–5 hrs	N/A	N/A

Rapidly, completely absorbed from GI tract. Protein binding: greater than 99%. Undergoes first-pass metabolism in liver. Primarily excreted in urine. Not removed by hemodialysis. **Half-life:** 11–16 hrs.

USES

Management of hypertension. May be used alone or with other antihypertensives. **OFF-LABEL:** Treatment of CHF, chronic angina pectoris, Raynaud's phenomenon.

PRECAUTIONS

CONTRAINDICATIONS: None known. **CAUTIONS:** Severe left ventricular dysfunction, CHF, hepatic/renal impairment, hypertrophic cardiomyopathy, edema, concomitant administration with beta-blockers/digoxin.

LIFESPAN CONSIDERATIONS:

Pregnancy/Lactation: Unknown if drug crosses placenta or is distributed in breast milk. **Pregnancy Category C. Children:** Safety and efficacy not established. **Elderly:** May experience greater hypotension response. Constipation may be more problematic.

INTERACTIONS

DRUG: Beta-blockers may have additive effect. May increase **digoxin** concentration. **Erythromycin** may increase concentration, risk of toxicity. **Agents producing hypokalemia (e.g., furosemide)** may increase risk of arrhythmias. **Procainamide, quinidine** may increase risk of QT-interval prolongation. **HERBAL: DHEA** may increase concentration. **St. John's wort** may decrease concentration. **Ephedra, ginseng, yohimbe** may worsen hypertension. **Garlic** may increase antihypertensive effect. **FOOD: Grapefruit, grapefruit juice** may increase absorption, concentration. **LAB VALUES:** None known.

AVAILABILITY (Rx)

TABLETS (EXTENDED-RELEASE): 2.5 mg, 5 mg, 10 mg.

ADMINISTRATION/HANDLING

PO

• Give without regard to food. • Do not crush, break tablets.

INDICATIONS/ROUTES/DOSAGE

HYPERTENSION

PO: ADULTS: Initially, 5 mg/day as single dose. **ELDERLY, PTS WITH HEPATIC IMPAIRMENT:** Initially, 2.5 mg/day. Adjust dosage at no less than 2-wk intervals. Maintenance: 2.5–10 mg/day. Range: 2.5–20 mg/day.

SIDE EFFECTS

FREQUENT (22%–18%): Headache, peripheral edema. **OCCASIONAL (6%–4%):** Flushing, respiratory infection, dizziness, light-headedness, asthenia (loss of strength, weakness). **RARE (less than 3%):** Paresthesia, abdominal discomfort, anxiety, muscle cramping, cough, diarrhea, constipation.

ADVERSE EFFECTS/ TOXIC REACTIONS

Overdose produces nausea, drowsiness, confusion, slurred speech, hypotension, bradycardia.

NURSING CONSIDERATIONS

BASELINE ASSESSMENT

Assess B/P, apical pulse immediately before drug administration (if pulse is 60 or less/min or systolic B/P is less than 90 mm Hg, withhold medication, contact physician).

INTERVENTION/EVALUATION

Assist with ambulation if lightheadedness, dizziness occur. Assess for peripheral edema behind media malleolus (sacral area in bedridden pts). Monitor pulse rate for bradycardia. Assess skin for flushing. Monitor hepatic enzyme tests. Question for headache, asthenia.

PATIENT/FAMILY TEACHING

• Do not abruptly discontinue medication. • Compliance with therapy regimen is essential to control hypertension. • To avoid hypotensive effect, rise slowly from lying to sitting position. Wait momentarily before standing. • Avoid tasks that require alertness, motor skills until response to drug is established. • Contact physician if palpitations, shortness of breath, pronounced dizziness, nausea occurs. • Swallow tablet whole; do not crush, chew. • Avoid grapefruit, grapefruit juice.

fenofibrate

fen-oh-**figh**-brate

(Antara, Apo-Fenofibrate ✤, Lipidil Supra, Lipofen, Lofibra, Novo-Fenofibrate ✤, Tricor, Triglide)

Do not confuse Tricor with Tracleer.

CLASSIFICATION

CLINICAL: Antihyperlipidemic (see p. 55C).

ACTION

Enhances synthesis of lipoprotein lipase (VLDL). **Therapeutic Effect:** Increases VLDL catabolism, reduces total plasma triglycerides.

PHARMACOKINETICS

Well absorbed from GI tract. Absorption increased when given with food. Protein binding: 99%. Rapidly metabolized in liver to active metabolite. Excreted primarily in urine with lesser amount in feces. Not removed by hemodialysis. **Half-life:** 20 hrs.

USES

Adjunct to diet for reduction of low density lipoprotein cholesterol (LDL-C), total cholesterol, triglycerides, apolipoprotein B in pts with primary hypercholesterolemia, mixed dyslipidemia. Treatment of hyperlipidemia in combination with ezetimibe.

PRECAUTIONS

CONTRAINDICATIONS: Gallbladder disease, severe renal/hepatic dysfunction (including primary biliary cirrhosis, unexplained persistent hepatic function abnormality). **CAUTIONS:** Anticoagulant therapy, history of hepatic disease, substantial alcohol consumption.

LIFESPAN CONSIDERATIONS:

Pregnancy/Lactation: Safety in pregnancy not established. Avoid use in breast-feeding mothers. **Pregnancy Category C.** **Children:** Safety and efficacy not established. **Elderly:** No age-related precautions noted.

INTERACTIONS

DRUG: Potentiates effects of **anticoagulants. Bile acid sequestrants** may impede absorption. **Cyclosporine** may increase risk of nephrotoxicity. **HMG-CoA reductase inhibitors** may increase risk of severe myopathy, rhabdomyolysis, acute renal failure. **HERBAL:** None significant. **FOOD: All foods** increase absorption. **LAB VALUES:** May increase BUN, serum creatine kinase (CK), AST, ALT. May decrease Hgb, Hct, serum uric acid, WBC count.

AVAILABILITY (Rx)

CAPSULES: 43 mg (Antara), 50 mg (Lipofen), 67 mg (Lofibra), 87 mg (Antara), 100 mg (Lipofen), 130 mg (Antara), 134 mg (Lofibra), 150 mg (Lipofen), 200 mg (Lipidil Supra, Lofibra). **TABLETS:** 48 mg (Tricor), 50 mg (Triglide), 54 mg (Lofibra), 145 mg (Tricor), 160 mg (Lofibra, Triglide).

ADMINISTRATION/HANDLING

PO

• Give Lofibra with meals. • Antara, Tricor, and Triglide may be given without regard to food.

INDICATIONS/ROUTES/DOSAGE

HYPERTRIGLYCERIDEMIA

PO (ANTARA): ADULTS, ELDERLY: 43–130 mg/day.

PO (LIPOFEN): ADULTS, ELDERLY: 50–160 mg/day.

PO (LOFIBRA): ADULTS, ELDERLY: 67–200 mg/day with meals.

PO (TRICOR): ADULTS, ELDERLY: 48–145 mg/day.

PO (TRIGLIDE): ADULTS, ELDERLY: 50–160 mg/day.

HYPERCHOLESTEROLEMIA

PO (ANTARA): ADULTS, ELDERLY: 130 mg/day.

PO (LIPOFEN): ADULTS, ELDERLY: 150 mg/day.

PO (LOFIBRA): ADULTS, ELDERLY: 200 mg/day with meals.

PO (TRICOR): ADULTS, ELDERLY: 145 mg/day.

PO (TRIGLIDE): ADULTS, ELDERLY: 160 mg/day.

SIDE EFFECTS

FREQUENT (8%–4%): Pain, rash, headache, asthenia, fatigue, flu-like symptoms, dyspepsia, nausea/vomiting, rhinitis. **OCCASIONAL (3%–2%):** Diarrhea, abdominal pain, constipation, flatulence, arthralgia, decreased libido, dizziness, pruritus. **RARE (less than 2%):** Increased appetite, insomnia, polyuria, cough, blurred vision, eye floaters, earache.

F

ADVERSE EFFECTS/ TOXIC REACTIONS

May increase cholestrol excretion into bile, leading to cholelithiasis. Pancreatitis, hepatitis, thrombocytopenia, agranulocytosis occur rarely.

NURSING CONSIDERATIONS

BASELINE ASSESSMENT

Obtain serum cholesterol, triglycerides, hepatic function tests (including ALT), blood counts during initial therapy and periodically during treatment. Treatment should be discontinued if hepatic enzyme levels persist greater than 3 times normal limit.

INTERVENTION/EVALUATION

For pts on concurrent therapy with hydroxamethylglutaryl-CoA (HMG-CoA) reductase inhibitors, monitor for complaints of myopathy (muscle pain, weakness). Monitor serum CK. Monitor serum cholesterol, triglyceride for therapeutic response.

PATIENT/FAMILY TEACHING

• Take with food. • Inform physician if diarrhea, constipation, nausea becomes severe. • Report skin rash/irritation, insomnia, muscle pain, tremors, dizziness.

fenoldopam

phen-**ole**-doe-pam
(Corlopam)

CLASSIFICATION

PHARMACOTHERAPEUTIC: Vasodilator (dopamine receptor agonist). **CLINICAL:** Antihypertensive.

F

ACTION

Rapid-acting vasodilator. Agonist for D_1-like dopamine receptors, produces vasodilation in coronary, renal, mesenteric, peripheral arteries. **Therapeutic Effect:** Reduces systolic, diastolic B/P, increases heart rate.

PHARMACOKINETICS

After IV administration, metabolized in the liver. Primarily excreted in urine. Unknown if removed by hemodialysis. **Half-life:** Approximately 5 min.

USES

Short-term (48 hrs or less) management of severe hypertension when rapid, but quickly reversible, emergency reduction of B/P is clinically indicated, including malignant hypertension with deteriorating end-organ function. **OFF-LABEL:** Prevention of contrast media-induced nephrotoxicity.

PRECAUTIONS

CONTRAINDICATIONS: None known. **CAUTIONS:** Glaucoma, intraocular hypertension, tachycardia, hypotension, hypokalemia, sulfite sensitivity.

LIFESPAN CONSIDERATIONS:

Pregnancy/Lactation: Unknown if distributed in breast milk. **Pregnancy Category B. Children:** Safety and efficacy not established. **Elderly:** No age-related precautions noted.

INTERACTIONS

DRUG: Beta-blockers may produce excessive hypotension. **HERBAL:** None significant. **FOOD:** None known. **LAB VALUES:** May elevate BUN, serum glucose, LDH, transaminase. May decrease serum potassium.

AVAILABILITY (Rx)

INJECTION, SOLUTION: 10 mg/ml.

ADMINISTRATION/HANDLING

◀ **ALERT** ▶ Must give by continuous IV infusion, not as bolus injection. B/P must be monitored diligently during infusion.

IV

Reconstitution • Each 10 mg (1 ml) must be diluted with 250 ml 0.9% NaCl or D_5W to provide a concentration of 40 mcg/ml.

Rate of administration • Administer as IV infusion at initial rate of 0.1 mcg/kg/min. • Use infusion pump.

Storage • Store ampules at room temperature. • Diluted solution is stable for 24 hrs. Discard any solution not used within 24 hrs.

IV INCOMPATIBILITIES

Bumetanide (Bumex), furosemide (Lasix).

IV COMPATIBILITIES

Amiodarone (Cordarone), calcium gluconate, diltiazem (Cardizem), dobutamine, dopamine, epinephrine, heparin, hydromorphone (Dilaudid), lidocaine, lorazepam (Ativan), magnesium, midazolam (Versed), milrinone (Primacor), morphine, nitroglycerin, nonepinephrine, potassium chloride, propofol (Diprivan).

INDICATIONS/ROUTES/DOSAGE

SHORT-TERM MANAGEMENT OF SEVERE HYPERTENSION

IV INFUSION (CONTINUOUS): ADULTS, ELDERLY: Initially, 0.1 mcg/kg/min. May increase in increments of 0.05–0.1 mcg/kg/min until target B/P is achieved. Usual length of treatment is 1–6 hrs with tapering of dose q15–30min. Average rate: 0.25–0.5 mcg/kg/min. **Maximum rate:** 1.6 mcg/kg/min. **CHILDREN:** Initially, 0.2 mcg/kg/min. May increase in increments of 0.3–0.5 mcg/kg/min q20–30min. Dosage greater than 0.8 mcg/kg/min has resulted in tachycardia with no additional benefit.

SIDE EFFECTS

◀ **ALERT** ▶ Avoid concurrent use of beta-blockers (may cause unforseen hypotension).

OCCASIONAL: Headache (7%), flushing (3%), nausea (4%), hypotension (2%). **RARE (2% or less):** Anxiety, vomiting, constipation, nasal congestion, diaphoresis, back pain.

ADVERSE EFFECTS/ TOXIC REACTIONS

Excessive hypotension occurs occasionally. Substantial tachycardia may lead to ischemic cardiac events worsened heart failure. Allergic-type reactions, including anaphylaxis and life-threatening asthmatic exacerbation, may occur in pts with sulfite sensitivity.

NURSING CONSIDERATIONS

BASELINE ASSESSMENT

Determine initial B/P, apical pulse. It is essential to diligently monitor B/P, EKG during infusion to avoid hypotension and too-rapid decrease of B/P. Assess medication history (esp. for beta-blockers). Obtain baseline serum electrolytes, particularly potassium, and monitor periodically thereafter during infusion. Question asthmatic pts for history of sulfite sensitivity. Check with physician for desired B/P parameters.

INTERVENTION/EVALUATION

Monitor rate of infusion frequently. Monitor EKG for tachycardia (may lead to ischemic heart disease, MI, angina, arrhythmias, worsening heart failure). Monitor closely for symptomatic hypotension.

fenoprofen

fen-oh-**proe**-fen

(Nalfon)

Do not confuse Nalfon with Naldecon.

CLASSIFICATION

PHARMACOTHERAPEUTIC: NSAID. **CLINICAL:** Nonsteroidal anti-inflammatory, analgesic, antigout, vascular headache prophylactic/suppressant (see p. 123C).

ACTION

Analgesic, anti-inflammatory effects by inhibiting prostaglandin synthesis. **Therapeutic Effect:** Reduces inflammatory response, intensity of pain.

PHARMACOKINETICS

Rapidly absorbed following PO administration. Protein binding: 99%. Metabolized in liver. Primarily excreted in urine; small amount excreted in feces. **Half-life:** 3 hrs.

USES

Treatment of acute or long-term mild to moderate pain, symptomatic treatment of acute and/or chronic rheumatoid arthritis, osteoarthritis. **OFF-LABEL:** Treatment of ankylosing spondylitis, psoriatic arthritis, vascular headaches.

PRECAUTIONS

CONTRAINDICATIONS: Active peptic ulcer disease, chronic inflammation of GI tract, GI bleeding/ulceration, history of hypersensitivity to aspirin/NSAIDs, significant renal impairment. **CAUTIONS:** Renal/hepatic impairment, history of GI

F

tract diseases, predisposition to fluid retention.

LIFESPAN CONSIDERATIONS:

Pregnancy/Lactation: Crosses placenta; distributed in breast milk. **Pregnancy Category C (D if used in third trimester or near delivery).** **Children:** Safety and efficacy not established. **Elderly:** Age-related renal, hepatic impairment may increase risk of hepatotoxicity, renal toxicity.

F

INTERACTIONS

DRUG: May decrease the effects of **antihypertensives, diuretics. Aspirin, other salicylates** may increase risk of GI side effects, bleeding. **Bone marrow depressants** may increase risk of hematologic reactions. May increase effects of **heparin, oral anticoagulants, thrombolytics**. May increase concentration, risk of toxicity of **lithium.** May increase risk of **methotrexate** toxicity. **Probenecid** may increase concentration. **HERBAL:** None significant. **FOOD:** None known. **LAB VALUES:** May increase bleeding time, BUN, serum glucose, protein, alkaline phosphatase, LDH, creatinine, AST, ALT.

AVAILABILITY (Rx)

TABLETS: 600 mg.

CAPSULES: 200 mg, 300 mg.

ADMINISTRATION/HANDLING

◄ **ALERT** ► Do not exceed dosage of 3.2 g/day. Do not crush, open, or break capsules.

INDICATIONS/ROUTES/DOSAGE

MILD TO MODERATE PAIN

PO: ADULTS, ELDERLY: 200 mg q4–6h as needed.

RHEUMATOID ARTHRITIS, OSTEOARTHRITIS

PO: ADULTS, ELDERLY: 300–600 mg 3–4 times a day.

SIDE EFFECTS

FREQUENT (9%–3%): Headache, somnolence, dyspepsia (heartburn, indigestion, epigastric pain), nausea, vomiting, constipation. **OCCASIONAL (2%–1%):** Dizziness, pruritus, anxiety, asthenia, diarrhea, abdominal cramps, flatulence, tinnitus, blurred vision, peripheral edema, fluid retention.

ADVERSE EFFECTS/ TOXIC REACTIONS

Overdose may result in acute hypotension, tachycardia. Peptic ulcer, GI bleeding, gastritis, severe hepatic reaction (jaundice), nephrotoxicity (hematuria, dysuria, proteinuria), severe hypersensitivity reaction (bronchospasm, angioedema) occur rarely.

NURSING CONSIDERATIONS

BASELINE ASSESSMENT

Assess onset, type, location, duration of pain, inflammation. Inspect appearance of affected joints for immobility, deformities, skin condition.

INTERVENTION/EVALUATION

Assist with ambulation if somnolence, drowsiness, dizziness occurs. Monitor for evidence of dyspepsia. Monitor daily pattern of bowel activity/stool consistency. Check behind medial malleolus for fluid retention (usually first area noted). Evaluate for therapeutic response (relief of pain, stiffness, swelling; increased joint mobility; reduced joint tenderness; improved grip strength).

PATIENT/FAMILY TEACHING

• Swallow capsule whole; do not crush, chew. • Avoid tasks that require alertness, motor skills until response to drug is established. • If GI upset occurs, take with food, milk. • Avoid aspirin, alcohol during therapy (increases risk of GI bleeding).

fentanyl

fen-ta-nill

(Actiq, Duragesic, Fentora, Ionsys, Sublimaze)

Do not confuse fentanyl with alfentanil.

CLASSIFICATION

PHARMACOTHERAPEUTIC: Opioid, narcotic agonist **(Schedule II)**. **CLINICAL:** Analgesic (see p. 136C).

ACTION

Binds to opioid receptors in CNS, reducing stimuli from sensory nerve endings, inhibits ascending pain pathways. **Therapeutic Effect:** Alters pain reception, increases pain threshold.

PHARMACOKINETICS

Route	Onset	Peak	Duration
IV	1–2 min	3–5 min	0.5–1 hr
IM	7–15 min	20–30 min	1–2 hrs
Transdermal	6–8 hrs	24 hrs	72 hrs
Transmucosal	5–15 min	20–30 min	1–2 hrs

Well absorbed after IM or topical administration. Transmucosal form absorbed through buccal mucosa and GI tract. Protein binding: 80%–85%. Metabolized in liver. Primarily eliminated by biliary system. **Half-life:** 2–4 hrs IV; 17 hrs transdermal; 6.6 hrs transmucosal.

USES

For sedation, pain relief, preop medication; adjunct to general or regional anesthesia. **Duragesic:** Management of chronic pain *(transdermal)*. **Actiq:** Treatment breakthrough for pain in chronic cancer or AIDS-related pain. **Ionsys:** Short-term management of acute postoperative pain during hospitalization. **Fentora:** Breakthrough pain in pts on chronic opioids.

PRECAUTIONS

CONTRAINDICATIONS: Increased intracranial pressure, severe hepatic/renal impairment, severe respiratory depression. **CAUTIONS:** Bradycardia; renal, hepatic, respiratory disease; head injuries; altered level of consciousness (LOC); use of MAOIs within 14 days; transdermal not recommended in those younger than 12 yrs or younger than 18 yrs and weighing less than 50 kg.

LIFESPAN CONSIDERATIONS:

Pregnancy/Lactation: Readily crosses placenta. Unknown if distributed in breast milk. May prolong labor if administered in latent phase of first stage of labor or before cervical dilation of 4–5 cm has occurred. Respiratory depression may occur in neonate if mother received opiates during labor. **Pregnancy Category C (D if used for prolonged periods or at high dosages at term). Children:** PATCH: Safety and efficacy not established in those younger than 12 yrs. Neonates more susceptible to respiratory depressant effects. **Elderly:** May be more susceptible to respiratory depressant effects. Age-related renal impairment may require dosage adjustment.

INTERACTIONS

DRUG: Benzodiazepines may increase the risk of hypotension, respiratory depression. **Buprenorphine** may decrease the effects of fentanyl. **Alcohol, CNS depressant medications** may increase CNS depression. **Erythromycin, itraconazole, ketoconazole, protease inhibitors (e.g., ritonavir)** may increase effects of transmucosal fentanyl. **MAOIs** may potentiate effects. **HERBAL: Gotu kola, kava kava, St. John's wort, valerian** may increase CNS depression. **FOOD:** None known. **LAB VALUES:** May increase serum amylase, lipase.

F

AVAILABILITY (Rx)

BUCCAL TABLET (FENTORA): 100 mcg, 200 mcg, 400 mcg, 600 mcg, 800 mcg. **INJECTION SOLUTION (SUBLIMAZE):** 50 mcg/ml. **TRANSDERMAL IONTOPHORETIC SYSTEM (IONSYS):** Provides up to 80 doses fentanyl (40 mcg/activation). Each dose delivered over 10 min. **TRANSDERMAL PATCH (DURAGESIC):** 12 mcg/hr, 25 mcg/hr, 50 mcg/hr, 75 mcg/hr, 100 mcg/hr. **TRANSMUCOSAL LOZENGES (ACTIQ):** 200 mcg, 400 mcg, 600 mcg, 800 mcg, 1,200 mcg, 1,600 mcg.

ADMINISTRATION/HANDLING

IV

Rate of administration • For initial anesthesia induction dosage, give small amount, via tuberculin syringe. • Give by slow IV injection (over 1–2 min). • Too-rapid IV increases risk of severe adverse reactions (skeletal, thoracic muscle rigidity resulting in apnea, laryngospasm, bronchospasm, peripheral circulatory collapse, anaphylactoid effects, cardiac arrest).

Storage • Store parenteral form at room temperature. • Opiate antagonist (naloxone) should be readily available.

TRANSDERMAL

• Apply to hairless area of intact skin of upper torso. • Use flat, nonirritated site. • Firmly press evenly for 10–20 sec, ensuring adhesion is in full contact with skin and edges are completely sealed. • Use only water to cleanse site before application (soaps, oils, may irritate skin). • Rotate sites of application. • Carefully fold used patches so that system adheres to itself; discard in toilet.

BUCCAL TABLETS

• Place tablet above a rear molar between upper cheek and gum. • Dissolve over 30 min. • Swallow remaining pieces. • Do not split tablet.

TRANSMUCOSAL

• Suck lozenge vigorously.

IONTOPHORETIC SYSTEM

• Apply to intact, nonirritated skin on chest or upper outer arm (do not apply on abdomen). • Clip (do not shave) excessive hair before system application.

IV INCOMPATIBILITY

Phenytoin (Dilantin).

IV COMPATIBILITIES

Atropine, bupivacaine (Marcaine, Sensorcaine), clonidine (Duraclon), diltiazem (Cardizem), diphenhydramine (Benadryl), dobutamine (Dobutrex), dopamine (Intropin), droperidol (Inapsine), heparin, hydromorphone (Dilaudid), ketorolac (Toradol), lipids, lorazepam (Ativan), metoclopramide (Reglan), midazolam (Versed), milrinone (Primacor), morphine, nitroglycerin, norepinephrine (Levophed), ondansetron (Zofran), potassium chloride, propofol (Diprivan).

INDICATIONS/ROUTES/DOSAGE

ACUTE PAIN MANAGEMENT:

IM/IV: ADULTS, ELDERLY: 50–100 mcg/dose q1–2h as needed.

PREOPERATIVE SEDATION, POSTOPERATIVE PAIN, ADJUNCT TO REGIONAL ANESTHESIA

IV, IM: ADULTS, ELDERLY, CHILDREN 12 YRS AND OLDER: 50–100 mcg/dose.

ADJUNCT TO GENERAL ANESTHESIA

IV: ADULTS, ELDERLY, CHILDREN 12 YRS AND OLDER: 2–50 mcg/kg.

USUAL BUCCAL DOSE

ADULTS, ELDERLY: Initially, 100 mcg. Titrate dose providing adequate analgesia with tolerable side effects.

USUAL TRANSDERMAL DOSE

ADULTS, ELDERLY, CHILDREN 12 YRS AND OLDER: Initially, 25 mcg/hr. May increase after 3 days.

USUAL TRANSMUCOSAL DOSE

ADULTS, CHILDREN: 200–400 mcg for breakthrough pain.

USUAL IONTOPHORETIC DOSE

TRANSDERMAL: ADULTS, ELDERLY: 40 mcg/activation. Maximum of six 40-mcg doses/hr (eighty 40-mcg doses/24 hrs). Each on-demand dose delivered over 10-minute period.

USUAL EPIDURAL DOSE

ADULTS, ELDERLY: Bolus dose of 100 mcg, followed by continuous infusion of 10 mcg/ml concentration at 4–12 ml/hr.

DOSAGE IN RENAL IMPAIRMENT

Dosage is modified based on creatinine clearance.

Creatinine Clearance	Dosage
10–50 ml/min	75% of usual dose
Less than 10 ml/min	50% of usual dose

SIDE EFFECTS

FREQUENT: IV: Postoperative drowsiness, nausea, vomiting. **Transdermal (10%–3%):** Headache, pruritus, nausea, vomiting, diaphoresis, dyspnea, confusion, dizziness, somnolence, diarrhea, constipation, decreased appetite. **OCCASIONAL: IV:** Postoperative confusion, blurred vision, chills, orthostatic hypotension, constipation, difficulty urinating. **Transdermal (3%–1%):** Chest pain, arrhythmias, erythema, pruritus, syncope, agitation, skin irritations.

ADVERSE EFFECTS/ TOXIC REACTIONS

Overdose or too-rapid IV administration may produce severe respiratory depression, skeletal/thoracic muscle rigidity (may lead to apnea, laryngospasm, bronchospasm, cold/clammy skin, cyanosis, coma). Tolerance to analgesic effect may occur with repeated use.

NURSING CONSIDERATIONS

BASELINE ASSESSMENT

Resuscitative equipment, opiate antagonist (naloxone 0.5 mcg/kg) must be available. Establish baseline B/P, respirations. Assess type, location, intensity, duration of pain.

INTERVENTION/EVALUATION

Assist with ambulation. Encourage postoperative pt to turn, cough, deep breathe q2h. Monitor respiratory rate, B/P, heart rate, oxygen saturation. Assess for relief of pain.

PATIENT/FAMILY TEACHING

• Avoid alcohol; do not take other medications without consulting physician. • Do not perform activities requiring alertness, coordination. • Teach pt proper transdermal application. • Use as directed to avoid overdosage; potential for physical dependence with prolonged use. • After long-term use, must be discontinued slowly.

Feosol, *see ferrous sulfate*

Fergon, *see ferrous gluconate*

Fer-In-Sol, *see ferrous sulfate*

Ferrlicit, *see sodium ferric gluconate complex*

ferrous fumarate

fair-us **fume**-ah-rate
(Femiron, Feostat, Ferro-Sequels, Nephro-Fer, Palafer ✽)

ferrous gluconate

fair-us **glue**-kuh-nate
(Apo-Ferrous Gluconate ✽, Fergon)

ferrous sulfate

fair-us **sul**-fate
(Apo-Ferrous Sulfate ✽, Fer-In-Sol, Fer-Iron, Slow-Fe)

FIXED-COMBINATION(S)

Ferro-Sequels: ferrous fumarate/docusate (stool softener): 150 mg/100 mg.

◆CLASSIFICATION

PHARMACOTHERAPEUTIC: Enzymatic mineral. **CLINICAL:** Iron preparation (see p. 105C).

ACTION

Essential component in formation of Hgb, myoglobin, enzymes. Promotes effective erythropoiesis and transport, utilization of oxygen. **Therapeutic Effect:** Prevents iron deficiency.

PHARMACOKINETICS

Absorbed in duodenum and upper jejunum. Ten percent absorbed in pts with normal iron stores; increased to 20%–30% in those with inadequate iron stores. Primarily bound to serum transferrin. Excreted in urine, sweat, sloughing of intestinal mucosa, by menses. **Half-life:** 6 hrs.

USES

Prevention, treatment of iron deficiency anemia due to inadequate diet, malabsorption, pregnancy, blood loss.

PRECAUTIONS

CONTRAINDICATIONS: Hemochromatosis, hemosiderosis, hemolytic anemias, peptic ulcer disease, regional enteritis, ulcerative colitis. **CAUTIONS:** Bronchial asthma, iron hypersensitivity, GI tract inflammation.

⌛ LIFESPAN CONSIDERATIONS:

Pregnancy/Lactation: Crosses placenta. Excreted in breast milk. **Pregnancy Category A. Children/Elderly:** No age-related precautions noted.

INTERACTIONS

DRUG: **Antacids, calcium supplements, pancreatin, pancrelipase** may decrease absorption of ferrous compounds. May decrease absorption of **etidronate, quinolones, tetracyclines.** **HERBAL:** None significant. **FOOD:** **Eggs, milk** inhibit ferrous fumarate absorption. **LAB VALUES:** May increase serum bilirubin, iron. May decrease serum calcium. May obscure occult blood in stools.

AVAILABILITY (OTC)

FERROUS FUMARATE

TABLETS: 63 mg (20 mg elemental iron) (Femiron), 350 mg (115 mg elemental iron) (Nephro-Fer). **TABLETS (CHEWABLE [FEOSTAT]):** 100 mg (33 mg elemental iron).

TABLETS (TIMED-RELEASE [FERRO-SEQUELS]): 150 mg (50 mg elemental iron).

FERROUS GLUCONATE

TABLETS: 240 mg (27 mg elemental iron) (Fergon), 325 mg (36 mg elemental iron).

FERROUS SULFATE

ORAL DROPS (FER-IN-SOL, FER-IRON): 75 mg/0.6 ml. **TABLETS:** 325 mg (65 mg elemental iron). **ELIXIR:** 220 mg/5 ml (44 mg elemental iron per 5 ml).

TABLETS (TIMED-RELEASE [SLOW-FE]): 160 mg (50 mg elemental iron).

ADMINISTRATION/HANDLING

PO

• Store all forms (tablets, capsules, suspension, drops) at room temperature. • Ideally, give between meals with water but may give with meals if GI discomfort occurs. • Transient staining of mucous membranes, teeth occurs with liquid iron preparation. To avoid staining, place liquid on back of tongue with dropper or straw. • Avoid simultaneous administration of antacids, tetracycline. • Do not crush timed-release preparations.

INDICATIONS/ROUTES/DOSAGE

IRON DEFICIENCY ANEMIA

Dosage is expressed in terms of milligrams of elemental iron, degree of anemia, pt weight, presence of any bleeding. Expect to use periodic hematologic determinations as guide to therapy.

PO (FERROUS FUMARATE): ADULTS, ELDERLY: 60–100 mg twice a day. **CHILDREN:** 3–6 mg/kg/day in 2–3 divided doses.

PO (FERROUS GLUCONATE): ADULTS, ELDERLY: 60 mg 2–4 times a day. **CHILDREN:** 3–6 mg/kg/day in 2–3 divided doses.

PO (FERROUS SULFATE): ADULTS, ELDERLY: 325 mg 2–4 times a day. **CHILDREN:** 3–6 mg/kg/day in 2–3 divided doses.

PREVENTION OF IRON DEFICIENCY

PO (FERROUS FUMARATE): ADULTS, ELDERLY: 60–100 mg/day. **CHILDREN:** 1–2 mg/kg/day.

PO (FERROUS GLUCONATE): ADULTS, ELDERLY: 60 mg/day. **CHILDREN:** 1–2 mg/kg/day.

PO (FERROUS SULFATE): ADULTS, ELDERLY: 325 mg/day. **CHILDREN:** 1–2 mg/kg/day.

SIDE EFFECTS

OCCASIONAL: Mild, transient nausea. **RARE:** Heartburn, anorexia, constipation, diarrhea.

ADVERSE EFFECTS/ TOXIC REACTIONS

Large doses may aggravate existing GI tract disease (peptic ulcer, regional enteritis, ulcerative colitis). Severe iron poisoning occurs most often in children, manifested as vomiting, severe abdominal pain, diarrhea, dehydration, followed by hyperventilation, pallor, cyanosis, cardiovascular collapse.

F

NURSING CONSIDERATIONS

BASELINE ASSESSMENT

To prevent mucous membrane and teeth staining with liquid preparation, use dropper or straw and allow solution to drop on back of tongue. Eggs, milk inhibit absorption.

INTERVENTION/EVALUATION

Monitor serum iron, total iron-binding capacity, reticulocyte count, Hgb, ferritin. Monitor daily pattern of bowel activity/stool consistency. Assess for clinical improvement, record relief of iron deficiency symptoms (fatigue, irritability, pallor, paresthesia of extremities, headache).

PATIENT/FAMILY TEACHING

• Expect stool color to darken. • If GI discomfort occurs, take after meals or with food. • Do not take within 2 hrs of antacids (prevents absorption).

feverfew

Also known as bachelor's button, featherfew, midsummer daisy, Santa maria.

CLASSIFICATION

HERBAL: See Appendix G.

ACTION

May inhibit platelet aggregation, serotonin release from platelets, leukocytes.

Inhibits/blocks prostaglandin synthesis. **Effect:** Reduces pain intensity, vomiting, noise sensitivity with severe migraine headaches.

USES

Fever, headache, prevention of migraine and menstrual irregularities, arthritis, psoriasis, allergies, asthma, vertigo.

PRECAUTIONS

CONTRAINDICATIONS: Pregnancy/lactation (may cause uterine contraction/abortion). Allergies to ragweed, chrysanthemums, marigolds, daisies. **CAUTIONS:** None known.

LIFESPAN CONSIDERATIONS:

Pregnancy/Lactation: Contraindicated. **Children:** Safety and efficacy not established; avoid use. **Elderly:** No age-related precautions noted.

INTERACTIONS

DRUG: **Anticoagulants, antiplatelet agents** may increase risk of bleeding. **NSAIDs** may decrease effectiveness. **HERBAL:** **Garlic, ginger, ginkgo** may increase risk of bleeding. **FOOD:** None known. **LAB VALUES:** None known.

AVAILABILITY (Rx)

CAPSULES: 100 mg. **FEVERFEW LEAF:** 380 mg.

INDICATIONS/ROUTES/DOSAGE

MIGRAINE HEADACHE

PO: ADULTS, ELDERLY: 50–100 mg extract a day. **Leaf:** 50–125 mg a day.

SIDE EFFECTS

ORAL: Abdominal pain, muscle stiffness, pain, indigestion, diarrhea, flatulence, nausea, vomiting. **Chewing Leaf:** Mouth ulceration, inflammation of oral mucosa and tongue, swelling of lips, loss of taste.

ADVERSE EFFECTS/ TOXIC REACTIONS

Hypersensitivity reaction occurs rarely.

NURSING CONSIDERATIONS

BASELINE ASSESSMENT

Assess if pt is pregnant or breast-feeding (contraindicated).

INTERVENTION/EVALUATION

Assess for hypersensitivity reaction, mouth ulcers, muscle/joint pain.

PATIENT/FAMILY TEACHING

• Do not use during pregnancy or lactation. • Avoid use in children.

fexofenadine

fex-**oh**-fen-eh-deen

(Allegra)

FIXED-COMBINATION(S)

Allegra-D 12 Hour: fexofenadine/pseudoephedrine (sympathomimetic): 60 mg/120 mg. **Allegra-D 24 Hour:** fexofenadine/pseudoephedrine (sympathomimetic):180 mg/240 mg.

CLASSIFICATION

PHARMACOTHERAPEUTIC: Piperidine. **CLINICAL:** Antihistamine (see p. 52C).

ACTION

Prevents, antagonizes most histamine effects (urticaria, pruritus). **Therapeutic Effect:** Relieves allergic rhinitis symptoms.

PHARMACOKINETICS

Rapidly absorbed after PO administration. Protein binding: 60%–70%. Does not cross blood-brain barrier. Minimally metabolized. Eliminated in feces, urine. Not removed by hemodialysis. **Half-life:** 14.4 hrs (increased in renal impairment).

USES

Relief of seasonal allergic rhinitis, chronic idiopathic urticaria.

PRECAUTIONS

CONTRAINDICATIONS: None known. **CAUTIONS:** Severe renal impairment.

LIFESPAN CONSIDERATIONS:

Pregnancy/Lactation: Unknown if drug crosses placenta or is distributed in breast milk. **Pregnancy Category C.** **Children:** Safety and efficacy not established in those younger than 12 yrs. **Elderly:** No age-related precautions noted.

INTERACTIONS

DRUG: **Antacids** may decrease absorption if given within 15 min of fexofenadine. **HERBAL:** None significant. **FOOD:** None known. **LAB VALUES:** May suppress wheal, flare reactions to antigen skin testing unless drug is discontinued at least 4 days before testing.

AVAILABILITY (Rx)

ORAL SUSPENSION: 6 mg/ml. **TABLETS:** 30 mg, 60 mg, 180 mg.

ADMINISTRATION/HANDLING

PO

- Give without regard to food.

INDICATIONS/ROUTES/DOSAGE

ALLERGIC RHINITIS

PO: ADULTS, ELDERLY, CHILDREN 12 YRS AND OLDER: 60 mg twice a day or 180 mg once a day. **CHILDREN 2–11 YRS:** 30 mg twice a day.

URTICARIA

PO: ADULTS, ELDERLY, CHILDREN 12 YRS AND OLDER: 60 mg twice a day or 180 mg once a day. **CHILDREN 2–11 YRS:** 30 mg twice a day. **CHILDREN 6 MOS–2 YRS:** 15 mg twice a day.

DOSAGE IN RENAL IMPAIRMENT

PO: ADULTS, ELDERLY, CHILDREN 12 YRS AND OLDER: 60 mg once daily. **CHILDREN 2–11 YRS:** 30 mg once daily. **CHILDREN 6 MOS–2 YRS:** 15 mg once daily.

SIDE EFFECTS

RARE (less than 2%): Drowsiness, headache, fatigue, nausea, vomiting, abdominal distress, dysmenorrhea.

ADVERSE EFFECTS/ TOXIC REACTIONS

Hypersensitivity reaction occurs rarely.

NURSING CONSIDERATIONS

BASELINE ASSESSMENT

If pt is having an allergic reaction, obtain history of recently ingested foods, drugs, environmental exposure, emotional stress. Monitor rate, depth, rhythm, type of respiration; quality, rate of pulse. Assess lung sounds for rhonchi, wheezing, rales.

INTERVENTION/EVALUATION

Assess for therapeutic response; relief from allergy: itching, red, watery eyes, rhinorrhea, sneezing.

PATIENT/FAMILY TEACHING

• Avoid tasks that require alertness, motor skills until response to drug is established. • Avoid alcohol during antihistamine therapy. • Coffee, tea may help reduce drowsiness.

filgrastim

fill-**grass**-tim

(Neupogen)

Do not confuse Neupogen with Epogen or Nutramigen.

CLASSIFICATION

PHARMACOTHERAPEUTIC: Biologic modifier. **CLINICAL:** Granulocyte colony-stimulating factor (GCSF).

ACTION

Stimulates production, maturation, activation of neutrophils. **Therapeutic Effect:** Increases migration, activation of neutrophils.

PHARMACOKINETICS

Readily absorbed after subcutaneous administration. Not removed by hemodialysis. **Half-life:** 3.5 hrs.

USES

Decrease infection incidence in pts with malignancies receiving myelosuppressive therapy associated with severe neutropenia, fever. Reduce neutropenia duration, sequelae, in pts with nonmyeloid malignancies having myeloablative therapy followed by bone marrow transplant (BMT). Mobilization of hematopoietic progenitor cells into peripheral blood for collection by leukapheresis. Treatment of chronic, severe neutropenia. **OFF-LABEL:** Treatment of AIDS-related neutropenia, drug-induced neutropenia, myelodysplastic syndrome.

PRECAUTIONS

CONTRAINDICATIONS: Hypersensitivity to *Escherichia coli*–derived proteins, 24 hrs before or after cytotoxic chemotherapy, concurrent use of other drugs that may result in lowered platelet count. **CAUTIONS:** Malignancy with myeloid characteristics (due to a GCSF's potential to act as growth factor), gout, psoriasis, preexisting cardiac conditions, those taking lithium.

LIFESPAN CONSIDERATIONS:

Pregnancy/Lactation: Unknown if drug crosses placenta or is distributed in breast milk. **Pregnancy Category C.** **Children/Elderly:** No age-related precautions noted.

INTERACTIONS

DRUG: None significant. **HERBAL:** None significant. **FOOD:** None known. **LAB VALUES:** May increase LDH, leukocyte alkaline phosphatase (LAP) scores, serum alkaline phosphatase, uric acid.

AVAILABILITY (Rx)

INJECTION SOLUTION: 300 mcg/ml, 480 mcg/0.8 ml, 600 mcg/ml.

ADMINISTRATION/HANDLING

◄ ALERT ► May be given by subcutaneous injection, short IV infusion (15–30 min), or continuous IV infusion.

IV

Reconstitution • Use single-dose vial, do not reenter vial. Do not shake. • Dilute with 10–50 ml D_5W to concentration of 15 mcg/ml or greater. For concentration from 5–14 mcg/ml, add 2 ml of 5% albumin to each 50 ml D_5W to provide a final concentration of 2 mg/ml. Do not dilute to final concentration less than 5 mcg/ml.

Rate of administration • For intermittent infusion (piggyback), infuse over 15–30 min. • For continuous infusion, give single dose over 4–24 hrs. • In all situations, flush IV line with D_5W before and after administration.

Storage • Refrigerate vials. • Stable for up to 24 hrs at room temperature (provided vial contents are clear and contain no particulate matter). Remains stable if accidentally exposed to freezing temperature.

SUBCUTANEOUS

Aspirate syringe before injection (avoid intra-arterial administration).

Storage • Store in refrigerator, but remove before use and allow to warm to room temperature.

IV INCOMPATIBILITIES

Amphotericin (Fungizone), cefepime (Maxipime), cefotaxime (Claforan), cefoxitin (Mefoxin), ceftizoxime (Cefizox), ceftriaxone (Rocephin), cefuroxime (Zinacef), clindamycin (Cleocin), dactinomycin (Cosmegen), etoposide (VePesid), fluorouracil, furosemide (Lasix), heparin, mannitol, methylprednisolone (Solu-Medrol), mitomycin (Mutamycin), prochlorperazine (Compazine), total parenteral nutrition (TPN).

IV COMPATIBILITIES

Bumetanide (Bumex), calcium gluconate, hydromorphone (Dilaudid), lorazepam (Ativan), morphine, potassium chloride.

INDICATIONS/ROUTES/DOSAGE

◄ **ALERT** ► Begin therapy at least 24 hrs after last dose of chemotherapy and at least 24 hrs after bone marrow infusion.

MYELOSUPPRESSION

IV OR SUBCUTANEOUS INFUSION, SUBCUTANEOUS INJECTION: ADULTS, ELDERLY: Initially, 5 mcg/kg/day. May increase by 5 mcg/ kg for each chemotherapy cycle based on duration/severity of absolute neutrophil count (ANC) nadir.

BONE MARROW TRANSPLANT

IV OR SUBCUTANEOUS INFUSION: ADULTS, ELDERLY, CHILDREN: 5–10 mcg/kg/day. Adjust dosage daily during period of neutrophil recovery based on neutrophil response.

MOBILIZATION OF PROGENITOR CELLS

IV OR SUBCUTANEOUS INFUSION: ADULTS: 10 mcg/kg/day beginning at least 4 days before first leukapheresis and continuing until last leukapheresis.

CHRONIC NEUTROPENIA, CONGENITAL NEUTROPENIA

SUBCUTANEOUS: ADULTS, CHILDREN: 6 mcg/kg/dose twice a day.

IDIOPATHIC OR CYCLIC NEUTROPENIA

SUBCUTANEOUS: ADULTS, CHILDREN: 5 mcg/kg/dose once a day.

SIDE EFFECTS

FREQUENT: Nausea/vomiting (57%), mild to severe bone pain (22%) (more frequent with high-dose IV form, less frequent with low-dose subcutaneous form), alopecia (18%), diarrhea (14%), fever (12%), fatigue (11%). **OCCASIONAL (9%–5%):** Anorexia, dyspnea, headache, cough, rash. **RARE (less than 5%):** Psoriasis, hematuria, proteinuria, osteoporosis.

ADVERSE EFFECTS/ TOXIC REACTIONS

Long-term administration occasionally produces chronic neutropenia, splenomegaly. Thrombocytopenia, MI, arrhythmias occur rarely. Adult respiratory distress syndrome may occur in septic pts.

NURSING CONSIDERATIONS

BASELINE ASSESSMENT

CBC, platelet count (differential) should be obtained before therapy initiation and twice weekly thereafter.

INTERVENTION/EVALUATION

In septic pts, be alert to adult respiratory distress syndrome. Closely monitor those with preexisting cardiac conditions. Monitor B/P (transient decrease in B/P may occur), temperature, CBC with differential, platelet count, Hct, serum uric acid, hepatic function tests.

PATIENT/FAMILY TEACHING

- Inform physician of fever, chills, severe bone pain, chest pain, palpitations.

finasteride

fin-**ah**-stir-eyd

(Propecia, Proscar)

Do not confuse Proscar with Posicor, ProSom, Prozac, or Psorcon.

CLASSIFICATION

PHARMACOTHERAPEUTIC: Androgen hormone inhibitor. **CLINICAL:** Benign prostatic hyperplasia agent.

ACTION

Inhibits 5-alpha reductase, an intracellular enzyme that converts testosterone into dihydrotestosterone (DHT) in prostate gland, resulting in decreased serum DHT. **Therapeutic Effect:** Reduces size of prostate gland.

PHARMACOKINETICS

Route	Onset	Peak	Duration
PO	24 hrs	1–2 days	5–7 days

Rapidly absorbed from GI tract. Protein binding: 90%. Widely distributed. Metabolized in liver. **Half-life:** 6–8 hrs. Onset of clinical effect: 3–6 mos of continued therapy.

USES

Proscar: Reduces risk of acute urinary retention, need for surgery in symptomatic benign prostatic hypertrophy (BPH alone or in combination with doxazosin [Cardura]). Most improvement noted in hesitancy, feeling of incomplete bladder emptying, interruption of urinary stream, difficulty initiating flow, dysuria, impaired volume, force of urinary stream. **Propecia:** Treatment of hair loss. **OFF-LABEL:** Adjuvant monotherapy after radical prostatectomy in treatment of prostate cancer, female hirsutism.

PRECAUTIONS

CONTRAINDICATIONS: Exposure to semen of treated pt or handling of finasteride tablets by those who are or may be pregnant. **CAUTIONS:** Hepatic function abnormalities.

LIFESPAN CONSIDERATIONS:

Pregnancy/Lactation: Physical handling of tablet in those who are or may become pregnant may produce abnormalities of external genitalia of male fetus. **Pregnancy Category X. Children:** Not indicated in children. **Elderly:** Efficacy not established.

INTERACTIONS

DRUG: None significant. **HERBAL:** **St. John's wort** may decrease concentration. Avoid concurrent use with **saw palmetto** (not adequately studied). **FOOD:** None known. **LAB VALUES:** Decreases serum prostate-specific antigen (PSA) level, even in presence of prostate cancer.

AVAILABILITY (Rx)

TABLETS: 1 mg (Propecia), 5 mg (Proscar).

ADMINISTRATION/HANDLING

PO

• Do not break, crush film-coated tablets. • Give without regard to meals.

INDICATIONS/ROUTES/DOSAGE

BENIGN PROSTATIC HYPERPLASIA (BPH)

PO: ADULTS, ELDERLY: 5 mg once a day (for minimum of 6 mos).

HAIR LOSS

PO: ADULTS: 1 mg/day.

SIDE EFFECTS

RARE (4%–2%): Gynecomastia, sexual dysfunction (impotence, decreased libido, decreased volume of ejaculate).

ADVERSE EFFECTS/ TOXIC REACTIONS

Hypersensitivity reaction, circumoral swelling, testicular pain occur rarely.

NURSING CONSIDERATIONS

BASELINE ASSESSMENT

Digital rectal exam, serum PSA determination should be performed in those with BPH before initiating therapy and periodically thereafter.

INTERVENTION/EVALUATION

Diligent monitoring of I&O, esp. in those with large residual urinary volume, severely diminished urinary flow for obstructive uropathy.

PATIENT/FAMILY TEACHING

• Pt should be aware of potential for impotence. • May not notice improved urinary flow even if prostate gland shrinks. • Need to take medication longer than 6 mos, and it is unknown if medication decreases need for surgery. • Because of potential risk to male fetus, women who are or may become pregnant should not handle tablets or be exposed to pt's semen. • Volume of ejaculate may be decreased during treatment.

Fioricet, *see acetaminophen*

Fiorinal, *see aspirin*

Flagyl, *see metronidazole*

flavocoxid

flay-**vox**-ah-sid
(Limbrel)

CLASSIFICATION

PHARMACOTHERAPEUTIC: Oral nutritional supplement. **CLINICAL:** Antiarthritis.

ACTION

Inhibits prostaglandin synthesis, arachidonic acid metabolism, reducing production of leukotrienes. Acts through antioxidant mechanism. **Therapeutic Effect:** Produces anti-inflammatory, analgesic effects, increases mobility.

PHARMACOKINETICS

Undergoes hydrolysis at intestinal mucosal border. Food decreases absorption. Little hepatic metabolism.

USES

For clinical dietary management of mild to moderate osteoarthritis, including associated inflammation.

PRECAUTIONS

CONTRAINDICATIONS: History of peptic ulcer. **CAUTIONS:** None known.

LIFESPAN CONSIDERATIONS:

Pregnancy/Lactation: Unknown if drug crosses placenta or is distributed in breast milk. **Pregnancy Category not classified. Children:** Safety and efficacy not established in children younger than 18 yrs. **Elderly:** No age-related precautions noted.

INTERACTIONS

DRUG: None significant. **HERBAL:** None significant. **FOOD:** **All foods** decrease absorption. **LAB VALUES:** None known.

AVAILABILITY (Rx)

CAPSULES: 250 mg, 500 mg.

ADMINISTRATION/HANDLING

PO

• Pt should not consume food 1 hr before or after taking flavocoxid (limits drug absorption).

INDICATIONS/ROUTES/DOSAGE

OSTEOARTHRITIS

PO: ADULTS 18 YRS AND OLDER, ELDERLY: 250–500 mg q12h.

SIDE EFFECTS

RARE (2%): Increase in varicose veins, psoriasis, mild hypertension.

ADVERSE EFFECTS/ TOXIC REACTIONS

GI bleeding, perforation, ulceration occur rarely in pts currently or previously treated with NSAIDs, COX-2 inhibitors.

NURSING CONSIDERATIONS

BASELINE ASSESSMENT

Assess onset, type, location, duration of pain, inflammation. Inspect appearance of affected joint for immobility, deformities, skin condition.

INTERVENTION/EVALUATION

Assess for therapeutic response (relief of pain, stiffness, swelling; increased joint mobility, reduced joint tenderness, improved grip strength).

PATIENT/FAMILY TEACHING

- Food should not be consumed 1 hr before or after taking flavocoxid.

flavoxate

fla-vox-ate

(Urispas)

Do not confuse Urispas with Urised.

CLASSIFICATION

PHARMACOTHERAPEUTIC: Anticholinergic. **CLINICAL:** Antispasmodic.

F

ACTION

Relaxes detrusor, other smooth muscle by cholinergic blockade, counteracting muscle spasm in urinary tract. **Therapeutic Effect:** Produces anticholinergic, local anesthetic, analgesic effects, relieving urinary symptoms.

PHARMACOKINETICS

Unknown absorption, distribution, metabolism. Protein binding: 50%–80%. Excreted in urine. **Half-life:** 10–20 hrs.

USES

Urinary analgesic, anesthetic for symptomatic relief of dysuria, urgency, nocturia, frequency, incontinence associated with cystitis, prostatitis, urethritis, urethrocystitis, urethrotrigonitis.

PRECAUTIONS

CONTRAINDICATIONS: Duodenal, pyloric obstruction; GI hemorrhage, obstruction; ileus; lower urinary tract obstruction. **CAUTIONS:** Glaucoma.

LIFESPAN CONSIDERATIONS:

Pregnancy/Lactation: Unknown if drug crosses placenta or is distributed in breast milk. **Pregnancy Category B. Children:** Safety and efficacy not established in children younger than 12 yrs. **Elderly:** Higher risk of confusion.

INTERACTIONS

DRUG: None significant. **HERBAL:** None significant. **FOOD:** None known. **LAB VALUES:** None known.

AVAILABILITY (Rx)

TABLETS: 100 mg.

INDICATIONS/ROUTES/DOSAGE

URINARY ANALGESIC, ANESTHETIC

PO: ADULTS, ELDERLY, ADOLESCENTS: 100–200 mg 3–4 times a day.

SIDE EFFECTS

FREQUENT: Drowsiness, dry mouth/throat. **OCCASIONAL:** Constipation, difficult urination, blurred vision, dizziness, headache, photosensitivity, nausea, vomiting, abdominal pain. **RARE:** Confusion (primarily in elderly), hypersensitivity, increased intraocular pressure (IOP), leukopenia.

ADVERSE EFFECTS/ TOXIC REACTIONS

Overdose may produce anticholinergic effects (unsteadiness, severe dizziness, drowsiness, fever, facial flushing, dyspnea, anxiety, irritability).

NURSING CONSIDERATIONS

BASELINE ASSESSMENT

Assess for dysuria, urgency, frequency, incontinence, suprapubic pain.

INTERVENTION/EVALUATION

Monitor for symptomatic relief. Observe elderly, esp. for mental confusion.

PATIENT/ FAMILY TEACHING

- Avoid tasks that require alertness motor skills until response to drug is established.

flecainide

(Tambocor)

See Antiarrhythmics (p. 15C)

Flexeril, *see cyclobenzaprine*

Flomax, *see tamsulosin*

Flonase, *see fluticasone*

Flovent, *see fluticasone*

Floxin Otic, *see ofloxacin*

fluconazole

flu-**con**-ah-zole

(Apo-Fluconazole ♣, Diflucan, Novo-Fluconazole ♣)

Do not confuse Diflucan with diclofenac.

CLASSIFICATION

CLINICAL: Antifungal.

ACTION

Interferes with cytochrome P-450, an enzyme necessary for ergosterol formation. **Therapeutic Effect:** Directly damages fungal membrane, altering its function. Fungistatic.

PHARMACOKINETICS

Well absorbed from GI tract. Widely distributed, including to CSF. Protein binding: 11%. Partially metabolized in liver. Excreted unchanged primarily in urine. Partially removed by hemodialysis. **Half-life:** 20–30 hrs (increased in renal impairment).

USES

Prevention of candidiasis in pts undergoing bone marrow transplant receiving chemotherapy and/or radiation therapy, treatment of esophageal, oropharyngeal, disseminated, vulvovaginal, urinary tract candidiasis, treatment and suppression of cryptococcal meningitis. **OFF-LABEL:** Treatment of coccidioidomycosis, cryptococcosis, fungal pneumonia, onychomycosis, ringworm of the hand, septicemia.

PRECAUTIONS

CONTRAINDICATIONS: None known. **CAUTIONS:** Hepatic/renal impairment, hypersensitivity to other triazoles (e.g., itraconazole, terconazole), imidazoles (e.g., butoconazole, ketoconazole).

LIFESPAN CONSIDERATIONS:

Pregnancy/Lactation: Unknown if excreted in breast milk. **Pregnancy Category C. Children:** No age-related precautions noted. **Elderly:** Age-related renal impairment may require dosage adjustment.

INTERACTIONS

DRUG: High fluconazole dosages increase **cyclosporine, sirolimus, tacrolimus** concentrations. **Isoniazid, rifampin** may increase drug metabolism. May increase concentration, effects of **oral antidiabetic medication.** May decrease metabolism of **phenytoin, warfarin. HERBAL:** None significant. **FOOD:** None known. **LAB VALUES:** May increase serum alkaline phosphatase, bilirubin, AST, ALT.

AVAILABILITY (Rx)

INJECTION, SOLUTION: 2 mg/ml (in 100- or 200-ml containers). **POWDER FOR ORAL SUSPENSION:** 10 mg/ml, 40 mg/ml. **TABLETS:** 50 mg, 100 mg, 150 mg, 200 mg.

ADMINISTRATION/HANDLING

IV

Rate of administration • Do not exceed maximum flow rate 200 mg/hr.

Storage • Store at room temperature. • Do not remove from outer wrap until ready to use. • Squeeze inner bag to check for leaks. • Do not use parenteral form if solution is cloudy, precipitate forms, seal is not intact, or it is discolored. • Do not add supplementary medication.

PO

• Give without regard to meals. • PO and IV therapy equally effective; IV therapy for pt intolerant of drug or unable to take orally.

IV INCOMPATIBILITIES

Amphotericin B (Fungizone), amphotericin B complex (Abelcet, Ambisome, Amphotec), ampicillin (Polycillin), calcium gluconate, cefotaxime (Claforan), ceftazidime (Fortaz), ceftriaxone (Rocephin), cefuroxime (Zinacef), chloramphenicol (Chloromycetin), clindamycin (Cleocin), co-trimoxazole (Bactrim), diazepam (Valium), digoxin (Lanoxin), erythromycin (Erythrocin), furosemide (Lasix), haloperidol (Haldol), hydroxyzine (Vistaril), imipenem and cilastatin (Primaxin), total parenteral nutrition (TPN).

IV COMPATIBILITIES

Diltiazem (Cardizem), dobutamine (Dobutrex), dopamine (Intropin), heparin, lipids, lorazepam (Ativan), midazolam (Versed), propofol (Diprivan).

INDICATIONS/ROUTES/DOSAGE

OROPHARYNGEAL CANDIDIASIS

PO, IV: ADULTS, ELDERLY: 200 mg once, then 100 mg/day for at least 14 days. **CHILDREN:** 6 mg/kg/day once, then 3 mg/kg/day.

ESOPHAGEAL CANDIDIASIS

PO, IV: ADULTS, ELDERLY: 200 mg once, then 100 mg/day (up to 400 mg/day) for 21 days and at least 14 days following resolution of symptoms. **CHILDREN:** 6 mg/kg/day once, then 3 mg/kg/day (up to 12 mg/kg/day) for 21 days at at least 14 days following resolution of symptoms.

URINARY CANDIDIASIS

PO, IV: ADULTS, ELDERLY: 50–200 mg/day.

VAGINAL CANDIDIASIS

PO: ADULTS: 150 mg once.

PREVENTION OF CANDIDIASIS IN PTS UNDERGOING BONE MARROW TRANSPLANTATION

PO: ADULTS: 400 mg/day.

SYSTEMIC CANDIDIASIS

PO, IV: ADULTS, ELDERLY: 400 mg once, then 200 mg/day (up to 400 mg/day) for at least 28 days and at least 14 days following resolution of symptoms. **CHILDREN:** 6–12 mg/kg/day.

CRYPTOCOCCAL MENINGITIS

PO, IV: ADULTS, ELDERLY: 400 mg once, then 200 mg/day (up to 800 mg/day) for 10–12 wks after CSF becomes negative (200 mg/day for suppression of relapse in pts with AIDS). **CHILDREN:** 12 mg/kg/day once, then 6–12 mg/kg/day (6 mg/kg/day for suppression of relapse).

ONYCHOMYCOSIS

PO: ADULTS: 150 mg/wk.

DOSAGE IN RENAL IMPAIRMENT

After a loading dose of 400 mg, daily dosage is based on creatinine clearance.

Creatinine Clearance	% of Recommended Dose
Greater than 50 ml/min	100
21–50 ml/min	50
11–20 ml/min	25
Dialysis	Dose after dialysis

SIDE EFFECTS

OCCASIONAL (4%–1%): Hypersensitivity reaction (chills, fever, pruritus, rash), dizziness, drowsiness, headache, constipation, diarrhea, nausea, vomiting, abdominal pain.

ADVERSE EFFECTS/ TOXIC REACTIONS

Exfoliative skin disorders, serious hepatic effects, blood dyscrasias (eosinophilia, thrombocytopenia, anemia, leukopenia) have been reported rarely.

NURSING CONSIDERATIONS

BASELINE ASSESSMENT

Establish baselines for CBC, serum potassium, hepatic function studies.

INTERVENTION/EVALUATION

Assess for hypersensitivity reaction (chills, fever). Monitor serum hepatic/renal function tests, potassium, CBC, platelet count. Report rash, itching promptly. Monitor temperature at least daily. Monitor daily pattern of bowel activity/stool consistency. Assess for dizziness; provide assistance as needed.

PATIENT/FAMILY TEACHING

• Avoid tasks that require alertness, motor skills until response to drug is established (dizziness, drowsiness). • Notify physician of dark urine, pale stool, jaundiced skin or sclera of eyes, rash, pruritus. • Pts with oropharyngeal infections should be taught appropriate oral hygiene. • Consult physician before taking any other medication.

fludarabine

flew-**dare**-ah-bean

(Fludara)

Do not confuse Fludara with FUDR.

CLASSIFICATION

PHARMACOTHERAPEUTIC: Antimetabolite. **CLINICAL:** Antineoplastic (see p. 79C).

ACTION

Inhibits DNA synthesis by interfering with DNA polymerase alpha, ribonucleotide reductase, DNA primase. **Therapeutic Effect:** Induces cell death.

PHARMACOKINETICS

Rapidly dephosphorylated in serum, then phosphorylated intracellularly to active triphosphate. Primarily excreted in urine. **Half-life:** 7–20 hrs.

USES

Treatment of chronic lymphocytic leukemia (CLL) in those who have not responded to or have not progressed with another standard alkylating agent. Treatment of non-Hodgkin's lymphoma.

PRECAUTIONS

CONTRAINDICATIONS: Concurrent use with pentostatin. **CAUTIONS:** Preexisting neurologic problems, renal insufficiency, myelosuppression.

LIFESPAN CONSIDERATIONS:

Pregnancy/Lactation: If possible, avoid use during pregnancy, esp. first trimester. May cause fetal harm. Not known whether distributed in breast milk. Breast-feeding not recommended. **Pregnancy Category D. Children:** Safety and efficacy not established. **Elderly:** Age-related renal impairment may require dosage adjustment.

F

INTERACTIONS

DRUG: May decrease effects of **antigout medications. Bone marrow depressants** may increase risk of myelosuppression. **Live virus vaccines** may potentiate virus replication, increase vaccine side effects, decrease pt's antibody response to vaccine. **HERBAL:** None significant. **FOOD:** None known. **LAB VALUES:** May increase serum alkaline phosphatase, uric acid, AST.

AVAILABILITY (Rx)

INJECTION POWDER FOR RECONSTITUTION: 50 mg.

ADMINISTRATION/HANDLING

◀ **ALERT** ▶ Give by IV infusion. Do not add to other IV infusions. Avoid small veins, swollen, edematous extremities; areas overlying joints, tendons.

IV

Reconstitution • Reconstitute 50-mg vial with 2 ml Sterile Water for Injection to provide concentration of 25 mg/ml. • Further dilute with 100–125 ml 0.9% NaCl or D_5W.

Rate of administration • Infuse over 30 min.

Storage • Store in refrigerator. • Handle with extreme care during preparation/administration. If contact with skin or mucous membranes occurs, wash thoroughly with soap and water; rinse eyes profusely with plain water. • After reconstitution, use within 8 hrs; discard unused portion.

IV INCOMPATIBILITIES

Acyclovir (Zovirax), amphotericin B (Fungizone), hydroxyzine (Vistaril), prochlorperazine (Compazine).

IV COMPATIBILITIES

Heparin, hydromorphone (Dilaudid), lorazepam (Ativan), magnesium sulfate, morphine, multivitamins, potassium chloride.

INDICATIONS/ROUTES/DOSAGE

CHRONIC LYMPHOCYTIC LEUKEMIA

IV: ADULTS: 25 mg/m^2 daily for 5 consecutive days. Continue for up to 3 additional cycles. Begin each course of treatment every 28 days.

NON-HODGKIN'S LYMPHOMA

IV: ADULTS, ELDERLY: Initially, 20 mg/m^2, then 30 mg/m^2/day for 48 hrs.

DOSAGE IN RENAL IMPAIRMENT

Creatinine Clearance	Dosage
30–70 ml/min	Decrease dose by 20%
Less than 30 ml/min	Not recommended

SIDE EFFECTS

FREQUENT: Fever (60%), nausea/vomiting (36%), chills (11%). **OCCASIONAL (20%–10%):** Fatigue, generalized pain, rash, diarrhea, cough, asthenia, stomatitis, dyspnea, peripheral edema. **RARE (7%–3%):** Anorexia, sinusitis, dysuria, myalgia, paresthesia, headache, visual disturbances.

ADVERSE EFFECTS/ TOXIC REACTIONS

Pneumonia occurs frequently. Severe hematologic toxicity (anemia, thrombocytopenia, neutropenia), GI bleeding may occur. Tumor lysis syndrome may begin with flank pain, hematuria; may also include hypercalcemia, hyperphosphatemia, hyperuricemia, resulting in renal failure. High-dosage therapy may produce acute leukemia, blindness, coma.

NURSING CONSIDERATIONS

BASELINE ASSESSMENT

Assess baseline CBC, platelet, serum creatinine. Drug should be discontinued if intractable vomiting, diarrhea, stomatitis, GI bleeding occurs.

INTERVENTION/EVALUATION

Assess for fatigue, visual disturbances, peripheral edema. Assess for onset of pneumonia. Monitor for dyspnea, cough, rapid decrease in WBC count, intractable vomiting, diarrhea, GI bleeding (bright red or tarry stool). Assess oral mucosa for erythema, ulceration at inner margin of lips, sore throat, difficulty swallowing (stomatitis). Assess skin for rash. Be alert to possible tumor lysis syndrome (onset of flank pain, hematuria).

PATIENT/FAMILY TEACHING

• Avoid crowds, exposure to infection. • Maintain fastidious oral hygiene. • Promptly report fever, sore throat, signs of local infection, unusual bruising/bleeding from any site. • Contact physician if nausea/vomiting continues.

fludrocortisone

floo-droe-**kor**-ti-sone

(Florinef)

Do not confuse Florinef with Fioricet or Florinal.

CLASSIFICATION

PHARMACOTHERAPEUTIC: Mineralocorticoid. **CLINICAL:** Glucocorticosteroid (see p. 92C).

ACTION

Acts at distal tubules. **Therapeutic Effect:** Increases potassium, hydrogen ion excretion. Replaces sodium loss, raises blood pressure (with low dosages).

PHARMACOKINETICS

Well absorbed from GI tract. Protein binding: 42%. Widely distributed. Metabolized in liver, kidney. Primarily excreted in urine. **Half-life:** 3.5 hrs.

USES

Partial replacement therapy for primary and secondary adrenocortical insufficiency in Addison's disease. Adjunctive treatment of sodium-wasting forms of congenital adrenogenital syndrome. **OFF-LABEL:** Treatment of acidosis in renal tubular disorders, idiopathic orthostatic hypotension.

PRECAUTIONS

CONTRAINDICATIONS: CHF, systemic fungal infection. **CAUTIONS:** Hypertension, edema, renal impairment.

LIFESPAN CONSIDERATIONS:

Pregnancy/Lactation: Unknown whether drug crosses placenta or is distributed in breast milk. **Pregnancy Category C. Children:** May cause growth suppression, inhibition of endogenous steroid production. **Elderly:** Studies not performed.

INTERACTIONS

DRUG: May increase risk of **digoxin** toxicity (hypokalemia). **Hepatic enzyme inducers (e.g., phenytoin)** may increase metabolism. **Medications causing hypokalemia** may increase effects. **Sodium-containing medications** may increase B/P, incidence of edema, serum sodium. **HERBAL:** None significant. **FOOD:** None known. **LAB VALUES:** May increase serum sodium. May decrease Hct, serum potassium.

AVAILABILITY (Rx)

TABLETS: 0.1 mg.

ADMINISTRATION/HANDLING

PO

• Give with food, milk.

INDICATIONS/ROUTES/DOSAGE

ADDISON'S DISEASE

PO: ADULTS, ELDERLY: 0.05–0.1 mg/day. Range: 0.1 mg 3 times a wk to 0.2

mg/day. Administration with cortisone, hydrocortisone preferred.

SODIUM-WASTING ADRENOGENITAL SYNDROME

PO: ADULTS, ELDERLY: 0.1–0.2 mg/day.

USUAL PEDIATRIC DOSAGE

CHILDREN: 0.05–0.1 mg/day.

F

SIDE EFFECTS

FREQUENT: Increased appetite, exaggerated sense of well-being, abdominal distention, weight gain, insomnia, mood swings. **High dosages, prolonged therapy, too-rapid withdrawal:** Increased susceptibility to infection (signs/symptoms masked), delayed wound healing, hypokalemia, hypocalcemia, GI distress, diarrhea or constipation, hypertension. **OCCASIONAL:** Headache, dizziness, menstrual difficulty/amenorrhea, gastric ulcer development. **RARE:** Hypersensitivity reaction.

ADVERSE EFFECTS/ TOXIC REACTIONS

LONG-TERM THERAPY: Muscle wasting (esp. in arms, legs), osteoporosis, spontaneous fractures, amenorrhea, cataracts, glaucoma, peptic ulcer disease, CHF. **ABRUPT WITHDRAWAL AFTER LONG-TERM THERAPY:** Anorexia, nausea, fever, headache, joint pain, rebound inflammation, fatigue, weakness, lethargy, dizziness, orthostatic hypotension.

NURSING CONSIDERATIONS

BASELINE ASSESSMENT

Obtain baselines for weight, B/P, serum glucose, electrolytes, chest X-ray, EKG.

INTERVENTION/EVALUATION

Monitor serum electrolytes, renin, glucose, B/P. Taper dosage slowly if medication is to be discontinued.

PATIENT/FAMILY TEACHING

• Do not change dose/schedule or stop taking drug; must taper off gradually. • Report fever, sore throat, muscle aches, sudden weight gain, swelling, continual headaches. • Maintain fastidious personal hygiene, avoid exposure to disease, trauma. • Severe stress (serious infection, surgery, trauma) may require increased dosage.

flumazenil

flew-**maz**-ah-nil
(Anexate ✦, Romazicon)

CLASSIFICATION

PHARMACOTHERAPEUTIC: Benzodiazepine receptor antagonist. **CLINICAL:** Antidote.

ACTION

Antagonizes effect of benzodiazepines on gamma-aminobutyric acid (GABA) receptor complex in CNS. **Therapeutic Effect:** Reverses sedative effect of benzodiazepines.

PHARMACOKINETICS

Route	Onset	Peak	Duration
IV	1–2 min	6–10 min	Less than 1 hr

Duration, degree of benzodiazepine reversal directly related to dosage, plasma concentration. Protein binding: 50%. Metabolized by liver; excreted in urine.

USES

Complete or partial reversal of sedative effects of benzodiazepines when general anesthesia has been induced and/or maintained with benzodiazepines, when sedation has been produced with benzodiazepines for diagnostic and therapeutic procedures, management of benzodiazepine overdosage.

PRECAUTIONS

CONTRAINDICATIONS: History of hypersensitivity to benzodiazepines; pts who have been administered benzodiazepines for control of a potentially life-threatening condition (increased intracranial pressure [ICP], status epilepticus); pts exhibiting signs/symptoms of tricyclic antidepressant overdose (anticholinergic signs [mydriasis, dry mucosa, hypoperistalsis], arrhythmias, motor abnormalities, cardiovascular collapse). **CAUTIONS:** Head injury, hepatic impairment, alcoholism, drug dependency.

LIFESPAN CONSIDERATIONS:

Pregnancy/Lactation: Unknown whether drug crosses placenta or is distributed in breast milk. Not recommended during labor, delivery. **Pregnancy Category C.** **Children:** No age-related precautions noted. **Elderly:** Benzodiazepine-induced sedation tends to be deeper, more prolonged, requiring careful monitoring.

INTERACTIONS

DRUG: Toxic effects (e.g., seizures, arrhythmias) of other drugs taken in overdosage (esp. **tricyclic antidepressants**) may emerge with reversal of sedative effects of **benzodiazepines.** **HERBAL:** None significant. **FOOD:** None known. **LAB VALUES:** None known.

AVAILABILITY (Rx)

INJECTION SOLUTION: 0.1 mg/ml.

ADMINISTRATION/HANDLING

◄ ALERT ► Compatible with D_5W, lactated Ringer's, 0.9% NaCl.

Rate of administration • **Reversal of conscious sedation or general anesthesia:** Give over 15 sec. • **Reversal of benzodiazepine overdose:** Give over 30 sec. • Administer through freely running IV infusion into large vein (local injection produces pain, inflammation at injection site).

Storage • Store parenteral form at room temperature. • Discard after 24 hrs once medication is drawn into syringe, is mixed with any solutions, or if particulate/discoloration is noted. • Rinse spilled medication from skin with cool water.

IV INCOMPATIBILITIES

No information available for Y-site administration.

IV COMPATIBILITIES

Aminophylline, cimetidine (Tagamet), dobutamine (Dobutrex), dopamine (Intropin), famotidine (Pepcid), heparin, lidocaine, procainamide (Pronestyl), ranitidine (Zantac).

INDICATIONS/ROUTES/DOSAGE

REVERSAL OF CONSCIOUS SEDATION OR GENERAL ANESTHESIA

IV: ADULTS, ELDERLY: Initially, 0.2 mg (2 ml) over 15 sec; may repeat dose in 45 sec; then at 60-sec intervals. **Maximum:** 1 mg (10-ml) total dose. **CHILDREN, NEONATES:** Initially, 0.01 mg/kg; may repeat in 45 sec, then at 60-sec intervals. **Maximum:** 0.2 mg single dose.

BENZODIAZEPINE OVERDOSE

IV: ADULTS, ELDERLY: Initially, 0.2 mg (2 ml) over 30 sec; if desired level of consciousness (LOC) is not achieved after 30 sec, 0.3 mg (3 ml) may be given over 30 sec. Additional doses of 0.5 mg (5 ml) may be administered over 30 sec at 60-sec intervals. **Maximum:** 1 mg/dose or 3 mg/hr. **CHILDREN, NEONATES:** Initially, 0.01 mg/kg; may repeat in 45 sec, then at 60-sec intervals. **Maximum:** 0.2 mg single dose.

◄ ALERT ► If resedation occurs, repeat dose at 20-min intervals. **Maximum dose in reversal of sedation, anesthesia:** 0.2 mg/min up to cumulative dose of 1 mg or up to 3 mg in any 1 hr. **Maximum dose in benzodiazepine overdose:** 0.5 mg/min up to cumulative dose of 1 mg or up to 3 mg in any 1 hr.

SIDE EFFECTS

FREQUENT (11%–3%): Agitation, anxiety, dry mouth, dyspnea, insomnia, palpitations, tremors, headache, blurred vision, dizziness, ataxia, nausea, vomiting, pain at injection site, diaphoresis. **OCCASIONAL (2%–1%):** Fatigue, flushing, auditory disturbances, thrombophlebitis, rash. **RARE (less than 1%):** Urticaria, pruritus, hallucinations.

ADVERSE EFFECTS/ TOXIC REACTIONS

Toxic effects (seizures, arrhythmias), of other drugs taken in overdose, (esp. tricyclic antidepressants) may emerge with reversal of sedative effect of benzodiazepines. May provoke panic attack in those with a history of panic disorder.

NURSING CONSIDERATIONS

BASELINE ASSESSMENT

ABGs should be obtained prior to and at 30-min intervals during IV administration. Prepare to intervene in reestablishing airway, assisting ventilation (drug may not fully reverse ventilatory insufficiency induced by benzodiazepines). Note that effects of flumazenil may dissipate before effects of benzodiazepines.

INTERVENTION/EVALUATION

Properly manage airway, assist breathing, maintain circulatory access and support, perform internal decontamination by lavage and charcoal as indicated, provide adequate clinical evaluation. Monitor for reversal of benzodiazepine effect. Assess for possible resedation, respiratory depression, hypoventilation. Assess closely for return of unconsciousness (narcosis) for at least 1 hr after pt is fully alert.

PATIENT/FAMILY TEACHING

- Avoid ingestion of alcohol, tasks that require alertness, motor skills or taking nonprescription drugs until at least 18–24 hrs after discharge.

flunisolide

floo-**niss**-oh-lide

(AeroBid, AeroBid-M, Aerospan, Apo-Flunisolide ♣, Bronalide ♣, Nasalide, Nasarel, Rhinalar ♣)

Do not confuse flunisolide with fluocinonide, or Nasalide with Nasalcrom.

♦ CLASSIFICATION

PHARMACOTHERAPEUTIC: Adrenocorticosteroid. **CLINICAL:** Antiasthmatic, anti-inflammatory (see pp. 71C, 92C).

ACTION

Controls rate of protein synthesis, depresses migration of polymorphonuclear leukocytes, reverses capillary permeability, stabilizes lysosomal membranes. **Therapeutic Effect:** Prevents, controls inflammation.

PHARMACOKINETICS

Rapidly absorbed from lungs and GI tract following inhalation. About 50% of dose is absorbed from nasal mucosa following intranasal administration. Metabolized in liver. Partially excreted in urine and feces. **Half-life:** 1–2 hrs.

USES

Inhalation: Long-term control of persistent bronchial asthma. Assists in reducing, discontinuing oral corticosteroid therapy. **Intranasal:** Relieves symptoms of seasonal, perennial rhinitis. **OFF-LABEL:** Prevents recurrence of nasal polyps after surgery.

PRECAUTIONS

CONTRAINDICATIONS: Hypersensitivity to any corticosteroid, persistently positive sputum cultures for *Candida albicans,* primary treatment of status asthmaticus, systemic fungal infections. **CAUTIONS:** Adrenal insufficiency.

LIFESPAN CONSIDERATIONS:

Pregnancy/Lactation: Unknown if distributed in breast milk. **Pregnancy Category C. Children:** Safety and efficacy not established. **Elderly:** No age-related cautions noted.

INTERACTIONS

DRUG: Bupropion may lower seizure threshold. **HERBAL:** None significant. **FOOD:** None known. **LAB VALUES:** None known.

AVAILABILITY (Rx)

AEROSOL WITH ADAPTER (AEROBID): 250 mcg/activation. **AEROSOL (AEROBID-M):** 250 mcg/activation. **AEROSPAN:** 80 mcg/activation. **NASAL SPRAY (NASALIDE, NASAREL):** 25 mcg/activation.

ADMINISTRATION/HANDLING

INHALATION

• Shake container well; instruct pt to exhale as completely as possible. • Place mouthpiece fully into mouth; holding inhaler upright, instruct pt to inhale deeply, slowly while pressing top of canister and hold breath as long as possible before exhaling; then exhale slowly. • Wait 1 min between inhalations when multiple inhalations ordered (allows for deeper bronchial penetration). • Rinse mouth with water immediately after inhalation (prevents mouth/throat dryness).

INTRANASAL

• Clear nasal passages before use (topical nasal decongestants may be needed 5–15 min before use). • Instruct pt to tilt head slightly forward. • Insert spray tip up in one nostril, pointing toward inflamed nasal turbinates, away from nasal septum. • Pump medication into one nostril while the pt holds other nostril closed and concurrently inspires through nose. • Discard opened nasal solution after 3 mos.

INDICATIONS/ROUTES/DOSAGE

USUAL INHALATION DOSAGE

INHALATION: ADULTS, ELDERLY: 2 inhalations twice a day, morning and evening. **Maximum:** 4 inhalations twice a day. **CHILDREN 6–15 YRS:** 2 inhalations twice a day.

USUAL INTRANASAL DOSAGE

◄ **ALERT** ► Improvement usually seen within a few days; may take up to 3 wks. Discontinue use after 3 wks if no significant improvement occurs.

INTRANASAL: ADULTS, ELDERLY: Initially, 2 sprays each nostril twice a day, may increase at 4–7 day intervals to 2 sprays 3 times a day. **Maximum:** 8 sprays in each nostril daily. **CHILDREN 6–14 YRS:** Initially, 1 spray 3 times a day or 2 sprays twice a day. **Maximum:** 4 sprays in each nostril daily. Maintenance: 1 spray into each nostril daily.

SIDE EFFECTS

FREQUENT: Inhalation (25%–10%): Unpleasant taste, nausea, vomiting, sore throat, diarrhea, cold symptoms, nasal congestion. **OCCASIONAL: Inhalation (9%–3%):** Dizziness, irritability, anxiety, tremors, abdominal pain, heartburn, oropharyngeal candidiasis, edema. **Nasal:** Mild nasopharyngeal irritation/dryness, rebound congestion, bronchial asthma, rhinorrhea, altered taste.

ADVERSE EFFECTS/ TOXIC REACTIONS

Acute hypersensitivity reaction (urticaria, angioedema, severe bronchospasm) occurs rarely. Transfer from systemic to local steroid therapy may unmask previously suppressed bronchial asthma condition.

NURSING CONSIDERATIONS

BASELINE ASSESSMENT

Establish baseline assessment of asthma, rhinitis.

INTERVENTION/EVALUATION

Advise pts receiving bronchodilators by inhalation concomitantly with steroid inhalation therapy to use bronchodilator several min before corticosteroid aerosol (enhances penetration of steroid into bronchial tree). Monitor rate, depth, rhythm, type of respiration; quality/rate of pulse. Assess lung sounds for rhonchi, wheezing, rales. Monitor ABGs.

PATIENT/FAMILY TEACHING

• Do not change dose/schedule or stop taking drug; must taper off gradually under medical supervision. • Maintain fastidious oral hygiene. • Rinse mouth with water immediately after inhalation (prevents mouth/throat dryness, fungal infection oral). • Increase fluid intake (decreases lung secretion viscosity). • **Intranasal:** Teach proper use of nasal spray. • Clear nasal passages before use. • Contact physician if no improvement in symptoms, sneezing or nasal irritation occurs. • Improvement usually noted in several days.

fluocinolone

(Flurosyn, Synalar, Synemol)

fluocinonide

(Lidex, Vanos, Vasoderm)

See Corticosteroids: topical (p. 94C)

fluorouracil, 5-FU

flur-oh-**your**-ah-sill

(Adrucil, Carac, Efudex, Fluoroplex)

Do not confuse Efudex with Efidac.

CLASSIFICATION

PHARMACOTHERAPEUTIC: Antimetabolite. **CLINICAL:** Antineoplastic (see p. 79C).

ACTION

Blocks formation of thymidylic acid. Cell cycle-specific for S phase of cell division. **Therapeutic Effect:** Inhibits DNA, RNA synthesis. **Topical:** Destroys rapidly proliferating cells.

PHARMACOKINETICS

Widely distributed. Crosses blood-brain barrier. Rapidly metabolized in tissues to active metabolite, which is localized intracellularly. Primarily excreted by lungs as carbon dioxide. Removed by hemodialysis. **Half-life:** 20 hrs.

USES

Parenteral: Treatment of carcinoma of colon, rectum, breast, stomach, pancreas. Used in combination with levamisole after surgical resection in pts with Duke's stage C colon cancer. **Topical:** Treatment of multiple actinic or solar keratoses, superficial basal cell carcinomas. **OFF-LABEL: Parenteral:** Treatment of bladder, cervical, endometrial, head/neck, liver, lung, ovarian, prostate carcinomas; treatment of pericardial, peritoneal, pleural effusions. **Topical:** Treatment of actinic cheilitis, radiodermatitis.

PRECAUTIONS

CONTRAINDICATIONS: Major surgery within previous mo, myelosuppression, poor nutritional status, potentially serious infections. **CAUTIONS:** History of high-dose pelvic irradiation, metastatic cell infiltration of bone marrow, hepatic/renal impairment.

LIFESPAN CONSIDERATIONS:

Pregnancy/Lactation: If possible, avoid use during pregnancy, esp. first trimester. May cause fetal harm. Unknown whether distributed in breast milk. Breast-feeding not recommended. **Pregnancy Category D. (X: Topical) Children:** No age-related precautions noted. **Elderly:** Age-related renal impairment may require dosage adjustment.

INTERACTIONS

DRUG: Bone marrow depressants may increase risk of myelosuppression. **Live virus vaccines** may potentiate virus replication, increase vaccine side effects, decrease pt's antibody response to vaccine. **HERBAL:** Avoid use of **black cohosh, dong quai** in pts with estrogen-dependent tumors. **FOOD:** None known. **LAB VALUES:** May decrease serum albumin. May increase excretion of 5-hydroxyindoleacetic acid (5-HIAA) in urine. **Topical:** May cause eosinophilia, leukocytosis, thrombocytopenia, toxic granulation.

AVAILABILITY (Rx)

CREAM, TOPICAL: (CARAC) 0.5%, **(EFUDEX)** 5%, **(FLUOROPLEX)** 1%. **INJECTION SOLUTION: (ADRUCIL):** 50 mg/ml. **SOLUTION, TOPICAL: (EFUDEX)** 2%.

ADMINISTRATION/HANDLING

◄ ALERT ► Give by IV injection or IV infusion. Do not add to other IV infusions. Avoid small veins, swollen/edematous extremities, areas overlying joints, tendons. May be carcinogenic, mutagenic, teratogenic. Handle with extreme care during preparation/administration.

IV

Reconstitution • IV push does not need to be diluted or reconstituted. • Inject through Y-tube or 3-way stopcock of free-flowing solution. • For IV infusion, further dilute with D_5W or 0.9% NaCl.

Rate of administration • Give IV push slowly over 1–2 min. • IV infusion is administered over 30 min–24 hrs. • Extravasation produces immediate pain, severe local tissue damage. • Follow protocol.

Storage • Solution appears colorless to faint yellow. Slight discoloration does not adversely affect potency or safety. • If precipitate forms, redissolve by heating, shaking vigorously; allow to cool to body temperature.

IV INCOMPATIBILITIES

Amphotericin B complex (Abelcet, AmBisome, Amphotec), droperidol (Inapsine), filgrastim (Neupogen), ondansetron (Zofran), vinorelbine (Navelbine).

IV COMPATIBILITIES

Granisetron (Kytril), heparin, hydromorphone (Dilaudid), leucovorin, morphine, potassium chloride, propofol (Diprivan), total parenteral nutrition (TPN).

INDICATIONS/ROUTES/DOSAGE

USUAL THERAPY

IV: ADULTS, ELDERLY, CHILDREN: Initially, 12 mg/kg/day for 4–5 days. **Maximum:** 800 mg/day. Maintenance: 6 mg/kg every other day for 4 doses repeated in 4 wks; or 15 mg/kg as a single bolus dose; or 5–15 mg/kg/wk as a single dose, not to exceed 1 g.

MULTIPLE ACTINIC OR SOLAR KERATOSES

TOPICAL (CARAC): ADULTS, ELDERLY: Apply once a day.

TOPICAL (EFUDEX, FLUOROPLEX): **ADULTS, ELDERLY:** Apply twice a day.

BASAL CELL CARCINOMA
TOPICAL (EFUDEX): **ADULTS, ELDERLY:** Apply twice a day for 3–6 wks up to 10–12 wks.

SIDE EFFECTS

OCCASIONAL: Parenteral: Anorexia, diarrhea, minimal alopecia, fever, dry skin, skin fissures, scaling, erythema. **Topical:** Pain, pruritus, hyperpigmentation, irritation, inflammation, burning at application site, photosensitivity. **RARE:** Nausea, vomiting, anemia, esophagitis, proctitis, GI ulcer, confusion, headache, lacrimation, visual disturbances, angina, allergic reaction.

ADVERSE EFFECTS/ TOXIC REACTIONS

Earliest sign of toxicity (4–8 days after beginning therapy) is stomatitis (dry mouth, burning sensation, mucosal erythema, ulceration at inner margin of lips). Most common dermatologic toxicity is pruritic rash (generally on extremities, less frequently on trunk). Leukopenia generally occurs within 9–14 days after drug administration but may occur as late as 25th day. Thrombocytopenia occasionally occurs within 7–17 days after administration. Pancytopenia, agranulocytosis occur rarely.

NURSING CONSIDERATIONS

BASELINE ASSESSMENT

Obtain CBC with differential, platelet count, serum renal/hepatic function tests.

INTERVENTION/EVALUATION

Monitor for rapidly falling WBC count, intractable diarrhea, GI bleeding (bright red or tarry stool). Assess oral mucosa for stomatitis. Drug should be discontinued if intractable diarrhea, stomatitis, GI bleeding occurs. Assess skin for rash.

PATIENT/FAMILY TEACHING

• Maintain fastidious oral hygiene. • Inform physician of signs/symptoms of infection, unusual bruising/bleeding, visual changes, nausea, vomiting, diarrhea, chest pain, palpitations. • Avoid sunlight, artificial light sources; wear protective clothing, sunglasses, sunscreen. • **Topical:** Apply only to affected area. • Do not use occlusive coverings. • Be careful near eyes, nose, mouth. • Wash hands thoroughly after application. • Treated areas may be unsightly for several weeks after therapy.

fluoxetine

floo-**ox**-e-teen
(Apo-Fluoxetine ✱, Novo-Fluoxetine ✱, Prozac, Prozac Weekly, Sarafem)

Do not confuse fluoxetine with fluvastatin, Prozac with Prilosec, Proscar, or ProSom; or Sarafem with Serophene.

FIXED-COMBINATION(S)

Symbyax: fluoxetine/olanzapine (an antipsychotic): 25 mg/6 mg, 50 mg/6 mg, 25 mg/12 mg, 50 mg/12 mg.

CLASSIFICATION

PHARMACOTHERAPEUTIC: Psychotherapeutic. **CLINICAL:** Antidepressant, antiobsessional agent, antibulimic (see p. 37C).

ACTION

Selectively inhibits serotonin uptake in CNS, enhancing serotonergic function. **Therapeutic Effect:** Relieves depression; reduces obsessive-compulsive, bulimic behavior.

PHARMACOKINETICS

Well absorbed from GI tract. Crosses blood-brain barrier. Protein binding: 94%. Metabolized in liver to active metabolite. Primarily excreted in urine. Not removed by hemodialysis. **Half-life:** 2–3 days; metabolite 7–9 days.

USES

Treatment of clinical depression, obsessive-compulsive disorder (OCD), bulimia nervosa, premenstrual dysphoric disorder (PMDD), panic disorder. **OFF-LABEL:** Treatment of body dysmorphic disorder, fibromyalgia, hot flashes, post-traumatic stress disorder (PTSD), Raynaud's phenomena.

PRECAUTIONS

CONTRAINDICATIONS: Use within 14 days of MAOIs. **CAUTIONS:** Seizure disorder, cardiac dysfunction, diabetes, those at high risk for suicide.

LIFESPAN CONSIDERATIONS:

Pregnancy/Lactation: Unknown whether drug crosses placenta or is distributed in breast milk. **Pregnancy Category C. Children:** May be more sensitive to behavioral side effects (e.g., insomnia, restlessness). **Elderly:** No age-related precautions noted.

INTERACTIONS

DRUG: Aspirin, NSAIDs may increase risk of bleeding. **Alcohol, other CNS depressants** may increase CNS depression. **Highly protein-bound medications (e.g., oral anticoagulants)** may increase adverse effects. **MAOIs** may produce serotonin syndrome and neuroleptic malignant syndrome. May increase **phenytoin** concentration, risk of toxicity. May increase concentration/toxicity of **tricyclic antidepressants. HERBAL: Gotu kola, kava kava, St. John's wort, valerian** may increase CNS depression. **St. John's wort** may increase effects, risk of toxicity. **FOOD:** None known. **LAB VALUES:** None known.

AVAILABILITY (Rx)

CAPSULES: 10 mg (Prozac, Sarafem), 20 mg (Prozac, Sarafem), 40 mg (Prozac). **TABLETS (PROZAC):** 10 mg, 20 mg. **ORAL SOLUTION (PROZAC):** 20 mg/5 ml.

CAPSULES (DELAYED-RELEASE [PROZAC WEEKLY]): 90 mg.

ADMINISTRATION/HANDLING

PO

- Give with food, milk if GI distress occurs.

INDICATIONS/ROUTES/DOSAGE

◀ **ALERT** ▶ Use lower or less frequent doses in pts with renal/hepatic impairment, those with concurrent disease or multiple medications, the elderly.

DEPRESSION

PO: ADULTS: Initially, 20 mg each morning. If therapeutic improvement does not occur after 2 wks, gradually increase to maximum of 80 mg/day in 2 equally divided doses in morning and at noon. **ELDERLY:** Initially, 10 mg/day. May increase by 10–20 mg q2wk. **CHILDREN 7–17 YRS:** Initially, 5–10 mg/day. Titrate upward as needed. Usual dosage: 20 mg/day. **Prozac Weekly:** 90 mg/wk, begin 7 days after last dose of 20 mg.

PANIC DISORDER

PO: ADULTS, ELDERLY: Initially, 10 mg/day. May increase to 20 mg/day after 1 wk. **Maximum:** 60 mg/day.

BULIMIA NERVOSA

PO: ADULTS: 60–80 mg each morning.

OBSESSIVE-COMPULSIVE DISORDER (OCD)

PO: ADULTS, ELDERLY: 40–80 mg/day. **CHILDREN 7–18 YRS:** Initially, 10 mg/day. May increase to 20 mg/day after 2 wks. Range: 10–80 mg/day.

PREMENSTRUAL DYSPHORIC DISORDER (SARAFEM)

PO: ADULTS: 20 mg/day **or** 20 mg/day beginning 14 days prior to menstruation and continuing through first full day of menses (repeated with each cycle).

SIDE EFFECTS

FREQUENT (greater than 10%): Headache, asthenia (loss of strength), insomnia, anxiety, drowsiness, nausea, diarrhea, decreased appetite. **OCCASIONAL (9%–2%):** Dizziness, tremor, fatigue, vomiting, constipation, dry mouth, abdominal pain, nasal congestion, diaphoresis, rash. **RARE (less than 2%):** Flushed skin, lightheadedness, impaired concentration.

ADVERSE EFFECTS/ TOXIC REACTIONS

Overdose may produce seizures, nausea, vomiting, excessive agitation, restlessness.

NURSING CONSIDERATIONS

BASELINE ASSESSMENT

For pts on long-term therapy, baseline hepatic/renal function tests, blood counts; testing should be performed periodically thereafter.

INTERVENTION/EVALUATION

Supervise suicidal-risk pt closely during early therapy (as energy level improves, suicide potential increases). Assess appearance, behavior, speech pattern, level of interest, mood. Monitor daily pattern of bowel activity/stool consistency. Assess skin for rash. Monitor serum hepatic function tests, glucose, sodium, weight.

PATIENT/FAMILY TEACHING

• Maximum therapeutic response may require 4 or more wks of therapy. • Do not abruptly discontinue medication. • Avoid tasks that require alertness, motor skills until response to drug is established. • Avoid alcohol. • To avoid insomnia, take last dose of drug before 4 PM.

fluphenazine hydrochloride (oral)

fluphenazine decanoate (injection)

floo-**fen**-a-zeen

(Apo-Fluphenazine ✤, Modecate ✤, Moditen ✤, Prolixin, Prolixin Decanoate)

Do not confuse Moditen with Modane or Mobidin.

CLASSIFICATION

PHARMACOTHERAPEUTIC: Phenothiazine. **CLINICAL:** Antipsychotic (see p. 62C).

ACTION

Antagonizes dopamine neurotransmission at synapses by blocking postsynaptic dopaminergic receptors in brain. **Therapeutic Effect:** Decreases psychotic behavior. Produces weak anticholinergic, sedative, antiemetic effects; strong extrapyramidal effects.

PHARMACOKINETICS

Erratic absorption. Protein binding: greater than 90%. Metabolized in liver. Excreted in urine. **Half-life:** 33 hrs.

USES

Management of psychotic disturbances (schizophrenia, delusions, hallucinations). **OFF-LABEL:** Treatment of neurogenic pain (adjunct to tricyclic antidepressants).

PRECAUTIONS

CONTRAINDICATIONS: Narrow-angle glaucoma, myelosuppression, severe cardiac/hepatic disease, severe hypertension/hypotension, subcortical brain damage. **CAUTIONS:** Seizures, Parkinson's disease.

LIFESPAN CONSIDERATIONS:

Pregnancy/Lactation: Crosses placenta; distributed in breast milk. **Pregnancy Category C. Children:** Those with acute illnesses (e.g., chickenpox, measles, gastroenteritis, CNS infection) are at risk for developing neuromuscular, extrapyramidal symptoms (EPS), particularly dystonias. **Elderly:** Susceptible to anticholinergic effects.

INTERACTIONS

DRUG: Alcohol, other CNS depressants, may increase hypotensive, CNS, respiratory depressant effects. **Antithyroid agents** may increase risk of agranulocytosis. EPS may increase with **medications producing EPS. Hypotensive agents, antihypertensive medications** may increase hypotension. May decrease effects of **levodopa. Lithium** may decrease absorption, produce adverse neurologic effects. **MAOIs, tricyclic antidepressants** may increase anticholinergic, sedative effects. **Medications prolonging QT interval (e.g., erythromycin)** may have additive effect. **HERBAL:St. John's wort, dong quai** may increase photosensitization. **Gotu kola, kava kava, St. John's wort, valerian** may increase CNS depression. **FOOD:** None known. **LAB VALUES:** May produce false-positive pregnancy, phenylketonuria test results. May cause EKG changes, including Q- and T-wave disturbances.

AVAILABILITY (Rx)

ELIXIR (PROLIXIN): 2.5 mg/5 ml. **INJECTION SOLUTION:** 2.5 mg/ml (Prolixin), 25 mg/ml (Prolixin Decanoate). **ORAL CONCENTRATE (PROLIXIN):** 5 mg/ml. **TABLETS (PROLIXIN):** 1 mg, 2.5 mg, 5 mg, 10 mg.

ADMINISTRATION/HANDLING

- Avoid skin contact with fluphenazine solution (prevents contact dermatitis).

INDICATIONS/ROUTES/DOSAGE

PSYCHOSIS

PO: ADULTS, ELDERLY: 0.5–10 mg/day in divided doses q6–8h.

IM: (DECANOATE) ADULTS, ELDERLY: 2.5–10 mg/day in divided doses q6–8h or 12.5 mg q2wk.

SIDE EFFECTS

FREQUENT: Hypotension, dizziness, syncope (occur frequently after first injection, occasionally after subsequent injections, rarely with oral doses). **OCCASIONAL:** Somnolence (during early therapy), dry mouth, blurred vision, lethargy, constipation or diarrhea, nasal congestion, peripheral edema, urinary retention. **RARE:** Ocular changes, altered skin pigmentation (with prolonged use of high doses).

ADVERSE EFFECTS/ TOXIC REACTIONS

EPS appear dose related (particularly high dosage), divided into 3 categories: akathisia (inability to sit still, tapping of feet, urge to move around), parkinsonian symptoms (hypersalivation, mask-like facial expression, shuffling gait, tremors), acute dystonias (torticollis [neck muscle spasm], opisthotonos [rigidity of back muscles], oculogyric crisis [rolling back of eyes]). Dystonic reaction may produce diaphoresis, pallor. Tardive dyskinesia (tongue protrusion, puffing of cheeks, chewing/puckering of the mouth) occurs rarely but may be irreversible. Abrupt withdrawal after long-term therapy may precipitate dizziness, gastritis, nausea, vomiting, tremors. Blood dyscrasias, particularly agranulocytosis, mild leukopenia, may occur. May lower seizure threshold.

NURSING CONSIDERATIONS

BASELINE ASSESSMENT

Avoid skin contact with solution (contact dermatitis). Assess behavior, appearance, emotional status, response to environment, speech pattern, thought content.

F

INTERVENTION/EVALUATION

Monitor B/P for hypotension. Monitor CBC for blood dyscrasias. Monitor for fine tongue movement (may be early sign of tardive dyskinesia). Supervise suicidal-risk pt closely during early therapy (as depression lessens, energy level improves, increasing suicide potential). Assess for therapeutic response (interest in surroundings, improvement in self-care, increased ability to concentrate, relaxed facial expression).

PATIENT/FAMILY TEACHING

• Full therapeutic effect may take up to 6 wks. • Urine may darken. • Do not abruptly withdraw from long-term drug therapy. • Drowsiness generally subsides during continued therapy. • Avoid tasks that require alertness, motor skills until response to drug is established.

flurandrenolide

(Cordran)

See Corticosteroids: topical (p. 95C)

flurazepam

flure-**az**-e-pam

(Apo-Flurazepam ✤, Dalmane)

Do not confuse Dalmane with Dialume.

◆CLASSIFICATION

PHARMACOTHERAPEUTIC: Benzodiazepine (**Schedule IV**). **CLINICAL:** Sedative-hypnotic (see p. 140C).

ACTION

Enhances action of inhibitory neurotransmitter gamma-aminobutyric acid (GABA). **Therapeutic Effect:** Produces hypnotic effect due to CNS depression.

PHARMACOKINETICS

Route	Onset	Peak	Duration
PO	15–20 min	3–6 hrs	7–8 hrs

Well absorbed from GI tract. Protein binding: 97%. Crosses blood-brain barrier. Widely distributed. Metabolized in liver to active metabolite. Primarily excreted in urine. Not removed by hemodialysis. **Half-life:** 2.3 hrs; metabolite: 40–114 hrs.

USES

Short-term treatment of insomnia (4 wks or less). Reduces sleep-induction time, number of nocturnal awakenings; increases length of sleep.

PRECAUTIONS

CONTRAINDICATIONS: Acute alcohol intoxication, narrow angle glaucoma, hypersensitivity to other benzodiazepines, pregnancy, breast-feeding. **CAUTIONS:** Renal/hepatic impairment.

⧖ LIFESPAN CONSIDERATIONS:

Pregnancy/Lactation: Crosses placenta. May be distributed in breast milk. Chronic ingestion during pregnancy may produce withdrawal symptoms, CNS depression in neonates. **Pregnancy Category X. Children:** Safety and efficacy not established in those younger than 15 yrs. **Elderly:** Use small initial doses with gradual dose increases to avoid ataxia, excessive sedation.

INTERACTIONS

DRUG: **Alcohol, CNS depressants** may increase CNS depression. **Azole antifungals** may increase concentration, risk of toxicity. **HERBAL:** **Gotu kola, kava kava, St. John's wort, valerian** may increase CNS depression. **FOOD:** None known. **LAB VALUES:** None known.

AVAILABILITY (Rx)

CAPSULES: 15 mg, 30 mg.

ADMINISTRATION/HANDLING

PO

• Give without regard to meals. • Capsules may be emptied and mixed with food.

INDICATIONS/ROUTES/DOSAGE

INSOMNIA

PO: **ELDERLY, DEBILITATED, HEPATIC DISEASE, LOW SERUM ALBUMIN:** 15 mg at bedtime. **ADULTS:** 15–30 mg at bedtime. **CHILDREN OLDER THAN 15 YRS:** 15 mg at bedtime.

SIDE EFFECTS

FREQUENT: Drowsiness, dizziness, ataxia, sedation. Morning drowsiness occurs initially. **OCCASIONAL:** GI disturbances, anxiety, blurred vision, dry mouth, headache, confusion, skin rash, irritability, slurred speech. **RARE:** Paradoxical CNS excitement, restlessness (esp. in elderly, debilitated).

ADVERSE EFFECTS/ TOXIC REACTIONS

Abrupt or too-rapid withdrawal after long-term use may result in pronounced restlessness/irritability, insomnia, hand tremors, abdominal/muscle cramps, vomiting, diaphoresis, seizures. Overdose results in drowsiness, confusion, diminished reflexes, coma.

NURSING CONSIDERATIONS

BASELINE ASSESSMENT

Assess B/P, pulse, respirations immediately before administration. Provide safe environment conducive to sleep (back rub, quiet environment, low lighting raise bed rails).

INTERVENTION/EVALUATION

Assess for paradoxical reaction, particularly during early therapy. Evaluate for therapeutic response (decrease in number of nocturnal awakenings, increase in sleep duration).

PATIENT/FAMILY TEACHING

• Smoking reduces drug effectiveness. • Do not abruptly withdraw medication after long-term use. • May have disturbed sleep pattern 1–2 nights after discontinuing. • Notify physician if pregnant or planning to become pregnant (Pregnancy Category X). • Avoid alcohol, other CNS depressants. • May be habit forming.

flurbiprofen

flure-bi-proe-fen

(Apo-Flurbiprofen ✤, Ansaid, Froben ✤, Froben SR ✤, Ocufen)

Do not confuse Ocufen with Ocuflox.

CLASSIFICATION

PHARMACOTHERAPEUTIC: Phenylalkanoic acid. **CLINICAL:** Nonsteroidal anti-inflammatory, antidysmenorrheal (see p. 124C).

ACTION

Produces analgesic, anti-inflammatory effect by inhibiting prostaglandin synthesis. Relaxes iris sphincter. **Therapeutic Effect:** Reduces inflammatory response, intensity of pain. Prevents, decreases miosis during cataract surgery.

PHARMACOKINETICS

Well absorbed from GI tract; ophthalmic solution penetrates cornea after administration (may be systemically absorbed). Protein binding: 99%. Widely distributed. Metabolized in liver. Primarily excreted in urine. **Half-life:** 3–4 hrs.

USES

Oral: Symptomatic treatment of acute and/or chronic rheumatoid arthritis, osteoarthritis, dysmenorrhea, pain. **Ophthalmic:** Inhibits intraoperative miosis. **OFF-LABEL: Oral:** Ankylosing spondylitis, dental pain, postoperative gynecologic pain.

PRECAUTIONS

CONTRAINDICATIONS: Active peptic ulcer; chronic inflammation of GI tract; GI bleeding, ulceration; history of hypersensitivity to aspirin, NSAIDs. **CAUTIONS:** Renal/hepatic impairment, history of GI tract disease, predisposition to fluid retention, soft contact lens wearers, surgical pts with bleeding tendencies.

LIFESPAN CONSIDERATIONS:

Pregnancy/Lactation: Crosses placenta. Unknown whether distributed in breast milk. Avoid use during last trimester (may adversely affect fetal cardiovascular system: premature closure of ductus arteriosus). **Pregnancy Category C (D if used in third trimester or near delivery) Ophthalmic: Pregnancy Category C. Children:** Safety and efficacy not established. **Elderly:** GI bleeding/ulceration more likely to cause serious adverse effects. Age-related renal impairment may increase risk of hepatic/renal toxicity; decreased dosage recommended.

INTERACTIONS

DRUG: May decrease effects of **acetylcholine, carbachol** (with ophthalmic flurbiprofen). May decrease effects of **antihypertensives, diuretics. Aspirin, other salicylates** may increase risk of GI side effects, bleeding. **Bone marrow depressants** may increase risk of hematologic reactions. May decrease antiglaucoma effect of **epinephrine, other antiglaucoma medications.** May increase the effects of **heparin, oral anticoagulants, thrombolytics.** May increase concentration, risk of toxicity of **lithium, cyclosporine.** May increase risk of **methotrexate** toxicity. **Probenecid** may increase concentration. **HERBAL: Cat's claw, dong quai, evening primrose, feverfew, garlic, ginger, ginkgo, red clover, ginseng, horse chestnut, SAMe** may increase antiplatelet activity. **FOOD:** None known. **LAB VALUES:** May increase bleeding time, serum alkaline phosphatase, LDH, AST, ALT.

AVAILABILITY (Rx)

OPHTHALMIC SOLUTION (OCUFEN): 0.03%.

TABLETS (ANSAID): 50 mg, 100 mg.

ADMINISTRATION/HANDLING

PO

• Do not crush, break enteric-coated tablets. • May give with food, milk, antacids if GI distress occurs.

OPHTHALMIC

• Place finger on lower eyelid, pull out until pocket is formed between eye and lower lid. • Hold dropper above pocket, place prescribed number of drops into pocket. Close eye gently. • Apply digital pressure to lacrimal sac for 1–2 min (minimizes drainage into nose/throat, reducing risk of systemic effects). • Remove excess solution with tissue.

INDICATIONS/ROUTES/DOSAGE

RHEUMATOID ARTHRITIS, OSTEOARTHRITIS

PO: ADULTS, ELDERLY: 200–300 mg/day in 2–4 divided doses. **Maximum:** 100 mg/dose or 300 mg/day.

DYSMENORRHEA, PAIN

PO: ADULTS: 50 mg 4 times a day.

USUAL OPHTHALMIC DOSAGE

ADULTS, ELDERLY, CHILDREN: Apply 1 drop q30min starting 2 hrs before surgery for total of 4 doses.

SIDE EFFECTS

OCCASIONAL: PO (9%–3%): Headache, abdominal pain, diarrhea, indigestion, nausea, fluid retention. **Ophthalmic:** Burning/stinging on instillation, keratitis, elevated intraocular pressure. **RARE (less than 3%): PO:** Blurred vision, flushed skin, dizziness, drowsiness, anxiety, insomnia, unusual fatigue, constipation, decreased appetite, vomiting, confusion.

ADVERSE EFFECTS/ TOXIC REACTIONS

Overdose may result in acute renal failure. Rare reactions with long-term use include peptic ulcer, GI bleeding, gastritis, severe hepatic reaction (jaundice), nephrotoxicity (hematuria, dysuria, proteinuria), severe hypersensitivity reaction (angioedema, bronchospasm), cardiac arrhythmias.

NURSING CONSIDERATIONS

BASELINE ASSESSMENT

Anti-inflammatory: Assess onset, type, location, duration of pain/inflammation. Inspect appearance of affected joints for immobility, deformities, skin condition.

INTERVENTION/EVALUATION

Monitor for headache, dyspepsia, dizziness. Monitor daily pattern of bowel activity/stool consistency. **Systemic Use:** Monitor CBC, platelet count, BUN, serum creatinine, hepatic function tests. Monitor stool for occult blood loss. **Ocular:** Periodic eye exams. **Anti-inflammatory:** Evaluate for therapeutic response (relief of pain, stiffness, swelling; increased joint mobility; reduced joint tenderness; improved grip strength).

PATIENT/FAMILY TEACHING

• Swallow tablet whole; do not crush, chew. • Avoid aspirin, alcohol (increases risk of GI bleeding). • If GI upset occurs, take with food, milk. • Report GI distress, visual disturbances, rash, edema, headache. • **Ophthalmic:** Eye burning may occur with instillation.

F

flutamide

flew-tah-myd

(Apo-Flutamide ♣, Euflex ♣, Eulexin, Novo-Flutamide ♣)

Do not confuse flutamide with Flumadine.

CLASSIFICATION

PHARMACOTHERAPEUTIC: Antiandrogen, hormone. **CLINICAL:** Antineoplastic (see p. 79C).

ACTION

Inhibits androgen uptake and/or binding of androgen in target tissue. Used in conjunction with leuprolide to inhibit stimulant effects of flutamide on serum testosterone. **Therapeutic Effect:** Suppresses testicular androgen production, decreases growth of prostate carcinoma.

PHARMACOKINETICS

Completely absorbed from GI tract. Protein binding: 94%–96%. Metabolized in liver to active metabolite. Primarily excreted in urine. Not removed by hemodialysis. **Half-life:** 6 hrs (increased in elderly).

USES

Treatment of metastatic carcinoma of prostate (in combination with luteinizing hormone-releasing hormone [LHRH] analogues, e.g., leuprolide). Management of locally confined stages B_2-C, D_2 carcinoma. **OFF-LABEL:** Female hirsutism.

PRECAUTIONS

CONTRAINDICATIONS: Severe hepatic impairment. **CAUTIONS:** None known.

⌛ LIFESPAN CONSIDERATIONS:

Pregnancy/Lactation: Not used in this pt population. **Pregnancy Category D.** **Children:** Not used in children. **Elderly:** No age-related precautions noted.

INTERACTIONS

DRUG: May increase effects of **oral anticoagulants.** **HERBAL: St. John's wort** may decrease concentration. **FOOD:** None known. **LAB VALUES:** May increase serum glucose, estradiol, testosterone, bilirubin, creatinine, AST, ALT.

AVAILABILITY (Rx)

CAPSULES: 125 mg.

ADMINISTRATION/HANDLING

PO

- Give without regard to food.

INDICATIONS/ROUTES/DOSAGE

PROSTATIC CARCINOMA

PO: ADULTS, ELDERLY: 250 mg q8h.

SIDE EFFECTS

FREQUENT: Hot flashes (50%); decreased libido, diarrhea (24%); generalized pain (23%); asthenia (17%); constipation (12%); nausea, nocturia (11%). **OCCASIONAL (8%–6%):** Dizziness, paresthesia, insomnia, impotence, peripheral edema, gynecomastia. **RARE (5%–4%):** Rash, diaphoresis, hypertension, hematuria, vomiting, urinary incontinence, headache, flu-like syndrome, photosensitivity.

ADVERSE EFFECTS/ TOXIC REACTIONS

Hepatoxicity (including hepatic encephalopathy), hemolytic anemia may be noted.

NURSING CONSIDERATIONS

INTERVENTION/EVALUATION

Periodically monitor hepatic function tests in long-term therapy.

PATIENT/FAMILY TEACHING

• Do not stop taking medication (both drugs must be continued). • Urine color may change to amber or yellow-green. • Avoid prolonged exposure to sun, tanning beds. Wear clothing to protect from ultraviolet exposure until tolerance is determined.

fluticasone

flew-**tih**-cah-sewn

(Cutivate, Flonase, Flovent, Flovent Diskus, Flovent HFA)

FIXED-COMBINATION(S)

Advair: Advair HFA fluticasone/salmeterol (bronchodilator): 100 mcg/50 mcg; 250 mcg/50 mcg; 500 mcg/50 mcg.

CLASSIFICATION

PHARMACOTHERAPEUTIC: Corticosteroid. **CLINICAL:** Anti-inflammatory, antipruritic (see pp. 71C, 92C, 95C).

ACTION

Controls rate of protein synthesis, depresses migration of polymorphonuclear leukocytes, reverses capillary permeability, stabilizes lysosomal membranes. **Therapeutic Effect:** Prevents, controls inflammation.

PHARMACOKINETICS

Inhalation/intranasal: Protein binding: 91%. Undergoes extensive first-pass metabolism in liver. Excreted in urine. **Half-life:** 3–7.8 hrs. **Topical:** Amount absorbed depends on affected area and skin condition (absorption increased with fever, hydration, inflamed or denuded skin).

USES

Nasal: Relief of seasonal/perennial allergic rhinitis. **Topical:** Relief of inflammation/pruritus associated with steroid-responsive disorders (e.g., contact dermatitis, eczema). **Inhalation:** Long-term control of persistent bronchial asthma. Assists in reducing, discontinuing oral corticosteroid therapy.

PRECAUTIONS

CONTRAINDICATIONS: Untreated localized infection of nasal mucosa. **Inhalation:** Primary treatment of status asthmaticus, acute excacerbation of asthma, other acute asthmatic conditions. **CAUTIONS:** Untreated systemic ocular herpes simplex viral infection; untreated fungal, bacterial infection; active or quiescent tuberculosis.

⌛ LIFESPAN CONSIDERATIONS:

Pregnancy/Lactation: Unknown if drug crosses placenta or is distributed in breast milk. **Pregnancy Category C. Children:** Safety and efficacy not established in those younger than 4 yrs. Children 4 yrs and older may experience growth suppression with prolonged or high doses. **Elderly:** No age-related precautions noted.

INTERACTIONS

DRUG: Bupropion may lower seizure threshold. **HERBAL:** None significant. **FOOD:** None known. **LAB VALUES:** None known.

AVAILABILITY (Rx)

AEROSOL FOR ORAL INHALATION (FLOVENT, FLOVENT HFA): 44 mcg/inhalation, 110 mcg/inhalation, 220 mcg/inhalation. **CREAM (CUTIVATE):** 0.05%. **OINTMENT (CUTIVATE):** 0.005%. **POWDER FOR ORAL INHALATION (FLOVENT DISKUS):** 50 mcg, 100 mcg, 250 mcg. **SUSPENSION INTRANASAL SPRAY (FLONASE):** 50 mcg/inhalation.

F

ADMINISTRATION/HANDLING

INHALATION

• Shake container well; exhale as completely as possible. • Place mouthpiece fully into mouth; holding inhaler upright, inhale deeply, slowly while pressing top of canister, hold breath as long as possible before exhaling, then exhale slowly. • Wait 1 min between inhalations when multiple inhalations ordered (allows for deeper bronchial penetration). • Rinse mouth with water immediately after inhalation (prevents mouth/throat dryness).

INTRANASAL

• Clear nasal passages before use (topical nasal decongestants may be needed 5–15 min before use). • Tilt head slightly forward. • Insert spray tip up in 1 nostril, pointing toward inflamed nasal turbinates, away from nasal septum. • Pump medication into 1 nostril while holding other nostril closed, concurrently inspire through nose.

INDICATIONS/ROUTES/DOSAGE

ALLERGIC RHINITIS

INTRANASAL: ADULTS, ELDERLY: Initially, 200 mcg (2 sprays in each nostril once daily or 1 spray in each nostril q12h). Maintenance: 1 spray in each nostril once daily. **Maximum:** 200 mcg/day. **CHILDREN 4 YRS AND OLDER:** Initially, 100 mcg (1 spray in each nostril once daily). **Maximum:** 200 mcg/day.

F

USUAL TOPICAL DOSAGE

TOPICAL: ADULTS, ELDERLY, CHILDREN 3 MOS AND OLDER: Apply sparingly to affected area once or twice a day.

MAINTENANCE TREATMENT FOR ASTHMA (PREVIOUSLY TREATED WITH BRONCHODILATORS)

INHALATION POWDER (FLOVENT DISKUS): ADULTS, ELDERLY, CHILDREN 12 YRS AND OLDER: Initially, 100 mcg q12h. **Maximum:** 500 mcg/day.

INHALATION (ORAL [FLOVENT]): ADULTS, ELDERLY, CHILDREN 12 YRS AND OLDER: 88 mcg twice a day. **Maximum:** 440 mcg twice a day.

MAINTENANCE TREATMENT FOR ASTHMA (PREVIOUSLY TREATED WITH INHALED STEROIDS)

INHALATION POWDER (FLOVENT DISKUS): ADULTS, ELDERLY, CHILDREN 12 YRS AND OLDER: Initially, 100–250 mcg q12h. **Maximum:** 500 mcg q12h.

INHALATION (ORAL [FLOVENT]): ADULTS, ELDERLY, CHILDREN 12 YRS AND OLDER: 88–220 mcg twice a day. **Maximum:** 440 mcg twice a day.

MAINTENANCE TREATMENT FOR ASTHMA (PREVIOUSLY TREATED WITH ORAL STEROIDS)

INHALATION POWDER (FLOVENT DISKUS): ADULTS, ELDERLY, CHILDREN 12 YRS AND OLDER: 500–1,000 mcg twice a day.

INHALATION (ORAL [FLOVENT]): ADULTS, ELDERLY, CHILDREN 12 YRS AND OLDER: 880 mcg twice a day.

SIDE EFFECTS

FREQUENT: Inhalation: Throat irritation, hoarseness, dry mouth, cough, temporary wheezing, oropharyngeal candidiasis (particularly if mouth is not rinsed with water after each administration). **Intranasal:** Mild nasopharyngeal irritation; nasal burning, stinging, dryness; rebound congestion; rhinorrhea; altered sense of taste. **OCCASIONAL: Inhalation:** Oral candidiasis. **Intranasal:** Nasal/pharyngeal candidiasis, headache. **Topical:** Stinging, burning of skin.

ADVERSE EFFECTS/ TOXIC REACTIONS

None known.

NURSING CONSIDERATIONS

BASELINE ASSESSMENT

Establish baseline history of skin disorder, asthma, rhinitis.

INTERVENTION/EVALUATION

Monitor rate, depth, rhythm, type of respiration; quality/rate of pulse. Assess lung sounds for rhonchi, wheezing, rales. Monitor ABGs. Assess oral mucous membranes for evidence of candidiasis. Monitor growth in pediatric pts. **Topical:** Assess involved area for therapeutic response to irritation.

PATIENT/FAMILY TEACHING

• Advise pts receiving bronchodilators by inhalation concomitantly with steroid inhalation therapy to use bronchodilator several min before corticosteroid aerosol (enhances penetration of steroid into bronchial tree). • Do not change dose/schedule or stop taking drug; must taper off gradually under medical supervision. • Maintain fastidious oral hygiene. • Rinse mouth with water immediately after inhalation (prevents mouth/throat dryness, oral fungal infection). • Increase fluid intake (decreases lung secretion viscosity). • **Intranasal:** Teach proper use of nasal spray. • Clear nasal passages before use. • Contact physician if no improvement in symptoms or sneezing/nasal irritation occurs. • Improvement noted in several days. • **Topical:** Rub thin film gently into affected area. • Use only for prescribed area and no longer than ordered. • Avoid contact with eyes.

fluvastatin

flu-vah-**stah**-tin

(Lescol, Lescol XL)

Do not confuse fluvastatin with fluoxetine.

CLASSIFICATION

PHARMACOTHERAPEUTIC: Hydroxamethylglutaryl-CoA (HMG-CoA) reductase inhibitor. **CLINICAL:** Antihyperlipidemic (see p. 56C).

ACTION

Inhibits HMG-CoA reductase, the enzyme that catalyzes the early step in cholesterol synthesis. **Therapeutic Effect:** Decreases LDL cholesterol, VLDL, plasma triglyceride. Slightly increases HDL cholesterol.

PHARMACOKINETICS

Well absorbed from GI tract. Unaffected by food. Does not cross blood-brain barrier. Protein binding: greater than 98%. Primarily eliminated in feces. **Half-life:** 1.2 hrs.

USES

Adjunct to diet therapy to decrease elevated total, LDL cholesterol in those with primary hypercholesterolemia (types IIa, IIb); those with combined hypercholesterolemia and hypertriglyceridemia. Treatment of elevated triglycerides, apolipoprotein; secondary prevention of coronary events.

PRECAUTIONS

CONTRAINDICATIONS: Active hepatic disease, lactation, pregnancy, unexplained increased serum transaminase. **CAUTIONS:** Anticoagulant therapy; history of hepatic disease; substantial alcohol consumption; major surgery; severe acute infection; trauma; hypotension; severe metabolic, endocrine, electrolyte disorders; uncontrolled seizures. Withholding/discontinuing fluvastatin may be necessary when pt is at risk for renal failure (secondary to rhabdomyolysis).

LIFESPAN CONSIDERATIONS:

Pregnancy/Lactation: Contraindicated in pregnancy (suppression of cholesterol biosynthesis may cause fetal toxicity), lactation. Unknown whether drug is distributed in breast milk. **Pregnancy Category X. Children:** Safety and efficacy not established. **Elderly:** No age-related precautions noted.

INTERACTIONS

DRUG: Increased risk of acute renal failure, rhabdomyolysis with **cyclosporine, erythromycin, gemfibrozil, immunosuppressants, niacin. Cholestyramine** may reduce effects. May increase concentration/toxicity of **digoxin. Phenytoin** may increase maximum concentration. **HERBAL: Kava kava, SAMe, St. John's wort, valerian** may increase risk of serotonin syndrome, increase CNS depression. **FOOD:** None Known. **LAB VALUES:** May increase serum creatine kinase (CK), transaminase.

AVAILABILITY (Rx)

CAPSULES (LESCOL): 20 mg, 40 mg.

TABLETS (EXTENDED-RELEASE [LESCOL XL]): 80 mg.

ADMINISTRATION/HANDLING

PO

- Give without regard to food.

INDICATIONS/ROUTES/DOSAGE

HYPERLIPOPROTEINEMIA

PO: ADULTS, ELDERLY: Initially, 20 mg/day (capsule) in the evening. May increase up to 40 mg/day. Maintenance: 20–40 mg/day in a single dose or divided doses. **PATIENTS REQUIRING MORE THAN 25% DECREASE IN LDL CHOLESTEROL:** 40 mg 1–2 times a day or 80 mg tablet once a day.

SIDE EFFECTS

FREQUENT (8%–5%): Headache, dyspepsia, back pain, myalgia, arthralgia, diarrhea, abdominal cramping, rhinitis. **OCCASIONAL (4%–2%):** Nausea, vomiting, insomnia, constipation, flatulence, rash, pruritus, fatigue, cough, dizziness.

F

ADVERSE EFFECTS/ TOXIC REACTIONS

Myositis (inflammation of voluntary muscle) with or without increased CK, muscle weakness, occur rarely. May progress to frank rhabdomyolysis, renal impairment.

NURSING CONSIDERATIONS

BASELINE ASSESSMENT

Question for possibility of pregnancy before initiating therapy (Pregnancy Category X). Assess baseline lab results (serum cholesterol, triglycerides, hepatic function test).

INTERVENTION/EVALUATION

Monitor daily pattern of bowel activity/ stool consistency. Assess for headache, dizziness. Assess for rash, pruritus. Monitor serum cholesterol, triglyceride lab results for therapeutic response. Be alert for malaise, muscle cramping, weakness.

PATIENT/FAMILY TEACHING

• Follow special diet (important part of treatment). • Periodic lab tests are essential part of therapy. • Report promptly any muscle pain/weakness, esp. if accompanied by fever, malaise.

fluvoxamine

floo-**vox**-a-meen
(Luvox)

CLASSIFICATION

PHARMACOTHERAPEUTIC: Serotonin reuptake inhibitor. **CLINICAL:** Antidepressant, antiobsessive (see p. 37C).

ACTION

Selectively inhibits neuronal reuptake of serotonin. **Therapeutic Effect:** Relieves depression, symptoms of obsessive-compulsive disorder (OCD).

PHARMACOKINETICS

Well absorbed following PO administration. Protein binding: 77%. Metabolized in liver. Excreted in urine. **Half-life:** 15.6 hrs.

USES

Treatment of OCD. **OFF-LABEL:** Treatment of anxiety disorders in children, depression, panic disorder.

PRECAUTIONS

CONTRAINDICATIONS: Use within 14 days of MAOIs. **CAUTIONS:** Renal/hepatic impairment, elderly.

LIFESPAN CONSIDERATIONS:

Pregnancy/Lactation: Unknown if drug crosses the placenta; distributed in breast milk. **Pregnancy Category C.** **Children:** Safety and efficacy not established **Elderly:** Potential for reduced serum clearance; maintain caution.

INTERACTIONS

DRUG: May increase concentration, risk of toxicity of **benzodiazepines, carbamazepine, clozapine, theophylline. Cisapride** may increase risk of cardiotoxicity. **Lithium, tryptophan** may enhance fluvoxamine's serotonergic effects. **MAOIs** may produce serious reactions (hyperthermia, rigidity, myoclonus). **Tricyclic antidepressants** may increase concentration. May increase effects of **warfarin.** **HERBAL:** **St. John's wort** may increase pharmacologic effects, risk of toxicity. **FOOD:** None known. **LAB VALUES:** May decrease serum sodium.

AVAILABILITY (Rx)

TABLETS: 25 mg, 50 mg, 100 mg.

INDICATIONS/ROUTES/DOSAGE

OCD

PO: ADULTS: 50 mg at bedtime; may increase by 50 mg every 4–7 days. Dosages greater than 100 mg/day given in 2 divided doses. **Maximum:** 300 mg/day. **CHILDREN 8–17 YRS:** 25 mg at bedtime; may increase by 25 mg every 4–7 days. Dosages greater than 50 mg/day given in 2 divided doses. **Maximum:** 200 mg/day.

SIDE EFFECTS

FREQUENT: Nausea (40%), headache, somnolence, insomnia (22%–21%). **OCCASIONAL (14%–8%):** Dizziness, diarrhea, dry mouth, asthenia, weakness, dyspepsia, constipation, abnormal ejaculation. **RARE (6%–3%):** Anorexia, anxiety, tremor, vomiting, flatulence, urinary frequency, sexual dysfunction, altered taste.

ADVERSE EFFECTS/ TOXIC REACTIONS

Overdose may produce seizures, nausea, vomiting, excessive agitation, extreme restlessness.

NURSING CONSIDERATIONS

INTERVENTION/EVALUATION

Supervise suicidal-risk pt closely during early therapy (as energy level improves, suicide potential increases). Assess appearance, behavior, speech pattern, level of interest, mood. Assist with ambulation if dizziness, somnolence occurs. Monitor daily pattern of bowel activity/stool consistency.

PATIENT/FAMILY TEACHING

• Maximum therapeutic response may require 4 wks or more of therapy. • Dry mouth may be relieved by sugarless gum, sips of tepid water. • Do not abruptly discontinue medication. • Avoid tasks that require alertness, motor skills until response to drug is established.

F

folic acid

(Apo-Folic ✤, Folvite)

foe-lik

Do not confuse Folvite with Florvite.

CLASSIFICATION

PHARMACOTHERAPEUTIC: Coenzyme. **CLINICAL:** Nutritional supplement.

ACTION

Stimulates production of platelets, RBCs, WBCs. **Therapeutic Effect:** Essential for nucleoprotein synthesis, maintenance of normal erythropoiesis.

PHARMACOKINETICS

PO form almost completely absorbed from GI tract (upper duodenum). Protein binding: High. Metabolized in liver and plasma to active form. Excreted in urine. Removed by hemodialysis.

USES

Treatment of megaloblastic and macrocytic anemias due to folate deficiency (e.g., pregnancy, inadequate dietary intake). Supplement to prevent neural tube defects. **OFF-LABEL:** Decrease risk of colon cancer.

PRECAUTIONS

CONTRAINDICATIONS: Anemias (aplastic, normocytic, pernicious, refractory). **CAUTIONS:** None known.

LIFESPAN CONSIDERATIONS:

Pregnancy/Lactation: Distributed in breast milk. **Pregnancy Category A (C if more than recommended daily allowance). Children/Elderly:** No age-related precautions noted.

INTERACTIONS

DRUG: **Analgesics, carbamazepine, estrogens** may increase folic acid requirements. **Antacids, cholestyramine** may decrease absorption. May decrease the effects of **hydantoin anticonvulsants. Methotrexate, triamterene, trimethoprim** may antagonize effects. **HERBAL:** None significant. **FOOD:** None known. **LAB VALUES:** May decrease vitamin B_{12} concentration.

AVAILABILITY (Rx)

INJECTION SOLUTION: 5 mg/ml. **TABLETS:** 0.4 mg (OTC), 0.8 mg (OTC), 1 mg.

ADMINISTRATION/HANDLING

◄ **ALERT** ► Parenteral form used in acutely ill, parenteral/enteral alimentation, those unresponsive to oral route in GI malabsorption syndrome. Dosage greater than 0.1 mg a day may conceal pernicious anemia.

INDICATIONS/ROUTES/DOSAGE

ANEMIA

IM/IV/SUBCUTANEOUS/PO: ADULTS, ELDERLY, CHILDREN 4 YRS AND OLDER: 0.4 mg/day. **CHILDREN YOUNGER THAN 4 YRS:** Up to 0.3 mg/day. **INFANTS:** 0.1 mg/day. **PREGNANT/LACTATING WOMEN:** 0.8 mg/day.

PREVENTION OF NEURAL TUBE DEFECTS

PO: WOMEN OF CHILD-BEARING AGE: 400 mcg/day. **WOMEN AT HIGH RISK OR FAMILY HISTORY OF NEURAL TUBE DEFECTS:** 4 mg/day.

SIDE EFFECTS

None known.

ADVERSE EFFECTS/ TOXIC REACTIONS

Allergic hypersensitivity occurs rarely with parenteral form. Oral folic acid is nontoxic.

NURSING CONSIDERATIONS

BASELINE ASSESSMENT

Pernicious anemia should be ruled out with Schilling test and vitamin B_{12} blood level before initiating therapy (may produce irreversible neurologic damage). Resistance to treatment may occur if decreased hematopoiesis, alcoholism, antimetabolic drugs, deficiency of vitamin B_6, B_{12}, C, E is evident.

INTERVENTION/EVALUATION

Assess for therapeutic improvement: improved sense of well-being, relief from iron deficiency symptoms (fatigue, shortness of breath, sore tongue, headache, pallor).

PATIENT/FAMILY TEACHING

- Eat foods rich in folic acid, including fruits, vegetables, organ meats.

follitropin alpha

(Gonal-F)

See Fertility agents (p. 100C)

fomepizole

(Antizol)

See Appendix M

fondaparinux

fond-dah-**pear**-in-ux
(Arixtra)

CLASSIFICATION

PHARMACOTHERAPEUTIC: Factor Xa inhibitor, pentasaccharide. **CLINICAL:** Antithrombotic.

ACTION

Factor Xa inhibitor and pentasaccharide that selectively binds to antithrombin, and increases its affinity for factor Xa, inhibiting factor Xa, stopping blood coagulation cascade. **Therapeutic Effect:** Indirectly prevents formation of thrombin and subsequently fibrin clot.

PHARMACOKINETICS

Well absorbed after subcutaneous administration. Undergoes minimal, if any, metabolism. Highly bound to antithrombin III. Distributed mainly in blood and to a minor extent in extravascular fluid. Excreted unchanged in urine. Removed by hemodialysis. **Half-life:** 17–21 hrs (prolonged in renal impairment).

USES

Prevention of venous thromboembolism in pts undergoing total hip replacement, hip fracture surgery, knee replacement surgery. Treatment of acute deep vein thrombosis (DVT), acute pulmonary embolism. Used concurrently with warfarin therapy. Prevention of DVT in pts undergoing abdominal surgery.

PRECAUTIONS

CONTRAINDICATIONS: Active major bleeding, bacterial endocarditis, body weight less than 50 kg, severe renal impairment (creatinine clearance less than 30 ml/min), thrombocytopenia associated with antiplatelet antibody formation in presence of fondaparinux. **CAUTIONS:** Conditions with increased risk of hemorrhage (GI ulceration, hemophilia, concurrent use of antiplatelet agents, severe uncontrolled hypertension, history of cerebrovascular accident [CVA]), history of heparin-induced thrombocytopenia, renal impairment, elderly, neuraxial anesthesia, indwelling epidural catheter use.

LIFESPAN CONSIDERATIONS: **Pregnancy/Lactation:** Use with caution, particularly during last trimester, immediate postpartum period (increased risk of maternal hemorrhage). Unknown if excreted in breast milk. **Pregnancy Category B. Children:** Safety and efficacy not established. **Elderly:** Age-related renal impairment may increase risk of bleeding.

INTERACTIONS

DRUG: **Anticoagulants, antiplatelet medications, drotecogin alfa, NSAIDs, thrombolytics, aspirin** may increase risk of bleeding. **HERBAL:** **Cat's claw, dong quai, evening primrose, feverfew, garlic, ginger, ginkgo, red clover, ginseng, horse chestnut, SAMe** may increase antiplatelet activity. **FOOD:** None known. **LAB VALUES:** Reversible increases in serum creatinine, AST, ALT. May decrease Hgb, Hct, platelet count.

AVAILABILITY (Rx)

INJECTION, SOLUTION: 2.5 mg/0.5 ml, 5 mg/0.4 ml, 7.5 mg/0.6 ml, 10 mg/0.8 ml.

ADMINISTRATION/HANDLING

SUBCUTANEOUS

• Parenteral form appears clear, colorless. Discard if discoloration or particulate matter is noted. • Store at room temperature. • Do not expel air bubble from prefilled syringe before injection. • Pinch fold of skin at injection site between thumb and forefinger. Introduce entire length of subcutaneous needle into skin fold during injection. Inject into fatty tissue between left and right anterolateral or left and right posterolateral abdominal wall. • Rotate injection sites.

F

INDICATIONS/ROUTES/DOSAGE

PREVENTION OF VENOUS THROMBOEMBOLISM

SUBCUTANEOUS: ADULTS: 2.5 mg once a day for 5–9 days after surgery. Initial dose should be given 6–8 hrs after surgery. Dosage should be adjusted in elderly and those with renal impairment.

TREATMENT OF VENOUS THROMBOEMBOLISM, PULMONARY EMBOLISM

SUBCUTANEOUS: ADULTS, ELDERLY WEIGHING GREATER THAN 100 KG: 10 mg once daily. **ADULTS, ELDERLY WEIGHING 50–100 KG:** 7.5 mg once daily. **ADULTS, ELDERLY WEIGHING LESS THAN 50 KG:** 5 mg once daily.

DOSAGE IN RENAL IMPAIRMENT

Creatinine clearance 30–50 ml/min: use caution. **Creatinine clearance less than 30 ml/min:** contraindicated.

SIDE EFFECTS

OCCASIONAL (14%): Fever. **RARE (4%–1%):** Injection site hematoma, nausea, peripheral edema.

ADVERSE EFFECTS/ TOXIC REACTIONS

Accidental overdose may lead to bleeding complications ranging from local ecchymoses to major hemorrhage. Thrombocytopenia occurs rarely.

NURSING CONSIDERATIONS

BASELINE ASSESSMENT

Assess CBC, including platelet count, baseline BUN, creatinine clearance.

INTERVENTION/EVALUATION

Periodically monitor CBC, platelet count, stool for occult blood (no need for daily monitoring in pts with normal presurgical coagulation parameters). Assess for any signs of bleeding: bleeding at surgical site, hematuria, blood in stool, bleeding from gums, petechiae, ecchymosis, bleeding from injection sites. Monitor B/P, pulse; hypotension, tachycardia may indicate bleeding, hypovolemia.

PATIENT/FAMILY TEACHING

• Usual length of therapy is 5–9 days. • Do not take any OTC medication (esp. aspirin, NSAIDs). • Consult physician if swelling of hands/feet, unusual back pain, unusual bleeding, bruising, weakness, sudden or severe headache occurs.

formoterol

for-**moe**-ter-ol
(Foradil Aerolizer)

FIXED COMBINATION(S)

Symbicort: formoterol/budesonide. **(glucocorticoid):** 4.5 mcg/80 mcg, 4.5 mcg/160 mcg.

CLASSIFICATION

PHARMACOTHERAPEUTIC: Sympathomimetic (beta$_2$-adrenergic agonist). **CLINICAL:** Bronchodilator (see p. 70C).

ACTION

Stimulates beta$_2$-adrenergic receptors in lungs, resulting in relaxation of bronchial smooth muscle. Inhibits release of mediators from various cells in lungs, including mast cells, with little effect on heart rate. **Therapeutic Effect:** Relieves bronchospasm, reduces airway resistance. Improves bronchodilation, nighttime asthma control, peak flow rates.

PHARMACOKINETICS

Route	Onset	Peak	Duration
Inhalation	1–3 min	0.5–1 hr	12 hrs

Absorbed from bronchi after inhalation. Metabolized in liver. Primarily excreted in urine. Unknown if removed by hemodialysis. **Half-life:** 10 hrs.

USES

For long-term maintenance treatment of asthma, prevention of exercise-induced bronchospasm, treatment of bronchoconstriction in pts with chronic obstructive pulmonary disease (COPD). Can be used concomitantly with short-acting beta-agonists, inhaled or systemic corticosteroids, theophylline therapy.

PRECAUTIONS

CONTRAINDICATIONS: None known. **CAUTIONS:** Hypertension, cardiovascular disease, seizure disorder, thyrotoxicosis. May increase risk of severe excacerbation of asthma.

LIFESPAN CONSIDERATIONS:

Pregnancy/Lactation: Unknown if drug crosses placenta or is distributed in breast milk. **Pregnancy Category C.** **Children:** Safety and efficacy not established in children younger than 5 yrs. **Elderly:** May be more sensitive to tremor, tachycardia due to age-related increased sympathetic sensitivity.

INTERACTIONS

DRUG: **Beta-blockers** may antagonize bronchodilating effects. **Diuretics, steroids, xanthine derivatives** may increase risk of hypokalemia. **Drugs that can prolong QT interval (e.g., erythromycin, quinidine, thioridazine), MAOIs, tricyclic antidepressants** may potentiate cardiovascular effects. **HERBAL:** None significant. **FOOD:** None known. **LAB VALUES:** May decrease serum potassium. May increase serum glucose.

AVAILABILITY (Rx)

INHALATION POWDER IN CAPSULES: 12 mcg.

ADMINISTRATION/HANDLING

INHALATION

• Pull off Aerolizer Inhaler cover, twisting mouthpiece in direction of arrow to open. • Place capsule in chamber. Capsule is pierced by pressing and releasing buttons on side of Aerolizer, once only. • Exhale completely; place mouthpiece into mouth, close lips. • Inhale quickly, deeply through mouth (this causes capsule to spin, dispensing the drug). Hold breath as long as possible before exhaling slowly. • Check capsule to ensure all the powder is gone. If not, inhale again to receive rest of the dose. Rinse mouth with water immediately after inhalation (prevents mouth/throat dryness).

Storage • Maintain capsules in individual blister pack until immediately before use. • Do not swallow capsules. • Do not use with a spacer.

INDICATIONS/ROUTES/DOSAGE

ASTHMA, COPD

INHALATION: ADULTS, ELDERLY, CHILDREN 5 YRS AND OLDER: 12 mcg capsule q12h.

EXERCISE-INDUCED BRONCHOSPASM

INHALATION: ADULTS, ELDERLY, CHILDREN 5 YRS AND OLDER: 12 mcg capsule at least 15 min before exercise. Do not repeat for another 12 hrs.

SIDE EFFECTS

OCCASIONAL: Tremor, muscle cramps, tachycardia, insomnia, headache, irritability, mouth/throat irritation.

ADVERSE EFFECTS/ TOXIC REACTIONS

Excessive sympathomimetic stimulation may produce palpitations, extrasystoles, chest pain.

NURSING CONSIDERATIONS

INTERVENTION/EVALUATION

Assess rate, depth, rhythm, type of respiration; quality/rate of pulse. Monitor EKG, serum potassium, ABG determinations. Assess lung sounds for wheezing (bronchoconstriction), rales.

PATIENT/FAMILY TEACHING

• Instruct pt in proper use of inhaler. • Increase fluid intake (decreases lung secretion viscosity). • Rinsing mouth with water immediately after inhalation may prevent mouth/throat irritation. • Avoid excessive use of caffeine derivatives (chocolate, coffee, tea, cola).

Fortaz, *see ceftazidime*

Fortovase, *see saquinavir*

Fosamax, *see alendronate*

fosamprenavir

foss-am-**pren**-ah-vur
(Lexiva, Telzir ✦)

◆CLASSIFICATION

PHARMACOTHERAPEUTIC: Antiretroviral. **CLINICAL:** Protease inhibitor.

ACTION

Rapidly converted to amprenavir, inhibiting HIV-1 protease by binding to enzyme's active site, preventing processing of viral precursors, forming immature, noninfectious viral particles. **Therapeutic Effect:** Impairs HIV replication, proliferation.

PHARMACOKINETICS

Rapidly absorbed after PO administration. Protein binding: 90%. Metabolized in liver. Excreted in urine, feces. **Half-life:** 7.7 hrs.

USES

Treatment of HIV infection in combination with other antiretroviral agents.

PRECAUTIONS

CONTRAINDICATIONS: Concurrent use of amprenavir, dihydroergotamine, ergonovine, ergotamine, methylergonovine, midazolam, pimozide, triazolam. If fosamprenavir is given concurrently with ritonavir, then flecainide and propafenone are also contraindicated. **EXTREME CAUTION:** Hepatic impairment. **CAUTIONS:** Diabetes mellitus, elderly, renal impairment, known sulfonamide allergy.

⌛ LIFESPAN CONSIDERATIONS:

Pregnancy/Lactation: Unknown if drug crosses placenta or is distributed in breast milk. **Pregnancy Category C.** **Children:** Safety and efficacy not established in children younger than 4 yrs. **Elderly:** Age-related hepatic impairment may require decreased dosage.

INTERACTIONS

DRUG: May interfere with metabolism of **amiodarone, bepridil, ergotamine, lidocaine, midazolam, oral**

contraceptives, quinidine, triazolam, tricyclic antidepressants. Antacids, didanosine may decrease absorption. **Carbamazepine, phenobarbital, phenytoin, rifampin** may decrease concentration. May increase concentrations of **clozapine, hydroxamethylglutaryl-CoA (HMG-CoA) reductase inhibitors (statins), warfarin.** HERBAL: **St. John's wort** may decrease concentration. FOOD: None known. LAB VALUES: May increase serum lipase, triglycerides, AST, ALT.

AVAILABILITY (Rx)

TABLETS: 700 mg (equivalent to 600 mg amprenavir).

ADMINISTRATION/HANDLING

PO

• Give without regard to meals. • Do not crush, break film-coated tablets.

INDICATIONS/ROUTES/DOSAGE

HIV INFECTION WITHOUT PREVIOUS PROTEASE INHIBITOR THERAPY

PO: ADULTS, ELDERLY: 1,400 mg twice daily without ritonavir; or 1,400 mg once daily plus ritonavir 200 mg once daily; or 700 mg twice daily plus ritonavir 100 mg twice daily.

HIV INFECTION WITH PREVIOUS PROTEASE INHIBITOR THERAPY

PO: ADULTS, ELDERLY: 700 mg twice daily plus ritonavir 100 mg twice daily.

CONCURRENT THERAPY WITH EFAVIRENZ

PO: ADULTS, ELDERLY: In pts receiving fosamprenavir plus once-daily ritonavir in combination with efavirenz, an additional 100 mg/day ritonavir (300 mg total/day) should be given.

DOSAGE IN HEPATIC IMPAIRMENT:

Mild to moderate impairment: Reduce fosamprenavir to 700 mg twice daily (without concurrent ritonavir). **Severe impairment:** Not recommended.

SIDE EFFECTS

FREQUENT (39%–35%): Nausea, rash, diarrhea. OCCASIONAL (19%–8%): Headache, vomiting, fatigue, depression. RARE (7%–2%): Pruritus, abdominal pain, perioral paresthesia.

ADVERSE EFFECTS/ TOXIC REACTIONS

Severe or life-threatening dermatologic reactions, including Stevens-Johnson syndrome, occur rarely.

NURSING CONSIDERATIONS

BASELINE ASSESSMENT

Obtain baseline lab testing, esp. hepatic function tests, before beginning therapy and at periodic intervals during therapy. Offer emotional support. Obtain medication history.

INTERVENTION/EVALUATION

Closely monitor for evidence of GI discomfort. Monitor daily pattern of bowel activity/stool consistency. Assess skin for rash. Monitor serum chemistry tests for marked abnormalities, particularly hepatic profile. Assess for opportunistic infections (onset of fever, oral mucosa changes, cough, other respiratory symptoms).

PATIENT/FAMILY TEACHING

• Eat small, frequent meals to offset nausea, vomiting. • Continue therapy for full length of treatment. • Doses should be evenly spaced. • Medication is not a cure for HIV infection, nor does it reduce risk of transmission to others. • Pt may continue to experience illnesses, including opportunistic infections. • Diarrhea can be controlled with OTC medication.

foscarnet

foss-**car**-net
(Foscavir)

CLASSIFICATION

CLINICAL: Antiviral (see p. 65C).

F

ACTION

Selectively inhibits binding sites on virus-specific DNA polymerase, reverse transcriptase. **Therapeutic Effect:** Inhibits replication of herpes virus.

PHARMACOKINETICS

Sequestered into bone, cartilage. Protein binding: 14%–17%. Primarily excreted unchanged in urine. Removed by hemodialysis. **Half-life:** 3.3–6.8 hrs (increased in renal impairment).

USES

Treatment of herpes virus infections suspected to be caused by acyclovir-resistant or ganciclovir-resistant strains. Treatment of cytomegalovirus (CMV) retinitis.

PRECAUTIONS

CONTRAINDICATIONS: None known. **CAUTIONS:** Neurologic/cardiac abnormalities, history of renal impairment, altered calcium, other electrolyte imbalances.

LIFESPAN CONSIDERATIONS:

Pregnancy/Lactation: Unknown if distributed in breast milk. **Pregnancy Category C. Children:** Safety and efficacy not established. **Elderly:** Age-related renal impairment may require dosage adjustment.

INTERACTIONS

DRUG: Nephrotoxic medications may increase risk of renal toxicity. **Pentamidine (IV)** may cause reversible hypocalcemia, hypomagnesemia, nephrotoxicity. **Zidovudine (AZT)** may increase risk of anemia. **HERBAL:** None significant. **FOOD:** None known. **LAB VALUES:** May increase serum alkaline phosphatase, bilirubin, creatinine, AST, ALT. May decrease serum magnesium, potassium. May alter serum calcium, phosphate concentrations.

AVAILABILITY (Rx)

INJECTION SOLUTION: 24 mg/ml.

ADMINISTRATION/HANDLING

IV

Reconstitution • Standard 24 mg/ml solution may be used without dilution when central venous catheter is used for infusion; 24 mg/ml solution *must* be diluted to 12 mg/ml when peripheral vein catheter is being used. • Dilute only with D_5W or 0.9% NaCl solution.

Rate of administration • Because dosage is calculated on body weight, unneeded quantity may be removed before start of infusion to avoid overdosage. Aseptic technique must be used and solution administered within 24 hrs of first entry into sealed bottle. • Do not give by IV injection or rapid infusion (increases toxicity). • Administer by IV infusion at rate not faster than 1 hr for doses up to 60 mg/kg and 2 hrs for doses greater than 60 mg/kg. • To minimize toxicity and phlebitis, use central venous lines or veins with adequate blood flow to permit rapid dilution, dissemination of foscarnet. • Use IV infusion pump to prevent accidental overdose.

Storage • Store parenteral vials at room temperature. • After dilution, stable for 24 hrs at room temperature. • Do not use if solution is discolored or particulate forms.

IV INCOMPATIBILITIES

Acyclovir (Zovirax), amphotericin B (Fungizone), co-trimoxazole (Bactrim), diazepam (Valium), digoxin (Lanoxin), diphenhydramine (Benadryl), dobutamine (Dobutrex), droperidol (Inapsine), ganciclovir (Cytovene), haloperidol (Haldol), leucovorin, midazolam (Versed), pentamidine (Pentam IV), prochlorperazine (Compazine), vancomycin (Vancocin).

IV COMPATIBILITIES

Dopamine (Intropin), heparin, hydromorphone (Dilaudid), lorazepam (Ativan), morphine, potassium chloride, total parenteral nutrition (TPN).

INDICATIONS/ROUTES/DOSAGE

CYTOMEGALOVIRUS (CMV) RETINITIS

IV: ADULTS, ELDERLY: Initially, 60 mg/kg q8h or 100 mg/kg q12h for 2–3 wks. Maintenance: 90–120 mg/kg/day as a single IV infusion.

HERPES INFECTION

IV: ADULTS: 40 mg/kg q8–12h for 2–3 wks or until healed.

DOSAGE IN RENAL IMPAIRMENT

Dosages are individualized based on creatinine clearance. Refer to dosing guide provided by manufacturer.

SIDE EFFECTS

FREQUENT: Fever (65%); nausea (47%); vomiting, diarrhea (30%). **OCCASIONAL (5% or greater):** Anorexia, pain/inflammation at injection site, fever, rigors, malaise, altered B/P, headache, paresthesia, dizziness, rash, diaphoresis, abdominal pain. **RARE (5%–1%):** Back/chest pain, edema, flushing, pruritus, constipation, dry mouth.

ADVERSE EFFECTS/ TOXIC REACTIONS

Nephrotoxicity occurs to some extent in most pts. Seizures, serum mineral/electrolyte imbalances may be life-threatening.

NURSING CONSIDERATIONS

BASELINE ASSESSMENT

Obtain baseline serum mineral and electrolyte levels, vital signs, CBC values, renal function tests. Risk of renal impairment can be reduced by sufficient fluid intake to assure diuresis prior to and during therapy.

INTERVENTION/EVALUATION

Monitor serum creatinine, calcium, phosphorus, potassium, magnesium, Hgb, Hct. Obtain periodic ophthalmologic exams. Assess for signs of serum electrolyte imbalance, esp. hypocalcemia (perioral paresthesia, paresthesia of extremities), hypokalemia (weakness, muscle cramps, paresthesia of extremities, irritability). Monitor renal function tests. Assess for tremors; provide safety measures for potential seizures. Assess for bleeding, anemia, developing superinfections.

PATIENT/FAMILY TEACHING

• Important to report perioral tingling, numbness in extremities, paresthesias during or following infusion (may indicate electrolyte abnormalities). • Tremors should be reported promptly due to potential for seizures.

fosfomycin

foss-fo-**mye**-sin

(Monurol)

Do not confuse Monurol with Monopril.

CLASSIFICATION

PHARMACOTHERAPEUTIC: Antibiotic. **CLINICAL:** UTI agent.

ACTION

Prevents bacterial cell wall formation by inhibiting synthesis of peptidoglycan. **Therapeutic Effect:** Bactericidal.

PHARMACOKINETICS

Rapidly absorbed following PO administration. Not bound to plasma proteins. Not metabolized. Partially excreted in urine; minimal elimination in feces. **Half-life:** 4–8 hrs.

F

USES

Single-dose treatment for uncomplicated UTI in women. **OFF-LABEL:** Serious UTI in men.

PRECAUTIONS

CONTRAINDICATIONS: None known. **CAUTIONS:** Renal impairment.

LIFESPAN CONSIDERATIONS:

Pregnancy/Lactation: Unknown if drug crosses placenta or is distributed is breast milk. **Pregnancy Category B. Children:** Safety and efficacy not established in children younger than 12 yrs. **Elderly:** Age-related renal impairment may require dosage adjustment.

INTERACTIONS

DRUG: **Metoclopramide** lowers concentration, urinary excretion. **HERBAL:** None significant. **FOOD:** None known. **LAB VALUES:** May increase eosinophil count, serum alkaline phosphatase, bilirubin, AST, ALT. May alter platelet, WBC counts. May decrease serum Hct, Hgb levels.

AVAILABILITY (Rx)

POWDER FOR ORAL SOLUTION: 3 g.

ADMINISTRATION/HANDLING

- Give without regard to food.

INDICATIONS/ROUTES/DOSAGE

UTI

PO (UNCOMPLICATED): FEMALES: 3 g mixed in 4 oz water as a single dose.

PO (COMPLICATED): MALES: 3 g/day q2–3days for 3 doses.

SIDE EFFECTS

OCCASIONAL (9%–3%): Diarrhea, nausea, headache, back pain. **RARE (less than 2%):** Dysmenorrhea, pharyngitis, abdominal pain, rash.

ADVERSE EFFECTS/ TOXIC REACTIONS

None known.

NURSING CONSIDERATIONS

PATIENT/FAMILY TEACHING

• Symptoms should improve in 2–3 days. • Always mix medication with water before taking.

fosinopril

fo-**sin**-o-pril

(Monopril, Novo-Fosinopril ✱)

Do not confuse Monopril with Monurol.

CLASSIFICATION

PHARMACOTHERAPEUTIC: Angiotensin-converting enzyme (ACE) inhibitor. **CLINICAL:** Antihypertensive (see p. 7C).

ACTION

Suppresses renin-angiotensin-aldosterone system (prevents conversion of angiotensin I to angiotensin II, a potent vasoconstrictor; may inhibit angiotensin II at local vascular, renal sites). Decreases plasma angiotensin II, increases plasma renin activity, decreases aldosterone secretion. **Therapeutic Effect:** Reduces peripheral arterial resistance, pulmonary capillary wedge pressure; improves cardiac output, exercise tolerance.

PHARMACOKINETICS

Route	Onset	Peak	Duration
PO	1 hr	2–6 hrs	24 hrs

Slowly absorbed from GI tract. Protein binding: 97%–98%. Metabolized in liver and GI mucosa to active metabolite. Primarily excreted in urine. Minimal removal by hemodialysis. **Half-life:** 11.5 hrs.

USES

Treatment of hypertension. Used alone or in combination with other antihypertensives. Treatment of heart failure. **OFF-LABEL:** Treatment of diabetic, nondiabetic nephropathy; post-MI left ventricular dysfunction; renal crisis in scleroderma.

PRECAUTIONS

CONTRAINDICATIONS: History of angioedema from previous treatment with ACE inhibitors. **CAUTIONS:** Renal impairment, those with sodium depletion or on diuretic therapy, dialysis, hypovolemia, coronary/cerebrovascular insufficiency.

⌛ LIFESPAN CONSIDERATIONS:

Pregnancy/Lactation: Crosses placenta. Distributed in breast milk. May cause fetal or neonatal mortality or morbidity. **Pregnancy Category C (D if used in second or third trimester). Children:** Safety and efficacy not established. Neonates, infants may be at increased risk for oliguria, neurologic abnormalities. **Elderly:** May be more sensitive to hypotensive effects.

INTERACTIONS

DRUG: Alcohol, diuretics, antihypertensive agents may increase effect. **NSAIDs** may decrease effect. **Potassium-sparing diuretics, potassium supplements** may cause hyperkalemia. May increase **lithium** concentration/toxicity. **HERBAL: Ephedra, ginseng, yohimbe** may worsen hypertension. **Garlic** may increase antihypertensive effect. **Licorice** may cause sodium/water retention, loss of potassium. **FOOD:** None known. **LAB VALUES:** May increase BUN, serum alkaline phosphatase, bilirubin, creatinine, potassium, AST, ALT. May decrease serum sodium. May cause positive antinuclear antibody titer (ANA).

F

AVAILABILITY (Rx)

TABLETS: 10 mg, 20 mg, 40 mg.

ADMINISTRATION/HANDLING

PO

• Give without regard to food. • Tablets may be crushed.

INDICATIONS/ROUTES/DOSAGE

HYPERTENSION

PO: ADULTS, ELDERLY: Initially, 10 mg/day. Maintenance: 20–40 mg/day as a single or 2 divided doses. **Maximum:** 80 mg/day. **CHILDREN 6–16 YRS WEIGHING MORE THAN 50 KG:** Initially, 5–10 mg/day.

HEART FAILURE

PO: ADULTS, ELDERLY: Initially, 10 mg/day. Maintenance: 20–40 mg/day. **Maximum:** 40 mg/day.

SIDE EFFECTS

FREQUENT (12%–9%): Dizziness, cough. **OCCASIONAL (4%–2%):** Hypotension, nausea, vomiting, upper respiratory tract infection.

ADVERSE EFFECTS/ TOXIC REACTIONS

Excessive hypotension ("first-dose syncope") may occur in pts with CHF, severely salt/volume depleted. Angioedema (swelling of face/lips), hyperkalemia occur rarely. Agranulocytosis, neutropenia may be noted in those with renal impairment, collagen vascular disease (scleroderma, systemic lupus erythematosus). Nephrotic syndrome may be noted in those with history of renal disease.

NURSING CONSIDERATIONS

BASELINE ASSESSMENT

Obtain B/P immediately before each dose, in addition to regular monitoring (be alert to fluctuations). Renal function tests should be performed before beginning therapy. In pts with renal impairment, autoimmune disease, or taking drugs that affect leukocytes or immune response, CBC, differential count should be performed before therapy begins and q2wks for 3 mos, then periodically thereafter.

INTERVENTION/EVALUATION

If excessive reduction in B/P occurs, place pt in supine position with legs elevated. Assist with ambulation if dizziness occurs. Assess for urinary frequency. Auscultate lung sounds for rales, wheezing in those with CHF. Monitor urinalysis for proteinuria. Monitor serum potassium in those on concurrent diuretic therapy.

PATIENT/FAMILY TEACHING

• Report any sign of infection (sore throat, fever). • Several wks may be needed for full therapeutic effect of B/P reduction. • Skipping doses or voluntarily discontinuing drug may produce severe, rebound hypertension. • To reduce hypotensive effect, rise slowly from lying to sitting position, permit legs to dangle from bed momentarily before standing. • Inform physician if vomiting, excessive perspiration, persistent cough develops.

fosphenytoin

fos-phen-ih-**toyn**

(Cerebyx)

Do not confuse Cerebyx with Celebrex or Celexa.

CLASSIFICATION

PHARMACOTHERAPEUTIC: Hydantoin. **CLINICAL:** Anticonvulsant (see p. 34C).

ACTION

Stabilizes neuronal membranes, limits spread of seizure activity. Decreases sodium, calcium ion influx into neurons. Decreases post-tetanic potentiation, repetitive discharge. **Therapeutic Effect:** Decreases seizure activity.

PHARMACOKINETICS

Completely absorbed after IM administration. Protein binding: 95%–99%. Rapidly and completely hydrolyzed to phenytoin after IM or IV administration. Time of complete conversion to phenytoin: 4 hrs after IM injection; 2 hrs after IV infusion. **Half-life:** 8–15 min (for conversion to phenytoin).

USES

Acute treatment, control of generalized convulsive status epilepticus; prevention, treatment of seizures occurring during neurosurgery; short-term substitution of oral phenytoin.

PRECAUTIONS

CONTRAINDICATIONS: Adams-Stokes syndrome; hypersensitivity to ethotoin, phosphenytoin, phenytoin, mephenytoin; second- or third-degree AV block; severe bradycardia; SA block. **CAUTIONS:** Porphyria, hypotension, severe myocardial insufficiency, renal/hepatic disease, hypoalbuminemia.

LIFESPAN CONSIDERATIONS:

Pregnancy/Lactation: May increase frequency of seizures during pregnancy. Increased risk of congenital malformations. Unknown if excreted in breast milk. **Pregnancy Category D.** **Children:** Safety not established. **Elderly:** Lower dosage recommended.

INTERACTIONS

DRUG: **Alcohol, other CNS depressants** may increase CNS depression. **Amiodarone, anticoagulants, cimetidine, disulfiram, fluoxetine, isoniazid, sulfonamides** may increase concentration, effects, risk of toxicity. **Antacids** may decrease absorption. **Fluconazole, ketoconazole, miconazole** may increase concentration. May decrease effects of **glucocorticoids. Lidocaine, propranolol** may increase cardiac depressant effects. **Valproic acid** may increase concentration, decrease metabolism. May increase metabolism of **xanthines.** **HERBAL:** None significant. **FOOD:** None known. **LAB VALUES:** May increase serum glucose, GGT, alkaline phosphatase.

AVAILABILITY (Rx)

INJECTION SOLUTION: 75 mg/ml (equivalent to 50 mg/ml phenytoin).

ADMINISTRATION/HANDLING

IV

Reconstitution • Dilute in D_5W or 0.9% NaCl to a concentration ranging from 1.5–25 mg PE/ml.

Rate of administration • Administer at rate less than 150 mg PE/min (decreases risk of hypotension, arrhythmias).

Storage • Refrigerate. Do not store at room temperature for longer than 48 hrs. • After dilution, solution is stable for 8 hrs at room temperature or 24 hrs if refrigerated.

IV INCOMPATIBILITY

Midazolam (Versed).

IV COMPATIBILITIES

Lorazepam (Ativan), phenobarbital, potassium chloride.

INDICATIONS/ROUTES/DOSAGE

◀ **ALERT** ▶ 150 mg fosphenytoin yields 100 mg phenytoin. Dosage, concentration solution, infusion rate of fosphenytoin are expressed in terms of phenytoin equivalents (PE).

STATUS EPILEPTICUS

IV: ADULTS: Loading dose: 15–20 mg PE/kg infused at rate of 100–150 mg PE/min.

NONEMERGENT SEIZURES

IV, IM: ADULTS: Loading dose: 10–20 mg PE/kg. Maintenance: 4–6 mg PE/kg/day.

SHORT-TERM SUBSTITUTION FOR ORAL PHENYTOIN

IV, IM: ADULTS: May substitute for oral phenytoin at same total daily dose.

SIDE EFFECTS

FREQUENT: Dizziness, paresthesia, tinnitus, pruritus, headache, somnolence. **OCCASIONAL:** Morbilliform rash.

ADVERSE EFFECTS/ TOXIC REACTIONS

Too high fosphenytoin blood concentration may produce ataxia (muscular incoordination), nystagmus (rhythmic oscillation of eyes), diplopia, lethargy, slurred speech, nausea, vomiting, hypotension. As drug level increases, extreme lethargy may progress to coma.

NURSING CONSIDERATIONS

BASELINE ASSESSMENT

Review history of seizure disorder (intensity, frequency, duration, level of consciousness [LOC]). Initiate seizure precautions. Obtain vital signs, medication history (esp. use of phenytoin, other anticonvulsants). Observe clinically.

INTERVENTION/EVALUATION

Monitor EKG, measure cardiac function, respiratory function, B/P during and immediately following infusion (10–20 min). Discontinue if skin rash appears.

Interrupt or decrease rate if hypotension, arrhythmias are detected. Assess pt postinfusion (may feel dizzy, ataxic, drowsy). Assess blood levels of fosphenytoin (2 hrs post IV infusion or 4 hrs post IM injection).

PATIENT/FAMILY TEACHING

• Teach pt about his seizure condition and role in its management. • If noncompliance is an issue in causing acute seizures, discuss and address reasons for noncompliance. • Avoid tasks that require alertness, motor skills until response to drug is established.

Fragmin, *see dalteparin*

frovatriptan

fro-va-**trip**-tan

(Frova)

CLASSIFICATION

PHARMACOTHERAPEUTIC: Serotonin receptor agonist. **CLINICAL:** Antimigraine (see p. 60C).

ACTION

Binds selectively to vascular receptors, producing vasoconstrictive effect on cranial blood vessels. **Therapeutic Effect:** Relieves migraine headache.

PHARMACOKINETICS

Well absorbed after PO administration. Metabolized by liver to inactive metabolite. Eliminated in urine. **Half-life:** 26 hrs (increased in hepatic impairment).

USES

Treatment of acute migraine headache with or without aura in adults.

PRECAUTIONS

CONTRAINDICATIONS: Basilar or hemiplegic migraine, cerebrovascular or peripheral vascular disease, coronary artery disease, ischemic heart disease (angina pectoris, history of MI, silent ischemia, Prinzmetal's angina), severe hepatic impairment (Child-Pugh grade C), uncontrolled hypertension, use within 24 hrs of ergotamine-containing preparations or another serotonin receptor agonist, use within 14 days of MAOIs. **CAUTIONS:** Mild to moderate hepatic impairment, pt profile suggesting cardiovascular risks.

LIFESPAN CONSIDERATIONS:

Pregnancy/Lactation: Unknown if drug is excreted in breast milk. **Pregnancy Category C.** **Children:** Safety and efficacy not established. **Elderly:** Not recommended in the elderly.

INTERACTIONS

DRUG: **Ergotamine-containing medications** may produce vasospastic reaction. **Fluoxetine, fluvoxamine, paroxetine, sertraline** may produce weakness, hyperreflexia, uncoordination. **Oral contraceptives** decrease frovatriptan clearance, volume of distribution. **Propranolol** may dramatically increase plasma concentration. **HERBAL:** None significant. **FOOD:** None known. **LAB VALUES:** None known.

AVAILABILITY (Rx)

TABLETS: 2.5 mg.

ADMINISTRATION/HANDLING

PO

• Do not crush, chew film-coated tablets.

INDICATIONS/ROUTES/DOSAGE

ACUTE MIGRAINE HEADACHE

PO: ADULTS, ELDERLY: Initially 2.5 mg. If headache improves but then returns, dose may be repeated after 2 hrs. **Maximum:** 7.5 mg/day.

SIDE EFFECTS

OCCASIONAL (8%–4%): Dizziness, paresthesia, fatigue, flushing. **RARE (3%–2%):** Hot/cold sensation, dry mouth, dyspepsia (heartburn, epigastric distress).

ADVERSE EFFECTS/ TOXIC REACTIONS

Cardiac reactions (ischemia, coronary artery vasospasm, MI), noncardiac vasospasm-related reactions (cerebral hemorrhage, cerebrovascular accident [CVA]), occur rarely, particularly in pts with hypertension, obesity, smokers, diabetes, strong family history of coronary artery disease; males older than 40 yrs; postmenopausal women.

NURSING CONSIDERATIONS

BASELINE ASSESSMENT

Question for history of peripheral vascular disease, renal/hepatic impairment, possibility of pregnancy. Question regarding onset, location, duration of migraine, possible precipitating symptoms.

INTERVENTION/EVALUATION

Assess for relief of migraine headache, potential for photophobia, phonophobia (sound sensitivity), nausea, vomiting.

PATIENT/FAMILY TEACHING

• Take a single dose as soon as symptoms of an actual migraine attack appear. • Medication is intended to relieve migraine headaches, not to prevent or reduce number of attacks. • Avoid tasks that require alertness, motor skills until response to drug is established. • Contact physician immediately if palpitations, pain, tightness in chest or throat, sudden or severe abdominal pain, pain or weakness of extremities occurs.

fulvestrant

full-**ves**-trant

(Faslodex)

Do not confuse Faslodex with Fosamax.

CLASSIFICATION

PHARMACOTHERAPEUTIC: Estrogen antagonist. **CLINICAL:** Antineoplastic (see p. 79C).

ACTION

Competes with endogenous estrogen at estrogen receptor binding sites. **Therapeutic Effect:** Inhibits tumor growth.

PHARMACOKINETICS

Extensively, rapidly distributed after IM administration. Protein binding: 99%. Metabolized in liver. Eliminated by hepatobiliary route; excreted in feces. **Half-life:** 40 days in postmenopausal women. Peak serum levels occur in 7–9 days.

USES

Treatment of hormone receptor–positive metastatic breast cancer in postmenopausal women with disease progression following antiestrogen therapy. **OFF-LABEL:** Endometriosis, uterine bleeding.

PRECAUTIONS

CONTRAINDICATIONS: Known or suspected pregnancy. **CAUTIONS:** Thrombocytopenia, bleeding diathesis, anticoagulant therapy, hepatic disease, reduced hepatic blood flow, estrogen receptor–negative breast cancer.

LIFESPAN CONSIDERATIONS:

Pregnancy/Lactation: Do not administer to pregnant women. Unknown if excreted in breast milk. May cause fetal harm. **Pregnancy Category D. Children:** Not for use in children. **Elderly:** No age-related precautions noted.

INTERACTIONS

DRUG: None significant. **HERBAL:** None significant. **FOOD:** None known. **LAB VALUES:** None known.

F

AVAILABILITY (Rx)

INJECTION, SOLUTION: 50 mg/ml in 2.5-ml and 5-ml syringes.

ADMINISTRATION/HANDLING

IM

• Administer slowly into upper, outer quadrant or ventro-gluteal area of buttock as a single 5-ml injection or 2 concurrent 2.5-ml injections.

INDICATIONS/ROUTES/DOSAGE

BREAST CANCER

IM: ADULTS, ELDERLY: 250 mg given once monthly.

SIDE EFFECTS

FREQUENT (26%–13%): Nausea, hot flashes, pharyngitis, asthenia (loss of strength, energy), vomiting, vasodilatation, headache. **OCCASIONAL (12%–5%):** Injection site pain, constipation, diarrhea, abdominal pain, anorexia, dizziness, insomnia, paresthesia, bone/back pain, depression, anxiety, peripheral edema, rash, diaphoresis, fever. **RARE (2%–1%):** Vertigo, weight gain.

ADVERSE EFFECTS/ TOXIC REACTIONS

UTI occurs occasionally. Vaginitis, anemia, thromboembolic phenomena, leukopenia occur rarely.

NURSING CONSIDERATIONS

BASELINE ASSESSMENT

Estrogen receptor assay should be done before beginning therapy. Baseline CT should be performed initially and periodically thereafter for evidence of tumor regression.

INTERVENTION/EVALUATION

Monitor blood chemistry, plasma lipids. Be alert to increased bone pain, ensure adequate pain relief. Check for edema, esp. of dependent areas. Monitor for and assist with ambulation if asthenia or dizziness occurs. Assess for headache. Offer antiemetic for nausea/vomiting.

PATIENT/FAMILY TEACHING

• Notify physician if nausea/vomiting, asthenia, hot flashes become unmanageable.

furosemide

feur-**oh**-sah-mide

(Apo-Furosemide ✱, Lasix, Novo-Semide ✱)

Do not confuse Lasix with Lidex, Luvox, or Luxiq, or furosemide with Torsemide.

CLASSIFICATION

PHARMACOTHERAPEUTIC: Loop. **CLINICAL:** Diuretic (see p. 97C).

ACTION

Enhances excretion of sodium, chloride, potassium by direct action at ascending limb of loop of Henle. **Therapeutic Effect:** Produces diuresis, lowers B/P.

PHARMACOKINETICS

Route	Onset	Peak	Duration
PO	30–60 min	1–2 hrs	6–8 hrs
IV	5 min	20–60 min	2 hrs
IM	30 min	N/A	N/A

Well absorbed from GI tract. Protein binding: 91%–97%. Partially metabolized in liver. Primarily excreted in urine (nonrenal clearance increases in severe renal impairment). Not removed by hemodialysis. **Half-life:** 30–90 min (increased in renal/hepatic impairment, neonates).

USES

Treatment of edema associated with CHF, chronic renal failure (including nephrotic syndrome), hepatic cirrhosis, acute pulmonary edema. Treatment of hypertension, either alone or in combination with other antihypertensives. **OFF-LABEL:** Treatment of hypercalcemia.

PRECAUTIONS

CONTRAINDICATIONS: Anuria, hepatic coma, severe electrolyte depletion. **CAUTIONS:** Hepatic cirrhosis.

LIFESPAN CONSIDERATIONS:

Pregnancy/Lactation: Crosses placenta. Distributed in breast milk. **Pregnancy Category C. Children:** Half-life increased in neonates; may require increased dosage interval. **Elderly:** May be more sensitive to hypotensive, electrolyte effects, developing circulatory collapse, thromboembolic effect. Age-related renal impairment may require dosage adjustment.

INTERACTIONS

DRUG: **Amphotericin B, nephrotoxic, ototoxic medications** may increase risk of nephrotoxicity, ototoxicity. May decrease the effects of **anticoagulants, heparin.** May increase risk of **lithium** toxicity. **Other medications causing hypokalemia** may increase risk of hypokalemia. **Probenecid** may increase concentration. **HERBAL:** None significant. **FOOD:** None known. **LAB VALUES:** May increase serum glucose, BUN, uric acid. May decrease serum calcium, chloride, magnesium, potassium, sodium.

AVAILABILITY (Rx)

INJECTION, SOLUTION: 10 mg/ml. **ORAL SOLUTION:** 10 mg/ml, 40 mg/5 ml. **TABLETS:** 20 mg, 40 mg, 80 mg.

F

ADMINISTRATION/HANDLING

IV

Rate of administration • May give undiluted but is compatible with D_5W, 0.9% NaCl, or lactated Ringer's solutions. • Administer each 40 mg or fraction by IV push over 1–2 min. Do not exceed administration rate of 4 mg/min in those with renal impairment.

Storage • Solution appears clear, colorless. • Discard yellow solutions.

IM

• Temporary pain at injection site may be noted.

PO

• Give with food to avoid GI upset, preferably with breakfast (may prevent nocturia).

IV INCOMPATIBILITIES

Ciprofloxacin (Cipro), diltiazem (Cardizem), dobutamine (Dobutrex), dopamine (Intropin), doxorubicin (Adriamycin), droperidol (Inapsine), esmolol (Brevibloc), famotidine (Pepcid), filgrastim (Neupogen), fluconazole (Diflucan), gemcitabine (Gemzar), gentamicin (Garamycin), idarubicin (Idamycin), labetalol (Trandate), meperidine (Demerol), metoclopramide (Reglan), midazolam (Versed), milrinone (Primacor), nicardipine (Cardene), ondansetron (Zofran), quinidine, thiopental (Pentothal), vecuronium (Norcuron), vinblastine (Velban), vincristine (Oncovin), vinorelbine (Navelbine).

IV COMPATIBILITIES

Aminophylline, amiodarone (Cordarone), bumetanide (Bumex), calcium gluconate, cimetidine (Tagamet), heparin, hydromorphone (Dilaudid), lidocaine, lipids, morphine, nitroglycerin, norepinephrine (Levophed), potassium chloride, propofol (Diprivan).

F

INDICATIONS/ROUTES/DOSAGE

EDEMA, HYPERTENSION

PO: ADULTS, ELDERLY: Initially, 20–80 mg/dose; may increase by 20–40 mg/dose q6–8h. May titrate up to 600 mg/day in severe edematous states. **CHILDREN:** 1–6 mg/kg/day in divided doses q6–12h. **NEONATES:** 1–4 mg/kg/dose 1–2 times a day.

IV, IM: ADULTS, ELDERLY: 20–40 mg/dose; may increase by 20 mg/dose q1–2h. **Maximum Single Dose:** 160–200 mg. **CHILDREN:** 1–2 mg/kg/dose q6–12h. **Maximum:** 6 mg/kg/dose. **NEONATES:** 1–2 mg/kg/dose q12–24h.

IV INFUSION: ADULTS, ELDERLY: Bolus of 0.1 mg/kg, followed by infusion of 0.1 mg/kg/hr; may double q2h. **Maximum:** 0.4 mg/kg/hr. **CHILDREN:** 0.05 mg/kg/hr; titrate to desired effect.

SIDE EFFECTS

EXPECTED: Increased urinary frequency/volume. **FREQUENT:** Nausea, dyspepsia, abdominal cramps, diarrhea or constipation, electrolyte disturbances. **OCCASIONAL:** Dizziness, light-headedness, headache, blurred vision, paresthesia, photosensitivity, rash, fatigue, bladder spasm, restlessness, diaphoresis. **RARE:** Flank pain.

ADVERSE EFFECTS/ TOXIC REACTIONS

Vigorous diuresis may lead to profound water loss/electrolyte depletion, resulting in hypokalemia, hyponatremia, dehydration. Sudden volume depletion may result in increased risk of thrombosis, circulatory collapse, sudden death. Acute hypotensive episodes may occur, sometimes several days after beginning therapy. Ototoxicity (deafness, vertigo, tinnitus) may occur, esp. in pts with severe renal impairment. Can exacerbate diabetes mellitus, systemic lupus erythematosus, gout, pancreatitis. Blood dyscrasias have been reported.

NURSING CONSIDERATIONS

BASELINE ASSESSMENT

Check vital signs, esp. B/P for hypotension before administration. Assess baseline serum electrolytes, esp. for hypokalemia. Assess skin turgor, mucous membranes for hydration status; observe for edema. Assess muscle strength, mental status. Note skin temperature, moisture. Obtain baseline weight. Initiate I&O monitoring.

INTERVENTION/EVALUATION

Monitor B/P, vital signs, serum electrolytes, I&O, weight. Note extent of diuresis. Watch for changes from initial assessment (hypokalemia may result in changes in muscle strength, tremor, muscle cramps, altered in mental status, cardiac arrhythmias). Hyponatremia may result in confusion, thirst, cold/clammy skin.

PATIENT/FAMILY TEACHING

• Expect increased frequency, volume of urination. • Report palpitations, signs of electrolyte imbalances (noted previously), hearing abnormalities (sense of fullness in ears, tinnitus). • Eat foods high in potassium such as whole grains (cereals), legumes, meat, bananas, apricots, orange juice, potatoes (white, sweet), raisins. • Avoid sunlight, sunlamps.

gabapentin

gah-bah-**pen**-tin
(Apo-Gabapentin ♣, Neurontin, Novo-Gabapentin ♣)

Do not confuse Neurontin with Neoral, Noroxin.

CLASSIFICATION

CLINICAL: Anticonvulsant, antineuralgic (see p. 34C).

ACTION

May increase synthesis or accumulation of gamma-aminobutyric acid (GABA) by binding to as-yet-undefined receptor sites in brain tissue. **Therapeutic Effect:** Reduces seizure activity, neuropathic pain.

PHARMACOKINETICS

Well absorbed from GI tract (not affected by food). Protein binding: less than 5%. Widely distributed. Crosses blood-brain barrier. Primarily excreted unchanged in urine. Removed by hemodialysis. **Half-life:** 5–7 hrs (increased in renal impairment, elderly).

USES

Adjunct in treatment of partial seizures in children 12 yrs and older and adults (with or without secondary generalized seizures, partial seizures in children 3–12 yrs); adjunct in treatment of neuropathic pain, postherpetic neuralgia. **OFF-LABEL:** Treatment of bipolar disorder, chronic pain, diabetic peripheral neuropathy, essential tremor, hot flashes, hyperhidrosis, migraines, psychiatric disorders (social phobia), agitation in dementia.

PRECAUTIONS

CONTRAINDICATIONS: None known. **CAUTIONS:** Renal impairment.

LIFESPAN CONSIDERATIONS:

Pregnancy/Lactation: Unknown whether it is distributed in breast milk. **Pregnancy Category C. Children:** Safety and efficacy not established in those 3 yrs and younger. **Elderly:** Age-related renal impairment may require dosage adjustment.

INTERACTIONS

DRUG: **Antacids** decrease absorption. **Morphine** may increase CNS depression. **HERBAL:** **Evening primrose** may decrease seizure threshold. **Gotu kola, kava kava, St. John's wort, valerian** may increase CNS depression. **FOOD:** None known. **LAB VALUES:** May decrease serum WBC count.

AVAILABILITY (Rx)

CAPSULES (NEURONTIN): 100 mg, 300 mg, 400 mg. **ORAL SOLUTION (NEURONTIN):** 250 mg/5 ml. **TABLETS (NEURONTIN):** 100 mg, 300 mg, 400 mg, 600 mg, 800 mg.

ADMINISTRATION/HANDLING

PO

• Give without regard to meals; may give with food to avoid, reduce GI upset. • If treatment is discontinued or anticonvulsant therapy is added, do so gradually over at least 1 wk (reduces risk of loss of seizure control).

INDICATIONS/ROUTES/DOSAGE

ADJUNCTIVE THERAPY FOR SEIZURE CONTROL

PO: ADULTS, ELDERLY, CHILDREN OLDER THAN 12 YRS: Initially, 300 mg 3 times a day. May titrate dosage. Range: 900–1,800 mg/day in 3 divided doses. **Maximum:** 3,600 mg/day. **CHILDREN 3–12 YRS:** Initially, 10–15 mg/kg/day in 3 divided doses. May titrate up to 25–35 mg/kg/day (for children 5–12 yrs) and 40 mg/kg/day (for children 3–4 yrs). **Maximum:** 50 mg/kg/day.

ADJUNCTIVE THERAPY FOR NEUROPATHIC PAIN

PO: ADULTS, ELDERLY: Initially, 100 mg 3 times a day; may increase by 300 mg/day

G

at weekly intervals. **Maximum:** 3,600 mg/day in 3 divided doses. **CHILDREN:** Initially, 5 mg/kg/dose at bedtime, followed by 5 mg/kg/dose for 2 doses on day 2, then 5 mg/kg/dose for 3 doses on day 3. Range: 8–35 mg/kg/day in 3 divided doses.

POSTHERPETIC NEURALGIA

PO: ADULTS, ELDERLY: 300 mg on day 1, 300 mg twice a day on day 2, and 300 mg 3 times a day on day 3. Titrate up to 1,800 mg/day.

DOSAGE IN RENAL IMPAIRMENT

Dosage and frequency are modified based on creatinine clearance:

Creatinine Clearance	Dosage
60 ml/min or higher	300–1,200 mg tid
30–59 ml/min	200–700 mg q12h
16–29 ml/min	200–700 mg/day
Less than 16 ml/min	100–300 mg/day
Hemodialysis	125–300 mg after each 4-hr hemodialysis session

SIDE EFFECTS

FREQUENT (19%–10%): Fatigue, drowsiness, dizziness, ataxia. **OCCASIONAL (8%–3%):** Nystagmus (rapid eye movements), tremor, diplopia (blurred vision) rhinitis, weight gain. **RARE (less than 2%):** Anxiety, dysarthria (speech difficulty), memory loss, dyspepsia, pharyngitis, myalgia.

ADVERSE EFFECTS/ TOXIC REACTIONS

Abrupt withdrawal may increase seizure frequency. Overdosage may result in slurred speech, drowsiness, lethargy, diarrhea.

NURSING CONSIDERATIONS

BASELINE ASSESSMENT

Review history of seizure disorder (type, onset, intensity, frequency, duration, level of consciousness [LOC]). Routine laboratory monitoring of serum levels unnecessary for safe use.

INTERVENTION/EVALUATION

Provide safety measures as needed. Monitor seizure frequency/duration, renal function, weight, behavior in children.

PATIENT/FAMILY TEACHING

• Take gabapentin only as prescribed; do not abruptly stop taking drug (may increase seizure frequency). • Avoid tasks that require alertness, motor skills until response to drug is established. • Avoid alcohol. • Carry identification card/bracelet to note seizure disorder/ anticonvulsant therapy.

galantamine

gal-**an**-tah-mine

(Razadyne, Razadyne ER)

Do not confuse Razadyne with Rozerem.

◆CLASSIFICATION

PHARMACOTHERAPEUTIC: Cholinesterase inhibitor. **CLINICAL:** Antidementia.

ACTION

Elevates acetylcholine concentrations by slowing degeneration of acetylcholine released by still intact cholinergic neurons (Alzheimer's disease involves degeneration of cholinergic neuronal pathways). **Therapeutic Effect:** Slows progression of Alzheimer's disease.

PHARMACOKINETICS

Rapidly absorbed from GI tract. Protein binding: 18%. Distributed to blood cells; binds to plasma proteins, mainly albumin. Metabolized in liver. Excreted in urine. **Half-life:** 7 hrs.

USES

Treatment of mild to moderate dementia of Alzheimer's type.

PRECAUTIONS

CONTRAINDICATIONS: Severe hepatic renal impairment. **CAUTIONS:** Moderate renal/hepatic impairment, history of ulcer disease, those on concurrent NSAIDs, asthma, chronic obstructive pulmonary disease (COPD), bladder outflow obstruction, supraventricular cardiac conduction conditions.

LIFESPAN CONSIDERATIONS:

Pregnancy/Lactation: Unknown if drug crosses placenta or is distributed in breast milk. **Pregnancy Category B. Children:** Not prescribed for this pt population. **Elderly:** No age-related precautions noted, but use is not recommended in those with severe hepatic/renal impairment (creatinine clearance less than 9 ml/min).

INTERACTIONS

DRUG: May interfere with the effects of **bethanechol, succinylcholine. Cimetidine, erythromycin, ketoconazole, paroxetine** may increase concentration. **HERBAL: St. John's wort** may decrease concentration. **FOOD:** None known. **LAB VALUES:** None known.

AVAILABILITY (Rx)

ORAL SOLUTION (RAZADYNE): 4 mg/ml. **TABLETS (RAZADYNE):** 4 mg, 8 mg, 12 mg.

CAPSULES (EXTENDED-RELEASE [RAZADYNE ER]): 8 mg, 16 mg, 24 mg.

ADMINISTRATION/HANDLING

PO

- Give with morning and evening meals.

INDICATIONS/ROUTES/DOSAGE

ALZHEIMER'S DISEASE

PO: ADULTS, ELDERLY: Initially, 4 mg twice a day (8 mg/day). After a minimum of 4 wks (if well tolerated), may increase to 8 mg twice a day (16 mg/day). After another 4 wks, may increase to 12 mg twice daily (24 mg/day). Range: 16–24 mg/day in 2 divided doses.

PO (EXTENDED-RELEASE): ADULTS, ELDERLY: Initially, 8 mg once daily for 4 wks; then increase to 16 mg once daily for 4 wks or longer. If tolerated, may increase to 24 mg once daily. **Range:** 16–24 mg once daily.

DOSAGE IN RENAL IMPAIRMENT

For moderate impairment, maximum dosage is 16 mg/day. Drug is not recommended for pts with severe impairment.

SIDE EFFECTS

FREQUENT (17%–5%): Nausea, vomiting, diarrhea, anorexia, weight loss. **OCCASIONAL (9%–4%):** Abdominal pain, insomnia, depression, headache, dizziness, fatigue, rhinitis. **RARE (less than 3%):** Tremors, constipation, confusion, cough, anxiety, urinary incontinence.

ADVERSE EFFECTS/ TOXIC REACTIONS

Overdose may cause cholinergic crisis (increased salivation, lacrimation, urination, defecation, bradycardia, hypotension, muscle weakness). Treatment aimed at generally supportive measures, use of anticholinergics (e.g., atropine).

NURSING CONSIDERATIONS

BASELINE ASSESSMENT

Assess cognitive, behavioral, functional deficits of pt. Assess serum hepatic/renal function tests.

INTERVENTION/EVALUATION

Monitor cognitive, behavioral, functional status of pt. Evaluate EKG, periodic rhythm strips in pts with underlying arrhythmias. Assess for evidence of GI disturbances (nausea, vomiting, diarrhea, anorexia, weight loss).

G

PATIENT/FAMILY TEACHING

• Take with morning and evening meals (reduces risk of nausea). • Avoid tasks that require alertness, motor skills until response to drug is established. • Report persistent GI disturbances, excessive salivation, diaphoresis, excessive tearing, excessive fatigue, insomnia, depression, dizziness, increased muscle weakness.

G

Gamimune N, *see immune globulin IV*

Gammagard S/D, *see immune globulin IV*

Gammar-P IV, *see immune globulin IV*

ganciclovir

gan-**sy**-clo-ver

(Cytovene, Vitrasert)

Do not confuse Cytovene with Cytosar.

✦CLASSIFICATION

PHARMACOTHERAPEUTIC: Synthetic nucleoside. **CLINICAL:** Antiviral (see p. 65C).

ACTION

Competes with viral DNA polymerase and incorporation into growing viral DNA chains. **Therapeutic Effect:** Interferes with DNA synthesis, viral replication.

PHARMACOKINETICS

Widely distributed. Protein binding: 1%–2%. Undergoes minimal metabolism. Excreted unchanged primarily in urine. Removed by hemodialysis. **Half-life:** 2.5–3.6 hrs (increased in renal impairment).

USES

Parenteral: Treatment of cytomegalovirus (CMV) retinitis in immunocompromised pts (e.g., HIV), prophylaxis of CMV infection in transplant pts. **Oral:** Maintenance treatment of CMV retinitis. **Implant:** Treatment of CMV retinitis. **OFF-LABEL:** Treatment of other CMV infections (gastroenteritis, hepatitis, pneumonitis).

PRECAUTIONS

CONTRAINDICATIONS: Absolute neutrophil count less than 500/mm^3, platelet count less than 25,000/mm^3, hypersensitivity to acyclovir, ganciclovir, immunocompetent pts, pts with congenital or neonatal CMV disease. **CAUTIONS:** Pts with neutropenia, thrombocytopenia, renal impairment; children (long-term safety not determined due to potential for long-term carcinogenic, adverse reproductive effects).

⌛ LIFESPAN CONSIDERATIONS:

Pregnancy/Lactation: Effective contraception should be used during therapy; ganciclovir should not be used during pregnancy. Breast-feeding should be discontinued; may be resumed no sooner than 72 hrs after the last dose of ganciclovir. **Pregnancy Category C.** **Children:** Safety and efficacy not established in those younger than 12 yrs. **Elderly:** Age-related renal impairment may require dosage adjustment.

INTERACTIONS

DRUG: Bone marrow depressants may increase myelosuppression. **Imipenem/cilastatin** may increase risk of seizures. **Nephrotoxic medications** may increase risk of renal impairment, increase concentration/toxicity. **Zidovudine (AZT)** may increase risk of hepatotoxicity. **HERBAL:** None significant. **FOOD:** None known. **LAB VALUES:** May increase serum alkaline phosphatase, bilirubin, AST, ALT.

AVAILABILITY (Rx)

CAPSULES (CYTOVENE): 250 mg, 500 mg. **IMPLANT (VITRASERT):** 4.5 mg. **INJECTION, POWDER FOR RECONSTITUTION (CYTOVENE):** 500 mg.

ADMINISTRATION/HANDLING

IV

Reconstitution • Reconstitute 500-mg vial with 10 ml Sterile Water for Injection to provide concentration of 50 mg/ml; do **not** use Bacteriostatic Water (contains parabens, which is incompatible with ganciclovir). • Further dilute with 100 ml D_5W, 0.9% NaCl, lactated Ringer's, or any combination thereof to provide a concentration of 5 mg/ml.

Rate of administration • Administer only by IV infusion over 1 hr. • Do not give by IV push or rapid IV infusion (increases risk of toxicity); protect from infiltration (high pH causes severe tissue irritation). • Use large veins to permit rapid dilution, dissemination of ganciclovir (minimizes phlebitis); central venous ports may reduce catheter-associated infection.

Storage • Store vials at room temperature. Do not refrigerate. • Reconstituted solution in vial is stable for 12 hrs at room temperature. • After dilution, refrigerate, use within 24 hrs. • Discard if precipitate forms, discoloration occurs. • Avoid exposure to skin, eyes, mucous membranes. • Use latex gloves, safety glasses during preparation/handling of solution. • Avoid inhalation. • If solution contacts skin or mucous membranes, wash thoroughly with soap and water; rinse eyes thoroughly with plain water.

PO

• Give with food.

IV INCOMPATIBILITIES

Aldesleukin (Proleukin), amifostine (Ethyol), aztreonam (Azactam), cefepime (Maxipime), cytarabine (ARA-C), doxorubicin (Adriamycin), fludarabine (Fludara), foscarnet (Foscavir), gemcitabine (Gemzar), lipids, ondansetron (Zofran), piperacillin and tazobactam (Zosyn), sargramostim (Leukine), total parenteral nutrition (TPN), vinorelbine (Navelbine).

IV COMPATIBILITIES

Amphotericin B, enalapril (Vasotec), filgrastim (Neupogen), fluconazole (Diflucan), propofol (Diprivan).

INDICATIONS/ROUTES/DOSAGE

CMV RETINITIS

IV: ADULTS, CHILDREN 3 MOS AND OLDER: 10 mg/kg/day in divided doses q12h for 14–21 days, then 5 mg/kg/day as a single daily dose or 6 mg/kg 5 days a wk.
PO: ADULTS, ELDERLY: 1,000 mg 3 times/day or 500 mg 6 times/day.

PREVENTION OF CMV DISEASE IN TRANSPLANT PTS

IV: ADULTS, CHILDREN: 10 mg/kg/day in divided doses q12h for 7–14 days, then 5 mg/kg/day as a single daily dose.

OTHER CMV INFECTIONS

IV: ADULTS: Initially, 10 mg/kg/day in divided doses q12h for 14–21 days, then 5 mg/kg/day as a single daily dose. Maintenance: 1,000 mg 3 times a day or 500 mg q3h (6 times a day). **CHILDREN:** Initially, 10 mg/kg/day in divided doses q12h for 14–21 days, then 5 mg/kg/day as a single daily dose. Maintenance: 30 mg/kg/dose q8h.
INTRAVITREAL IMPLANT: ADULTS: 1 implant q6–9mo plus oral ganciclovir. **CHILDREN 9 YRS AND OLDER:** 1 implant

q6–9mo plus oral ganciclovir (30 mg/dose q8h).

ADULT DOSAGE IN RENAL IMPAIRMENT

Dosage and frequency are modified based on creatinine clearance.

CrCl	Induction Dosage	Maintenance Dosage	Oral
50–69 ml/min	2.5 mg/kg q12h	2.5 mg/kg q24h	1,500 mg/day
25–49 ml/min	2.5 mg/kg q24h	1.25 mg/kg q24h	1,000 mg/day
10–24 ml/min	1.25 mg/kg q24h	0.625 mg/kg q24h	500 mg/day
Less than 10 ml/min	1.25 mg/kg 3 times/wk	0.625 mg/kg 3 times/wk	500 mg 3 times/wk

CrCl = creatinine clearance

SIDE EFFECTS

FREQUENT: Diarrhea (41%), fever (40%), nausea (25%), abdominal pain (17%), vomiting (13%). **OCCASIONAL (11%–6%):** Diaphoresis, infection, paresthesia, flatulence, pruritus. **RARE (4%–2%):** Headache, stomatitis, dyspepsia, phlebitis.

ADVERSE EFFECTS/ TOXIC REACTIONS

Hematologic toxicity occurs commonly: leukopenia (41%–29%), anemia (25%–19%). Intraocular implant occasionally results in visual acuity loss, vitreous hemorrhage, retinal detachment. GI hemorrhage occurs rarely.

NURSING CONSIDERATIONS

BASELINE ASSESSMENT

Evaluate hematologic baseline. Obtain specimens for support of differential diagnosis (urine, feces, blood, throat) because retinal infection is usually due to hematogenous dissemination.

INTERVENTION/EVALUATION

Monitor I&O, ensure adequate hydration (minimum 1,500 ml/24 hrs). Diligently evaluate hematology reports for neutropenia, thrombocytopenia, decreased platelets. Question pt regarding visual acuity, therapeutic improvement, complications. Assess for rash, pruritus.

PATIENT/FAMILY TEACHING

• Ganciclovir provides suppression, not cure, of CMV retinitis. • Frequent blood tests, eye exams are necessary during therapy because of toxic nature of drug. • Report any new symptom promptly. • May temporarily or permanently inhibit sperm production in men, suppress fertility in women. • Barrier contraception should be used during and for 90 days after therapy because of mutagenic potential.

ganirelix

(Antagon)

See Fertility agents (p. 101C)

garlic

Also known as ail, allium, nectar of the gods, poor man's treacle, stinking rose.

CLASSIFICATION

HERBAL: See Appendix G.

ACTION

Possesses antithrombotic properties, can increase fibrinolytic activity, decrease platelet aggregation, increase PT. Acts as HMG-CoA reductase inhibitor (statins). **Effect:** Lowers serum cholesterol. Causes smooth muscle relaxation/vasodilation , reducing B/P. Reduces oxidative stress and LDL oxidation, preventing age-related vascular changes, atherosclerosis. Prevents endothelial cell depletion, producing antioxidant effect.

USES

Treatment of hypertension, hyperlipidemia; prevention of coronary artery disease, age-related vascular changes, atherosclerosis.

PRECAUTIONS

CONTRAINDICATIONS: Pts with bleeding disorders. **CAUTIONS:** Diabetes (may decrease blood glucose levels), inflammatory GI conditions (may irritate GI tract). Hypothyroidism (may reduce iodine uptake). May prolong bleeding time (discontinue 1–2 wks before surgery).

LIFESPAN CONSIDERATIONS:

Pregnancy/Lactation: **Caution:** May stimulate labor and cause colic in infants. **Children:** Safety and efficacy not established (may be beneficial in children with hypercholesterolemia). **Elderly:** No age-related precautions noted.

INTERACTIONS

DRUG: May enhance effects of **anticoagulants, antiplatelets** (e.g., **aspirin, clopidogrel, enoxaparin, warfarin).** May decrease effects of **cyclosporine, oral contraceptives. Insulin, oral antidiabetic agents** may increase hypoglycemic effects. **Saquinavir, other antiretrovirals** may decrease concentration, effect of garlic. **HERBAL: Feverfew, ginger, ginkgo, ginseng** may increase risk of bleeding. **FOOD:** None known. **LAB VALUES:** May decrease serum glucose, cholesterol. May increase INR.

AVAILABILITY (OTC)

CAPSULES: 100 mg, 300 mg, 500 mg, 1,000 mg, 1.5 g. **EXTRACT. OIL. POWDER. TABLETS:** 400 mg, 1,250 mg. **TEA.**

INDICATIONS/ROUTES/DOSAGE

HYPERLIPIDEMIA, HYPERTENSION

PO (CAPSULES, POWDER, TEA): ADULTS, ELDERLY: 600–1,200 mg a day in divided doses 3 times a day.

◀ **ALERT** ▶ Appropriate doses for other conditions vary depending on the preparation used.

SIDE EFFECTS

Breath/body odor, oropharyngeal/esophageal burning, heartburn, nausea, vomiting, diarrhea, allergic reactions (rhinitis, urticaria, angioedema).

ADVERSE EFFECTS/ TOXIC REACTIONS

None known.

NURSING CONSIDERATIONS

BASELINE ASSESSMENT

Assess serum lipid levels, determine whether pt is taking anticoagulants, antiplatelets. Assess if diabetic, taking insulin or oral hypoglycemic agents.

INTERVENTION/EVALUATION

Monitor CBC, coagulation studies, serum lipid, glucose levels. Assess for hypersensitivity reaction, contact dermatitis.

PATIENT/FAMILY TEACHING

• Avoid use in pregnancy or breastfeeding. • Inform all health care providers of garlic use. • Discontinue 1–2 wks before any procedure in which excessive bleeding may occur.

gefitinib

geh-**fih**-tih-nib
(Iressa)

CLASSIFICATION

PHARMACOTHERAPEUTIC: Epidermal growth factor receptor antibody. **CLINICAL:** Antineoplastic.

G

ACTION

Blocks signaling pathway that binds to epidermal growth factor receptor (EGFR) on surface of normal and cancer cells. EGFR activates the enzyme tyrosine kinase, which sends signals instructing cells to grow. **Therapeutic Effect:** Inhibits growth signal within the cancer cell.

PHARMACOKINETICS

Slowly absorbed, extensively distributed throughout the body. Protein binding: 90%. Undergoes extensive metabolism in liver. Excreted in feces. **Half-life:** 48 hrs.

USES

Treatment in pts with locally advanced or metastatic non–small cell lung cancer after failure of platinum-based and docetaxel chemotherapies.

PRECAUTIONS

CONTRAINDICATIONS: None known. **CAUTIONS:** Severe renal impairment, hepatic impairment.

LIFESPAN CONSIDERATIONS:

Pregnancy/Lactation: Has potential to cause fetal harm, potential abortifacient. Substitute formula feedings for breast-feedings. Those with child-bearing potential should use contraceptive methods during treatment and up to 12 mos following therapy. **Pregnancy Category D.** **Children:** Safety and efficacy not established. **Elderly:** No age-related precautions noted.

INTERACTIONS

DRUG: **Cimetidine, phenytoin, ranitidine, rifampin** may decrease concentration/effectiveness. **Itraconazole, ketoconazole** increase gefitinib concentration. Increases effect of **metoprolol. Warfarin** increases risk of bleeding. **HERBAL:** None significant. **FOOD:** **Grapefruit, grapefruit juice** may increase concentration. **LAB VALUES:** May increase serum alkaline phosphatase, bilirubin, AST, ALT.

AVAILABILITY (Rx)

TABLETS: 250 mg.

ADMINISTRATION/HANDLING

PO

• Give without regard to food. • Do not crush, break film-coated tablet. • For pts unable to swallow, or to give via G-tube: • Drop whole tablet in ½ glass water. Do not crush. • Stir until dispersed (10 min). • Drink immediately, rinse with ½ glass water or administer via G-tube, flush with 50 ml water.

INDICATIONS/ROUTES/DOSAGE

NON-SMALL CELL LUNG CANCER

PO: ADULTS, ELDERLY: 250 mg/day; may increase to 500 mg/day for pts receiving drugs that may decrease gefitinib blood concentrations (e.g., rifampin, phenytoin).

SIDE EFFECTS

FREQUENT (48%–25%): Diarrhea, rash, acne. **OCCASIONAL (13%–8%):** Dry skin, nausea, vomiting, pruritus. **RARE (7%–2%):** Anorexia, asthenia, weight loss, peripheral edema, eye pain.

ADVERSE EFFECTS/ TOXIC REACTIONS

Pancreatitis, ocular hemorrhage occur rarely. Hypersensitivity reaction produces angioedema, urticaria. Interstitial lung disease has been reported.

NURSING CONSIDERATIONS

BASELINE ASSESSMENT

Antiemetics, antidiarrheals may be effective in preventing and treating nausea, vomiting, diarrhea. Pts with poorly tolerated diarrhea may be helped by briefly interrupting drug therapy (up to 14 days).

INTERVENTION/EVALUATION

Encourage adequate fluid intake. Assess bowel sounds for hyperactivity. Monitor daily pattern of bowel activity/stool consistency. Assess skin for rash. Assess hepatic function test results.

PATIENT/FAMILY TEACHING

• Do not have immunizations without physician's approval (drug lowers resistance). • Avoid crowds, persons with known infections. • Report signs of infection at once (fever, flu-like symptoms). • Contact physician if severe or persistent diarrhea, nausea, vomiting, anorexia occurs. • Avoid pregnancy during therapy.

gemcitabine

gem-**cih**-tah-bean
(Gemzar)

CLASSIFICATION

PHARMACOTHERAPEUTIC: Antimetabolite. **CLINICAL:** Antineoplastic (see p. 79C).

ACTION

Inhibits ribonucleotide reductase, the enzyme necessary for catalyzing DNA synthesis. **Therapeutic Effect:** Produces death of cells undergoing DNA synthesis.

PHARMACOKINETICS

Not extensively distributed after IV infusion (increased with length of infusion). Protein binding: less than 10%. Excreted primarily in urine as metabolite. **Half-life:** 42–94 min (influenced by gender of pt, duration of infusion).

USES

Metastatic breast cancer in combination with paclitaxel. Treatment of locally advanced (stage II, III) or metastatic (stage IV) adenocarcinoma of pancreas. Indicated for pts previously treated with 5-fluorouracil. Monotherapy or in combination with cisplatin for treatment for locally advanced or metastatic non–small cell lung cancer, ovarian cancer. **OFF-LABEL:** Treatment of biliary tract carcinoma, bladder carcinoma, gall bladder carcinoma, germ cell tumors (e.g., testicular), Hodgkin's lymphoma, non-Hodgkin's lymphoma.

PRECAUTIONS

CONTRAINDICATIONS: None known. **CAUTIONS:** Renal/hepatic impairment.

LIFESPAN CONSIDERATIONS:

Pregnancy/Lactation: If possible, avoid use during pregnancy, esp. first trimester. May cause fetal harm. Unknown if distributed in breast milk. Breast-feeding not recommended. **Pregnancy Category D. Children:** Safety and efficacy not established. **Elderly:** Increased risk of hematologic toxicity.

INTERACTIONS

DRUG: Bone marrow depressants may increase the risk of myelosuppression. **Immunosuppressants (e.g., cyclosporine, tacrolimus)** may increase risk of infection. **Live virus vaccines** may potentiate virus replication, increase vaccine side effects, decrease pt's antibody response to vaccine. **HERBAL:** None significant. **FOOD:** None known. **LAB VALUES:** May increase BUN, serum alkaline phosphatase, bilirubin, creatinine, AST, ALT.

AVAILABILITY (Rx)

INJECTION, POWDER FOR RECONSTITUTION: 200 mg, 1-g vials.

ADMINISTRATION/HANDLING

IV

Reconstitution • Use gloves when handling/preparing gemcitabine. • Reconstitute 200-mg or 1-g vial with 0.9% NaCl injection without preservative (5 ml or 25 ml, respectively) to provide concentration of 40 mg/ml. • Shake to dissolve.

Rate of administration • May give without further dilution. • May be further diluted with 0.9% NaCl to a

concentration as low as 0.1 mg/ml.
• Infuse over 30 min.

Storage • Store at room temperature (refrigeration may cause crystallization). • Reconstituted solution is stable for 24 hrs at room temperature.

IV INCOMPATIBILITIES
Acyclovir (Zovirax), amphotericin B (Fungizone), cefoperazone (Cefobid), furosemide (Lasix), ganciclovir (Cytovene), imipenem and cilastatin (Primaxin), irinotecan (Camptosar), methotrexate, methylprednisolone (Solu-Medrol), mitomycin (Mutamycin), piperacillin/tazobactam (Zosyn), prochlorperazine (Compazine).

IV COMPATIBILITIES
Bumetanide (Bumex), calcium gluconate, dexamethasone (Decadron), diphenhydramine (Benadryl), dobutamine (Dobutrex), dopamine (Intropin), granisetron (Kytril), heparin, hydrocortisone (Solu-Cortef), lorazepam (Ativan), ondansetron (Zofran), potassium.

INDICATIONS/ROUTES/DOSAGE
◀ **ALERT** ▶ Dosage is individualized based on clinical response, tolerance to adverse effects. When used in combination therapy, consult specific protocols for optimum dosage, sequence of drug administration.

BREAST CANCER
IV: ADULTS, ELDERLY: 1,250 mg/m^2 over 30 min on days 1 and 8 of each 21-day cycle.

NON–SMALL CELL LUNG CANCER
IV: ADULTS, ELDERLY, CHILDREN: 1,000 mg/m^2 on days 1, 8, and 15, repeated every 28 days; or 1,250 mg/m^2 on days 1 and 8. Repeat every 21 days.

OVARIAN CANCER
IV: ADULTS, ELDERLY: 1,000 mg/m^2 on days 1 and 8 of each 21-day cycle (in combination with carboplatin).

PANCREATIC CANCER
IV: ADULTS: 1,000 mg/m^2 once weekly for up to 7 wks or until toxicity necessitates decreasing dosage or withholding the dose, followed by 1 wk of rest. Subsequent cycles should consist of once-weekly dose for 3 consecutive wks out of every 4 wks. For pts completing cycles at 1,000 mg/m^2, increase dose to 1,250 mg/m^2 as tolerated. Dose for next cycle may be increased to 1,500 mg/m^2.

DOSAGE REDUCTION GUIDELINES
PANCREATIC CANCER, NON–SMALL CELL LUNG CANCER: Dosage adjustments should be based on granulocyte count and platelet count, as follows:

Absolute Granulocyte Counts (cells/mm^3)	Platelet Count (cells/mm^3)	% of Full Dose
1,000 and	100,000	100
500–999 or	50,000–99,000	75
Less than 500 or	Less than 50,000	Hold

BREAST CANCER

Absolute Granulocyte Counts (cells/mm^3)	Platelet Count (cells/mm^3)	% of Full Dose
Equal to or greater than 1,200 and	Greater than 75,000	100
1,000–1,199 or	50,000–75,000	75
700–999 and	Equal to or greater than 50,000	50
Less than 700	Less than 50,000	Hold

OVARIAN CANCER

Absolute Granulocyte Counts (cells/mm^3)	Platelet Count (cells/mm^3)	% of Full Dose
1,500 or greater and	100,000 or greater	100
1,000–1,499	and/or 75,000–99,999	50
Less than 1,000	and/or less than 75,000	Hold

SIDE EFFECTS

FREQUENT: Nausea, vomiting (69%); generalized pain (48%); fever (41%); mild to moderate pruritic rash (30%); mild to moderate dyspnea, constipation (23%); peripheral edema (20%). **OCCASIONAL (19%–10%):** Diarrhea, petechiae, alopecia, stomatitis, infection, somnolence, paresthesia. **RARE:** Diaphoresis, rhinitis, insomnia, malaise.

ADVERSE EFFECTS/ TOXIC REACTIONS

Severe myelosuppression (anemia, thrombocytopenia, leukopenia) occurs commonly.

NURSING CONSIDERATIONS

BASELINE ASSESSMENT

CBC, renal/hepatic function tests should be performed before starting therapy and periodically thereafter. Drug should be suspended or dosage modified if myelosuppression is detected.

INTERVENTION/EVALUATION

Assess all lab results before giving each dose. Monitor for dyspnea, fever, pruritic rash, dehydration. Assess oral mucosa for erythema, ulceration at inner margin of lips, sore throat, difficulty swallowing (stomatitis). Assess skin for rash. Monitor for, report diarrhea. Provide antiemetics as needed.

PATIENT/FAMILY TEACHING

• Avoid crowds, exposure to infection. • Maintain fastidious oral hygiene. • Promptly report fever, sore throat, signs of local infection, easy bruising, rash. • Contact physician if nausea or vomiting continues at home.

gemfibrozil

gem-**fi**-broe-zil

(Apo-Gemfibrozil ✤, Lopid, Novo-Gemfibrozil ✤)

Do not confuse Lopid with Lorabid or Levbid.

◆ CLASSIFICATION

PHARMACOTHERAPEUTIC: Fibric acid derivative. **CLINICAL:** Antihyperlipoproteinemic (see p. 55C).

ACTION

Inhibits lipolysis of fat in adipose tissue; decreases hepatic uptake of free fatty acids (reduces hepatic triglyceride production). Inhibits synthesis of VLDL carrier apolipoprotein B. **Therapeutic Effect:** Lowers serum cholesterol, triglycerides (decreases VLDL, LDL; increases HDL).

PHARMACOKINETICS

Well absorbed from GI tract. Protein binding: 99%. Metabolized in liver. Primarily excreted in urine. Not removed by hemodialysis. **Half-life:** 1.5 hrs.

USES

Treatment of hypertriglyceridemia in types IV and V hyperlipidemia for pts who are at greater risk for pancreatitis and those who have not responded to dietary intervention.

PRECAUTIONS

CONTRAINDICATIONS: Hepatic dysfunction (including primary biliary cirrhosis), preexisting gallbladder disease, severe renal dysfunction. **CAUTIONS:** Hypothyroidism, diabetes mellitus, estrogen or anticoagulant therapy.

⧖ LIFESPAN CONSIDERATIONS:

Pregnancy/Lactation: Unknown if drug crosses placenta or is distributed in breast milk. Decision to discontinue nursing or drug should be based on potential for serious adverse effects. **Pregnancy Category C. Children:** Not recommended in those younger than 2 yrs (cholesterol necessary for normal development). **Elderly:** Age-related renal impairment may require dosage adjustment.

G

INTERACTIONS

DRUG: Lovastatin may cause rhabdomyolysis, leading to acute renal failure. May increase effect of **pioglitazone, repaglinide, warfarin**. **HERBAL:** None significant. **FOOD:** None known. **LAB VALUES:** May increase serum alkaline phosphatase, bilirubin, creatinine kinase, LDH, AST, ALT. May decrease Hgb, Hct, leukocyte counts, serum potassium.

AVAILABILITY (Rx)

TABLETS: 600 mg.

ADMINISTRATION/HANDLING

PO

• Give 30 min before morning and evening meals.

INDICATIONS/ROUTES/DOSAGE

HYPERLIPIDEMIA

PO: ADULTS, ELDERLY: 1,200 mg/day in 2 divided doses 30 min before breakfast and dinner.

SIDE EFFECTS

FREQUENT (20%): Dyspepsia. **OCCASIONAL (10%–2%):** Abdominal pain, diarrhea, nausea, vomiting, fatigue. **RARE (less than 2%):** Constipation, acute appendicitis, vertigo, headache, rash, pruritus, altered taste.

ADVERSE EFFECTS/ TOXIC REACTIONS

Cholelithiasis, cholecystitis, acute appendicitis, pancreatitis, malignancy occur rarely.

NURSING CONSIDERATIONS

BASELINE ASSESSMENT

Assess baseline lab results: serum glucose, triglyceride, cholesterol, hepatic function tests; CBC.

INTERVENTION/EVALUATION

Determine daily pattern of bowel activity/stool consistency. Monitor LDL, VLDL, serum triglyceride, cholesterol lab results for therapeutic response. Assess for rash, pruritus. Check for headache, dizziness. Monitor hepatic function, hematology tests. Assess for pain, esp. right upper quadrant or epigastric pain suggestive of adverse gallbladder effects. Monitor serum glucose for those receiving insulin, oral antihyperglycemics.

PATIENT/FAMILY TEACHING

• Follow special diet (important part of treatment). • Take before meals. • Periodic lab tests are essential part of therapy. • Notify physician if dizziness, blurred vision, abdominal pain, diarrhea, nausea, vomiting becomes pronounced.

gemifloxacin

gem-ih-**flocks**-ah-sin
(Factive)

CLASSIFICATION

PHARMACOTHERAPEUTIC: Fluoroquinolone. **CLINICAL:** Antibacterial.

ACTION

Inhibits the enzyme DNA gyrase in susceptible microorganisms, interfering with bacterial cell replication, repair. **Therapeutic Effect:** Bactericidal.

PHARMACOKINETICS

Rapidly, well absorbed from GI tract. Protein binding: 70%. Widely distributed.

Penetrates well into lung tissue and fluid. Undergoes limited metabolism in the liver. Primarily excreted in feces; lesser amount eliminated in urine. Partially removed by hemodialysis. **Half-life:** 4–12 hrs.

USES

Treatment of susceptible infections due to *S. pneumoniae, H. influenzae, H. parainfluenzae, M. catarrhalis, M. pneumoniae, C. pneumoniae, K. pneumoniae* including acute bacterial exacerbation of chronic bronchitis, community-acquired pneumonia of mild to moderate severity.

PRECAUTIONS

CONTRAINDICATIONS: Concurrent use of amiodarone, quinidine, procainamide, sotalol; history of prolonged QT interval; hypersensitivity to fluoroquinolones; uncorrected electrolyte disorders (esp. hypokalemia, hypomagnesemia). **CAUTIONS:** Hepatic/renal impairment, clinically significant bradycardia, acute myocardial ischemia.

⌛ LIFESPAN CONSIDERATIONS:

Pregnancy/Lactation: Has potential for teratogenic effects. Substitute formula feedings for breast-feedings. **Pregnancy Category C. Children:** Safety and efficacy not established in those 18 yrs and younger. **Elderly:** Age-related renal impairment may require dosage adjustment.

INTERACTIONS

DRUG: **Aluminum-, magnesium-containing antacids, bismuth subsalicylate, didanosine, iron preparations and other metals, sucralfate, zinc preparations** may decrease absorption of gemifloxacin. **Antipsychotics, class 1A and class III antiarrhythmics, erythromycin, tricyclic antidepressants** may increase risk of prolonged QT interval, life-threatening arrhythmias. **Cyclosporine** increases risk of nephrotoxicity. **Probenecid** increases concentration. **HERBAL:** **Dong quai, St. John's wort** may increase risk of photosensitization. **FOOD:** None known. **LAB VALUES:** May increase BUN, serum alkaline phosphatase, bilirubin, LDH, creatinine, AST, ALT.

AVAILABILITY (Rx)

TABLETS: 320 mg.

ADMINISTRATION/HANDLING

PO

• Give without regard to meals. • Do not crush, break tablet. • Do not administer antacids with or within 2 hrs of gemifloxacin.

INDICATIONS/ROUTES/DOSAGE

ACUTE BACTERIAL EXACERBATION OF CHRONIC BRONCHITIS

PO: ADULTS, ELDERLY: 320 mg once a day for 5 days.

COMMUNITY-ACQUIRED PNEUMONIA

PO: ADULTS, ELDERLY: 320 mg once a day for 7 days.

DOSAGE IN RENAL IMPAIRMENT

Dosage and frequency are modified based on creatinine clearance.

Creatinine Clearance	Dosage
Greater than 40 ml/min	320 mg once a day
40 ml/min or less	160 mg once a day

SIDE EFFECTS

OCCASIONAL (4%–2%): Diarrhea, rash, nausea. **RARE (1% or less):** Headache, abdominal pain, dizziness.

ADVERSE EFFECTS/ TOXIC REACTIONS

Antibiotic-associated colitis (severe abdominal pain/tenderness, severe watery diarrhea) may result from altered bacterial balance. Hypersensitivity reaction, including photosensitivity (rash, pruritus, blisters, edema, burning skin) may occur.

G

NURSING CONSIDERATIONS

BASELINE ASSESSMENT

Question for history of hypersensitivity to fluoroquinolone antibiotics.

INTERVENTION/EVALUATION

Monitor for signs/symptoms of infection. Assess WBC count, hepatic function tests. Encourage adequate fluid intake. Monitor daily pattern of bowel activity/stool consistency. Assess skin for rash. Be alert for superinfection (oral candidiasis, genital pruritus).

PATIENT/FAMILY TEACHING

• Take with 8 oz of water, without regard to food. • Drink several glasses of water between meals. • Complete full course of therapy. • Do not take antacids with or within 2 hrs of gemifloxacin dose (reduces or destroys effectiveness).

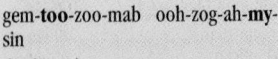

gemtuzumab ozogamicin

gem-**too**-zoo-mab ooh-zog-ah-**my**-sin

(Mylotarg)

CLASSIFICATION

PHARMACOTHERAPEUTIC: Monoclonal antibody. **CLINICAL:** Antineoplastic (see p. 79C).

ACTION

Binds to antigen on surface of leukemic blast cells, resulting in formation of complex that leads to release of antibiotic inside myeloid cells. Antibiotic then binds to DNA, resulting in DNA double-strand breaks, cell death. **Therapeutic Effect:** Inhibits colony formation in leukemic bone marrow cells.

PHARMACOKINETICS

Elimination half-life: 45 hrs after first infusion; 60 hrs after second infusion.

USES

Treatment of pts with CD33 acute myloid leukemia (AML) in first relapse who are 60 yrs and older and not considered candidates for cytotoxic chemotherapy.

PRECAUTIONS

CONTRAINDICATIONS: Hypersensitivity to any component of formulation, pts with anti-CD33 antibody, pregnancy. **CAUTIONS:** Hepatic impairment.

LIFESPAN CONSIDERATIONS:

Pregnancy/Lactation: May cause fetal harm. Unknown if excreted in breast milk. **Pregnancy Category D. Children:** Safety and efficacy not established. **Elderly:** No age-related precautions noted.

INTERACTIONS

DRUG: Bone marrow depressants may have additive effect on myelosuppression. **Live virus vaccines** may potentiate virus replication, increase vaccine side effects, decrease pt's antibody response to vaccine. **HERBAL:** None significant. **FOOD:** None known. **LAB VALUES:** May increase serum bilirubin, AST, ALT. May decrease Hgb, Hct, platelet count, WBC count, serum magnesium, potassium.

AVAILABILITY (Rx)

INJECTION, POWDER FOR RECONSTITUTION: 5 mg.

ADMINISTRATION/HANDLING

IV

Reconstitution • Allow vials to come to room temperature. • Reconstitute each vial with 5 ml Sterile Water for Injection using sterile syringes to provide concentration of 1 mg/ml. • Gently swirl; inspect for particulate matter/discoloration. • Withdraw desired volume from each vial and inject into 100 ml 0.9% NaCl and place into a UV protectant bag.

Rate of administration • Do not give IV push or bolus. • Infuse over 2 hrs. • Use separate line equipped with a low protein binding 1.2-micron filter. • May give through peripheral or central line.

Storage • Protect from direct/indirect sunlight, unshielded fluorescent light during preparation/administration. • Refrigerate; do not freeze. • Following reconstitution in vial, stable for 8 hrs if refrigerated and protected from light. • Once diluted with 100 ml 0.9% NaCl, use immediately.

IV INCOMPATIBILITIES

Do not mix with any other medications.

INDICATIONS/ROUTES/DOSAGE

CD33 POSITIVE ACUTE MYELOID LEUKEMIA (AML)

IV: ADULTS 60 YRS AND OLDER: 9 mg/m^2 infused over 2 hrs repeated in 14 days for a total of 2 doses.

SIDE EFFECTS

◀ **ALERT** ▶ Most pts experience a postinfusion symptom complex of fever (85%), chills (73%), nausea (70%), vomiting (63%) that resolves within 2–4 hrs with supportive therapy.

FREQUENT (44%–31%): Asthenia, diarrhea, abdominal pain, headache, stomatitis, dyspnea, epistaxis. **OCCASIONAL (25%–15%):** Constipation, neutropenic fever, nonspecific rash, herpes simplex infection, hypertension, hypotension, petechiae, peripheral edema, dizziness, insomnia, back pain. **RARE (14%–10%):** Pharyngitis, ecchymosis, dyspepsia, tachycardia, hematuria, rhinitis.

ADVERSE EFFECTS/ TOXIC REACTIONS

Severe myelosuppression, (neutropenia, anemia, thrombocytopenia) occurs in 98% of all pts. Sepsis occurs in 25% of pts. Hepatotoxicity may occur.

NURSING CONSIDERATIONS

BASELINE ASSESSMENT

Obtain baseline CBC, hepatic function studies, serum chemistry for comparison to expected myelosuppression. Use strict aseptic technique to protect pt from infection.

INTERVENTION/EVALUATION

Monitor CBC, blood chemistries, WBC, hepatic function studies. Monitor for myelosuppression (fever, sore throat, signs of local infection, unusual bruising/bleeding from any site), symptoms of anemia (excessive fatigue, weakness). Assess for impending stomatitis. Monitor B/P for hypertension/hypotension.

PATIENT/FAMILY TEACHING

• Do not have immunizations without physician's approval (drug lowers resistance). • Avoid contact with those who have recently received live virus vaccine. • Promptly report fever, sore throat, signs of local infection, unusual bruising/bleeding from any site.

Gemzar, *see gemcitabine*

gentamicin

jen-ta-**mye**-sin

(Alcomicin ✤, Garamycin, Genoptic, Gentak)

CLASSIFICATION

PHARMACOTHERAPEUTIC: Aminoglycoside. **CLINICAL:** Antibiotic (see p. 19C).

G

ACTION

Irreversibly binds to protein of bacterial ribosomes. **Therapeutic Effect:** Interferes with protein synthesis of susceptible microorganisms. Bactericidal.

PHARMACOKINETICS

Rapid, complete absorption after IM administration. Protein binding: less than 30%. Widely distributed (does not cross blood-brain barrier, low concentrations in CSF). Excreted unchanged in urine. Removed by hemodialysis. **Half-life:** 2–4 hrs (increased in renal impairment, neonates; decreased in cystic fibrosis, burn or febrile pts).

USES

Parenteral: Treatment of infections susceptible to *Pseudomonas* and other gram-negative organisms including skin/skin-structure, bone, joint, respiratory tract, intra-abdominal, complicated urinary tract, acute pelvic infections; burns; septicemia; meningitis. **Ophthalmic:** Ointment or solution for superficial eye infections. **Topical:** Cream or ointment for superficial skin infections. Ophthalmic or topical applications may be combined with systemic administration for serious, extensive infections. **OFF-LABEL: Topical:** Prophylaxis of minor bacterial skin infections, treatment of dermal ulcer.

PRECAUTIONS

CONTRAINDICATIONS: Hypersensitivity to other aminoglycosides (cross-sensitivity) or their components. Sulfite sensitivity may result in anaphylaxis, esp. in asthmatic pts. **CAUTIONS:** Elderly, neonates due to renal insufficiency or immaturity; neuromuscular disorders (potential for respiratory depression), prior hearing loss, vertigo, renal impairment. Cumulative effects may occur with concurrent systemic administration and topical application to large areas.

LIFESPAN CONSIDERATIONS:

Pregnancy/Lactation: Readily crosses placenta; unknown if distributed in breast milk. **Pregnancy Category C. Children:** Caution in neonates: Immature renal function increases half-life and toxicity. **Elderly:** Age-related renal impairment may require dosage adjustment.

INTERACTIONS

DRUG: Nephrotoxic, ototoxic medications may increase risk of nephrotoxicity, ototoxicity. May increase neuromuscular blockade with concurrent use of **neuromuscular blockers. HERBAL:** None significant. **FOOD:** None known. **LAB VALUES:** May increase serum creatinine, bilirubin, BUN, LDH, AST, ALT. May decrease serum calcium, magnesium, potassium, sodium. Therapeutic peak serum level is 6–10 mcg/ml, trough is 0.5–2 mcg/ml. Toxic peak serum level is greater than 10 mcg/ml, trough is greater than 2 mcg/ml.

AVAILABILITY (Rx)

CREAM, TOPICAL: 0.1%. **INJECTION, INFUSION:** 40 mg/50 ml; 60 mg/50 ml; 60 mg/100 ml; 80 mg/50 ml; 80 mg/100 ml; 100 mg/50 ml; 100 mg/100 ml. **INJECTION, SOLUTION:** 10 mg/ml, 40 mg/ml. **OINTMENT, OPHTHALMIC:** 0.3%. **OINTMENT, TOPICAL:** 0.1%. **SOLUTION, OPHTHALMIC: (GENOPTIC, GENTAK)** 0.3%.

ADMINISTRATION/HANDLING

IV

Reconstitution • Dilute with 50–200 ml D_5W or 0.9% NaCl. Amount of diluent for infants, children depends on individual needs.

Rate of administration • Infuse over 30–60 min for adults, older children; over 60–120 min for infants, young children.

Storage • Store vials at room temperature. • Solution appears clear or slightly yellow. • Intermittent IV infusion (piggyback) is stable for 24 hrs at room temperature. • Discard if precipitate forms.

IM

• To minimize discomfort, give deep IM slowly. • Less painful if injected into gluteus maximus than lateral aspect of thigh.

INTRATHECAL

• Use only 2 mg/ml intrathecal preparation without preservative. • Mix with 10% estimated CSF volume or NaCl. • Use intrathecal forms immediately after preparation. Discard unused portion. • Give over 3–5 min.

OPHTHALMIC

• Place finger on lower eyelid, pull out until a pocket is formed between eye and lower lid. • Hold dropper above pocket, place correct number of drops (¼–½ inch ointment) into pocket. Close eye gently. • **Solution:** Apply digital pressure to lacrimal sac for 1–2 min (minimizes drainage into nose/throat, reducing risk of systemic effects). • **Ointment:** Close eye for 1–2 min, rolling eyeball (increases contact area of drug to eye). • Remove excess solution or ointment around eye with tissue.

TOPICAL

• Wash affected area with soap and water; allow to dry before applying. • Apply a small amount of gentamicin to the affected area and rub in gently.

IV INCOMPATIBILITIES

Allopurinol (Aloprim), amphotericin B complex (Abelcet, AmBisome, Amphotec), furosemide (Lasix), heparin, hetastarch (Hespan), idarubicin (Idamycin), indomethacin (Indocin), propofol (Diprivan).

IV COMPATIBILITIES

Amiodarone (Cordarone), diltiazem (Cardizem), enalapril (Vasotec), filgrastim (Neupogen), hydromorphone (Dilaudid), insulin, lipids, lorazepam (Ativan), magnesium sulfate, midazolam (Versed), morphine, multivitamins, total parenteral nutrition (TPN).

INDICATIONS/ROUTES/DOSAGE

◄ **ALERT** ► Space parenteral doses evenly around the clock. Dosage based on ideal body weight. Peak, trough levels are determined periodically to maintain desired serum concentrations and minimize risk of toxicity.

USUAL PARENTERAL DOSAGE

IV, IM: ADULTS, ELDERLY: 3–6 mg/kg/day in divided doses q8h or 4–7 mg/kg once a day. **CHILDREN 5–12 YRS:** 2–2.5 mg/kg/dose q8h. **CHILDREN YOUNGER THAN 5 YRS:** 2.5 mg/kg/dose q8h. **NEONATES:** 2.5–3.5 mg/kg/dose q8–12h.

HEMODIALYSIS

IV, IM: ADULTS, ELDERLY: 0.5–0.7 mg/kg/dose after dialysis. **CHILDREN:** 1.25–1.75 mg/kg/dose after dialysis.

INTRATHECAL: ADULTS: 4–8 mg/day. **CHILDREN 3 MOS–12 YRS:** 1–2 mg/day. **NEONATES:** 1 mg/day.

USUAL OPHTHALMIC DOSAGE

OPHTHALMIC OINTMENT: ADULTS, ELDERLY: Apply thin strip to conjunctiva 2–3 times a day.

OPHTHALMIC SOLUTION: ADULTS, ELDERLY, CHILDREN: 1–2 drops q2–4h up to 2 drops/hr.

USUAL TOPICAL DOSAGE

TOPICAL: ADULTS, ELDERLY: Apply 3–4 times/day.

DOSAGE IN RENAL IMPAIRMENT

Creatinine Clearance	Dosage Interval
41–60 ml/min	q12h
20–40 ml/min	q24h
Less than 20 ml/min	Monitor levels to determine dosage interval

SIDE EFFECTS

OCCASIONAL: IM: Pain, induration at injection site. **IV:** Phlebitis, thrombophlebitis, hypersensitivity reactions (fever, pruritus, rash, urticaria). **Ophthalmic:** Burning, tearing, itching, blurred vision. **Topical:** Redness, itching. **RARE:** Alopecia, hypertension, fatigue.

ADVERSE EFFECTS/ TOXIC REACTIONS

Nephrotoxicity (increased BUN, serum creatinine; decreased creatinine clearance) may be reversible if drug is stopped at first sign of symptoms. Irreversible ototoxicity (tinnitus, dizziness, diminished hearing), neurotoxicity (headache, dizziness, lethargy, tremor, visual disturbances) occur occasionally. Risk increases with higher dosages, prolonged therapy, or if solution is applied directly to mucosa. Superinfections, particularly with fungi, may result from bacterial imbalance via any route of administration. Ophthalmic application may cause paresthesia of conjunctiva, mydriasis.

NURSING CONSIDERATIONS

BASELINE ASSESSMENT

Dehydration must be treated before beginning parenteral therapy. Establish baseline hearing acuity. Question for history of allergies, esp. aminoglycosides, sulfites (parabens for topical/ ophthalmic routes).

INTERVENTION/EVALUATION

Monitor I&O (maintain hydration), urinalysis (casts, RBCs, WBCs, decrease in specific gravity). Be alert to ototoxic, neurotoxic symptoms (see Adverse Effects/Toxic Reactions). Check IM injection site for induration. Evaluate IV site for phlebitis (heat, pain, red streaking over vein). Assess for rash (**Ophthalmic:** redness, burning, itching, tearing; **Topical:** redness, itching). Be alert for superinfection (genital/anal pruritus, changes in oral mucosa, diarrhea). When treating pts with neuromuscular disorders, assess respiratory response carefully. Therapeutic serum level: Peak 6–10 mcg/ml; trough: 0.5–2 mcg/ml. Toxic serum level: Peak: greater than 10 mcg/ml; trough: greater than 2 mcg/ml.

PATIENT/FAMILY TEACHING

• Discomfort may occur with IM injection. • Blurred vision, tearing may occur briefly after each ophthalmic dose. • Notify physician if hearing, visual, balance, urinary problems occur, even after therapy is completed. • **Ophthalmic:** Contact physician if tearing, redness, irritation continues. • **Topical:** Cleanse area gently before applying; notify physician if redness, itching occurs.

Geodon, *see ziprasidone*

ginger

Also known as black ginger, race ginger, zingiber.

CLASSIFICATION

HERBAL: See Appendix G.

ACTION

Possesses antipyretic, analgesic, antitussive, sedative properties. Increases GI motility; may act on serotonin receptors, primarily 5-HT_3. **Effect:** Reduces nausea/vomiting.

USES

Prevention of nausea/vomiting caused by motion sickness, early pregnancy, dyspepsia; treatment of rheumatoid arthritis.

PRECAUTIONS

CONTRAINDICATIONS: None known. **CAUTIONS:** Pregnancy; pts with bleeding conditions, diabetes (may cause hypoglycemia).

LIFESPAN CONSIDERATIONS:

Pregnancy/Lactation: Use during pregnancy is controversial (large amounts act as an abortifacient). **Children:** Safety and efficacy not established. **Elderly:** No age-related precautions noted.

INTERACTIONS

DRUG: Large amounts may increase risk of bleeding with **anticoagulants, antiplatelets**. **HERBAL: Feverfew, garlic, ginkgo, ginseng** may increase risk of bleeding. **FOOD:** None known. **LAB VALUES:** None known.

AVAILABILITY (Rx)

CAPSULES: 470 mg, 550 mg. **EXTRACT. POWDER. ROOT:** 470 mg, 550 mg. **TEA. TABLETS. TINCTURE.**

INDICATIONS/ROUTES/DOSAGE

MORNING SICKNESS

PO: ADULTS: 250 mg 4 times a day. **Maximum:** 4 g a day.

MOTION SICKNESS

PO: ADULTS: 1 g (dried powder root) 30 min before travel.

NAUSEA

PO: ADULTS: 550–1,100 mg 3 times a day.

ARTHRITIS

PO: ADULTS: 170 mg 3 times a day or 255 mg twice a day.

SIDE EFFECTS

Abdominal discomfort, heartburn, diarrhea, hypersensitivity reaction, nausea.

ADVERSE EFFECTS/ TOXIC REACTIONS

CNS depression, arrhythmias.

NURSING CONSIDERATIONS

BASELINE ASSESSMENT

Assess for use of anticoagulants, antiplatelets (may increase risk of bleeding).

INTERVENTION/EVALUATION

Monitor for hypersensitivity reaction.

PATIENT/FAMILY TEACHING

- Use cautiously during pregnancy or breast-feeding.

ginkgo biloba

Also known as fossil tree, maidenhair tree, tanakan.

CLASSIFICATION

HERBAL: See Appendix G.

ACTION

Possesses antioxidant, free radical scavenging properties. **Effect:** Protects tissues from oxidative damage, prevents progression of tissue degeneration in pts with dementia. Inhibits platelet-activating factor bonding at numerous sites, decreasing platelet aggregation, smooth muscle contraction; may increase cardiac contractility, coronary blood flow. Decreases blood viscosity, improving circulation by relaxing vascular smooth muscle. Increases cerebral, peripheral blood flow, reduces vascular permeability. May influence neurotransmitter system (e.g., cholinergic).

USES

Treatment of dementia syndromes, including Alzheimer's. Improves cerebral, peripheral circulation. Improves conditions associated with cerebral vascular insufficiency (memory loss, difficulty concentrating, vertigo, tinnitus). Improves cognitive behavior, sleep patterns in pts with depression. Acts as antioxidant.

PRECAUTIONS

CONTRAINDICATIONS: Pregnancy, lactation. **CAUTIONS:** Pts with bleeding disorders, diabetes, epilepsy, or those prone to seizures. Avoid use in couples having difficulty conceiving.

LIFESPAN CONSIDERATIONS:

Pregnancy/Lactation: Contraindicated. **Children:** Safety and efficacy not established. Avoid use. **Elderly:** No age-related precautions noted.

INTERACTIONS

DRUG: **Anticoagulants, antiplatelets (warfarin, aspirin, heparin, clopidogrel)** may increase risk of bleeding. Effects may be increased with concurrent use of **MAOIs**. **HERBAL:** **Feverfew, ginger, garlic, ginseng** may increase risk of bleeding. **FOOD:** None known. **LAB VALUES:** May alter glucose.

AVAILABILITY (OTC)

CAPSULES: 40 mg, 60 mg. **FLUID EXTRACT. TABLETS:** 40 mg, 60 mg. **TINCTURE.**

INDICATIONS/ROUTES/DOSAGE

DEMENTIA

PO: ADULTS, ELDERLY: 120–240 mg a day (extract) in 2–3 doses.

VERTIGO, TINNITUS

PO: ADULTS, ELDERLY: 120–160 mg a day.

COGNITIVE FUNCTION

PO: ADULTS, ELDERLY: 120–600 mg a day.

◄ **ALERT** ► Appropriate doses for other conditions vary; should be started at low doses, titrated to higher doses as needed.

SIDE EFFECTS

Headache, dizziness, palpitations, constipation, allergic skin reactions. Large doses may cause nausea, vomiting, diarrhea, fatigue, diminished muscle tone.

ADVERSE EFFECTS/ TOXIC REACTIONS

None known.

NURSING CONSIDERATIONS

BASELINE ASSESSMENT

Assess for use of anticoagulants, antiplatelets, MAOIs. Assess for history of bleeding disorders, diabetes, seizures.

INTERVENTION/EVALUATION

Monitor for hypersensitivity reaction, serum glucose.

PATIENT/FAMILY TEACHING

• Avoid use with anticoagulants antiplatelets. • May take up to 6 mos before effectiveness is noted. • Do not use during pregnancy, breast-feeding. • Avoid use in children.

ginseng

Also known as Asian ginseng, Chinese ginseng, red ginseng.

CLASSIFICATION

HERBAL: See Appendix G.

ACTION

Affects hypothalamic-pituitary-adrenal axis. Appears to stimulate lymphocytic action. **Effect:** Reduces stress. Affects immune function.

USES

Increases resistance to stress. Boosts energy level. Enhances brain activity. Increases physical endurance. Aids in serum glucose control. Improves cognitive function, concentration, memory, work efficiency.

PRECAUTIONS

CONTRAINDICATIONS: Pts with bleeding tendencies, thrombosis. Avoid use during pregnancy, lactation. **CAUTIONS:** Pts with cardiac disorders, diabetes, hormone-sensitive cancers (breast, uterine, ovarian), endometriosis, uterine fibroids.

LIFESPAN CONSIDERATIONS:

Pregnancy/Lactation: Insufficient information. Do not use. **Children:** Safety and efficacy not established. **Elderly:** No age-related precautions noted.

INTERACTIONS

DRUG: **Anticoagulants, antiplatelets (aspirin, clopidogrel, enoxaparin, heparin, warfarin)** may increase risk of bleeding. May increase effects of **oral antidiabetic agents, insulin.** Effects may be decreased with concurrent use of **furosemide**. Ginseng may interfere with effects of **immunosuppressants (e.g., cyclosporine, prednisone).** **HERBAL:** **Chamomile, feverfew, garlic, ginger, ginkgo** may increase risk of bleeding. **FOOD:** **Coffee, tea** may increase effect. **LAB VALUES:** May prolong activated partial thromboplastin time (aPTT), decrease serum glucose.

AVAILABILITY (OTC)

CAPSULES: 100 mg, 250 mg, 410 mg, 500 mg. **DRIED ROOT. EXTRACT. POWDER. TABLETS:** 250 mg, 1,000 mg. **TEA** (usually 1,500 mg/bag). **TINCTURE.**

INDICATIONS/ROUTES/DOSAGE

USUAL DOSAGE

PO: ADULTS, ELDERLY: **(Tablets/capsules):** 200–600 mg a day. **(Powder root):** 0.6–3 g 1–3 times a day. **(Tea—1,500 mg):** 1–3 times a day.

SIDE EFFECTS

FREQUENT: Insomnia. **OCCASIONAL:** Vaginal bleeding, amenorrhea, palpitations, hypertension, diarrhea, headache, allergic reactions.

ADVERSE EFFECTS/ TOXIC REACTIONS

None known.

NURSING CONSIDERATIONS

BASELINE ASSESSMENT

Assess if pt is pregnant, breast-feeding. Assess if pt is diabetic, taking oral hypoglycemic agents, insulin. Assess for anticoagulant, immunosuppressant use. Determine baseline serum glucose.

INTERVENTION/EVALUATION

Monitor coagulation studies, serum glucose. Assess for hypersensitivity reaction, rash.

PATIENT/FAMILY TEACHING

• Avoid use in pregnancy or breast-feeding, children. • Avoid continuous use for longer than 3 mos.

G

glatiramer

glah-**tie**-rah-mir

(Copaxone)

Do not confuse Copaxone with Compazine.

♦CLASSIFICATION

PHARMACOTHERAPEUTIC: Immunosuppressive. **CLINICAL:** Neurologic agent.

ACTION

May act by modifying immune processes thought to be responsible for pathogenesis of multiple sclerosis. **Therapeutic Effect:** Slows progression of multiple sclerosis.

PHARMACOKINETICS

Substantial fraction of glatiramer is hydrolyzed locally. Some fraction of injected material enters lymphatic circulation, reaching regional lymph nodes; some may enter systemic circulation intact.

USES

Treatment of relapsing, remitting multiple sclerosis.

PRECAUTIONS

CONTRAINDICATIONS: Hypersensitivity to glatiramer, mannitol. **CAUTIONS:** Pts exhibiting immediate postinjection reaction (flushing, chest pain, palpitations, anxiety, dyspnea, urticaria).

LIFESPAN CONSIDERATIONS:

Pregnancy/Lactation: Unknown if drug is distributed in breast milk. **Pregnancy Category B. Children:** Safety and efficacy not established. **Elderly:** Information not available.

INTERACTIONS

DRUG: None significant. **HERBAL:** None significant. **FOOD:** None known. **LAB VALUES:** None known.

AVAILABILITY (Rx)

INJECTION SOLUTION: 20 mg/ml in prefilled syringes.

ADMINISTRATION/HANDLING

SUBCUTANEOUS

- Refrigerate syringes. • Inject into deltoid region, abdomen, gluteus maximus, or lateral aspect of thigh. • Prefilled syringe suitable for single use only; discard unused portions.

INDICATIONS/ROUTES/DOSAGE

MULTIPLE SCLEROSIS

SUBCUTANEOUS: ADULTS, ELDERLY: 20 mg once a day.

SIDE EFFECTS

EXPECTED (73%–40%): Pain, erythema, inflammation, pruritus at injection site; asthenia. **FREQUENT (27%–18%):** Arthralgia, vasodilation, anxiety, hypertonia, nausea, transient chest pain, dyspnea, flu-like symptoms, rash, pruritus. **OCCASIONAL (17%–10%):** Palpitations, back pain, diaphoresis, rhinitis, diarrhea, urinary urgency. **RARE (8%–6%):** Anorexia, fever, neck pain, peripheral edema, ear pain, facial edema, vertigo, vomiting.

ADVERSE EFFECTS/ TOXIC REACTIONS

Infection occurs commonly. Lymphadenopathy occurs occasionally.

NURSING CONSIDERATIONS

INTERVENTION/EVALUATION

Observe injection site for reaction. Monitor for fever, chills (evidence of infection).

PATIENT/FAMILY TEACHING

- Report difficulty in breathing/swallowing, rash, itching, swelling of lower extremities, fatigue. • Avoid pregnancy.

Gleevec, *see imatinib*

glimepiride

glim-**eh**-purr-eyd

(Amaryl)

Do not confuse glimepiride with glipizide or glyburide, Avandaryl with Benadryl.

FIXED-COMBINATION(S)

Avandaryl: glimepiride, rosiglitazone (an antidiabetic): 1 mg/4 mg, 2 mg/4 mg, 4 mg/4 mg.
Duetact: glimepiride, pioglitazone (an antidiabetic) 2 mg/30 mg; 4 mg/30 mg.

CLASSIFICATION

PHARMACOTHERAPEUTIC: Second-generation sulfonylurea. **CLINICAL:** Hypoglycemic (see p. 41C).

ACTION

Promotes release of insulin from beta cells of pancreas, increases insulin sensitivity at peripheral sites. **Therapeutic Effect:** Lowers serum glucose.

PHARMACOKINETICS

Route	Onset	Peak	Duration
PO	N/A	2–3 hrs	24 hrs

Completely absorbed from GI tract. Protein binding: greater than 99%. Metabolized in liver. Excreted in urine, eliminated in feces. **Half-life:** 5–9.2 hrs.

USES

Adjunct to diet, exercise in management of non–insulin dependent diabetes mellitus (type 2, NIDDM). Use in combination with insulin or metformin in pts whose diabetes is not controlled by diet, exercise in conjunction with oral hypoglycemic agent.

PRECAUTIONS

CONTRAINDICATIONS: Diabetic complications, (ketosis, acidosis, diabetic coma); monotherapy for type 1 diabetes mellitus; severe hepatic/renal impairment; stress situations (severe infection, trauma, surgery). **CAUTIONS:** Severe diarrhea, intestinal obstruction, prolonged vomiting, hepatic disease, hyperthyroidism (uncontrolled), renal impairment, adrenal insufficiency, debilitation, malnutrition, pituitary insufficiency.

LIFESPAN CONSIDERATIONS: **Pregnancy/Lactation:** Not recommended for use during pregnancy. Unknown if distributed in breast milk. **Pregnancy Category C. Children:** Safety and efficacy not established. **Elderly:** Hypoglycemia may be difficult to recognize. Age-related renal impairment may increase sensitivity to glucose-lowering effect.

INTERACTIONS

DRUG: Beta-blockers may increase hypoglycemic effect, mask signs of hypoglycemia. **Cimetidine, ciprofloxacin, fluconazole, MAOIs, quinidine, ranitidine, large doses of salicylates** may increase effect. **Corticosteroids, lithium, thiazide diuretics** may decrease effect. May increase effects of **oral anticoagulants**. **HERBAL: Garlic** may worsen hypoglycemia. **FOOD:** None known. **LAB VALUES:** May increase BUN, LDH concentrations, serum alkaline phosphatase, creatinine, AST.

AVAILABILITY (Rx)

TABLETS: 1 mg, 2 mg, 4 mg.

ADMINISTRATION/HANDLING

PO

- Give with breakfast or first main meal.

INDICATIONS/ROUTES/DOSAGE

DIABETES MELLITUS

PO: ADULTS, ELDERLY: Initially, 1–2 mg once a day, with breakfast or first main meal. Maintenance: 1–4 mg once a day. After dose of 2 mg is reached, dosage should be increased in increments of up to 2 mg q1–2wks, based on serum glucose response. **Maximum:** 8 mg/day. **ELDERLY:** Initially, 1 mg/day. Titrate dose to avoid hypoglycemia.

DOSAGE IN RENAL IMPAIRMENT

PO: ADULTS: Initially, 1 mg/day, then titrate dose based on fasting serum glucose levels.

SIDE EFFECTS

FREQUENT: Altered taste, dizziness, somnolence, weight gain, constipation, diarrhea, heartburn, nausea, vomiting, stomach fullness, headache. **OCCASIONAL:** Increased sensitivity of skin to sunlight, peeling of skin, pruritus, rash.

ADVERSE EFFECTS/ TOXIC REACTIONS

Overdose or insufficient food intake may produce hypoglycemia, (esp. with increased glucose demands). GI hemorrhage, cholestatic hepatic jaundice, leukopenia, thrombocytopenia, pancytopenia, agranulocytosis, aplastic or hemolytic anemia occur rarely.

NURSING CONSIDERATIONS

BASELINE ASSESSMENT

Check serum glucose level. Discuss lifestyle to determine extent of learning,

G

emotional needs. Ensure follow-up instruction if pt or family does not thoroughly understand diabetes management or serum glucose testing technique.

INTERVENTION/EVALUATION

Monitor serum glucose level, food intake. Assess for hypoglycemia (cool/wet skin, tremors, dizziness, anxiety, headache, tachycardia, perioral numbness, hunger, diplopia), hyperglycemia (polyuria, polyphagia, polydipsia, nausea, vomiting, dim vision, fatigue, deep or rapid breathing). Be alert to conditions that alter glucose requirements (fever, increased activity or stress, trauma, surgical procedure).

PATIENT/FAMILY TEACHING

• Prescribed diet is principal part of treatment; do not skip or delay meals. • Carry candy, sugar packets, other sugar supplements for immediate response to hypoglycemia. • Wear medical alert identification. • Check with physician when glucose demands are altered (fever, infection, trauma, stress, heavy physical activity).

*glipiZIDE

glip-ih-zide

(Glucotrol, Glucotrol XL)

Do not confuse glipizide with glimepiride or glyburide.

FIXED-COMBINATION(S)

Metaglip: glipizide/metformin (an antidiabetic): 2.5 mg/250 mg; 2.5 mg/500 mg; 5 mg/500 mg.

CLASSIFICATION

PHARMACOTHERAPEUTIC: Second-generation sulfonylurea. **CLINICAL:** Hypoglycemic (see p. 41C).

ACTION

Promotes release of insulin from beta cells of pancreas, increases insulin sensitivity at peripheral sites. **Therapeutic Effect:** Lowers serum glucose.

PHARMACOKINETICS

Route	Onset	Peak	Duration
PO	15–30 min	2–3 hrs	12–24 hrs
Extended-release	2–3 hrs	6–12 hrs	24 hrs

Well absorbed from GI tract. Protein binding: 99%. Metabolized in liver. Excreted in urine. **Half-life:** 2–4 hrs.

USES

Adjunct to diet, exercise in management of stable, mild to moderately severe non–insulin dependent diabetes mellitus (type 2, NIDDM). May be used to supplement insulin in those with type 1 diabetes mellitus. May be used concomitantly with insulin or metformin to improve glycemic control.

PRECAUTIONS

CONTRAINDICATIONS: Diabetic ketoacidosis with or without coma, type 1 diabetes mellitus. **CAUTIONS:** Adrenal/pituitary insufficiency, hypoglycemic reactions, hepatic/renal impairment.

LIFESPAN CONSIDERATIONS:

Pregnancy/Lactation: Insulin is drug of choice during pregnancy; glipizide given within 1 mo of delivery may produce neonatal hypoglycemia. Drug crosses placenta. Distributed in breast milk. **Pregnancy Category C. Children:** Safety and efficacy not established. **Elderly:** Hypoglycemia may be difficult to recognize. Age-related renal impairment may increase sensitivity to glucose-lowering effect.

INTERACTIONS

DRUG: Beta-blockers may increase hypoglycemic effect, mask signs of hypoglycemia. **Cimetidine, ciprofloxacin, fluconazole, MAOIs, quinidine, ranitidine, large doses of salicylates** may increase effect. **Corticosteroids, lithium, thiazide diuretics** may decrease the effect. May increase effects of **oral anticoagulants.** **HERBAL: Garlic** may worsen hypoglycemia. **FOOD:** None known. **LAB VALUES:** May increase BUN, serum alkaline phosphatase, creatinine, LDH, AST.

AVAILABILITY (Rx)

TABLETS (GLUCOTROL): 5 mg, 10 mg.

TABLETS (EXTENDED-RELEASE [GLUCOTROL XL]): 2.5 mg, 5 mg, 10 mg.

ADMINISTRATION/HANDLING

PO

• May give with food (response better if taken 15–30 min before meals). • Do not crush extended-release tablets.

INDICATIONS/ROUTES/DOSAGE

DIABETES MELLITUS

PO: ADULTS: Initially, 5 mg/day or 2.5 mg in elderly or those with hepatic disease. Adjust dosage in 2.5- to 5-mg increments at intervals of several days. Immediate-release tablet: **Maximum single dose:** 15 mg. **Maximum dose/day:** 40 mg. Maintenance (extended-release tablet): 20 mg/day. Extended-release tablet: **Maximum dose:** 20 mg/day. **ELDERLY:** Initially, 2.5–5 mg/day. May increase by 2.5–5 mg/day q1–2wks.

SIDE EFFECTS

FREQUENT: Altered taste, dizziness, somnolence, weight gain, constipation, diarrhea, heartburn, nausea, vomiting, stomach fullness, headache. **OCCASIONAL:** Increased sensitivity of skin to sunlight, peeling of skin, pruritus, rash.

ADVERSE EFFECTS/ TOXIC REACTIONS

Overdose or insufficient food intake may produce hypoglycemia, (esp. with increased glucose demands). GI hemorrhage, cholestatic hepatic jaundice, leukopenia, thrombocytopenia, pancytopenia, agranulocytosis, aplastic or hemolytic anemia occur rarely.

NURSING CONSIDERATIONS

BASELINE ASSESSMENT

Check serum glucose level. Discuss lifestyle to determine extent of learning, emotional needs. Ensure follow-up instruction if pt or family does not thoroughly understand diabetes management or serum glucose testing technique.

INTERVENTION/EVALUATION

Monitor serum glucose level, food intake. Assess for hypoglycemia (cool/wet skin, tremors, dizziness, anxiety, headache, tachycardia, perioral numbness, hunger, diplopia), hyperglycemia (polyuria, polyphagia, polydipsia, nausea, vomiting, dim vision, fatigue, deep or rapid breathing). Be alert to conditions that alter glucose requirements (fever, increased activity or stress, trauma, surgical procedure).

PATIENT/FAMILY TEACHING

• Prescribed diet is principal part of treatment; do not skip or delay meals. • Carry candy, sugar packets, other sugar supplements for immediate response to hypoglycemia. • Wear medical alert identification. • Check with physician when glucose demands are altered (fever, infection, trauma, stress, heavy physical activity).

glucagon

glue-ka-gon

(GlucaGen, GlucaGen Diagnostic Kit, Glucagon, Glucagon Diagnostic Kit, Glucagon Emergency Kit)

Do not confuse glucagon with Glaucon.

G

CLASSIFICATION

PHARMACOTHERAPEUTIC: Glucose elevating agent. **CLINICAL:** Antihypoglycemic, antispasmodic, antidote.

ACTION

Promotes hepatic glycogenolysis, gluconeogenesis. Stimulates cAMP, an enzyme, resulting in increased serum glucose concentration, smooth muscle relaxation, and exerts inotropic myocardial effect. **Therapeutic Effect:** Increases serum glucose level.

PHARMACOKINETICS

Onset of action occurs within 4–10 min following IM administration. Recovery occurs within 12–32 min. **Half-life:** 8–18 min.

USES

Treatment of severe hypoglycemia in diabetic pts. Not for use in chronic hypoglycemia or hypoglycemia due to starvation, adrenal insufficiency (hepatic glycogen unavailable). Diagnostic aid in radiographic examination of GI tract. **OFF-LABEL:** Treatment of esophageal obstruction due to foreign bodies; toxicity associated with beta-blockers, calcium channel blockers.

PRECAUTIONS

CONTRAINDICATIONS: Hypersensitivity to glucagon, beef/pork proteins, known pheochromocytoma. **CAUTIONS:** History of insulinoma, pheochromocytoma.

LIFESPAN CONSIDERATIONS:

Pregnancy/Lactation: Unknown if drug crosses placenta or is distributed in breast milk. **Pregnancy Category B.** **Children/Elderly:** No age-related precautions noted.

INTERACTIONS

DRUG: May increase effects of **anticoagulants**. **HERBAL:** None significant. **FOOD:** None known. **LAB VALUES:** May decrease serum potassium.

AVAILABILITY (Rx)

INJECTION POWDER (GLUCAGEN, GLUCAGEN DIAGNOSTIC KIT, GLUCAGON, GLUCAGON DIAGNOSTIC KIT, GLUCAGON EMERGENCY KIT): 1 mg.

ADMINISTRATION/HANDLING

◄ ALERT ► Place pt on side to prevent aspiration (glucagon, hypoglycemia may produce nausea/vomiting).

IV, IM, SUBCUTANEOUS

Reconstitution • Reconstitute powder with manufacturer's diluent when preparing doses of 2 mg or less. For doses greater than 2 mg, dilute with Sterile Water for Injection. • To provide 1 mg glucagon/ml, use 1 ml diluent. For 1-mg vial of glucagon, use 10 ml diluent for 10-mg vial.

Rate of administration • Pt usually awakens in 5–20 min. Although 1–2 additional doses may be administered, concern for effects of continuing cerebral hypoglycemia requires consideration of parenteral glucose. • When pt awakens, give supplemental carbohydrate to restore hepatic glycogen and prevent secondary hypoglycemia. If pt fails to respond to glucagon, IV glucose is necessary.

Storage • Store vial at room temperature. • After reconstitution, is stable for 48 hrs if refrigerated. If reconstituted with Sterile Water for Injection, use immediately. Do not use glucagon solution unless clear.

IV INCOMPATIBILITIES

Do not mix glucagon with any other medications.

INDICATIONS/ROUTES/DOSAGE

HYPOGLYCEMIA

◄ ALERT ► Administer IV dextrose if pt fails to respond to glucagon.

IV, IM, SUBCUTANEOUS: ADULTS, ELDERLY, CHILDREN WEIGHING MORE THAN

20 KG: 0.5–1 mg. May give 1 or 2 additional doses if response is delayed. **CHILDREN WEIGHING 20 KG OR LESS:** 0.5 mg.

DIAGNOSTIC AID

IV, IM: ADULTS, ELDERLY: 0.25–2 mg 10 min prior to procedure.

SIDE EFFECTS

OCCASIONAL: Nausea, vomiting. **RARE:** Allergic reaction (urticaria, respiratory distress, hypotension).

ADVERSE EFFECTS/ TOXIC REACTIONS

Overdose may produce persistent nausea/vomiting, hypokalemia (severe fatigue, decreased appetite, palpitations, muscle cramps).

NURSING CONSIDERATIONS

BASELINE ASSESSMENT

Obtain immediate assessment, including history, clinical signs/symptoms. If presence of hypoglycemic coma is established, give glucagon promptly.

INTERVENTION/EVALUATION

Monitor response time carefully. Have IV dextrose readily available in event pt does not awaken within 5–20 min. Assess for possible allergic reaction (urticaria, respiratory difficulty, hypotension). When pt is conscious, give oral carbohydrate.

PATIENT/FAMILY TEACHING

• Recognize significance of identifying symptoms of hypoglycemia: pale, cool skin; anxiety, difficulty concentrating, headache, hunger, nausea, shakiness, diaphoresis, unusual fatigue, unusual weakness, unconsciousness. • If symptoms of hypoglycemia develop, instruct pt, family, or friend to give sugar form first (orange juice, honey, hard candy, sugar cubes, table sugar dissolved in water or juice) followed by cheese and crackers, half a sandwich, glass of milk.

Glucophage, *see metformin*

Glucophage XR, *see metformin*

glucosamine/ chondroitin

◆CLASSIFICATION

HERBAL: See Appendix G.

ACTION

Glucosamine: Necessary for synthesis of mucopolysaccharides, which comprise body's tendons, ligaments, cartilage, synovial fluid. May decrease glucose-induced insulin secretion. **Effect:** Relieves symptoms of osteoarthritis. **Chondroitin:** Endogenously found in cartilage tissue, substrate for forming joint matrix structure. May possess anticoagulant properties. **Effect:** Relieves symptoms of osteoarthritis.

USES

Treatment of osteoarthritis.

PRECAUTIONS

CONTRAINDICATIONS: None known. **CAUTIONS: Glucosamine:** Diabetes (may increase insulin resistance). **Chondroitin:** None known.

INTERACTIONS

DRUG: Warfarin may increase effect. Monitor **anticoagulant therapy** closely; may increase risk of bleeding with chondroitin. **HERBAL:** None significant. **FOOD:** None known. **LAB VALUES:** May increase serum glucose, antifactor Xa.

AVAILABILITY (OTC)

GLUCOSAMINE
CAPSULES: 500 mg. **TABLETS:** 500 mg.
CHONDROITIN
CAPSULES: 250 mg.
◀ **ALERT** ▶ Many combination products are available.

INDICATIONS/ROUTES/DOSAGE

OSTEOARTHRITIS
PO: ADULTS, ELDERLY: (Glucosamine): 500 mg 3 times a day or 1–2 g a day. **(Chondroitin):** 200–400 mg 2–3 times a day.

SIDE EFFECTS

GLUCOSAMINE: Mild GI symptoms (gas, bloating, cramps). **CHONDROITIN:** Well tolerated. May cause nausea, diarrhea, constipation, edema, alopecia, allergic reactions.

ADVERSE EFFECTS/ TOXIC REACTIONS

None known.

NURSING CONSIDERATIONS

BASELINE ASSESSMENT

Determine whether pt is taking anticoagulants, antiplatelets, antidiabetic drugs. Assess if pt is pregnant or breast-feeding.

INTERVENTION/EVALUATION

Monitor effectiveness of therapy in relieving osteoarthritis symptoms. Monitor serum glucose levels.

PATIENT/FAMILY TEACHING

• Avoid use in pregnancy, breast-feeding, children. • May take several mos of therapy to be effective. • Glucosamine may alter serum glucose levels.

Glucotrol, *see glipizide*

Glucovance, *see glyburide and metformin*

*glyBURIDE

glye-byoo-ride
(Apo-Glyburide ✱, Daonil ✱, DiaBeta, Euglucon ✱, Glycron, Glynase, Glynase Pres-Tab, Micronase, Novo-Glyburide ✱)

Do not confuse glyburide with glimepiride or glipizide, or Micronase with Micro-K, Micronor.

FIXED-COMBINATION(S)

Glucovance: glyburide/metformin (an antidiabetic): 1.25 mg/250 mg; 2.5 mg/500 mg; 5 mg/500 mg.

◆ CLASSIFICATION

PHARMACOTHERAPEUTIC: Second-generation sulfonylurea. **CLINICAL:** Hypoglycemic (see p. 41C).

ACTION

Promotes release of insulin from beta cells of pancreas, increases insulin sensitivity at peripheral sites. **Therapeutic Effect:** Lowers serum glucose level.

PHARMACOKINETICS

Route	Onset	Peak	Duration
PO	0.25–1 hr	1–2 hrs	12–24 hrs

Well absorbed from GI tract. Protein binding: 99%. Metabolized in liver to weakly active metabolite. Primarily excreted in urine. Not removed by hemodialysis. **Half-life:** 1.4–1.8 hrs.

USES

Adjunct to diet, exercise in management of stable, mild to moderately severe non–insulin dependent diabetes mellitus (type 2, NIDDM). May be used to supplement insulin in those with type 1 diabetes mellitus. May be used concomitantly with insulin or metformin to improve glycemic control.

PRECAUTIONS

CONTRAINDICATIONS: Diabetic ketoacidosis with or without coma, monotherapy for type 1 diabetes mellitus. **CAUTIONS:** Adrenal or pituitary insufficiency, hypoglycemic reactions, hepatic or renal impairment.

LIFESPAN CONSIDERATIONS:

Pregnancy/Lactation: Crosses placenta. Distributed in breast milk. May produce neonatal hypoglycemia if given within 2 wks of delivery. **Pregnancy Category C. Children:** Safety and efficacy not established. **Elderly:** Hypoglycemia may be difficult to recognize. Age-related renal impairment may increase sensitivity to glucose-lowering effect.

INTERACTIONS

DRUG: **Beta-blockers** may increase hypoglycemic effect, mask signs of hypoglycemia. **Cimetidine, ciprofloxacin, fluconazole, MAOIs, quinidine, ranitidine, large doses of salicylates** may increase effect. **Corticosteroids, lithium, thiazide diuretics** may decrease effect. May increase effects of **oral anticoagulants. HERBAL: Garlic** may worsen hypoglycemia. **FOOD:** None known. **LAB VALUES:** May increase BUN, serum alkaline phosphatase, creatinine, LDH, AST.

AVAILABILITY (Rx)

TABLETS (DIABETA, MICRONASE): 1.25 mg, 2.5 mg, 5 mg. **TABLETS (MICRONIZED [GLYCRON, GLYNASE]):** 1.5 mg, 3 mg, 6 mg.

ADMINISTRATION/HANDLING

PO

- May give with food (response better if taken 15–30 min before meals).

INDICATIONS/ROUTES/DOSAGE

DIABETES MELLITUS

PO: ADULTS: Initially 2.5–5 mg. May increase by 2.5 mg/day at weekly intervals. Maintenance: 1.25–20 mg/day. **Maximum:** 20 mg/day. **ELDERLY:** Initially, 1.25–2.5 mg/day. May increase by 1.25–2.5 mg/day at 1- to 3-wk intervals.

PO (MICRONIZED TABLETS): ADULTS, ELDERLY: Initially 0.75–3 mg/day. May increase by 1.5 mg/day at weekly intervals. Maintenance: 0.75–12 mg/day as a single dose or in divided doses.

DOSAGE IN RENAL IMPAIRMENT

Not recommended in pts with creatinine clearance less than 50 ml/min.

SIDE EFFECTS

FREQUENT: Altered taste, dizziness, somnolence, weight gain, constipation, diarrhea, heartburn, nausea, vomiting, stomach fullness, headache. **OCCASIONAL:** Increased sensitivity of skin to sunlight, peeling of skin, pruritus, rash.

ADVERSE EFFECTS/ TOXIC REACTIONS

Overdose or insufficient food intake may produce hypoglycemia, (esp. in pts with increased glucose demands). Cholestatic jaundice, leukopenia, thrombocytopenia, pancytopenia, agranulocytosis, aplastic or hemolytic anemia occur rarely.

NURSING CONSIDERATIONS

BASELINE ASSESSMENT

Check serum glucose level. Discuss lifestyle to determine extent of learning, emotional needs. Ensure follow-up instruction if pt or family does not thoroughly understand diabetes management or glucose testing technique.

INTERVENTION/EVALUATION

Monitor serum glucose level, food intake. Assess for hypoglycemia (cool, wet skin; tremors, dizziness, anxiety, headache, tachycardia, perioral numbness,

G

hunger, diplopia) hyperglycemia (polyuria, polyphagia, polydipsia, nausea, vomiting, dim vision, fatigue, deep or rapid breathing). Be alert to conditions that alter glucose requirements (fever, increased activity or stress, trauma, surgical procedure).

PATIENT/FAMILY TEACHING

• Prescribed diet is principal part of treatment; do not skip or delay meals. • Carry candy, sugar packets, other sugar supplements for immediate response to hypoglycemia. • Wear medical alert identification. • Check with physician when glucose demands are altered (fever, infection, trauma, stress, heavy physical activity).

G

glycopyrrolate

glye-koe-**pye**-roe-late

(Robinul)

Do not confuse Robinul with Reminyl.

CLASSIFICATION

PHARMACOTHERAPEUTIC: Quaternary anticholinergic. **CLINICAL:** Antimuscarinic, antiarrhythmic, cholinergic adjunct.

ACTION

Inhibits action of acetylcholine at postganglionic parasympathetic sites in smooth muscle, secretory glands, CNS. **Therapeutic Effect:** Reduces salivation/excessive secretions of respiratory tract; reduces gastric secretions, acidity.

USES

Inhibits salivation/excessive secretions of respiratory tract. Reverses muscarinic effects of cholinergic agents (e.g., neostigmine).

PRECAUTIONS

CONTRAINDICATIONS: Acute hemorrhage, myasthenia gravis, narrow-angle glaucoma, obstructive uropathy, paralytic ileus, tachycardia, ulcerative colitis. **CAUTIONS:** Those with fever, hyperthyroidism, hepatic/renal disease, hypertension, CHF, GI infection, diarrhea, reflux esophagitis. **Pregnancy Category B.**

INTERACTIONS

DRUG: **Antacids, antidiarrheals** may decrease absorption. May decrease absorption of **ketoconazole**. **Other anticholinergics** may increase effect. May increase severity of GI lesions with wax matrix formulation of **potassium chloride**. **HERBAL:** None known. **FOOD:** None known. **LAB VALUES:** May decrease serum uric acid.

AVAILABILITY (Rx)

INJECTION SOLUTION (ROBINUL): 0.2 mg/ml.

ADMINISTRATION/HANDLING

IV

• Administer undiluted as IV push through tubing of free-flowing compatible IV solution.

IM

• Administer undiluted or dilute with D_5W, $D_{10}W$, or 0.9% NaCl.

IV INCOMPATIBILITY

None known.

IV COMPATIBILITIES

Diphenhydramine (Benadryl), droperidol (Inapsine), hydromorphone (Dilaudid), hydroxyzine (Vistaril), lidocaine, midazolam (Versed), morphine, promethazine (Phenergan).

INDICATIONS/ROUTES/DOSAGE

PREOPERATIVE INHIBITION OF SALIVATION, EXCESSIVE RESPIRATORY TRACT SECRETIONS

IM: ADULTS, ELDERLY: 4 mcg/kg 30–60 min before procedure. **CHILDREN 2 YRS**

AND OLDER: 4 mcg/kg. **CHILDREN YOUNGER THAN 2 YRS:** 4–9 mcg/kg.

BLOCK EFFECTS OF ANTICHOLINESTERASE AGENTS

IV: ADULTS, ELDERLY: 0.2 mg for each 1 mg neostigmine or 5 mg pyridostigmine.

SIDE EFFECTS

FREQUENT: Dry mouth, decreased sweating, constipation. **OCCASIONAL:** Blurred vision, gastric bloating, urinary hesitancy, drowsiness (with high dosage), headache, photosensitivity, altered taste, anxiety, flushing, insomnia, impotence, mental confusion or excitement (particularly in elderly, children), temporary light-headedness (with parenteral form), local irritation (with parenteral form). **RARE:** Dizziness, faintness.

ADVERSE EFFECTS/ TOXIC REACTIONS

Overdose may produce temporary paralysis of ciliary muscle, pupillary dilation, tachycardia, palpitations, hot/dry/flushed skin, absence of bowel sounds, hyperthermia, increased respiratory rate, EKG abnormalities, nausea, vomiting, rash over face/upper trunk, CNS stimulation, psychosis (agitation, restlessness, rambling speech, visual hallucinations, paranoid behavior, delusions, followed by depression).

NURSING CONSIDERATIONS

BASELINE ASSESSMENT

Before giving medication, instruct pt to void (reduces risk of urinary retention).

INTERVENTION/EVALUATION

Monitor daily pattern of bowel activity/ stool consistency. Palpate bladder for urinary retention. Monitor heart rate, changes in B/P, temperature. Assess skin turgor, mucous membranes to evaluate hydration status (encourage adequate fluid intake), bowel sounds for peristalsis. Be alert for fever (increased risk of hyperthermia).

PATIENT/FAMILY TEACHING

• May cause dry mouth. • Take 30 min before meals (food decreases absorption of medication). • Use care not to become overheated during exercise in hot weather (may result in heat stroke). • Avoid hot baths, saunas. • Avoid tasks that require alertness, motor skills until response to drug is established. • Do not take antacids or medicine for diarrhea within 1 hr of taking this medication (decreased effectiveness).

gonadorelin

go-nad-oh-**rell**-in

(Factrel, Lutrepulse ✱)

Do not confuse gonadorelin with gonadotropin, Factrel with guanadrel or Sectral.

CLASSIFICATION

PHARMACOTHERAPEUTIC: Gonadotropin-releasing hormone. **CLINICAL:** Diagnostic agent.

ACTION

Stimulates release of luteinizing hormone (LH) from anterior pituitary gland. **Therapeutic Effect:** Stimulates release of gonadotropin-releasing hormone from hypothalamus.

PHARMACOKINETICS

	Onset	Peak	Duration
IV	NA	20 min	3–5 hrs

Half-life: 4 min.

USES

Evaluation of hypothalamic pituitary gonadotropic function, evaluation of abnormal gonadotropin regulation as in precocious or delayed puberty, treatment of primary hypothalamic amenorrhea.

PRECAUTIONS

CONTRAINDICATIONS: None known. **CAUTIONS:** None known. **Pregnancy Category B.**

INTERACTIONS

DRUG: Androgens, estrogens, progestins, glucocorticoids, spironolactone may increase effect/toxicity. **Oral contraceptives, digoxin** may decrease effect. **HERBAL:** None significant. **FOOD:** None known. **LAB VALUES:** None known.

G

AVAILABILITY (Rx)

INJECTION, POWDER FOR RECONSTITUTION: 100 mcg (Factrel), 0.8 mg (Lutrepulse), 3.2 mg (Lutrepulse).

INDICATIONS/ROUTES/DOSAGE

◀ **ALERT** ▶ Test should be conducted in absence of other drugs that affect pituitary secretion of gonadotropins.

GONADORELIN ACETATE
PRIMARY HYPOTHALAMIC AMENORRHEA

IV (LUTREPULSE) PUMP: ADULTS: 5 mcg q90min (range 1–20 mcg); treatment interval 21 days. Refer to manufacturer's manual for proper dilutions/settings on pump. Response usually occurs 2–3 wks after initiation. Continue additional 2 wks after ovulation occurs (maintains corpus luteum). **Note:** Pump will pulsate q90min for 7 days.

GONADORELIN HYDROCHLORIDE
DIAGNOSTIC AGENT

IV, SUBCUTANEOUS: ADULTS: 100 mcg. In females, perform test in early follicular phase of menstrual cycle.

SIDE EFFECTS

OCCASIONAL: Swelling, pain, itching at injection site with subcutaneous administration. Local or generalized skin rash with chronic subcutaneous administration. **RARE:** Headache, nausea, lightheadedness, abdominal discomfort, hypersensitivity reactions (bronchospasm, tachycardia, flushing, urticaria), induration at injection site.

ADVERSE EFFECTS/ TOXIC REACTIONS

Anaphylactic reaction occurs rarely.

NURSING CONSIDERATIONS

BASELINE ASSESSMENT

Ensure pt understands procedure before starting test. **Gonadorelin Acetate:** Pt instructions included with kit from manufacturer. **Gonadorelin Hydrochloride:** Draw venous blood sample (for LH) immediately before admini-stration.

INTERVENTION/EVALUATION

Gonadorelin Acetate: With baseline pelvic ultrasound, perform follow-up studies. **Gonadorelin Hydrochloride:** Change cannula, IV site at 48-hr intervals. Ensure that protocol for test is maintained: usually venous blood samples (for LH) drawn after administration at intervals of 15, 30, 45, 60, 120 min.

goserelin

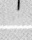

gos-**er**-ah-lin
(Zoladex, Zoladex LA ✱)

◆CLASSIFICATION

PHARMACOTHERAPEUTIC: Gonadotropin-releasing hormone analogue. **CLINICAL:** Antineoplastic (see pp. 79C, 101C).

ACTION

Stimulates release of luteinizing hormone (LH) and follicle-stimulating hormone (FSH) from anterior pituitary. **Therapeutic Effect:** In females, reduces ovarian, uterine, mammary gland size, regresses hormone-responsive tumors. In males, decreases testosterone level, reduces growth of abnormal prostate tissue.

PHARMACOKINETICS

Protein binding: 27%. Metabolized in liver. Excreted in urine. **Half-life:** 4.2 hrs (male); 2.3 hrs (female).

USES

Treatment of advanced carcinoma of prostate as alternative when orchiectomy, estrogen therapy is either not indicated or unacceptable to pt. In combination with flutamide before and during radiation therapy for early stages of prostate cancer. Management of endometriosis. Treatment of advanced breast cancer in premenopausal and perimenopausal women. Endometrial thinning before ablation for dysfunctional uterine bleeding.

PRECAUTIONS

CONTRAINDICATIONS: Pregnancy. **CAUTIONS:** None known.

LIFESPAN CONSIDERATIONS:

Pregnancy/Lactation: Crosses placenta; unknown if distributed in breast milk. **Pregnancy Category D (advanced breast cancer), X (endometriosis, endometrial thinning). Children:** Safety and efficacy not established. **Elderly:** No age-related precautions noted.

INTERACTIONS

DRUG: None significant. **HERBAL:** None significant. **FOOD:** None known. **LAB VALUES:** May increase serum prostatic acid phosphatase, testosterone.

AVAILABILITY (Rx)

INJECTION, SOLUTION (ZOLADEX): 3.6 mg, 10.8 mg.

ADMINISTRATION/HANDLING

INJECTION

• Clean area of skin on upper abdominal wall with alcohol swab. • Stretch or pinch pt's skin with one hand, and insert needle into subcutaneous tissue. • Direct needle so that it parallels the abdominal wall. Push needle in until barrel hub touches pt's skin. Withdraw needle 1 cm to create a space to discharge goserelin. Fully depress plunger. • Withdraw needle, bandage site.

INDICATIONS/ROUTES/DOSAGE

PROSTATIC CARCINOMA

IMPLANT: ADULTS OLDER THAN 18 YRS, ELDERLY: 3.6 mg every 28 days or 10.8 q12wks subcutaneously into upper abdominal wall.

BREAST CARCINOMA, ENDOMETRIOSIS

IMPLANT: ADULTS: 3.6 mg every 28 days subcutaneously into upper abdominal wall.

ENDOMETRIAL THINNING

IMPLANT: ADULTS: 3.6 mg subcutaneously into upper abdominal wall as a single dose or in 2 doses 4 wks apart.

SIDE EFFECTS

FREQUENT: Headache (60%), hot flashes (55%), depression (54%), diaphoresis (45%), sexual dysfunction (21%), impotence (18%), lower urinary tract symptoms (13%). **OCCASIONAL (10%–5%):** Pain, lethargy, dizziness, insomnia, anorexia, nausea, rash, upper respiratory tract infection, hirsutism, abdominal pain. **RARE:** Pruritus.

ADVERSE EFFECTS/ TOXIC REACTIONS

Arrhythmias, CHF, hypertension occur rarely. Ureteral obstruction, spinal cord compression observed (immediate orchiectomy may be necessary).

NURSING CONSIDERATIONS

INTERVENTION/EVALUATION

Monitor pt closely for worsening signs/symptoms of prostatic cancer, esp. during first mo of therapy.

PATIENT/FAMILY TEACHING

• Use contraceptive measures during therapy. • Inform physician if pt becomes pregnant or regular menstruation persists. • Breakthrough menstrual bleeding may occur if dose is missed.

• Use nonhormonal methods of contraception.

granisetron

gran-**is**-eh-tron
(Kytril)

CLASSIFICATION

PHARMACOTHERAPEUTIC: Serotonin receptor antagonist. **CLINICAL:** Antiemetic.

ACTION

Selectively blocks serotonin stimulation at receptor sites at chemoreceptor trigger zone, vagal nerve terminals. **Therapeutic Effect:** Prevents nausea/vomiting.

PHARMACOKINETICS

Route	Onset	Peak	Duration
IV	1–3 min	N/A	24 hrs

Rapidly, widely distributed to tissues. Protein binding: 65%. Metabolized in liver to active metabolite. Eliminated in urine, feces. **Half-life:** 10–12 hrs (increased in elderly).

USES

Prevents nausea/vomiting associated with emetogenic cancer therapy (includes high-dose cisplatin). Prevention, treatment of postop nausea, vomiting. Prophylaxis of nausea/vomiting associated with cancer radiation therapy. **OFF-LABEL: PO:** Prophylaxis of nausea/vomiting associated with radiation therapy.

PRECAUTIONS

CONTRAINDICATIONS: None known. **CAUTIONS:** Safety in children younger than 2 yrs not established.

LIFESPAN CONSIDERATIONS:

Pregnancy/Lactation: Unknown if drug is distributed in breast milk. **Pregnancy Category B. Children:** Safety and efficacy not established in children younger than 2 yrs. **Elderly:** No age-related precautions noted.

INTERACTIONS

DRUG: Hepatic enzyme inducers may decrease effect. **HERBAL:** None significant. **FOOD:** None known. **LAB VALUES:** May increase AST, ALT.

AVAILABILITY (Rx)

INJECTION SOLUTION: 0.1 mg/ml, 1 mg/ml. **ORAL SOLUTION:** 2 mg/10 ml. **TABLETS:** 1 mg.

ADMINISTRATION/HANDLING

IV

Reconstitution • May be given undiluted or dilute with 20–50 ml 0.9% NaCl or D_5W. Do not mix with other medications.

Rate of administration • May give undiluted as IV push over 30 sec. • For IV piggyback, infuse over 5–20 min depending on volume of diluent used.

Storage • Appears as a clear, colorless solution. • Store at room temperature. • After dilution, stable for at least 24 hrs at room temperature. • Inspect for particulates, discoloration.

PO

• Give 30 min to 1 hr prior to initiating chemotherapy.

IV INCOMPATIBILITY

Amphotericin B (Fungizone).

IV COMPATIBILITIES

Allopurinol (Aloprim), bumetanide (Bumex), calcium gluconate, carboplatin (Paraplatin), cisplatin (Platinol), cyclophosphamide (Cytoxan), cytarabine (Ara-C), dacarbazine (DTIC-Dome), dexamethasone (Decadron), diphenhydramine (Benadryl), docetaxel (Taxotere), doxorubicin (Adriamycin), etoposide (VePesid), gemcitabine (Gemzar), lipids, magnesium, mitoxantrone (Novantrone), paclitaxel (Taxol), potassium.

INDICATIONS/ROUTES/DOSAGE

PREVENTION OF CHEMOTHERAPY-INDUCED NAUSEA/VOMITING

PO: ADULTS, ELDERLY: 2 mg 1 hr before chemotherapy or 1 mg 1 hr before and 12 hrs after chemotherapy.

IV: ADULTS, ELDERLY, CHILDREN 2 YRS AND OLDER: 10 mcg/kg/dose (or 1 mg/dose) within 30 min of chemotherapy.

PREVENTION OF RADIATION-INDUCED NAUSEA/VOMITING

PO: ADULTS, ELDERLY: 2 mg once a day, given 1 hr before radiation therapy.

POSTOPERATIVE NAUSEA/VOMITING

PO: ADULTS, ELDERLY, CHILDREN 4 YRS AND OLDER: 20–40 mcg/kg as a single postoperative dose.

IV: ADULTS, ELDERLY: 1 mg as a single postoperative dose. **CHILDREN OLDER THAN 4 YRS:** 20–40 mcg/kg. **Maximum:** 1 mg.

SIDE EFFECTS

FREQUENT (21%–14%): Headache, constipation, asthenia. **OCCASIONAL (8%–6%):** Diarrhea, abdominal pain. **RARE (less than 2%):** Altered taste, fever.

ADVERSE EFFECTS/ TOXIC REACTIONS

Hypersensitivity reaction, hypertension, hypotension, arrhythmias (sinus bradycardia, atrial fibrillation, AV block, ventricular ectopy), EKG abnormalities occur rarely.

NURSING CONSIDERATIONS

BASELINE ASSESSMENT

Ensure that granisetron is given within 30 min of starting chemotherapy.

INTERVENTION/EVALUATION

Monitor for therapeutic effect. Assess for headache. Monitor daily pattern of bowel activity/stool consistency.

PATIENT/FAMILY TEACHING

• Granisetron is effective shortly following administration; prevents nausea/vomiting. • Explain that transitory taste disorder may occur.

griseofulvin

griz-ee-oh-**full**-vin

(Fulvicin P/G, Fulvicin U/F, Grifulvin V, Grisactin 500, Griseofulicin, Gris-PEG)

CLASSIFICATION

CLINICAL: Antifungal.

ACTION

Inhibits fungal cell mitosis by disrupting mitotic spindle structure. **Therapeutic Effect:** Fungistatic.

PHARMACOKINETICS

Ultramicrosize is almost completely absorbed. Absorption is significantly enhanced after a fatty meal. Extensively metabolized in liver. Minimal excretion in urine. **Half-life:** 24 hrs.

USES

Treatment of susceptible tinea (ringworm) infections of the skin, hair, and nails: t. capitis, t. corporis, t. cruris, t. pedis, t. unguium.

PRECAUTIONS

CONTRAINDICATIONS: Hepatocellular failure, porphyria. **CAUTIONS:** Exposure to sun/ultraviolet light (photosensitivity), hypersensitivity to penicillins.

LIFESPAN CONSIDERATIONS:

Pregnancy/Lactation: Crosses placenta; unknown if distributed in breast milk. **Pregnancy Category C. Children:** Safety and efficacy not established in children younger than 2 yrs. **Elderly:** No age-related precautions noted.

INTERACTIONS

DRUG: May decrease effects of **oral contraceptives, warfarin.** **HERBAL:** None significant. **FOOD: High-fat foods** enhance absorption. **LAB VALUES:** None known.

AVAILABILITY (Rx)

ORAL SUSPENSION (GRIFULVIN V): 125 mg/5 ml. **TABLETS (MICROSIZE [FULVICIN -U/F, GRISACTIN 500, GRIFULVIN V]):** 250 mg, 500 mg. **TABLETS (ULTRAMICROSIZE):** 125 mg (Fulvicin P/G, Gris-PEG), 165 mg (Fulvicin P/G), 250 mg (Fulvicin P/G, Gris-PEG), 330 mg (Fulvicin P/G, Griseofulicin).

G

INDICATIONS/ROUTES/DOSAGE

USUAL DOSAGE

◀ **ALERT** ▶ Duration of therapy depends on site of infection.

PO (MICROSIZE TABLETS, ORAL SUSPENSION): ADULTS: 500–1,000 mg as a single dose or in divided doses. **CHILDREN 2 YRS AND OLDER:** 10–20 mg/kg/day.

PO (ULTRAMICROSIZE TABLETS): ADULTS: 330–750 mg/day as a single dose or in divided doses. **CHILDREN 2 YRS AND OLDER:** 5–10 mg/kg/day.

SIDE EFFECTS

OCCASIONAL: Hypersensitivity reaction (pruritus, rash, urticaria), headache, nausea, diarrhea, excessive thirst, flatulence, oral thrush, dizziness, insomnia. **RARE:** Paresthesia of hands/feet, proteinuria, photosensitivity reaction.

ADVERSE EFFECTS/ TOXIC REACTIONS

Granulocytopenia occurs rarely and should necessitate discontinuation of drug.

NURSING CONSIDERATIONS

BASELINE ASSESSMENT

Question for history of allergies, esp. to griseofulvin, penicillins.

INTERVENTION/EVALUATION

Assess skin for rash, response to therapy. Determine daily pattern of bowel activity/stool consistency. Question presence of headache: onset, location, type of discomfort. Assess for dizziness.

PATIENT/FAMILY TEACHING

• Prolonged therapy (wks or mos) usually is necessary. • Do not miss a dose; continue therapy as long as ordered. • Avoid alcohol (may produce tachycardia, flushing). • May cause photosensitivity reaction; avoid exposure to sunlight. • Maintain good hygiene (prevents superinfection). • Separate personal items in direct contact with affected areas. • Keep affected areas dry; wear light clothing for ventilation. • Take with foods high in fat such as milk, ice cream (reduces GI upset, assists absorption).

guaifenesin

gwye-**fen**-e-sin

(Guiatuss, Humibid, Mucinex, Organidin, Phanasin, Robitussin)

Do not confuse guaifenesin with guanfacine or Mucinex with Mucomyst.

FIXED-COMBINATION(S)

Mucinex D: guaifenesin/pseudoephedrine (a sympathomimetic): 600 mg/60 mg; 1,200 mg/120 mg. **Mucinex DM:** guaifenesin/dextromethorphan (a cough suppressant): 600 mg/30 mg; 1,200 mg/60 mg. **Robitussin AC:** guaifenesin/codeine (a narcotic analgesic): 100 mg/10 mg; 75 mg/2.5 mg per 5 ml. **Robitussin DM:** guaifenesin/dextromethorphan (a cough suppressant): 100 mg/10 mg per 5 ml.

◆ CLASSIFICATION

CLINICAL: Expectorant.

ACTION

Stimulates respiratory tract secretions by decreasing adhesiveness, viscosity of phlegm. **Therapeutic Effect:** Promotes removal of viscous mucus.

PHARMACOKINETICS

Well absorbed from GI tract. Metabolized in liver. Excreted in urine. **Half-life:** 1 hr.

USES

Expectorant for symptomatic treatment of coughs.

PRECAUTIONS

CONTRAINDICATIONS: None known. **CAUTIONS:** None known.

⌛ LIFESPAN CONSIDERATIONS:

Pregnancy/Lactation: Unknown if drug crosses placenta or is distributed in breast milk. **Pregnancy Category C.** **Children:** Caution advised in children younger than 2 yrs with persistent cough. **Elderly:** No age-related precautions noted.

INTERACTIONS

DRUG: None significant. **HERBAL:** None significant. **FOOD:** None known. **LAB VALUES:** None known.

AVAILABILITY (OTC)

LIQUID: 100 mg/5 ml. **SYRUP:** 100 mg/5 ml. **SYRUP, ORAL DROPS:** 50 mg/ml. **TABLETS:** 200 mg, 400 mg.

TABLETS EXTENDED-RELEASE: (MUCINEX): 600 mg.

ADMINISTRATION/HANDLING

PO

• Store syrup, liquid, tablets at room temperature. • Give without regard to meals. • Do not crush, break extended-release tablet. May sprinkle contents on soft food, then swallow without crushing/chewing.

INDICATIONS/ROUTES/DOSAGE

EXPECTORANT

PO: ADULTS, ELDERLY, CHILDREN OLDER THAN 12 YRS: 200–400 mg q4h. **CHILDREN 6–12 YRS:** 100–200 mg q4h. **Maximum:** 1.2 g/day. **CHILDREN 2–5 YRS:** 50–100 mg q4h. **Maximum:** 600 mg/day. **CHILDREN, 6 MOS–2 YRS:** 25–50 mg of q4h. **Maximum:** 300 mg/day.

PO (EXTENDED-RELEASE): ADULTS, ELDERLY, CHILDREN OLDER THAN 12 YRS: 600–1,200 mg q12h. **Maximum:** 2.4 g/day. **CHILDREN 6–12 YRS:** 600 mg q12h. **Maximum:** 1.2 g/day.

SIDE EFFECTS

RARE: Dizziness, headache, rash, diarrhea, nausea, vomiting, abdominal pain.

ADVERSE EFFECTS/ TOXIC REACTIONS

Overdose may produce nausea, vomiting.

NURSING CONSIDERATIONS

BASELINE ASSESSMENT

Assess type, severity, frequency of cough. Increase fluid intake, environmental humidity to lower viscosity of lung secretions.

INTERVENTION/EVALUATION

Initiate deep breathing, coughing exercises, particularly in pts with pulmonary impairment. Assess for clinical improvement; record onset of relief of cough.

PATIENT/FAMILY TEACHING

• Avoid tasks that require alertness, motor skills until response to drug is established. • Do not take for chronic cough. • Inform physician if cough persists or if fever, rash, headache, sore throat is present with cough. • Maintain adequate hydration.

halcinonide

(Halog)

See Corticosteroids: topical

Haldol, *see haloperidol*

halobetasol

(Ultravate)

See Corticosteroids: topical (p. 95C)

haloperidol

hal-oh-**pear**-ih-dawl

(Apo-Haloperidol ✤, Haldol, Haldol Decanoate, Novoperidol ✤, Peridol ✤)

Do not confuse Haldol with Halcion, Halog, or Stadol.

CLASSIFICATION

CLINICAL: Antipsychotic, antiemetic, antidyskinetic (see p. 62C).

ACTION

Competitively blocks postsynaptic dopamine receptors, interrupts nerve impulse movement, increases turnover of dopamine in brain. **Therapeutic Effect:** Produces tranquilizing effect. Strong extrapyramidal, antiemetic effects; weak anticholinergic, sedative effects.

PHARMACOKINETICS

Readily absorbed from GI tract. Protein binding: 92%. Extensively metabolized in liver. Primarily excreted in urine. Not removed by hemodialysis. **Half-life:** 12–37 hrs PO; 10–19 hrs IV; 17–25 hrs IM.

USES

Treatment of psychoses, Tourette's disorder, severe behavioral problems in children, emergency sedation of severely agitated/psychotic pts. **OFF-LABEL:** Treatment of Huntington's chorea, infantile autism, nausea/vomiting associated with cancer chemotherapy.

PRECAUTIONS

CONTRAINDICATIONS: Narrow-angle glaucoma, CNS depression, myelosuppression, Parkinson's disease, severe cardiac, hepatic disease. **CAUTIONS:** Renal/hepatic impairment, cardiovascular disease, history of seizures.

LIFESPAN CONSIDERATIONS:

Pregnancy/Lactation: Crosses placenta. Distributed in breast milk. **Pregnancy Category C. Children:** More susceptible to dystonias; not recommended in those younger than 3 yrs. **Elderly:** More susceptible to orthostatic hypotension, anticholinergic effects, sedation; increased risk for extrapyramidal effects. Decreased dosage recommended.

INTERACTIONS

DRUG: **Alcohol, other CNS depressants** may increase CNS depression. **Epinephrine** may block alpha-adrenergic effects. **Medications producing extrapyramidal symptoms (EPS)** may increase extrapyramidal symptoms. **Lithium** may increase neurologic toxicity. **HERBAL:** **Gotu kola, kava kava, St. John' wort, valerian** may increase CNS depression. **FOOD:** None known. **LAB VALUES:** None known. Therapeutic serum level is 0.2–1 mcg/ml; toxic serum level is greater than 1 mcg/ml.

AVAILABILITY (Rx)

INJECTION, SOLUTION (LACTATE [HALDOL]): 5 mg/ml. **INJECTION, SOLUTION**

(DECANOATE [HALDOL DECANOATE]): 50 mg/ml, 100 mg/ml. **ORAL CONCENTRATE:** 2 mg/ml. **TABLETS (HALDOL):** 0.5 mg, 1 mg, 2 mg, 5 mg, 10 mg, 20 mg.

ADMINISTRATION/HANDLING

IV

◀ **ALERT** ▶ Only haloperidol lactate is given IV.

Reconstitution • May give undiluted. • Flush with at least 2 ml 0.9% NaCl before and after administration. • May add to 30–50 ml of most solutions (D_5W preferred).

Rate of administration • Give IV push at rate of 5 mg/min. • Infuse IV piggyback over 30 min. • For IV infusion, up to 25 mg/hr has been used (titrated to pt response).

Storage • Discard if precipitate forms, discoloration occurs. • Store at room temperature; do not freeze. • Protect from light.

IM

Parenteral administration • Pt should remain recumbent for 30–60 min in head-low position with legs raised to minimize hypotensive effect. • Prepare Decanoate IM injection using 21-gauge needle. • Do not exceed maximum volume of 3 ml per IM injection site. • Inject slow, deep IM into upper outer quadrant of gluteus maximus.

PO

• Give without regard to meals. • Scored tablets may be crushed.

IV INCOMPATIBILITIES

Allopurinol (Aloprim), amphotericin B complex (Abelcet, AmBisome, Amphotec), cefepime (Maxipime), fluconazole (Diflucan), foscarnet (Foscavir), heparin, lipids, nitroprusside (Nipride), piperacillin/tazobactam (Zosyn).

IV COMPATIBILITIES

Dobutamine (Dobutrex), dopamine (Intropin), fentanyl (Sublimaze), hydromorphone (Dilaudid), lidocaine, lorazepam (Ativan), midazolam (Versed), morphine, nitroglycerin, norepinephrine (Levophed), propofol (Diprivan).

INDICATIONS/ROUTES/DOSAGE

ACUTE PSYCHOSIS, DELIRIUM

IV: ADULTS, ELDERLY: 0.5–50 mg at a rate of 5 mg/min. May repeat as needed.

PSYCHOTIC DISORDERS

IM: ADULTS, ELDERLY, CHILDERN 12 YRS AND OLDER: Initially, 2–5 mg. May repeat at 1-hr intervals as needed. **Maximum:** 100 mg/day.

IM (decanoate): ADULTS, ELDERLY, CHILDREN 12 YRS AND OLDER: Initially, 10–15 times previous daily oral dose up to maximum initial dose of 100 mg. **Maximum:** 300 mg/mo.

PO: ADULTS, ELDERLY, CHILDREN 12 YRS AND OLDER: Initially, 0.5–5 mg 2–3 times/day. Dosage gradually adjusted as needed. **ELDERELY:** 0.5–2 mg 2–3 times/day. Doasge gradually adjusted as needed. **CHILDREN, 3–12 YRS OR 15–40 KG:** Initially 0.05 mg/kg/day in 2–3 divided doses. May increase by 0.5-mg increments at 5- to 7-day intervals. **Maximum:** 0.15 mg/kg/day in divided doses.

SEVERE BEHAVIORAL PROBLEMS

PO: CHILDREN 3–12 YRS, WEIGHING 15–40 KG: 0.05–0.075 mg/kg/day. Initially, 0.5 mg/day. May increase by 0.5 mg/day q5–7days divided into 2–3 doses a day. Maintenance: Up to 6 mg/day.

TOURETTE'S DISORDER

PO: ADULTS, ELDERLY: 6–15 mg/day. May increase by 2 mg increments as needed. Maintenance: 9 mg/day. **CHILDREN 3–12 YRS, WEIGHING 15–40 KG:** 0.05–0.075 mg/kg/day. Initially, 0.5 mg/day. May increase by 0.5 mg/day q5–7days divided into 2–3 doses a day. Maintenance: Up to 6 mg/day.

SIDE EFFECTS

FREQUENT: Blurred vision, constipation, orthostatic hypotension, dry mouth, swelling or soreness of female breasts, peripheral edema. **OCCASIONAL:** Allergic reaction, difficulty urinating, decreased thirst, dizziness, diminished sexual function, drowsiness, nausea, vomiting, photosensitivity, lethargy.

ADVERSE EFFECTS/ TOXIC REACTIONS

Extrapyramidal symptoms appear to be dose related and typically occur in first few days of therapy. Marked drowsiness/lethargy, excessive salivation, fixed stare may be mild to severe in intensity. Less frequently noted are severe akathisia (motor restlessness), acute dystonias: torticollis (neck muscle spasm), opisthotonos (rigidity of back muscles), oculogyric crisis (rolling back of eyes). Tardive dyskinesia (tongue protrusion, puffing of cheeks, chewing/puckering of the mouth) may occur during long-term therapy or after drug discontinuance, and may be irreversible. Elderly female pts have greater risk of developing this reaction.

NURSING CONSIDERATIONS

BASELINE ASSESSMENT

Assess behavior, appearance, emotional status, response to environment, speech pattern, thought content.

INTERVENTION/EVALUATION

Supervise suicidal-risk pt closely during early therapy (as depression lessens, energy level improves, causing increased suicide potential). Monitor for rigidity, tremor, mask-like facial expression, fine tongue movement. Assess for therapeutic response (interest in surroundings, improvement in self-care, increased ability to concentrate, relaxed facial expression). Therapeutic serum level: 0.2–1 mcg/ml. Toxic serum level: greater than 1 mcg/ml.

PATIENT/FAMILY TEACHING

• Full therapeutic effect may take up to 6 wks. • Do not abruptly withdraw from long-term drug therapy. • Sugarless gum, sips of tepid water may relieve dry mouth. • Drowsiness generally subsides during continued therapy. • Avoid tasks that require alertness, motor skills until response to drug is established. • Avoid alcohol. • Report muscle stiffness. • Avoid exposure to sunlight, overheating, dehydration (increased risk of heat stroke).

haloprogin

(Halotex)

See Antifungals: topical

heparin

hep-a-rin

(Hep-Lock, Hep-Pak CVC, Hepalean ✤, Hepalean Leo ✤)

Do not confuse heparin with Hespan.

CLASSIFICATION

PHARMACOTHERAPEUTIC: Blood modifier. **CLINICAL:** Anticoagulant (see p. 30C).

ACTION

Interferes with blood coagulation by blocking conversion of prothrombin to thrombin and fibrinogen to fibrin. **Therapeutic Effect:** Prevents further extension of existing thrombi or new clot formation. No effect on existing clots.

PHARMACOKINETICS

Well absorbed following subcutaneous administration. Protein binding: Very high. Metabolized in liver. Removed from circulation via uptake by reticuloendothelial system. Primarily excreted in urine. Not removed by hemodialysis. **Half-life:** 1–6 hrs.

USES

Prophylaxis, treatment of thromboembolic disorders, including venous thrombosis, pulmonary embolism, peripheral arterial embolism, atrial fibrillation with embolism. Prevention of thromboembolus in cardiac and vascular surgery, dialysis procedures, blood transfusions, blood sampling for laboratory purposes. Adjunct in treatment of coronary occlusion with acute MI. Maintains patency of indwelling intravascular devices. Diagnosis, treatment of acute/chronic consumptive coagulation pathology (e.g., disseminated intravascular coagulation [DIC]). Prevents cerebral thrombosis in progressive strokes.

PRECAUTIONS

CONTRAINDICATIONS: Intracranial hemorrhage, severe hypotension, severe thrombocytopenia, subacute bacterial endocarditis, uncontrolled bleeding. **CAUTIONS:** IM injections, peptic ulcer disease, menstruation, recent surgery or invasive procedures, severe hepatic or renal disease.

LIFESPAN CONSIDERATIONS:

Pregnancy/Lactation: Use with caution, particularly during last trimester, immediate postpartum period (increased risk of maternal hemorrhage). Does not cross placenta. Not distributed in breast milk. **Pregnancy Category C. Children:** No age-related precautions noted. Benzyl alcohol preservative may cause gasping syndrome in infants. **Elderly:** More susceptible to hemorrhage. Age-related renal impairment may increase risk of bleeding.

INTERACTIONS

DRUG: Antithyroid medications, valproic acid may cause hypoprothrombinemia. **Other anticoagulants, platelet aggregation inhibitors, thrombolytics** may increase risk of bleeding. **Probenecid** may increase effect. **HERBAL: Cat's claw, dong quai, evening primrose, feverfew, red clover, horse chestnut, garlic, ginseng, ginkgo** may increase antiplatelet activity. **FOOD:** None known. **LAB VALUES:** May increase free fatty acids, serum AST, ALT. May decrease serum cholesterol, triglycerides.

AVAILABILITY (Rx)

INJECTION SOLUTION: 10 units/ml (Hep-Lock), 100 units/ml, 1,000 units/ml, 2,500 units/ml, 5,000 units/ml, 7,500 units/ml, 10,000 units/ml, 20,000 units/ml, 25,000 units/250 ml infusion, 25,000 units/500 ml infusion. **INJECTABLE KIT (HEP-PAK CVC):** 20 units/ml, 100 units/ml.

ADMINISTRATION/HANDLING

◀ **ALERT** ▶ Do **not** give by IM injection (pain, hematoma, ulceration, erythema).

IV

◀ **ALERT** ▶ Used in full-dose therapy. Intermittent IV dosage produces higher incidence of bleeding abnormalities. Continuous IV route preferred.

Reconstitution • Dilute IV infusion in isotonic sterile saline, D_5W, or lactated Ringer's. • Invert container at least 6 times (ensures mixing, prevents pooling of medication).

Rate of administration • Use constant-rate IV infusion pump.

Storage • Store at room temperature.

SUBCUTANEOUS

◀ **ALERT** ▶ Used in low-dose therapy.

• After withdrawal of heparin from vial, change needle before injection (prevents leakage along needle track). • Inject above iliac crest or in abdominal fat layer. Do not inject within 2 inches of umbilicus or any scar tissue. • Withdraw needle rapidly, apply prolonged pressure at injection site. Do not massage. • Rotate injection sites.

IV INCOMPATIBILITIES

Amiodarone (Cordarone), amphotericin B complex (Abelcet, AmBisome, Amphotec), ciprofloxacin (Cipro), dacarbazine (DTIC), diazepam (Valium), dobutamine (Dobutrex), doxorubicin (Adriamycin), droperidol (Inapsine), filgrastim (Neupogen), gentamicin (Garamycin), haloperidol (Haldol), idarubicin (Idamycin), labetalol (Trandate), lipids, nicardipine (Cardene), phenytoin (Dilantin), quinidine, tobramycin (Nebcin), vancomycin (Vancocin).

IV COMPATIBILITIES

Aminophylline, ampicillin/sulbactam (Unasyn), aztreonam (Azactam), calcium gluconate, cefazolin (Ancef), ceftazidime (Fortaz), ceftriaxone (Rocephin), digoxin (Lanoxin), diltiazem (Cardizem), dopamine (Intropin), enalapril (Vasotec), famotidine (Pepcid), fentanyl (Sublimaze), furosemide (Lasix), hydromorphone (Dilaudid), insulin, lidocaine, lorazepam (Ativan), magnesium sulfate, methylprednisolone (Solu-Medrol), midazolam (Versed), milrinone (Primacor), morphine, nitroglycerin, norepinephrine (Levophed), oxytocin (Pitocin), piperacillin/tazobactam (Zosyn), procainamide (Pronestyl), propofol (Diprivan), total parenteral nutrition (TPN).

INDICATIONS/ROUTES/DOSAGE

LINE FLUSHING

IV: ADULTS, ELDERLY, CHILDREN: 100 units q6–8h. **INFANTS WEIGHING LESS THAN 10 KG:** 10 units q6–8h.

TREATMENT OF THROMBOEMBOLIC DISORDERS

INTERMITTENT IV: ADULTS, ELDERLY: Initially, 10,000 units, then 50–70 units/kg (5,000–10,000 units) q4–6h. **CHILDREN 1 YR AND OLDER:** Initially, 50–100 units/kg, then 50–100 units q4h.

IV INFUSION: Weight-based dosing per institutional nomogram is recommended. 20,000–40,000 units administered over 24 hrs; dose usually preceeded by loading dose of 35–70 units/kg or 5,000 units. Dosage must be adjusted as determined by aPTT results.

PREVENTION OF THROMBOEMBOLIC DISORDERS

SUBCUTANEOUS: ADULT, ELDERLY: 5,000 units q8–12h.

SIDE EFFECTS

OCCASIONAL: Pruritus, burning (particularly on soles of feet) caused by vasospastic reaction. **RARE:** Pain, cyanosis of extremity 6–10 days after initial therapy lasting 4–6 hrs, hypersensitivity reaction (chills, fever, pruritus, urticaria, asthma, rhinitis, lacrimation, headache).

ADVERSE EFFECTS/ TOXIC REACTIONS

Bleeding complications ranging from local ecchymoses to major hemorrhage occur more frequently in high-dose therapy, intermittent IV infusion, women 60 yrs and older. **Antidote:** Protamine sulfate 1–1.5 mg, IV, for every 100 units heparin subcutaneous within 30 min of overdose, 0.5–0.75 mg for every 100 units heparin subcutaneous if within 30–60 min of overdose, 0.25–0.375 mg for every 100 units heparin subcutaneous if 2 hrs have elapsed since overdose, 25–50 mg if heparin was given by IV infusion.

NURSING CONSIDERATIONS

BASELINE ASSESSMENT

Cross-check dose with co-worker. Determine aPTT before administration and 24 hrs following initiation of therapy, then q24–48hrs for first wk of therapy or until maintenance dose is established. Follow with aPTT determinations 1–2 times weekly for 3–4 wks. In long-term therapy, monitor 1–2 times/mo.

INTERVENTION/EVALUATION

Monitor aPTT (therapeutic dosage at 1.5–2.5 times normal) diligently. Assess Hct, platelet count, AST, ALT, urine and stool for occult blood, regardless of route of administration. Assess for decrease in B/P, increase in pulse rate, complaint of abdominal/back pain, severe headache (may be evidence of hemorrhage). Question for increase in amount of discharge during menses. Assess peripheral pulses; skin for ecchymosis, petechiae. Check for excessive bleeding from minor cuts, scratches. Assess gums for erythema, gingival bleeding. Assess urine output for hematuria. Avoid IM injections of other medications due to potential for hematomas. When converting to warfarin (Coumadin) therapy, monitor prothrombin time (PT) results (will be 10%–20% higher while heparin is given concurrently).

PATIENT/FAMILY TEACHING

• Use electric razor, soft toothbrush to prevent bleeding. • Report any sign of red or dark urine, black or red stool, coffee-ground vomitus, blood-tinged mucus from cough. • Do not use any OTC medication without physician approval (may interfere with platelet aggregation). • Wear or carry identification that notes anticoagulant therapy. • Inform dentist, other physicians of heparin therapy.

Hepsera, *see adefovir*

Herceptin, *see trastuzumab*

hetastarch

het-ah-starch
(Hespan, Hextend)

CLASSIFICATION

CLINICAL: Plasma volume expander.

ACTION

Exerts osmotic pull on tissue fluids. **Therapeutic Effect:** Reduces hemoconcentration, blood viscosity; increases circulating blood volume.

PHARMACOKINETICS

Smaller molecules, less than 50,000 molecular weight, rapidly excreted by kidneys; larger molecules, 50,000 molecular weight and greater, slowly degraded to smaller-sized molecules, then excreted. **Half-life:** 17 days.

USES

Fluid replacement, plasma volume expansion in treatment of shock due to hemorrhage, burns, surgery, sepsis, trauma; leukapheresis.

PRECAUTIONS

CONTRAINDICATIONS: Anuria, oliguria, severe bleeding disorders, severe CHF. **CAUTIONS:** Thrombocytopenia, elderly, very young, pulmonary edema, CHF, renal impairment, hepatic disease, those on sodium restriction.

LIFESPAN CONSIDERATIONS: **Pregnancy/Lactation:** Unknown if drug crosses placenta or is distributed in breast milk. **Pregnancy Category C.** **Children:** Safety and efficacy not established. **Elderly:** Age-related renal impairment may require dosage adjustment.

INTERACTIONS

DRUG: None significant. **HERBAL:** None significant. **FOOD:** None known. **LAB**

VALUES: May prolong bleeding/clotting times, aPTT, PT. May decrease Hct.

AVAILABILITY (Rx)

INJECTION SOLUTION (HESPAN, HEXTEND): 6 g/100 ml 0.9% NaCl (500 ml infusion container).

ADMINISTRATION/HANDLING

IV

Rate of administration • Administer only by IV infusion. • Do not add drugs or mix with other IV fluids. • In acute hemorrhagic shock, administer at rate approaching 1.2 g/kg (20 ml/kg) per hour. Use slower rates for burns, septic shock. • Monitor central venous pressure (CVP) when given by rapid infusion. If there is a precipitous rise in CVP, immediately discontinue drug (overexpansion of blood volume).

Storage • Store solutions at room temperature. • Solution should appear clear, pale yellow to amber. Do not use if discolored (deep turbid brown) or if precipitate forms.

IV INCOMPATIBILITIES

Amikacin (Amikin), ampicillin (Polycillin), cefazolin (Ancef, Kefzol), cefotaxime (Claforan), cefoxitin (Mefoxin), gentamicin (Garamycin), ranitidine (Zantac), tobramycin (Nebcin).

INDICATIONS/ROUTES/DOSAGE

PLASMA VOLUME EXPANDER

IV: ADULTS, ELDERLY: 500–1,000 ml (30–60 g) per dose. **Maximum total daily dose:** 1.2 g/kg or 1,500 ml (90 g). **CHILDREN:** 10 ml/kg/dose. **Maximum total daily dose:** 20 ml/kg.

LEUKAPHERESIS

IV: ADULTS, ELDERLY: 250–700 ml infused at constant rate, usually 1:8 to venous whole blood.

SIDE EFFECTS

RARE: Allergic reaction resulting in vomiting, mild temperature elevation, chills, pruritus, submaxillary/parotid gland enlargement, peripheral edema of lower extremities, mild flu-like symptoms, headache, muscle aches.

ADVERSE EFFECTS/ TOXIC REACTIONS

Fluid overload may occur (increased B/P, distended neck veins). Neurologic changes in fluid overload include headache, weakness, blurred vision, behavioral changes, incoordination, isolated muscle twitching. Pulmonary edema may occur (tachypnea, rales/crackles, wheezing, coughing). Anaphylactic reaction (periorbital edema, urticaria, wheezing) may occur.

NURSING CONSIDERATIONS

INTERVENTION/EVALUATION

Monitor for fluid overload (peripheral and/or pulmonary edema, impending CHF symptoms). Assess lung sounds for wheezing, rales/crackles. During leukapheresis, monitor leukocyte, platelet count, Hgb, Hct, PT, PTT, I&O. Monitor central venous B/P (detects overexpansion of blood volume). Monitor urine output closely (increase in output generally occurs in oliguric pts following administration). Assess for periorbital edema, pruritus, wheezing, urticaria (allergic reaction). Monitor for oliguria, anuria, any change in output ratio. Monitor for bleeding from surgical/ trauma sites.

Hivid, *see zalcitabine*

Humalog, *see insulin*

Humalog Mix 75 and 25 Pen, *see insulin*

Humira, *see adalimumab*

Humulin 70 and 30, *see insulin*

Humulin N, *see insulin*

Humulin R, *see insulin*

Hycamtin, *see topotecan*

*hydrALAZINE

hye-**dral**-a-zeen
(Apo-Hydralazine ✤, Apresoline, Novohylazin ✤)

Do not confuse hydralazine with hydroxyzine.

FIXED-COMBINATION(S)

Apresazide: hydralazine/hydrochlorothiazide (a diuretic): 25 mg/25 mg; 50 mg/50 mg; 100 mg/50 mg. **BiDil:** hydralazine/isosorbide (a nitrate): 37.5 mg/20 mg.

CLASSIFICATION

PHARMACOTHERAPEUTIC: Vasodilator. **CLINICAL:** Antihypertensive (see p. 59C).

ACTION

Direct vasodilating effects on arterioles. **Therapeutic Effect:** Decreases B/P, systemic resistance.

PHARMACOKINETICS

Route	Onset	Peak	Duration
PO	20–30 min	N/A	2–4 hrs
IV	5–20 min	N/A	2–6 hrs

Well absorbed from GI tract. Widely distributed. Protein binding: 85%–90%. Metabolized in liver to active metabolite. Primarily excreted in urine. Not removed by hemodialysis. **Half-life:** 3–7 hrs (increased with renal impairment).

USES

Management of moderate to severe hypertension. **OFF-LABEL:** Treatment of CHF, hypertension secondary to eclampsia, preeclampsia, primary pulmonary hypertension.

PRECAUTIONS

CONTRAINDICATIONS: Coronary artery disease, lupus erythematosus, rheumatic heart disease. **CAUTIONS:** Renal impairment, cerebrovascular disease.

LIFESPAN CONSIDERATIONS:

Pregnancy/Lactation: Drug crosses placenta. Unknown if drug is distributed in breast milk. Thrombocytopenia, leukopenia, petechial bleeding, hematomas have occurred in newborns (resolved within 1–3 wks). **Pregnancy Category C.** **Children:** No age-related precautions noted. **Elderly:** More sensitive to hypotensive effects. Age-related renal impairment may require dosage adjustment.

INTERACTIONS

DRUG: Diuretics, other antihypertensives may increase hypotensive effect. **HERBAL: Ephedra, ginseng, yohimbe** may worsen hypertension. **Garlic** may increase antihypertensive effect. **FOOD:** None known. **LAB VALUES:** May produce positive direct Coombs' test.

AVAILABILITY (Rx)

INJECTION SOLUTION: 20 mg/ml. **TABLETS:** 10 mg, 25 mg, 50 mg, 100 mg.

H

ADMINISTRATION/HANDLING

IV

Rate of administration • May give undiluted. • Give single dose over 1 min.

Storage • Store at room temperature.

PO

• Best given with food at regularly spaced meals. • Tablets may be crushed.

IV INCOMPATIBILITIES

Aminophylline, ampicillin (Polycillin), furosemide (Lasix).

IV COMPATIBILITIES

Dobutamine (Dobutrex), heparin, hydrocortisone (Solu-Cortef), nitroglycerin, potassium.

INDICATIONS/ROUTES/DOSAGE

MODERATE TO SEVERE HYPERTENSION

PO: ADULTS: Initially, 10 mg 4 times a day. May increase by 10–25 mg/dose q2–5 days. **Maximum:** 300 mg/day. **ELDERLY:** Initially, 10 mg 2–3 times a day. May increase by 10–25 mg q2–3 days. **CHILDREN:** Initially, 0.75–1 mg/kg/day in 2–4 divided doses, not to exceed 25 mg/dose. May increase over 3–4 wks. **Maximum:** 7.5 mg/kg/day (5 mg/kg/day in infants). **Maximum daily dose:** 200 mg.

IV, IM: ADULTS, ELDERLY: Initially, 10–20 mg/dose q4–6h. May increase to 40 mg/dose. **CHILDREN:** Initially, 0.1–0.2 mg/kg/dose (**Maximum:** 20 mg) q4–6h, as needed, up to 1.7–3.5 mg/kg/day in divided doses q4–6h.

DOSAGE IN RENAL IMPAIRMENT

Dosage interval is based on creatinine clearance.

Creatinine Clearance	Dosage Interval
10–50 ml/min	q8h
Less than 10 ml/min	q8–24h

SIDE EFFECTS

FREQUENT: Headache, palpitations, tachycardia (generally disappears in 7–10 days). **OCCASIONAL:** GI disturbance (nausea, vomiting, diarrhea), paraesthesia, fluid retention, peripheral edema, dizziness, flushed face, nasal congestion.

ADVERSE EFFECTS/ TOXIC REACTIONS

High dosage may produce lupus erythematosus–like reaction (fever, facial rash, muscle/joint aches, splenomegaly). Severe orthostatic hypotension, skin flushing, severe headache, myocardial ischemia, cardiac arrhythmias may develop. Profound shock may occur with severe overdosage.

NURSING CONSIDERATIONS

BASELINE ASSESSMENT

Obtain B/P, pulse immediately before each dose, in addition to regular monitoring (be alert to fluctuations).

INTERVENTION/EVALUATION

Monitor for headache, palpitations, tachycardia. Assess for peripheral edema of hands, feet. Monitor daily pattern of bowel activity/stool consistency.

PATIENT/FAMILY TEACHING

• To reduce hypotensive effect, rise slowly from lying to sitting position, permit legs to dangle from bed momentarily before standing. • Unsalted crackers, dry toast may relieve nausea. • If taking high-dose therapy, report muscle/joint aches, fever (lupus-like reaction).

hydrochlorothiazide

high-drow-chlor-oh-**thigh**-ah-zide

(Apo-Hydro, Aquazide H, Esidrix, HydroDIURIL, Microzide, Oretic)

FIXED-COMBINATION(S)

Accuretic: hydrochlorothiazide/quinapril (an angiontensin-converting enzyme [ACE] inhibitor): 12.5 mg/10 mg; 12.5 mg/20 mg; 25 mg/20 mg. **Aldactazide:** hydrochlorothiazide/spironolactone (a potassium-sparing diuretic): 25 mg/25 mg; 50 mg/50 mg. **Aldoril:** hydrochlorothiazide/methyldopa (an antihypertensive): 15 mg/250 mg; 25 mg/250 mg; 30 mg/500 mg; 50 mg/500 mg. **Apresazide:** hydrochlorothiazide/hydralazine (a vasodilator): 25 mg/25 mg; 50 mg/50 mg; 50 mg/100 mg. **Atacand HCT:** hydrochlorothiazide/candesartan (an angiotensin II receptor antagonist): 12.5 mg/16 mg; 12.5 mg/32 mg. **Avalide:** hydrochlorothiazide/irbesartan (an angiotensin II receptor antagonist): 12.5 mg/150 mg; 12.5 mg/300 mg, 25 mg/300 mg. **Benicar HCT:** hydrochlorothiazide/olmesartan (an angiotensin II receptor antagonist): 12.5 mg/20 mg; 12.5 mg/40 mg; 25 mg/40 mg. **Capozide:** hydrochlorothiazide/captopril (an ACE inhibitor): 15 mg/25 mg; 15 mg/50 mg; 25 mg/25 mg; 25 mg/50 mg. **Diovan HCT:** hydrochlorothiazide/valsartan (an angiotensin II receptor antagonist): 12.5 mg/80 mg; 12.5 mg/160 mg. **Dyazide/Maxide:** hydrochlorothiazide/triamterene (a potassium-sparing diuretic): 25 mg/37.5 mg; 25 mg/50 mg; 50 mg/75 mg. **Hyzaar:** hydrochlorothiazide/losartan (an angiotensin II receptor antagonist): 12.5 mg/50 mg; 12.5 mg/100 mg; 25 mg/100 mg. **Inderide:** hydrochlorothiazide/propranolol (a beta-blocker): 25 mg/40 mg; 25 mg/80 mg; 50 mg/80 mg; 50 mg/120 mg; 50 mg/160 mg. **Lopressor HCT:** hydrochlorothiazide/metoprolol (a beta-blocker): 25 mg/50 mg; 25 mg/100 mg; 50 mg/100 mg. **Lotensin HCT:** hydrochlorothiazide/bepridil (a calcium channel blocker): 6.25 mg/5 mg; 12.5 mg/10 mg; 12.5 mg/20 mg; 25 mg/20 mg. **Micardis HCT:** hydrochlorothiazide/telmisartan (an angiotensin II receptor antagonist): 12.5 mg/40 mg; 12.5 mg/80 mg. **Moduretic:** hydrochlorothiazide/amiloride (a potassium-sparing diuretic): 50 mg/5 mg. **Normozide:** hydrochlorothiazide/labetalol (a beta-blocker): 25 mg/100 mg; 25 mg/300 mg. **Prinzide/Zestoretic:** hydrochlorothiazide/lisinopril (an ACE inhibitor): 12.5 mg/10 mg; 12.5 mg/20 mg; 25 mg/20 mg. **Teveten HCT:** hydrochlorothiazide/eprosartan (an angiotensin II receptor antagonist): 12.5 mg/600 mg; 25 mg/600 mg. **Timolide:** hydrochlorothiazide/timolol (a beta-blocker): 25 mg/10 mg. **Uniretic:** hydrochlorothiazide/moexipril (an ACE inhibitor): 12.5 mg/7.5 mg; 25 mg/15 mg. **Vaseretic:** hydrochlorothiazide/enalapril (an ACE inhibitor): 12.5 mg/5 mg; 25 mg/10 mg. **Ziac:** hydrochlorothiazide/bisoprolol (a beta-blocker): 6.25 mg/5 mg; 6.25 mg/10 mg.

CLASSIFICATION

PHARMACOTHERAPEUTIC: Sulfonamide derivative. **CLINICAL:** Thiazide diuretic, antihypertensive (see p. 97C).

ACTION

Diuretic: Blocks reabsorption of water, sodium, potassium at cortical diluting segment of distal tubule. **Antihypertensive:** Reduces plasma, extracellular fluid volume, peripheral vascular resistance by direct effect on blood vessels. **Therapeutic Effect:** Promotes diuresis; reduces B/P.

H

PHARMACOKINETICS

Route	Onset	Peak	Duration
PO (diuretic)	2 hrs	4–6 hrs	6–12 hrs

Variably absorbed from GI tract. Primarily excreted unchanged in urine. Not removed by hemodialysis. **Half-life:** 5.6–14.8 hrs.

USES

Treatment of mild to moderate hypertension, edema in CHF, nephrotic syndrome. **OFF-LABEL:** Treatment of diabetes insipidus, prevention of calcium-containing renal calculi.

PRECAUTIONS

CONTRAINDICATIONS: Anuria, history of hypersensitivity to sulfonamides or thiazide diuretics, renal decompensation, concurrent use with dofetilide. **CAUTIONS:** Severe renal disease, hepatic impairment, diabetes mellitus, elderly or debilitated, thyroid disorders.

⧖ LIFESPAN CONSIDERATIONS:

Pregnancy/Lactation: Crosses placenta. Small amount distributed in breast milk; breast-feeding not advised. **Pregnancy Category B (D if used in pregnancy-induced hypertension). Children:** No age-related precautions noted, except jaundiced infants may be at risk for hyperbilirubinemia. **Elderly:** May be more sensitive to hypotensive, electrolyte effects. Age-related renal impairment may require dosage adjustment.

INTERACTIONS

DRUG: Cholestyramine, colestipol may decrease absorption, effects. May increase risk of **digoxin** toxicity associated with hydrochlorothiazide-induced hypokalemia. May increase risk of **lithium** toxicity. **HERBAL: Ephedra, ginseng, yohimbe** may worsen hypertension. **Garlic** may increase antihypertensive effect. **FOOD:** None known. **LAB VALUES:** May increase serum glucose, cholesterol, LDL, bilirubin, calcium, creatinine, uric acid, triglycerides. May decrease urinary calcium, serum magnesium, potassium, sodium.

AVAILABILITY (Rx)

CAPSULES (MICROZIDE): 12.5 mg. **ORAL SOLUTION:** 50 mg/5 ml. **TABLETS (AQUAZIDE, ORETIC):** 25 mg, 50 mg, 100 mg.

ADMINISTRATION/HANDLING

PO

• If GI upset occurs, give with food or milk, preferably with breakfast (may prevent nocturia).

INDICATIONS/ROUTES/DOSAGE

EDEMA

PO: ADULTS: 25–100 mg/day in 1–2 divided doses. **Maximum:** 200 mg/day.

HYPERTENSION

PO: ADULTS: 12.5–50 mg/day.

USUAL ELDERLY DOSAGE

PO: 12.5–25 mg once daily.

USUAL PEDIATRIC DOSAGE

PO: CHILDREN OLDER THAN 6 MOS: 2 mg/kg/day in 2 divided doses. **CHILDREN 6 MOS AND YOUNGER:** 2–3 mg/kg/day in 2 divided doses.

SIDE EFFECTS

EXPECTED: Increased urinary frequency, urine volume. **FREQUENT:** Potassium depletion. **OCCASIONAL:** Orthostatic hypotension, headache, GI disturbances, photosensitivity.

ADVERSE EFFECTS/ TOXIC REACTIONS

Vigorous diuresis may lead to profound water loss/electrolyte depletion, resulting in hypokalemia, hyponatremia, dehydration. Acute hypotensive episodes may occur. Hyperglycemia may occur during prolonged therapy. Pancreatitis, blood dyscrasias, pulmonary edema, allergic pneumonitis, dermatologic reactions occur rarely. Overdose can lead to lethargy, coma without changes in electrolytes or hydration.

NURSING CONSIDERATIONS

BASELINE ASSESSMENT

Check vital signs, esp. B/P for hypotension before administration. Assess baseline electrolytes; esp. for hypokalemia. Evaluate skin turgor, mucous membranes for hydration status. Evaluate for peripheral edema. Assess muscle strength, mental status. Note skin temperature, moisture. Obtain baseline weight. Initiate I&O.

INTERVENTION/EVALUATION

Continue to monitor B/P, vital signs, electrolytes, I&O, daily weight. Note extent of diuresis. Watch for changes from initial assessment (hypokalemia may result in weakness, tremor, muscle cramps, nausea, vomiting, altered mental status, tachycardia; hyponatremia may result in confusion, thirst, cold/clammy skin). Be esp. alert for potassium depletion in pts taking digoxin (cardiac arrhythmias). Potassium supplements are frequently ordered. Check for constipation (may occur with exercise diuresis).

PATIENT/FAMILY TEACHING

• Expect increased frequency, volume of urination. • To reduce hypotensive effect, rise slowly from lying to sitting position, permit legs to dangle momentarily before standing. • Eat foods high in potassium, such as whole grains (cereals), legumes, meat, bananas, apricots, orange juice, potatoes (white, sweet), raisins. • Protect skin from sun, ultraviolet rays (photosensitivity may occur).

hydrocodone ⚑

high-drough-**koe**-doan
(Hycodan ✤, Robidone ✤)

FIXED-COMBINATION(S)

Anexsia: hydrocodone/acetaminophen (a non-narcotic analgesic): 5 mg/500 mg; 7.5 mg/650 mg; 10 mg/650 mg. **Duocet:** hydrocodone/acetaminophen: 5 mg/500 mg. **Hycet:** hydrocodone/acetaminophen: 7.5 mg/325 mg per 15 ml. **Hycodan:** hydrocodone/homatropine (an anticholinergic): 5 mg/1.5 mg. **Hycotuss, Vitussin:** hydrocodone/guaifenesin (an expectorant): 5 mg/100 mg. **Lorcet:** hydrocodone/acetaminophen: 7.5 mg/650 mg; 10 mg/650 mg. **Lortab Elixer:** hydrocodone/acetaminophen: 2.5 mg/167 mg per 5 ml. **Lortab with ASA:** hydrocodone/aspirin: 5 mg/500 mg. **Lortab:** hydrocodone/acetaminophen: 2.5 mg/500 mg; 5 mg/500 mg; 7.5 mg/500 mg; 10 mg/500 mg. **Norco:** hydrocodone/acetaminophen: 10 mg/325 mg. **Reprexain CIII:** hydrocodone/ibuprofen (an NSAID): 5 mg/200 mg. **Tussend:** hydrocodone/pseudoephedrine (a sympathomimetic)/guaifenesin (an expectorant): 2.5 mg/30 mg/100 mg per 5 ml. **Vicodin ES:**hydrocodone/acetaminophen: 7.5 mg/750 mg. **Vicodin HP:** hydrocodone/acetaminophen: 10 mg/650 mg. **Vicodin:** hydrocodone/acetaminophen: 5 mg/500 mg. **Vicoprofen:** hydrocodone/ibuprofen (an NSAID): 7.5 mg/200 mg. **Xodol:** hydrocodone/acetaminophen: 5 mg/300 mg. **Zydone:** hydrocodone/acetaminophen: 5 mg/400 mg; 7.5 mg/400 mg; 10 mg/400 mg.

◆ CLASSIFICATION

PHARMACOTHERAPEUTIC: Opioid agonist (**Schedule III**). **CLINICAL:**

Narcotic analgesic, antitussive (see p. 136C).

ACTION

Binds with opioid receptors in CNS. **Therapeutic Effect:** Reduces intensity of pain stimuli incoming from sensory nerve endings, altering pain perception, emotional response to pain; suppresses cough reflex.

PHARMACOKINETICS

Route	Onset	Peak	Duration
PO (analgesic)	10–20 min	30–60 min	4–6 hrs
PO (antitussive)	N/A	N/A	4–6 hrs

Well absorbed from GI tract. Metabolized in liver. Primarily excreted in urine. **Half-life:** 3.8 hrs. (increased in elderly).

USES

Relief of moderate to moderately severe pain, nonproductive cough.

PRECAUTIONS

CONTRAINDICATIONS: None known. **EXTREME CAUTION:** CNS depression, anoxia, hypercapnia, respiratory depression, seizures, acute alcoholism, shock, untreated myxedema, respiratory dysfunction. **CAUTIONS:** Increased intracranial pressure (ICP), hepatic impairment, acute abdominal conditions, hypothyroidism, prostatic hypertrophy, Addison's disease, urethral stricture, chronic obstructive pulmonary disease (COPD).

LIFESPAN CONSIDERATIONS:

Pregnancy/Lactation: Readily crosses placenta. Distributed in breast milk. May prolong labor if administered in latent phase of first stage of labor or before cervical dilation of 4–5 cm has occurred. Respiratory depression may occur in neonate if mother received opiates during labor. Regular use of opiates during pregnancy may produce withdrawal symptoms (irritability, excessive crying, tremors, hyperactive reflexes, fever, vomiting, diarrhea, yawning, sneezing, seizures) in the neonate. **Pregnancy Category C (D if used for prolonged periods or at high dosages at term).** **Children:** Those younger than 2 yrs may be more susceptible to respiratory depression. **Elderly:** May be more susceptible to respiration depression, may cause paradoxical excitement. Age-related renal impairment, prostatic hypertrophy or obstruction may increase risk of urinary retention; dosage adjustment recommended.

INTERACTIONS

DRUG: **Alcohol, other CNS depressants** may increase CNS or respiratory depression, hypotension. **MAOIs** may produce a severe, sometimes fatal reaction with hydrocodone; plan to administer ¼ of usual hydrocodone dose. **HERBAL:** **Gotu kola, kava kava, St. John's wort, valerian** may increase CNS depression. **FOOD:** None known. **LAB VALUES:** May increase serum amylase, lipase.

ADMINISTRATION/HANDLING

PO

• Give without regard to meals. • Tablets may be crushed.

INDICATIONS/ROUTES/DOSAGE

ANALGESIA

PO: ADULTS, CHILDREN OLDER THAN 12 YRS: 5–15 mg q4–6h. **ELDERLY:** 2.5–10 mg q4–6h.

COUGH

PO: ADULTS, ELDERLY: 5–10 mg q4–6h as needed. **Maximum:** 15 mg/dose. **CHILDREN:** 0.6 mg/kg/day in 3–4 divided doses at intervals of at least 4 hrs. **Maximum single dose:** 10 mg (children older than 12 yrs), 5 mg (children 2–12 yrs), 1.25 mg (children younger than 2 yrs).

PO (EXTENDED-RELEASE): ADULTS: 10 mg q12h. **CHILDREN 6–12 YRS:** 5 mg q12h.

SIDE EFFECTS

FREQUENT: Sedation, hypotension, diaphoresis, facial flushing, dizziness, somnolence. **OCCASIONAL:** Urine retention, blurred vision, constipation, dry mouth, headache, nausea, vomiting, difficult/painful urination, euphoria, dysphoria.

ADVERSE EFFECTS/ TOXIC REACTIONS

Overdose results in respiratory depression, skeletal muscle flaccidity, cold/clammy skin, cyanosis, extreme drowsiness progressing to seizures, stupor, coma. Tolerance to analgesic effect, physical dependence may occur with repeated use. Prolonged duration of action, cumulative effect may occur in those with hepatic/renal impairment.

NURSING CONSIDERATIONS

BASELINE ASSESSMENT

Obtain vital signs before giving medication. If respirations are 12/min or less (20/min or less in children), withhold medication, contact physician. **Analgesic:** Assess onset, type, location, duration of pain. Effect of medication is reduced if full pain recurs before next dose. **Antitussive:** Assess type, severity, frequency of cough.

INTERVENTION/EVALUATION

Palpate bladder for urinary retention. Monitor daily pattern of bowel activity/stool consistency. Initiate deep breathing and coughing exercises, particularly in pts with pulmonary impairment. Assess for clinical improvement; record onset of relief of pain, cough.

PATIENT/FAMILY TEACHING

• Change positions slowly to avoid orthostatic hypotension. • Avoid tasks that require alertness, motor skills until response to drug is established. • Tolerance or dependence may occur with prolonged use at high dosages. • Avoid alcohol. • Report nausea, vomiting, constipation, shortness of breath, difficulty breathing. • May take with food.

hydrocortisone

hye-dro-**kor**-ti-sone

(Anusol HC, Caldecort, Colocort, Cortaid, Cortef, Cortenema ✤, Cortizone-10, Hytone, Nupercainal Hydrocortisone Cream, Preparation H Hydrocortisone, Proctocort, Solu-Cortef, Westcort).

FIXED-COMBINATION(S)

Cortisporin: hydrocortisone/neomycin/polymyxin (anti-infective): 5 mg/10,000 units/5 mg; 10 mg/10,000 units/5 mg.

CLASSIFICATION

PHARMACOTHERAPEUTIC: Adrenal corticosteroid. **CLINICAL:** Glucocorticoid (see pp. 92C, 95C).

ACTION

Inhibits accumulation of inflammatory cells at inflammation sites, phagocytosis, lysosomal enzyme release, synthesis and/or release of mediators of inflammation. **Therapeutic Effect:** Prevents/suppresses cell-mediated immune reactions. Decreases/prevents tissue response to inflammatory process.

PHARMACOKINETICS

Route	Onset	Peak	Duration
IV	N/A	4–6 hrs	8–12 hrs

Well absorbed after IM administration. Widely distributed. Metabolized in liver.

Half-life: Plasma, 1.5–2 hrs; biologic, 8–12 hrs.

USES

Management of adrenocortical insufficiency; relief of inflammation of corticosteroid-responsive dermatoses; adjunctive treatment of ulcerative colitis, status asthmaticus, shock.

PRECAUTIONS

CONTRAINDICATIONS: Fungal, tuberculosis, viral skin lesions; serious infections. **CAUTIONS:** Hyperthyroidism, cirrhosis, ulcerative colitis, hypertension, osteoporosis, thromboembolic tendencies, CHF, seizure disorders, thrombophlebitis, peptic ulcer, diabetes.

H

LIFESPAN CONSIDERATIONS:

Pregnancy/Lactation: Crosses placenta, distributed in breast milk. May produce cleft palate if used chronically during first trimester. Breast-feeding contraindicated. **Pregnancy Category C (D if used in first trimester). Children:** Prolonged treatment or high dosages may decrease short-term growth rate, cortisol secretion. **Elderly:** May be more susceptible to developing hypertension or osteoporosis.

INTERACTIONS

DRUG: Amphotericin may worsen hypokalemia. **Bupropion** may lower seizure threshold. May increase risk of **digoxin** toxicity caused by hypokalemia. May decrease effects of **diuretics, insulin, oral hypoglycemics, potassium supplements. Hepatic enzyme inducers** may decrease effects. **Live virus vaccines** may decrease pt's antibody response to vaccine, increase vaccine side effects, potentiate virus replication. **HERBAL: St. John's wort** may decrease concentration. **Cat's claw, echinacea** may increase immunostimulant properties. **FOOD:** None known. **LAB VALUES:** May increase serum glucose, lipids, amylase, sodium. May decrease serum calcium, potassium, thyroxine.

AVAILABILITY (Rx)

CREAM, RECTAL: (Cortizone-10, Nupercainal Hydrocortisone Cream, Preparation H Hydrocortisone):1%. **CREAM, TOPICAL:** 0.2%, 0.5%, 1%, 2.5%. **INJECTION, POWDER FOR RECONSTITUTION: (SOLU-CORTEF):** 100 mg, 250 mg, 500 mg, 1 g. **OINTMENT, TOPICAL:** 0.2%, 0.5%, 1%, 2.5%. **SUPPOSITORY: (ANUSOL HC):** 25 mg. **SUSPENSION, RECTAL: (COLOCORT):** 100 mg/60 ml. **TABLET: (CORTEF):** 5 mg, 10 mg, 20 mg.

ADMINISTRATION/HANDLING

IV

HYDROCORTISONE SODIUM SUCCINATE

• After reconstitution, use solution within 72 hrs. Use immediately if further diluted with D_5W, 0.9% NaCl, or other compatible diluent. • Once reconstituted, solution is stable for 72 hrs at room temperature.

Reconstitution • May further dilute with D_5W or 0.9% NaCl. For IV push, dilute to 50 mg/ml; for intermittent infusion, dilute to 1 mg/ml.

Rate of administration • Administer IV push over 3–5 min. Give intermittent infusion over 20–30 min.

Storage • Store at room temperature.

PO

• Give with food if GI distress occurs.

RECTAL

• Shake homogeneous suspension well. • Instruct pt to lie on left side with left leg extended, right leg flexed. • Gently insert applicator tip into rectum, pointed slightly toward navel (umbilicus). Slowly instill medication.

TOPICAL

• Gently cleanse area before application. • Use occlusive dressings only as ordered. • Apply sparingly; rub into area thoroughly.

IV INCOMPATIBILITIES

Ciprofloxacin (Cipro), diazepam (Valium), idarubicin (Idamycin), midazolam (Versed), phenytoin (Dilantin).

IV COMPATIBILITIES

Aminophylline, amphotericin, calcium gluconate, cefepime (Maxipime), digoxin (Lanoxin), diltiazem (Cardizem), diphenhydramine (Benadryl), dopamine (Intropin), insulin, lidocaine, lipids, lorazepam (Ativan), magnesium sulfate, morphine, norepinephrine (Levophed), procainamide (Pronestyl), potassium chloride, propofol (Diprivan).

INDICATIONS/ROUTES/DOSAGE

ACUTE ADRENAL INSUFFICIENCY

IV: ADULTS, ELDERLY: 100 mg IV bolus; then 300 mg/day in divided doses q8h. **CHILDREN:** 1–2 mg/kg IV bolus; then 150–250 mg/day in divided doses q6–8h. **INFANTS:** 1–2 mg/kg/dose IV bolus; then 25–150 mg/day in divided doses q6–8h.

ANTI-INFLAMMATION, IMMUNOSUPPRESSION

IV, IM: ADULTS, ELDERLY: 15–240 mg q12h. **CHILDREN:** 1–5 mg/kg/day in divided doses q12h.

PO: ADULTS, ELDERLY: 15–240 mg q12h. **CHILDREN:** 2.5–10 mg/kg/day.

PHYSIOLOGIC REPLACEMENT

PO: CHILDREN: 0.5–0.75 mg/kg/day in divided doses q8h.

IM: CHILDREN: 0.25–0.35 mg/kg/day as a single dose.

STATUS ASTHMATICUS

IV: ADULTS, ELDERLY: 100–500 mg q6h. **CHILDREN:** 2 mg/kg/dose q6h.

SHOCK

IV: ADULTS, ELDERLY, CHILDREN 12 YRS AND OLDER: 500 mg–2 g q2–6h. **CHILDREN YOUNGER THAN 12 YRS:** 50 mg/kg. May repeat in 4 hrs, then q24h as needed.

ADJUNCTIVE TREATMENT OF ULCERATIVE COLITIS

RECTAL: ADULTS, ELDERLY: 100 mg at bedtime for 21 nights or until clinical and proctologic remission occurs (may require 2–3 mos of therapy).

RECTAL (CORTIFOAM): ADULTS, ELDERLY: 1 applicator 1–2 times a day for 2–3 wks, then every second day until therapy ends.

USUAL TOPICAL DOSAGE: ADULTS, ELDERLY: Apply sparingly 2–4 times a day.

SIDE EFFECTS

FREQUENT: Insomnia, heartburn, anxiety, abdominal distention, diaphoresis, acne, mood swings, increased appetite, facial flushing, delayed wound healing, increased susceptibility to infection, diarrhea or constipation. **OCCASIONAL:** Headache, edema, change in skin color, frequent urination. **Topical:** Pruritus, redness, irritation. **RARE:** Tachycardia, allergic reaction (rash, hives), psychological changes, hallucinations, depression. **Topical:** Allergic contact dermatitis, purpura. **Systemic:** Absorption more likely with use of occlusive dressings or extensive application in young children.

ADVERSE EFFECTS/ TOXIC REACTIONS

Long-term therapy: Hypocalcemia, hypokalemia, muscle wasting (esp. arms, legs), osteoporosis, spontaneous fractures, amenorrhea, cataracts, glaucoma, peptic ulcer, CHF. **Abrupt withdrawal after long-term therapy:** Nausea, fever, headache, sudden severe joint pain, rebound inflammation, fatigue, weakness, lethargy, dizziness, orthostatic hypotension.

NURSING CONSIDERATIONS

BASELINE ASSESSMENT

Obtain baseline values for weight, B/P, serum glucose, cholesterol, electrolytes.

Check results of initial tests (tuberculosis [TB] skintest, x-rays, EKG).

INTERVENTION/EVALUATION

Assess for edema. Be alert to infection (reduced immune response): sore throat, fever, vague symptoms. Monitor daily pattern of bowel activity/stool consistency. Monitor electrolytes. Watch for hypocalcemia (muscle twitching, cramps), hypokalemia (weakness, paresthesias [esp. lower extremities], nausea/vomiting, irritability, EKG changes). Assess emotional status, ability to sleep.

PATIENT/FAMILY TEACHING

• Notify physician of fever, sore throat, muscle aches, sudden weight gain, swelling. • Do not take aspirin or any other medication without consulting physician. • Limit caffeine, avoid alcohol. • Inform dentist, other physicians of cortisone therapy now or within past 12 mos. • Caution against overusing joints injected for symptomatic relief. • **Topical:** Apply after shower or bath for best absorption. • Do not cover unless physician orders; do not use tight diapers, plastic pants, coverings. • Avoid contact with eyes.

Hydrodiuril, *see hydrochlorothiazide*

hydromorphone

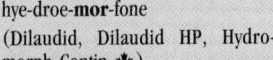

hye-droe-**mor**-fone

(Dilaudid, Dilaudid HP, Hydromorph Contin ✦)

Do not confuse hydromorphone with hydrocodone or Dilaudid with Dilantin.

CLASSIFICATION

PHARMACOTHERAPEUTIC: Opioid agonist (**Schedule II**). **CLINICAL:** Narcotic analgesic, antitussive (see p. 136C).

ACTION

Binds to opioid receptors in CNS, reducing intensity of pain stimuli from sensory nerve endings. **Therapeutic Effect:** Alters perception, emotional response to pain; suppresses cough reflex.

PHARMACOKINETICS

Route	Onset	Peak	Duration
PO	30 min	90–120 min	4 hrs
IV	10–15 min	15–30 min	2–3 hrs
IM	15 min	30–60 min	4–5 hrs
Subcutaneous	15 min	30–90 min	4 hrs
Rectal	15–30 min	N/A	N/A

Well absorbed from GI tract after IM administration. Widely distributed. Metabolized in liver. Excreted in urine. **Half-life:** 1–3 hrs.

USES

Relief of moderate to severe pain, persistent nonproductive cough.

PRECAUTIONS

CONTRAINDICATIONS: Obstetrical analgesia, respiratory depression in absence of resuscitative equipment, status asthmaticus. **EXTREME CAUTION:** CNS depression, anoxia, hypercapnia, respiratory depression, seizures, acute alcoholism, shock, untreated myxedema, respiratory dysfunction. **CAUTIONS:** Increased intracranial pressure (ICP), hepatic impairment, acute abdominal conditions, hypothyroidism, prostatic hypertrophy, Addison's disease, urethral stricture, chronic obstructive pulmonary disease (COPD).

LIFESPAN CONSIDERATIONS:

Pregnancy/Lactation: Readily crosses placenta. Unknown if distributed in breast milk. May prolong labor if administered in latent phase of first stage of labor or before cervical dilation of 4–5 cm has occurred. Respiratory depression may occur in neonate if mother receives opiates during labor. Regular use of opiates during pregnancy may produce withdrawal symptoms in the neonate (irritability, excessive crying, tremors, hyperactive reflexes, fever, vomiting, diarrhea, yawning, sneezing, seizures). **Pregnancy Category C (D if used for prolonged periods or at high dosages at term). Children:** Those younger than 2 yrs may be more susceptible to respiratory depression. **Elderly:** May be more susceptible to respiratory depression, may cause paradoxical excitement. Age-related renal impairment, prostatic hypertrophy or obstruction may increase risk of urinary retention; dosage adjustment recommended.

INTERACTIONS

DRUG: **Alcohol, other CNS depressants** may increase CNS, respiratory depression, hypotension. **MAOIs** may produce a severe, sometimes fatal reaction with hydromorphone; plan to administer ¼ of usual hydromorphone dose. **HERBAL:** **Gotu kola, kava kava, St. John's wort, valerian** may increase CNS depression. **FOOD:** None known. **LAB VALUES:** May increase serum amylase, lipase.

AVAILABILITY (Rx)

INJECTION, POWDER FOR RECONSTITUTION: (DILAUDID HP): 250 mg. **INJECTION, SOLUTION: (DILAUDID):** 1 mg/ml, 2 mg/ml, 4 mg/ml, 10mg/ml. **LIQUID, ORAL:** 1 mg/ml. **SUPPOSITORY: (DILAUDID):** 3 mg. **TABLET: (DILAUDID):** 2 mg, 4 mg, 8 mg.

ADMINISTRATION/HANDLING

IV

◄ **ALERT** ► High concentration injection (10 mg/ml) should be used only in those tolerant to opiate agonists, currently receiving high doses of another opiate agonist for severe, chronic pain due to cancer.

Reconstitution • May give undiluted. • May further dilute with 5 ml Sterile Water for Injection or 0.9% NaCl.

Rate of administration • Administer IV push very slowly (over 2–5 min). • Rapid IV increases risk of severe adverse reactions (chest wall rigidity, apnea, peripheral circulatory collapse, anaphylactoid effects, cardiac arrest).

Storage • Store at room temperature; protect from light. • Slight yellow discoloration of parenteral form does not indicate loss of potency.

IM, SUBCUTANEOUS

• Use short 25- to 30-gauge needle for subcutaneous injection. • Administer slowly; rotate injection sites. • Pts with circulatory impairment experience higher risk of overdosage due to delayed absorption of repeated administration.

PO

• Give without regard to meals. • Tablets may be crushed.

RECTAL

• Refrigerate suppositories. • Moisten suppository with cold water before inserting well up into rectum.

IV INCOMPATIBILITIES

Amphotericin B complex (Abelcet, AmBisome, Amphotec), cefazolin (Ancef, Kefzol), diazepam (Valium), lipids, phenobarbital, phenytoin (Dilantin), total parenteral nutrition (TPN).

H

IV COMPATIBILITIES

Diltiazem (Cardizem), diphenhydramine (Benadryl), dobutamine (Dobutrex), dopamine (Intropin), fentanyl (Sublimaze), furosemide (Lasix), heparin, lorazepam (Ativan), magnesium sulfate, metoclopramide (Reglan), midazolam (Versed), milrinone (Primacor), morphine, propofol (Diprivan).

INDICATIONS/ROUTES/DOSAGE

ANALGESIA

PO: ADULTS, ELDERLY, CHILDREN WEIGHING 50 KG AND MORE: 2–4 mg q3–4h. Range: 2–8 mg/dose. **CHILDREN OLDER THAN 6 MOS AND WEIGHING LESS THAN 50 KG:** 0.03–0.08 mg/kg/dose q3–4h.

IV: ADULTS, ELDERLY, CHILDREN WEIGHING MORE THAN 50 KG (FOR OPIATE-NAIVE PT): 0.2–0.6 mg q2–3h. **USUAL DOSAGE:** 1–2 mg q3–4h. **CHILDREN WEIGHING 50 KG OR LESS:** 0.015 mg/kg/dose q3–6h as needed.

RECTAL: ADULTS, ELDERLY: 3 mg q4–8h.

PATIENT-CONTROLLED ANALGESIA (PCA) IV: ADULTS, ELDERLY: 0.05–0.5 mg at 5–15 min lockout. **Maximum (4-hr):** 4–6 mg.

EPIDURAL: ADULTS, ELDERLY: Bolus dose of 1–1.5 mg infusion at rate of 0.04–0.4 mg/hr. Demand dose of 0.15 mg at 30 min lockout.

COUGH

PO: ADULTS, ELDERLY, CHILDREN OLDER THAN 12 YRS: 1 mg q3–4h. **CHILDREN 6–12 YRS:** 0.5 mg q3–4h.

SIDE EFFECTS

FREQUENT: Drowsiness, dizziness, hypotension (including orthostatic hypotension), decreased appetite. **OCCASIONAL:** Confusion, diaphoresis, facial flushing, urinary retention, constipation, dry mouth, nausea, vomiting, headache, pain at injection site. **RARE:** Allergic reaction, depression.

ADVERSE EFFECTS/ TOXIC REACTIONS

Overdose results in respiratory depression, skeletal muscle flaccidity, cold/clammy skin, cyanosis, extreme drowsiness progressing to seizures, stupor, coma. Tolerance to analgesic effect, physical dependence may occur with repeated use. Prolonged duration of action, cumulative effect may occur in those with hepatic/renal impairment.

NURSING CONSIDERATIONS

BASELINE ASSESSMENT

Obtain vital signs before giving medication. If respirations are 12/min or less (20/min or less in children), withhold medication, contact physician. **Analgesic:** Assess onset, type, location, duration of pain. Effect of medication is reduced if full pain recurs before next dose. **Antitussive:** Assess type, severity, frequency of cough.

INTERVENTION/EVALUATION

Monitor vital signs; assess for pain relief, cough. Assess breath sounds. Increase fluid intake, environmental humidity to decrease viscosity of lung secretions. To prevent pain cycles, instruct pt to request pain medication as soon as discomfort begins. Monitor daily pattern of bowel activity/stool consistency (esp. in long-term use). Initiate deep breathing and coughing exercises, particularly in pts with pulmonary impairment. Assess for clinical improvement; record onset of relief of pain, cough.

PATIENT/FAMILY TEACHING

• Avoid alcohol, tasks that require alertness/motor skills until response to drug is established. • Tolerance or dependence may occur with prolonged use at high dosages. • Change positions slowly to avoid orthostatic hypotension.

hydroxychloroquine

hye-drox-ee-**klor**-oh-kwin

(Apo-Hydroxyquine ✤, Plaquenil)

Do not confuse hydroxychloroquine with hydrocortisone or hydroxyzine.

CLASSIFICATION

CLINICAL: Antimalarial, antirheumatic.

ACTION

Concentrates in parasite acid vesicles, interfering with parasite protein synthesis. Antirheumatic action may involve suppressing formation of antigens responsible for hypersensitivity reactions. **Therapeutic Effect:** Inhibits parasite growth.

PHARMACOKINETICS

Variable rate of absorption. Widely distributed in body tissues (eyes, kidneys, liver, lungs). Protein binding: 45%. Partially metabolized in liver. Partially excreted in urine. **Half-life:** 32 days (in plasma); 50 days (in blood).

USES

Treatment of falciparum malaria (terminates acute attacks, cures nonresistant strains); suppression of acute attacks, prolongation of interval between treatment/relapse in vivax, ovale, malariae malaria. Treatment of discoid or systematic lupus erythematosus, acute and chronic rheumatoid arthritis. **OFF-LABEL:** Treatment of juvenile arthritis, sarcoid-associated hypercalcemia.

PRECAUTIONS

CONTRAINDICATIONS: Long-term therapy for children, porphyria, psoriasis, retinal or visual field changes. **CAUTIONS:** Alcoholism, hepatic disease, G6PD deficiency. Children are esp. susceptible to hydroxychloroquine fatalities.

LIFESPAN CONSIDERATIONS:

Pregnancy/Lactation: Crosses placenta; distributed in breast milk. **Pregnancy Category C. Children:** Long-term therapy not recommended. **Elderly:** No age-related precautions noted.

INTERACTIONS

DRUG: May increase **penicillamine** concentration, risk of hematologic, renal, severe skin reactions. **HERBAL:** None significant. **FOOD:** None known. **LAB VALUES:** None known.

AVAILABILITY (Rx)

TABLETS: 200 mg (155 mg base).

INDICATIONS/ROUTES/DOSAGE

TREATMENT OF ACUTE ATTACK OF MALARIA (DOSAGE IN MG BASE)

PO

Dose	Times	Adults	Children
Initial	Day 1	620 mg	10 mg/kg
Second	6 hrs later	310 mg	5 mg/kg
Third	Day 2	310 mg	5 mg/kg
Fourth	Day 3	310 mg	5 mg/kg

SUPPRESSION OF MALARIA

PO: ADULTS: 310 mg base weekly on same day each wk, beginning 2 wks before entering an endemic area and continuing for 4–6 wks after leaving the area. **CHILDREN:** 5 mg base/kg/wk, beginning 2 wks before entering an endemic area and continuing for 4–6 wks after leaving the area. If therapy is not begun before exposure, administer a loading dose of 10 mg base/kg in 2 equally divided doses 6 hrs apart, followed by the usual dosage regimen.

RHEUMATOID ARTHRITIS

PO: ADULTS: Initially, 400–600 mg (310–465 mg base) daily for 5–10 days, gradually increased to optimum response level. Maintenance (usually within 4–12 wks): Dosage decreased by 50% and then continued at maintenance dose of 200–400 mg/day. Maximum effect may not be seen for several mos.

LUPUS ERYTHEMATOSUS

PO: ADULTS: Initially, 400 mg once or twice a day for several wks or mos. Maintenance: 200–400 mg/day.

SIDE EFFECTS

FREQUENT: Transient headache, anorexia, nausea, vomiting. **OCCASIONAL:** Visual disturbances, anxiety, fatigue, pruritus (esp. palms, soles, scalp), irritability, personality changes, diarrhea. **RARE:** Stomatitis, dermatitis, impaired hearing.

ADVERSE EFFECTS/ TOXIC REACTIONS

Ocular toxicity (esp. retinopathy) may progress even after drug is discontinued. **Prolonged therapy:** Peripheral neuritis, neuromyopathy, hypotension, EKG changes, agranulocytosis, aplastic anemia, thrombocytopenia, seizures, psychosis. **Overdosage:** Headache, vomiting, visual disturbances, drowsiness, seizures, hypokalemia followed by cardiovascular collapse, death.

NURSING CONSIDERATIONS

BASELINE ASSESSMENT

Evaluate CBC, hepatic function.

INTERVENTION/EVALUATION

Monitor, report any visual disturbances promptly. Evaluate for GI distress. Give dose with food (for malaria). Monitor hepatic function tests. Assess skin/buccal mucosa; inquire about pruritus. Report impaired vision/hearing immediately.

PATIENT/FAMILY TEACHING

• Continue drug for full length of treatment. • In long-term therapy, therapeutic response may not be evident for up to 6 mos. • Immediately notify physician of **any** new symptom of visual difficulties, muscular weakness, impaired hearing, tinnitus.

hydroxyurea

high-**drocks**-ee-your-e-ah
(Apo-Hydroxyurea ♣, Droxia, Hydrea, Mylocel)

CLASSIFICATION

PHARMACOTHERAPEUTIC: Synthetic urea analogue. **CLINICAL:** Antineoplastic (see p. 80C).

ACTION

Inhibits DNA synthesis without interfering with RNA synthesis or protein. **Therapeutic Effect:** Interferes with normal repair process of cancer cells damaged by irradiation.

PHARMACOKINETICS

Well absorbed from GI tract. Protein binding: 75%–80%. Metabolized in liver. Excreted in urine as urea and unchanged drug. **Half-life:** 3–4 hrs.

USES

Treatment of melanoma; resistant chronic myelocytic leukemia; recurrent, metastatic, inoperable ovarian carcinoma. Used in combination with radiation therapy for local control of primary squamous cell carcinoma of head/neck, excluding lip. Treatment of sickle cell anemia. **OFF-LABEL:** Treatment of HIV, psoriasis, hematologic conditions (e.g., polycythemia vera), uterine, cervical, non-small cell lung cancer, primary brain tumors, renal cell cancer, prostate cancer.

PRECAUTIONS

CONTRAINDICATIONS: WBC count less than 2,500/mm^3 or platelet count less than 100,000/mm^3. **CAUTIONS:** Previous irradiation therapy, other cytoxic drugs, renal/hepatic impairment.

⌛ LIFESPAN CONSIDERATIONS:

Pregnancy/Lactation: Crosses placenta; distributed in breast milk. May be harmful to fetus. **Pregnancy Category D.** **Children:** Safety and efficacy not established. **Elderly:** More sensitive to hydroxyurea effects; may require lower dosage.

INTERACTIONS

DRUG: May decrease effects of **antigout medications. Antiretroviral agents (e.g., didanosine, stavudine)** may cause pancreatitis, hepatotoxicity, peripheral neuropathy. **Bone marrow depressants** may increase myelosuppression. **Live virus vaccines** may potentiate virus replication, increase vaccine side effects, decrease the pt's antibody response to vaccine. **HERBAL:** None significant. **FOOD:** None known. **LAB VALUES:** May increase BUN, serum creatinine, uric acid.

AVAILABILITY (Rx)

CAPSULES: 200 mg (Droxia), 300 mg (Droxia), 400 mg (Droxia), 500 mg (Hydrea). **TABLETS (MYLOCEL):** 1,000 mg.

ADMINISTRATION/HANDLING

Capsules may be opened and emptied into water (will not dissolve completely).

INDICATIONS/ROUTES/DOSAGE

◄ **ALERT** ► Therapy interrupted when platelet count falls below 100,000/mm^3 or WBC count falls below 2,500/mm^3. Resume when counts return to normal.

MELANOMA; RECURRENT, METASTATIC, OR INOPERABLE OVARIAN CARCINOMA

PO: ADULTS, ELDERLY: 80 mg/kg every 3 days or 20–30 mg/kg/day as a single dose.

CONTROL OF PRIMARY SQUAMOUS CELL CARCINOMA OF THE HEAD/NECK, EXCLUDING LIPS (IN COMBINATION WITH RADIATION THERAPY)

PO: ADULTS, ELDERLY: 80 mg/kg every 3 days, beginning at least 7 days before starting radiation therapy.

RESISTANT CHRONIC MYELOCYTIC LEUKEMIA

PO: ADULTS, ELDERLY: 20–30 mg/kg once a day. **CHILDREN:** 10–20 mg/kg once a day.

HIV INFECTION

PO: ADULTS, ELDERLY: 1,000–1,500 mg/day as single dose or in divided doses.

SICKLE CELL ANEMIA

PO: ADULTS, ELDERLY, CHILDREN: Initially, 15 mg/kg once a day. May increase by 5 mg/kg/day. **Maximum:** 35 mg/kg/day.

SIDE EFFECTS

FREQUENT: Nausea, vomiting, anorexia, constipation or diarrhea. **OCCASIONAL:** Mild, reversible rash; facial flushing; pruritus; fever; chills; malaise. **RARE:** Alopecia, headache, drowsiness, dizziness, disorientation.

ADVERSE EFFECTS/ TOXIC REACTIONS

Myelosuppression manifested as hematologic toxicity (leukopenia and to a lesser extent, thrombocytopenia, anemia).

NURSING CONSIDERATIONS

BASELINE ASSESSMENT

Obtain bone marrow studies, hepatic/renal function tests before therapy begins, periodically thereafter. Obtain Hgb, WBC, platelet count, serum uric acid at baseline, and weekly during therapy. Those with marked renal impairment may develop visual or auditory hallucinations, marked hematologic toxicity.

H

INTERVENTION/EVALUATION

Monitor daily pattern of bowel activity/stool consistency. Monitor for hematologic toxicity (fever, sore throat, signs of local infection, unusual bleeding/bruising from any site), symptoms of anemia (excessive fatigue, weakness). Assess skin for rash, erythema. Monitor CBC with differential, platelet count, Hgb, renal/hepatic function, uric acid.

PATIENT/FAMILY TEACHING

- Promptly report fever, sore throat, signs of local infection, unusual bleeding/bruising from any site.

H

*hydrOXYzine

high-**drox**-ih-zeen

(Apo-Hydroxyzine ♣, Atarax, Novo-hydroxyzin ♣)

Do not confuse hydroxyzine with hydralazine or hydroxyurea.

CLASSIFICATION

PHARMACOTHERAPEUTIC: Piperazine derivative. **CLINICAL:** Antihistamine, antianxiety, antispasmodic, antiemetic, antipruritic (see pp. 12C, 52C).

ACTION

Competes with histamine for receptor sites in GI tract, blood vessels, respiratory tract. Diminishes vestibular stimulation, depresses labyrinthine function. **Therapeutic Effect:** Produces anxiolytic, anticholinergic, antihistaminic, analgesic effects; relaxes skeletal muscle; controls nausea, vomiting.

PHARMACOKINETICS

Route	Onset	Peak	Duration
PO	15–30 min	N/A	4–6 hrs

Well absorbed from GI tract and after parenteral administration. Metabolized in liver. Primarily excreted in urine. Not removed by hemodialysis. **Half-life:** 20–25 hrs (increased in the elderly).

USES

Treatment of anxiety, preoperative sedation, antipruritic.

PRECAUTIONS

CONTRAINDICATIONS: None known. **CAUTIONS:** Narrow-angle glaucoma, prostatic hypertrophy, bladder neck obstruction, asthma, chronic obstructive pulmonary disorder (COPD).

LIFESPAN CONSIDERATIONS:

Pregnancy/Lactation: Unknown if drug crosses placenta or is distributed in breast milk. **Pregnancy Category C. Children:** Not recommended in newborns or premature infants (increased risk of anticholinergic effects). Paradoxical excitement may occur. **Elderly:** Increased risk of dizziness, sedation, confusion. Hypotension, hyperexcitability may occur.

INTERACTIONS

DRUG: Alcohol, other CNS depressants may increase CNS depressant effects. **MAOIs** may increase anticholinergic, CNS depressant effects. **HERBAL: Gotu kola, kava kava, St. John's wort, valerian** may increase CNS depression. **FOOD:** None known. **LAB VALUES:** May cause false-positive urine 17-hydroxycorticosteroid determinations.

AVAILABILITY (Rx)

INJECTION SOLUTION (HYZINE, VISTACOT, VISTAJECT-50, VISTARIL IM): 25 mg/ml, 50 mg/ml. **ORAL SUSPENSION (VISTARIL):** 25 mg/5 ml. **SYRUP (ATARAX):** 10 mg/5 ml. **TABLETS (ATARAX):** 10 mg, 25 mg, 50 mg, 100 mg.

CAPSULES (VISTARIL): 25 mg, 50 mg, 100 mg.

ADMINISTRATION/HANDLING

IM

◄ **ALERT** ► Significant tissue damage, thrombosis, gangrene may occur if injection is given subcutaneous, intra-arterial, or by IV.

• IM may be given undiluted. • Use Z-track technique of injection to prevent subcutaneous infiltration. • Inject deep IM into gluteus maximus or midlateral thigh in adults, midlateral thigh in children.

PO

• Shake oral suspension well. • Scored tablets may be crushed; do not crush/break capsule.

INDICATIONS/ROUTES/DOSAGE

ANXIETY

PO: ADULTS, ELDERLY: 25–100 mg 4 times a day. **Maximum:** 600 mg/day. **CHILDREN 6 YRS AND OLDER:** 50–100 mg/day in divided doses. **CHILDREN, YOUNGER THAN 6 YEARS:** 50 mg/day in divided doses.

NAUSEA/VOMITING

IM: ADULTS, ELDERLY: 25–100 mg/dose q4–6h.

PRURITUS

PO: ADULTS, ELDERLY: 25 mg 3–4 times a day. **CHILDREN 6 YRS AND OLDER:** 50–100 mg/day in divided doses. **CHILDREN, YOUNGER THAN 6 YEARS:** 50 mg/day in divided doses.

PREOPERATIVE SEDATION

PO: ADULTS, ELDERLY: 50–100 mg. **CHILDREN:** 2 mg/kg/day in divided doses q6–8h.

IM: ADULTS, ELDERLY: 25–100 mg. **CHILDREN:** 0.5–1 mg/kg/dose q4–6h.

SIDE EFFECTS

Side effects are generally mild, transient. **FREQUENT:** Drowsiness, dry mouth, marked discomfort with IM injection. **OCCASIONAL:** Dizziness, ataxia, asthenia, slurred speech, headache, agitation, increased anxiety. **RARE:** Paradoxical reactions (hyperactivity, anxiety in children; excitement, restlessness in elderly or debilitated pts) generally noted during first 2 wks of therapy, particularly in presence of uncontrolled pain.

ADVERSE EFFECTS/ TOXIC REACTIONS

Hypersensitivity reaction (wheezing, dyspnea, chest tightness) may occur.

NURSING CONSIDERATIONS

BASELINE ASSESSMENT

Anxiety: Offer emotional support to anxious pt. Assess motor responses (agitation, trembling, tension), autonomic responses (cold/clammy hands, diaphoresis). **Antiemetic:** Assess for dehydration (poor skin turgor, dry mucous membranes, longitudinal furrows in tongue).

INTERVENTION/EVALUATION

For those on long-term therapy, hepatic/renal function tests, blood counts should be performed periodically. Monitor lung sounds for signs of hypersensitivity reaction. Monitor serum electrolytes in pts with severe vomiting. Assess for paradoxical reaction, particularly during early therapy. Assist with ambulation if drowsiness, lightheadedness occurs.

PATIENT/FAMILY TEACHING

• Marked discomfort may occur with IM injection. • Sugarless gum, sips of tepid water may relieve dry mouth. • Drowsiness usually diminishes with continued therapy. • Avoid tasks that require alertness, motor skills until response to drug is established.

H

hyoscyamine

hye-oh-**sye**-a-meen

(Anaspaz, Cystospaz, Cystospaz-M, Hyosine, Levbid, Levsin, Levsin S/L, Levsinex, NuLev, Spacol, Spacol T/S, Symax SL, Symax SR)

Do not confuse Anaspaz with Anaprox.

FIXED COMBINATIONS

Donnatal: hyoscyamine/atropine (anticholinergic)/phenobarbital (sedative)/scopolamine (anticholinergic): 0.1037 mg/0.0194 mg/16.2 mg/0.0065 mg.

CLASSIFICATION

PHARMACOTHERAPEUTIC: Anticholinergic. **CLINICAL:** Antimuscarinic, antispasmodic.

ACTION

Inhibits action of acetylcholine at postganglionic (muscarinic) receptor sites. **Therapeutic Effect:** Decreases secretions (bronchial, salivary, sweat gland, gastric juices). Reduces motility of GI, urinary tracts.

PHARMACOKINETICS

Completely absorbed following PO administration. Partially hydrolyzed. Majority excreted unchanged in urine. Removed by hemodialysis. **Half-life:** 3.5 hrs (immediate-release); 7 hrs (sustained-release).

USES

Oral: Adjunctive therapy for peptic ulcer disease, irritable bowel syndrome, neurogenic bladder or bowel; treatment of infantile colic, GI tract disorders caused by spasm; reduce abdominal rigidity; reduce tremors associated with Parkinson's disease; drying agent in acute rhinitis. **Parenteral:** Preoperatively to reduce secretions, block cardiac vagal inhibitory reflexes; relief of biliary, renal colic; reduce GI motility to facilitate diagnostic procedures; reduce pain, hypersecretion in pancreatitis; reversal of neuromuscular blockade.

PRECAUTIONS

CONTRAINDICATIONS: GI/GU obstruction, myasthenia gravis, narrow-angle glaucoma, paralytic ileus, severe ulcerative colitis. **CAUTIONS:** Hyperthyroidism, CHF, cardiac arrhythmias, prostatic hypertrophy, neuropathy, chronic lung disease.

LIFESPAN CONSIDERATIONS:

Pregnancy/Lactation: Crosses placenta; distributed in breast milk. **Pregnancy Category C. Children:** Safety and efficacy not established. **Elderly:** No age-related precautions noted.

INTERACTIONS

DRUG: Antacids, antidiarrheals may decrease absorption. May decrease absorption of **ketoconazole. Other anticholinergics** may increase effects. May increase severity of GI lesions with matrix formulation of **potassium chloride. HERBAL:** None significant. **FOOD:** None known. **LAB VALUES:** None known.

AVAILABILITY (Rx)

CAPSULES, TIMED-RELEASE: (CYSTOSPAZ-M, LEVSINEX): 0.375 mg. **ELIXI-R: (HYOSINE, LEVSIN):** 0.125 mg/5 ml. **INJECTION, SOLUTION:** (Levsin): 0.5 mg/ml. **SOLUTION, ORAL DROPS: (HYOSINE, LEVSIN):** 0.125 mg/ml. **TABLET: (ANASPAZ, LEVSIN):** 0.125 mg. **(CYSTOSPAZ):** 0.15 mg. **TABLET, ORAL DISINTEGRATING: (NULEV):** 0.125 mg. **TABLET, SUBLINGUAL: (LEVSIN/SL, SYMAX/SL):** 0.125 mg.

TABLET, EXTENDED-RELEASE: (LEVBID, SYMAX SR): 0.375 mg.

ADMINISTRATION/HANDLING

PO

• Give without regard to meals. • Tablets may be crushed, chewed. • Extended-release capsule should be swallowed whole. • Allow oral disintegrating tablet placed on tongue to dissolve before swallowing; may give with or without water.

PARENTERAL

• May give undiluted.

INDICATIONS/ROUTES/DOSAGE

GI TRACT DISORDERS

PO, SUBLINGUAL: ADULTS, ELDERLY, CHILDREN 12 YRS AND OLDER: 0.125–0.25 mg q4h as needed. Extended-release: 0.375–0.75 mg q12h. **Maximum:** 1.5 mg/day. **CHILDREN 2–11 YRS:** 0.0625–0.125 mg q4h as needed. **Maximum:** 0.75 mg/day.

IV, IM: ADULTS, ELDERLY, CHILDREN 12 YRS AND OLDER: 0.25–0.5 mg q4h for 1–4 doses.

HYPERMOTILITY OF LOWER URINARY TRACT

PO: SUBLINGUAL: ADULTS, ELDERLY: 0.15–0.3 mg 4 times a day; or extended-release 0.375 mg q12h.

INFANT COLIC

PO: INFANTS: Drops dosed q4h as needed (based on weight): 2.3 kg: 3 drops, 3.4 kg: 4 drops, 5 kg: 5 drops, 7 kg: 6 drops, 10 kg: 8 drops, 15 kg: 11 drops.

SIDE EFFECTS

FREQUENT: Dry mouth (sometimes severe), decreased diaphoresis, constipation. **OCCASIONAL:** Blurred vision, bloated feeling, urinary hesitancy, somnolence (with high dosage), headache, intolerance to light, loss of taste, anxiety, flushing, insomnia, impotence, mental confusion or excitement (particularly in elderly, children), temporary lightheadedness (with parenteral form), local irritation (with parenteral form). **RARE:** Dizziness, faintness.

ADVERSE EFFECTS/ TOXIC REACTIONS

Overdose may produce temporary paralysis of ciliary muscle, pupillary dilation, tachycardia, palpitations, hot/dry/flushed skin, absence of bowel sounds, hyperthermia, increased respiratory rate, EKG abnormalities, nausea, vomiting; rash over face/upper trunk, CNS stimulation, psychosis (agitation, restlessness, rambling speech, visual hallucinations, paranoid behavior, delusions) followed by depression.

NURSING CONSIDERATIONS

BASELINE ASSESSMENT

Before giving medication, instruct pt to void (reduces risk of urinary retention).

INTERVENTION/EVALUATION

Monitor daily pattern of bowel activity/stool consistency. Palpate bladder for urinary retention. Monitor changes in B/P, temperature. Assess skin turgor, mucous membranes to evaluate hydration status (encourage adequate fluid intake), bowel sounds for peristalsis. Be alert for fever (increased risk of hyperthermia).

PATIENT/FAMILY TEACHING

• May cause dry mouth; maintain good oral hygiene habits (lack of saliva may increase risk of cavities). • Inform physician of rash, eye pain, difficulty in urinating, constipation. • Avoid tasks that require alertness, motor skills until response to drug is established. • Avoid hot baths, saunas.

Hyzaar, *see*

hydrochlorothiazide and losartan

H

ibandronate

eye-**band**-droh-nate
(Bondronal ✱, Boniva)

CLASSIFICATION

PHARMACOTHERAPEUTIC: Bisphosphonate. **CLINICAL:** Calcium regulator.

ACTION

Binds to bone hydroxyapatite (part of mineral matrix of bone), inhibits osteoclast activity. **Therapeutic Effect:** Reduces rate of bone turnover, bone resorption, resulting in net gain in bone mass.

PHARMACOKINETICS

Absorbed in upper GI tract. Extent of absorption impaired by food, beverages (other than plain water). Rapidly binds to bone. Unabsorbed portion eliminated in urine. Protein binding: 90%. **Half-life:** 10–60 hrs.

USES

Treatment/prevention of osteoporosis in postmenopausal women.

PRECAUTIONS

CONTRAINDICATIONS: Hypersensitivity to other bisphosphonates (e.g., alendronate, etidronate, pamidronate, risedronate, tiludronate), inability to stand or sit upright for at least 60 min, severe renal impairment with creatinine clearance less than 30 ml/min, uncorrected hypocalcemia. **CAUTIONS:** GI diseases (duodenitis, dysphagia, esophagitis, gastritis, ulcers [drug may exacerbate these conditions]), mild to moderate renal impairment.

LIFESPAN CONSIDERATIONS:

Pregnancy/Lactation: Potential for teratogenic effects. Unknown if excreted in breast milk. Do not breast-feed. **Pregnancy Category C. Children:** Safety and efficacy not established. **Elderly:** No age-related precautions noted.

INTERACTIONS

DRUG: **Antacids containing aluminum, calcium, magnesium; vitamin D** decrease absorption. **Aspirin, NSAIDs** may increase GI irritation. **HERBAL:** None significant. **FOOD:** **Beverages (other than plain water), dietary supplements, food** interfere with absorption. **LAB VALUES:** May decrease serum alkaline phosphatase. May increase serum cholesterol.

AVAILABILITY (Rx)

INJECTION SOLUTION: 3 mg/3 ml syringe. **TABLETS:** 2.5 mg, 150 mg.

ADMINISTRATION/HANDLING

PO

• Give 60 min before first food, beverage of the day, on an empty stomach with 6–8 oz plain water (not mineral water) while pt is standing or sitting in upright position. • Pt cannot lie down for 60 min following drug administration. • Pt should not chew, suck tablet (potential for oropharyngeal ulceration).

IV

• Give over 15–20 sec.

INDICATIONS/ROUTES/DOSAGE

OSTEOPOROSIS

PO: ADULTS, ELDERLY: 2.5 mg daily. Alternatively, 150 mg once monthly.
IV: ADULTS, ELDERLY: 3 mg q3mo.

DOSAGE IN RENAL IMPAIRMENT

Creatinine clearance less than 30 ml/min: Not recommended.

SIDE EFFECTS

FREQUENT (13%–6%): Back pain, dyspepsia (epigastric distress, heartburn), peripheral discomfort, diarrhea, headache, myalgia. **IV:** Abdominal pain, dyspepsia, constipation, nausea, diarrhea. **OCCASIONAL (4%–3%):** Dizziness, arthralgia, asthenia. **RARE (2% or less):** Vomiting, hypersensitivity reaction.

ADVERSE EFFECTS/ TOXIC REACTIONS

Upper respiratory infection occurs occasionally. Overdose results in hypocalcemia, hypophosphatemia, significant GI disturbances.

NURSING CONSIDERATIONS

BASELINE ASSESSMENT

Hypocalcemia, vitamin D deficiency must be corrected before beginning therapy. Obtain laboratory baselines, esp. serum electrolytes, renal function. Obtain results of bone density study.

INTERVENTION/EVALUATION

Monitor electrolytes, esp. serum calcium, alkaline phosphatase. Monitor renal function tests.

PATIENT/FAMILY TEACHING

• Instruct pt that expected benefits occur only when medication is taken with full glass (6–8 oz) of plain water, first thing in the morning and at least 60 min before first food, beverage, medication of the day. Any other beverage (mineral water, orange juice, coffee) significantly reduces absorption of medication. • Do not lie down for at least 60 min after taking medication (potentiates delivery to stomach, reduces risk of esophageal irritation). • Consider weight-bearing exercises, modify behavioral factors (e.g., cigarette smoking, alcohol consumption).

ibritumomab

ih-brit-uh-**moe**-mab
(Zevalin)

CLASSIFICATION

PHARMACOTHERAPEUTIC: Monoclonal antibody. **CLINICAL:** Antineoplastic (see p. 80C).

ACTION

Combines targeting power of monoclonal antibodies (MAbs) with cancer-killing ability of radiation. **Therapeutic Effect:** Targets CD antigen (present in greater than 90% of pts with B-cell non-Hodgkin's lymphoma) inducing cellular damage.

PHARMACOKINETICS

Tumor uptake is greater than normal tissue in non-Hodgkin's lymphoma. Most of dose cleared by binding to tumor. Minimally excreted in urine. **Half-life:** 27–30 hrs.

USES

Treatment of non-Hodgkin's lymphoma in combination with rituxumab in pts with relapsed or refractory low-grade, follicular, or CD20-positive transformed B-cell non-Hodgkin's lymphoma.

PRECAUTIONS

CONTRAINDICATIONS: Platelet count less than 100,000 cells/mm^3, neutrophil count less than 1,500 cells/mm^3, history of failed stem cell collection. **CAUTIONS:** Mild thrombocytopenia, prior external beam radiation, cardiovascular disease, hypertension/hypotension.

LIFESPAN CONSIDERATIONS:

Pregnancy/Lactation: Has potential to cause fetal harm. Those with childbearing potential should use contraceptive methods during and up to 12 mos after therapy. **Pregnancy Category D.**

I

Children: Safety and efficacy not established. **Elderly:** No age-related precautions noted.

INTERACTIONS

DRUG: **Any medication that interferes with platelet function, anticoagulants** increase potential for prolonged/severe thrombocytopenia. **Bone marrow depressants** may increase myelosuppression. **Live virus vaccines** may potentiate virus replication, increase vaccine side effects, decrease pt's antibody response to vaccine. **HERBAL:** **Cat's claw, dong quai, evening primrose, feverfew, red clover, horse chestnut, garlic, ginseng, ginkgo** may increase antiplatelet activity. **FOOD:** None known. **LAB VALUES:** Severe reduction of Hgb, Hct, platelet count, WBC count.

AVAILABILITY (Rx)

INJECTION SOLUTION: 3.2-mg vial (1.6 mg/ml).

ADMINISTRATION/HANDLING

Rate of administration • Give IV push over 10 min.

IV INCOMPATIBILITIES

Do not mix with any medications.

INDICATIONS/ROUTES/DOSAGE

NON-HODGKIN'S LYMPHOMA

IV: ADULTS, ELDERLY: Regimen consists of two steps: STEP 1: Single infusion of 250 mg/m^2 rituximab preceding (4 hrs or less) a fixed dose of 5 mCi (1.6 mg total antibody dose) of indium-111 ibritumomab administered IV push over 10 min. STEP 2: Follows step 1 by 7–9 days and consists of a second infusion of 250 mg/m^2 rituximab preceding (4 hrs or less) a fixed dose of 0.4 mCi/kg of Y-90 ibritumomab administered IV push over 10 min.

◀ **ALERT** ▶ Reduce dosage to 0.3 mCi/kg if platelet count is 100,000–149,000 cells/mm^3. Do not administer if platelet count is less than 100,000 cells/mm^3.

SIDE EFFECTS

FREQUENT (43%–24%): Asthenia (loss of strength, energy), nausea, chills. **OCCASIONAL (17%–10%):** Fever, abdominal pain, dyspnea, headache, vomiting, dizziness, cough, oral candidiasis. **RARE (9%–5%):** Pruritus, diarrhea, back pain, peripheral edema, anorexia, rash, flushing, arthralgia, myalgia, ecchymosis, rhinitis, constipation, insomnia.

ADVERSE EFFECTS/ TOXIC REACTIONS

Thrombocytopenia (95%), neutropenia (77%), anemia (61%) may be severe and prolonged; may be followed by infection (29%). Hypersensitivity reaction produces hypotension, bronchospasm, angioedema. Severe cutaneous or mucocutaneous reactions.

NURSING CONSIDERATIONS

BASELINE ASSESSMENT

Pretreatment with acetaminophen and diphenhydramine before each infusion may prevent infusion-related effects. Offer emotional support. Use strict asepsis. CBC, blood chemistries should be obtained as baseline before beginning therapy. ANC nadir is 62 days before recovery begins.

INTERVENTION/EVALUATION

Diligently monitor lab values for possibly severe/prolonged thrombocytopenia, neutropenia, anemia. Monitor for hematologic toxicity (fever, sore throat, signs of local infections, unusual bruising/bleeding), symptoms of anemia (excessive fatigue, weakness). Assess for GI symptoms (nausea, vomiting, abdominal pain, diarrhea).

PATIENT/FAMILY TEACHING

• Do not have immunizations without physician's approval (drug lowers resistance). • Avoid crowds, persons with known infections. • Report signs of infection at once (fever, flu-like symptoms). • Contact physician if nausea/vomiting continues at home. • Avoid pregnancy during therapy.

ibuprofen

eye-**byoo**-pro-fen

(Advil, Advil Children's, Advil Infants', Advil Junior, Advil Migraine, Apo-Ibuprofen ✱, Genpril, Ibu-200, Motrin, Motrin Children's, Motrin IB, Motrin Infants', Motrin Junior Strength, Neo Profen, Novo-profen ✱)

FIXED-COMBINATION(S)

Children's Advil Cold: ibuprofen/pseudoephedrine (a nasal decongestant): 100 mg/15 mg per 5 ml. **Combunox:** ibuprofen/oxycodone (a narcotic analgesic): 400 mg/5 mg. **Reprexain CIII:** ibuprofen/hydrocodone: 200 mg/5 mg. **Vicoprofen:** ibuprofen/hydrocodone (a narcotic analgesic): 200 mg/7.5 mg.

CLASSIFICATION

PHARMACOTHERAPEUTIC: Nonsteroidal anti-inflammatory. **CLINICAL:** Antirheumatic, analgesic, antipyretic, antidysmenorrheal, vascular headache suppressant (see p. 124C).

ACTION

Inhibits prostaglandin synthesis. Produces vasodilation acting on heat-regulating center of hypothalamus. **Therapeutic Effect:** Produces analgesic, anti-inflammation effects, decreases fever.

PHARMACOKINETICS

Route	Onset	Peak	Duration
PO (analgesic)	0.5 hr	N/A	4–6 hrs
PO (anti-rheumatic)	2 days	1–2 wks	N/A

Rapidly absorbed from GI tract. Protein binding: greater than 90%. Metabolized in liver. Primarily excreted in urine. Not removed by hemodialysis. **Half-life:** 2–4 hrs.

USES

Treatment of fever, juvenile rheumatoid arthritis, osteoarthritis, minor pain, mild to moderate pain, primary dysmenorrhea. **NeoProfen:** Close clinically significant patent ductus arteriosus (PDA) in premature infants weighing between 500–1,500 g who are no more than 32 wks gestational age when usual medical management is ineffective. **OFF-LABEL:** Treatment of psoriatic arthritis, vascular headaches, cystic fibrosis, ankylosing spondylitis.

PRECAUTIONS

CONTRAINDICATIONS: Active peptic ulcer, chronic inflammation of GI tract, GI bleeding disorders/ulceration, history of hypersensitivity to aspirin, NSAIDs. **NeoProfen:** Infants with proven or suspected untreated infection, congenital heart disease where patency of the PDA is necessary for satisfactory pulmonary or systemic blood flow (e.g., pulmonary atresia), bleeding, thrombocytopenia, coagulation defects, suspected necrotizing enterocolitis, significant renal impairment. **CAUTIONS:** CHF, hypertension, renal/hepatic impairment, dehydration, GI disease (e.g., bleeding, ulcers), concurrent anticoagulant use. **NeoProfen:** Presence of controlled infection or infants at risk for infection.

LIFESPAN CONSIDERATIONS:

Pregnancy/Lactation: Unknown if drug crosses placenta or is distributed

I

in breast milk. Avoid use during third trimester (may adversely affect fetal cardiovascular system: premature closure of ductus arteriosus). **Pregnancy Category B (D if used in third trimester or near delivery). Children:** Safety and efficacy not established in those younger than 6 mos. **Elderly:** GI bleeding, ulceration more likely to cause serious adverse effects. Age-related renal impairment may increase risk of hepatic/renal toxicity; reduced dosage recommended.

INTERACTIONS

DRUG: May decrease effects of **antihypertensives, diuretics. Aspirin, other salicylates** may increase risk of GI side effects, bleeding. **Bone marrow depressants** may increase risk of hematologic reactions. May increase concentration/nephrotoxicity with **cyclosporine**. May increase effects of **heparin, oral anticoagulants, thrombolytics.** May increase concentration, risk of toxicity of **lithium.** May increase risk of **methotrexate** toxicity. **Probenecid** may increase concentration. **HERBAL: Cat's claw, dong quai, evening primrose, feverfew, red clover, horse chestnut, garlic, ginseng, ginkgo** may increase antiplatelet activity. **FOOD:** None known. **LAB VALUES:** May prolong bleeding time. May alter serum glucose level. May increase BUN, serum creatinine, potassium, AST, ALT. May decrease Hgb, Hct.

AVAILABILITY (Rx)

CAPLET: (ADVIL, IBU-200, MOTRIN IB: 200 mg. **CAPSULE: (ADVIL, ADVIL MIGRAINE):** 200 mg. **GELCAP: (ADVIL, MOTRIN IB):** 200 mg. **INJECTION, SOLUTION:** 10 mg/ml. **SUSPENSION, ORAL: (ADVIL CHILDREN'S, MOTRIN CHILDREN'S):** 100 mg/5 ml. **SUSPENSION, ORAL DROPS: (ADVIL INFANTS', MOTRIN INFANTS'):** 40 mg/ml. **TABLET: (ADVIL JUNIOR, MOTRIN JUNIOR):** 100 mg. **(ADVIL, GENPRIL):** 200 mg. **(MOTRIN):** 400 mg, 600 mg, 800 mg. **TABLET, CHEWABLE: (ADVIL CHILDRENS', MOTRIN CHILDRENS'):** 50 mg. **(ADVIL JUNIOR, MOTRIN JUNIOR STRENGTH):** 100 mg.

ADMINISTRATION/HANDLING

IV (NEOPROFEN)

Reconstitution • Dilute to appropriate volume with D_5W or 0.9% NaCl. • Discard any remaining medication after first withdrawal from vial.

Rate of administration • Administer via IV port nearest the insertion site. • Infuse continuously over 15 min.

Storage • Store at room temperature. • Stable for 30 min after dilution.

PO

• Give with food, milk, antacids if GI distress occurs.

INDICATIONS/ROUTES/DOSAGE

FEVER

PO: ADULTS, ELDERLY, CHILDREN 12 YRS AND OLDER: 200–400 mg q4–6h prn. Maximum: 1,200 mg/day. **CHILDREN, 6 MOS–12 YRS:** 5–10 mg/kg q6–8h prn. Maximum: 40 mg/kg/day.

OSTEOARTHRITIS, RHEUMATOID ARTHRITIS

PO: ADULTS, ELDERLY: 1,200–3,200 mg/day in 3–4 divided doses.

MINOR PAIN

PO: ADULTS, ELDERLY, CHILDREN 12 YRS AND OLDER: 200–400 mg q4–6h prn. Maximum: 1,200 mg/day. **CHILDREN, 6 MOS–12 YRS:** 5–10 mg/kg q6–8h prn. Maximum: 40 mg/kg/day.

MILD TO MODERATE PAIN

PO: ADULTS, ELDERLY: 400 mg q4h prn.

PRIMARY DYSMENORRHEA

PO: ADULTS: 400 mg q4h prn.

JUVENILE RHEUMATOID ARTHRITIS

PO: CHILDREN: 30–50 mg/kg/day in 3–4 divided doses. Maximum: 2.4 g/day.

PATENT DUCTUS ARTERIOSUS

IV: INFANTS: Initially, 10 mg/kg then 2 doses of 5 mg/kg, after 24 hrs and 48 hrs. All doses based on birth weight.

SIDE EFFECTS

OCCASIONAL (9%–3%): Nausea with or without vomiting, dyspepsia, dizziness, rash. **RARE (less than 3%):** Diarrhea or constipation, flatulence, abdominal cramps or pain, pruritus.

ADVERSE EFFECTS/ TOXIC REACTIONS

Acute overdose may result in metabolic acidosis. Rare reactions with long-term use include peptic ulcer, GI bleeding, gastritis, severe hepatic reaction (cholestasis, jaundice), nephrotoxicity (dysuria, hematuria, proteinuria, nephrotic syndrome), severe hypersensitivity reaction (particularly in pts with systemic lupus erythematosus or other collagen diseases). **NeoProfen:** Hypoglycemia, hypocalcemia, respiratory failure, UTI, edema, atelectasis may occur.

NURSING CONSIDERATIONS

BASELINE ASSESSMENT

Assess onset, type, location, duration of pain, inflammation. Inspect appearance of affected joints for immobility, deformities, skin condition. Assess temperature.

INTERVENTION/EVALUATION

Monitor for evidence of nausea, dyspepsia. Monitor CBC, hepatic/renal function tests. Monitor daily pattern of bowel activity/stool consistency. Assess skin for rash. Evaluate for therapeutic response (relief of pain, stiffness, swelling; increased joint mobility; reduced joint tenderness; improved grip strength). Monitor temperature for fever.

PATIENT/FAMILY TEACHING

• Avoid aspirin, alcohol during therapy (increases risk of GI bleeding). • If GI upset occurs, take with food, milk, antacids. • Do not crush, chew enteric-coated tablet. • May cause dizziness. • Avoid tasks that require alertness, motor skills until response to drug is established.

idarubicin

eye-dah-**roo**-bi-sin

(Idamycin PFS, Zavedos)

Do not confuse idarubicin with doxorubicin, or Idamycin with Adriamycin.

CLASSIFICATION

PHARMACOTHERAPEUTIC: Anthracycline antibiotic. **CLINICAL:** Antineoplastic (see p. 80C).

ACTION

Inhibits nucleic acid synthesis by interacting with enzyme topoisomerase II, promoting DNA strand supercoiling. **Therapeutic Effect:** Produces death of rapidly dividing cells.

PHARMACOKINETICS

Widely distributed. Protein binding: 97%. Rapidly metabolized in liver to active metabolite. Primarily eliminated by biliary excretion. Not removed by hemodialysis. **Half-life:** 4–46 hrs; metabolite: 8–92 hrs.

USES

Treatment of acute leukemias (AML, ANLL, ALL) accelerated phase or blast phase of chronic myelogenous leukemia (CML), breast cancer. **OFF-LABEL:** Autologous hematopoietic stem cell transplantation (in combination with busulfan).

PRECAUTIONS

CONTRAINDICATIONS: Arrhythmias, cardiomyopathy, preexisting myelosuppression, pregnancy, severe CHF. **CAUTIONS:**

Renal/hepatic impairment, concurrent radiation therapy.

LIFESPAN CONSIDERATIONS:

Pregnancy/Lactation: If possible, avoid use during pregnancy (may be embryotoxic). Unknown if drug is distributed in breast milk (advise to discontinue breast-feeding before drug initiation). **Pregnancy Category D.** **Children:** Safety and efficacy not established. **Elderly:** Cardiotoxicity may be more frequent. Caution in those with inadequate bone marrow reserves. Age-related renal impairment may require dosage adjustment.

I

INTERACTIONS

DRUG: May decrease effects of **antigout medications. Bone marrow depressants** may increase myelosuppression. **Live virus vaccines** may potentiate virus replication, increase vaccine side effects, decrease pt's antibody response to vaccine. **HERBAL:** None significant. **FOOD:** None known. **LAB VALUES:** May increase serum alkaline phosphatase, bilirubin, uric acid, AST, ALT. May cause EKG changes.

AVAILABILITY (Rx)

INJECTION SOLUTION: 1 mg/ml in 5 ml, 10 ml vials.

ADMINISTRATION/HANDLING

◄ **ALERT** ► Give by free-flowing IV infusion (**never** subcutaneous or IM). Gloves, gowns, eye goggles recommended during preparation/administration of medication. If powder/solution comes in contact with skin, wash thoroughly. Avoid small veins, swollen/edematous extremities, areas overlying joints/tendons.

IV

Reconstitution • Reconstitute each 10-mg vial with 10 ml 0.9% NaCl (5 ml/5-mg vial) to provide a concentration of 1 mg/ml.

Rate of administration • Administer into tubing of freely running IV infusion of D_5W or 0.9% NaCl, preferably via butterfly needle, **slowly** (longer than 10–15 min). • Extravasation produces immediate pain, severe local tissue damage. Terminate infusion immediately. Apply cold compresses for 30 min immediately, then q30min 4 times a day for 3 days. Keep extremity elevated.

Storage • Reconstituted solution is stable for 72 hrs (3 days) at room temperature or 168 hrs (7 days) if refrigerated. • Discard unused solution.

IV INCOMPATIBILITIES

Acyclovir (Zovirax), allopurinol (Aloprim), ampicillin and sulbactam (Unasyn), cefazolin (Ancef, Kefzol), cefepime (Maxipime), ceftazidime (Fortaz), clindamycin (Cleocin), dexamethasone (Decadron), furosemide (Lasix), hydrocortisone (Solu-Cortef), lorazepam (Ativan), meperidine (Demerol), methotrexate, piperacillin and tazobactam (Zosyn), sodium bicarbonate, teniposide (Vumon), vancomycin (Vancocin), vincristine (Oncovin).

IV COMPATIBILITIES

Diphenhydramine (Benadryl), granisetron (Kytril), magnesium, potassium.

INDICATIONS/ROUTES/DOSAGE

USUAL DOSAGE

IV: ADULTS: 8–12 mg/m^2/day for 3 days in combination with Ara-C. **CHILDREN (SOLID TUMOR):** 5 mg/m^2 once a day for 3 days. **CHILDREN (LEUKEMIA):** 10–12 mg/m^2 once a day for 3 days.

DOSAGE IN HEPATIC/RENAL IMPAIRMENT

Dosage is modified based on serum creatinine or bilirubin level.

Serum Level	Dose Reduction
Serum creatinine 2 mg/dl or more	25%
Serum bilirubin greater than 2.5 mg/dl	50%
Serum bilirubin greater than 5 mg/dl	Do not give

SIDE EFFECTS

FREQUENT: Nausea, vomiting (82%), complete alopecia (scalp, axillary, pubic hair) (77%), abdominal cramping, diarrhea (73%), mucositis (50%). **OCCASIONAL:** Hyperpigmentation of nailbeds, phalangeal, dermal creases (46%), fever (36%), headache (20%). **RARE:** Conjunctivitis, neuropathy.

ADVERSE EFFECTS/ TOXIC REACTIONS

Myelosuppression manifested as hematologic toxicity (principally leukopenia and, to lesser extent, anemia, thrombocytopenia), generally occurs within 10–15 days after starting therapy, returns to normal levels by third wk. Cardiotoxicity (either acute, manifested as transient EKG abnormalities, or chronic, manifested as CHF) may occur.

NURSING CONSIDERATIONS

BASELINE ASSESSMENT

Determine baseline renal/hepatic function, CBC results. Obtain EKG before therapy. Antiemetic medication before and during therapy may prevent or relieve nausea, vomiting. Inform pt of high potential for alopecia.

INTERVENTION/EVALUATION

Monitor CBC with differential, platelet count, EKG, renal/hepatic function tests. Monitor for hematologic toxicity (fever, sore throat, signs of local infection, unusual bruising/bleeding from any site), symptoms of anemia (excessive fatigue, weakness). Avoid IM injections, rectal temperatures, other trauma that may precipitate bleeding. Check infusion site frequently for extravasation (causes severe local necrosis). Assess for potentially fatal CHF (dyspnea, rales, pulmonary edema), life-threatening arrhythmias.

PATIENT/FAMILY TEACHING

• Total body alopecia is frequent but reversible. • Assist with ways to cope with hair loss. • New hair growth resumes 2–3 mos after last therapy dose and may have different color, texture. • Maintain fastidious oral hygiene. • Avoid crowds, those with infections. • Teach pt, family the early signs of bleeding, infection. • Inform physician of fever, sore throat, bleeding, bruising. • Urine may turn pink or red. • Use contraceptive measures during therapy.

ifosfamide ⚑

eye-**fos**-fah-mide
(Ifex)

CLASSIFICATION

PHARMACOTHERAPEUTIC: Alkylating agent. **CLINICAL:** Antineoplastic (see p. 80C).

ACTION

Inhibits DNA, RNA protein synthesis by cross-linking with DNA, RNA strands, preventing cell growth. Cell cycle-phase nonspecific. **Therapeutic Effect:** Interferes with DNA, RNA function.

PHARMACOKINETICS

Metabolized in liver to active metabolite. Crosses blood-brain barrier (to a limited extent). Primarily excreted in urine. Removed by hemodialysis. **Half-life:** 15 hrs.

USES

Chemotherapy of germ cell testicular carcinoma (used in combination with agents that protect against hemorrhagic cystitis). **OFF-LABEL:** Head/neck, breast, cervical, small cell lung, non–small cell lung, ovarian, epithelial, bladder, endometrial carcinomas, soft tissue sarcomas, Hodgkin's, non-Hodgkin's lymphomas, neuroblastoma, osteosarcoma, germ cell ovarian tumors, Wilms' tumor.

PRECAUTIONS

CONTRAINDICATIONS: Pregnancy, severe myelosuppression. **CAUTIONS:** Renal/hepatic impairment, compromised bone marrow function.

LIFESPAN CONSIDERATIONS:

Pregnancy/Lactation: If possible, avoid use during pregnancy, esp. first trimester. May cause fetal harm. Drug is distributed in breast milk. Breast-feeding not recommended. **Pregnancy Category D. Children:** Not intended for this pt population. **Elderly:** Age-related renal impairment may require dosage adjustment.

INTERACTIONS

DRUG: Bone marrow depressants may increase myelosuppression. **Live-virus vaccines** may potentiate virus replication, increase vaccine side effects, decrease pt's antibody response to vaccine. **HERBAL: St. John's wort** may decrease concentration. **FOOD:** None known. **LAB VALUES:** May increase BUN, serum bilirubin, creatinine, uric acid, AST, ALT.

AVAILABILITY (Rx)

INJECTION, POWDER FOR RECONSTITUTION (IFEX): 1 g, 3 g.

ADMINISTRATION/HANDLING

◀ **ALERT** ▶ Hemorrhagic cystitis occurs if mesna is not given concurrently. Mesna should always be given with ifosfamide.

IV

Reconstitution • Reconstitute 1-g vial with 20 ml Sterile Water for Injection or Bacteriostatic Water for Injection to provide concentration of 50 mg/ml. Shake to dissolve. • Further dilute with D_5W or 0.9% NaCl to provide concentration of 0.6–20 mg/ml.

Rate of administration • Infuse over minimum of 30 min. • Give with at least 2,000 ml PO or IV fluid (prevents bladder toxicity). • Give with protectant against hemorrhagic cystitis (i.e., mesna).

Storage • Store vial at room temperature. • After reconstitution with Bacteriostatic Water for Injection, solution is stable for 1 wk at room temperature, 3 wks if refrigerated (further diluted solution is stable for 6 wks if refrigerated). • Solution prepared with other diluents should be used within 6 hrs.

IV INCOMPATIBILITIES

Cefepime (Maxipime), methotrexate.

IV COMPATIBILITIES

Granisetron (Kytril), ondansetron (Zofran).

INDICATIONS/ROUTES/DOSAGE

◀ **ALERT** ▶ Dosage individualized based on clinical response, tolerance to adverse effects. When used in combination therapy, consult specific protocols for optimum dosage, sequence of drug administration.

GERM CELL TESTICULAR CARCINOMA

IV: ADULTS: 700–2,000 mg/m^2/day for 5 consecutive days. Repeat q3wk or after recovery from hematologic toxicity. Administer with mesna. **CHILDREN:** 1,200–1,800 mg/m^2/day for 3–5 days q21–28 days.

SIDE EFFECTS

FREQUENT: Alopecia (83%); nausea, vomiting (58%). **OCCASIONAL (15%–5%):** Confusion, drowsiness, hallucinations, infection. **RARE (less than 5%):** Dizziness, seizures, disorientation, fever, malaise, stomatitis (mucosal irritation, glossitis, gingivitis).

ADVERSE EFFECTS/ TOXIC REACTIONS

Hemorrhagic cystitis with hematuria, dysuria occurs frequently if protective agent (mesna) is not used. Myelosuppression, characterized by leukopenia and, to a lesser extent, thrombocytopenia occurs frequently. Pulmonary toxicity, hepatotoxicity, nephrotoxicity, cardiotoxicity, CNS toxicity (confusion, hallucinations, somnolence, coma) may require discontinuation of therapy.

NURSING CONSIDERATIONS

BASELINE ASSESSMENT

Obtain urinalysis before each dose. If hematuria occurs (greater than 10 RBCs per field), therapy should be withheld until resolution occurs. Obtain WBC, platelet count, Hgb before each dose.

INTERVENTION/EVALUATION

Monitor hematologic studies, urinalysis diligently. Assess for fever, sore throat, signs of local infection, unusual bruising/bleeding from any site, symptoms of anemia (excessive fatigue, weakness).

PATIENT/FAMILY TEACHING

• Alopecia is reversible, but new hair growth may have a different color or texture. • Maintain copious daily fluid intake (protects against cystitis). • Do not have immunizations without physician's approval (drug lowers resistance). • Avoid contact with those who have recently received live virus vaccine. • Avoid crowds, those with infections. • Report unusual bleeding/bruising, fever, chills, sore throat, joint pain, sores in mouth or on lips, yellowing skin or eyes.

iloprost

eye-low-prost
(Ventavis)

◆ CLASSIFICATION

PHARMACOTHERAPEUTIC: Prostaglandin. **CLINICAL:** Vasodilator.

ACTION

Dilates systemic, pulmonary arterial vascular beds, alters pulmonary vascular resistance, suppresses vascular smooth muscle proliferation. **Therapeutic Effect:** Improves symptoms, exercise tolerance in pts with pulmonary hypertension; delays deterioration of condition.

PHARMACOKINETICS

Protein binding: 60%. Metabolized in liver. Primarily excreted in urine; minimal elimination in feces. **Half-life:** 20–30 min.

USES

Treatment of pulmonary arterial hypertension in pts with NYHA class III, IV symptoms. May be used in combination with bosentan for treatment of pulmonary arterial hypertension.

PRECAUTIONS

CONTRAINDICATIONS: None known. **CAUTIONS:** Hepatic impairment, concurrent conditions or medications that may increase risk of syncope.

⌛ LIFESPAN CONSIDERATIONS:

Pregnancy/Lactation: Unknown if drug crosses placenta or is distributed is breast milk. **Pregnancy Category C.**

Children: Safety and efficacy not established. **Elderly:** No age-related precautions noted.

INTERACTIONS

DRUG: Anticoagulants, antiplatelet agents may increase risk of bleeding. **Antihypertensives, other vasodilators** may increase hypotensive effects. **HERBAL:** None significant. **FOOD:** None known. **LAB VALUES:** May increase serum alkaline phosphatase, GGT.

AVAILABILITY (Rx)

SOLUTION FOR ORAL INHALATION: 10 mcg/ml (2-ml ampule).

ADMINISTRATION/HANDLING

ORAL INHALATION

• For inhalation only, using Prodose ADD system. • Transfer entire contents of ampule into the medication chamber. • After use, discard remainder of medicine.

INDICATIONS/ROUTES/DOSAGE

PULMONARY HYPERTENSION

ORAL INHALATION: ADULTS: Initially, 2.5 mcg/dose; if tolerated, increased to 5 mcg/dose. Administer 6–9 times a day at intervals of 2 hrs or longer while pt is awake. Maintenance: 5 mcg/dose. **Maximum daily dose:** 45 mcg.

SIDE EFFECTS

FREQUENT (39%–27%): Increased cough, headache, flushing. **OCCASIONAL (13%–11%):** Flu-like symptoms, nausea, lockjaw, jaw pain, hypotension. **RARE (8%–2%):** Insomnia, syncope, palpitations, vomiting, back pain, muscle cramps.

ADVERSE EFFECTS/ TOXIC REACTIONS

Hemoptysis, pneumonia occur occasionally. CHF, renal failure, dyspnea, chest pain occur rarely.

NURSING CONSIDERATIONS

BASELINE ASSESSMENT

Assess B/P, pulse.

INTERVENTION/EVALUATION

Monitor pulse, B/P during therapy. Assess for signs of pulmonary venous hypertension.

PATIENT/FAMILY TEACHING

• Instruct on proper administration of medication using supplied inhalation system. • Advise pt to discard any remaining solution in the medication chamber after each inhalation session.

imatinib

ih-**mah**-tin-ib
(Gleevec)

CLASSIFICATION

PHARMACOTHERAPEUTIC: Protein tyrosine kinase inhibitor. **CLINICAL:** Antineoplastic (see p. 80C).

ACTION

Inhibits Bcr-Abl tyrosine kinase, an enzyme created by Philadelphia chromosome abnormality found in pts with chronic myeloid leukemia (CML). **Therapeutic Effect:** Suppresses tumor growth during the three stages of CML: blast crisis, accelerated phase, chronic phase.

PHARMACOKINETICS

Well absorbed after PO administration. Binds to plasma proteins, particularly albumin. Metabolized in liver. Eliminated mainly in feces as metabolites. **Half-life:** 18 hrs.

USES

Treatment of CML in blast crisis, accelerated phase, chronic phase after failure of interferon-alpha therapy. Treatment of GI stromal tumors (GIST).

PRECAUTIONS

CONTRAINDICATIONS: Pregnancy. **CAUTIONS:** Hepatic/renal impairment.

LIFESPAN CONSIDERATIONS:

Pregnancy/Lactation: Has potential for severe teratogenic effects. Avoid breast-feeding. **Pregnancy Category D.** **Children:** Safety and efficacy not established. **Elderly:** Increased frequency of fluid retention.

INTERACTIONS

DRUG: **Carbamazepine, dexamethasone, phenobarbital, phenytoin, rifampicin** decrease concentration. **Clarithromycin, erythromycin, itraconazole, ketoconazole** increase concentration. May alter therapeutic effects of **cyclosporine, pimozide.** May increase concentration of **dihydropyridine, calcium channel blockers, simvastatin, triazolodiazepines, benzodiazepines. Live virus vaccines** may potentiate viral replication, increase vaccine side effects, decrease pt's antibody response to vaccine. Reduces effect of **warfarin.** **HERBAL:** **St. John's wort** decreases concentration. **FOOD:** None known. **LAB VALUES:** May increase serum bilirubin, AST, ALT. May decrease platelet count, WBC count, serum potassium.

AVAILABILITY (Rx)

CAPSULES: 100 mg. **TABLETS:** 100 mg, 400 mg.

ADMINISTRATION/HANDLING

PO

- Give with a meal and large glass of water.

INDICATIONS/ROUTES/DOSAGE

CML

PO: ADULTS, ELDERLY: 400 mg/day for pts in chronic-phase CML; 600 mg/day for pts in accelerated phase or blast crisis. May increase dosage from 400 to 600 mg/day for pts in chronic phase or from 600 to 800 mg (given as 300–400 mg twice a day) for pts in accelerated phase or blast crisis in the absence of a severe drug reaction or severe neutropenia or thrombocytopenia in the following circumstances: progression of the disease, failure to achieve a satisfactory hematologic response after 3 mos or more of treatment, or loss of a previously achieved hematologic response. **CHILDREN:** 260 mg/m^2 a day as a single daily dose or in 2 divided doses.

GI STROMAL TUMORS

PO: ADULTS, ELDERLY: 400 or 600 mg once daily.

SIDE EFFECTS

FREQUENT (68%–24%): Nausea, diarrhea, vomiting, headache, fluid retention (periorbital, lower extremities), rash, musculoskeletal pain, muscle cramps, arthralgia. **OCCASIONAL (23%–10%):** Abdominal pain, cough, myalgia, fatigue, fever, anorexia, dyspepsia, constipation, night sweats, pruritus. **RARE (less than 10%):** Nasopharyngitis, petechiae, asthenia, epistaxis.

ADVERSE EFFECTS/ TOXIC REACTIONS

Severe fluid retention (pleural effusion, pericardial effusion, pulmonary edema, ascites), hepatotoxicity occur rarely. Neutropenia, thrombocytopenia are expected responses to the drug. Respiratory toxicity is manifested as dyspnea, pneumonia. Heart damage (left ventricular dysfunction, CHF) may occur.

I

NURSING CONSIDERATIONS

BASELINE ASSESSMENT

Obtain CBC weekly for first mo, biweekly for second mo, periodically thereafter. Monitor hepatic function tests (serum transaminase, bilirubin, alkaline phosphatase) before beginning treatment, monthly thereafter.

INTERVENTION/EVALUATION

Assess periorbital area, lower extremities for early evidence of fluid retention. Monitor for unexpected, rapid weight gain. Offer antiemetics to control nausea, vomiting. Monitor daily pattern of bowel activity/stool consistency. Monitor CBC for evidence of neutropenia, thrombocytopenia; assess hepatic function tests for hepatotoxicity. Duration of neutropenia or thrombocytopenia ranges from 2–4 wks.

PATIENT/FAMILY TEACHING

• Avoid crowds, those with known infection. • Avoid contact with anyone who recently received live virus vaccine; do not receive vaccinations. • Take with food and a full glass of water.

Imdur, *see isosorbide*

imipenem/cilastatin

im-ih-**peh**-nem/sill-as-**tah**-tin
(Primaxin IM, Primaxin IV)

CLASSIFICATION

PHARMACOTHERAPEUTIC: Fixed-combination carbapenem. **CLINICAL:** Antibiotic.

ACTION

Imipenem: Penetrates bacterial cell membrane, inhibiting cell wall synthesis. **Cilastatin:** Competitively inhibits the enzyme dehydropeptidase, preventing renal metabolism of imipenem. **Therapeutic Effect:** Produces bacterial cell death.

PHARMACOKINETICS

Readily absorbed after IM administration. Protein binding: 13%–21%. Widely distributed. Metabolized in kidneys. Primarily excreted in urine. Removed by hemodialysis. **Half-life:** 1 hr (increased in renal impairment).

USES

Treatment of susceptible infections due to gram-negative, gram-positive, anaerobic organisms including respiratory tract, skin/skin structure, gynecologic, bone, joint, intra-abdominal, complicated or uncomplicated UTIs; endocarditis; polymicrobic infections; septicemia; serious nosocomial infections.

PRECAUTIONS

CONTRAINDICATIONS: IM: Severe shock, heart block, hypersensitivity to local anesthetics of the amide type. **IV:** Pts with meningitis. **CAUTIONS:** History of seizures, sensitivity to penicillins, renal impairment.

LIFESPAN CONSIDERATIONS:

Pregnancy/Lactation: Crosses placenta. Distributed in cord blood, amniotic fluid, breast milk. **Pregnancy Category C.** **Children:** No precautions noted. **Elderly:** Age-related renal impairment may require dosage adjustment.

INTERACTIONS

DRUG: None significant. **HERBAL:** None significant. **FOOD:** None known. **LAB VALUES:** May increase BUN, serum alkaline phosphatase, bilirubin, creatinine, LDH, AST, ALT. May decrease Hgb, Hct.

AVAILABILITY (Rx)

IM INJECTION, POWDER FOR RECONSTITUTION (PRIMAXIN IM): 500 mg, 750 mg. **IV INJECTION, POWDER FOR RECONSTITUTION (PRIMAXIN IV):** 250 mg, 500 mg.

ADMINISTRATION/HANDLING

IV

Reconstitution • Dilute each 250- or 500-mg vial with 100 ml D_5W; 0.9% NaCl.

Rate of administration • Give by intermittent IV infusion (piggyback). Do not give IV push. • Infuse over 20–30 min (1-g dose over 40–60 min). • Observe pt during initial 30 min of first-time infusion for possible hypersensitivity reaction.

Storage • Solution appears colorless to yellow; discard if solution turns brown. • IV infusion (piggyback) is stable for 4 hrs at room temperature, 24 hrs if refrigerated. • Discard if precipitate forms.

IM

• Prepare with 1% lidocaine without epinephrine; 500-mg vial with 2 ml, 750-mg vial with 3 ml lidocaine HCl. • Administer suspension within 1 hr of preparation. • Do not mix with any other medications. • Inject deep in large muscle mass.

IV INCOMPATIBILITIES

Allopurinol (Aloprim), amphotericin B complex (Abelcet, AmBisome, Amphotec), fluconazole (Diflucan).

IV COMPATIBILITIES

Diltiazem (Cardizem), insulin, lipids, propofol (Diprivan), total parenteral nutrition (TPN).

INDICATIONS/ROUTES/DOSAGE

SERIOUS INFECTIONS

IV: ADULTS, ELDERLY: 2–4 g/day in divided doses q6h.

MILD TO MODERATE INFECTIONS

IV: ADULTS, ELDERLY: 1–2 g/day in divided doses q6–8h. **CHILDREN OLDER THAN 3 MOS–12 YRS:** 60–100 mg/kg/day in divided doses q6h. **Maximum:** 4 g/day. **CHILDREN 1–3 MOS:** 100 mg/kg/day in divided doses q6h. **CHILDREN YOUNGER THAN 1 MO:** 20–25 mg/kg/dose q8–24h. **IM: ADULTS, ELDERLY:** 500–750 mg q12h.

DOSAGE IN RENAL IMPAIRMENT

Dosage and frequency are modified based on creatinine clearance and severity of infection.

Creatinine Clearance	Dosage (IV)
31–70 ml/min	500 mg q8h
21–30 ml/min	500 mg q12h
5–20 ml/min	250 mg q12h

SIDE EFFECTS

OCCASIONAL (3%–2%): Diarrhea, nausea, vomiting. **RARE (2%–1%):** Rash.

ADVERSE EFFECTS/ TOXIC REACTIONS

Antibiotic-associated colitis, other superinfections may occur. Anaphylactic reactions have been reported.

NURSING CONSIDERATIONS

BASELINE ASSESSMENT

Question for history of allergies, particularly to beta-lactams, penicillins, cephalosporins. Inquire about history of seizures.

INTERVENTION/EVALUATION

Monitor renal, hepatic, hematologic function tests. Evaluate for phlebitis (heat, pain, red streaking over vein), pain at IV injection site. Assess for GI discomfort, nausea, vomiting. Monitor daily pattern of bowel activity/stool consistency. Assess skin for rash. Be alert to tremors, possible seizures.

imipramine

ih-**mih**-prah-meen

(Apo-Imipramine ♣, Novo-Pramine ♣, Tofranil, Tofranil-PM)

Do not confuse imipramine with desipramine.

CLASSIFICATION

PHARMACOTHERAPEUTIC: Tricyclic. **CLINICAL:** Antidepressant, antineuritic, antipanic, antineuralgic, antinarcoleptic adjunct, anticataplectic, antibulimic (see p. 37C).

ACTION

Blocks reuptake of neurotransmitters (norepinephrine, serotonin) at presynaptic membranes, increasing their concentration at postsynaptic receptor sites. **Therapeutic Effect:** Relieves depression, controls nocturnal enuresis.

USES

Treatment of various forms of depression, often in conjunction with psychotherapy. Treatment of nocturnal enuresis in children older than 6 yrs. **OFF-LABEL:** Treatment of attention-deficit hyperactivity disorder, cataplexy associated with narcolepsy, neurogenic pain, panic disorder.

PRECAUTIONS

CONTRAINDICATIONS: Acute recovery period after MI, use within 14 days of MAOIs. **CAUTIONS:** Prostatic hypertrophy; history of urinary retention, obstruction; glaucoma; diabetes mellitus; history of seizures; hyperthyroidism; cardiac, hepatic, renal disease; schizophrenia; increased intraocular pressure; hiatal hernia. **Pregnancy Category D.**

INTERACTIONS

DRUG: **Alcohol, other CNS depressants** may increase hypotensive effects, CNS and respiratory depression caused by imipramine. **Antithyroid agents** may increase risk of agranulocytosis. **Cimetidine** may increase concentration, risk of toxicity. May decrease the effects of **clonidine. MAOIs** may increase risk of neuroleptic malignant syndrome, hyperpyrexia, hypertensive crisis, seizures. **Phenothiazines** may increase anticholinergic, sedative effects. **Phenytoin** may decrease concentration. **Sympathomimetics** may increase risk of cardiac effects. **HERBAL:** **Kava kava, SAMe, St. John's wort, valerian** may increase risk of serotonin syndrome, CNS depression. **FOOD:** **Grapefruit, grapefruit juice** may increase concentration/toxicity. **LAB VALUES:** May alter serum glucose, EKG readings. Therapeutic serum level is 225–300 ng/ml; toxic serum level is greater than 500 ng/ml.

AVAILABILITY (Rx)

CAPSULES (TOFRANIL-PM): 75 mg, 100 mg, 125 mg, 150 mg. **TABLETS (TOFRANIL):** 10 mg, 25 mg, 50 mg.

ADMINISTRATION/HANDLING

PO

- Give with food, milk if GI distress occurs.

INDICATIONS/ROUTES/DOSAGE

DEPRESSION

PO: ADULTS: Initially, 75–100 mg/day. May gradually increase to 300 mg/day then reduce dosage to effective maintenance level 50–150 mg/day. **ELDERLY:** Initially, 10–25 mg/day at bedtime. May increase by 10–25 mg every 3–7 days. Range: 50–150 mg/day. **CHILDREN:** 1.5 mg/kg/day. May increase by 1 mg/kg every 3–4 days. **Maximum:** 5 mg/kg/day.

ENURESIS

PO: CHILDREN, 6 YRS AND OLDER: Initially, 25 mg at bedtime. May increase by 25 mg if inadequate response seen after 1 wk. **Maximum:** 2.5 mg/kg/day or 50 mg at bedtime for ages 6–12 yrs; 75 mg at bedtime for ages over 12 yrs.

SIDE EFFECTS

FREQUENT: Drowsiness, fatigue, dry mouth, blurred vision, constipation, delayed micturition, orthostatic hypotension, diaphoresis, impaired concentration, increased appetite, urinary retention, photosensitivity. **OCCASIONAL:** GI disturbances (nausea, metallic taste). **RARE:** Paradoxical reactions, (agitation, restlessness, nightmares, insomnia), extrapyramidal symptoms (particularly fine hand tremor).

ADVERSE EFFECTS/ TOXIC REACTIONS

Overdose may produce seizures; cardiovascular effects (severe orthostatic hypotension, dizziness, tachycardia, palpitations, arrhythmias). May result in altered temperature regulation (hyperpyrexia, hypothermia). Abrupt withdrawal from prolonged therapy may produce headache, malaise, nausea, vomiting, vivid dreams.

NURSING CONSIDERATIONS

BASELINE ASSESSMENT

For pts on long-term therapy, hepatic/renal function tests, blood counts should be performed periodically.

INTERVENTION/EVALUATION

Supervise suicidal-risk pt closely during early therapy (as depression lessens, energy level improves, causing increased suicide potential). Assess appearance, behavior, speech pattern, level of interest, mood. Monitor daily pattern of bowel activity/stool consistency. Monitor B/P, pulse for hypotension, arrhythmias. Assess for urinary retention by bladder palpation. Therapeutic serum level: 225–300 ng/ml; toxic serum level: greater than 500 ng/ml.

PATIENT/FAMILY TEACHING

• Change positions slowly to avoid hypotensive effect. • Tolerance to postural hypotension, sedative, anticholinergic effects usually develops during early therapy. • Therapeutic effect may be noted within 2–5 days, maximum effect within 2–3 wks. • Sugarless gum, sips of tepid water may relieve dry mouth. • Do not abruptly discontinue medication. • Avoid tasks that require alertness, motor skills until response to drug is established.

Imitrex, *see sumatriptan*

immune globulin IV (IGIV)

ih-**mewn glah**-byew-lin

(Carimune NF, Cytogam, Flebogamma 5%, Gammagard Liquid 10%, Gammagard S/D, Gamunex, Octagam 5%, Polygam S/D)

CLASSIFICATION

CLINICAL: Immune serum.

ACTION

Blocks Fc receptor on macrophages in pts with idiopathic thrombocytopenia purpura (ITP). Immunomodulatory effects on T cells and macrophages, esp. cytokine synthesis, B-cell immune function. Provides antibodies that neutralize bacteria, viral toxins. **Therapeutic Effect:** Provides passive immunity against infection; induces rapid increase in platelet count; produces anti-inflammatory effect.

PHARMACOKINETICS

Evenly distributed between intravascular and extravascular space. **Half-life:** 21–23 days.

USES

Treatment of pts with primary immunodeficiency syndromes, ITP, Kawasaki disease, prevention of recurrent bacterial infections in pts with hypogammaglobulinemia associated with B-cell chronic lymphocytic leukemia (CLL). Treatment adjunct in bone marrow transplantation. **OFF-LABEL:** Control/prevention of infections in infants, children with immunosuppression due to AIDS or AIDS-related complex; prevention of acute infections in immunosuppressed pts; prevention, treatment of infection in high-risk, preterm, low-birth-weight neonates; treatment of chronic inflammatory demyelinating polyneuropathies, multiple sclerosis.

PRECAUTIONS

CONTRAINDICATIONS: Hypersensitivity to gamma globulin, thimerosal, anti-IgA antibodies; isolated IgA deficiency. **CAUTIONS:** Cardiovascular disease, history of thrombosis, renal impairment, diabetes, volume depletion, sepsis, concomitant nephrotoxic drugs.

LIFESPAN CONSIDERATIONS:

Pregnancy/Lactation: Unknown if drug crosses placenta or is distributed in breast milk. **Pregnancy Category C.** **Children/Elderly:** No age-related precautions noted.

INTERACTIONS

DRUG: **Live virus vaccines** may increase vaccine side effects, potentiate virus replication, decrease pt's antibody response to vaccine. **HERBAL:** None significant. **FOOD:** None known. **LAB VALUES:** None known.

AVAILABILITY (Rx)

INJECTION, POWDER FOR RECONSTITUTION: CARIMUNE NF: 3 g, 6 g, 12 g. **GAMMAGARD S/D:** 2.5 g, 5 g, 10 g. **POLYGAM S/D:** 5 g, 10 g. **INJECTION, SOLUTION: CYTOGAM:** 1 g, 2.5 g. **FLEBOGAMMA 5%:** 0.5 g, 2.5 g, 5 g, 10 g. **GAMMAGARD LIQUID 10%, GAMUNEX:** 1 g, 2.5 g, 5 g, 10 g, 20 g. **OCTAGAM 5%:** 1 g, 2.5 g, 5 g, 10 g.

ADMINISTRATION/HANDLING

IV

Reconstitution • Reconstitute only with diluent provided by manufacturer. • Discard partially used or turbid preparations.

Rate of administration • Give by infusion only. • After reconstituted, administer via separate tubing. • Avoid mixing with other medication or IV infusion fluids. • Rate of infusion varies with product used. • Monitor vital signs, B/P diligently during and immediately after IV administration (precipitous fall in B/P may indicate anaphylactic reaction). Stop infusion immediately. Epinephrine should be readily available.

Storage • Refer to individual IV preparations for storage requirements, stability after reconstitution.

IV INCOMPATIBILITIES

Do not mix with any other medications.

INDICATIONS/ROUTES/DOSAGE

PRIMARY IMMUNODEFICIENCY SYNDROME

IV: ADULTS, ELDERLY, CHILDREN: 200–400 mg/kg once monthly.

SUBCUTANEOUS: ADULTS, ELDERLY: 100–200 mg/kg once weekly.

ITP

IV: ADULTS, ELDERLY, CHILDREN: 400–1,000 mg/kg/day for 2–5 days.

KAWASAKI DISEASE

IV: ADULTS, ELDERLY, CHILDREN: 2 g/kg as a single dose.

CLL

IV: ADULTS, ELDERLY, CHILDREN: 400 mg/kg q3–4wk.

BONE MARROW TRANSPLANT

IV: ADULTS, ELDERLY, CHILDREN: 400–500 mg/kg/dose every wk for 12 wks, then every mo.

SIDE EFFECTS

FREQUENT: Tachycardia, backache, headache, arthralgia, myalgia. **OCCASIONAL:** Fatigue, wheezing, injection site rash/pain, leg cramps, urticaria, bluish color of lips/nailbeds, light-headedness.

ADVERSE EFFECTS/ TOXIC REACTIONS

Anaphylactic reactions occur rarely but incidence increases with repeated injections. Epinephrine should be readily available. Overdose may produce chest tightness, chills, diaphoresis, dizziness, facial flushing, nausea, vomiting, fever, hypotension. Hypersensitivity reaction (anxiety, arthralgia, dizziness, flushing, myalgia, palpitations, pruritus) occurs rarely.

NURSING CONSIDERATIONS

BASELINE ASSESSMENT

Inquire about history of exposure to disease for pt/family as appropriate. Have epinephrine readily available. Pt should be well hydrated prior to administration.

INTERVENTION/EVALUATION

Control rate of IV infusion carefully; too-rapid infusion increases risk of precipitous fall in B/P, signs of anaphylaxis (facial flushing, chest tightness, chills, fever, nausea, vomiting, diaphoresis). Assess pt closely during infusion, esp. first hr; monitor vital signs continuously. Stop infusion temporarily if aforementioned signs noted. For treatment of ITP, monitor platelet count.

PATIENT/FAMILY TEACHING

• Explain rationale for therapy. • Rapid response, lasts 1–3 mos. • Inform physician if sudden weight gain, fluid retention, edema, decreased urine output, shortness of breath occur.

immune globulin subcutaneous

Ih-**mewn-glah**-byew-lin
(Vivaglobulin)

CLASSIFICATION

CLINICAL: Immune globulin.

ACTION

Immune globulin replacement therapy for IgG antibodies against bacteria/viruses. **Therapeutic Effect:** Provides immunity against infection.

PHARMACOKINETICS

Bioavailability 73 (compared to IGIV), time to peak plasma levels: 2.5 days.

USES

Treatment of primary immune deficiency.

PRECAUTIONS

CONTRAINDICATIONS: History of anaphylactic or severe systemic reaction to immune globulins, selective IgA deficiency with known antibody against IgA. **CAUTIONS:** Cardiovascular disease, renal impairment, diabetes, sepsis, concomitant nephrotoxic medications.

LIFESPAN CONSIDERATIONS: **Pregnancy/Lactation:** Unknown if drug crosses placenta or is distributed in breast milk. **Pregnancy Category C. Children/Elderly:** No age-related precautions noted.

INTERACTIONS

DRUG: **Live virus vaccines** may potentiate viral replication, increase vaccine side effects, decrease pt's antibody response to vaccine. **HERBAL:** None significant. **FOOD:** None known. **LAB VALUES:** None known.

AVAILABILITY (Rx)

INJECTION, SOLUTION: (VIVAGLOBULIN): IgG 160 mg/ml (3 ml, 10 ml, 20 ml).

ADMINISTRATION/HANDLING

• Refrigerate; do not freeze; do not shake. • Allow vial to reach room temperature prior to use. • Do not use if cloudy or precipitate forms. • Follow manufacturer's instructions for filling reservoir, preparing pump. • Inject via infusion pump into abdomen, thigh, upper arm, lateral hip. Maximum rate: 20 ml/hr.

INDICATIONS/ROUTES/DOSAGE

PRIMARY IMMUNE DEFICIENCY

SUBCUTANEOUS INFUSION: ADULTS, ELDERLY, CHILDREN 2 YRS AND OLDER: 100–200 mg/kg/wk. Adjust dose over time to achieve desired clinical response or target IgG levels

SIDE EFFECTS

FREQUENT: Local injection site reactions (92%), headache (48%), fever (25%), nausea (18%), sore throat, rash (17%). **OCCASIONAL:** Pain, diarrhea, cough (10%), weakness (5%), tachycardia, skin disorder, urine abnormality (3%).

ADVERSE EFFECTS/ TOXIC REACTIONS

Anaphylactic reactions are rare, but epinephrine should be readily available. Overdose may produce chest tightness, chills, diaphoresis, dizziness, facial flushing, nausea, vomiting, fever, hypotension. Hypersensitivity reaction (anxiety, arthralgia, dizziness, flushing, myalgia, palpitations, pruritus) occurs rarely.

NURSING CONSIDERATIONS

BASELINE ASSESSMENT

Inquire about history of exposure to disease for pt/family. Epinephrine should be readily available.

INTERVENTION/EVALUATION

Monitor for infusion-related adverse reaction, clinical response, anaphylaxis. Monitor Ig level.

PATIENT/FAMILY TEACHING

Explain rationale for therapy. Report to physician any sudden weight gain, fluid retention, edema, decreased urine output, shortness of breath, unusual reactions.

Imodium A-D, *see loperamide*

Increlex, *see mecasermin*

indapamide

in-**dap**-a-mide
(Apo-Indapamide ✤, Lozide ✤, Lozol, Novo-Indapamide ✤)

Do not confuse indapamide with iodamide or iopamidol.

CLASSIFICATION

PHARMACOTHERAPEUTIC: Thiazide. **CLINICAL:** Diuretic, antihypertensive (see p. 97C).

ACTION

Diuretic: Blocks reabsorption of water, sodium, potassium at cortical diluting segment of distal tubule. **Antihypertensive:** Reduces plasma, extracellular fluid volume and peripheral vascular resistance by direct effect on blood vessels. **Therapeutic Effect:** Promotes diuresis, reduces B/P.

PHARMACOKINETICS

Almost completely absorbed following PO administration. Protein binding: 71%–79%. Extensively metabolized in liver. Excreted in urine. **Half-life:** 14–15 hrs.

USES

Management of hypertension. Treatment of edema associated with CHF, nephrotic syndrome.

PRECAUTIONS

CONTRAINDICATIONS: None known. **CAUTIONS:** History of hypersensitivity to sulfonamides or thiazide diuretics, renal decompensation, anuria. Severe renal disease, hepatic impairment, diabetes mellitus, elderly, debilitated, thyroid disorders.

LIFESPAN CONSIDERATIONS:

Pregnancy/Lactation: Unknown if drug crosses placenta or is distributed in breast milk. **Pregnancy Category B (D if used in pregnancy-induced hypertension). Children:** Safety and efficacy not established. **Elderly:** May be more sensitive to hypotensive, electrolyte effects.

INTERACTIONS

DRUG: May increase risk of **digoxin** toxicity associated with indapamide-induced hypokalemia. May increase risk of **lithium** toxicity. **HERBAL: Ephedra, ginseng, yohimbe** may worsen hypertension. **Garlic** may increase antihypertensive effect. **FOOD:** None known. **LAB VALUES:** May increase plasma renin activity. May decrease protein-bound iodine, serum calcium, potassium, sodium.

AVAILABILITY (Rx)

TABLETS: 1.25 mg, 2.5 mg.

ADMINISTRATION/HANDLING

PO

• Give with food, milk if GI upset occurs, preferably with breakfast (may prevent nocturia).

INDICATIONS/ROUTES/DOSAGE

EDEMA

PO: ADULTS: Initially, 2.5 mg/day, may increase to 5 mg/day after 1 wk.

HYPERTENSION

PO: ADULTS, ELDERLY: Initially, 1.25 mg, may increase to 2.5 mg/day after 4 wks or 5 mg/day after additional 4 wks.

SIDE EFFECTS

FREQUENT (5% and greater): Fatigue, paresthesia of extremities, tension, irritability, agitation, headache, dizziness, light-headedness, insomnia, muscle cramps. **OCCASIONAL (less than 5%):** Urinary frequency, urticaria, rhinorrhea, flushing, weight loss, orthostatic hypotension, depression, blurred vision, nausea, vomiting, diarrhea, constipation, dry mouth, impotence, rash, pruritus.

ADVERSE EFFECTS/ TOXIC REACTIONS

Vigorous diuresis may lead to profound water and electrolyte depletion, resulting in hypokalemia, hyponatremia, dehydration. Acute hypotensive episodes may occur. Hyperglycemia may be noted during prolonged therapy. Pancreatitis, blood dyscrasias, pulmonary edema, allergic pneumonitis, dermatologic reactions occur rarely. Overdose can lead to lethargy, coma without changes in electrolytes or hydration.

NURSING CONSIDERATIONS

BASELINE ASSESSMENT

Check vital signs, esp. B/P for hypotension, before administration. Assess baseline electrolytes, particularly check for hypokalemia. Observe for edema; assess skin turgor, mucous membranes for

I

hydration status. Assess muscle strength, mental status. Note skin temperature, moisture. Obtain baseline weight. Initiate I&O.

INTERVENTION/EVALUATION

Continue to monitor B/P, vital signs, electrolytes, I&O, weight. Note extent of diuresis. Watch for electrolyte disturbances (hypokalemia may result in weakness, tremor, muscle cramps, nausea, vomiting, altered mental status, tachycardia; hyponatremia may result in confusion, thirst, cold/clammy skin).

PATIENT/FAMILY TEACHING

• Expect increased frequency, volume of urination. • To reduce hypotensive effect, rise slowly from lying to sitting position, permit legs to dangle momentarily before standing. • Eat foods high in potassium such as whole grains (cereals), legumes, meat, bananas, apricots, orange juice, potatoes (white, sweet), raisins. • Take early in the day to avoid nocturia.

Inderal, *see propranolol*

Inderal LA, *see propranolol*

indinavir

in-**din**-oh-vir

(Crixivan)

Do not confuse indinavir with Denavir.

CLASSIFICATION

PHARMACOTHERAPEUTIC: Protease inhibitor. **CLINICAL:** Antiviral (see pp. 65C, 112C).

ACTION

Suppresses HIV protease, an enzyme necessary for splitting viral polyprotein precursors into mature infectious viral particles. **Therapeutic Effect:** Interrupts HIV replication, slowing progression of HIV infection.

PHARMACOKINETICS

Rapidly absorbed after PO administration. Protein binding: 60%. Metabolized in liver. Primarily excreted in urine. Unknown if removed by hemodialysis. **Half-life:** 1.8 hrs (increased in hepatic impairment).

USES

Treatment of HIV infection as part of a multidrug regimen (at least 3 anti-retroviral agents). **OFF-LABEL:** Prophylaxis following occupational exposure to HIV.

PRECAUTIONS

CONTRAINDICATIONS: Concurrent use with terfenadine, cisapride, astemizole, triazolam, midazolam, pimozide, ergot derivatives, nephrolithiasis. **CAUTIONS:** Renal/hepatic impairment.

LIFESPAN CONSIDERATIONS:

Pregnancy/Lactation: Unknown if excreted in breast milk. Breast-feeding not recommended in HIV-infected women. **Pregnancy Category C. Children:** Safety and efficacy not established. **Elderly:** Information not available.

INTERACTIONS

DRUG: May increase concentration/toxicity of **midazolam, triazolam, sildenafil. Efavirenz, rifabutin, rifampin** may decrease concentration/effect. **HMG-CoA inhibitors (e.g., lovastatin, simvastatin)** may increase risk of myopathy. **Itraconazole, ketoconazole, delavirdine** may increase concentration. **HERBAL: St. John's wort** may decrease concentration, effect. **FOOD: Grapefruit, grapefruit juice**

may decrease concentration, effect. **High-fat, high-calorie, and high-protein meals** may decrease concentration. **LAB VALUES:** May increase serum bilirubin (in 10% of pts), AST, ALT.

AVAILABILITY (Rx)

CAPSULES: 100 mg, 200 mg, 333 mg, 400 mg.

ADMINISTRATION/HANDLING

PO

• Store at room temperature. • Protect from moisture (capsules sensitive to moisture; keep in original bottle). • Best given without food 1 hr before or 2 hrs following a meal but may give with water, skim milk, juice, coffee, tea, light meal (e.g., dry toast with jelly). • Do not give with meal high in fat, calories, protein. • If indinavir and didanosine are given concurrently, give at least 1 hr apart on an empty stomach.

INDICATIONS/ROUTES/DOSAGE

HIV INFECTION (IN COMBINATION WITH OTHER ANTIRETROVIRALS)

PO: ADULTS: 800 mg (two 400-mg capsules) q8h.

DOSAGE ADJUSTMENTS WHEN GIVEN CONCOMITANTLY: DELAVIRDINE, ITRACONAZOLE, KETOCONAZOLE: Reduce dose to 600 mg q8h. **EFAVIRENZ:** Increase dose to 1,000 mg q8h. **LOPINAVIR/RITONAVIR:** Reduce dose to 600 mg twice a day. **NEVIRAPINE:** Increase dose to 1,000 mg q8h. **RIFABUTIN:** Reduce rifabutin by ½ and increase indinavir to 1,000 mg q8h. **RITONAVIR:** 100–200 mg twice a day and indinavir 800 mg twice a day or ritonavir 400 mg twice a day and indinavir 400 mg twice a day.

HIV INFECTION IN PTS WITH HEPATIC INSUFFICIENCY

PO: ADULTS: 600 mg q8h.

SIDE EFFECTS

FREQUENT: Nausea (12%), abdominal pain (9%), headache (6%), diarrhea (5%). **OCCASIONAL:** Vomiting, asthenia, fatigue (4%); insomnia; accumulation of fat in waist, abdomen, back of neck. **RARE:** Altered taste, heartburn, symptomatic urinary tract disease, transient renal dysfunction.

ADVERSE EFFECTS/ TOXIC REACTIONS

Nephrolithiasis (flank pain with or without hematuria) occurs in 4% of pts.

NURSING CONSIDERATIONS

BASELINE ASSESSMENT

Offer emotional support. Establish baseline lab values. Emphasize need for close monitoring of renal function (urinalysis, serum creatinine) during therapy.

INTERVENTION/EVALUATION

Encourage adequate hydration. Pt should drink 48 oz (1.5 L) of liquid for each 24 hrs during therapy. Monitor for evidence of nephrolithiasis (flank pain, hematuria), contact physician if symptoms occur (therapy should be interrupted for 1–3 days). Monitor daily pattern of bowel activity/stool consistency. Assess for abdominal discomfort, headache. Monitor serum bilirubin, glucose, cholesterol, triglycerides, amylase, lipase, hepatic function tests, CD4 cell count, CBC.

PATIENT/FAMILY TEACHING

• Advise that indinavir is not a cure for HIV; condition may progress despite treatment. • If dose is missed, take next dose at regularly scheduled time (do **not** double the dose). • Best taken without food but water only (optimal absorption) 1 hr before or 2 hrs following a meal but may take with water, skim milk, juice, coffee, tea, light carbohydrate meal. • Avoid St. John's wort, grapefruit, grapefruit juice.

indomethacin

in-doe-**meth**-a-sin

(Apo-Indomethacin ♣, Indocid ♣, Indocin, Indocin-IV, Indocin-SR, Novomethacin ♣)

Do not confuse Indocin with Imodium or Vicodin.

CLASSIFICATION

PHARMACOTHERAPEUTIC: Nonsteroidal anti-inflammatory. **CLINICAL:** Anti-inflammatory, analgesic (see p. 124C).

I

ACTION

Produces analgesic, anti-inflammatory effects by inhibiting prostaglandin synthesis. Increases sensitivity of premature ductus to dilating effects of prostaglandins. **Therapeutic Effect:** Reduces inflammatory response, intensity of pain. Closure of patent ductus arteriosus.

PHARMACOKINETICS

Rectal absorption more rapid than oral administration. Protein binding: 99%. Metabolized in liver. Excreted in urine. **Half-life:** 4.5 hrs.

USES

Treatment of active stages of rheumatoid arthritis, osteoarthritis, ankylosing spondylitis, acute gouty arthritis. Relieves acute bursitis, tendonitis. For closure of hemodynamically significant patent ductus arteriosus of premature infants weighing 500–1,750 g. **OFF-LABEL:** Treatment of fever due to malignancy, pericarditis, psoriatic arthritis, rheumatic complications associated with Paget's disease of bone, vascular headache.

PRECAUTIONS

CONTRAINDICATIONS: Active GI bleeding, ulcerations; hypersensitivity to aspirin, indomethacin, other NSAIDs; renal impairment; thrombocytopenia. **CAUTIONS:** Cardiac dysfunction, hypertension, decreased renal/hepatic function, epilepsy, concurrent anticoagulant therapy.

⌛ LIFESPAN CONSIDERATIONS:

Pregnancy/Lactation: Crosses placenta; distributed in breast milk. **Pregnancy Category C (D if used after 34 wks gestation, close to delivery, or for longer than 48 hrs). Children:** Safety and efficacy not established in those younger than 14 yrs. **Elderly:** GI bleeding, ulceration increase risk of serious adverse effects.

INTERACTIONS

DRUG: May increase concentration of **aminoglycosides** in neonates. May decrease effects of **antihypertensives, diuretics. Aspirin, other salicylates** may increase risk of GI side effects, bleeding. **Bone marrow depressants** may increase risk of hematologic reactions. May increase effects of **heparin, oral anticoagulants, thrombolytics.** May increase concentration, risk of toxicity of **lithium.** May increase risk of **methotrexate** toxicity. **Probenecid** may increase concentration. Do not give **triamterene** concurrently as it may potentiate renal failure. **HERBAL: Cat's claw, dong quai, evening primrose, feverfew, red clover, horse chestnut, garlic, ginseng, ginkgo** may increase antiplatelet activity. **FOOD:** None known. **LAB VALUES:** May prolong bleeding time. May alter serum glucose. May increase BUN, serum creatinine, potassium, AST, ALT. May decrease serum sodium, platelet count.

AVAILABILITY (Rx)

CAPSULES (INDOCIN): 25 mg, 50 mg. **INJECTION, POWDER FOR RECONSTITUTION (INDOCIN IV):** 1 mg. **ORAL SUSPENSION (INDOCIN):** 25 mg/5 ml. **SUPPOSITORIES:** 50 mg.

CAPSULES (SUSTAINED-RELEASE [INDOCIN SR]): 75 mg.

ADMINISTRATION/HANDLING

IV

Reconstitution • To 1-mg vial, add 1–2 ml preservative-free Sterile Water for Injection or 0.9% NaCl to provide concentration of 1 mg or 0.5 mg/ml, respectively. • Do not further dilute.

Rate of administration • Administer over 5–10 sec. • Restrict fluid intake.

Storage • IV solutions made without preservatives should be used immediately. • Use IV immediately following reconstitution. • IV solution appears clear; discard if cloudy or precipitate forms. • Discard unused portion.

PO

• Give after meals or with food, antacids. • Do not crush sustained-release capsules.

RECTAL

◀ **ALERT** ▶ IV injection preferred for patent ductus arteriosus in neonate (but may give dose PO via NG tube or rectally). • If suppository is too soft, chill for 30 min in refrigerator or run cold water over foil wrapper. • Moisten suppository with cold water before inserting well into rectum.

IV INCOMPATIBILITIES

Amino acid injection, calcium gluconate, cimetidine (Tagamet), dobutamine (Dobutrex), dopamine (Intropin), gentamicin (Garamycin), tobramycin (Nebcin).

IV COMPATIBILITIES

Insulin, potassium.

INDICATIONS/ROUTES/DOSAGE

MODERATE TO SEVERE RHEUMATOID ARTHRITIS, OSTEOARTHRITIS, ANKYLOSING SPONDYLITIS

PO: ADULTS, ELDERLY: Initially, 25 mg 2–3 times a day; increased by 25–50 mg/wk up to 150–200 mg/day. Or 75 mg/day (extended-release) up to 75 mg twice a day. **CHILDREN:** 1–2 mg/kg/day. **Maximum:** 150–200 mg/day.

ACUTE GOUTY ARTHRITIS

PO: ADULTS, ELDERLY: Initially, 100 mg, then 50 mg 3 times a day for 3–5 days.

ACUTE BURSITIS, TENDONITIS

PO: ADULTS, ELDERLY: 75–150 mg/day in 3–4 divided doses.

USUAL RECTAL DOSAGE

ADULTS, ELDERLY: 50 mg 4 times a day. **CHILDREN:** Initially, 1.5–2.5 mg/kg/day, increased up to 4 mg/kg/day. **Maximum:** 150–200 mg/day.

PATENT DUCTUS ARTERIOSUS

IV: NEONATES: Initially, 0.2 mg/kg. Subsequent doses are based on age, as follows: **NEONATES OLDER THAN 7 DAYS:** 0.25 mg/kg for 2nd and 3rd doses. **NEONATES 2–7 DAYS:** 0.2 mg/kg for 2nd and 3rd doses. **NEONATES LESS THAN 48 HRS:** 0.1 mg/kg for 2nd and 3rd doses. In general, dosing interval is 12 hrs if urine output is greater than 1 ml/kg/hr after prior dose, 24 hrs if urine output is less than 1 ml/kg/hr but greater than 0.6 ml/kg/hr. Dose is held if urine output is less than 0.6. ml/kg/hr or if neonate is anuric.

SIDE EFFECTS

FREQUENT (11%–3%): Headache, nausea, vomiting, dyspepsia (heatburn, indigestion, epigastric pain), dizziness. **OCCASIONAL (less than 3%):** Depression, tinnitus, diaphoresis, drowsiness, constipation, diarrhea. **Patent ductus arteriosus:** Bleeding abnormalities. **RARE:** Hypertension, confusion, urticaria, pruritus, rash, blurred vision.

ADVERSE EFFECTS/ TOXIC REACTIONS

Paralytic ileus, ulceration of esophagus, stomach, duodenum, small intestine may occur. Pts with renal impairment may develop hyperkalemia with worsening of renal impairment. May aggravate depression or other psychiatric disturbances, epilepsy, parkinsonism. Nephrotoxicity (dysuria, hematuria, proteinuria, nephrotic syndrome) occurs rarely. Metabolic acidosis/alkalosis, bradycardia occur rarely in pts with patent ductus arteriosus.

NURSING CONSIDERATIONS

BASELINE ASSESSMENT

May mask signs of infection. Assess onset, type, location, duration of pain, fever, inflammation. Inspect appearance of affected joints for immobility, deformities, skin condition.

INTERVENTION/EVALUATION

Monitor for evidence of nausea, dyspepsia. Assist with ambulation if dizziness occurs. Evaluate for therapeutic response: relief of pain, stiffness, swelling; increased joint mobility; reduced joint tenderness; improved grip strength. Monitor BUN, serum creatinine, potassium, hepatic function tests. In neonates, also monitor heart rate, heart sounds for murmur, B/P, urine output, EKG, serum sodium, glucose, platelets.

PATIENT/FAMILY TEACHING

• Avoid aspirin, alcohol during therapy (increases risk of GI bleeding). • If GI upset occurs, take with food, milk. • Avoid tasks that require alertness, motor skills until response to drug is established. • Swallow capsule whole; do not crush or chew sustained-release capsule.

infliximab

in-**flicks**-ih-mab
(Remicade)

Do not confuse Remicade with Reminyl.

CLASSIFICATION

PHARMACOTHERAPEUTIC: Monoclonal antibody. **CLINICAL:** GI anti-inflammatory.

ACTION

Binds to tumor necrosis factor (TNF), inhibiting functional activity of TNF. Reduces infiltration of inflammatory cells. **Therapeutic Effect:** Decreases inflamed areas of intestine.

PHARMACOKINETICS

Route	Onset	Peak	Duration
IV (Crohn's disease)	1–2 wks	N/A	8–48 wks
IV (Rheumatoid arthritis [RA])	3–7 days	N/A	6–12 wks

Absorbed into GI tissue; primarily distributed in vascular compartment. **Half-life:** 9.5 days.

USES

In combination with methotrexate, reduces signs/symptoms, inhibits progression of structural damage, improves physical function in moderate to severe active rheumatoid arthritis, psoriatic arthritis. Reduces signs/symptoms, induces and maintains remission in moderate to severe active Crohn's disease. Reduces number of draining enterocutaneous/rectovaginal fistulas, maintains fistula closure in fistulizing Crohn's disease. Reduces sign/symptoms of active ankylosing spondylitis. Treatment of chronic severe plaque psoriasis in pts who are candidates for systemic therapy. Reduces sign/symptoms, induces and maintains clinical remission and mucosal healing, eliminates corticosteroid use in moderate to severe active ulcerative colitis. **OFF-LABEL:** CHF, juvenile arthritis, psoriasis, reactive arthritis, sciatica.

PRECAUTIONS

CONTRAINDICATIONS: Sensitivity to murine proteins, sepsis, serious active infection. **CAUTIONS:** History of recurrent infections.

LIFESPAN CONSIDERATIONS:

Pregnancy/Lactation: Unknown if distributed in breast milk. **Pregnancy Category B. Children:** Safety and efficacy not established. **Elderly:** Use cautiously due to higher rate of infection.

INTERACTIONS

DRUG: **Anakinra** may increase risk of infection. **Immunosuppressants** may reduce frequency of infusion reactions, antibodies to infliximab. **Live virus vaccines** may decrease immune response. **HERBAL:** None significant. **FOOD:** None known. **LAB VALUES:** None known.

AVAILABILITY (Rx)

INJECTION, POWDER FOR RECONSTITUTION: 100 mg.

ADMINISTRATION/HANDLING

IV

Reconstitution • Reconstitute each vial with 10 ml Sterile Water for Injection, using 21-gauge or smaller needle. Direct stream of Sterile Water to glass wall of vial. • Swirl vial gently to dissolve contents (do not shake). • Allow solution to stand for 5 min and inject into 250 ml bag 0.9% NaCl; gently mix. Concentration should range between 0.4 and 4 mg/ml. • Begin infusion within 3 hrs after reconstitution.

Rate of administration • Administer IV infusion over 2 hrs, using a low protein-binding filter.

Storage • Refrigerate vials. • Solution should appear colorless to light yellow and opalescent; do not use if discolored or particulate forms.

IV INCOMPATIBILITIES

Do not infuse in same IV line with other agents.

INDICATIONS/ROUTES/DOSAGE

RHEUMATOID ARTHRITIS

IV INFUSION: ADULTS, ELDERLY: 3 mg/kg followed by additional doses at 2 and 6 wks after first infusion, then q8wk thereafter.

CROHN'S DISEASE

IV INFUSION: ADULTS, ELDERLY, CHILDREN: 5 mg/kg followed by additional doses at 2 and 6 wks after first infusion, then q8wk thereafter. For adults who respond then lose response, consideration may be given to treatment with 10 mg/kg.

FISTULIZING CROHN'S DISEASE

IV INFUSION: ADULTS, ELDERLY: 5 mg/kg followed by additional doses at 2 and 6 wks after first infusion, then q8wk thereafter. For pts who respond then lose response, consideration may be given to treatment with 10 mg/kg.

ANKYLOSING SPONDYLITIS

IV INFUSION: ADULTS, ELDERLY: 5 mg/kg followed by additional doses at 2 and 6 wks after first infusion, then q6wk thereafter.

PSORIATRIC ARTHRITIS

IV INFUSION: ADULTS, ELDERLY: 5 mg/kg followed by additional doses at 2 and 6 wks after first infusion, then q8wk thereafter. May be used with or without methotrexate.

PLAQUE PSORIASIS

IV INFUSION: ADULTS, ELDERLY: 5 mg/kg followed by additional doses at 2 and 6 wks after first infusion, then q8wk thereafter.

ULCERATIVE COLITIS

IV INFUSION: ADULTS, ELDERLY: 5 mg/kg followed by additional doses at 2 and 6 wks after first infusion, then q8wk thereafter.

SIDE EFFECTS

FREQUENT (22%–10%): Headache, nausea, fatigue, fever. **OCCASIONAL (9%–5%):** Fever/chills during infusion, pharyngitis, vomiting, pain, dizziness, bronchitis, rash, rhinitis, cough, pruritus, sinusitis, myalgia, back pain. **RARE (4%–1%):** Hypotension or hypertension, paresthesia,

I

anxiety, depression, insomnia, diarrhea, UTI.

ADVERSE EFFECTS/ TOXIC REACTIONS

Serious infections, including sepsis, occur rarely. Potential for hypersensitivity reaction, lupus-like syndrome, severe hepatic reaction.

NURSING CONSIDERATIONS

BASELINE ASSESSMENT

Monitor daily pattern of bowel activity/stool consistency. Check baseline hydration status (skin turgor for tenting mucous membranes, urinary status).

INTERVENTION/EVALUATION

Monitor urinalysis, erythrocyte sedimentation rate (ESR), B/P. Monitor for signs of infection. **Crohn's Disease:** Monitor C-reactive protein, frequency of stools. Assess for abdominal pain. **Rheumatoid Arthritis:** Monitor C-reactive protein. Assess for decreased pain, swollen joints, stiffness.

insulin

in-sull-in

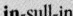

Rapid-acting: INSULIN LISPRO: (Humalog), **INSULIN ASPART:** (Novolog), **INSULIN GLULISINE:** (Apidra), **Short-acting: REGULAR INSULIN:** (Humulin R, Novolin R) **Intermediate-acting: NPH:** (Humulin N, Novolin N) **Long-acting: INSULIN DETEMIR:** (Levemir), **INSULIN GLARGINE:** (Lantus)

FIXED-COMBINATION(S)

Novolog Mix 70/30: aspart suspension 70% and aspart solution 30%. **Humalog Mix 75/25:** lispro suspension 75% and lispro solution 25%. **Humulin Mix 50/50:** NPH 50% and regular 50%. **Humulin 70/30, Novolin 70/30:** NPH 70% and rapid acting regular 30%.

CLASSIFICATION

PHARMACOTHERAPEUTIC: Exogenous insulin. **CLINICAL:** Antidiabetic (see p. 40C).

ACTION

Facilitates passage of glucose, potassium, magnesium across cellular membranes of skeletal/cardiac muscle, adipose tissue. Controls storage, metabolism of carbohydrates, protein, fats. Promotes conversion of glucose to glycogen in liver. **Therapeutic Effect:** Controls glucose levels in diabetic pts.

PHARMACOKINETICS

RAPID-ACTING

	Onset (min)	Peak (hrs)	Duration (hrs)
Aspart (Novolog)	10–20	1–3	3–5
Glulisine (Apidra)	10–15	1–1.5	3–5
Lispro (Humalog)	15–30	0.5–2.5	3–6.5

SHORT-ACTING

	Onset (min)	Peak (hrs)	Duration (hrs)
Regular (Humulin R)	30–60	1–5	6–10
Regular (Novolin R)	30–60	1–5	6–10

INTERMEDIATE-ACTING

	Onset (hrs)	Peak (hrs)	Duration (hrs)
NPH (Humulin N)	1–2	6–14	16–24+
NPH (Novolin N)	1–2	6–14	16–24+

LONG-ACTING

	Onset (hrs)	Peak (hrs)	Duration (hrs)
Detemir (Levemir)	0.8–2	Relatively flat	12 (0.2 units/kg) 24 (0.4 units/kg)
Glargine (Lantus)	1.1	No peak	24

USES

Treatment of insulin-dependent type 1 diabetes mellitus; non–insulin-dependent type 2 diabetes mellitus when diet and weight control therapy has failed to maintain satisfactory serum glucose levels or in event of pregnancy, surgery, trauma, infection, fever, severe renal, hepatic, endocrine dysfunction. Regular insulin used for emergency treatment of ketoacidosis, to promote passage of glucose across cell membrane in hyperalimentation, to facilitate intracellular shift of potassium in hyperkalemia.

PRECAUTIONS

CONTRAINDICATIONS: Hypersensitivity, insulin resistance may require change of type or species source of insulin.

LIFESPAN CONSIDERATIONS:
Pregnancy/Lactation: Insulin is drug of choice for diabetes in pregnancy; close medical supervision is needed. Following delivery, insulin needs may drop for 24–72 hrs, then rise to pre-pregnancy levels. Not secreted in breast milk; lactation may decrease insulin requirements. **Pregnancy Category B. Children:** No age-related precautions noted. **Elderly:** Decreased vision, fine motor tremors may lead to inaccurate self-dosing.

INTERACTIONS

DRUG: Alcohol may increase effects. **Beta-adrenergic blockers** may increase risk of hyperglycemia, hypoglycemia; may mask signs, prolong periods of hypoglycemia. **Glucocorticoids, thiazide diuretics** may increase serum glucose. **HERBAL:** None significant. **FOOD:** None known. **LAB VALUES:** May decrease serum magnesium, phosphate, potassium.

AVAILABILITY

RAPID-ACTING
ASPART (NOVOLOG): 100 units/ml vial, 3 ml cartridge, 3 ml Flex-Pen. **GLULISINE (APIDRA):** 100 units/ml vial, 3 ml cartridge. **LISPRO (HUMALOG):** 100 units/ml vial, 3 ml cartridge, 3 ml pen.
SHORT-ACTING
REGULAR (HUMULIN R): 100 units/ml vial. **REGULAR (NOVOLIN R):** 100 units/ml vial, 3 ml cartridge, 3 ml Innolet.
INTERMEDIATE-ACTING
NPH (HUMULIN N): 100 units/ml vial, 3 ml pen. **NPH (NOVOLIN N):** 100 units/ml vial, 3 ml cartridge, 3 ml Innolet.
LONG-ACTING
DETEMIR (LEVEMIR): 100 units/ml vial, 3 ml Flex-Pen. **GLARGINE (LANTUS):** 100 units/ml vial, 3 ml cartridge. **INTERMEDIATE- AND SHORT-ACTING MIXTURES:** Humulin 50/50, Humulin 70/30, Humalog Mix 75/25, Humalog Mix 50/50, Novolin 70/30, Novolog Mix 70/30.

ADMINISTRATION/HANDLING

IV (REGULAR)
• Use only if solution is clear. • May give undiluted.

RAPID-ACTING
Aspart (Novolog) • May give subcutaneous, IV infusion. • Can mix with NPH (draw aspart into syringe first; inject immediately after mixing). • After first use, stable at room temperature for 28 days. • Administer 5–10 min before meals.
Glulisine (Apidra) • For subcutaneous use only. • May mix with NPH (draw glulisine into syringe first; inject immediately after mixing). • After first use, stable at room temperature for

28 days. • Administer 15 min before or within 20 min after starting a meal.
Lispro (Humalog) • For subcutaneous use only. • May mix with NPH. Stable for 28 days at room temperature; syringe is stable for 14 days if refrigerated. • After first use, stable at room temperature for 28 days. • Administer 15 min before or immediately after meals.

SHORT-ACTING
Regular (Humulin R, Novolin R) • May give subcutaneous, IM, IV. • May mix with NPH for immediate use or for storage for future use. Stable for 1 mo at room temperature, 3 mos if refrigerated. • Can mix with Sterile Water for Injection or 0.9% NaCl. • After first use, stable at room temperature for 28 days. • Administer 30 min before meals.

INTERMEDIATE-ACTING
NPH (Humulin N, Novolin N) • For subcutaneous use only. • May mix with aspart (Novolog) or lispro (Humalog). Draw aspart or lispro first and use immediately. • May mix with regular (Humulin R, Novolin R) insulin. Draw regular insulin first, use immediately or may store for future use (up to 28 days). • After first use, stable at room temperature for 28 days. • Administer 15 min before meals when mixed with aspart or lispro; 30 min before meals when mixed with regular.

LONG-ACTING
Detemir (Levemir) • For subcutaneous use only. • Do not mix with other insulins. • After first use, stable at room temperature for 42 days. • Evening dose given at dinner or at bedtime. Twice daily regimens can be given 12 hrs after morning dose.
Glargine (Lantus) • For subcutaneous use only. • Do not mix with other insulins. • After first use, stable at room temperature for 28 days. • Administer once daily at same time. Meal timing is not applicable.

SUBCUTANEOUS
• Check serum glucose concentration before administration; dosage highly individualized. • Subcutaneous injections may be given in thigh, abdomen, upper arm, buttocks, upper back if there is adequate adipose tissue. • Rotation of injection sites is essential; maintain careful record. • Prefilled syringes should be stored in vertical or oblique position to avoid plugging; plunger should be pulled back slightly and syringe rocked to remix solution before injection.

IV INCOMPATIBILITIES
Diltiazem (Cardizem), dopamine (Intropin), nafcillin (Nafcil).

IV COMPATIBILITIES
Amiodarone (Cordarone), ampicillin/sulbactam (Unasyn), cefazolin (Ancef), cimetidine (Tagamet), digoxin (Lanoxin): (physically compatible for 3 hrs in 0.9% NaCl. In D_5W, water, a slight haze develops within 1 hr), dobutamine (Dobutrex), famotidine (Pepcid), gentamicin, heparin, magnesium sulfate, metoclopramide (Reglan), midazolam (Versed), milrinone (Primacor), morphine, nitroglycerin, potassium chloride, propofol (Diprivan), vancomycin (Vancocin).

INDICATIONS/ROUTES/DOSAGE
USUAL DOSAGE
◄ **ALERT** ► Adjust dosage to achieve premeal and bedtime serum glucose of 80–140 mg/dl (children younger than 5 yrs: 100–200 mg/dl).

SUBCUTANEOUS: ADULTS, ELDERLY, CHILDREN: 0.5–1 unit/kg/day. **ADOLESCENTS (DURING GROWTH SPURT):** 0.8–1.2 unit/kg/day.

DIABETIC KETOACIDOSIS
IV ADULTS, ELDERLY: 0.1 unit/kg/hr. Titration based on serum glucose level.

SIDE EFFECTS
OCCASIONAL: Localized redness, swelling, itching (due to improper insulin

injection technique) allergy to insulin cleansing solution. **INFREQUENT:** Somogyi effect, (rebound hyperglycemia) with chronically excessive insulin dosages. Systemic allergic reaction (rash, angioedema, anaphylaxis), lipodystrophy (depression at injection site due to breakdown of adipose tissue), lipohypertrophy (accumulation of subcutaneous tissue at injection site due to inadequate site rotation). **RARE:** Insulin resistance.

ADVERSE EFFECTS/ TOXIC REACTIONS

Severe hypoglycemia (due to hyperinsulinism) may occur with insulin overdose, decrease/delay of food intake, excessive exercise, those with brittle diabetes. Diabetic ketoacidosis may result from stress, illness, omission of insulin dose, long-term poor insulin control.

NURSING CONSIDERATIONS

BASELINE ASSESSMENT

Check serum glucose level. Discuss lifestyle to determine extent of learning, emotional needs.

INTERVENTION/EVALUATION

Assess for hypoglycemia (refer to pharmacokinetics table for peak times and duration): cool, wet skin, tremors, dizziness, headache, anxiety, tachycardia, numbness in mouth, hunger, diplopia. Check sleeping pt for restlessness, diaphoresis. Check for hyperglycemia: polyuria (excessive urine output), polyphagia (excessive food intake), polydipsia (excessive thirst), nausea/vomiting, dim vision, fatigue, deep and rapid breathing (Kussmaul respirations). Be alert to conditions altering glucose requirements: fever, increased activity/stress, surgical procedure.

PATIENT/FAMILY TEACHING

• Prescribed diet is an essential part of treatment; do not skip/delay meals. • Carry candy, sugar packets, other sugar supplements for immediate response to hypoglycemia. • Wear or carry medical alert identification. • Check with physician when insulin demands are altered (e.g., fever, infection, trauma, stress, heavy physical activity). • Do not take other medication without consulting physician. • Weight control, exercise, hygiene (including foot care), not smoking are integral parts of therapy. • Protect skin, limit sun exposure. • Inform dentist, physician, surgeon of medication before any treatment is given.

I

insulin (oral inhalation)

(Exubera)

CLASSIFICATION

PHARMACOTHERAPEUTIC: Exogenous insulin. **CLINICAL:** Antidiabetic.

ACTION

Facilitates passage of glucose, potassium, magnesium across cellular membranes of skeletal/cardiac muscle, adipose tissue. Controls storage/metabolism of carbohydrates, protein, fats. Promotes conversion of glucose to glycogen in liver. **Therapeutic Effect:** Controls serum glucose levels in diabetic pts.

PHARMACOKINETICS

Onset	Peak	Duration
0.5–1 hr	2–4 hrs	5–7 hrs

Onset of action is similar to rapid-acting analogs, duration similar to regular insulin. Dry powder is deposited in alveoli of lungs, absorbed into alveolar capillary bloodstream, delivered to site of action.

USES

Treatment of type 1 diabetes mellitus (DM) in combination with a longer-acting insulin. Treatment of type 2 DM as monotherapy or in combination with oral agents or longer-acting insulin.

PRECAUTIONS

CONTRAINDICATIONS: Hypersensitivity to human insulin, smokers or those who have smoked within 6 mos, unstable or poorly controlled lung disease. **CAUTIONS:** Pts with asthma, emphysema, COPD, renal/hepatic impairment. **Pregnancy Category C.**

INTERACTIONS

DRUG: Alcohol may increase insulin effect. **Beta-adrenergic blockers** may increase risk of hypoglycemia/hyperglycemia, mask signs of hypoglycemia, prolong period of hypoglycemia. **Glucocorticoids, thiazide diuretics** may increase serum glucose levels. **HERBAL:** None significant. **FOOD:** None known. **LAB VALUES:** May decrease serum potassium, magnesium, phosphate.

AVAILABILITY (Rx)

BLISTER PACKS: 1 mg (equivalent to 3 units regular insulin), 3 mg (equivalent to 8 units regular insulin).

ADMINISTRATION/HANDLING

INHALATION

• Store at room temperature; do not freeze or refrigerate. • Use within 3 mos after opening foil wrapper. • Blister pack placed into slot on inhaler and dispersed by inhaler into aerosol cloud that is captured in a holding chamber for delivery. • Pt inhales aerosol at beginning of a slow deep breath in which air is drawn into chamber, releasing aerosol into pulmonary system. • Administer immediately prior to meals.

INDICATIONS/ROUTES/DOSAGE

DM

INHALATION: ADULTS, ELDERLY: 0.05 mg/kg, with dose rounded down to nearest whole number of milligrams.

SIDE EFFECTS

FREQUENT: Hypoglycemia, cough (mild, nonproductive) within seconds to min of inhalation, dry mouth.

ADVERSE EFFECTS/ TOXIC REACTIONS

Severe hypoglycemia may occur in overdose in insulin, decrease/delay of food intake, excessive exercise, or in pts with brittle diabetes. Diabetic ketoacidosis may result from stress, illness, omission of insulin dose, long-term poor insulin control.

NURSING CONSIDERATIONS

BASELINE ASSESSMENT

Check serum glucose level. Discuss lifestyle to determine extent of learning, emotional needs.

INTERVENTION/EVALUATION

Assess for hypoglycemia: cool/wet skin, tremors, dizziness, headache, anxiety, tachycardia, numbness in mouth, hunger, diplopia. Check sleeping pt for restlessness, diaphoresis. Check for hyperglycemia, polyuria, polyphagia, polydipsia, nausea/vomiting, dim vision, fatigue, deep rapid breathing (Kussmaul respirations). Be alert for conditions altering glucose requirements: fever, increased activity/stress, trauma.

PATIENT/FAMILY TEACHING

• Diet is essential part of treatment, do not skip/delay meals. • Carry candy, sugar packets, other sugar supplements for immediate response to hypoglycemia. • Wear/carry medical alert identification. • Check with physician when insulin demands are altered. • Do not take other medication without consulting physician. • Weight control, exercise, hygiene, not smoking are integral parts of therapy. • Protect skin, limit sun exposure. • Inform dentist, physician, surgeon of medication before any treatment is given.

Integrillin, *see eptifibatide*

interferon alfa-2a

inn-ter-**fear**-on

(Roferon-A)

Do not confuse interferon alfa-2a with interferon alfa-2b.

CLASSIFICATION

PHARMACOTHERAPEUTIC: Biologic response modifier. **CLINICAL:** Antineoplastic (see p. 80C).

ACTION

Inhibits viral replication in virus-infected cells, suppresses cell proliferation, increases phagocytic action of macrophage, augments specific lymphocytic cell toxicity. **Therapeutic Effect:** Prevents rapid growth of malignant cells; inhibits hepatitis virus.

PHARMACOKINETICS

Well absorbed after IM, subcutaneous administration. Undergoes proteolytic degradation during reabsorption in kidneys. **Half-life:** 2 hrs (IM); 3 hrs (subcutaneous).

USES

Treatment of hairy cell leukemia, AIDS-related Kaposi's sarcoma, chronic myelogenous leukemia (CML), chronic hepatitis C. **OFF-LABEL:** Treatment of active, chronic hepatitis; bladder, renal carcinoma; malignant melanoma; multiple myeloma; mycosis fungoides; non-Hodgkin's lymphoma.

PRECAUTIONS

CONTRAINDICATIONS: Autoimmune hepatitis. **CAUTIONS:** Renal/hepatic impairment, seizure disorders, compromised CNS function, cardiac disease, history of cardiac abnormalities, myelosuppression.

LIFESPAN CONSIDERATIONS:

Pregnancy/Lactation: If possible, avoid use during pregnancy. Breastfeeding not recommended. **Pregnancy Category C. Children:** Safety and efficacy not established. **Elderly:** Neurotoxicity, cardiotoxicity may occur more frequently. Age-related renal impairment may require dosage adjustment.

INTERACTIONS

DRUG: Bone marrow depressants may increase myelosuppression. **HERBAL:** None significant. **FOOD:** None known. **LAB VALUES:** May increase serum alkaline phosphatase, LDH, AST, ALT. May decrease Hgb, Hct, leukocyte, platelet counts.

AVAILABILITY (Rx)

INJECTION SOLUTION (PRE-FILLED SYRINGE): 3 million units/0.5 ml, 6 million units/0.5 ml, 9 million units/0.5 ml. **INJECTION (SINGLE DOSE VIAL):** 36 million units/ml.

ADMINISTRATION/HANDLING

IM, SUBCUTANEOUS

• Refrigerate. • Do not shake vial. • Solution appears colorless. • Do not use if discolored or precipitate forms.

INDICATIONS/ROUTES/DOSAGE

HAIRY CELL LEUKEMIA

IM, SUBCUTANEOUS: ADULTS: Initially, 3 million units/day for 16–24 wks. Maintenance: 3 million units 3 times a wk. Do not use 36-million-unit vial.

CHRONIC MYELOGENOUS LEUKEMIA

IM, SUBCUTANEOUS: ADULTS: 9 million units/day. Continue treatment until disease progression is noted.

AIDS-RELATED KAPOSI'S SARCOMA

IM, SUBCUTANEOUS: ADULTS: Initially, 36 million units/day for 10–12 wks, may give 3 million units on day 1, 9 million units on day 2, 18 million units on day 3, then 36 million units/day for remaining of 10–12 wks. Maintenance: 36 million units/day 3 times a wk.

CHRONIC HEPATITIS C

IM, SUBCUTANEOUS: ADULTS, ELDERLY: 3 million units 3 times a wk for 12 mos.

SIDE EFFECTS

FREQUENT (greater than 20%): Flu-like symptoms (fever, fatigue, headache, myalgia, anorexia, chills), nausea, vomiting, cough, dyspnea, hypotension, edema, chest pain, dizziness, diarrhea, weight loss, altered taste, abdominal discomfort, confusion, paresthesia, depression, visual/sleep disturbances, diaphoresis, lethargy. **OCCASIONAL (20%–5%):** Alopecia (partial), rash, dry throat/skin, pruritus, flatulence, constipation, hypertension, palpitations, sinusitis. **RARE (less than 5%):** Hot flashes, hypermotility, Raynaud's syndrome, bronchospasm, earache, ecchymosis.

ADVERSE EFFECTS/ TOXIC REACTIONS

Arrhythmias, CVA, transient ischemic attacks, CHF, pulmonary edema, MI occur rarely.

NURSING CONSIDERATIONS

BASELINE ASSESSMENT

CBC, platelet count, blood chemistries, urinalysis, renal/hepatic function tests should be performed before initial therapy and routinely thereafter.

INTERVENTION/EVALUATION

Offer emotional support. Monitor all levels of clinical function (numerous side effects). Encourage ample fluid intake, particularly during early therapy.

PATIENT/FAMILY TEACHING

• Clinical response may take 1–3 mos. • Flu-like symptoms tend to diminish with continued therapy. • Contact physician if nausea/vomiting continues at home. • Avoid alcohol while taking medication. • Avoid tasks that require alertness, motor skills until response to drug is established.

interferon alfa-2b

inn-ter-**fear**-on

(Intron-A)

Do not confuse interferon alfa-2b with interferon alfa-2a.

FIXED-COMBINATION(S)

Rebetron: interferon alfa-2b/ribavirin (an antiviral): 3 million units/ 200 mg.

CLASSIFICATION

PHARMACOTHERAPEUTIC: Biologic response modifier. **CLINICAL:** Antineoplastic (see p. 80C).

ACTION

Inhibits viral replication in virus-infected cells, suppresses cell proliferation, augments specific cytotoxicity of lymphocytes. **Therapeutic Effect:** Prevents rapid growth of malignant cells; inhibits hepatitis virus.

PHARMACOKINETICS

Well absorbed after IM, subcutaneous administration. Undergoes proteolytic degradation during reabsorption in kidneys. **Half-life:** 2–3 hrs.

USES

Treatment of hairy cell leukemia, condylomata acuminata (genital, venereal warts), AIDS-related Kaposi's sarcoma, chronic hepatitis (non-A, non-B/C), chronic hepatitis B (including children 1 yr and older), follicular lymphoma. **OFF-LABEL:** Treatment of bladder, cervical, renal carcinoma; chronic myelocytic leukemia; laryngeal papillomatosis; multiple myeloma; mycosis fungoides.

PRECAUTIONS

CONTRAINDICATIONS: Autoimmune hepatitis. **CAUTIONS:** Renal/hepatic impairment, seizure disorders, compromised CNS function, cardiac diseases, history of cardiac abnormalities, myelosuppression.

LIFESPAN CONSIDERATIONS:

Pregnancy/Lactation: If possible, avoid use during pregnancy. Breastfeeding not recommended. **Pregnancy Category C.** **Children:** Safety and efficacy not established. **Elderly:** Neurotoxicity, cardiotoxicity may occur more frequently. Age-related renal impairment may require dosage adjustment.

INTERACTIONS

DRUG: **Bone marrow depressants** may increase myelosuppression. **HERBAL:** None significant. **FOOD:** None known. **LAB VALUES:** May increase prothrombin time (PT), activated partial thromboplastin time (aPTT), serum LDH, alkaline phosphatase, AST, ALT. May decrease Hgb, Hct, leukocyte, platelet counts.

AVAILABILITY (Rx)

INJECTION, POWDER FOR RECONSTITUTION: 10 million units, 18 million units, 50 million units. **INJECTION, SOLUTION (MULTIDOSE PRE-FILLED PEN):** 3 million units/0.2 ml (6 doses-18 million units), 5 million units/0.2 ml (6 doses-30 million units), 10 million units/0.2 mg (6 doses-60 million units). **INJECTION, SOLUTION (MULTIDOSE VIAL):** 6 million units/ml, 10 million units/ml. **INJECTION, SOLUITON (SINGLE DOSE VIAL):** 10 million units/ml.

ADMINISTRATION/HANDLING

IV

Reconstitution • Prepare immediately before use. • Reconstitute with diluent provided by manufacturer. • Withdraw desired dose and further dilute with 100 ml 0.9% NaCl to provide final concentration at least 10 million international units/100 ml.

Rate of administration • Administer over 20 min.

Storage • Refrigerate unopened vials (stable for 7 days at room temperature).

IM, SUBCUTANEOUS

• Do not give IM if platelets are less than 50,000/m^3; give subcutaneous. • For hairy cell leukemia, reconstitute each 3 million international units vial with 1 ml Bacteriostatic Water for Injection to provide concentration of 3 million international units/ml (1 ml to 5 million-international units vial; 2 ml to 10 million-international units vial; 5 ml to 25 million-international units vial provides concentration of 5 million international units/ml). • For condylomata acuminata, reconstitute each 10 million international units vial with 1 ml Bacteriostatic Water for Injection to provide concentration of 10 million international units/ml. • For AIDS-related Kaposi's sarcoma, reconstitute 50 million international units vial with 1 ml Bacteriostatic Water for Injection to provide concentration of 50 million international units/ml. • Agitate vial gently, withdraw with sterile syringe.

IV INCOMPATIBILITIES

Do not mix with other medications via Y-site administration.

INDICATIONS/ROUTES/DOSAGE

HAIRY CELL LEUKEMIA

IM, SUBCUTANEOUS: ADULTS: 2 million units/m^2 3 times a wk. If severe adverse reactions occur, modify dose or temporarily discontinue drug.

CONDYLOMATA ACCUMINATA

INTRALESIONAL: ADULTS: 1 million units/lesion 3 times a wk for 3 wks. Use only 10-million-unit vial, and reconstitute with no more than 1 ml diluent.

AIDS-RELATED KAPOSI'S SARCOMA

IM, SUBCUTANEOUS: ADULTS: 30 million units/m^2 3 times a wk. Use only 50-million-unit vials. If severe adverse reactions occur, modify dose or temporarily discontinue drug.

CHRONIC HEPATITIS C

IM, SUBCUTANEOUS: ADULTS: 3 million units 3 times a wk for up to 6 mos. For pts who tolerate therapy and whose ALT level normalizes within 16 wks, therapy may be extended for up to 18–24 mos.

CHRONIC HEPATITIS B

IM, SUBCUTANEOUS: ADULTS: 30–35 million units weekly, either as 5 million units/day or 10 million units 3 times a wk.

MALIGNANT MELANOMA

IV: ADULTS: Initially, 20 million units/m^2 5 times a wk for 4 wks. Maintenance: 10 million units IM or subcutaneously 3 times a wk for 48 wks.

FOLLICULAR LYMPHOMA

SUBCUTANEOUS: ADULTS: 5 million units 3 times a wk for up to 18 mos.

SIDE EFFECTS

FREQUENT: Flu-like symptoms, (fever, fatigue, headache, myalgia, anorexia, chills), rash (hairy cell leukemia, Kaposi's sarcoma only). **Pts with Kaposi's sarcoma**: All previously mentioned side effects plus depression, dyspepsia, dry mouth or thirst, alopecia, rigors. **OCCASIONAL:** Dizziness, pruritus, dry skin, dermatitis, altered taste. **RARE:** Confusion, leg cramps, back pain, gingivitis, flushing, tremor, anxiety, eye pain.

ADVERSE EFFECTS/ TOXIC REACTIONS

Hypersensitivity reactions occur rarely. Severe flu-like symptoms appear dose-related.

NURSING CONSIDERATIONS

BASELINE ASSESSMENT

CBC, platelet count, blood chemistries, urinalysis, renal/hepatic function tests should be performed before initial therapy and routinely thereafter.

INTERVENTION/EVALUATION

Offer emotional support. Monitor all levels of clinical function (numerous side effects). Encourage ample fluid intake, particularly during early therapy.

PATIENT/FAMILY TEACHING

• Clinical response occurs in 1–3 mos. • Flu-like symptoms tend to diminish with continued therapy. • Some symptoms may be alleviated or minimized by bedtime doses. • Do not have immunizations without physician's approval (drug lowers resistance). • Avoid contact with those who have recently received live virus vaccine. • Avoid tasks that require alertness, motor skills until response to drug is established. • Sips of tepid water may relieve dry mouth.

interferon beta-1a

inn-ter-**fear**-on

(Avonex, Avonex Prefilled Syringe, Rebif)

Do not confuse interferon beta-1a with interferon beta-1b or Avonex with Avelox.

◆ **CLASSIFICATION**

PHARMACOTHERAPEUTIC: Biologic response modifier. **CLINICAL:** Multiple sclerosis agent.

ACTION

Interacts with specific cell receptors found on surface of cells. **Therapeutic Effect:** Produces antiviral, immunoregulatory effects.

PHARMACOKINETICS

Peak serum levels attained 3–15 hrs after IM administration. Biological markers increase within 12 hrs and remain elevated for 4 days. **Half-life:** 10 hrs (Avonex); 69 hrs (Rebif).

USES

Treatment of relapsing multiple sclerosis to slow progression of physical disability, decrease frequency of clinical exacerbations. **OFF-LABEL:** Treatment of AIDS, AIDS-related Kaposi's sarcoma, condylomata accuminata, malignant melanoma, renal cell carcinoma.

PRECAUTIONS

CONTRAINDICATIONS: **Avonex:** Hypersensitivity to natural or recombinant interferon beta, human albumin. **Rebif:** Hypersensitivity to natural or recombinant interferon, human albumin. **CAUTIONS:** Chronic progressive multiple sclerosis, children younger than 18 yrs, depression.

LIFESPAN CONSIDERATIONS:

Pregnancy/Lactation: Has abortifacient potential. Unknown if drug is distributed in breast milk. **Pregnancy Category C. Children:** Safety and efficacy not established. **Elderly:** No information available.

INTERACTIONS

DRUG: None significant. **HERBAL:** None significant. **FOOD:** None known. **LAB VALUES:** May increase serum glucose, BUN, alkaline phosphatase, bilirubin, calcium, AST, ALT. May decrease Hgb, neutrophil, platelet, WBC counts.

AVAILABILITY (Rx)

INJECTION, POWDER FOR RECONSTITUTION (AVONEX): 30 mcg. **INJECTION SOLUTION (PREFILLED SYRINGE):** 22 mcg/ml (Rebif), 30 mcg/0.5 ml (Avonex Prefilled Syringe), 44 mcg/ml (Rebif). **TITRATION PACK (PREFILLED SYRINGE [REBIF]):** 8.8 mcg, 22 mcg.

ADMINISTRATION/HANDLING

IM (AVONEX) SYRINGE

• Refrigerate syringe. • Allow to warm to room temperature before use. • May store up to 7 days at room temperature.

IM (AVONEX) VIAL

• Refrigerate vials. • Following reconstitution, may refrigerate again but use within 6 hrs if refrigerated. • Reconstitute 30 mcg *MicroPin* (6.6 million international units) vial with 1.1 ml diluent (supplied by manufacturer). • Gently swirl to dissolve medication; do not shake. • Discard if discolored or particulate forms. • Discard unused portion (contains no preservative).

SUBCUTANEOUS (REBIF)

• Refrigerate. May store at room temperature up to 30 days. Avoid heat, light. Administer at same time of day 3 days each wk. Separate doses by at least 48 hrs.

INDICATIONS/ROUTES/DOSAGE

RELAPSING MULTIPLE SCLEROSIS

IM (AVONEX): ADULTS: 30 mcg once weekly.

SUBCUTANEOUS (REBIF): ADULTS: **(Target dose 44 mcg 3 times/wk)** Initially, 8.8 mcg 3 times/wk for 8 wks, then 22 mcg 3 times/wk for 8 wks, then 44 mcg 3 times/wk thereafter. **(Target dose 22 mcg 3 times/wk)** Initially, 4.4 mcg 3 times/wk for 8 wks, then 11 mcg

3 times/wk for 8 wks, then 22 mcg 3 times/wk thereafter.

DOSAGE IN HEPATIC IMPAIRMENT (REBIF)

Increased hepatic function test results, leukopenia: Decrease dose 20–50% until toxicity resolves.

SIDE EFFECTS

FREQUENT: Headache (67%), flu-like symptoms (61%), myalgia (34%), upper respiratory tract infection (31%), depression with suicidal thoughts (25%), generalized pain (24%), asthenia, chills (21%), sinusitis (18%), infection (11%). **OCCASIONAL:** Abdominal pain, arthralgia (9%), chest pain, dyspnea (6%), malaise, syncope (4%). **RARE:** Injection site reaction, hypersensitivity reaction (3%).

ADVERSE EFFECTS/ TOXIC REACTIONS

Anemia occurs in 8% of pts. Hepatic failure has been reported.

NURSING CONSIDERATIONS

BASELINE ASSESSMENT

Obtain Hgb, CBC, platelet count, blood chemistries including hepatic function tests. Assess home situation for support of therapy.

INTERVENTION/EVALUATION

Assess for headache, flu-like symptoms, myalgia. Periodically monitor lab results, reevaluate injection technique. Assess for depression, suicidal ideation.

PATIENT/FAMILY TEACHING

• Do not change schedule, dosage without consultation with physician. • Instruct on correct reconstitution of product and administration, including aseptic technique. • Provide puncture-resistant container for used needles, syringes; explain proper disposal. • Explain that injection site reactions may occur. These do not require discontinuation of therapy, but type and extent should be carefully noted.

interferon beta-1b

inn-ter-**fear**-on

(Betaseron)

Do not confuse interferon beta-1b with interferon beta-1a.

CLASSIFICATION

PHARMACOTHERAPEUTIC: Biologic response modifier. **CLINICAL:** Multiple sclerosis, cancer, AIDS agent.

ACTION

Interacts with specific cell receptors found on surface of cells. **Therapeutic Effect:** Produces antiviral, immunoregulatory effects.

PHARMACOKINETICS

Slowly absorbed following subcutaneous administration. **Half-life:** 8 min–4.3 hrs.

USES

Reduces frequency of clinical exacerbations in pts with relapsing-remitting multiple sclerosis (recurrent attacks of neurologic dysfunction). Treatment of early stages of multiple sclerosis. **OFF-LABEL:** Treatment of acute non-A and non-B hepatitis, AIDS, AIDS-related Kaposi's sarcoma, malignant melanoma, renal cell carcinoma.

PRECAUTIONS

CONTRAINDICATIONS: Hypersensitivity to albumin, interferon. **CAUTIONS:** Chronic progressive multiple sclerosis, children younger than 18 yrs.

LIFESPAN CONSIDERATIONS:

Pregnancy/Lactation: Unknown if distributed in breast milk. **Pregnancy Category C.** **Children:** Safety and efficacy not established. **Elderly:** No information available.

INTERACTIONS

DRUG: None significant. **HERBAL:** None significant. **FOOD:** None known. **LAB VALUES:** May increase serum glucose, BUN, alkaline phosphatase, bilirubin, calcium, AST, ALT. May decrease Hgb level, neutrophil, platelet, WBC counts.

AVAILABILITY (Rx)

INJECTION POWDER FOR RECONSTITUTION: 0.3 mg (9.6 million units).

ADMINISTRATION/HANDLING

SUBCUTANEOUS

• Store vials at room temperature. • After reconstitution, stable for 3 hrs if refrigerated. • Use within 3 hrs of reconstitution. • Discard if discolored or precipitate forms. • Reconstitute 0.3-mg (9.6 million international units) vial with 1.2 ml diluent (supplied by manufacturer) to provide concentration of 0.25 mg/ml (8 million units/ml). • Gently swirl to dissolve medication; do not shake. • Discard if discolored or particulate forms. • Withdraw 1 ml solution and inject subcutaneous into arms, abdomen, hips, thighs using 27-gauge needle. • Discard unused portion (contains no preservative).

INDICATIONS/ROUTES/DOSAGE

RELAPSING-REMITTING MULTIPLE SCLEROSIS

SUBCUTANEOUS: ADULTS: 0.25 mg (8 million units) every other day.

SIDE EFFECTS

FREQUENT: Injection site reaction (85%), headache (84%), flu-like symptoms (76%), fever (59%), asthenia (49%), myalgia (44%), sinusitis (36%), diarrhea, dizziness (35%), altered mental status (29%), constipation (24%), diaphoresis (23%), vomiting (21%). **OCCASIONAL:** Malaise (15%), drowsiness (6%), alopecia (4%).

ADVERSE EFFECTS/ TOXIC REACTIONS

Seizures occur rarely.

NURSING CONSIDERATIONS

BASELINE ASSESSMENT

Obtain Hgb, CBC, platelet count, blood chemistries (including hepatic function tests). Assess home situation for support of therapy.

INTERVENTION/EVALUATION

Periodically monitor lab results, reevaluate injection technique. Assess for nausea (high incidence). Monitor sleep pattern. Monitor daily pattern of bowel activity/stool consistency. Assist with ambulation if dizziness occurs. Monitor food intake.

PATIENT/FAMILY TEACHING

• Inform physician of flu-like symptoms (occur commonly but decrease over time). • Wear sunscreens, protective clothing if exposed to sunlight, ultraviolet light until tolerance known.

interferon gamma-1b

inn-ter-**fear**-on

(Actimmune)

CLASSIFICATION

PHARMACOTHERAPEUTIC: Biologic response modifier. **CLINICAL:** Immunologic agent.

ACTION

Induces activation of macrophages in blood monocytes to phagocytes, (necessary in cellular immune response to intracellular, extracellular pathogens). Enhances phagocytic function, antimicrobial activity of monocytes. **Therapeutic Effect:** Decreases signs/

symptoms of serious infections in chronic granulomatous disease.

PHARMACOKINETICS

Slowly absorbed after subcutaneous administration. **Half-life:** 0.5–1 hr.

USES

Reduces frequency, severity of serious infections due to chronic granulomatous disease. Delays time to disease progression in pts with severe, malignant osteopetrosis.

PRECAUTIONS

CONTRAINDICATIONS: Hypersensitivity to *Escherichia coli*-derived products. **CAUTIONS:** Seizure disorders, compromised CNS function, preexisting cardiac disease (e.g., ischemia, CHF, arrhythmias), myelosuppression.

⧖ LIFESPAN CONSIDERATIONS:

Pregnancy/Lactation: Unknown if drug crosses placenta or is distributed in breast milk. **Pregnancy Category C.** **Children:** Safety and efficacy not established in those younger than 1 yr. Flu-like symptoms may occur more frequently. **Elderly:** No information available.

INTERACTIONS

DRUG: Bone marrow depressants may increase myelosuppression. **HERBAL:** None significant. **FOOD:** None known. **LAB VALUES:** None known.

AVAILABILITY (Rx)

INJECTION SOLUTION: 100 mcg (2 million units).

ADMINISTRATION/HANDLING

◀ **ALERT** ▶ Avoid excessive agitation of vial; do not shake.

SUBCUTANEOUS

• Refrigerate vials. Do not freeze. • Do not keep at room temperature for more than 12 hrs; discard after 12 hrs. • Vials are single dose; discard unused portion. • Solution is clear, colorless. Do not use if discolored or precipitate forms. • When given 3 times/wk, rotate injection sites.

INDICATIONS/ROUTES/DOSAGE

CHRONIC GRANULOMATOUS DISEASE; SEVERE, MALIGNANT OSTEOPETROSIS

SUBCUTANEOUS: ADULTS, ELDERLY, CHILDREN OLDER THAN 1 YR: 50 mcg/m^2 (1.5 million units/m^2) in pts with body surface area (BSA) greater than 0.5 m^2; 1.5 mcg/kg/dose in pts with BSA 0.5 m^2 or less. Give 3 times/wk.

SIDE EFFECTS

FREQUENT: Fever (52%), headache (33%), rash (17%), chills, fatigue, diarrhea (14%). **OCCASIONAL (13%–10%):** Vomiting, nausea. **RARE (6%–3%):** Weight loss, myalgia, anorexia.

ADVERSE EFFECTS/ TOXIC REACTIONS

May exacerbate preexisting CNS dysfunction (manifested as decreased mental status, gait disturbance, dizziness), cardiac abnormalities.

NURSING CONSIDERATIONS

BASELINE ASSESSMENT

CBC, platelet count, blood chemistries, urinalysis, renal/hepatic function tests should be performed before initial therapy and at 3-mo intervals during course of treatment.

INTERVENTION/EVALUATION

Monitor for flu-like symptoms (fever, chills, fatigue, myalgia). Assess skin for evidence of rash.

PATIENT/FAMILY TEACHING

• Flu-like symptoms (fever, chills, fatigue, muscle aches) are generally mild and tend to disappear as treatment continues. Symptoms may be minimized with bedtime administration. • Avoid tasks that require alertness, motor skills until response to drug is established. • If home use prescribed, instruct in proper technique of administration; care in proper disposal of needles, syringes. • Vials should remain refrigerated.

interleukin-2 (aldesleukin)

in-tur-**lew**-kin
(IL-2, Proleukin)

Do not confuse interleukin-2 with interferon 2.

CLASSIFICATION

PHARMACOTHERAPEUTIC: Biologic response modifier. **CLINICAL:** Antineoplastic (see p. 75C).

ACTION

Promotes proliferation, differentiation, recruitment of T and B cells, lymphokine-activated and natural killer cells, thymocytes. **Therapeutic Effect:** Enhances cytolytic activity in lymphocytes.

PHARMACOKINETICS

Primarily distributed into plasma, lymphocytes, lungs, liver, kidney, spleen. Metabolized to amino acids in cells lining the kidneys. **Half-life:** 85 min.

USES

Treatment of metastatic renal cell carcinoma, metastatic melanoma. **OFF-LABEL:** Treatment of colorectal cancer, Kaposi's sarcoma, non-Hodgkin's lymphoma.

PRECAUTIONS

CONTRAINDICATIONS: Abnormal pulmonary function or thallium stress test results, bowel ischemia or perforation, coma or toxic psychosis lasting longer than 48 hrs, GI bleeding requiring surgery, intubation lasting more than 72 hrs, organ allografts, pericardial tamponade, renal dysfunction requiring dialysis for longer than 72 hrs, repetitive or difficult-to-control seizures; retreatment in those who experience any of the following toxicities: angina, MI, recurrent chest pain with EKG changes, sustained ventricular tachycardia, uncontrolled or unresponsive cardiac rhythm disturbances. **EXTREME CAUTION:** Pts with normal thallium stress tests and pulmonary function tests who have history of cardiac or pulmonary disease. **CAUTIONS:** Pts with fixed requirements for large volumes of fluid (e.g., those with hypercalcemia), history of seizures.

LIFESPAN CONSIDERATIONS:

Pregnancy/Lactation: Avoid use in those of either sex not practicing effective contraception. **Pregnancy Category C.** **Children:** Safety and efficacy not established. **Elderly:** Age-related renal impairment may require dosage adjustment; will not tolerate toxicity.

INTERACTIONS

DRUG: **Antihypertensives** may increase hypotensive effect. **Cardiotoxic, hepatotoxic, myelotoxic, nephrotoxic medications** may increase risk of toxicity. **Glucocorticoids** may decrease effects. **HERBAL:** None significant. **FOOD:** None known. **LAB VALUES:** May increase BUN, serum alkaline phosphatase, bilirubin, creatinine, AST, ALT. May decrease serum calcium, magnesium, phosphorus, potassium, sodium.

AVAILABILITY (Rx)

INJECTION, POWDER FOR RECONSTITUTION (PROLEUKIN): 22 million units (1.3 mg) (18 million units/ml when reconstituted).

ADMINISTRATION/HANDLING

◄ **ALERT** ► Hold administration in pts who develop moderate to severe lethargy or somnolence (continued administration may result in coma).

IV

Reconstitution • Reconstitute 22 million units vial with 1.2 ml Sterile Water for Injection to provide concentration of 18 million units/ml. Bacteriostatic Water for Injection or NaCl should not be used to reconstitute because of increased aggregation. • During reconstitution, direct Sterile Water for Injection at the side of vial. Swirl contents gently to avoid foaming. Do not shake.

Rate of administration • Further dilute dose in 50 ml D_5W and infuse over 15 min. Do not use an in-line filter. • Solution should be warmed to room temperature before infusion. • Monitor diligently for drop in mean arterial B/P (sign of capillary leak syndrome [CLS]). Continued treatment may result in significant hypotension (less than 90 mm Hg or a 20 mm Hg drop from baseline systolic pressure), edema, pleural effusion, altered mental status.

Storage • Refrigerate vials; do not freeze. • Reconstituted solution is stable for 48 hrs refrigerated or at room temperature (refrigeration preferred).

IV INCOMPATIBILITIES

Ganciclovir (Cytovene), pentamidine (Pentam), prochlorperazine (Compazine), promethazine (Phenergan).

IV COMPATIBILITIES

Calcium gluconate, dopamine (Intropin), heparin, lorazepam (Ativan), magnesium, potassium.

INDICATIONS/ROUTES/DOSAGE

METASTATIC MELANOMA, METASTATIC RENAL CELL CARCINOMA

IV: ADULTS 18 YRS AND OLDER: 600,000 units/kg q8h for 14 doses; followed by 9 days of rest, then another 14 doses for a total of 28 doses per course. Course may be repeated after rest period of at least 7 wks from date of hospital discharge.

MELANOMA (IN COMBINATION WITH CYTOTOXIC AGENTS)

IV: ADULTS: 24 million international units/m^2 days 12–16 and 19–23.

SIDE EFFECTS

Side effects are generally self-limiting and reversible within 2–3 days after discontinuing therapy. **FREQUENT (89%–48%):** Fever, chills, nausea, vomiting, hypotension, diarrhea, oliguria/anuria, altered mental status, irritability, confusion, depression, sinus tachycardia, pain (abdominal, chest, back), fatigue, dyspnea, pruritus. **OCCASIONAL (47%–17%):** Edema, erythema, rash, stomatitis, anorexia, weight gain, infection (UTI, injection site, catheter tip), dizziness. **RARE (15%–4%):** Dry skin, sensory disorders (vision, speech, taste), dermatitis, headache, arthralgia, myalgia, weight loss, hematuria, conjunctivitis, proteinuria.

ADVERSE EFFECTS/ TOXIC REACTIONS

Anemia, thrombocytopenia, leukopenia occur commonly. GI bleeding pulmonary edema occur occasionally. Capillary leak syndrome results in hypotension (systolic pressure less than 90 mm Hg or a 20 mm Hg drop from baseline systolic pressure), extravasation of plasma proteins and fluid into extravascular space, loss of vascular tone. May result in cardiac arrhythmias, angina, MI, respiratory insufficiency. Fatal malignant hyperthermia, cardiac arrest, cerebrovascular accident (CVA), pulmonary emboli, bowel perforation/gangrene, severe depression leading to suicide occur in less than 1% of pts.

NURSING CONSIDERATIONS

BASELINE ASSESSMENT

Pts with bacterial infection and with indwelling central lines should be treated with antibiotic therapy before treatment begins. All pts should be neurologically stable with a negative CT scan before treatment begins. CBC, blood chemistries (including electrolytes), renal/hepatic function tests, chest x-ray should be performed before therapy begins and daily thereafter.

INTERVENTION/EVALUATION

Monitor CBC with differential, platelets, electrolytes, renal/hepatic functions, weight, pulse oximetry. Determine serum amylase frequently during therapy. Discontinue medication at first sign of hypotension and hold for moderate to severe lethargy (physician must decide whether therapy should continue). Assess altered mental status (irritability, confusion, depression), weight gain/loss. Maintain strict I&O. Assess for extravascular fluid accumulation (rales in lungs, edema in dependent areas).

PATIENT/FAMILY TEACHING

• Nausea may decrease during therapy. • At home, increase fluid intake (protects against renal impairment). • Do not have immunizations without physician's approval (drug lowers resistance). • Avoid exposure to persons with infection. • Contact physician if fever, chills, lower back pain, difficulty with urination, unusual bleeding/bruising, black tarry stools, blood in urine, petechial rash (pinpoint red spots on skin) occur. • Report symptoms of depression or suicidal ideation immediately.

ipratropium

ih-prah-**trow**-pea-um

(Apo-Ipravent ♣, Atrovent, Atrovent HFA, Novo-Ipramide ♣, Nu-Ipratropium ♣, PMS-Ipratropium ♣)

Do not confuse Atrovent with Alupent.

FIXED-COMBINATION(S)

Combivent, Duoneb: ipratropium/albuterol (a bronchodilator): *Aerosol:* 18 mcg/103 mcg per actuation. *Solution:* 0.5 ml/2.5 ml per 3 ml.

CLASSIFICATION

PHARMACOTHERAPEUTIC: Anticholinergic. **CLINICAL:** Bronchodilator.

ACTION

Blocks action of acetylcholine at parasympathetic sites in bronchial smooth muscle. **Therapeutic Effect:** Causes bronchodilation, inhibits nasal secretions.

PHARMACOKINETICS

Route	Onset	Peak	Duration
Inhalation	1–3 min	1 hr	4–6 hrs

Minimal systemic absorption after inhalation. Metabolized in liver (systemic absorption). Primarily eliminated in feces. **Half-life:** 1.5–4 hrs.

USES

Inhalation: Maintenance treatment of bronchospasm due to chronic obstructive pulmonary disease (COPD), bronchitis, emphysema, asthma. Not to be used for immediate bronchospasm relief. **Nasal Spray:** Rhinorrhea (0.03% associated with perennial rhinitis, 0.06% associated with common cold), seasonal allergy.

PRECAUTIONS

CONTRAINDICATIONS: History of hypersensitivity to atropine. **CAUTIONS:** Narrow-angle glaucoma, prostatic hypertrophy, bladder neck obstruction.

LIFESPAN CONSIDERATIONS:

Pregnancy/Lactation: Unknown if distributed in breast milk. **Pregnancy Category B. Children/Elderly:** No age-related precautions noted.

INTERACTIONS

DRUG: **Anticholinergics, medications with anticholinergic properties** may increase toxicity. **HERBAL:** None significant. **FOOD:** None known. **LAB VALUES:** None known.

AVAILABILITY (Rx)

SOLUTION, INTRANASAL SPRAY: 0.03%; 0.06%. **SOLUTION FOR NEBULIZATION:** 0.02%. **SOLUTION FOR ORAL INHALATION:** (ATROVENT) 18 mcg/actuation; (ATROVENT HFA) 17 mcg/actuation.

ADMINISTRATION/HANDLING

INHALATION

• Shake container well. • Exhale completely through mouth; place mouthpiece into mouth, close lips, holding inhaler upright. • Inhale deeply through mouth while fully depressing top of canister. Hold breath as long as possible before exhaling slowly. • Wait 2 min before inhaling second dose (allows for deeper bronchial penetration). • Rinse mouth with water immediately after inhalation (prevents mouth/throat dryness).

NASAL

• Store at room temperature. • Initial pump priming requires 7 actuations of pump. • If used regularly as recommended, no further priming is required. If not used for more than 24 hrs, pump will require 2 actuations, or if not used for more than 7 days, the pump will require 7 actuations to reprime.

INDICATIONS/ROUTES/DOSAGE

BRONCHOSPASM

INHALATION: ADULTS, ELDERLY, CHILDREN OLDER THAN 12 YRS: 2 inhalations 4 times a day. **Maximum:** 12 inhalations/day. **CHILDREN 3–12 YRS:** 1–2 inhalations 3 times a day. **Maximum:** 6 inhalations/day.

NEBULIZATION: ADULTS, ELDERLY, CHILDREN OLDER THAN 12 YRS: 500 mcg 3–4 times a day. **CHILDREN 3–12 YRS:** 125–250 mcg 3 times a day.

RHINORRHEA (PERENNIAL ALLERGIC/NON-ALLERGIC RHINITIS)

INTRANASAL (0.03%): ADULTS, ELDERLY, CHILDREN 6 YRS AND OLDER: 2 sprays per nostril 2–3 times a day.

RHINORRHEA (COMMON COLD)

INTRANASAL (0.06%): ADULTS, ELDERLY CHILDREN 12 YRS AND OLDER: 2 sprays per nostril 3–4 times a day for up to 4 days. **CHILDREN 5–11 YRS:** 2 sprays per nostril 3 times a day for up to 4 days.

RHINORRHEA (SEASONAL ALLERGY)

INTRANASAL (0.06%): ADULTS, ELDERLY, CHILDREN 5 YRS AND OLDER: 2 sprays per nostril 4 times a day for up to 3 wks.

SIDE EFFECTS

FREQUENT: **Inhalation (6%–3%):** Cough, dry mouth, headache, nausea. **Nasal:** Dry nose/mouth, headache, nasal irritation. **OCCASIONAL:** **Inhalation (2%):** Dizziness, transient increased bronchospasm. **RARE (less than 1%):** **Inhalation:** Hypotension, insomnia, metallic/unpleasant taste, palpitations, urinary retention. **Nasal:** Diarrhea, constipation, dry throat, abdominal pain, nasal congestion.

ADVERSE EFFECTS/ TOXIC REACTIONS

Worsening of angle-closure glaucoma, acute eye pain, hypotension occur rarely.

NURSING CONSIDERATIONS

BASELINE ASSESSMENT

Offer emotional support (high incidence of anxiety due to difficulty in breathing, sympathomimetic response to drug).

INTERVENTION/EVALUATION

Monitor rate, depth, rhythm, type of respiration; quality, rate of pulse. Assess lung sounds for rhonchi, wheezing, rales. Monitor ABGs. Observe lips, fingernails for cyanosis (blue or dusky color in light-skinned pts; gray in dark-skinned pts). Observe for retractions (clavicular, sternal, intercostal), hand tremor. Evaluate for clinical improvement (quieter, slower respirations, relaxed facial expression, cessation of retractions).

PATIENT/FAMILY TEACHING

• Increase fluid intake (decreases lung secretion viscosity). • Do not take more than 2 inhalations at any one time (excessive use may produce paradoxical bronchoconstriction, decreased bronchodilating effect). • Rinsing mouth with water immediately after inhalation may prevent mouth and throat dryness. • Avoid excessive use of caffeine derivatives (chocolate, coffee, tea, cola, cocoa).

irbesartan

ir-beh-**sar**-tan
(Avapro)

FIXED-COMBINATION(S)

Avalide: irbesartan/hydrochlorothiazide (a diuretic): 150 mg/12.5 mg; 300 mg/12.5 mg, 300 mg/25 mg.

◆ CLASSIFICATION

PHARMACOTHERAPEUTIC: Angiotensin II receptor antagonist. **CLINICAL:** Antihypertensive (see p. 8C).

ACTION

Blocks vasoconstrictor, aldosterone-secreting effects of angiotensin II, inhibiting binding of angiotensin II to AT_1 receptors. **Therapeutic Effect:** Produces vasodilation, decreases peripheral resistance, decreases B/P.

PHARMACOKINETICS

Rapidly, completely absorbed after PO administration. Protein binding: 90%. Undergoes hepatic metabolism to inactive metabolite. Recovered primarily in feces and, to a lesser extent, in urine. Not removed by hemodialysis. **Half-life:** 11–15 hrs.

USES

Treatment of hypertension alone or in combination with other antihypertensives. Treatment of diabetic nephropathy. **OFF-LABEL:** Treatment of atrial fibrillation, CHF.

PRECAUTIONS

CONTRAINDICATIONS: Bilateral renal artery stenosis, biliary cirrhosis/obstruction, primary hyperaldosteronism, severe hepatic insufficiency. **CAUTIONS:** Mild to moderate hepatic dysfunction, sodium/water depletion, CHF, unilateral renal artery stenosis, coronary artery disease.

⌛ LIFESPAN CONSIDERATIONS:

Pregnancy/Lactation: Unknown if drug is distributed in breast milk. May cause fetal or neonatal morbidity or mortality. **Pregnancy Category C (D if used in second or third trimester).** **Children:** Safety and efficacy not established. **Elderly:** No age-related precautions noted.

INTERACTIONS

DRUG: **Diuretics** produce additive hypotensive effects. **HERBAL:** **Ephedra, ginseng, yohimbe** may worsen hypertension. **Garlic** may increase antihypertensive effect. **FOOD:** None known. **LAB VALUES:** May slightly increase BUN, serum creatinine. May decrease Hgb.

AVAILABILITY (Rx)

TABLETS: 75 mg, 150 mg, 300 mg.

ADMINISTRATION/HANDLING

PO

- Give without regard to meals.

INDICATIONS/ROUTES/DOSAGE

HYPERTENSION

PO: ADULTS, ELDERLY, CHILDREN 13 YRS AND OLDER: Initially, 75–150 mg/day. May increase to 300 mg/day. **CHILDREN 6–12 YRS:** Initially, 75 mg/day. May increase to 150 mg/day.

NEPHROPATHY

PO: ADULTS, ELDERLY: Target dose of 300 mg/day.

SIDE EFFECTS

OCCASIONAL (9%–3%): Upper respiratory tract infection, fatigue, diarrhea, cough. **RARE (2%–1%):** Heartburn, dizziness, headache, nausea, rash.

ADVERSE EFFECTS/ TOXIC REACTIONS

Overdose may manifest as hypotension, tachycardia. Bradycardia occurs less often.

NURSING CONSIDERATIONS

BASELINE ASSESSMENT

Obtain B/P, apical pulse immediately before each dose, in addition to regular monitoring (be alert to fluctuations). If excessive reduction in B/P occurs, place pt in supine position, feet slightly elevated. Question possibility of pregnancy (see Pregnancy Category). Assess medication history (esp. diuretic therapy).

INTERVENTION/EVALUATION

Maintain hydration (offer fluids frequently). Assess for evidence of upper respiratory infection. Assist with ambulation if dizziness occurs. Monitor electrolytes, renal/hepatic function tests, urinalysis, B/P, pulse. Assess for hypotension.

PATIENT/FAMILY TEACHING

- Inform female pt regarding consequences of second- and third-trimester exposure to irbesartan.
- Avoid tasks that require alertness, motor skills until response to drug is established (possible dizziness effect).
- Report any sign of infection (sore throat, fever).
- Caution against exercising during hot weather (risk of dehydration, hypotension).

irinotecan

eye-rin-**oh**-teh-can
(Camptosar)

◆CLASSIFICATION

PHARMACOTHERAPEUTIC: DNA topoisomerase inhibitor. **CLINICAL:** Antineoplastic (see p. 80C).

ACTION

Interacts with topoisomerase I, an enzyme that relieves torsional strain in DNA by inducing reversible single-strand breaks. Prevents religation of these single-stranded breaks resulting in damage to double-strand DNA, cell death. **Therapeutic Effect:** Produces cytotoxic effect on cancer cells.

PHARMACOKINETICS

Metabolized to active metabolite in liver after IV administration. Protein binding: 95% (metabolite). Excreted in urine and eliminated by biliary route. **Half-life:** 6 hrs; metabolite, 10 hrs.

USES

Treatment of metastatic carcinoma of colon, rectum in pts whose disease has recurred or progressed after 5-fluorouracil-based therapy. **OFF-LABEL:** Non–small cell lung cancer, refractory solid tumor configuration, untreated rhabdomyosarcoma.

PRECAUTIONS

CONTRAINDICATIONS: None known. **CAUTIONS:** Pt previously receiving pelvic, abdominal irradiation (increased risk of myelosuppression), elderly older than 65 yrs.

LIFESPAN CONSIDERATIONS:

Pregnancy/Lactation: May cause fetal harm. Unknown if distributed in breast milk; discontinue breast-feeding. **Pregnancy Category D. Children:** Safety and efficacy not established. **Elderly:** Risk of diarrhea significantly increased.

INTERACTIONS

DRUG: Diuretics may increase risk of dehydration (due to vomiting, diarrhea associated with irinotecan therapy). **Laxatives** may increase severity of diarrhea. **Live virus vaccines** may potentiate virus replication, increase vaccine side effects, decrease pt's antibody response to vaccine. **Other bone marrow depressants** may increase risk of myelosuppression. **Prochlorperazine** may increase akathisia. **HERBAL: St. John's wort** may decrease irinotecan effectiveness. **FOOD:** None known. **LAB VALUES:** May increase serum alkaline phosphatase, AST.

AVAILABILITY (Rx)

INJECTION SOLUTION: 20 mg/ml.

ADMINISTRATION/HANDLING

IV

Reconstitution • Dilute in D_5W (preferred) or 0.9% NaCl to concentration of 0.12 to 1.1 mg/ml.

Rate of administration • Administer all doses as IV infusion over 90 min. • Assess for extravasation (flush site with Sterile Water, apply ice if extravasation occurs).

Storage • Store vials at room temperature, protect from light. • Solution diluted in D_5W is stable for 48 hrs if refrigerated. • Use within 24 hrs if refrigerated or 6 hrs if kept at room temperature. • Do not refrigerate solution if diluted with 0.9% NaCl.

IV INCOMPATIBILITY

Gemcitabine (Gemzar).

INDICATIONS/ROUTES/DOSAGE

CARCINOMA OF THE COLON, RECTUM

IV: ADULTS, ELDERLY: Initially, 125 mg/m^2 once weekly for 4 wks, followed by a rest period of 2 wks. Additional courses may be repeated q6wks. Dosage may be adjusted in 25–50 mg/m^2 increments to as high as 150 mg/m^2 or as low as 50 mg/m^2.

SIDE EFFECTS

EXPECTED: Nausea (64%), alopecia (49%), vomiting (45%), diarrhea (32%). **FREQUENT:** Constipation, fatigue (29%); fever (28%); asthenia (loss of strength, energy) (25%); skeletal pain (23%); abdominal pain, dyspnea (22%). **OCCASIONAL:** Anorexia (19%); headache, stomatitis (18%); rash (16%).

ADVERSE EFFECTS/ TOXIC REACTIONS

Myelosuppression characterized as neutropenia occurs in 97% of pts; neutrophil count less than 50/mm^3 occurs in 78% of pts. Thrombocytopenia, anemia, sepsis occur frequently.

NURSING CONSIDERATIONS

BASELINE ASSESSMENT

Offer emotional support to pt, family. Assess hydration status, electrolytes, CBC before each dose. Premedicate with antiemetics on day of treatment, starting at least 30 min before administration.

INTERVENTION/EVALUATION

Assess for early signs of diarrhea (preceded by complaints of diaphoresis, abdominal cramping). Monitor hydration status, I&O, electrolytes, CBC, Hgb, platelets. Monitor infusion site for signs of inflammation. Inform pt of possibility of alopecia. Assess skin for rash.

PATIENT/FAMILY TEACHING

• Inform pt of possible diarrhea causing dehydration, electrolyte depletion. • Provide antiemetic, antidiarrheal regimen for subsequent use. • Do not have immunizations without physician's approval (drug lowers resistance). • Avoid contact with those who have recently received live virus vaccine. • Avoid crowds, those with infections.

iron dextran

iron **dex**-tran

(DexFerrum, Dexiron ✤, Infed, Infufer ✤)

CLASSIFICATION

PHARMACOTHERAPEUTIC: Trace element. **CLINICAL:** Hematinic iron preparation.

ACTION

Essential component in formation of Hgb. Necessary for effective erythropoiesis, transport and utilization of oxygen. Serves as cofactor of several essential enzymes. **Therapeutic Effect:** Replenishes Hgb, depleted iron stores.

PHARMACOKINETICS

Readily absorbed after IM administration. Most absorption occurs within 72 hrs; remainder within 3–4 wks. Bound to protein to form hemosiderin, ferritin, or transferrin. No physiologic system of elimination. Small amounts lost daily in shedding of skin, hair, nails and in feces, urine, perspiration. **Half-life:** 5–20 hrs.

USES

Treatment of established iron deficiency anemia. Use only when PO administration is not feasible or when rapid replenishment of iron is warranted.

PRECAUTIONS

CONTRAINDICATIONS: All anemias except iron deficiency anemia (pernicious, aplastic, normocytic, refractory). **EXTREME CAUTION:** Serious hepatic impairment. **CAUTIONS:** History of allergies, bronchial asthma, rheumatoid arthritis.

LIFESPAN CONSIDERATIONS:

Pregnancy/Lactation: May cross placenta in some form (unknown). Trace distributed in breast milk. **Pregnancy Category C. Children/Elderly:** No age-related precautions noted.

INTERACTIONS

DRUG: None significant. **HERBAL:** None significant. **FOOD:** None known. **LAB VALUES:** None known.

AVAILABILITY (Rx)

INJECTION SOLUTION (DEXFERRUM, INFED): 50 mg/ml.

ADMINISTRATION/HANDLING

◀ **ALERT** ▶ Test dose is generally given before full dosage; monitor pt for several min after injection due to potential for anaphylactic reaction.

IV

Reconstitution • May give undiluted or dilute in 0.9% NaCl for infusion.

Rate of administration • Do not exceed IV administration rate of 50 mg/min (1 ml/min). Too-rapid IV rate may produce flushing, chest pain, hypotension, tachycardia, shock. • Pt must remain recumbent 30–45 min after IV administration (minimizes postural hypotension).

Storage • Store at room temperature.

IM

• Draw up medication with one needle; use new needle for injection (minimizes skin staining). • Administer deep IM in upper outer quadrant of buttock only. • Use Z-tract technique (displacement of subcutaneous tissue lateral to injection site before inserting needle) to minimize skin staining.

IV INCOMPATIBILITIES

Do not mix with other medications.

INDICATIONS/ROUTES/DOSAGE

◀ **ALERT** ▶ Discontinue oral iron preparations before administering iron dextran. Dosage expressed in terms of milligrams of elemental iron. Dosage individualized based on degree of anemia, pt weight, presence of any bleeding. Use periodic hematologic determinations as guide to therapy.

◀ **ALERT** ▶ Not normally given in first 4 mos of life.

IRON DEFICIENCY ANEMIA (NO BLOOD LOSS)

IV, IM: ADULTS, ELDERLY: Mg iron = 0.66 × weight (kg) × (100 – Hgb [g/dl]/14.8.

IRON REPLACEMENT SECONDARY TO BLOOD LOSS

IV, IM: ADULTS, ELDERLY: Replacement iron (mg) = blood loss (ml) times Hct.

MAXIMUM DAILY DOSAGES

ADULTS WEIGHING MORE THAN 50 KG: 100 mg. **CHILDREN WEIGHING MORE THAN 15 KG:** 100 mg. **CHILDREN 5–15 KG:** 50 mg. **CHILDREN WEIGHING LESS THAN 5 KG:** 25 mg.

SIDE EFFECTS

FREQUENT: Allergic reaction (rash, pruritus), backache, myalgia, chills, dizziness, headache, fever, nausea, vomiting, flushed skin, pain/redness at injection site, brown discoloration of skin, metallic taste.

ADVERSE EFFECTS/ TOXIC REACTIONS

Anaphylaxis occurs rarely in first few min following injection. Leukocytosis, lymphadenopathy occur rarely.

NURSING CONSIDERATIONS

BASELINE ASSESSMENT

Do not give concurrently with oral iron form (excessive iron may produce excessive iron storage [hemosiderosis]). Be alert to pts with rheumatoid arthritis, iron deficiency anemia (acute exacerbation of joint pain, swelling may occur). Inguinal lymphadenopathy may occur with IM injection. Assess for adequate muscle mass before injecting medication.

INTERVENTION/EVALUATION

Monitor IM site for abscess formation, necrosis, atrophy, swelling, brownish color to skin. Question pt regarding soreness, pain, inflammation at/near IM injection site. Check IV site for phlebitis. Monitor serum ferritin.

PATIENT/FAMILY TEACHING

• Pain, brown staining may occur at injection site. • Oral iron should not be taken when receiving iron injections. • Stools often become black with iron therapy but is harmless unless accompanied by red streaking, sticky consistency of stool, abdominal pain/cramping, which should be reported to physician.

I

• Oral hygiene, hard candy, gum may reduce metallic taste. • Notify physician immediately if fever, back pain, headache occur.

iron sucrose

iron **sue**-crose
(Venofer)

CLASSIFICATION

PHARMACOTHERAPEUTIC: Trace element. **CLINICAL:** Hematinic iron preparation.

I

ACTION

Essential component in formation of Hgb. Necessary for effective erythropoiesis, transport and utilization of oxygen. Serves as cofactor of several essential enzymes. **Therapeutic Effect:** Replenishes body iron stores in pts on chronic hemodialysis who have iron deficiency anemia and are receiving erythropoietin.

PHARMACOKINETICS

Distributed mainly in blood and to some extent in extravascular fluid. Iron sucrose is dissociated into iron and sucrose by reticuloendothelial system. Sucrose component is eliminated mainly by urinary excretion. **Half-life:** 6 hrs.

USES

Treatment of iron deficiency anemia in pts undergoing chronic hemodialysis or peritoneal dialysis who are receiving supplemental erythropoietin therapy. Treatment of iron deficiency anemia in pts with chronic kidney disease who are not undergoing dialysis. **OFF-LABEL:** Treatment of dystrophic epidermolysis bullosa.

PRECAUTIONS

CONTRAINDICATIONS: All anemias except iron deficiency anemia (pernicious, aplastic, normocytic, refractory anemia), evidence of iron overload. **CAUTIONS:** History of allergies, bronchial asthma; hepatic/renal/cardiac dysfunction.

LIFESPAN CONSIDERATIONS:

Pregnancy/Lactation: Unknown if drug crosses placenta or is distributed in breast milk. **Pregnancy Category B.** **Children:** Safety and efficacy not established. **Elderly:** Age-related renal impairment may require dosage adjustment.

INTERACTIONS

DRUG: None significant. **HERBAL:** None significant. **FOOD:** None known. **LAB VALUES:** Increases Hgb, Hct, serum ferritin, transferrin.

AVAILABILITY (Rx)

INJECTION SOLUTION: 20 mg/ml or 100 mg elemental iron in 5-ml single-dose vial.

ADMINISTRATION/HANDLING

◄ **ALERT** ► Administer directly into dialysis line during hemodialysis.

IV

Reconstitution • May give undiluted as slow IV injection or IV infusion. For IV infusion, dilute each vial in maximum of 100 ml 0.9% NaCl immediately before infusion.

Rate of administration • For IV injection, administer into the dialysis line at a rate of 1 ml (20 mg iron) undiluted solution per min (5 min per vial). Do not exceed 1 vial per injection. • For IV infusion, administer into dialysis line (reduces risk of hypotensive episodes) at a rate of 100 mg iron over at least 15 min.

Storage • Store at room temperature.

IV INCOMPATIBILITIES

Do not mix with other medications or add to parenteral nutrition solution for IV infusion.

INDICATIONS/ROUTES/DOSAGE

IRON DEFICIENCY ANEMIA

Dosage is expressed in terms of milligrams of elemental iron.

IV: ADULTS, ELDERLY: 5 ml iron sucrose (100 mg elemental iron) delivered during dialysis; administer 1–3 times a wk to total dose of 1,000 mg in 10 doses. Give no more than 3 times a wk.

SIDE EFFECTS

FREQUENT (36%–23%): Hypotension, leg cramps, diarrhea.

ADVERSE EFFECTS/ TOXIC REACTIONS

Too-rapid IV administration may produce severe hypotension, headache, vomiting, nausea, dizziness, paresthesia, abdominal/muscle pain, edema, cardiovascular collapse. Hypersensitivity reaction occurs rarely.

NURSING CONSIDERATIONS

INTERVENTION/EVALUATION

Initially, monitor Hgb, Hct, serum ferritin, transferrin monthly then q2–3mo thereafter. Reliable serum iron values can be obtained 48 hrs following administration.

isoetharine

(Bronkosol)

See Bronchodilators

isoflurophate

(Floropryl)

See Antiglaucoma agents

isoniazid

eye-**soe**-nye-a-zid

(INH, Isotamine ✤, Nydrazid, PMS Isoniazid ✤)

FIXED-COMBINATION(S)

Rifamate: isoniazid/rifampin (antitubercular): 150 mg/300 mg. **Rifater:** isoniazid/pyrazinamide/ rifampin (antitubercular): 50 mg/ 300 mg/120 mg.

CLASSIFICATION

PHARMACOTHERAPEUTIC: Isonicotinic acid derivative. **CLINICAL:** Antitubercular.

ACTION

Inhibits mycolic acid synthesis. Causes disruption of bacterial cell wall, loss of acid-fast properties in susceptible mycobacteria. Active only during bacterial cell division. **Therapeutic Effect:** Bactericidal against actively growing intracelleluar, extracellular susceptible mycobacteria.

PHARMACOKINETICS

Readily absorbed from GI tract. Protein binding: 10%–15%. Widely distributed (including to CSF). Metabolized in liver. Primarily excreted in urine. Removed by hemodialysis. **Half-life:** 0.5-5 hrs.

USES

Treatment of susceptible mycobacterial infection due to *M. tuberculosis*. Drug of choice in tuberculosis prophylaxis. Used in combination with one or more other antitubercular agents for treatment of active tuberculosis.

PRECAUTIONS

CONTRAINDICATIONS: Acute hepatic disease, history of hypersensitivity reactions, hepatic injury with previous isoniazid therapy. **CAUTIONS:** Chronic hepatic disease, alcoholism, severe renal impairment. May be cross-sensitive with nicotinic acid, other chemically related medications.

LIFESPAN CONSIDERATIONS:

Pregnancy/Lactation: Prophylaxis usually postponed until after delivery. Crosses placenta. Distributed in breast milk. **Pregnancy Category C. Children:** No age-related precautions noted. **Elderly:** More susceptible to developing hepatitis.

INTERACTIONS

DRUG: **Alcohol** may increase isoniazid metabolism, risk of hepatotoxicity. May increase toxicity of **carbamazepine, phenytoin. Disulfiram** may increase CNS effects. **Hepatotoxic medications** may increase risk of hepatotoxicity. May decrease **ketoconazole** concentration. **HERBAL:** None significant. **FOOD:** **Foods containing tyramine** may cause hypertensive crisis. **LAB VALUES:** May increase serum bilirubin, AST, ALT.

AVAILABILITY (Rx)

INJECTION SOLUTION (NYDRAZID): 100 mg/ml. **SYRUP:** 50 mg/5 ml. **TABLETS:** 100 mg, 300 mg.

ADMINISTRATION/HANDLING

PO

• Give 1 hr before or 2 hrs following meals (may give with food to decrease GI upset, but will delay absorption). • Administer at least 1 hr before antacids, those containing esp. aluminum.

INDICATIONS/ROUTES/DOSAGE

ACTIVE TUBERCULOSIS (IN COMBINATION WITH ONE OR MORE ANTITUBERCULARS)

PO, IM: ADULTS, ELDERLY: 5 mg/kg/day as a single dose. **Maximum:** 300 mg/day. **CHILDREN:** 10–15 mg/kg/day as a single dose or 2 divided doses. **Maximum:** 300 mg/day.

TUBERCULOSIS PROPHYLAXIS

PO, IM: ADULTS, ELDERLY: 300 mg/day as a single dose. **CHILDREN:** 10 mg/kg/day as a single dose or 2 divided doses. **Maximum:** 300 mg/day.

SIDE EFFECTS

FREQUENT: Nausea, vomiting, diarrhea, abdominal pain. **RARE:** Pain at injection site, hypersensitivity reaction.

ADVERSE EFFECTS/ TOXIC REACTIONS

Neurotoxicity (ataxia, paraesthesia), optic neuritis, hepatotoxicity occur rarely.

NURSING CONSIDERATIONS

BASELINE ASSESSMENT

Question for history of hypersensitivity reactions, hepatic injury from isoniazid, sensitivity to nicotinic acid or chemically related medications. Ensure collection of specimens for culture, sensitivity. Evaluate initial hepatic function results.

INTERVENTION/EVALUATION

Monitor hepatic function test results, assess for hepatitis: anorexia, nausea, vomiting, weakness, fatigue, dark urine, jaundice (hold concurrent INH therapy and inform physician promptly). Assess for paraesthesia of extremities (those esp. at risk for neuropathy may be given pyridoxine prophylactically: malnourished, elderly, diabetics, pts with chronic hepatic disease [including alcoholics]). Be alert for fever, skin eruptions (hypersensitivity reaction).

PATIENT/FAMILY TEACHING

• Do not skip doses; continue taking isoniazid for full length of therapy (6–24 mos). • Take preferably 1 hr before or 2 hrs following meals (with food if GI upset). • Avoid alcohol during treatment. • Do not take any other medications, including antacids, without consulting physician. • Must take isoniazid at least 1 hr before antacid.

• Avoid tuna, sauerkraut, aged cheeses, smoked fish (provide list of tyramine-containing foods) that may cause hypertensive reaction (red/itching skin, palpitations, lightheadedness, hot or clammy feeling, headache). • Notify physician of any new symptom, immediately for vision difficulties, nausea/vomiting, dark urine, yellowing of skin/eyes (jaundice), fatigue, paraesthesia of extremities.

isoproterenol

(Isuprel)

See Sympathomimetics

isosorbide dinitrate

eye-sew-**sore**-bide

(Apo-ISDN ✱, Cedocard ✱, Dilatrate-SR, Isochron, Isordil, Isordil Tembids)

isosorbide mononitrate

(Imdur, ISMO, Monoket)

Do not confuse Isordil with Isuprel or Plendil, or Imdur with Inderal or K-Dur.

FIXED-COMBINATION(S)

BiDil: isosorbide/hydralazine, (a vasodilator): 20 mg/37.5 mg.

CLASSIFICATION

PHARMACOTHERAPEUTIC: Nitrate. **CLINICAL:** Antianginal (see p. 121C).

ACTION

Stimulates intracellular cyclic guanosine monophosphate. **Therapeutic Effect:** Relaxes vascular smooth muscle of arterial, venous vasculature. Decreases preload, afterload.

PHARMACOKINETICS

Route	Onset	Peak	Duration
Dinitrate			
Sublingual	2–5 min	N/A	1–2 hrs
Oral (Chewable)	2–5 min	N/A	1–2 hrs
Oral	15–40 min	N/A	4–6 hrs
Oral (Sustained-Release)	30 min	N/A	12 hrs
Mononitrate			
Oral (Extended-Release)	60 min	N/A	N/A

Dinitrate poorly absorbed and metabolized in liver to its activate metabolite isosorbide mononitrate. Mononitrate well absorbed after PO administration. Excreted in urine and feces. **Half-life:** Dinitrate, 1–4 hrs; mononitrate, 4 hrs.

USES

Prophylaxis, treatment of angina pectoris. **OFF-LABEL:** CHF, dysphagia, pain relief, relief of esophageal spasm with gastroesophageal reflux.

PRECAUTIONS

CONTRAINDICATIONS: Closed-angle glaucoma, head trauma, hypersensitivity to nitrates, increased intracranial pressure, orthostatic hypotension, concurrent use of sildenafil, tadalafil, vardenafil. **Extended-Release Tablets:** GI hypermotility, GI malabsorption, severe anemia. **CAUTIONS:** Acute MI, hepatic/renal disease, glaucoma (contraindicated in closed-angle glaucoma), blood volume depletion from diuretic therapy, systolic B/P less than 90 mm Hg.

LIFESPAN CONSIDERATIONS:

Pregnancy/Lactation: Unknown if drug crosses placenta or is distributed in breast milk. **Pregnancy Category C. Children:** Safety and efficacy not established. **Elderly:** May be more sensitive to hypotensive effects. Age-related renal impairment may require dosage adjustment.

INTERACTIONS

DRUG: **Alcohol, antihypertensives, vasodilators** may increase risk of orthostatic hypotension. **Sildenafil, tadalafil, vardenafil** may potentiate hypotensive effects (concurrent use of these agents is contraindicated). **HERBAL:** None significant. **FOOD:** None known. **LAB VALUES:** May increase urine catecholamine, urine vanillylmandelic acid levels.

I

AVAILABILITY (Rx)

Dinitrate

TABLETS: (ISORDIL): 5 mg, 10 mg, 20 mg, 30 mg, 40 mg.

CAPSULE, SUSTAINED-RELEASE (DILATRATE SR): 40 mg. **TABLET, EXTENDED-RELEASE: (ISOCHRON):** 40 mg. **TABLET, SUBLINGUAL: (ISORDIL):** 2.5 mg, 5 mg.

Moninitrate

TABLETS (ISMO): 20 mg. **(MONOKET):** 10 mg, 20 mg.

TABLET, EXTENDED-RELEASE (IMDUR): 30 mg, 60 mg, 120 mg.

ADMINISTRATION/HANDLING

PO

• Best if taken on an empty stomach. • Oral tablets may be crushed. • Do not crush/break sublingual, sustained-, extended-release form. • Do not crush chewable form before administering.

SUBLINGUAL

• Do not crush/chew sublingual tablets. • Dissolve tablets under tongue; do not swallow.

INDICATIONS/ROUTES/DOSAGE

ANGINA

PO (ISOSORBIDE DINITRATE): ADULTS, ELDERLY: 5–40 mg 4 times a day. **Sustained-release:** 40 mg q8–12h. **PO (ISOSORBIDE MONONITRATE): ADULTS, ELDERLY:** 5–10 mg twice a day given 7 hrs apart. **Sustained-release:** Initially, 30–60 mg/day in morning as a single dose. May increase dose at 3 day intervals. **Maximum:** 240 mg/day.

SIDE EFFECTS

FREQUENT: Headache (may be severe) occurs mostly in early therapy, diminishes rapidly in intensity, usually disappears during continued treatment, transient flushing of face/neck, dizziness (esp. if pt is standing immobile or is in a warm environment), weakness, orthostatic hypotension, nausea, vomiting, restlessness. **OCCASIONAL:** GI upset, blurred vision, dry mouth. **SUBLINGUAL: FREQUENT:** Burning, tingling at oral point of dissolution.

ADVERSE REACTIONS/ TOXIC EFFECTS

Drug should be discontinued if blurred vision occurs. Severe orthostatic hypotension manifested by syncope, pulselessness, cold/clammy skin, diaphoresis. Tolerance may occur with repeated, prolonged therapy, but may not occur with extended-release form. Minor tolerance with intermittent use of sublingual tablets. High dosage tends to produce severe headache.

NURSING CONSIDERATIONS

BASELINE ASSESSMENT

Record onset, type (sharp, dull, squeezing), radiation, location, intensity, duration of anginal pain; precipitating factors (exertion, emotional stress). If headache occurs during management therapy, administer medication with meals.

INTERVENTION/EVALUATION

Assist with ambulation if light-headedness, dizziness occurs. Assess for facial/neck flushing. Monitor number of anginal episodes, orthostatic B/P.

PATIENT/FAMILY TEACHING

• Do not chew/crush sublingual, extended-, sustained-release forms. • Take sublingual tablets while sitting down. • Notify physician if angina persists for longer than 20 min. • Rise slowly from lying to sitting position, dangle legs momentarily before standing (prevents dizziness effect). • Take oral form on empty stomach (however, if headache occurs during management therapy, take medication with meals). • Dissolve sublingual tablet under tongue; do not swallow. • Take at first signal of angina. • If pain not relieved within 5 min, dissolve second tablet under tongue. • Repeat if no relief in another 5 min. • If pain continues, contact physician. • Expel from mouth any remaining sublingual tablet after pain is completely relieved. • Do not change from one brand of drug to another. • Avoid alcohol (intensifies hypotensive effect). • If alcohol is ingested soon after taking nitrates, possible acute hypotensive episode (marked drop in B/P, vertigo, pallor) may occur.

isotretinoin

evolve

eye-so-**tret**-ah-noyn

(Accutane, Amnesteem, Claravis, Isotrex ♣, Sotret)

Do not confuse Accutane with Accupril or Accurbron.

CLASSIFICATION

PHARMACOTHERAPEUTIC: Keratinization stabilizer. **CLINICAL:** Antiacne, antirosacea agent.

ACTION

Reduces sebaceous gland size, inhibiting gland activity. **Therapeutic Effect:** Produces antikeratinizing, anti-inflammatory effects.

USES

Treatment of severe, recalcitrant cystic acne unresponsive to conventional acne therapies. **OFF-LABEL:** Treatment of gram-negative folliculitis, severe rosacea, severe keratinization disorders.

PRECAUTIONS

CONTRAINDICATIONS: Hypersensitivity to isotretinoin, parabens (component of capsules). **CAUTIONS:** Renal/hepatic dysfunction.

LIFESPAN CONSIDERATIONS:

Pregnancy/Lactation: Contraindicated in females who are or may become pregnant while undergoing treatment (very high risk of fetal harm, major fetal birth defects/deformities). Unknown if crosses placenta or distributed in breast milk; breast-feeding not recommended. **Pregnancy Category X.** **Children:** Safety and efficacy not established in children younger than 12 yrs. Careful consideration must be given to children 12–17 yrs, esp. those with known metabolic disease, structural bone disease. **Elderly:** No age-related precautions noted.

INTERACTIONS

DRUG: **Etretinate, tretinoin, vitamin A** may increase toxic effects. **Tetracycline** may increase potential for pseudotumor cerebri. **HERBAL:** **Dong quai, St. John's wort** may cause photosensitization. **FOOD:** None known. **LAB VALUES:** May increase serum triglycerides, cholesterol, AST, ALT, alkaline phosphatase, LDH, fasting serum glucose, uric acid, sedimentation rate. May decrease HDL.

AVAILABILITY (Rx)

CAPSULES: **Accutane, Amnesteem, Claravis:** 10 mg, 20 mg, 40 mg; **Sotret:** 10 mg, 20 mg, 30 mg, 40 mg.

INDICATIONS/ROUTES/DOSAGE

RECALCITRANT CYSTIC ACNE

PO: ADULTS: Initially, 0.5–2 mg/kg/day divided in 2 doses for 15–20 wks. May repeat after at least 2 mos of therapy.

SIDE EFFECTS

FREQUENT: Cheilitis (inflammation of lips) (90%), skin/mucous membrane dryness (80%), skin fragility, pruritus, epistaxis, dry nose/mouth, conjunctivitis (40%), hypertriglyceridemia (25%), nausea, vomiting, abdominal pain (20%). **OCCASIONAL (3%–2%):** Musculoskeletal symptoms (16%) including bone/joint pain, arthralgia, generalized muscle aches; photosensitivity (10%–5%). **RARE:** Diminished night vision, depression.

ADVERSE EFFECTS/ TOXIC REACTIONS

Inflammatory bowel disease, pseudotumor cerebri (benign intracranial hypertension) have been associated with isotretinoin therapy.

NURSING CONSIDERATIONS

BASELINE ASSESSMENT

Assess baselines for serum glucose, lipids.

INTERVENTION/EVALUATION

Assess acne for decreased cysts. Evaluate skin/mucous membranes for excessive dryness. Monitor serum glucose, lipids.

PATIENT/FAMILY TEACHING

• Transient exacerbation of acne may occur during initial period. • May have decreased tolerance to contact lenses during and following therapy. • Do not take vitamin supplements with vitamin A due to additive effects. • Immediately notify physician of onset of abdominal pain, severe diarrhea, rectal bleeding (possible inflammatory bowel disease), headache, nausea/vomiting, visual disturbances (possible pseudotumor cerebri). • Diminished night vision may occur suddenly; take caution with night driving. • Avoid prolonged exposure to sunlight; use sunscreens, protective clothing. • Do not donate blood during or for 1 mo following treatment. • **Women:** Explain serious risk to fetus if pregnancy occurs (give both oral and written warnings, with pt acknowledging in writing that she understands the warnings and consents to treatment). • Must have negative serum pregnancy test within 2 wks before starting therapy; therapy will begin on the second or third day of next normal menstrual period. • Effective contraception (using 2 reliable forms of contraception simultaneously) must be used for at least 1 mo before, during, and for at least 1 mo after therapy.

isradipine

iss-**rah**-dih-peen

(DynaCirc, DynaCirc CR)

Do not confuse DynaCirc with Dynabac or Dynacin.

CLASSIFICATION

PHARMACOTHERAPEUTIC: Calcium channel blocker. **CLINICAL:** Antihypertensive (see p. 73C).

ACTION

Inhibits calcium movement across cardiac, vascular smooth-muscle cell membranes. Potent peripheral vasodilator (does not depress SA, AV nodes). **Therapeutic Effect:** Produces relaxation of coronary vascular smooth muscle, coronary vasodilation. Increases myocardial oxygen delivery in those with vasospastic angina.

PHARMACOKINETICS

Route	Onset	Peak	Duration
PO	2–3 hrs	2–4 wks (multiple doses) 8–16 hrs (single dose)	N/A

PO (Controlled-release)	2 hrs	8–10 hrs	N/A

Well absorbed from GI tract. Protein binding: 95%. Metabolized in liver (undergoes first-pass effect). Primarily excreted in urine. Not removed by hemodialysis. **Half-life:** 8 hrs.

USES

Management of hypertension. May be used alone or with other antihypertensives. **OFF-LABEL:** Treatment of chronic angina pectoris, Raynaud's phenomenon.

PRECAUTIONS

CONTRAINDICATIONS: Cardiogenic shock, CHF, heart block, hypotension, sinus bradycardia, ventricular tachycardia. **CAUTIONS:** Sick sinus syndrome, severe left ventricular dysfunction, hepatic disease, edema, concurrent therapy with beta-blockers.

LIFESPAN CONSIDERATIONS:

Pregnancy/Lactation: Unknown if drug crosses placenta or is distributed in breast milk. **Pregnancy Category C.** **Children:** Safety and efficacy not established. **Elderly:** Age-related renal impairment may require dosage adjustment.

INTERACTIONS

DRUG: **Beta blockers** may have additive effect. **HERBAL:** **Ephedra, ginseng, yohimbe** may worsen hypertension. **Garlic** may increase antihypertensive effect. **FOOD:** **Grapefruit, grapefruit juice** may increase absorption. **LAB VALUES:** None known.

AVAILABILITY (Rx)

CAPSULES (CONTROLLED-RELEASE [DYNACIRC-CR]): 5 mg, 10 mg.

CAPSULES (DYNACIRC): 2.5 mg, 5 mg.

ADMINISTRATION/HANDLING

PO

- May open capsules, but avoid crushing contents.

INDICATIONS/ROUTES/DOSAGE

HYPERTENSION

PO: ADULTS, ELDERLY: Initially 2.5 mg twice a day. May increase by 2.5 mg at 2- to 4-wk intervals. Range: 5–20 mg/day.

SIDE EFFECTS

FREQUENT (7%–4%): Peripheral edema, palpitations (higher frequency in females). **OCCASIONAL (3%):** Facial flushing, cough. **RARE (2%–1%):** Angina, tachycardia, rash, pruritus.

ADVERSE EFFECTS/ TOXIC REACTIONS

Overdose produces nausea, drowsiness, confusion, slurred speech. CHF occurs rarely.

NURSING CONSIDERATIONS

BASELINE ASSESSMENT

Assess baseline renal/hepatic function tests. Assess B/P, apical pulse immediately before drug is administered (if pulse is 60 beats/min or less or systolic B/P is less than 90 mm Hg, withhold medication, contact physician).

INTERVENTION/EVALUATION

Assess for peripheral edema behind medial malleolus (sacral area in bedridden pts). Monitor pulse rate for bradycardia. Monitor B/P; observe for signs, symptoms of CHF. Assess skin for flushing.

PATIENT/FAMILY TEACHING

- Do not abruptly discontinue medication. Compliance with therapy regimen is essential to control hypertension. • To avoid hypotensive effect, rise slowly from lying to sitting position, wait momentarily before standing. • Contact physician if palpitations, shortness of breath, pronounced dizziness, nausea occurs.
- Avoid grapefruit, grapefruit juice.

itraconazole

eye-tra-**con**-ah-zoll
(Sporanox)
Do not confuse Sporanox with Suprax.

◆CLASSIFICATION

CLINICAL: Antifungal.

ACTION

Inhibits synthesis of ergosterol (vital component of fungal cell formation). **Therapeutic Effect:** Damages fungal cell membrane, altering its function. Fungistatic.

PHARMACOKINETICS

Moderately absorbed from GI tract. Absorption is increased if drug is taken with food. Protein binding: 99%. Widely distributed, primarily in fatty tissue, liver, kidneys. Metabolized in liver to active metabolite. Primarily excreted in urine. Not removed by hemodialysis. **Half-life:** 21 hrs; metabolite, 12 hrs.

USES

Treatment of aspergillosis, blastomycosis, esophageal and oropharyngeal candidiasis, empiric treatment in febrile neutropenia, histoplasmosis, onychomycosis. **OFF-LABEL:** Suppression of histoplasmosis; treatment of disseminated sporotrichosis, fungal pneumonia/septicemia, tinea infection (ringworm) of the hand.

PRECAUTIONS

CONTRAINDICATIONS: Hypersensitivity to fluconazole, ketoconazole, miconazole. **CAUTIONS:** Hepatitis, HIV-infected pts, pts with achlorhydria, hypochlorhydria (decreases absorption), hepatic impairment.

⌛ LIFESPAN CONSIDERATIONS:

Pregnancy/Lactation: Distributed in breast milk. **Pregnancy Category C. Children:** Safety and efficacy not established. **Elderly:** Age-related renal impairment may require dosage adjustment.

INTERACTIONS

DRUG: May increase concentration/toxicity of **midazolam, triazolam, oral antidiabetic agents (e.g., glyburide, glipizide), HMG-CoA reductase inhibitors (e.g., lovastatin, simvastatin), calcium channel-blocking agents (e.g., felodipine, nifedipine), carbamazepine, cyclosporine, sirolimus, tacrolimus, digoxin, protease inhibitors (e.g., indinavir, ritonavir, saquinavir), ergot alkaloids, warfarin. Carbamazepine, isoniazid, rifampin, phenobarbital, phenytoin** may decrease concentration/effect. May inhibit metabolism of **busulfan, docetaxel, vinca alkaloids. Erythromycin** may increase risk of cardiac toxicity. **Antacids, H_2 antagonists, proton pump inhibitors (e.g., omeprazole)** may decrease absorption. **HERBAL: St. John's wort** may decrease concentration. **FOOD: Grapefruit, grapefruit juice** may alter absorption. **LAB VALUES:** May increase LDH, serum alkaline phosphatase, bilirubin, AST, ALT. May decrease serum potassium.

AVAILABILITY (Rx)

CAPSULES: 100 mg. **INJECTION SOLUTION:** 10 mg/ml (25-ml ampule). **ORAL SOLUTION:** 10 mg/ml.

ADMINISTRATION/HANDLING

IV

Reconstitution • Use only components provided by manufacturer. • Do not dilute with any other diluent. • Add full contents of ampule (250 mg/10 ml) to infusion bag provided (50 ml 0.9% NaCl). • Mix gently.

Rate of administration • Infuse over 60 min using extension line and infusion set provided. • After administration, flush infusion set with 15–20 ml 0.9% NaCl over 30 sec to 15 min. • Discard entire infusion line.

Storage • Store at room temperature. Do not freeze.

PO

• Give capsules with food (increases absorption). • Give solution on empty stomach.

IV INCOMPATIBILITIES

◀ ALERT ▶ Dilution compatibility other than 0.9% NaCl is unknown. Do not mix with D_5W or lactated Ringer's. Not for IV bolus administration. Do not administer any medication in same bag or through same IV line as itraconazole. Do not mix with any other medication.

INDICATIONS/ROUTES/DOSAGE

BLASTOMYCOSIS, HISTOPLASMOSIS

PO: ADULTS, ELDERLY: Initially, 200 mg once a day. **Maximum:** 400 mg/day in 2 divided doses.

IV: ADULTS, ELDERLY: 200 mg twice a day for 4 doses, then 200 mg once a day.

ASPERGILLOSIS

PO: ADULTS, ELDERLY: 600 mg/day in 3 divided doses for 3–4 days, then 200–400 mg/day in 2 divided doses.

IV: ADULTS, ELDERLY: 200 mg twice a day for 4 doses, then 200 mg once a day.

ESOPHAGEAL CANDIDIASIS

PO: ADULTS, ELDERLY: Swish 100–200 mg (10–20 ml) in mouth for several seconds, then swallow. **Maximum:** 200 mg/day.

OROPHARYNGEAL CANDIDIASIS

PO: ADULTS, ELDERLY: 200 mg (10 ml) oral solution, swish and swallow once a day for 7–14 days.

FEBRILE NEUTROPENIA

IV: ADULTS, ELDERLY: 200 mg twice a day for 4 doses, then 200 mg for up to 14 days. Then give PO 200 mg twice a day until neutropenia resolves.

ONYCHOMYCOSIS (FINGERNAIL)

PO: ADULTS, ELDERLY: 200 mg twice a day for 7 days, off for 21 days, repeat 200 mg twice a day for 7 days.

ONYCHOMYCOSIS (TOENAIL)

PO: ADULTS, ELDERLY: 200 mg once daily for 12 wks.

SIDE EFFECTS

FREQUENT (11%–9%): Nausea, rash. **OCCASIONAL (5%–3%):** Vomiting, headache, diarrhea, hypertension, peripheral edema, fatigue, fever. **RARE (2% or less):** Abdominal pain, dizziness, anorexia, pruritus.

ADVERSE EFFECTS/ TOXIC REACTIONS

Hepatitis (anorexia, abdominal pain, unusual fatigue/weakness, jaundiced skin/ sclera, dark urine) occurs rarely.

NURSING CONSIDERATIONS

BASELINE ASSESSMENT

Determine baseline temperature, hepatic function tests. Assess allergies.

INTERVENTION/EVALUATION

Assess for signs, symptoms of hepatic dysfunction. Monitor hepatic enzyme test results in pts with preexisting hepatic dysfunction.

PATIENT/ FAMILY TEACHING

• Take capsules with food, liquids if GI distress occurs. • Therapy will continue for at least 3 mos, until lab tests, clinical presentation indicate infection is controlled. • Immediately report unusual fatigue, yellow skin, dark urine, pale stool, anorexia, nausea, vomiting. • Avoid grapefruit, grapefruit juice.

Ivanz, *see ertapenem*

I

Kadian, *see morphine*

Kaletra, *see lopinavir and ritonavir*

kaolin/pectin

kay-oh-lyn

(Kaodene, Kao-Spen, Kapectolin)

Do not confuse kaolin, Kaodene, or Kapectolin with Kayexalate.

FIXED-COMBINATION(S)

Parepectolin: kaolin/pectin/opium: 5.5 g/162 mg/15 mg.

CLASSIFICATION

PHARMACOTHERAPEUTIC: Magnesium/aluminum silicate. **CLINICAL:** Antidiarrheal (see p. 43C).

ACTION

Adsorbent, protectant. **Therapeutic Effect:** Adsorbs bacteria, toxins; reduces water loss.

PHARMACOKINETICS

Not absorbed orally. Up to 90% of pectin decomposed in GI tract.

USES

Symptomatic treatment of mild to moderate acute diarrhea.

PRECAUTIONS

CONTRAINDICATIONS: None known. **CAUTIONS:** None known.

LIFESPAN CONSIDERATIONS:

Pregnancy/Lactation: Unknown if drug crosses placenta or is distributed in breast milk. **Pregnancy Category C.** **Children:** Not recommended in those younger than 3 yrs. **Elderly:** More sensitive to fluid and electrolyte loss; use caution.

INTERACTIONS

DRUG: May decrease absorption of **digoxin** when given concurrently with kaolin. **HERBAL:** None significant. **FOOD:** None known. **LAB VALUES:** None known.

AVAILABILITY (OTC)

ORAL SUSPENSION.

ADMINISTRATION/HANDLING

PO

- Shake suspension well before administration.

INDICATIONS/ROUTES/DOSAGE

ANTIDIARRHEAL

PO: ADULTS, ELDERLY: 60–120 ml after each loose bowel movement (LBM). **CHILDREN 12 YRS AND OLDER:** 60 ml after each LBM. **CHILDREN 6–12 YRS:** 30–60 ml after each LBM. **CHILDREN 3–5 YRS:** 15–30 ml after each LBM.

SIDE EFFECTS

RARE: Constipation.

ADVERSE EFFECTS/ TOXIC REACTIONS

None known.

NURSING CONSIDERATIONS

INTERVENTION/EVALUATION

Encourage adequate fluid intake. Assess bowel sounds for peristalsis, stools for frequency, consistency.

PATIENT/FAMILY TEACHING

- Do not use for more than 2 days or in presence of high fever.

kava kava

Also known as ava, kew, sakau, tonga, yagona.

◄ **ALERT** ► May be removed from market.

♦CLASSIFICATION

HERBAL: See Appendix G.

ACTION

Exact mechanism of action unknown but possesses CNS effects. **Effect:** Anxiolytic, sedative, analgesic effects.

USES

Treatment of anxiety disorders, stress, restlessness. Used for sedation, sleep enhancement.

PRECAUTIONS

CONTRAINDICATIONS: Pregnancy, lactation (may cause loss of uterine tone). **CAUTIONS:** Depression, history of recurrent hepatitis.

LIFESPAN CONSIDERATIONS:

Pregnancy/Lactation: Contraindicated. **Children:** Safety and efficacy not established. **Elderly:** No age-related precautions noted.

INTERACTIONS

DRUG: Alcohol, benzodiazepines may increase risk of drowsiness. **HERBAL: Chamomile, goldenseal, melatonin, St. John's wort, ginseng, valerian** may increase risk of excessive drowsiness. **FOOD:** None known. **LAB VALUES:** May increase hepatic function tests.

AVAILABILITY (OTC)

CAPSULES: 140 mg, 150 mg, 250 mg, 300 mg, 425 mg, 500 mg. **LIQUID. EXTRACT. TINCTURE.**

INDICATIONS/ROUTES/DOSAGE

USUAL DOSAGE

PO: ADULTS, ELDERLY: 100 mg 3 times a day or 1 cup of the tea 3 times a day.

SIDE EFFECTS

GI upset, headache, dizziness, vision changes (blurred vision, red eyes), allergic skin reactions, dermopathy (dry, flaky skin), yellowing of skin, hair, nails, sclera of eyes, nausea, vomiting, weight loss, shortness of breath.

ADVERSE EFFECTS/ TOXIC REACTIONS

None known.

NURSING CONSIDERATIONS

BASELINE ASSESSMENT

Assess if pt is pregnant or breast-feeding (contraindicated). Determine baseline hepatic function tests. Assess for use of other CNS depressants.

INTERVENTION/EVALUATION

Monitor hepatic function tests. Assess for allergic skin reactions.

PATIENT/FAMILY TEACHING

• Avoid use if pregnant, planning to become pregnant, or breast-feeding; not for use in children 12 yrs and younger. • Avoid tasks that require alertness, motor skills until response to herbal is established. • Do not use for more than 3 mos (may be habit forming).

Keflex, *see cephalexin*

Kefzol, *see cefazolin*

K

Keppra, *see levetiracetam*

ketamine

key-tah-meen
(Ketalar)

CLASSIFICATION

CLINICAL: Rapid-acting general anesthetic (see p. 2C).

ACTION

Selectively blocks afferent impulses, interacts with CNS transmitter systems. **Therapeutic Effect:** Produces anesthetic state characterized by profound analgesia, normal pharyngeal-laryngeal reflexes.

PHARMACOKINETICS

Route	Onset	Peak	Duration
IM (anesthetic)	3–4 min	N/A	12–25 min
IM (analgesic)	30 min	N/A	15–30 min
IV (anesthetic)	30 sec	N/A	5–10 min
IV (analgesic)	10–15 min	N/A	N/A

Rapidly distributed. Metabolized in liver. Primarily excreted in urine. **Half-life:** Distribution: 10–15 min, elimination: 2–3 hrs.

USES

Induction, maintenance of general anesthesia (esp. when cardiovascular depression to be avoided), sedation.

PRECAUTIONS

CONTRAINDICATIONS: Aneurysms, angina, CHF, elevated intracranial pressure (ICP), hypertension, psychotic disorders, thyrotoxicosis. **CAUTIONS:** Gastroesophageal reflux disease (GERD), hepatic impairment, pts with recent food intake (large meal), chronic alcoholism, acute intoxication.

LIFESPAN CONSIDERATIONS:

Pregnancy/Lactation: Not recommended; safety not established. **Pregnancy Category D. Children/Elderly:** No age-related precautions noted.

INTERACTIONS

DRUG: Paroxetine, sertraline, ketoconazole, NSAIDS, clarithromycin, propofol, protease inhibitors may increase concentration/effect. **Barbiturates, narcotics** may prolong recovery from sedation. **HERBAL:** None significant. **FOOD:** None known. **LAB VALUES:** May increase intraocular pressure (IOP).

AVAILABILITY (Rx)

INJECTION SOLUTION: 10 mg/ml, 50 mg/ml, 100 mg/ml.

ADMINISTRATION/HANDLING

IV

Reconstitution • For induction anesthesia using IV push, dilute 100 mg/ml with equal volume Sterile Water for Injection, D_5W, or 0.9% NaCl. • For maintenance IV infusion, dilute 50 mg/ml vial (10 ml) or 100 mg/ml vial (5 ml) to 250–500 ml D_5W or 0.9% NaCl to provide a concentration of 1–2 mg/ml.

Rate of administration • Administer IV push slowly over 60 sec (too-rapid IV may produce severe hypotension, respiratory depression). • Administer IV infusion at rate of 0.5 mg/kg/min.

IM

• Use 10 mg/ml vial.

IV INCOMPATIBILITIES

Doxapram (Dopram).

IV COMPATIBILITIES

Bupivacaine (Marcaine), clonidine (Duraclon), fentanyl (Sublimaze), lidocaine, morphine, propofol (Diprivan).

INDICATIONS/ROUTES/DOSAGE

INDUCTION/MAINTENANCE OF GENERAL ANESTHESIA, SEDATION, ANALGESIA

IV: ADULTS, ELDERLY: 1–4.5 mg/kg. Usual induction dose: 1–2 mg/kg. **CHILDREN:** 0.5–2 mg/kg. Usual induction dose: 1–2 mg/kg.

IM: ADULTS, ELDERLY: 3–8 mg/kg. **CHILDREN:** 3–7 mg/kg.

SIDE EFFECTS

FREQUENT: Increased B/P, pulse. Emergence reaction occurs frequently (12%), resulting in dreamlike state, vivid imagery, hallucinations, delirium, and occasionally accompanied by confusion, excitement, irrational behavior; lasts from few hrs to 24 hrs after administration. **OCCASIONAL:** Pain at injection site. **RARE:** Rash.

ADVERSE EFFECTS/ TOXIC REACTIONS

Continuous/repeated intermittent infusion may result in extreme somnolence, circulatory/respiratory depression. Too-rapid IV administration may produce severe hypotension, respiratory depression, irregular muscle movements.

NURSING CONSIDERATIONS

BASELINE ASSESSMENT

Resuscitative equipment, O_2 must be available. Obtain vital signs before induction.

INTERVENTION/EVALUATION

Monitor vital signs q3–5min during and after administration until recovery is achieved. Assess for emergence reaction (hypnotic or barbiturate may be needed). Keep verbal, tactile, visual stimulation at minimum during recovery.

PATIENT/FAMILY TEACHING

• Avoid tasks that require alertness, motor skills for 24 hrs after anesthesia.

Ketek, *see telithromycin*

K

ketoconazole

kee-toe-**koe**-na-zole

(Apo-Ketoconazole ✤, Nizoral, Nizoral AD, Nizoral Topical, Novo-Ketoconazole ✤, Xolegel)

Do not confuse Nizoral with Nasarel.

CLASSIFICATION

PHARMACOTHERAPEUTIC: Imidazole derivative. **CLINICAL:** Antifungal (see p. 45C).

ACTION

Inhibits synthesis of ergosterol, a vital component of fungal cell formation. **Therapeutic Effect:** Damages fungal cell membrane, altering its function Fungistatic.

PHARMACOKINETICS

Well absorbed from GI tract following PO administration. Protein binding: 91%–99%. Metabolized in liver.

Primarily excreted in bile with minimal elimination in urine. Negligible systemic absorption following topical absorption. Ketoconazole is not detected in plasma after shampooing, topical administration. **Half-life:** 2–12 hrs.

USES

Oral: Treatment of histoplasmosis, blastomycosis, candidiasis, chronic mucocutaneous candidiasis, coccidioidomycosis, paracoccidioidomycosis, chromomycosis, seborrheic dermatitis, tineas (ringworm): corporis, capitis, manus, cruris, pedis, unguium (onychomycosis), oral thrush, candiduria. **Shampoo:** Reduces scaling due to dandruff. Treatment of tinea versicolor. **Topical:** Treatment of tineas, pityriasis versicolor, cutaneous candidiasis, seborrhea dermatitis, dandruff. **Xolegel:** Treatment of seborrheic dermatitis. **OFF-LABEL: Systemic:** Treatment of fungal pneumonia, prostate cancer, septicemia.

K

PRECAUTIONS

CONTRAINDICATIONS: None known. **CAUTIONS:** Hepatic impairment.

LIFESPAN CONSIDERATIONS:

Pregnancy/Lactation: Oral form distributed in breast milk. Unknown if topical form crosses placena or is distributed in breast milk. **Pregnancy Category C. Children:** **Cream, shampoo:** Safety and efficacy not established. **Oral form:** Safety and efficacy not established in those younger than 2 yrs. **Elderly:** No age-related precautions noted.

INTERACTIONS

DRUG: May increase concentration/toxicity of **midazolam, triazolam, cyclosporine, sirolimus, tacrolimus, digoxin, protease inhibitors (e.g., indinavir, ritonavir, saquinavir), ergot alkaloids, warfarin. Isoniazid, rifampin** may decrease concentration/effect. **Erythromycin** may increase risk of cardiac toxicity. **Antacids, H_2 antagonists, proton pump inhibitors (e.g., omeprazole)** may decrease absorption. **HERBAL: Echinacea** may have additive hepatotoxic effects. **St. John's wort** may decrease concentration. **FOOD:** None known. **LAB VALUES:** May increase serum alkaline phosphatase, bilirubin, AST, ALT. May decrease serum corticosteroid, testosterone.

AVAILABILITY (Rx)

CREAM (NIZORAL TOPICAL): 2%. **GEL (XOLEGEL):** 2%. **SHAMPOO (NIZORAL AD [OTC]):** 1%. **TABLETS (NIZORAL):** 200 mg.

ADMINISTRATION/HANDLING

PO

• Give with food to minimize GI irritation. • Tablets may be crushed. • Ketoconazole requires acidity; give antacids, anticholinergics, H_2 blockers **at least** 2 hrs following dosing.

SHAMPOO

• Apply to wet hair, massage for 1 min, rinse thoroughly, reapply for 3 min, rinse.

TOPICAL

• Apply, rub gently into affected/surrounding area.

INDICATIONS/ROUTES/DOSAGE

USUAL DOSAGE

PO: ADULTS, ELDERLY: 200–400 mg/day. **CHILDREN:** 3.3–6.6 mg/kg/day. **Maximum:** 800 mg/day in 2 divided doses.

TOPICAL: ADULTS, ELDERLY: Apply to affected area 1–2 times a day for 2–4 wks.

SHAMPOO: ADULTS, ELDERLY: Use twice weekly for 4 wks, allowing at least 3 days between shampooing. Use intermittently to maintain control.

SIDE EFFECTS

OCCASIONAL (10%–3%): Nausea, vomiting. **RARE (less than 2%):** Abdominal pain, diarrhea, headache, dizziness, photophobia. **Topical:** Burning, irritation, pruritus.

ADVERSE EFFECTS/ TOXIC REACTIONS

Hematologic toxicity (thrombocytopenia, hemolytic anemia, leukopenia) occurs occasionally. Hepatotoxicity may occur within first wk to several mos after starting therapy. Anaphylaxis occurs rarely.

NURSING CONSIDERATIONS

BASELINE ASSESSMENT

Confirm that culture or histologic test was done for accurate diagnosis; therapy may begin before results known.

INTERVENTION/EVALUATION

Monitor hepatic function tests; be alert for hepatotoxicity: dark urine, pale stools, jaundice, fatigue, anorexia, nausea, or vomiting (unrelieved by giving medication with food). Monitor CBC for hematologic toxicity. Monitor daily pattern of bowel activity/stool consistency. Assess for dizziness, provide assistance as needed. Evaluate skin for rash, urticaria, pruritus. **Topical:** Check for localized burning, pruritus, irritation.

PATIENT/FAMILY TEACHING

• Prolonged therapy (wks or mos) is usually necessary. • Do not miss a dose; continue therapy as long as directed. • Avoid alcohol (potential for hepatotoxicity). • May cause dizziness; avoid tasks that require alertness, motor skills until response to drug is established. • Take antacids, antiulcer medications at least 2 hrs after ketoconazole. • Notify physician of dark urine, pale stool, yellow skin or eyes, increased irritation in topical use, onset of other new symptoms. • **Topical:** Rub well into affected areas. • Avoid contact with eyes. • Keep skin clean, dry; wear light clothing for ventilation. • Separate personal items in direct contact with affected area. • **Shampoo:** Initially, use 2 times a wk for 4 wks with at least 3 days between shampooing; frequency then determined by response to medication.

ketoprofen

kee-toe-**proe**-fen

(Apo-Keto ✽, Novo-Keto-EC ✽, Orudis KT, Oruvail, Rhodis ✽)

CLASSIFICATION

PHARMACOTHERAPEUTIC: Nonsteroidal anti-inflammatory. **CLINICAL:** Antirheumatic, analgesic, antidysmenorrheal, vascular headache suppressant (see p. 124C).

ACTION

Produces analgesic, anti-inflammatory effects by inhibiting prostaglandin synthesis. **Therapeutic Effect:** Reduces inflammatory response, intensity of pain.

PHARMACOKINETICS

Immediate-release capsules are rapidly, well absorbed following PO administration; extended-release capsules are well-absorbed. Protein binding: 99%. Metabolized in liver. Excreted in urine; less than 10% excreted as unchanged (unconjugated) drug. **Half-life:** 2.4 hrs.

K

USES

Symptomatic treatment of acute and chronic rheumatoid arthritis, osteoarthritis. Relief of mild to moderate pain, primary dysmenorrhea. **OFF-LABEL:** Treatment of acute gouty arthritis, psoriatic arthritis, ankylosing spondylitis, vascular headache.

PRECAUTIONS

CONTRAINDICATIONS: Active peptic ulcer disease, chronic inflammation of GI tract, GI bleeding/ulceration, history of hypersensitivity to aspirin, NSAIDs. **CAUTIONS:** Renal/hepatic impairment, history of GI tract disease, predisposition to fluid retention.

K

LIFESPAN CONSIDERATIONS:

Pregnancy/Lactation: Crosses placenta; unknown if distributed in breast milk. Avoid during late pregnancy (ductus arteriosis). **Pregnancy Category C. (D if used in third trimester or near delivery).** **Children:** Safety and efficacy not established. **Elderly:** Age-related renal impairment may require dosage adjustment.

INTERACTIONS

DRUG: May decrease effects of **antihypertensives, diuretics. Aspirin, other salicylates** may increase risk of GI side effects, bleeding. **Bone marrow depressants** may increase risk of hematologic reactions. May increase effects of **heparin, oral anticoagulants, thrombolytics.** May increase concentration, risk of toxicity of **lithium.** May increase risk of **methotrexate** toxicity. **Probenecid** may increase concentration. **HERBAL: Cat's claw, dong quai, evening primrose, feverfew, red clover, horse chestnut, garlic, ginseng, ginkgo** may increase antiplatelet acitivity, risk of bleeding. **FOOD:** None known. **LAB VALUES:** May prolong bleeding time. May increase serum alkaline phosphatase, hepatic function test results. May decrease Hgb, Hct, serum sodium.

AVAILABILITY (OTC)

CAPSULES: 25 mg, 50 mg, 75 mg. **TABLETS (ORUDIS KT):** 12.5 mg (OTC).

CAPSULES (EXTENDED-RELEASE [ORUVAIL]): 200 mg.

ADMINISTRATION/HANDLING

PO

• May give with food, milk, full glass (8 oz) of water (minimizes potential GI distress). • Do not break, chew extended-release capsules.

INDICATIONS/ROUTES/DOSAGE

ACUTE OR CHRONIC RHEUMATOID ARTHRITIS AND OSTEOARTHRITIS

PO: ADULTS: Initially, 75 mg 3 times a day or 50 mg 4 times a day. **ELDERLY:** Initially, 25–50 mg 3–4 times a day. Maintenance: 150–300 mg/day in 3–4 divided doses.

PO (EXTENDED-RELEASE): ADULTS, ELDERLY: 200 mg once a day.

MILD TO MODERATE PAIN, DYSMENORRHEA

PO: ADULTS, ELDERLY: 25–50 mg q6–8h. **Maximum:** 300 mg/day.

OVER-THE-COUNTER (OTC) DOSAGE

PO: ADULTS, ELDERLY: 12.5 mg q4–6h. **Maximum:** 6 tabs/day.

DOSAGE IN RENAL IMPAIRMENT

MILD: 150 mg/day maximum. **SEVERE:** 100 mg/day maximum.

SIDE EFFECTS

FREQUENT (11%): Dyspepsia (heartburn, indigestion, epigastric pain). **OCCASIONAL (more than 3%):** Nausea, diarrhea/constipation, flatulence, abdominal cramps, headache. **RARE (less than 2%):** Anorexia, vomiting, visual disturbances, fluid retention.

ADVERSE EFFECTS/ TOXIC REACTIONS

Peptic ulcer, GI bleeding, gastritis, severe hepatic reaction (cholestasis, jaundice) occur rarely. Nephrotoxicity (dysuria, hematuria, proteinuria, nephrotic syndrome), severe hypersensitivity reaction (bronchospasm, angioedema) occur rarely.

NURSING CONSIDERATIONS

BASELINE ASSESSMENT

Assess onset, type, location, duration of pain/inflammation. Inspect appearance of affected joints for immobility, deformities, skin condition.

INTERVENTION/EVALUATION

Monitor for evidence of nausea, dyspepsia. Monitor for therapeutic response (relief of pain, improved range of motion, grip strength, mobility). Monitor renal/hepatic function tests, mental status.

PATIENT/FAMILY TEACHING

• Avoid aspirin, alcohol during therapy (increases risk of GI bleeding). • If GI upset occurs, take with food, milk. • Swallow capsule whole; do not crush/chew.

ketorolac

key-**tore**-oh-lack

(Acular, Acular LS, Acular PF, Toradol, Toradol IM, Toradol IV/IM)

Do not confuse Acular with Acthar or Ocular.

♦CLASSIFICATION

PHARMACOTHERAPEUTIC: Nonsteroidal anti-inflammatory. **CLINICAL:** Analgesic, intraocular anti-inflammatory (see p. 124C).

ACTION

Inhibits prostaglandin synthesis, reduces prostaglandin levels in aqueous humor. **Therapeutic Effect:** Reduces intensity of pain stimulus, reduces intraocular inflammation.

PHARMACOKINETICS

Route	Onset	Peak	Duration
PO	30–60 min	1.5–4 hrs	4–6 hrs
IV/IM	30 min	1–2 hrs	4–6 hrs

Readily absorbed from GI tract after IM administration. Protein binding: 99%. Largely metabolized in liver. Primarily excreted in urine. Not removed by hemodialysis. **Half-life:** 3.8–6.3 hrs (increased with renal impairment, in elderly).

USES

Short-term relief of mild to moderate pain. **Ophthalmic:** Relief of ocular itching due to seasonal allergic conjunctivitis. Treatment postop for inflammation following cataract extraction, pain following incisional refractive surgery. **OFF-LABEL:** Prevention, treatment of ocular inflammation (ophthalmic form).

PRECAUTIONS

CONTRAINDICATIONS: Active peptic ulcer disease, chronic inflammation of GI tract, GI bleeding/ulceration, history of hypersensitivity to aspirin, NSAIDs. **CAUTIONS:** Renal/hepatic impairment, history of GI tract disease, predisposition to fluid retention.

⌛ LIFESPAN CONSIDERATIONS:

Pregnancy/Lactation: Unknown if drug is excreted in breast milk. Avoid

K

use during third trimester (may adversely affect fetal cardiovascular system: premature closure of ductus arteriosus). **Pregnancy Category C (D if used in third trimester)**. **Children:** Safety and efficacy not established, but doses of 0.5 mg/kg have been used. **Elderly:** GI bleeding, ulceration more likely to cause serious adverse effects. Age-related renal impairment may increase risk of hepatic/renal toxicity; decreased dosage recommended.

INTERACTIONS

DRUG: May decrease effects of **antihypertensives, diuretics. Aspirin, other salicylates** may increase risk of GI side effects, bleeding. **Bone marrow depressants** may increase risk of hematologic reactions. May increase effects of **heparin, oral anticoagulants, thrombolytics.** May increase concentration, risk of toxicity of **lithium.** May increase risk of **methotrexate** toxicity. **Probenecid** may increase concentration. **HERBAL:** **Cat's claw, dong quai, evening primrose, feverfew, red clover, horse chestnet, garlic, ginseng, ginkgo** may decrease antiplatelet activity, risk of bleeding. **FOOD:** None known. **LAB VALUES:** May prolong bleeding time. May increase hepatic function test results.

AVAILABILITY (Rx)

INJECTION SOLUTION (TORADOL, TORADOL IM, TORADOL IV/IM): 15 mg/ml, 30 mg/ml. **OPHTHALMIC SOLUTION:** 0.4% (Acular LS), 0.5% (Acular, Acular PF). **TABLETS (TORADOL):** 10 mg.

ADMINISTRATION/HANDLING

IV

• Give undiluted as IV push. • Give over at least 15 sec.

IM

• Give deep IM slowly into large muscle mass.

PO

• Give with food, milk, antacids if GI distress occurs.

OPHTHALMIC

• Place finger on lower eyelid, pull out until pocket is formed between eye and lower lid. Hold dropper above pocket, place prescribed number of drops in pocket. • Close eye gently. Apply digital pressure to lacrimal sac for 1–2 min (minimizes drainage into nose/throat, reducing risk of systemic effects).

IV INCOMPATIBILITY

Promethazine (Phenergan).

IV COMPATIBILITIES

Fentanyl (Sublimaze), hydromorphone (Dilaudid), morphine, nalbuphine (Nubain).

INDICATIONS/ROUTES/DOSAGE

SHORT-TERM RELIEF OF MILD TO MODERATE PAIN (MULTIPLE DOSES)

PO: ADULTS, ELDERLY: 10 mg q4–6h. **Maximum:** 40 mg/24 hrs.

IV, IM: ADULTS YOUNGER THAN 65 YRS: 30 mg q6h. **Maximum:** 120 mg/24 hrs. **ADULTS 65 YRS AND OLDER, THOSE WITH RENAL IMPAIRMENT, THOSE WEIGHING LESS THAN 50 KG:** 15 mg q6h. **Maximum:** 60 mg/24 hrs. **CHILDREN 2–16 YRS:** 0.5 mg/kg q6h.

SHORT-TERM RELIEF OF MILD TO MODERATE PAIN (SINGLE DOSE)

IV: ADULTS YOUNGER THAN 65 YRS, CHILDREN 17 YRS AND OLDER WEIGHING MORE THAN 50 KG: 30 mg. **ADULTS 65 YRS AND OLDER, WITH RENAL IMPAIRMENT, WEIGHING LESS THAN 50 KG:** 15 mg. **CHILDREN 2–16 YRS:** 0.5 mg/kg. **Maximum:** 15 mg.

IM: ADULTS YOUNGER THAN 65 YRS, CHILDREN 17 YRS AND OLDER, WEIGHING

MORE THAN 50 KG: 60 mg. **ADULTS 65 YRS AND OLDER, WITH RENAL IMPAIRMENT, WEIGHING LESS THAN 50 KG:** 30 mg. **CHILDREN 2–16 YRS:** 1 mg/kg. **Maximum:** 15 mg.

ALLERGIC CONJUNCTIVITIS

OPHTHALMIC: ADULTS, ELDERLY, CHILDREN 3 YRS AND OLDER: 1 drop 4 times a day.

CATARACT EXTRACTION

OPHTHALMIC: ADULTS, ELDERLY: 1 drop 4 times a day. Begin 24 hrs after surgery and continue for 2 wks.

REFRACTIVE SURGERY

OPHTHALMIC: ADULTS, ELDERLY: 1 drop 4 times a day for 3 days.

SIDE EFFECTS

FREQUENT (17%–12%): Headache, nausea, abdominal cramps/pain, dyspepsia (heartburn, indigestion, epigastric pain). **OCCASIONAL (9%–3%):** Diarrhea. **Ophthalmic:** Transient stinging, burning. **RARE (3%–1%):** Constipation, vomiting, flatulence, stomatitis. **Ophthalmic:** Ocular irritation, allergic reactions (manifested by pruritus, stinging), superficial ocular infection, keratitis.

ADVERSE EFFECTS/ TOXIC REACTIONS

Peptic ulcer, GI bleeding, gastritis, severe hepatic reaction (cholestasis, jaundice) occur rarely. Nephrotoxicity (glomerular nephritis, interstitial nephritis, nephrotic syndrome) may occur in pts with preexisting renal impairment. Acute hypersensitivity reaction (fever, chills, joint pain) occurs rarely.

NURSING CONSIDERATIONS

BASELINE ASSESSMENT

Assess onset, type, location, duration of pain.

INTERVENTION/EVALUATION

Monitor renal/hepatic function tests, urinary output. Monitor daily pattern of bowel activity/stool consistency. Observe for occult blood loss. Evaluate for therapeutic response: relief of pain, stiffness, swelling; increased joint mobility, reduced joint tenderness, improved grip strength. Be alert to signs of bleeding (may also occur with ophthalmic route due to systemic absorption).

PATIENT/FAMILY TEACHING

• Avoid aspirin, alcohol during therapy with oral or ophthalmic ketorolac (increases tendency to bleed). • If GI upset occurs, take with food, milk. • Avoid tasks that require alertness, motor skills until response to drug is established. • **Ophthalmic:** Transient stinging, burning may occur upon instillation. • Do not administer while wearing soft contact lenses.

K

Klonopin, *see clonazepam*

Klor-Con, *see potassium chloride*

Kytril, *see granisetron*

labetalol

lah-**bet**-ah-lol
(Apo-Labetolol ♣, Normodyne, Trandate)

Do not confuse Trandate with tramadol or Trental.

FIXED-COMBINATION(S)

Normozide: labetalol/hydrochlorothiazide (a diuretic): 100 mg/25 mg; 200 mg/25 mg; 300 mg/25 mg.

CLASSIFICATION

PHARMACOTHERAPEUTIC: Alpha-, beta-adrenergic blocker. **CLINICAL:** Antihypertensive.

ACTION

Blocks alpha$_1$-, beta$_1$-, beta$_2$- (large doses) adrenergic receptor sites. Large doses increase airway resistance. **Therapeutic Effect:** Slows sinus heart rate; decreases peripheral vascular resistance, cardiac output B/P.

PHARMACOKINETICS

Route	Onset	Peak	Duration
PO	0.5–2 hrs	2–4 hrs	8–12 hrs
IV	2–5 min	5–15 min	2–4 hrs

Completely absorbed from GI tract. Protein binding: 50%. Undergoes first-pass metabolism. Metabolized in liver. Primarily excreted in urine. Not removed by hemodialysis. **Half-life:** PO, 6–8 hrs; IV, 5.5 hrs.

USES

Management of mild to severe hypertension. May be used alone or in combination with other antihypertensives. **OFF-LABEL:** Control of hypotension during surgery, treatment of chronic angina pectoris.

PRECAUTIONS

CONTRAINDICATIONS: Bronchial asthma, cardiogenic shock, overt cardiac failure, second- or third-degree heart block, severe bradycardia, uncontrolled CHF, other conditions associated with severe, prolonged hypotension. **CAUTIONS:** Medication-controlled CHF, nonallergic bronchospastic disease (chronic bronchitis, emphysema), hepatic or cardiac impairment, pheochromocytoma, diabetes mellitus.

LIFESPAN CONSIDERATIONS:

Pregnancy/Lactation: Drug crosses placenta. Small amount distributed in breast milk. **Pregnancy Category C (D if used in second or third trimester).** **Children:** Safety and efficacy not established. **Elderly:** Age-related peripheral vascular disease may increase susceptibility to decreased peripheral circulation.

INTERACTIONS

DRUG: Diuretics, other antihypertensives may increase hypotensive effect. **Insulin, oral hypoglycemics** may mask symptoms of hypoglycemia, prolong hypoglycemic effect of these drugs. **MAOIs** may produce hypertension. **Sympathomimetics, xanthines** may mutually inhibit effects. **HERBAL: Ephedra, ginseng, yohimbe** may worsen hypertension. **Garlic** may increase antihypertensive effect. **Licorice** may cause water retention, increased serum sodium, decreased serum potassium. **FOOD:** None known. **LAB VALUES:** May increase serum antinuclear antibody titer (ANA), BUN, serum LDH, lipoprotein, alkaline phosphatase, bilirubin, creatinine, potassium, triglyceride, uric acid, AST, ALT.

AVAILABILITY (Rx)

INJECTION SOLUTION (TRANDATE): 5 mg/ml. **TABLETS (NORMODYNE, TRANDATE):** 100 mg, 200 mg, 300 mg.

ADMINISTRATION/HANDLING

IV

◀ ALERT ▶ Pt must be in supine position for IV administration and for

3 hrs after receiving medication (substantial drop in B/P upon standing should be expected).

Reconstitution • For IV infusion, dilute 200 mg in 160 ml D_5W, 0.9% NaCl, lactated Ringer's, or any combination thereof to provide concentration of 1 mg/ml.

Rate of administration • For IV push, give over 2 min at 10-min intervals. • For IV infusion, administer at rate of 2 mg/min (2 ml/min) initially. Rate is adjusted according to B/P. • Monitor B/P immediately before and q5–10min during IV administration (maximum effect occurs within 5 min).

Storage • Store at room temperature. • After dilution, IV solution is stable for 24 hrs. • Solution appears clear, colorless to light yellow. • Discard if discolored or precipitate forms.

PO

• Give without regard to food. • Tablets may be crushed.

IV INCOMPATIBILITIES

Amphotericin B complex (Abelcet, AmBisome, Amphotec), ceftriaxone (Rocephin), furosemide (Lasix), heparin, nafcillin (Nafcil), thiopental.

IV COMPATIBILITIES

Aminophylline, amiodarone (Cordarone), calcium gluconate, diltiazem (Cardizem), dobutamine (Dobutrex), dopamine (Intropin), enalapril (Vasotec), fentanyl (Sublimaze), hydromorphone (Dilaudid), lidocaine, lorazepam (Ativan), magnesium sulfate, midazolam (Versed), milrinone (Primacor), morphine, nitroglycerin, norepinephrine (Levophed), potassium chloride, potassium phosphate, propofol (Diprivan).

INDICATIONS/ROUTES/DOSAGE

HYPERTENSION

PO: ADULTS: Initially, 100 mg twice a day adjusted in increments of 100 mg twice a day q2–3 days. Maintenance: 200–400 mg twice a day. **Maximum:** 2.4 g/day. **ELDERLY:** Initially, 100 mg 1–2 times a day. May increase as needed.

SEVERE HYPERTENSION, HYPERTENSIVE CRISIS

IV: ADULTS: Initially, 20 mg. Additional doses of 20–80 mg may be given at 10-min intervals, up to total dose of 300 mg.

IV INFUSION: ADULTS: Initially, 2 mg/min up to total dose of 300 mg.

PO (AFTER IV THERAPY): ADULTS: Initially, 200 mg; then, 200–400 mg in 6–12 hrs. Increase dose at 1-day intervals to desired level.

SIDE EFFECTS

FREQUENT: Drowsiness, difficulty sleeping, excessive fatigue, weakness, diminished sexual function, transient scalp tingling. **OCCASIONAL:** Dizziness, dyspnea, peripheral edema, depression, anxiety, constipation, diarrhea, nasal congestion, nausea, vomiting, abdominal discomfort. **RARE:** Altered taste, dry eyes, increased urination, paresthesia.

ADVERSE EFFECTS/ TOXIC REACTIONS

May precipitate, aggravate CHF due to decreased myocardial stimulation. Abrupt withdrawal may precipitate myocardial ischemia, producing chest pain, diaphoresis, palpitations, headache, tremor. May mask signs, symptoms of acute hypoglycemia (tachycardia, B/P changes) in diabetic pts.

NURSING CONSIDERATIONS

BASELINE ASSESSMENT

Assess baseline renal/hepatic function tests. Assess B/P, apical pulse immediately before drug administration (if pulse is 60/min or less or systolic B/P is lower than 90 mm Hg, withhold medication, contact physician).

L

INTERVENTION/EVALUATION

Monitor B/P for hypotension. Assess pulse for quality, irregular rate, bradycardia. Monitor EKG for cardiac arrhythmias. Monitor daily pattern of bowel activity/stool consistency. Assist with ambulation if dizziness occurs. Assess for evidence of CHF: dyspnea (particularly on exertion or lying down), night cough, peripheral edema, distended neck veins. Monitor I&O (increase in weight, decrease in urine output may indicate CHF).

PATIENT/FAMILY TEACHING

• Do not discontinue drug except upon advice of physician (abrupt discontinuation may precipitate heart failure). • Compliance with therapy regimen is essential to control hypertension, arrhythmias. • Avoid tasks that require alertness, motor skills until response to drug is established. • Report shortness of breath, excessive fatigue, weight gain, prolonged dizziness, headache. • Do not use nasal decongestants, OTC cold preparations (stimulants) without physician approval.

L

lactulose

lak-tyoo-lose

(Acilac ♣, Apo-Lactulose ♣, Constulose, Enulose, Generlac, Kristalose, Laxilose ♣)

Do not confuse lactulose with lactose.

CLASSIFICATION

PHARMACOTHERAPEUTIC: Lactose derivative. **CLINICAL:** Hyperosmotic laxative, ammonia detoxicant (see p. 118C).

ACTION

Retains ammonia in colon (decreases serum ammonia concentration) producing osmotic effect. **Therapeutic Effect:** Promotes increased peristalsis, bowel evacuation, expelling ammonia from colon.

PHARMACOKINETICS

Route	Onset	Peak	Duration
PO	24–48 hrs	N/A	N/A
Rectal	30–60 min	N/A	N/A

Poorly absorbed from GI tract. Extensively metabolized in colon. Primarily excreted in feces.

USES

Prevention, treatment of portal systemic encephalopathy (including hepatic precoma, coma); treatment of constipation.

PRECAUTIONS

CONTRAINDICATIONS: Abdominal pain, appendicitis, nausea, pts on galactose-free diet, vomiting. **CAUTIONS:** Diabetes mellitus.

LIFESPAN CONSIDERATIONS:

Pregnancy/Lactation: Unknown if drug crosses placenta or is distributed in breast milk. **Pregnancy Category B.** **Children:** Avoid use in children younger than 6 yrs (usually unable to describe symptoms). **Elderly:** No age-related precautions noted.

INTERACTIONS

DRUG: May decrease transit time of concurrently administered **oral medications,** decreasing absorption. **HERBAL:** None significant. **FOOD:** None known. **LAB VALUES:** May decrease serum potassium.

AVAILABILITY (Rx)

PACKETS (KRISTALOSE): 10 g, 20 g. **SYRUP (CONSTULOSE, ENULOSE, GENERLAC):** 10 g/15 ml.

ADMINISTRATION/HANDLING

PO

• Store solution at room temperature. • Solution appears pale yellow to yellow, viscous liquid. Cloudiness, darkened solution does not indicate potency loss. • Drink water, juice, milk with each dose (aids stool softening, increases palatability).

RECTAL

• Lubricate anus with petroleum jelly before enema insertion. • Insert carefully (prevents damage to rectal wall) with nozzle toward navel. • Squeeze container until entire dose expelled. • Retain until definite lower abdominal cramping felt.

INDICATIONS/ROUTES/DOSAGE

CONSTIPATION

PO: ADULTS, ELDERLY: 15–30 ml (10–20 g)/day, up to 60 ml (40 g)/day. **CHILDREN:** 7.5 ml (5 g)/day after breakfast.

PORTAL-SYSTEMIC ENCEPHALOPATHY

PO: ADULTS, ELDERLY: Initially, 30–45 ml every hr to induce rapid laxation. Then, 30–45 ml (20–30 g) 3–4 times a day. Adjust dose q1–2 days to produce 2–3 soft stools a day. Usual daily dose: 90–150 ml (60–100 g). **CHILDREN:** 40–90 ml/day in divided doses 3–4 times a day. **INFANTS:** 2.5–10 ml/day in 3–4 divided doses.

RECTAL (AS RETENTION ENEMA): ADULTS, ELDERLY: 300 ml (200 g) with 700 ml water or saline solution; pt should retain 30–60 min. Repeat q4–6h. If evacuation occurs too promptly, repeat immediately.

SIDE EFFECTS

OCCASIONAL: Abdominal cramping, flatulence, increased thirst, abdominal discomfort. **RARE:** Nausea, vomiting.

ADVERSE EFFECTS/ TOXIC REACTIONS

Diarrhea indicates overdose. Long-term use may result in laxative dependence, chronic constipation, loss of normal bowel function.

NURSING CONSIDERATIONS

INTERVENTION/EVALUATION

Encourage adequate fluid intake. Assess bowel sounds for peristalsis. Monitor daily pattern of bowel activity/stool consistency; record time of evacuation. Assess for abdominal disturbances. Monitor serum electrolytes in pts exposed to prolonged, frequent, excessive use of medication.

PATIENT/FAMILY TEACHING

• Evacuation occurs in 24–48 hrs of initial dose. • Institute measures to promote defecation: increase fluid intake, exercise, high-fiber diet.

Lamictal, *see lamotrigine*

Lamisil Oral, *see terbinafine*

lamivudine

lah-**mih**-view-deen

(Epivir, Epivir-HBV, Heptovir ✤)

Do not confuse lamivudine with lamotrigine.

FIXED-COMBINATION(S)

Combivir: lamivudine/zidovudine (an antiviral): 150 mg/300 mg. **Epzicom:** lamivudine/abacavir (an antiviral): 300 mg/600 mg. **Trizivir:** lamivudine/zidovudine/abacavir (an antiviral): 150 mg/300 mg/300 mg.

CLASSIFICATION

PHARMACOTHERAPEUTIC: Nucleoside reverse transcriptase inhibitors. **CLINICAL:** Antiviral (see pp. 65C, 111C).

ACTION

Inhibits HIV reverse transcriptase by viral DNA chain termination. Inhibits

RNA-, DNA-dependent DNA polymerase, an enzyme necessary for HIV replication. **Therapeutic Effect:** Slows HIV replication, reduces progression of HIV infection.

PHARMACOKINETICS

Rapidly, completely absorbed from GI tract. Protein binding: less than 36%. Widely distributed (crosses blood-brain barrier). Primarily excreted unchanged in urine. Not removed by hemodialysis or peritoneal dialysis. **Half-life:** 11–15 hrs (intracellular), 2–11 hrs (serum, adults), 1.7–2 hrs (serum, children) (increased in renal impairment).

USES

Epivir: Treatment of HIV infection in combination with other antiretroviral agents. **Epivir HBV:** Treatment of chronic hepatitis B. **OFF-LABEL:** Prophylaxis in health care workers at risk of acquiring HIV after occupational exposure to virus.

L

PRECAUTIONS

CONTRAINDICATIONS: None known. **CAUTIONS:** Peripheral neuropathy, history of peripheral neuropathy, history of pancreatitis in children, renal impairment.

LIFESPAN CONSIDERATIONS:

Pregnancy/Lactation: Drug crosses placenta. Unknown if distributed in breast milk. Breast-feeding not recommended (possibility of HIV transmission). **Pregnancy Category C. Children:** Safety and efficacy not established in those younger than 3 mos. **Elderly:** Age-related renal impairment may require dosage adjustment.

INTERACTIONS

DRUG: Co-trimoxazole increases concentration. **Zalcitabine** may inhibit intracellular phosphorylation of both drugs; avoid concurrent administration. **HERBAL: St. John's wort** may decrease concentration, effect. **FOOD:** None known. **LAB VALUES:** May increase Hgb, neutrophil count, serum amylase, AST, ALT.

AVAILABILITY (Rx)

ORAL SOLUTION: 5 mg/ml (Epivir-HBV), 10 mg/ml (Epivir). **TABLETS:** 100 mg (Epivir-HBV), 150 mg (Epivir), 300 mg (Epivir).

ADMINISTRATION/HANDLING

PO

- Give without regard to meals.

INDICATIONS/ROUTES/DOSAGE

HIV INFECTION

PO: ADULTS, CHILDREN 12–16 YRS, WEIGHING 50 KG (100 LB) OR MORE: 150 mg twice a day or 300 mg once a day. **ADULTS WEIGHING LESS THAN 50 KG:** 2 mg/kg twice a day. **CHILDREN 3 MOS–11 YRS:** 4 mg/kg twice a day (up to 150 mg/dose).

CHRONIC HEPATITIS B

PO: ADULTS, CHILDREN 17 YRS AND OLDER: 100 mg/day. **CHILDREN YOUNGER THAN 17 YRS:** 3 mg/kg/day. **Maximum:** 100 mg/day.

DOSAGE IN RENAL IMPAIRMENT

Dosage and frequency are modified based on creatinine clearance.

Creatinine Clearance (ml/min)	Dosage
50 ml/min or higher	150 mg twice a day
30–49 ml/min	150 mg once a day
15–29 ml/min	150 mg first dose, then 100 mg once a day
5–14 ml/min	150 mg first dose, then 50 mg once a day
Less than 5 ml/min	50 mg first dose, then 25 mg once a day

SIDE EFFECTS

FREQUENT: Headache (35%), nausea (33%), malaise, fatigue (27%), nasal disturbances (20%), diarrhea, cough

(18%), musculoskeletal pain, neuropathy (12%), insomnia (11%), anorexia, dizziness, fever, chills (10%). **OCCASIONAL:** Depression (9%), myalgia (8%), abdominal cramps (6%), dyspepsia, arthralgia (5%).

ADVERSE EFFECTS/ TOXIC REACTIONS

Pancreatitis occurs in 13% of pediatric pts. Anemia, neutropenia, thrombocytopenia occur rarely. Lactic acidosis, severe hepatomegaly with steatosis have been reported.

NURSING CONSIDERATIONS

BASELINE ASSESSMENT

Establish baseline lab values, esp. renal function.

INTERVENTION/EVALUATION

Monitor serum creatinine, amylase, lipase, BUN. Assess for headache, nausea, cough. Monitor daily pattern of bowel activity/stool consistency. Modify diet or administer laxative as needed. Assess for dizziness, sleep pattern. If pancreatitis in children occurs, movement aggravates abdominal pain; sitting up, flexing at the waist relieves the pain.

PATIENT/FAMILY TEACHING

• Continue therapy for full length of treatment. • Doses should be evenly spaced. • Inform pt lamivudine is not a cure for HIV/AIDS nor does it reduce risk of transmission to others; pt may continue to experience illnesses, including opportunistic infections. • Avoid tasks requiring alertness, motor skills until response to drug is established. • Advise parents to closely monitor pediatric pts for symptoms of pancreatitis (severe, steady abdominal pain often radiating to the back, clammy skin, hypotension; nausea/vomiting may accompany abdominal pain).

lamotrigine

lam-**oh**-trih-jeen

(Apo-Lamotrigine ✤, Lamictal, Lamictal CD, Novo-Lamotrigine ✤)

Do not confuse lamotrigine with lamivudine.

◆CLASSIFICATION

CLINICAL: Anticonvulsants (see p. 34C).

ACTION

May block voltage-sensitive sodium channels, stabilizing neuronal membranes, regulating presynaptic transmitter release of excitatory amino acids. **Therapeutic Effect:** Produces anticonvulsant activity.

USES

Adjunctive therapy in adults and children with partial seizures, treatment of adults and children with generalized seizures of Lennox-Gastaut syndrome. Conversion to monotherapy in adults treated with another enzyme-inducing antiepileptic drug (EIAED). Long-term maintenance treatment of bipolar disorder. Treatment of pts 2 yrs and older with primary generalized tonic-clonic seizures.

PRECAUTIONS

CONTRAINDICATIONS: None known. **CAUTIONS:** Renal, hepatic, cardiac impairment.

⌛ LIFESPAN CONSIDERATIONS:

Pregnancy/Lactation: Distributed in breast milk. Breast-feeding not recommended. Increased fetal risk of oral cleft formation has been noted with use during pregnancy. **Pregnancy Category C. Children:** Safety and efficacy in pts 18 yrs and younger with bipolar disorder, 16 yrs and younger with epilepsy has not been established. **Elderly:** Age-related renal impairment may require dosage adjustment.

INTERACTIONS

DRUG: **Carbamazepine, phenobarbital, primidone, valproic acid** decrease concentration. May increase concentration of **carbamazepine, valproic acid.** **HERBAL:** **Evening primrose** may decrease seizure threshold. **FOOD:** None known. **LAB VALUES:** None known.

AVAILABILITY (Rx)

TABLETS: 25 mg, 100 mg, 150 mg, 200 mg. **TABLETS (CHEWABLE):** 2 mg, 5 mg, 25 mg.

ADMINISTRATION/HANDLING

PO

- Give without regard to food.

INDICATIONS/ROUTES/DOSAGE

SEIZURE CONTROL IN PTS RECEIVING ENZYME-INDUCING ANTIEPILEPTIC DRUGS (EIAEDs), WITHOUT VALPROIC ACID

PO: ADULTS, ELDERLY, CHILDREN OLDER THAN 12 YRS: Recommended as add-on therapy: 50 mg once a day for 2 wks, followed by 100 mg/day in 2 divided doses for 2 wks. Maintenance: Dosage may be increased by 100 mg/day every wk, up to 300–500 mg/day in 2 divided doses. **CHILDREN 2–12 YRS:** 0.6 mg/kg/day in 2 divided doses for 2 wks, then 1.2 mg/kg/day in 2 divided doses for wks 3 and 4. Maintenance: 5–15 mg/kg/day. **Maximum:** 400 mg/day.

SEIZURE CONTROL IN PTS RECEIVING COMBINATION THERAPY OF EIAEDs AND VALPROIC ACID

PO: ADULTS, ELDERLY, CHILDREN OLDER THAN 12 YRS: 25 mg every other day for 2 wks, followed by 25 mg once a day for 2 wks. Maintenance: Dosage may be increased by 25–50 mg/day q1–2wk, up to 150 mg/day in 2 divided doses. **CHILDREN 2–12 YRS:** 0.15 mg/kg/day in 2 divided doses for 2 wks, then 0.3 mg/kg/day in 2 divided doses for wks 3 and 4. Maintenance: 1–5 mg/kg/day in 2 divided doses. **Maximum:** 200 mg/day.

CONVERSION TO MONOTHERAPY FOR PTS RECEIVING EIAEDs

PO: ADULTS, ELDERLY, CHILDREN 16 YRS AND OLDER: 500 mg/day in 2 divided doses. Titrate to desired dose while maintaining EIAED at fixed level, then withdraw EIAED by 20% each wk over a 4-wk period.

CONVERSION TO MONOTHERAPY FOR PTS RECEIVING VALPROIC ACID

PO: ADULTS, ELDERLY, CHILDREN 16 YRS AND OLDER: Titrate lamotrigine to 200 mg/day, maintaining valproic acid dose. Maintain lamotrigine dose and decrease valproic acid to 500 mg/day, no greater than 500 mg/day/wk, then maintain 500 mg/day for 1 wk. Increase lamotrigine to 300 mg/day and decrease valproic acid to 250 mg/day. Maintain for 1 wk, then discontinue valproic acid and increase lamotrigine by 100 mg/day each wk until maintenance dose of 500 mg/day reached.

BIPOLAR DISORDER IN PTS RECEIVING EIAEDs

PO: ADULTS, ELDERLY: 50 mg/day for 2 wks, then 100 mg/day for 2 wks, then 200 mg/day for 1 wk, then 300 mg/day for 1 wk, then up to usual maintenance dose 400 mg/day in divided doses.

BIPOLAR DISORDER IN PTS RECEIVING VALPROIC ACID

PO: ADULTS, ELDERLY: 25 mg/day every other day for 2 wks, then 25 mg/day for 2 wks, then 50 mg/day for 1 wk, then 100 mg/day. Usual maintenance dose with valproic acid: 100 mg/day.

DISCONTINUATION THERAPY

◄ ALERT ► A dosage reduction of approximately 50% per wk over at least 2 wks is recommended.

DOSAGE IN RENAL IMPAIRMENT

◄ ALERT ► Decreased dosage may be effective in pts with significant renal impairment.

SIDE EFFECTS

FREQUENT: Dizziness (38%), headache (29%), diplopia (double vision) (28%), ataxia (22%), nausea (19%), blurred vision (16%), somnolence, rhinitis (14%). **OCCASIONAL (10%–5%):** Rash, pharyngitis, vomiting, cough, flu-like symptoms, diarrhea, dysmenorrhea, fever, insomnia, dyspepsia. **RARE:** Constipation, tremor, anxiety, pruritus, vaginitis, hypersensitivity reaction.

ADVERSE EFFECTS/ TOXIC REACTIONS

Abrupt withdrawal may increase seizure frequency. Serious rashes, including Stevens-Johnson syndrome have been reported.

NURSING CONSIDERATIONS

BASELINE ASSESSMENT

Review history of seizure disorder (type, onset, intensity, frequency, duration, level of consciousness [LOC]), drug history (esp. other anticonvulsants), other medical conditions (e.g., renal impairment). Provide safety precautions; quiet, dark environment.

INTERVENTION/EVALUATION

Report to physician promptly if rash occurs (drug discontinuation may be necessary). Assist with ambulation if dizziness, ataxia occurs. Assess for clinical improvement (decreased intensity/frequency of seizures). Assess for visual abnormalities, headache.

PATIENT/FAMILY TEACHING

• Take medication only as prescribed; do not abruptly withdraw medication after long-term therapy. • Avoid alcohol, tasks that require alertness, motor skills until response to drug is established. • Carry identification card/bracelet to note anticonvulsant therapy. • Strict maintenance of drug therapy is essential for seizure control. • Report to physician any rash, fever, swelling of glands. • May cause photosensitivity reaction; avoid exposure to sunlight, artificial light.

Lanoxin, *see digoxin*

lansoprazole

lan-so-**prah**-zoll

(Prevacid, Prevacid IV, Prevacid Solu-Tab)

Do not confuse Prevacid with Pepcid, Pravachol, or Prevpac.

FIXED-COMBINATION(S)

Prevacid NapraPac: lansoprazole/naproxen (an NSAID): 15 mg/375 mg; 15 mg/500 mg.

CLASSIFICATION

CLINICAL: Proton pump inhibitor (see p. 139C).

ACTION

Selectively inhibits parietal cell membrane enzyme system (hydrogen-potassium adenosine triphosphatase), proton pump. **Therapeutic Effect:** Suppresses gastric acid secretion.

PHARMACOKINETICS

Route	Onset	Peak	Duration
PO (15 mg)	2–3 hrs	N/A	24 hrs
PO (30 mg)	1–2 hrs	N/A	Longer than 24 hrs

Rapid, complete absorption (food may decrease absorption) once drug has left stomach. Protein binding: 97%. Distributed primarily to gastric parietal cells and converted to two active metabolites. Extensively metabolized in liver. Eliminated in bile and urine. Not removed by hemodialysis. **Half-life:** 1.5 hrs (increased in hepatic impairment, the elderly).

USES

Short-term treatment (4 wks and less) of healing, symptomatic relief of active duodenal ulcer, short-term treatment (8 wks and less) for healing, symptomatic relief of erosive esophagitis. Long-term treatment of pathologic hypersecretory conditions, including Zollinger-Ellison syndrome. Short-term treatment (8 wks and less) of active gastric ulcer, *H. pylori*–associated duodenal ulcer, maintenance treatment for healed duodenal ulcer. Treatment of gastroesophageal reflux disease (GERD), NSAID-associated gastric ulcer. **IV:** Short-term treatment of erosive esophagitis.

PRECAUTIONS

CONTRAINDICATIONS: None known. **CAUTIONS:** Hepatic impairment.

LIFESPAN CONSIDERATIONS:

Pregnancy/Lactation: Unknown if distributed in breast milk. **Pregnancy Category B. Children:** Safety and efficacy not established. **Elderly:** No age-related precautions noted but doses greater than 30 mg not recommended.

INTERACTIONS

DRUG: May interfere with absorption of **ampicillin, digoxin, iron salts, ketoconazole. Sucralfate** may delay absorption. **HERBAL:** None significant. **FOOD: Food** may decrease absorption. **LAB VALUES:** May increase LDH, serum alkaline phosphatase, bilirubin, cholesterol, creatinine, AST, ALT, triglycerides, uric acid. May produce abnormal albumin/globulin ratio, electrolyte balance, platelet, RBC, WBC counts. May increase Hgb, Hct.

AVAILABILITY (Rx)

GRANULES FOR ORAL SUSPENSION (PREVACID): 15 mg/pack; 30 mg/pack. **INJECTION POWDER FOR RECONSTITUTION (PREVACID IV):** 30 mg. **TABLETS, ORALLY-DISINTEGRATING (PREVACID SOLU-TAB):** 15 mg, 30 mg.

CAPSULES (DELAYED-RELEASE [PREVACID]): 15 mg, 30 mg.

ADMINISTRATION/HANDLING

IV

Reconstitution • Reconstitute with 5 ml Sterile Water for Injection. • Further dilute with 50 ml 0.9% NaCl or D_5W.

Rate of administration • Infuse over 30 min. • Use in-line filter.

Storage • Store at room temperature. • After reconstitution, stable for 1 hr prior to further dilution. • Following dilution, stable for 24 hrs in 0.9% NaCl, 12 hrs in D_5W.

PO

• Give while fasting or before meals (food diminishes absorption). • Do not chew/crush delayed-release capsules. • If pt has difficulty swallowing capsules, open capsules, sprinkle granules on 1 tbsp of applesauce, swallow immediately.

PO (SOLU-TAB)

• May give via oral syringe or nasogastric tube. • May dissolve in 4 ml (15 mg) or 10 ml (30 mg) water.

IV INCOMPATIBILITIES

Aminophylline, amphotericin B, ampicillin, ampicillin-sulbactam (Unasyn), aztreonam (Azactam), calcium gluconate, cefazolin (Ancef), cefepime (Maxipime), ciprofloxacin (Cipro), clindamycin (Cleocin), digoxin, diltiazem (Cardizem), diphenhydramine (Benadryl), dobutamine, dopamine, furosemide (Lasix), hydromorphone (Dilaudid), imipenem (Primaxin), lidocaine, lorazepam (Ativan), magnesium, midazolam (Versed), morphine, nitroglycerin, potassium chloride.

IV COMPATIBILITIES

Acyclovir (Zovirax), amikacin (Amikin), ceftriaxone (Rocephin), dexamethasone (Decadron), fluconazole (Diflucan), gentamicin, heparin, piperacillin/tazobactam (Zosyn).

INDICATIONS/ROUTES/DOSAGE

DUODENAL ULCER

PO: ADULTS, ELDERLY: 15 mg/day, before eating, preferably in the morning, for up to 4 wks. Maintenance: 15 mg/day.

EROSIVE ESOPHAGITIS

PO: ADULTS, ELDERLY: 30 mg/day, before eating, for up to 8 wks. If healing does not occur within 8 wks (in 5%–10% of cases), may give for additional 8 wks. Maintenance: 15 mg/day. **CHILDREN 12–17 YRS:** 30 mg/day up to 8 wks. **CHILDREN 1–11 YRS OF AGE, GREATER THAN 30 KG:** 30 mg/day; **30 KG OR LESS:** 15 mg/day.

IV: ADULTS, ELDERLY: 30 mg once a day for up to 7 days. Switch to oral lansoprazole therapy as soon as pt can tolerate oral route.

GASTRIC ULCER

PO: ADULTS: 30 mg/day for up to 8 wks.

NSAID GASTRIC ULCER

PO: ADULTS, ELDERLY: (Healing): 30 mg/day for up to 8 wks. (Prevention): 15 mg/day for up to 12 wks.

GASTROESOPHAGEAL REFLUX DISEASE

PO: ADULTS: 15 mg/day for up to 8 wks.

***H. PYLORI* INFECTION**

PO: ADULTS, ELDERLY: (triple drug therapy) 30 mg q12h for 10–14 days; (dual drug therapy) 30 mg q8h for 14 days.

PATHOLOGIC HYPERSECRETORY CONDITIONS (INCLUDING ZOLLINGER-ELLISON SYNDROME)

PO: ADULTS, ELDERLY: 60 mg/day. Individualize dosage according to pt needs and for as long as clinically indicated. Administer up to 120 mg/day in divided doses.

SIDE EFFECTS

OCCASIONAL (3%–2%): Diarrhea, abdominal pain, rash, pruritus, altered appetite. **RARE (1%):** Nausea, headache.

ADVERSE EFFECTS/ TOXIC REACTIONS

Bilirubinemia, eosinophilia, hyperlipemia occur rarely.

NURSING CONSIDERATIONS

BASELINE ASSESSMENT

Obtain baseline lab values. Assess drug history, esp. use of sucralfate.

INTERVENTION/EVALUATION

Monitor ongoing laboratory results. Assess for therapeutic response (relief of GI symptoms). Question if diarrhea, abdominal pain, nausea occurs.

PATIENT/ FAMILY TEACHING

• Do not chew/crush delayed-release capsules. • For pts who have difficulty swallowing capsules, open capsules, sprinkle granules on 1 tbsp of applesauce, swallow immediately.

lanthanum

lan-**thah**-num

(Fosrenol)

◆CLASSIFICATION

CLINICAL: Phosphate regulator.

ACTION

Dissociates in acidic environment of upper GI tract to lanthanum ions that bind to dietary phosphate released from food during digestion, forming highly insoluble lanthanum phosphate complexes. **Therapeutic Effect:** Reduces phosphate absorption.

PHARMACOKINETICS

Very low absorption following PO administration. Protein binding: greater than 99%. Not metabolized. Phosphate complexes are eliminated in urine. **Half-Life:** 53 hrs (in plasma); 2–3.6 yrs (from bone).

USES

Reduce serum phosphate levels in pts with end-stage renal disease.

PRECAUTIONS

CONTRAINDICATIONS: None known. **CAUTIONS:** Acute peptic ulcer disease, ulcerative colitis, Crohn's disease, bowel obstruction.

LIFESPAN CONSIDERATIONS:

Pregnancy/Lactation: Unknown if drug crosses placenta or is distributed in breast milk; do not breast-feed. **Pregnancy Category C. Children:** Safety and efficacy not established; not recommended for children. **Elderly:** No age-related precautions noted.

INTERACTIONS

DRUG: Antacids interact with lanthanum carbonate; separate administration by 2 hrs. **HERBAL:** None significant. **FOOD:** None known. **LAB VALUES:** None known.

L

AVAILABILITY (Rx)

TABLETS, CHEWABLE: 250 mg, 500 mg, 750 mg, 1 g (Fosrenol).

ADMINISTRATION/HANDLING

PO

• Tablets should be chewed thoroughly before swallowing and given during or immediately after meals.

INDICATIONS/ROUTES/DOSAGE

PHOSPHATE CONTROL

PO: ADULTS, ELDERLY: 750 mg–1,500 mg in divided doses, taken with or immediately after a meal. Dose can be titrated at 2- to 3-wk intervals in 750 mg increments, based on serum phosphate levels.

SIDE EFFECTS

FREQUENT: Nausea (11%), vomiting (9%), dialysis graft occlusion (8%), abdominal pain (5%). Nausea, vomiting decrease over time.

ADVERSE EFFECTS/ TOXIC REACTIONS

None known.

NURSING CONSIDERATIONS

BASELINE ASSESSMENT

Obtain baseline serum phosphorus.

INTERVENTION/EVALUATION

Monitor serum phosphate (target concentration is less than 6 mg/dL).

PATIENT/FAMILY TEACHING

• Take with or immediately after a meal. • Do not take lanthanum within 2 hrs of antacids. • Nausea, vomiting usually diminish over time.

Lantus, *see insulin*

Lasix, *see furosemide*

latanoprost

See Antiglaucoma agents (p. 49C)

leflunomide

lee-**flew**-no-mide

(Apo-Leflunomide ✱, Arava, Novo-Leflunomide ✱)

CLASSIFICATION

PHARMACOTHERAPEUTIC: Immunomodulatory agent. **CLINICAL:** Anti-inflammatory.

ACTION

Inhibits dihydroorotate dehydrogenase, the enzyme involved in autoimmune process that leads to rheumatoid arthritis. **Therapeutic Effect:** Reduces signs/symptoms of rheumatoid arthritis, retards structural damage.

PHARMACOKINETICS

Well absorbed after PO administration. Protein binding: greater than 99%. Metabolized to active metabolite in GI wall, liver. Excreted through renal, biliary systems. Not removed by hemodialysis. **Half-life:** 16 days.

USES

Treatment of active rheumatoid arthritis. Improve physical function in pts with rheumatoid arthritis. **OFF-LABEL:** Treatment of cytomegalovirus (CMV) disease.

PRECAUTIONS

CONTRAINDICATIONS: Pregnant or planning to become pregnant. **CAUTIONS:** Hepatic/renal impairment, positive hepatitis B or C serology, those with immunodeficiency or bone marrow dysplasias, breast-feeding mothers.

LIFESPAN CONSIDERATIONS:

Pregnancy/Lactation: Can cause fetal harm. Unknown if excreted in breast milk. Avoid use in breast-feeding mothers. **Pregnancy Category X. Children:** Safety and efficacy not established in those younger than 18 yrs. **Elderly:** No age-related precautions noted.

INTERACTIONS

DRUG: **Hepatotoxic medications** may increase risk of side effects, hepatotoxicity. May increase effects of **warfarin. HERBAL:** None significant. **FOOD:** None known. **LAB VALUES:** May increase hepatic enzyme levels, esp. AST, ALT.

AVAILABILITY (Rx)

TABLETS: 10 mg, 20 mg.

ADMINISTRATION/HANDLING

PO

- Give without regard to food.

INDICATIONS/ROUTES/DOSAGE

RHEUMATOID ARTHRITIS

PO: ADULTS, ELDERLY: Initially, 100 mg/day for 3 days, then 10–20 mg/day.

SIDE EFFECTS

FREQUENT (20%–10%): Diarrhea, respiratory tract infection, alopecia, rash, nausea.

ADVERSE EFFECTS/ TOXIC REACTIONS

Transient thrombocytopenia, leukopenia, hepatotoxicity occur rarely.

NURSING CONSIDERATIONS

BASELINE ASSESSMENT

Question for possibility of pregnancy (Pregnancy Category X). Assess limitations in activities of daily living due to rheumatoid arthritis.

INTERVENTION/EVALUATION

Monitor tolerance to medication. Assess symptomatic relief of rheumatoid arthritis (relief of pain; improved range of motion, grip strength, mobility). Monitor hepatic function tests.

PATIENT/FAMILY TEACHING

• May take without regard to food. • Improvement may take longer than 8 wks. • Avoid pregnancy (Pregnancy Category X).

lenalidomide

len-ah-**lid**-oh-mide
(Revlimid)

CLASSIFICATION

PHARMACOTHERAPEUTIC: Immunomodulator. **CLINICAL:** Immunosuppressive.

L

ACTION

Inhibits secretion of pro-inflammatory cytokines, increases secretion of anti-inflammatory cytokines. **Therapeutic Effect:** Prevents growth of B-cell lymphoma cell line, myeloblastic cell line.

PHARMACOKINETICS

Well absorbed following PO administration. Protein binding: 30%. Eliminated in urine. **Half-life:** 3 hrs (increased in renal impairment).

USES

Treatment of transfusion-dependent anemia due to myelodysplastic syndromes. Treatment of multiple myeloma (in combination with dexamethasone).

PRECAUTIONS

CONTRAINDICATIONS: Pregnancy **(Pregnancy Category X)**, women capable of becoming pregnant. **CAUTIONS:** Renal function impairment.

LIFESPAN CONSIDERATIONS:

Pregnancy/Lactation: Contraindicated in women who are or may become pregnant and who are not using two required types of birth control or who are not continually abstaining from heterosexual sexual contact. Can cause severe birth defects, fetal death. Unknown if distributed in breast milk; do not breast-feed. **Pregnancy Category X. Children:** Safety and efficacy not established in children younger than 18 yrs. **Elderly:** Age-related renal impairment may require care in dosage selection. Risk of toxic reactions greater in those with renal insufficiency.

INTERACTIONS

DRUG: None significant. **HERBAL:** None significant. **FOOD:** None known. **LAB VALUES:** May decrease WBC count, Hgb, Hct, thrombocytes, troponin I, serum creatinine, sodium, T_3, T_4. May decrease bilirubin, glucose, potassium, magnesium.

AVAILABILITY (Rx)

CAPSULES: 5 mg, 10 mg, 15 mg, 25 mg.

ADMINISTRATION/HANDLING

• Store at room temperature. • Do not crush/open capsules.

INDICATIONS/ROUTES/DOSAGE

MYELODYSPLASTIC SYNDROME

PO: ADULTS, ELDERLY: 10 mg once daily.

DOSAGE ADJUSTMENTS

PLATELETS:

Thrombocytopenia within 4 wks with 10 mg/day

Baseline platelets 100,000/mcl or greater: Platelets less than 50,000/mcl, hold treatment. Resume at 5 mg/day when platelets return to 50,000/mcl or greater. **Baseline platelets less than 100,000/mcl:** Platelets fall to 50% of baseline, hold treatment. Resume at 5 mg/day if baseline is 60,000/mcl or greater and platelets return to 50,000/mcl or greater. Resume at 5 mg/day if baseline is less than 60,000/mcl and platelets return to 30,000/mcl or greater.

Thrombocytopenia after 4 wks with 10 mg/day Platelets less than 30,000/mcl OR less than 50,000/mcl with platelet transfusion, hold treatment. Resume at 5 mg/day when platelets return to 30,000/mcl or greater.

Thrombocytopenia developing with 5 mg/day Platelets less than 30,000/mcl OR less than 50,000/mcl with platelet transfusion, hold treatment. Resume at 5 mg every other day when platelets return to 30,000/mcl or greater.

NEUTROPHILS:

Neutropenia within 4 wks with 10 mg/day

Baseline absolute neutrophil count (ANC) 1,000/mcl or greater: ANC less than 750/mcl, hold treatment. Resume at 5 mg/day when ANC 1,000/mcl or greater. **Baseline ANC less than 1,000/mcl:** ANC less than 500/mcl, hold treatment. Resume at 5 mg/day when ANC 500/mcl or greater.

Neutropenia after 4 wks with 10 mg/day ANC less than 500/mcl for 7 days or longer or associated with fever, hold treatment. Resume at 5 mg/day when ANC 500/mcl or greater.

Neutropenia developing with 5 mg/day ANC less than 500/mcl for 7 days or longer or associated with fever, hold treatment. Resume at 5 mg every other day when ANC 500/mcl or greater.

MULTIPLE MYELOMA

PO: ADULTS, ELDERLY: 25 mg/day on days 1–21 of repeated 28-day cycle. (Dexamethasone 40 mg/day on days 1–4, 9–12, 17–20 of each 28-day cycle for first 4 cycles, then 40 mg/day on days 1–4 every 28 days.)

DOSAGE ADJUSTMENTS

PLATELETS:

Thrombocytopenia Platelets fall to less than 30,000/mcl, hold treatment, monitor CBC. Resume at 15 mg/day when platelets 30,000/mcl or greater. For each subsequent fall to less than 30,000/mcl, hold treatment and resume at 5 mg/day less than previous dose when platelets return to 30,000/mcl or greater. Do not dose to less than 5 mg/day.

NEUTROPHILS:

Neutropenia Neutrophils fall to less than 1,000/mcl, hold treatment, add G-CSF, follow CBC weekly. Resume at 25 mg/day when neutrophils return to 1,000/mcl and neutropenia is the only toxicity. Resume at 15 mg/day if other toxicity is present. For each subsequent fall to less than 1,000/mcl, hold treatment and resume at 5 mg/day less than previous dose when neutrophils return to 1,000/mcl or greater. Do not dose to less than 5 mg/day.

SIDE EFFECTS

FREQUENT (49%–31%): Diarrhea, pruritus, rash, fatigue. **OCCASIONAL (24%–12%):** Constipation, nausea, arthralgia, fever, back pain, peripheral edema, cough, dizziness, headache, muscle cramps, epistaxis, asthenia, dry skin, abdominal pain. **RARE (10%–5%):** Extremity pain, vomiting, generalized edema, anorexia, insomnia, night sweats, myalgia, dry mouth, ecchymosis, rigors, depression, dysgeusia, palpitations.

ADVERSE EFFECTS/ TOXIC REACTIONS

Significant increased risk of deep vein thrombosis, pulmonary embolism. Thrombocytopenia occurs in 62% of pts, neutropenia in 59% of pts, and anemia in 12% of pts. Upper respiratory infection (nasopharyngitis, pneumonia, sinusitis, bronchitis, rhinitis), UTI occur occasionally. Cellulitis, peripheral neuropathy, hypertension, hypothyroidism occur in approximately 6% of pts.

NURSING CONSIDERATIONS

BASELINE ASSESSMENT

Due to high potential for human birth defects/fetal death, female pts must avoid pregnancy 4 wks before therapy, during therapy, during dose interruptions and 4 wks following therapy. Contraception must be used even if pt has history of infertility unless it is due to hysterectomy or menopause that has occurred for at least 24 consecutive mos. Two reliable forms of contraception must be used. Females of childbearing potential must have two negative pregnancy tests before therapy initiation.

INTERVENTION/EVALUATION

Perform pregnancy tests on women of childbearing potential. Perform test weekly during the first 4 wks of use, then at 4-wk intervals in women with regular menstrual cycles or q2wk in women with irregular menstrual cycles. Monitor for hematologic toxicity; obtain CBC weekly during first 8 wks of therapy and at least monthly thereafter. Observe for signs, symptoms of thromboembolism (shortness of breath, chest pain, extremity pain, swelling).

L

PATIENT/FAMILY TEACHING

• Two approved birth control methods must be used before, during, and after therapy for female pts. • A pregnancy test must be performed within 10–14 days and 24 hrs before therapy begins. • Males must always use a latex condom during any sexual contact with females of childbearing potential even if they have undergone a successful vasectomy.

lepirudin

leh-**peer**-u-din
(Refludan)

CLASSIFICATION

PHARMACOTHERAPEUTIC: Thrombin inhibitor. **CLINICAL:** Anticoagulant.

ACTION

Inhibits thrombogenic action of thrombin (independent of antithrombin II, not inhibited by platelet factor 4). **Therapeutic Effect:** Produces dose-dependent increases in activated partial thromboplastin time (aPTT).

PHARMACOKINETICS

Distributed primarily in extracellular fluid. Primarily eliminated by kidneys. **Half-life:** 1.3 hrs (increased in renal impairment).

USES

Anticoagulant in pts with heparin-induced thrombocytopenia or associated thromboembolic disease to prevent further thromboembolic complications. **OFF-LABEL:** Acute coronary syndromes with history of heparin-induced thrombocytopenia; acute MI; percutaneous coronary intervention with history of heparin-induced thrombocytopenia; prevention/reduction of ischemic complications associated with unstable angina.

PRECAUTIONS

CONTRAINDICATIONS: Hypersensitivity to hirudins or to any of the components in Refludan [lepirudin (rDNA)] for injection. **CAUTIONS:** Conditions associated with increased risk of bleeding (bacterial endocarditis, recent major bleeding, cerebrovascular accident [CVA], stroke, intracranial surgery, hemorrhagic diathesis, severe hypertension, severe renal/hepatic impairment, recent major surgery).

LIFESPAN CONSIDERATIONS:

Pregnancy/Lactation: Unknown if drug is distributed in breast milk or crosses placenta. **Pregnancy Category B.** **Children:** Safety and efficacy not established. **Elderly:** Age-related renal impairment may require dosage adjustment.

INTERACTIONS

DRUG: **Platelet aggregation inhibitors, thrombolytics, warfarin** may increase risk of bleeding complications. **HERBAL:** **Cats's claw, dong quai, evening primrose, feverfew, red clover, horse chestnut, garlic, ginseng, ginkgo** may increase antiplatelet activity. **FOOD:** None known. **LAB VALUES:** Increases aPTT, thrombin time.

AVAILABILITY (Rx)

INJECTION, POWDER FOR RECONSTITUTION: 50 mg.

ADMINISTRATION/HANDLING

IV

Reconstitution • Add 1 ml Sterile Water for Injection or 0.9% NaCl to 50-mg vial. • Shake gently. • Produces a clear, colorless solution (do not use if cloudy). • For IV push, further dilute by transferring to syringe and adding sufficient Sterile Water for Injection,

0.9% NaCl, or D_5W to produce concentration of 5 mg/ml. • For IV infusion, add contents of 2 vials (100 mg) to 250 ml or 500 ml 0.9% NaCl or D_5W, providing concentration of 0.4 or 0.2 mg/ml, respectively.

Rate of administration • IV push given over 15–20 sec. • Adjust IV infusion based on aPTT or pt's body weight.

Storage • Store unreconstituted vials at room temperature. • Reconstituted solution to be used immediately. • IV infusion stable for up to 24 hrs at room temperature.

IV INCOMPATIBILITIES

Do not mix with other medications.

INDICATIONS/ROUTES/DOSAGE

ANTICOAGULATION

◀ **ALERT** ▶ Dosage adjusted according to aPTT ratio with target range of 1.5–2.5 times normal.

IV: ADULTS, ELDERLY: 0.2–0.4 mg/kg, IV slowly over 15–20 sec, followed by IV infusion of 0.1–0.15 mg/kg/hr for 2–10 days or longer.

◀ **ALERT** ▶ For pts weighing more than 110 kg, maximum initial dose is 44 mg, with maximum IV rate of 16.5 mg/hr.

DOSAGE IN RENAL IMPAIRMENT

Initial dose is decreased to 0.2 mg/kg, with infusion rate adjusted based on creatinine clearance.

Creatinine Clearance (ml/min)	% of Standard Infusion Rate	Infusion Rate (mg/kg/hr)
45–60	50	0.075
30–44	30	0.045
15–29	15	0.0225

SIDE EFFECTS

FREQUENT (14%–5%): Bleeding from gums, puncture sites, wounds; hematuria; fever; GI, rectal bleeding. **OCCASIONAL (3%–1%):** Epistaxis, allergic reaction (rash, pruritus), vaginal bleeding.

ADVERSE EFFECTS/ TOXIC REACTIONS

Overdose is characterized by excessively high aPTT. Intracranial bleeding occurs rarely. Abnormal hepatic function in 6% of pts.

NURSING CONSIDERATIONS

BASELINE ASSESSMENT

Assess CBC, including platelet count. Determine initial B/P. Assess renal/hepatic function.

INTERVENTION/EVALUATION

Monitor aPTT diligently. Assess Hct, platelet count, urine/stool specimen for occult blood, AST, ALT, renal function studies. Assess for decrease in B/P, increase in pulse rate, complaint of abdominal/back pain, severe headache (may be evidence of hemorrhage). Question for increased discharge during menses. Check peripheral pulses; skin for ecchymosis, petechiae. Check for excessive bleeding from minor cuts, scratches. Assess gums for erythema, gingival bleeding. Assess urine output for hematuria.

PATIENT/FAMILY TEACHING

- Report bleeding, bruising, dizziness, light-headedness, rash, pruritus, fever, edema, breathing difficulty.

Lescol, *see fluvastatin*

Lescol XL, *see fluvastatin*

L

letrozole

leh-troe-zoll
(Femara)

Do not confuse Femara with Femhrt.

CLASSIFICATION

PHARMACOTHERAPEUTIC: Aromatase inhibitor, hormone. **CLINICAL:** Antineoplastic (see p. 80C).

ACTION

Decreases circulating estrogen by inhibiting aromatase, an enzyme that catalyzes the final step in estrogen production. **Therapeutic Effect:** Inhibits growth of breast cancers stimulated by estrogens.

PHARMACOKINETICS

Rapidly, completely absorbed. Metabolized in liver. Primarily eliminated by kidneys. Unknown if removed by hemodialysis. **Half-life:** Approximately 2 days.

USES

First line treatment of locally advanced or metastatic breast cancer. Treatment of advanced breast cancer in postmenopausal women with disease progression following anti-estrogen therapy. Postsurgical treatment for postmenopausal women with hormone sensitive early breast cancer. Prevention of recurrent breast cancer.

PRECAUTIONS

CONTRAINDICATIONS: None known. **CAUTIONS:** Renal/hepatic impairment.

LIFESPAN CONSIDERATIONS:

Pregnancy/Lactation: Unknown if distributed in breast milk. **Pregnancy Category D. Children:** Safety and efficacy not established. **Elderly:** No age-related precautions noted.

INTERACTIONS

DRUG: **Tamoxifen** may reduce concentration. **HERBAL:** None significant. **FOOD:** None known. **LAB VALUES:** May increase serum calcium, cholesterol, GGT, AST, ALT.

AVAILABILITY (Rx)

TABLETS: 2.5 mg.

ADMINISTRATION/HANDLING

PO

- Give without regard to food.

INDICATIONS/ROUTES/DOSAGE

BREAST CANCER

PO: ADULTS, ELDERLY: 2.5 mg/day. Continue until tumor progression is evident.

DOSAGE IN SEVERE HEPATIC IMPAIRMENT

PO: ADULTS, ELDERLY: 2.5 mg every other day.

SIDE EFFECTS

FREQUENT (21%–9%): Musculoskeletal pain (back, arm, leg), nausea, headache. **OCCASIONAL (8%–5%):** Constipation, arthralgia, fatigue, vomiting, hot flashes, diarrhea, abdominal pain, cough, rash, anorexia, hypertension, peripheral edema. **RARE (4%–1%):** Asthenia (loss of strength, energy), somnolence, dyspepsia (heartburn, indigestion, epigastric pain), weight gain, pruritus.

ADVERSE EFFECTS/ TOXIC REACTIONS

Pleural effusion, pulmonary embolism, bone fracture, thromboembolic disorder, MI occur rarely.

NURSING CONSIDERATIONS

INTERVENTION/EVALUATION

Monitor for, assist with ambulation if asthenia, dizziness occurs. Assess for headache. Offer antiemetic for nausea, vomiting. Monitor CBC, thyroid function, electrolytes, hepatic/renal function tests. Monitor for evidence of musculoskeletal pain; offer analgesics for pain relief.

PATIENT/FAMILY TEACHING

- Notify physician if nausea, asthenia, hot flashes become unmanageable.

leucovorin calcium (folinic acid, citrovorum factor)

loo-**koe**-vor-in

CLASSIFICATION

PHARMACOTHERAPEUTIC: Folic acid antagonist. **CLINICAL:** Antidote.

ACTION

Competes with methotrexate for same transport processes into cells (limits methotrexate action on normal cells). **Therapeutic Effect:** Reverses toxic effects of folic acid antagonists. Reverses folic acid deficiency.

PHARMACOKINETICS

Readily absorbed from GI tract. Widely distributed. Primarily concentrated in liver. Metabolized in liver, intestinal mucosa to active metabolite. Primarily excreted in urine. **Half-life:** 15 min; metabolite, 30–35 min.

USES

Antidote for folic acid antagonists (methotrexate, trimethoprim, pyrimethoamine). Treatment of megaloblastic anemias when folate deficient (e.g., infancy, celiac disease, pregnancy, when oral therapy not possible). Treatment of colon cancer (with fluorouracil). Methotrexate rescue, after high-dose methotrexate for osteosarcoma. **OFF-LABEL:** Treatment of Ewing's sarcoma, gestational trophoblastic neoplasms, non-Hodgkin's lymphoma; treatment adjunct for head/neck carcinoma.

PRECAUTIONS

CONTRAINDICATIONS: Pernicious anemia, other megaloblastic anemias secondary to vitamin B_{12} deficiency. **CAUTIONS:** History of allergies, bronchial asthma. **With 5-fluorouracil:** Those with GI toxicities (more common/severe).

LIFESPAN CONSIDERATIONS:

Pregnancy/Lactation: Unknown if drug crosses placenta or is distributed in breast milk. **Pregnancy Category C. Children:** May increase risk of seizures by counteracting anticonvulsant effects of barbiturate, hydantoins. **Elderly:** Age-related renal impairment may require dosage adjustment when used in rescue from effects of high-dose methotrexate therapy.

INTERACTIONS

DRUG: May decrease effects of **anticonvulsants.** May increase **5-fluorouracil** toxicity/effect when taken in combination. **HERBAL:** None significant. **FOOD:** None known. **LAB VALUES:** None known.

AVAILABILITY (Rx)

INJECTION POWDER FOR RECONSTITUTION: 50 mg, 100 mg, 200 mg, 350 mg, 500 mg. **INJECTION, SOLUTION:** 10 mg/ml. **TABLETS:** 5 mg, 10 mg, 15 mg, 25 mg.

L

ADMINISTRATION/HANDLING

IV

◀ **ALERT** ▶ Strict adherence to timing of 5-fluorouracil following leucovorin therapy must be maintained.

Reconstitution • Reconstitute each 50-mg vial with 5 ml Sterile Water for Injection or Bacteriostatic Water for Injection containing benzyl alcohol to provide concentration of 10 mg/ml. • Due to benzyl alcohol in 1-mg ampule and in Bacteriostatic Water for Injection, reconstitute doses greater than 10 mg/m^2 with Sterile Water for Injection. • Further dilute with D_5W or 0.9% NaCl.

Rate of administration • Do not exceed 160 mg/min if given by IV infusion (due to calcium content).

Storage • Store vials for parenteral use at room temperature. • Injection appears as clear, yellowish solution. • Use immediately if reconstituted with Sterile Water for Injection; is stable for 7 days if reconstituted with Bacteriostatic Water for Injection.

PO

• Scored tablets may be crushed.

IV INCOMPATIBILITIES

Amphotericin B complex (Abelcet, AmBisome, Amphotec), droperidol (Inapsine), foscarnet (Foscavir).

IV COMPATIBILITIES

Cisplatin (Platinol AQ), cyclophosphamide (Cytoxan), doxorubicin (Adriamycin), etoposide (VePesid), filgrastim (Neupogen), 5-fluorouracil, gemcitabine (Gemzar), granisetron (Kytril), heparin, methotrexate, metoclopramide (Reglan), mitomycin (Mutamycin), piperacillin and tazobactam (Zosyn), vinblastine (Velban), vincristine (Oncovin).

INDICATIONS/ROUTES/DOSAGE

CONVENTIONAL RESCUE DOSAGE IN HIGH-DOSE METHOTREXATE THERAPY

PO, IV, IM: ADULTS, ELDERLY, CHILDREN: 10 mg/m^2 IM or IV one time, then PO q6h until serum methotrexate level is less than 10^{-8} M. If 24-hr serum creatinine level increases by 50% or greater over baseline or methotrexate level exceeds 5×10^{-6} M or 48-hr level exceeds 9×10^{-7} M, increase to 100 mg/m^2 IV q3h until methotrexate level is less than 10^{-8} M.

FOLIC ACID ANTAGONIST OVERDOSE

PO: ADULTS, ELDERLY, CHILDREN: 2–15 mg/day for 3 days or 5 mg every 3 days.

MEGALOBLASTIC ANEMIA SECONDARY TO FOLATE DEFICIENCY

IM: ADULTS, ELDERLY, CHILDREN: 1 mg/day.

COLON CANCER

◀ **ALERT** ▶ For rescue therapy in cancer chemotherapy, refer to specific protocols used for optimal dosage and sequence of leucovorin administration.

IV: ADULTS, ELDERLY: 200 mg/m^2 followed by 370 mg/m^2 fluorouracil daily for 5 days. Repeat course at 4-wk intervals for 2 courses then 4–5 wk intervals or 20 mg/m^2 followed by 425 mg/m^2 fluorouracil daily for 5 days. Repeat course at 4-wk intervals for 2 courses then 4–5 wk intervals.

SIDE EFFECTS

FREQUENT: When combined with chemotherapeutic agents: diarrhea, stomatitis, nausea, vomiting, lethargy, malaise, fatigue, alopecia, anorexia. **OCCASIONAL:** Urticaria, dermatitis.

ADVERSE EFFECTS/ TOXIC REACTIONS

Excessive dosage may negate chemotherapeutic effects of folic acid antagonists. Anaphylaxis occurs rarely. Diarrhea may cause rapid clinical deterioration.

NURSING CONSIDERATIONS

BASELINE ASSESSMENT

Give as soon as possible, preferably within 1 hr, for treatment of accidental overdosage of folic acid antagonists.

INTERVENTION/EVALUATION

Monitor for vomiting—may need to change from oral to parenteral therapy. Observe elderly, debilitated closely due to risk for severe toxicities. Assess CBC with differential, platelet count (also electrolytes, hepatic function tests if used in combination with chemotherapeutic agents).

PATIENT/FAMILY TEACHING

• Explain purpose of medication in treatment of cancer. • Report allergic reaction, vomiting.

leuprolide

loo-proe-lide

(Eligard, Lupron, Lupron Depot, Lupron Depot-Gyn, Lupron Depot-Ped, Viadur)

Do not confuse leuprolide or Lupron with Lopurin or Nuprin.

CLASSIFICATION

PHARMACOTHERAPEUTIC: Gonadotropin-releasing hormone analogue. **CLINICAL:** Antineoplastic (see pp. 81C, 101C).

ACTION

Stimulates release of luteinizing hormone (LH), follicle-stimulating hormone (FSH) from anterior pituitary gland. **Therapeutic Effect:** Produces pharmacologic castration, decreases growth of abnormal prostate tissue in males; causes endometrial tissue to become inactive, atrophic in females; decreases rate of pubertal development in children with central precocious puberty.

PHARMACOKINETICS

Rapidly, well absorbed after subcutaneous administration. Absorbed slowly after IM administration. Protein binding: 43%–49%. **Half-life:** 3–4 hrs.

USES

Palliative treatment of advanced prostate carcinoma. Initial management of endometriosis or treatment of recurrent symptoms. Preoperative treatment of anemia caused by uterine leiomyomata (fibroids). Treatment of central precocious puberty.

PRECAUTIONS

CONTRAINDICATIONS: Lactation, pernicious anemia, pregnancy, undiagnosed vaginal bleeding. Eligard 7.5 mg is contraindicated in pts with hypersensitivity to GnRH, GnRH agonist analogs or any of the components. 30 mg Lupron Depot contraindicated in women; implant form is contraindicated in women, children. **CAUTIONS:** Long-term use in children.

LIFESPAN CONSIDERATIONS:

Pregnancy/Lactation: Depot: Contraindicated in pregnancy. May cause spontaneous abortion. **Pregnancy Category X. Children:** Long-term safety not established. **Elderly:** No age-related precautions noted.

INTERACTIONS

DRUG: None significant. **HERBAL:** None significant. **FOOD:** None known. **LAB VALUES:** May increase serum prostatic acid phosphatase (PAP). Initially increases, then decreases, serum testosterone.

AVAILABILITY (Rx)

IMPLANT (VIADUR): 65 mg. **INJECTION DEPOT FORMULATION:** 3.75 mg (Lupron Depot), 7.5 mg (Eligard, Lupron Depot,

Lupron Depot-Ped), 11.25 mg (Lupron Depot, Lupron Depot-Ped, Lupron Depot-Gyn), 15 mg (Lupron Depot-Ped), 22.5 mg (Eligard, Lupron Depot), 30 mg (Lupron Depot), 45 mg (Eligard). **INJECTION SOLUTION (LUPRON):** 5 mg/ml.

ADMINISTRATION/HANDLING

◀ ALERT ▶ May be carcinogenic, mutagenic, teratogenic. Handle with extreme care during preparation/administration.

IM

Lupron Depot • Store at room temperature. • Protect from light, heat. • Do not freeze vials. • Reconstitute only with diluent provided. Follow manufacturer's instructions for mixing. • Do not use needles less than 22 gauge; use syringes provided by the manufacturer (0.5 ml low-dose insulin syringes may be used as an alternative). • Administer immediately.

Eligard • Refrigerate. • Allow to warm to room temperature before reconstitution. • Follow manufacturer's instructions for mixing. • Following reconstitution, administer within 30 min.

SUBCUTANEOUS

Lupron • Refrigerate vials. • Injection appears clear, colorless. • Discard if discolored or precipitate forms. • Administer into deltoid muscle, anterior thigh, abdomen.

INDICATIONS/ROUTES/DOSAGE

ADVANCED PROSTATIC CARCINOMA

IM (LUPRON DEPOT): ADULTS, ELDERLY: 7.5 mg every mo or 22.5 mg q3mos or 30 mg q4mos.

SUBCUTANEOUS (ELIGARD): ADULTS, ELDERLY: 7.5 mg every mo or 22.5 mg q3mos or 30 mg q4mos.

SUBCUTANEOUS (LUPRON): ADULTS, ELDERLY: 1 mg/day.

SUBCUTANEOUS (VIADUR): ADULTS, ELDERLY: 65 mg implanted q12mos.

ENDOMETRIOSIS

IM (LUPRON DEPOT): ADULTS, ELDERLY: 3.75 mg/mo for up to 6 mos or 11.25 mg q3mo for up to 2 doses.

UTERINE LEIOMYOMATA

IM (WITH IRON [LUPRON DEPOT]): ADULTS, ELDERLY: 3.75 mg/mos for up to 3 mos or 11.25 mg as a single injection.

PRECOCIOUS PUBERTY

IM (LUPRON DEPOT): CHILDREN: 0.3 mg/kg/dose every 28 days. Minimum: 7.5 mg. If down regulation is not achieved, titrate upward in 3.75-mg increments q4wks.

SUBCUTANEOUS (LUPRON): CHILDREN: 20–45 mcg/kg/day. Titrate upward by 10 mcg/kg/day if down regulation is not achieved.

SIDE EFFECTS

FREQUENT: Hot flashes (ranging from mild flushing to diaphoresis). **Females:** Amenorrhea, spotting. **OCCASIONAL:** Arrhythmias; palpitations; blurred vision; dizziness; edema; headache; burning, pruritus, swelling at injection site; nausea; insomnia; weight gain. **Females:** Deepening voice, hirsutism, decreased libido, increased breast tenderness, vaginitis, altered mood. **Males:** Constipation, decreased testicle size, gynecomastia, impotence, decreased appetite, angina. **RARE: Males:** Thrombophlebitis.

ADVERSE EFFECTS/ TOXIC REACTIONS

Occasionally, signs/symptoms of prostatic carcinoma worsen 1–2 wks after initial dosing (subsides during continued therapy). Increased bone pain and, less frequently, dysuria, hematuria, weakness, paresthesia of lower extremities may be noted. Myocardial infarction, pulmonary embolism occur rarely.

NURSING CONSIDERATIONS

BASELINE ASSESSMENT

Question for possibility of pregnancy before initiating therapy (Pregnancy

Category X). Obtain serum testosterone, PAP periodically during therapy. Serum testosterone, PAP should increase during first wk of therapy. Serum testosterone then should decrease to baseline level or less within 2 wks, PAP within 4 wks.

INTERVENTION/EVALUATION

Monitor for arrhythmias, palpitations. Assess for peripheral edema. Assess sleep pattern. Monitor for visual difficulties. Assist with ambulation if dizziness occurs. Offer antiemetics if nausea occurs.

PATIENT/FAMILY TEACHING

• Hot flashes tend to decrease during continued therapy. • Temporary exacerbation of signs/symptoms of disease may occur during first few wks of therapy. • Use contraceptive measures during therapy. • Inform physician if regular menstruation persists, pregnancy occurs. • Avoid tasks that require alertness, motor skills until response to drug is established (potential for dizziness).

levalbuterol

lee-val-**bwet**-err-all

(Xopenex, Xopenex HFA)

Do not confuse Xopenex with Xanax.

CLASSIFICATION

PHARMACOTHERAPEUTIC: Sympathomimetic. **CLINICAL:** Bronchodilator (see p. 70C).

ACTION

Stimulates beta_2-adrenergic receptors in lungs, resulting in relaxation of bronchial smooth muscle. **Therapeutic Effect:** Relieves bronchospasm, reduces airway resistance.

PHARMACOKINETICS

Route	Onset	Peak	Duration
Inhalation	10–17 min	1.5 hrs	5–6 hrs

Metabolized in liver to inactive metabolite. **Half-life:** 3.3–4 hrs.

USES

Treatment, prevention of bronchospasm due to reversible obstructive airway disease.

PRECAUTIONS

CONTRAINDICATIONS: History of hypersensitivity to sympathomimetics. **CAUTIONS:** Cardiovascular disorders (cardiac arrhythmias), seizures, hypertension, hyperthyroidism, diabetes mellitus.

LIFESPAN CONSIDERATIONS:

Pregnancy/Lactation: Crosses placenta. Unknown if distributed in breast milk. **Pregnancy Category C. Children:** Safety and efficacy not established in those younger than 12 yrs. **Elderly:** Lower initial dosages recommended.

INTERACTIONS

DRUG: Beta-adrenergic blocking agents (beta-blockers) antagonize effects. **Digoxin** may increase risk of arrhythmias. **MAOIs, tricyclic antidepressants** may potentiate cardiovascular effects. **HERBAL:** None significant. **FOOD:** None known. **LAB VALUES:** May increase serum potassium.

AVAILABILITY (Rx)

INHALATION AEROSOL: 45 mcg/activation. **SOLUTION FOR NEBULIZATION:** 0.31 in 3-ml vials, 0.63 mg in 3-ml vials, 1.25 mg in 3-ml vials.

ADMINISTRATION/HANDLING

NEBULIZATION

• No diluent necessary. • Protect from light, excessive heat. Store at room temperature. • Once foil is opened, use within 2 wks. • Discard if solution is not colorless. • Do not mix with other medications. • Give over 5–15 min.

INHALATION

• Shake well before inhalation. • Wait 2 min before inhaling second dose (allows for deeper bronchial penetration). • Rinse mounth with water immediately after inhalation (prevents mouth/throat dryness).

INDICATIONS/ROUTES/DOSAGE

TREATMENT/PREVENTION OF BRONCHOSPASM

NEBULIZATION: ADULTS, ELDERLY, CHILDREN 12 YRS AND OLDER: Initially, 0.63 mg 3 times a day 6–8 hrs apart. May increase to 1.25 mg 3 times a day with dose monitoring. **CHILDREN 6–11 YRS:** Initially 0.31 mg 3 times a day. **Maximum:** 0.63 mg 3 times a day.

INHALATION: ADULTS, ELDERLY, CHILDREN 4 YRS AND OLDER: 1–2 inhalations q4–6h.

SIDE EFFECTS

FREQUENT: Tremor, anxiety, headache, throat dryness or irritation. **OCCASIONAL:** Cough, bronchial irritation. **RARE:** Drowsiness, diarrhea, dry mouth, flushing, diaphoresis, anorexia.

ADVERSE EFFECTS/ TOXIC REACTIONS

Excessive sympathomimetic stimulation may produce palpitations, extrasystoles, tachycardia, chest pain, slight increase in B/P followed by substantial decrease, chills, diaphoresis, blanching of skin. Too-frequent or excessive use may decrease bronchodilating effectiveness, lead to severe, paradoxical bronchoconstriction.

NURSING CONSIDERATIONS

BASELINE ASSESSMENT

Offer emotional support (high incidence of anxiety due to difficulty in breathing, sympathomimetic response to drug).

INTERVENTION/EVALUATION

Monitor rate, depth, rhythm, type of respiration; quality/rate of pulse, EKG, serum potassium, ABG determinations. Assess lung sounds for wheezing (bronchoconstriction), rales.

PATIENT/FAMILY TEACHING

• Increase fluid intake (decreases lung secretion viscosity). • Rinsing mouth with water immediately after inhalation may prevent mouth/throat dryness. • Avoid excessive use of caffeine derivatives (chocolate, coffee, tea, cola, cocoa). • Notify physician if palpitations, tachycardia, chest pain, tremors, dizziness, headache occurs.

Levaquin, *see levofloxacin*

levetiracetam evolve

leva-tir-**ass** eh-tam

(Keppra)

Do not confuse Keppra with Kaletra.

CLASSIFICATION

CLINICAL: Anticonvulsant.

ACTION

Inhibits burst firing without affecting normal neuronal excitability. **Therapeutic Effect:** Prevents seizure activity.

PHARMACOKINETICS

Rapidly, completely absorbed following PO administration. Protein binding: less than 10%. Metabolized primarily by enzymatic hydrolysis. Primarily excreted in urine as unchanged drug. **Half-life:** 6–8 hrs.

USES

Oral: Adjunctive therapy in treatment of partial-onset seizures in adults and children with epilepsy. Treatment of myoclonic seizures in adults and adolescents. **Injection:** Treatment of partial-onset seizures in adults.

PRECAUTIONS

CONTRAINDICATIONS: None known. **CAUTIONS:** Renal impairment. **Pregnancy Category C.**

LIFESPAN CONSIDERATIONS:

Pregnancy/Lactation: Distributed in breast milk. Breast-feeding not recommended. **Pregnancy Category C.** **Children:** Safety and efficacy not established. **Elderly:** Age-related renal impairment may require dosage adjustment.

INTERACTIONS

DRUG: None significant. **HERBAL:** **Ginkgo biloba** may decrease anticonvulsant effectiveness. **FOOD:** None known. **LAB VALUES:** May increase Hgb, Hct, RBC, WBC counts.

AVAILABILITY (Rx)

INJECTION, SOLUTION: 100 mg/ml. **ORAL SOLUTION:** 100 mg/ml. **TABLETS:** 250 mg, 500 mg, 750 mg, 1,000 mg.

ADMINISTRATION/HANDLING

IV

Rate of infusion • Infuse over 15 mins.

Reconstitution • Dilute with 100 ml. 0.9% NaCl or D_5W.

Storage • Store at room temperature.
• Stable for 24 hrs following dilution.

IV INCOMPATIBILITY

Data not available.

PO

• Give without regard to food.

IV COMPATIBILITY

Diazepam (Valium), Lorazepan (Ativan), Valproate (Depacon).

INDICATIONS/ROUTES/DOSAGE

PARTIAL-ONSET SEIZURES

IV/PO: ADULTS, ELDERLY, CHILDREN 17 YRS AND OLDER: Initially, 500 mg q12h. May increase by 1,000 mg/day q2wk. **Maximum:** 3,000 mg/day.

PO: CHILDREN 4–16 YRS: 10–20 mg/kg/day in 2 divided doses. May increase at weekly intervals by 10–20 mg/kg. **Maximum:** 60 mg/kg/day.

MYOCLONIC SEIZURES

PO: ADULTS, ELDERLY, CHILDREN 12 YRS AND OLDER: Initially, 500 mg q12h. May increase by 1,000 mg/day q2wk. **Maximum:** 3,000 mg/day.

DOSAGE IN RENAL IMPAIRMENT

Dosage is modified based on creatinine clearance.

Creatinine Clearance (ml/min)	Dosage
Higher than 80 ml/min	500–1,500 mg q12h
50–80 ml/min	500–1,000 mg q12h
30–49 ml/min	250–750 mg q12h
Less than 30 ml/min	250–500 mg q12h
End-stage renal disease using dialysis	500–1,000 mg q24h, after dialysis, a 250- to 500-mg supplemental dose is recommended.

SIDE EFFECTS

FREQUENT (15%–10%): Drowsiness, asthenia (loss of strength, energy), headache, infection. **OCCASIONAL (9%–3%):** Dizziness, pharyngitis, pain, depression, anxiety, vertigo, rhinitis, anorexia. **RARE (less than 3%):** Amnesia, emotional lability, cough, sinusitis, anorexia, diplopia.

ADVERSE EFFECTS/ TOXIC REACTIONS

Acute psychosis, seizures have been reported. Sudden discontinuance increases risk of seizure activity.

NURSING CONSIDERATIONS

BASELINE ASSESSMENT

Review history of seizure disorder (intensity, frequency, duration, level of consciousness [LOC]). Initiate seizure precautions. Assess for hypersensitivity to levetiracetam, renal function tests.

INTERVENTION/EVALUATION

Observe for recurrence of seizure activity. Assess for clinical improvement (decrease in intensity/frequency of seizures). Monitor renal function tests. Assist with ambulation if dizziness occurs.

PATIENT/FAMILY TEACHING

• Drowsiness usually diminishes with continued therapy. • Avoid tasks that require alertness, motor skills until response to drug is established. • Do not abruptly discontinue medication (may precipitate seizures). • Strict maintenance of drug therapy is essential for seizure control.

L

levobunolol hydrochloride

(Betagan Liquifilm)

See Antiglaucoma agents (p. 50C)

levobupivacaine

(Chirocaine)

See Anesthetics: local

levofloxacin

levo-**flox**-a-sin

(Iquix, Levaquin, Levaquin Leva-Pak, Novo-Levofloxacin ✱, Quixin)

◆CLASSIFICATION

PHARMACOTHERAPEUTIC: Fluoroquinolone. **CLINICAL:** Antibiotic (see p. 24C).

ACTION

Inhibits DNA enzyme gyrase in susceptible microorganisms, interfering with bacterial cell replication, repair. **Therapeutic Effect:** Bactericidal.

PHARMACOKINETICS

Well absorbed after PO, IV administration. Protein binding: 24%–8%. Penetrates rapidly, extensively into leukocytes, epithelial cells, macrophages. Lung concentrations are 2–5 times higher than those of plasma. Eliminated unchanged in urine. Partially removed by hemodialysis. **Half-life:** 8 hrs.

USES

Treatment of susceptible infections due to *S. pneumoniae, S. aureus, E. faecalis, H. influenzae, M. catarrhalis, serratia marcescens, K. pneumoniae, E. coli, P. mirabilis, P. aeruginosa, C. pneumoniae, Legionella pneumophila, Mycoplasma pneumoniae.* Treatment of acute bacterial exacerbation of chronic bronchitis, acute bacterial sinusitus, community-acquired pneumonia, nosocomial pneumonia, acute maxillary sinusitis, complicated UTI, acute pyelonephritis, uncomplicated mild to moderate skin/skin structure infections, prostatitis. **Ophthalmic:** Treatment of superficial infections to conjunctiva (0.5%), cornea (1.5%). **OFF-LABEL:** Anthrax, gonorrhea, pelvic inflammatory disease (PID).

PRECAUTIONS

CONTRAINDICATIONS: Hypersensitivity to other fluoroquinolones, cinoxacin, nalidixic acid. **CAUTIONS:** Suspected CNS disorders, seizure disorder, renal impairment, bradycardia, cardiomyopathy, hypokalemia, hypomagnesemia.

LIFESPAN CONSIDERATIONS:

Pregnancy/Lactation: Excreted in breast milk. Avoid use in pregnancy. **Pregnancy Category C. Children:** Safety and efficacy not established in those younger than 18 yrs. **Elderly:** Age-related renal impairment may require dosage adjustment.

INTERACTIONS

DRUG: Antacids, iron preparations, sucralfate, zinc decrease absorption. **NSAIDs** may increase risk of CNS stimulation, seizures. May increase effects of **warfarin. HERBAL:** None significant. **FOOD:** None known. **LAB VALUES:** May alter serum glucose.

AVAILABILITY (Rx)

INFUSION PREMIX: 250 mg/50 ml, 500 mg/100 ml, 750 mg/150 ml. **INJECTION, SOLUTION:** 25 mg/ml. **OPHTHALMIC SOLUTION:** (IQUIX) 1.5%; (QUIXIN) 0.5%. **ORAL SOLUTION:** 25 mg/ml. **TABLETS:** 250 mg, 500 mg, 750 mg.

ADMINISTRATION/HANDLING

IV

Reconstitution • For infusion using single-dose vial, withdraw desired amount (10 ml for 250 mg, 20 ml for 500 mg). Dilute each 10 ml (250 mg) with minimum 40 ml 0.9% NaCl, D_5W.

Rate of administration • Administer slowly, over not less than 60 min.

Storage • Available in single-dose 20-ml (500-mg) vials and premixed with D_5W, ready to infuse.

PO

• Do not administer antacids (aluminum, magnesium), sucralfate, iron or multivitamin preparations with zinc within 2 hrs of levofloxacin administration (significantly reduces levofloxacin absorption). • Encourage intake of cranberry juice, citrus fruits (acidifies urine). • Give without regard to food.

OPHTHALMIC

• Place a gloved finger on lower eyelid, pull out until a pocket is formed between eye and lower lid. Hold dropper above pocket, place correct number of drops into pocket. • Close eye gently. Apply digital pressure to lacrimal sac for 1–2 min (minimizes drainage into nose/throat, reducing risk of systemic effects).

IV INCOMPATIBILITIES

Furosemide (Lasix), heparin, insulin, nitroglycerin, propofol (Diprivan).

IV COMPATIBILITIES

Aminophylline, dobutamine (Dobutrex), dopamine (Intron), fentanyl (Sublimaze), lidocaine, lorazepam (Ativan), morphine.

INDICATIONS/ROUTES/DOSAGE

BACTERIAL SINUSITIS

PO: ADULTS, ELDERLY: 500 mg once daily for 10 days or 750 mg once daily for 5 days.

BRONCHITIS

PO, IV: ADULTS, ELDERLY: 500 mg q24h for 7 days.

COMMUNITY-ACQUIRED PNEUMONIA

PO: ADULTS, ELDERLY: 750 mg/day for 5 days or 500 mg for 7–14 days.

PNEUMONIA, NOSOCOMIAL

PO, IV: ADULTS, ELDERLY: 750 mg q24h for 7–14 days.

ACUTE MAXILLARY SINUSITIS

PO, IV: ADULTS, ELDERLY: 500 mg q24h for 10–14 days.

SKIN/SKIN STRUCTURE INFECTIONS

PO, IV: ADULTS, ELDERLY: (Uncomplicated) 500 mg q24h for 7–10 days. (Complicated) 750 mg q24h for 7–14 days.

PROSTATITIS

IV, PO: ADULTS, ELDERLY: 500 mg q24h for 28 days.

UNCOMPLICATED UTI

IV, PO: ADULTS, ELDERLY: 250 mg q24h for 3 days.

UTI, ACUTE PYELONEPHRITIS

PO, IV: ADULTS, ELDERLY: 250 mg q24h for 10 days.

BACTERIAL CONJUNCTIVITIS

OPHTHALMIC: ADULTS, ELDERLY, CHILDREN 1 YR AND OLDER (QUIXIN): 1–2 drops q2h for 2 days (up to 8 times a day), then 1–2 drops q4h for 5 days.

CORNEAL ULCER

OPHTHALMIC: ADULTS, ELDERLY, CHILDREN OLDER THAN 5 YRS (IQUIX): Days 1–3: Instill 1–2 drops q30min to 2 hrs while awake and 4–6 hrs after retiring. **Days 4 through completion:** 1–2 drops q1–4h while awake.

DOSAGE IN RENAL IMPAIRMENT

For bronchitis, pneumonia, sinusitis, skin/skin structure infections, dosage and frequency are modified based on creatinine clearance.

Creatinine Clearance	Dosage
50–80 ml/min	No change
20–49 ml/min	500 mg initially, then 250 mg q24h
10–19 ml/min	500 mg initially, then 250 mg q48h

For pts undergoing dialysis, 500 mg initially, then 250 mg q48h. For UTI, pyelonephritis, dosage and frequency are modified based on creatinine clearance.

Creatinine Clearance	Dosage
20 ml/min	No change
10–19 ml/min	250 mg initially, then 250 mg q48h

For complicated skin infection, acute bacterial sinusitis, community-acquired pneumonia or nosocomial pneumonia, dosage based on creatinine clearance.

Creatinine Clearance	Dosage
50–80 ml/min	No change
20–49 ml/min	Initiallly, 750 mg, then 750 mg q48h
10–19 ml/min	Initiallly 750 mg, then 500 mg q48h
Dialysis	500 mg q48h

SIDE EFFECTS

OCCASIONAL (3%–1%): Diarrhea, nausea, abdominal pain, dizziness, drowsiness, headache, light-headedness. **Ophthalmic:** Local burning/discomfort, margin crusting, crystals/scales, foreign body sensation, ocular itching, altered taste. **RARE (less than 1%):** Flatulence; pain, inflammation, swelling in calves, hands, shoulder; chest pain; difficulty breathing; palpitations; edema; tendon pain. **Ophthalmic:** Corneal staining, keratitis, allergic reaction, eyelid swelling, tearing, reduced visual acuity.

ADVERSE EFFECTS/ TOXIC REACTIONS

Antibiotic-associated colitis (severe abdominal pain/cramps, severe watery diarrhea, fever) may occur. Superinfection (genital/anal pruritus, ulceration/changes in oral mucosa, moderate to severe diarrhea) may occur from altered bacterial balance. Hypersensitivity reactions, including photosensitivity (rash, pruritus, blisters, edema, sensation of burning skin) have occurred in pts receiving fluoroquinolones.

NURSING CONSIDERATIONS

BASELINE ASSESSMENT

Question for hypersensitivity to levofloxacin, other fluoroquinolones.

INTERVENTION/EVALUATION

Monitor serum glucose, renal/hepatic function tests. Report hypersensitivity reaction: skin rash, urticaria, pruritus, photosensitivity promptly. Be alert for superinfection (genital/anal pruritus, ulceration/changes in oral mucosa, moderate to severe diarrhea, new or increased fever). Provide symptomatic relief for nausea. Evaluate food tolerance, altered taste.

PATIENT/FAMILY TEACHING

• Drink 6–8 glasses of fluid a day (citrus, cranberry juice acidifies urine). • Avoid tasks that require alertness, motor skills until response to drug is established (may cause dizziness, drowsiness). • Notify physician if tendon pain/swelling, palpitations, chest pain, difficulty breathing, persistent diarrhea occurs.

levorphanol tartrate

leh-**vor**-phan-ole

(Levo-Dromoran)

See Opioid analgesics (p. 136C)

Levothroid, *see levothyroxine*

levothyroxine

lee-voe-thye-**rox**-een

(Eltroxin ✤, Levothroid, Levoxyl, Synthroid, Unithroid)

Do not confuse levothyroxine with liothyronine.

FIXED-COMBINATION(S)

With liothyronine, T_3 **(Thyrolar).**

CLASSIFICATION

PHARMACOTHERAPEUTIC: Synthetic isomer of thyroxine. **CLINICAL:** Thyroid hormone (T_4) (see p. 149C).

ACTION

Involved in normal metabolism, growth, development, esp. of CNS in infants. Possesses catabolic, anabolic effects. **Therapeutic Effect:** Increases basal metabolic rate, enhances gluconeogenesis, stimulates protein synthesis.

PHARMACOKINETICS

Variable, incomplete absorption from GI tract. Protein binding: greater than 99%. Widely distributed. Deiodinated in peripheral tissues, minimal metabolism in liver. Eliminated by biliary excretion. **Half-life:** 6–7 days.

USES

Treatment of hypothyroidism, myxedema coma, pituitary thyroid-stimulating hormone (TSH) suppression.

PRECAUTIONS

CONTRAINDICATIONS: Hypersensitivity to tablet components (e.g., tartrazine); allergy to aspirin; lactose intolerance; MI, thyrotoxicosis uncomplicated by hypothyroidism; treatment of obesity. **CAUTIONS:** Elderly, angina pectoris, hypertension, other cardiovascular disease.

LIFESPAN CONSIDERATIONS:

Pregnancy/Lactation: Drug does not cross placenta. Minimal excretion in breast milk. **Pregnancy Category A.** **Children:** No age-related precautions noted. Caution in neonates in interpreting thyroid function tests. **Elderly:** May be more sensitive to thyroid effects; individualized dosage recommended.

INTERACTIONS

DRUG: Cholestyramine, colestipol may decrease absorption. **Estrogens** may cause decrease in serum-free thyroxine. May alter effect of **oral anticoagulants. Sympathomimetics** may increase risk of coronary insufficiency, effects of levothyroxine. **H_2 antagonists, proton pump inhibitors** may decrease effect. **HERBAL:** None significant. **FOOD:** None known. **LAB VALUES:** None known.

L

AVAILABILITY (Rx)

INJECTION, POWDER FOR RECONSTITUTION (SYNTHROID): 200 mcg, 500 mcg. **TABLETS: (LEVOTHROID, LEVOXYL, SYNTHROID, UNITHROID):** 0.025 mg, 0.05 mg, 0.075 mg, 0.088 mg, 0.1 mg, 0.112 mg, 0.125 mg, 0.137 mg, 0.15 mg, 0.175 mg, 0.2 mg, 0.3 mg.

ADMINISTRATION/HANDLING

◀ **ALERT** ▶ Do not interchange brands (problems with bioequivalence between manufacturers).

IV

Reconstitution • Reconstitute 200-mcg or 500-mcg vial with 5 ml 0.9% NaCl to provide concentration of 40 or 100 mcg/ml, respectively; shake until clear.

Rate of administration • Use immediately; discard unused portions. • Give each 100 mcg or less over 1 min.

Storage • Store vials at room temperature.

PO

• Give at same time each day to maintain hormone levels. • Administer before breakfast to prevent insomnia. • Tablets may be crushed.

IV INCOMPATIBILITIES

Do not use or mix with other IV solutions.

INDICATIONS/ROUTES/DOSAGE

HYPOTHYROIDISM

PO: ADULTS, ELDERLY, CHILDREN OLDER THAN 12 YRS, GROWTH AND PUBERTY COMPLETE: 1.7 mcg/kg/day as single daily dose. Usual maintenance: 100–200 mcg/day. **CHILDREN OLDER THAN 12 YRS, GROWTH AND PUBERTY INCOMPLETE:** 2–3 mcg/kg/day. **CHILDREN 6–12 YRS:** 4–5 mcg/kg/day. **CHILDREN 1–5 YRS:** 5–6 mcg/kg/day. **CHILDREN 6–12 MOS:** 6–8 mcg/kg/day. **CHILDREN 3–6 MOS:** 8–10 mcg/kg/day. **CHILDREN YOUNGER THAN 3 MOS:** 10–15 mcg/kg/day.

MYXEDEMA COMA

IV: ADULTS, ELDERLY: Initially, 300–500 mcg. Maintenance: 75–100 mcg/day.

PITUITARY TSH SUPPRESSION

PO: ADULTS, ELDERLY: Doses greater than 2 mcg/kg/day usually required to suppress TSH below 0.1 milliunits/liter.

SIDE EFFECTS

OCCASIONAL: Reversible hair loss at start of therapy in children. **RARE:** Dry skin, GI intolerance, rash, urticaria, pseudotumor cerebri, severe headache in children.

ADVERSE EFFECTS/ TOXIC REACTIONS

Excessive dosage produces signs/symptoms of hyperthyroidism (weight loss, palpitations, increased appetite, tremors, anxiety, tachycardia, hypertension, headache, insomnia, menstrual irregularities). Cardiac arrhythmias occur rarely.

NURSING CONSIDERATIONS

BASELINE ASSESSMENT

Question for hypersensitivity to tartrazine, aspirin, lactose. Obtain baseline weight, vital signs. Signs/symptoms of diabetes mellitus, diabetes insipidus, adrenal insufficiency, hypopituitarism may become intensified. Treat with adrenocortical steroids before thyroid therapy in coexisting hypothyroidism and hypoadrenalism.

INTERVENTION/EVALUATION

Monitor pulse for rate, rhythm (report pulse of 100 or marked increase). Observe for tremors, anxiety. Assess appetite, sleep pattern.

PATIENT/FAMILY TEACHING

• Do not discontinue drug therapy; replacement for hypothyroidism is lifelong. • Follow-up office visits, thyroid function tests are essential. • Take medication at the same time each day, preferably in the morning. • Monitor pulse for rate, rhythm; report irregular rhythm or pulse rate over 100 beats/min. • Do not change brands. • Notify physician promptly of chest pain, weight loss, anxiety, tremors, insomnia. • Children may have reversible hair loss, increased aggressiveness during first few mos of therapy. • Full therapeutic effect may take 1–3 wks.

Levoxyl, *see levothyroxine*

Lexapro, *see escitalopram*

Lexiva, *see fosamprenavir*

lidocaine

lye-doe-kane

(Anestacon, Betacaine ✦, Lidoderm, Xylocaine)

FIXED-COMBINATION(S)

EMLA: lidocaine/prilocaine (an anesthetic): 2.5%/2.5%. **Lidocaine with epinephrine:** lidocaine/epinephrine (a sympathomimetic): 2%/1:50,000; 1%/1:100,000; 1%/1:200,000; 0.5%/1:200,000. **Lidosite:** lidocaine/epinephrine, (a sympathomimetic): 10%/0.1%. **Synéra:** lidocaine/tetracaine (an anesthetic) 70 mg/70 mg.

CLASSIFICATION

PHARMACOTHERAPEUTIC: Amide anesthetic. **CLINICAL:** Antiarrhythmic, anesthetic (see pp. 4C, 5C, 14C).

ACTION

Anesthetic: Inhibits conduction of nerve impulses. **Therapeutic Effect:** Causes temporary loss of feeling/sensation. **Antiarrhythmic:** Decreases depolarization, automaticity, excitability of ventricle during diastole by direct action. **Therapeutic Effect:** Inhibits ventricular arrhythmias.

PHARMACOKINETICS

Route	Onset	Peak	Duration
IV	30–90 sec	N/A	10–20 min
Local anesthetic	2.5 min	N/A	30–60 min

Completely absorbed after IM administration. Protein binding: 60% to 80%. Widely distributed. Metabolized in liver. Primarily excreted in urine. Minimally removed by hemodialysis. **Half-life:** 1–2 hrs.

USES

Antiarrhythmic: Rapid control of acute ventricular arrhythmias following MI, cardiac catheterization, cardiac surgery, digitalis-induced ventricular arrhythmias. **Local Anesthetic:** Infiltration/nerve block for dental/surgical procedures, childbirth. **Topical Anesthetic:** Local skin disorders (minor burns, insect bites, prickly heat, skin manifestations of chickenpox, abrasions). Mucous membranes (local anesthesia of oral, nasal, laryngeal mucous membranes; local anesthesia of respiratory, urinary tracts; relief of discomfort of pruritus ani, hemorrhoids, pruritus vulvae). **Dermal patch:** Relief of chronic pain in postherpetic neuralgia.

PRECAUTIONS

CONTRAINDICATIONS: Adams-Stokes syndrome, hypersensitivity to amide-type local anesthetics, supraventricular arrhythmias, Wolff-Parkinson-White syndrome. Spinal anesthesia contraindicated

L

in septicemia. **CAUTIONS:** Hepatic disease, marked hypoxia, severe respiratory depression, hypovolemia, heart block, bradycardia, atrial fibrillation.

LIFESPAN CONSIDERATIONS:

Pregnancy/Lactation: Crosses placenta. Distributed in breast milk. **Pregnancy Category B. Children:** No age-related precautions noted. **Elderly:** More sensitive to adverse effects. Dose, rate of infusion should be reduced. Age-related renal impairment may require dosage adjustment.

INTERACTIONS

DRUG: Anticonvulsants may increase cardiac depressant effects. **Beta-adrenergic blockers** may increase risk of toxicity. **Other antiarrhythmics** may increase cardiac effects. **HERBAL: St. John's wort** may decrease concentration. **FOOD:** None known. **LAB VALUES:** IM lidocaine may increase creatine kinase (CK) level (used to diagnose acute MI). Therapeutic serum level: 1.5 to 6 mcg/ml; toxic serum level: greater than 6 mcg/ml.

AVAILABILITY (Rx)

CREAM, TOPICAL: 4%. **INFUSION PREMIX:** 0.4% (4 mg/ml in 250 ml, 500 ml); 0.8% (8 mg/ml in 250 ml, 500 ml). **INJECTION, SOLUTION:** 0.5% (5 mg/ml), 1% (10 mg/ml), 2% (20 mg/ml). **JELLY, TOPICAL:** 2%. **SOLUTION, TOPICAL:** 4%. **SOLUTION, VISCOUS:** 2%. **TRANSDERMAL, TOPICAL (LIDODERM):** 5%.

ADMINISTRATION/HANDLING

◄ **ALERT** ► Resuscitative equipment, drugs (including O_2) must always be readily available when administering lidocaine by any route.

IV

◄ **ALERT** ► Use only lidocaine without preservative, clearly marked **for IV use**

Reconstitution • For IV infusion, prepare solution by adding 1 g to 1 L D_5W to provide concentration of 1 mg/ml (0.1%). • Commercially available preparations of 0.2%, 0.4%, and 0.8% may be used for IV infusion. **Maximum concentration:** 4 g/250 ml.

Rate of administration • For IV push, use 1% (10 mg/ml) or 2% (20 mg/ml). • Administer IV push at rate of 25–50 mg/min. • Administer for IV infusion at rate of 1–4 mg/min (1–4 ml); use volume control IV set.

Storage • Store at room temperature.

IM

• Use 10% (100 mg/ml); clearly identify lidocaine that is **for IM use.** • Give in deltoid muscle (serum level is significantly higher than if injection is given in gluteus muscle or lateral thigh).

TOPICAL

• Not for ophthalmic use. • For skin disorders, apply directly to affected area or put on gauze or bandage, which is then applied to the skin. • For mucous membrane use, apply to desired area per manufacturer's insert. • Administer lowest dosage possible that still provides anesthesia.

IV INCOMPATIBILITIES

Amphotericin B complex (Abelcet, AmBisome, Amphotec), thiopental.

IV COMPATIBILITIES

Aminophylline, amiodarone (Cordarone), calcium gluconate, digoxin (Lanoxin), diltiazem (Cardizem), dobutamine (Dobutrex), dopamine (Intropin), enalapril (Vasotec), furosemide (Lasix), heparin, insulin, lipids, nitroglycerin, potassium chloride.

INDICATIONS/ROUTES/DOSAGE

VENTRICULAR ARRHYTHMIAS

IM: ADULTS, ELDERLY: 300 mg (or 4.3 mg/kg). May repeat in 60–90 min.

IV: ADULTS, ELDERLY: Initially, 50–100 mg (1 mg/kg) IV bolus at rate of 25–50 mg/min. May repeat in 5 min. Give no more than 200–300 mg in 1 hr. Maintenance: 20–50 mcg/kg/min (1–4 mg/min) as IV infusion. **CHILDREN, INFANTS:** Initially, 0.5–1 mg/kg IV bolus; may repeat but total dose not to exceed 3–5 mg/kg. Maintenance: 10–50 mcg/kg/min as IV infusion.

LOCAL ANESTHESIA

INFILTRATION, NERVE BLOCK: ADULTS: Local anesthetic dosage varies with procedure, degree of anesthesia, vascularity, duration. **Maximum dose:** 4.5 mg/kg. Do not repeat within 2 hrs.

TOPICAL LOCAL ANESTHESIA

TOPICAL: ADULTS, ELDERLY: Apply to affected areas as needed.

TREATMENT OF POST-HERPETIC NEURALGIA

TOPICAL (DERMAL PATCH): ADULTS, ELDERLY: Apply to intact skin over most painful area (up to 3 applications once for up to 12 hrs in a 24-hr period).

SIDE EFFECTS

CNS effects generally dose-related and of short duration. **OCCASIONAL: IM:** Pain at injection site. **Topical:** Burning, stinging, tenderness at application site. **RARE:** Generally with high dose: Drowsiness; dizziness; disorientation; light-headedness; tremors; apprehension; euphoria; sensation of heat, cold, numbness; blurred or double vision; tinnitus (ringing in ears); nausea.

ADVERSE EFFECTS/ TOXIC REACTIONS

Serious adverse reactions lidocaine are uncommon, but high dosage by any route may produce cardiovascular depression, bradycardia, hypotension, arrhythmias, heart block, cardiovascular collapse, cardiac arrest. Potential for malignant hyperthermia. CNS toxicity may occur, esp. with regional anesthesia use, progressing rapidly from mild side effects to tremors, somnolence, seizures, vomiting, respiratory depression. Methemoglobinemia (evidenced by cyanosis) has occurred following topical application of lidocaine for teething discomfort and laryngeal anesthetic spray.

NURSING CONSIDERATIONS

BASELINE ASSESSMENT

Question for hypersensitivity to lidocaine, amide anesthetics. Obtain baseline B/P, pulse, respiratory rate, EKG, serum electrolytes.

INTERVENTION/EVALUATION

Monitor EKG, vital signs closely during and following drug administration for cardiac performance. If EKG shows arrhythmias, prolongation of PR interval or QRS complex, inform physician immediately. Assess pulse for rhythm, rate, quality. Assess B/P for evidence of hypotension. Monitor for therapeutic serum level (1.5–6 mcg/ml). For lidocaine given by all routes, monitor vital signs, pt's level of consciousness (LOC). Drowsiness should be considered a warning sign of high serum levels of lidocaine. Therapeutic serum level: 1.5–6 mcg/ml; toxic serum level: greater than 6 mcg/ml.

PATIENT/FAMILY TEACHING

• **Local anesthesia:** Ensure that pt understands loss of feeling/sensation, need for protection until anesthetic wears off (no ambulation, including special positions for some regional anesthesia). • **Oral mucous membrane anesthesia:** Do not eat, drink, chew gum for 1 hr after application (swallowing reflex may be impaired, increasing risk of aspiration; numbness of tongue, buccal mucosa may lead to bite trauma).

Lidoderm, *see lidocaine*

L

linezolid

lyn-eh-**zoe**-lid
(Zyvox, Zyvoxam ✦)

Do not confuse Zyvox with Zovirax.

CLASSIFICATION

PHARMACOTHERAPEUTIC: Oxalodinone. **CLINICAL:** Antibiotic.

ACTION

Binds to site on bacterial 23S ribosomal RNA, preventing formation of a complex essential for bacterial translation. **Therapeutic Effect:** Bacteriostatic against enterococci, staphylococci; bactericidal against streptococci.

PHARMACOKINETICS

Rapidly, extensively absorbed after PO administration. Protein binding: 31%. Metabolized in liver by oxidation. Excreted in urine. **Half-life:** 4–5.4 hrs.

USES

Treatment of susceptible infections due to aerobic and facultative, gram-positive microorganisms, including *E. faecium* (vancomycin-resistant strains only), *S. aureus* (including methicillin-resistant strains), *S. agalactiae, S. pneumoniae* (including multidrug-resistant strains) *S. pyogenes*. Treatment of pneumonia, skin, soft tissue infections (including diabetic foot infections), bacteremia caused by susceptible vancomycin-resistant organisms.

PRECAUTIONS

CONTRAINDICATIONS: None known. **CAUTIONS:** Uncontrolled hypertension, pheochromocytoma, carcinoid syndrome, severe renal/hepatic impairment, untreated hyperthyroidism.

LIFESPAN CONSIDERATIONS:

Pregnancy/Lactation: Unknown if distributed in breast milk. **Pregnancy Category C. Children:** Safety and efficacy not established. **Elderly:** No age-related precautions noted.

INTERACTIONS

DRUG: **Bone marrow depressants** may increase risk of leukopenia, thrombocytopenia. **Adrenergic medications (sympathomimetics)** may increase effect. **SSRIs** may increase risk of serotonin syndrome. **HERBAL:** None significant. **FOOD:** Excessive amounts of **tyramine-containing foods, beverages** may cause significant hypertension. **LAB VALUES:** May decrease Hgb, platelet count, WBC count, serum ALT.

AVAILABILITY (Rx)

INJECTION PREMIX: 2 mg/ml in 100-ml, 200-ml, 300-ml bags. **POWDER FOR ORAL SUSPENSION:** 100 mg/5 ml. **TABLETS:** 600 mg.

ADMINISTRATION/HANDLING

IV

Rate of administration • Infuse over 30–120 min.

Storage • Store at room temperature. • Protect from light. • Yellow color does not affect potency.

PO

• Give without regard to meals. • Use suspension within 21 days after reconstitution.

IV INCOMPATIBILITIES

Amphotericin B complex (Abelcet, AmBisome, Amphotec), chlorpromazine (Thorazine), co-trimoxazole (Bactrim), diazepam (Valium), erythromycin (Erythrocin), pentamidine (Pentam IV), phenytoin (Dilantin), total parenteral nutrition (TPN).

INDICATIONS/ROUTES/DOSAGE

VANCOMYCIN-RESISTANT INFECTIONS (VRI)

PO, IV: ADULTS, ELDERLY, CHILDREN OLDER THAN 11 YRS: 600 mg q12h for 14–28 days. **CHILDREN 11 YRS AND YOUNGER:** 10 mg/kg q8–12h for 14–28 days.

PNEUMONIA, COMPLICATED SKIN/SKIN STRUCTURE INFECTIONS

PO, IV: ADULTS, ELDERLY, CHILDREN OLDER THAN 11 YRS: 600 mg q12h for 10–14 days. **CHILDREN 11 YRS AND YOUNGER:** 10 mg/kg q8h for 10–14 days.

UNCOMPLICATED SKIN/SKIN STRUCTURE INFECTIONS

PO: ADULTS, ELDERLY: 400 mg q12h for 10–14 days. **CHILDREN OLDER THAN 11 YRS:** 600 mg q12h for 10–14 days. **CHILDREN 5–11 YRS:** 10 mg/kg/dose q12h for 10–14 days. **CHILDREN YOUNGER THAN 5 YRS:** 10 mg/kg q8h for 10–14 days.

USUAL NEONATE DOSAGE

PO IV: NEONATES: 10 mg/kg/dose q8–12h.

SIDE EFFECTS

OCCASIONAL (5%–2%): Diarrhea, nausea, headache. **RARE (less than 2%):** Altered taste, vaginal candidiasis, fungal infection, dizziness, tongue discoloration.

ADVERSE EFFECTS/ TOXIC REACTIONS

Thrombocytopenia, myelosuppression occur rarely. Antibiotic-associated colitis (severe abdominal pain/tenderness, fever, severe watery diarrhea) may result from altered bacterial balance.

NURSING CONSIDERATIONS

INTERVENTION/EVALUATION

Monitor daily pattern of bowel activity/stool consistency; mild GI effects may be tolerable, but increasing severity may indicate onset of antibiotic-associated colitis. Be alert for superinfection (severe genital/anal pruritus, abdominal pain, severe mouth soreness, moderate to severe diarrhea). Monitor CBC weekly.

PATIENT/FAMILY TEACHING

• Continue therapy for full length of treatment. • Doses should be evenly spaced. • May cause GI upset (may take with food, milk). • Excessive amounts of tyramine-containing foods (red wine, aged cheese) may cause severe reaction (severe headache, neck stiffness, diaphoresis, palpitations).

liothyronine (T_3)

lye-oh-**thye**-roe-neen

(Cytomel, Triostat)

Do not confuse liothyronine with levothyroxine.

FIXED-COMBINATION(S)

With levothyroxine, T_4 **(Thyrolar).**

CLASSIFICATION

PHARMACOTHERAPEUTIC: Synthetic form thyroid hormone T_3. **CLINICAL:** Thyroid hormone (see p. 149C).

ACTION

Involved in normal metabolism, growth, development, esp. of CNS in infants. Possesses catabolic, anabolic effects. **Therapeutic Effect:** Increases basal metabolic rate, enhances gluconeogenesis, stimulates protein synthesis.

PHARMACOKINETICS

Almost completely absorbed following PO administration. Absorption reduced to 43% in congestive heart failure (CHF) pts. Not firmly bound to serum protein. Excreted in urine. **Half-life:** 25 hrs.

USES

PO: Replacement in decreased, absent thyroid function (partial, complete absence of gland; primary atrophy; functional deficiency; effects of surgery, radiation, antithyroid agents; pituitary, hypothalamic hypothyroidism). Management of simple (nontoxic) goiter; diagnostically in T_3 suppression test (differentiates hyperthyroidism from euthyroidism). **IV:** Myxedema coma, precoma.

PRECAUTIONS

CONTRAINDICATIONS: MI, thyrotoxicosis uncomplicated by hypothyroidism; obesity. **CAUTIONS:** Cardiovascular disease, adrenal insufficiency, coronary artery disease, diabetes mellitus, diabetes insipidus.

LIFESPAN CONSIDERATIONS:

Pregnancy/Lactation: Does not cross placenta; is distributed in breast milk. Avoid during late pregnancy (ductus arteriosis). **Pregnancy Category A. Children:** Safety and efficacy not established. **Elderly:** Age-related increased sensitivity to thyroid effects may require dosage adjustment.

L

INTERACTIONS

DRUG: Cholestyramine, colestipol may decrease absorption. May alter effects of **oral anticoagulants. Sympathomimetics** may increase risk of coronary insufficiency, effects. **HERBAL:** None significant. **FOOD:** None known. **LAB VALUES:** None known.

AVAILABILITY (Rx)

INJECTION SOLUTION (TRIOSTAT): 10 mcg/ml. **TABLETS (CYTOMEL):** 5 mcg, 25 mcg, 50 mcg.

ADMINISTRATION/HANDLING

◄ **ALERT** ► Do not use different brands of liothyronine interchangeably because of problems with bioequivalence among manufacturers.

IV

• Administer IV dose over 4 hrs but no longer than 12 hrs apart.

INDICATIONS/ROUTES/DOSAGE

HYPOTHYROIDISM

PO: ADULTS, ELDERLY: Initially, 25 mcg/day. May increase in increments of 12.5–25 mcg/day q1–2wk. **Maximum:** 100 mcg/day. **CHILDREN:** Initially, 5 mcg/day. May increase by 5 mcg/day q3–4 days. Maintenance: 100 mcg/day (children older than 3 yrs); 50 mcg/day (children 1–3 yrs); 20 mcg/day (infants).

MYXEDEMA

PO: ADULTS, ELDERLY: Initially, 5 mcg/day. Increase by 5–10 mcg q1–2wk (after 25 mcg/day has been reached, may increase in 12.5-mcg increments). Maintenance: 50–100 mcg/day.

NONTOXIC GOITER

PO: ADULTS, ELDERLY: Initially, 5 mcg/day. Increase by 5–10 mcg/day q1–2wk. When 25 mcg/day has been reached, may increase by 12.5–25 mcg/day q1–2wk. Maintenance: 75 mcg/day. **CHILDREN:** 5 mcg/day. May increase by 5 mcg q1–2wk. Maintenance: 15–20 mcg/day.

CONGENITAL HYPOTHYROIDISM

PO: CHILDREN: Initially, 5 mcg/day. Increase by 5 mcg/day q3–4 days. Maintenance: Full adult dosage (children older than 3 yrs); 50 mcg/day (children 1–3 yrs); 20 mcg/day (infants).

T_3 SUPPRESSION TEST

PO: ADULTS, ELDERLY: 75–100 mcg/day for 7 days; then repeat I^{131} thyroid uptake test.

MYXEDEMA COMA, PRECOMA

◄ **ALERT** ► Initial and subsequent dosages are based on the pt's clinical status and response.

IV: ADULTS, ELDERLY: Initially, 25–50 mcg (10–20 mcg in pts with cardiovascular disease). Total dose at least 65 mcg/day.

SIDE EFFECTS

OCCASIONAL: Reversible hair loss at start of therapy in children. **RARE:** Dry skin, GI intolerance, rash, urticaria, pseudotumor cerebri, severe headache in children.

ADVERSE EFFECTS/ TOXIC REACTIONS

Excessive dosage produces signs/symptoms of hyperthyroidism (weight loss, palpitations, increased appetite, tremors, anxiety, tachycardia, hypertension, headache, insomnia, menstrual irregularities). Cardiac arrhythmias occur rarely.

NURSING CONSIDERATIONS

BASELINE ASSESSMENT

Question for hypersensitivity to tartrazine, aspirin. Obtain baseline weight, vital signs. Signs/symptoms of diabetes mellitus, diabetes insipidus, adrenal insufficiency, hypopituitarism may become intensified. Treat with adrenocortical steroids prior to thyroid therapy in coexisting hypothyroidism and hypoadrenalism.

INTERVENTION/EVALUATION

Monitor pulse for rate, rhythm. Report irregular pulse or rate over 100 beats/min. Assess for tremors, anxiety. Assess appetite, sleep pattern.

PATIENT/FAMILY TEACHING

• Do not discontinue drug therapy; replacement for hypothyroidism is lifelong. • Follow-up office visits, thyroid function tests are essential. • Take medication at the same time each day, preferably in morning. • Teach pt, family to take pulse correctly, report marked increase, pulse of 100 beats/min or over, change of rhythm. • Notify physician promptly of chest pain, weight loss, anxiety, tremors, insomnia. • Children may have reversible hair loss, increased aggressiveness during first few mos of therapy.

Lipitor, *see atorvastatin*

lisinopril

ly-**sin**-oh-pril

(Apo-Lisinopril ✦, Prinivil, Zestril)

Do not confuse lisinopril with fosinopril; Prinivil with Desyrel, Plendil, Proventil, or Restoril; Fibsol with Lioresal; or Zestril with Zetia, Zostrix. Do not confuse lisinopril's combination form Zestoretic with Prilosec.

FIXED-COMBINATION(S)

Prinzide/Zestoretic: lisinopril/hydrochlorothiazide (a diuretic): 10 mg/12.5 mg; 20 mg/12.5 mg; 20 mg/25 mg.

CLASSIFICATION

PHARMACOTHERAPEUTIC: Angiotensin-converting enzyme (ACE) inhibitor. **CLINICAL:** Antihypertensive (see p. 7C).

ACTION

Suppresses renin-angiotensin-aldosterone system (prevents conversion of angiotensin I to angiotensin II, a potent vasoconstrictor; may inhibit angiotensin II at local vascular, renal sites). Decreases plasma angiotensin II, increases plasma renin activity, decreases aldosterone secretion. **Therapeutic Effect:** Reduces peripheral arterial resistance, B/P (afterload), pulmonary capillary wedge pressure (preload), pulmonary vascular resistance. In those with heart failure, decreases heart size, increases cardiac output, exercise tolerance time.

PHARMACOKINETICS

Route	Onset	Peak	Duration
PO	1 hr	6 hrs	24 hrs

Incompletely absorbed from GI tract. Protein binding: 25%. Primarily excreted unchanged in urine. Removed by hemodialysis. **Half-life:** 12 hrs (increased in renal impairment).

USES

Treatment of hypertension. Used alone or in combination with other antihypertensives. Adjunctive therapy in management of heart failure. Treatment of acute myocardial infarction within 24 hrs in hemodynamically stable pts to improve survival. Treatment of left ventricular dysfuction following myocardial infarction. **OFF-LABEL:** Treatment of hypertension, renal crises with scleroderma.

PRECAUTIONS

CONTRAINDICATIONS: History of angioedema from treatment with ACE inhibitors. **CAUTIONS:** Renal impairment, those with sodium depletion or on diuretic therapy, dialysis, hypovolemia, coronary/cerebrovascular insufficiency, severe CHF.

LIFESPAN CONSIDERATIONS:

Pregnancy/Lactation: Crosses placenta. Unknown if distributed in breast milk. **Pregnancy Category C (D if used in second or third trimester). Children:** Safety and efficacy not established. **Elderly:** May be more sensitive to hypotensive effects.

INTERACTIONS

DRUG: **Alcohol, diuretics, hypotensive agents** may increase effects. May increase concentration, risk of toxicity of **lithium. NSAIDs** may decrease effects. **Potassium-sparing diuretics, potassium supplements** may cause hyperkalemia. **HERBAL:** **Ephedra, ginseng, yohimbe** may worsen hypertension. **Garlic** may increase antihypertensive effect. **FOOD:** None known. **LAB VALUES:** May increase BUN, serum alkaline phosphatase, bilirubin, creatinine, potassium, AST, ALT. May decrease serum sodium. May cause positive ANA titer.

AVAILABILITY (Rx)

TABLETS (PRINIVIL, ZESTRIL): 2.5 mg, 5 mg, 10 mg, 20 mg, 30 mg, 40 mg.

ADMINISTRATION/HANDLING

PO

• Give without regard to food. • Tablets may be crushed.

INDICATIONS/ROUTES/DOSAGE

HYPERTENSION (USED ALONE)

PO: ADULTS: Initially, 10 mg/day. May increase by 5–10 mcg/day at 1- to 2-wk intervals. **Maximum:** 40 mg/day. **ELDERLY:** Initially, 2.5–5 mg/day. May increase by 2.5–5 mg/day at 1- to 2-wk intervals. **Maximum:** 40 mg/day.

HYPERTENSION (IN COMBINATION WITH OTHER ANTIHYPERTENSIVES)

◄ **ALERT** ► Discontinue diuretics 48–72 hrs prior to initiating lisinopril therapy.

PO: ADULTS: Initially, 2.5–5 mg/day titrated to pt's needs.

ADJUNCTIVE THERAPY FOR MANAGEMENT OF HEART FAILURE

PO: ADULTS, ELDERLY: Initially, 2.5–5 mg/day. May increase by no more than 10 mg/day at intervals of at least 2 wks. Maintenance: 5–40 mg/day.

IMPROVE SURVIVAL IN PTS AFTER MYOCARDIAL INFARCTION (MI)

PO: ADULTS, ELDERLY: Initially, 5 mg, then 5 mg after 24 hrs, 10 mg after 48 hrs, then 10 mg/day for 6 wks. For pts with low systolic B/P, give 2.5 mg/day for 5 days, then 2.5–5 mg/day. Pt should continue with thrombolytics, aspirin, beta-blockers.

DOSAGE IN RENAL IMPAIRMENT

Titrate to pt's needs after giving the following initial dose:

Creatinine Clearance	% Normal Dose
10–50 ml/min	50–75
Less than 10 ml/min	25–50

SIDE EFFECTS

FREQUENT (12%–5%): Headache, dizziness, postural hypotension. **OCCASIONAL (4%–2%):** Chest discomfort, fatigue, rash, abdominal pain, nausea, diarrhea, upper respiratory infection. **RARE (1% or less):** Palpitations, tachycardia, peripheral edema, insomnia, paresthesia, confusion, constipation, dry mouth, muscle cramps.

ADVERSE EFFECTS/ TOXIC REACTIONS

Excessive hypotension ("first-dose syncope") may occur in pts with CHF, severe salt/volume depletion. Angioedema (swelling of face and lips), hyperkalemia occur rarely. Agranulocytosis, neutropenia may be noted in pts with collagen vascular disease (scleroderma, systemic lupus erythematosus). Nephrotic syndrome may be noted in pts with history of renal disease.

NURSING CONSIDERATIONS

BASELINE ASSESSMENT

Obtain B/P, apical pulse immediately before each dose, in addition to regular monitoring (be alert to fluctuations). If excessive reduction in B/P occurs, place pt in supine position, feet slightly elevated. In pts with renal impairment, autoimmune disease, taking drugs that affect leukocytes or immune response, CBC and differential count should be performed before beginning therapy and q2wks for 3 mos, then periodically thereafter.

INTERVENTION/EVALUATION

Assess for edema. Auscultate lungs for rales. Monitor I&O; weigh daily. Monitor daily pattern of bowel activity/stool consistency. Assist with ambulation if dizziness occurs. Monitor B/P, renal function tests, WBC, serum potassium.

PATIENT/FAMILY TEACHING

• To reduce hypotensive effect, rise slowly from lying to sitting position, permit legs to dangle from bed momentarily before standing. • Limit alcohol intake. • Inform physician if vomiting, diarrhea, diaphoresis, swelling of face/lips/tongue, difficulty in breathing occur.

lithium carbonate

lith-ee-um

(Apo-Lithium ✦, Duralith ✦, Eskalith, Eskalith CR, Lithobid)

lithium citrate

(Cibalith-S)

Do not confuse Lithobid with Levbid, Lithostat, or Lithotabs.

◆CLASSIFICATION

PHARMACOTHERAPEUTIC: Psychotherapeutic. **CLINICAL:** Antimanic, antidepressant, vascular headache prophylactic.

ACTION

Affects storage, release, reuptake of neurotransmitters. Antimanic effect may result from increased norepinephrine reuptake, serotonin receptor sensitivity. **Therapeutic Effect:** Produces antimanic, antidepressant effects.

PHARMACOKINETICS

Rapidly, completely absorbed from GI tract. Primarily excreted unchanged in urine. Removed by hemodialysis. **Half-life:** 18–24 hrs (increased in elderly).

USES

Prophylaxis, treatment of acute mania, manic phase of bipolar disorder (manic depressive illness). **OFF-LABEL:** Prevention of vascular headache; treatment of depression, neutropenia.

PRECAUTIONS

CONTRAINDICATIONS: Debilitated pts, severe cardiovascular disease, severe dehydration, severe renal disease, severe sodium depletion. **CAUTIONS:** Cardiovascular disease, thyroid disease, elderly.

LIFESPAN CONSIDERATIONS:

Pregnancy/Lactation: Freely crosses placenta. Distributed in breast milk. **Pregnancy Category D. Children:** May increase bone formation or density (alter parathyroid hormone concentrations). **Elderly:** More susceptible to develop lithium-induced goiter or clinical hypothyroidism, CNS toxicity. Increased thirst, urination noted more frequently; lower dosage recommended.

INTERACTIONS

DRUG: May increase effects of **antithyroid medications, iodinated glycerol, potassium iodide. Diuretics, NSAIDs** may increase lithium concentration, risk of toxicity. **Haloperidol** may increase extrapyramidal symptoms (EPS), risk of neurologic toxicity. **Molindone** may increase risk of neurotoxicity. May decrease absorption of **phenothiazines. Phenothiazines** may increase intracellular concentration, increase renal excretion of lithium. **Phenothiazines** may increase delirium, EPS when given concurrently with lithium. Antiemetic effect of some **phenothiazines** may mask early signs of lithium toxicity. **HERBAL:** None significant. **FOOD:** None known. **LAB VALUES:** May increase serum glucose, immunoreactive parathyroid hormone, calcium. Therapeutic serum level is 0.6–1.2 mEq/L; toxic serum level is greater than 1.5 mEq/L.

AVAILABILITY (Rx)

CAPSULES: 150 mg, 300 mg, 600 mg. **SYRUP:** 300 mg/5 ml. **TABLETS:** 300 mg.

TABLETS (CONTROLLED-RELEASE): 450 mg. **TABLETS (SLOW-RELEASE):** 300 mg.

ADMINISTRATION/HANDLING

PO

• Preferable to administer with meals, milk. • Do not crush, chew, break slow-release or film-coated tablets.

INDICATIONS/ROUTES/DOSAGE

◄ **ALERT** ► During acute phase, a therapeutic serum lithium concentration of 1–1.4 mEq/L is required. For long-term control, desired level is 0.5–1.3 mEq/L. Monitor serum drug concentration, clinical response to determine proper dosage.

USUAL DOSAGE

PO: ADULTS: 300 mg 3–4 times a day or 450–900 mg slow-release form twice a day. **Maximum:** 2.4 g/day. **ELDERLY:** 900–1,200 mg/day. Maintenance: 300 mg twice a day. May increase by 300 mg/day q1wk. **CHILDREN 12 YRS AND OLDER:** 600–1,800 mg/day in 3–4 divided doses (2 doses/day for slow-release). **CHILDREN 6–11 YRS:** 15–60 mg/kg/day in 3–4 divided doses not to exceed usual adult dose.

SIDE EFFECTS

◄ **ALERT** ► Side effects are dose related and seldom occur at lithium serum levels less than 1.5 mEq/L.

OCCASIONAL: Fine hand tremor, polydipsia, polyuria, mild nausea. **RARE:** Weight gain, bradycardia, tachycardia, acne, rash, muscle twitching, peripheral cyanosis, pseudotumor cerebri (eye pain, headache, tinnitus, vision disturbances).

ADVERSE EFFECTS/ TOXIC REACTIONS

Lithium serum concentration of 1.5–2.0 mEq/L may produce vomiting, diarrhea, drowsiness, confusion, incoordination, coarse hand tremor, muscle twitching, T-wave depression on EKG. Lithium serum concentration of 2.0–2.5 mEq/L may result in ataxia, giddiness, tinnitus, blurred vision, clonic movements, severe hypotension. Acute toxicity may be characterized by seizures, oliguria, circulatory failure, coma, death.

NURSING CONSIDERATIONS

BASELINE ASSESSMENT

Serum lithium levels should be tested q3–4 days during initial phase of therapy, q1–2mo thereafter, and weekly if there is no improvement of disorder or adverse effects occur.

INTERVENTION/EVALUATION

Serum lithium testing should be performed as close as possible to 12th hr following last dose. Clinical assessment of therapeutic effect, tolerance to drug effect is also necessary for correct dosing-level management. Assess behavior, appearance, emotional status, response to environment, speech pattern, thought content. Monitor serum lithium concentrations, CBC with differential, urinalysis, creatinine clearance. Monitor renal, hepatic, thyroid, cardiovascular function; serum electrolytes. Assess for increased urinary output, persistent thirst. Report polyuria, prolonged vomiting, diarrhea, fever to physician (may need to temporarily reduce or discontinue dosage). Monitor for signs of lithium toxicity. Assess for therapeutic response (interest in surroundings, improvement in self-care, increased ability to concentrate, relaxed facial expression). Monitor lithium levels q3–4 days at initiation of therapy (then q1–2mos). Obtain lithium levels 8–12 hrs postdose. Therapeutic serum level: 0.6–1.2 mEq/L; toxic serum level: greater than 1.5 mEq/L.

PATIENT/FAMILY TEACHING

• Limit alcohol, caffeine intake. • Avoid tasks requiring coordination until CNS effects of drug are known. • May cause dry mouth. • Maintain steady salt, fluid intake (avoid dehydration). • Inform physician if vomiting, diarrhea, muscle weakness, tremors, drowsiness, ataxia occurs. • Serum level monitoring is necessary to determine proper dose.

lomefloxacin

low-meh-**flocks**-ah-sin
(Maxaquin)

CLASSIFICATION

PHARMACOTHERAPEUTIC: Quinolone. **CLINICAL:** Antibiotic (see p. 24C).

ACTION

Inhibits the enzyme DNA-gyrase in susceptible microorganisms. **Therapeutic Effect:** Interferes with bacterial cell replication and repair. Bactericidal.

PHARMACOKINETICS

Well absorbed from GI tract. Protein binding: 10%. Widely distributed. Metabolized in liver. Primarily excreted in urine. Not removed by hemodialysis. **Half-life:** 4–6 hrs (increased in renal impairment, elderly).

USES

Treatment of susceptible infecitons due to *H. influenzae, M. catarrhalis, E. coli, K. pneumoniae, P. mirabilis, S. saprophyticus, P. aeruginosa* including urinary tract, lower respiratory tract infections; postop prophylaxis in pts undergoing transurethral procedures.

PRECAUTIONS

CONTRAINDICATIONS: Hypersensitivity to quinolones. **CAUTIONS:** Renal impairment, CNS disorders, seizures, those taking theophylline, caffeine.

LIFESPAN CONSIDERATIONS:

Pregnancy/Lactation: Unknown if distributed in breast milk. If possible, do not use during pregnancy/lactation (risk of arthropathy to fetus/infant). **Pregnancy Category C. Children:** Safety and efficacy not established. **Elderly:** Age-related renal impairment may require dosage adjustment.

INTERACTIONS

DRUG: Antacids, iron preparations, sucralfate may decrease absorption. May increase effects of **caffeine, oral anticoagulants.** Decreases **theophylline** clearance, may increase concentration, risk of toxicity of **theophylline.** **HERBAL: Dong quai, St. John's wort** may increase risk of photosensitization. **FOOD:** None known. **LAB VALUES:** May increase BUN, serum alkaline phosphatase, bilirubin, creatinine, LDH, AST, ALT.

AVAILABILITY (Rx)

TABLETS: 400 mg.

ADMINISTRATION/HANDLING

PO

• May be given without regard to meals (preferred dosing time: 2 hrs after meals). • Do not administer antacids (aluminum, magnesium) within 2 hrs of lomefloxacin. • Encourage intake of cranberry juice, citrus fruits (acidifies urine).

INDICATIONS/ROUTES/DOSAGE

COMPLICATED UTI

PO: ADULTS, ELDERLY: 400 mg/day for 10–14 days.

UNCOMPLICATED UTI

PO: ADULTS, ELDERLY: 400 mg/day for 3 days.

LOWER RESPIRATORY TRACT INFECTIONS

PO: ADULTS, ELDERLY: 400 mg/day for 10 days.

SURGICAL PROPHYLAXIS

PO: ADULTS, ELDERLY: 400 mg 2–6 hrs before surgery.

DOSAGE IN RENAL IMPAIRMENT

Dosage and frequency are modified based on creatinine clearance.

Creatinine Clearance	Dosage
41 ml/min and higher	No change
10–40 ml/min	400 mg initially, then 200 mg/day for 10–14 days

SIDE EFFECTS

OCCASIONAL (3%–2%): Nausea, headache, moderate to severe photosensitivity, dizziness. **RARE (1%):** Diarrhea.

ADVERSE EFFECTS/ TOXIC REACTIONS

Antibiotic-associated colitis (severe abdominal pain, tenderness, fever, severe watery diarrhea), other superinfections may result from altered bacterial balance.

NURSING CONSIDERATIONS

BASELINE ASSESSMENT

Question for history of hypersensitivity to quinolones.

INTERVENTION/EVALUATION

Monitor signs/symptoms of infection, WBC count. Assess mental status. Check for dizziness, headache. Be alert for superinfection (genital pruritus, vaginitis, fever, oral candidiasis).

PATIENT/FAMILY TEACHING

• Do not skip doses; take full course of therapy. • Do not take antacids (reduces/destroys effectiveness). • Avoid sunlight, ultraviolet exposure; wear sunscreen, protective clothing if photosensitivity develops.

Lomotil, *see diphenoxylate with atropine*

lomustine

low-**meuw**-steen
(CeeNU)

◆ CLASSIFICATION

PHARMACOTHERAPEUTIC: Alkylating agent (nitrosourea). **CLINICAL:** Antineoplastic (see p. 81C).

ACTION

Inhibits DNA, RNA protein synthesis by cross-linking with DNA and RNA strands, preventing cell division. Cell cycle–phase nonspecific. **Therapeutic Effect:** Interferes with DNA, RNA function.

PHARMACOKINETICS

Rapidly absorbed following PO administration. Highly lipid soluble. Metabolized in liver. Excreted in urine. **Half-life:** 16 hrs.

USES

Treatment of primary/metastatic brain tumors, disseminated Hodgkin's lymphoma. **OFF-LABEL:** Breast, colorectal, GI, non–small cell lung, renal carcinoma; malignant melanoma, multiple myeloma.

PRECAUTIONS

CONTRAINDICATIONS: Pregnancy. **CAUTIONS:** Depressed platelet, leukocyte, erythrocyte counts.

⌛ LIFESPAN CONSIDERATIONS:

Pregnancy/Lactation: May be harmful to fetus. Distributed in breast milk. Avoid breast-feeding. **Pregnancy Category D. Children:** Safety and efficacy not established. **Elderly:** Age-related renal impairment may require dosage adjustment.

INTERACTIONS

DRUG: Bone marrow depressants may increase myelosuppression. **Live virus vaccines** may potentiate virus replication, increase vaccine side effects, decrease pt's antibody response to vaccine. **HERBAL:** None significant. **FOOD:** None known. **LAB VALUES:** May increase hepatic function test results.

AVAILABILITY (Rx)

CAPSULES: 10 mg, 40 mg, 100 mg.

ADMINISTRATION/HANDLING

◀ **ALERT** ▶ Lomustine dosage is individualized based on clinical response and tolerance of adverse effects. When used in combination therapy, consult specific protocols for optimum dosage, sequence of drug administration.

INDICATIONS/ROUTES/DOSAGE

USUAL DOSAGE

PO: ADULTS, ELDERLY: 100–130 mg/m^2 as single dose. Repeat dose at intervals of at least 6 wks but not until circulating blood elements have returned to acceptable levels. Adjust dose based on hematologic response to previous dose. **CHILDREN:** 75–150 mg/m^2 as a single dose every 6 wks.

DOSAGE IN RENAL IMPAIRMENT

Creatinine Clearance	Dosage
10–50 ml/min	75% of normal dosage
Less than 10 ml/min	50% of normal dosage

SIDE EFFECTS

FREQUENT: Nausea, vomiting (occurs 45 min–6 hrs after dose, lasting 12–24 hrs); anorexia (often follows for 2–3 days).

L

OCCASIONAL: Neurotoxicity (confusion, slurred speech), stomatitis, darkening of skin, diarrhea, rash, pruritus, alopecia.

ADVERSE EFFECTS/ TOXIC REACTIONS

Myelosuppression may result in hematologic toxicity (principally leukopenia, mild anemia, thrombocytopenia). Leukopenia occurs about 6 wks after a dose, thrombocytopenia about 4 wks after a dose; both persist for 1–2 wks. Refractory anemia, thrombocytopenia occur commonly if lomustine therapy continues for more than 1 yr. Hepatotoxicity occurs infrequently. Large cumulative doses of lomustine may result in renal damage.

NURSING CONSIDERATIONS

BASELINE ASSESSMENT

Manufacturer recommends weekly blood counts; experts recommend first blood count obtained 2–3 wks following initial therapy, subsequent blood counts indicated by prior toxicity. Antiemetics can reduce duration, frequency of nausea, vomiting.

INTERVENTION/EVALUATION

Monitor CBC with differential; platelet count; hepatic, renal, pulmonary function tests. Monitor for stomatitis. Monitor for hematologic toxicity (fever, sore throat, signs of local infection, unusual bruising/bleeding from any site), symptoms of anemia (excessive fatigue, weakness).

PATIENT/FAMILY TEACHING

• Nausea, vomiting generally abates in less than 1 day. • Fasting before therapy can reduce frequency/duration of GI effects. • Maintain fastidious oral hygiene. • Do not have immunizations without physician's approval (drug lowers resistance). • Avoid crowds, those with known illness. • Promptly report fever, sore throat, signs of local infection, unusual bruising/bleeding from any site, swelling of legs or feet, jaundice.

loperamide

loe-**per**-a-mide

(Apo-Loperamide ✦, Diarr-Eze ✦, Diamode, Imodium, Imodium A-D, Loperacap ✦, Novo-Loperamide ✦)

Do not confuse Imodium with Indocin or Ionamin.

FIXED-COMBINATION(S)

Imodium Advanced: loperamide/simethicone (an antiflatulant): 2 mg/125 mg.

CLASSIFICATION

CLINICAL: Antidiarrheal (see p. 43C).

ACTION

Directly affects intestinal wall muscles. **Therapeutic Effect:** Slows intestinal motility, prolongs transit time of intestinal contents by reducing fecal volume, diminishing loss of fluid, electrolytes, increasing viscosity, bulk of stool.

PHARMACOKINETICS

Poorly absorbed from GI tract. Protein binding: 97%. Metabolized in liver. Eliminated in feces; excreted in urine. Not removed by hemodialysis. **Half-life:** 9.1–14.4 hrs.

USES

Controls, provides symptomatic relief of acute nonspecific diarrhea, chronic diarrhea associated with inflammatory bowel disease, traveler's diarrhea.

PRECAUTIONS

CONTRAINDICATIONS: Acute ulcerative colitis (may produce toxic megacolon), diarrhea associated with pseudomembranous enterocolitis due to broad-spectrum antibiotics or to organisms that invade intestinal mucosa (e.g., *Escherichia coli,* shigella, salmonella), pts who must avoid constipation. **CAUTIONS:** Those with fluid or electrolyte depletion, hepatic impairment.

LIFESPAN CONSIDERATIONS:

Pregnancy/Lactation: Unknown if drug crosses placenta or is distributed in breast milk. **Pregnancy Category C.** **Children:** Not recommended in those younger than 6 yrs (infants younger than 3 mos more susceptible to CNS effects). **Elderly:** May mask dehydration, electrolyte depletion.

INTERACTIONS

DRUG: **Opioid (narcotic) analgesics** may increase risk of constipation. **HERBAL:** None significant. **FOOD:** None known. **LAB VALUES:** None known.

AVAILABILITY (Rx)

CAPLETS: 2 mg. **CAPSULES:** 2 mg. **LIQUID:** 1 mg/5 ml (OTC). **TABLETS:** 2 mg (OTC).

ADMINISTRATION/HANDLING

LIQUID

• When administering to children, use accompanying plastic dropper to measure the liquid.

INDICATIONS/ROUTES/DOSAGE

ACUTE DIARRHEA

PO (CAPSULES): ADULTS, ELDERLY: Initially, 4 mg; then 2 mg after each unformed stool. **Maximum:** 16 mg/day. **CHILDREN 9–12 YRS, WEIGHING MORE THAN 30 KG:** Initially, 2 mg 3 times a day for 24 hrs. **CHILDREN 6–8 YRS, WEIGHING 20–30 KG:** Initially, 2 mg twice a day for 24 hrs. **CHILDREN 2–5 YRS, WEIGHING 13–20 KG:** Initially, 1 mg 3 times a day for 24 hrs. Maintenance: 1 mg/10 kg only after loose stool.

CHRONIC DIARRHEA

PO: ADULTS, ELDERLY: Initially, 4 mg; then 2 mg after each unformed stool until diarrhea is controlled. **CHILDREN:** 0.08–0.24 mg/kg/day in 2–3 divided doses. **Maximum:** 2 mg/dose.

TRAVELER'S DIARRHEA

PO: ADULTS, ELDERLY: Initially, 4 mg; then 2 mg after each loose bowel movement. **Maximum:** 8 mg/day for 2 days. **CHILDREN 9–11 YRS:** Initially, 2 mg; then 1 mg after each loose bowel movement. **Maximum:** 6 mg/day for 2 days. **CHILDREN 6–8 YRS:** Initially, 1 mg; then 1 mg after each loose bowel movement. **Maximum:** 4 mg/day for 2 days.

SIDE EFFECTS

RARE: Dry mouth, drowsiness, abdominal discomfort, allergic reaction (rash, pruritus).

ADVERSE EFFECTS/ TOXIC REACTIONS

Toxicity results in constipation, GI irritation (nausea, vomiting), CNS depression. Activated charcoal is used to treat loperamide toxicity.

NURSING CONSIDERATIONS

BASELINE ASSESSMENT

Do not administer in presence of bloody diarrhea, temperature greater than 101°F.

INTERVENTION/EVALUATION

Encourage adequate fluid intake. Assess bowel sounds for peristalsis. Monitor daily pattern of bowel activity/stool consistency. Withhold drug, notify physician promptly in event of abdominal pain, distention, fever.

PATIENT/FAMILY TEACHING

• Do not exceed prescribed dose. • May cause dry mouth. • Avoid alcohol. • Avoid tasks that require alertness, motor skills until response to drug is established. • Notify physician if diarrhea does not stop within 3 days, abdominal distention, pain occurs, fever develops.

lopinavir/ritonavir

low-**pin**-ah-veer/rih-**ton**-ah-veer
(Kaletra)

Do not confuse Kaletra with Keppra.

CLASSIFICATION

PHARMACOTHERAPEUTIC: Protease inhibitor combination. **CLINICAL:** Antiretroviral (see pp. 65C, 113C).

L

ACTION

Lopinavir inhibits activity of protease, an enzyme, late in HIV replication process; ritonavir increases plasma levels of lopinavir. **Therapeutic Effect:** Formation of immature, noninfectious viral particles.

PHARMACOKINETICS

Readily absorbed after PO administration (absorption increased when taken with food). Protein binding: 98%–99%. Metabolized in liver. Eliminated primarily in feces. Not removed by hemodialysis. **Half-life:** 5–6 hrs.

USES

In combination with other antiretroviral agents for treatment of HIV infection.

PRECAUTIONS

CONTRAINDICATIONS: Concomitant use of ergot derivatives (causes vasospasm, peripheral ischemia of extremities), flecainide, midazolam, pimozide, propafenone (increased risk of serious cardiac arrhythmias), triazolam (increased sedation, respiratory depression); hypersensitivity to lopinavir, ritonavir. **CAUTIONS:** Hepatic impairment, hepatitis B or C. High-dose itraconazole, ketoconazole not recommended. Metronidazole may cause disulfiram-type reaction with oral solution (contains alcohol).

LIFESPAN CONSIDERATIONS:

Pregnancy/Lactation: Unknown if excreted in breast milk. Not recommended that HIV-infected mothers breast-feed. **Pregnancy Category C. Children:** Safety and efficacy not established in those younger than 6 mos. **Elderly:** Age-related renal/hepatic/cardiac impairment requires caution.

INTERACTIONS

DRUG: May increase concentration/toxicity of **amiodarone, bepridil, lidocaine, atorvastatin, lovastatin, simvastatin, clarithromycin, cyclosporine, tacrolimus, sirolimus, felodipine, nicardipine, nifedipine, fluticasone, itraconazole, ketoconazole, midazolam, triazolam, nelfinavir, sildenafil, trazodone, warfarin.** May decrease concentration /effect of **atovaquone, oral contraceptives. Carbamazepine, phenobarbital, phenytoin, rifampin** may decrease concentration/effect. May cause acute ergot toxicity with **dihydroergotamine, ergotamine.** May cause disulfiram-like reaction with **metronidazole. HERBAL: St. John's wort** may decrease concentration/effect. **FOOD:** None known. **LAB VALUES:** May increase serum glucose, GGT, total cholesterol, triglycerides, uric acid, AST, ALT.

AVAILABILITY (Rx)

ORAL SOLUTION: 80 mg/ml lopinavir/20 mg/ml ritonavir.

TABLETS: 200 mg lopinavir/50 mg ritonavir.

ADMINISTRATION/HANDLING

PO

• Swallow tablets whole; do not chew, break, crush. • Does not require refrigeration. • Give tablets without regard to food. • Solution must be given with food.

INDICATIONS/ROUTES/ DOSAGE

HIV INFECTION

PO: ADULTS: 2 tablets (400 mg lopinavir/ 100 mg ritonavir) or 5 ml twice a day. Increase to 3 tablets (600 mg lopinavir/ 100 mg ritonavir) or 6.5 ml when taken with efavirenz or nevirapine. **CHILDREN WEIGHING 15–40 KG WHO ARE NOT TAKING EFAVIRENZ OR NEVIRAPINE:** 10 mg/kg twice a day. **CHILDREN WEIGHING 7–14 KG WHO ARE NOT TAKING ALPRENAVIR, EFAVIRENZ, NELFINAVIR, NEVIRAPINE:** 12 mg/kg twice a day. **CHILDREN WEIGHING 15–40 KG WHO ARE TAKING EFAVIRENZ OR NEVIRAPINE:** 11 mg/kg twice a day. **CHILDREN WEIGHING 7–14 KG WHO ARE TAKING EFAVIRENZ OR NEVIRAPINE:** 13 mg/kg twice a day.

PO (ONCE DAILY):

◄ ALERT ► Once-daily dosing is not recommended in therapy-experienced pts and has not been evaluated in children.

ADULTS: 4 tablets (800 mg lopinavir/ 200 mg ritonavir) or 10 ml once daily.

SIDE EFFECTS

FREQUENT (14%): Mild to moderate diarrhea. **OCCASIONAL (6%–2%):** Nausea, asthenia, abdominal pain, headache, vomiting. **RARE (less than 2%):** Insomnia, rash.

ADVERSE EFFECTS/ TOXIC REACTIONS

Anemia, leukopenia, lymphadenopathy, deep vein thrombosis, Cushing's syndrome, pancreatitis, hemorrhagic colitis occur rarely.

NURSING CONSIDERATIONS

BASELINE ASSESSMENT

Obtain baseline CBC, renal/hepatic function tests, weight.

INTERVENTION/EVALUATION

Monitor daily pattern of bowel activity/ stool consistency. Assess for opportunistic infections: onset of fever, oral mucosa changes, cough, other respiratory symptoms. Check weight at least 2 times a wk. Assess for nausea, vomiting. Monitor for signs/symptoms of pancreatitis (nausea, vomiting, abdominal pain), electrolytes, serum glucose, cholesterol, hepatic function, CBC with differential, platelets, CD4 cell count, viral load.

PATIENT/FAMILY TEACHING

• Explain correct administration of medication. • Eat small, frequent meals to offset nausea, vomiting. • Medication is not a cure for HIV infection, nor does it reduce risk of transmission to others.

L

Lopressor, *see metoprolol*

loratadine

low-**rah**-tah-deen

(Alavert, Claritin, Claritin RediTab, Dimetapp, Tavist ND)

FIXED-COMBINATION(S)

Claritin-D: loratadine/pseudoephedrine (a sympathomimetic): 5 mg/120 mg; 10 mg/240 mg.

CLASSIFICATION

PHARMACOTHERAPEUTIC: H_1 antagonist. **CLINICAL:** Antihistamine (see p. 53C).

ACTION

Competes with histamine for H_1 receptor sites on effector cells. **Therapeutic Effect:** Prevents allergic responses mediated by histamine, (e.g., rhinitis, urticaria, pruritus).

PHARMACOKINETICS

Route	Onset	Peak	Duration
PO	1–3 hrs	8–12 hrs	Longer than 24 hrs

Rapidly, almost completely absorbed from GI tract. Protein binding: 97%; metabolite, 73%–77%. Distributed mainly to liver, lungs, GI tract, bile. Metabolized in liver to active metabolite; undergoes extensive first-pass metabolism. Eliminated in urine and feces. Not removed by hemodialysis. **Half-life:** 8.4 hrs; metabolite, 28 hrs (increased in elderly, hepatic impairment).

L

USES

Relief of nasal, non-nasal symptoms of seasonal allergic rhinitis (hayfever). Treatment of idiopathic chronic urticaria (hives). **OFF-LABE\L:** Adjunct treatment of bronchial asthma.

PRECAUTIONS

CONTRAINDICATIONS: Hypersensitivity to loratadine or its ingredients. **CAUTIONS:** Hepatic impairment, breast-feeding women.

LIFESPAN CONSIDERATIONS:

Pregnancy/Lactation: Excreted in breast milk. **Pregnancy Category B. Children:** Safety and efficacy not established in children younger than 2 yrs. **Elderly:** More sensitive to anticholinergic effects (e.g., dry mouth, nose, throat).

INTERACTIONS

DRUG: Clarithromycin, erythromycin, fluconazole, ketoconazole may increase concentration. **HERBAL:** None significant. **FOOD: All foods** delay absorption. **LAB VALUES:** May suppress wheal, flare reactions to antigen skin testing unless drug is discontinued 4 days before testing.

AVAILABILITY (Rx)

SYRUP (CLARITIN): 10 mg/10 ml. **TABLETS (ALAVERT, CLARITIN, TAVIST ND):** 10 mg. **TABLETS (RAPIDLY-DISINTEGRATING [ALAVERT, CLARITIN REDITAB]):** 10 mg.

ADMINISTRATION/HANDLING

PO

• Preferably give on empty stomach (food delays absorption).

RAPIDLY DISINTEGRATING TABLETS

• Place under tongue. • Disintegration occurs within seconds, after which tablet contents may be swallowed with or without water.

INDICATIONS/ROUTES/DOSAGE

ALLERGIC RHINITIS, URTICARIA

PO: ADULTS, ELDERLY, CHILDREN 6 YRS AND OLDER: 10 mg once a day. **CHILDREN 2–5 YRS:** 5 mg once a day.

DOSAGE IN RENAL/HEPATIC IMPAIRMENT

PO: ADULTS, ELDERLY, CHILDREN 6 YRS AND OLDER: 10 mg every other day. **CHILDREN 2–5 YRS:** 5 mg every other day.

SIDE EFFECTS

FREQUENT (12%–8%): Headache, fatigue, drowsiness. **OCCASIONAL (3%):** Dry mouth, nose, throat. **RARE:** Photosensitivity.

ADVERSE EFFECTS/ TOXIC REACTIONS

None significant.

NURSING CONSIDERATIONS

BASELINE ASSESSMENT

Assess lung sounds for wheezing, skin for urticaria, other allergy symptoms.

INTERVENTION/EVALUATION

For upper respiratory allergies, increase fluids to decrease viscosity of secretions, offset thirst, replenish loss of fluids from increased diaphoresis. Monitor symptoms for therapeutic response.

PATIENT/FAMILY TEACHING

• Drink plenty of water (may cause dry mouth). • Avoid alcohol. • Avoid tasks that require alertness, motor skills until response to drug is established (may cause drowsiness). • May cause photosensitivity reactions (avoid direct exposure to sunlight.)

lorazepam

low-**raz**-ah-pam

(Apo-Lorazepam ✤, Ativan, Lorazepam Intensol, Novo-Lorazem ✤)

Do not confuse lorazepam with Alprazolam.

CLASSIFICATION

PHARMACOTHERAPEUTIC: Benzodiazepine **(Schedule IV). CLINICAL:** Antianxiety, sedative-hypnotic, antiemetic, skeletal muscle relaxant, amnesiac, anticonvulsant, antitremor (see p. 12C).

ACTION

Enhances action of inhibitory neurotransmitter gamma-aminobutyric acid (GABA) in CNS, affecting memory, motor, sensory, cognitive function. **Therapeutic Effect:** Produces anxiolytic, anticonvulsant, sedative, muscle relaxant, antiemetic effects.

PHARMACOKINETICS

Route	Onset	Peak	Duration
PO	60 min	N/A	8–12 hrs
IV	15–30 min	N/A	8–12 hrs
IM	30–60 min	N/A	8–12 hrs

Well absorbed after PO, IM administration. Protein binding: 85%. Widely distributed. Metabolized in liver. Primarily excreted in urine. Not removed by hemodialysis. **Half-life:** 10–20 hrs.

USES

Oral: Management of anxiety disorders, short-term relief of symptoms of anxiety, anxiety associated with depressive symptoms. Treatment of nausea, vomiting. **IV:** Status epilepticus, pre-anesthesia for amnesia, antiemetic adjunct. **OFF-LABEL:** Treatment of alcohol withdrawal, panic disorders, skeletal muscle spasms, chemotherapy-induced nausea/vomiting, tension headache, tremors. Adjunctive treatment before endoscopic procedures (diminishes pt recall).

PRECAUTIONS

CONTRAINDICATIONS: Narrow-angle glaucoma, preexisting CNS depression, severe hypotension, severe uncontrolled pain. **CAUTIONS:** Neonates, renal/hepatic impairment, compromised pulmonary function, concomitant CNS depressant use.

LIFESPAN CONSIDERATIONS:

Pregnancy/Lactation: May cross placenta. May be distributed in breast milk. May increase risk of fetal abnormalities if administered during first trimester of pregnancy. Chronic ingestion during pregnancy may produce fetal toxicity, withdrawal symptoms, CNS depression in neonates. **Pregnancy Category D.** **Children:** Safety and efficacy not established in those younger than 12 yrs. **Elderly:** Use small initial doses with gradual increases to avoid ataxia, excessive sedation.

INTERACTIONS

DRUG: Alcohol, other CNS depressants may increase CNS depression. **HERBAL: Gotu kola, kava kava, St. John's wort, valerian** may increase

L

CNS depression. **FOOD:** None known. **LAB VALUES:** None known. Therapeutic serum level: 50–240 ng/ml; toxic serum level: unknown.

AVAILABILITY (Rx)

INJECTION SOLUTION: 2 mg/ml, 4 mg/ml. **ORAL SOLUTION (LORAZEPAM INTENSOL):** 2 mg/ml. **TABLETS:** 0.5 mg, 1 mg, 2 mg.

ADMINISTRATION/HANDLING

IV

Reconstitution • Dilute with equal volume of Sterile Water for Injection. To dilute prefilled 0.9% NaCl or D_5W syringe, remove air from half-filled syringe, aspirate equal volume of diluent, pull plunger back slightly to allow for mixing, gently invert syringe several times (do not shake vigorously).

Rate of administration • Give by IV push into tubing of free-flowing IV infusion (0.9% NaCl, D_5W) at a rate not to exceed 2 mg/min.

Storage • Refrigerate parenteral form. • Do not use if discolored or precipitate forms. • Avoid freezing.

IM

• Give deep IM into large muscle mass.

PO

• Give with food. • Tablets may be crushed.

IV INCOMPATIBILITIES

Aldesleukin (Proleukin), aztreonam (Azactam), idarubicin (Idamycin), ondansetron (Zofran), sufentanil (Sufenta).

IV COMPATIBILITIES

Bumetanide (Bumex), cefepime (Maxipime), diltiazem (Cardizem), dobutamine (Dobutrex), dopamine (Intropin), heparin, labetalol (Normodyne, Trandate), lipids, milrinone (Primacor), norepinephrine (Levophed), piperacillin and tazobactam (Zosyn), potassium, propofol (Diprivan).

INDICATIONS/ROUTES/DOSAGE

ANXIETY

PO: ADULTS: 1–10 mg/day in 2–3 divided doses. Average: 2–6 mg/day. **ELDERLY:** Initially, 0.5–1 mg/day. May increase gradually. Range: 0.5–4 mg.
IV: ADULTS, ELDERLY: 0.02–0.06 mg/kg q2–6h.
IV INFUSION: ADULTS, ELDERLY: 0.01–0.1 mg/kg/h.
PO, IV: CHILDREN: 0.05 mg/kg/dose q4–8h. Range: 0.02–0.1 mg/kg. **Maximum:** 2 mg/dose.

INSOMNIA DUE TO ANXIETY

PO: ADULTS: 2–4 mg at bedtime. **ELDERLY:** 0.5–1 mg at bedtime.

ANTIEMETIC

IV: ADULTS, ELDERLY: 0.5–2 mg q4–6h as needed. **CHILDREN 2–15 YRS:** 0.05 mg/kg (up to 2 mg) prior to chemotherapy.
PO: ADULTS, ELDERLY: 0.5–2 mg q4–6h as needed.

PREOPERATIVE SEDATION

IV: ADULTS, ELDERLY: 0.044 mg/kg 15–20 min before surgery. **Maximum total dose:** 2 mg.
IM: ADULTS, ELDERLY: 0.05 mg/kg 2 hrs before procedure. **Maximum total dose:** 4 mg.

STATUS EPILEPTICUS

IV: ADULTS, ELDERLY: 4 mg over 2–5 min. May repeat in 10–15 min. **Maximum:** 8 mg in 12-hr period. **CHILDREN:** 0.1 mg/kg over 2–5 min. May give second dose of 0.05 mg/kg in 15–20 min. **Maximum:** 4 mg. **NEONATES:** 0.05 mg/kg. May repeat in 10–15 min.

SIDE EFFECTS

FREQUENT: Drowsiness (initially in the morning), ataxia, confusion. **OCCASIONAL:** Blurred vision, slurred speech, hypotension, headache. **RARE:** Paradoxical CNS restlessness, excitement in elderly/debilitated.

ADVERSE EFFECTS/ TOXIC REACTIONS

Abrupt or too-rapid withdrawal may result in pronounced restlessness, irritability, insomnia, hand tremor, abdominal cramping, muscle cramps, diaphoresis, vomiting, seizures. Overdose results in somnolence, confusion, diminished reflexes, coma.

NURSING CONSIDERATIONS

BASELINE ASSESSMENT

Offer emotional support to anxious pt. Pt must remain recumbent for up to 8 hrs (individualized) following parenteral administration to reduce hypotensive effect. Assess motor responses (agitation, trembling, tension), autonomic responses (cold or clammy hands, diaphoresis).

INTERVENTION/EVALUATION

Monitor B/P, respiratory rate, heart rate, CBC with differential, hepatic function tests. For those on long-term therapy, hepatic/renal function tests, blood counts should be performed periodically. Assess for paradoxical reaction, particularly during early therapy. Evaluate for therapeutic response: calm facial expression, decreased restlessness, insomnia. Therapeutic serum level: 50–240 ng/ml; toxic serum level: N/A.

PATIENT/FAMILY TEACHING

• Drowsiness usually disappears during continued therapy. • Avoid tasks that require alertness, motor skills until response to drug is established. • Smoking reduces drug effectiveness. • Do not abruptly withdraw medication after long-term therapy. • Do not use alcohol, CNS depressants. • Contraception recommended for long-term therapy. • Notify physician at once if pregnancy is suspected.

losartan

lo-**sar** tan
(Cozaar)

Do not confuse Cozaar with Zocor.

FIXED-COMBINATION(S)

Hyzaar: losartan/hydrochlorothiazide (a diuretic): 50 mg/12.5 mg; 100 mg/12.5 mg; 100 mg/25 mg.

◆CLASSIFICATION

PHARMACOTHERAPEUTIC: Angiotensin II receptor antagonist. **CLINICAL:** Antihypertensive (see p. 8C).

ACTION

Potent vasodilator. Blocks vasoconstrictor, aldosterone-secreting effects of angiotensin II, inhibiting binding of angiotensin II to AT_1 receptors. **Therapeutic Effect:** Causes vasodilation, decreases peripheral resistance, decreases B/P.

PHARMACOKINETICS

Route	Onset	Peak	Duration
PO	N/A	6 hrs	24 hrs

Well absorbed after PO administration. Protein binding: 98%. Undergoes first-pass metabolism in liver to active metabolites. Excreted in urine and via the biliary system. Not removed by hemodialysis. **Half-life:** 2 hrs, metabolite: 6–9 hrs.

USES

Treatment of hypertension. Used alone or in combination with other antihypertensives. Treatment of diabetic nephropathy, prevention of stroke. **OFF-LABEL:** CHF, erythrocytosis.

PRECAUTIONS

CONTRAINDICATIONS: None known. **CAUTIONS:** Renal/hepatic impairment, renal arterial stenosis.

LIFESPAN CONSIDERATIONS:

Pregnancy/Lactation: Has caused fetal/neonatal morbidity, mortality. Potential for adverse effects on breast-fed infant. Do not breast-feed. **Pregnancy Category C (D if used in second or third trimester). Children:** Safety and efficacy not established. **Elderly:** No age-related precautions noted.

INTERACTIONS

DRUG: NSAIDs may decrease effect. **Cyclosporine, potassium-sparing diuretics, potassium supplements** may increase serum potassium. **Diuretics, other antihypertensive medications** may produce additive hypotension. **HERBAL: Ephedra, ginseng, yohimbe** may worsen hypertension. **Garlic** may increase antihypertensive effect. **FOOD: Grapefruit, grapefruit juice** may alter absorption. **LAB VALUES:** May increase BUN, serum alkaline phosphatase, bilirubin, creatinine, AST, ALT. May decrease Hgb, Hct.

AVAILABILITY (Rx)

TABLETS: 25 mg, 50 mg, 100 mg.

ADMINISTRATION/HANDLING

PO

- May give without regard to food.

INDICATIONS/ROUTES/DOSAGE

HYPERTENSION

PO: ADULTS, ELDERLY: Initially, 50 mg once a day. **Maximum:** May be given once or twice a day, with total daily doses ranging from 25–100 mg. **CHILDREN 6–16 YRS:** 0.7 mg/kg once daily. **Maximum:** 50 mg/day.

NEPHROPATHY

PO: ADULTS, ELDERLY: Initially, 50 mg/day. May increase to 100 mg/day based on B/P response.

STROKE PREVENTION

PO: ADULTS, ELDERLY: 50 mg/day. **Maximum:** 100 mg/day.

HYPERTENSION IN PTS WITH HEPATIC IMPAIRMENT

PO: ADULTS, ELDERLY: Initially, 25 mg/day in 2 divided doses.

SIDE EFFECTS

FREQUENT (8%): Upper respiratory tract infection. **OCCASIONAL (4%–2%):** Dizziness, diarrhea, cough. **RARE (1% or less):** Insomnia, dyspepsia, heartburn, back/leg pain, muscle cramps, myalgia, nasal congestion, sinusitis.

ADVERSE EFFECTS/ TOXIC REACTIONS

Overdosage may manifest as hypotension and tachycardia. Bradycardia occurs less often. Institute supportive measures.

NURSING CONSIDERATIONS

BASELINE ASSESSMENT

Obtain B/P, apical pulse immediately before each dose, in addition to regular monitoring (be alert to fluctuations). If excessive reduction in B/P occurs, place pt in supine position, feet slightly elevated. Question for possibility of pregnancy (see Pregnancy/Lactation). Assess medication history (esp. diuretic).

INTERVENTION/EVALUATION

Maintain hydration (offer fluids frequently). Assess for evidence of upper respiratory infection, cough. Assist with ambulation if dizziness occurs. Monitor daily pattern of bowel activity/stool consistency. Monitor B/P, pulse.

PATIENT/FAMILY TEACHING

• Inform female pt regarding consequences of second- and third-trimester exposure to losartan. • Report pregnancy to physician as soon as possible. • Avoid tasks that require alertness, motor skills until response to drug is established (possible dizziness effect). • Report any sign of infection (sore throat, fever), chest pain. • Do not take OTC cold preparations, nasal decongestants. • Do not stop taking medication.

Lotensin, *see benazepril*

Lotensin HCT,
see benazepril and hydrochlorothiazide

Lotrel, *see amlodipine and benazepril*

lovastatin

lo-va-**sta**-tin

(Altoprev, Apo-Lovastatin ✤, Mevacor, Novo-Lovastatin ✤)

Do not confuse lovastatin with Leustatin or Livostin, or Mevacor with Mivacron.

FIXED-COMBINATION(S)

Advicor: lovastatin/niacin: 20 mg/500 mg; 20 mg/750 mg; 20 mg/1,000 mg.

CLASSIFICATION

PHARMACOTHERAPEUTIC: HMG-CoA reductase inhibitor. **CLINICAL:** Antihyperlipidemic (see p. 56C).

ACTION

Inhibits HMG-CoA reductase, the enzyme that catalyzes the early step in cholesterol synthesis. **Therapeutic Effect:** Decreases LDL cholesterol, VLDL cholesterol, triglycerides; increases HDL cholesterol.

PHARMACOKINETICS

Route	Onset	Peak	Duration
PO	3 days	4–6 wks	N/A

Incompletely absorbed from GI tract (increased on empty stomach). Protein binding: 95%. Hydrolyzed in liver to active metabolite. Primarily eliminated in feces. Not removed by hemodialysis. **Half-life:** 1.1–1.7 hrs.

USES

Decreases elevated serum total and LDL cholesterol in primary hypercholesterolemia; primary prevention of coronary artery disease. Slows progression of coronary atherosclerosis in pts with coronary heart disease. Adjunct to diet in adolescent pts (10–17 yrs) with heterozygous familial hypercholesterolemia.

PRECAUTIONS

CONTRAINDICATIONS: Active hepatic disease, pregnancy, unexplained elevated hepatic function tests. **CAUTIONS:** History of heavy/chronic alcohol use; renal impairment; concomitant use of cyclosporine, fibrates, gemfibrozil, niacin.

⧖ LIFESPAN CONSIDERATIONS:

Pregnancy/Lactation: Contraindicated in pregnancy (suppression of cholesterol biosynthesis may cause fetal toxicity) and lactation. Unknown if drug is distributed in breast milk. **Pregnancy Category X.** **Children:** Safety and efficacy not established. **Elderly:** No age-related precautions noted.

L

INTERACTIONS

DRUG: **Cyclosporine, gemfibrozil, fibrates, niacin** may increase risk of rhabdomyolysis, acute renal failure. May increase concentration/toxicity of **digoxin. Erythromycin, itraconazole, ketoconazole** may increase concentration causing severe muscle inflammation, myalgia, weakness. **HERBAL:** None significant. **FOOD:** Large amounts of **grapefruit juice** may increase risk of side effects (e.g., myalgia, weakness). **LAB VALUES:** May increase serum creatine kinase, transaminase.

AVAILABILITY (Rx)

TABLETS (MEVACOR): 10 mg, 20 mg, 40 mg.

TABLETS (EXTENDED-RELEASE [ALTOPREV]): 20 mg, 40 mg, 60 mg.

ADMINISTRATION/HANDLING

PO

- Give with meals.

INDICATIONS/ROUTES/DOSAGE

ATHEROSCLEROSIS, CORONARY ARTERY DISEASE

PO: ADULTS, ELDERLY: Initially, 20 mg/day. Maintenance: 10–80 mg once daily or in 2 divided doses. **Maximum:** 80 mg/day.

HYPERCHOLESTEROLEMIA

PO: ADULTS, ELDERLY: Initially, 20 mg/day. Maintenance: 10–80 mg once daily or in 2 divided doses. **Maximum:** 80 mg/day.

PO (EXTENDED-RELEASE): ADULTS, ELDERLY: Initially, 20–60 mg once daily at bedtime. Maintenance: 10–60 mg once daily at bedtime.

HETEROZYGOUS FAMILIAL HYPERCHOLESTEROLEMIA

PO: CHILDREN 10–17 YRS: Initially, 10 mg/day. May increase to 20 mg/day after 8 wks and 40 mg/day after 16 wks if needed.

SIDE EFFECTS

Generally well tolerated. Side effects usually mild and transient. **FREQUENT (9%–5%):** Headache, flatulence, diarrhea, abdominal pain, abdominal cramping, rash, pruritus. **OCCASIONAL (4%–3%):** Nausea, vomiting, constipation, dyspepsia. **RARE (2%–1%):** Dizziness, heartburn, myalgia, blurred vision, eye irritation.

ADVERSE EFFECTS/ TOXIC REACTIONS

Potential for cataract development. Occasionally produces myopathy manifested as muscle pain, tenderness, weakness with elevated creatine kinase. Severe myopathy may lead to rhabdomyolysis.

NURSING CONSIDERATIONS

BASELINE ASSESSMENT

Question for possibility of pregnancy before initiating therapy (Pregnancy Category X). Assess baseline lab results: serum cholesterol, triglycerides, hepatic function tests.

INTERVENTION/EVALUATION

Monitor daily pattern of bowel activity/stool consistency. Monitor for headache, dizziness, blurred vision. Assess for rash, pruritus. Monitor serum cholesterol, triglycerides for therapeutic response. Be alert for malaise, muscle cramping/weakness.

PATIENT/FAMILY TEACHING

• Take with meals. • Follow special diet (important part of treatment). • Periodic lab tests are essential part of therapy. • Avoid grapefruit juice. • Inform physician of severe gastric upset, vision changes, myalgia, weakness, changes in color of urine/stool, yellowing of eyes/skin, unusual bruising.

Lovenox, *see enoxaparin*

loxapine hydrochloride

lox-ah-peen
(Apo-Loxapine ✦, Loxapac ✦, Loxitane)

loxapine succinate

(Loxitane)
See Antipsychotics (p. 62C)

lubiprostone

loo-bi-**pros**-tone
(Amitiza)

◆ CLASSIFICATION

PHARMACOTHERAPEUTIC: Chloride channel activator. **CLINICAL:** Constipation agent.

ACTION

Secretes fluid into abdominal lumen through activation of chloride channels in apical membranes of GI epithelium. **Therapeutic Effect:** Increases intestinal motility, thereby increasing passage of stool, alleviating symptoms associated with chronic idiopathic constipation.

PHARMACOKINETICS

Rapidly, extensively metabolized within stomach and jejunum. Minimal distribution beyond GI tissue. Protein binding: 94%. Excreted mainly in urine with trace amount eliminated in feces. **Half-life:** 0.9–1.4 hrs.

USES

Treatment of chronic idiopathic constipation in adults.

PRECAUTIONS

CONTRAINDICATIONS: History of mechanical GI obstruction. **CAUTIONS:** Diarrhea.

⌛ LIFESPAN CONSIDERATIONS:

May have potential for teratogenic effects. **Pregnancy/Lactation:** Unknown if distributed in breast milk. **Pregnancy Category C. Children:** Safety and efficacy not established. **Elderly:** No age-related precautions noted.

INTERACTIONS

DRUG: None significant. **HERBAL:** None significant. **FOOD:** None known. **LAB VALUES:** None known.

AVAILABILITY (Rx)

CAPSULES: 24 mcg.

ADMINISTRATION/HANDLING

PO
- Give with food.

INDICATIONS/ROUTES/DOSAGE

CHRONIC IDIOPATHIC CONSTIPATION
PO: ADULTS, ELDERLY: 24 mcg twice daily with food.

SIDE EFFECTS

FREQUENT (31%): Nausea. **OCCASIONAL (13%–4%):** Headache, diarrhea, abdominal distention, abdominal pain, flatulence, vomiting, peripheral edema, dizziness. **RARE (3%–2%):** Dyspepsia (hearburn, indigestion, epigastric distress), loose stools, fatigue, dry mouth, arthralgia, back pain, cough.

ADVERSE EFFECTS/ TOXIC REACTIONS

UTI, upper respiratory tract infection occurs in 4% of pts.

NURSING CONSIDERATIONS

BASELINE ASSESSMENT

Women should have negative pregnancy test prior to beginning therapy and comply with effective contraceptive measures during therapy. Assess for diarrhea (avoid use in these pts).

INTERVENTION/EVALUATION

Assess for improvement in symptoms (relief from bloating, cramping, urgency, abdominal discomfort).

PATIENT/FAMILY TEACHING

Inform physician of new/worsening episodes of abdominal pain, severe diarrhea. Avoid tasks that require alertness, motor skills until response to drug is established.

L

Lupron, *see leuprolide*

lymphocyte immune globulin N

lym-phow-site ih-**mewn glah**-byew-lin **N**

(Atgam)

Do not confuse Atgam with Ativan.

CLASSIFICATION

PHARMACOTHERAPEUTIC: Biologic response modifier. **CLINICAL:** Immunosuppressant.

ACTION

Acts as lymphocyte selective immunosuppressant, reducing number/altering function of T lymphocytes, which are responsible for cell-mediated and humoral immunity. Stimulates release of hematopoietic growth factors. **Therapeutic Effect:** Prevents allograft rejection; treats aplastic anemia.

PHARMACOKINETICS

Unknown absorption, metabolism, elimination. **Half-life:** Approximately 5–7 days.

USES

Prevention/treatment of renal allograft rejection. Treatment of moderate to severe aplastic anemia in pts not candidates for bone marrow transplant. **OFF-LABEL:** Immunosuppressant in bone marrow, heart, liver transplants; treatment of pure red cell aplasia, multiple sclerosis, myasthenia gravis, scleroderma.

PRECAUTIONS

CONTRAINDICATIONS: Systemic hypersensitivity reaction to previous injection of lymphocyte immune globulin N. **CAUTIONS:** Concurrent immunosuppressive therapy.

LIFESPAN CONSIDERATIONS:

Pregnancy/Lactation: Unknown if drug crosses placenta; or is distributed in breast milk. **Pregnancy Category C. Children:** Safety and efficacy not established. **Elderly:** No age-related precautions noted.

INTERACTIONS

DRUG: Corticosteroids, other immunosuppresants mask reaction to lymphocyte immune globulin. **HERBAL:** None significant. **FOOD:** None known. **LAB VALUES:** May alter renal function test results.

AVAILABILITY

INJECTION SOLUTION: 250 mg/5 ml.

ADMINISTRATION/HANDLING

IV

Reconstitution • Total daily dose must be further diluted with 0.9% NaCl (do not use D_5W). • Gently rotate diluted solution. Do not shake. • Final concentration must not exceed 4 mg/ml.

Rate of administration • Use 0.2- to 1-micron filter. • Give total daily dose over minimum of 4 hrs.

Storage • Keep refrigerated before and after dilution. • Discard diluted solution after 24 hrs.

IV INCOMPATIBILITIES

No information is available for Y-site administration.

INDICATIONS/ROUTES/DOSAGE

PREVENTION OF RENAL ALLOGRAFT REJECTION

IV: ADULTS, ELDERLY, CHILDREN: 15 mg/kg/day for 14 days, then every other day for 14 days. First dose within 24 hrs before or after transplantation.

TREATMENT OF RENAL ALLOGRAFT REJECTION

IV: ADULTS, ELDERLY, CHILDREN: 10–15 mg/kg/day for 14 days, then every other day for 14 more days. **Maximum:** 21 doses in 28 days.

APLASTIC ANEMIA

IV: ADULTS, ELDERLY, CHILDREN: 10–20 mg/kg once a day for 8–14 days, then every other day. **Maximum:** 21 doses.

SIDE EFFECTS

FREQUENT: Fever (51%), thrombocytopenia (30%), rash (2%), chills (16%), leukopenia (14%), systemic infection (13%). **OCCASIONAL (10%–5%):** Serum sickness-like reaction, dyspnea, apnea, arthralgia, chest pain, back pain, flank pain, nausea, vomiting, diarrhea, phlebitis.

ADVERSE EFFECTS/ TOXIC REACTIONS

Thrombocytopenia may occur but is generally transient. Severe hypersensitivity reaction, including anaphylaxis, occurs rarely.

NURSING CONSIDERATIONS

BASELINE ASSESSMENT

Use of high-flow vein (CVL, PICC, Groshong catheter) may prevent chemical phlebitis that may occur if peripheral vein is used.

INTERVENTION/EVALUATION

Monitor frequently for chills, fever, erythema, pruritus. Obtain order for prophylactic antihistamines or corticosteroids.

Lyrica, *see pregabalin*

L

Macrobid, *see nitrofurantoin*

magnesium

mag-**knee**-see-um

magnesium chloride

(Mag-Delay SR, Slow-Mag)

magnesium citrate

(Citrate of Magnesia, Citro-Mag ♣)

magnesium hydroxide

(Phillips Milk of Magnesia)

magnesium oxide

(Mag-Ox 400, Uro-Mag)

magnesium protein complex

(Mg-PLUS)

magnesium sulfate

(Epsom salt, magnesium sulfate injection, Sulfamag)

Do not confuse magnesium sulfate with manganese sulfate.

FIXED-COMBINATION(S)

With aluminum, an antacid **(Aludrox, Delcid, Gaviscon, Maalox)**; with aluminum and simethicone, an antiflatulent **(Di-Gel, Gelusil, Maalox Plus, Mylanta)**; with aluminum and calcium, an antacid **(Camalox)**; with mineral oil, a lubricant laxative **(Haley's MO)**; with magnesium oxide and aluminum oxide, an antacid **(Riopan)**.

◆CLASSIFICATION

CLINICAL: Antacid, anticonvulsant, electrolyte, laxative (see pp. 10C, 117C, 118C).

ACTION

Antacid: Acts in stomach to neutralize gastric acid. **Therapeutic Effect:** Increases pH. **Laxative:** Osmotic effect primarily in small intestine, draws water into intestinal lumen. **Therapeutic Effect:** Promotes peristalsis, bowel evacuation. **Systemic (dietary supplement replacement):** Found primarily in intracellular fluids. **Therapeutic Effect:** Essential for enzyme activity, nerve conduction, muscle contraction. Maintains and restores magnesium levels. **Anticonvulsant:** Blocks neuromuscular transmission, amount of acetylcholine released at motor end plate. **Therapeutic Effect:** Produces seizure control.

PHARMACOKINETICS

Antacid, laxative: Minimal absorption through intestine. Absorbed dose primarily excreted in urine. **Systemic:** Widely distributed. Primarily excreted in urine.

USES

Magnesium Chloride: Dietary supplement. **Magnesium Citrate:** Evacuation of bowel before surgical, diagnostic procedures. **Magnesium Hydroxide:** Short-term treatment of constipation, symptoms of hyperacidity, magnesium replacement. **Magnesium Oxide:** Magnesium replacement. **Magnesium Sulfate:** Treatment/prevention of hypomagnesemia, prevention of seizures, treatment of cardiac arrhythmias, treatment of constipation. **OFF-LABEL: Magnesium sulfate:** Premature labor, torsades de pointes, acute asthma, MI, tocolysis.

PRECAUTIONS

CONTRAINDICATIONS: Antacid: Appendicitis, symptoms of appendicitis, ileostomy, intestinal obstruction, severe renal impairment. **Laxative:** Appendicitis, CHF, colostomy, hypersensitivity, ileostomy, intestinal obstruction, undiagnosed rectal bleeding. **Systemic:** Heart block, myocardial damage, renal failure. **CAUTIONS:** Safety in children younger than 6 yrs not known. **Antacids:** Undiagnosed GI/rectal bleeding, ulcerative colitis, colostomy, diverticulitis, chronic diarrhea. **Laxative:** Diabetes mellitus, pts on low-salt diet (some products contain sugar, sodium). **Systemic:** Severe renal impairment.

LIFESPAN CONSIDERATIONS:

Pregnancy/Lactation: **Antacid:** Unknown if distributed in breast milk. **Parenteral:** Readily crosses placenta. Distributed in breast milk for 24 hrs after magnesium therapy is discontinued. Continuous IV infusion increases risk of magnesium toxicity in neonate. IV administration should not be used 2 hrs preceding delivery. **Pregnancy Category B.** **Children:** No age-related precautions noted. **Elderly:** Increased risk of developing magnesium deficiency (e.g., poor diet, decreased absorption, medications).

INTERACTIONS

DRUG: **Antacids** may decrease absorption of **ketoconazole, tetracyclines, fluoroquinolones.** May decrease effect of **methenamine. Antacids, laxatives** may decrease effects of **digoxin, oral anticoagulants, phenothiazines.** May reduce absorption of **ciprofloxacin. Sodium polystyrene sulfonate**may bind with magnesium, preventing neutralization of bicarbonate ions, leading to systemic alkalosis. May form nonabsorbable complex with **tetracyclines. Calcium** may neutralize effects of magnesium. **CNS depressant medications** may increase CNS depression. May alter cardiac conduction, increase degree of heart block with **digoxin.** **HERBAL:** None significant. **FOOD:** None known. **LAB VALUES:** **Antacid:** May increase gastrin production, pH. **Laxative:** May decrease serum potassium. **Systemic:** None known.

AVAILABILITY

MAGNESIUM CHLORIDE
TABLETS (MAG DELAY SR, SLO-MAG): 64 mg.
MAGNESIUM CITRATE
ORAL SOLUTION (CITRATE OF MAGNESIA): 290 mg/5 ml.
MAGNESIUM HYDROXIDE
ORAL LIQUID (PHILLIPS MILK OF MAGNESIA): 400 mg/5 ml, 800 mg/5 ml. **TABLETS (CHEWABLE [PHILLIPS MILK OF MAGNESIA]):** 311 mg.
MAGNESIUM OXIDE
CAPSULES (URO-MAG): 140 mg. **TABLETS (MAG-OX 400):** 400 mg.
MAGNESIUM SULFATE
INFUSION SOLUTION: 10 mg/ml, 20 mg/ml, 40 mg/ml, 80 mg/ml. **INJECTION SOLUTION:** 125 mg/ml, 500 mg/ml.

M

ADMINISTRATION/HANDLING

IV

Reconstitution • Must dilute (do not exceed 20 mg/ml concentration).

Rate of administration • For IV infusion, do not exceed magnesium sulfate concentration 200 mg/ml (20%). • Do not exceed IV infusion rate of 150 mg/min.

Storage • Store at room temperature.

IM

• For adults, elderly, use 250 mg/ml (25%) or 500 mg/ml (50%) magnesium sulfate concentration. • For infants, children, do not exceed 200 mg/ml (20%).

PO (ANTACID)

• Shake suspension well before use. • Chewable tablets should be chewed thoroughly before swallowing, followed by full glass of water.

PO (LAXATIVE)
• Drink full glass of liquid (8 oz) with each dose (prevents dehydration). • Flavor may be improved by following with fruit juice, citrus carbonated beverage. • Refrigerate citrate of magnesia (retains potency, palatability).

IV INCOMPATIBILITIES

Amphotericin B complex (Abelcet, AmBisome, Amphotec), cefepime (Maxipime).

IV COMPATIBILITIES

Amikacin (Amikin), cefazolin (Ancef), ciprofloxacin (Cipro), dobutamine (Dobutrex), enalapril (Vasotec), gentamicin, heparin, hydromorphone (Dilaudid), insulin, lipids, milrinone (Primacor), morphine, piperacillin/tazobactam (Zosyn), potassium chloride, propofol (Diprivan), tobramycin (Nebcin), vancomycin (Vancocin).

M

INDICATIONS/ROUTES/DOSAGE

HYPOMAGNESEMIA
PO (MAGNESIUM SULFATE): **ADULTS, ELDERLY:** 3 g q6h for 4 doses as needed. IV, IM: **ADULTS, ELDERLY:** 1–12 g/day in divided doses. **CHILDREN:** 25–50 mg/kg/dose q4–6h for 3–4 doses. Maintenance: 30–60 mg/kg/day.

HYPERTENSION, SEIZURES
IV, IM (MAGNESIUM SULFATE): **CHILDREN:** 20–100 mg/kg/dose q4–6h as needed.
IV: **ADULTS:** Initially, 4 g then 1–4 g/hr by continuous infusion.

ARRHYTHMIAS
IV (MAGNESIUM SULFATE): **ADULTS, ELDERLY:** Initially, 1–2 g then infusion of 0.5–1 g/hr.

CONSTIPATION
PO (MAGNESIUM SULFATE): **ADULTS, ELDERLY, CHILDREN 12 YRS AND OLDER:** 10–30 g/day in divided doses. **CHILDREN 6–11 YRS:** 5–10 g/day in divided doses. **CHILDREN 2–5 YRS:** 2.5–5 g/kg/day in divided doses.
PO (MAGNESIUM HYDROXIDE): **ADULTS, ELDERLY, CHILDREN 12 YRS AND OLDER:** 6–8 tablets or 30–60 ml/day. **CHILDREN 6–11 YRS:** 3–4 tablets or 7.5–15 ml/day. **CHILDREN 2–5 YRS:** 1–2 tablets or 2.5–7.5 ml/day.

HYPERACIDITY
PO (MAGNESIUM HYDROXIDE): **ADULTS, ELDERLY:** 2–4 tablets or 5–15 ml as needed up to 4 times a day. **CHILDREN 7–14 YRS:** 1 tablet or 2.5–5 ml as needed up to 4 times a day.

MAGNESIUM DEFICIENCY
PO (MAGNESIUM OXIDE): **ADULTS, ELDERLY:** 1–2 tablets 2–3 times a day.

DIETARY SUPPLEMENT
PO (MAGNESIUM CHLORIDE): **ADULTS, ELDERLY:** 54–483 mg/day in 2–4 divided doses.

CATHARTIC
PO (MAGNESIUM CITRATE): **ADULTS, ELDERLY, CHILDREN 12 YRS AND OLDER:** 120–300 ml. **CHILDREN 6–11 YRS:** 100–150 ml. **CHILDREN YOUNGER THAN 6 YRS:** 0.5 ml/kg up to maximum of 200 ml.

SIDE EFFECTS

FREQUENT: Antacid: Chalky taste, diarrhea, laxative effect. **OCCASIONAL: Antacid:** Nausea, vomiting, stomach cramps. **Antacid, laxative:** Prolonged use or large doses in renal impairment may cause hypermagnesemia (dizziness, palpitations, altered mental status, fatigue, weakness). **Laxative:** Cramping, diarrhea, increased thirst, flatulence. **Systemic (dietary supplement, electrolyte replacement):** Reduced respiratory rate, decreased reflexes, flushing, hypotension, decreased heart rate.

ADVERSE EFFECTS/ TOXIC REACTIONS

Magnesium as antacid, laxative has no known adverse reactions. Systemic use may produce prolonged PR interval, widening of QRS interval. Magnesium toxicity may cause loss of deep tendon reflexes, heart block, respiratory paralysis, cardiac arrest. Antidote: 10–20 ml 10% calcium gluconate (5–10 mEq of calcium).

NURSING CONSIDERATIONS

BASELINE ASSESSMENT

Assess if pt is sensitive to magnesium. **Antacid:** Assess GI pain (duration, location, quality, time of occurrence, relief with food, causative/excacerbative factors). **Laxative:** Monitor daily pattern of bowel activity/stool consistency, bowel sounds for peristalsis. Assess pt for weight loss, nausea, vomiting, history of recent abdominal surgery. **Systemic:** Assess renal function, serum magnesium.

INTERVENTION/EVALUATION

Antacid: Assess for relief of gastric distress. Monitor renal function (esp. if dosing is long-term or frequent). **Laxative:** Monitor daily pattern of bowel activity/stool consistency. Maintain adequate fluid intake. **Systemic:** Monitor renal function, magnesium levels, EKG for cardiac function. Test patellar reflexes (knee jerk reflexes) before giving repeat parenteral doses (used as indication of CNS depression; suppressed reflexes may be sign of impending respiratory arrest). Patellar reflex must be present, respiratory rate should be 16/min or over before each parenteral dose. Provide seizure precautions.

PATIENT/FAMILY TEACHING

• **Antacid:** Give at least 2 hrs apart from other medication. • Do not take longer than 2 wks unless directed by physician. • For peptic ulcer, take 1 and 3 hrs after meals and at bedtime for 4–6 wks. • Chew tablets thoroughly, followed by glass of water; shake suspensions well. Repeat dosing or large doses may have laxative effect. • **Laxative:** Drink full glass (8 oz) liquid to aid stool softening. • Use only for short term. Do not use if abdominal pain, nausea, vomiting is present. • **Systemic:** Inform physician of any signs of hypermagnesemia (dizziness, palpitations, altered mental status, fatigue, weakness).

mannitol

man-i-tall

(Osmitrol, Resectisol)

CLASSIFICATION

CLINICAL: Osmotic diuretic, antiglaucoma, antihemolytic.

ACTION

Elevates osmotic pressure of glomerular filtrate, inhibiting tubular reabsorption of water and electrolytes, resulting in increased flow of water into interstitial fluid/plasma. **Therapeutic Effect:** Produces diuresis; reduces intraocular pressure (IOP), intracranial pressure (ICP), cerebral edema.

PHARMACOKINETICS

Route	Onset	Peak	Duration
IV (diuresis)	15–30 min	N/A	2–8 hrs
IV (reduced ICP)	15–30 min	N/A	3–8 hrs
IV (reduced IOP)	N/A	30–60 min	4–8 hrs

Remains in extracellular fluid. Primarily excreted in urine. Removed by hemodialysis. **Half-life:** 100 min.

USES

Prevention, treatment of oliguric phase of acute renal failure (before evidence of permanent renal failure). Reduces increased ICP due to cerebral edema, spinal cord edema, IOP due to acute glaucoma. Promotes urinary excretion of toxic substances (aspirin, bromides, imipramine, barbiturates).

PRECAUTIONS

CONTRAINDICATIONS: Dehydration, intracranial bleeding, severe pulmonary edema, congestion; several renal disease (anuria), increasing oliguria, azotemia. **CAUTIONS:** None known.

LIFESPAN CONSIDERATIONS:

Pregnancy/Lactation: Unknown if drug crosses placenta or is distributed in breast milk. **Pregnancy Category C.** **Children:** Safety and efficacy not established in those younger than 12 yrs. **Elderly:** Age-related renal impairment may require dosage adjustment.

INTERACTIONS

DRUG: May increase risk of **digoxin** toxicity associated with mannitol-induced hypokalemia. **HERBAL:** None significant. **FOOD:** None known. **LAB VALUES:** May decrease serum phosphate, potassium, sodium.

AVAILABILITY (Rx)

INJECTION (OSMITROL): 5%, 10%, 15%, 20%, 25%. **IRRIGATION SOLUTION (RESECTISOL):** 5%.

ADMINISTRATION/HANDLING

◄ ALERT ► Assess IV site for patency before each dose. Pain, thrombosis noted with extravasation.

IV

Rate of administration • In-line filter (less than 5 microns) used for concentrations over 20%. • Administer test dose for pts with oliguria. • Give IV push over 3–5 min; over 20–30 min for cerebral edema, elevated ICP. Maximum concentration: 25%. • Do not add KCl or NaCl to mannitol 20% or greater. Do not add to whole blood for transfusion.

Storage • Store at room temperature. • If crystals are noted in solution, warm bottle in hot water, shake vigorously at intervals. Cool to body temperature before administration. Do not use if crystals remain after warming procedure.

IV INCOMPATIBILITIES

Cefepime (Maxipime), doxorubicin liposomal (Doxil), filgrastim (Neupogen).

IV COMPATIBILITIES

Cisplatin (Platinol), lipids, ondansetron (Zofran), propofol (Diprivan).

INDICATIONS/ROUTES/DOSAGE

ICP

IV: ADULTS, ELDERLY: 0.25–1 g/kg q6–8h. **Maximum:** 6 g/24 hrs. **CHILDREN:** 0.25–1 g/kg as needed. **Maximum:** 2 g/kg/dose.

IOP

IV: ADULTS, ELDERLY: 1.5–2 g/kg as a 15%–20% solution. **Maximum:** 6 g/24 hrs. **CHILDREN:** 1–2 g/kg. **Maximum:** 2 g/kg/dose.

RENAL IMPAIRMENT, OLIGURIA

IV: ADULTS, ELDERLY: Use test dose. 300–400 mg/kg or up to 100 g given as a single dose. **CHILDREN:** 0.25–2 g/kg. **Maximum:** 6 g/kg/24 hrs.

TOXICITY, POISONING

IV: ADULTS, ELDERLY: Continuous infusion as a 5%–20% solution. **CHILDREN:** Up to 2 g/kg as 5%–10% solution.

SIDE EFFECTS

FREQUENT: Dry mouth, thirst. **OCCASIONAL:** Blurred vision, increased urinary frequency/volume, headache, arm pain, backache, nausea, vomiting, urticaria, dizziness, hypotension, hypertension, tachycardia, fever, angina-like chest pain.

ADVERSE EFFECTS/ TOXIC REACTIONS

Fluid, electrolyte imbalance may occur due to rapid administration of large doses or inadequate urine output resulting in overexpansion of extracellular fluid. Circulatory overload may produce pulmonary edema, CHF. Excessive diuresis may produce hypokalemia, hyponatremia. Fluid loss in excess of electrolyte excretion may produce hypernatremia, hyperkalemia.

NURSING CONSIDERATIONS

BASELINE ASSESSMENT

Check B/P, pulse before giving medication. Assess skin turgor, mucous membranes, mental status, muscle strength. Obtain baseline weight. Assess I&O.

INTERVENTION/EVALUATION

Monitor urinary output to ascertain therapeutic response. Monitor serum electrolytes, BUN, renal/hepatic reports. Assess vital signs, skin turgor, mucous membranes. Weigh daily. Signs of hyponatremia include confusion, drowsiness, thirst, dry mouth, cold/clammy skin. Signs of hypokalemia include changes in muscle strength, tremors, muscle cramps, altered mental status, cardiac arrhythmias. Signs of hyperkalemia include colic, diarrhea, muscle twitching followed by weakness, paralysis, arrhythmias.

PATIENT/FAMILY TEACHING

• Expect increased urinary frequency/volume. • May cause dry mouth.

maprotiline hydrochloride

(Ludiomil)

See Antidepressants

Mavik, *see trandolapril*

Maxalt, *see rizatriptan*

Maxipine, *see cefepime*

mecasermin

meh-cah-**sir**-min

(Increlex, Iplex)

◆CLASSIFICATION

PHARMACOTHERAPEUTIC: Human insulin-like growth factor-1. **CLINICAL:** Growth hormone.

ACTION

Recombinant DNA-engineered human insulin-like growth factor-1 (rhIGF-1), designed to replace natural IGF-1 in pediatric pts who are deficient, leading to decreased growth (skeletal, cell, organ). **Therapeutic Effect:** Promotes normalized statural growth, cartilage/organ growth.

PHARMACOKINETICS

Extensively bound to albumin. Protein binding: greater than 80%. Metabolized in liver, kidney. **Half-life:** 5.8 hrs.

USES

Long-term treatment of growth failure in children with severe primary IGF-1 deficiency or with growth hormone (GH) gene deletions who have developed neutralizing antibodies to GH.

PRECAUTIONS

CONTRAINDICATIONS: Closed epiphyses; active or suspected neoplasia. **CAUTIONS:** Uncorrected thyroid, nutritional deficiencies.

⌛ LIFESPAN CONSIDERATIONS:

Pregnancy/Lactation: Unknown if distributed in breast milk. **Pregnancy**

Category C. Children: Safety and efficacy not established in children younger than 2 yrs. **Elderly:** Safety and efficacy not established.

INTERACTIONS

DRUG: None significant. **HERBAL:** None significant. **FOOD:** None known. **LAB VALUES:** May increase AST, ALT, serum cholesterol, triglycerides, LDH. May decrease serum glucose.

AVAILABILITY (Rx)

INJECTION SOLUTION: 10 mg/ml (40 mg vial) (Increlex); 36 mg/0.6 ml (Iplex).

ADMINISTRATION/HANDLING

SUBCUTANEOUS

◀ ALERT ▶ Must be administered within 20 min before or after meal, snack. Omit dose and do not make up for omitted dose if pt is unable to eat. Rotate injection sites. May be given in thigh, abdomen, upper arm.

Storage • Refrigerate vials. • After initial needle entry, refrigerated vial is stable for 30 days only. • Discard if cloudy or contains precipitate.

INDICATIONS/ROUTES/DOSAGE

◀ ALERT ▶ Give subcutaneous only; do not give IM, IV. Assess preprandial glucose during treatment initiation and dosage adjustment until well-tolerated dose is established.

INITIAL DOSE

SUBCUTANEOUS (INCRELEX): CHILDREN 2 YRS AND OLDER: Initial dose is 0.04–0.08 mg/kg (40–80 mcg/kg) twice a day. If tolerated for 7 days, dose can be increased in 0.04 mg/kg/dose (40 mcg/kg/dose)-increments, to a maximum dose of 0.12 mg/kg (120 mcg/kg) twice a day. Reduce dose if hypoglycemia occurs despite adequate food intake.

(IPLEX): CHILDREN 3 YRS AND OLDER: Initially, 0.05 mg/kg once daily. May increase to 1–2 mg/kg/day given once daily. Withhold dose if hypoglycemia is present.

SIDE EFFECTS

FREQUENT (42%): Hypoglycemia. **OCCASIONAL (15%):** Snoring, tonsillar hypertrophy. **RARE (5% or greater):** Vomiting, injection site bruising, arthralgia, extremity pain, otitis media with associated ear pain, headache, dizziness.

ADVERSE EFFECTS/ TOXIC REACTIONS

Intracranial hypertension has been reported. Thickening of soft facial tissue occurs rarely. Hypoglycemic seizure has occurred.

NURSING CONSIDERATIONS

BASELINE ASSESSMENT

Must be administered within 20 min before or after meal, snack. If pt is unable to eat, omit dose; drug must be given within 20 min parameter. Obtain preprandial serum glucose level. Pts should avoid high-risk activities within 2–3 hrs of dosing until a tolerated dose is established.

INTERVENTION/EVALUATION

Monitor serum glucose for hypoglycemia, take appropriate measures to maintain pt within glucose parameters. Monitor small children closely due to potentially erratic food intake. Monitor facial features, growth.

PATIENT/FAMILY TEACHING

• Contact physician if limp, complaint of hip/knee pain occurs.

mechlorethamine

(Mustargen)

See Cancer chemotherapeutic agents (p. 81C)

M

meclizine

mek-li-zeen

(Antivert, Bonamine ✤, Bonine, Dramamine Less Drowsy Formula)

Do not confuse Antivert with Axert.

CLASSIFICATION

PHARMACOTHERAPEUTIC: Anticholinergic. **CLINICAL:** Antiemetic, antivertigo.

ACTION

Reduces labyrinthine excitability, diminishes vestibular stimulation of labyrinth, affecting chemoreceptor trigger zone. **Therapeutic Effect:** Reduces nausea, vomiting, vertigo.

PHARMACOKINETICS

Route	Onset	Peak	Duration
PO	30–60 min	N/A	12–24 hrs

Well absorbed from GI tract. Widely distributed. Metabolized in liver. Primarily excreted in urine. **Half-life:** 6 hrs.

USES

Prevention/treatment of nausea, vomiting, vertigo due to motion sickness. Treatment of vertigo associated with diseases affecting vestibular system.

PRECAUTIONS

CONTRAINDICATIONS: None known. **CAUTIONS:** Narrow-angle glaucoma, obstructive diseases of GI/GU tract.

LIFESPAN CONSIDERATIONS:

Pregnancy/Lactation: Unknown if drug crosses placenta or is distributed in breast milk (may produce irritability in nursing infants). **Pregnancy Category B.** **Children/Elderly:** May be more sensitive to anticholinergic effects (e.g., dry mouth).

INTERACTIONS

DRUG: Alcohol, CNS depressant medications may increase CNS depressant effect. **HERBAL:** None significant. **FOOD:** None known. **LAB VALUES:** May produce false-negative results in antigen skin testing unless meclizine is discontinued 4 days before testing.

AVAILABILITY (Rx)

TABLETS (ANTIVERT): 12.5 mg, 25 mg, 50 mg **(DRAMAMINE LESS DROWSY FORMULA):** 25 mg. **TABLETS (CHEWABLE [BONINE]):** 25 mg.

ADMINISTRATION/HANDLING

PO

• Give without regard to meals. • Scored tablets may be crushed.

INDICATIONS/ROUTES/DOSAGE

MOTION SICKNESS

PO: ADULTS, ELDERLY, CHILDREN 12 YRS AND OLDER: 12.5–25 mg 1 hr before travel. May repeat q12–24h. May require a dose of 50 mg.

VERTIGO

PO: ADULTS, ELDERLY, CHILDREN 12 YRS AND OLDER: 25–100 mg/day in divided doses, as needed.

SIDE EFFECTS

FREQUENT: Drowsiness. **OCCASIONAL:** Blurred vision; dry mouth, nose, throat.

ADVERSE EFFECTS/ TOXIC REACTIONS

Hypersensitivity reaction (eczema, pruritus, rash, cardiac disturbances, photosensitivity) may occur. Overdose may vary from CNS depression (sedation, apnea, cardiovascular collapse, death) to severe paradoxical reaction (hallucinations, tremor, seizures). Children may experience paradoxical reaction (restlessness, insomnia, euphoria, anxiety, tremors). Overdose in children may result in hallucinations, seizures, death.

M

NURSING CONSIDERATIONS

INTERVENTION/EVALUATION

Monitor B/P, esp. in elderly (increased risk of hypotension). Monitor children closely for paradoxical reaction. Monitor serum electrolytes in those with severe vomiting. Assess skin turgor, mucous membranes to evaluate hydration status.

PATIENT/FAMILY TEACHING

• Tolerance to sedative effect may occur. • Avoid tasks that require alertness, motor skills until response to drug is established. • Dry mouth, drowsiness, dizziness may be an expected response of drug. • Avoid alcoholic beverages during therapy. • Sugarless gum, sips of tepid water may relieve dry mouth. • Coffee, tea may help reduce drowsiness.

M

meclofenamate

(Meclodium, Meclomen)

See Nonsteroidal Anti-Inflammatory Drugs (NSAIDs)

*medroxy-PROGESTERone

me-**drox**-ee-proe-**jess**-te-rone

(Apo-Medroxy ✤, Depo-Provera, Depo-Provera Contraceptive, Depo-SubQ-Provera 104, Novo-Medrone ✤, Provera)

Do not confuse medroxyprogesterone with hydroxyprogesterone, methylprednisolone, or methyltestosterone.

FIXED-COMBINATION(S)

Prempro, Premphase: medroxy-progesterone/conjugated estrogens: 1.5 mg/0.3 mg; 1.5 mg/0.45 mg; 2.5 mg/0.625 mg; 5 mg/0.625 mg.

CLASSIFICATION

PHARMACOTHERAPEUTIC: Hormone. **CLINICAL:** Progestin, antineoplastic.

ACTION

Transforms endometrium from proliferative to secretory (in estrogen-primed endometrium). Inhibits secretion of pituitary gonadotropins. **Therapeutic Effect:** Prevents follicular maturation, ovulation. Stimulates growth of mammary alveolar tissue; relaxes uterine smooth muscle. Corrects hormonal imbalance.

PHARMACOKINETICS

Slowly absorbed after IM administration. Protein binding: 90%. Metabolized in liver. Primarily excreted in urine. **Half-life:** 30 days.

USES

PO: Prevention of endometrial hyperplasia (concurrently given with estrogen to women with intact uterus), treatment of secondary amenorrhea, abnormal uterine bleeding. **IM:** Adjunctive therapy, palliative treatment of inoperable, recurrent, metastatic endometrial carcinoma, renal carcinoma; prevention of pregnancy. **OFF-LABEL:** Hormone replacement therapy in estrogen-treated menopausal women, treatment of endometriosis.

PRECAUTIONS

CONTRAINDICATIONS: Carcinoma of breast; estrogen-dependent neoplasm; history of or active thrombotic disorders (cerebral apoplexy, thrombophlebitis, thromboembolic disorders) hypersensitivity to progestins; known or suspected pregnancy; missed abortion; severe hepatic dysfunction; undiagnosed abnormal genital bleeding; use as pregnancy test. **CAUTIONS:** Those with conditions aggravated by fluid retention (asthma, seizures, migraine, cardiac/renal dysfunction), diabetes, history of mental depression.

LIFESPAN CONSIDERATIONS:

Pregnancy/Lactation: Avoid use during pregnancy, esp. first 4 mos (congenital heart, limb reduction defects may occur). Distributed in breast milk. **Pregnancy Category X. Children:** Safety and efficacy not established. **Elderly:** No age-related precautions noted.

INTERACTIONS

DRUG: **Hepatic enzyme inducers (e.g., carbamazepine, phenytoin, rifampin)** may decrease effect. May interfere with effects of **bromocriptine**. **HERBAL:** **St. John's wort** may decrease effect. **FOOD:** None known. **LAB VALUES:** May alter serum thyroid, hepatic function tests, prothrombin time (PT), metapyrone test.

AVAILABILITY (Rx)

INJECTION SUSPENSION: 104 mg/0.65 ml prefilled syringe (Depo-SubQ-Provera 104), 150 mg/ml (Depo-Provera Contraceptive), 400 mg/ml (Depo-Provera). **TABLETS (PROVERA):** 2.5 mg, 5 mg, 10 mg.

ADMINISTRATION/HANDLING

IM

• Shake vial immediately before administering (ensures complete suspension). • Rarely, a residual lump, change in skin color, sterile abscess occurs at injection site. • Inject IM only in upper arm, upper outer aspect of buttock.

PO

• Give without regard to meals.

INDICATIONS/ROUTES/DOSAGE

HORMONE REPLACEMENT THERAPY

PO: ADULTS: 5–10 mg for 12–14 consecutive days a mo, beginning on day 1 or 16 of cycle given as part of regimen with conjugated estrogens.

ENDOMETRIAL HYPERPLASIA

PO: ADULTS: 2.5–10 mg/day for 14 days.

SECONDARY AMENORRHEA

PO: ADULTS: 5–10 mg/day for 5–10 days, beginning at any time during menstrual cycle.

ABNORMAL UTERINE BLEEDING

PO: ADULTS: 5–10 mg/day for 5–10 days, beginning on calculated day 16 or day 21 of menstrual cycle.

ENDOMETRIAL, RENAL CARCINOMA

IM: ADULTS, ELDERLY: Initially, 400–1,000 mg; repeat at 1-wk intervals. If improvement occurs and disease is stabilized, begin maintenance with as little as 400 mg/mo.

PREGNANCY PREVENTION

IM (DEPO-PROVERA): ADULTS: 150 mg q3mo.

SUBCUTANEOUS (DEPO-SUBQ-PROVERA 104): ADULTS: 104 mg q3mo (q12–14wk).

SIDE EFFECTS

FREQUENT: Transient menstrual abnormalities (spotting, change in menstrual flow/cervical secretions, amenorrhea) at initiation of therapy. **OCCASIONAL:** Edema, weight change, breast tenderness, anxiety, insomnia, fatigue, dizziness. **RARE:** Alopecia, depression, dermatologic changes, headache, fever, nausea.

ADVERSE EFFECTS/ TOXIC REACTIONS

Thrombophlebitis, pulmonary/cerebral embolism, retinal thrombosis occur rarely.

NURSING CONSIDERATIONS

BASELINE ASSESSMENT

Question for hypersensitivity to progestins, possibility of pregnancy before initiating therapy (Pregnancy Category X). Obtain baseline weight, serum glucose, B/P.

M

INTERVENTION/EVALUATION

Check weight daily; report weekly gain of 5 lb or more. Check B/P periodically. Assess skin for rash, urticaria. Report development of chest pain, sudden shortness of breath, sudden decrease in vision, migraine headache, pain (esp. with swelling, warmth, redness) in calves, numbness of arm/leg (thrombotic disorders) immediately.

PATIENT/FAMILY TEACHING

• Inform physician of sudden loss of vision, severe headache, chest pain, coughing up of blood (hemoptysis), numbness in arm/leg, severe pain/swelling in calf, unusual heavy vaginal bleeding, severe abdominal pain/tenderness. • Depo-Provera Contraceptive injection should be used as long-term birth control method (e.g., longer than 2 yrs) only if other birth control methods are inadequate.

megestrol

me-**jess**-trole

(Apo-Megestrol ✦, Megace, Megace ES, Megace OS ✦)

CLASSIFICATION

PHARMACOTHERAPEUTIC: Hormone. **CLINICAL:** Antineoplastic (see p. 81C).

ACTION

Suppresses release of luteinizing hormone from anterior pituitary by inhibiting pituitary function. **Therapeutic Effect:** Reduces tumor size. Increases appetite.

PHARMACOKINETICS

Well absorbed from GI tract. Metabolized in liver; excreted in urine. **Half-life:** 13–105 hrs (mean 34 hrs).

USES

Palliative management of recurrent, inoperable, metastatic endometrial or breast carcinoma. Treatment of anorexia, cachexia, unexplained significant weight loss in pts with AIDS. **OFF-LABEL:** Appetite stimulant, treatment of hormone-dependent or advanced prostate carcinoma, treatment of uterine bleeding.

PRECAUTIONS

CONTRAINDICATIONS: **Suspension:** Known or suspected pregnancy. **CAUTIONS:** History of thrombophlebitis.

LIFESPAN CONSIDERATIONS:

Pregnancy/Lactation: If possible, avoid use during pregnancy, esp. first 4 mos. Breast-feeding not recommended. **Pregnancy Category X. Children:** Safety and efficacy not established. **Elderly:** No age-related precautions noted.

INTERACTIONS

DRUG: **Dofetilide** may increase risk of cardiotoxicity (QT prolongation, torsades de pointes, cardiac arrest). **HERBAL:** Avoid **black cohosh, dong quai** in estrogen-dependent tumors. **FOOD:** None known. **LAB VALUES:** May increase serum glucose.

AVAILABILITY (Rx)

ORAL SUSPENSION: 40 mg/ml (Megace), 625 mg/5 ml (equivalent to 800 mg/20 ml) (Megace ES). **TABLETS (MEGACE):** 20 mg, 40 mg.

ADMINISTRATION/HANDLING

PO

• Store tablets, oral suspension at room temperature. • Shake suspension well before use.

INDICATIONS/ROUTES/DOSAGE

PALLIATIVE TREATMENT OF ADVANCED BREAST CANCER

PO: ADULTS, ELDERLY: 160 mg/day in 4 equally divided doses.

PALLIATIVE TREATMENT OF ADVANCED ENDOMETRIAL CARCINOMA
PO: ADULTS, ELDERLY: 40–320 mg/day in divided doses. **Maximum:** 800 mg/day in 1–4 divided doses.
ANOREXIA, CACHEXIA, WEIGHT LOSS
PO: ADULTS, ELDERLY: 800 mg (20 ml)/day.
PO (MEGACE ES): ADULTS, ELDERLY: 625 mg/day.

SIDE EFFECTS

FREQUENT: Weight gain secondary to increased appetite. **OCCASIONAL:** Nausea, breakthrough bleeding, backache, headache, breast tenderness, carpal tunnel syndrome. **RARE:** Feeling of coldness.

ADVERSE EFFECTS/ TOXIC REACTIONS

Thrombophlebitis, pulmonary embolism occur rarely.

NURSING CONSIDERATIONS

BASELINE ASSESSMENT

Question for possibility of pregnancy before initiating therapy (Pregnancy Category X. Provide support to pt, family, recognizing this drug is palliative, not curative.

INTERVENTION/EVALUATION

Monitor for tumor response.

PATIENT/FAMILY TEACHING

• Contraception is imperative. • Report calf pain, difficulty breathing, vaginal bleeding. • May cause headache, nausea, vomiting, breast tenderness, backache.

melatonin

Also known as pineal hormone.

CLASSIFICATION

HERBAL: See Appendix G.

ACTION

Hormone synthesized endogenously by pineal gland. Interacts with melatonin receptors in brain. **Effect:** Regulates body's circadian rhythm, sleep patterns. Acts as antioxidant, protecting cells from oxidative damage by free radicals.

USES

Treatment for insomnia, jet lag. Used as antioxidant.

PRECAUTIONS

CONTRAINDICATIONS: Pregnancy or lactation. **CAUTIONS:** Depression (may worsen dysphoria), seizures (may increase incidence), cardiovascular/hepatic disease.

LIFESPAN CONSIDERATIONS:

Pregnancy/Lactation: Contraindicated. **Children:** Safety and efficacy not established. **Elderly:** No age-related precautions noted.

INTERACTIONS

DRUG: **Alcohol, benzodiazepines** may have additive effects. Melatonin may interfere with effects of **immunosuppressants.** May enhance effects of **isoniazid.** **HERBAL:** **Chamomile, ginseng, goldenseal, kava kava, valerian** may increase sedative effects. **FOOD:** None known. **LAB VALUES:** May increase human growth hormone levels. May decrease luteinizing hormone (LH) levels.

AVAILABILITY (OTC)

LOZENGES: 3 mg. **POWDER. TABLETS:** 0.5 mg, 3 mg.

INDICATIONS/ROUTES/DOSAGE

INSOMNIA
PO: ADULTS, ELDERLY: 0.5–5 mg at bedtime.
JET LAG
PO: ADULTS, ELDERLY: 5 mg a day beginning 3 days before flight and continuing until 3 days after flight.

SIDE EFFECTS

Headache, transient depression, fatigue, drowsiness, dizziness, abdominal cramps/irritability, decreased alertness, hypersensitivity reaction, tachycardia, nausea, vomiting, anorexia, altered sleep patterns, confusion.

ADVERSE EFFECTS/ TOXIC REACTIONS

None known.

NURSING CONSIDERATIONS

BASELINE ASSESSMENT

Assess if pt is pregnant or breast-feeding (avoid use). Determine whether pt has history of seizures, depression. Assess sleep patterns if used for insomnia. Determine medication usage (esp. CNS depressants).

INTERVENTION/EVALUATION

Monitor effectiveness in improving insomnia. Assess for hypersensitivity reactions, CNS effects.

PATIENT/FAMILY TEACHING

• Do not use if pregnant, planning to become pregnant, breast-feeding. • Avoid tasks that require mental alertness, motor skills (e.g., driving).

meloxicam

meh-**locks**-ih-cam
(Mobic)

CLASSIFICATION

PHARMACOTHERAPEUTIC: Nonsteroidal anti-inflammatory. **CLINICAL:** Anti-inflammatory, analgesic (see p. 124C).

ACTION

Produces analgesic, anti-inflammatory effects by inhibiting prostaglandin synthesis. **Therapeutic Effect:** Reduces inflammatory response, intensity of pain.

PHARMACOKINETICS

Route	Onset	Peak	Duration
PO (analgesic)	30 min	4–5 hrs	N/A

Well absorbed after PO administration. Protein binding: 99%. Metabolized in liver. Eliminated in urine, feces. Not removed by hemodialysis. **Half-life:** 15–20 hrs.

USES

Relief of signs/symptoms of osteoarthritis, rheumatoid arthritis. Treatment of juvenile rheumatoid arthritis. **OFF-LABEL:** Ankylosing spondylitis.

PRECAUTIONS

CONTRAINDICATIONS: Aspirin-induced nasal polyps associated with bronchospasm. **CAUTIONS:** History of GI disease (e.g., ulcers), renal/hepatic impairment, CHF, dehydration, hypertension, asthma, hemostatic disease. Concurrent use of anticoagulants.

LIFESPAN CONSIDERATIONS:

Pregnancy/Lactation: Excreted in breast milk. **Pregnancy Category C (D if used in third trimester or near delivery).** **Children:** Safety and efficacy not established. **Elderly:** Age-related renal impairment may require dosage adjustment. More susceptible to GI toxicity; lower dosage recommended.

INTERACTIONS

DRUG: **Aspirin** may increase risk of epigastric distress (heartburn, indigestion). May increase concentration, risk of toxicity of **lithium.** **HERBAL:** **Cat's claw, dong quai, evening primrose, feverfew, garlic, ginger, ginkgo, red clover, green tea, SAMe** may increase antiplatelet activity, risk of bleeding.

FOOD: None known. **LAB VALUES:** May increase serum creatinine, AST, ALT.

AVAILABILITY (Rx)

ORAL SUSPENSION: 7.5 mg/5 ml. **TABLETS:** 7.5 mg, 15 mg.

ADMINISTRATION/HANDLING

PO

- Give without regard to meals.

INDICATIONS/ROUTES/DOSAGE

OSTEOARTHRITIS, RHEUMATOID ARTHRITIS

PO: ADULTS: Initially, 7.5 mg/day. **Maximum:** 15 mg/day.

JUVENILE RHEUMATOID ARTHRITIS

PO: CHILDREN, 2 YRS AND OLDER: 0.125 mg/kg once daily. **Maximum:** 7.5 mg.

SIDE EFFECTS

FREQUENT (9%–7%): Dyspepsia, headache, diarrhea, nausea. **OCCASIONAL (4%–3%):** Dizziness, insomnia, rash, pruritus, flatulence, constipation, vomiting. **RARE (less than 2%):** Somnolence (drowsiness), urticaria, photosensitivity, tinnitus.

ADVERSE EFFECTS/ TOXIC REACTIONS

In those treated chronically, peptic ulcer, GI bleeding, gastritis, severe hepatic reaction (jaundice), nephrotoxicity (hematuria, dysuria, proteinuria), severe hypersensitivity reaction (bronchospasm, angioedema) occur rarely.

NURSING CONSIDERATIONS

BASELINE ASSESSMENT

Assess onset, type, location, duration of pain/inflammation. Inspect appearance of affected joints for immobility, deformities, skin condition.

INTERVENTION/EVALUATION

Monitor CBC, hepatic/renal function tests. Evaluate for therapeutic response (relief of pain, stiffness, swelling, increased joint mobility, reduced joint tenderness, improved grip strength).

PATIENT/FAMILY TEACHING

- Take with food, milk to reduce GI upset. • Inform physician of tinnitus, persistent abdominal pain/cramping, severe nausea/vomiting, difficulty breathing, unusual bruising/bleeding, rash, peripheral edema, chest pain, palpitations.

melphalan

mel-fah-lan

(Alkeran, Alkeran I.V.)

Do not confuse Alkeran with Leukeran, or melphalan with Mephyton or Myleran.

CLASSIFICATION

PHARMACOTHERAPEUTIC: Alkylating agent. **CLINICAL:** Antineoplastic (see p. 81C).

ACTION

Inhibits protein synthesis primarily by cross-linking strands of DNA, RNA. Cell cycle–phase nonspecific. **Therapeutic Effect:** Disrupts nucleic acid function producing cell death.

PHARMACOKINETICS

Oral administration is highly variable. Incomplete intestinal absorption, variable first-pass metabolism, rapid hydrolysis may result. Protein binding: 60%–90%. Extensively metabolized in blood. Eliminated from plasma primarily by chemical hydrolysis. Partially excreted in feces; minimal elimination in urine. **Half-life:** 38–108 min.

USES

Treatment of epithelial ovarian carcinoma, multiple myeloma. **OFF-LABEL:** Treatment of breast, endometrial, testicular carcinoma; chronic myelocytic leukemia, Hodgkin's lymphoma, malignant melanoma, neuroblastoma, rhabdomyosarcoma.

PRECAUTIONS

CONTRAINDICATIONS: Pregnancy, severe myelosuppression. **CAUTIONS:** Leukocyte count less than 3,000/mm^3 or platelet count less than 100,000/mm^3, bone marrow suppression, renal impairment.

LIFESPAN CONSIDERATIONS:

Pregnancy/Lactation: May cause fetal harm. Unknown if distributed in breast milk. **Pregnancy Category D. Children:** Safety and efficacy not established. **Elderly:** Age-related renal impairment may require dosage adjustment.

INTERACTIONS

DRUG: May decrease effects of **antigout medications. Bone marrow depressants** may increase myelosuppression. **Live virus vaccines** may potentiate virus replication, increase vaccine side effects, decrease pt's antibody response to vaccine. **HERBAL:** None significant. **FOOD:** None known. **LAB VALUES:** May increase serum uric acid. May cause positive direct Coombs' test.

AVAILABILITY (Rx)

INJECTION, POWDER FOR RECONSTITUTION (ALKERAN I.V.): 50 mg. **TABLETS (ALKERAN):** 2 mg.

ADMINISTRATION/HANDLING

IV

Reconstitution • Reconstitute 50-mg vial with diluent supplied by manufacturer to yield 5 mg/ml solution. • Further dilute with 0.9% NaCl to final concentration not exceeding 2 mg/ml (central line) or 0.45 mg/ml (peripheral line).

Rate of administration • Infuse over 15–30 min at rate not to exceed 10 mg/min.

Storage • Store at room temperature; protect from light. • Once reconstituted, stable for 90 min at room temperature (do not refrigerate).

PO

• Store tablets in refrigerator; protect from light.

IV INCOMPATIBILITIES

Do not mix melphalan with any other medications.

INDICATIONS/ROUTES/DOSAGE

OVARIAN CARCINOMA

PO: ADULTS, ELDERLY: 0.2 mg/kg/day for 5 successive days. Repeat at 4- to 6-wk intervals.

MULTIPLE MYELOMA

PO: ADULTS: Initially, 6 mg once a day, adjusted as indicated; or 0.15 mg/kg/day for 7 days or 0.25 mg/kg/day for 4 days. Repeat at 4- to 6-wk intervals.

IV: ADULTS: 16 mg/m^2/dose every 2 wks for 4 doses, then repeated monthly according to protocol.

DOSAGE IN RENAL IMPAIRMENT

PO, IV: BUN LEVEL GREATER THAN 30 MG/DL: Decrease melphalan dosage by 50%. **SERUM CREATININE LEVEL GREATER THAN 1.5 MG/DL:** Decrease melphalan dosage by 50%.

SIDE EFFECTS

FREQUENT: Nausea, vomiting (may be severe with large dose). **OCCASIONAL:** Diarrhea, stomatitis, rash, pruritus, alopecia.

ADVERSE EFFECTS/ TOXIC REACTIONS

Myelosuppression manifested as hematologic toxicity (principally leukopenia, thrombocytopenia, and, to lesser extent, anemia, pancytopenia, agranulocytosis). Leukopenia may occur as early as 5 days after drug initiation. WBC, platelet counts return to normal during 5th wk after therapy, but leukopenia, thrombocytopenia may last more than 6 wks after discontinuing drug. Hyperuricemia noted by hematuria, crystalluria, flank pain.

NURSING CONSIDERATIONS

BASELINE ASSESSMENT

Obtain CBC weekly. Dosage may be decreased or discontinued if WBC falls below 3,000/mm^3 or platelet count falls below 100,000/mm^3. Antiemetics may be effective in preventing/treating nausea, vomiting.

INTERVENTION/EVALUATION

Monitor CBC with diffferential, platelet count, serum electrolytes, Hgb. Monitor for stomatitis. Monitor for hematologic toxicity (fever, sore throat, signs of local infection, unusual bruising/bleeding from any site), symptoms of anemia (excessive fatigue, weakness), signs of hyperuricemia (hematuria, flank pain). Avoid IM injections, rectal temperatures, other traumas that may induce bleeding.

PATIENT/FAMILY TEACHING

• Increase fluid intake (may protect against hyperuricemia). • Maintain fastidious oral hygiene. • Alopecia is reversible, but new hair growth may have different color, texture. • Avoid crowds, those with infections. • Inform physician if fever, shortness of breath, cough, sore throat, bleeding, bruising occurs.

memantine

meh-**man**-teen
(Ebixa ✦, Namenda)

CLASSIFICATION

PHARMACOTHERAPEUTIC: Neurotransmitter inhibitor. **CLINICAL:** Anti-Alzheimer's agent.

ACTION

Decreases effects of glutamate, the principle excitatory neurotransmitter in the brain. Persistent CNS excitation by glutamate is thought to cause symptoms of Alzheimer's disease. **Therapeutic Effect:** May reduce clinical deterioration in moderate to severe Alzheimer's disease.

PHARMACOKINETICS

Rapidly, completely absorbed after PO administration. Protein binding: 45%. Undergoes little metabolism; most of dose is excreted unchanged in urine. **Half-life:** 60–80 hrs.

USES

Treatment of moderate to severe Alzheimer's disease.

PRECAUTIONS

CONTRAINDICATIONS: Severe renal impairment. **CAUTIONS:** Moderate renal impairment, seizure disorder, GU conditions that raise urine pH level.

LIFESPAN CONSIDERATIONS:

Pregnancy/Lactation: Unknown if drug crosses placenta or is distributed in breast milk. **Pregnancy Category B.** **Children:** Not prescribed for this pt population. **Elderly:** No age-related precautions noted, but use is not recommended in those with severe renal impairment (creatinine clearance less than 9 ml/min).

INTERACTIONS

DRUG: **Carbonic anhydrase inhibitors, sodium bicarbonate** may decrease renal elimination of memantine. **Cimetidine, hydrochlorothiazide, nicotine, quinidine, ranitidine** may alter plasma levels. **HERBAL:** None significant. **FOOD:** None known. **LAB VALUES:** None known.

M

AVAILABILITY (Rx)

ORAL SOLUTION: 2 mg/ml. **TABLETS:** 5 mg, 10 mg.

ADMINISTRATION/HANDLING

PO

- Give without regard to food.

INDICATIONS/ROUTES/DOSAGE

ALZHEIMER'S DISEASE

PO: ADULTS, ELDERLY: Initially, 5 mg once a day. May increase dosage at intervals of at least 1 wk in 5-mg increments to 10 mg/day (5 mg twice a day), then 15 mg/day (5 mg and 10 mg as separate doses), and finally 20 mg/day (10 mg twice a day). Target dose: 20 mg/day.

DOSAGE IN RENAL IMPAIRMENT

Creatinine Clearance	Dosage
30 ml/min or greater	No adjustments needed
5–29 ml/min	5 mg twice daily

SIDE EFFECTS

OCCASIONAL (7%–4%): Dizziness, headache, confusion, constipation, hypertension, cough. **RARE (3%–2%):** Back pain, nausea, fatigue, anxiety, peripheral edema, arthralgia, insomnia.

ADVERSE EFFECTS/ TOXIC REACTIONS

None known.

NURSING CONSIDERATIONS

BASELINE ASSESSMENT

Assess cognitive, behavioral, functional deficits of pt. Assess renal function.

INTERVENTION/EVALUATION

Monitor cognitive, behavioral, functional status of pt. Monitor urine pH (alterations of urine pH toward the alkaline condition may lead to accumulation of the drug with possible increase in side effects). Monitor BUN, creatinine clearance lab values.

PATIENT/FAMILY TEACHING

- Do not reduce or stop medication; do not increase dosage without physician direction. • Ensure adequate fluid intake. • If therapy is interrupted for several days, restart at lowest dose, titrate to current dose at minimum of 1-wk intervals. • Inform family of local chapter of Alzheimer's Disease Association (provides a guide to services for these pts).

menotropins

(Humegon, Pergonal, Repronex)

See Fertility agents (p. 102C)

meperidine

me-**per**-i-deen

(Demerol, Meperitab)

Do not confuse with Demulen or Dymelor.

CLASSIFICATION

PHARMACOTHERAPEUTIC: Narcotic agonist. **CLINICAL:** Opiate analgesic **(Schedule II)** (see p. 136C).

ACTION

Binds to opioid receptors within CNS. **Therapeutic Effect:** Alters pain perception, emotional response to pain.

PHARMACOKINETICS

Route	Onset	Peak	Duration
PO	15 min	60 min	2–4 hrs
IV	Less than 5 min	5–7 min	2–3 hrs
IM	10–15 min	30–50 min	2–4 hrs
Subcutaneous	10–15 min	30–50 min	2–4 hrs

Variably absorbed from GI tract; well absorbed after IM administration. Protein binding: 60%–80%. Widely distributed. Metabolized in liver to active metabolite. Primarily excreted in urine. Not removed by hemodialysis. **Half-life:** 2.4–4 hrs; metabolite 8–16 hrs (increased in hepatic impairment/ disease).

USES

Relief of moderate to severe pain. **OFF-LABEL:** Reduces postoperative shivering. Reduces rigors from amphotericin.

PRECAUTIONS

CONTRAINDICATIONS: Delivery of premature infant, diarrhea due to poisoning, use of MAOIs within 14 days. **CAUTIONS:** Renal/hepatic impairment, elderly, debilitated, supraventricular tachycardia, cor pulmonale, history of seizures, acute abdominal conditions, increased intracranial pressure (ICP), respiratory abnormalities.

LIFESPAN CONSIDERATIONS:

Pregnancy/Lactation: Crosses placenta. Distributed in breast milk. Respiratory depression may occur in neonate if mother received opiates during labor. Regular use of opiates during pregnancy may produce withdrawal symptoms in neonate (irritability, excessive crying, tremors, hyperactive reflexes, fever, vomiting, diarrhea, yawning, sneezing, seizures). **Pregnancy Category B (D if used for prolonged periods or at high dosages at term). Children:** Paradoxical excitement may occur. Those younger than 2 yrs more susceptible to respiratory depressant effects. **Elderly:** More susceptible to respiratory depressant effects. Age-related renal impairment may increase risk of urinary retention.

INTERACTIONS

DRUG: Alcohol, other CNS depressants may increase CNS, respiratory depression, hypotension. **MAOIs** may produce severe, sometimes fatal reaction; meperidine use is contraindicated. **HERBAL: Gotu kola, kava kava, St. John's wort, valerian** may increase CNS depression, sedation. **FOOD:** None known. **LAB VALUES:** May increase serum amylase, lipase. Therapeutic serum level: 100–550 ng/ml; toxic serum level: greater than 1,000 ng/ml.

AVAILABILITY (Rx)

INJECTION, SOLUTION: 25 mg/ml, 50 mg/ml, 75 mg/ml, 100 mg/ml. **INJECTION, SOLUTION (FOR PCA):** 10 mg/ml. **SYRUP (DEMEROL):** 50 mg/5 ml. **TABLET (DEMEROL, MEPERITAB):** 50 mg, 100 mg.

ADMINISTRATION/HANDLING

IV

Reconstitution • May give undiluted or dilute in D_5W, dextrose-saline combination (2.5%, 5%, 10% dextrose in water—0.45%, 0.9% NaCl), Ringer's, lactated Ringer's, molar sodium lactate diluent for IV injection or infusion.

Rate of administration • IV dosage must always be administered very slowly, over 2–3 min. • Rapid IV increases risk of severe adverse reactions (chest wall rigidity, apnea, peripheral circulatory collapse, anaphylactoid effects, cardiac arrest).

Storage • Store at room temperature.

IM, SUBCUTANEOUS

◄ ALERT ► IM preferred over subcutaneous route (subcutaneous produces pain, local irritation, induration). • Administer slowly. • Those with circulatory impairment at higher risk for overdosage due to delayed absorption of repeated administration.

PO

• Give without regard to meals. • Dilute syrup in glass of water (prevents anesthetic effect on mucous membranes).

IV INCOMPATIBILITIES

Allopurinol (Aloprim), amphotericin B complex (Abelcet, AmBisome, Amphotec), cefepime (Maxipime), cefoperazone (Cefobid), doxorubicin liposomal (Doxil), furosemide (Lasix), idarubicin (Idamycin), nafcillin (Nafcil).

IV COMPATIBILITIES

Atropine, bumetanide (Bumex), diltiazem (Cardizem), diphenhydramine (Benadryl), dobutamine (Dobutrex), dopamine (Intropin), glycopyrrolate (Robinul), heparin, hydroxyzine (Vistaril), insulin, lidocaine, lipids, magnesium, midazolam (Versed), oxytocin (Pitocin), potassium, total parenteral nutrition (TPN).

INDICATIONS/ROUTES/DOSAGE

ANALGESIA

IV: ADULTS: 5–25 mg q2–4h as needed. IM: ADULTS: 50–75 mg q3–4h as needed. ELDERLY: 25 mg q4h as needed. CHILDREN: 1–1.5 mg/kg/dose q3–4h as needed.

PO: ADULTS: 50 mg q3–4h as needed. **Range:** 50–150 mg q2–4h as needed. ELDERLY: 50 mg q4h as needed. CHILDREN: 1–1.5 mg/kg/dose q3–4h as needed.

PATIENT-CONTROLLED ANALGESIA (PCA)

IV: ADULTS: **Initial dose:** 10 mg. **Demand dose:** 5–25 mg. **Lockout Interval:** 5–10 min.

DOSAGE IN RENAL IMPAIRMENT

Dosage is based on creatinine clearance.

Creatinine Clearance	Dosage
10–50 ml/min	75% of usual dose
Less than 10 ml/min	50% of usual dose

SIDE EFFECTS

FREQUENT: Sedation, hypotension (including orthostatic hypotension), diaphoresis, facial flushing, dizziness, nausea, vomiting, constipation. OCCASIONAL: Confusion, arrhythmias, tremors, urinary retention, abdominal pain, dry mouth, headache, irritation at injection site, euphoria, dysphoria. RARE: Allergic reaction (rash, pruritus), insomnia.

ADVERSE EFFECTS/ TOXIC REACTIONS

Overdose results in respiratory depression, skeletal muscle flaccidity, cold/clammy skin, cyanosis, extreme somnolence progressing to seizures, stupor, coma. **Antidote:** 0.4 mg naloxone (Narcan). Tolerance to analgesic effect, physical dependence may occur with repeated use.

NURSING CONSIDERATIONS

BASELINE ASSESSMENT

Pt should be in recumbent position before drug is administered by parenteral route. Assess onset, type, location, duration of pain. Obtain vital signs before giving medication. If respirations are 12/min or less (20/min or less in children), withhold medication, contact physician. Effect of medication is reduced if full pain recurs before next dose.

INTERVENTION/EVALUATION

Monitor vital signs 15–30 min after subcutaneous/IM dose, 5–10 min after IV dose (monitor for decreased B/P, change in rate/quality of pulse). Monitor pain level, sedation response. Monitor daily pattern of bowel activity/stool consistency; avoid constipation. Check for adequate voiding. Initiate deep breathing, coughing exercises, particularly in pts with pulmonary impairment. Therapeutic serum level: 100–550 ng/ml; toxic serum level: higher than 1,000 ng/ml.

PATIENT/FAMILY TEACHING

• Medication should be taken before pain fully returns, within ordered intervals. • Discomfort may occur with injection. • Change positions slowly to avoid orthostatic hypotension. • Increase fluids, bulk to prevent constipation. • Tolerance, dependence may occur with prolonged use of high doses. • Avoid alcohol, other CNS depressants. • Avoid tasks requiring mental alertness, motor control until response to drug is established.

mepivacaine

(Carbocaine, Polocaine)

FIXED-COMBINATION(S)

With levonordefrin, a vasoconstrictor **(Isocaine)**

See Anesthetics: local (p. 5C)

mercaptopurine

(Purinethol)

See Cancer chemotherapeutic agents (p. 81C)

meropenem

murr-oh-**peh**-nem

(Merrem IV)

CLASSIFICATION

PHARMACOTHERAPEUTIC: Carbapenem. **CLINICAL:** Antibiotic.

ACTION

Binds to penicillin-binding proteins. Inhibits bacterial cell wall synthesis. **Therapeutic Effect:** Bactericidal.

PHARMACOKINETICS

After IV administration, widely distributed into tissues and body fluids, including CSF. Protein binding: 2%. Primarily excreted unchanged in urine. Removed by hemodialysis. **Half-life:** 1 hr.

USES

Treatment of intra-abdominal infections caused by *viridans group streptococci, E. coli, K. pneumoniae, P. aeruginosa, B. fragilis*, peptostreptococcus species; bacterial meningitis caused by *S. pneumoniae, H. influenzae, N. meningitidis*. **OFF-LABEL:** Lower respiratory tract infections, febrile neutropenia, gynecologic/obstetric infections, sepsis.

PRECAUTIONS

CONTRAINDICATIONS: History of seizures, CNS abnormality, hypersensitivity to penicillins. **CAUTIONS:** Hypersensitivity to penicillins, cephalosporins, other allergens; renal impairment; CNS disorders, particularly with history of seizures, concurrent probenecid use.

LIFESPAN CONSIDERATIONS:

Pregnancy/Lactation: Unknown if distributed in breast milk. **Pregnancy Category B.** **Children:** Safety and efficacy not established in those younger than 3 mos. **Elderly:** Age-related renal impairment may require dosage adjustment.

INTERACTIONS

DRUG: **Probenecid** may increase concentration, risk of toxicity (reduces renal excretion of meropenem). **HERBAL:** None significant. **FOOD:** None known. **LAB VALUES:** May increase BUN, serum alkaline phosphatase, bilirubin, creatinine, LDH, AST, ALT. May decrease Hgb, Hct, serum potassium.

AVAILABILITY (Rx)

INJECTION, POWDER FOR RECONSTITUTION: 500 mg, 1 g.

ADMINISTRATION/HANDLING

IV

Reconstitution • Reconstitute each 500 mg with 10 ml Sterile Water for Injection to provide concentration of

M

50 mg/ml. • Shake to dissolve until clear. • May further dilute with 100 ml 0.9% NaCl or D_5W.

Rate of administration • May give by IV push or IV intermittent infusion (piggyback). • If administering as IV intermittent infusion (piggyback), give over 15–30 min; if administered by IV push (5–20 ml), give over 3–5 min.

Storage • Store vials at room temperature. • After reconstitution with 0.9% NaCl, stable for 2 hrs at room temperature or 18 hrs if refrigerated (with D_5W, stable for 1 hr at room temperature, 8 hrs if refrigerated).

IV INCOMPATIBILITIES

Acyclovir (Zovirax), amphotericin B (Fungizone), diazepam (Valium), doxycycline (Vibramycin), metronidazole (Flagyl), ondansetron (Zofran).

IV COMPATIBILITIES

Dobutamine (Dobutrex), dopamine (Intropin), heparin, lipids, magnesium.

INDICATIONS/ROUTES/DOSAGE

INTRA-ABDOMINAL INFECTIONS

IV: ADULTS, ELDERLY, CHILDREN WEIGHING MORE THAN 50 KG: 1 g q8h. **CHILDREN 3 MOS AND OLDER, WEIGHING 50 KG AND LESS:** 20 mg/kg q8h. **Maximum:** 1 g q8h.

MENINGITIS

IV: ADULTS, ELDERLY, CHILDREN WEIGHING 50 KG OR MORE: 2 g q8h. **CHILDREN 3 MOS AND OLDER WEIGHING LESS THAN 50 KG:** 40 mg/kg q8h. **Maximum:** 2 g/dose.

DOSAGE IN RENAL IMPAIRMENT

Dosage and frequency are modified based on creatinine clearance.

Creatinine Clearance	Dosage	Interval
26–49 ml/min	Recommended dose (1,000 mg)	q12h
10–25 ml/min	½ of recommended dose	q12h
Less than 10 ml/min	½ of recommended dose	q24h

SIDE EFFECTS

FREQUENT (5%–3%): Diarrhea, nausea, vomiting, headache, inflammation at injection site. **OCCASIONAL (2%):** Oral candidiasis, rash, pruritus. **RARE (less than 2%):** Constipation, glossitis.

ADVERSE EFFECTS/ TOXIC REACTIONS

Antibiotic-associated colitis, other superinfections may occur. Anaphylactic reactions have been reported. Seizures may occur in those with CNS disorders (e.g., brain lesions, history of seizures), bacterial meningitis, renal impairment.

NURSING CONSIDERATIONS

BASELINE ASSESSMENT

Inquire about history of seizures.

INTERVENTION/EVALUATION

Monitor daily pattern of bowel activity/ stool consistency. Monitor for nausea, vomiting. Evaluate for inflammation at IV injection site. Assess skin for rash. Evaluate hydration status. Monitor I&O, renal function tests. Check mental status; be alert to tremors, possible seizures. Assess temperature, B/P 2 times/day, more often if necessary. Monitor serum electrolytes, esp. potassium.

Merrem, *see meropenem*

mesalamine (5-aminosalicylic acid, 5-ASA)

mez-**al**-a-meen

(Asacol, Canasa, FIV-ASA, Lialda, Mesasal ♣, Pentasa, Rowasa, Salofalk ♣)

Do not confuse Asacol with Os-Cal.

CLASSIFICATION

PHARMACOTHERAPEUTIC: Salicylic acid derivative. **CLINICAL:** Anti-inflammatory agent.

ACTION

Locally inhibits arachidonic acid metabolite production (increased in chronic inflammatory bowel disease). **Therapeutic Effect:** Blocks prostaglandin production, diminishes inflammation in colon.

PHARMACOKINETICS

Poorly absorbed from colon. Moderately absorbed from GI tract. Metabolized in liver to active metabolite. Unabsorbed portion eliminated in feces; absorbed portion excreted in urine. Unknown if removed by hemodialysis. **Half-life:** 0.5–1.5 hrs; metabolite, 5–10 hrs.

USES

Oral: Treatment, maintenance of remission of mild to moderate active ulcerative colitis. **Rectal:** Treatment of active mild to moderate distal ulcerative colitis, proctosigmoiditis or proctitis.

PRECAUTIONS

CONTRAINDICATIONS: None known. **CAUTIONS:** Preexisting renal disease, sulfasalazine sensitivity.

LIFESPAN CONSIDERATIONS:

Pregnancy/Lactation: Unknown if drug crosses placenta or is distributed in breast milk. **Pregnancy Category B. Children:** Safety and efficacy not established. **Elderly:** Age-related renal impairment may require dosage adjustment.

INTERACTIONS

DRUG: Anticoagulants may increase risk of bleeding. **Varicella virus vaccine** may increase risk of developing Reye's syndrome. **HERBAL:** None significant. **FOOD:** None known. **LAB VALUES:** May increase BUN, serum alkaline phosphatase, creatinine, AST, ALT.

AVAILABILITY (Rx)

RECTAL SUSPENSION (ROWASA): 4 g/60 ml. **SUPPOSITORIES (CANASA):** 500 mg, 1 g.

CAPSULES (CONTROLLED-RELEASE [PENTASA]): 250 mg, 500 mg. **TABLETS (DELAYED-RELEASE [ASACOL]):** 400 mg. **(LIALDA):** 1.2 g.

ADMINISTRATION/HANDLING

◀ **ALERT** ▶ Store rectal suspension, suppository, oral forms at room temperature.

PO

• Have pt swallow whole; do not break outer coating of tablet. • Give without regard to food.

RECTAL

• Shake bottle well. • Instruct pt to lie on left side with lower leg extended, upper leg flexed forward. • Knee-chest position may also be used. • Insert applicator tip into rectum, pointing toward umbilicus. • Squeeze bottle steadily until contents are emptied.

INDICATIONS/ROUTES/DOSAGE

TREATMENT OF ULCERATIVE COLITIS

PO (CAPSULE): ADULTS, ELDERLY: 1 g 4 times a day. **CHILDREN:** 50 mg/kg/day divided q6–12h.

PO (TABLET): ADULTS, ELDERLY: 800 mg 3 times a day. **CHILDREN:** 50 mg/kg/day divided q8–12h.

PO (LIALDA): ADULTS, ELDERLY: 1.2–2.4 g once daily.

MAINTENANCE OF REMISSION IN ULCERATIVE COLITIS

PO (CAPSULE): ADULTS, ELDERLY: 1 g 4 times a day.

PO (TABLET): ADULTS, ELDERLY: 1.6 g/day in divided doses.

DISTAL ULCERATIVE COLITIS, PROCTOSIGMOIDITIS, PROCTITIS

RECTAL (RETENTION ENEMA): ADULTS, ELDERLY: 60 ml (4 g) at bedtime; retained overnight for approximately 8 hrs for 3–6 wks.

M

RECTAL: (500 MG SUPPOSITORY) **ADULTS, ELDERLY:** Twice a day. May increase to 3 times a day.
RECTAL (1,000 MG SUPPOSITORY): **ADULTS, ELDERLY:** Once daily at bedtime. Continue therapy for 3–6 wks.

SIDE EFFECTS

Mesalamine is generally well tolerated, with only mild, transient effects. **FREQUENT (greater than 6%): PO:** Abdominal cramps/pain, diarrhea, dizziness, headache, nausea, vomiting, rhinitis, unusual fatigue. **Rectal:** Abdominal/stomach cramps, flatulence, headache, nausea. **OCCASIONAL (6%–2%): PO:** Hair loss, decreased appetite, back/joint pain, flatulence, acne. **Rectal:** Hair loss. **RARE (less than 2%): Rectal:** Anal irritation.

ADVERSE EFFECTS/ TOXIC REACTIONS

Sulfite sensitivity may occur in susceptible pts, manifested as cramping, headache, diarrhea, fever, rash, urticaria, pruritus, wheezing. Discontinue drug immediately. Hepatitis, pancreatitis, pericarditis occur rarely with oral forms.

NURSING CONSIDERATIONS

INTERVENTION/EVALUATION

Encourage adequate fluid intake. Assess bowel sounds for peristalsis. Monitor daily pattern of bowel activity/stool consistency; record time of evacuation. Assess for abdominal disturbances. Assess skin for rash, urticaria. Discontinue medication if rash, fever, cramping, diarrhea occurs.

PATIENT/FAMILY TEACHING

• Avoid tasks that require alertness, motor skills until response to drug is established. • May discolor urine yellow-brown. • Suppositories stain fabrics.

M

mesna

mess-na
(Mesnex, Uromitexan ✱)

CLASSIFICATION

PHARMACOTHERAPEUTIC: Cytoprotective agent. **CLINICAL:** Antineoplastic adjunct, antidote.

ACTION

Binds with and detoxifies urotoxic metabolites of ifosfamide/cyclophosphamide. **Therapeutic Effect:** Inhibits ifosfamide/cyclophosphamide-induced hemorrhagic cystitis.

PHARMACOKINETICS

Rapidly metabolized after IV administration to mesna disulfide, which is reduced to mesna in kidney. Excreted in urine. **Half-life:** 24 min.

USES

Detoxifying agent used as protectant against hemorrhagic cystitis induced by ifosamide, cyclophosphamide.

PRECAUTIONS

CONTRAINDICATIONS: None known. **CAUTIONS:** None known.

LIFESPAN CONSIDERATIONS:

Pregnancy/Lactation: Unknown if drug crosses placenta or is distributed in breast milk. **Pregnancy Category B.** **Children:** Safety and efficacy not established. **Elderly:** Information not available.

INTERACTIONS

DRUG: Warfarin may increase risk of bleeding. **HERBAL:** None significant. **FOOD:** None known. **LAB VALUES:** May produce false-positive test result for urinary ketones.

AVAILABILITY (Rx)

INJECTION SOLUTION: 100 mg/ml. **TABLETS:** 400 mg.

ADMINISTRATION/HANDLING

IV

Reconstitution • May dilute with D_5W or 0.9% NaCl to concentration of 1–20 mg/ml. • May add to solutions containing ifosfamide or cyclophosphamide.

Rate of administration • Administer by IV infusion over 15–30 min or by continuous infusion.

Storage • Store parenteral form at room temperature. • After dilution, is stable for 24 hrs at room temperature (recommended use within 6 hrs). Discard unused medication.

PO

• Dilute mesna solution before PO administration to decrease sulfur odor. Can be diluted in carbonated cola drinks, fruit juices, milk.

IV INCOMPATIBILITIES

Amphotericin B complex (Abelcet, AmBisome, Amphotec).

IV COMPATIBILITIES

Allopurinol (Aloprim), docetaxel (Taxotere), doxorubicin (Adriamycin), etoposide (VePesid), gemcitabine (Gemzar), granisetron (Kytril), lipids, methotrexate, ondansetron (Zofran), paclitaxel (Taxol), vinorelbine (Navelbine).

INDICATIONS/ROUTES/DOSAGE

PREVENTION OF HEMORRHAGIC CYSTITIS IN PTS RECEIVING IFOSFAMIDE

IV: ADULTS, ELDERLY: 20% of ifosfamide dose at time of ifosfamide administration and 4 and 8 hrs after each dose of ifosfamide. Total dose: 60% of ifosfamide dosage. Range: 60%–160% of the daily ifosfamide dose.

PREVENTION OF HEMORRHAGIC CYSTITIS IN PTS RECEIVING LOW-DOSE CYCLOPHOSPHAMIDE

PO: ADULTS, ELDERLY: 20 mg/kg q3–4h.

PREVENTION OF HEMORRHAGIC CYSTITIS IN PTS RECEIVING HIGH-DOSE CYCLOPHOSPHAMIDE

IV: ADULTS, ELDERLY: 40% of cyclophosphamide dose at 0, 3, 6, 9 hrs and IV fluids.

SIDE EFFECTS

FREQUENT (more than 17%): Altered taste, soft stools. **Large doses:** Diarrhea, myalgia, headache, fatigue, nausea, hypotension, allergic reaction.

ADVERSE EFFECTS/ TOXIC REACTIONS

Hematuria occurs rarely.

NURSING CONSIDERATIONS

BASELINE ASSESSMENT

◄ ALERT ► Each dose must be administered with ifosfamide.

INTERVENTION/EVALUATION

Assess morning urine specimen for hematuria. If such occurs, dosage reduction or discontinuation may be necessary. Monitor daily pattern of bowel activity/stool consistency; record time of evacuation. Monitor B/P for hypotension.

PATIENT/FAMILY TEACHING

• Inform physician if headache, myalgia, nausea occurs.

M

mesoridazine

mez-oh-**rid**-a-zeen

(Serentil)

Do not confuse Serentil with Proventil, Serevent, or sertraline.

◆ **CLASSIFICATION**

PHARMACOTHERAPEUTIC: Phenothiazine. **CLINICAL:** Antipsychotic (see p. 62C).

ACTION

Blocks dopamine at postsynaptic receptor in brain. Possesses anticholinergic, sedative effects. **Therapeutic Effect:** Diminishes behavioral response in psychosis, schizophrenia.

PHARMACOKINETICS

Absorption may be erratic. Protein binding: 75%–91%. Undergoes first-pass metabolism. Small portions are metabolized in liver. Excreted in urine, feces. **Half-life:** Unknown.

M

USES

Treatment of schizophrenia in pts who fail to respond to other antipsychotic medication. Treatment of behavioral problems.

PRECAUTIONS

CONTRAINDICATIONS: Coma, concurrent administration of drugs that cause QT-interval prolongation, myelosuppression, severe cardiovascular disease, severe CNS depression, subcortical brain damage. **CAUTIONS:** Respiratory, hepatic, renal, cardiac impairment, alcohol withdrawal, history of seizures, urinary retention, glaucoma, prostatic hypertrophy.

LIFESPAN CONSIDERATIONS:

Pregnancy/Lactation: Crosses placenta; distributed in breast milk. **Pregnancy Category C.** **Children:** Increased risk of developing extrapyramidal symptoms (EPS), dystonias. **Elderly:** Increased risk of anticholinergic effects, EPS, orthostatic hypotension, sedation symptoms.

INTERACTIONS

DRUG: **Alcohol, other CNS depressants** may increase CNS effects, respiratory depression, hypotensive effects. **Antithyroid agents** may increase risk of agranulocytosis. **EPS-producing medications** may increase EPS. **Antihypertensives, hypotension-producing medications** may increase hpotension. May decrease effects of **levodopa. Lithium** may decrease absorption, produce adverse neurologic effects. **MAOIs, tricyclic antidepressants** may increase anticholinergic, sedative effects. **HERBAL:** **Gotu kola, kava kava, St. John's wort, valerian** may increase CNS depression. **FOOD:** None known. **LAB VALUES:** May produce false-positive pregnancy, phenylketonuria (PKU) test results. May produce EKG changes, including prolonged QT interval, T-wave depression or inversion.

AVAILABILITY (Rx)

INJECTION SOLUTION: 25 mg/ml. **ORAL SOLUTION:** 25 mg/ml. **TABLETS:** 10 mg, 25 mg, 50 mg, 100 mg.

ADMINISTRATION/HANDLING

- Avoid skin contact with oral solution (may irritate skin).

INDICATIONS/ROUTES/DOSAGE

SCHIZOPHRENIA

PO: ADULTS, ELDERLY: 25–50 mg 3 times a day. **Maximum:** 400 mg/day.
IM: ADULTS, ELDERLY: Initially, 25 mg. May repeat in 30–60 min. Range: 25–200 mg.

SEVERE BEHAVIORAL PROBLEMS (COMBATIVENESS OR EXPLOSIVE, HYPEREXCITABLE BEHAVIOR)

PO: ELDERLY: Initially, 10 mg once or twice a day. May increase at 4–7 day intervals. **Maximum:** 250 mg.
IM: ADULTS, ELDERLY: Initially, 25 mg. May repeat in 30–60 min. Range: 25–200 mg.

SIDE EFFECTS

FREQUENT: Orthostatic hypotension, dizziness, syncope occur frequently after first injection, occasionally after subsequent injections, rarely with oral form. **OCCASIONAL:** Drowsiness (during early therapy), dry mouth, blurred vision, lethargy, constipation, diarrhea, nasal congestion, peripheral edema, urinary retention. **RARE:** Ocular changes, altered skin pigmentation (in those taking high doses for prolonged periods), darkening of urine.

ADVERSE EFFECTS/ TOXIC REACTIONS

Abrupt withdrawal following long-term therapy may precipitate nausea, vomiting, gastritis, dizziness, tremors. Blood dyscrasias, particularly agranulocytosis, mild leukopenia may occur. May lower seizure threshold.

NURSING CONSIDERATIONS

BASELINE ASSESSMENT

Avoid skin contact with solution (contact dermatitis). Assess behavior, appearance, emotional status, response to environment, speech pattern, thought content.

INTERVENTION/EVALUATION

Assess for orthostatic hypotension. Monitor daily pattern of bowel activity/stool consistency. Supervise suicidal-risk pt closely during early therapy (as depression lessens, energy level improves, increasing suicide potential). Assess for therapeutic response (interest in surroundings, improvement in self-care, increased ability to concentrate, relaxed facial expression).

PATIENT/FAMILY TEACHING

• Full therapeutic effect may take up to 6 wks. • Urine may become dark. • Do not abruptly withdraw from long-term drug therapy. • Report visual disturbances. • Drowsiness generally subsides during continued therapy. • Do not use alcohol, other CNS depressants.

metaproterenol

met-a-proe-**ter**-e-nole

(Alupent)

Do not confuse metaproterenol with metipranolol or metoprolol, or Alupent with Atrovent.

CLASSIFICATION

PHARMACOTHERAPEUTIC: Sympathomimetic (an adrenergic agonist). **CLINICAL:** Bronchodilator (see p. 70C).

ACTION

Stimulates beta$_2$-adrenergic receptors, resulting in relaxation of bronchial smooth muscle. **Therapeutic Effect:** Relieves bronchospasm, reduces airway resistance.

PHARMACOKINETICS

Systemic absorption is rapid following aerosol administration; however, serum concentrations at recommended doses are very low. Metabolized in liver. Excreted in urine primarily as glucoside metabolite. **Half-life:** Unknown.

USES

Treatment of reversible airway obstruction caused by asthma, chronic obstructive pulmonary disease (COPD).

PRECAUTIONS

CONTRAINDICATIONS: Narrow-angle glaucoma, preexisting arrhythmias associated with tachycardia. **CAUTIONS:** Ischemic heart disease, hypertension, hyperthyroidism, seizure disorder, CHF, diabetes, arrhythmias.

M

LIFESPAN CONSIDERATIONS:

Pregnancy/Lactation: Unknown if drug crosses placenta or is distributed in breast milk. **Pregnancy Category C. Children:** Safety and efficacy not established. **Elderly:** No age-related precautions noted.

INTERACTIONS

DRUG: May decrease effects of **beta-blockers. Digoxin, other sympathomimetics** may increase risk of arrhythmias. **MAOIs** may increase risk of hypertensive crisis. **Tricyclic antidepressants** may increase cardiovascular effects. **HERBAL:** None significant. **FOOD:** None known. **LAB VALUES:** May decrease serum potassium.

AVAILABILITY (Rx)

AEROSOL ORAL INHALATION: 0.65 mg/inhalation. **SOLUTION FOR ORAL INHALATION:** 0.4%, 0.6%. **SYRUP:** 10 mg/5 ml. **TABLETS:** 10 mg, 20 mg.

INDICATIONS/ROUTES/DOSAGE

TREATMENT OF BRONCHOSPASM

PO: ADULTS, CHILDREN 10 YRS AND OLDER: 20 mg 3–4 times a day. **ELDERLY:** 10 mg 3–4 times a day. May increase to 20 mg/dose. **CHILDREN 6–9 YRS:** 10 mg 3–4 times a day. **CHILDREN 2–5 YRS:** 1–2.6 mg/kg/day in 3–4 divided doses. **CHILDREN YOUNGER THAN 2 YRS:** 0.4 mg/kg 3–4 times a day.

INHALATION: ADULTS, ELDERLY, CHILDREN 12 YRS AND OLDER: 2–3 inhalations q3–4h. **Maximum:** 12 inhalations/24 hrs.

NEBULIZATION: ADULTS, ELDERLY, CHILDREN 12 YRS AND OLDER: 10–15 mg (0.2–0.3 ml) of 5% q4–6h. **CHILDREN YOUNGER THAN 12 YRS, INFANTS:** 0.5–1 mg/kg (0.01–0.02 ml/kg) of 5% q4–6h.

SIDE EFFECTS

FREQUENT (over 10%): Rigors, tremors, anxiety, nausea, dry mouth. **OCCASIONAL (9%–1%):** Dizziness, vertigo, asthenia, headache, GI distress, vomiting, cough, dry throat. **RARE (less than 1%):** Drowsiness, diarrhea, altered taste.

ADVERSE EFFECTS/ TOXIC REACTIONS

Excessive sympathomimetic stimulation may cause palpitations, extrasystoles, tachycardia, chest pain, slight increase in B/P followed by substantial decrease, chills, diaphoresis, blanching of skin. Too-frequent or excessive use may lead to loss of bronchodilating effectiveness and/or severe, paradoxical bronchoconstriction.

NURSING CONSIDERATIONS

BASELINE ASSESSMENT

Offer emotional support (high incidence of anxiety because of difficulty in breathing, sympathomimetic response to drug).

INTERVENTION/EVALUATION

Monitor rate, depth, rhythm, type of respiration; quality/rate of pulse. Assess lung sounds for rhonchi, wheezing, rales. Monitor ABGs, pulmonary function tests. Observe lips, fingernails for cyanosis (blue or dusky color in light-skinned pts; gray in dark-skinned pts). Evaluate for clinical improvement (quieter, slower respirations; relaxed facial expression; cessation of clavicular, sternal, intercostal retractions).

PATIENT/FAMILY TEACHING

• Increase fluid intake (decreases lung secretion viscosity). • Do not exceed recommended dosage. • May cause anxiety, restlessness, insomnia. • Inform physician if palpitations, tachycardia, chest pain, tremors, dizziness, headache, flushing, difficulty in breathing persists. • Avoid excessive use of caffeine derivatives (chocolate, coffee, tea, cola, cocoa).

metformin

met-**for**-min

(Fortamet, Glucophage, Glucophage XR, Glumetza ✤, Glycon ✤, Novo-Metformin ✤, Riomet)

FIXED-COMBINATION(S)

Actoplus Met: metformin/pioglitazone (an antidiabetic): 500 mg/15 mg, 850 mg/15 mg. **Avandamet:** metformin/rosiglitazone (an antidiabetic): 500 mg/1 mg; 500 mg/2 mg; 500 mg/4 mg; 1,000 mg/2 mg; 1,000 mg/4 mg. **Glucovance:** metformin/glyburide (an antidiabetic): 250 mg/1.25 mg; 500 mg/2.5 mg; 500 mg/5 mg. **Metaglip:** metformin/glipizide (an antidiabetic): 250 mg/2.5 mg; 500 mg/2.5 mg; 500 mg/5 mg.

CLASSIFICATION

PHARMACOTHERAPEUTIC: Antihyperglycemic. **CLINICAL:** Antidiabetic (see p. 42C).

ACTION

Decreases hepatic production of glucose. Decreases absorption of glucose, improves insulin sensitivity. **Therapeutic Effect:** Improves glycemic control, stabilizes/decreases body weight, improves lipid profile.

PHARMACOKINETICS

Slowly, incompletely absorbed after PO administration. Food delays, decreases extent of absorption. Protein binding: Negligible. Primarily distributed to intestinal mucosa, salivary glands. Primarily excreted unchanged in urine. Removed by hemodialysis. **Half-life:** 3–6 hrs.

USES

Management of type 2 diabetes mellitus as monotherapy or concomitantly with oral sulfonylurea or insulin. **OFF-LABEL:** Treatment of HIV lipodystrophy syndrome, metabolic complications of AIDS, polycystic ovary syndrome, prediabetes, weight reduction.

PRECAUTIONS

◀ **ALERT** ▶ Lactic acidosis is rare but potentially severe consequence of metformin therapy. Withhold in pts with conditions that may predispose to lactic acidosis (e.g., hypoxemia, dehydration, hypoperfusion, sepsis).

CONTRAINDICATIONS: Acute CHF, MI, cardiovascular collapse, renal disease/dysfunction, respiratory failure, septicemia. **CAUTIONS:** Conditions delaying food absorption (e.g., diarrhea, high fever, malnutrition, gastroparesis, vomiting), causing hyperglycemia, hypoglycemia, uncontrolled hypothyroidism, hyperthyroidism, cardiovascular pts, concurrent drugs that affect renal function, hepatic impairment, elderly, malnourished/debilitated pts with renal impairment, CHF, excessive alcohol intake, chronic respiratory difficulty.

LIFESPAN CONSIDERATIONS:

Pregnancy/Lactation: Insulin is drug of choice during pregnancy. Distributed in breast milk in animals. **Pregnancy Category B. Children:** Safety and efficacy not established. **Elderly:** Age-related renal impairment or peripheral vascular disease may require dosage adjustment or discontinuation.

INTERACTIONS

DRUG: Furosemide, cimetidine may increase concentration. **Cationic medications (e.g., digoxin, morphine, quinine, ranitidine, vancomycin)** may increase concentration, effect. **Contrast agents** may increase risk of metformin-induced lactic acidosis, acute renal failure (discontinue metformin 48 hrs prior to contrast exposure). **HERBAL: Garlic** may cause hypoglycemia. **FOOD:** None known. **LAB VALUES:** None known.

M

AVAILABILITY (Rx)

ORAL SOLUTION (RIOMET): 100 mg/ml. **TABLETS (GLUCOPHAGE):** 500 mg, 850 mg, 1,000 mg.

TABLETS (EXTENDED-RELEASE): 500 mg (Fortamet, Glucophage XL, Glumetza), 750 mg (Glucophage XL), 1,000 mg (Fortamet, Glumetza).

ADMINISTRATION/HANDLING

PO

- Do not crush extended-release tablets.
- Give with meals.

INDICATIONS/ROUTES/DOSAGE

DIABETES MELLITUS

PO (IMMEDIATE-RELEASE TABLETS, SOLUTION): ADULTS, ELDERLY: Initially, 500 mg twice a day or 850 mg once daily. Maintenance: 1–2.55 g/day in 2–3 divided doses. **Maximum:** 2,500 mg/day. **CHILDREN 10–16 YRS:** Initially, 500 mg twice a day. Maintenance: Titrate in 500 mg increments weekly. **Maximum:** 2,000 mg/day.

PO (EXTENDED-RELEASE TABLETS [GLUCOPHAGE XL]): ADULTS, ELDERLY: Initially, 500 mg once daily. Maintenance: 1–2 g daily. **Maximum:** 2,000 mg/day.

PO (EXTENDED-RELEASE TABLETS [FORTAMET, GLUMETZA]): ADULTS, ELDERLY: 500 mg–1 g once daily. Maintenance: 1–2.5 g once daily. **Maximum:** 2,500 mg/day.

SIDE EFFECTS

OCCASIONAL (greater than 3%): GI disturbances (diarrhea, nausea, vomiting, abdominal bloating, flatulence, anorexia) that are transient and resolve spontaneously during therapy. **RARE (3%–1%):** Unpleasant/metallic taste that resolves spontaneously during therapy.

ADVERSE EFFECTS/ TOXIC REACTIONS

Lactic acidosis occurs rarely (0.03 cases/ 1,000 pts) but is a serious but often fatal (50%) complication. Lactic acidosis is characterized by increase in blood lactate levels (greater than 5 mmol/L), decrease in blood pH, electrolyte disturbances. Symptoms include unexplained hyperventilation, myalgia, malaise, somnolence. May advance to cardiovascular collapse (shock), acute CHF, acute MI, prerenal azotemia.

NURSING CONSIDERATIONS

BASELINE ASSESSMENT

Inform pt of potential risks/advantages of therapy, of alternative modes of therapy. Before initiation of therapy and annually thereafter, assess Hgb, Hct, RBC, serum creatinine.

INTERVENTION/EVALUATION

Monitor fasting serum glucose, Hgb A, renal function. Monitor folic acid, renal function tests for evidence of early lactic acidosis. If pt is on concurrent oral sulfonylureas, assess for hypoglycemia (cool/wet skin, tremors, dizziness, anxiety, headache, tachycardia, numbness in mouth, hunger, diplopia). Be alert to conditions that alter glucose requirements: fever, increased activity, stress, surgical procedure.

PATIENT/ FAMILY TEACHING

• Discontinue metformin, contact physician immediately if evidence of lactic acidosis appears (unexplained hyperventilation, muscle aches, extreme fatigue, unusual drowsiness). • Prescribed diet is principal part of treatment; do not skip, delay meals. • Diabetes mellitus requires lifelong control. • Avoid alcohol. • Inform physician if headache, nausea, vomiting, diarrhea persist or skin rash, unusual bruising/bleeding, change in color of urine or stool occurs.

methadone

meth-a-done

(Dolophine, Metadol ♣, Methadone Intensol, Methadose)

CLASSIFICATION

PHARMACOTHERAPEUTIC: Narcotic agonist. **CLINICAL:** Opioid analgesic (**Schedule II**) (see p. 136C).

ACTION

Binds with opioid receptors within CNS. **Therapeutic Effect:** Alters processes affecting analgesia, emotional response to pain; reduces withdrawal symptoms from other opioid drugs.

PHARMACOKINETICS

Route	Onset	Peak	Duration
Oral	0.5–1 hr	1.5–2 hrs	6–8 hrs
IM	10–20 min	1–2 hrs	4–5 hrs
IV	N/A	15–30 min	3–4 hrs

Well absorbed after IM injection. Protein binding: 80%–85%. Metabolized in liver. Primarily excreted in urine. Not removed by hemodialysis. **Half-life:** 15–25 hrs.

USES

Relief of severe pain, detoxification, temporary maintenance treatment of narcotic abstinence syndrome.

PRECAUTIONS

CONTRAINDICATIONS: Delivery of premature infant, diarrhea due to poisoning, hypersensitivity to narcotics, labor. **EXTREME CAUTION:** Renal/hepatic impairment, elderly/debilitated, supraventricular tachycardia, cor pulmonale, history of seizures, acute abdominal conditions, increased intracranial pressure (ICP), respiratory abnormalities.

LIFESPAN CONSIDERATIONS:

Pregnancy/Lactation: Crosses placenta. Distributed in breast milk. Respiratory depression may occur in neonate if mother received opiates during labor. Regular use of opiates during pregnancy may produce withdrawal symptoms in neonate (irritability, excessive crying, tremors, hyperactive reflexes, fever, vomiting, diarrhea, yawning, sneezing, seizures). **Pregnancy Category B (D if used for prolonged periods or at high dosages at term).** **Children:** Paradoxical excitement may occur. Those younger than 2 yrs more susceptible to respiratory depressant effects. **Elderly:** More susceptible to respiratory depressant effects. Age-related renal impairment may increase risk of urinary retention.

INTERACTIONS

DRUG: Alcohol, other CNS depressants may increase CNS effects, respiratory depression, hypotension. **Clarithromycin** may increase concentration/toxicity. **Amiodarone, erythromycin** may prolong QT interval. **MAOIs** may produce severe, sometimes fatal reaction (reduce dose to ¼ of usual methadone dose). **HERBAL: Gotu kola, kava kava, St. John's wort, valerian** may increase CNS depression. **FOOD: Grapefruit, grapefruit juice** may alter concentration, effect. **LAB VALUES:** May increase serum amylase, lipase.

AVAILABILITY (Rx)

INJECTION SOLUTION (DOLOPHINE): 10 mg/ml. **ORAL CONCENTRATE (METHADONE INTENSOL, METHADOSE):** 10 mg/ml. **ORAL SOLUTION:** 5 mg/5 ml, 10 mg/5 ml. **TABLETS (DISPERSIBLE [METHADOSE]):** 40 mg. **TABLETS (DOLOPHINE, METHADOSE):** 5 mg, 10 mg.

ADMINISTRATION/HANDLING

IM, SUBCUTANEOUS

◀ ALERT ▶ IM preferred over subcutaneous route (subcutaneous produces pain, local irritation, induration). • Do not use if solution appears cloudy or contains a precipitate. • Administer slowly. • Those with circulatory impairment

M

experience higher risk of overdosage due to delayed absorption of repeated administration.

PO

• Give without regard to meals. • Dilute syrup in glass of water (prevents anesthetic effect on mucous membranes).

INDICATIONS/ROUTES/DOSAGE

ANALGESIA

PO: ADULTS, ELDERLY: Initially, 5–10 mg q3–4h. **CHILDREN:** 0.1–0.2 mg/kg q6–12h as needed. **Maximum:** 10 mg/dose.
IV, IM, SUBCUTANEOUS: ADULTS, ELDERLY: Initially, 2.5–10 mg q3–4h.

DETOXIFICATION

PO: ADULTS, ELDERLY: Initially, dose should not exceed 30 mg. An additional 5–10 mg may be provided if withdrawal symptoms have not been suppressed or if symptoms reappear after 2–4 hrs. Total daily dose not to exceed 40 mg. **Range:** 80–120 mg/day with titration occurring cautiously. Withdrawal should be less than 10% of the maintenance dose every 10–14 days. **Short-term:** Initially, titrate to 40 mg/day in 2 divided doses. Continue 40 mg dose for 2–3 days. Decrease dose every day or every other day.

SIDE EFFECTS

FREQUENT: Sedation, decreased B/P (orthostatic hypotension), diaphoresis, facial flushing, constipation, dizziness, nausea, vomiting. **OCCASIONAL:** Confusion, urinary retention, palpitations, abdominal cramps, visual changes, dry mouth, headache, decreased appetite, anxiety, insomnia. **RARE:** Allergic reaction (rash, pruritus).

ADVERSE EFFECTS/ TOXIC REACTIONS

Overdose results in respiratory depression, skeletal muscle flaccidity, cold/clammy skin, cyanosis, extreme somnolence progressing to seizures, stupor, coma. Early sign of toxicity presents as increased sedation after being on a stable dose. Cardiac toxicity manifested as QT prolongation, torsades de pointes. **ANTIDOTE:** 0.4 mg naloxone (Narcan). Tolerance to analgesic effect, physical dependence may occur with repeated use.

NURSING CONSIDERATIONS

BASELINE ASSESSMENT

Pt should be in recumbent position before drug administration by parenteral route. Obtain vital signs before giving medication. If respirations are 12/min or less (20/min or less in children), withhold medication, contact physician.

INTERVENTION/EVALUATION

Monitor vital signs 15–30 min after subcutaneous/IM dose, 5–10 min following IV dose. Oral medication is 50% as potent as parenteral. Assess for adequate voiding. Assess for clinical improvement, record onset of relief of pain. Provide support to pt in detoxification program; monitor for withdrawal symptoms.

PATIENT/FAMILY TEACHING

• Methadone may produce drug dependence, has potential for being abused. • Avoid alcohol. • Do not stop taking abruptly after prolonged use. • May cause dry mouth, drowsiness; avoid tasks that require alertness, motor skills until response to drug is established. Call physician if increased sedation occurs after being on a stable dose.

methimazole

meth-**im**-a-zole
(Tapazole)

CLASSIFICATION

PHARMACOTHERAPEUTIC: Thiomidazole derivative. **CLINICAL:** Antithyroid.

ACTION

Inhibits synthesis of thyroid hormone by interfering with incorporation of iodine into tyrosyl residues. **Therapeutic Effect:** Decreases thyroid hormone levels.

USES

Treatment of hyperthyroidism. Used to attain a normal metabolic state before thyroidectomy, to control thyrotoxic crisis that may accompany thyroidectomy.

PRECAUTIONS

CONTRAINDICATIONS: None known. **CAUTIONS:** Pts older than 40 yrs or in combination with other agranulocytosis-inducing drugs, hepatic impairment.

⌛ LIFESPAN CONSIDERATIONS:

Pregnancy/Lactation: Crosses placenta; distributed in breast milk. Avoid breast-feeding. **Pregnancy Category D.** **Children:** Safety and efficacy not established. **Elderly:** No age-related precautions noted.

INTERACTIONS

DRUG: **Amiodarone, iodinated glycerol, iodine, potassium iodide** may decrease response. May increase concentration of **digoxin** as pt becomes euthyroid. May decrease thyroid uptake of I^{131}. May decrease effect of **oral anticoagulants.** **HERBAL:** None significant. **FOOD:** None known. **LAB VALUES:** May increase LDH, serum alkaline phosphatase, bilirubin, AST, ALT. May decrease prothrombin time (PT), WBC count.

AVAILABILITY (Rx)

TABLETS: 5 mg, 10 mg, 20 mg.

ADMINISTRATION/HANDLING

• Store at room temperature. • Give with food if GI symptoms occur.

INDICATIONS/ROUTES/DOSAGE

HYPERTHYROIDISM

PO: ADULTS, ELDERLY: Initially, 15–60 mg/day in 3 divided doses. Maintenance: 5–15 mg/day. **CHILDREN:** Initially, 0.4 mg/kg/day in 3 divided doses. Maintenance: ⅓–⅔ the initial dose.

SIDE EFFECTS

FREQUENT (5%–4%): Fever, rash, pruritus. **OCCASIONAL (3%–1%):** Dizziness, loss of taste, nausea, vomiting, stomach pain, peripheral neuropathy, numbness in fingers, toes, face. **RARE (less than 1%):** Swollen lymph nodes, salivary glands.

ADVERSE EFFECTS/ TOXIC REACTIONS

Agranulocytosis (may occur as long as 4 mos after therapy), pancytopenia, hepatitis have occurred.

NURSING CONSIDERATIONS

BASELINE ASSESSMENT

Obtain baseline weight, pulse.

INTERVENTION/EVALUATION

Monitor pulse; weigh daily. Assess skin for rash, pruritus, lymphadenopathy. Monitor CBC with differential, hepatic function, prothrombin time. Assess for signs of infection, bleeding.

PATIENT/FAMILY TEACHING

• Do not exceed ordered dose. • Space doses evenly around the clock. • Take resting pulse daily to monitor therapeutic results. • Seafood, iodine products may be restricted. • Report illness, unusual bleeding/bruising immediately.

methocarbamol

(Robaxin)

FIXED-COMBINATION(S)

With aspirin, an analgesic **(Robaxisal)**

See Skeletal muscle relaxants.

M

methohexital

(Brevital)

See Anesthetics: general (p. 2C)

methotrexate

meth-oh-**trex**-ate

(Apo-Methotrexate ✦, Rheumatrex, Trexall)

Do not confuse Trexall with Trexan.

CLASSIFICATION

PHARMACOTHERAPEUTIC: Antimetabolite. **CLINICAL:** Antineoplastic, antiarthritic, antipsoriatic (see p. 81C).

M

ACTION

Competes with enzymes necessary to reduce folic acid to tetrahydrofolic acid, a component essential to DNA, RNA, protein synthesis. **Therapeutic Effect:** Inhibits DNA, RNA, protein synthesis.

PHARMACOKINETICS

Variably absorbed from GI tract. Completely absorbed after IM administration. Protein binding: 50%–60%. Widely distributed. Metabolized intracellularly in liver. Primarily excreted in urine. Removed by hemodialysis but not by peritoneal dialysis. **Half-life:** 8–12 hrs (large doses, 8–15 hrs).

USES

Treatment of breast, head/neck, non–small lung, small cell lung carcinomas, trophoblastic tumors, acute lymphocytic, meningeal leukemias, non-Hodgkin's lymphomas (lymphosarcoma, Burkitt's lymphoma), mycosis fungoides, osteosarcoma, psoriasis, rheumatoid arthritis. **OFF-LABEL:** Treatment of acute myelocytic leukemia; bladder, cervical, ovarian, prostatic, renal, testicular carcinomas; psoriatic arthritis; systemic dermatomyositis. Treatment of and maintenance of remission in Crohn's disease.

PRECAUTIONS

CONTRAINDICATIONS: Hepatic disease, renal impairment, preexisting myelosuppression, psoriasis, rheumatoid arthritis with alcoholism. **CAUTIONS:** Peptic ulcer, ulcerative colitis, myelosuppression, ascites, pleural effusion.

LIFESPAN CONSIDERATIONS:

Pregnancy/Lactation: Avoid pregnancy during methotrexate therapy and minimum 3 mos after therapy in males or at least one ovulatory cycle after therapy in females. May cause fetal death, congenital anomalies. Drug is distributed in breast milk. Breast-feeding not recommended. **Pregnancy Category D (X for patients with psoriasis or rheumatoid arthritis). Children/Elderly:** Renal or hepatic impairment may require dosage adjustment.

INTERACTIONS

DRUG: Acyclovir (parenteral) may increase risk of neurotoxicity. **Alcohol, hepatotoxic medications** may increase risk of hepatotoxicity. **Asparaginase** may decrease effect. **Bone marrow depressants** may increase myelosuppression. **Live virus vaccines** may potentiate virus replication, increase vaccine side effects, decrease pt's antibody response to vaccine. **NSAIDs** may increase risk of toxicity. **Probenecid, salicylates** may increase concentration, risk of toxicity. **HERBAL: Echinacea, cat's claw** possess immunostimulant properties. **FOOD:** None known. **LAB VALUES:** May increase serum uric acid, AST.

AVAILABILITY (Rx)

INJECTION, POWDER FOR RECONSTITUTION: 20 mg, 50 mg, 1 g. **INJECTION**

SOLUTION: 25 mg/ml. **TABLETS:** 2.5 mg (Rheumatrex), 5 mg (Trexall), 7.5 mg (Trexall), 10 mg (Trexall), 15 mg (Trexall).

ADMINISTRATION/HANDLING

◀ **ALERT** ▶ May be carcinogenic, mutagenic, teratogenic. Handle with extreme care during preparation/ administration. Wear gloves when preparing solution. If powder or solution comes in contact with skin, wash immediately, thoroughly with soap, water. May give IM, IV, intra-arterially, intrathecally.

IV

Reconstitution • Reconstitute each 5 mg with 2 ml Sterile Water for Injection or 0.9% NaCl to provide concentration of 2.5 mg/ml. Maximum concentration 25 mg/ml. • May further dilute with D_5W or 0.9% NaCl. • For intrathecal use, dilute with preservative-free 0.9% NaCl to provide 1 mg/ml concentration.

Rate of administration • Give IV push at rate of 10 mg/min. • Give IV infusion over 0.5–4 hrs.

Storage • Store vials at room temperature.

IV INCOMPATIBILITIES

Chlorpromazine (Thorazine), droperidol (Inapsine), gemcitabine (Gemzar), idarubicin (Idamycin), midazolam (Versed), nalbuphine (Nubain).

IV COMPATIBILITIES

Cisplatin (Platinol AQ), cyclophosphamide (Cytoxan), daunorubicin (DaunoXome), doxorubicin (Adriamycin), etoposide (VePesed), 5-fluorouracil, granisetron (Kytril), leucovorin, lipids, mitomycin (Mutamycin), ondansetron (Zofran), paclitaxel (Taxol), vinblastine (Velban), vincristine (Oncovin), vinorelbine (Navelbine).

INDICATIONS/ROUTES/DOSAGE

◀ **ALERT** ▶ Refer to individual specific protocols for optimum dosage, sequence of administration.

TROPHOBLASTIC NEOPLASMS

PO, IM: ADULTS, ELDERLY: 15–30 mg/day for 5 days; repeat in 7 days for 3–5 courses.

IV: 11 mg/m^2 on days 1–5, repeat every 3 wks.

HEAD/NECK CANCER

PO, IV, IM: ADULTS, ELDERLY: 25–50 mg/m^2 once weekly.

CHORIOCARCINOMA, CHORIOADENOMA DESTRUENS, HYDATIDIFORM MOLE

PO, IV: ADULTS, ELDERLY: 15–30 mg/day for 5 days; repeat 3–5 times with 1–2 wks between courses.

BREAST CANCER

IV: ADULTS, ELDERLY: 30–60 mg/m^2 days 1 and 8 q3–4wk.

ACUTE LYMPHOCYTIC LEUKEMIA

PO, IV, IM: ADULTS, ELDERLY: Induction: 3.3 mg/m^2/day in combination with other chemotherapeutic agents. Maintenance: 30 mg/m^2/wk PO or IM in divided doses or 2.5 mg/kg IV every 14 days.

BURKITT'S LYMPHOMA

PO: ADULTS: 10–25 mg/day for 4–8 days; repeat with 7- to 10-day rest between courses.

LYMPHOSARCOMA

PO: ADULTS, ELDERLY: 0.625–2.5 mg/kg/day.

MYCOSIS FUNGOIDES

PO: ADULTS, ELDERLY: 2.5–10 mg/day.

IM: ADULTS, ELDERLY: 5–50 mg once weekly. If refractory, 15–37.5 mg 2 times/wk.

RHEUMATOID ARTHRITIS

PO: ADULTS, ELDERLY: 7.5 mg once weekly or 2.5 mg q12h for 3 doses once weekly. **Maximum:** 20 mg/wk.

JUVENILE RHEUMATOID ARTHRITIS

PO, IM, SUBCUTANEOUS: CHILDREN: 5–15 mg/m^2/wk as a single dose or in 3 divided doses given q12h.

M

PSORIASIS

PO: ADULTS, ELDERLY: 10–25 mg once weekly or 2.5–5 mg q12h for 3 doses once weekly.

IM: ADULTS, ELDERLY: 10–25 mg once weekly.

ANTINEOPLASTIC DOSAGE FOR CHILDREN

PO, IM: CHILDREN: 7.5–30 mg/m^2/wk or q2wk.

IV: CHILDREN: 10–33,000 mg/m^2 bolus or continuous infusion over 6–42 hrs.

DOSAGE IN RENAL IMPAIRMENT

Creatinine Clearance	Dosage
61–80 ml/min	Reduce by 25%
51–60 ml/min	Reduce by 33%
10–50 ml/min	Reduce by 50%–70%

SIDE EFFECTS

FREQUENT (10%–3%): Nausea, vomiting, stomatitis; burning/erythema at psoriatic site (in pts with psoriasis). **OCCASIONAL (3%–1%):** Diarrhea, rash, dermatitis, pruritus, alopecia, dizziness, anorexia, malaise, headache, drowsiness, blurred vision.

ADVERSE EFFECTS/ TOXIC REACTIONS

High potential for various, severe toxicities. GI toxicity may produce gingivitis, glossitis, pharyngitis, stomatitis, enteritis, hematemesis. Hepatotoxicity more likely to occur with frequent small doses than with large intermittent doses. Pulmonary toxicity characterized by interstitial pneumonitis. Hematologic toxicity, resulting from marked myelosuppression, may manifest as leukopenia, thrombocytopenia, anemia, hemorrhage. Dermatologic toxicity may produce rash, pruritus, urticaria, pigmentation, photosensitivity, petechiae, ecchymosis, pustules. Severe nephrotoxicity produces azotemia, hematuria, renal failure.

NURSING CONSIDERATIONS

BASELINE ASSESSMENT

Question for possibility of pregnancy before initiating therapy (Pregnancy Category X) in pts with psoriasis, rheumatoid arthritis. Obtain all functional tests before therapy, repeat throughout therapy. Antiemetics may prevent nausea, vomiting.

INTERVENTION/EVALUATION

Monitor hepatic/renal function tests, Hgb, Hct, WBC, differential, platelet count, urinalysis, chest x-rays, serum uric acid. Monitor for hematologic toxicity (fever, sore throat, signs of local infection, unusual bruising/bleeding from any site), symptoms of anemia (excessive fatigue, weakness). Assess skin for evidence of dermatologic toxicity. Keep pt well hydrated, urine alkaline. Avoid IM injections, rectal temperatures, traumas that induce bleeding. Apply 5 full min of pressure to IV sites.

PATIENT/FAMILY TEACHING

• Maintain fastidious oral hygiene. • Do not have immunizations without physician's approval (drug lowers resistance). • Avoid crowds, those with infection. • Avoid alcohol, salicylates. • Avoid sunlamp, sunlight exposure. • Use contraceptive measures during therapy and for 3 mos (males) or 1 ovulatory cycle (females) after therapy. • Promptly report fever, sore throat, signs of local infection, unusual bruising/bleeding from any site. • Alopecia is reversible, but new hair growth may have different color, texture. • Contact physician if nausea/vomiting continues at home.

methylcellulose

meth-ill-**cell**-you-los
(Citrucel, Cologel)

Do not confuse Citrucel with Citracal.

CLASSIFICATION

CLINICAL: Bulk-forming laxative.

ACTION

Dissolves and expands in water. **Therapeutic Effect:** Increases bulk, moisture content in stool, increasing peristalsis, bowel motility.

PHARMACOKINETICS

Route	Onset	Peak	Duration
PO	12–24 hrs	N/A	N/A

Acts in small, large intestines. Full effect may not be evident for 2–3 days.

USES

Prophylaxis in those who should not strain during defecation. Facilitates defecation in those with diminished colonic motor response.

PRECAUTIONS

CONTRAINDICATIONS: Abdominal pain, dysphagia, nausea, partial bowel obstruction, symptoms of appendicitis, vomiting. **CAUTIONS:** None known.

LIFESPAN CONSIDERATIONS:

Pregnancy/Lactation: Safe for use in pregnancy. **Pregnancy Category C. Children:** Safety and efficacy not established in those younger than 6 yrs. Not recommended in this age group. **Elderly:** No age-related precautions noted.

INTERACTIONS

DRUG: May decrease effects of **digoxin, oral anticoagulants, salicylates** by decreasing their absorption. May interfere with effects of **potassium-sparing diuretics, potassium supplements. HERBAL:** None significant. **FOOD:** None known. **LAB VALUES:** May increase serum glucose. May decrease serum potassium.

AVAILABILITY (OTC)

POWDER (CITRUCEL, COLOGEL).

ADMINISTRATION/HANDLING

PO

- Instruct pt to drink 6–8 glasses of water/day (aids stool softening).
- Do not swallow in dry form; mix with at least 1 full glass (8 oz) of liquid.

INDICATIONS/ROUTES/DOSAGE

CONSTIPATION

PO: ADULTS, ELDERLY: 1 tbsp (15 ml) in 8 oz water 1–3 times a day. **CHILDREN 6–12 YRS:** 1 tsp (5 ml) in 4 oz water 3–4 times a day.

SIDE EFFECTS

RARE: Some degree of abdominal discomfort, nausea, mild cramps, griping, faintness.

ADVERSE EFFECTS/ TOXIC REACTIONS

Esophageal/bowel obstruction may occur if drug is administered with insufficient liquid (less than 250 ml or 1 full [8 oz] glass).

NURSING CONSIDERATIONS

INTERVENTION/EVALUATION

Encourage adequate fluid intake. Assess bowel sounds for peristalsis. Monitor daily pattern of bowel activity/stool consistency; record time of evacuation. Monitor serum electrolytes in those exposed to prolonged, frequent, excessive use of medication.

PATIENT/FAMILY TEACHING

- Institute measures to promote defecation: increase fluid intake, exercise, high-fiber diet.

M

methyldopa

meth-ill-**doe**-pa
(Aldomet, Apo-Methyldopa ✤, Methyldopate, Novomedopa ✤)
Do not confuse Aldomet with Anzemet.

FIXED-COMBINATION(S)

Aldoril: methyldopa/hydrochlorothiazide (a diuretic): 250 mg/15 mg; 250 mg/25 mg; 500 mg/30 mg; 500 mg/50 mg.

◆CLASSIFICATION

PHARMACOTHERAPEUTIC: Alpha-adrenergic agonist. **CLINICAL:** Antihypertensive (see p. 58C).

ACTION

Stimulates central inhibitory alpha-adrenergic receptors, lowers arterial pressure, reduces plasma renin activity. **Therapeutic Effect:** Reduces B/P.

PHARMACOKINETICS

Variable absorption from GI tract. Protein binding: Negligible. Metabolized in liver. Excreted in urine. Removed by hemodialysis. **Half-life:** 1.7 hrs.

USES

Management of moderate to severe hypertension.

PRECAUTIONS

CONTRAINDICATIONS: Hepatic disease, hepatic disorders previously associated with methyldopa therapy, MAOIs, pheochromocytoma. **CAUTIONS:** Renal impairment.

LIFESPAN CONSIDERATIONS:

Pregnancy/Lactation: Unknown if drug crosses placenta; distributed in breast milk. **Pregnancy Category B.** **Children:** Safety and efficacy not established. **Elderly:** Age-related renal impairment may require dosage adjustment.

INTERACTIONS

DRUG: **Hypotensive medications, antihypertensives, diuretics** may increase effects. May increase risk of **lithium** toxicity. **MAOIs** may cause hyperexcitability. **NSAIDs, tricyclic antidepressants** may decrease effects. May decrease effects of **sympathomimetics.** **HERBAL:** None significant. **FOOD:** None known. **LAB VALUES:** May increase BUN, serum prolactin, alkaline phosphatase, bilirubin, creatinine, potassium, sodium, uric acid, AST, ALT. May produce false-positive Coombs' test, prolong prothrombin time (PT).

AVAILABILITY (Rx)

INJECTION SOLUTION: 50 mg/ml. **ORAL SUSPENSION (METHYLDOPATE):** 250 mg/5 ml. **TABLETS (ALDOMET):** 125 mg, 250 mg, 500 mg.

ADMINISTRATION/HANDLING

IV

Reconstitution • For IV infusion, add prescribed dose to 100 ml D_5W. • Alternatively, add prescribed dose to D_5W to make final concentration of 100 mg per 10 ml.

Rate of administration • Infuse over 30–60 min.

Storage • Discard if solution contains precipitate or is discolored.

INDICATIONS/ROUTES/DOSAGE

HYPERTENSION

IV: ADULTS, ELDERLY: 250–500 mg q6h. **Maximum:** 1 g q6h. **CHILDREN:** 5–10 mg/kg/dose q6–8h. **Maximum:** 65 mg/kg/day or 3 g/24 hrs.

PO: ADULTS, ELDERLY: Initially, 250 mg 2–3 times a day. May increase at 2-day intervals up to 3 g/day. Range: 250–1,000 mg/day in 2 divided doses.

CHILDREN: Initially, 10 mg/kg/day in 2–4 divided doses. May increase at 2-day intervals up to 65 mg/kg/day. **Maximum:** 3 g/day.

SIDE EFFECTS

FREQUENT: Peripheral edema, drowsiness, headache, dry mouth. **OCCASIONAL:** Altered mental status (anxiety, depression), decreased sexual function/libido, diarrhea, swelling of breasts, nausea, vomiting, lightheadedness, paresthesia, rhinitis.

ADVERSE EFFECTS/ TOXIC REACTIONS

Hepatotoxicity (abnormal hepatic function tests, jaundice, hepatitis), hemolytic anemia, unexplained fever/flu-like symptoms may occur. If these conditions appear, discontinue medication, contact physician.

NURSING CONSIDERATIONS

BASELINE ASSESSMENT

Obtain baseline B/P, pulse, weight.

INTERVENTION/EVALUATION

Monitor B/P, pulse closely q30min until stabilized. Monitor weight daily during initial therapy. Monitor hepatic function tests. Assess for peripheral edema.

PATIENT/FAMILY TEACHING

- Avoid alcohol; may cause drowsiness.
- Avoid tasks requiring mental alertness, motor skills until response to drug is established.

methylergonovine

meth-ill-er-goe-**noe**-veen
(Methergine)

CLASSIFICATION

PHARMACOTHERAPEUTIC: Ergot alkaloid. **CLINICAL:** Uterine stimulant.

ACTION

Stimulates alpha-adrenergic, serotonin receptors, producing arterial vasoconstriction. Causes vasospasm of coronary arteries. Directly stimulates uterine muscle. **Therapeutic Effect:** Increases strength, frequency of uterine contractions, decreases uterine bleeding.

PHARMACOKINETICS

Route	Onset	Peak	Duration
PO	5–10 min	N/A	N/A
IV	Immediate	N/A	3 hrs
IM	2–5 min	N/A	N/A

Rapidly absorbed from GI tract after IM administration. Distributed rapidly to plasma, extracellular fluid, tissues. Metabolized in liver, undergoes first-pass effect. Primarily excreted in urine. **Half-life:** IV (alpha phase), 2–3 min or less; IV (beta phase), 20–30 min or longer.

M

USES

Prevention/treatment of postpartum, postabortion hemorrhage due to atony, involution (not for induction, augmentation of labor). **OFF-LABEL:** Treatment of incomplete abortion.

PRECAUTIONS

CONTRAINDICATIONS: Hypertension, pregnancy, toxemia, untreated hypocalcemia. **CAUTIONS:** Renal/hepatic impairment, coronary artery disease, occlusive peripheral vascular disease, sepsis.

LIFESPAN CONSIDERATIONS:

Pregnancy/Lactation: Contraindicated during pregnancy. Small amounts distributed in breast milk. **Pregnancy Category C. Children/Elderly:** No information available.

INTERACTIONS

DRUG: Vasoconstrictors, vasopressors may increase effects. **HERBAL:** None significant. **FOOD:** None known. **LAB VALUES:** May decrease serum prolactin.

AVAILABILITY (Rx)

INJECTION SOLUTION: 0.2 mg/ml. **TABLETS:** 0.2 mg.

ADMINISTRATION/HANDLING

Reconstitution • Dilute to volume of 5 ml with 0.9% NaCl.

Rate of administration • Give over at least 1 min, carefully monitoring B/P.

Storage • Refrigerate ampules. • Initial dose may be given parenterally, followed by oral regimen. • IV use in life-threatening emergencies only.

IV INCOMPATIBILITIES

None known.

IV COMPATIBILITIES

Heparin, potassium.

M

INDICATIONS/ROUTES/DOSAGE

PREVENTION/TREATMENT OF POSTPARTUM, POSTABORTION HEMORRHAGE

PO: ADULTS: 0.2 mg 3–4 times a day. Continue for up to 7 days.

IV, IM: ADULTS: Initially, 0.2 mg. May repeat q2–4h as needed.

SIDE EFFECTS

FREQUENT: Nausea, uterine cramping, vomiting. **OCCASIONAL:** Abdominal pain, diarrhea, dizziness, diaphoresis, tinnitus, bradycardia, chest pain. **RARE:** Allergic reaction (rash, pruritus), dyspnea; severe or sudden hypertension.

ADVERSE EFFECTS/ TOXIC REACTIONS

Severe hypertensive episodes may result in cerebrovascular accident (CVA), serious arrhythmias, seizures. Hypertensive effects are more frequent with pt susceptibility, rapid IV administration, concurrent use of regional anesthesia, vasoconstrictors. Peripheral ischemia may lead to gangrene.

NURSING CONSIDERATIONS

BASELINE ASSESSMENT

Determine baseline serum calcium level, B/P, pulse. Assess bleeding before administration.

INTERVENTION/EVALUATION

Monitor uterine tone, bleeding, B/P, pulse q15min until stable (about 1–2 hrs). Assess extremities for color, warmth, movement, pain. Report chest pain promptly. Provide support with ambulation if dizziness occurs.

PATIENT/FAMILY TEACHING

• Avoid smoking because of added vasoconstriction. • Report increased cramping, bleeding, foul-smelling lochia. • Report pale, cold hands/feet (possibility of diminished circulation).

methylphenidate

meth-ill-**fen**-i-date

(Concerta, Daytrana, Metadate CD, Metadate ER, Methylin, Methylin ER, PMS-Methylphenidate 🍁, Riphenidate 🍁, Ritalin, Ritalin LA, Ritalin SR)

Do not confuse Ritalin with Rifadin.

CLASSIFICATION

CLINICAL: **(Schedule II)** CNS stimulant.

ACTION

Blocks reuptake of norepinephrine, dopamine into presynaptic neurons. **Therapeutic Effect:** Decreases motor restlessness, fatigue. Increases motor activity, attention span, mental alertness. Produces mild euphoria.

PHARMACOKINETICS

Onset	Peak	Duration
Immediate-release	2 hrs	3–5 hrs
Sustained-release	4–7 hrs	3–8 hrs
Extended-release	N/A	8–12 hrs

Slowly, incompletely absorbed from GI tract. Protein binding: 15%. Metabolized in liver. Eliminated in urine, in feces by biliary system. Unknown if removed by hemodialysis. **Half-life:** 2–4 hrs.

USES

Adjunct to treatment of attention deficit hyperactivity disorder (ADHD) with moderate to severe distractibility, short attention spans, hyperactivity, emotional impulsivity in children older than 6 yrs. Management of narcolepsy in adults. **OFF-LABEL:** Treatment of disease-related fatigue, secondary mental depression.

PRECAUTIONS

CONTRAINDICATIONS: Use of MAOIs within 14 days, marked anxiety, tension, agitation, motor tics, family history or diagnosis of Tourette's syndrome, glaucoma. **CAUTIONS:** Hypertension, seizures, acute stress reaction, emotional instability, history of drug dependence, heart failure, recent MI, hyperthyroidism, known structural cardiac abnormality, psychosis.

LIFESPAN CONSIDERATIONS:

Pregnancy/Lactation: Unknown if drug crosses placenta or is distributed in breast milk. **Pregnancy Category C.** **Children:** May be more susceptible to developing anorexia, insomnia, stomach pain, decreased weight. Chronic use may inhibit growth. **Elderly:** No age-related precautions noted.

INTERACTIONS

DRUG: **MAOIs** may increase effects. **Other CNS stimulants** may have additive effect. **HERBAL:** **Ephedra** may cause hypertension, arrhythmias. **Yohimbe** may increase CNS stimulation. **FOOD:** None known. **LAB VALUES:** None known.

AVAILABILITY (Rx)

ORAL SOLUTION (METHYLIN): 5 mg/5 ml, 10 mg/5 ml. **TABLETS (CHEWABLE [METHYLIN]):** 2.5 mg, 5 mg, 10 mg. **TABLETS (METHYLIN, RITALIN):** 5 mg, 10 mg, 20 mg. **TOPICAL PATCH (DAYTRANA):** 10 mg/9 hrs, 15 mg/9 hrs, 20 mg/9 hrs, 30 mg/9 hrs.

CAPSULES (EXTENDED-RELEASE [METADATE CD]): 10 mg, 20 mg, 30 mg, 40 mg, 50 mg, 60 mg. **CAPSULES (EXTENDED-RELEASE [RITALIN LA]):** 10 mg, 20 mg, 30 mg, 40 mg. **TABLETS (EXTENDED-RELEASE [CONCERTA]):** 18 mg, 27 mg, 36 mg, 54 mg, 72 mg. **TABLETS (EXTENDED-RELEASE [MENTADATE ER, METHYLIN ER]):** 10 mg, 20 mg. **TABLETS (SUSTAINED-RELEASE [RITALIN SR]):** 20 mg.

ADMINISTRATION/HANDLING

◄ **ALERT** ► Sustained-release, extended-release tablets may be given in place of regular tablets, once daily dose is titrated using regular tablets, and titrated dosage corresponds to sustained-release or extended-release tablet strength.

PO

• Do not give drug in afternoon or evening (drug may cause insomnia). • Do not crush, break extended-release capsules, extended- or sustained-release tablets. • Tablets may be crushed. • Give dose 30–45 min before meals.

• **METADATE CD:** May be opened, sprinkled on applesauce.

PATCH

• To be worn daily for 9 hrs. • Replace daily in morning. • Apply to dry, clean area of hip. • Avoid applying to waistline (clothing may cause patch to rub off). • Alternate application site daily. • Press firmly in place for 30 sec to ensure patch is in good contact with skin.

M

INDICATIONS/ROUTES/DOSAGE

ADHD

PO: ADULTS, CHILDREN 6 YRS AND OLDER: Initially, 0.3 mg/kg/dose or 2.5–5 mg before breakfast and lunch. May increase by 0.1 mg/kg/dose or by 5–10 mg/day at weekly intervals. **Usual dose:** 0.5–1 mg/kg/day. **Maximum:** 2 mg/kg/day or 90 mg/day.

PO (CONCERTA): CHILDREN 6 YRS AND OLDER: Initially, 18 mg once a day; may increase by 18 mg/day at weekly intervals. **Maximum:** 72 mg/day.

PO (METADATE CD): CHILDREN 6 YRS AND OLDER: Initially, 20 mg/day. May increase by 20 mg/day at weekly intervals. **Maximum:** 60 mg/day.

PO (RITALIN LA): CHILDREN 6 YRS AND OLDER: Initially, 20 mg/day. May increase by 10 mg/day at weekly intervals. **Maximum:** 60 mg/day.

PO (METADATE ER, METHYLIN ER, RITALIN SR): CHILDREN 6 YRS AND OLDER: May replace regular tablets after daily dose is titrated and 8-hr dosage corresponds to sustained-release or extended-release tablet strength.

PATCH (DAYTRANA): CHILDREN: 10–30 mg daily (applied and worn for 9 hrs).

NARCOLEPSY

PO: ADULTS, ELDERLY: 10 mg 2–3 times a day. Range: 10–60 mg/day.

SIDE EFFECTS

FREQUENT: Anxiety, insomnia, anorexia. **OCCASIONAL:** Dizziness, drowsiness, headache, nausea, abdominal pain, fever, rash, arthralgia, vomiting. **RARE:** Blurred vision, Tourette's syndrome (uncontrolled vocal outbursts, repetitive body movements, tics), palpitations.

ADVERSE EFFECTS/ TOXIC REACTIONS

Prolonged administration to children with ADHD may delay normal weight gain pattern. Overdose may produce tachycardia, palpitations, arrhythmias, chest pain, psychotic episode, seizures, coma. Hypersensitivity reactions, blood dyscrasias occur rarely.

NURSING CONSIDERATIONS

INTERVENTION/EVALUATION

CBC with differential, platelet count should be performed routinely during therapy. If paradoxical return of attention deficit occurs, dosage should be reduced or discontinued. Monitor growth.

PATIENT/ FAMILY TEACHING

• Avoid tasks that require alertness, motor skills until response to drug is established. • Sugarless gum, sips of tepid water may relieve dry mouth. • Report any increase in seizures. • Take daily dose early in morning to avoid insomnia. • Report anxiety, palpitations, fever, vomiting, skin rash. • Avoid caffeine. • Do not abruptly stop taking after prolonged use.

*methylPREDNISolone

(Medrol)

*methylPREDNISolone acetate

(DepoMedrol)

*methylPREDNISolone sodium succinate

(Solu-Medrol)

meth-il-pred-**niss**-oh-lone

Do not confuse methylprednisolone with medroxyprogesterone or Medrol with Mebaral.

CLASSIFICATION

PHARMACOTHERAPEUTIC: Adrenal corticosteroid. **CLINICAL:** Glucocorticoid (see p. 92C).

ACTION

Suppresses migration of polymorphonuclear leukocytes, reverses increased capillary permeability. **Therapeutic Effect:** Decreases inflammation.

PHARMACOKINETICS

Route	Onset	Peak	Duration
PO	N/A	1–2 hrs	30–36 hrs
IM	N/A	4–8 days	1–4 wks

Well absorbed from GI tract after IM administration. Widely distributed. Metabolized in liver. Excreted in urine. Removed by hemodialysis. **Half-life:** 3.5 hrs.

USES

Endocrine Disorders: Substitution therapy for deficiency states: (acute or chronic adrenal insufficiency, congenital adrenal hyperplasia, adrenal insufficiency secondary to pituitary insufficiency). **Nonendocrine Disorders:** Arthritis; rheumatic carditis; allergic reaction; collagen, intestinal tract, hepatic, ocular, renal, skin diseases; bronchial asthma; cerebral edema; malignancies, spinal cord injury.

PRECAUTIONS

CONTRAINDICATIONS: Administration of live virus vaccines, systemic fungal infection. **CAUTIONS:** Hypothyroidism, cirrhosis, hypertension, diabetes, CHF, ulcerative colitis, thromboembolic disorders.

LIFESPAN CONSIDERATIONS:

Pregnancy/Lactation: Crosses placenta. Distributed in breast milk. May cause cleft palate (chronic use first trimester). Breast-feeding contraindicated. **Pregnancy Category C. Children:** Prolonged treatment or high dosages may decrease short-term growth rate, cortisol secretion. **Elderly:** No age-related precaution noted.

INTERACTIONS

DRUG: **Amphotericin** may increase hypokalemia. May increase risk of **digoxin** toxicity caused by hypokalemia. May decrease effects of **diuretics, insulin, oral hypoglycemics, potassium supplements. Hepatic enzyme inducers** may decrease effects. **Live virus vaccines** may decrease pt's antibody response to vaccine, increase vaccine side effects, potentiate virus replication. **HERBAL:** **Echinacea, cat's claw** possess immunostimulant properties. **St. John's wort** may decrease concentration. **FOOD:** None known. **LAB VALUES:** May increase serum glucose, cholesterol, lipid, amylase, sodium. May decrease serum calcium, potassium, thyroxine.

AVAILABILITY (Rx)

INJECTION POWDER FOR RECONSTITUTION (SOLU-MEDROL): 40 mg, 125 mg, 500 mg, 1 g. **INJECTION SUSPENSION:** 20 mg/ml, 40 mg/ml, 80 mg/ml. **TABLETS (MEDROL):** 2 mg, 4 mg, 8 mg, 16 mg, 32 mg.

ADMINISTRATION/HANDLING

IV

Reconstitution • For infusion, add to D_5W, 0.9% NaCl.

Rate of administration • Give IV push over 2–3 min. • Give IV piggyback over 10–20 min. • Do **not** give methylprednisolone acetate IV.

Storage • Store vials at room temperature.

IM

• Methylprednisolone acetate should not be further diluted. • Methylprednisolone sodium succinate should be reconstituted with Bacteriostatic Water for Injection. • Give deep IM in gluteus maximus.

M

PO

• Give with food, milk. • Give single doses before 9 AM; give multiple doses at evenly spaced intervals.

IV INCOMPATIBILITIES

Ciprofloxacin (Cipro), diltiazem (Cardizem), docetaxel (Taxotere), etoposide (VePesid), filgrastim (Neupogen), gemcitabine (Gemzar), paclitaxel (Taxol), potassium chloride, propofol (Diprivan), vinorelbine (Navelbine).

IV COMPATIBILITIES

Dopamine (Intropin), heparin, lipids, midazolam (Versed), theophylline.

INDICATIONS/ROUTES/DOSAGE

ANTI-INFLAMMATORY, IMMUNOSUPPRESSIVE

IV: ADULTS, ELDERLY: 10–40 mg. May repeat as needed. **CHILDREN:** 0.5–1.7 mg/kg/day or 5–25 mg/m^2/day in 2–4 divided doses.

PO: ADULTS, ELDERLY: 2–60 mg/day in 1–4 divided doses. **CHILDREN:** 0.5–1.7 mg/kg/day or 5–25 mg/m^2/day in 2–4 divided doses.

STATUS ASTHMATICUS

IV: ADULTS, ELDERLY, CHILDREN: Initially, 2 mg/kg/dose, then 0.5–1 mg/kg/dose q6h for up to 5 days.

SPINAL CORD INJURY

IV BOLUS: ADULTS, ELDERLY: 30 mg/kg over 15 min. Maintenance dose: 5.4 mg/kg/h over 23 hrs, to be given within 45 min of bolus dose.

IM (METHYLPREDNISOLONE ACETATE): ADULTS, ELDERLY: 10–80 mg/day. **CHILDREN:** 0.5–1.7 mg/kg/day or 5–25 mg/m^2/day in 2–4 divided doses.

INTRA-ARTICULAR, INTRALESIONAL: ADULTS, ELDERLY: 4–40 mg, up to 80 mg q1–5wk.

SIDE EFFECTS

FREQUENT: Insomnia, heartburn, anxiety, abdominal distention, diaphoresis, acne, mood swings, increased appetite, facial flushing, GI distress, delayed wound healing, increased susceptibility to infection, diarrhea, constipation. **OCCASIONAL:** Headache, edema, tachycardia, change in skin color, frequent urination, depression. **RARE:** Psychosis, increased blood coagulability, hallucinations.

ADVERSE EFFECTS/ TOXIC REACTIONS

Long-term therapy: Hypocalcemia, hypokalemia, muscle wasting (esp. in arms, legs), osteoporosis, spontaneous fractures, amenorrhea, cataracts, glaucoma, peptic ulcer, CHF. **Abrupt withdrawal after long-term therapy:** Anorexia, nausea, fever, headache, severe arthralgia, rebound inflammation, fatigue, weakness, lethargy, dizziness, orthostatic hypotension.

NURSING CONSIDERATIONS

BASELINE ASSESSMENT

Question for hypersensitivity to any of the corticosteroids, components. Obtain baselines for height, weight, B/P, serum glucose, electrolytes. Check results of initial tests (tuberculosis [TB] skin test, x-rays, EKG).

INTERVENTION/EVALUATION

Monitor I&O, daily weight; assess for edema. Monitor daily pattern of bowel activity/stool consistency. Check vital signs at least 2 times a day. Be alert for infection (sore throat, fever, vague symptoms). Monitor serum electrolytes. Monitor for hypocalcemia (muscle twitching, cramps, positive Trousseau's or Chvostek's signs), hypokalemia (weakness, muscle cramps, numbness, tingling [esp. lower extremities], nausea/vomiting, irritability, EKG changes). Assess emotional status, ability to sleep. Check lab results for blood coagulability, clinical evidence of thromboembolism.

PATIENT/ FAMILY TEACHING

• Take oral dose with food, milk. • Do not change dose/schedule or stop taking

M

drug; must taper off gradually under medical supervision. • Notify physician of fever, sore throat, muscle aches, sudden weight gain, edema. • Maintain' fastidious personal hygiene, avoid exposure to disease, trauma. • Severe stress (serious infection, surgery, trauma) may require increased dosage. • Follow-up visits, lab tests are necessary. • Children must be assessed for growth retardation. • Inform dentist, other physicians of methylprednisolone therapy now or within past 12 mos.

methysergide

(Sansert)

See Antimigraine agents

metipranolol

(OptiPranolol)

See Antiglaucoma agents (p. 50C)

metoclopramide

meh-tah-**klo**-prah-myd

(Apo-Metoclop ♣, Reglan)

Do not confuse Reglan with Renagel.

CLASSIFICATION

PHARMACOTHERAPEUTIC: Dopamine receptor antagonist. **CLINICAL:** GI emptying adjunct, peristaltic stimulant, antiemetic.

ACTION

Stimulates motility of upper GI tract. Decreases reflux into esophagus. Raises threshold activity in chemoreceptor trigger zone. **Therapeutic Effect:** Accelerates intestinal transit, gastric emptying. Relieves nausea, vomiting.

PHARMACOKINETICS

Route	Onset	Peak	Duration
PO	30–60 min	N/A	N/A
IV	1–3 min	N/A	N/A
IM	10–15 min	N/A	N/A

Well absorbed from GI tract. Metabolized in liver. Protein binding: 30%. Primarily excreted in urine. Not removed by hemodialysis. **Half-life:** 4–6 hrs.

USES

Facilitates intestinal intubation, stimulates gastric emptying, intestinal transit in conjunction with radiography; treatment of gastroparesis, gastroesophageal reflux disease (GERD); prevents cancer chemotherapy-induced nausea, vomiting; prevents postoperative nausea, vomiting. **OFF-LABEL:** Prevention of aspiration pneumonia; treatment of drug-related postoperative nausea/vomiting, gastric stasis in preterm infants, persistent hiccups, slow gastric emptying, vascular headaches.

PRECAUTIONS

CONTRAINDICATIONS: Concurrent use of medications likely to produce extrapyramidal reactions, GI hemorrhage, GI obstruction/perforation, history of seizure disorders, pheochromocytoma. **CAUTIONS:** Renal impairment, CHF, cirrhosis.

LIFESPAN CONSIDERATIONS:

Pregnancy/Lactation: Crosses placenta. Distributed in breast milk. **Pregnancy Category B.** **Children:** More susceptible to having dystonic reactions. **Elderly:** More likely to have parkinsonian dyskinesias after long-term therapy.

INTERACTIONS

DRUG: **Alcohol, other CNS depressants** may increase CNS depressant

M

effect. **HERBAL:** None significant. **FOOD:** None known. **LAB VALUES:** May increase serum aldosterone, prolactin.

AVAILABILITY (Rx)

INJECTION SOLUTION: 5 mg/ml. **SYRUP:** 5 mg/5 ml. **TABLETS:** 5 mg, 10 mg.

ADMINISTRATION/HANDLING

IV

Reconstitution • Dilute doses greater than 10 mg in 50 ml D_5W, 0.9% NaCl, or lactated Ringer's.

Rate of administration • Infuse over 15 min. • May give slow IV push at rate of 10 mg over 1–2 min. • Too rapid IV injection may produce intense feeling of anxiety, restlessness, followed by drowsiness.

Storage • Store vials at room temperature. • After dilution, IV infusion (piggyback) is stable for 48 hrs.

PO

• Give 30 min before meals and at bedtime. • Tablets may be crushed.

IV INCOMPATIBILITIES

Allopurinol (Aloprim), cefepime (Maxipime), doxorubicin liposomal (Doxil), furosemide (Lasix), propofol (Diprivan).

IV COMPATIBILITIES

Dexamethasone, diltiazem (Cardizem), diphenhydramine (Benadryl), fentanyl (Sublimaze), heparin, hydromorphone (Dilaudid), lipids, morphine, potassium chloride, total parenteral nutrition (TPN).

INDICATIONS/ROUTES/DOSAGE

PREVENTION OF CHEMOTHERAPY-INDUCED NAUSEA/VOMITING

IV: ADULTS, ELDERLY, CHILDREN: 1–2 mg/kg 30 min before chemotherapy; repeat q2h for 2 doses, then q3h as needed for total of 5 doses/day.

POSTOPERATIVE NAUSEA/VOMITING

IV: ADULTS, ELDERLY: 10–20 mg q4–6h as needed. **CHILDREN:** 0.25 mg/kg/dose q6–8h as needed.

DIABETIC GASTROPARESIS

PO, IV: ADULTS: 10 mg 30 min before meals and at bedtime for 2–8 wks.

PO: ELDERLY: Initially, 5 mg 30 min before meals and at bedtime. May increase to 10 mg.

IV: ELDERLY: 5 mg over 1–2 min. May increase to 10 mg.

SYMPTOMATIC GASTROESOPHAGEAL REFLUX

PO: ADULTS: 10–15 mg up to 4 times a day, or single doses up to 20 mg as needed. **ELDERLY:** Initially, 5 mg 4 times a day. May increase to 10 mg. **CHILDREN:** 0.4–0.8 mg/kg/day in 4 divided doses.

FACILITATE SMALL BOWEL INTUBATION (SINGLE DOSE)

IV: ADULTS, ELDERLY: 10 mg as a single dose. **CHILDREN 6–14 YRS:** 2.5–5 mg as a single dose. **CHILDREN YOUNGER THAN 6 YRS:** 0.1 mg/kg as a single dose.

DOSAGE IN RENAL IMPAIRMENT

Dosage is modified based on creatinine clearance.

Creatinine Clearance	% of Normal Dose
40–50 ml/min	75%
10–40 ml/min	50%
Less than 10 ml/min	25%–50%

SIDE EFFECTS

◄ **ALERT** ► Doses of 2 mg/kg or greater, or increased length of therapy, may result in a greater incidence of side effects.

FREQUENT (10%): Drowsiness, restlessness, fatigue, lethargy. **OCCASIONAL (3%):** Dizziness, anxiety, headache, insomnia, breast tenderness, altered menstruation, constipation, rash, dry mouth, galactorrhea, gynecomastia. **RARE (less than 3%):** Hypotension, hypertension, tachycardia.

ADVERSE EFFECTS/ TOXIC REACTIONS

Extrapyramidal reactions occur most frequently in children, young adults (18–30 yrs) receiving large doses (2 mg/kg) during chemotherapy and usually are limited to akathisia (involuntary limb movement, facial grimacing, motor restlessness).

NURSING CONSIDERATIONS

BASELINE ASSESSMENT

Antiemetic: Assess for dehydration (poor skin turgor, dry mucous membranes, longitudinal furrows in tongue).

INTERVENTION/EVALUATION

Monitor for anxiety, restlessness, extrapyramidal symptoms (EPS) during IV administration. Monitor daily pattern of bowel activity/stool consistency. Assess skin for rash. Evaluate for therapeutic response from gastroparesis (nausea, vomiting, bloating). Monitor renal function, B/P, heart rate.

PATIENT/FAMILY TEACHING

• Avoid tasks that require alertness, motor skills until drug response is established. • Report involuntary eye, facial, limb movement (extrapyramidal reaction). • Avoid alcohol.

metolazone

me-**toh**-lah-zone

(Mykrox, Zaroxolyn)

Do not confuse metolazone with methazolamide or metoprolol, or Zaroxolyn with Zarontin.

CLASSIFICATION

PHARMACOTHERAPEUTIC: Thiazide-like. **CLINICAL:** Diuretic, antihypertensive (see p. 97C).

ACTION

Diuretic: Blocks reabsorption of sodium, potassium, chloride at distal convoluted tubule, promoting delivery of sodium to potassium side, increasing sodium-potassium (Na-K) exchange. **Therapeutic Effect:** Produces renal excretion. **Antihypertensive:** Reduces plasma and extracellular fluid volume, peripheral vascular resistance. **Therapeutic Effect:** Reduces B/P.

PHARMACOKINETICS

Route	Onset	Peak	Duration
PO (diuretic)	1 hr	2 hrs	12–24 hrs

Incompletely absorbed from GI tract. Protein binding: 95%. Primarily excreted unchanged in urine. Not removed by hemodialysis. **Half-life:** 14 hrs.

USES

Zaroxolyn: Treatment of mild to moderate essential hypertension, edema due to renal disease, edema due to CHF. **Mykrox:** Treatment of mild to moderate hypertension.

PRECAUTIONS

CONTRAINDICATIONS: Anuria, hepatic coma/precoma, history of hypersensitivity to sulfonamides, thiazide diuretics, renal decompensation. **CAUTIONS:** Severe renal disease, hepatic impairment, gout, lupus erythematosus, diabetes, elevated serum cholesterol, triglycerides.

LIFESPAN CONSIDERATIONS:

Pregnancy/Lactation: Crosses placenta. Small amount distributed in breast milk; breast-feeding not advised. **Pregnancy Category B (D if used in pregnancy-induced hypertension). Children:** No age-related precautions noted. **Elderly:** May be more sensitive to hypotensive or electrolyte effects. Age-related renal impairment may require dosage adjustment.

INTERACTIONS

DRUG: **Cholestyramine, colestipol** may decrease absorption/effect. May increase risk of **digoxin** toxicity associated with metolazone-induced hypokalemia. May increase risk of **lithium** toxicity. **HERBAL:** **Dong quai, St. John's wort** may increase photosensitization. **Ephedra, yohimbe, ginseng** may worsen hypertension. **Garlic** may increase antihypertensive effect. **FOOD:** None known. **LAB VALUES:** May increase serum glucose, cholesterol, LDL, bilirubin, calcium, creatinine, uric acid, triglycerides. May decrease urinary calcium, serum magnesium, potassium, sodium.

AVAILABILITY (Rx)

TABLETS (EXTENDED-RELEASE [ZAROXOLYN]): 2.5 mg, 5 mg, 10 mg. **TABLETS (PROMPT-RELEASE [MYKROX]):** 0.5 mg.

M

ADMINISTRATION/HANDLING

PO

- May give with food, milk if GI upset occurs, preferably with breakfast (may prevent nocturia).

INDICATIONS/ROUTES/DOSAGE

EDEMA

PO (ZAROXOLYN): ADULTS, ELDERLY: 2.5–10 mg/day. May increase to 20 mg/day in edema associated with renal disease or heart failure. **CHILDREN:** 0.2–0.4 mg/kg/day in 1–2 divided doses.

HYPERTENSION

PO (ZAROXOLYN): ADULTS, ELDERLY: 2.5–5 mg/day.

PO (MYKROX): ADULTS, ELDERLY: Initially, 0.5 mg/day. May increase up to 1 mg/day.

SIDE EFFECTS

EXPECTED: Increased urinary frequency/volume. **FREQUENT (10%–9%):** Dizziness, lightheadedness, headache. **OCCASIONAL (6%–4%):** Muscle cramps/spasm, fatigue, lethargy. **RARE (less than 2%):** Asthenia (loss of strength, energy), palpitations, depression, nausea, vomiting, abdominal bloating, constipation, diarrhea, urticaria.

ADVERSE EFFECTS/ TOXIC REACTIONS

Vigorous diuresis may lead to profound water loss and electrolyte depletion, resulting in hypokalemia, hyponatremia, dehydration. Acute hypotensive episodes may occur. Hyperglycemia may occur during prolonged therapy. Pancreatitis, paresthesia, blood dyscrasias, pulmonary edema, allergic pneumonitis, dermatologic reactions occur rarely. Overdose can lead to lethargy, coma without changes in electrolytes, hydration.

NURSING CONSIDERATIONS

BASELINE ASSESSMENT

Check vital signs, esp. B/P for hypotension, before administration. Assess baseline serum electrolytes, particularly check for hypokalemia. Assess skin turgor, mucous membranes for hydration status. Assess for peripheral edema. Assess muscle strength, mental status. Note skin temperature, moisture. Obtain baseline weight. Monitor I&O.

INTERVENTION/EVALUATION

Continue to monitor B/P, vital signs, serum electrolytes, I&O, weight. Note extent of diuresis. Monitor for electrolyte disturbances (hypokalemia may result in weakness, tremors, muscle cramps, nausea, vomiting, altered mental status, tachycardia; hyponatremia may result in confusion, thirst, cold/clammy skin).

PATIENT/FAMILY TEACHING

• Expect increased urinary frequency/volume. • Rise slowly from lying to sitting position, permit legs to dangle momentarily before standing to reduce hypotensive effect. • Eat foods high in potassium, such as whole grains (cereals), legumes, meat, bananas, apricots, orange juice, potatoes (white, sweet), raisins.

metoprolol

me-**toe**-pro-lole

(Apo-Metoprolol ✦, Betaloc ✦, Lopressor, Novo-Metoprolol ✦, Nu-Metop ✦, Toprol XL)

Do not confuse metoprolol with metaproterenol or metolazone, or Toprol XL with Topamax, Tegretol, Tegretol XR.

FIXED-COMBINATION(S)

Lopressor HCT: metoprolol/hydrochlorothiazide (a diuretic): 50 mg/25 mg; 100 mg/25 mg; 100 mg/50 mg.

CLASSIFICATION

PHARMACOTHERAPEUTIC: $Beta_1$-adrenergic blocker. **CLINICAL:** Antianginal, antihypertensive, MI adjunct (see p. 68C).

ACTION

Selectively blocks $beta_1$-adrenergic receptors; high dosages may block $beta_2$-adrenergic receptors. Decreases oxygen requirements. Large doses increase airway resistance. **Therapeutic Effect:** Slows heart rate, decreases cardiac output, reduces B/P. Decreases myocardial ischemia severity.

PHARMACOKINETICS

Route	Onset	Peak	Duration
PO	10–15 min	N/A	6 hrs
PO (extended release)	N/A	6–12 hrs	24 hrs
IV	Immediate	20 min	5–8 hrs

Well absorbed from GI tract. Protein binding: 12%. Widely distributed. Metabolized in liver (undergoes significant first-pass metabolism). Primarily excreted in urine. Removed by hemodialysis. **Half-life:** 3–7 hrs.

USES

Lopressor: Treatment of acute myocardial infarction (AMI), angina pectoris, hypertension. **Toprol XL:** Treatment of angina pectoris, CHF, hypertension. **OFF-LABEL:** To increase survival rate in diabetic pts with coronary artery disease (CAD). Treatment/prevention of anxiety, cardiac arrhythmias, hypertrophic cardiomyopathy, mitral valve prolapse syndrome, pheochromocytoma, tremors, thyrotoxicosis, vascular headache.

PRECAUTIONS

CONTRAINDICATIONS: Cardiogenic shock, MI with heart rate less than 45 beats/min or systolic B/P less than 100 mm Hg, overt heart failure, second- or third-degree heart block, sinus bradycardia. **CAUTIONS:** Bronchospastic disease, renal impairment, peripheral vascular disease, hyperthyroidism, diabetes mellitus, inadequate cardiac function.

LIFESPAN CONSIDERATIONS:

Pregnancy/Lactation: Crosses placenta. Distributed in breast milk. Avoid use during first trimester. May produce bradycardia, apnea, hypoglycemia, hypothermia during delivery, low birth-weight infants. **Pregnancy Category C (D if used in second or third trimester). Children:** Safety and efficacy not established. **Elderly:** Age-related peripheral vascular disease may increase susceptibility to decreased peripheral circulation.

INTERACTIONS

DRUG: Cimetidine may increase concentration. **Diuretics, other antihypertensives** may increase hypotensive

M

effect. May mask symptoms of hypoglycemia, prolong hypoglycemic effect of **insulin, oral hypoglycemics. NSAIDs** may decrease antihypertensive effect. **Sympathomimetics, xanthines** may mutually inhibit effects. **HERBAL: Ephedra, yohimbe, ginseng** may worsen hypertension. **Garlic** may increase antihypertensive effect. **FOOD:** None known. **LAB VALUES:** May increase serum antinuclear antibody titer (ANA), BUN, serum lipoprotein, LDH, alkaline phosphatase, bilirubin, creatinine, potassium, uric acid, AST, ALT, triglycerides.

AVAILABILITY (Rx)

INJECTION SOLUTION (LOPRESSOR): 1 mg/ml. **TABLETS (LOPRESSOR):** 25 mg, 50 mg, 100 mg.

TABLETS (EXTENDED-RELEASE [TOPROL XL]): 25 mg, 50 mg, 100 mg, 200 mg.

ADMINISTRATION/HANDLING

IV

Rate of administration • May give undiluted. • Administer IV injection over 1 min. • Monitor EKG, B/P during administration.

Storage • Store at room temperature.

PO

• Tablets may be crushed; do not crush/break extended-release tablets. • Give at same time each day. • May be given with or immediately after meals (enhances absorption).

IV INCOMPATIBILITIES

Amphotericin B complex (Abelcet, AmBisome, Amphotec).

IV COMPATIBILITY

Alteplase (Activase).

INDICATIONS/ROUTES/DOSAGE

HYPERTENSION

PO: ADULTS: Initially, 100 mg/day as single or divided dose. Increase at weekly (or longer) intervals. Maintenance: 100–450 mg/day. **ELDERLY:** Initially, 25 mg/day. Range: 25–300 mg/day.

PO (EXTENDED-RELEASE): ADULTS: 50–100 mg/day as single dose. May increase at least at weekly intervals until optimum B/P attained. **Maximum:** 200 mg/day. **ELDERLY:** Initially, 25–50 mg/day as a single dose. May increase at 1–2 wk intervals.

ANGINA PECTORIS

PO: ADULTS: Initially, 100 mg/day as single or divided dose. Increase at weekly (or longer) intervals. Maintenance: 100–450 mg/day.

PO (EXTENDED-RELEASE): ADULTS: Initially, 100 mg/day as single dose. May increase at least at weekly intervals until optimum clinical response achieved. **Maximum:** 400 mg/day.

CHF

PO (EXTENDED-RELEASE): ADULTS: Initially, 25 mg/day. May double dose q2wk. **Maximum:** 200 mg/day.

EARLY TREATMENT OF MI

IV: ADULTS: 5 mg q5min for 3 doses, followed by 50 mg orally q6h for 48 hrs. Begin oral dose 15 min after last IV dose. In pts who do not tolerate full IV dose, give 25–50 mg orally q6h, 15 min after last IV dose.

LATE TREATMENT, MAINTENANCE AFTER MI

PO: ADULTS: 100 mg twice a day for at least 3 mos.

SIDE EFFECTS

Metoprolol is generally well tolerated, with transient and mild side effects. **FREQUENT:** Diminished sexual function, drowsiness, insomnia, unusual fatigue/weakness. **OCCASIONAL:** Anxiety, diarrhea, constipation, nausea, vomiting, nasal congestion, abdominal discomfort, dizziness, difficulty breathing, cold hands/feet. **RARE:** Altered taste, dry eyes, nightmares, paresthesia, allergic reaction (rash, pruritus).

ADVERSE EFFECTS/ TOXIC REACTIONS

Overdose may produce profound bradycardia, hypotension, bronchospasm. Abrupt withdrawal may result in diaphoresis, palpitations, headache, tremulousness, exacerbation of angina, MI, ventricular arrhythmias. May precipitate CHF, MI in pts with heart disease; thyroid storm in those with thyrotoxicosis; peripheral ischemia in those with existing peripheral vascular disease. Hypoglycemia may occur in pts with previously controlled diabetes mellitus.

NURSING CONSIDERATIONS

BASELINE ASSESSMENT

Assess baseline renal/hepatic function tests. Assess B/P, apical pulse immediately before drug administration (if pulse is 60/min or less or systolic B/P is less than 90 mm Hg, withhold medication, contact physician). **Antianginal:** Record onset, type (sharp, dull, squeezing), radiation, location, intensity, duration of anginal pain, precipitating factors (exertion, emotional stress).

INTERVENTION/EVALUATION

Assess for paradoxical reactions. Measure B/P near end of dosing interval (determines whether B/P is controlled throughout day). Monitor B/P for hypotension, respiration for shortness of breath. Assess pulse for quality, irregular rate, bradycardia. Assess for evidence of CHF: dyspnea (esp. on exertion, lying down), night cough, peripheral edema, distended neck veins. Monitor I&O (increased weight, decreased urinary output may indicate CHF). Therapeutic response to hypertension noted in 1–2 wks.

PATIENT/FAMILY TEACHING

• Do not abruptly discontinue medication. • Compliance with therapy regimen is essential to control hypertension, arrhythmias. • If dose is missed, take next scheduled dose (do not double dose). • To avoid hypotensive effect, rise slowly from lying to sitting position, wait momentarily before standing. • Report excessive fatigue, dizziness. • Avoid tasks that require alertness, motor skills until response to drug is established. • Do not use nasal decongestants, OTC cold preparations (stimulants) without physician approval. • Monitor B/P, pulse before taking medication. • Restrict salt, alcohol intake.

MetroGel-Vaginal,

see metronidazole

metronidazole

me-troe-**ni**-da-zole

(Apo-Metronidazole ♣, Flagyl, Flagyl ER, Flagyl I.V. RTU, MetroCream, MetroGel, MetroGel-Vaginal, MetroLotion, NidaGel ♣, Noritate, Vandazole)

FIXED-COMBINATION(S)

Helidac: metronidazole/bismuth/tetracycline (an anti-infective): 250 mg/262 mg/500 mg.

CLASSIFICATION

PHARMACOTHERAPEUTIC: Nitroimidazole derivative. **CLINICAL:** Antibacterial, antiprotozoal.

ACTION

Disrupts DNA, inhibiting nucleic acid synthesis. **Therapeutic Effect:** Produces bactericidal, antiprotozoal, amebicidal, trichomonacidal effects. Produces

M

anti-inflammatory, immunosuppressive effects when applied topically.

PHARMACOKINETICS

Well absorbed from GI tract; minimally absorbed after topical application. Protein binding: less than 20%. Widely distributed; crosses blood-brain barrier. Metabolized in liver to active metabolite. Primarily excreted in urine; partially eliminated in feces. Removed by hemodialysis. **Half-life:** 8 hrs (increased in alcoholic hepatic disease, in neonates).

USES

Treatment of anaerobic infections (skin/skin structure, CNS, lower respiratory tract, bone/joints, intra-abdominal, gynocologic, endocarditis, septicemia). Treatment of trichomoniasis, amebiasis, antibiotic-associated pseudomembranous colitis (AAPC). Topical treatment of acne rosacea. **OFF-LABEL:** Treatment of bacterial vaginosis, grade III-IV decubitus ulcers with anaerobic infection, *H. pylori* associated gastritis and duodenal ulcer, inflammatory bowel disease.

M

PRECAUTIONS

CONTRAINDICATIONS: Hypersensitivity to other nitroimidazole derivatives (also parabens with topical application). **CAUTIONS:** Blood dyscrasias, severe hepatic dysfunction, CNS disease, predisposition to edema, concurrent corticosteroid therapy.

LIFESPAN CONSIDERATIONS:

Pregnancy/Lactation: Readily crosses placenta. Distributed in breast milk. Contraindicated during first trimester in those with trichomoniasis. Topical use during pregnancy, lactation discouraged. **Pregnancy Category B. Children:** Safety and efficacy of topical administration in those younger than 21 yrs not established. **Elderly:** Age-related hepatic impairment may require dosage adjustment.

INTERACTIONS

DRUG: **Alcohol** may cause disulfiram-type reaction. **Disulfiram** may increase risk of toxicity. May increase effects of **oral anticoagulants.** **HERBAL:** None significant. **FOOD:** None known. **LAB VALUES:** May increase serum LDH, AST, ALT.

AVAILABILITY (Rx)

CAPSULES (FIAGYL 375): 375 mg. **INJECTION (INFUSION [FIAGYL I.V. RTU]):** 500 mg/100 ml. **TABLETS (FIAGYL):** 250 mg, 500 mg. **TOPICAL CREAM:** 0.75% (MetroCream, Rozex), 1% (Noritate). **TOPICAL GEL (METROGEL):** 0.75%, 1%. **TOPICAL LOTION (METROLOTION):** 0.75%. **VAGINAL GEL (METROGEL-VAGINAL, VANDAZOLE):** 0.75%.

TABLETS (EXTENDED-RELEASE [FLAGYL ER]): 750 mg.

ADMINISTRATION/HANDLING

IV

Rate of administration • Infuse IV over 30–60 min. Do not give by IV bolus. • Avoid prolonged use of indwelling catheters.

Storage • Store at room temperature (ready-to-use infusion bags).

PO

• Give without regard to meals. Give with food to decrease GI irritation.

IV INCOMPATIBILITIES

Amphotericin B complex (Abelcet, AmBisome, Amphotec), filgrastim (Neupogen), total parenteral nutrition (TPN).

IV COMPATIBILITIES

Diltiazem (Cardizem), dopamine (Intropin), heparin, hydromorphone (Dilaudid), lipids, lorazepam (Ativan), magnesium sulfate, midazolam (Versed), morphine.

INDICATIONS/ROUTES/DOSAGE

ANAEROBIC INFECTIONS

PO, IV: ADULTS, ELDERLY, CHILDREN: Initially, 15 mg/kg once, then 7.5 mg/kg/dose q6h. **Maximum:** 4 g/day.

AMEBIC DYSENTERY

PO: ADULTS, ELDERLY: 500–750 mg 3 times a day for 5–10 days. **CHILDREN:** 35–50 mg/kg/day in 3 divided doses for 10 days. **Maximum:** 750 mg/dose.

AMEBIC LIVER ABSCESS

PO: ADULTS, ELDERLY: 500–750 mg 3 times a day for 5–10 days. **CHILDREN:** 50 mg/kg/day in 3 divided doses. **Maximum:** 750 mg/dose.

GIARDIASIS

PO: ADULTS, ELDERLY: 250 mg 3 times a day for 5 days. **CHILDREN:** 15 mg/kg/day in 3 divided doses for 7–10 days. **Maximum:** 250 mg/dose.

PSEUDOMEMBRANOUS COLITIS

PO: ADULTS, ELDERLY: 500–750 mg 3 times a day or 250–500 mg 4 times a day. **CHILDREN:** 7.5 mg/kg q6h for 7–10 days.

TRICHOMONIASIS

PO: ADULTS, ELDERLY: 250 mg 3 times a day or 375 mg twice a day or 500 mg twice a day or 2 g as a single dose. **CHILDREN:** 15 mg/kg/day in 3 divided doses for 7 days.

BACTERIAL VAGINOSIS

PO: ADULTS: (NON-PREGNANT): 500 mg twice a day for 7 days or 750 mg (extended-release) once daily for 7 days or 2 g as a single dose. **(PREGNANT):** 250 mg 3 times a day for 7 days.

INTRAVAGINAL: ADULTS: (PREGNANT, NON-PREGNANT): 0.75% apply twice a day for 5 days.

◄ **ALERT** ► Centers for Disease Control (CDC) does not recommend the use of topical agents during pregnancy.

ROSACEA

TOPICAL: ADULTS, ELDERLY: (1%): Apply to affected area once daily. **(0.75%):** Apply to affected area twice a day.

SIDE EFFECTS

FREQUENT: Systemic: Anorexia, nausea, dry mouth, metallic taste. **Vaginal:** Symptomatic cervicitis/vaginitis, abdominal cramps, uterine pain. **OCCASIONAL: Systemic:** Diarrhea, constipation, vomiting, dizziness, erythematous rash, urticaria, reddish brown urine. **Topical:** Transient erythema, mild dryness, burning, irritation, stinging, tearing when applied too close to eyes. **Vaginal:** Vaginal, perineal, vulvar itching; vulvar swelling. **RARE:** Mild, transient leukopenia; thrombophlebitis with IV therapy.

ADVERSE EFFECTS/ TOXIC REACTIONS

Oral therapy may result in furry tongue, glossitis, cystitis, dysuria, pancreatitis, flattening of T waves on EKG. Peripheral neuropathy (manifested as numbness, tingling of hands/feet) usually is reversible if treatment is stopped immediately upon appearance of neurologic symptoms. Seizures occur occasionally.

M

NURSING CONSIDERATIONS

BASELINE ASSESSMENT

Question for history of hypersensitivity to metronidazole, other nitroimidazole derivatives (and parabens with topical). Obtain specimens for diagnostic tests, cultures before giving first dose (therapy may begin before results are known).

INTERVENTION/EVALUATION

Monitor daily pattern of bowel activity/stool consistency. Monitor I&O, assess for urinary problems. Be alert to neurologic symptoms (dizziness; paresthesia of extremities). Assess for rash, urticaria. Watch for onset of superinfection (ulceration/change of oral mucosa, furry tongue, vaginal discharge, genital/anal pruritus).

PATIENT/FAMILY TEACHING

- Urine may be red-brown or dark.
- Avoid alcohol, alcohol-containing preparations (cough syrups, elixirs).

• Avoid tasks that require alertness, motor skills until response to drug established (may cause dizziness). • If taking metronidazole for trichomoniasis, refrain from sexual intercourse until full treatment is completed. • For amebiasis, frequent stool specimen checks will be necessary. • **Topical:** Avoid contact with eyes. • May apply cosmetics after application. • Metronidazole acts on erythema, papules, pustules but has no effect on rhinophyma (hypertrophy of nose), telangiectasia, ocular problems (conjunctivitis, keratitis, blepharitis). • Other recommendations for rosacea include avoidance of hot/spicy foods, alcohol, extremes of hot/cold temperatures, excessive sunlight.

Mevacor, *see lovastatin*

M

mexiletine

(Mexitil)

See Antiarrhythmics (p. 14C)

Miacalcin, *see calcitonin*

Miacalcin Nasal, *see calcitonin*

micafungin

my-cah-**fun**-gin

(Mycamine)

CLASSIFICATION

CLINICAL: Antifungal.

ACTION

Inhibits synthesis of glucan (vital component of fungal cell formation), damaging fungal cell membrane. **Therapeutic Effect:** Decreased glucon content leads to cellular lysis.

PHARMACOKINETICS

Extensively bound to albumin. Protein binding: greater than 99%. Slowly metabolized in liver to active metabolite. Primarily excreted in feces and, to a lesser extent, in urine. Not removed by hemodialysis. **Half-life:** 11–21 hrs.

USES

Treatment of esophageal candidiasis, prophylaxis of *Candida* infection in pts undergoing hematopoietic stem cell transplant. **OFF-LABEL:** Treatment of infections due to *Aspergillus*, prophylaxis of HIV-related esophageal candidiasis.

PRECAUTIONS

CONTRAINDICATIONS: None known. **CAUTIONS:** Hepatic/renal impairment.

LIFESPAN CONSIDERATIONS:

Pregnancy/Lactation: May reduce sperm count. May be embryotoxic. Unknown if distributed in breast milk. **Pregnancy Category C. Children:** Safety and efficacy not established. **Elderly:** No age-related precautions noted.

INTERACTIONS

DRUG: May increase concentration of **nifedipine, sirolimus. HERBAL:** None significant. **FOOD:** None known. **LAB VALUES:** May increase BUN, serum creatinine, alkaline phosphatase, bilirubin, LDH, transaminase, AST, ALT. May decrease serum albumin, calcium, magnesium, phosphorus, potassium, Hgb, Hct, WBC, platelet count.

AVAILABILITY (Rx)

INJECTION POWDER FOR RECONSTITUTION: 50 mg vials (Mycamine).

ADMINISTRATION/HANDLING

IV

Reconstitution • Add 5 ml 0.9% NaCl (without bacteriostatic agent) to each 50 mg vial to yield micafungin 10 mg/ml. • Gently swirl to dissolve; do not shake. • Further dilute 50–150 mg micafungin to 100 ml 0.9% NaCl and infuse as piggyback. • Alternatively, D_5W may be used for reconstitution and dilution. • Flush existing IV line with 0.9% NaCl or D_5W before infusion.

Rate of administration • Infuse over 60 min.

Storage • Reconstituted solution is stable for 24 hrs at room temperature. • Discard if precipitate is present.

IV INCOMPATIBILITIES

Do not mix with any other medication.

INDICATIONS/ROUTES/DOSAGE

ESOPHAGEAL CANDIDIASIS

IV: ADULTS, ELDERLY: Give 150 mg a day as a single dose.

CANDIDA PROPHYLAXIS IN STEM CELL PTS

IV: ADULTS, ELDERLY: Give 50 mg a day as a single dose.

SIDE EFFECTS

OCCASIONAL (3%–2%): Nausea, headache, diarrhea, vomiting, pyrexia. **RARE (1%):** Dizziness, drowsiness, pruritus, abdominal pain, dyspepsia (heartburn, indigestion, epigastric pain).

ADVERSE EFFECTS/ TOXIC REACTIONS

Hypersensitivity reaction characterized by rash, pruritus, facial edema occurs rarely. Anaphylaxis, hemoglobinuria, hemolytic anemia have been reported.

NURSING CONSIDERATIONS

BASELINE ASSESSMENT

Determine baseline hepatic/renal function tests and periodically thereafter.

INTERVENTION/EVALUATION

Monitor serum chemistry results for evidence of hepatic/renal impairment.

Micardis, *see telmisartan*

miconazole

mih-**kon**-nah-zoll

(Micatin, Micozole ✦, Mitrazol, Monistat ✦, Monistat 3, Monistat 7, Monistat-Derm, Vusion)

Do not confuse miconazole with Micronase, or Mitrazol with Micronor.

CLASSIFICATION

PHARMACOTHERAPEUTIC: Imidazole derivative. **CLINICAL:** Antifungal (see p. 46C).

ACTION

Inhibits synthesis of ergosterol (vital component of fungal cell formation), damaging fungal cell membrane. **Therapeutic Effect:** Fungistatic; may be fungicidal, depending on concentration.

PHARMACOKINETICS

Small amounts absorbed systemically after vaginal administration. Protein binding: 91%–93%. Primarily excreted in feces. **Half-life:** 24 hrs.

USES

Vaginal: Vulvovaginal candidiasis. **Topical:** Cutaneous candidiasis, tinea cruris, t. corporis, t. pedis, t. versicolor. **Vusion:** Treatment of diaper rash.

PRECAUTIONS

CONTRAINDICATIONS: Avoid vaginal preparations during first trimester of pregnancy. **CAUTIONS:** Sensitivity to other antifungals (clotrimazole, ketoconazole).

LIFESPAN CONSIDERATIONS:

Pregnancy/Lactation: Unknown if drug crosses placenta or is distributed in breast milk. **Pregnancy Category C. Children:** Safety in those younger than 1 yr not established. **Elderly:** No age-related precautions noted.

INTERACTIONS

DRUG: None significant. **HERBAL:** None significant. **FOOD:** None known. **LAB VALUES:** None known.

AVAILABILITY (Rx)

CREAM (TOPICAL): Micatin, Monistat-Derm: 2%; **Vusion:** 0.25%. **CREAM (VAGINAL): Monistat-7:** 2%; **Monistat-3:** 4%; **TOPICAL POWDER: Mitrazol:** 2%; **VAGINAL SUPPOSITORY: Monistat-7:**100 mg; **Monistat-3:** 200 mg, 1,200 mg.

M

INDICATIONS/ROUTES/DOSAGE

VULVOVAGINAL CANDIDIASIS

INTRAVAGINAL SUPPOSITORY: ADULTS, ELDERLY: 100 mg suppository at bedtime for 7 days, or 200 mg suppository at bedtime for 3 days, or 1,200 mg suppository once at bedtime or during the day.

INTRAVAGINAL CREAM: ADULTS, ELDERLY: 2% cream: 1 applicatorful at bedtime for 7 days. 4% cream: 1 applicatorful at bedtime for 3 days.

TOPICAL FUNGAL INFECTIONS, CUTANEOUS CANDIDIASIS

TOPICAL: ADULTS, ELDERLY: Apply liberally twice per day, morning and evening.

DIAPER RASH

TOPICAL: INFANTS: As needed.

SIDE EFFECTS

Topical: Pruritus, burning, stinging, erythema, urticaria. **Vaginal (2%):** Vulvovaginal burning, pruritus, irritation; headache; skin rash.

ADVERSE EFFECTS/ TOXIC REACTIONS

None known.

NURSING CONSIDERATIONS

BASELINE ASSESSMENT

Topical: Avoid occlusive dressings. Apply only small amount to cover area completely. **Spray:** Shake well before using.

INTERVENTION/EVALUATION

Topical/Vaginal: Assess for burning, pruritus, irritation.

PATIENT/FAMILY TEACHING

• **Vaginal Preparation:** Base interacts with certain latex products such as contraceptive diaphragm. • Ask physician about douching, sexual intercourse. • **Topical:** Rub well into affected areas. • Avoid getting in eyes. • Keep areas clean, dry; wear light clothing for ventilation. • Separate personal items in contact with affected areas.

midazolam

my-**dah**-zoe-lam

(Apo-Midazolam ✱, Versed)

Do not confuse Versed with VePesid.

CLASSIFICATION

PHARMACOTHERAPEUTIC: Benzodiazepine (**Schedule IV**). **CLINICAL:** Sedative (see p. 3C).

ACTION

Enhances action of gamma-aminobutyric acid (GABA), one of the major inhibitory neurotransmitters in the brain. **Therapeutic Effect:** Produces anxiolytic, hypnotic, anticonvulsant, muscle relaxant, amnestic effects.

PHARMACOKINETICS

Route	Onset	Peak	Duration
PO	10–20 min	N/A	N/A
IV	1–5 min	5–7 min	20–30 min
IM	5–15 min	15–60 min	2–6 hrs

Well absorbed after IM administration. Protein binding: 97%. Metabolized in liver to active metabolite. Primarily excreted in urine. Not removed by hemodialysis. **Half-life:** 1–5 hrs.

USES

Sedation, anxiolytic, amnesia before procedure or induction of anesthesia, conscious sedation before diagnostic/radiographic procedure, continuous IV sedation of intubated or mechanically ventilated pts. **OFF-LABEL:** Anxiety, status epilepticus.

PRECAUTIONS

CONTRAINDICATIONS: Acute alcohol intoxication, acute narrow-angle glaucoma, allergies to cherries, coma, shock. **CAUTIONS:** Acute illness, severe fluid electrolyte imbalance, renal/hepatic/pulmonary impairment, CHF, treated open-angle glaucoma.

LIFESPAN CONSIDERATIONS:

Pregnancy/Lactation: Crosses placenta. Unknown if drug is distributed in breast milk. **Pregnancy Category D.** **Children:** Neonates more likely to have respiratory depression. **Elderly:** Age-related renal impairment may require dosage adjustment.

INTERACTIONS

DRUG: Alcohol, other CNS depressants may increase CNS effects, respiratory depression, hypotensive effects. **Hypotensive medications, antihypertensives** may increase hypotensive effects. **HERBAL: Kava kava, gotu kola, St. John's wort, valerian** may increase CNS depression. **FOOD: Grapefruit, grapefruit juice** increases oral absorption, systemic availability. **LAB VALUES:** None known.

AVAILABILITY (Rx)

INJECTION SOLUTION: 1 mg/ml, 5 mg/ml. **INJECTION SOLUTION (PRESERVATIVE-FREE):** 1 mg/ml, 5 mg/ml. **SYRUP:** 2 mg/ml.

ADMINISTRATION/HANDLING

IV

Rate of administration • May give undiluted or as infusion. • Resuscitative equipment, O_2 must be readily available before IV administration. • Administer by slow IV injection, in incremental dosages. Give each incremental dose over 2 min or longer at intervals of at least 2 min. • Reduce IV rate in those older than 60 yrs, debilitated pts with chronic disease states, pulmonary impairment. • Too-rapid IV rate, excessive doses, or single large dose increases risk of respiratory depression/arrest.

Storage • Store vials at room temperature.

IM

• Give deep IM into large muscle mass.

IV INCOMPATIBILITIES

Albumin, ampicillin and sulbactam (Unasyn), amphotericin B complex (Abelcet, AmBisome, Amphotec), ampicillin (Polycillin), bumetanide (Bumex), co-trimoxazole (Bactrim), dexamethasone (Decadron), fosphenytoin (Cerebyx), furosemide (Lasix), hydrocortisone (Solu-Cortef), lipids, methotrexate, nafcillin (Nafcil), sodium bicarbonate, sodium pentothal (Thiopental).

IV COMPATIBILITIES

Amiodarone (Cordarone), atropine, calcium gluconate, diltiazem (Cardizem), diphenhydramine (Benadryl), dobutamine (Dobutrex), dopamine (Intropin),

M

etomidate (Amidate), fentanyl (Sublimaze), glycopyrrolate (Robinul), heparin, hydromorphone (Dilaudid), hydroxyzine (Vistaril), insulin, lorazepam (Ativan), milrinone (Primacor), morphine, nitroglycerin, norepinephrine (Levophed), potassium chloride, propofol (Diprivan).

INDICATIONS/ROUTES/DOSAGE

PREOPERATIVE SEDATION

PO: CHILDREN: 0.25–0.5 mg/kg. **Maximum:** 20 mg.

IV: ADULTS, ELDERLY: 0.02–0.04 mg/kg. **CHILDREN 6–12 YRS:** 0.025–0.05 mg/kg. **CHILDREN 6 MOS–5 YRS:** 0.05–0.1 mg/kg.

IM: ADULTS, ELDERLY: 0.07–0.08 mg/kg 30–60 min before surgery. **CHILDREN:** 0.1–0.15 mg/kg 30–60 min before surgery. **Maximum:** 10 mg.

CONSCIOUS SEDATION FOR DIAGNOSTIC, THERAPEUTIC, ENDOSCOPIC PROCEDURES

IV: ADULTS, ELDERLY: 1–2.5 mg over 2 min. Titrate as needed. **Maximum total dose:** 2.5–5 mg. **CHILDREN 6–12 YRS:** 0.025–0.05 mg/kg. Total dose of 0.4 mg/kg may be necessary. **Maximum total dose:** 10 mg. **CHILDREN 6 MOS–5 YRS:** 0.05–0.1 mg/kg. Total dose of 0.6 mg/kg may be necessary. **Maximum total dose:** 6 mg.

CONTINUOUS SEDATION DURING MECHANICAL VENTILATION

IV: ADULTS, ELDERLY: Initially, 0.02–0.08 mg/kg. May repeat at 5- to 15-min intervals or continuous infusion rate of 0.04–0.2 mg/kg/hr and titrated to desired effect. **CHILDREN:** Initially, 0.05–0.2 mg/kg followed by a continuous infusion of 0.06–0.12 mg/kg/hr (1–2 mcg/kg/min) titrated to desired effect.

STATUS EPILEPTICUS

IV: CHILDREN OLDER THAN 2 MOS: Loading dose of 0.15 mg/kg followed by continuous infusion of 1 mcg/kg/min. Titrate as needed. Range: 1–18 mcg/kg/min.

SIDE EFFECTS

FREQUENT (10%–4%): Decreased respiratory rate, tenderness at IM or IV injection site, pain during injection, oxygen desaturation, hiccups. **OCCASIONAL (3%–2%):** Hypotension, paradoxical CNS reaction. **RARE (less than 2%):** Nausea, vomiting, headache, coughing.

ADVERSE EFFECTS/ TOXIC REACTIONS

Inadequate or excessive dosage, improper administration may result in cerebral hypoxia, agitation, involuntary movements, hyperactivity, combativeness. Too-rapid IV rate, excessive doses, or single large dose increases risk of respiratory depression/arrest. Respiratory depression/apnea may produce hypoxia, cardiac arrest.

NURSING CONSIDERATIONS

BASELINE ASSESSMENT

Resuscitative equipment, oxygen must be available. Obtain vital signs before administration.

INTERVENTION/EVALUATION

Monitor respiratory rate, oxygen saturation continuously during parenteral administration for underventilation, apnea. Monitor vital signs, level of sedation q3–5min during recovery period.

midodrine

my-doe-dreen

(Amatine ✤, Orvalen, ProAmatine)

Do not confuse Amatine or ProAmatine with amantadine or protamine.

CLASSIFICATION

PHARMACOTHERAPEUTIC: Vasopressor. **CLINICAL:** Orthostatic hypotension adjunct.

ACTION

Forms active metabolite desglymidodrine, an alpha$_1$-agonist, activating alpha receptors of arteriolar, venous vasculature. **Therapeutic Effect:** Increases vascular tone, B/P.

PHARMACOKINETICS

Rapid absorption from GI tract following PO administration. Protein binding: Low. Undergoes enzymatic hydrolysis (deglycination) in systemic circulation. Excreted in urine. **Half-life:** 0.5 hr.

USES

Treatment of symptomatic orthostatic hypotension. **OFF-LABEL:** Infection-related hypotension, intradialytic hypotension, psychotropic agent-induced hypotension, urinary incontinence.

PRECAUTIONS

CONTRAINDICATIONS: Acute renal impairment, persistent hypertension, pheochromocytoma, severe cardiac disease, thyrotoxicosis, urine retention. **CAUTIONS:** Renal/hepatic impairment, history of visual problems.

LIFESPAN CONSIDERATIONS:

Pregnancy/Lactation: Unknown if drug crosses placenta or is distributed is breast milk. **Pregnancy Category C. Children:** Safety and efficacy not established. **Elderly:** Age-related renal impairment may require dosage adjustment.

INTERACTIONS

DRUG: **Digoxin** may have additive bradycardic effects. **Sodium-retaining steroids (e.g., fludrocortisone)** may increase sodium retention. **Vasoconstrictors** may have additive effects. **HERBAL:** None significant. **FOOD:** None known. **LAB VALUES:** None known.

AVAILABILITY (Rx)

TABLETS: 2.5 mg, 5 mg, 10 mg.

ADMINISTRATION/HANDLING

• Give without regard to food. • Last dose of day should be given 3–4 hrs before bedtime.

INDICATIONS/ROUTES/DOSAGE

ORTHOSTATIC HYPOTENSION

PO: ADULTS, ELDERLY: 10 mg 3 times a day. Give during the day when pt is upright, such as upon arising, midday, and late afternoon. Do not give later than 6 PM. **Maximum:** 40 mg/day.

DOSAGE IN RENAL IMPAIRMENT

For adults and elderly pts, give 2.5 mg 3 times a day; increase gradually, as tolerated.

SIDE EFFECTS

FREQUENT (20%–7%): Paresthesia, piloerection, pruritus, dysuria, supine hypertension. **OCCASIONAL (less than 7%–1%):** Pain, rash, chills, headache, facial flushing, confusion, dry mouth, anxiety.

ADVERSE EFFECTS/ TOXIC REACTIONS

Increased systolic arterial pressure has been noted.

NURSING CONSIDERATIONS

BASELINE ASSESSMENT

Assess sensitivity to midodrine, other medications (esp. digoxin, sodium-retaining vasoconstrictors). Assess medical history, esp. renal impairment, severe hypertension, cardiac disease.

INTERVENTION/EVALUATION

Monitor B/P, renal, hepatic, cardiac function.

PATIENT/FAMILY TEACHING

• Do not take last dose of the day after evening meal or less than 4 hrs before bedtime. • Do not give if pt will be supine. • Use caution with OTC medications that may affect B/P (e.g., cough and cold, diet medications).

M

mifepristone

miff-eh-**pris**-tone
(Mifeprex)

Do not confuse Mifeprex with Mirapex or mifepristone with misoprostol.

CLASSIFICATION

CLINICAL: Abortifacient.

ACTION

Has antiprogestational activity resulting from competitive interaction with progesterone. Inhibits activity of endogenous, exogenous progesterone. Has antiglucocorticoid, weak antiandrogenic activity. **Therapeutic Effect:** Terminates pregnancy.

PHARMACOKINETICS

Protein binding: 98%. Metabolized in liver. Primarily eliminated in feces; minimal excretion in urine. **Half-life:** 20–54 hrs.

USES

Termination of intrauterine pregnancy. **OFF-LABEL:** Breast/ovarian cancer, Cushing's syndrome, endometriosis, intrauterine fetal death, nonviable early pregnancy, postcoital contraception/contragestation, unresectable meningioma.

PRECAUTIONS

CONTRAINDICATIONS: Chronic adrenal failure, concurrent long-term steroid or anticoagulant therapy, confirmed or suspected ectopic pregnancy, intrauterine device (IUD) in place, hemorrhagic disorders, concurrent anticoagulant therapy, inherited porphyria, hypersensitivity to misoprostol, other prostaglandins. **CAUTIONS:** Treatment of women older than 35 yrs, smoke more than 10 cigarettes/day, cardiovascular disease, hypertension, hepatic/renal impairment, diabetes, severe anemia. **Pregnancy Category X.**

INTERACTIONS

DRUG: Anticoagulants may increase risk of bleeding. **Carbamazepine, phenobarbital, phenytoin, rifampin** may increase metabolism. **Erythromycin, itraconazole, ketoconazole** may inhibit metabolism. **HERBAL: St. John's wort** may increase metabolism. **FOOD: Grapefruit, grapefruit juice** may inhibit metabolism. **LAB VALUES:** May decrease Hgb, Hct, RBC count.

AVAILABILITY (Rx)

TABLETS: 200 mg.

INDICATIONS/ROUTES/DOSAGE

TERMINATION OF PREGNANCY

PO: ADULTS: Day 1: 600 mg as single dose. **Day 3:** 400 mcg misoprostol. **Day 14:** Post-treatment examination.

SIDE EFFECTS

FREQUENT (greater than 10%): Headache, dizziness, abdominal pain, nausea, vomiting, diarrhea, fatigue. **OCCASIONAL (10%–3%):** Uterine hemorrhage, insomnia, vaginitis, dyspepsia (heartburn, indigestion, epigastric pain), back pain, fever, viral infections, rigors. **RARE (2%–1%):** Anxiety, syncope, anemia, asthenia (loss of strength, energy), leg pain, sinusitis, leukorrhea.

ADVERSE EFFECTS/ TOXIC REACTIONS

None known.

NURSING CONSIDERATIONS

BASELINE ASSESSMENT

Assess for use of ketoconazole, itraconazole, erythromycin, rifampin, anticonvulsants (affects metabolism).

INTERVENTION/EVALUATION

◄ **ALERT** ► If mifepristone results in an incomplete abortion, surgical intervention may be necessary.

Monitor Hgb/Hct. Confirm pregnancy is completely terminated at approximately 14 days after drug administration. Assess degree of vaginal bleeding.

PATIENT/FAMILY TEACHING

• Advise pts of treatment procedure and effects, need for follow-up visit. • Vaginal bleeding, uterine cramping may occur.

milrinone

mill-re-none

(Primacor, Primacor I.V.)

CLASSIFICATION

PHARMACOTHERAPEUTIC: Cardiac inotropic agent. **CLINICAL:** Vasodilator (see p. 74C).

ACTION

Inhibits phosphodiesterase, which increases cyclic adenosine monophosphate (cAMP), potentiating delivery of calcium to myocardial contractile systems. **Therapeutic Effect:** Relaxes vascular muscle, causing vasodilation. Increases cardiac output; decreases pulmonary capillary wedge pressure, vascular resistance.

PHARMACOKINETICS

Route	Onset	Peak	Duration
IV	5–15 min	N/A	N/A

Protein binding: 70%. Primarily excreted unchanged in urine. **Half-life:** 2.4 hrs.

USES

Short-term management of congestive heart failure (CHF).

PRECAUTIONS

CONTRAINDICATIONS: None known. **CAUTIONS:** Severe obstructive aortic or pulmonic valvular disease, history of ventricular arrhythmias, atrial fibrillation/flutter, renal impairment.

LIFESPAN CONSIDERATIONS:

Pregnancy/Lactation: Unknown if drug crosses placenta or is distributed in breast milk. **Pregnancy Category C.** **Children:** Safety and efficacy not established. **Elderly:** Age-related renal impairment may require dosage adjustment.

INTERACTIONS

DRUG: Other cardiac glycosides produce additive inotropic effects. **HERBAL:** None significant. **FOOD:** None known. **LAB VALUES:** None known.

AVAILABILITY (Rx)

INJECTION SOLUTION (PRIMACOR, PRIMACOR I.V.): 1 mg/ml, 10-ml single-dose vial, 20-ml single-dose vial, 50-ml single-dose vial, 5-ml sterile cartridge unit. **INJECTION SOLUTION (PREMIX [PRIMACOR]):** 200 mcg/ml.

ADMINISTRATION/HANDLING

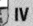

IV

Reconstitution • For IV infusion, dilute 20-mg (20-ml) vial with 80 or 180 ml diluent (0.9% NaCl, D_5W) to provide concentration of 200 or 100 mcg/ml, respectively. Maximum concentration: 100 mg/250 ml.

Rate of administration • For IV injection (loading dose), administer undiluted slowly over 10 min. • Monitor for arrhythmias, hypotension during IV therapy; reduce or temporarily discontinue infusion until condition stabilizes.

Storage • Store at room temperature.

IV INCOMPATIBILITY

Furosemide (Lasix).

IV COMPATIBILITIES

Calcium gluconate, digoxin (Lanoxin), diltiazem (Cardizem), dobutamine (Dobutrex), dopamine (Intropin), heparin, lidocaine, magnesium, midazolam (Versed), nitroglycerin, potassium, propofol (Diprivan).

INDICATIONS/ROUTES/DOSAGE

MANAGEMENT OF CHF

IV: ADULTS: Initially, 50 mcg/kg over 10 min. Continue with maintenance infusion rate of 0.375–0.75 mcg/kg/min based on hemodynamic and clinical response. Total daily dosage: 0.59–1.13 mg/kg.

DOSAGE IN RENAL IMPAIRMENT

For pts with severe renal impairment, reduce dosage to 0.2–0.43 mcg/kg/min.

SIDE EFFECTS

OCCASIONAL (3%–1%): Headache, hypotension. **RARE (less than 1%):** Angina, chest pain.

ADVERSE EFFECTS/ TOXIC REACTIONS

Supraventricular/ventricular arrhythmias (12%), nonsustained ventricular tachycardia (2%), sustained ventricular tachycardia (1%) may occur.

NURSING CONSIDERATIONS

BASELINE ASSESSMENT

Offer emotional support (difficulty breathing may produce anxiety). Assess B/P, apical pulse rate before treatment begins and during IV therapy. Assess lung sounds; observe for edema.

INTERVENTION/EVALUATION

Monitor B/P, heart rate, cardiac output, EKG, serum potassium, renal function, signs/symptoms of CHF.

minocycline

mi-noe-**sye**-kleen

(Arestin, Dynacin, Minocin, Myrac, Novo Minocycline ✦, Solodyn, Vectrin)

Do not confuse Dynacin with Dynabac or Minocin with Mithracin or niacin.

CLASSIFICATION

PHARMACOTHERAPEUTIC: Tetracycline. **CLINICAL:** Antibiotic.

ACTION

Inhibits bacterial protein synthesis by binding to ribosomes. **Therapeutic Effect:** Bacteriostatic.

PHARMACOKINETICS

Protein binding: 76%. Partial elimination in feces; minimal excretion in urine. Not removed by hemodialysis. **Half-life:** 11–12 hrs (oral capsule).

USES

Treatment of susceptible infections due to *Rickettsiae, M. pneumoniae, C. trachomatis, C. psittaci, H. ducreyi, Yersinia pestis, Francisella tularensis, Bivrio cholerae,* Brucella species, gram-negative organisms. Treatment of prostate, urinary tract, CNS infections (not meningitis), uncomplicated gonorrhea, inflammatory acne, brucellosis, skin granulomas, cholera, trachoma, nocardiasis, yaws, syphilis (when penicillins are contraindicated). **Solodyn:** Treatment of inflammatory lesions of non-nodular moderate to severe acne. **OFF-LABEL:** Treatment of atypical mycobacterial infection, rheumatoid arthritis, scleroderma.

PRECAUTIONS

CONTRAINDICATIONS: Children younger than 8 yrs, hypersensitivity to tetracyclines, last half of pregnancy. **CAUTIONS:** Renal impairment, sun/ultraviolet exposure (severe photosensitivity reaction).

⧗ LIFESPAN CONSIDERATIONS:

Pregnancy/Lactation: Readily crosses placenta; distributed in breast milk. May inhibit fetal skeletal growth.

Pregnancy Category D. Children: May cause permanent discoloration of teeth, enamel hypoplasia. Not recommended in children younger than 8 yrs. **Elderly:** No age-related precautions noted.

INTERACTIONS

DRUG: Antacids may decrease absorption, effect. **Carbamazepine, phenytoin** may decrease concentration. **Cholestyramine, colestipol** may decrease absorption. **Ergot** may increase risk of ergotism. May decrease the effects of **oral contraceptives. HERBAL: St. John's wort** may increase risk of photosensitivity. **FOOD:** None known. **LAB VALUES:** May increase serum alkaline phosphatase, amylase, bilirubin, AST, ALT.

AVAILABILITY (Rx)

CAPSULES (DYNACIN, MINOCIN, VECTRIN): 50 mg, 75 mg, 100 mg. **CAPSULES (PELLET-FILLED [MINOCIN]):** 50 mg, 100 mg. **TABLETS (MINOCIN, MYRAC):** 50 mg, 75 mg, 100 mg.

TABLETS, (EXTENDED RELEASE [SOLODYN]): 45 mg, 90 mg, 135 mg.

ADMINISTRATION/HANDLING

PO

• Store at room temperature. • Give capsules, tablets with full glass of water.

INDICATIONS/ROUTES/DOSAGE

USUAL DOSAGE

PO: ADULTS, ELDERLY: Initially, 100–200 mg, then 100 mg q12h or 50 mg q6h. **Maximum:** 400 mg/day. **CHILDREN OLDER THAN 8 YRS:** Initially, 4 mg/kg, then 2 mg/kg q12h.

ACNE

PO: CHILDREN 12 YRS AND OLDER: 1 mg/kg once daily for 12 wks.

SIDE EFFECTS

FREQUENT: Dizziness, light-headedness, diarrhea, nausea, vomiting, abdominal cramps, possibly severe photosensitivity, drowsiness, vertigo. **OCCASIONAL:** Altered pigmentation of skin, mucous membranes; rectal/genital pruritus, stomatitis.

ADVERSE EFFECTS/ TOXIC REACTIONS

Superinfection (esp. fungal), anaphylaxis, increased intracranial pressure (ICP) may occur. Bulging fontanelles occur rarely in infants.

NURSING CONSIDERATIONS

BASELINE ASSESSMENT

Question for history of allergies, esp. tetracyclines, sulfite.

INTERVENTION/EVALUATION

Assess ability to ambulate (may cause vertigo, dizziness). Monitor daily pattern of bowel activity/stool consistency. Assess skin for rash. Observe for signs of increased intracranial pressure (altered level of consciousness, widened pulse pressure). Be alert for superinfection (diarrhea, stomatitis, anal/genital pruritus).

PATIENT/FAMILY TEACHING

• Continue antibiotic for full length of treatment. • Space doses evenly. • Drink full glass of water with capsules or tablets, avoid bedtime doses. • Avoid tasks that require alertness, motor skills until response to drug is established. • Notify physician if diarrhea, rash, other new symptom occurs. • Protect skin from sun exposure.

minoxidil

min-**ox**-i-dill

(Apo-Gain ✤, Loniten, Milnox ✤, Rogaine, Rogaine Extra Strength)

Do not confuse Loniten with Lotensin.

CLASSIFICATION

CLINICAL: Antihypertensive, hair growth stimulant (see p. 59C).

ACTION

Acts directly on vascular smooth muscle, producing vasodilation of arterioles. **Therapeutic Effect:** Decreases peripheral vascular resistance, B/P; increases cutaneous blood flow; stimulates hair follicle epithelium, hair follicle growth.

PHARMACOKINETICS

Route	Onset	Peak	Duration
PO	0.5 hr	2–8 hrs	2–5 days

Well absorbed from GI tract; minimal absorption after topical application. Protein binding: None. Widely distributed. Metabolized in liver to active metabolite. Primarily excreted in urine. Removed by hemodialysis. **Half-life:** 4.2 hrs.

M

USES

Treatment of severe symptomatic hypertension, hypertension associated with organ damage. Used for pts who fail to respond to maximal therapeutic dosages of diuretic and two other antihypertensive agents. Treatment of alopecia androgenetica (**males:** baldness of vertex of scalp; **females:** diffuse hair loss or thinning of frontoparietal areas).

PRECAUTIONS

CONTRAINDICATIONS: Pheochromocytoma. **CAUTIONS:** Severe renal impairment, chronic CHF, coronary artery disease, recent MI (1 mo).

LIFESPAN CONSIDERATIONS:

Pregnancy/Lactation: Crosses placenta. Distributed in breast milk. **Pregnancy Category C. Children:** No age-related precautions noted. **Elderly:** More sensitive to hypotensive effects. Age-related renal impairment may require dosage adjustment.

INTERACTIONS

DRUG: NSAIDs may decrease hypotensive effects. **Parenteral antihypertensives, nitrates** may increase hypotensive effect. **HERBAL: Licorice** may cause increased serum sodium, water retention. **FOOD:** None known. **LAB VALUES:** May increase plasma renin activity, BUN, alkaline phosphatase, creatinine, sodium. May decrease Hgb, Hct, erythrocyte count.

AVAILABILITY

TABLETS (LONITEN): 2.5 mg, 10 mg. **TOPICAL SOLUTION (OTC):** 2% (20 mg/ml) (Rogaine), 5% (50 mg/ml) (Rogaine ExtraStrength).

ADMINISTRATION/HANDLING

PO

• Give without regard to food. Give with food if GI upset occurs. • Tablets may be crushed.

TOPICAL

• Shampoo, dry hair before applying medication. • Wash hands immediately after application. • Do not use hair dryer after application (reduces effectiveness).

INDICATIONS/ROUTES/DOSAGE

HYPERTENSION

PO: ADULTS, CHILDREN 12 YRS AND OLDER: Initially, 5 mg/day. Increase in at least 3-day intervals to 10 mg, then 20 mg, then up to 40 mg/day in 1–2 doses. **ELDERLY:** Initially, 2.5 mg/day. May increase gradually. Maintenance: 10–40 mg/day. Maximum: 100 mg/day. **CHILDREN YOUNGER THAN 12 YRS:** Initially, 0.1–0.2 mg/kg (5 mg maximum) daily. Gradually increase at a minimum of 3-day intervals. Maintenance: 0.25–1 mg/kg/day in 1–2 doses. **Maximum:** 50 mg/day.

HAIR REGROWTH

TOPICAL: ADULTS: 1 ml to affected areas of scalp 2 times per day. Total daily dose not to exceed 2 ml.

SIDE EFFECTS

FREQUENT: PO: Edema with concurrent weight gain, hypertrichosis (elongation, thickening, increased pigmentation of fine body hair; develops in 80% of pts within 3–6 wks after beginning therapy). **OCCASIONAL: PO:** EKG T-wave changes (usually revert to pretreatment state with continued therapy or drug withdrawal). **Topical:** Pruritus, rash, dry/flaking skin, erythema. **RARE: PO:** Breast tenderness, headache, photosensitivity reaction. **Topical:** Allergic reaction, alopecia, burning sensation at scalp, soreness at hair root, headache, visual disturbances.

ADVERSE EFFECTS/ TOXIC REACTIONS

Tachycardia, angina pectoris may occur due to increased oxygen demands associated with increased heart rate, cardiac output. Fluid/electrolyte imbalance, CHF may occur, esp. if a diuretic is not given concurrently. Too-rapid reduction in B/P may result in syncope, cerebrovascular accident (CVA), MI, ocular/vestibular ischemia. Pericardial effusion, tamponade may be seen in pts with renal impairment not on dialysis.

NURSING CONSIDERATIONS

BASELINE ASSESSMENT

Assess B/P in both arms and take pulse for 1 full min immediately before giving medication. If pulse increases 20 beats or more/min over baseline or systolic or diastolic B/P decreases more than 20 mm Hg, withhold drug, contact physician.

INTERVENTION/EVALUATION

Monitor fluids/electrolytes, body weight, B/P. Assess for peripheral edema. Assess for signs of CHF (cough, rales at base of lungs, cool extremities, dyspnea on exertion). Monitor fluid, serum electrolytes. Assess for distant or muffled heart sounds by auscultation (pericardial effusion, tamponade).

PATIENT/FAMILY TEACHING

• Maximum B/P response occurs in 3–7 days. • Reversible growth of fine body hair may begin 3–6 wks following initiation of treatment. • When used topically for stimulation of hair growth, treatment must continue on a permanent basis—cessation of treatment will begin reversal of new hair growth. • Avoid exposure to sunlight, artificial light sources.

mirtazapine

mir-**taz**-a-peen

(Novo-Mirtazapine ✱, Remeron, Remeron Soltab)

Do not confuse Remeron with Premarin.

◆CLASSIFICATION

PHARMACOTHERAPEUTIC: Tetracyclic compound. **CLINICAL:** Antidepressant (see p. 38C).

ACTION

Acts as antagonist at presynaptic $alpha_2$-adrenergic receptors, increasing norepinephrine, serotonin neurotransmission. Has low anticholinergic activity. **Therapeutic Effect:** Relieves depression, produces sedative effects.

PHARMACOKINETICS

Rapidly, completely absorbed after PO administration; absorption not affected by food. Protein binding: 85%. Metabolized in liver. Primarily excreted in urine. Unknown if removed by hemodialysis. **Half-life:** 20–40 hrs (longer in males [37 hrs] than females [26 hrs]).

M

USES

Treatment of depression.

PRECAUTIONS

CONTRAINDICATIONS: Use of MAOIs within 14 days. **CAUTIONS:** Cardiovascular/GI disorders, prostatic hyperplasia, urinary retention, narrow-angle glaucoma, renal/hepatic impairment.

LIFESPAN CONSIDERATIONS:

Pregnancy/Lactation: Unknown if distributed in breast milk. **Pregnancy Category C. Children:** Safety and efficacy not established. **Elderly:** Age-related renal impairment may require dosage adjustment.

INTERACTIONS

DRUG: Alcohol, CNS depressant medications may increase impairment of cognition, motor skills. **MAOIs** may increase risk of neuroleptic malignant syndrome, hypertensive crisis, severe seizures. **HERBAL: Gotu kola, kava kava, St. John's wort, valerian** may increase CNS depression. **FOOD:** None known. **LAB VALUES:** May increase serum cholesterol, triglycerides, AST, ALT.

AVAILABILITY (Rx)

TABLETS (REMERON): 15 mg, 30 mg, 45 mg. **TABLETS (ORALLY-DISINTEGRATING [REMERON SOLTAB]):** 15 mg, 30 mg, 45 mg.

ADMINISTRATION/HANDLING

PO

• Give without regard to food. • May crush/break scored tablets.

ORALLY-DISINTEGRATING TABLETS

• Do not split tablet. • Place on tongue; dissolves without water.

INDICATIONS/ROUTES/DOSAGE

DEPRESSION

PO: ADULTS: Initially, 15 mg at bedtime. May increase by 15 mg/day q1–2wk. **Maximum:** 45 mg/day. **ELDERLY:** Initially, 7.5 mg at bedtime. May increase by 7.5–15 mg/day q1–2wk. **Maximum:** 45 mg/day.

SIDE EFFECTS

FREQUENT: Drowsiness (54%), dry mouth (25%), increased appetite (17%), constipation (13%), weight gain (12%). **OCCASIONAL:** Asthenia (8%), dizziness (7%), flu-like symptoms (5%), abnormal dreams (4%). **RARE:** Abdominal discomfort, vasodilation, paresthesia, acne, dry skin, thirst, arthralgia.

ADVERSE EFFECTS/ TOXIC REACTIONS

Higher incidence of seizures than with tricyclic antidepressants, (esp. in those with no history of seizures). Overdose may produce cardiovascular effects (severe orthostatic hypotension, dizziness, tachycardia, palpitations, arrhythmias). Abrupt discontinuation from prolonged therapy may produce headache, malaise, nausea, vomiting, vivid dreams. Agranulocytosis occurs rarely.

NURSING CONSIDERATIONS

BASELINE ASSESSMENT

For pts on long-term therapy, hepatic/renal function tests, blood counts should be performed periodically.

INTERVENTION/EVALUATION

Supervise suicidal-risk pt closely during early therapy (as depression lessens, energy level improves, increasing suicide potential). Children, adolescents are at increased risk for suicidal thoughts/behavior and worsening of depression, esp. during first few mos of therapy. Assess appearance, behavior, speech pattern, level of interest, mood. Monitor for hypotension, arrhythmias.

PATIENT/FAMILY TEACHING

• Take as single bedtime dose.
• Avoid alcohol, depressant/sedating

medications. • Avoid tasks requiring mental alertness, motor skills until response to drug established.

misoprostol

mis-oh-**pros**-toll

(Apo-Misoprostol ✤, Cytotec, Novo-Misoprostol ✤)

Do not confuse misoprostol with mifepristone, or Cytotec with Cytoxan.

FIXED-COMBINATION(S)

Arthrotec: misoprostol/diclofenac (an NSAID): 200 mcg/50 mg; 200 mcg/75 mg.

CLASSIFICATION

PHARMACOTHERAPEUTIC: Prostaglandin. **CLINICAL:** Antisecretory, gastric protectant.

ACTION

Replaces protective prostaglandins consumed with prostaglandin-inhibiting therapies (e.g., NSAIDs). **Therapeutic Effect:** Reduces acid secretion from gastric parietal cells, stimulates bicarbonate production from gastric/duodenal mucosa.

PHARMACOKINETICS

Route	Onset	Peak	Duration
PO	30 min	1–1.5 hrs	3–6 hrs

Rapidly absorbed from GI tract. Protein binding: 80%–90%. Rapidly converted to active metabolite. Primarily excreted in urine. Unknown if removed by hemodialysis. **Half-life:** 20–40 min.

USES

Prevention of NSAID-induced gastric ulcers and in pts at high risk for developing gastric ulcer/gastric ulcer complications. **OFF-LABEL:** Treatment of therapeutic second-trimester abortion, cervical ripening, duodenal ulcer, treatment/prevention of NSAID-associated gastric ulcer, induction of labor.

PRECAUTIONS

CONTRAINDICATIONS: Pregnancy (produces uterine contractions). **CAUTIONS:** Renal impairment.

LIFESPAN CONSIDERATIONS:

Pregnancy/Lactation: Unknown if distributed in breast milk. Produces uterine contractions, uterine bleeding, expulsion of products of conception (abortifacient property). **Pregnancy Category X.** **Children:** Safety and efficacy not established. **Elderly:** No age-related precautions noted.

INTERACTIONS

DRUG: **Antacids containing magnesium** worsen diarrhea associated with misoprostol. **HERBAL:** None significant. **FOOD:** None known. **LAB VALUES:** None known.

AVAILABILITY (Rx)

TABLETS: 100 mcg, 200 mcg.

ADMINISTRATION/HANDLING

PO

• Give with or after meals (minimizes diarrhea).

INDICATIONS/ROUTES/DOSAGE

PREVENTION OF NSAID-INDUCED GASTRIC ULCER

PO: ADULTS: 200 mcg 4 times a day with food (last dose at bedtime). Continue for duration of NSAID therapy. May reduce dosage to 100 mcg if 200-mcg dose is not tolerated. **ELDERLY:** 100–200 mcg 4 times a day with food.

SIDE EFFECTS

FREQUENT (40%–20%): Abdominal pain, diarrhea. **OCCASIONAL (3%–2%):** Nausea, flatulence, dyspepsia, headache. **RARE (1%):** Vomiting, constipation.

ADVERSE EFFECTS/ TOXIC REACTIONS

Overdosage may produce sedation, tremor, seizures, dyspnea, palpitations, hypotension, bradycardia.

NURSING CONSIDERATIONS

BASELINE ASSESSMENT

Question for possibility of pregnancy before initiating therapy (Pregnancy Risk Category X).

PATIENT/FAMILY TEACHING

• Avoid magnesium-containing antacids (minimizes potential for diarrhea). • Women of childbearing potential must not be pregnant before or during medication therapy (may result in hospitalization, surgery, infertility, fetal death). • Incidence of diarrhea may be lessened by taking immediately following meals.

M

mitomycin

my-toe-**my**-sin
(Mutamycin)

CLASSIFICATION

PHARMACOTHERAPEUTIC: Antibiotic. **CLINICAL:** Antineoplastic (see p. 81C).

ACTION

Alkylating agent, cross-linking with strands of DNA. **Therapeutic Effect:** Inhibits DNA, RNA synthesis.

PHARMACOKINETICS

Widely distributed. Does not cross blood-brain barrier. Primarily metabolized in liver, excreted in urine. **Half-life:** 50 min.

USES

Treatment of disseminated adenocarcinoma of stomach, pancreas. **OFF-LABEL:** Treatment of biliary, bladder, breast, cervical, colorectal, head/neck, lung carcinomas; chronic myelocytic leukemia, esophageal cancer.

PRECAUTIONS

CONTRAINDICATIONS: Coagulation disorders, bleeding tendencies, platelet count less than 75,000/mm^3, serious infection, serum creatinine greater than 1.7 mg/dl, WBC count less than 3,000/mm^3. **CAUTIONS:** Myelosuppression, renal/hepatic impairment.

LIFESPAN CONSIDERATIONS:

Pregnancy/Lactation: If possible, avoid use during pregnancy, esp. first trimester. Breast-feeding not recommended. Safety in pregnancy not established. **Pregnancy Category: D. Children:** No age-related precautions noted. **Elderly:** Age-related renal impairment may require dosage adjustment.

INTERACTIONS

DRUG: Bone marrow depressants may increase myelosuppression. **Live virus vaccines** may potentiate virus replication, increase vaccine side effects, decrease pt's antibody response to vaccine. **HERBAL:** Avoid **black cohosh, dong quai** in estrogen-dependent tumors. **FOOD:** None known. **LAB VALUES:** May increase BUN, serum creatinine.

AVAILABILITY (Rx)

INJECTION, POWDER FOR RECONSTITUTION: 5 mg, 20 mg, 40 mg.

ADMINISTRATION/HANDLING

◄ ALERT ► May be carcinogenic, mutagenic, teratogenic. Handle with extreme care during preparation/administration. Give via IV push, IV infusion.

Extremely irritating to vein. Injection may produce pain with induration, thrombophlebitis, paresthesia.

IV

Reconstitution • Reconstitute 5-mg vial with 10 ml Sterile Water for Injection (40 ml for 20-mg vial) to provide solution containing 0.5 mg/ml. • Do not shake vial to dissolve. • Allow vial to stand at room temperature until complete dissolution occurs. • For IV infusion, further dilute with 50–100 ml D_5W or 0.9% NaCl.

Rate of administration • Give IV push over 5–10 min. • Extravasation may produce cellulitis, ulceration, tissue sloughing. Terminate administration immediately, inject ordered antidote. Apply ice intermittently for up to 72 hrs; keep area elevated.

Storage • Use only clear, blue-gray solutions. • Concentration of 0.5 mg/ml is stable for 7 days at room temperature or 2 wks if refrigerated. Further diluted solution with D_5W is stable for 3 hrs, 24 hrs if diluted with 0.9% NaCl.

IV INCOMPATIBILITIES

Aztreonam (Azactam), bleomycin (Blenoxane), cefepime (Maxipime), filgrastim (Neupogen), heparin, piperacillin/tazobactam (Zosyn), sargramostin (Leukine), vinorelbine (Navelbine).

IV COMPATIBILITIES

Cisplatin (Platinol AQ), cyclophosphamide (Cytoxan), doxorubicin (Adriamycin), 5-fluorouracil, granisetron (Kytril), leucovorin, methotrexate, ondansetron (Zofran), vinblastine (Velban), vincristine (Oncovin).

INDICATIONS/ROUTES/DOSAGE

USUAL DOSAGE

IV: ADULTS, ELDERLY, CHILDREN: Initially, 10–20 mg/m^2 as single dose. Repeat q6–8wk. Give additional courses only after platelet, WBC counts are within acceptable levels, as shown below.

Leukocytes/ mm^3	Platelets/ mm^3	% of Prior Dose to Give
4,000	More than 100,000	100%
3,000–3,999	75,000–99,000	100%
2,000–2,999	25,000–74,999	70%
1,999 or less	Less than 25,000	50%

DOSAGE IN RENAL IMPAIRMENT

Pts with creatinine clearance less than 10 ml/min should receive 75% of normal dose.

SIDE EFFECTS

FREQUENT (greater than 10%): Fever, anorexia, nausea, vomiting. **OCCASIONAL (10%–2%):** Stomatitis, paresthesia, purple colored bands on nails; rash, alopecia, unusual fatigue. **RARE (less than 1%):** Thrombophlebitis, cellulitis with extravasation.

ADVERSE EFFECTS/ TOXIC REACTIONS

Marked myelosuppression results in hematologic toxicity manifested as leukopenia, thrombocytopenia, and, to a lesser extent, anemia (generally occurs within 2–4 wks after initial therapy). Renal toxicity may be evidenced by increased BUN, serum creatinine levels. Pulmonary toxicity manifested as dyspnea, cough, hemoptysis, pneumonia. Long-term therapy may produce hemolytic uremic syndrome, characterized by hemolytic anemia, thrombocytopenia, renal failure, hypertension.

NURSING CONSIDERATIONS

BASELINE ASSESSMENT

Obtain CBC with differential, PT, bleeding time, before and periodically during therapy. Antiemetics before and during therapy may alleviate nausea/vomiting.

M

INTERVENTION/EVALUATION

Monitor hematologic status, renal function studies. Assess IV site for phlebitis, extravasation. Monitor for hematologic toxicity (fever, sore throat, signs of local infection, unusual bruising/bleeding from any site), symptoms of anemia (excessive fatigue, weakness). Assess for renal toxicity (foul odor from urine, elevated BUN, serum creatinine).

PATIENT/FAMILY TEACHING

• Maintain fastidious oral hygiene. • Immediately report any stinging, burning, pain at injection site. • Do not have immunizations without physician's approval (drug lowers resistance to infection). • Avoid contact with those who have recently received live virus vaccine. • Alopecia is reversible, but new hair growth may have different color, texture. • Contact physician if nausea/vomiting, fever, sore throat, bruising, bleeding, shortness of breath, painful urination occur.

M

mitotane

(Lysodren)

See Cancer chemotherapeutic agents (p. 81C)

mitoxantrone

my-toe-**zan**-trone

(Novantrone)

CLASSIFICATION

PHARMACOTHERAPEUTIC: Anthracenedione. **CLINICAL:** Nonvesicant, antineoplastic (see p. 81C).

ACTION

Inhibits B-cell, T-cell, macrophage proliferation, DNA, RNA synthesis. Active throughout entire cell cycle. **Therapeutic Effect:** Causes cell death.

PHARMACOKINETICS

Protein binding: 78%. Widely distributed. Metabolized in liver. Primarily eliminated in feces by biliary system. Not removed by hemodialysis. **Half-life:** 2.3–13 days.

USES

Treatment of acute, nonlymphocytic leukemia (monocytic, myelogenous, promyelocytic), late-stage hormone-resistant prostate cancer, multiple sclerosis. **OFF-LABEL:** Treatment of acute lymphocytic leukemia; breast, hepatic carcinoma; non-Hodgkin's lymphoma.

PRECAUTIONS

CONTRAINDICATIONS: Baseline left ventricular ejection fraction less than 50%, cumulative lifetime mitoxantrone dose of 140 mg/m^2 or more, multiple sclerosis with hepatic impairment. **CAUTIONS:** Preexisting bone marrow suppression, previous treatment with cardiotoxic medications, hepatobiliary impairment.

LIFESPAN CONSIDERATIONS:

Pregnancy/Lactation: If possible, avoid use during pregnancy, esp. first trimester. May cause fetal harm. Breastfeeding not recommended. **Pregnancy Category D. Children:** Safety and efficacy not established. **Elderly:** No age-related precautions noted.

INTERACTIONS

DRUG: May decrease effect of **antigout medications. Bone marrow depressants** may increase myelosuppression. **Live virus vaccines** may potentiate virus replication, increase vaccine side effects, decrease pt's antibody response to vaccine. **HERBAL:** Avoid **black cohosh, dong quai** in estrogen-dependent tumors. **FOOD:** None known. **LAB VALUES:** May increase serum bilirubin, uric acid, AST, ALT.

AVAILABILITY (Rx)

INJECTION SOLUTION: 2 mg/ml.

ADMINISTRATION/HANDLING

◀ **ALERT** ▶ May be carcinogenic, mutagenic, teratogenic. Handle with extreme care during preparation/administration. Give by IV injection, IV infusion. Must dilute before administration.

IV

Reconstitution • Dilute with at least 50 ml D_5W or 0.9% NaCl.

Rate of administration • Do not administer by subcutaneous, IM, intrathecal, or intra-arterial injection. • Do not give IV push over less than 3 min. • Give IV bolus over at least 3 min, IV intermittent infusion over 15–60 min, or IV continuous infusion (0.02–0.5 mg/ml) in D_5W or 0.9% NaCl.

Storage • Store vials at room temperature.

IV INCOMPATIBILITIES

Aztreonam (Azactam), cefepime (Maxipime), heparin, paclitaxel (Taxol), piperacillin/tazobactam (Zosyn).

IV COMPATIBILITIES

Allopurinol (Aloprim), etoposide (VePesid), gemcitabine (Gemzar), granisetron (Kytril), ondansetron (Zofran), potassium chloride.

INDICATIONS/ROUTES/DOSAGE

LEUKEMIAS

IV: ADULTS, ELDERLY, CHILDREN 2 YRS AND OLDER: 12 mg/m^2 once a day for 2–3 days. **CHILDREN YOUNGER THAN 2 YRS:** 0.4 mg/kg once a day for 3–5 days.

SOLID TUMORS

IV: ADULTS, ELDERLY: 12–14 mg/m^2 once q3–4wk. **CHILDREN:** 18–20 mg/m^2 once q3–4 wk.

PROSTATE CANCER

IV: ADULTS, ELDERLY: 12–14 mg/m^2 every 21 days.

MULTIPLE SCLEROSIS

IV: ADULTS, ELDERLY: 12 mg/m^2/dose q3mo.

SIDE EFFECTS

FREQUENT (greater than 10%): Nausea, vomiting, diarrhea, cough, headache, stomatitis, abdominal discomfort, fever, alopecia. **OCCASIONAL (9%–4%):** Ecchymosis, fungal infection, conjunctivitis, UTI. **RARE (3%):** Arrhythmias.

ADVERSE EFFECTS/ TOXIC REACTIONS

Myelosuppression may be severe, resulting in GI bleeding, sepsis, pneumonia. Renal failure, seizures, jaundice, CHF may occur. Cardiotoxicity has been reported.

NURSING CONSIDERATIONS

BASELINE ASSESSMENT

Offer emotional support. Establish baseline for CBC with differential, temperature, pulse rate/quality, respiratory status.

INTERVENTION/EVALUATION

Monitor hematologic status, pulmonary function studies, hepatic/renal function tests. Monitor for stomatitis, fever, signs of local infection, unusual bruising/bleeding from any site. Extravasation produces swelling, pain, burning, blue discoloration of skin.

PATIENT/FAMILY TEACHING

• Urine will appear blue/green for 24 hrs after administration. Blue tint to sclera may appear. • Maintain adequate daily fluid intake (may protect against renal impairment). • Do not have

M

immunizations without physician's approval (drug lowers resistance to infection). • Avoid crowds, those with infection. • Contraceptive measures recommended during therapy.

mivacurium

(Mivacron)

See Neuromuscular blockers (p. 120C)

Mobic, *see meloxicam*

modafinil

mode-ah-**feen**-awl

(Alertec ✱, Provigil, Sparlon)

CLASSIFICATION

PHARMACOTHERAPEUTIC: Alpha$_1$-agonist. **CLINICAL:** Wakefulness-promoting agent, antinarcoleptic.

ACTION

Binds to dopamine reuptake carrier sites, increasing alpha activity, decreasing delta, theta, beta brain wave activity. **Therapeutic Effect:** Reduces number of sleep episodes, total daytime sleep.

PHARMACOKINETICS

Well absorbed. Protein binding: 60%. Widely distributed. Metabolized in liver. Excreted by kidneys. Unknown if removed by hemodialysis. **Half-life:** 8–10 hrs.

USES

Treatment of excessive daytime sleepiness associated with narcolepsy, other sleep disorders. **OFF-LABEL:** Treatment of attention deficit hyperactivity disorder, brain injury–related underarousal, depression, endozepine stupor, multiple sclerosis-related fatigue, parkinson-related fatigue, seasonal affective disorder.

PRECAUTIONS

CONTRAINDICATIONS: None known. **CAUTIONS:** History of clinically significant mitral valve prolapse, left ventricular hypertrophy, hepatic impairment, history of seizures.

LIFESPAN CONSIDERATIONS:

Pregnancy/Lactation: Unknown if drug is excreted in breast milk. Use caution if given to pregnant women. **Pregnancy Category C. Children:** Safety and efficacy not established in those younger than 16 yrs. **Elderly:** Age-related renal or hepatic impairment may require decreased dosage.

INTERACTIONS

DRUG: May decrease concentrations of **cyclosporine, oral contraceptives, theophylline.** May increase concentrations of **diazepam, phenytoin, propranolol, tricyclic antidepressants, warfarin. Other CNS stimulants** may increase CNS stimulation. **HERBAL:** None significant. **FOOD:** None known. **LAB VALUES:** None known.

AVAILABILITY (Rx)

TABLETS (PROVIGIL): 100 mg, 200 mg. **(SPARLON):** 85 mg, 170 mg, 255 mg, 340 mg, 425 mg.

ADMINISTRATION/HANDLING

PO

- Give without regard to meals.

INDICATIONS/ROUTES/DOSAGE

NARCOLEPSY, OTHER SLEEP DISORDERS

PO: ADULTS, ELDERLY: 200 mg/day. **(SPARLON):** 85–425 mg once daily.

SIDE EFFECTS

FREQUENT: Anxiety, insomnia, nausea. **OCCASIONAL:** Anorexia, diarrhea, dizziness, dry mouth/skin, muscle stiffness, polydipsia, rhinitis, paresthesia, tremor, headache, vomiting.

ADVERSE EFFECTS/ TOXIC REACTIONS

Agitation, excitation, increased B/P, insomnia may occur.

NURSING CONSIDERATIONS

BASELINE ASSESSMENT

Obtain baseline evidence of narcolepsy or other sleep disorders, including pattern, environmental situations, length of sleep episodes. Question for sudden loss of muscle tone (cataplexy) precipitated by strong emotional responses before sleep episode. Assess frequency/severity of sleep episodes before drug therapy.

INTERVENTION/EVALUATION

Monitor sleep pattern, evidence of restlessness during sleep, length of insomnia episodes at night. Assess for dizziness, anxiety; initiate fall precautions. Sugarless gum, sips of tepid water may relieve dry mouth.

PATIENT/FAMILY TEACHING

• Avoid tasks that require alertness, motor skills until response to drug is established. • Do not increase dose without physician approval. • Use alternative contraceptives during therapy and 1 mo after discontinuing modafinil (reduces effectiveness of oral contraceptives).

moexipril

moe-**ex**-a-prile
(Univasc)

FIXED-COMBINATION(S)

Uniretic: moexipril/hydrochlorothiazide (a diuretic): 7.5 mg/12.5 mg, 15 mg/12.5 mg, 15 mg/25 mg.

CLASSIFICATION

PHARMACOTHERAPEUTIC: Angiotensin-converting enzyme (ACE) inhibitor. **CLINICAL:** Antihypertensive (see p. 7C).

ACTION

Suppresses renin-angiotensin-aldosterone system (prevents conversion of angiotensin I to angiotensin II, a potent vasoconstrictor; may inhibit angiotensin II at local vascular, renal sites). **Therapeutic Effect:** Reduces peripheral arterial resistance, B/P.

PHARMACOKINETICS

Route	Onset	Peak	Duration
PO	1 hr	3–6 hrs	24 hrs

Incompletely absorbed from GI tract. Food decreases drug absorption. Rapidly converted to active metabolite. Protein binding: 50%. Primarily recovered in feces, partially excreted in urine. Unknown if removed by dialysis. **Half-life:** 1 hr, metabolite 2–9 hrs.

USES

Treatment of hypertension. Used alone or in combination with thiazide diuretics. **OFF-LABEL:** Treatment of left ventricular dysfunction after myocardial infarction.

PRECAUTIONS

CONTRAINDICATIONS: History of angioedema from previous treatment with ACE inhibitors. **CAUTIONS:** Renal impairment,

M

dialysis, hypovolemia, coronary or cerebrovascular insufficiency, hyperkalemia, aortic stenosis, ischemic heart disease, angina, severe CHF, cerebrovascular disease, those with sodium depletion or on diuretic therapy.

LIFESPAN CONSIDERATIONS:

Pregnancy/Lactation: Crosses placenta. Unknown if distributed in breast milk. **Pregnancy Category C (D if used in second or third trimesters). Children:** Safety and efficacy not established. **Elderly:** Age-related renal impairment may require dosage adjustment.

INTERACTIONS

DRUG: Alcohol, antihypertensives, diuretics may increase effect. May increase **lithium** concentration, risk of toxicity. **NSAIDs** may decrease effects. **Potassium-sparing diuretics, potassium supplements** may cause hyperkalemia. **HERBAL: Ephedra, yohimbe, ginseng** may worsen hypertension. **Garlic** may increase antihypertensive effect. **FOOD:** None known. **LAB VALUES:** May increase BUN, serum alkaline phosphatase, bilirubin, creatinine, potassium, AST, ALT. May decrease serum sodium. May cause positive serum antinuclear antibody (ANA) titer.

AVAILABILITY (Rx)

TABLETS: 7.5 mg, 15 mg.

ADMINISTRATION/HANDLING

PO

• Give 1 hr before meals. • Tablets may be crushed.

INDICATIONS/ROUTES/DOSAGE

HYPERTENSION

PO: ADULTS, ELDERLY: For pts not receiving diuretics, initial dose is 7.5 mg once a day or 3.75 mg (when combined with thiazide diuretic) 1 hr before meals. Adjust according to B/P effect. Maintenance: 7.5–30 mg a day in 1–2 divided doses 1 hr before meals.

DOSAGE IN RENAL IMPAIRMENT

PO: ADULTS, ELDERLY: 3.75 mg once a day in pts with creatinine clearance of 40 ml/min. **Maximum:** May titrate up to 15 mg/day.

SIDE EFFECTS

OCCASIONAL: Cough, headache (6%), dizziness (4%), fatigue (3%). **RARE:** Flushing, rash, myalgia, nausea, vomiting.

ADVERSE EFFECTS/ TOXIC REACTIONS

Excessive hypotension ("first-dose syncope") may occur in pts with CHF, severely salt/volume depleted. Angioedema (swelling of face/lips), hyperkalemia occur rarely. Agranulocytosis, neutropenia may be noted in those with collagen vascular disease (scleroderma, systemic lupus erythematosus), renal impairment. Nephrotic syndrome may be noted in those with history of renal disease.

NURSING CONSIDERATIONS

BASELINE ASSESSMENT

Obtain B/P, apical pulse immediately before each dose, in addition to regular monitoring (be alert to fluctuations). If excessive reduction in B/P occurs, place pt in supine position, feet slightly elevated. Renal function tests should be performed before therapy begins. In pts with renal impairment, autoimmune disease, taking drugs that affect leukocytes or immune response, CBC with differential count should be performed before therapy, q2wk for 3 mos, then periodically thereafter.

INTERVENTION/EVALUATION

Monitor B/P, serum potassium, renal function, WBC count. Observe for hypotensive effect within 1–3 hrs of first dose or increase in dose. Assist with ambulation if dizziness occurs.

PATIENT/FAMILY TEACHING

• Do not abruptly stop medication. • Inform physician of sore throat, fever, difficulty breathing, chest pain, cough. • Notify physician of signs of angioedema. • Arrhythmias may occur. • To reduce hypotensive effect, rise slowly from lying to sitting position, permit legs to dangle momentarily before standing.

molindone

(Moban)

See Antipsychotics

mometasone

mo-**met**-a-sone

(Elocon)

mometasone furoate monohydrate

(Asmanex Twisthaler, Nasonex)

CLASSIFICATION

PHARMACOTHERAPEUTIC: Adrenocorticosteroid. **CLINICAL:** Anti-inflammatory.

ACTION

Inhibits release of inflammatory cells into nasal tissue, preventing early activation of allergic reaction. **Therapeutic Effect:** Decreases response to seasonal/perennial rhinitis.

PHARMACOKINETICS

Undetectable in plasma. Protein binding: 98%–99%. Swallowed portion undergoes extensive metabolism. Excreted primarily through bile and, to a lesser extent, urine. **Half-life:** 5.8 hrs (nasal).

USES

Nasal: Treatment of nasal symptoms of seasonal/perennial allergic rhinitis in adults, children over 2 yrs. Prophylaxis of nasal symptoms of seasonal allergic rhinitis in adults, adolescents over 12 yrs. Treatment of nasal polyps. **Inhalation:** Maintenance treatment of asthma as prophylactic therapy or supplement in pts requiring oral steroids for purpose of decreasing oral steroid requirement. **Topical:** Relief of inflammatory, pruritic manifestations of steroid-responsive dermatoses.

PRECAUTIONS

CONTRAINDICATIONS: Hypersensitivity to any corticosteroid, persistently positive sputum cultures for *Candida albicans*, status asthmaticus (inhalation), systemic fungal infections, untreated localized infection involving nasal mucosa. **CAUTIONS:** Adrenal insufficiency, cirrhosis, glaucoma, hypothyroidism, untreated infection, osteoporosis, tuberculosis.

LIFESPAN CONSIDERATIONS:

Pregnancy/Lactation: Unknown if drug crosses placenta or is distributed in breast milk. **Pregnancy Category C. Children:** Prolonged treatment/high doses may decrease short-term growth rate, cortisol secretion. **Elderly:** No age-related precautions noted.

INTERACTIONS

DRUG: Ketoconazole may increase concentration (inhalation). **HERBAL:** None significant. **FOOD:** None known. **LAB VALUES:** None known.

AVAILABILITY (Rx)

CREAM (ELOCON): 0.1%. **LOTION (ELOCON):** 0.1%. **NASAL SPRAY (NASONEX):**

50 mcg/spray. **OINTMENT (ELOCON):** 0.1%. **ORAL INHALER (ASMANEX TWISTHALER): 220 mcg.**

ADMINISTRATION/HANDLING

INHALATION

• Hold twisthaler straight up with pink portion (base) on bottom, remove cap. • Exhale fully. • Firmly close lips around mouthpiece and inhale a fast, deep breath. • Hold breath for 10 secs.

INTRANASAL

• Shake well before each use. • Clear nasal passages as much as possible prior to administration of nasal spray. • Insert spray tip into nostril, pointing toward nasal passages, away from nasal septum. • Spray into nostril while holding other nostril closed, concurrently inspire through nose to permit medication as high into nasal passages as possible.

M

TOPICAL

• Apply thin layer of cream, lotion, ointment to cover affected area. Rub in gently. • Do not cover area with occlusive dressing.

INDICATIONS/ROUTES/DOSAGE

ALLERGIC RHINITIS

NASAL SPRAY: ADULTS, ELDERLY, CHILDREN 12 YRS AND OLDER: 2 sprays in each nostril once a day. **CHILDREN 2–11 YRS:** 1 spray in each nostril once a day.

ASTHMA

INHALATION: ADULTS, ELDERLY, CHILDREN 12 YRS AND OLDER: Initially, inhale 220 mcg (1 puff) once a day. **Maximum:** 880 mcg once a day.

SKIN DISEASE

TOPICAL: ADULTS, ELDERLY, CHILDREN 12 YRS AND OLDER: Apply cream, lotion, or ointment to affected area once a day.

NASAL POLYP

NASAL SPRAY: ADULTS, ELDERLY: 2 sprays in each nostril twice a day.

SIDE EFFECTS

OCCASIONAL: Inhalation: Headache, allergic rhinitis, upper respiratory infection, muscle pain, fatigue. **Nasal:** Nasal irritation, stinging. **Topical:** Burning. **RARE: Inhalation:** Abdominal pain, dyspepsia, nausea. **Nasal:** Nasal/pharyngeal candidiasis. **Topical:** Pruritus.

ADVERSE EFFECTS/ TOXIC REACTIONS

Acute hypersensitivity reaction (urticaria, angioedema, severe bronchospasm) occurs rarely. Transfer from systemic to local steroid therapy may unmask previously suppressed bronchial asthma condition.

NURSING CONSIDERATIONS

BASELINE ASSESSMENT

Question for hypersensitivity to any corticosteroids.

INTERVENTION/EVALUATION

Teach proper use of nasal spray. Clear nasal passages before use. Contact physician if no improvement in symptoms, sneezing, nasal irritation occur.

PATIENT/FAMILY TEACHING

• Do not change dose schedule or stop taking drug; must taper off gradually under medical supervision. • Contact physician if symptoms do not improve; sneezing, nasal irritation occur. • Clear nasal passages prior to use. • Inhale rapidly, deeply; rinse mouth after inhalation. • With topical form, do not cover affected area with bandage, dressing.

Monopril, *see fosinopril*

montelukast

mon-**tee**-leu-cast
(Singulair)

CLASSIFICATION

PHARMACOTHERAPEUTIC: Leukotriene receptor inhibitor. **CLINICAL:** Antiasthmatic (see p. 72C).

ACTION

Binds to cysteinyl leukotriene receptors, inhibiting effects of leukotrienes on bronchial smooth muscle. **Therapeutic Effect:** Decreases bronchoconstriction, vascular permeability, mucosal edema, mucus production.

PHARMACOKINETICS

Route	Onset	Peak	Duration
PO	N/A	N/A	24 hrs
PO (chewable)	N/A	N/A	24 hrs

Rapidly absorbed from GI tract. Protein binding: 99%. Extensively metabolized in liver. Excreted almost exclusively in feces. **Half-life:** 2.7–5.5 hrs (slightly longer in elderly).

USES

Prophylaxis, chronic treatment of asthma. Not for use in reversal of bronchospasm in acute asthma attacks, status asthmaticus, exercise-induced bronchospasm. Treatment of seasonal allergic rhinitis (hay fever). Relief of perennial allergic rhinitis. **OFF-LABEL:** Acute asthma.

PRECAUTIONS

CONTRAINDICATIONS: None known. **CAUTIONS:** Systemic corticosteroid treatment reduction during montelukast therapy, hepatic impairment.

LIFESPAN CONSIDERATIONS:

Pregnancy/Lactation: Unknown if excreted in breast milk. Use during pregnancy only if necessary. **Pregnancy Category B. Children/Elderly:** No age-related precautions noted in those older than 6 yrs or the elderly.

INTERACTIONS

DRUG: **Phenobarbital, rifampin** may decrease duration of action. **Prednisone** may decrease bioavailability. **HERBAL:** **St. John's wort** may decrease concentration, effect. **FOOD:** None known. **LAB VALUES:** May increase serum AST, ALT.

AVAILABILITY (Rx)

ORAL GRANULES: 4 mg. **TABLETS:** 10 mg. **TABLETS (CHEWABLE):** 4 mg, 5 mg.

ADMINISTRATION/HANDLING

PO

- Administer in evening without regard to meals.

M

INDICATIONS/ROUTES/DOSAGE

BRONCHIAL ASTHMA, PERENNIAL ALLERGIC RHINITIS, SEASONAL ALLERGIC RHINITIS

PO: ADULTS, ELDERLY, ADOLESCENTS OLDER THAN 14 YRS: One 10-mg tablet a day, taken in the evening. **CHILDREN 6–14 YRS:** One 5-mg chewable tablet a day, taken in the evening. **CHILDREN 1–5 YRS:** One 4-mg chewable tablet a day, taken in the evening.

SIDE EFFECTS

Adults, adolescents 15 yrs and older: **FREQUENT (18%):** Headache. **OCCASIONAL (4%):** Influenza. **RARE (3%–2%):** Abdominal pain, cough, dyspepsia, dizziness, fatigue, dental pain. **Children 6–14 yrs:** **RARE (less than 2%):** Diarrhea, laryngitis, pharyngitis, nausea, otitis media, sinusitis, viral infection.

ADVERSE EFFECTS/ TOXIC REACTIONS

None known.

NURSING CONSIDERATIONS

BASELINE ASSESSMENT

Chewable tablet contains phenylalanine (component of aspartame); parents of phenylketonuric pts should be informed. Montelukast should not be abruptly substituted for inhaled or oral corticosteroids.

INTERVENTION/EVALUATION

Monitor rate, depth, rhythm, type of respirations; quality/rate of pulse. Assess lung sounds for rhonchi, wheezing, rales. Observe lips, fingernails for cyanosis (blue/dusky color in light-skinned pts, gray in dark-skinned pts).

PATIENT/FAMILY TEACHING

• Increase fluid intake (decreases lung secretion viscosity). • Take as prescribed, even during symptom-free periods as well as during excacerbations of asthma. • Do not alter/stop other asthma medications. • Drug is not for treatment of acute asthma attacks. • Pts with aspirin sensitivity should avoid aspirin, NSAIDs while taking montelukast.

M

moricizine

(Ethmozine)

See Antiarrhythmics (p. 15C)

morphine

mor-feen

(Astramorph PF, Avinza, DepoDur, Duramorph PF, Infumorph, Kadian, M-Eslon ♣, MS Contin, MSIR, Oramorph SR, RMS, Roxanol, Roxanol-T, Statex ♣)

Do not confuse morphine with hydromorphone, or Roxanol with Roxicet.

CLASSIFICATION

PHARMACOTHERAPEUTIC: Narcotic agonist. **CLINICAL:** Opiate analgesic (**Schedule II**) (see p. 136C).

ACTION

Binds with opioid receptors within CNS. **Therapeutic Effect:** Alters pain perception, emotional response to pain.

PHARMACOKINETICS

Route	Onset	Peak	Duration
Oral solution	N/A	1 hr	3–5 hrs
Tablets	N/A	1 hr	3–5 hrs
Tablets (ER)	N/A	3–4 hrs	8–12 hrs
IV	Rapid	0.3 hr	3–5 hrs
IM	5–30 min	0.5–1 hr	3–5 hrs
Epidural	N/A	1 hr	12–20 hrs
Subcutaneous	N/A	1.1–5 hrs	3–5 hrs
Rectal	N/A	0.5–1 hr	3–7 hrs

Variably absorbed from GI tract. Readily absorbed after IM, subcutaneous administration. Protein binding: 20%–35%. Widely distributed. Metabolized in liver. Primarily excreted in urine. Removed by hemodialysis. **Half-life:** 2–3 hrs. (Increased in hepatic disease.)

USES

Relief of severe, acute, or chronic pain; analgesia during labor. Drug of choice for pain due to MI, dyspnea from pulmonary edema not resulting from chemical respiratory irritant.

PRECAUTIONS

CONTRAINDICATIONS: Acute or severe asthma, GI obstruction, paralytic ileus, severe hepatic/renal impairment, severe respiratory depression. **EXTREME CAUTION:** Chronic obstructive pulmonary disease (COPD), cor pulmonale, hypoxia, hypercapnia preexisting respiratory depression, head injury, increased intracranial pressure (ICP), severe hypotension. **CAUTIONS:** Biliary tract disease, pancreatitis, Addison's disease, hypothyroidism, urethral stricture, prostatic hypertrophy, debilitated pts, those with CNS depression, toxic psychosis, seizure disorders, alcoholism.

LIFESPAN CONSIDERATIONS:

Pregnancy/Lactation: Crosses placenta. Distributed in breast milk. May prolong labor if administered in latent phase of first stage of labor or before cervical dilation of 4–5 cm has occurred. Respiratory depression may occur in neonate if mother received opiates during labor. Regular use of opiates during pregnancy may produce withdrawal symptoms in neonate (irritability, excessive crying, tremors, hyperactive reflexes, fever, vomiting, diarrhea, yawning, sneezing, seizures). **Pregnancy Category C (D if used for prolonged periods or at high dosages at term). Children:** Paradoxical excitement may occur; those younger than 2 yrs are more susceptible to respiratory depressant effects. **Elderly:** Paradoxical excitement may occur. Age-related renal impairment may increase risk of urinary retention.

INTERACTIONS

DRUG: Alcohol, other CNS depressants may increase CNS effects, respiratory depression, hypotension. **MAOIs** may produce severe, sometimes fatal reaction (reduce dosage to ¼ of usual morphine dose). **HERBAL: Gotu kola, kava kava, St. John's wort, valerian** may increase CNS depression. **FOOD:** None known. **LAB VALUES:** May increase serum amylase, lipase.

AVAILABILITY (Rx)

INJECTION, LIPOSOMAL SUSPENSION (DEPODUR): 10 mg/ml. **INJECTION, SOLUTION:** 2 mg/ml, 4 mg/ml, 5 mg/ml, 10 mg/ml, 15 mg/ml, 25 mg/ml, 50 mg/ml. **INJECTION, SOLUTION (EPIDURAL, INTRATHECAL, IV INFUSION) (ASTRAMORPH, DURAMORPH):** 0.5 mg/ml, 1 mg/ml. **INJECTION, SOLUTION (EPIDURAL OR INTRATHECAL) (INFUMORPH):** 10 mg/ml, 25 mg/ml. **INJECTION, SOLUTION (PCA PUMP):** 0.5 mg/ml, 1 mg/ml, 2 mg/ml, 5 mg/ml. **SOLUTION ORAL (ROXANOL):** 20 mg/ml. **SUPPOSITORY (RMS):** 5 mg, 10 mg, 20 mg, 30 mg. **TABLETS:** 15 mg, 30 mg.

CAPSULES, EXTENDED-RELEASE (AVINZA): 30 mg, 60 mg, 90 mg, 120 mg. **CAPSULES, SUSTAINED-RELEASE (KADIAN):** 20 mg, 30 mg, 50 mg, 60 mg, 80 mg, 100 mg. **TABLETS, EXTENDED-RELEASE (MS CONTIN, ORAMORPH SR):** 15 mg, 30 mg, 60 mg, 100 mg, 200 mg.

ADMINISTRATION/HANDLING

IV

Reconstitution • May give undiluted. • For IV injection, may dilute 2.5–15 mg morphine in 4–5 ml Sterile Water for Injection. • For continuous IV infusion, dilute to concentration of 0.1–1 mg/ml in D_5W and give through controlled infusion device.

Rate of administration • Always administer very slowly. Rapid IV increases risk of severe adverse reactions (apnea, chest wall rigidity, peripheral circulatory collapse, cardiac arrest, anaphylactoid effects).

Storage • Store at room temperature.

EPIDURAL, LIPOSOMAL

• May give either diluted or undiluted. • Do not use an in-line filter. • Astramorph, Duramorph, Infumorph are not for IV or IM administration. • Store solution in refrigerator; do not freeze. May store at room temperature for 7 days. • Following withdrawal from vial, use within 4 hrs. • Gently invert vial to resuspend drug; avoid aggressive agitation.

M

IM, SUBCUTANEOUS

• Administer slowly, rotating injection sites. • Pts with circulatory impairment experience higher risk of overdosage due to delayed absorption of repeated administration.

PO

• Mix liquid form with fruit juice to improve taste. • Do not crush, break extended-release capsule. • **Kadian:** May mix with applesauce immediately prior to administration.

RECTAL

• If suppository is too soft, chill for 30 min in refrigerator or run cold water over foil wrapper. • Moisten suppository with cold water before inserting well into rectum.

IV INCOMPATIBILITIES

Amphotericin B complex (Abelcet, AmBisome, Amphotec), cefepime (Maxipime), doxorubicin liposomal (Doxil), lipids, thiopental.

IV COMPATIBILITIES

Amiodarone (Cordarone), atropine, bumetanide (Bumex), bupivacaine (Marcaine, Sensorcaine), diltiazem (Cardizem), diphenhydramine (Benadryl), dobutamine (Dobutrex), dopamine (Intropin), glycopyrrolate (Robinul), heparin, hydroxyzine (Vistaril), lidocaine, lorazepam (Ativan), magnesium, midazolam (Versed), milrinone (Primacor), nitroglycerin, potassium, propofol (Diprivan), total parenteral nutrition (TPN).

INDICATIONS/ROUTES/DOSAGE

◀ **ALERT** ▶ Dosage should be titrated to desired effect.

ANALGESIA

PO (IMMEDIATE-RELEASE): ADULTS, ELDERLY: 10–30 mg q3–4h as needed. **CHILDREN:** 0.2–0.5 mg/kg q3–4h as needed.

◀ **ALERT** ▶ For the Avinza dosage below, be aware that this drug is to be administered once a day only.

◀ **ALERT** ▶ For the Kadian dosage information below, be aware that this drug is to be administered q12h or once a day only.

◀ **ALERT** ▶ Be aware that pediatric dosages of extended-release preparations Kadian and Avinza have not been established.

◀ **ALERT** ▶ For the MS Contin and Oramorph SR dosage information below, be aware that the daily dosage is divided and given q8h or q12h.

PO (EXTENDED-RELEASE [AVINZA]): ADULTS, ELDERLY: Dosage requirement should be established using prompt-release formulations and is based on total daily dose. Avinza is given once a day only.

PO (EXTENDED-RELEASE [KADIAN]): ADULTS, ELDERLY: Dosage requirement should be established using prompt-release formulations and is based on total daily dose. Dose is given once a day or divided and given q12h.

PO (EXTENDED-RELEASE [MS CONTIN, ORAMORPH SR]): ADULTS, ELDERLY: Dosage requirement should be established using prompt-release formulations and is based on total daily dose. Daily dose is divided and given q8h or q12h. **CHILDREN:** 0.3–0.6 mg/kg/dose q12h.

IV: ADULTS, ELDERLY: 2.5–5 mg q3–4h as needed. Note: Repeated doses (e.g., 1–2 mg) may be given more frequently (e.g., every hour) if needed. **CHILDREN:** 0.05–0.1 mg/kg q3–4h as needed.

IV CONTINUOUS INFUSION: ADULTS, ELDERLY: 0.8–10 mg/hr. Range: Up to 80 mg/hr. **CHILDREN:** 10–30 mcg/kg/hr.

IM: ADULTS, ELDERLY: 5–10 mg q3–4h as needed. **CHILDREN:** 0.1 mg/kg q3–4h as needed.

EPIDURAL: ADULTS, ELDERLY: Initially, 1–6 mg bolus, infusion rate: 0.1–1 mg/hr. **Maximum:** 10 mg/24 hrs.

INTRATHECAL: ADULTS, ELDERLY: One-tenth of the epidural dose: 0.2–1 mg/dose.

PCA

IV: ADULTS, ELDERLY: Loading dose: 5–10 mg. **Intermittent bolus:** 0.5–3 mg. **Lockout interval:** 5–12 min. **Continuous infusion:** 1–10 mg/hr. **4-hr limit:** 20–30 mg.

SIDE EFFECTS

◄ **ALERT** ► Ambulatory pts, those not in severe pain may experience nausea, vomiting more frequently than those in supine position or who have severe pain. **FREQUENT:** Sedation, decreased B/P (including orthostatic hypotension), diaphoresis, facial flushing, constipation, dizziness, drowsiness, nausea, vomiting. **OCCASIONAL:** Allergic reaction (rash, pruritus), dyspnea, confusion, palpitations, tremors, urinary retention, abdominal cramps, vision changes, dry mouth, headache, decreased appetite, pain/burning at injection site. **RARE:** Paralytic ileus.

ADVERSE EFFECTS/ TOXIC REACTIONS

Overdose results in respiratory depression, skeletal muscle flaccidity, cold/clammy skin, cyanosis, extreme somnolence progressing to seizures, stupor, coma. Tolerance to analgesic effect, physical dependence may occur with repeated use. Prolonged duration of action, cumulative effect may occur in those with hepatic/renal impairment.

NURSING CONSIDERATIONS

BASELINE ASSESSMENT

Pt should be in recumbent position before drug is given by parenteral route. Assess onset, type, location, duration of pain. Obtain vital signs before giving medication. If respirations are 12/min or less (20/min or less in children), withhold medication, contact physician. Effect of medication is reduced if full pain recurs before next dose.

INTERVENTION/EVALUATION

Monitor vital signs 5–10 min after IV administration, 15–30 min after subcutaneous, IM. Be alert for decreased respirations, B/P. Check for adequate voiding. Monitor daily pattern of bowel activity/stool consistency; avoid constipation. Initiate deep breathing, coughing exercises, particularly in those with pulmonary impairment. Assess for clinical improvement, record onset of pain relief. Consult physician if pain relief is not adequate.

PATIENT/FAMILY TEACHING

• Discomfort may occur with injection. • Change positions slowly to avoid orthostatic hypotension. • Avoid tasks that require alertness, motor skills until response to drug is established. • Avoid alcohol, CNS depressants. • Tolerance, dependence may occur with prolonged use of high doses.

Motrin, *see ibuprofen*

moxifloxacin

moks-i-**floks**-a-sin

(Avelox, Avelox IV, Vigamox)

Do not confuse Avelox with Avonex.

CLASSIFICATION

PHARMACOTHERAPEUTIC: Fluoroquinolone. **CLINICAL:** Antibacterial (see p. 24C).

M

ACTION

Inhibits two enzymes, topoisomerase II and IV, in susceptible microorganisms. **Therapeutic Effect:** Interferes with bacterial DNA replication. Prevents/delays emergence of resistant organisms. Bactericidal.

PHARMACOKINETICS

Well absorbed from GI tract after PO administration. Protein binding: 50%. Widely distributed throughout body with tissue concentration often exceeding plasma concentration. Metabolized in liver. Primarily excreted in urine, with lesser amount in feces. **Half-life:** 10.7–13.3 hrs.

USES

Treatment of susceptible infections due to *S. pneumoniae, S. pyogenes, S. aureus, H. influenzae, M. catarrhalis, K. pneumoniae, M. pneumoniae, C. pneumoniae* including acute bacterial exacerbation of chronic bronchitis, acute bacterial sinusitis, intra-abdominal infection, community-acquired pneumonia, uncomplicated skin/skin structure infections. **Ophthalmic:** Topical treatment of bacterial conjunctivitis due to susceptible strains of bacteria.

PRECAUTIONS

CONTRAINDICATIONS: Hypersensitivity to quinolones. **CAUTIONS:** Renal/hepatic impairment, CNS disorders, cerebral arthrosclerosis, seizures, those with prolonged QT interval, uncorrected hypokalemia, those receiving quinidine, procainamide, amiodarone, sotalol.

LIFESPAN CONSIDERATIONS:

Pregnancy/Lactation: May be distributed in breast milk. May produce teratogenic effects. **Pregnancy Category C.** **Children:** Safety and efficacy not established. **Elderly:** No age-related precautions noted.

INTERACTIONS

DRUG: **Antacids, didanosine (chewable, buffered tablets, pediatric powder for oral solution), iron preparations, sucralfate** may decrease absorption. **HERBAL:** None significant. **FOOD:** None known. **LAB VALUES:** None known.

AVAILABILITY (Rx)

INJECTION INFUSION (AVELOX IV): 400 mg (250 ml). **OPHTHALMIC SOLUTION (VIGAMOX):** 0.5%. **TABLETS (AVELOX):** 400 mg.

ADMINISTRATION/HANDLING

IV

Reconstitution • Available in ready-to-use containers.

Rate of administration • Give by IV infusion only. • Avoid rapid or bolus IV infusion. • Infuse over 60 min.

Storage • Store at room temperature. • Do not refrigerate.

PO

• Give without regard to meals. • Oral moxifloxacin should be administered 4 hrs before or 8 hrs after antacids, multivitamins, iron preparations, sucralfate, didanosine chewable/buffered tablets, pediatric powder for oral solution.

OPHTHALMIC

• Tilt head backward, have pt look up. • Gently pull lower eye-lid down until pocket formed. • Hold dropper above pocket. • Without touching eyelid or conjunctival sac, place drops into center of pocket. • Close eyes gently, apply gentle finger pressure to lacrimal sac at inner canthus. • Remove excess solution around eye with a tissue.

IV INCOMPATIBILITIES

Do not add or infuse other drugs simultaneously through the same IV line.

Flush line before and after use if same IV line is used with other medications.

INDICATIONS/ROUTES/DOSAGE

ACUTE BACTERIAL SINUSITIS

PO, IV: ADULTS, ELDERLY: 400 mg q24h for 10 days.

ACUTE BACTERIAL EXACERBATION OF CHRONIC BRONCHITIS

PO, IV: ADULTS, ELDERLY: 400 mg q24h for 5 days.

COMMUNITY-ACQUIRED PNEUMONIA

PO, IV: ADULTS, ELDERLY: 400 mg q24h for 7–14 days.

INTRA-ABDOMINAL INFECTION

PO/IV: ADULTS, ELDERLY: 400 mg q24h for 5–14 days.

SKIN/SKIN STRUCTURE INFECTION

PO, IV: ADULTS, ELDERLY: 400 mg once a day for 7–21 days.

TOPICAL TREATMENT OF BACTERIAL CONJUNCTIVITIS DUE TO SUSCEPTIBLE STRAINS OF BACTERIA

OPHTHALMIC: ADULTS, ELDERLY CHILDREN 1 YR AND OLDER: 1 drop 3 times a day for 7 days.

SIDE EFFECTS

FREQUENT (8%–6%): Nausea, diarrhea. **OCCASIONAL: PO, IV (3%–2%):** Dizziness, headache, abdominal pain, vomiting. **Ophthalmic (6%–1%):** Conjunctival irritation, reduced visual acuity, dry eye, keratitis, eye pain, ocular itching, swelling of tissue around cornea, eye discharge, fever, cough, pharyngitis, rash, rhinitis. **RARE (1%):** Change in sense of taste, dyspepsia (heartburn, epigastric pain, indigestion), photosensitivity.

ADVERSE EFFECTS/ TOXIC REACTIONS

Pseudomembranous colitis (severe abdominal cramps/pain, severe watery diarrhea, fever) may occur. Superinfection (anal/genital pruritus, moderate to severe diarrhea, stomatitis) may occur.

NURSING CONSIDERATIONS

BASELINE ASSESSMENT

Question for history of hypersensitivity to moxifloxacin, quinolones.

INTERVENTION/EVALUATION

Monitor daily pattern of bowel activity/stool consistency. Assist with ambulation if dizziness occurs. Assess for headache, abdominal pain, vomiting, altered taste, dyspepsia (heartburn, indigestion). Monitor WBC, signs of infection.

PATIENT/FAMILY TEACHING

• May be taken without regard to food. • Drink plenty of fluids. • Avoid exposure to direct sunlight; may cause photosensitivity reaction. • Do not take antacids 4 hrs before or 8 hrs after dosing. • Take full course of therapy.

M

MS Contin, *see morphine*

mupirocin

mew-pie-ro-sin

(Bactroban, Bactroban Nasal, Centany)

Do not confuse Bactroban or Bactroban Nasal with bacitracin, baclofen, or Bactrim.

CLASSIFICATION

PHARMACOTHERAPEUTIC: Anti-infective. **CLINICAL:** Topical antibacterial.

ACTION

Inhibits bacterial protein, RNA synthesis. Less effective on DNA synthesis. **Nasal:** Eradicates nasal colonization of methicillin-resistant *Staphylococcus aureus* (MRSA). **Therapeutic Effect:** Prevents bacterial growth, replication. Bacteriostatic.

PHARMACOKINETICS

Following topical administration, penetrates outer layer of skin (minimal through intact skin). Protein binding: 95%. Metabolized in liver; excreted in urine. **Half-life:** 17–36 min.

USES

Ointment: Topical treatment of impetigo caused by *S. aureus*, *S. pyogenes;* treatment of folliculitis, furunculosis, minor wounds, burns, ulcers caused by susceptible organisms. **Cream:** Treatment of traumatic skin lesions due to *S. aureus*, *S. pyogenes*, prophylactic agent applied to IV catheter exit sites. **Intranasal ointment:** Eradication of *S. aureus* from nasal, perineal carriage sites. **OFF-LABEL:** Treatment of infected eczema, folliculitis, minor bacterial skin infections.

M

PRECAUTIONS

CONTRAINDICATIONS: None known. **CAUTIONS:** Renal impairment, burn pts.

LIFESPAN CONSIDERATIONS:

Pregnancy/Lactation: Unknown if distributed in breast milk. Temporarily discontinue breast-feeding while using mupirocin. **Pregnancy Category B.** **Children:** Safety and efficacy not established. **Elderly:** No age-related precautions noted.

INTERACTIONS

DRUG: None significant. **HERBAL:** None significant. **FOOD:** None known. **LAB VALUES:** None known.

AVAILABILITY (Rx)

CREAM, TOPICAL (BACTROBAN): 2%. **OINTMENT, INTRANASAL (BACTROBAN, NASAL):** 2%. **OINTMENT, TOPICAL (BACTROBAN, CENTANY):** 2%.

ADMINISTRATION/HANDLING

TOPICAL

CREAM, OINTMENT • For topical use only. • May cover with gauze dressing. • Avoid contact with eyes.

INTRANASAL

• Apply ½ ointment from single-use tube into each nostril. • Avoid contact with eyes.

INDICATIONS/ROUTES/DOSAGE

USUAL TOPICAL DOSAGE

TOPICAL: ADULTS, ELDERLY, CHILDREN: **Cream:** Apply small amount 3 times a day for 10 days. **Ointment:** Apply small amount 3–5 times a day for 5–14 days.

USUAL NASAL DOSAGE

INTRANASAL: ADULTS, ELDERLY, CHILDREN: Apply small amount 2 times/day for 5 days.

SIDE EFFECTS

FREQUENT: Nasal (9%–3%): Headache, rhinitis, upper respiratory congestion, pharyngitis, altered taste. **OCCASIONAL: Nasal (2%):** Burning, stinging, cough. **Topical (2%–1%):** Pain, burning, stinging, pruritus. **RARE: Nasal (less than 1%):** Pruritus, diarrhea, dry mouth, epistaxis, nausea, rash. **Topical (less than 1%):** Rash, nausea, dry skin, contact dermatitis.

ADVERSE EFFECTS/ TOXIC REACTIONS

Superinfection may result in bacterial, fungal infections, esp. with prolonged, repeated therapy.

NURSING CONSIDERATIONS

BASELINE ASSESSMENT

Assess skin for type, extent of lesions.

INTERVENTION/EVALUATION

Isolate neonates, pts with poor hygiene. Wear gloves, gown if necessary when contact with discharges is likely; continue until 24 hrs after therapy is effective. Cleanse/dispose of articles soiled with discharge according to institutional guidelines. In event of skin reaction, stop applications, cleanse area gently, notify physician.

PATIENT/FAMILY TEACHING

• For external use only. • Avoid contact with eyes. • Explain precautions to avoid spread of infection; teach how to apply medication. • If skin reaction, irritation develops, notify physician. • If no improvement is noted in 3–5 days, pt should be reevaluated.

muromonab-CD3

mur-oo-**mon**-ab
(Orthoclone OKT3)

CLASSIFICATION

PHARMACOTHERAPEUTIC: Murine monoclonal antibody. **CLINICAL:** Immunosuppressant.

ACTION

Monoclonal antibody derived from purified IgG_2 immune globulin that reacts with T-3 (CD3) antigen of human T-cell membranes. Blocks production, function of T cells (have major role in acute organ rejection). **Therapeutic Effect:** Reverses organ rejection.

PHARMACOKINETICS

Binds to lymphocytes. **Half-life:** Approximately 18 hrs.

USES

Treatment of acute allograft rejection in renal transplant pts; steroid-resistant acute allograft rejection in cardiac, hepatic transplant pts.

PRECAUTIONS

CONTRAINDICATIONS: History of hypersensitivity to any murine-derived product, fluid overload (as evidenced by chest x-ray, weight gain of more than 3%) in wk before initial treatment. **CAUTIONS:** Hepatic, renal, cardiac impairment.

LIFESPAN CONSIDERATIONS:

Pregnancy/Lactation: Crosses placenta; unknown if distributed in breast milk. **Pregnancy Category C. Children:** Safety and efficacy not established. **Elderly:** No age-related precautions noted.

INTERACTIONS

DRUG: Live virus vaccines may potentiate virus replication, increase vaccine's side effects, decrease pt's response to vaccine. **Other immunosuppressants** may increase risk of infection, lymphoproliferative disorders. **HERBAL: Echinacea** may decrease effects. **FOOD:** None known. **LAB VALUES:** None known.

AVAILABILITY (Rx)

INJECTION SOLUTION: 1 mg/ml.

ADMINISTRATION/HANDLING

IV

Reconstitution • Draw solution into syringe through 0.22-micron filter. Discard filter; use needle for IV administration.

Rate of administration • Administer IV push over less than 1 min. • Give methylprednisolone 1 mg/kg before and 100 mg hydrocortisone 30 min after dose (decreases adverse reaction to first dose).

Storage • Refrigerate ampule. Do not use if left unrefrigerated for over 4 hrs. • Do not shake ampule before using. • Fine translucent particles may develop; does not affect potency.

IV INCOMPATIBILITIES

Do not mix with any other medications.

INDICATIONS/ROUTES/DOSAGE

TREATMENT OF ACUTE ALLOGRAFT REJECTION

IV: ADULTS, ELDERLY, CHILDREN 12 YRS AND OLDER: 5 mg/day for 10–14 days, beginning as soon as acute renal rejection is diagnosed. **CHILDREN YOUNGER THAN 12 YRS:** 0.1 mg/kg/day for 10–14 days, beginning as soon as acute renal rejection is diagnosed.

SIDE EFFECTS

FREQUENT: Fever, chills, dyspnea, malaise frequently occur 30 min–6 hrs after first dose. This reaction markedly diminishes after second day of treatment. **OCCASIONAL:** Chest pain, nausea, vomiting, diarrhea, tremor.

ADVERSE EFFECTS/ TOXIC REACTIONS

Cytokine release syndrome, a frequent occurrence, may range from mild flu-like symptoms to a life-threatening, shock-like reaction. Infection due to immunosuppression generally occurs within 45 days after initial treatment. Cytomegalovirus occurs in 19% of pts, herpes simplex occurs in 27%. Severe, life-threatening infection occurs in fewer than 5%. Severe pulmonary edema occurs in less than 2%. Fatal hypersensitivity reactions occur occasionally.

NURSING CONSIDERATIONS

BASELINE ASSESSMENT

Chest x-ray must be taken within 24 hrs of initiation of therapy and be clear of fluid. Weight should be at least 3% above minimum weight the wk before beginning treatment (pulmonary edema occurs when fluid overload is present before treatment). Have resuscitative drugs, equipment immediately available.

INTERVENTION/EVALUATION

Monitor WBC, differential, platelet count, renal/hepatic function tests, immunologic tests (plasma levels, quantitative T-lymphocyte surface phenotyping) before and during therapy. If fever exceeds 100°F, antipyretics should be instituted. Monitor for fluid overload by chest x-ray and weight gain of more than 3% over weight before treatment. Assess lung sounds for evidence of fluid overload. Monitor I&O. Monitor daily pattern of bowel activity/stool consistency.

PATIENT/FAMILY TEACHING

• Inform pt of first-dose reaction (fever, chills, chest tightness, wheezing, nausea, vomiting, diarrhea). • Avoid crowds, those with infections. • Do not receive immunizations.

Mycamine, *see micafungin*

mycophenolate

my-co-**feno**-late
(CellCept, Myfortic)

CLASSIFICATION

PHARMACOTHERAPEUTIC: Immunologic agent. **CLINICAL:** Immunosuppressant (see p. 115C).

ACTION

Suppresses immunologically mediated inflammatory response by inhibiting inosine monophosphate dehydrogenase, an enzyme that deprives lymphocytes of nucleotides necessary for DNA, RNA synthesis, thus inhibiting proliferation of T and B lymphocytes. **Therapeutic Effect:** Prevents transplant rejection.

PHARMACOKINETICS

Rapidly, extensively absorbed after PO administration (food decreases drug plasma concentration but does not affect absorption). Protein binding: 97%. Completely hydrolyzed to active metabolite mycophenolic acid. Primarily excreted in urine. Not removed by hemodialysis. **Half-life:** 17.9 hrs.

USES

Cellcept: Prophylaxis of organ rejection in pts receiving allogeneic hepatic/renal/cardiac transplants (**Myfortic:** Renal transplants). Should be used concurrently with cyclosporine and corticosteroids. **OFF-LABEL:** Treatment of liver transplantation rejection, mild heart transplant rejection, moderate to severe psoriasis.

PRECAUTIONS

CONTRAINDICATIONS: Hypersensitivity to mycophenolic acid or polysorbate 80 (IV formulation). **CAUTIONS:** Active serious digestive disease, renal impairment, neutropenia, women of childbearing potential.

LIFESPAN CONSIDERATIONS:

Pregnancy/Lactation: Unknown if drug crosses placenta or is distributed in breast milk. Avoid breast-feeding. **Pregnancy Category C. Children:** Safety and efficacy not established. **Elderly:** Age-related renal impairment may require dosage adjustment.

INTERACTIONS

DRUG: May increase concentrations of **acyclovir, ganciclovir** in pts with renal impairment. **Antacids (aluminum and magnesium-containing), cholestyramine** may decrease absorption. **Live virus vaccines** may potentiate virus replication, increase vaccine side effects, decrease pt's antibody response to vaccine. **Other immunosuppressants** may increase risk of infection, lymphomas. **Probenecid** may increase concentration. **HERBAL: Cat's claw, echinacea** may decrease effects. **FOOD: All foods** may decrease concentration. **LAB VALUES:** May increase serum cholesterol, alkaline phosphatase, creatinine, AST, ALT. May alter serum glucose, lipids, calcium, potassium, phosphate, uric acid.

AVAILABILITY (Rx)

CAPSULES (CELLCEPT): 250 mg. **INJECTION, POWER FOR RECONSTITUTION (CELLCEPT):** 500 mg. **ORAL SUSPENSION (CELLCEPT):** 200 mg/ml. **TABLETS (CELLCEPT):** 500 mg.

TABLETS (DELAYED-RELEASE [MYFORTIC]): 180 mg, 360 mg.

ADMINISTRATION/HANDLING

IV

Reconstitution • Reconstitute each 500-mg vial with 14 ml D_5W. Gently agitate. • For 1-g dose, further dilute with 140 ml D_5W; for 1.5-g dose further dilute with 210 ml D_5W, providing a concentration of 6 mg/ml.

Rate of administration • Infuse over at least 2 hrs.

Storage • Store at room temperature.

PO

• Give on empty stomach. • Do not open capsules or crush delayed-release tablets. Avoid inhalation of powder in capsules, direct contact of powder on skin/mucous membranes. If contact occurs, wash thoroughly, with soap, water. Rinse eyes profusely with plain water. • May store reconstituted

M

suspension in refrigerator or at room temperature. • Suspension is stable for 60 days after reconstitution. • Suspension can be administered orally or via a nasogastric tube (minimum size 8 French).

IV INCOMPATIBILITIES

Mycophenolate is compatible only with D_5W. Do not infuse concurrently with other drugs or IV solutions.

INDICATIONS/ROUTES/DOSAGE

PREVENTION OF RENAL TRANSPLANT REJECTION

PO, IV (CELLCEPT): ADULTS, ELDERLY: 1 g twice a day. **CHILDREN:** 600 mg/m^2/dose 2 times/day. **Maximum:** 1 g 2 times/day.

PO (MYFORTIC): ADULTS, ELDERLY: 720 mg twice a day. **CHILDREN 5–16 YRS:** 400 mg/m^2 twice a day. **Maximum:** 720 mg twice a day.

M

PREVENTION OF HEART TRANSPLANT REJECTION

PO, IV (CELLCEPT): ADULTS, ELDERLY: 1.5 g twice a day.

PREVENTION OF LIVER TRANSPLANT REJECTION

PO (CELLCEPT): ADULTS, ELDERLY: 1.5 g twice a day.

IV (CELLCEPT): ADULTS, ELDERLY: 1 g twice a day.

USUAL PEDIATRIC DOSAGE

PO (CELLCEPT): CHILDREN: 600 mg/m^2/dose twice a day. **Maximum:** 2 g/day.

SIDE EFFECTS

FREQUENT (37%–20%): UTI, hypertension, peripheral edema, diarrhea, constipation, fever, headache, nausea. **OCCASIONAL (18%–10%):** Dyspepsia; dyspnea; cough; hematuria; asthenia; vomiting; edema; tremors; abdominal, chest, back pain; oral candidiasis; acne. **RARE (9%–6%):** Insomnia, respiratory tract infection, rash, dizziness.

ADVERSE EFFECTS/ TOXIC REACTIONS

Significant anemia, leukopenia, thrombocytopenia, neutropenia, leukocytosis may occur, particularly in those undergoing renal transplant rejection. Sepsis, infection occur occasionally. GI tract hemorrhage occurs rarely. There is an increased risk of developing neoplasms. Immunosuppression results in increased susceptibility to infection.

NURSING CONSIDERATIONS

BASELINE ASSESSMENT

Women of childbearing potential should have a negative serum or urine pregnancy test within 1 wk before initiation of drug therapy. Assess medical history, esp. renal function, existence of active digestive system disease, drug history, esp. other immunosuppressants.

INTERVENTION/EVALUATION

CBC should be performed weekly during first mo of therapy, twice monthly during second and third mos of treatment, then monthly throughout the first yr. If rapid fall in WBC occurs, dosage should be reduced or discontinued. Assess particularly for delayed bone marrow suppression. Report any major change in assessment of pt.

PATIENT/FAMILY TEACHING

• Effective contraception should be used before, during, and for 6 wks after discontinuing therapy, even if pt has a history of infertility, other than hysterectomy. • Two forms of contraception must be used concurrently unless abstinence is absolute. • Contact physician if unusual bleeding/bruising, sore throat, mouth sores, abdominal pain, fever occurs. • Inform pts of need for laboratory follow-up while taking medication. • Inform pts of risk of malignancies that may occur.

nabilone

nab-ah-lone
(Cesamet)

◆CLASSIFICATION

PHARMACOTHERAPEUTIC: Synthetic cannabinoid. **CLINICAL:** Antiemetic **(Schedule II)**.

ACTION

Interacts with cannabinoid receptor system (CB 1 receptor) found in neural tissue. **Therapeutic Effect:** Produces antinausea, antiemetic effect.

PHARMACOKINETICS

Completely absorbed from GI tract. Distributed into tissue. Extensively metabolized in liver. Primarily excreted in feces, with lesser amount eliminated in urine. **Half-life:** 2 hrs.

USES

Treatment of nausea/vomiting associated with cancer chemotherapy in those who have failed to respond to other antiemetic therapy.

PRECAUTIONS

CONTRAINDICATIONS: None known. **CAUTIONS:** Elderly, history of hypertension, heart disease, psychiatric disorders, history of substance abuse, including alcohol, orthostatic hypotension.

⌛ LIFESPAN CONSIDERATIONS:

Pregnancy/Lactation: Unknown if distributed in breast milk; do not breastfeed. **Pregnancy Category C. Children:** Safety and efficacy not established in those younger than 18 yrs. **Elderly:** Age-related renal, hepatic, cardiac impairment may require dosage adjustment.

INTERACTIONS

DRUG: Antihistamines, anticholinergics, atropine, scopolamine, sympathomimetics may produce additive hypertensive, tachycardiac effects. **Ethanol, lithium, muscle relaxants, other CNS depressants, tricyclic antidepressants** may produce additive drowsiness, CNS depressant effects. **HERBAL:** None significant. **FOOD:** None known. **LAB VALUES:** None known.

AVAILABILITY (Rx)

CAPSULES: 1 mg.

ADMINISTRATION/HANDLING

PO

- Store at room temperature.

INDICATIONS/ROUTES/DOSAGE

PREVENTION OF CHEMOTHERAPY-INDUCED NAUSEA/VOMITING

PO: ADULTS: 1 or 2 mg twice daily, 1–3 hrs before chemotherapy is given. **Maximum daily dose:** 6 mg in divided doses 3 times daily. May give 2–3 times/day during entire chemotherapy cycle and for 48 hrs after last dose of chemotherapy is given.

SIDE EFFECTS

FREQUENT (52%–36%): Vertigo, drowsiness, dry mouth. **OCCASIONAL (14%–6%):** Change in mood (anxiety, depression, detachment, euphoria, dysphoria), ataxia, sleep disturbance, headache. **RARE (4%–2%):** Nausea, disorientation, depersonalization.

ADVERSE EFFECTS/ TOXIC REACTIONS

Drug has abuse potential, psychological dependence. Pt may experience decrease in cognitive memory, decreased ability to concentrate, distortion in sense of time. Overdose manifested as hypertension, hypotension, tachycardia, orthostatic hypotension, psychosis, hallucinations, respiratory depression.

N

NURSING CONSIDERATIONS

BASELINE ASSESSMENT

Offer emotional support. Assess hydration status if excessive vomiting occurs (skin turgor, mucous membranes, urinary output).

INTERVENTION/EVALUATION

Monitor for therapeutic relief from nausea/vomiting. Maintain quiet, supportive atmosphere. Supervise closely for serious mood, behavior responses, esp. in pts with history of psychiatric illness. Monitor serum electrolytes in pts with severe vomiting. Monitor B/P, heart rate.

PATIENT/FAMILY TEACHING

Avoid tasks that require alertness, motor skills until response to drug is established. Avoid alcohol. Sugarless gum, sips of tepid water may relieve dry mouth.

N

nabumetone

na-**byu**-me-tone
(Apo-Nabumetone ✤, Novo-Nabumetone ✤, Relafen)

CLASSIFICATION

PHARMACOTHERAPEUTIC: Nonsteroidal anti-inflammatory. **CLINICAL:** Analgesic, anti-inflammatory (see p. 125C).

ACTION

Produces analgesic anti-inflammatory effects by inhibiting prostaglandin synthesis. **Therapeutic Effect:** Reduces inflammatory response, intensity of pain.

PHARMACOKINETICS

Readily absorbed from GI tract. Protein binding: 99%. Widely distributed. Metabolized in liver to active metabolite. Primarily excreted in urine. Not removed by hemodialysis. **Half-life:** 22–30 hrs.

USES

Acute, chronic treatment of osteoarthritis, rheumatoid arthritis.

PRECAUTIONS

CONTRAINDICATIONS: Active peptic ulcer disease, chronic inflammation of GI tract, GI bleeding/ulceration, history of hypersensitivity to aspirin or NSAIDs, history of significant renal impairment. **CAUTIONS:** CHF, hypertension, decreased hepatic/renal function, concurrent use of anticoagulants.

⌛ LIFESPAN CONSIDERATIONS:

Pregnancy/Lactation: Distributed in low concentration in breast milk. Avoid use during last trimester (may adversely affect fetal cardiovascular system: premature closing of ductus arteriosus). **Pregnancy Category C (D if used in third trimester or near delivery). Children:** Safety and efficacy not established. **Elderly:** Age-related renal impairment may increase risk of hepatic/renal toxicity; reduced dosage recommended. More likely to have serious adverse effects with GI bleeding/ulceration.

INTERACTIONS

DRUG: May decrease effects of **antihypertensives, diuretics. Aspirin, other salicylates** may increase risk of GI side effects, bleeding. **Bone marrow depressants** may increase risk of hematologic reactions. May increase concentration of **cyclosporine,** risk of cyclosporine-induced nephropathy. May increase effects of **heparin, oral anticoagulants, thrombolytics.** May increase concentration/risk of **lithium** toxicity. May increase risk of **methotrexate** toxicity. **Probenecid** may increase concentration. **HERBAL: Cat's claw, dong quai, evening primrose, feverfew, garlic, ginger, ginkgo,**

red clover, horse chestnut, ginseng possess antiplatelet activity, may increase risk of bleeding. **FOOD:** None known. **LAB VALUES:** May increase urine protein levels, BUN, serum LDH, alkaline phosphatase, creatinine, potassium, AST, ALT. May decrease serum uric acid.

AVAILABILITY (Rx)

TABLETS (RELAFEN): 500 mg, 750 mg.

ADMINISTRATION/HANDLING

PO

• Give with food, milk, antacids if GI distress occurs. • Do not crush; swallow whole.

INDICATIONS/ROUTES/DOSAGE

RHEUMATOID ARTHRITIS, OSTEOARTHRITIS

PO: ADULTS, ELDERLY: Initially, 1,000 mg as a single dose or in 2 divided doses. May increase up to 2,000 mg/day as a single or in 2 divided doses.

SIDE EFFECTS

FREQUENT (14%–12%): Diarrhea, abdominal cramps/pain, dyspepsia. **OCCASIONAL (9%–4%):** Nausea, constipation, flatulence, dizziness, headache. **RARE (3%–1%):** Vomiting, stomatitis, confusion.

ADVERSE EFFECTS/ TOXIC REACTIONS

Overdose may result in acute hypotension, tachycardia. Rare reactions with long-term use include peptic ulcer, GI bleeding, gastritis, nephrotoxicity (dysuria, cystitis, hematuria, proteinuria, nephrotic syndrome), severe hepatic reactions (cholestasis, jaundice), severe hypersensitivity reactions (bronchospasm, angioedema).

NURSING CONSIDERATIONS

BASELINE ASSESSMENT

Assess onset, type, location, duration of pain/inflammation. Inspect appearance of affected joints for immobility, deformities, skin condition.

INTERVENTION/EVALUATION

Assist with ambulation if drowsiness, dizziness occurs. Monitor for evidence of dyspepsia, pattern of daily bowel activity/stool consistency. Evaluate for therapeutic response: relief of pain, stiffness, swelling. Assess for increase in joint mobility, reduced joint tenderness; improved grip strength.

PATIENT/FAMILY TEACHING

• May cause serious GI bleeding with or without pain. • Avoid aspirin. • May take with food if GI upset occurs. • Avoid tasks requiring mental alertness, motor skills until response to drug is established (may cause dizziness, confusion).

nadolol

nay-**doe**-lole

(Apo-Nadol, Corgard, Novo-Nadolol)

FIXED-COMBINATION(S)

Corzide: nadolol/bendroflumethiazide (a diuretic): 40 mg/5 mg, 80 mg/5 mg.

CLASSIFICATION

PHARMACOTHERAPEUTIC: Betaadrenergic blocker. **CLINICAL:** Antianginal, antihypertensive (see p. 68C).

ACTION

Blocks beta$_1$- and beta$_2$-adrenergenic receptors. Large doses increase airway resistance. **Therapeutic Effect:** Slows heart rate, decreases cardiac output, B/P. Decreases myocardial ischemia severity by decreasing oxygen requirements.

N

PHARMACOKINETICS

Variable absorption after PO administration. Protein binding: 28%–30%. Not metabolized. Excreted unchanged in feces. **Half-life:** 20–24 hrs.

USES

Management of mild to moderate hypertension. Used alone or in combination with diuretics, esp. thiazide type. Management of chronic stable angina pectoris. **OFF-LABEL:** Treatment of arrhythmias, hypertrophic cardiomyopathy, MI, mitral valve prolapse syndrome, neuroleptic-induced akathisia, pheochromocytoma, tremors, thyrotoxicosis, vascular headaches.

PRECAUTIONS

CONTRAINDICATIONS: Bronchial asthma, cardiogenic shock, CHF secondary to tachyarrhythmias, chronic obstructive pulmonary disease (COPD), pts receiving MAOI therapy, second- or third-degree heart block, sinus bradycardia, uncontrolled cardiac failure. **CAUTIONS:** Inadequate cardiac function, renal/hepatic impairment, diabetes mellitus, hyperthyroidism.

LIFESPAN CONSIDERATIONS:

Pregnancy/Lactation: Crosses placenta; distributed in breast milk. **Pregnancy Category C (D if used in second or third trimester). Children:** Safety and efficacy not established. **Elderly:** No age-related precautions noted.

INTERACTIONS

DRUG: Cimetidine may increase concentration. **Diuretics, other antihypertensives** may increase hypotensive effect. May mask symptoms of hypoglycemia, prolong hypoglycemic effect of **insulin, oral hypoglycemics. NSAIDs** may decrease antihypertensive effect. **Sympathomimetics, xanthines** may mutually inhibit effects. **HERBAL: Ephedra, garlic, yohimbe, ginseng** may increase hypertension. **Licorice** may cause increased serum sodium, water retention, decreased serum potassium. **FOOD:** None known. **LAB VALUES:** May increase serum antinuclear antibody titer, BUN, serum LDH, lipoprotein, alkaline phosphatase, bilirubin, creatinine, potassium, uric acid, AST, ALT, triglycerides.

AVAILABILITY (Rx)

TABLETS: 20 mg, 40 mg, 80 mg, 120 mg, 160 mg.

ADMINISTRATION/HANDLING

PO

• Give without regard to meals. • Tablets may be crushed.

INDICATIONS/ROUTES/DOSAGE

HYPERTENSION, ANGINA

PO: ADULTS: Initially, 40 mg/day. May increase by 40–80 mg at 3–7 day intervals. **Maximum: (Hypertension)** 240–360 mg/day. **(Angina):** 160–240 mg. **ELDERLY:** Initially, 20 mg/day. May increase gradually. Range: 20–240 mg/day.

DOSAGE IN RENAL IMPAIRMENT

Dosage is modified based on creatinine clearance.

Creatinine Clearance	% Usual Dosage
10–50 ml/min	50
Less than 10 ml/min	25

SIDE EFFECTS

Nadolol is generally well tolerated, with transient and mild side effects. **FREQUENT:** Diminished sexual function, drowsiness, unusual fatigue/weakness. **OCCASIONAL:** Bradycardia, difficulty breathing, depression, cold hands/feet, diarrhea, constipation, anxiety, nasal congestion, nausea, vomiting. **RARE:** Altered taste, dry eyes, pruritus.

ADVERSE EFFECTS/ TOXIC REACTIONS

Overdose may produce profound bradycardia, hypotension. Abrupt withdrawal may result in diaphoresis, palpitations, headache, tremors, exacerbation of angina, MI ventricular arrhythmias. May precipitate CHF, MI in pts with cardiac disease; thyroid storm in those with thyrotoxicosis; peripheral ischemia in those with existing peripheral vascular disease. Hypoglycemia may occur in pts with previously controlled diabetes.

NURSING CONSIDERATIONS

BASELINE ASSESSMENT

Assess baseline renal/hepatic function tests. Assess B/P, apical pulse immediately before drug administration (if pulse is 60/min or less or systolic B/P is less than 90 mm Hg, withhold medication, contact physician). **Antianginal:** Record onset, type (sharp, dull, squeezing), radiation, location, intensity, duration of anginal pain; precipitating factors (exertion, emotional stress).

INTERVENTION/EVALUATION

Monitor B/P for hypotension, respiratory effort for dyspnea. Assess pulse for quality, irregular rate, bradycardia. Assess hands/feet for coldness, tingling, numbness. Assess for evidence of CHF: dyspnea (particularly on exertion, lying down), night cough, peripheral edema, distended neck veins. Monitor I&O (increase in weight, decrease in urinary output may indicate CHF).

PATIENT/FAMILY TEACHING

• Do not discontinue abruptly (may precipitate angina). • Inform physician if difficulty breathing, night cough, swelling of arms/legs, slow pulse, dizziness, confusion, depression, rash, fever, sore throat, unusual bleeding/bruising occurs. • Avoid tasks that require mental alertness, motor skills until response to drug is established.

nafarelin

naf-ah-**rell**-in

(Synarel)

Do not confuse nafarelin with Anafranil, or Synarel with Symmetrel.

CLASSIFICATION

PHARMACOTHERAPEUTIC: Gonadotropin inhibitor. **CLINICAL:** Hormone agonist (see p. 102C).

ACTION

Initially stimulates release of pituitary gonadotropins, luteinizing hormone (LH) and follicle stimulating hormone (FSH). **Therapeutic Effect:** Results in temporary increase of ovarian steroidogenesis. Continued dosing abolishes stimulatory effect on pituitary gland and, after about 4 wks, leads to decreased secretion of gonadal steroids.

USES

Management of endometriosis, including dysmenorrhea, dyspareunia, pelvic pain. Treatment of central precocious puberty.

PRECAUTIONS

CONTRAINDICATIONS: Hypersensitivity to nafarelin, other agonist analogues; undiagnosed abnormal vaginal bleeding. **CAUTIONS:** History of osteoporosis, chronic alcohol/tobacco use, intercurrent rhinitis. **Pregnancy Category X.**

INTERACTIONS

DRUG: None significant. **HERBAL:** None significant. **FOOD:** None known. **LAB VALUES:** None known.

AVAILABILITY (Rx)

NASAL SOLUTION: 2 mg/ml (each spray delivers 200 mcg).

N

INDICATIONS/ROUTES/DOSAGE

ENDOMETRIOSIS

◀ **ALERT** ▶ Initiate treatment between days 2 and 4 of menstrual cycle. Duration of therapy is 6 mos.

INTRANASAL: ADULTS: 400 mcg a day: 200 mcg (1 spray) into 1 nostril in morning, 1 spray into other nostril in evening. For pts with persistent regular menstruation following initial treatment, increase dosage to 800 mcg a day (1 spray into each nostril in morning and evening).

CENTRAL PRECOCIOUS PUBERTY

INTRANASAL: CHILDREN: 1,600 mcg a day: 400 mcg (2 sprays into each nostril in morning and evening; total 8 sprays). May increase dose to 1,800 mcg a day: 600 mcg (3 sprays) into alternating nostrils 3 times a day.

SIDE EFFECTS

COMMON (90%): Hot flashes. **OCCASIONAL (22%–10%):** Decreased libido, vaginal dryness, headache, emotional lability, acne, myalgia, decreased breast size, nasal irritation. **RARE (8%–2%):** Insomnia, edema, weight gain, seborrhea, depression.

ADVERSE EFFECTS/ TOXIC REACTIONS

None known.

NURSING CONSIDERATIONS

BASELINE ASSESSMENT

Inquire about menstrual cycle; therapy should begin between days 2 and 4 of cycle.

INTERVENTION/EVALUATION

Check for pain relief as result of therapy. Inquire about menstrual cessation, other decreased estrogen effects.

PATIENT/FAMILY TEACHING

• Pt should use nonhormonal contraceptive during therapy. • Do not take drug if pregnancy is suspected **(Pregnancy Category X)**. • Discuss importance of full length of therapy, regular visits to physician's office. • Notify physician if regular menstruation continues (menstruation should stop with therapy).

nafcillin

naf-**sill**-in

(Nallpen ♣, Unipen ♣)

Do not confuse Unipen with Unicap.

CLASSIFICATION

PHARMACOTHERAPEUTIC: Penicillinase-resistant penicillin. **CLINICAL:** Antibiotic (see p. 27C).

ACTION

Binds to bacterial membranes. **Therapeutic Effect:** Inhibits cell wall synthesis. Bactericidal.

USES

Treatment of respiratory tract, skin/skin structure infections, osteomyelitis, endocarditis; meningitis, perioperatively, esp. in cardiovascular, orthopedic procedures. Predominant treatment of infections caused by penicillinase-producing staphylococci.

PRECAUTIONS

CONTRAINDICATIONS: Hypersensitivity to any penicillin. **CAUTIONS:** History of allergies, particularly cephalosporins, severe renal/hepatic impairment.

⌛ LIFESPAN CONSIDERATIONS:

Pregnancy/Lactation: Readily crosses placenta; appears in cord blood, amniotic fluid. Distributed in breast milk. May lead to rash, diarrhea, candidiasis in neonate, infant. **Pregnancy Category B.** **Children:** Immature renal function in neonate may delay renal excretion.

Elderly: Age-related renal impairment may require dosage adjustment.

INTERACTIONS

DRUG: Probenecid may increase concentration, risk of toxicity. **HERBAL:** None significant. **FOOD:** None known. **LAB VALUES:** May cause false-positive Coombs' test.

AVAILABILITY (Rx)

INJECTION, POWDER FOR RECONSTITUTION: 1 g, 2 g.

ADMINISTRATION/HANDLING

◀ **ALERT** ▶ Space doses evenly around the clock.

IV

Reconstitution • For IV push, reconstitute each vial with 15–30 ml Sterile Water for Injection or 0.9% NaCl. Administer over 5–10 min. • For intermittent IV infusion (piggyback), further dilute with 50–100 ml D_5W, $D_{10}W$, 0.9% NaCl, 0.45% NaCl, 0.2% NaCl, Ringer's solution, lactated Ringer's solution, or any combination thereof.

Rate of administration • Infuse over 30–60 min. • Because of potential for hypersensitivity/anaphylaxis, start initial dose at few drops per min, increase slowly to ordered rate; stay with pt first 10–15 min, then check q10min. • Limit IV therapy to less than 48 hrs, if possible. Stop infusion if pt complains of pain at IV site.

Storage (IV Infusion [piggyback]) • Stable for 24 hrs at room temperature, 96 hrs if refrigerated. • Discard if precipitate forms.

IM

• Reconstitute each 500 mg with 1.7 ml Sterile Water for Injection or 0.9% NaCl to provide concentration of 250 mg/ml. • Inject IM into large muscle mass.

IV INCOMPATIBILITIES

Diltiazem (Cardizem), droperidol (Inapsine), fentanyl, insulin, labetalol (Normodyne, Trandate), midazolam (Versed), nalbuphine (Nubain), vancomycin (Vancocin), verapamil (Isoptin).

IV COMPATIBILITIES

Heparin, lidocaine, lipids, magnesium, potassium chloride, propofol (Diprivan).

INDICATIONS/ROUTES/DOSAGE

USUAL DOSAGE

IV: ADULTS, ELDERLY: 0.5–2 g q4–6h. **CHILDREN:** 50–200 mg/kg/day in divided doses q4–6h. **Maximum:** 12 g a day. **NEONATES:** 50–75 mg/kg/day in divided doses q6–12h.

IM: ADULTS, ELDERLY: 500 mg q4–6h. **CHILDREN:** 50–200 mg/kg/day in divided doses q4–6h. **Maximum:** 12 g a day.

SIDE EFFECTS

FREQUENT: Mild hypersensitivity reaction (fever, rash, pruritus), GI effects (nausea, vomiting, diarrhea). **OCCASIONAL:** Hypokalemia with high IV dosages, phlebitis, thrombophlebitis (common in elderly). **RARE:** Extravasation with IV administration.

ADVERSE EFFECTS/ TOXIC REACTIONS

Superinfections, potentially fatal antibiotic-associated colitis may result from altered bacterial balance. Hematologic effects (esp. involving platelets, WBCs), severe hypersensitivity reactions, anaphylaxis occur rarely.

NURSING CONSIDERATIONS

BASELINE ASSESSMENT

Question for history of allergies, esp. penicillins, cephalosporins.

INTERVENTION/EVALUATION

Hold medication, promptly report rash (possible hypersensitivity), diarrhea

N

(fever, abdominal pain, mucus/blood in stool may indicate antibiotic-associated colitis). Evaluate IV site frequently for phlebitis (heat, pain, red streaking over vein), infiltration (potential extravasation). Monitor periodic CBC, urinalysis, serum potassium, renal/hepatic function. Be alert for superinfection: increased fever, onset of sore throat, vomiting, diarrhea, stomatitis, anal/genital pruritus. Check hematology reports (esp. WBCs), periodic serum renal/hepatic reports in prolonged therapy.

PATIENT/FAMILY TEACHING

• Continue antibiotic for full length of treatment. • Doses should be evenly spaced. • Discomfort may occur with IM injection. • Report IV discomfort immediately. • Notify physician in event of diarrhea, rash, other new symptoms.

naftifine

(Naftin)

See Antifungals: topical

nalbuphine

nal-**byoo**-feen

(Nubain)

Do not confuse Nubain with Navane.

CLASSIFICATION

PHARMACOTHERAPEUTIC: Narcotic agonist, antagonist. **CLINICAL:** Opioid analgesic (see p. 136C).

ACTION

Binds with opioid receptors within CNS. May displace opioid agonists, competitively inhibiting their action; may precipitate withdrawal symptoms. **Therapeutic Effect:** Alters pain perception, emotional response to pain.

PHARMACOKINETICS

Route	Onset	Peak	Duration
IV	2–3 min	30 min	3–6 hrs
IM	Less than 15 min	60 min	3–6 hrs
Subcutaneous	Less than 15 min	N/A	3–6 hrs

Well absorbed after IM, subcutaneous administration. Protein binding: 50%. Metabolized in liver. Primarily eliminated in feces by biliary secretion. **Half-life:** 3.5–5 hrs.

USES

Relief of moderate to severe pain, preop sedation, obstetric analgesia, adjunct to anesthesia.

PRECAUTIONS

CONTRAINDICATIONS: Respiratory rate less than 12 breaths/min. **CAUTIONS:** Hepatic/renal impairment, respiratory depression, recent MI, recent biliary tract surgery, head trauma, increased intracranial pressure (ICP), pregnancy, those suspected of being opioid dependent.

LIFESPAN CONSIDERATIONS: **Pregnancy/Lactation:** Readily crosses placenta. Distributed in breast milk (breast-feeding not recommended). May cause fetal, neonatal adverse effects during labor/delivery (e.g., fetal bradycardia). **Pregnancy Category B (D if used for prolonged periods or at high dosages at term).** **Children:** Paradoxical excitement may occur. Those younger than 2 yrs more susceptible to respiratory depression. **Elderly:** More susceptible to respiratory depression. Age-related renal impairment may increase risk of urinary retention.

INTERACTIONS

DRUG: **Alcohol, other CNS depressants** may increase CNS effects, respiratory depression, hypotension. **Buprenorphine** may decrease effects. **MAOIs** may produce a severe, possibly fatal reaction; (reduce dose to 25% of the usual nalbuphine dose). **HERBAL:** **Gotu kola, kava kava, St. John's wort, valerian** may increase CNS depression. **FOOD:** None known. **LAB VALUES:** May increase serum amylase, lipase.

AVAILABILITY (Rx)

INJECTION SOLUTION: 10 mg/ml, 20 mg/ml.

ADMINISTRATION/HANDLING

IV

Reconstitution • May give undiluted.

Rate of administration • For IV push, administer each 10 mg over 3–5 min.

Storage • Store parenteral form at room temperature.

IM

• Rotate IM injection sites.

IV INCOMPATIBILITIES

Amphotericin B complex (Abelcet, AmBisome, Amphotec), cefepime (Maxipime), docetaxel (Doxil), lipids, methotrexate, nafcillin (Nafcil), piperacillin and tazobactam (Zosyn), sargramostim (Leukine, Prokine), sodium bicarbonate.

IV COMPATIBILITIES

Diphenhydramine (Benadryl), droperidol (Inapsine), glycopyrrolate (Robinul), hydroxyzine (Vistaril), ketorolac (Toradol), lidocaine, midazolam (Versed), propofol (Diprivan).

INDICATIONS/ROUTES/DOSAGE

ANALGESIA

IV, IM, SUBCUTANEOUS: ADULTS, ELDERLY: 10 mg q3–6h as needed. Do not exceed maximum single dose of 20 mg or daily dose of 160 mg. For pts receiving long-term narcotic analgesics of similar duration of action, give 25% of usual dose. **CHILDREN 1 YR AND OLDER:** 0.1–0.15 mg/kg q3–6h as needed.

SUPPLEMENT TO ANESTHESIA

IV: ADULTS, ELDERLY: Induction: 0.3–3 mg/kg over 10–15 min. Maintenance: 0.25–0.5 mg/kg as needed.

SIDE EFFECTS

FREQUENT (35%): Sedation. **OCCASIONAL (9%–3%):** Diaphoresis, cold/clammy skin, nausea, vomiting, dizziness, vertigo, dry mouth, headache. **RARE (less than 1%):** Restlessness, emotional lability, paresthesia, flushing, paradoxical reaction.

ADVERSE EFFECTS/ TOXIC REACTIONS

Abrupt withdrawal after prolonged use may produce symptoms of narcotic withdrawal (abdominal cramping, rhinorrhea, lacrimation, anxiety, fever, piloerection [goose bumps]). Overdose results in severe respiratory depression, skeletal muscle flaccidity, cyanosis, extreme somnolence progressing to seizures, stupor, coma. Tolerance to analgesic effect, physical dependence may occur with chronic use.

NURSING CONSIDERATIONS

BASELINE ASSESSMENT

Raise bed rails. Obtain vital signs before giving medication. If respirations are 12/min or less (20/min or less in children), withhold medication, contact physician. Assess onset, type, location, duration of pain. Effect of medication is reduced if full pain recurs before next dose. Low abuse potential.

INTERVENTION/EVALUATION

Monitor for change in respirations, B/P, rate/quality of pulse. Monitor daily pattern of bowel activity/stool consistency. Initiate deep breathing, coughing

N

exercises, particularly in pts with pulmonary impairment. Assess for clinical improvement, record onset of relief of pain. Consult physician if pain relief is not adequate.

PATIENT/FAMILY TEACHING

• Avoid alcohol. • Avoid tasks that require alertness, motor skills until response to drug is established. • May cause dry mouth. • May be habit forming.

naloxone

nay-**lox**-own

(Narcan)

Do not confuse naltrexone or Narcan with Norcuron.

CLASSIFICATION

PHARMACOTHERAPEUTIC: Narcotic antagonist. **CLINICAL:** Antidote.

N

ACTION

Displaces opioids at opioid-occupied receptor sites in CNS. **Therapeutic Effect:** Reverses opioid-induced sleep/sedation, increases respiratory rate, raises B/P to normal range.

PHARMACOKINETICS

Route	Onset	Peak	Duration
IV	1–2 min	N/A	20–60 min
IM	2–5 min	N/A	20–60 min
Subcutaneous	2–5 min	N/A	20–60 min

Well absorbed after IM, subcutaneous administration. Metabolized in liver. Primarily excreted in urine. **Half-life:** 60–100 min.

USES

Diagnosis, treatment of opioid toxicity, treatment of opioid-induced respiratory depression, other effects (e.g., sedation, coma, seizures). Used in neonates to reverse respiratory depression caused by opioids given to mother during labor or delivery. **OFF-LABEL:** Treatment of ethanol ingestion, *Pneumocystitis carinii* pneumonia (PCP).

PRECAUTIONS

CONTRAINDICATIONS: Respiratory depression due to nonopioid drugs. **CAUTIONS:** Chronic cardiac/pulmonary disease, coronary artery disease. Those suspected of being opioid dependent, postop pts (to avoid cardiovascular changes).

LIFESPAN CONSIDERATIONS:

Pregnancy/Lactation: Unknown if drug crosses placenta or is distributed in breast milk. **Pregnancy Category B.** **Children/Elderly:** No age-related precautions noted.

INTERACTIONS

DRUG: Reverses analgesic properties, side effects, may precipitate withdrawal symptoms of **butorphanol, nalbuphine, pentazocine, opioid agnonist analgesics.** **HERBAL:** None significant. **FOOD:** None known. **LAB VALUES:** None known.

AVAILABILITY (Rx)

INJECTION SOLUTION: 0.02 mg/ml, 0.4 mg/ml, 1 mg/ml.

ADMINISTRATION/HANDLING

IV

Reconstitution • May dilute 1 mg/ml with 50 ml Sterile Water for Injection to provide concentration of 0.02 mg/ml. • For continuous IV infusion, dilute each 2 mg of naloxone with 500 ml of D_5W in water or 0.9% NaCl, producing solution containing 0.004 mg/ml.

Rate of administration • May administer undiluted. • Give each 0.4 mg as IV push over 15 sec. • Use the 0.4 mg/ml and 1 mg/ml for injection for adults, the 0.02 mg/ml concentration for neonates.

Storage • Store parenteral form at room temperature. • Use mixture within 24 hrs; discard unused solution. • Protect from light. Stable in D_5W or 0.9% NaCl at 4 mcg/ml for 24 hrs.

IM

- Give deep IM in large muscle mass.

IV INCOMPATIBILITIES

Amphotericin B complex (Abelcet, AmBisome, Amphotec).

IV COMPATIBILITIES

Heparin, ondansetron (Zofran), propofol (Diprivan).

INDICATIONS/ROUTES/DOSAGE

OPIOID TOXICITY

IV, IM, SUBCUTANEOUS: ADULTS, ELDERLY: 0.4–2 mg q2–3min as needed. May repeat q20–60min. **CHILDREN 5 YRS AND OLDER AND WEIGHING 20 KG AND MORE:** 2 mg/dose; if no response, may repeat q2–3min. May need to repeat dose q20–60min. **CHILDREN YOUNGER THAN 5 YRS AND WEIGHING LESS THAN 20 KG:** 0.1 mg/kg; if no response, repeat q2–3min. May need to repeat dose q20–60min.

POSTANESTHESIA NARCOTIC REVERSAL

IV: CHILDREN: 0.01 mg/kg; may repeat q2–3min.

NEONATAL OPIOID-INDUCED DEPRESSION

IV: NEONATES: 0.01 mg/kg. May repeat q2–3min as needed. May need to repeat dose q1–2h.

SIDE EFFECTS

None known; little or no pharmacologic effect in absence of narcotics.

ADVERSE EFFECTS/ TOXIC REACTIONS

Too-rapid reversal of narcotic-induced respiratory depression may result in nausea, vomiting, tremors, increased B/P, tachycardia. Excessive dosage in postop pts may produce significant reversal of analgesia, tremors. Hypotension or hypertension, ventricular tachycardia/fibrillation, pulmonary edema may occur in those with cardiovascular disease.

NURSING CONSIDERATIONS

BASELINE ASSESSMENT

Maintain clear airway. Obtain weight of children to calculate drug dosage.

INTERVENTION/EVALUATION

Monitor vital signs, esp. rate, depth, rhythm of respiration, during and frequently following administration. Carefully observe pt after satisfactory response (duration of opiate may exceed duration of naloxone, resulting in recurrence of respiratory depression). Assess for increased pain with reversal of opiate.

N

naltrexone

nal-**trex**-own

(ReVia, Vivitrol)

Do not confuse ReVia with Revex, Vivitrol with Vivactil.

CLASSIFICATION

PHARMACOTHERAPEUTIC: Opioid receptor antagonist. **CLINICAL:** Ethanol detoxification agent, antidote.

ACTION

Blocks effects of endogenous opioid peptides by competitively binding at opioid receptors. **Therapeutic Effect: Alcohol Deterrent:** Decreases craving, drinking days, relapse rate. **Antidote:** Blocks physical dependence of morphine, heroin, other opioids.

PHARMACOKINETICS

Route	Onset	Peak	Duration
PO	N/A	N/A	24–72 hrs
IM	N/A	2 hrs	2–4 wks

Well absorbed following PO administration. Protein binding: 31%. Metabolized in liver; undergoes first-pass metabolism. Reduction in first-pass hepatic metabolism when given by intramuscular route. Excreted primarily in urine; partial elimination in feces. **Half-life:** 4 hrs (PO), 5–10 days (IM).

USES

Vivitrol: Treatment of alcohol dependence in pts able to abstain from alcohol in outpatient setting prior to initiation of treatment. **ReVia:** Blocks effects of exogenously administered opioids. **OFF-LABEL:** Treatment of postconcussional syndrome unresponsive to other treatments; eating disorders.

PRECAUTIONS

CONTRAINDICATIONS: Opioid dependence, acute opioid withdrawal, failed naloxone challenge, positive urine screen for opioids, acute hepatitis, hepatic failure. **CAUTIONS:** Active hepatic disease. History of suicide attempts, depression.

LIFESPAN CONSIDERATIONS:

Pregnancy/Lactation: Unknown if drug crosses placenta or is distributed in breast milk. **Pregnancy Category C.** **Children:** Safety and efficacy not established in children younger than 18 yrs. **Elderly:** No age-related precautions noted.

INTERACTIONS

DRUG: Concurrent use with **thioridazine** may produce lethargy, drowsiness. Benefits of opioid-containing products **(cough and cold preparations, antidiarrheal preparations, opioid analgesics)** are negated. **HERBAL:** None significant. **FOOD:** None known. **LAB VALUES:** May increase serum transaminase, AST, ALT, eosinophil count. May decrease platelet count.

AVAILABILITY (Rx)

INJECTION SUSPENSION, EXTENDED-RELEASE KIT (VIVITROL): 380 mg/4 ml vial. **TABLETS (REVIA):** 50 mg.

ADMINISTRATION/HANDLING

◀ **ALERT** ▶ In those with narcotic dependence, do not attempt treatment until pt has remained opioid free for 7–10 days. Test urine for opioids for verification. Pt should not be experiencing withdrawal symptoms.

IV/SUBCUTANEOUS

• Administer naloxone challenge test (see Indications/Routes/Dosage). • If pt experiences any signs/symptoms of withdrawal, withhold treatment (challenge test can be repeated in 24 hrs). • Naloxone challenge test must be negative before naltrexone therapy is initiated.

IM

• Give in gluteal region, alternating buttocks • Vivitrol must be suspended only in diluent supplied in kit. • All components (microspheres, diluent, preparation needle, administration needle with safety device) are required for administration. Spare administration needle is provided in case of clogging.

STORAGE

• Store entire diluent supplied in the kit. • All components (microspheres, diluent, preparation needle, administration needle with safety device) are required for preparation administration. Spare administration needle is provided in case of clogging.

INDICATIONS/ROUTES/DOSAGE

ADJUNCT IN TREATMENT OF ALCOHOL DEPENDENCE

IM: ADULTS, ELDERLY: (Vivitrol): 380 mg once every 4 wks or once/mo.

NALOXONE CHALLENGE TEST

IV: ADULTS, ELDERLY: Draw 2 ampules naloxone, 2 ml (0.8 mg) into syringe. Inject 0.5 ml (0.2 mg); while needle is still in vein, observe for 30 sec for withdrawal signs/symptoms (see Adverse Effects/Toxic Reactions). If no evidence of withdrawal, inject remaining 1.5 ml (0.6 mg); observe for additional 20 min for withdrawal signs/symptoms.

SUBCUTANEOUS: ADULTS, ELDERLY: Give 2 ml (0.8 mg); observe for 45 min for withdrawal signs/symptoms.

OPIOID-FREE STATE

PO: ADULTS, ELDERLY: Initially, 25 mg. Observe pt for 1 hr. If no withdrawal signs appear, give another 25 mg. Maintenance regimen is flexible, variable, and individualized. May be given as 50 mg daily, 100 mg q.o.d., or 150 mg every 3 days for 12 wks.

SIDE EFFECTS

COMMON: IM Route: (69%): Injection site reaction (induration, tenderness, pain, nodules, swelling, pruritus, ecchymosis). **FREQUENT: Alcohol Deterrent: (33%–10%):** Nausea, headache, depression. **NARCOTIC ADDICTION (10%–5%):** Insomnia, anxiety, headache, low energy, abdominal cramps, nausea, vomiting, joint/muscle pain. **OCCASIONAL: Alcohol Deterrent (4%-2%):** Dizziness, anxiety, fatigue, insomnia, vomiting, suicidal ideation. **NARCOTIC ADDICTION (10%):** Irritability, increased energy, dizziness, anorexia, diarrhea, constipation, rash, chills, increased thirst.

ADVERSE EFFECTS/ TOXIC REACTIONS

Signs/symptoms of opioid withdrawal include stuffy/runny nose, tearing, yawning, diaphoresis, tremor, vomiting, piloerection (goose bumps), feeling of temperature change, arthralgia, myalgia, abdominal cramps, feeling of skin crawling. Accidental naltrexone overdosage produces withdrawal symptoms within 5 min of ingestion, lasts up to 48 hrs. Symptoms present as confusion, visual hallucinations, drowsiness, significant vomiting, diarrhea. Hepatotoxicity may occur with large doses.

NURSING CONSIDERATIONS

BASELINE ASSESSMENT

Treatment with naltrexone should not be instituted unless pt is opioid free for 7–10 days, alcohol free for 3–5 days before therapy begins. Obtain medication history (esp. opioids), other medical conditions (esp. hepatitis, other hepatic disease). If there is any question of opioid dependence, a naloxone challenge test (see Indications/Routes/Dosage) should be performed.

INTERVENTION/EVALUATION

Monitor closely for evidence of hepatotoxicity (abdominal pain that lasts longer than a few days, white bowel movements, dark urine, jaundice), serum AST, ALT, bilirubin.

PATIENT/FAMILY TEACHING

If heroin, other opiates are self-administered, there will be no effect. However, any attempt to overcome naltrexone's prolonged 24–72 hr blockade of opioid effect by taking large amounts of opioids is dangerous and may result in coma, serious injury, fatal overdose. Naltrexone blocks effects of opioid-containing medicine (cough/cold preparations, antidiarrheal preparations, opioid analgesics). Contact physician if abdominal pain lasting longer than 3 days, white bowel movement, dark-colored urine, yellow eyes occurs.

Naprosyn, *see naproxen*

naproxen

na-**prox**-en
(EC-Naprosyn, Naprelan, Naprelan 375, Naprelan 500)

naproxen sodium

(Aleve, Anaprox, Anaprox DS, Apo-Naproxen ✤, Novo-Naprox ✤, Nu-Naprox ✤, Pamprin)

Do not confuse Aleve with Allese or Anaprox with Anaspaz.

FIXED-COMBINATION(S)

Prevacid NapraPac: naproxen/lansoprazole (proton pump inhibitor): 375 mg/15 mg, 500 mg/15 mg.

CLASSIFICATION

PHARMACOTHERAPEUTIC: Nonsteroidal anti-inflammatory. **CLINICAL:** Analgesic, anti-inflammatory (see p. 125C).

N

ACTION

Produces analgesic, anti-inflammatory effects by inhibiting prostaglandin synthesis. **Therapeutic Effect:** Reduces inflammatory response, intensity of pain.

PHARMACOKINETICS

Route	Onset	Peak	Duration
PO (analgesic)	Less than 1 hr	N/A	7 hrs or less
PO (anti-rheumatic)	Less than 14 days	2–4 wks	N/A

Completely absorbed from GI tract. Protein binding: 99%. Metabolized in liver. Primarily excreted in urine. Not removed by hemodialysis. **Half-life:** 13 hrs.

USES

Treatment of acute or long-term mild to moderate pain, primary dysmenorrhea, rheumatoid arthritis, juvenile rheumatoid arthritis, osteoarthritis, ankylosing spondylitis, acute gouty arthritis, bursitis, tendinitis. **OFF-LABEL:** Treatment of vascular headaches.

PRECAUTIONS

CONTRAINDICATIONS: Hypersensitivity to aspirin, naproxen, other NSAIDs. **CAUTIONS:** GI/cardiac disease, renal/hepatic impairment. Concurrent use of anticoagulants.

LIFESPAN CONSIDERATIONS:

Pregnancy/Lactation: Crosses placenta. Distributed in breast milk. Avoid use during third trimester (may adversely affect fetal cardiovascular system: premature closing of ductus arteriosus). **Pregnancy Category C (D if used in third trimester or near delivery). Children:** Safety and efficacy not established in those younger than 2 yrs. Children older than 2 yrs at increased risk of skin rash. **Elderly:** Age-related renal impairment may increase risk of hepatic/renal toxicity; reduced dosage recommended. More likely to have serious adverse effects with GI bleeding/ulceration.

INTERACTIONS

DRUG: May decrease effects of **antihypertensives, diuretics. Aspirin, other salicylates** may increase risk of GI side effects, bleeding. **Bone marrow depressants** may increase risk of hematologic reactions. May increase effects of **heparin, oral anticoagulants, thrombolytics.** May increase concentration, risk of toxicity of **lithium.** May increase risk of **methotrexate** toxicity. **Probenecid** may increase concentration. **HERBAL:** **Cat's claw, dong quai, evening primrose, feverfew, garlic, ginger, ginkgo, red clover, horse chestnut, ginseng** possess antiplatelet activity, may increase risk of bleeding. **FOOD:** None known. **LAB VALUES:** May prolong bleeding time, alter serum glucose. May increase serum hepatic function test results. May decrease serum sodium, uric acid.

AVAILABILITY (Rx)

GELCAPS (ALEVE [OTC]): 220 mg naproxen sodium (equivalent to 200 mg naproxen). **ORAL SUSPENSION (NAPROSYN):** 125 mg/5 ml naproxen. **TABLETS:** 220 mg naproxen (Aleve [OTC]), 250 mg (Naprosyn), 275 mg naproxen sodium (equivalent to 250 mg naproxen) (Anaprox), 550 mg naproxen sodium (equivalent to 500 mg naproxen) (Anaprox DS).

TABLETS (CONTROLLED-RELEASE): 375 mg naproxen (EC-Naprosyn), 421 mg naproxen (Naprelan), 500 mg naproxen (EC-Naprosyn), 550 mg naproxen sodium (equivalent to 500 mg naproxen) (Naprelan).

ADMINISTRATION/HANDLING

PO

- Swallow enteric-coated form whole; scored tablets may be broken/crushed.
- May give with food, milk, antacids if GI distress occurs.

INDICATIONS/ROUTES/DOSAGE

RHEUMATOID ARTHRITIS, OSTEOARTHRITIS, ANKYLOSING SPONDYLITIS

PO: ADULTS, ELDERLY: 250–500 mg naproxen (275–550 mg naproxen sodium) twice a day or 250 mg naproxen (275 mg naproxen sodium) in morning and 500 mg naproxen (550 mg naproxen sodium) in evening. **Naprelan:** 750–1,000 mg once a day.

ACUTE GOUTY ARTHRITIS

PO: ADULTS, ELDERLY: Initially, 750 mg naproxen (825 mg naproxen sodium), then 250 mg naproxen (275 mg naproxen sodium) q8h until attack subsides. **Naprelan:** Initially, 1,000–1,500 mg, then 1,000 mg once a day until attack subsides.

MILD TO MODERATE PAIN, DYSMENORRHEA, BURSITIS, TENDINITIS

PO: ADULTS, ELDERLY: Initially, 500 mg naproxen (550 mg naproxen sodium), then 250 mg naproxen (275 mg naproxen sodium) q6–8h as needed. **Maximum:** 1.25 g/day naproxen (1.375 g/day naproxen sodium). **Naprelan:** 1,000 mg once a day.

JUVENILE RHEUMATOID ARTHRITIS

PO (NAPROXEN ONLY): CHILDREN: 10–15 mg/kg/day in 2 divided doses. **Maximum:** 1,000 mg/day.

OTC USES

PO: ADULTS 65 YRS AND YOUNGER, CHILDREN 12 YRS AND OLDER: 220 mg (200 mg naproxen sodium) q8–12h. May take 440 mg (200 mg naproxen sodium) as initial dose. **ADULTS OLDER THAN 65 YRS:** 220 mg (200 mg naproxen sodium) q12h.

SIDE EFFECTS

FREQUENT (9%–4%): Nausea, constipation, abdominal cramps/pain, heartburn, dizziness, headache, drowsiness. **OCCASIONAL (3%–1%):** Stomatitis, diarrhea, indigestion. **RARE (less than 1%):** Vomiting, confusion.

ADVERSE EFFECTS/ TOXIC REACTIONS

Rare reactions with long-term use include peptic ulcer, GI bleeding, gastritis, severe hepatic reactions (cholestasis, jaundice), nephrotoxicity (dysuria, hematuria, proteinuria, nephrotic syndrome), and severe hypersensitivity reaction (fever, chills, bronchospasm).

NURSING CONSIDERATIONS

BASELINE ASSESSMENT

Assess onset, type, location, duration of pain/inflammation. Inspect appearance of affected joints for immobility, deformities, skin condition.

N

INTERVENTION/EVALUATION

Assist with ambulation if dizziness occurs. Monitor CBC, platelet count, serum renal/hepatic function tests, Hgb, daily pattern of bowel activity/stool consistency. Evaluate for therapeutic response: relief of pain, stiffness, swelling; increased joint mobility; reduced joint tenderness; improved grip strength.

PATIENT/FAMILY TEACHING

• Avoid tasks that require alertness, motor skills until response to drug is established. • If GI upset occurs, take with food, milk. • Avoid aspirin, alcohol during therapy (increases risk of GI bleeding). • Report headache, rash, visual disturbances, weight gain, black or tarry stools, persistent headache.

naratriptan

nare-a-**trip**-tan

(Amerge)

Do not confuse Amerge with Amaryl.

CLASSIFICATION

PHARMACOTHERAPEUTIC: Serotonin receptor agonist. **CLINICAL:** Antimigraine (see p. 60C).

ACTION

Binds selectively to vascular receptors, producing vasoconstrictive effect on cranial blood vessels. **Therapeutic Effect:** Relieves migraine headache.

PHARMACOKINETICS

Well absorbed after PO administration. Protein binding: 28%–31%. Metabolized by liver to inactive metabolite. Eliminated primarily in urine and, to lesser extent, in feces. **Half-life:** 6 hrs (increased in hepatic/renal impairment).

USES

Treatment of acute migraine headache with or without aura in adults.

PRECAUTIONS

CONTRAINDICATIONS: Basilar/hemiplegic migraine, cerebrovascular, peripheral vascular disease, coronary artery disease, ischemic heart disease (including angina pectoris, history of MI, silent ischemia, Prinzmetal's angina), severe hepatic impairment (Child-Pugh grade C), severe renal impairment (serum creatinine less than 15 ml/min), uncontrolled hypertension, use within 24 hrs of ergotamine-containing preparations or another serotonin receptor agonist, MAOIs use within 14 days. **CAUTIONS:** Mild to moderate renal/hepatic impairment, pt profile suggesting cardiovascular risks.

LIFESPAN CONSIDERATIONS:

Pregnancy/Lactation: Unknown if drug is excreted in breast milk. **Pregnancy Category C.** **Children:** Safety and efficacy not established. **Elderly:** Not recommended in the elderly.

INTERACTIONS

DRUG: **Ergotamine-containing medications** may produce vasospastic reaction. **Fluoxetine, fluvoxamine, paroxetine, sertraline** may produce hyperreflexia, incoordination, weakness. **Oral contraceptives** decrease naratriptan clearance, volume of distribution. **HERBAL:** None significant. **FOOD:** None known. **LAB VALUES:** None known.

AVAILABILITY (Rx)

TABLETS: 1 mg, 2.5 mg.

ADMINISTRATION/HANDLING

PO

• Give without regard to food. • Do not crush tablets.

INDICATIONS/ROUTES/DOSAGE

ACUTE MIGRAINE ATTACK

PO: ADULTS: 1 mg or 2.5 mg. If headache improves but then returns, dose may be repeated after 4 hrs. **Maximum:** 5 mg/24 hrs.

DOSAGE IN MILD TO MODERATE HEPATIC/RENAL IMPAIRMENT

Lower starting dose is recommended. Do not exceed 2.5 mg/24 hrs.

SIDE EFFECTS

OCCASIONAL (5%): Nausea. **RARE (2%):** Paresthesia; dizziness; fatigue; drowsiness; jaw, neck, throat pressure.

ADVERSE EFFECTS/ TOXIC REACTIONS

Corneal opacities, other ocular defects may occur. Cardiac events (ischemia, coronary artery vasospasm, MI), noncardiac vasospasm-related reactions (hemorrhage, cerebrovascular accident [CVA]), occur rarely, particularly in pts with hypertension, diabetes, strong family history of coronary artery disease; obese pts; smokers; males older than 40 yrs; postmenopausal women.

NURSING CONSIDERATIONS

BASELINE ASSESSMENT

Question for history of peripheral vascular disease, renal/hepatic impairment, possibility of pregnancy. Question pt regarding onset, location, duration of migraine; possible precipitating symptoms.

INTERVENTION/EVALUATION

Assess for relief of migraine headache; potential for photophobia, phonophobia (sound sensitivity), nausea, vomiting.

PATIENT/FAMILY TEACHING

• Do not crush, chew tablet; swallow whole with water. • May repeat dose after 4 hrs (maximum of 5 mg/24 hrs). • May cause dizziness, fatigue, drowsiness. • Avoid tasks that require alertness, motor skills until response to drug is established. • Inform physician of any chest pain, palpitations, tightness in throat, rash, hallucinations, anxiety, panic.

Nasacort AQ, *see triamcinolone*

Nasonex, *see mometasone*

natalizumab

nat-ah-**liz**-zoo-mab
(Tysabri)

CLASSIFICATION

PHARMACOTHERAPEUTIC: Monoclonal antibody. **CLINICAL:** Multiple sclerosis agent.

ACTION

Binds to surface of leukocytes, inhibiting adhesion of leukocytes to vascular endothelial cells of GI tract, preventing migration of leukocytes across endothelium into inflamed parenchymal tissue. **Therapeutic Effect:** Inhibits inflammatory activity of activated immune cells, reduces clinical exacerbations of multiple sclerosis.

PHARMACOKINETICS

Half-life: 11 days.

USES

Treatment of relapsing forms of multiple sclerosis to reduce frequency of clinical exacerbations.

PRECAUTIONS

CONTRAINDICATIONS: None known. **CAUTIONS:** Chronic progressive multiple sclerosis, children younger than 18 yrs. Concomitant immunosuppressants (may increase risk of infection).

LIFESPAN CONSIDERATIONS:

Pregnancy/Lactation: Unknown if drug crosses placenta or is distributed

N

in breast milk. **Pregnancy Category C. Children:** Safety and efficacy not established in those younger than 18 yrs. **Elderly:** No age-related precautions noted.

INTERACTIONS

DRUG: None significant. **HERBAL:** None significant. **FOOD:** None known. **LAB VALUES:** May alter hepatic enzyme levels. Increases lymphocytes, monocytes, eosinophils, basophils, red blood cells, usually reversible within 16 wks after last dose.

AVAILABILITY (Rx)

INJECTION SOLUTION: 300 mg/15 ml concentrate.

ADMINISTRATION/HANDLING

IV

Reconstitution • Withdraw 15 ml natalizumab from vial; inject concentrate into 100 ml 0.9% NaCl. • Invert solution to mix completely; do not shake. • Discard if solution is discolored or particulate forms.

Rate of administration • Infuse over 1 hr. • Following completion of infusion, flush with 0.9% NaCl.

Storage • Refrigerate vials. • Do not shake, freeze. Protect from light. • After reconstitution, solution is stable for 8 hrs if refrigerated.

IV INCOMPATIBILITIES

Do not mix with any other medications or diluent other than 0.9% NaCl.

INDICATIONS/ROUTES/DOSAGE

RELAPSED MULTIPLE SCLEROSIS

IV INFUSION: ADULTS 18 YRS AND OLDER, ELDERLY: 300 mg every 4 wks.

SIDE EFFECTS

FREQUENT (35%–15%): Headache, fatigue, depression, arthralgia. **OCCASIONAL (10%–5%):** Abdominal discomfort, rash, urinary urgency/frequency, irregular menstruation/dysmenorrhea, dermatitis. **RARE (4%–2%):** Pruritus, chest discomfort, local bleeding, rigors, tremor, syncope.

ADVERSE EFFECTS/ TOXIC REACTIONS

UTI, lower respiratory tract infection, gastroenteritis, vaginitis, allergic reaction, tonsillitis occur occasionally.

NURSING CONSIDERATIONS

BASELINE ASSESSMENT

Obtain CBC, serum chemistries including hepatic enzyme levels. Assess home situation for support of therapy.

INTERVENTION/EVALUATION

Periodically monitor lab results and reevaluate injection technique. Assess for arthralgia, depression, urinary changes, menstrual irregularities. Assess skin for evidence of rash, pruritus, dermatitis. Monitor for signs/symptoms of urinary, respiratory infection.

natamycin

(Natacyn)

See Antifungals: topical

nateglinide

nah-**teh**-glih-nide

(Starlix)

CLASSIFICATION

PHARMACOTHERAPEUTIC: Antihyperglycemic. **CLINICAL:** Antidiabetic (see p. 42C).

ACTION

Stimulates insulin release from beta cells of pancreas by depolarizing beta cells, leading to opening of calcium channels. Resulting calcium influx induces insulin secretion. **Therapeutic Effect:** Lowers serum glucose concentration.

PHARMACOKINETICS

Absolute bioavailability is approximately 73%. Protein binding: 98%. Extensive metabolism in liver. Primarily excreted in urine; minimal elimination in feces. **Half-life:** 1.5 hrs.

USES

Treatment of type 2 diabetes mellitus in pts whose disease cannot be adequately controlled with diet and exercise and in pts who have not been chronically treated with other antidiabetic agents. Used as monotherapy or in combination with other drugs.

PRECAUTIONS

CONTRAINDICATIONS: Diabetic ketoacidosis, type 1 diabetes mellitus. **CAUTIONS:** Hepatic/renal impairment.

LIFESPAN CONSIDERATIONS:

Pregnancy/Lactation: Unknown if drug crosses placenta or is distributed is breast milk. **Pregnancy Category C.** **Children:** Safety and efficacy not established. **Elderly:** Increased susceptibility to hypoglycemia.

INTERACTIONS

DRUG: **Beta-blockers, MAOIs, NSAIDs, salicylates** may increase hypoglycemic effect. **Corticosteroids, thiazide diuretics, thyroid medications, sympathomimetics** may decrease hypoglycemic effect. **HERBAL:** None significant. **FOOD:** Peak plasma levels may be significantly reduced if administered within 10 min prior to a **liquid meal.** **LAB VALUES:** None known.

AVAILABILITY (Rx)

TABLETS: 60 mg, 120 mg.

ADMINISTRATION/HANDLING

PO

- Ideally, give within 15 min of a meal, but may be given immediately before a meal to as long as 30 min before a meal.

INDICATIONS/ROUTES/DOSAGE

DIABETES MELLITUS

PO: ADULTS, ELDERLY: 120 mg 3 times a day before meals. Initially, 60 mg may be given.

SIDE EFFECTS

FREQUENT (10%): Upper respiratory tract infection. **OCCASIONAL (4%–3%):** Back pain, flu symptoms, dizziness, arthropathy, diarrhea. **RARE (3% or less):** Bronchitis, cough.

ADVERSE EFFECTS/ TOXIC REACTIONS

Hypoglycemia occurs in less than 2% of pts.

NURSING CONSIDERATIONS

BASELINE ASSESSMENT

Check fasting serum glucose, glycosylated Hgb (HbA_{1C}) periodically to determine minimum effective dose. Discuss lifestyle to determine extent of learning, emotional needs. Ensure follow-up instruction if pt, family do not thoroughly understand diabetes management, glucose-testing technique. At least 1 wk should elapse to assess response to drug before new dose adjustment is made.

INTERVENTION/EVALUATION

Monitor serum glucose, food intake. Assess for hypoglycemia (cool, wet skin, tremors, dizziness, anxiety, headache, tachycardia, numbness in mouth, hunger, diplopia), hyperglycemia (polyuria, polyphagia, polydipsia, nausea, vomiting, dim vision, fatigue, deep rapid breathing). Be alert to conditions that alter glucose requirements: fever,

N

increased activity, stress, surgical procedures.

PATIENT/FAMILY TEACHING

• Diabetes mellitus requires lifelong control. • Prescribed diet, exercise are principal parts of treatment; do not skip, delay meals. • Continue to adhere to dietary instructions, regular exercise program, regular testing of serum glucose.

Natrecor, *see nesiritide*

Nebcin, *see tobramycin*

nedocromil

ned-oh-**crow**-mil
(Alocril, Tilade)

CLASSIFICATION

PHARMACOTHERAPEUTIC: Mast cell stabilizer. **CLINICAL:** Respiratory inhalant anti-inflammatory (see p. 71C).

ACTION

Prevents activation, release of inflammation mediators (histamine, leukotrienes, mast cells, eosinophils, monocytes). **Therapeutic Effect:** Prevents early, late asthmatic responses.

USES

Inhalation: Maintenance therapy for preventing airway inflammation, bronchoconstriction in pts with mild to moderate bronchial asthma. **Ophthalmic:** Treatment of pruritus associated with allergic conjunctivitis. **OFF-LABEL:** Prevention of bronchospasm in pts with reversible obstructive airway disease.

PRECAUTIONS

CONTRAINDICATIONS: None known. **CAUTIONS:** Not used for reversing acute bronchospasm.

LIFESPAN CONSIDERATIONS:

Pregnancy/Lactation: Unknown if distributed in breast milk. **Pregnancy Category B. Children:** Safety and efficacy of ophthalmic form not established in children younger than 3 yrs; safety and efficacy of inhaled form not established in children younger than 6 yrs. **Elderly:** No age-related precautions noted.

INTERACTIONS

DRUG: None significant. **HERBAL:** None significant. **FOOD:** None known. **LAB VALUES:** None known.

AVAILABILITY (Rx)

AEROSOL FOR INHALATION (TILADE): 1.75 mg/activation. **OPHTHALMIC SOLUTION (ALOCRIL):** 2%.

INDICATIONS/ROUTES/DOSAGE

MILD TO MODERATE ASTHMA

ORAL INHALATION: ADULTS, ELDERLY, CHILDREN 6 YRS AND OLDER: 2 inhalations 4 times a day. May decrease to 3 times a day then twice a day as asthma becomes controlled.

ALLERGIC CONJUNCTIVITIS

OPHTHALMIC: ADULTS, ELDERLY, CHILDREN 3 YRS AND OLDER: 1–2 drops in each eye twice a day.

SIDE EFFECTS

FREQUENT (10%–6%): Inhalation: Cough, pharyngitis, bronchospasm, headache, altered taste. **Ophthalmic:** Burning sensation in eye. **OCCASIONAL (5%–1%): Inhalation:** Rhinitis, upper respiratory tract infection, abdominal pain, fatigue.

RARE (less than 1%): Inhalation: Diarrhea, dizziness. **Ophthalmic:** Conjunctivitis, light intolerance.

ADVERSE EFFECTS/ TOXIC REACTIONS

None known.

NURSING CONSIDERATIONS

INTERVENTION/EVALUATION

Evaluate therapeutic response: reduced dependence on antihistamine, less frequent, less severe asthmatic attacks.

PATIENT/FAMILY TEACHING

• Increase fluid intake (decreases lung secretion viscosity). • Must be administered at regular intervals (even when symptom free) to achieve optimal results of therapy. • Unpleasant taste after inhalation may be relieved by rinsing mouth with water immediately.

nelarabine

nel-**ay**-reh-bean
(Arranon)

CLASSIFICATION

PHARMACOTHERAPEUTIC: DNA demethylation agent. **CLINICAL:** Antineoplastic; antimetabolite.

ACTION

Incorporates into DNA, leading to inhibition of DNA synthesis. Exerts cytotoxic effect on rapidly dividing cells by causing demethylation of DNA. **Therapeutic Effect:** Produces cell death.

PHARMACOKINETICS

Rapidly eliminated from plasma. Extensive distribution. Protein binding: Less than 25%. Partially eliminated in urine. **Half-Life:** 30 min.

USES

Treatment of T-cell acute lymphoblastic leukemia, T-cell lymphoblastic lymphoma in pts whose disease has not responded to or has relapsed following treatment with at least two chemotherapy regimens. **OFF-LABEL:** Chronic myelocytic leukemia (CML) T-cell blast phase.

PRECAUTIONS

CONTRAINDICATIONS: None known. **CAUTIONS:** Previous or current intrathecal chemotherapy, craniospinal radiation therapy, hepatic disease, renal impairment.

LIFESPAN CONSIDERATIONS:

Pregnancy/Lactation: May cause developmental abnormalities of the fetus. Mothers should avoid breast-feeding. **Pregnancy Category D. Children:** No age-related precautions noted. **Elderly:** Increased risk of neurologic toxicities.

INTERACTIONS

DRUG: Live virus vaccines may potentiate virus replication, increase vaccine side effects, decrease pt's antibody response to vaccine. **HERBAL:** None significant. **FOOD:** None known. **LAB VALUES:** May decrease Hgb, Hct, WBCs, RBCs, platelets, serum albumin, calcium, glucose, magnesium, potassium. May increase serum, bilirubin, transaminase, creatinine, AST.

AVAILABILITY (Rx)

INJECTION SOLUTION: 250 mg (5 mg/ml) in 50 ml vials (Arranon).

ADMINISTRATION/HANDLING

IV

Reconstitution • Do not dilute before administration. • Transfer appropriate dose into polyvinylchloride infusion bag or glass container before administration.

N

Rate of administration • Administer as 2-hr infusion for adults, 1-hr infusion for pediatric pts.

Storage • Store vials at room temperature. • Solution should appear colorless, free of precipitate.

INDICATIONS/ROUTES/DOSAGE

T-CELL LEUKEMIA, LYMPHOMA

IV: ADULTS, ELDERLY: 1,500 mg/m^2 infused over 2 hrs on day 1, 3, and 5 repeated q21days. **CHILDREN 21 YRS AND YOUNGER:** 650 mg/m^2 infused over 1 hr daily for 5 consecutive days repeated q21days.

SIDE EFFECTS

ADULTS

FREQUENT (50%–41%): Fatigue, nausea. **OCCASIONAL (25%–11%):** Cough, fever, drowsiness, vomiting, dyspnea, diarrhea, constipation, dizziness, asthenia (loss of strength, energy), peripheral edema, paresthesia, headache, peripheral neuropathy, myalgia, petechiae, generalized edema. **RARE (9%–4%):** Anorexia, abdominal pain, arthralgia, hypertension, tachycardia, confusion, rigors, stomatitis, back pain, epistaxis, insomnia, dehydration, extremity pain, depression, abdominal distention, blurred vision.

CHILDREN

FREQUENT (17%): Headache. **OCCASIONAL (10%–6%):** Vomiting, drowsiness, asthenia (loss of strength, energy), peripheral neuropathy. **RARE (4%–2%):** Paresthesia, tremor, ataxia.

ADVERSE EFFECTS/ TOXIC REACTIONS

Overdose may result in severe neurotoxicity, myelosuppression. Hematologic toxicity manifested as thrombocytopenia, neutropenia, anemia occurs in most cases. Pleural effusion occurs in 10% of pts, pneumonia in 8% of pts, seizures in 6% of pts.

NURSING CONSIDERATIONS

BASELINE ASSESSMENT

Give emotional support to pt, family. Use strict asepsis, protect pt from infection. Hydration, urine alkalization, prophylaxis with allopurinol must be given to prevent hyperuricemia of tumor lysis syndrome. Perform blood counts as needed to monitor response and toxicity but esp. before each dosing cycle.

INTERVENTION/EVALUATION

Monitor for hematologic toxicity (fever, sore throat, signs of local infections, unusual bruising/bleeding), symptoms of anemia (excessive fatigue, weakness). Assess response to medication; monitor and report nausea, vomiting, diarrhea. Avoid rectal temperatures, other traumas that may induce bleeding.

PATIENT/FAMILY TEACHING

• Do not have immunizations without physician's approval (drug lowers resistance). • Avoid crowds, persons with known infections. • Report signs of infection at once (fever, flu-like symptoms). • Contact physician if nausea/vomiting continues at home. • Advise men to use barrier contraception while receiving treatment. • Women should use effective contraceptive measures to avoid pregnancy. • Contact physician if new or worsening symptoms of peripheral neuropathy occur.

nelfinavir

nel-**fin**-eh-veer
(Viracept)

CLASSIFICATION

PHARMACOTHERAPEUTIC: Protease inhibitor. **CLINICAL:** Antiviral (see pp. 65C, 113C).

ACTION

Inhibits activity of HIV-1 protease, the enzyme necessary for formation of infectious HIV. **Therapeutic Effect:** Formation of immature noninfectious viral particles rather than HIV replication.

PHARMACOKINETICS

Well absorbed after PO administration (absorption increased with food). Protein binding: 98%. Metabolized in liver. Highly bound to plasma proteins. Eliminated primarily in feces. Unknown if removed by hemodialysis. **Half-life:** 3.5–5 hrs.

USES

Treatment of HIV infection in combination with other antiretrovirals. **OFF-LABEL:** HIV, postexposure prophylaxis.

PRECAUTIONS

CONTRAINDICATIONS: Concurrent administration with amiodarone, midazolam, rifampin, triazolam. **CAUTIONS:** Hepatic impairment.

⌛ LIFESPAN CONSIDERATIONS:

Pregnancy/Lactation: Unknown if distributed in breast milk. **Pregnancy Category B.** **Children:** No age-related precautions noted in those older than 2 yrs. **Elderly:** No information available.

INTERACTIONS

DRUG: **Anticonvulsants, rifabutin, rifampin** decrease concentration. Increases concentration of **indinavir, saquinavir.** Decreases effects of **oral contraceptives. Ritonavir** increases concentration. **Lovastatin, simvastatin** may increase risk of adverse effects. **HERBAL:** **St. John's wort** may decrease concentration/effects. **FOOD:** **All foods** increase concentration. **LAB VALUES:** May decrease Hgb, neutrophil, WBC counts. May increase serum creatine kinase (CK), AST, ALT.

AVAILABILITY (Rx)

POWDER FOR ORAL SUSPENSION: 50 mg/g. **TABLETS:** 250 mg, 625 mg.

ADMINISTRATION/HANDLING

PO

• Give with food (light meal, snack). • Mix oral powder with small amount of water, milk, formula, soy formula, soy milk, dietary supplement. • Entire contents must be consumed in order to ingest full dose. • Do not mix with acidic food, orange juice, apple juice, applesauce (bitter taste), or with water in original oral powder container.

INDICATIONS/ROUTES/DOSAGE

HIV INFECTION

PO: ADULTS: 750 mg (three 250-mg tablets) 3 times a day or 1,250 mg twice a day in combination with nucleoside analogues (enhances antiviral activity). **CHILDREN 2–13 YRS:** 45–55 mg/kg twice a day or 25–35 mg/kg 3 times a day. **Maximum:** 2,500 mg/day.

SIDE EFFECTS

FREQUENT (20%): Diarrhea. **OCCASIONAL (7%–3%):** Nausea, rash. **RARE (2%–1%):** Flatulence, asthenia.

ADVERSE EFFECTS/ TOXIC REACTIONS

Diabetes mellitus, hyperglycemia occur rarely.

NURSING CONSIDERATIONS

BASELINE ASSESSMENT

Check hematology, hepatic function tests for accurate baseline.

INTERVENTION/EVALUATION

Monitor daily pattern of bowel activity/ stool consistency. Monitor hepatic enzyme studies for abnormalities. Be alert to development of opportunistic infections (fever, chills, cough, myalgia).

N

PATIENT/FAMILY TEACHING

• Take with food (optimizes absorption). • Take medication every day as prescribed. • Doses should be evenly spaced around the clock. • Do not alter dose, discontinue medication without informing physician. • Medication is not a cure for HIV infection nor does it reduce risk of transmission to others; pt may continue to experience illnesses, including opportunistic infections.

neomycin

nee-oh-**mye**-sin

(Myciguent, Neo-Fradin, Neo-Rx, Neo-Tab)

FIXED-COMBINATION(S)

Neosporin GU Irrigant: neomycin/polymyxin B: 40 mg/200,000 units/ml. **Neosporin Ointment, Triple Antibiotic:** neomycin/polymyxin B/bacitracin: 3.5 mg/5,000 units/400 units/g; 3.5 mg/10,000 units/400 units/g.

CLASSIFICATION

PHARMACOTHERAPEUTIC: Aminoglycoside. **CLINICAL:** Antibiotic (see p. 19C).

ACTION

Binds to bacterial microorganisms. **Therapeutic Effect:** Interferes with bacterial protein synthesis.

PHARMACOKINETICS

Poorly absorbed from GI tract following PO administration. Protein binding: Low. Primarily eliminated unchanged in feces; minimal excretion in urine. Removed by hemodialysis. **Half-life:** 3 hrs.

USES

Preparation of GI tract for surgery. Treatment of minor skin infections, diarrhea caused by *E. coli*. Adjunct in treatment of hepatic encephalopathy.

PRECAUTIONS

CONTRAINDICATIONS: Hypersensitivity to neomycin, other aminoglycosides (cross-sensitivity), or their components. **CAUTIONS:** Elderly, infants with renal insufficiency/immaturity; neuromuscular disorders, prior hearing loss, vertigo, renal impairment.

LIFESPAN CONSIDERATIONS:

Pregnancy/Lactation: Unknown if distributed in breast milk. Avoid breastfeeding. **Pregnancy Category C. Children:** Safety and efficacy not established in children younger than 18 yrs. **Elderly:** Age-related renal impairment may require dosage adjustment.

INTERACTIONS

DRUG: Nephrotoxic medications, other aminoglycosides, ototoxic medications may increase nephrotoxicity, ototoxicity if significant systemic absorption occurs. **HERBAL:** None significant. **FOOD:** None known. **LAB VALUES:**None known.

AVAILABILITY

CREAM: 0.5%. **OINTMENT:** 0.5%. **ORAL SOLUTION (NEO-FRADIN):** 125 mg/5 ml. **TABLETS:** 500 mg.

INDICATIONS/ROUTES/DOSAGE

PREOPERATIVE BOWEL ANTISEPSIS

PO: ADULTS, ELDERLY: 1 g/hr for 4 doses; then 1 g q4h for 5 doses or 1 g at 1 PM, 2 PM, and 10 PM. (with erythromycin) on day before surgery. **CHILDREN:** 90 mg/kg/day in divided doses q4h for 2 days or 25 mg/kg at 1 PM, 2 PM, and 10 PM. on day before surgery.

HEPATIC ENCEPHALOPATHY

PO: ADULTS, ELDERLY: 4–12 g/day in divided doses q4–6h. **CHILDREN:** 2.5–7 g/m^2/day in divided doses q4–6h.

DIARRHEA CAUSED BY *ESCHERICHIA COLI*

PO: ADULTS, ELDERLY: 3 g/day in divided doses q6h. **CHILDREN:** 50 mg/kg/day in divided doses q6h.

MINOR SKIN INFECTIONS

TOPICAL: ADULTS, ELDERLY, CHILDREN: Apply to affected area 1–3 times a day.

SIDE EFFECTS

FREQUENT: Systemic: Nausea, vomiting, diarrhea, irritation of mouth, rectal area. **Topical:** Pruritus, redness, swelling, rash. **RARE: Systemic:** Malabsorption syndrome, neuromuscular blockade (difficulty breathing, drowsiness, weakness).

ADVERSE EFFECTS/ TOXIC REACTIONS

Nephrotoxicity (evidenced by increased BUN, serum creatinine, decreased creatinine clearance) may be reversible if drug is stopped at first sign of nephrotoxic symptoms. Irreversible ototoxicity (tinnitus, dizziness, reduced hearing) and neurotoxicity (headache, dizziness, lethargy, tremor, visual disturbances) occur occasionally. Severe respiratory depression, anaphylaxis occur rarely. Superinfections, particularly fungal infections, may occur.

NURSING CONSIDERATIONS

BASELINE ASSESSMENT

Dehydration must be treated before aminoglycoside therapy. Establish pt's baseline hearing acuity before beginning therapy.

INTERVENTION/EVALUATION

Be alert to ototoxic, neurotoxic symptoms. Assess for hypersensitivity reaction (**topical:** assess for rash, redness, pruritus). Be alert for superinfection, particularly genital/anal pruritus, stomatitis, diarrhea.

PATIENT/FAMILY TEACHING

• Continue antibiotic for full length of treatment. • Space doses evenly. • **Topical:** Cleanse area gently before application; report redness, pruritus. • Inform physician if tinnitus, impaired hearing, dizziness occurs.

neostigmine

nee-oh-**stig**-meen

(Prostigmin, Prostigmin Bromide)

Do not confuse neostigmine with physostigmine.

CLASSIFICATION

PHARMACOTHERAPEUTIC: Cholinergic. **CLINICAL:** Antimyasthenic, antidote (see p. 86C).

ACTION

Prevents destruction of acetylcholine by attaching to enzyme acetylcholinesterase, enhancing impulse transmission across myoneural junction. **Therapeutic Effect:** Improves intestinal/skeletal muscle tone; stimulates salivary, sweat gland secretions.

USES

Improvement of muscle strength in control of myasthenia gravis, diagnosis of myasthenia gravis, prevention/treatment of postop distention, urinary retention, antidote for reversal of effects of nondepolarizing neuromuscular blocking agents after surgery.

PRECAUTIONS

CONTRAINDICATIONS: GI/GU obstruction, history of hypersensitivity reaction to bromides, peritonitis. **CAUTIONS:** Epilepsy, asthma, bradycardia, hyperthyroidism, arrhythmias, peptic ulcer,

N

recent coronary occlusion. **Pregnancy Category C.**

INTERACTIONS

DRUG: **Anticholinergics** reverse, prevent effects. **Cholinesterase inhibitors** may increase risk of toxicity. Antagonizes effects of **neuromuscular blockers. Procainamide, quinidine** may antagonize action. **HERBAL:** None significant. **FOOD:** None known. **LAB VALUES:** None known.

AVAILABILITY (Rx)

INJECTION SOLUTION (PROSTIGMIN): 0.25 mg/ml, 0.5 mg/ml, 1 mg/ml. **TABLETS (PROSTIGMIN BROMIDE):** 15 mg.

ADMINISTRATION/HANDLING

◀ **ALERT** ▶ Discontinue all anticholinesterase therapy at least 8 hrs prior to testing for diagnosis of myasthenia gravis. Give 0.011 mg/kg atropine sulfate IV simultaneously with neostigmine or IM 30 min before administering neostigmine to prevent adverse effects.

IV INCOMPATIBILITY

None known.

IV COMPATIBILITIES

Glycopyrrolate (Robinul), heparin, ondansetron (Zofran), potassium chloride, thiopental (Pentothal).

INDICATIONS/ROUTES/DOSAGE

MYASTHENIA GRAVIS

PO: ADULTS, ELDERLY: Initially, 15–30 mg 3–4 times a day. Increase as necessary. Maintenance: 150 mg/day (range of 15–375 mg). **CHILDREN:** 2 mg/kg/day or 60 mg/m^2/day divided q3–4h.

IV, IM, SUBCUTANEOUS: ADULTS: 0.5–2.5 mg as needed. **CHILDREN:** 0.01–0.04 mg/kg q2–4h.

DIAGNOSIS OF MYASTHENIA GRAVIS

IM: ADULTS, ELDERLY: 0.022 mg/kg. If cholinergic reaction occurs, discontinue tests and administer 0.4–0.6 mg or more atropine sulfate IV. **CHILDREN:** 0.025–0.04 mg/kg preceded by atropine sulfate 0.011 mg/kg subcutaneously.

PREVENTION OF POSTOPERATIVE URINARY RETENTION

IM, SUBCUTANEOUS: ADULTS, ELDERLY: 0.25 mg q4–6h for 2–3 days.

POSTOPERATIVE ABDOMINAL DISTENTION, URINARY RETENTION

IM, SUBCUTANEOUS: ADULTS, ELDERLY: 0.5–1 mg. Catheterize pt if voiding does not occur within 1 hr. After voiding, administer 0.5 mg q3h for 5 injections.

REVERSAL OF NEUROMUSCULAR BLOCKADE

IV: ADULTS, ELDERLY: 0.5–2.5 mg given slowly. **CHILDREN:** 0.025–0.08 mg/kg/dose. **INFANTS:** 0.025–0.1 mg/kg/dose.

SIDE EFFECTS

FREQUENT: Muscarinic effects (diarrhea, diaphoresis, increased salivation, nausea, vomiting, abdominal cramps/pain). **OCCASIONAL:** Muscarinic effects (urinary urgency/frequency, increased bronchial secretions, miosis, lacrimation).

ADVERSE EFFECTS/ TOXIC REACTIONS

Overdose produces cholinergic crisis manifested as abdominal discomfort/cramps, nausea, vomiting, diarrhea, flushing, facial warmth, excessive salivation, diaphoresis, lacrimation, pallor, bradycardia, tachycardia, hypotension, bronchospasm, urinary urgency, blurred vision, miosis, fasciculation (involuntary muscular contractions visible under skin).

NURSING CONSIDERATIONS

BASELINE ASSESSMENT

Larger doses should be given at time of greatest fatigue. Avoid large doses in those with megacolon, reduced GI motility.

INTERVENTION/EVALUATION

Monitor muscle strength, vital signs. Monitor for therapeutic response to medication (increased muscle strength, decreased fatigue, improved chewing, swallowing functions).

PATIENT/FAMILY TEACHING

• Report nausea, vomiting, diarrhea, diaphoresis, increased salivary secretions, palpitations, muscle weakness, severe abdominal pain, difficulty breathing.

Neo-Synephrine, *see phenylephrine*

nesiritide

ness-**ear**-ih-tide
(Natrecor)

CLASSIFICATION

PHARMACOTHERAPEUTIC: Brain natriuretic peptide. **CLINICAL:** Endogenous hormone.

ACTION

Facilitates cardiovascular homeostasis, fluid status through counterregulation of renin-angiotensin-aldosterone system, stimulating cyclic guanosine monophosphate, thereby leading to smooth-muscle cell relaxation. **Therapeutic Effect:** Promotes vasodilation, natriuresis, diuresis, correcting CHF.

PHARMACOKINETICS

Route	Onset	Peak	Duration
IV	15–30 min	1–2 hrs	4 hrs

Excreted primarily in heart by left ventricle. Metabolized by natriuretic neutral endopeptidase enzymes on vascular luminal surface. **Half-life:** 18–23 min.

USES

Treatment of acutely decompensated CHF in pts who have dyspnea at rest or with minimal activity.

PRECAUTIONS

CONTRAINDICATIONS: Cardiogenic shock, systolic B/P less than 90 mm Hg. **CAUTIONS:** Significant valvular stenosis, restrictive/obstructive cardiomyopathy, constrictive pericarditis, pericardial tamponade, suspected low cardiac filling pressures, atrial/ventricular arrhythmias/conduction defects, hypotension, hepatic/renal insufficiency.

LIFESPAN CONSIDERATIONS:

Pregnancy/Lactation: Unknown if drug crosses placenta or is distributed in breast milk. **Pregnancy Category C. Children:** Safety and efficacy not established. **Elderly:** No age-related precautions noted.

INTERACTIONS

DRUG: ACE inhibitors, IV nitroglycerin, milrinone, nitroprusside may increase risk of hypotension. **HERBAL:** None significant. **FOOD:** None known. **LAB VALUES:** None known.

AVAILABILITY (Rx)

INJECTION POWDER FOR RECONSTITUTION: 1.5 mg/5-ml vial.

ADMINISTRATION/HANDLING

◄ **ALERT** ► Do not mix with other injections, infusions. Do not give IM.

IV

Reconstitution • Reconstitute one 1.5-mg vial with 5 ml D_5W or 0.9% NaCl, 0.2% NaCl or any combination thereof. Swirl or rock gently, add to 250-ml bag D_5W or 0.9% NaCl, 0.2% NaCl, or any combination thereof, yielding a solution of 6 mcg/ml.

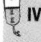

N

Rate of administration • Give as an IV bolus over approximately 60 secs initially, followed by continuous IV infusion.

Storage • Store vial at room temperature. Once reconstituted, use within 24 hrs at room temperature or refrigerated.

IV INCOMPATIBILITIES

Bumetanide (Bumex), enalapril (Vasotec), ethacrynic acid (Edecrin), furosemide (Lasix), heparin, hydralazine (Apresoline), insulin, sodium metabisulfite.

INDICATIONS/ROUTES/DOSAGE

TREATMENT OF ACUTE CHF

IV BOLUS: ADULTS, ELDERLY: 2 mcg/kg followed by a continuous IV infusion of 0.01 mcg/kg/min. At intervals of 3 hrs or longer, may be increased by 0.005 mcg/kg/min (preceded by a bolus of 1 mcg/kg), up to a maximum of 0.03 mcg/kg/min.

SIDE EFFECTS

FREQUENT (11%): Hypotension. **OCCASIONAL (8%–2%):** Headache, nausea, bradycardia. **RARE (1% or less):** Confusion, paresthesia, somnolence, tremor.

ADVERSE EFFECTS/ TOXIC REACTIONS

Ventricular arrhythmias, (ventricular tachycardia, atrial fibrillation, AV node conduction abnormalities), angina pectoris occur rarely.

NURSING CONSIDERATIONS

BASELINE ASSESSMENT

Obtain B/P immediately before each dose, in addition to regular monitoring (be alert to fluctuations). If excessive reduction in B/P occurs, place pt in supine position with legs elevated.

INTERVENTION/EVALUATION

Monitor B/P, pulse rate for hypotension frequently during therapy. Hypotension is dose-limiting and dose-dependent. With physician, establish parameters for adjusting rate, stopping infusion. Maintain accurate I&O; measure urinary output frequently. Immediately notify physician of decreased urinary output, cardiac arrhythmias, significant decrease in B/P, heart rate.

PATIENT/FAMILY TEACHING

- Report chest pain, palpitations.

Neulasta, *see pegfilgrastim*

Neupogen, *see filgrastim*

Neurontin, *see gabapentin*

nevirapine

neh-**veer**-a-peen
(Viramune)

CLASSIFICATION

PHARMACOTHERAPEUTIC: Non-nucleoside reverse transcriptase inhibitor. **CLINICAL:** Antiviral (see p. 112C).

ACTION

Binds directly to HIV-1 reverse transcriptase, changing shape of enzyme, blocking RNA-, DNA-dependent polymerase activity. **Therapeutic Effect:** Interferes with HIV replication, slowing progression of HIV infection.

PHARMACOKINETICS

Readily absorbed after PO administration. Protein binding: 60%. Widely distributed. Extensively metabolized in liver. Excreted primarily in urine. **Half-life:** 45 hrs (single dose), 25–30 hrs (multiple doses).

USES

Used in combination with other antiretroviral agents for treatment of HIV-1 infected adults who have experienced clinical, immunologic deterioration. **OFF-LABEL:** Reduce risk of transmitting HIV from infected mother to newborn.

PRECAUTIONS

CONTRAINDICATIONS: None known. **CAUTIONS:** Renal/hepatic dysfunction, elevated AST, ALT levels, history of chronic hepatitis (B or C), higher CD4+ cell counts.

LIFESPAN CONSIDERATIONS:

Pregnancy/Lactation: Crosses placenta. Distributed in breast milk. Breast-feeding not recommended (possibility of HIV transmission). **Pregnancy Category C. Children:** Granulocytopenia occurs more frequently. **Elderly:** No information available.

INTERACTIONS

DRUG: May alter effect of **clarithromycin.** May decrease effect of **methadone, warfarin.** Concurrent use of **prednisone** may increse incidence, severity of rash in first 6 wks of nevirapine therapy. May decrease concentrations of **ketoconazole, oral contraceptives, protease inhibitors. Rifabutin, rifampin** may decrease concentration. **HERBAL: St. John's wort** may decrease concentration, effects. **FOOD:** None known. **LAB VALUES:** May significantly increase serum bilirubin, GGT, AST, ALT. May significantly decrease Hgb, neutrophil, platelet counts.

AVAILABILITY (Rx)

ORAL SUSPENSION: 50 mg/5 ml. **TABLETS:** 200 mg.

ADMINISTRATION/HANDLING

PO

- Give without regard to meals.

INDICATIONS/ROUTES/DOSAGE

HIV INFECTION

PO: ADULTS: 200 mg once a day for 14 days (to reduce risk of rash). Maintenance: 200 mg twice a day in combination with nucleoside analogues. **CHILDREN OLDER THAN 8 YRS:** 4 mg/kg once a day for 14 days; then 4 mg/kg twice a day. **Maximum:** 400 mg/day. **CHILDREN 2 MOS–8 YRS:** 4 mg/kg once a day for 14 days; then 7 mg/kg twice a day.

SIDE EFFECTS

FREQUENT (8%–3%): Rash, fever, headache, nausea, granulocytopenia (more common in children). **OCCASIONAL (3%–1%):** Stomatitis (burning, erythema, ulceration of oral mucosa; dysphagia). **RARE (less than 1%):** Paresthesia, myalgia, abdominal pain.

ADVERSE EFFECTS/ TOXIC REACTIONS

Skin reactions, hepatitis may become severe, life-threatening.

NURSING CONSIDERATIONS

BASELINE ASSESSMENT

Establish baseline lab values, esp. hepatic function tests, before initiating therapy and at intervals during therapy. Obtain medication history (esp. use of oral contraceptives).

INTERVENTION/EVALUATION

Closely monitor for evidence of rash (usually appears on trunk, face, extremities; occurs within first 6 wks of drug initiation). Observe for rash accompanied by fever, blistering, oral lesions,

N

conjunctivitis, swelling, muscle/joint aches, general malaise.

PATIENT/FAMILY TEACHING

• If nevirapine therapy is missed for longer than 7 days, restart by using one 200 mg tablet daily for first 14 days, followed by one 200 mg tablet 2 times/day. • Continue therapy for full length of treatment. • Doses should be evenly spaced. • Nevirapine is not a cure for HIV infection, nor does it reduce risk of transmission to others. • If rash appears, contact physician before continuing therapy.

Nexium, *see esomeprazole*

niacin, nicotinic acid

nye-a-sin

(Niacor, Niaspan, Slo-Niacin)

Do not confuse niacin, Niacor, or Niaspan with minocin or Nitro-Bid.

FIXED-COMBINATION(S)

Advicor: niacin/lovastatin: 500 mg/20 mg; 750 mg/20 mg; 1,000 mg/20 mg.

CLASSIFICATION

CLINICAL: Antihyperlipidemic, water-soluble vitamin (see p. 55C).

ACTION

Component of two coenzymes needed for tissue respiration, lipid metabolism, glycogenolysis. Inhibits synthesis of very-low-density lipoproteins (VLDL). **Therapeutic Effect:** Reduces total, LDL, VLDL cholesterol levels and triglyceride levels; increases HDL cholesterol concentration.

PHARMACOKINETICS

Readily absorbed from GI tract. Widely distributed. Metabolized in liver. Primarily excreted in urine. **Half-life:** 45 min.

USES

Adjunct in treatment of hyperlipidemias, peripheral vascular disease; treatment of pellagra; dietary supplement.

PRECAUTIONS

CONTRAINDICATIONS: Active peptic ulcer disease, arterial hemorrhaging, hepatic dysfunction, hypersensitivity to niacin, tartrazine (frequently seen in pts sensitive to aspirin), severe hypotension. **CAUTIONS:** Diabetes mellitus, gallbladder disease, gout, history of jaundice/hepatic disease.

LIFESPAN CONSIDERATIONS:

Pregnancy/Lactation: Not recommended for use during pregnancy/lactation. Distributed in breast milk. **Pregnancy Category A (C if used at dosages above the recommended daily allowance). Children:** No age-related precautions noted. Not recommended in those younger than 2 yrs. **Elderly:** No age-related precautions noted.

INTERACTIONS

DRUG: Alcohol may increase risk of side effects. May alter effect of **anticoagulants.** May increase effect of **antihypertensives. Lovastatin, pravastatin, simvastatin** may increase risk of acute renal failure, rhabdomyolysis. **HERBAL:** None significant. **FOOD:** None known. **LAB VALUES:** May increase serum uric acid.

AVAILABILITY (OTC)

TABLETS (NIACOR): 50 mg, 100 mg, 250 mg, 500 mg. **TABLETS (IMMEDIATE-RELEASE):** 50 mg, 100 mg, 250 mg, 500 mg.

CAPSULES (EXTENDED-RELEASE): 125 mg, 250 mg, 400 mg, 500 mg. **TABLETS (CONTROLLED-RELEASE [SLO-NIACIN]):** 250 mg, 500 mg, 750 mg. **TABLETS (EXTENDED-RELEASE [NIASPAN]):** 500 mg, 750 mg, 1,000 mg.

ADMINISTRATION/HANDLING

PO

• For pts switching from immediate-release niacin to extended-release niacin, initiate extended-release form with low doses and titrate to therapeutic response. • Give at bedtime after low-fat snack. • Give aspirin 30 min before taking extended-release niacin to minimize flushing.

INDICATIONS/ROUTES/DOSAGE

HYPERLIPIDEMIA

PO (IMMEDIATE-RELEASE): ADULTS, ELDERLY: Initially, 50–100 mg twice a day for 7 days. Increase gradually by doubling dose qwk up to 1–1.5 g/day in 2–3 doses. **Maximum:** 3 g/day. **CHILDREN:** Initially, 100–250 mg/day (**maximum:** 10 mg/kg/day) in 3 divided doses. May increase by 100 mg/wk or 250 mg q2–3wk. **Maximum:** 2,250 mg/day.

PO (CONTROLLED-RELEASE): ADULTS, ELDERLY: Initially, 500 mg/day in 2 divided doses for 1 wk; then increase to 500 mg twice a day. Maintenance: 2 g/day.

NUTRITIONAL SUPPLEMENT

PO: ADULTS, ELDERLY: 10–20 mg/day. **Maximum:** 100 mg/day.

PELLAGRA

PO (IMMEDIATE-RELEASE): ADULTS, ELDERLY: 50–100 mg 3–4 times a day. **Maximum:** 500 mg/day. **CHILDREN:** 50–100 mg 3 times a day.

SIDE EFFECTS

FREQUENT: Flushing (esp. face, neck) occurring within 20 min of drug administration and lasting for 30–60 min, GI upset, pruritus. **OCCASIONAL:** Dizziness, hypotension, headache, blurred vision, burning/tingling of skin, flatulence, nausea, vomiting, diarrhea. **RARE:** Hyperglycemia, glycosuria, rash, hyperpigmentation, dry skin.

ADVERSE EFFECTS/ TOXIC REACTIONS

Arrhythmias occur rarely.

NURSING CONSIDERATIONS

BASELINE ASSESSMENT

Question for history of hypersensitivity to niacin, tartrazine, aspirin. Assess serum baselines, cholesterol, triglyceride, glucose, hepatic function tests.

INTERVENTION/EVALUATION

Evaluate flushing, degree of GI discomfort. Check for headache, dizziness, blurred vision. Monitor daily pattern of bowel activity/stool consistency. Monitor hepatic function, serum cholesterol, triglycerides. Check serum glucose carefully in those on insulin, oral antihyperglycemics. Assess skin for rash, dryness. Monitor serum uric acid.

PATIENT/FAMILY TEACHING

• Transient flushing of the skin, sensation of warmth, pruritus, tingling may occur. • Notify physician if dizziness occurs (avoid sudden changes in posture). • Inform physician if nausea, vomiting, loss of appetite, yellowing of skin, dark urine, feeling of weakness occurs. • Advise pt to take aspirin 30 min before taking extended-release niacin to minimize flushing.

N

Niaspan, *see niacin, nicotinic acid*

*niCARdipine

nigh-**car**-dih-peen

(Cardene, Cardene IV, Cardene SR)

Do not confuse nicardipine with nifedipine, Cardene with codeine, or Cardene SR with Cardizem SR or codeine.

CLASSIFICATION

PHARMACOTHERAPEUTIC: Calcium channel blocker. **CLINICAL:** Antianginal, antihypertensive (see p. 73C).

ACTION

Inhibits calcium ion movement across cell membranes, depressing contraction of cardiac, vascular smooth muscle. **Therapeutic Effect:** Increases heart rate, cardiac output. Decreases systemic vascular resistance, B/P.

PHARMACOKINETICS

Route	Onset	Peak	Duration
PO	N/A	1–2 hrs	8 hrs

Rapidly, completely absorbed from GI tract. Protein binding: 95%. Undergoes first-pass metabolism in liver. Primarily excreted in urine. Not removed by hemodialysis. **Half-life:** 2–4 hrs.

USES

PO: Treatment of chronic stable (effort-associated) angina, essential hypertension. **Sustained-Release:** Treatment of essential hypertension. **Parenteral:** Short-term treatment of hypertension when oral therapy not feasible or desirable. **OFF-LABEL:** Treatment of associated neurologic deficits, Raynaud's phenomenon, subarachnoid hemorrhage, vasospastic angina.

PRECAUTIONS

CONTRAINDICATIONS: Atrial fibrillation/flutter associated with accessory conduction pathways, cardiogenic shock, CHF, second- or third-degree heart block, severe hypotension, sinus bradycardia, ventricular tachycardia, within several hours of IV beta-blocker therapy. **CAUTIONS:** Sick sinus syndrome, severe left ventricular dysfunction, renal/hepatic impairment, cardiomyopathy, edema, concomitant beta-blocker or digoxin therapy.

LIFESPAN CONSIDERATIONS:

Pregnancy/Lactation: Unknown if distributed in breast milk. **Pregnancy Category C. Children:** Safety and efficacy not established. **Elderly:** Age-related renal impairment may require dosage adjustment.

INTERACTIONS

DRUG: **Beta-blockers** may have additive effect. **Digoxin** may increase concentration. **Hypokalemia-producing agents (e.g., furosemide, other diuretics)** may increase risk of arrhythmias. **Procainamide, quinidine** may increase risk of QT-interval prolongation. **HERBAL:** **Ephedra, garlic, yohimbe, ginseng** may increase hypertension. **Licorice** may cause retention of sodium, water; may increase loss of potassium. **FOOD:** **Grapefruit, grapefruit juice** may alter absorption. **LAB VALUES:** None known.

AVAILABILITY (Rx)

CAPSULES (CARDENE): 20 mg, 30 mg. **INJECTION SOLUTION (CARDENE IV):** 2.5 mg/ml.

CAPSULES (SUSTAINED-RELEASE [CARDENE SR]): 30 mg, 45 mg, 60 mg.

ADMINISTRATION/HANDLING

IV

Reconstitution • Dilute each 25-mg ampule with 250 ml D_5W, 0.9% NaCl, 0.45% NaCl, or any combination thereof to provide concentration of 1 mg/10 ml. **Maximum Concentration:** 4 mg/10 ml.

Rate of administration • Give by slow IV infusion. • Change IV site q12h if administered peripherally.

Storage • Store at room temperature. • Diluted IV solution is stable for 24 hrs at room temperature.

PO

• Do not crush/break sustained-release capsules. • Give without regard to food.

IV INCOMPATIBILITIES

Furosemide (Lasix), heparin, thiopental (Pentothal).

IV COMPATIBILITIES

Diltiazem (Cardizem), dobutamine (Dobutrex), dopamine (Intropin), epinephrine, hydromorphone (Dilaudid), labetalol (Trandate), lorazepam (Ativan), midazolam (Versed), milrinone (Primacor), morphine, nitroglycerin, norepinephrine (Levophed).

INDICATIONS/ROUTES/DOSAGE

CHRONIC STABLE ANGINA

PO: ADULTS, ELDERLY: Initially, 20 mg 3 times a day. Range: 20–40 mg 3 times a day.

ESSENTIAL HYPERTENSION

PO: ADULTS, ELDERLY: Initially, 20 mg 3 times a day. Range: 20–40 mg 3 times a day.

PO (SUSTAINED-RELEASE): ADULTS, ELDERLY: Initially, 30 mg twice a day. Range: 30–60 mg twice a day.

SHORT-TERM TREATMENT OF HYPERTENSION (PARENTERAL DOSAGE AS SUBSTITUTE FOR ORAL NICARDIPINE)

IV: ADULTS, ELDERLY: 0.5 mg/hr (for pt receiving 20 mg PO q8h); 1.2 mg/hr (for pt receiving 30 mg PO q8h); 2.2 mg/hr (for pt receiving 40 mg PO q8h).

PTS NOT ALREADY RECEIVING NICARDIPINE

IV: ADULTS, ELDERLY (GRADUAL B/P DECREASE): Initially, 5 mg/hr. May increase by 2.5 mg/hr q15min. After B/P goal is achieved, decrease rate to 3 mg/hr. **ADULTS, ELDERLY (RAPID B/P DECREASE):** Initially, 5 mg/hr. May increase by 2.5 mg/hr q5min. **Maximum:** 15 mg/hr until desired B/P attained. After B/P goal achieved, decrease rate to 3 mg/hr.

CHANGING FROM IV TO ORAL ANTIHYPERTENSIVE THERAPY

ADULTS, ELDERLY: Begin antihypertensives other than nicardipine when IV has been discontinued; for nicardipine, give first dose 1 hr before discontinuing IV.

DOSAGE IN HEPATIC IMPAIRMENT

For adults and elderly pts, initially give 20 mg twice a day; then titrate.

DOSAGE IN RENAL IMPAIRMENT

For adults and elderly pts, initially give 20 mg q8h (30 mg twice a day [sustained-release capsules]); then titrate.

SIDE EFFECTS

FREQUENT (10%–7%): Headache, facial flushing, peripheral edema, light-headedness, dizziness. **OCCASIONAL (6%–3%):** Asthenia (loss of strength, energy), palpitations, angina, tachycardia. **RARE (less than 2%):** Nausea, abdominal cramps, dyspepsia (heartburn, indigestion, epigastric pain), dry mouth, rash.

ADVERSE EFFECTS/ TOXIC REACTIONS

Overdose produces confusion, slurred speech, drowsiness, marked hypotension, bradycardia.

NURSING CONSIDERATIONS

BASELINE ASSESSMENT

Concurrent therapy of sublingual nitroglycerin may be used for relief of anginal pain. Record onset, type (sharp, dull, squeezing), radiation, location, intensity, duration of anginal pain, precipitating factors (exertion, emotional stress).

N

INTERVENTION/EVALUATION

Monitor B/P during and following IV infusion. Assess for peripheral edema behind medial malleolus. Assess skin for facial flushing, dermatitis, rash. Question for asthenia, headache. Monitor serum hepatic enzyme results. Assess EKG, pulse for tachycardia.

PATIENT/FAMILY TEACHING

• Take sustained-release capsule with food; do not crush. • Avoid alcohol, limit caffeine. • Inform physician if angina pains not relieved or palpitations, shortness of breath, swelling, dizziness, constipation, nausea, hypotension occurs.

nicotine

nik-o-teen

(Commit, Habitrol ✤, NicoDerm ✤, NicoDerm CQ, Nicorette, Nicorette Plus ✤, Nicotrol, Nicotrol Inhaler, Nicotrol NS, Nicotrol Patch)

Do not confuse Nicoderm with Nitroderm.

CLASSIFICATION

PHARMACOTHERAPEUTIC: Cholinergic-receptor agonist. **CLINICAL:** Smoking deterrent.

ACTION

Binds to acetylcholine receptors, producing both stimulating, depressant effects on peripheral, central nervous systems. **Therapeutic Effect:** Provides source of nicotine during nicotine withdrawal, reduces withdrawal symptoms.

PHARMACOKINETICS

Absorbed slowly after transdermal administration. Protein binding: 5%. Metabolized in liver. Excreted primarily in urine. **Half-life:** 4 hrs.

USES

Alternative, less potent form of nicotine (without tar, carbon monoxide, carcinogenic substances of tobacco) used as part of smoking cessation program.

PRECAUTIONS

CONTRAINDICATIONS: Immediate post-MI period, life-threatening arrhythmias, severe or worsening angina. **CAUTIONS:** Hyperthyroidism, pheochromocytoma, insulin-dependent diabetes mellitus, severe renal impairment, eczematous dermatitis, oral/pharyngeal inflammation, esophagitis, peptic ulcer (delays healing in peptic ulcer disease).

⌛ LIFESPAN CONSIDERATIONS:

Pregnancy/Lactation: Passes freely into breast milk. Use of cigarettes, nicotine gum associated with decrease in fetal breathing movements. **Pregnancy Category D (transdermal) X (chewing gum). Children:** Not recommended. **Elderly:** Age-related decrease in cardiac function may require dosage adjustment.

INTERACTIONS

DRUG: Smoking cessation, decreased dosage of nicotine may increase effects of **beta-adrenergic blockers, bronchodilators (e.g., theophylline), insulin, propoxyphene. HERBAL:** None significant. **FOOD:** None known. **LAB VALUES:** None known.

AVAILABILITY (OTC)

CHEWING GUM (NICORETTE): 2 mg, 4 mg. **INHALATION (NICOTROL INHALER):** 10 mg cartridge. **LOZENGE (COMMIT):** 2 mg, 4 mg. **NASAL SPRAY (NICOTROL NS):** 0.5 mg/spray. **TRANSDERMAL PATCH (NICODERM CQ, NICOTROL PATCH):** 5 mg/16 hrs, 7 mg/24 hrs, 10 mg/16 hrs, 14 mg/24 hrs, 21 mg/24 hrs mg.

ADMINISTRATION/HANDLING

GUM

• Do not swallow. • Chew 1 piece when urge to smoke present. • Chew slowly and intermittently for 30 min. • Chew until distinctive nicotine taste (peppery) or slight tingling in mouth perceived, then stop; when tingling almost gone (about 1 min) repeat chewing procedure (this allows constant slow buccal absorption). • Too-rapid chewing may cause excessive release of nicotine, resulting in adverse effects similar to oversmoking (e.g., nausea, throat irritation).

INHALER

• Insert cartridge into mouthpiece. • Puff on nicotine cartridge mouthpiece for 20 min.

TRANSDERMAL

• Apply promptly upon removal from protective pouch (prevents evaporation, loss of nicotine). Use only intact pouch. Do not cut patch. • Apply only once/day to hairless, clean, dry skin on upper body, outer arm. • Replace daily; rotate sites; do not use same site within 7 days; do not use same patch longer than 24 hrs. • Wash hands with water alone after applying patch (soap may increase nicotine absorption). • Discard used patch by folding patch in half (sticky side together), placing in pouch of new patch, and throwing away in such a way as to prevent child or pet accessibility.

INDICATIONS/ROUTES/DOSAGE

SMOKING CESSATION AID TO RELIEVE NICOTINE WITHDRAWAL SYMPTOMS

PO (CHEWING GUM): ADULTS, ELDERLY: Usually, 10–12 pieces/day. **Maximum:** 30 pieces/day.

PO (LOZENGE):

◄ **ALERT** ► For those who smoke the first cigarette within 30 min of waking, administer the 4-mg lozenge; otherwise administer the 2-mg lozenge.

ADULTS, ELDERLY: One 4-mg or 2-mg lozenge q1–2h for the first 6 wks; 1 lozenge q2–4h for wks 7–9; and 1 lozenge q4–8h for wks 10–12. **Maximum:** 1 lozenge at a time, 5 lozenges/6 hrs, 20 lozenges/day.

TRANSDERMAL: ADULTS, ELDERLY WHO SMOKE 10 CIGARETTES OR MORE PER DAY: Follow the guidelines below. **Step 1:** 21 mg/day for 4–6 wks. **Step 2:** 14 mg/day for 2 wks. **Step 3:** 7 mg/day for 2 wks. **ADULTS, ELDERLY WHO SMOKE LESS THAN 10 CIGARETTES PER DAY:** Follow the guidelines below. **Step 1:** 14 mg/day for 6 wks. **Step 2:** 7 mg/day for 2 wks. **PTS WEIGHING LESS THAN 100 LB, PTS WITH A HISTORY OF CARDIOVASCULAR DISEASE:** Initially, 14 mg/day for 4–6 wks, then 7 mg/day for 2–4 wks.

TRANSDERMAL (NICOTROL): ADULTS, ELDERLY: One patch a day for 6 wks.

NASAL: ADULTS, ELDERLY: 1–2 doses/hr (1 dose = 2 sprays [1 in each nostril] = 1 mg). **Maximum:** 5 doses (5 mg)/hr; 40 doses (40 mg)/day.

INHALER (NICOTROL): ADULTS, ELDERLY: Puff on nicotine cartridge mouthpiece for about 20 min as needed.

SIDE EFFECTS

FREQUENT: All forms: Hiccups, nausea. **Gum:** Mouth/throat soreness, nausea, hiccups. **Transdermal:** Erythema, pruritus, burning at application site. **OCCASIONAL: All forms:** Eructation, GI upset, dry mouth, insomnia, diaphoresis, irritability. **Gum:** Hiccups, hoarseness. **Inhaler:** Mouth/throat irritation, cough. **RARE: All forms:** Dizziness, myalgia, arthralgia.

ADVERSE EFFECTS/ TOXIC REACTIONS

Overdose produces palpitations, tachyarrhythmias, seizures, depression, confusion, diaphoresis, hypotension, rapid/weak pulse, dyspnea. Lethal dose for adults is 40–60 mg. Death results from respiratory paralysis.

NURSING CONSIDERATIONS

BASELINE ASSESSMENT

Screen, evaluate those with coronary heart disease (history of MI, angina pectoris), serious cardiac arrhythmias, Buerger's disease, Prinzmetal's variant angina.

INTERVENTION/EVALUATION

Monitor smoking habit, B/P, pulse, sleep pattern, skin for erythema, pruritus, burning at application site if transdermal system used.

PATIENT/FAMILY TEACHING

• Instruct pt on proper application of transdermal system. • Inform pt to chew gum slowly to avoid jaw ache, maximize benefit. • Inform physician if persistent rash, pruritus occurs with patch. • Do not smoke while wearing patches.

*NIFEdipine

nye-**fed**-i-peen

(Adalat CC, Adalat XL ♣, Apo-Nifed ♣, Nifediac CC, Nifedical XL, Novo-Nifedin ♣, Procardia, Procardia XL)

Do not confuse nifedipine with nicardipine or nimodipine.

◆CLASSIFICATION

PHARMACOTHERAPEUTIC: Calcium channel blocker. **CLINICAL:** Antianginal, antihypertensive (see p. 73C).

ACTION

Inhibits calcium ion movement across cell membranes, depressing contraction of cardiac, vascular smooth muscle. **Therapeutic Effect:** Increases heart rate, cardiac output. Decreases systemic vascular resistance, B/P.

PHARMACOKINETICS

Route	Onset	Peak	Duration
Sublingual	1–5 min	N/A	N/A
PO	20–30 min	N/A	4–8 hrs
PO (extended release)	2 hrs	N/A	24 hrs

Rapidly, completely absorbed from GI tract. Protein binding: 92%–98%. Undergoes first-pass metabolism in liver. Primarily excreted in urine. Not removed by hemodialysis. **Half-life:** 2–5 hrs.

USES

Treatment of angina due to coronary artery spasm (Prinzmetal's variant angina), chronic stable angina (effort-associated angina). **Extended-Release:** Treatment of essential hypertension. **OFF-LABEL:** Treatment of Raynaud's phenomenon, pulmonary hypertension.

PRECAUTIONS

CONTRAINDICATIONS: Advanced aortic stenosis, severe hypotension. **CAUTIONS:** Renal/hepatic impairment.

⧗ LIFESPAN CONSIDERATIONS:

Pregnancy/Lactation: Insignificant amount distributed in breast milk. **Pregnancy Category C. Children:** Safety and efficacy not established. **Elderly:** Age-related renal impairment may require dosage adjustment.

INTERACTIONS

DRUG: Beta-blockers may have additive effect. May increase **digoxin** concentration, risk of toxicity. **Hypokalemia-producing agents (e.g., furosemide, other diuretics)** may increase risk of arrhythmias. **HERBAL: Ephedra, garlic, yohimbe, ginseng** may increase hypertension. **Licorice** may cause retention of sodium, water; may increase loss of potassium. **FOOD: Grapefruit, grapefruit juice** may increase concentration. **LAB VALUES:** May cause positive ANA, direct Coombs' test.

AVAILABILITY (Rx)

CAPSULES (PROCARDIA): 10 mg.

TABLETS, EXTENDED-RELEASE: (Adalat CC, Nifediac CC, Nifedical XL, Procardia XL): 30 mg, 60 mg, 90 mg.

ADMINISTRATION/HANDLING

PO

• Do not crush/break extended-release tablet. • Give without regard to meals. • Grapefruit juice may alter absorption.

SUBLINGUAL

• Capsule must be punctured, chewed, and/or squeezed to express liquid into mouth.

INDICATIONS/ROUTES/DOSAGE

PRINZMETAL'S VARIANT ANGINA, CHRONIC STABLE (EFFORT-ASSOCIATED) ANGINA

PO: ADULTS, ELDERLY: Initially, 10 mg 3 times a day. Increase at 7- to 14-day intervals. Maintenance: 10 mg 3 times a day up to 30 mg 4 times a day.
PO (EXTENDED-RELEASE): ADULTS, ELDERLY: Initially, 30–60 mg/day. May increase at 7- to 14-day intervals. **Maximum:** 120–180 mg/day.

ESSENTIAL HYPERTENSION

PO (EXTENDED-RELEASE): ADULTS, ELDERLY: Initially, 30–60 mg/day. May increase at 7- to 14-day intervals. **Maximum:** 120–180 mg/day.

SIDE EFFECTS

FREQUENT (30%–11%): Peripheral edema, headache, flushed skin, dizziness. **OCCASIONAL (12%–6%):** Nausea, shakiness, muscle cramps/pain, drowsiness, palpitations, nasal congestion, cough, dyspnea, wheezing. **RARE (5%–3%):** Hypotension, rash, pruritus, urticaria, constipation, abdominal discomfort, flatulence, sexual dysfunction.

ADVERSE EFFECTS/ TOXIC REACTIONS

May precipitate CHF, MI in pts with cardiac disease, peripheral ischemia. Overdose produces nausea, drowsiness, confusion, slurred speech.

NURSING CONSIDERATIONS

BASELINE ASSESSMENT

Concurrent therapy of sublingual nitroglycerin may be used for relief of anginal pain. Record onset, type (sharp, dull, squeezing), radiation, location, intensity, duration of anginal pain; precipitating factors (exertion, emotional stress). check B/P for hypotension immediately before giving medication.

INTERVENTION/EVALUATION

Assist with ambulation if lightheadedness, dizziness occurs. Assess for peripheral edema. Assess skin for flushing. Monitor serum hepatic enzymes.

PATIENT/ FAMILY TEACHING

• Rise slowly from lying to sitting position, permit legs to dangle from bed momentarily before standing to reduce hypotensive effect. • Contact physician if palpitations, shortness of breath, pronounced dizziness, nausea occurs. • Avoid alcohol, concomitant grapefruit, grapefruit juice use.

nilutamide

nih-**lute**-ah-myd
(Anandron 🍁, Nilandron)

CLASSIFICATION

PHARMACOTHERAPEUTIC: Hormone.
CLINICAL: Antineoplastic (see p. 82C).

ACTION

Competitively inhibits androgen activity by binding to androgen receptors in target tissue. **Therapeutic Effect:** Decreases growth of abnormal prostate tissue.

PHARMACOKINETICS

Well absorbed following PO administration. Protein binding: 80%–84%.

Metabolized in liver. Primarily excreted in urine. **Half-life:** 38–59 hrs.

USES

Treatment of metastatic prostatic carcinoma (stage D_2) in combination with surgical castration. For maximum benefit, begin on same day or day after surgical castration.

PRECAUTIONS

CONTRAINDICATIONS: Severe hepatic impairment, severe respiratory insufficiency. **CAUTIONS:** Hepatitis, marked increase in serum hepatic enzymes.

LIFESPAN CONSIDERATIONS:

Children: Safety and efficacy not established. **Elderly:** No age-related precautions noted.

INTERACTIONS

DRUG: May increase effect of **warfarin.** May increase concentration, risk of toxicity with **fosphenytoin, phenytoin, theophylline. HERBAL: St. John's wort** may decrease concentration. **FOOD:** None known. **LAB VALUES:** May increase serum bilirubin, creatinine, AST, ALT.

AVAILABILITY (Rx)

TABLETS: 150 mg.

INDICATIONS/ROUTES/DOSAGE

PROSTATIC CARCINOMA

PO: ADULTS, ELDERLY: 300 mg once a day for 30 days, then 150 mg once a day. Begin on day of, or day after, surgical castration.

SIDE EFFECTS

FREQUENT (greater than 10%): Hot flashes, delay in recovering vision after bright illumination (e.g., sun, television, bright lights), decreased libido, diminished sexual function, mild nausea, gynecomastia, alcohol intolerance. **OCCASIONAL (less than 10%):** Constipation, hypertension, dizziness, dyspnea, UTI.

ADVERSE EFFECTS/ TOXIC REACTIONS

Interstitial pneumonitis occurs rarely.

NURSING CONSIDERATIONS

BASELINE ASSESSMENT

Baseline chest x-ray, hepatic enzymes should be obtained before beginning therapy.

INTERVENTION/EVALUATION

Monitor B/P periodically and hepatic function tests in long-term therapy.

PATIENT/FAMILY TEACHING

• Contact physician if any side effects occur at home, esp. signs of hepatic toxicity (jaundice, dark urine, fatigue, abdominal pain). • Caution about driving at night (tinted glasses may help).

nimodipine

nye-**mode**-i-peen
(Nimotop)

Do not confuse nimodipine with nifedipine.

CLASSIFICATION

PHARMACOTHERAPEUTIC: Calcium channel blocker. **CLINICAL:** Cerebral vasospasm agent (see p. 73C).

ACTION

Inhibits movement of calcium ions across vascular smooth-muscle cell membranes. **Therapeutic Effect:** Produces favorable effect on severity of neurologic deficits due to cerebral vasospasm. Exerts greatest effect on cerebral arteries; may prevent cerebral spasm.

PHARMACOKINETICS

Rapidly absorbed from GI tract. Protein binding: 95%. Metabolized in liver. Excreted in urine; eliminated in feces. Not removed by hemodialysis. **Half-life:** terminal, 3 hrs.

USES

Improvement of neurologic deficits due to cerebral vasospasm following subarachnoid hemorrhage from ruptured congenital intracranial aneurysms in pts in satisfactory neurologic condition. **OFF-LABEL:** Treatment of chronic and classic migraine, chronic cluster headaches.

PRECAUTIONS

CONTRAINDICATIONS: Atrial fibrillation/flutter, cardiogenic shock, CHF, heart block, sinus bradycardia, ventricular tachycardia, within several hours of IV beta-blocker therapy. **CAUTIONS:** Renal/hepatic impairment.

LIFESPAN CONSIDERATIONS:

Pregnancy/Lactation: Unknown if drug crosses placenta or is distributed in breast milk. **Pregnancy Category C.** **Children:** Safety and efficacy not established. **Elderly:** Age-related renal impairment may require dosage adjustment. May experience greater hypotensive response, constipation.

INTERACTIONS

DRUG: Beta-blockers may have additive effect, increase depression of cardiac SA/AV conduction. May increase **digoxin** concentration. **Agents inducing hypokalemia** may increase risk of arrhythmias. **Erythromycin, itraconazole, ketoconazole, protease inhibitors** may inhibit metabolism. **Rifabutin, rifampin** may increase metabolism. **HERBAL: Ephedra, garlic, yohimbe, ginseng** may increase hypertension. **Licorice** may cause retention of sodium, water; may increase loss of potassium. **FOOD: Grapefruit juice** may increase concentration, risk of toxicity. **LAB VALUES:** None known.

AVAILABILITY (Rx)

CAPSULES: 30 mg.

ADMINISTRATION/HANDLING

PO

- If pt unable to swallow, place hole in both ends of capsule with 18-gauge needle to extract contents into syringe.
- Empty into NG tube; flush tube with 30 ml normal saline.

INDICATIONS/ROUTES/DOSAGE

SUBARACHNOID HEMORRHAGE

PO: ADULTS, ELDERLY: 60 mg q4h for 21 days. Begin within 96 hrs of subarachnoid hemorrhage.

DOSAGE IN HEPATIC FAILURE

PO: ADULTS, ELDERLY: 30 mg q4h.

SIDE EFFECTS

OCCASIONAL (6%–2%): Hypotension, peripheral edema, diarrhea, headache. **RARE (less than 2%):** Allergic reaction (rash, urticaria), tachycardia, flushing of skin.

ADVERSE EFFECTS/ TOXIC REACTIONS

Overdose produces nausea, weakness, dizziness, somnolence, confusion, slurred speech.

NURSING CONSIDERATIONS

BASELINE ASSESSMENT

Assess level of consciousness (LOC), neurologic response, initially and throughout therapy. Monitor baseline hepatic function tests. Assess B/P, apical pulse immediately before drug administration (if pulse is 60/min or less or systolic B/P is less than 90 mm Hg, withhold medication, contact physician).

N

INTERVENTION/EVALUATION

Monitor CNS response, heart rate, B/P for evidence of hypotension, signs/symptoms of CHF.

PATIENT/FAMILY TEACHING

• Do not crush/chew capsules. • Inform physician if palpitations, shortness of breath, swelling, constipation, nausea, dizziness occurs.

nisoldipine

(Sular)

See Calcium channel blockers

nitazoxanide

nye-tah-**zocks**-ah-nide

(Alinia)

CLASSIFICATION

PHARMACOTHERAPEUTIC: Antiparasitic. **CLINICAL:** Antiprotozoal.

ACTION

Interferes with body's reaction to pyruvate ferredoxin oxidoreductase, an enzyme essential for anaerobic energy metabolism. **Therapeutic Effect:** Produces antiprotozoal activity, reducing/terminating diarrheal episodes.

PHARMACOKINETICS

Rapidly hydrolyzed to active metabolite. Protein binding: 99%. Excreted in urine, bile, feces. **Half-life:** 2–4 hrs.

USES

Treatment of diarrhea caused by *Cryptosporidium parvum, Giardia lamblia* in children 12 mos and older, adults.

PRECAUTIONS

CONTRAINDICATIONS: History of sensitivity to aspirin, salicylates. **CAUTIONS:** GI disorders, hepatic/biliary disease, renal impairment.

LIFESPAN CONSIDERATIONS:

Pregnancy/Lactation: Unknown if distributed in breast milk. **Pregnancy Category B. Children:** Safety and efficacy in children older than 11 yrs has not been established. **Elderly:** Not for use in this age group.

INTERACTIONS

DRUG: None significant. **HERBAL:** None significant. **FOOD:** None known. **LAB VALUES:** May increase serum creatinine, ALT.

AVAILABILITY (Rx)

POWDER FOR ORAL SUSPENSION: 100 mg/5 ml. **TABLETS:** 500 mg.

ADMINISTRATION/HANDLING

PO, ORAL SUSPENSION

• Store unreconstituted powder at room temperature. • Reconstitute oral suspension with 48 ml water to provide concentration of 100 mg/5 ml. • Shake vigorously to suspend powder. • Reconstituted solution is stable for 7 days at room temperature. • Give with food.

PO (TABLETS)

• Give with food.

INDICATIONS/ROUTES/DOSAGE

DIARRHEA CAUSED BY *C. PARVUM*

PO: ADULTS, ELDERLY, CHILDREN 4 YRS AND OLDER: 200 mg q12h for 3 days. **CHILDREN 12–47 MOS:** 100 mg q12h for 3 days.

DIARRHEA CAUSED BY *G. LAMBLIA*

PO: ADULTS, ELDERLY, CHILDREN 12 YRS AND OLDER: 500 mg q12h for 3 days. **CHILDREN 4–11 YRS:** 200 mg q12h for 3 days. **CHILDREN 12–47 MOS:** 100 mg q12h for 3 days.

SIDE EFFECTS

OCCASIONAL (8%): Abdominal pain. **RARE (2%–1%):** Diarrhea, vomiting, headache.

ADVERSE EFFECTS/ TOXIC REACTIONS

None known.

NURSING CONSIDERATIONS

BASELINE ASSESSMENT

Establish baseline B/P, weight, serum glucose, electrolytes. Assess for dehydration.

INTERVENTION/EVALUATION

Evaluate serum glucose in diabetics, electrolytes (therapy generally reduces abnormalities). Weigh pt daily. Encourage adequate fluid intake. Assess bowel sounds for peristalsis. Monitor daily pattern of bowel activity/stool consistency.

PATIENT/FAMILY TEACHING

• Parents of children with diabetes should be aware that the oral suspension contains 1.48 g of sucrose per 5 ml. • Therapy should provide significant improvement of diarrhea.

nitrofurantoin

ny-tro-feur-**an**-toyn
(Apo-Nitrofurantoin ✦, Furadantin, Macrobid, Macrodantin, Novo-Furantoin ✦)

CLASSIFICATION

PHARMACOTHERAPEUTIC: Antibacterial. **CLINICAL:** UTI prophylaxis.

ACTION

Inhibits synthesis of bacterial DNA, RNA, proteins, cell walls by altering, inactivating ribosomal proteins. **Therapeutic Effect:** Bacteriostatic (bactericidal at high concentrations).

PHARMACOKINETICS

Microcrystalline form rapidly, completely absorbed; macrocrystalline form more slowly absorbed. Food increases absorption. Protein binding: 40%. Primarily concentrated in urine, kidneys. Metabolized in most body tissues. Primarily excreted in urine. Removed by hemodialysis. **Half-life:** 20–60 min.

USES

Prevention/treatment of UTI caused by susceptible gram-negative, gram-positive organisms.

PRECAUTIONS

CONTRAINDICATIONS: Anuria, oliguria, substantial renal impairment (creatinine clearance less than 40 ml/min); infants younger than 1 mo because of risk of hemolytic anemia. **CAUTIONS:** Renal impairment, diabetes mellitus, electrolyte imbalance, anemia, vitamin B deficiency, debilitated (greater risk of peripheral neuropathy), G6PD deficiency (greater risk of hemolytic anemia).

LIFESPAN CONSIDERATIONS:

Pregnancy/Lactation: Readily crosses placenta. Distributed in breast milk. Contraindicated at term and during lactation when infant suspected of having G6PD deficiency. **Pregnancy Category B (contraindicated at term). Children:** No age-related precautions noted in those older than 1 mo. **Elderly:** More likely to develop acute pneumonitis, peripheral neuropathy. Age-related renal impairment may require dosage adjustment.

INTERACTIONS

DRUG: Hemolytics may increase risk of toxicity. **Neurotoxic medications** may increase risk of neurotoxicity.

N

Probenecid may increase concentration, risk of toxicity. **HERBAL:** None significant. **FOOD:** None known. **LAB VALUES:** None known.

AVAILABILITY (Rx)

CAPSULES (MACROCRYSTALLINE, MONOHYDRATE [MACROBID]): 100 mg. **CAPSULES (MACROCRYSTALLINE [MACRODANTIN, NITRO MACRO]):** 25 mg, 50 mg, 100 mg. **ORAL SUSPENSION (MICROCRYSTALLINE [FURADANTIN]):** 25 mg/5 ml.

ADMINISTRATION/HANDLING

PO

• Give with food, milk to enhance absorption, reduce GI upset.

INDICATIONS/ROUTES/DOSAGE

UTI

PO (FURADANTIN, MACRODANTIN): ADULTS, ELDERLY: 50–100 mg q6h. **Maximum:** 400 mg/day. **CHILDREN:** 5–7 mg/kg/day in divided doses q6h. **Maximum:** 400 mg/day.

PO (MACROBID): ADULTS, ELDERLY: 100 mg twice a day. **Maximum:** 400 mg/day.

LONG-TERM PREVENTION OF UTI

PO: ADULTS, ELDERLY: 50–100 mg at bedtime. **CHILDREN:** 1–2 mg/kg/day as a single dose. **Maximum:** 100 mg/day.

SIDE EFFECTS

FREQUENT: Anorexia, nausea, vomiting, dark urine. **OCCASIONAL:** Abdominal pain, diarrhea, rash, pruritus, urticaria, hypertension, headache, dizziness, drowsiness. **RARE:** Photosensitivity, transient alopecia, asthmatic exacerbation in those with history of asthma.

ADVERSE EFFECTS/ TOXIC REACTIONS

Superinfection, hepatotoxicity, peripheral neuropathy (may be irreversible), Stevens-Johnson syndrome, permanent pulmonary function impairment, anaphylaxis occur rarely.

NURSING CONSIDERATIONS

BASELINE ASSESSMENT

Question for history of asthma. Evaluate lab test results for renal/hepatic baseline values.

INTERVENTION/EVALUATION

Monitor I&O, renal function results. Monitor daily pattern of bowel activity/stool consistency. Assess skin for rash, urticaria. Be alert for numbness/tingling, esp. of lower extremities (may signal onset of peripheral neuropathy). Observe for signs of hepatotoxicity (fever, rash, arthralgia, hepatomegaly). Perform respiratory assessment: auscultate lungs, check for cough, chest pain, difficulty breathing.

PATIENT/FAMILY TEACHING

• Urine may become dark yellow/brown. • Take with food, milk for best results, reduce GI upset. • Complete full course of therapy. • Avoid sun, ultraviolet light; use sunscreens, wear protective clothing. • Notify physician if cough, fever, chest pain, difficult breathing, numbness/tingling of fingers, toes occurs. • Rare occurrence of alopecia is transient.

nitroglycerin

nye-troe-**gli**-ser-in

(Minitran, Nitrek, Nitro-Bid, Nitro-Dur, Nitrolingual, Nitrong, Nitro-Quick, Nitrostat, Nitro-Tab, Nitro-Time)

Do not confuse nitroglycerin with nitroprusside; Nitro-Bid with Nicobid; Nitro-Dur with Nicoderm; Nitrostat with Hyperstat, or Nilstat, or Nystatin.

CLASSIFICATION

PHARMACOTHERAPEUTIC: Nitrate. **CLINICAL:** Antianginal, antihypertensive, coronary vasodilator (see p. 122C).

ACTION

Decreases myocardial oxygen demand. Reduces left ventricular preload, afterload. **Therapeutic Effect:** Dilates coronary arteries, improves collateral blood flow to ischemic areas within myocardium. IV form produces peripheral vasodilation.

PHARMACOKINETICS

Route	Onset	Peak	Duration
Sublingual	1–3 min	4–8 min	30–60 min
Translingual spray	2 min	4–10 min	30–60 min
Buccal tablet	2–5 min	4–10 min	2 hrs
PO (extended-release)	20–45 min	45–120 min	4–8 hrs
Topical	15–60 min	30–120 min	2–12 hrs
Transdermal patch	40–60 min	60–180 min	18–24 hrs
IV	1–2 min	Immediate	3–5 min

Well absorbed after PO, sublingual, topical administration. Undergoes extensive first-pass metabolism. Metabolized in liver, by enzymes in bloodstream. Primarily excreted in urine. Not removed by hemodialysis. **Half-life:** 1–4 min.

USES

Lingual, sublingual, buccal dose used for acute relief of angina pectoris. Extended-release, topical forms used for prophylaxis, long-term angina management. IV form used in treatment of CHF, acute MI.

PRECAUTIONS

CONTRAINDICATIONS: Allergy to adhesives (transdermal), closed-angle glaucoma, constrictive pericarditis (IV), early MI (sublingual), GI hypermotility/malabsorption (extended-release), head trauma, hypotension (IV), inadequate cerebral circulation (IV), increased intracranial pressure (ICP), nitrates, orthostatic hypotension, pericardial tamponade (IV), severe anemia, uncorrected hypovolemia (IV). **CAUTIONS:** Acute MI, hepatic/renal disease, glaucoma (contraindicated in closed-angle glaucoma), blood volume depletion from diuretic therapy, systolic B/P less than 90 mm Hg.

LIFESPAN CONSIDERATIONS:

Pregnancy/Lactation: Unknown if drug crosses placenta or is distributed in breast milk. **Pregnancy Category B.** **Children:** Safety and efficacy not established. **Elderly:** More susceptible to hypotensive effects. Age-related renal impairment may require dosage adjustment.

INTERACTIONS

DRUG: **Alcohol, other antihypertensives, vasodilators** may increase risk of orthostatic hypotension. Concurrent use of **sildenafil, tadalafil, vardenafil** produces significant hypotension. **HERBAL:** None significant. **FOOD:** None known. **LAB VALUES:** May increase serum methemoglobin, urine catecholamine, urine vanillylmandelic acid concentrations.

AVAILABILITY (Rx)

INFUSION, PRE-MIX: 25 mg/250 ml, 50 mg/500 ml (0.1 mg/ml), 50 mg/250 ml (0.2 mg/ml), 100 mg/250 ml, 200 mg/500 ml (0.4 mg/ml). **INJECTION, SOLUTION:** 5 mg/ml. **OINTMENT: (NITRO-BID):** 2%. **SOLUTION, TRANSLINGUAL SPRAY: (NITROLINGUAL):** 0.4 mg/spray. **TRANSDERMAL PATCH: (MINITRAN, NITREK, NITRO-DUR):** 0.1 mg/hr, 0.2 mg/hr, 0.3 mg/hr, 0.4 mg/hr, 0.6 mg/hr, 0.8 mg/hr.

CAPSULE, EXTENDED-RELEASE: (NITRO-TIME): 2.5 mg, 6 mg, 9 mg.

TABLET, SUBLINGUAL: (NITROQUICK, NITROSTAT, NITRO-TAB): 0.4 mg.

ADMINISTRATION/HANDLING

◀ **ALERT** ▶ Cardioverter/defibrillator must not be discharged through paddle electrode overlying nitroglycerin (transdermal, ointment) system (may cause burns to pt or damage to paddle via arcing).

IV

Reconstitution • Available in ready-to-use injectable containers. • Dilute vials in 250 or 500 ml D_5W or 0.9% NaCl. Maximum concentration: 250 mg/250 ml.

Rate of administration • Use microdrop or infusion pump.

Storage • Store at room temperature.

PO

• Do not chew extended-release form. • Do not shake oral aerosol canister before lingual spraying.

SUBLINGUAL

• Do not swallow. • Dissolve under tongue. • Administer while seated. • Slight burning sensation under tongue may be lessened by placing tablet in buccal pouch. • Keep sublingual tablets in original container.

TOPICAL

• Spread thin layer on clean, dry, hairless skin of upper arm or body (not below knee or elbow), using applicator or dose-measuring papers. Do not use fingers; do not rub/massage into skin.

TRANSDERMAL

• Apply patch on clean, dry, hairless skin of upper arm or body (not below knee or elbow).

IV INCOMPATIBILITY

Alteplase (Activase).

IV COMPATIBILITIES

Amiodarone (Cordarone), diltiazem (Cardizem), dobutamine (Dobutrex), dopamine (Intropin), epinephrine, famotidine (Pepcid), fentanyl (Sublimaze), furosemide (Lasix), heparin, hydromorphone (Dilaudid), insulin, labetalol (Trandate), lidocaine, lipids, lorazepam (Ativan), midazolam (Versed), milrinone (Primacor), morphine, nicardipine (Cardene), nitroprusside (Nipride), norepinephrine (Levophed), propofol (Diprivan).

INDICATIONS/ROUTES/DOSAGE

ACUTE TREATMENT/PROPHYLAXIS OF ANGINA PECTORIS

LINGUAL SPRAY: ADULTS, ELDERLY: 1 spray onto or under tongue q3–5min until relief is noted (no more than 3 sprays in 15-min period).

SUBLINGUAL: ADULTS, ELDERLY: One tablet under tongue. If chest pain has not improved in 5 min, call 911. After the call, may take additional tablet. A third tablet may be taken 5 min after second dose (Maximum of 3 tablets).

LONG-TERM PROPHYLAXIS OF ANGINA

PO (EXTENDED-RELEASE): ADULTS, ELDERLY: 2.5–9 mg 2–4 times a day. **Maximum:** 26 mg 4 times a day.

TOPICAL: ADULTS, ELDERLY: Initially, ½ inch q8h. Increase by ½ inch with each application. Range: 1–2 inches q8h up to 4–5 inches q4h.

TRANSDERMAL PATCH: ADULTS, ELDERLY: Initially, 0.2–0.4 mg/hr. Maintenance: 0.4–0.8 mg/hr. Consider patch on for 12–14 hrs, patch off for 10–12 hrs (prevents tolerance).

CHF, ACUTE MI

IV: ADULTS, ELDERLY: Initially, 5 mcg/min via infusion pump. Increase in 5-mcg/min increments at 3- to 5-min intervals until B/P response is noted or until dosage reaches 20 mcg/min; then increase as needed by 10 mcg/min. Dosage may be further titrated according to clinical, therapeutic response up to

200 mcg/min. **CHILDREN:** Initially, 0.25–0.5 mcg/kg/min; titrate by 0.5–1 mcg/kg/min up to 20 mcg/kg/min.

SIDE EFFECTS

FREQUENT: Headache (possibly severe; occurs mostly in early therapy, diminishes rapidly in intensity, usually disappears during continued treatment), transient flushing of face/neck, dizziness (esp. if pt is standing immobile or is in a warm environment), weakness, orthostatic hypotension. **Sublingual:** Burning, tingling sensation at oral point of dissolution. **Ointment:** Erythema, pruritus. **OCCASIONAL:** GI upset. **Transdermal:** Contact dermatitis.

ADVERSE EFFECTS/ TOXIC REACTIONS

Discontinue drug if blurred vision, dry mouth occurs. Severe orthostatic hypotension may occur, manifested by syncope, pulselessness, cold/clammy skin, diaphoresis. Tolerance may occur with repeated, prolonged therapy; minor tolerance may occur with intermittent use of sublingual tablets. High doses tend to produce severe headache.

NURSING CONSIDERATIONS

BASELINE ASSESSMENT

Record onset, type (sharp, dull, squeezing), radiation, location, intensity, duration of anginal pain; precipitating factors (exertion, emotional stress). Assess B/P, apical pulse before administration and periodically following dose. Pt must have continuous EKG monitoring for IV administration.

INTERVENTION/EVALUATION

Monitor B/P, heart rate. Assess for facial, neck flushing. Cardioverter/defibrillator must not be discharged through paddle electrode overlying nitroglycerin system (may cause burns to pt or damage to paddle via arcing).

PATIENT/FAMILY TEACHING

• Rise slowly from lying to sitting position, dangle legs momentarily before standing. • Take oral form on empty stomach (however, if headache occurs during therapy, take medication with meals). • Use spray only when lying down. • Dissolve sublingual tablet under tongue; do not swallow. • Take at first sign of angina. • May take another dose q5min if needed up to a total of 3 doses. • If not relieved within 5 min, contact physician or immediately go to emergency room. • Do not change brands. • Keep container away from heat, moisture. • Do not inhale lingual aerosol but spray onto or under tongue (avoid swallowing after spray is administered). • Expel from mouth any remaining lingual, sublingual, intrabuccal tablet after pain is completely relieved. • Place transmucosal tablets under upper lip or buccal pouch (between cheek and gum); do not chew/swallow tablet. • Avoid alcohol (intensifies hypotensive effect). If alcohol is ingested soon after taking nitroglycerin, possible acute hypotensive episode (marked drop in B/P, vertigo, diaphoresis, pallor) may occur.

nitroprusside ⚑

nye-troe-**pruss**-ide

(Nipride ✤, Nitropress)

Do not confuse nitroprusside with nitroglycerin or Nitrostat.

CLASSIFICATION

PHARMACOTHERAPEUTIC: Hypertensive emergency agent. **CLINICAL:** Antihypertensive, vasodilator, CHF/MI adjunct, antidote.

N

ACTION

Direct vasodilating action on arterial, venous smooth muscle. Decreases peripheral vascular resistance, preload, afterload; improves cardiac output. **Therapeutic Effect:** Dilates coronary arteries, decreases oxygen consumption, relieves persistent chest pain.

PHARMACOKINETICS

Route	Onset	Peak	Duration
IV	1–10 min	Dependent on infusion rate	Dissipates rapidly after stopping IV

Reacts with Hgb in erythrocytes, producing cyanmethemoglobin, cyanide ions. Primarily excreted in urine. **Half-life:** less than 10 min.

USES

Immediate reduction of B/P in hypertensive crisis. Produces controlled hypotension in surgical procedures to reduce bleeding. Treatment of acute CHF. **OFF-LABEL:** Control of paroxysmal hypertension before, during surgery for pheochromocytoma, peripheral vasospasm caused by ergot alkaloid overdose, treatment adjunct for MI, valvular regurgitation.

PRECAUTIONS

CONTRAINDICATIONS: Compensatory hypertension (AV shunt, coarctation of aorta), congenital (Leber's) optic atrophy, inadequate cerebral circulation, moribund pts, tobacco amblyopia. **CAUTIONS:** Severe hepatic/renal impairment, hypothyroidism, hyponatremia, elderly.

LIFESPAN CONSIDERATIONS:

Pregnancy/Lactation: Unknown if drug crosses placenta or is distributed in breast milk. **Pregnancy Category C.** **Children:** Safety and efficacy not established. **Elderly:** More sensitive to hypotensive effect. Age-related renal impairment may require dosage adjustment.

INTERACTIONS

DRUG: Dobutamine may increase cardiac output, decrease pulmonary wedge pressure. **Antihypertensives** may increase hypotensive effect. **HERBAL:** None significant. **FOOD:** None known. **LAB VALUES:** None known.

AVAILABILITY (Rx)

INJECTION SOLUTION: 25 mg/ml.

ADMINISTRATION/HANDLING

IV

Reconstitution • Dilute with 250–1,000 ml D_5W to provide concentration of 200 mcg, 50 mcg/ml, respectively. Maximum concentration: 200 mg/250 ml. • Wrap infusion bottle in aluminum foil immediately after mixing.

Rate of administration • Give by IV infusion only, using infusion rate chart provided by manufacturer or protocol. • Administer using IV infusion pump and lock in rate. • Be alert for extravasation (produces severe pain, sloughing).

Storage • Protect solution from light. • Solution should appear very faint brown. • Use only freshly prepared solution. Once prepared, do not keep or use longer than 24 hrs. • Deterioration evidenced by color change from brown to blue, green, dark red. • Discard unused portion.

IV INCOMPATIBILITY

Cisatracurium (Nimbex).

IV COMPATIBILITIES

Diltiazem (Cardizem), dobutamine (Dobutrex), dopamine (Intropin), enalapril (Vasotec), heparin, insulin, labetalol (Normodyne, Trandate), lidocaine, midazolam (Versed), milrinone (Primacor), nitroglycerin, propofol (Diprivan).

INDICATIONS/ROUTES/DOSAGE

USUAL PARENTERAL DOSAGE

IV INFUSION: ADULTS, ELDERLY: Initially, 0.3–0.5 mcg/kg/min. May increase by 0.5 mcg/kg/min to desired hemodynamic effect or appearance of headache, nausea. Usual dose: 3 mcg/kg/min. **Maximum:** 10 mcg/kg/min.

SIDE EFFECTS

OCCASIONAL: Flushing of skin, increased intracranial pressure, pruritus, pain/redness at injection site.

ADVERSE EFFECTS/ TOXIC REACTIONS

Too-rapid IV infusion rate reduces B/P too quickly. Nausea, vomiting, diaphoresis, apprehension, headache, restlessness, muscle twitching, dizziness, palpitations, retrosternal pain, abdominal pain may occur. Symptoms disappear rapidly if rate of administration is slowed or temporarily discontinued. Overdose produces metabolic acidosis, tolerance to therapeutic effect.

NURSING CONSIDERATIONS

BASELINE ASSESSMENT

Monitor EKG, B/P continuously. Check with physician for desired B/P parameters (B/P is normally maintained approximately 30%–40% below pretreatment levels). Medication should be discontinued if therapeutic response is not achieved within 10 min after IV infusion at 10 mcg/kg/min.

INTERVENTION/EVALUATION

Monitor rate of infusion frequently. Monitor blood acid-base balance, electrolytes, laboratory results, I&O. Assess for metabolic acidosis (weakness, disorientation, headache, nausea, hyperventilation, vomiting). Assess for therapeutic response to medication. Monitor B/P for potential rebound hypertension after infusion is discontinued.

nizatidine

ni-**za**-ti-deen

(Apo-Nizatidine ✤, Axid, Axid AR, Novo-Nizatidine ✤)

Do not confuse Axid with Ansaid.

CLASSIFICATION

PHARMACOTHERAPEUTIC: H_2 receptor antagonist. **CLINICAL:** Antiulcer, gastric acid secretion inhibitor (see p. 104C).

ACTION

Inhibits histamine action at histamine-2 (H_2) receptors of parietal cells. **Therapeutic Effect:** Inhibits basal/nocturnal gastric acid secretion.

PHARMACOKINETICS

Rapidly, well absorbed from GI tract. Protein binding: 35%. Metabolized in liver. Primarily excreted in urine. Not removed by hemodialysis. **Half-life:** 1–2 hrs (increased with renal impairment).

USES

Short-term treatment of active duodenal ulcer, active benign gastric ulcer. Prevention of duodenal ulcer recurrence. Treatment of gastroesophageal reflux disease (GERD), including erosive esophagitis. OTC for prevention of meal-induced heartburn, acid indigestion, sour stomach. **OFF-LABEL:** Gastric hypersecretory conditions, multiple endocrine adenoma, Zollinger-Ellison syndrome, weight gain reduction in pts taking Zyprexa. Part of multidrug therapy for *H. pylori* eradication used to reduce risk of duodenal ulcer recurrence.

PRECAUTIONS

CONTRAINDICATIONS: Hypersensitivity to other H_2-antagonists. **CAUTIONS:** Renal/hepatic impairment.

LIFESPAN CONSIDERATIONS:

Pregnancy/Lactation: Unknown if drug crosses placenta or is distributed in breast milk. **Pregnancy Category B.** **Children:** Safety and efficacy not established in those younger than 12 yrs. **Elderly:** No age-related precautions noted.

INTERACTIONS

DRUG: **Antacids** may decrease absorption (do not give within 1 hr). May decrease absorption of **itraconazole, ketoconazole** (separate by 2 hrs). **HERBAL:** None significant. **FOOD:** None known. **LAB VALUES:** Interferes with skin tests using allergen extracts. May increase serum alkaline phosphatase, AST, ALT.

AVAILABILITY (Rx)

CAPSULES: 75 mg (Axid AR [OTC]), 150 mg (Axid), 300 mg (Axid). **ORAL SOLUTION (AXID):** 15 mg/ml.

ADMINISTRATION/HANDLING

PO

• Give without regard to meals. Best given after meals or at bedtime. • Do not administer within 1 hr of magnesium- or aluminum-containing antacids (decreases absorption). • May give immediately before eating for heartburn prevention.

INDICATIONS/ROUTES/DOSAGE

ACTIVE DUODENAL ULCER

PO: ADULTS, ELDERLY: 300 mg at bedtime or 150 mg twice a day.

PREVENTION OF DUODENAL ULCER RECURRENCE

PO: ADULTS, ELDERLY: 150 mg at bedtime.

GASTROESOPHAGEAL REFLUX DISEASE

PO: ADULTS, ELDERLY: 150 mg twice a day.

ACTIVE BENIGN GASTRIC ULCER

PO: ADULTS, ELDERLY: 150 mg twice a day or 300 mg at bedtime.

PO, ORAL SOLUTION: CHILDREN 12 YRS AND OLDER: 150 mg twice a day.

DYSPEPSIA

PO: ADULTS, ELDERLY: 75 mg 30–60 min before meals; no more than 2 tablets a day.

DOSAGE IN RENAL IMPAIRMENT

Dosage adjustment is based on creatinine clearance.

Creatinine Clearance	Active Ulcer	Maintenance Therapy
20–50 ml/min	150 mg at bedtime	150 mg every other day
Less than 20 ml/min	150 mg every other day	150 mg q3days

SIDE EFFECTS

OCCASIONAL (2%): Somnolence, fatigue. **RARE (1%):** Diaphoresis, rash.

ADVERSE EFFECTS/ TOXIC REACTIONS

Asymptomatic ventricular tachycardia, hyperuricemia not associated with gout, nephrolithiasis occur rarely.

NURSING CONSIDERATIONS

INTERVENTION/EVALUATION

Assess for abdominal pain, GI bleeding (overt blood in emesis/stool, tarry stools). Monitor blood tests for elevated AST, ALT, serum alkaline phosphatase (hepatocellular injury).

PATIENT/ FAMILY TEACHING

• Avoid tasks that require alertness, motor skills until drug response is established. • Avoid alcohol, aspirin, smoking. • Inform physician if symptoms of heartburn, acid indigestion, sour stomach persist after 2 wks of continuous use of nizatidine.

Nolvadex, *see tamoxifen*

norepinephrine

nor-eh-pih-**nef**-rin
(Levophed)

Do not confuse Levophed with Levid, or norepinephrine with epinephrine.

CLASSIFICATION

PHARMACOTHERAPEUTIC: Sympathomimetic. **CLINICAL:** Vasopressor (see p. 148C).

ACTION

Stimulates $beta_1$-adrenergic receptors, alpha-adrenergic receptors, increasing peripheral resistance. Enhances contractile myocardial force, increases cardiac output. Constricts resistance, capacitance vessels. **Therapeutic Effect:** Increases systemic B/P, coronary blood flow.

PHARMACOKINETICS

Route	Onset	Peak	Duration
IV	Rapid	1–2 min	N/A

Localized in sympathetic tissue. Metabolized in liver. Primarily excreted in urine.

USES

Corrects hypotension unresponsive to adequate fluid volume replacement (as part of shock syndrome) caused by MI, bacteremia, open heart surgery, renal failure.

PRECAUTIONS

CONTRAINDICATIONS: Hypovolemic states (unless as an emergency measure), mesenteric/peripheral vascular thrombosis, profound hypoxia. **CAUTIONS:** Severe cardiac disease, hypertensive or hypothyroid pts, those taking MAOIs.

LIFESPAN CONSIDERATIONS:

Pregnancy/Lactation: Readily crosses placenta. May produce fetal anoxia due to uterine contraction, constriction of uterine blood vessels. **Pregnancy Category C.** **Children/Elderly:** No age-related precautions noted.

INTERACTIONS

DRUG: Beta-blockers may have mutually inhibitory effects. **Digoxin** may increase risk of arrhythmias. **Ergonovine, oxytocin** may increase vasoconstriction. **MAOIs** may cause prolonged hypertension. **Maprotiline, tricyclic antidepressants** may increase cardiovascular effects. May decrease effects of **methyldopa.** **HERBAL:** None significant. **FOOD:** None known. **LAB VALUES:** None known.

AVAILABILITY (Rx)

INJECTION SOLUTION: 1-mg/ml ampules.

ADMINISTRATION/HANDLING

◄ **ALERT** ► Blood, fluid volume depletion should be corrected before drug is administered.

IV

Reconstitution • Add 4 ml (4 mg) to 250 ml (16 mcg/ml). Maximum concentration: 32 ml (32 mg) to 250 ml (128 mcg/ml).

Rate of administration • Closely monitor IV infusion flow rate (use infusion pump). • Monitor B/P q2min during IV infusion until desired therapeutic response is achieved, then q5min during remaining IV infusion. • Never leave pt unattended. • Maintain B/P at

N

80–100 mm Hg in previously normotensive pts, and 30–40 mm Hg below preexisting B/P in previously hypertensive pts. • Reduce IV infusion gradually. Avoid abrupt withdrawal. • If using peripherally inserted catheter, it is imperative to check the IV site frequently for free flow and infused vein for blanching, hardness to vein, coldness, pallor to extremity. • If extravasation occurs, area should be infiltrated with 10–15 ml sterile saline containing 5–10 mg phentolamine (does not alter pressor effects of norepinephrine).

Storage • Do not use if brown or contains precipitate. • Store ampules at room temperature.

IV INCOMPATIBILITY

Regular insulin.

IV COMPATIBILITIES

Amiodarone (Cordarone), calcium gluconate, diltiazem (Cardizem), dobutamine (Dobutrex), dopamine (Intropin), epinephrine, esmolol (Brevibloc), fentanyl (Sublimaze), furosemide (Lasix), haloperidol (Haldol), heparin, hydromorphone (Dilaudid), labetalol (Trandate), lipids, lorazepam (Ativan), magnesium, midazolam (Versed), milrinone (Primacor), morphine, nicardipine (Cardene), nitroglycerin, potassium chloride, propofol (Diprivan).

INDICATIONS/ROUTES/DOSAGE

ACUTE HYPOTENSION UNRESPONSIVE TO FLUID VOLUME REPLACEMENT

IV: ADULTS, ELDERLY: Initially, administer at 0.5–1 mcg/min. Adjust rate of flow to establish and maintain desired B/P (40 mm Hg below preexisting systolic pressure). Average maintenance dose: 8–30 mcg/min. **CHILDREN:** Initially, 0.05–0.1 mcg/kg/min; titrate to desired effect. **Maximum:** 1–2 mcg/kg/min. Range: 0.5–3 mcg/min.

SIDE EFFECTS

Norepinephrine produces less pronounced, less frequent side effects than epinephrine. **OCCASIONAL (5%–3%):** Anxiety, bradycardia, palpitations. **RARE (2%–1%):** Nausea, anginal pain, shortness of breath, fever.

ADVERSE EFFECTS/ TOXIC REACTIONS

Extravasation may produce tissue necrosis, sloughing. Overdose manifested as severe hypertension with violent headache (may be first clinical sign of overdose), arrhythmias, photophobia, retrosternal or pharyngeal pain, pallor, diaphoresis, vomiting. Prolonged therapy may result in plasma volume depletion. Hypotension may recur if plasma volume is not maintained.

NURSING CONSIDERATIONS

BASELINE ASSESSMENT

Assess EKG, B/P continuously (be alert to precipitous B/P drop). Never leave pt alone during IV infusion. Be alert to pt complaint of headache.

INTERVENTION/EVALUATION

Monitor IV flow rate diligently. Assess for extravasation characterized by blanching of skin over vein, coolness (results from local vasoconstriction); color, temperature of IV site extremity (pallor, cyanosis, mottling). Assess nailbed capillary refill. Monitor I&O; measure output hourly, report urine output less than 30 ml/hr. IV should not be reinstated unless systolic B/P falls below 70–80 mm Hg.

norfloxacin

nor-**flox**-a-sin
(Apo-Norflox ✤, Norfloxacine ✤, Noroxin, Novo-Norfloxacin ✤, PMS-Norfloxacin ✤)

CLASSIFICATION

PHARMACOTHERAPEUTIC: Quinolone. **CLINICAL:** Anti-infective (see p. 24C).

ACTION

Interferes with bacterial cell replication by inhibiting DNA-gyrase in susceptible microorganisms. **Therapeutic Effect:** Bactericidal.

USES

Treatment of susceptible infections due to *E. faecalis, E. coli, K. pneumoniae, P. mirabilis, P. aeruginosa, S. epidermidis, S. saprophyticus,* including UTIs, uncomplicated gonococcal infections, acute or chronic prostatitis.

PRECAUTIONS

CONTRAINDICATIONS: Children younger than 18 yrs (increased risk of arthropathy), hypersensitivity to other quinolones or their components. **CAUTIONS:** Renal impairment, predisposition to seizures.

LIFESPAN CONSIDERATIONS:

Pregnancy/Lactation: Unknown if drug crosses placenta or is distributed in breast milk. **Pregnancy Category C.** **Children:** Safety and efficacy not established. **Elderly:** Age-related renal impairment may require dosage adjustment.

INTERACTIONS

DRUG: **Antacids, sucralfate** may decrease absorption. May increase effects of **oral anticoagulants. Didanosine** may decrease absorption, effect. Decreases clearance of **theophylline,** may increase concentration, risk of toxicity. **HERBAL:** **Dong quai, St. John's wort** may increase risk of photosensitization. **FOOD:** None known. **LAB VALUES:** May increase BUN, serum alkaline phosphatase, bilirubin, creatinine, LDH, AST, ALT.

AVAILABILITY (Rx)

TABLETS: 400 mg.

ADMINISTRATION/HANDLING

PO

• Give 1 hr before or 2 hrs after meals with 8 oz of water. • Encourage additional glasses of water between meals. • Do not administer antacids with or within 2 hrs of norfloxacin dose. • Encourage cranberry juice, citrus fruits (to acidify urine).

INDICATIONS/ROUTES/DOSAGE

UTI

PO: ADULTS, ELDERLY: 400 mg twice a day for 3–21 days.

PROSTATITIS

PO: ADULTS: 400 mg twice a day for 28 days.

GONORRHEA

PO: ADULTS, ELDERLY: 800 mg as a single dose.

DOSAGE IN RENAL IMPAIRMENT

Dosage and frequency are modified based on creatinine clearance.

Creatinine Clearance	Dosage
30 ml/min or higher	400 mg twice a day
Less than 30 ml/min	400 mg once a day

SIDE EFFECTS

FREQUENT: Nausea, headache, dizziness. **RARE:** Vomiting, diarrhea, dry mouth,

N

bitter taste, anxiety, drowsiness, insomnia, photosensitivity, tinnitus, crystalluria, rash, fever, seizures.

ADVERSE EFFECTS/ TOXIC REACTIONS

Superinfection, anaphylaxis, Stevens-Johnson syndrome, arthropathy occur rarely. Hypersensitivity reactions, including photosensitivity (rash, pruritus, blisters, edema, burning skin) may be noted.

NURSING CONSIDERATIONS

BASELINE ASSESSMENT

Question for history of hypersensitivity to norfloxacin, quinolones.

INTERVENTION/EVALUATION

Assess for nausea, headache, dizziness. Evaluate food tolerance. Assess for chest, joint pain.

PATIENT/FAMILY TEACHING

• Take 1 hr before or 2 hrs after meals. • Complete full course of therapy. • Take with 8 oz of water; drink several glasses of water between meals. • May cause dizziness, drowsiness. • Do not take antacids with or within 2 hrs of norfloxacin dose (reduces or destroys effectiveness).

Normodyne, *see labetalol*

nortriptyline

nor-**trip**-ti-leen

(Apo-Nortriptyline ✤, Aventyl ✤, Norventyl ✤, Novo-Nortriptyline ✤, Pamelor)

Do not confuse nortriptyline with amitriptyline, or Aventyl with Ambenyl or Bentyl.

CLASSIFICATION

PHARMACOTHERAPEUTIC: Tricyclic compound. **CLINICAL:** Antidepressant (see pp. 37C, 146C).

ACTION

Blocks reuptake of neurotransmitters (norepinephrine, serotonin) at neuronal presynaptic membranes, increasing their availability at postsynaptic receptor sites. **Therapeutic Effect:** Relieves depression, anxiety disorders, nocturnal enuresis.

USES

Treatment of various forms of depression, often in conjunction with psychotherapy. Treatment of nocturnal enuresis. **OFF-LABEL:** Treatment of neurogenic pain, panic disorder; prevention of migraine headache. Treatment of chronic pain, anxiety disorders, attention-deficit hyperactivity disorder (ADHD), adjunctive therapy for smoking cessation.

PRECAUTIONS

CONTRAINDICATIONS: Acute recovery period after MI, MAOI use within 14 days. **CAUTIONS:** Prostatic hypertrophy, history of urinary retention/obstruction, glaucoma, diabetes mellitus, history of seizures, hyperthyroidism, cardiac/hepatic/renal disease, schizophrenia, increased intraocular pressure (IOP), hiatal hernia. **Pregnancy Category D.**

INTERACTIONS

DRUG: Alcohol, other CNS depressants may increase CNS effects, respiratory depression, hypotensive effects. **Antithyroid agents** may increase risk of agranulocytosis. **Cimetidine** may increase concentration, risk of toxicity. May decrease effects of **clonidine. MAOIs** may increase risk of neuroleptic malignant syndrome, seizures, hyperpyrexia, hypertensive crisis. **Phenothiazines** may increase anticholinergic, sedative effects. **Sympathomimetics** may increase risk of cardiac effects. **HERBAL: Gotu kola, kava kava, St. John's wort, valerian** may increase CNS depression. **FOOD:** None known. **LAB VALUES:** May alter serum glucose, EKG readings. Therapeutic peak serum level: 6–10 mcg/ml; therapeutic trough serum level: 0.5–2 mcg/ml. Toxic peak serum level: greater than 12 mcg/ml; toxic trough serum level: greater than 2 mcg/ml.

AVAILABILITY (Rx)

CAPSULES (PAMELOR): 10 mg, 25 mg, 50 mg, 75 mg. **ORAL SOLUTION (PAMELOR):** 10 mg/5 ml.

ADMINISTRATION/HANDLING

◀ **ALERT** ▶ At least 14 days must elapse between use of MAOIs and nortriptyline.

PO

• Give with food, milk if GI distress occurs.

INDICATIONS/ROUTES/DOSAGE

DEPRESSION

PO: ADULTS: 75–100 mg/day in 1–4 divided doses until therapeutic response is achieved. Reduce dosage gradually to effective maintenance level. **ELDERLY:** Initially, 10–25 mg at bedtime. May increase by 25 mg every 3–7 days. **Maximum:** 150 mg/day. **CHILDREN 12 YRS AND OLDER:** 30–50 mg/day in 3–4 divided doses. **Maximum:** 150 mg/day. **CHILDREN 6–11 YRS:** 10–20 mg/day in 3–4 divided doses.

ENURESIS

PO: CHILDREN 12 YRS AND OLDER: 25–35 mg/day. **CHILDREN 8–11 YRS:** 10–20 mg/day. **CHILDREN 6–7 YRS:** 10 mg/day.

SIDE EFFECTS

FREQUENT: Drowsiness, fatigue, dry mouth, blurred vision, constipation, delayed micturition, orthostatic hypotension, diaphoresis, impaired concentration, increased appetite, urinary retention. **OCCASIONAL:** GI disturbances (nausea, GI distress, metallic taste), photosensitivity. **RARE:** Paradoxical reactions (agitation, restlessness, nightmares, insomnia), extrapyramidal symptoms (particularly fine hand tremor).

ADVERSE EFFECTS/ TOXIC REACTIONS

High dosage may produce cardiovascular effects (severe orthostatic hypotension, dizziness, tachycardia, palpitations, arrhythmias), altered temperature regulation (hyperpyrexia, hypothermia). Abrupt discontinuation from prolonged therapy may produce headache, malaise, nausea, vomiting, vivid dreams.

NURSING CONSIDERATIONS

BASELINE ASSESSMENT

For pts on long-term therapy, hepatic/renal function tests, blood counts should be performed periodically.

INTERVENTION/EVALUATION

Supervise suicidal-risk pt closely during early therapy (as depression lessens, energy level improves, increasing suicide potential). Assess appearance, behavior, speech pattern, level of interest, mood. Monitor daily pattern of bowel activity/stool consistency; avoid constipation with increased fluids, bulky foods. Monitor B/P, pulse for hypotension, arrhythmias. Assess for urinary retention, including output estimate, bladder palpation if indicated. Therapeutic serum level: Peak: 6–10 mcg/ml; trough: 0.5–2 mcg/ml. Toxic serum level: Peak: over 12 mcg/ml; trough: over 2 mcg/ml.

PATIENT/FAMILY TEACHING

• Change positions slowly to avoid hypotensive effect. • Tolerance to postural hypotension, sedative, anticholinergic effects usually develops during early therapy. • Avoid tasks that require alertness, motor skills until response to drug is established. • Therapeutic effect may be noted in 2 wks or longer. • Photosensitivity to sun may occur. • Use sunscreens, protective clothing. • Dry mouth may be relieved by sugarless gum, sips of tepid water. • Report visual disturbances. • Do not abruptly discontinue medication.

N

Norvasc, *see amlodipine*

Novantrone, *see mitoxantrone*

nystatin

nye-**stat**-in

(Bio-Statin, Mycostatin, Nilstat ✤, Nyaderm, Nystat-Rx, Nystop, Pedi-Dri)

Do not confuse nystatin or Mycostatin with Nitrostat.

FIXED-COMBINATION(S)

Mycolog, Myco-Triacet: nystatin/triamcinolone (a steroid): 100,000 units/0.1%.

CLASSIFICATION

CLINICAL: Antifungal (see p. 47C).

ACTION

Binds to sterols in cell membrane, increasing fungal cell-membrane permeability, permitting loss of potassium, other cellular components. **Therapeutic Effect:** Fungistatic.

PHARMACOKINETICS

PO: Poorly absorbed from GI tract. Eliminated unchanged in feces. **Topical:** Not absorbed systemically from intact skin.

USES

Treatment of cutaneous, oral cavity, vaginal fungal infections caused by *Candida sp.* **OFF-LABEL:** Prophylaxis, treatment of oropharyngeal candidiasis, tinea barbae, tinea capitis.

PRECAUTIONS

CONTRAINDICATIONS: None known. **CAUTIONS:** None known.

LIFESPAN CONSIDERATIONS:

Pregnancy/Lactation: Unknown if distributed in breast milk. Vaginal applicators may be contraindicated, requiring manual insertion of tablets during pregnancy. **Pregnancy Category B (C: oral). Children:** No age-related precautions noted for suspension, topical use. Lozenges not recommended in those younger than 5 yrs. **Elderly:** No age-related precautions noted.

INTERACTIONS

DRUG: None significant. **HERBAL:** None significant. **FOOD:** None known. **LAB VALUES:** None known.

AVAILABILITY (Rx)

CAPSULES (BIO-STATIN): 500,000 units, 1,000,000 units. **CREAM (MYCOSTATIN TOPICAL):** 100,000 units/g. **OINTMENT:** 100,000 units/g. **ORAL LOZENGES (MYCOSTATIN PASTILLES):** 200,000 units. **ORAL SUSPENSION (MYCOSTATIN):** 100,000 units/ml. **TABLETS (MYCOSTATIN):** 500,000 units. **TOPICAL POWDER (MYCOSTATIN TOPICAL, NYSTOP, PEDI-DRI):** 100,000 units/g. **VAGINAL TABLETS:** 100,000 units.

ADMINISTRATION/HANDLING

PO

• Dissolve lozenges (troches) slowly, completely in mouth (optimal therapeutic effect). Do not chew/swallow lozenges whole. • Shake suspension well before administration. • Place and hold suspension in mouth or swish throughout mouth as long as possible before swallowing.

INDICATIONS/ROUTES/DOSAGE

INTESTINAL INFECTION

PO: ADULTS, ELDERLY: 500,000–1,000,000 units q8h.

ORAL CANDIDIASIS

PO: ADULTS, ELDERLY, CHILDREN: 400,000–600,000 units 4 times/day. **INFANTS:** 200,000 units 4 times/day.

VAGINAL INFECTIONS

VAGINAL: ADULTS, ELDERLY, ADOLESCENTS: 1 tablet/day at bedtime for 14 days.

CUTANEOUS CANDIDAL INFECTIONS

TOPICAL: ADULTS, ELDERLY, CHILDREN: Apply 2–4 times/day.

SIDE EFFECTS

OCCASIONAL: PO: None known. **Topical:** Skin irritation. **Vaginal:** Vaginal irritation.

ADVERSE EFFECTS/ TOXIC REACTIONS

High dosages of oral form may produce nausea, vomiting, diarrhea, GI distress.

NURSING CONSIDERATIONS

BASELINE ASSESSMENT

Confirm that cultures, histologic tests were done for accurate diagnosis.

INTERVENTION/EVALUATION

Assess for increased irritation with topical, increased vaginal discharge with vaginal application.

PATIENT/FAMILY TEACHING

• Do not miss doses; complete full length of treatment (continue vaginal use during menses). • Notify physician if nausea, vomiting, diarrhea, stomach pain develops. • **Vaginal:** Insert high in vagina. • Check with physician regarding douching, sexual intercourse. • **Topical:** Rub well into affected areas. • Avoid contact with eyes. • Use cream (sparingly) or powder on erythematous areas. • Keep areas clean, dry; wear light clothing for ventilation. • Separate personal items in contact with affected areas.

N

octreotide

ok-**tree**-oh-tide

(Sandostatin, Sandostatin LAR Depot)

Do not confuse octreotide with OctreoScan, or Sandostatin with Sandimmune or Sandoglobulin.

CLASSIFICATION

CLINICAL: Secretory inhibitory, growth hormone suppressant.

ACTION

Suppresses secretion of serotonin, gastroenteropancreatic peptides. Enhances fluid/electrolyte absorption from GI tract. **Therapeutic Effect:** Prolongs intestinal transit time.

PHARMACOKINETICS

Route	Onset	Peak	Duration
Subcutaneous	N/A	N/A	Up to 12 hrs

Rapidly, completely absorbed from injection site. Excreted in urine. Removed by hemodialysis. **Half-life:** 1.5 hrs.

USES

Controls diarrhea in pts with metastatic carcinoid tumors, vasoactive intestinal peptic-secreting tumors (VIPomas), secretory diarrhea, acromegaly. **OFF-LABEL:** Control of bleeding esophageal varices, treatment of AIDS-associated secretory diarrhea, chemotherapy-induced diarrhea, insulinomas, small-bowel fistulas, control of bleeding esophageal varices.

PRECAUTIONS

CONTRAINDICATIONS: None known. **CAUTIONS:** Insulin-dependent diabetes, renal failure.

LIFESPAN CONSIDERATIONS:

Pregnancy/Lactation: Unknown if excreted in breast milk. **Pregnancy Category B. Children:** Dosage not established in children. **Elderly:** No age-related precautions noted.

INTERACTIONS

DRUG: May decrease effectiveness of **cyclosporine. Glucagon, growth hormone, insulin, oral antidiabetics** may alter glucose concentrations. **HERBAL:** None significant. **FOOD:** None known. **LAB VALUES:** May decrease serum thyroxine (T_4).

AVAILABILITY (Rx)

INJECTION SOLUTION (SANDOSTATIN): 0.05 mg/ml, 0.1 mg/ml, 0.2 mg/ml, 0.5 mg/ml, 1 mg/ml. **INJECTION SUSPENSION (SANDOSTATIN LAR DEPOT):** 10-mg, 20-mg, 30-mg vials.

ADMINISTRATION/HANDLING

◄ **ALERT** ► Sandostatin may be given IV, IM, subcutaneous. Sandostatin LAR Depot may be given only IM.

IM

• Give immediately after mixing. • Administer deep IM in large muscle mass at 4-wk intervals. • Avoid deltoid injections.

SUBCUTANEOUS

• Do not use if discolored or particulates form. • Avoid multiple injections at same site within short periods.

INDICATIONS/ROUTES/DOSAGE

DIARRHEA

IV (SANDOSTATIN): ADULTS, ELDERLY: Initially, 50–100 mcg q8h. May increase by 100 mcg/dose q48h. **Maximum:** 500 mcg q8h.

SUBCUTANEOUS (SANDOSTATIN): ADULTS, ELDERLY: 50 mcg 1–2 times a day.

IV, SUBCUTANEOUS (SANDOSTATIN): CHILDREN: 1–10 mcg/kg q12h.

CARCINOID TUMOR

IV, SUBCUTANEOUS (SANDOSTATIN): ADULTS, ELDERLY: 100–600 mcg/day in 2–4 divided doses.

IM (SANDOSTATIN LAR DEPOT): ADULTS, ELDERLY: 20 mg q4wk.

VIPOMA

IV, SUBCUTANEOUS (SANDOSTATIN): ADULTS, ELDERLY: 200–300 mcg/day in 2–4 divided doses.
IM (SANDOSTATIN LAR DEPOT): ADULTS, ELDERLY: 20 mg q4wk.

ESOPHAGEAL VARICES

IV (SANDOSTATIN): ADULTS, ELDERLY: Bolus of 25–50 mcg followed by IV infusion of 25–50 mcg/hr for 48 hrs.

ACROMEGALY

IV, SUBCUTANEOUS (SANDOSTATIN): ADULTS, ELDERLY: 50 mcg 3 times a day. Increase as needed. **Maximum:** 500 mcg 3 times a day.
IM (SANDOSTATIN LAR DEPOT): ADULTS, ELDERLY: 20 mg q4wk for 3 mos. **Maximum:** 40 mg q4wk.

SIDE EFFECTS

FREQUENT (10%–6%, 58%–30% in acromegaly pts): Diarrhea, nausea, abdominal discomfort, headache, injection site pain. **OCCASIONAL (5%–1%):** Vomiting, flatulence, constipation, alopecia, facial flushing, pruritus, dizziness, fatigue, arrhythmias, ecchymosis, blurred vision. **RARE (less than 1%):** Depression, diminished libido, vertigo, palpitations, dyspnea.

ADVERSE EFFECTS/ TOXIC REACTIONS

Increased risk of cholelithiasis. Prolonged high dose therapy may produce hypothyroidism. GI bleeding, hepatitis, seizures occur rarely.

NURSING CONSIDERATIONS

BASELINE ASSESSMENT

Establish baseline B/P, weight, serum glucose, electrolytes.

INTERVENTION/EVALUATION

Monitor serum glucose, thyroid function tests; fluid, electrolyte balance; fecal fat. In acromegaly, monitor growth hormone levels. Weigh every 2–3 days, report over 5 lb gain per wk. Monitor B/P, pulse, respirations periodically during treatment. Be alert for decreased urinary output, peripheral edema (esp. ankles). Monitor daily pattern of bowel activity/stool consistency.

PATIENT/FAMILY TEACHING

- Therapy should provide significant improvement of severe, watery diarrhea.

Ocuflox, *see ofloxacin*

ocular lubricant

ock-you-lar **lube**-rih-cant
(Hypotears, Lacrilube, Tears Naturale)

◆ CLASSIFICATION

PHARMACOTHERAPEUTIC: Topical ophthalmic. **CLINICAL:** Lubricant, toner, buffer, viscosity agent.

ACTION

Forms an occlusive film on eye surface. **Therapeutic Effect:** Lubricates/protects eye from drying.

USES

Protection/lubrication of eye in exposure keratitis, decreased corneal sensitivity, recurrent corneal erosions, keratitis sicca (particularly for nighttime use), after removal of foreign body, during and following surgery.

PRECAUTIONS

CONTRAINDICATIONS: None known. **CAUTIONS:** None known. **Pregnancy Category Unknown.**

O

INTERACTIONS

DRUG: None significant. **HERBAL:** None significant. **FOOD:** None known. **LAB VALUES:** None known.

AVAILABILITY (OTC)

OPHTHALMIC OINTMENT. SOLUTION.

ADMINISTRATION/HANDLING

OPHTHALMIC (OINTMENT)

• Do not use with contact lenses. • Hold tube in hand for a few minutes to warm ointment. • Avoid touching tip of tube or dropper to any surface. • Gently pull lower lid down to form pouch between eye and lower lid (conjunctival sac). • Place ordered amount of ointment into pouch with sweeping motion. • Instruct pt to close eye for 1–2 min and roll eyeball around in all directions. • Inform pt of temporary blurred vision. If possible, apply just before bedtime.

OPHTHALMIC (DROPS)

• Do not use with contact lenses. • Instruct pt to lie down or tilt head backward and look up. • Gently pull lower lid down to form pouch between eye and lower lid (conjunctival sac). • Hold dropper above pouch. Instill drop(s); have pt close eye gently for 1–2 min (placing drops directly onto eye may cause sudden squeezing of eyelid, with subsequent loss of solution). • Apply gentle pressure with fingers to bridge of nose (inside corner of eye) for 1–2 min (promotes absorption, minimizes drainage into nose/throat).

INDICATIONS/ROUTES/DOSAGE

USUAL OPHTHALMIC DOSAGE

OPHTHALMIC: ADULTS, ELDERLY: Small amount in conjunctival sac as needed.

SIDE EFFECTS

FREQUENT: Temporary blurred vision after administration, esp. with ointment.

ADVERSE EFFECTS/ TOXIC REACTIONS

None known.

NURSING CONSIDERATIONS

PATIENT/FAMILY TEACHING

• Teach proper application. • Do not use with contact lenses. • Do not touch tip of tube or dropper to any surface (may contaminate). • Temporary blurred vision will occur, esp. with administration of ointment. • Avoid activities requiring visual acuity until blurring clears. • Notify physician if eye pain, change of vision, worsening of condition occurs or if condition is unchanged after 72 hrs.

ofloxacin

o-**flox**-a-sin

(Apo-Oflox ♣, Apo-Ofloxacin ♣, Floxin, Floxin Otic, Novo-Ofloxacin ♣, Ocuflox)

Do not confuse Floxin with Flexeril or Flexon, or Ocuflox with Ocufen.

CLASSIFICATION

PHARMACOTHERAPEUTIC: Fluoroquinolone. **CLINICAL:** Antibiotic (see p. 24C).

ACTION

Interferes with bacterial cell replication, repair by inhibiting DNA-gyrase in susceptible microorganisms. **Therapeutic Effect:** Bactericidal.

PHARMACOKINETICS

Rapidly, well absorbed from GI tract. Protein binding: 20%–25%. Widely distributed (including to cerebrospinal fluid [CSF]). Metabolized in liver. Primarily excreted in urine. Removed by hemodialysis. **Half-life:** 4.7–7 hrs (increased in renal impairment, cirrhosis, elderly).

USES

Treatment of susceptible infections due to *S. pneumoniae, S. aureus, S. pyogenes, H. influenzae, P. mirabilis, N. gonorrhoeae, C. trachomatis, E. coli, K. pneumoniae, P. aeruginosa*, including infections of urinary tract, lower respiratory tract, skin/skin structure; sexually transmitted diseases; prostatitis due to *E. coli;* pelvic inflammatory disease (PID). **Ophthalmic:** Bacterial conjunctivitis, corneal ulcers. **Otic:** Otitis externa, acute or chronic otitis media.

PRECAUTIONS

CONTRAINDICATIONS: Children 18 yrs and younger, hypersensitivity to any quinolones. **CAUTIONS:** Renal impairment, CNS disorders, seizures, those taking theophylline, caffeine. May mask/delay symptoms of syphilis; serologic test for syphilis should be done at diagnosis and 3 mos after treatment.

LIFESPAN CONSIDERATIONS:

Pregnancy/Lactation: Distributed in breast milk; potentially serious adverse reactions in breast-feeding infants. Risk of arthropathy to fetus. **Pregnancy Category C. Children:** Safety and efficacy not established (otic not established in those younger than 1 yr). **Elderly:** No age-related precautions for otic. Age-related renal impairment may require dosage adjustment for oral administration.

INTERACTIONS

DRUG: **Antacids, sucralfate** may decrease absorption, effect. May increase effects of **caffeine. Didanosine** may decrease absorption, effect. May increase **theophylline** concentration, risk of toxicity. **HERBAL: Dong quai, St. John's wort** may increase photosensitization. **FOOD:** None known. **LAB VALUES:** None known.

AVAILABILITY (Rx)

OPHTHALMIC SOLUTION (OCUFLOX): 0.3%. **OTIC SOLUTION (FLOXIN):** 0.3%. **TABLETS (FLOXIN):** 200 mg, 300 mg, 400 mg.

ADMINISTRATION/HANDLING

PO

• Do not give with food; preferred dosing time is 1 hr before or 2 hrs following meals. • Do not administer antacids (aluminum, magnesium) or iron/zinc-containing products within 2 hrs of ofloxacin. • Encourage cranberry juice, citrus fruits (to acidify urine). • Give with 8 oz of water, encourage fluid intake.

OPHTHALMIC

• Place gloved finger on lower eyelid and pull out, forming pocket between eye and lower lid (conjuctival sac). Hold dropper above pocket and place prescribed number of drops into pocket. Instruct pt to close eye gently (placing drops directly onto eye may cause sudden squeezing of eye lids, with subsequent loss of solution). • Apply gentle pressure with fingers to bridge of nose at inner canthus for 1 min to minimize systemic absorption.

OTIC

• Instruct pt to lie down with head turned so affected ear is upright. • Instill toward canal wall, not directly on eardrum. • Pull auricle down and posterior in children; up and posterior in adults.

INDICATIONS/ROUTES/DOSAGE

UTI

PO: ADULTS: 200 mg q12h for 10 days.

PID

PO: ADULTS: 400 mg q12h for 10–14 days.

LOWER RESPIRATORY TRACT, SKIN/SKINSTRUCTURE INFECTION

PO: ADULTS: 400 mg q12h for 10 days.

PROSTATITIS, SEXUALLY TRANSMITTED DISEASE (CERVICITIS, URETHRITIS)

PO: ADULTS: 300 mg q12h.

O

ACUTE, UNCOMPLICATED GONORRHEA

PO: ADULTS: 400 mg 1 time.

USUAL ELDERLY DOSAGE

PO: ELDERLY: 200–400 mg q12–24h for 7 days up to 6 wks.

BACTERIAL CONJUNCTIVITIS

OPHTHALMIC: ADULTS, ELDERLY: 1–2 drops q2–4h for 2 days, then 4 times a day for 5 days.

CORNEAL ULCER

OPHTHALMIC: ADULTS: 1–2 drops q30min while awake for 2 days, then q60min while awake for 5–7 days, then 4 times a day.

ACUTE OTITIS MEDIA

OTIC: CHILDREN 1–12 YRS: 5 drops into affected ear 2 times/day for 10 days.

OTITIS EXTERNA

OTIC: ADULTS, ELDERLY, CHILDREN 12 YRS AND OLDER: 10 drops into the affected ear once a day for 7 days. **CHILDREN 6 MOS–11 YRS:** 5 drops into affected ear once a day for 7 days.

DOSAGE IN RENAL IMPAIRMENT

After normal initial dose, dosage and frequency are based on creatinine clearance.

Creatinine Clearance	Adjusted Dose	Dosage Interval
Greater than 50 ml/min	None	q12h
10–50 ml/min	None	q24h
Less than 10 ml/min		q24h

SIDE EFFECTS

FREQUENT (10%–7%): Nausea, headache, insomnia. **OCCASIONAL (5%–3%):** Abdominal pain, diarrhea, vomiting, dry mouth, flatulence, dizziness, fatigue, drowsiness, rash, pruritus, fever. **RARE (less than 1%):** Constipation, paresthesia.

ADVERSE EFFECTS/ TOXIC REACTIONS

Antibiotic-associated colitis, other superinfections may occur from altered bacterial balance. Hypersensitivity reaction (evidenced by rash, pruritus, blisters, edema, photosensitivity) occurs rarely. Arthropathy (swelling, pain, clubbing of fingers/toes, degeneration of stress-bearing portion of joint) may occur in children.

NURSING CONSIDERATIONS

BASELINE ASSESSMENT

Question for history of hypersensitivity to ofloxacin, other quinolones.

INTERVENTION/EVALUATION

Monitor signs/symptoms of infection, WBC, altered mental status. Assess skin, discontinue medication at first sign of rash, other allergic reaction. Monitor daily pattern of bowel activity/stool consistency. Assess for insomnia. Check for dizziness, headache, visual difficulties, tremors; provide assistance with ambulation as needed. Be alert for superinfection (genital pruritus, vaginitis, fever, stomatitis).

PATIENT/FAMILY TEACHING

• Do not take antacids within 6 hrs before or 2 hrs after taking ofloxacin. • Best taken 1 hr before or 2 hrs after meals. • May cause insomnia, headache, drowsiness, dizziness. • Avoid tasks requiring alertness, motor skills until response to drug is established.

olanzapine

oh-**lan**-za-peen

(Zyprexa, Zyprexa Intramuscular, Zyprexa Zydis)

Do not confuse olanzapine with olsalazine, or Zyprexa with Zyrtec.

FIXED-COMBINATION(S)

Symbyax: olanzapine/fluoxetine (an antidepressant): 6 mg/25 mg, 6 mg/50 mg, 12 mg/25 mg, 12 mg/50 mg.

CLASSIFICATION

PHARMACOTHERAPEUTIC: Dibenzapin derivative. **CLINICAL:** Antipsychotic (see p. 62C).

ACTION

Antagonizes alpha$_1$-adrenergic, dopamine, histamine, muscarinic, serotonin receptors. Produces anticholinergic, histaminic, CNS depressant effects. **Therapeutic Effect:** Diminishes psychotic symptoms.

PHARMACOKINETICS

Well absorbed after PO administration. Protein binding: 93%. Extensively distributed throughout body. Undergoes extensive first-pass metabolism in liver. Excreted primarily in urine and, to lesser extent, in feces. Not removed by dialysis. **Half-life:** 21–54 hrs.

USES

Oral: Management of manifestations of psychotic disorders. Treatment of acute mania associated with bipolar disorder. **IM:** Controls agitation in schizophrenia, bipolar disorder. **OFF-LABEL:** Treatment of anorexia, apathy, borderline personality disorder, Huntington's disease; maintenance of long-term treatment response in schizophrenic pts; nausea; vomiting.

PRECAUTIONS

CONTRAINDICATIONS: None known. **CAUTIONS:** Hypersensitivity to clozapine, pts who should avoid anticholinergics (e.g., pts with benign prostatic hypertrophy), hepatic impairment, elderly, concurrent use of potentially hepatotoxic drugs, dose escalation, known cardiovascular disease (history of MI, ischemia, heart failure, conduction abnormalities), cerebrovascular disease, conditions predisposing pts to hypotension (dehydration, hypovolemia, hypertensive medications), history of seizures, conditions lowering seizure threshold (e.g., Alzheimer's dementia), those at risk for aspiration pneumonia.

LIFESPAN CONSIDERATIONS:

Pregnancy/Lactation: Unknown if drug crosses placenta or is distributed in breast milk. **Pregnancy Category C.** **Children:** Safety and efficacy not established. **Elderly:** No age-related precautions noted.

INTERACTIONS

DRUG: **Alcohol, CNS depressants** may increase CNS depressant effects. **Anticholinergics** may increase anticholinergic effects. **Hepatotoxic medications** may increase hepatic function test levels. **HERBAL:** **Dong quai, St. John's wort** may increase photosensitization. **Gotu kola, kava kava, St. John's wort, valerian** may increase CNS depression. **FOOD:** None known. **LAB VALUES:** May significantly increase serum GGT, prolactin, AST, ALT.

AVAILABILITY (Rx)

INJECTION, POWDER FOR RECONSTITUTION (ZYPREXA INTRAMUSCULAR): 10 mg. **TABLETS (ZYPREXA):** 2.5 mg, 5 mg, 7.5 mg, 10 mg, 15 mg, 20 mg. **TABLETS (ORALLY DISINTEGRATING [ZYPREXA ZYDIS]):** 5 mg, 10 mg, 15 mg, 20 mg.

ADMINISTRATION/HANDLING

PO

• Give without regard to meals.

IM

• Reconstitute 10-mg vial with 2.1 ml Sterile Water for Injection to provide concentration of 5 mg/ml. • Use within 1 hr following reconstitution. • Discard unused portion.

INDICATIONS/ROUTES/DOSAGE

SCHIZOPHRENIA

PO: ADULTS: Initially, 5–10 mg once daily. May increase by 10 mg/day at 5–7 day intervals. If further adjustments are indicated, may increase by 5–10 mg/day at 7 day intervals. Range: 10–30 mg/day. **ELDERLY:** Initially, 2.5 mg/day. May increase as indicated. Range: 2.5–10 mg/day. **CHILDREN:** Initially, 2.5 mg/day. Titrate as necessary up to 20 mg/day.

BIPOLAR MANIA

PO: ADULTS: Initially, 10–15 mg/day. May increase by 5 mg/day at intervals of at least 24 hrs. **Maximum:** 20 mg/day. **CHILDREN:** Initially, 2.5 mg/day. Titrate as necessary up to 20 mg/day.

DOSAGE FOR ELDERLY, DEBILITATED PTS, THOSE PREDISPOSED TO HYPOTENSIVE REACTIONS

Initial dosage for these pts is 5 mg/day.

CONTROL OF AGITATION

IM: ADULTS, ELDERLY: 2.5–10 mg. May repeat 2 hrs after first dose and 4 hrs after 2nd dose. **Maximum:** 30 mg/day.

SIDE EFFECTS

FREQUENT: Drowsiness (26%), agitation (23%), insomnia (20%), headache (17%), nervousness (16%), hostility (15%), dizziness (11%), rhinitis (10%). **OCCASIONAL:** Anxiety, constipation (9%); nonaggressive atypical behavior (8%); dry mouth (7%); weight gain (6%); orthostatic hypotension, fever, arthralgia, restlessness, cough, pharyngitis, visual changes (dim vision) (5%). **RARE:** Tachycardia; back, chest, abdominal, or extremity pain; tremor.

ADVERSE EFFECTS/ TOXIC REACTIONS

Rare reactions include seizures, neuroleptic malignant syndrome a potentially fatal syndrome characterized by hyperpyrexia, muscle rigidity, irregular pulse or B/P, tachycardia, diaphoresis, cardiac arrhythmias. Extrapyramidal symptoms (EPS), dysphagia may occur. Overdose (300 mg) produces drowsiness, slurred speech.

NURSING CONSIDERATIONS

BASELINE ASSESSMENT

Obtain baseline hepatic function lab values before initiating treatment. Assess behavior, appearance, emotional status, response to environment, speech pattern, thought content.

INTERVENTION/EVALUATION

Monitor B/P. Assess for tremors, changes in gait, abnormal muscular movements, behavior. Supervise suicidal-risk pt closely during early therapy (as depression lessens, energy level improves, increasing suicide potential). Assess for therapeutic response (interest in surroundings, improvement in self-care, increased ability to concentrate, relaxed facial expression). Assist with ambulation if dizziness occurs. Assess sleep pattern. Notify physician if EPS occur.

PATIENT/FAMILY TEACHING

• Avoid dehydration, particularly during exercise, exposure to extreme heat, concurrent use of medication causing dry mouth, other drying effects. • Sugarless gum, sips of tepid water may relieve dry mouth. • Notify physician if pregnancy occurs or if there is intention to become pregnant during olanzapine therapy. • Take medication as ordered; do not stop taking or increase dosage. • Drowsiness generally subsides during continued therapy. • Avoid tasks that require alertness, motor skills until response to drug is established. • Monitor diet, exercise program to prevent weight gain.

olmesartan

ol-**mess**-er-tan
(Benicar)

CLASSIFICATION

PHARMACOTHERAPEUTIC: Angiotensin II receptor antagonist. **CLINICAL:** Antihypertensive (see p. 8C).

ACTION

Blocks vasoconstrictor, aldosterone-secreting effects of angiotensin II by inhibiting binding of angiotensin II to AT_1 receptors in vascular smooth muscle. **Therapeutic Effect:** Causes vasodilation, decreases peripheral resistance, decreases B/P.

PHARMACOKINETICS

Rapidly, completely absorbed after PO administration. Metabolized in liver. Recovered primarily in feces and, to lesser extent, in urine. Not removed by hemodialysis. **Half-life:** 13 hrs.

USES

Treatment of hypertension alone or in combination with other antihypertensives (diuretics, calcium channel blockers).

PRECAUTIONS

CONTRAINDICATIONS: Bilateral renal artery stenosis. **CAUTIONS:** Renal/hepatic impairment, renal arterial stenosis.

LIFESPAN CONSIDERATIONS:

Pregnancy/Lactation: Unknown if distributed in breast milk. **Pregnancy Category C (D if used in second or third trimester). Children:** Safety and efficacy not established. **Elderly:** No age-related precautions noted.

INTERACTIONS

DRUG: Diuretics have additive effects on B/P, may cause hypotension. **HERBAL: Ephedra, yohimbe, ginseng** may worsen hypertension. **Garlic** may increase antihypertensive effect. **FOOD:** None known. **LAB VALUES:** May increase Hgb, Hct.

AVAILABILITY (Rx)

TABLETS: 5 mg, 20 mg, 40 mg.

ADMINISTRATION/HANDLING

PO

- Give without regard to meals.

INDICATIONS/ROUTES/DOSAGE

HYPERTENSION

PO: ADULTS, ELDERLY: Initially, 20 mg/day. May increase to 40 mg/day after 2 wks. Lower initial dose may be necessary in pts receiving volume depleting medications (e.g., diuretics).

SIDE EFFECTS

OCCASIONAL (3%): Dizziness. **RARE (less than 2%):** Headache, diarrhea, upper respiratory tract infection.

ADVERSE EFFECTS/ TOXIC REACTIONS

Overdosage may manifest as hypotension, tachycardia. Bradycardia occurs less often. Rare cases of rhabdomyolysis have been reported.

NURSING CONSIDERATIONS

BASELINE ASSESSMENT

Obtain B/P, apical pulse immediately before each dose in addition to regular monitoring (be alert to fluctuations). If excessive reduction in B/P occurs, place pt in supine position, feet slightly elevated. Question for possibility of pregnancy (see Pregnancy Category). Assess medication history (esp. diuretics).

INTERVENTION/EVALUATION

Maintain hydration (offer fluids frequently). Assess for evidence of upper respiratory infection. Assist with ambulation if dizziness occurs. Monitor serum chemistry levels. Assess B/P for hypertension, hypotension.

PATIENT/FAMILY TEACHING

• Inform female pts regarding consequences of second- and third-trimester exposure to olmesartan. • Avoid tasks that require alertness, motor skills until response to drug is established (possible dizziness effect). • Report any signs of infection (sore throat, fever). • Discuss need for lifelong control, importance of diet, exercise. • Caution against exercise during hot weather (risk of dehydration, hypotension).

olsalazine

ohl-**sal**-ah-zeen
(Dipentum)

Do not confuse olsalazine with olanzapine.

CLASSIFICATION

PHARMACOTHERAPEUTIC: Salicylic acid derivative. **CLINICAL:** Anti-inflammatory.

ACTION

Converted to mesalamine in colon by bacterial action. Blocks prostaglandin production in bowel mucosa. **Therapeutic Effect:** Reduces colonic inflammation.

PHARMACOKINETICS

Small amount absorbed. Protein binding: 99%. Metabolized by bacteria in colon. Minimal elimination in urine, feces. **Half-life:** 0.9 hr.

O

USES

Maintenance of remission of ulcerative colitis in pts intolerant of sulfasalazine medication. **OFF-LABEL:** Treatment of inflammatory bowel disease.

PRECAUTIONS

CONTRAINDICATIONS: History of hypersensitivity to salicylates. **CAUTIONS:** Preexisting renal disease.

LIFESPAN CONSIDERATIONS:

Pregnancy/Lactation: Crosses placenta; distributed in breast milk. **Pregnancy Category C. Children:** Safety and efficacy not established. **Elderly:** Age-related renal impairment may require dosage adjustment.

INTERACTIONS

DRUG: Warfarin may increase prothrombin time (PT). **HERBAL:** None significant. **FOOD:** None known. **LAB VALUES:** May increase AST, ALT.

AVAILABILITY (Rx)

CAPSULES: 250 mg.

ADMINISTRATION/HANDLING

PO

- Give with food.

INDICATIONS/ROUTES/DOSAGE

MAINTENANCE OF CONTROLLED ULCERATIVE COLITIS

PO: ADULTS, ELDERLY: 1 g/day in 2 divided doses, preferably q12h.

SIDE EFFECTS

FREQUENT (10%–5%): Headache, diarrhea, abdominal pain/cramps, nausea. **OCCASIONAL (4%–1%):** Depression, fatigue, dyspepsia, upper respiratory tract infection, decreased appetite, rash, pruritus, arthralgia. **RARE (1%):** Dizziness, vomiting, stomatitis.

ADVERSE EFFECTS/ TOXIC REACTIONS

Sulfite sensitivity may occur in susceptible pts (manifested as cramping, headache, diarrhea, fever, rash, urticaria, pruritus, wheezing). Discontinue drug immediately. Excessive diarrhea associated with extreme fatigue is rarely noted.

NURSING CONSIDERATIONS

INTERVENTION/EVALUATION

Encourage adequate fluid intake. Assess bowel sounds for peristalsis. Monitor daily pattern of bowel activity/stool consistency; record time of evacuation. Assess for abdominal disturbances. Assess skin for rash, urticaria. Medication should be discontinued if rash, fever, cramping, diarrhea occurs.

PATIENT/FAMILY TEACHING

- Notify physician if diarrhea, cramping continues or worsens or if rash, fever, pruritus occurs.

omalizumab

oh-mah-**liz**-uw-mab
(Xolair)

CLASSIFICATION

PHARMACOTHERAPEUTIC: Monoclonal antibody. **CLINICAL:** Antiasthmatic.

ACTION

Selectively binds to human immunoglobulin E (IgE). Inhibits binding of IgE on surface of mast cells, basophiles. **Therapeutic Effect:** Prevents/reduces number of asthmatic attacks.

PHARMACOKINETICS

Absorbed slowly after subcutaneous administration, with peak concentration in 7–8 days. Excreted in liver, reticuloendothelial system, endothelial cells. **Half-life:** 26 days.

USES

Treatment of moderate to severe persistent asthma in pts reactive to perennial allergen and inadequately controlled asthma symptoms with inhaled corticosteroids. **OFF-LABEL:** Treatment of seasonal allergic rhinitis.

PRECAUTIONS

CONTRAINDICATIONS: None known. **CAUTIONS:** Not for use in reversing acute bronchospasm, status asthmaticus.

LIFESPAN CONSIDERATIONS:

Pregnancy/Lactation: Because IgE is present in breast milk, omalizumab is expected to be present in breast milk. Use only if clearly needed. **Pregnancy Category B. Children:** Safety and efficacy not established in children younger than 12 yrs. **Elderly:** No age-related precautions noted.

INTERACTIONS

DRUG: None significant. **HERBAL:** None significant. **FOOD:** None known. **LAB VALUES:** May increase serum IgE levels.

AVAILABILITY (Rx)

INJECTION, POWDER FOR RECONSTITUTION: 202.5 mg/1.2 ml or 150 mg/1.2 ml after reconstitution.

ADMINISTRATION/HANDLING

SUBCUTANEOUS

Reconstitution • Use only Sterile Water for Injection to prepare for subcutaneous administration. • Medication takes 15–20 min to dissolve. • Draw 1.4 ml Sterile Water for Injection into 3-ml syringe with 1-inch, 18-gauge needle; inject contents into powdered vial. • Swirl vial for approximately 1 min (do not shake) and again swirl vial for 5–10 sec every 5 min until no gel-like particles appear in the solution. • Do not use if contents do not dissolve completely within 40 min. • Invert vial for 15 sec (allows solution to drain toward the stopper). • Using new 3-ml syringe with 1-inch 18-gauge needle, obtain required 1.2-ml dose, replace 18-gauge needle with 25-gauge needle for subcutaneous administration.

Rate of administration • Subcutaneous administration may take 5–10 sec to administer due to its viscosity.

Storage • Use only clear or slightly opalescent solution; solution is slightly viscous. • Refrigerate. Reconstituted solution is stable for 8 hrs if refrigerated or within 4 hrs of reconstitution when stored at room temperature.

O

INDICATIONS/ROUTES/DOSAGE

◀ **ALERT** ▶ Retesting of IgE levels during treatment cannot be used as a guide for dosage determination (IgE levels remain elevated for up to 1 yr after discontinuation of treatment). Dosage is based on IgE levels obtained at initiation of treatment.

ASTHMA

SUBCUTANEOUS: ADULTS, ELDERLY, CHILDREN 12 YRS AND OLDER: 150–375 mg every 2 or 4 wks; dose and dosing frequency are individualized based on body weight and pretreatment IgE level (as shown below).

4-WK DOSING TABLE

Pretreatment Serum IgE Levels (units/ml)	Weight 30–60 kg	Weight 61–70 kg	Weight 71–90 kg	Weight 91–150 kg
30–100	150 mg	150 mg	150 mg	300 mg
101–200	300 mg	300 mg	300 mg	See next table
201–300	300 mg	See next table	See next table	See next table

2-WEEK DOSING TABLE

Pretreatment Serum IgE Levels (units/ml)	Weight 30–60 kg	Weight 61–70 kg	Weight 71–90 kg	Weight 91–150 kg
101–200	See preceding table	See preceding table	See preceding table	225 mg
201–300	See preceding table	225 mg	225 mg	300 mg
301–400	225 mg	225 mg	300 mg	Do not dose
401–500	300 mg	300 mg	375 mg	Do not dose
501–600	300 mg	375 mg	Do not dose	Do not dose
601–700	375 mg	Do not dose	Do not dose	Do not dose

SIDE EFFECTS

FREQUENT (45%–11%): Injection site ecchymosis, redness, warmth, stinging, urticaria; viral infection; sinusitis; headache; pharyngitis. **OCCASIONAL (8%–3%):** Arthralgia, leg pain, fatigue, dizziness. **RARE (2%):** Arm pain, earache, dermatitis, pruritus.

ADVERSE EFFECTS/ TOXIC REACTIONS

Anaphylaxis, occurring within 2 hrs of first dose or subsequent doses, occurs in 0.1% of pts. Malignant neoplasms occur in 0.5% of pts.

NURSING CONSIDERATIONS

BASELINE ASSESSMENT

Obtain baseline serum total IgE levels before initiation of treatment (dosage is based on pretreatment levels). Drug is not for treatment of acute exacerbations of asthma, acute bronchospasm, status asthmaticus.

INTERVENTION/EVALUATION

Monitor rate, depth, rhythm, type of respirations, quality/rate of pulse. Assess lung sounds for rhonchi, wheezing, rales. Observe lips, fingernails for cyanosis (blue/dusky color in light-skinned pts, gray in dark-skinned pts).

PATIENT/FAMILY TEACHING

• Increase fluid intake (decreases viscosity of pulmonary secretions). • Do not alter/stop other asthma medications.

omega-3 acid ethyl esters

oh-**meg**-ah 3 **ah**-sid **eth**-ill **eh**-stirs (Omacor)

Do not confuse Omacor with Amicar.

CLASSIFICATION

PHARMACOTHERAPEUTIC: Omega-3 fatty acid. **CLINICAL:** Antihypertriglyceridemia.

ACTION

Inhibits esterification of fatty acids, prevents hepatic enzymes from catalyzing final step of triglyceride synthesis. **Therapeutic Effect:** Reduces serum triglyceride levels.

PHARMACOKINETICS

Well absorbed following PO administration. Incorporated into phospholipids. **Half-life:** N/A.

USES

Adjunct to diet to reduce very high (500 mg/dL or higher) serum triglyceride levels in adult pts.

PRECAUTIONS

CONTRAINDICATIONS: None known. **CAUTIONS:** Known sensitivity, allergy to fish.

LIFESPAN CONSIDERATIONS:

Pregnancy/Lactation: Unknown if distributed in breast milk. **Pregnancy Category C. Children:** Safety and efficacy in children younger than 18 yrs not established. **Elderly:** No age-related precautions noted.

INTERACTIONS

DRUG: May increase bleeding time with **anticaogulants. Beta-blockers, estrogens, thiazide diuretics (e.g., hydrochlorothiazide)** may increase serum triglycerides (discontinue or change drug before therapy). **HERBAL:** None significant. **FOOD:** None known. **LAB VALUES:** May increase ALT, LDL.

AVAILABILITY (Rx)

CAPSULES, SOFT GELATIN (OIL-FILLED): 1 g.

ADMINISTRATION/HANDLING

PO

- Give without regard to meals.

INDICATIONS/ROUTES/DOSAGE

◀ **ALERT** ▶ Before initiating therapy, pt should be on standard cholesterol-lowering diet for minimum of 3–6 mos. Continue diet throughout therapy.

USUAL DOSAGE

PO: ADULTS, ELDERLY: 4 g/day, given as a single dose (4 capsules) or 2 capsules twice daily.

SIDE EFFECTS

OCCASIONAL (5%–3%): Eructation, altered taste, dyspepsia. **RARE (2%–1%):** Rash, back pain.

ADVERSE EFFECTS/TOXIC REACTIONS

None known.

NURSING CONSIDERATIONS

BASELINE ASSESSMENT

Assess baseline serum triglyceride level, hepatic function tests. Obtain diet history.

INTERVENTION/EVALUATION

Monitor serum triglyceride levels for therapeutic response. Monitor serum ALT, LDL periodically during therapy. Discontinue therapy if no response after 2 mos of treatment.

PATIENT/FAMILY TEACHING

- Continue to adhere to lipid-lowering diet (important part of treatment).

O

• Periodic lab tests are essential part of therapy to determine drug effectiveness.

omeprazole

oh-**mep**-rah-zole
(Apo-Omeprazole ♣, Losec ♣, Prilosec, Prilosec OTC, Zegerid)

Do not confuse Prilosec with prilocaine, Prinivil, or Prozac.

CLASSIFICATION

PHARMACOTHERAPEUTIC: Benzimidazole. **CLINICAL:** Gastric acid pump inhibitor (see p. 139C).

ACTION

Converted to active metabolites that irreversibly bind to, inhibit hydrogen-potassium adenosine triphosphatase, an enzyme on surface of gastric parietal cells. Inhibits hydrogen ion transport into gastric lumen. **Therapeutic Effect:** Increases gastric pH, reduces gastric acid production.

PHARMACOKINETICS

Route	Onset	Peak	Duration
PO	1 hr	2 hrs	72 hrs

Rapidly absorbed from GI tract. Protein binding: 99%. Primarily distributed into gastric parietal cells. Metabolized extensively in liver. Primarily excreted in urine. Unknown if removed by hemodialysis. **Half-life:** 0.5–1 hr (increased in hepatic impairment).

USES

Short-term treatment (4–8 wks) of erosive esophagitis (diagnosed by endoscopy), symptomatic gastroesophageal reflux disease (GERD) poorly responsive to other treatment. Long-term treatment of pathologic hypersecretory conditions; treatment of active duodenal ulcer. Maintenance healing of erosive esophagitis. **OFF-LABEL:** *H. pylori*–associated duodenal ulcer (with amoxicillin and clarithromycin), prevention/treatment of NSAID-induced ulcers, treatment of active benign gastric ulcers.

PRECAUTIONS

CONTRAINDICATIONS: None known. **CAUTIONS:** None known.

LIFESPAN CONSIDERATIONS:

Pregnancy/Lactation: Unknown if drug crosses placenta or is distributed in breast milk. **Pregnancy Category C. Children:** Safety and efficacy not established. **Elderly:** No age-related precautions noted.

INTERACTIONS

DRUG: May increase concentration of **diazepam, oral anticoagulants, phenytoin. HERBAL: Ginkgo biloba** may decrease effectiveness. **St. John's wort** may decrease concentration. **FOOD:** None known. **LAB VALUES:** May increase serum alkaline phosphatase, AST, ALT.

AVAILABILITY (Rx)

CAPSULES (DELAYED-RELEASE): (PRILOSEC): 10 mg, 20 mg, 40 mg. **(ZEGERID):** 20 mg, 40 mg.
TABLETS, DELAYED-RELEASE (PRILOSEC OTC): 20 mg.

ORAL SUSPENSION (ZEGERID): 20 mg, 40 mg.

ADMINISTRATION/HANDLING

PO

• Give before meals. • Do not crush delayed-release forms.

INDICATIONS/ROUTES/DOSAGE

EROSIVE ESOPHAGITIS, POORLY RESPONSIVE GERD, ACTIVE DUODENAL ULCER, PREVENTION/TREATMENT OF NSAID-INDUCED ULCERS

PO: ADULTS, ELDERLY: 20 mg/day.

MAINTENANCE HEALING OF EROSIVE ESOPHAGITIS

PO: ADULTS, ELDERLY: 20 mg/day.

PATHOLOGIC HYPERSECRETORY CONDITIONS

PO: ADULTS, ELDERLY: Initially, 60 mg/day up to 120 mg 3 times a day.

***H. PYLORI* DUODENAL ULCER**

PO: ADULTS, ELDERLY: 20 mg once daily or 40 mg/day as a single or in 2 divided doses in combination therapy with antibiotics. Dose varies with regimen used.

ACTIVE BENIGN GASTRIC ULCER

PO: ADULTS, ELDERLY: 40 mg/day for 4–8 wks.

OTC USE (FREQUENT HEARTBURN)

PO: ADULTS, ELDERLY: 20 mg/day for 14 days. May repeat after 4 mos if needed.

USUAL PEDIATRIC DOSAGE

CHILDREN OLDER THAN 2 YRS, WEIGHING 20 KG AND MORE: 20 mg/day. **CHILDREN OLDER THAN 2 YRS, WEIGHING LESS THAN 20 KG:** 10 mg/day.

SIDE EFFECTS

FREQUENT (7%): Headache. **OCCASIONAL (3%–2%):** Diarrhea, abdominal pain, nausea. **RARE (2%):** Dizziness, asthenia (loss of strength, energy), vomiting, constipation, upper respiratory tract infection, back pain, rash, cough.

ADVERSE EFFECTS/ TOXIC REACTIONS

Pancreatitis, hepatotoxicity, interstitial nephritis occur rarely.

NURSING CONSIDERATIONS

INTERVENTION/EVALUATION

Evaluate for therapeutic response (relief of GI symptoms). Question if GI discomfort, nausea, diarrhea occurs.

PATIENT/FAMILY TEACHING

• Report headache. • Swallow capsules whole; do not chew/crush. • Take before eating.

Omnicef, *see cefdinir*

ondansetron

on-**dan**-sah-tron

(Zofran, Zofran ODT)

Do not confuse Zofran with Zantac or Zosyn.

CLASSIFICATION

PHARMACOTHERAPEUTIC: Selective receptor antagonist. **CLINICAL:** Antinausea, antiemetic.

ACTION

Blocks serotonin, both peripherally on vagal nerve terminals, centrally in chemoreceptor trigger zone. **Therapeutic Effect:** Prevents nausea/vomiting.

PHARMACOKINETICS

Readily absorbed from GI tract. Protein binding: 70%–76%. Metabolized in liver. Primarily excreted in urine. Unknown if removed by hemodialysis. **Half-life:** 4 hrs.

USES

Prevention/treatment of nausea/vomiting due to cancer chemotherapy (including high-dose cisplatin). Prevention of postop nausea, vomiting. Prevention of radiation-induced nausea, vomiting. **OFF-LABEL:** Treatment of postoperative nausea, vomiting. Post-anesthetic shivering.

PRECAUTIONS

CONTRAINDICATIONS: None known. **CAUTIONS:** None known.

LIFESPAN CONSIDERATIONS:

Pregnancy/Lactation: Unknown if drug crosses placenta or is distributed in breast milk. **Pregnancy Category B.** **Children:** Safety and efficacy not established. **Elderly:** No age-related precautions noted.

INTERACTIONS

DRUG: Apomorphine may cause profound hypotension, alter level of consciousness. **HERBAL: St. John's wort** may decrease concentration. **FOOD:** None known. **LAB VALUES:** May transiently increase serum bilirubin, AST, ALT.

AVAILABILITY (Rx)

INJECTION (PREMIX): 32 mg/50 ml. **INJECTION SOLUTION (ZOFRAN):** 2 mg/ml. **ORAL SOLUTION (ZOFRAN):** 4 mg/5 ml. **TABLETS (ORALLY DISINTEGRATING [ZOFRAN ODT]):** 4 mg, 8 mg. **TABLETS (ZOFRAN):** 4 mg, 8 mg, 24 mg.

ADMINISTRATION/HANDLING

IV

Reconstitution • May give undiluted. • For IV infusion, dilute with 50 ml D_5W or 0.9% NaCl before administration.

Rate of administration • Give IV push over 2–5 min. • Give IV infusion over 15 min.

Storage • Store at room temperature. • Stable for 48 hrs following dilution.

IM

• Inject into large muscle mass.

PO

• Give without regard to food.

IV INCOMPATIBILITIES

Acyclovir (Zovirax), allopurinol (Aloprim), aminophylline, amphotericin B (Fungizone), amphotericin B complex (Abelcet, AmBisome, Amphotec), ampicillin (Polycillin), ampicillin and sulbactam (Unasyn), cefepime (Maxipime), cefoperazone (Cefobid), 5-fluorouracil, lipids, lorazepam (Ativan), meropenem (Merrem IV), methylprednisolone (Solu-Medrol).

IV COMPATIBILITIES

Carboplatin (Paraplatin), cisplatin (Platinol), cyclophosphamide (Cytoxan), cytarabine (Cytosar), dacarbazine (DTIC-Dome), daunorubicin (Cerubidine), dexamethasone (Decadron), diphenhydramine (Benadryl), docetaxel (Taxotere), dopamine (Intropin), etoposide (VePesid), gemcitabine (Gemzar), heparin, hydromorphone (Dilaudid), ifosfamide (Ifex), magnesium, mannitol, mesna (Mesnex), methotrexate, metoclopramide (Reglan), mitomycin (Mutamycin), mitoxantrone (Novantrone), morphine, paclitaxel (Taxol), potassium chloride, teniposide (Vumon), topotecan (Hycamtin), vinblastine (Velban), vincristine (Oncovin), vinorelbine (Navelbine).

INDICATIONS/ROUTES/DOSAGE

CHEMOTHERAPY-INDUCED EMESIS

IV: ADULTS, ELDERLY: 0.15 mg/kg 3 times a day beginning 30 min before chemotherapy or 0.45 mg/kg once daily or 8–10 mg 1–2 times/day or 24–32 mg once daily. **CHILDREN 6 MOS AND OLDER:** 0.15 mg/kg 3 times a day beginning 30 min before chemotherapy and again 4 and 8 hrs after first dose or 0.45 mg/kg as a single dose.

PO: ADULTS, ELDERLY: (highly emetogenic) 24 mg 30 min before start of chemotherapy, (moderately emetogenic) 8 mg q12h beginning 30 min before chemotherapy and continuing for 1–2 days after completion of chemotherapy.

PREVENTION OF POSTOPERATIVE NAUSEA/VOMITING

IV, IM: ADULTS, ELDERLY, CHILDREN OLDER THAN 12 YRS: 4 mg as a single dose. **CHILDREN 1 MO–12 YRS, WEIGHING MORE THAN 40 KG:** 4 mg. **CHILDREN 1 MO–12 YRS, WEIGHING 40 KG AND LESS:** 0.1 mg/kg.
PO: ADULTS, ELDERLY: 16 mg 1 hr before induction of anesthesia.

PREVENTION OF RADIATION-INDUCED NAUSEA/VOMITING

PO: ADULTS, ELDERLY: (total body irradiation) 8 mg 1–2 hrs daily before each fraction of radiotherapy, (single high-dose radiotherapy to abdomen) 8 mg

1–2 hrs before irradiation, then 8 mg q8h after first dose for 1–2 days after completion of radiotherapy, (daily fractionated radiotherapy to abdomen) 8 mg 1–2 hrs before irradiation, then 8 mg 8 hrs after first dose for each day of radiotherapy.

SIDE EFFECTS

FREQUENT (13%–5%): Anxiety, dizziness, drowsiness, headache, fatigue, constipation, diarrhea, hypoxia, urinary retention. **OCCASIONAL (4%–2%):** Abdominal pain, xerostomia, fever, feeling of cold, redness/pain at injection site, paresthesia, asthenia. **RARE (1%):** Hypersensitivity reaction (rash, pruritus), blurred vision.

ADVERSE EFFECTS/ TOXIC REACTIONS

Hypertension, acute renal failure, GI bleeding, respiratory depression, coma occur rarely.

NURSING CONSIDERATIONS

BASELINE ASSESSMENT

Assess for dehydration if excessive vomiting occurs (poor skin turgor, dry mucous membranes, longitudinal furrows in tongue). Provide emotional support.

INTERVENTION/EVALUATION

Monitor pt in environment. Assess bowel sounds for peristalsis. Provide supportive measures. Assess mental status. Monitor daily pattern of bowel activity/stool consistency; record time of evacuation.

PATIENT/FAMILY TEACHING

• Relief from nausea/vomiting generally occurs shortly after drug administration. • Avoid alcohol, barbiturates. • Report persistent vomiting (may cause drowsiness, dizziness). • Avoid tasks that require alertness, motor skills until response to drug is established.

Onxol, *see paclitaxel*

oprelvekin (interleukin-2, IL-2)

oh-**prel**-vee-kinn

(Neumega)

Do not confuse Neumega with Neupogen.

CLASSIFICATION

PHARMACOTHERAPEUTIC: Hematopoietic. **CLINICAL:** Platelet growth factor.

ACTION

Stimulates production of blood platelets, essential to blood-clotting process. **Therapeutic Effect:** Increases platelet production.

PHARMACOKINETICS

Renal elimination. **Half-life:** 5–8 hrs.

USES

Prevents severe thrombocytopenia, reduces need for platelet transfusions following myelosuppressive chemotherapy in pts with nonmyeloid malignancies.

PRECAUTIONS

CONTRAINDICATIONS: None known. **CAUTIONS:** CHF, those susceptible to developing CHF, history of heart failure, history of atrial arrhythmia.

LIFESPAN CONSIDERATIONS:

Pregnancy/Lactation: Unknown if drug crosses placenta or is distributed is breast milk. **Pregnancy Category C.** **Children:** Safety and efficacy not established. **Elderly:** No age-related precautions noted.

O

INTERACTIONS

DRUG: **Diuretics** may increase loss of potassium, worsen effects of hypokalemia. **HERBAL:** None significant. **FOOD:** None known. **LAB VALUES:** May decrease Hgb, Hct, usually within 3–5 days of initiation of therapy; reverses approximately 1 wk after discontinuance of therapy.

AVAILABILITY (Rx)

INJECTION, POWDER FOR RECONSTITUTION: 5 mg.

ADMINISTRATION/HANDLING

SUBCUTANEOUS

Reconstitution • Add 1 ml Sterile Water for Injection on side of vial; swirl contents gently (avoid excessive agitation) to provide concentration of 5 mg/ml oprelvekin. • Discard unused portion.

Storage • Store in refrigerator. Once reconstituted, use within 3 hrs. • Give single injection in abdomen, thigh, hip, upper arm.

INDICATIONS/ROUTES/DOSAGE

PREVENTION OF THROMBOCYTOPENIA

SUBCUTANEOUS: ADULTS: 50 mcg/kg once a day. **CHILDREN:** 75–100 mcg/kg once a day. Continue for 10–21 days or until platelet count reaches 50,000 cells/mcl after its nadir.

SIDE EFFECTS

FREQUENT: Nausea/vomiting (77%), fluid retention (59%), neutropenic fever (48%), diarrhea (43%), rhinitis (42%), headache (41%), dizziness (38%), fever (36%), insomnia (33%), cough (29%), rash, pharyngitis (25%), tachycardia (20%), vasodilation (19%).

ADVERSE EFFECTS/ TOXIC REACTIONS

Transient atrial fibrillation/flutter occurs in 10% of pts (may be due to increased plasma volume; oprelvekin is not directly arrhythmogenic). Arrhythmias usually are brief in duration and spontaneously convert to normal sinus rhythm. Papilledema may occur in children.

NURSING CONSIDERATIONS

BASELINE ASSESSMENT

Obtain CBC before chemotherapy and at regular intervals thereafter.

INTERVENTION/EVALUATION

Monitor platelet counts. Closely monitor fluid and electrolyte status, esp. in pts receiving diuretic therapy. Assess for fluid retention (peripheral edema, dyspnea on exertion, generally occurs during first wk of therapy and continues for duration of treatment). Monitor platelet count periodically to assess therapeutic duration of therapy. Dosing should continue until postnadir platelet count is more than 50,000 cells/mcl. Treatment should be stopped longer than 2 days before starting next round of chemotherapy.

Orapred, *see prednisolone*

orlistat

ohr-lih-stat

(Xenical)

Do not confuse Xenical with Xeloda.

CLASSIFICATION

PHARMACOTHERAPEUTIC: Gastric/pancreatic lipase inhibitor. **CLINICAL:** Obesity management agent (see p. 133C).

ACTION

Inhibits absorption of dietary fats by inactivating gastric, pancreatic enzymes. **Therapeutic Effect:** Resulting caloric deficit may have positive effects on weight control.

PHARMACOKINETICS

Minimal absorption after administration. Protein binding: 99%. Primarily eliminated unchanged in feces. Unknown if removed by hemodialysis. **Half-life:** 1–2 hrs.

USES

Management of obesity, including weight loss/maintenance, when used in conjunction with reduced-calorie diet. **OFF-LABEL:** Treatment of type 2 diabetes.

PRECAUTIONS

CONTRAINDICATIONS: Cholestasis, chronic malabsorption syndrome. **CAUTIONS:** None known.

LIFESPAN CONSIDERATIONS:

Pregnancy/Lactation: Unknown if excreted in breast milk. Not recommended during pregnancy or in breastfeeding women. **Pregnancy Category B.** **Children:** Safety and efficacy not established. **Elderly:** No age-related precautions noted.

INTERACTIONS

DRUG: May increase concentration of **pravastatin,** risk of rhabdomyolysis. May reduce absorption of **vitamin E.** May alter effect of **warfarin** by altering vitamin K level. **HERBAL:** None significant. **FOOD:** None known. **LAB VALUES:** Decreases serum glucose, cholesterol, LDL.

AVAILABILITY (Rx)

CAPSULES: 120 mg.

ADMINISTRATION/HANDLING

PO

- Give without regard to food.

INDICATIONS/ROUTES/DOSAGE

WEIGHT REDUCTION

PO: ADULTS, ELDERLY, CHILDREN 12–16 YRS: 120 mg 3 times a day with each main meal containing fat (omit if meal is occasionally missed or contains no fat).

SIDE EFFECTS

FREQUENT (30%–20%): Headache, abdominal discomfort, flatulence, fecal urgency, fatty/oily stool. **OCCASIONAL (14%–5%):** Back pain, menstrual irregularity, nausea, fatigue, diarrhea, dizziness. **RARE (less than 4%):** Anxiety, rash, myalgia, dry skin, vomiting.

ADVERSE EFFECTS/ TOXIC REACTIONS

Hypersensitivity reaction occurs rarely.

NURSING CONSIDERATIONS

INTERVENTION/EVALUATION

Monitor serum cholesterol, LDL, glucose, changes in coagulation parameters.

PATIENT/FAMILY TEACHING

• Maintain nutritionally balanced, reduced-calorie diet. • Daily intake of fat, carbohydrates, protein to be distributed over 3 main meals.

orphenadrine

(Norflex)

See Skeletal muscle relaxants

oseltamivir

ah-suhl-**tahm**-ah-veer

(Tamiflu)

O

◆ **CLASSIFICATION**

PHARMACOTHERAPEUTIC: Neuraminidase inhibitor. **CLINICAL:** Antiviral (see p. 65C).

ACTION

Selective inhibitor of influenza virus neuraminidase, an enzyme essential for viral replication. Acts against influenza A and B viruses. **Therapeutic Effect:** Suppresses spread of infection within respiratory system, reduces duration of clinical symptoms.

PHARMACOKINETICS

Readily absorbed. Protein binding: 3%. Extensively converted to active drug in liver. Primarily excreted in urine. **Half-life:** 6–10 hrs.

USES

Symptomatic treatment of uncomplicated acute illness caused by influenza A or B virus in adults and children 1 yr and older who are symptomatic no longer than 2 days. Prevention of influenza in adults, children 1 yr and older.

O

PRECAUTIONS

CONTRAINDICATIONS: None known. **CAUTIONS:** Renal impairment.

LIFESPAN CONSIDERATIONS: **Pregnancy/Lactation:** Unknown if excreted in breast milk. **Pregnancy Category C. Children:** Safety and efficacy not established in those younger than 1 yr. **Elderly:** No age-related precautions noted.

INTERACTIONS

DRUG: **Probenecid** increases concentration. **HERBAL:** None significant. **FOOD:** None known. **LAB VALUES:** None known.

AVAILABILITY (Rx)

CAPSULES: 75 mg. **ORAL SUSPENSION:** 12 mg/ml.

ADMINISTRATION/HANDLING

PO

- Give without regard to food.

INDICATIONS/ROUTES/DOSAGE

INFLUENZA

PO: ADULTS, ELDERLY: 75 mg 2 times a day for 5 days. **CHILDREN WEIGHING MORE THAN 40 KG:** 75 mg twice a day. **CHILDREN WEIGHING 24–40 KG:** 60 mg twice a day. **CHILDREN WEIGHING 15–23 KG:** 45 mg twice a day. **CHILDREN WEIGHING LESS THAN 15 KG:** 30 mg twice a day.

PREVENTION OF INFLUENZA

PO: ADULTS, ELDERLY, CHILDREN 13 YRS AND OLDER: 75 mg once daily for at least 7 days. **CHILDREN 1–12 YRS:** 30–60 mg once daily for 10 days.

DOSAGE IN RENAL IMPAIRMENT

PO: For adults, elderly pts, dosage is decreased to 75 mg once a day for at least 7 days and possibly up to 6 wks.

SIDE EFFECTS

FREQUENT (10%–7%): Nausea, vomiting, diarrhea. **RARE (2%–1%):** Abdominal pain, bronchitis, dizziness, headache, cough, insomnia, fatigue, vertigo.

ADVERSE EFFECTS/ TOXIC REACTIONS

Colitis, pneumonia, tympanic membrane disorder, pyrexia occur rarely.

NURSING CONSIDERATIONS

INTERVENTION/EVALUATION

Monitor serum glucose, renal function in pts with diabetes.

PATIENT/FAMILY TEACHING

• Begin as soon as possible from first appearance of flu symptoms. • Avoid contact with those who are at high risk for influenza. • Not a substitute for flu shot.

oxacillin

(Prostaphlin)

See Antibiotic: penicillins (p. 27C)

oxaliplatin

ox-**ale**-ee-plah-tin

(Eloxatin)

CLASSIFICATION

PHARMACOTHERAPEUTIC: Platinum-containing complex. **CLINICAL:** Antineoplastic (see p. 82C).

ACTION

Inhibits DNA replication by cross-linking with DNA strands. Cell cycle–phase nonspecific. **Therapeutic Effect:** Prevents cell division.

PHARMACOKINETICS

Rapidly distributed. Protein binding: 90%. Undergoes rapid, extensive nonenzymatic biotransformation. Excreted in urine. **Half-life:** 70 hrs.

USES

Combination treatment of metastatic carcinoma of colon, rectum with 5-fluorouracil (5-FU)/leucovorin in pts whose disease has recurred or progressed during or within 6 mos of completion of first-line therapy with bolus 5-FU/leucovorin and irinotecan. **OFF-LABEL:** Treatment of germ cell cancer, ovarian cancer, pancreatic cancer, renal cell cancer, solid tumors, head and neck cancer.

PRECAUTIONS

CONTRAINDICATIONS: History of allergy to other platinum compounds. **CAUTIONS:** Previous therapy with other antineoplastic agents, radiation, renal impairment, infection, pregnancy, immunosuppression, presence or history of peripheral neuropathy.

LIFESPAN CONSIDERATIONS:

Pregnancy/Lactation: If possible, avoid use during pregnancy, esp. first trimester. May cause fetal harm. Breastfeeding not recommended. **Pregnancy Category D. Children:** Safety and efficacy not established. **Elderly:** Increased incidence of diarrhea, dehydration, hypokalemia, fatigue.

INTERACTIONS

DRUG: Bone marrow depressants may increase myelosuppression, GI effects. **Live virus vaccines** may potentiate virus replication, increase vaccine side effects, decrease pt's antibody response to vaccine. **Nephrotic medications** may decrease clearance. **HERBAL:** None significant. **FOOD:** None known. **LAB VALUES:** May alter serum bilirubin, AST, ALT. May decrease Hgb, Hct, platelet count.

AVAILABILITY (Rx)

INJECTION SOLUTION: 50-mg, 100-mg vials 5 mg/ml.

ADMINISTRATION/HANDLING

◀ ALERT ▶ Wear protective gloves during handling of oxaliplatin. If solution comes in contact with skin, wash skin immediately with soap, water. Do not use aluminum needles or administration sets that may come in contact with drug; may cause degradation of platinum compounds.

◀ ALERT ▶ Pt to avoid ice, drinking, touching cold objects during infusion (can exacerbate acute neuropathy)

IV

Reconstitution • Dilute with 250–500 ml D_5W (never dilute with sodium chloride solution or other chloride-containing solutions).

Rate of administration • Infuse over 120 min.

Storage • Do not freeze; protect from light. • Store vials at room temperature. • After dilution, solution is stable for 6 hrs at room temperature, 24 hrs if refrigerated.

IV INCOMPATIBILITIES

Do not infuse oxaliplatin with alkaline medications.

INDICATIONS/ROUTES/DOSAGE

◀ **ALERT** ▶ Pretreat the pt with antiemetics (should be ordered). Repeat courses should not be given more frequently than every 2 wks.

COLO-RECTAL CANCER

IV: **ADULTS**: **Day 1:** Oxaliplatin 85 mg/m^2 in 250–500 ml D_5W and leucovorin 200 mg/m^2, both given simultaneously over more than 2 hrs in separate bags using a Y-line, followed by 5-FU 400 mg/m^2 IV bolus given over 2–4 min, followed by 5-FU 600 mg/m^2 in 500 ml D_5W as a 22-hr continuous IV infusion. **Day 2:** Leucovorin 200 mg/m^2 IV infusion given over more than 2 hrs, followed by 5-FU 400 mg/m^2 IV bolus given over 2–4 min, followed by 5-FU 600 mg/m^2 in 500 ml D_5W as a 22-hr continuous IV infusion. Repeat cycle every 2 wks for total of 6 mos. Prior to subsequent therapy cycles, evaluate pt for clinical toxicities and laboratory tests.

OVARIAN CANCER

IV: **ADULTS**: Cisplatin 100 mg/m^2 and oxaliplatin 130 mg/m^2 q3wk. Prior to subsequent therapy cycles, evaluate pt for clinical toxicities and laboratory tests.

SIDE EFFECTS

FREQUENT (76%–20%): Peripheral/sensory neuropathy (usually occurs in hands, feet, perioral area, throat but may present as jaw spasm, abnormal tongue sensation, eye pain, chest pressure, difficulty walking, swallowing, writing), nausea (64%), fatigue, diarrhea, vomiting, constipation, abdominal pain, fever, anorexia. **OCCASIONAL (14%–10%):** Stomatitis, earache, insomnia, cough, difficulty breathing, backache, edema. **RARE (7%–3%):** Dyspepsia, dizziness, rhinitis, flushing, alopecia.

ADVERSE EFFECTS/ TOXIC REACTIONS

Peripheral/sensory neuropathy can occur, without any prior event by drinking or holding a glass of cold liquid during IV infusion. Pulmonary fibrosis (characterized as nonproductive cough, dyspnea, crackles, radiologic pulmonary infiltrates) may warrant drug discontinuation. Hypersensitivity reaction (rash, urticaria, pruritus) occurs rarely.

NURSING CONSIDERATIONS

BASELINE ASSESSMENT

Pt to avoid ice or drinking, holding glass of cold liquid during IV infusion; can precipitate/exacerbate neurotoxicity (occurs within hrs or 1–2 days of dosing, lasts up to 14 days). Assess baseline BUN, serum creatinine, WBC, platelet count.

INTERVENTION/EVALUATION

Monitor for decrease in WBC, platelets (myelosuppression is minimal). Monitor for diarrhea, GI bleeding (bright red, tarry stool). Maintain strict I&O. Assess oral mucosa for stomatitis.

PATIENT/FAMILY TEACHING

• Promptly report fever, sore throat, signs of local infection, unusual bruising/bleeding from any site. • Do not have immunizations without physician's approval (drug lowers resistance). • Avoid contact with those who have recently taken oral polio vaccine. • Avoid cold drinks, ice, cold objects (may produce neuropathy).

O

oxaprozin

ox-a-**pro**-zin
(Apo-Oxaprozin ✤, Daypro)
Do not confuse oxaprozin with oxazepam.

CLASSIFICATION

PHARMACOTHERAPEUTIC: Nonsteroidal anti-inflammatory. **CLINICAL:** Analgesic, anti-inflammatory (see p. 125C).

ACTION

Produces analgesic, anti-inflammatory effects by inhibiting prostaglandin synthesis. **Therapeutic Effect:** Reduces inflammatory response, intensity of pain.

PHARMACOKINETICS

Well absorbed from GI tract. Protein binding: 99%. Widely distributed. Metabolized in liver. Primarily excreted in urine; partially eliminated in feces. Not removed by hemodialysis. **Half-life:** 42–50 hrs.

USES

Acute, chronic treatment of osteoarthritis, juvenile rheumatoid arthritis, rheumatoid arthritis.

PRECAUTIONS

CONTRAINDICATIONS: Active peptic ulcer disease, chronic inflammation of GI tract, GI bleeding/ulceration, history of hypersensitivity to aspirin, NSAIDs. **CAUTIONS:** Renal/hepatic impairment, history of GI tract disease, predisposition to fluid retention.

LIFESPAN CONSIDERATIONS:

Pregnancy/Lactation: Unknown if drug is excreted in breast milk. Avoid use during third trimester (may adversely affect fetal cardiovascular system: premature closure of ductus arteriosus). **Pregnancy Category C (D if used in third trimester or near delivery). Children:** Safety and efficacy not established. **Elderly:** Age-related renal impairment may increase risk of hepatic/renal toxicity; decreased dosage recommended. GI bleeding/ulceration more likely to cause serious adverse effects.

INTERACTIONS

DRUG: May decrease effects of **antihypertensives, diuretics. Aspirin, other salicylates** may increase risk of GI side effects, bleeding. **Bone marrow depressants** may increase risk of hematologic reactions. May increase effects of **heparin, oral anticoagulants, thrombolytics.** May increase concentration, risk of toxicity of **lithium.** May increase risk of **methotrexate** toxicity. **Probenecid** may increase concentration. **HERBAL: Cat's claw, dong quai, evening primrose, feverfew, garlic, ginger, ginkgo, red clover, horse chestnut, ginseng** possess antiplatelet activity, may increase risk of bleeding. **FOOD:** None known. **LAB VALUES:** May increase BUN, serum creatinine, AST, ALT.

AVAILABILITY (Rx)

TABLETS: 600 mg.

ADMINISTRATION/HANDLING

PO

- May give with food, milk, antacids if GI distress occurs.

INDICATIONS/ROUTES/DOSAGE

OSTEOARTHRITIS

PO: ADULTS, ELDERLY: 600–1,200 mg once a day (600 mg in pts with low body weight or mild disease).

RHEUMATOID ARTHRITIS

PO: ADULTS, ELDERLY: 1,200 mg once a day. Range: 600–1,800 mg/day.

JUVENILE RHEUMATOID ARTHRITIS

PO: CHILDREN WEIGHING MORE THAN 54 KG: 1,200 mg/day. **CHILDREN WEIGHING**

O

32–54 KG: 900 mg/day. **CHILDREN WEIGHING 22–31 KG:** 600 mg/day.

DOSAGE IN RENAL IMPAIRMENT

For adults, elderly pts with renal impairment, recommended initial dose is 600 mg/day; may be increased up to 1,200 mg/day.

SIDE EFFECTS

OCCASIONAL (9%–3%): Nausea, diarrhea, constipation, dyspepsia (heartburn, indigestion, epigastric pain), edema. **RARE (less than 3%):** Vomiting, abdominal cramps/pain, flatulence, anorexia, confusion, tinnitus, insomnia, drowsiness.

ADVERSE EFFECTS/ TOXIC REACTIONS

Hypertension, acute renal failure, respiratory depression, GI bleeding, coma occur rarely.

NURSING CONSIDERATIONS

BASELINE ASSESSMENT

Assess onset, type, location, duration of pain/inflammation.

INTERVENTION/EVALUATION

Observe for weight gain, edema, bleeding, ecchymoses, mental confusion. Monitor renal/hepatic function tests. Evaluate for therapeutic response (relief of pain, stiffness, swelling; increased joint mobility; reduced joint tenderness; improved grip strength).

PATIENT/FAMILY TEACHING

• Avoid aspirin, alcohol during therapy (increases risk of GI bleeding). • If gastric upset occurs, take with food, milk, antacids. • If GI effects persist, inform physician. • Avoid tasks that require alertness, motor skills until response to drug is established (may cause drowsiness, confusion).

oxazepam

ox-**az**-eh-pam

(Apo-Oxazepam ✦, Oxpram ✦, Serax)

Do not confuse oxazepam with oxaprozin, or Serax with Eurax or Xerac.

◆ CLASSIFICATION

PHARMACOTHERAPEUTIC: Benzodiazepine (**Schedule IV**). **CLINICAL:** Antianxiety (see p. 12C).

ACTION

Potentiates effects of gamma-aminobutyric acid (GABA) and other inhibitory neurotransmitters by binding to specific receptors in CNS. **Therapeutic Effect:** Produces anxiolytic effect, skeletal muscle relaxation.

PHARMACOKINETICS

Well absorbed from GI tract. Protein binding: 97%. Metabolized in liver. Primarily excreted in urine. Not removed by hemodialysis. **Half-life:** 5–20 hrs.

USES

Management of acute alcohol withdrawal symptoms (tremors, anxiety on withdrawal). Treatment of anxiety associated with depressive symptoms.

PRECAUTIONS

CONTRAINDICATIONS: Angle-closure glauccoma; preexisting CNS depression; severe, uncontrolled pain. **CAUTIONS:** History of drug dependence.

⌛ LIFESPAN CONSIDERATIONS:

Pregnancy/Lactation: Drug crosses placenta; is distributed in breast milk. May produce CNS depression in neonate. **Pregnancy Category D. Children:** Safety and efficacy not established.

Elderly: May produce excessive sedation, ataxia.

INTERACTIONS

DRUG: Alcohol, other CNS depressants may potentiate CNS depression. **HERBAL: Gotu kola, kava kava, St. John's wort, valerian** may increase CNS depression. **FOOD:** None known. **LAB VALUES:** May elevate serum alkaline phosphatase, bilirubin, LDH, AST, ALT. May produce abnormal renal function test results. Therapeutic serum drug level: 0.2–1.4 mcg/ml; toxic serum drug level: not established.

AVAILABILITY (Rx)

CAPSULES: 10 mg, 15 mg, 30 mg. **TABLETS:** 15 mg.

INDICATIONS/ROUTES/DOSAGE

ANXIETY

PO: ADULTS: 10–30 mg 3–4 times a day. **ELDERLY:** 10 mg 2–3 times a day. **CHILDREN:** 1 mg/kg/day.

ALCOHOL WITHDRAWAL

PO: ADULTS, ELDERLY: 15–30 mg 3–4 times a day.

SIDE EFFECTS

FREQUENT: Mild, transient drowsiness at beginning of therapy. **OCCASIONAL:** Dizziness, headache. **RARE:** Paradoxical CNS reactions, such as hyperactivity, nervousness in children and excitement, restlessness in elderly, debilitated (generally noted during first 2 wks of therapy).

ADVERSE EFFECTS/ TOXIC REACTIONS

Abrupt or too-rapid withdrawal may result in pronounced restlessness, irritability, insomnia, hand tremor, abdominal/muscle cramps, diaphoresis, vomiting, seizures. Overdose results in somnolence, confusion, diminished reflexes, coma.

NURSING CONSIDERATIONS

BASELINE ASSESSMENT

Offer emotional support to anxious pt. Assess motor responses (agitation, trembling, tension), autonomic responses (cold/clammy hands, diaphoresis).

INTERVENTION/EVALUATION

For those on long-term therapy, hepatic/renal function tests, blood counts should be performed periodically. Assess for paradoxical reaction, particularly during early therapy. Assist with ambulation if drowsiness, light-headedness occurs. Evaluate for therapeutic response (calm facial expression, decreased restlessness, diminished insomnia). Therapeutic serum level: 0.2–1.4 mcg/ml; toxic serum level: not established.

PATIENT/FAMILY TEACHING

• Avoid alcohol, other CNS depressants. • Avoid tasks requiring alertness, motor skills until response to drug is established (may cause drowsiness). • Avoid abrupt discontinuation.

O

oxcarbazepine

ox-car-**bah**-zeh-peen
(Trileptal)

CLASSIFICATION

CLINICAL: Anticonvulsant (see p. 34C).

ACTION

Blocks sodium channels, stabilizing hyperexcited neural membranes, inhibiting repetitive neuronal firing, diminishing synaptic impulses. **Therapeutic Effect:** Prevents seizures.

PHARMACOKINETICS

Completely absorbed from GI tract. Extensively metabolized in liver to active metabolite. Protein binding: 40%. Primarily excreted in urine. **Half-life:** 2 hrs; metabolite, 6–10 hrs.

USES

Monotherapy, adjunctive therapy in adults, children 2 yrs and older for treatment of partial seizures. **OFF-LABEL:** Atypical panic disorder, bipolar disorders, neuralgia/neuropathy.

PRECAUTIONS

CONTRAINDICATIONS: None known. **CAUTIONS:** Renal impairment, sensitivity to carbamazepine.

LIFESPAN CONSIDERATIONS:

Pregnancy/Lactation: Crosses placenta. Distributed in breast milk. **Pregnancy Category C.** **Children:** No age-related precautions in those older than 4 yrs. **Elderly:** Age-related renal impairment may require dosage adjustment.

INTERACTIONS

DRUG: **Carbamazepine, phenobarbital, phenytoin, valproic acid verapamil** may decrease concentration, effects. May decrease effectiveness of **felodipine, oral contraceptives, verapamil.** May increase concentration, risk of toxicity of **phenobarbital, phenytoin.** **HERBAL:** **Gotu kola, kava kava, St. John's wort, valerian** may increase CNS depression. **Evening primrose** may decrease seizure threshold. **St. John's wort** may decrease concentration. **FOOD:** None known. **LAB VALUES:** May increase GGT level, other hepatic function test results. May alter serum glucose. May decrease serum calcium, potassium, sodium.

AVAILABILITY (Rx)

ORAL SUSPENSION: 300 mg/5 ml. **TABLETS:** 150 mg, 300 mg, 600 mg.

ADMINISTRATION/HANDLING

PO

- Give without regard to food.

INDICATIONS/ROUTES/DOSAGE

ADJUNCTIVE TREATMENT OF SEIZURES

PO: ADULTS, ELDERLY: Initially, 600 mg/day in 2 divided doses. May increase by up to 600 mg/day at weekly intervals. **Maximum:** 2,400 mg/day. **CHILDREN 4–16 YRS:** 8–10 mg/kg. **Maximum:** 600 mg/day. Maintenance (based on weight): 1,800 mg/day for children weighing more than 39 kg; 1,200 mg/day for children weighing 29.1–39 kg; and 900 mg/day for children weighing 20–29 kg.

CONVERSION TO MONOTHERAPY

PO: ADULTS, ELDERLY: 600 mg/day in 2 divided doses (while decreasing concomitant anticonvulsant over 3–6 wks). May increase by 600 mg/day at weekly intervals up to 2,400 mg/day. **CHILDREN:** Initially, 8–10 mg/kg/day in 2 divided doses with simultaneous initial reduction of dose of concomitant antiepileptic.

INITIATION OF MONOTHERAPY

PO: ADULTS, ELDERLY: 600 mg/day in 2 divided doses. May increase by 300 mg/day every 3 days up to 1,200 mg/day. **CHILDREN:** Initially, 8–10 mg/kg/day in 2 divided doses. Increase at 3 day intervals by 5 mg/kg/day to achieve maintenance dose by weight as follows:

Weight	Dosage
70+ kg	1,500–2,100 mg/day
60–69 kg	1,200–2,100 mg/day
50–59 kg	1,200–1,800 mg/day
41–49 kg	1,200–1,500 mg/day
35–40 kg	900–1,500 mg/day
25–34 kg	900–1,200 mg/day
20–24 kg	600–900 mg/day

DOSAGE IN RENAL IMPAIRMENT

For pts with creatinine clearance less than 30 ml/min, give 50% of normal starting dose, then titrate slowly to desired dose.

SIDE EFFECTS

FREQUENT (22%–13%): Dizziness, nausea, headache. **OCCASIONAL (7%–5%):** Vomiting, diarrhea, ataxia (muscular incoordination), nervousness, dyspepsia, (heartburn, indigestion, epigastric pain), constipation. **RARE (4%):** Tremor, rash, back pain, epistaxis, sinusitis, diplopia.

ADVERSE EFFECTS/ TOXIC REACTIONS

Clinically significant hyponatremia may occur, manifested as leg cramping, hypotention, cold/clammy skin, increased pulse rate, headache, nausea, vomiting, diarrhea.

NURSING CONSIDERATIONS

BASELINE ASSESSMENT

Review history of seizure disorder (type, onset, intensity, frequency, duration, level of consciousness [LOC]), drug history (esp. other anticonvulsants). Provide safety precautions; quiet, dark environment.

INTERVENTION/EVALUATION

Assist with ambulation if dizziness, ataxia occurs. Assess for visual abnormalities, headache. Monitor serum sodium. Assess for signs of hyponatremia (nausea, malaise, headache, lethargy, confusion). Assess for clinical improvement (decrease in intensity, frequency of seizures).

PATIENT/FAMILY TEACHING

• Do not abruptly stop taking medication (may increase seizure activity). • Inform physician if rash, nausea, headache, dizziness occurs. • May need periodic blood tests.

oxiconazole

(Oxistat)

See Antifungals: topical (p. 47C)

oxybutynin

ox-i-**byoo**-ti-nin

(Ditropan, Ditropan XL, Novo-Oxybutynin ✤, Oxytrol, Urotrol)

Do not confuse oxybutynin with OxyContin, or Ditropan with diazepam.

CLASSIFICATION

PHARMACOTHERAPEUTIC: Anticholinergic. **CLINICAL:** Antispasmodic.

ACTION

Exerts antispasmodic (papaverine-like), antimuscarinic (atropine-like) action on detrusor smooth muscle of bladder. **Therapeutic Effect:** Increases bladder capacity, delays desire to void.

PHARMACOKINETICS

Route	Onset	Peak	Duration
PO	0.5–1 hr	3–6 hrs	6–10 hrs

Rapidly absorbed from GI tract. Metabolized in liver. Primarily excreted in urine. Unknown if removed by hemodialysis. **Half-life:** 1–2.3 hrs.

USES

Relief of symptoms (urgency, incontinence, frequency, nocturia, urge incontinence) associated with uninhibited neurogenic bladder, reflex neurogenic bladder.

PRECAUTIONS

CONTRAINDICATIONS: GI/GU obstruction, glaucoma, myasthenia gravis, toxic megacolon, ulcerative colitis. **CAUTIONS:** Renal/hepatic impairment, cardiovascular disease, hyperthyroidism, reflux esophagitis, hypertension, prostatic hypertrophy, neuropathy.

LIFESPAN CONSIDERATIONS:

Pregnancy/Lactation: Unknown if

drug crosses placenta or is distributed in breast milk. **Pregnancy Category B.** **Children:** No age-related precautions noted in those older than 5 yrs. **Elderly:** May be more sensitive to anticholinergic effects (e.g., dry mouth, urinary retention).

INTERACTIONS

DRUG: **Medications with anticholinergic effects (e.g., antihistamines)** may increase anticholinergic effects. **Ketoconazole, itraconazole, clarithromycin, erythromycin** may alter pharmacokinetic parameters. **HERBAL:** None significant. **FOOD:** None known. **LAB VALUES:** None known.

AVAILABILITY (Rx)

SYRUP (DITROPAN): 5 mg/5 ml. **TABLETS (DITROPAN, UROTROL):** 5 mg.

TABLETS (EXTENDED-RELEASE [DITRO-PAN XL]): 5 mg, 10 mg, 15 mg. **TRANSDERMAL (OXYTROL):** 3.9 mg.

ADMINISTRATION/HANDLING

PO

- Give without regard to meals.

TRANSDERMAL

- Apply patch to dry, intact skin on abdomen, hip, buttock. • Use new application site for each new patch; avoid reapplication to same site within 7 days.

INDICATIONS/ROUTES/DOSAGE

NEUROGENIC BLADDER

PO: ADULTS: 5 mg 2–3 times a day up to 5 mg 4 times a day. **ELDERLY:** 2.5–5 mg twice a day. May increase by 2.5 mg/day every 1–2 days. **CHILDREN 5 YRS AND OLDER:** 5 mg twice a day up to 5 mg 4 times a day. **CHILDREN 1–4 YRS:** 0.2 mg/kg/dose 2–4 times a day.

PO (EXTENDED-RELEASE): ADULTS, ELDERLY: 5–10 mg/day up to 30 mg/day. **CHILDREN 6 YRS AND OLDER:** Initially, 5–10 mg once daily. May increase in 5–10 mg increments. **Maximum:** 30 mg/day.

TRANSDERMAL: ADULTS: 3.9 mg applied twice a wk. Apply every 3–4 days.

SIDE EFFECTS

FREQUENT: Constipation, dry mouth, somnolence, decreased perspiration. **OCCASIONAL:** Decreased lacrimation/salivation, impotence, urinary hesitancy/retention, suppressed lactation, blurred vision, mydriasis, nausea/vomiting, insomnia.

ADVERSE EFFECTS/ TOXIC REACTIONS

Overdose produces CNS excitation (nervousness, restlessness, hallucinations, irritability), hypotension/hypertension, confusion, tachycardia, facial flushing, respiratory depression.

NURSING CONSIDERATIONS

BASELINE ASSESSMENT

Assess dysuria, urgency, frequency, incontinence.

INTERVENTION/EVALUATION

Monitor for symptomatic relief. Monitor I&O; palpate bladder for retention. Monitor daily pattern of bowel activity/stool consistency.

PATIENT/ FAMILY TEACHING

• Avoid alcohol. • May cause dry mouth. • Avoid tasks that require alertness, motor skills until response to drug is established (may cause drowsiness).

oxycodone

ox-ee-**koe**-done

(OxyContin, Oxydose, OxyFast, Oxy-IR, Roxicodone, Roxicodone Intensol, Supeudol ✤)

Do not confuse oxycodone with oxybutynin.

FIXED-COMBINATION(S)

Combunox: oxycodone/ibuprofen (an NSAID): 5 mg/400 mg. **Percocet, Roxicet, Tylox:** oxycodone/acetaminophen (a non-narcotic analgesic): 5 mg/500 mg. **Percocet:** oxycodone/acetaminophen: 2.5 mg/325 mg; 5 mg/325 mg; 5 mg/500 mg; 7.5 mg/325 mg; 7.5 mg/500 mg; 10 mg/325 mg; 10 mg/650 mg. **Percodan:** oxycodone/aspirin (a non-narcotic analgesic): 2.25 mg/325 mg; 4.5 mg/325 mg.

CLASSIFICATION

PHARMACOTHERAPEUTIC: Opioid analgesic (**Schedule II**). **CLINICAL:** Narcotic analgesic (see p. 136C).

ACTION

Binds with opioid receptors within CNS. **Therapeutic Effect:** Alters perception of and emotional response to pain.

PHARMACOKINETICS

Route	Onset	Peak	Duration
PO, Immediate-release	N/A	N/A	4–5 hrs
PO, Controlled-release	N/A	N/A	12 hrs

Moderately absorbed from GI tract. Protein binding: 38%–45%. Widely distributed. Metabolized in liver. Excreted in urine. Unknown if removed by hemodialysis. **Half-life:** 2–3 hrs (3.2 hrs controlled-release).

USES

Relief of mild to moderately severe pain.

PRECAUTIONS

CONTRAINDICATIONS: Acute bronchial asthma, hypercarbia, paralytic ileus, respiratory depression. **EXTREME CAUTION:** CNS depression, anoxia, hypercapnia, respiratory depression, seizures, acute alcoholism, shock, untreated myxedema, respiratory dysfunction. **CAUTIONS:** Increased intracranial pressure (ICP), hepatic impairment, acute abdominal conditions, hypothyroidism, prostatic hypertrophy, Addison's disease, urethral stricture, chronic obstructive pulmonary disease (COPD).

LIFESPAN CONSIDERATIONS:

Pregnancy/Lactation: Readily crosses placenta. Distributed in breast milk. Respiratory depression may occur in neonate if mother received opiates during labor. Regular use of opiates during pregnancy may produce withdrawal symptoms in neonate (irritability, excessive crying, tremors, hyperactive reflexes, fever, vomiting, diarrhea, yawning, sneezing, seizures). **Pregnancy Category B (D if used for prolonged periods or at high dosages at term). Children:** Paradoxical excitement may occur. Those younger than 2 yrs are more susceptible to respiratory depressant effects. **Elderly:** Age-related renal impairment may increase risk of urinary retention. May be more susceptible to respiratory depressant effects.

INTERACTIONS

DRUG: Alcohol, other CNS depressants may increase CNS effects, respiratory depression, hypotension. **MAOIs** may produce severe, sometimes fatal reaction (administer ¼ of usual oxycodone dose). **HERBAL: Gotu kola, kava kava, St. John's wort, valerian** may increase CNS depression. **FOOD:** None known. **LAB VALUES:** May increase serum amylase, lipase.

O

AVAILABILITY (Rx)

CAPSULES (IMMEDIATE-RELEASE [OXY-IR]): 5 mg. **ORAL CONCENTRATE (OXYDOSE, OXYFAST, ROXICODONE INTENSOL):** 20 mg/ml. **ORAL SOLUTION (ROXICODONE):** 5 mg/5 ml. **TABLETS (ROXICODONE):** 5 mg, 15 mg, 30 mg.

TABLETS (CONTROLLED-RELEASE [OXYCONTIN]): 10 mg, 20 mg, 40 mg, 80 mg, 160 mg.

ADMINISTRATION/HANDLING

PO

• Give without regard to meals. • Tablets may be crushed. • **Extended-release:** Swallow whole; do not crush, break, chew.

INDICATIONS/ROUTES/DOSAGE

ANALGESIA

PO (IMMEDIATE-RELEASE): **ADULTS, ELDERLY:** 5 mg q6h as needed. **CHILDREN OLDER THAN 12 YRS:** 2.5 mg q6h as needed. **CHILDREN 6–12 YRS:** 1.25 mg q6h as needed.

Opioid Naive

PO (CONTROLLED-RELEASE): **ADULTS, ELDERLY:** 10 mg q12h.

Currently on Opioid/ASA, Opioid/Acetaminophen, NSAIDs

PO: **ADULTS, ELDERLY:** *1–5 tablets:* 10–20 mg q12h. *6–9 tablets:* 20–30 mg q12h. *10–12 tablets:* 30–40 mg q12h.

◄ **ALERT** ► Dosages are reduced in pts with severe hepatic disease.

SIDE EFFECTS

◄ **ALERT** ► Effects are dependent on dosage amount. Ambulatory pts, those not in severe pain may experience dizziness, nausea, vomiting, hypotension more frequently than those in supine position or having severe pain.

FREQUENT: Drowsiness, dizziness, hypotension (including orthostatic hypotension), anorexia. **OCCASIONAL:** Confusion, diaphoresis, facial flushing, urinary retention, constipation, dry mouth, nausea, vomiting, headache. **RARE:** Allergic reaction, depression, paradoxical CNS hyperactivity, nervousness in children, paradoxical excitement, restlessness in elderly, debilitated pts.

ADVERSE EFFECTS/ TOXIC REACTIONS

Overdose results in respiratory depression, skeletal muscle flaccidity, cold/clammy skin, cyanosis, extreme somnolence progressing to seizures, stupor, coma. Hepatotoxicity may occur with overdose of acetaminophen component of fixed-combination product. Tolerance to analgesic effect, physical dependence may occur with repeated use.

NURSING CONSIDERATIONS

BASELINE ASSESSMENT

Assess onset, type, location, duration of pain. Effect of medication is reduced if full pain recurs before next dose. Obtain vital signs before giving medication. If respirations are 12/min or less (20/min or less in children), withhold medication, contact physician.

INTERVENTION/EVALUATION

Palpate bladder for urinary retention. Monitor daily pattern of bowel activity/stool consistency. Initiate deep breathing, coughing exercises, esp. in pts with pulmonary impairment. Monitor pain relief, respiratory rate, mental status, B/P.

PATIENT/FAMILY TEACHING

• May cause dry mouth, drowsiness. • Avoid tasks that require alertness, motor skills until response to drug is established. • Avoid alcohol. • May be habit forming. • Do not crush, chew, break extended-release tablets.

OxyContin, *see oxycodone*

OxyFast, *see oxycodone*

OxyIR, *see oxycodone*

oxymorphone

ox-ee-**more**-phone

(Opana, Opana ER, Opana Injectable)

CLASSIFICATION

PHARMACOTHERAPEUTIC: Opioid agonist **(Schedule II)**. **CLINICAL:** Narcotic analgesic, antianxiety, preoperative anesthetic.

ACTION

Binds to opiate receptors sites within CNS. **Therapeutic Effect:** Reduces intensity of pain stimuli, alters pain perception, emotional response to pain. Parenterally, 1 mg oxymorphone equivalent to 10 mg morphine.

PHARMACOKINETICS

	Onset	Peak	Duration
Parenteral	5–10 min	N/A	3–6 hrs

Well absorbed. Protein binding: 10–12%. Widely distributed. Extensive hepatic metabolism. Excreted in urine. **Half-life:** 0.6–2 hrs.

USES

Injection: Relief of moderate to severe pain, preoperative medication, anesthesia support, obstetric analgesia, relief of anxiety in those with dyspnea associated with pulmonary edema secondary to acute left ventricular dysfunction. **Oral:** Relief of moderate to severe acute pain, pts requiring continuous treatment for extended period of time.

PRECAUTIONS

CONTRAINDICATIONS: Hypersensitivity to morphine, acute asthma attack, acute respiratory depression, paralytic ileus, pulmonary edema secondary to chemical respiratory irritants. **EXTREME CAUTION:** Anoxia, hypercapnia, seizures, acute alcoholism, shock, untreated myxedema. **CAUTIONS:** Hepatic impairment, hypothyroidism, prostatic hypertrophy, Addison's disease, urethral stricture, COPD.

LIFESPAN CONSIDERATIONS:

Pregnancy/Lactation: Unknown if distributed in breast milk. May prolong labor if administered in latent phase of first stage of labor or before cervical dilation of 4–5 cm has occurred. Respiratory depression may occur in neonate if mother received opiates during labor. Regular use of opiates during pregnancy may produce withdrawal symptoms in the neonate (irritability, excessive crying, tremors, hyperactive reflexes, fever, vomiting, diarrhea, yawning, sneezing, seizures). **Pregnancy Category C. (Category D** if used for prolong periods or high doses at term.) **Children:** Safety and efficacy not established in those younger than 18 yrs. **Elderly:** May be more susceptible to respiration depression, may cause paradoxical excitement. Age-related hepatic impairment, debilitation may require dosage adjustment.

O

INTERACTIONS

DRUG: **Alcohol, other CNS depressants** may increase CNS effects, respiratory depression, hypotension. **Anticholinergics** may increase risk of urinary retention, severe constipation (may lead to paralytic ileus). **Propofol** increases risk of bradycardia. Decreased effect when given concurrently with **phenothiazines.** **HERBAL:** **Valerian, St. John's wort, kava kava, gotu kola** may produce CNS depressant effects. **FOOD:** None known. **LAB VALUES:** May increase serum amylase, lipase.

AVAILABILITY (Rx)

INJECTION: 1 mg/ml, 1.5 mg/ml. **TABLETS:** 5 mg, 10 mg. **TABLETS (EXTENDED-RELEASE):** 5 mg, 10 mg, 20 mg, 40 mg.

ADMINISTRATION/HANDLING

IV

Rate of administration • Administer IV push very slowly. • Rapid IV increases risk of severe adverse reactions (chest wall rigidity, apnea, peripheral circulatory collapse, anaphylactoid effects, cardiac arrest).

O

IM/SUBCUTANEOUS

• Inject deep IM, preferably in upper, outer quandrant of buttock. • Use short 30-gauge needle for subcutaneous injection. • Administer slowly, rotating injection sites. • Pts with circulatory impairment experience higher risk of overdosage due to delayed absorption of repeated administration.

ORAL • Give 1 hr before or 2 hrs after meals. • Do not chew, dissolve, or crush extended-release tablet.

Storage • Store parenteral form at room temperature. Refrigerate suppository form. • Discard parenteral form if discolored or particulate forms.

IV COMPATIBILITIES

Glycopyrrolate, hydroxyzine, ranitidine.

INDICATIONS/ROUTES/DOSAGE

ANALGESIA

IV: ADULTS 18 YRS AND OLDER, ELDERLY: 0.5 mg. Dose may be cautiously increased until satisfactory response is achieved.

◄ **ALERT** ► IM preferred over subcutaneous route (subcutaneous rate of absorption is less reliable).

IM/SUBCUTANEOUS: ADULTS 18 YRS AND OLDER, ELDERLY: Initially, 1–1.5 mg every 4–6 hrs as needed.

PO: ADULTS, ELDERLY: (IMMEDIATE-RELEASE): 10–20 mg q4–6hrs. **(EXTENDED-RELEASE):** Initially, 5 mg q12h. May increase by 5–10 mg q12h every 3–7 days.

ANALGESIA DURING LABOR

IM/SUBCUTANEOUS: ADULTS 18 YRS AND OLDER, ELDERLY: 0.5–1 mg.

SIDE EFFECTS

Note: Effects are dependent on dosage amount, route of administration. Ambulatory pts, those not in severe pain may experience dizziness, nausea, vomiting, hypotension more frequently than those in supine position or having severe pain. **FREQUENT (10% or higher):** Drowsiness, hypotension, dizziness, nausea, vomiting, constipation, weakness. **OCCASIONAL (Less than 10%):** Nervousness, headache, restlessness, malaise, confusion, anorexia, abdominal cramps, dry mouth, decreased urinary output, ureteral spasm, pain at injection site. **RARE (1% or less):** Depression, paradoxical CNS stimulation, hallucinations, rash, urticaria.

ADVERSE EFFECTS/ TOXIC REACTIONS

Overdosage results in respiratory depression, skeletal muscle flaccidity, cold/clammy skin, cyanosis, extreme somnolence progressing to convulsions, stupor, coma. Tolerance to analgesic effect, physical dependence may occur with repeated use. Prolonged duration of action, cumulative effect may occur in those with hepatic/renal impairment.

NURSING CONSIDERATIONS

BASELINE ASSESSMENT

Assess onset, type, location, duration of pain. Obtain vital signs before giving medication. If respirations are 12/min or lower, withhold medication, contact physician. Effect of medication is reduced if full pain recurs before next dose.

INTERVENTION/EVALUATION

Monitor vital signs 5–10 min after IV administration, 15–30 min after subcutaneous, IM. Be alert for decreased respirations, B/P. To prevent pain cycles, instruct pt to request pain medication as soon as discomfort begins. Assess for clinical improvement, record onset of pain relief. Consult physician if pain relief is not adequate.

PATIENT/FAMILY TEACHING

Discomfort may occur with injection. Change positions slowly to avoid postural hypotension. Avoid tasks that require alertness, motor skills until response to drug is established. Avoid alcohol. Tolerance/dependence may occur with prolonged use of high doses.

oxytocin

ox-ee-**toe**-sin

(Pitocin, Syntocinon)

Do not confuse Pitocin with Pitressin.

CLASSIFICATION

PHARMACOTHERAPEUTIC: Uterine smooth muscle stimulant. **CLINICAL:** Oxytocic.

ACTION

Affects uterine myofibril activity, stimulates mammary smooth muscle. **Therapeutic Effect:** Contracts uterine smooth muscle. Enhances lactation.

PHARMACOKINETICS

Route	Onset	Peak	Duration
IV	Immediate	N/A	1 hr
IM	3–5 min	N/A	2–3 hrs

Rapidly absorbed through nasal mucous membranes. Protein binding: 30%. Distributed in extracellular fluid. Metabolized in liver, kidney. Primarily excreted in urine. **Half-life:** 1–6 min.

USES

Induction of labor at term, control postpartum bleeding. Adjunct in management of abortion.

PRECAUTIONS

CONTRAINDICATIONS: Adequate uterine activity that fails to progress, cephalopelvic disproportion, fetal distress without imminent delivery, grand multiparity, hyperactive or hypertonic uterus, obstetric emergencies that favor surgical intervention, prematurity, unengaged fetal head, unfavorable fetal position/presentation, when vaginal delivery is contraindicated, (e.g., active genital herpes infection, placenta previa, cord presentation). **CAUTIONS:** Induction of labor should be for medical, not elective, reasons.

LIFESPAN CONSIDERATIONS:

Pregnancy/Lactation: Used as indicated, not expected to present risk of

O

fetal abnormalities. Small amounts in breast milk; breast-feeding not recommended. **Pregnancy Category X.** **Children/Elderly:** Not used in these pt populations.

INTERACTIONS

DRUG: **Caudal block anesthetics, vasopressors** may increase pressor effects. **Other oxytocics** may cause cervical lacerations, uterine hypertonus, uterine rupture. **HERBAL:** None significant. **FOOD:** None known. **LAB VALUES:** None known.

AVAILABILITY (Rx)

INJECTION (PITOCIN): 10 units/ml.

ADMINISTRATION/HANDLING

IV

Reconstitution • Dilute 10–40 units (1–4 ml) in 1,000 ml of 0.9% NaCl, lactated Ringer's, or D_5W to provide concentration of 10–40 milliunit/ml solution.

Rate of administration • Give by IV infusion (use infusion device to carefully control rate of flow as ordered by physician).

Storage • Store at room temperature.

IV INCOMPATIBILITIES

No known incompatibilities via Y-site administration.

IV COMPATIBILITIES

Heparin, insulin, multivitamins, potassium chloride.

INDICATIONS/ROUTES/DOSAGE

INDUCTION OR STIMULATION OF LABOR

IV: ADULTS: 0.5–1 milliunit/min. May gradually increase in increments of 1–2 milliunit/min. Rates of 9–10 milliunit/min are rarely required.

ABORTION

IV: ADULTS: 10–20 milliunit/min. **Maximum:** 30 unit/12 hr dose.

CONTROL OF POSTPARTUM BLEEDING

IV INFUSION: ADULTS: 10–40 units in 1,000 ml IV fluid at rate sufficient to control uterine atony.

IM: ADULTS: 10 units (total dose) after delivery.

SIDE EFFECTS

OCCASIONAL: Tachycardia, premature ventricular contractions, hypotension, nausea, vomiting. **RARE:** **Nasal:** Lacrimation/tearing, nasal irritation, rhinorrhea, unexpected uterine bleeding/contractions.

ADVERSE EFFECTS/ TOXIC REACTIONS

Hypertonicity may occur with tearing of uterus, increased bleeding, abruptio placentae (i.e., placental abruption), cervical/vaginal lacerations. **FETAL:** Bradycardia, CNS/brain damage, trauma due to rapid propulsion, low Apgar score at 5 min, retinal hemorrhage occur rarely. Prolonged IV infusion of oxytocin with excessive fluid volume has caused severe water intoxication with seizures, coma, death.

NURSING CONSIDERATIONS

BASELINE ASSESSMENT

Assess baselines for vital signs, B/P, fetal heart rate. Determine frequency, duration, strength of contractions.

INTERVENTION/EVALUATION

Monitor B/P, pulse, respirations, fetal heart rate, intrauterine pressure, contractions (duration, strength, frequency) q15min. Notify physician of contractions that last longer than 1 min, occur more frequently than every 2 min, or stop. Maintain careful I&O; be alert to potential water intoxication. Check for blood loss.

PATIENT/FAMILY TEACHING

- Keep pt, family informed of labor progress.

Pacerone, *see amiodarone*

paclitaxel

pass-leh-**tax**-ell
(Abraxane, Onxol, Taxol)

Do not confuse paclitaxel with Paxil, or Taxol with Taxotere.

CLASSIFICATION

PHARMACOTHERAPEUTIC: Taxoid, antimitotic agent. **CLINICAL:** Antineoplastic (see p. 82C).

ACTION

Disrupts microtubular cell network, essential for cellular function. Blocks cells in late G_2, M phases of cell cycle. **Therapeutic Effect:** Inhibits cellular mitosis, replication.

PHARMACOKINETICS

Does not readily cross blood-brain barrier. Protein binding: 89%–98%. Metabolized in liver to active metabolites; eliminated by bile. Not removed by hemodialysis. **Half-life:** 1.3–8.6 hrs.

USES

(ONXOL, TAXOL): First-line treatment of advanced ovarian cancer, treatment of metastatic ovarian cancer following failure of first-line or subsequent chemotherapy. Treatment of breast cancer, AIDS-related Kaposi's sarcoma, non–small cell lung cancer. **(ABRAXANE):** Treatment of breast cancer after failure of combination chemotherapy or relapse within 6 mos of adjuvant chemotherapy. **OFF-LABEL:** Treatment of upper GI tract adenocarcinoma, head and neck cancer, hormone-refractory prostate cancer, metastic breast cancer, non-Hodgkin's lymphoma, small-cell lung cancer, transitional cell cancer of urothelium.

PRECAUTIONS

CONTRAINDICATIONS: Baseline neutropenia (neutrophil count 1,500 cells/mm^3), (ONXOL, TAXOL) hypersensitivity to drugs developed with Cremophor EL (polyoxyethylated castor oil). **CAUTIONS:** Hepatic impairment, severe neutropenia, peripheral neuropathy.

LIFESPAN CONSIDERATIONS:

Pregnancy/Lactation: May produce fetal harm. Unknown if distributed in breast milk. Avoid use in pregnancy. **Pregnancy Category D. Children:** Safety and efficacy not established. **Elderly:** No age-related precautions noted.

INTERACTIONS

DRUG: Bone marrow depressants may increase myelosuppression. **Live virus vaccines** may potentiate virus replication, increase vaccine side effects, decrease pt's antibody response to vaccine. **HERBAL:** Avoid **black cohosh, dong quai** in estrogen-dependent tumors. **Gotu kola, kava kava, St. John's wort, valerian** may increase CNS depression. **FOOD:** None known. **LAB VALUES:** May elevate serum alkaline phosphatase, bilirubin, AST, ALT. Decreases Hgb, Hct, platelet, RBC, WBC counts.

AVAILABILITY (Rx)

INJECTION POWDER FOR RECONSTITUTION (ABRAXANE): 100-mg vial. **INJECTION SOLUTION (ONXOL, TAXOL):** 6 mg/ml.1

ADMINISTRATION/HANDLING

IV

◄ **ALERT** ► Wear gloves during handling; if contact with skin occurs, wash hands thoroughly with soap, water. If contact with mucous membranes occurs, flush with water.

P

ONXOL, TAXOL

Reconstitution • Dilute with 0.9% NaCl, D_5W to final concentration of 0.3–1.2 mg/ml.

Rate of administration • Administer at rate as ordered by physician through in-line filter not greater than 0.22 microns. • Monitor vital signs during infusion, esp. during first hour. • Discontinue administration if severe hypersensitivity reaction occurs.

Storage • Refrigerate unopened vials. • Prepared solution is stable at room temperature for 24 hrs. • Store diluted solutions in bottles or plastic bags. Administer through polyethylene-lined administration sets (avoid plasticized PVC equipment or devices).

ABRAXANE

Reconstitution • Reconstitute each vial with 20 ml 0.9% NaCl to provide concentration of 5 mg/ml. • Slowly inject onto inside wall of vial; gently swirl over 2 min to avoid foaming. • Inject appropriate amount into empty PVC-type bag.

Rate of administration • Infuse over 30 min.

Storage • Store unopened vials at room temperature • Once reconstituted, use immediately but may refrigerate for up to 8 hrs.

P

IV INCOMPATIBILITIES

◄ **ALERT** ► **IV Compatibility:** Data for Abraxane not known; avoid mixing with other medication.

Onxol, Taxol: Amphotericin B complex (Abelcet, AmBisome, Amphotec), chlorpromazine (Thorazine), doxorubicin liposomal (Doxil), hydroxyzine (Vistaril), methylprednisolone (Solu-Medrol), mitoxantrone (Novantrone).

IV COMPATIBILITIES

Onxol, Taxol: Carboplatin (Paraplatin), cisplatin (Platinol AQ), cyclophosphamide (Cytoxan), cytarabine (Cytosar), dacarbazine (DTIC-Dome), dexamethasone (Decadron), diphenhydramine (Benadryl), doxorubicin (Adriamycin), etoposide (VePesid), gemcitabine (Gemzar), granisetron (Kytril), hydromorphone (Dilaudid), lipids, magnesium sulfate, mannitol, methotrexate, morphine, ondansetron (Zofran), potassium chloride, vinblastine (Velban), vincristine (Oncovin).

INDICATIONS/ROUTES/DOSAGE

ONXOL, TAXOL

OVARIAN CANCER

IV: ADULTS: 135–175 mg/m^2/dose over 1–24 hrs q3wk or 50–80 mg/m^2 over 1–3 hrs weekly.

BREAST CARCINOMA

IV: ADULTS, ELDERLY: 175 mg/m^2 over 3 hrs q3wk or 50–80 mg/m^2 over 1–3 hrs weekly.

NON–SMALL-CELL LUNG CARCINOMA

IV: ADULTS, ELDERLY: 135 mg/m^2 over 24 hrs, followed by cisplatin 75 mg/m^2 q3wk.

KAPOSI'S SARCOMA

IV: ADULTS, ELDERLY: 135 mg/m^2/dose over 3 hrs q3wk or 100 mg/m^2/dose over 3 hrs q2wk.

DOSAGE IN HEPATIC IMPAIRMENT

Total Bilirubin	Total Dose
More than 3 mg/dl	Less than 50 mg/m^2
1.6–3 mg/dl	Less than 75 mg/m^2
1.5 mg/dl or less	Less than 135 mg/m^2

ABRAXANE

BREAST CANCER

IV INFUSION: ADULTS, ELDERLY: 260 mg/m^2 q3wks. For pts who experience severe neutropenia (neutrophils less than 500 cells/mm^3 for a wk or longer) or severe sensory neuropathy, reduce dosage to 220 mg/m^2 for subsequent courses. For recurrence of severe neutropenia or severe sensory neuropathy, reduce dosage to 180 mg/m^2 q3wks for subsequent courses. For grade 3 sensory neuropathy, hold until resolution to grade 1 or 2, followed by reduced dose for subsequent courses. Dosage of Abraxane for bilirubin greater than 1.5 mg/dl is not known.

SIDE EFFECTS

EXPECTED (90%–70%): Diarrhea, alopecia, nausea, vomiting. **FREQUENT (48%–46%):** Myalgia, arthralgia, peripheral neuropathy. **OCCASIONAL (20%–13%):** Mucositis, hypotension during infusion, pain/redness at injection site. **RARE (3%):** Bradycardia.

ADVERSE EFFECTS/ TOXIC REACTIONS

Neutropenic nadir occurs at median of 11 days. Anemia, leukopenia occur commonly; thrombocytopenia occurs occasionally. Severe hypersensitivity reaction (dyspnea, severe hypotension, angioedema, generalized urticaria) occurs rarely.

NURSING CONSIDERATIONS

BASELINE ASSESSMENT

Give emotional support to pt, family. Use strict asepsis, protect pt from infection. Check blood counts, particularly neutrophil, platelet count before each course of therapy or as clinically indicated.

INTERVENTION/EVALUATION

Monitor CBC, platelets, vital signs, hepatic enzymes. Monitor for hematologic toxicity (fever, sore throat, signs of local infections, unusual bleeding/ bruising), symptoms of anemia (excessive fatigue, weakness). Assess response to medication; monitor, report diarrhea. Avoid IM injections, rectal temperatures, other traumas that may induce bleeding. Hold pressure to injection sites for full 5 min.

PATIENT/FAMILY TEACHING

• Explain that alopecia is reversible, but new hair may have different color, texture. • Do not have immunizations without physician's approval (drug lowers resistance). • Avoid crowds, persons with known infections. • Report signs of infection at once (fever, flu-like symptoms). • Contact physician if nausea/vomiting continues at home. • Teach signs of peripheral neuropathy. • Avoid pregnancy during therapy.

palifermin

pal-ih-**fur**-min
(Kepivance)

CLASSIFICATION

PHARMACOTHERAPEUTIC: Keratinocyte growth factor. **CLINICAL:** Antineoplastic adjunct.

ACTION

Binds to keratinocyte growth factor receptor, present on epithelial cells of buccal mucosa, tongue, resulting in proliferation, differentiation, migration of epithelial cells. **Therapeutic Effect:** Reduces incidence, duration of severe oral mucositis.

PHARMACOKINETICS

Clearance is higher in cancer pts compared to healthy subjects. **Half-life:** 4.5 hrs.

USES

Reduces incidence, duration, severity of severe stomatitis in pts with hematologic malignancies receiving myelotoxic therapy requiring hematopoietic stem cell support.

PRECAUTIONS

CONTRAINDICATIONS: Pts allergic to *Escherichia coli*–derived proteins. **CAUTIONS:** Pregnant and breast-feeding pts.

P

LIFESPAN CONSIDERATIONS:

Pregnancy/Lactation: Unknown if drug crosses the placenta or is excreted in breast milk. Use palifermin only if potential benefit justifies fetal risk. **Pregnancy Category C. Children:** Safety and effectiveness have not been established. **Elderly:** No age-related precautions noted.

INTERACTIONS

DRUG: Binds to **heparin**, decreasing effectiveness. Administration during or within 24 hrs before or after **myelotoxic chemotherapy** results in increased severity, duration of oral mucositis. **HERBAL:** None significant. **FOOD:** None known. **LAB VALUES:** May elevate serum lipase, amylase.

AVAILABILITY (Rx)

INJECTION POWDER FOR RECONSTITUTION: 6.25-mg vials.

ADMINISTRATION/HANDLING

IV

Reconstitution • Reconstitute only with 1.2 ml Sterile Water for Injection, using aseptic technique. • Swirl gently to dissolve. Dissolution takes less than 3 min. Do not shake/agitate solution. • Yields final concentration of 5 mg/ml.

Rate of administration • If heparin is being used to maintain an IV line, use 0.9% NaCl to rinse IV line before and after palifermin administration. • Administer by IV bolus injection.

Storage • If reconstituted solution is not used immediately, may be refrigerated for up to 24 hrs. • Before administration, may be warmed to room temperature for up to 1 hr. • Discard if left at room temperature for more than 1 hr, if discolored or particulate forms. • Protect from light.

INDICATIONS/ROUTES/DOSAGE

MUCOSITIS (PREMYELOTOXIC THERAPY)

IV: ADULTS, ELDERLY: 60 mcg/kg/day for 3 consecutive days, with 3rd dose 24–48 hrs before chemotherapy.

MUCOSITIS (POSTMYELOTOXIC THERAPY)

IV: ADULTS, ELDERLY: Last 3 doses should be administered after myelotoxic therapy; first of these doses should be administered after, but on the same day of, hematopoietic stem cell infusion and at least 4 days after most recent administration of palifermin.

SIDE EFFECTS

FREQUENT: Rash (62%), fever (39%), pruritus (35%), erythema (32%), edema (28%). **OCCASIONAL:** Mouth, tongue thickness/discoloration (17%), altered taste (16%), dysesthesia manifested as hyperesthesia, hypoesthesia, paresthesia (12%), arthralgia (10%).

ADVERSE EFFECTS/ TOXIC REACTIONS

Transient hypertension occurs occasionally.

NURSING CONSIDERATIONS

BASELINE ASSESSMENT

Assess oral mucous membranes for stomatitis (erythema, white patches, ulceration, bleeding).

INTERVENTION/EVALUATION

Assess for oral inflammation, difficulty swallowing, mucosal bleeding. Offer sponge sticks to wash mouth with water. Monitor pt's pain level; medicate as necessary for improved pain control. Offer pt, family emotional support.

PATIENT/FAMILY TEACHING

• Offer bland meals; advise against eating any spicy food. • Rinse mouth often with tepid water; avoid hot, cold liquids. • Advise female pt to notify the physician if she is pregnant or breast-feeding.

P

paliperidone

pall-ih-**pear**-ih-doan
(Invega)

CLASSIFICATION

PHARMACOTHERAPEUTIC: Benzisoxazole derivative. **CLINICAL:** Antipsychotic.

ACTION:

May antagonize dopamine and serotonin receptors. **Therapeutic Effect:** Suppresses behavioral response in psychosis.

PHARMACOKINETICS

Absorbed from GI tract. Metabolized in liver to active metabolite. Primarily excreted in urine. **Half-life:** 23 hrs.

USES

Treatment of schizophrenia.

PRECAUTIONS

CONTRAINDICATIONS: Sensitivity to risperidone. Concomitant use with other medications that prolong QT interval (e.g., amiodarone, quinidine). **CAUTIONS:** History of cardiac arrhythmias, renal impairment, diabetes mellitus, heart failure, seizures, pts at risk for aspiration pneumonia. May increase risk of stroke in pts with dementia-related psychosis.

LIFESPAN CONSIDERATIONS:

Pregnancy/Lactation: Unknown if crosses placenta or is excreted in breast milk. **Pregnancy Category C. Children:** Safety and efficacy not established. **Elderly:** Potential for orthostatic hypotension. Age-related renal impairment may require dosage adjustment.

INTERACTIONS

DRUG: May decrease effects of **levodopa, dopamine agonists. Alcohol, CNS depressants** may increase CNS depression. **HERBAL:** None significant. **FOOD:** None known. **LAB VALUES:** May increase serum creatine phosphatase, uric acid, triglycerides, AST, ALT, prolactin. May decrease serum potassium, sodium, protein, glucose. May cause EKG changes.

AVAILABILITY (Rx)

TABLETS, EXTENDED-RELEASE: 3 mg, 6 mg, 9 mg, 12 mg.

ADMINISTRATION/HANDLING

PO

- May give without regard to food. Do not chew, divide, crush extended-release tablets.

INDICATIONS/ROUTES/DOSAGE

TREATMENT OF SCHIZOPHRENIA

PO: ADULTS, ELDERLY: 6 mg once daily. **RANGE:** 3–12 mg/day.

DOSAGE IN RENAL IMPAIRMENT

Creatinine Clearance	Maximum Daily Dosage
50–80 ml/min	6 mg/day
10–49 ml/min	3 mg/day

SIDE EFFECTS

OCCASIONAL: Tachycardia (14%), headache (12%), drowsiness (9%), akathesia (motor restlessness), anxiety (7%), dizziness (5%), dyspepsia, nausea (4%).

ADVERSE EFFECTS/ TOXIC REACTIONS

Neuroleptic malignant syndrome (NMS), hyperpyrexia, muscle rigidity, change in mental status, irregular pulse or B/P, tachycardia, diaphoresis, cardiac, arrhythmias, rhabdomyolysis, acute renal failure, tardive dyskinesia (protrusion of tongue, puffing of cheeks, chewing/puckering of mouth) may occur rarely.

P

NURSING CONSIDERATIONS

BASELINE ASSESSMENT

Renal function tests should be performed before therapy. Assess behavior, appearance, emotional status, response to environment, speech pattern, thought content.

INTERVENTION/EVALUATION

Monitor B/P, heart rate, weight, renal function tests, EKG. Monitor for fine tongue movement (may be first sign of tardive dyskinesia). Supervise suicidal-risk pt closely during early therapy. Assess for therapeutic response (greater interest in surroundings, improved self care, increased ability to concentrate, relaxed facial expression). Monitor for potential neuroleptic malignant syndrome (fever, muscle rigidity, irregular B/P or pulse, altered mental status).

PATIENT/FAMILY TEACHING

Avoid tasks that may require alertness, motor skills until response to drug is established (may cause drowsiness, dizziness). Use caution when changing position from lying or sitting to standing. Inform physician of trembling in fingers, altered gait, unusual muscle/skeletal movements, palpitations, severe dizziness, fainting, swelling/pain in breasts, visual changes, rash, difficulty in breathing.

palivizumab

pal-**iv**-ih-zoo-mab

(Synagis)

Do not confuse Synagis with Synalgos-DC.

CLASSIFICATION

PHARMACOTHERAPEUTIC: Monoclonal antibody. **CLINICAL:** Pediatric lower respiratory tract infection agent.

ACTION

Exhibits neutralizing activity against respiratory syncytial virus (RSV) in infants. **Therapeutic Effect:** Inhibits RSV replication in lower respiratory tract.

USES

Prevention of serious lower respiratory tract disease caused by RSV in pediatric pts at high risk for RSV disease (e.g., hemodynamically significant congenital heart disease).

PRECAUTIONS

CONTRAINDICATIONS: Children with cyanotic congenital heart disease. **CAUTIONS:** Thrombocytopenia, any coagulation disorder. Not to be used for treatment of established RSV disease. **Pregnancy Category C.**

INTERACTIONS

DRUG: None significant. **HERBAL:** None significant. **FOOD:** None known. **LAB VALUES:** None known.

AVAILABILITY (Rx)

INJECTION, SOLUTION: 50 mg/0.5 ml, 100 mg/ml.

INDICATIONS/ROUTES/DOSAGE

PREVENTION OF RSV

IM: CHILDREN: 15 mg/kg once/mo during RSV season.

SIDE EFFECTS

FREQUENT (49%–22%): Upper respiratory tract infection, otitis media, rhinitis, rash. **OCCASIONAL (10%–2%):** Pain, pharyngitis. **RARE (less than 2%):** Cough, diarrhea, vomiting, injection site reaction.

ADVERSE EFFECTS/ TOXIC REACTIONS

Anaphylaxis, severe acute hypersensitivity reaction occur very rarely.

NURSING CONSIDERATIONS

BASELINE ASSESSMENT

Assess for sensitivity to palivizumab.

INTERVENTION/EVALUATION

Monitor potential side effects, esp. otitis media, rhinitis, skin rash, upper respiratory tract infection.

PATIENT/FAMILY TEACHING

- Discuss with family the purpose, potential side effects of medication.

palonosetron

pal-oh-**noe**-seh-tron
(Aloxi)

CLASSIFICATION

PHARMACOTHERAPEUTIC: 5-HT_3 receptor antagonist. **CLINICAL:** Antinauseant, antiemetic.

ACTION

Acts centrally in chemoreceptor trigger zone, peripherally at vagal nerve terminals. **Therapeutic Effect:** Prevents nausea/vomiting associated with chemotherapy.

PHARMACOKINETICS

Protein binding: 52%. Metabolized in liver. Eliminated in urine. **Half-life:** 40 hrs.

USES

Prevention of acute, delayed nausea/vomiting associated with initial/repeated courses of moderately or highly ematogenic cancer chemotherapy. **OFF-LABEL:** Prevention of postop bleeding.

PRECAUTIONS

CONTRAINDICATIONS: None known. **CAUTIONS:** History of cardiovascular disease.

LIFESPAN CONSIDERATIONS:

Pregnancy/Lactation: Unknown if excreted in breast milk. **Pregnancy Category B. Children:** Safety and efficacy not established. **Elderly:** No age-related precautions noted.

INTERACTIONS

DRUG: Apomorphine may cause profound hypotension, altered consciousness. **HERBAL:** None significant. **FOOD:** None known. **LAB VALUES:** May transiently increase serum bilirubin, AST, ALT.

AVAILABILITY (Rx)

INJECTION SOLUTION: 0.25 mg/5 ml.

ADMINISTRATION/HANDLING

IV

Reconstitution • Give undiluted as IV push.

Rate of administration • Give IV push over 30 sec. • Flush infusion line with 0.9% NaCl before and following administration.

Storage • Store at room temperature. Solution should appear colorless, clear. Discard if cloudy precipitate forms.

IV INCOMPATIBILITIES

Do not mix with any other medications.

INDICATIONS/ROUTES/DOSAGE

CHEMOTHERAPY-INDUCED NAUSEA/VOMITING

IV: ADULTS, ELDERLY: 0.25 mg as a single dose 30 min before starting chemotherapy.

SIDE EFFECTS

OCCASIONAL (9%–5%): Headache, constipation. **RARE (less than 1%):** Diarrhea, dizziness, fatigue, abdominal pain, insomnia.

ADVERSE EFFECTS/ TOXIC REACTIONS

Overdose may produce combination of CNS stimulation, depressant effects.

P

NURSING CONSIDERATIONS

BASELINE ASSESSMENT

Assess for dehydration if excessive vomiting occurs (poor skin turgor, dry mucous membranes, longitudinal furrows in tongue). Provide emotional support.

INTERVENTION/EVALUATION

Monitor pt in environment. Provide supportive measures. Assess mental status. Monitor daily pattern of bowel activity/stool consistency; record time of evacuation.

PATIENT/FAMILY TEACHING

• Relief from nausea/vomiting generally occurs shortly after drug administration. • Avoid alcohol, barbiturates. • Report persistent vomiting.

pamidronate

pam-id-**row**-nate

(Aredia)

Do not confuse Aredia with Adriamcyin.

CLASSIFICATION

PHARMACOTHERAPEUTIC: Bisphosphonate. **CLINICAL:** Hypocalcemic.

ACTION

Binds to bone, inhibits osteoclast-mediated calcium resorption. **Therapeutic Effect:** Lowers serum calcium concentration.

PHARMACOKINETICS

Route	Onset	Peak	Duration
IV	24–48 hrs	5–7 days	N/A

After IV administration, rapidly absorbed by bone. Slowly excreted unchanged in urine. Unknown if removed by hemodialysis. **Half-life:** bone, 300 days; unmetabolized, 2.5 hrs.

USES

Treatment of moderate to severe hypercalcemia associated with malignancy (with/without bone metastases). Treatment of moderate to severe Paget's disease, osteolytic bone lesions of multiple myeloma, breast cancer.

PRECAUTIONS

CONTRAINDICATIONS: Hypersensitivity to other bisphosphonates, (e.g., etidronate, tiludronate, risedronate, alendronate). **CAUTIONS:** Cardiac failure, renal impairment.

LIFESPAN CONSIDERATIONS:

Pregnancy/Lactation: No adequate, well-controlled studies in pregnant women; unknown if fetal harm can occur. Unknown if excreted in breast milk. **Pregnancy Category D. Children:** Safety and efficacy not established. **Elderly:** May become overhydrated. Careful monitoring of fluid and electrolytes indicated; recommend dilution in smaller volume.

INTERACTIONS

DRUG: Calcium-containing medications, vitamin D may antagonize effects in treatment of hypercalcemia. **Nephrotoxic medications** may increase potential for nephrotoxicity. **HERBAL:** None significant. **FOOD:** None known. **LAB VALUES:** May decrease serum phosphate, magnesium, calcium, potassium.

AVAILABILITY (Rx)

INJECTION POWDER FOR RECONSTITUTION: 30 mg, 90 mg. **INJECTION SOLUTION:** 3 mg/ml, 6 mg/ml, 9 mg/ml.

ADMINISTRATION/HANDLING

IV

Reconstitution • Reconstitute each 30-mg vial with 10 ml Sterile Water for Injection to provide concentration of

3 mg/ml. • Allow drug to dissolve before withdrawing. • Further dilute with 1,000 ml sterile 0.45% or 0.9% NaCl or D_5W.

Rate of administration • Adequate hydration is essential in conjunction with pamidronate therapy (avoid overhydration in pts with potential for cardiac failure). • Administer as IV infusion over 2–24 hrs for treatment of hypercalcemia; over 2–4 hrs for other indications.

Storage • Store parenteral form at room temperature. • Reconstituted vial is stable for 24 hrs refrigerated; IV solution is stable for 24 hrs after dilution.

IV INCOMPATIBILITIES

Calcium-containing IV fluids.

INDICATIONS/ROUTES/DOSAGE

HYPERCALCEMIA

IV INFUSION: ADULTS, ELDERLY: Moderate hypercalcemia (corrected serum calcium level 12–13.5 mg/dl): 60–90 mg. Severe hypercalcemia (corrected serum calcium level greater than 13.5 mg/dl): 90 mg.

PAGET'S DISEASE

IV INFUSION: ADULTS, ELDERLY: 30 mg/day for 3 days.

OSTEOLYTIC BONE LESION

IV INFUSION: ADULTS, ELDERLY: 90 mg over 2–4 hrs once a mo.

SIDE EFFECTS

FREQUENT (greater than 10%): Temperature elevation (at least 1°C) 24–48 hrs after administration (27%); redness, swelling, induration, pain at catheter site in pts receiving 90 mg (18%); anorexia, nausea, fatigue. **OCCASIONAL (10%–1%):** Constipation, rhinitis.

ADVERSE EFFECTS/ TOXIC REACTIONS

Hypophosphatemia, hypokalemia, hypomagnesemia, hypocalcemia occur more frequently with higher dosages. Anemia, hypertension, tachycardia, atrial fibrillation, somnolence occur more frequently with 90-mg doses. GI hemorrhage occurs rarely.

NURSING CONSIDERATIONS

INTERVENTION/EVALUATION

Monitor serum calcium, potassium, magnesium, creatinine, Hgb, Hct, CBC. Provide adequate hydration; avoid overhydration. Monitor I&O carefully; check lungs for rales, dependent body parts for edema. Monitor B/P, temperature, pulse. Assess catheter site for redness, swelling, pain. Monitor food intake, daily pattern of bowel activity/stool consistency. Be alert for potential GI hemorrhage with 90-mg dosage.

pancreatin

evolve

pan-kree-**ah**-tin
(Ku-Zyme, Pancreatin)

pancrelipase

pan-kree-**lie**-pace
(Cotazym ✦, Cotazym-65 B ✦, Cotazym-S, Creon 5, Creon 10, Creon 20, Ilozyme, Kutrase, Ku-Zyme, Ku-Zyme HP, Lipram, Lipram-CR, Lipram-CR 5, Lipram-CR 20, Lipram-PN, Lipram-UL 12, Lipram-UL 18, Lipram-UL 20, Panase, Pancrease, Pancrease MT 4, Pancrease MT 10 ✦, Pancrease MT 16 ✦, Pancrease MT 20, Pancreatic EC, Pancreatil-UL 12, Pancrecarb MS-4, Pancrecarb MS-8, Pangestyme CN 10, Pangestyme CN 20, Pangestyme EC, Pangestyme MT 16, Pangestyme NL 18, Panokase, Plaretase, Protilase, Ultrase, Ultrase MT 12, Ultrase MT 18, Ultrase MT 20, Viokase, Viokase 8, Viokase 16, Zymase)

P

CLASSIFICATION

PHARMACOTHERAPEUTIC: Digestive enzyme. **CLINICAL:** Pancreatic enzyme replenisher.

ACTION

Replaces endogenous pancreatic enzymes. **Therapeutic Effect:** Assists in digestion of protein, starch, fats.

USES

Pancreatic enzyme replacement/supplement when enzymes are absent/deficient (chronic pancreatitis, cystic fibrosis, ductal obstruction from pancreatic cancer, common bile duct). Treatment of steatorrhea associated with postgastrectomy syndrome, bowel resection; reduces malabsorption. **OFF-LABEL:** Treatment of occluded feeding tubes.

PRECAUTIONS

CONTRAINDICATIONS: Acute pancreatitis, exacerbation of chronic pancreatitis, hypersensitivity to pork protein. **CAUTIONS:** Inhalation of powder may cause asthmatic attack. **Pregnancy Category C.**

P

INTERACTIONS

DRUG: **Antacids** may decrease effects. May decrease absorption of **iron supplements**. **HERBAL:** None significant. **FOOD:** None known. **LAB VALUES:** May increase serum uric acid.

AVAILABILITY (Rx)

CAPSULES: 15,000 units-12,000 units-15,000 units (Ku-Zyme), 30,000 units-24,000 units-30,000 units (Kutrase), 30,000 units-8,000 units-30,000 units (Panokase, Cotazym, Ku-Zyme HP). **POWDER FOR RECONSTITUTION, ORAL (VIOKASE):** 70,000 units-16,800 units-70,000 units/0.7 gm. **TABLETS:** 30,000 units-11,000 units-30,000 units (Ilozyme), 60,000 units-16,000 units-60,000 units (Viokase 16), 30,000 units-8,000 units-30,000 units (Panokase, Plaretase, Viokase 8).

CAPSULES (EXTENDED-RELEASE): 33,200 units-10,000 units-37,500 units (Creon 10, Lipram-CR), 30,000 units-10,000 units-30,000 units (Pangestyme CN 10, Lipram, Pancrease MT 10), 39,000 units-12,000 units-39,000 units (Lipram-UL 12, Pancreatil-UL 12, Ultrase MT 12), 12,000 units-4,000 units-12,000 units (Pancrease MT 4), 48,000 units-16,000 units-48,000 units (Lipram-PN, Pancrease MT 16, Pangestyme MT 16), 16,600 units-5,000 units-18,750 units (Creon 5, Lipram-CR5), 59,000 units-18,000 units-59,000 units (Pangestyme NL 18, Lipram-UL 18, Ultrase MT 18), 20,000 units-5,000 units-20,000 units (Cotazym-S), 66,400 units-20,000 units-75,000 units (Creon 20, Lipram-CR 20), 20,000 units-4,500 units-25,000 units (Lipram, Pancrease, Pangestyme EC, Ultrase), 56,000 units-20,000 units-44,000 units (Lipram-PN, Pancrease MT 20), 65,000 units-20,000 units-65,000 units (Lipram-UL 20, Pangestyme NL 18, Pangestyme CN 20, Ultrase MT 20), 20,000 units-4,000 units-25,000 units (Panase, Pancreatic EC, Protilase), 25,000 units-4,000 units-25,000 units (Pancrecarb MS-4), 40,000 units-8,000 units-45,000 units (Pancrecarb MS-8).

ADMINISTRATION/HANDLING

◀ **ALERT** ▶ Spilling powder (Viokase) on hands may irritate skin. Inhaling powder may irritate mucous membranes, produce bronchospasm.

PO

• Give before or with meals, snacks. • Tablets may be crushed. Do not crush extended-release form. • Instruct pt not to chew (minimizes irritation to mouth, lips, tongue). • May open capsule, spread over applesauce, mashed fruit, rice cereal.

INDICATIONS/ROUTES/DOSAGE

PANCREATIC ENZYME REPLACEMENT/ SUPPLEMENT

PO: ADULTS, ELDERLY: 1–3 capsules or tablets before or with meals, snacks. May increase to 8 tablets/dose. **CHILDREN:** 1–2 tablets with meals, snacks.

SIDE EFFECTS

RARE: Allergic reaction, mouth irritation, shortness of breath, wheezing.

ADVERSE EFFECTS/ TOXIC REACTIONS

Excessive dosage may produce nausea, cramping, diarrhea. Hyperuricosuria, hyperuricemia reported with extremely high dosages.

NURSING CONSIDERATIONS

INTERVENTION/EVALUATION

Question for therapeutic relief from GI symptoms. Do not change brands without consulting physician.

PATIENT/FAMILY TEACHING

• Do not chew capsules, tablets. • Instruct pts with trouble swallowing to open capsules, spread contents over applesauce, mashed fruit, rice cereal.

pancuronium bromide

(Pavulon)

See Neuromuscular blockers (p. 120C)

panitumumab

pan-ih-**tomb**-you-mab
(Vectibix)

CLASSIFICATION

PHARMACOTHERAPEUTIC: Monoclonal antibody. **CLINICAL:** Antineoplastic.

ACTION

Inhibits biologic activity of human vascular epidermal growth factor (EGFR) by binding to its receptors. **Therapeutic Effect:** Prevents cell growth, proliferation, transformation, survival.

PHARMACOKINETICS

Clearance varies by body weight, gender, tumor burden. **Half-life:** 3–10 days.

USES

Treatment of EGFR-expressing metastatic colorectal carcinoma with disease progression during or following fluoropyrimidine, oxaliplatin, irinotecan-containing chemotherapy regimens.

PRECAUTIONS

CONTRAINDICATIONS: None known. **CAUTIONS:** Interstitial pneumonitis, pulmonary fibrosis, pulmonary infiltrates.

LIFESPAN CONSIDERATIONS:

Pregnancy/Lactation: Teratogenic. Potential for fertility impairment. May decrease fetal body weight; increase risk of skeletal fetal abnormalities. Do not breast-feed. **Pregnancy Category C. Children:** Safety and efficacy not established. **Elderly:** No age-related precautions noted.

INTERACTIONS

DRUG: None significant. **HERBAL:** None significant. **FOOD:** None known. **LAB VALUES:** May decrease serum magnesium, calcium.

AVAILABILITY (Rx)

SOLUTION FOR INJECTION: 25 mg/ml vial (5 ml, 10 ml, 20 ml vials).

P

ADMINISTRATION/HANDLING

IV

◀ **ALERT** ▶ Do not give by IV push or bolus. Use low-protein-binding 0.2- or 0.22-micron in-line filter. Flush IV line before and after chemotherapy administration with 0.9% NaCl.

Reconstitution • Dilute in 100–250 ml 0.9% NaCl. • Do not shake solution. • Discard any unused portion.

Rate of administration • Give as IV infusion over 60 min. • Infuse doses greater than 1,000 mg over 90 min.

Storage • Refrigerate vials. • After dilution, solution may be stored for up to 6 hrs at room temperature, up to 24 hrs if refrigerated. • Discard if discolored but solution may contain visible, translucent-to-white particulates (will be removed by in-line filter).

IV INCOMPATIBILITY

Do not mix with dextrose solutions or any other medications.

INDICATIONS/ROUTES/DOSAGE

METASTATIC COLORECTAL CARCINOMA

IV INFUSION: ADULTS, ELDERLY: 6 mg/kg given over 60 min once every 14 days. Doses greater than 1,000 mg should be infused over 90 min.

SIDE EFFECTS

COMMON (65%–57%): Erythema, acneiform dermatitis, pruritus. **FREQUENT (26%–20%):** Fatigue, abdominal pain, skin exfoliation, paronychia (inflammation involving folds of tissue surrounding fingernail), nausea, rash, diarrhea, constipation, skin fissures. **OCCASIONAL (19%–10%):** Vomiting, acne, cough, peripheral edema, dry skin. **RARE (7%–2%):** Stomatitis, mucosal inflammation, eyelash growth, conjunctivitis, increased lacrimation.

ADVERSE EFFECTS/ TOXIC REACTIONS

Pulmonary fibrosis, severe dermatologic toxicity (complicated by infectious sequelae), sepsis occur rarely. Severe infusion reactions manifested as bronchospasm, fever, chills, hypotension occur rarely. Hypomagnesemia occurs in 39% of pts.

NURSING CONSIDERATIONS

BASELINE ASSESSMENT

Assess baseline serum magnesium, calcium prior to therapy, periodically during therapy, and for 8 wks after completion of therapy.

INTERVENTION/EVALUATION

Assess for skin, ocular, mucosal toxicity; report effects. Median time to development of skin/ocular toxicity is 14–15 days; resolution after last dosing is 84 days. Monitor serum electrolytes for hypomagnesemia, hypocalcemia. Offer antiemetic if nausea/vomiting occurs. Monitor daily pattern of bowel activity/stool consistency.

PATIENT/FAMILY TEACHING

Do not have immunizations without physician's approval (drug lowers resistance). Avoid contact with those who have recently received a live virus vaccine. Avoid crowds, those with infection. Warn female pt of childbearing age of potential risk for development of fetal abnormalities if pregnancy occurs.

pantoprazole

pan-toe-**pra**-zole

(Protonix, Protonix IV, Panto ✦)

Do not confuse Protonix with Lotronex.

◆ CLASSIFICATION

PHARMACOTHERAPEUTIC: Benzimidazole. **CLINICAL:** Proton pump inhibitor (see p. 139C).

ACTION

Irreversibly binds to, inhibits hydrogen-potassium adenosine triphosphate, an enzyme on surface of gastric parietal cells. Inhibits hydrogen ion transport into gastric lumen. **Therapeutic Effect:** Increases gastric pH, reduces gastric acid production.

PHARMACOKINETICS

Route	Onset	Peak	Duration
PO	N/A	N/A	24 hrs

Rapidly absorbed from GI tract. Protein binding: 98%. Primarily distributed into gastric parietal cells. Metabolized extensively in liver. Primarily excreted in urine. Not removed by hemodialysis. **Half-life:** 1 hr.

USES

Oral: Treatment, maintenance of healing of erosive esophagitis associated with gastroesophageal reflux disease (GERD). Treatment of hypersecretory conditions including Zollinger-Ellison syndrome. **IV:** Short-term treatment of erosive esophagitis associated with GERD, treatment of hypersecretory conditions. **OFF-LABEL:** Peptic ulcer disease, active ulcer bleeding (injection), adjunct in treatment of *H. pylori.*

PRECAUTIONS

CONTRAINDICATIONS: None known. **CAUTIONS:** History of chronic or current hepatic disease.

LIFESPAN CONSIDERATIONS:

Pregnancy/Lactation: Unknown if drug crosses placenta or is distributed in breast milk. **Pregnancy Category B. Children:** Safety and efficacy not established. **Elderly:** No age-related precautions noted.

INTERACTIONS

DRUG: May increase effect of **warfarin**. **HERBAL:** None significant. **FOOD:** None known. **LAB VALUES:** May increase serum creatinine, cholesterol, uric acid.

AVAILABILITY (Rx)

INJECTION POWDER FOR RECONSTITUTION (PROTONIX IV): 40 mg.

TABLETS (DELAYED-RELEASE [PROTONIX]): 20 mg, 40 mg.

ADMINISTRATION/HANDLING

IV

Reconstitution • Mix 40-mg vial with 10 ml 0.9% NaCl injection. • May be further diluted with 100 ml D_5W, 0.9% NaCl, or lactated Ringer's.

Rate of administration • Infuse 10 ml solution over at least 2 min. • Infuse 100 ml solution over at least 15 min.

Storage • Refrigerate vials. Store provided in-line filter at room temperature. • Once diluted with 10 ml 0.9% NaCl, stable for 2 hrs at room temperature; when further diluted with 100 ml, stable for 22 hrs at room temperature.

PO

• Give without regard to meals. • Do not crush, chew, split tablets; swallow whole.

IV INCOMPATIBILITIES

Do not mix with other medications. Flush IV with D_5W, 0.9% NaCl, or lactated Ringer's solution before and after administration.

INDICATIONS/ROUTES/DOSAGE

EROSIVE ESOPHAGITIS

PO: ADULTS, ELDERLY: 40 mg/day for up to 8 wks. If not healed after 8 wks, may continue an additional 8 wks.

IV: ADULTS, ELDERLY: 40 mg/day for 7–10 days.

MAINTENANCE OF HEALING OF EROSIVE ESOPHAGITIS

PO: ADULTS, ELDERLY: 40 mg once daily.

P

HYPERSECRETORY CONDITIONS

PO: ADULTS, ELDERLY: Initially, 40 mg twice a day. May increase to 240 mg/day. **IV: ADULTS, ELDERLY:** 80 mg twice a day. May increase to 80 mg q8h.

SIDE EFFECTS

RARE (less than 2%): Diarrhea, headache, dizziness, pruritus, rash.

ADVERSE EFFECTS/ TOXIC REACTIONS

Hyperglycemia occurs rarely.

NURSING CONSIDERATIONS

BASELINE ASSESSMENT

Obtain baseline lab values, including serum creatinine, cholesterol.

INTERVENTION/EVALUATION

Evaluate for therapeutic response (relief of GI symptoms). Question if GI discomfort, nausea occur.

PATIENT/FAMILY TEACHING

• Report headache. • Swallow tablets whole; do not chew, crush. • Take before eating.

Paraplatin, *see carboplatin*

paroxetine

par-**ox**-e-teen
(Paxil, Paxil CR, Pexeva)

Do not confuse paroxetine with pyridoxine, or Paxil with Doxil or Taxol.

CLASSIFICATION

PHARMACOTHERAPEUTIC: Serotonin uptake inhibitor. **CLINICAL:** Antidepressant, antiobsessive-compulsive, antianxiety (see pp. 12C, 38C).

ACTION

Selectively blocks uptake of neurotransmitter serotonin at CNS neuronal presynaptic membranes, increasing its availability at postsynaptic receptor sites. **Therapeutic Effect:** Relieves depression, reduces obsessive-compulsive behavior, decreases anxiety.

PHARMACOKINETICS

Well absorbed from GI tract. Protein binding: 95%. Widely distributed. Metabolized in liver. Excreted in urine. Not removed by hemodialysis. **Half-life:** 24 hrs.

USES

Treatment of major depression exhibited as persistent, prominent dysphoria (occurring nearly every day for at least 2 wks) manifested by 4 of 8 symptoms: change in appetite, change in sleep pattern, increased fatigue, impaired concentration, feelings of guilt/worthlessness, loss of interest in usual activities, psychomotor agitation/retardation, suicidal tendencies. Treatment of panic disorder, obsessive-compulsive disorder (OCD) manifested as repetitive tasks producing marked distress, time-consuming, or significant interference with social/occupational behavior. Treatment of social anxiety disorder (SAD), generalized anxiety disorder (GAD), premenstrual dysphoric disorder, post-traumatic stress disorder (PTSD). **OFF-LABEL:** Eating disorders, impulse disorders, menopause symptoms, premenstrual disorders, treatment of depression and OCD in children.

PRECAUTIONS

CONTRAINDICATIONS: Use of MAOIs within 14 days. **CAUTIONS:** History of seizures, mania, renal/hepatic impairment, cardiac disease, pts with suicidal tendencies, impaired platelet aggregation. Those who are volume depleted or using diuretics.

LIFESPAN CONSIDERATIONS:

Pregnancy/Lactation: May impair reproductive function. Not distributed in breast milk. May increase risk of congenital malformations. **Pregnancy Category D. Children:** Safety and efficacy not established. **Elderly:** Age-related renal impairment may require dosage adjustment.

INTERACTIONS

DRUG: May increase concentration, risk of toxicity of **tricyclic antidepressants. Aspirin, NSAIDs, warfarin** may increase risk of bleeding. **MAOIs** may cause confusion, agitation, severe seizures; increase risk of serotonin syndrome, hypertensive crises. **HERBAL: Kava kava, St. John's wort, valerian** may increase CNS depression. **St. John's wort** may increase effects, risk of toxicity. **FOOD:** None known. **LAB VALUES:** May increase serum hepatic enzyme levels. May decrease Hgb, Hct, WBC count.

AVAILABILITY (Rx)

ORAL SUSPENSION (PAXIL): 10 mg/5 ml. **TABLETS (PAXIL, PEXEVA):** 10 mg, 20 mg, 30 mg, 40 mg.

TABLETS (CONTROLLED-RELEASE [PAXIL CR]): 12.5 mg, 25 mg, 37.5 mg.

ADMINISTRATION/HANDLING

PO

• Give with food, milk if GI distress occurs. • Scored tablet may be crushed. • Do not crush controlled-release tablets. • Best if given as single morning dose.

INDICATIONS/ROUTES/DOSAGE

DEPRESSION

PO: ADULTS: Initially, 20 mg/day. May increase by 10 mg/day at intervals of more than 1 wk. **Maximum:** 50 mg/day.

PO (CONTROLLED-RELEASE): ADULTS: Initially, 25 mg/day. May increase by 12.5 mg/day at intervals of more than 1 wk. **Maximum:** 62.5 mg/day.

GAD

PO: ADULTS: Initially, 20 mg/day. May increase by 10 mg/day at intervals of more than 1 wk. Range: 20–50 mg/day.

OCD

PO: ADULTS: Initially, 20 mg/day. May increase by 10 mg/day at intervals of more than 1 wk. Range: 20–60 mg/day.

PANIC DISORDER

PO: ADULTS: Initially, 10–20 mg/day. May increase by 10 mg/day at intervals of more than 1 wk. Range: 10–60 mg/day.

PO (CONTROLLED-RELEASE): ADULTS, ELDERLY: Initially, 12.5 mg once daily. May increase by 12.5 mg/day at weekly intervals. **Maximum:** 75 mg/day.

SAD

PO: ADULTS: Initially 20 mg/day. Range: 20–60 mg/day.

PO (CONTROLLED-RELEASE): ADULTS, ELDERLY: Initially, 12.5 mg once daily. May increase by 12.5 mg/day at weekly intervals. **Maximum:** 37.5 mg/day.

PTSD

PO: ADULTS: Initially, 20 mg/day. May increase by 10 mg/day at intervals of more than 1 wk. Range: 20–50 mg/day.

PREMENSTRUAL DYSPHORIC DISORDER

PO (PAXIL CR): ADULTS: Initially, 12.5 mg/day. May increase by 12.5 mg at weekly intervals to a maximum of 25 mg/day.

USUAL ELDERLY DOSAGE

PO: Initially, 10 mg/day. May increase by 10 mg/day at intervals of more than 1 wk. **Maximum:** 40 mg/day.

PO (CONTROLLED-RELEASE): Initially, 12.5 mg/day. May increase by 12.5 mg/day at intervals of more than 1 wk. **Maximum:** 50 mg/day.

SIDE EFFECTS

FREQUENT: Nausea (26%); somnolence (23%); headache, dry mouth (18%); asthenia (15%); constipation (15%); dizziness, insomnia (13%); diarrhea (12%); diaphoresis (11%); tremor (8%). **OCCASIONAL:** Decreased appetite, respiratory

P

disturbance (e.g., increased cough) (6%); anxiety (5%); flatulence, paresthesia, yawning (4%); decreased libido, sexual dysfunction, abdominal discomfort (3%). **RARE:** Palpitations, vomiting, blurred vision, altered taste, confusion.

ADVERSE EFFECTS/ TOXIC REACTIONS

Hyponatremia, seizures, have been reported.

NURSING CONSIDERATIONS

BASELINE ASSESSMENT

Assess appearance, behavior, speech pattern, level of interest, mood.

INTERVENTION/EVALUATION

For those on long-term therapy, hepatic/renal function tests, blood counts should be performed periodically. Supervise suicidal-risk pt closely during early therapy (as depression lessens, energy level improves, increasing suicide potential). Assess appearance, behavior, speech pattern, level of interest, mood.

PATIENT/FAMILY TEACHING

• May cause dry mouth. • Avoid alcohol, St. John's wort. • Therapeutic effect may be noted within 1–4 wks. • Do not abruptly discontinue medication. • Avoid tasks that require alertness, motor skills until response to drug is established. • Inform physician of intention for pregnancy or if pregnancy occurs.

Paxil, *see paroxetine*

Paxil CR, *see paroxetine*

pegaspargase

(Oncaspar)

See Cancer chemotherapeutic agents (p. 82C)

Pegasys, *see peginterferon alfa-2a*

pegfilgrastim

pehg-phil-**gras**-tim

(Neulasta)

Do not confuse Neulasta with Neumega.

CLASSIFICATION

PHARMACOTHERAPEUTIC: Colony-stimulating factor. **CLINICAL:** Hematopoietic, antineutropenic.

ACTION

Regulates production of neutrophils within bone marrow. A glycoprotein, primarily affects neutrophil progenitor proliferation, differentiation, selected end-cell functional activation. **Therapeutic Effect:** Increases phagocytic ability, antibody-dependent destruction; decreases incidence of infection.

PHARMACOKINETICS

Readily absorbed after subcutaneous administration. **Half-life:** 15–80 hrs.

USES

Fights infection manifested by febrile neutropenia in cancer pts receiving moderately myelosuppressive chemotherapy. Stimulates WBC production in pts receiving myelosuppressive chemotherapy.

PRECAUTIONS

CONTRAINDICATIONS: Hypersensitivity to *Escherichia coli*–derived proteins, do not administer within 14 days before and 24 hrs after cytotoxic chemotherapy. **CAUTIONS:** Concurrent use with medications having mycoloid properties, sickle cell disease.

⌛ LIFESPAN CONSIDERATIONS:

Pregnancy/Lactation: Unknown if drug crosses placenta or is distributed in breast milk. **Pregnancy Category C. Children:** Safety and efficacy not established. **Elderly:** No age-related precautions noted.

INTERACTIONS

DRUG: Lithium may potentiate release of neutrophils. **HERBAL:** None significant. **FOOD:** None known. **LAB VALUES:** May increase serum LDH, alkaline phosphatase, uric acid.

AVAILABILITY (Rx)

INJECTION, SOLUTION: 6 mg/0.6 ml syringe.

ADMINISTRATION/HANDLING

SUBCUTANEOUS

Storage • Store in refrigerator, but may warm to room temperature up to maximum of 48 hrs before use. Discard if left at room temperature for more than 48 hrs. • Protect from light. • Avoid freezing; but if accidentally frozen, may allow to thaw in refrigerator before administration. Discard if freezing takes place a second time. • Discard if discolored or precipitate forms.

INDICATIONS/ROUTES/DOSAGE

MYELOSUPPRESSION

SUBCUTANEOUS: ADULTS, ELDERLY, CHILDREN 12–17 YRS, WEIGHING MORE THAN 45 KG: Give as single 6-mg injection once per chemotherapy cycle.

◀ **ALERT** ▶ Do not administer between 14 days before and 24 hrs after cytotoxic chemotherapy. Do not use in infants, children, adolescents weighing less than 45 kg.

SIDE EFFECTS

FREQUENT (72%–15%): Bone pain, nausea, fatigue, alopecia, diarrhea, vomiting, constipation, anorexia, abdominal pain, arthralgia, generalized weakness, peripheral edema, dizziness, stomatitis, mucositis, neutropenic fever.

ADVERSE EFFECTS/ TOXIC REACTIONS

Allergic reactions (anaphylaxis, rash, urticaria) occur rarely. Cytopenia resulting from antibody response to growth factors occurs rarely. Splenomegaly occurs rarely. Adult respiratory distress syndrome (ARDS) may occur in septic pts.

NURSING CONSIDERATIONS

BASELINE ASSESSMENT

CBC, platelet count should be obtained before initiating therapy and routinely thereafter.

INTERVENTION/EVALUATION

Monitor for allergic-type reactions. Assess for peripheral edema, particularly behind medial malleolus (usually first area showing peripheral edema). Assess mucous membranes for evidence of stomatitis, mucositis (red mucous membranes, white patches, extreme mouth soreness). Assess muscle strength. Monitor daily pattern of bowel activity/ stool consistency. ARDS may occur in septic pts.

PATIENT/FAMILY TEACHING

• Inform pts of possible side effects, signs/symptoms of allergic reactions. • Counsel pt on importance of compliance with pegfilgrastim treatment, including regular monitoring of blood counts.

P

peginterferon alfa-2a

peg-inn-ter-**fear**-on
(Pegasys)

CLASSIFICATION

PHARMACOTHERAPEUTIC: Immunomodulator. **CLINICAL:** Immunologic agent.

ACTION

Binds to specific membrane receptors on virus-infected cell surface, inhibiting viral replication. Suppresses cell proliferation, producing reversible decreases in leukocyte, platelet counts. **Therapeutic Effect:** Inhibits hepatitis C virus.

PHARMACOKINETICS

Readily absorbed after subcutaneous administration. Excreted by kidneys. **Half-life:** 80 hrs.

USES

Treatment of chronic hepatitis C alone or in combination with ribavirin in pts who have compensated hepatic disease.

P

PRECAUTIONS

CONTRAINDICATIONS: Autoimmune hepatitis, decompensated hepatic disease, infants, neonates. **EXTREME CAUTION:** History of neuropsychiatric disorders. **CAUTIONS:** Renal impairment (creatinine clearance less than 50 ml/min), elderly, pulmonary disorders, compromised CNS function, cardiac diseases, autoimmune disorders, endocrine abnormalities, colitis, ophthalmologic disorders, myelosuppression.

LIFESPAN CONSIDERATIONS:

Pregnancy/Lactation: May have abortifacient potential. Unknown if distributed in breast milk. **Pregnancy Category C (X when used with riboflavin). Children:** Safety and efficacy not established in those younger than 18 yrs. **Elderly:** CNS, cardiac, systemic effects may be more severe in the elderly, particularly in those with renal impairment.

INTERACTIONS

DRUG: Didanosine may cause hepatic failure, peripheral neuropathy, pancreatitis, lactic acidosis. May increase concentration, risk of toxicity of **methadone, theophylline.** Concurrent use of **ribavirin** may increase risk of hemolytic anemia. **HERBAL:** None significant. **FOOD:** None known. **LAB VALUES:** May increase ALT. May decrease absolute neutrophil, platelet, WBC counts. May cause slight decrease in Hgb, Hct.

AVAILABILITY (Rx)

INJECTION, PREFILLED SYRINGE: 180 mcg/0.5 ml. **INJECTION SOLUTION:** 180 mcg/ml.

ADMINISTRATION/HANDLING

SUBCUTANEOUS

• Refrigerate. • Vials are for single use only; discard unused portion. • Give subcutaneous in abdomen, thigh.

INDICATIONS/ROUTES/DOSAGE

HEPATITIS C

SUBCUTANEOUS: ADULTS 18 YRS AND OLDER, ELDERLY: 180 mcg (1 ml) injected in abdomen or thigh once weekly for 48 wks.

DOSAGE IN RENAL IMPAIRMENT

For pts who require hemodialysis, dosage is 135 mg injected in abdomen or thigh once weekly for 48 wks.

DOSAGE IN HEPATIC IMPAIRMENT

For pts with progressive ALT increases above baseline values, dosage is 135 mcg injected in abdomen or thigh once weekly for 48 wks.

SIDE EFFECTS

FREQUENT (54%): Headache. **OCCASIONAL (23%–13%):** Alopecia, nausea, insomnia, anorexia, dizziness, diarrhea, abdominal pain, flu-like symptoms, psychiatric reactions (depression, irritability, anxiety), injection site reaction. **RARE (8%–5%):** Impaired concentration, diaphoresis, dry mouth, nausea, vomiting.

ADVERSE EFFECTS/ TOXIC REACTIONS

Serious, acute hypersensitivity reactions, (urticaria, angioedema, bronchoconstriction, anaphylaxis), pancreatitis, colitis, endocrine disorders (diabetes mellitus, hyperthyroidism, hypothyroidism), ophthalmologic disorders, pulmonary abnormalities occur rarely.

NURSING CONSIDERATIONS

BASELINE ASSESSMENT

CBC, platelet count, blood chemistry, urinalysis, renal/hepatic function tests, EKG should be performed before initial therapy and routinely thereafter. Pts with diabetes, hypertension should have ophthalmologic exam before treatment begins.

INTERVENTION/EVALUATION

Monitor for evidence of depression. Offer emotional support. Monitor for abdominal pain, bloody diarrhea as evidence of colitis. Monitor chest x-ray for pulmonary infiltrates. Assess for pulmonary impairment. Encourage ample fluid intake, particularly during early therapy. Assess serum hepatitis C virus RNA levels after 24 wks of treatment.

PATIENT/FAMILY TEACHING

• Clinical response occurs in 1–3 mos. • Flu-like symptoms tend to diminish with continued therapy. • Immediately report symptoms of depression, suicidal ideation. • Avoid tasks requiring mental alertness, motor skills until response to drug is established.

peginterferon alfa-2b

peg-inn-ter-**fear**-on
(PEG-Intron)

CLASSIFICATION

PHARMACOTHERAPEUTIC: Immunomodulator. **CLINICAL:** Immunologic agent.

ACTION

Inhibits viral replication in virus-infected cells, suppresses cell proliferation, increases phagocytic action of macrophages, augments specific cytotoxicity of lymphocytes for target cells. **Therapeutic Effect:** Inhibits hepatitis C virus.

PHARMACOKINETICS

Bioavailability is increased after multiple weekly doses. Metabolized in liver. Excreted in urine. **Half-life:** 22–60 hrs.

USES

As monotherapy or in combination with ribavirin for treatment of chronic hepatitis C in pts not previously treated with interferon alfa who have compensated hepatic disease and are older than 18 yrs.

PRECAUTIONS

CONTRAINDICATIONS: Autoimmune hepatitis, decompensated hepatic disease, history of psychiatric disorders. **CAUTIONS:** Renal impairment (creatinine clearance less than 50 ml/min), elderly, pulmonary disorders, compromised CNS function, cardiac diseases, autoimmune disorders, endocrine disorders (diabetes, hyperthyroidism, hypothyroidism), ophthalmologic disorders, myelosuppression.

LIFESPAN CONSIDERATIONS:

Pregnancy/Lactation: May have abortifacient potential. Unknown if distributed in breast milk. **Pregnancy Category C (X when used with riboflavin).** **Children:** Safety and efficacy not established in those younger than 18 yrs. **Elderly:** CNS, cardiac, systemic effects may be more severe in the elderly, particularly in those with renal impairment.

INTERACTIONS

DRUG: None significant. **HERBAL:** None significant. **FOOD:** None known. **LAB VALUES:** May increase serum glucose, ALT. May decrease neutrophil, platelet counts.

AVAILABILITY (Rx)

INJECTION POWDER FOR RECONSTITUTION: 50 mcg, 80 mcg, 120 mcg, 150 mcg.

ADMINISTRATION/HANDLING

SUBCUTANEOUS

Reconstitution • To reconstitute, add 0.7 ml Sterile Water for Injection (supplied) to vial. Use immediately or after reconstituted, may be refrigerated for up to 24 hrs before use.

Storage • Store at room temperature.

P

INDICATIONS/ROUTES/DOSAGE

CHRONIC HEPATITIS C, MONOTHERAPY

SUBCUTANEOUS: ADULTS 18 YRS AND OLDER, ELDERLY: Administer appropriate dosage (see chart below) once weekly for 1 yr on same day each wk.

Vial Strength	Weight (kg)	mcg*	ml*
100 mcg/ml	37–45	40	0.4
	46–56	50	0.5
160 mcg/ml	57–72	64	0.4
	73–88	80	0.5
240 mcg/ml	89–106	96	0.4
	107–136	120	0.5
300 mcg/ml	137–160	150	0.5

*Of peginterferon alfa-2b to administer.

CHRONIC HEPATITIS C

SUBCUTANEOUS: COMBINATION THERAPY WITH RIBAVIRIN (400 MG TWICE A DAY): Initially, 1.5 mcg/kg/wk.

Weight	Dosage
Less than 40 kg	50 mcg
40–50 kg	64 mcg
51–60 kg	80 mcg
61–75 kg	96 mcg
76–85 kg	120 mcg
Greater than 85 kg	150 mcg

◄ **ALERT** ► Do not use in pts with creatinine clearance less than 50 ml/min. Dosage adjustments needed for hematologic toxicity (hemoglobin, white blood cells, neutrophils, platelets).

SIDE EFFECTS

FREQUENT (50%–47%): Flu-like symptoms; inflammation, bruising, pruritus, irritation at injection site. **OCCASIONAL (29%–18%):** Psychiatric reactions(depression, anxiety, emotional lability, irritability), insomnia, alopecia, diarrhea. **RARE:** Rash, diaphoresis, dry skin, dizziness, flushing, vomiting, dyspepsia.

ADVERSE EFFECTS/ TOXIC REACTIONS

Serious, acute hypersensitivity reactions (urticaria, angioedema, bronchoconstriction, anaphylaxis), pulmonary disorders, endocrine disorders (diabetes mellitus, hypothyroidism, hyperthyroidism) pancreatitis occur rarely. Ulcerative colitis may occur within 12 wks of starting treatment.

NURSING CONSIDERATIONS

BASELINE ASSESSMENT

CBC, platelet count, blood chemistry, urinalysis, renal/hepatic function tests, EKG should be performed before initial therapy and routinely thereafter. Pts with diabetes, hypertension should have ophthalmologic exam before treatment begins.

INTERVENTION/EVALUATION

Monitor for evidence of depression; offer emotional support. Monitor for abdominal pain, bloody diarrhea as evidence of colitis. Monitor chest x-ray for pulmonary infiltrates. Assess for pulmonary impairment. Encourage adequate fluid intake, particularly during early therapy. Assess serum hepatitis C virus RNA levels after 24 wks of treatment.

PATIENT/FAMILY TEACHING

• Maintain adequate hydration, avoid alcohol. • May experience flu-like syndrome (nausea, body aches, headache). • Inform physician of persistent abdominal pain, bloody diarrhea, fever, signs of depression or infection, unusual bruising/bleeding.

Peg-Intron, *see peginterferon alfa-2b*

pegvisomant

peg-**vis**-oh-mant

(Somavert)

Do not confuse Somavert with somatrem or somatropin.

CLASSIFICATION

PHARMACOTHERAPEUTIC: Protein. **CLINICAL:** Acromegaly agent.

ACTION

Selectively binds to growth hormone receptors on cell surfaces, blocking binding of endogenous growth hormones, interfering with growth hormone signal transduction. **Therapeutic Effect:** Decreases serum concentrations of IGF-1 serum protein, normalizing serum insulin-like growth factor 1 (IGF-1) levels.

PHARMACOKINETICS

Not distributed extensively into tissues after subcutaneous administration. Less than 1% excreted in urine. **Half-life:** 6 days.

USES

Treatment of acromegaly in pts with inadequate response to surgery, radiation, other medical therapies or those for whom these therapies are inappropriate.

PRECAUTIONS

CONTRAINDICATIONS: Latex allergy (stopper on vial contains latex). **CAUTIONS:** Elderly, diabetes mellitus.

LIFESPAN CONSIDERATIONS:

Pregnancy/Lactation: Unknown if excreted in breast milk. **Pregnancy Category B. Children:** Safety and efficacy not established. **Elderly:** Initiation of treatment should begin at low end of dosage range.

INTERACTIONS

DRUG: May enhance effects of **insulin, oral antidiabetics**, possibly resulting in hypoglycemia. Dosage should be decreased when initiating pegvisomant therapy. **Opioids** decrease serum pegvisomant. **HERBAL:** None significant. **FOOD:** None known. **LAB VALUES:** Interferes with measurement of serum growth hormone concentration. May increase AST, ALT, serum transaminase levels. Decreases effect of insulin on carbohydrate metabolism.

AVAILABILITY (Rx)

INJECTION POWDER FOR RECONSTITUTION: 10-mg, 15-mg, 20-mg vials.

ADMINISTRATION/HANDLING

SUBCUTANEOUS

Reconstitution • Withdraw 1 ml Sterile Water for Injection, inject into vial of pegvisomant, aiming stream against glass wall. • Hold vial between palms of both hands, roll to dissolve powder (do not shake).

Rate of administration • Administer subcutaneously only 1 dose from each vial.

Storage • Refrigerate unreconstituted vials. • Administer within 6 hrs following

P

reconstitution. • Solution should appear clear after reconstitution. Discard if cloudy or particulate forms.

INDICATIONS/ROUTES/DOSAGE

ACROMEGALY

SUBCUTANEOUS: ADULTS, ELDERLY: Initially, 40 mg, as a loading dose, then 10 mg daily. After 4–6 wks, adjust dosage in 5-mg increments if serum IGF-1 level is still elevated, or in 5-mg decrements if IGF-1 level has decreased below the normal range. **Maximum:** 30 mg daily.

DOSAGE IN HEPATIC IMPAIRMENT

BASELINE LFT GREATER THAN 3 TIMES UPPER LIMITS OF NORMAL (ULN): Do not initiate without comprehensive workup to determine cause.
HEPATIC FUNCTION TESTS 3 TIMES OR GREATER BUT LESS THAN 5 TIMES ULN: Continue treatment but monitor for hepatitis, hepatic injury.
HEPATIC FUNCTION TESTS 5 TIMES OR GREATER OR SERUM TRANSAMINASE GREATER THAN 3 TIMES ULN ASSOCIATED WITH ANY INCREASE IN TOTAL BILIRUBIN: Discontinue immediately, perform comprehensive hepatic workup.

P

SIDE EFFECTS

FREQUENT (23%): Infection (cold symptoms, upper respiratory tract infection, blister, ear infection). **OCCASIONAL (8%–5%):** Back pain, dizziness, injection site reaction, peripheral edema, sinusitis, nausea. **RARE (less than 4%):** Diarrhea, paresthesia.

ADVERSE EFFECTS/ TOXIC REACTIONS

May produce marked elevation of hepatic enzymes, including serum transaminase. Substantial weight gain occurs rarely.

NURSING CONSIDERATIONS

BASELINE ASSESSMENT

Obtain baseline AST, ALT, serum alkaline phosphatase, total bilirubin levels.

INTERVENTION/EVALUATION

Monitor all pts with tumors that secrete growth hormone with periodic imaging scans of sella turcica for progressive tumor growth. Monitor diabetic pts for hypoglycemia. Obtain IGF-1 serum concentrations 4–6 wks after therapy begins and periodically thereafter; dosage adjustment based on results; dosage adjustment should not be based on growth hormone assays.

PATIENT/FAMILY TEACHING

• Inform pt that routine monitoring of hepatic function tests is essential during treatment. • Contact physician if jaundice (yellowing of eyes, skin) occurs.

pemetrexed

pem-eh-**trex**-ed
(Alimta)

CLASSIFICATION

PHARMACOTHERAPEUTIC: Antimetabolite. **CLINICAL:** Antineoplastic.

ACTION

Disrupts folate-dependent enzymes essential for cell replication. **Therapeutic Effect:** Inhibits growth of mesothelioma cell lines.

PHARMACOKINETICS

Protein binding: 81%. Not metabolized. Excreted in urine. **Half-life:** 3.5 hrs.

USES

Combination chemotherapy with cisplatin for treatment of malignant pleural mesothelioma. Single agent in treatment of locally advanced or metastatic non–small cell lung cancer after prior chemotherapy. **OFF-LABEL:** Treatment of bladder, breast, cervical, colorectal, esophageal, gastric, head and neck, ovarian, pancreatic, renal cell carcinoma.

PRECAUTIONS

CONTRAINDICATIONS: None known. **CAUTIONS:** Hepatic/renal impairment.

LIFESPAN CONSIDERATIONS:

Pregnancy/Lactation: Unknown if drug crosses placenta or is distributed in breast milk. May cause fetal harm. Not recommended during pregnancy. **Pregnancy Category D. Children:** Safety and efficacy not established in children younger than 18 yrs. **Elderly:** Higher incidence of fatigue, leukopenia, neutropenia, thrombocytopenia in those 65 yrs and older.

INTERACTIONS

DRUG: Bone marrow depressants may increase risk of myelosuppression. **Live virus vaccines** may potentiate virus replication, increase vaccine side effects, decrease pt's antibody response to vaccine. **HERBAL:** None significant. **FOOD:** None known. **LAB VALUES:** May decrease platelet, RBC, WBC counts.

AVAILABILITY (Rx)

INJECTION POWDER FOR RECONSTITUTION: 500 mg.

ADMINISTRATION/HANDLING

IV INFUSION

Reconstitution • Dilute 500-mg vial with 20 ml 0.9% NaCl to provide concentration of 25 mg/ml. • Gently swirl each vial until powder is completely dissolved. • Solution appears clear and ranges in color from colorless to yellow or green-yellow. • Further dilute reconstituted solution with 100 ml 0.9% NaCl.

Rate of administration • Infuse over 10 min.

Storage • Store at room temperature. • Diluted solution is stable for up to 24 hrs at room temperature or if refrigerated.

IV INCOMPATIBILITIES

Use only 0.9% NaCl to reconstitute; flush line prior to and following infusion. Do not add any other medications to IV line.

INDICATIONS/ROUTES/DOSAGE

◄ **ALERT** ► Pretreatment with dexamethasone (or equivalent) will reduce risk, severity of cutaneous reaction; treatment with folic acid and vitamin B_{12} beginning 1 wk before treatment and continuing for 21 days after last pemetrexed dose will reduce risk of side effects.

MALIGNANT PLEURAL MESOTHELIOMA

IV: ADULTS, ELDERLY: 600 mg/m^2 q3wk when used as a single agent; 500 mg/m^2 q3wk when used in combination with cisplatin 75 mg/m^2.

NON–SMALL CELL LUNG CANCER

IV: ADULTS, ELDERLY: 500 mg/m^2 q3wk.

SIDE EFFECTS

FREQUENT (12%–10%): Fatigue, nausea, vomiting, rash, desquamation. **OCCASIONAL (8%–4%):** Stomatitis, pharyngitis, diarrhea, anorexia, hypertension, chest pain. **RARE (less than 3%):** Constipation, depression, dysphagia.

ADVERSE EFFECTS/ TOXIC REACTIONS

Myelosuppression, characterized as grade 1–4 neutropenia, thrombocytopenia, anemia, is noted.

NURSING CONSIDERATIONS

BASELINE ASSESSMENT

Question for possibility of pregnancy before initiating therapy (Pregnancy Category D). Do not breast-feed once treatment has been initiated. Obtain CBC, serum chemistry tests before therapy and repeat throughout therapy.

INTERVENTION/EVALUATION

Monitor Hgb, Hct, WBC, differential, platelet count. Monitor for hematologic toxicity (fever, sore throat, signs of local infection, unusual bruising/bleeding from any site), symptoms of anemia (excessive fatigue, weakness). Assess skin for evidence of dermatologic toxicity. Keep pt well hydrated, urine alkaline. Monitor WBC count for nadir, recovery.

PATIENT/FAMILY TEACHING

• Maintain fastidious oral hygiene. • Do not have immunizations without physician's approval (drug lowers resistance). • Avoid crowds, those with infection. • Use contraceptive measures during therapy. • Promptly report fever, sore throat, signs of local infection, unusual bruising/bleeding from any site.

penbutolol

(Levatol)

See Beta-adrenergic blockers (p. 68C)

penciclovir

pen-**sigh**-klo-vear

(Denavir)

CLASSIFICATION

PHARMACOTHERAPEUTIC: Anti-infective. **CLINICAL:** Topical antiviral.

ACTION

Inhibits antiviral activity against herpes simplex virus (HSV). **Therapeutic Effect:** Prevents DNA synthesis, HSV replication.

USES

Treatment of recurrent herpes labialis (cold sores).

PRECAUTIONS

CONTRAINDICATIONS: None known. **CAUTIONS:** None known.

LIFESPAN CONSIDERATIONS:

Pregnancy/Lactation: Unknown if distributed in breast milk. **Pregnancy Category B. Children:** Safety and efficacy not established. **Elderly:** No age-related precautions noted.

INTERACTIONS

DRUG: None significant. **HERBAL:** None significant. **FOOD:** None known. **LAB VALUES:** None known.

AVAILABILITY (Rx)

CREAM: 1%.

ADMINISTRATION/HANDLING

TOPICAL

• Store at room temperature. Do not freeze.

INDICATIONS/ROUTES/DOSAGE

◄ **ALERT** ► Begin treatment as soon as possible (as soon as symptom indicating immediate onset of virus is evident or lesions appear).

HERPES LABIALIS (COLD SORES)

TOPICAL: ADULTS, ELDERLY: Apply q2h during waking hours for 4 days.

SIDE EFFECTS

FREQUENT (greater than 5%): Headache, mild erythema. **OCCASIONAL (5%–1%):** Application site reaction. **RARE (less than 1%):** Altered taste, rash.

ADVERSE EFFECTS/ TOXIC REACTIONS

None known.

NURSING CONSIDERATIONS

BASELINE ASSESSMENT

Use only on lips/face. Do not apply to oral mucous membranes. Avoid application in, near eyes (produces irritation).

PATIENT/FAMILY TEACHING

• Observe precautions to avoid exposure of cold sores to direct sunlight.

penicillamine

pen-ih-**sill**-ah-mine

(Cuprimine, Depen)

Do not confuse penicillamine with penicillin.

CLASSIFICATION

PHARMACOTHERAPEUTIC: Heavy metal antagonist. **CLINICAL:** Chelating agent, anti-inflammatory.

ACTION

Chelates with lead, copper, mercury, iron to form soluble complexes; depresses circulating IgM rheumatoid factor levels; depresses T-cell activity; combines with cystine to form more soluble compound. **Therapeutic Effect:** Promotes excretion of heavy metals, acts as anti-inflammatory drug, prevents renal calculi, may dissolve existing stones.

USES

Promotes excretion of copper in treatment of Wilson's disease, decreases excretion of cystine, prevents renal calculi in cystinuria associated with nephrolithiasis. Treatment of active rheumatoid arthritis not controlled with conventional therapy. **OFF-LABEL:** Treatment of rheumatoid vasculitis, heavy metal toxicity.

PRECAUTIONS

CONTRAINDICATIONS: History of penicillamine-related aplastic anemia or agranulocytosis, rheumatoid arthritis, pts with history or evidence of renal insufficiency, pregnancy, breast-feeding. **CAUTIONS:** Elderly, debilitated, renal/hepatic impairment, penicillin allergy.

LIFESPAN CONSIDERATIONS:

Pregnancy/Lactation: Contraindicated in pregnancy. Teratogenic; may cause fetal death. **Pregnancy Category D. Children:** Efficacy not established. **Elderly:** Age-related renal/hepatic impairment may require dosage adjustment.

INTERACTIONS

DRUG: **Antacids, iron supplements** may decrease absorption. **Bone marrow depressants, gold compounds, immunosuppressants** may increase risk of hematologic, adverse renal effects. **HERBAL:** None significant. **FOOD:** **All foods** may decrease absorption. **LAB VALUES:** None known.

AVAILABILITY (Rx)

CAPSULES (CUPRIMINE): 125 mg, 250 mg. **TABLETS (DEPEN):** 250 mg.

INDICATIONS/ROUTES/DOSAGE

RHEUMATOID ARTHRITIS

PO: ADULTS, ELDERLY: 125–250 mg/day. **Maximum (adults):** May increase at 1- to 3-mo intervals up to 1–1.5 g/day. **Maximum (elderly):** 750 mg/day.

◄ **ALERT** ► Dose more than 500 mg/day should be in divided doses.

CHILDREN: Initially, 3 mg/kg/day (**Maximum:** 250 mg) for 3 mos, then 6 mg/kg/day (**Maximum:** 500 mg) in 2 divided doses for 3 mos. **Maximum:** 10 mg/kg/ day (750 mg/day) in 3–4 divided doses.

WILSON'S DISEASE

PO: ADULTS, CHILDREN, 12 YRS AND OLDER: 1 g/day in 4 divided doses. **Maximum:** 2 g/day. **ELDERLY:** 750 mg/day in 3–4 divided doses. **CHILDREN:** 20 mg/kg/day in 2–4 doses. **Maximum:** 1 g/day.

◄ **ALERT** ► Titrate to maintain urinary copper excretion more than 1 mg/day.

CYSTINURIA

◄ **ALERT** ► Doses titrated to maintain urinary cystine excretion at 100–200 mg/day.

PO: ADULTS, ELDERLY: Initially, 2 g/day in divided doses q6h. Range: 1–4 g/day.

CHILDREN: 30 mg/kg/day in 4 divided doses. **Maximum:** 4 g/day.

SIDE EFFECTS

FREQUENT: Rash (pruritic, erythematous, maculopapular, morbilliform), reduced/altered sense of taste (hypogeusia), GI disturbances (anorexia, epigastric pain, nausea, vomiting, diarrhea) oral ulcers, glossitis. **OCCASIONAL:** Proteinuria, hematuria, hot flashes, drug fever. **RARE:** Alopecia, tinnitus, pemphigoid rash (water blisters).

ADVERSE EFFECTS/ TOXIC REACTIONS

Aplastic anemia, agranulocytosis, thrombocytopenia, leukopenia, myasthenia gravis, bronchiolitis, erythematous-like syndrome, evening hypoglycemia, skin friability at sites of pressure/trauma producing extravasation or white papules at venipuncture, surgical sites reported. Iron deficiency may develop, particularly children, menstruating women.

NURSING CONSIDERATIONS

BASELINE ASSESSMENT

Baseline WBC, differential, Hgb, platelet count should be performed before beginning therapy, q2wk thereafter for first 6 mos, then monthly during therapy. Hepatic function tests (GGT, AST, ALT, LDH), CT scan for renal stones should also be ordered. A 2-hr interval is necessary between iron and penicillamine therapy. In event of upcoming surgery, dosage should be reduced to 250 mg/day until wound healing is complete.

INTERVENTION/EVALUATION

Encourage copious amounts of water in pts with cystinuria. Monitor WBC, differential, platelet count. If WBC less than 3,500, neutrophils less than 2,000/mm^3, monocytes more than 500/mm^3, or platelet counts less than 100,000, or if progressive fall in platelet count or WBC in 3 successive determinations noted, inform physician (drug withdrawal necessary). Assess for evidence of hematuria. Monitor urinalysis for hematuria, proteinuria (if proteinuria exceeds 1 g/24 hrs, inform physician).

PATIENT/FAMILY TEACHING

• Promptly report any missed menstrual periods/other indications of pregnancy. • Report fever, sore throat, chills, bruising, bleeding, difficulty breathing on exertion, unexplained cough or wheezing. • Take medication 1 hr before or 2 hrs after meals or at least 1 hr from any other drug, food, or milk.

penicillin G benzathine

pen-ih-**sil**-lin G **benz**-ah-thene
(Bicillin LA)

Do not confuse penicillin G benzathine with penicillin G potassium or penicillin G procaine.

FIXED-COMBINATION(S)

Bicillin CR: penicillin G benzathine/penicillin procaine: 600,000 units benzathine/600,000 units procaine.

◆CLASSIFICATION

PHARMACOTHERAPEUTIC: Penicillin. **CLINICAL:** Antibiotic (see p. 27C)

ACTION

Inhibits bacterial cell wall synthesis by binding to one or more of the penicillin-binding proteins of bacteria. **Therapeutic Effect:** Bactericidal.

USES

Treatment of mild to moderate severe infections caused by organisms susceptible to low concentrations of penicillin including streptococcal (Group A) upper respiratory infections, syphilis, yaws. Prophylaxis of infections caused by susceptible organisms (e.g., rheumatic fever prophylaxis).

PRECAUTIONS

CONTRAINDICATIONS: Hypersensitivity to any penicillin. **CAUTIONS:** Renal/cardiac impairment, seizure disorder, hypersensitivity to cephalosporins.

LIFESPAN CONSIDERATIONS:

Pregnancy/Lactation: Readily crosses placenta; distributed in breast milk. **Pregnancy Category B. Children:** May delay renal excretion in neonates, young infants. **Elderly:** Age-related renal impairment may require dosage adjustment.

INTERACTIONS

DRUG: **Probenecid** increases concentration. **HERBAL:** None significant. **FOOD:** None known. **LAB VALUES:** May cause positive Coombs' test.

AVAILABILITY (Rx)

INJECTION (PREFILLED SYRINGE [BICILLIN LA]): 600,000 units/ml.

ADMINISTRATION/HANDLING

◀ **ALERT** ▶ Do not give IV, intra-arterially, subcutaneously (may cause thrombosis, severe neurovascular damage, cardiac arrest, death).

IM

- Store in refrigerator. Do not freeze.
- Administer undiluted by deep IM injection.

INDICATIONS/ROUTES/DOSAGE

GROUP A STREPTOCOCCAL INFECTION

IM: ADULTS, ELDERLY: 1.2 million units as a single dose. **CHILDREN:** 25,000–50,000 units/kg as a single dose.

PREVENTION OF RHEUMATIC FEVER

IM: ADULTS, ELDERLY: 1.2 million units q3–4wk or 600,000 units twice monthly. **CHILDREN:** 25,000–50,000 units/kg q3–4wk.

EARLY SYPHILIS

IM: ADULTS, ELDERLY: 2.4 million units divided and administered in two separate injection sites.

CONGENITAL SYPHILIS

IM: CHILDREN: 50,000 units/kg weekly for 3 wks.

SYPHILIS OF MORE THAN 1 YR DURATION

IM: ADULTS, ELDERLY: 2.4 million units divided and administered in two separate injection sites weekly for 3 wks. **CHILDREN:** 50,000 units/kg weekly for 3 wks.

SIDE EFFECTS

OCCASIONAL: Lethargy, fever, dizziness, rash, pain at injection site. **RARE:** Seizures, interstitial nephritis.

ADVERSE EFFECTS/TOXIC REACTIONS

Hypersensitivity reactions, ranging from chills, fever, rash to anaphylaxis, may occur.

NURSING CONSIDERATIONS

BASELINE ASSESSMENT

Question for history of allergies, particularly penicillins, cephalosporins.

INTERVENTION/EVALUATION

Monitor CBC, urinalysis, renal function tests.

penicillin G potassium

pen-ih-**sil**-lin G

(Megacillin ✦, Novepen-G ✦, Pfizerpen)

Do not confuse penicillin G potassium with penicillin G benzathine or penicillin G procaine.

P

◆ **CLASSIFICATION**

PHARMACOTHERAPEUTIC: Penicillin. **CLINICAL:** Antibiotic (see p. 27C).

ACTION

Inhibits bacterial cell wall synthesis by binding to one or more of the penicillin-binding proteins of bacteria. **Therapeutic Effect:** Bactericidal.

PHARMACOKINETICS

Protein binding: 60%. Widely distributed. Metabolized in liver. Primarily excreted in urine. **Half-life:** 0.5 hr (increased in renal impairment).

USES

Treatment of susceptible infections due to gram-positive organisms, gram-negative organisms, actinomycosis, clostridium, diphtheria, Listeria, *N. meningitidis,* pasteurella including anthrax, endocarditis, respiratory tract infections, meningitis, neurosyphilis, skin/skin structure infections.

PRECAUTIONS

CONTRAINDICATIONS: Hypersensitivity to any penicillin. **CAUTIONS:** Renal/hepatic impairment, seizure disorder, hypersensitivity to cephalosporins.

LIFESPAN CONSIDERATIONS:

Pregnancy/Lactation: Readily crosses placenta; distributed in breast milk. **Pregnancy Category B. Children:** May delay renal excretion in neonates, young infants. **Elderly:** Age-related renal impairment may require dosage adjustment.

INTERACTIONS

DRUG: Concurrent use of **aminoglycosides** may cause mutual inactivation (must be given at least 1 hr apart). **ACE inhibitors, potassium-sparing diuretics, potassium supplements** may increase risk of hyperkalemia. May increase **methotrexate** concentration, toxicity. **Probenecid** increases concentration. **HERBAL:** None significant. **FOOD: Food, milk** decrease absorption. **LAB VALUES:** May cause positive Coombs' test.

AVAILABILITY (Rx)

INFUSION: 1 million units/50 ml, 2 million units/50 ml, 3 million units/50 ml. **INJECTION, POWDER FOR RECONSTITUTION:** 5 million units.

ADMINISTRATION/HANDLING

IV

Reconstitution • Follow dilution guide per manufacturer. • After reconstitution, further dilute with 50–100 ml D_5W or 0.9% NaCl for final concentration of 100–500,000 units/ml (50,000 units/ml for infants, neonates).

Rate of administration • Infuse over 15–60 min.

Storage • Reconstituted solution is stable for 7 days if refrigerated.

IV INCOMPATIBILITIES

Amikacin (Amikin), aminophylline, amphotericin B, dopamine (Intropin).

IV COMPATIBILITIES

Amiodarone (Cordarone), calcium gluconate, diltiazem (Cardizem), diphenhydramine (Benadryl), furosemide (Lasix), heparin, hydromorphone (Dilaudid), lidocaine, lipids, magnesium sulfate, methylprednisolone (Solu-Medrol), morphine, potassium chloride, total parenteral nutrition (TPN).

INDICATIONS/ROUTES/DOSAGE

USUAL DOSAGE

IV, IM: ADULTS, ELDERLY: 2–24 million units/day in divided doses q4–6h. **CHILDREN:** 25,000–400,000 units/kg/day in divided doses q4–6h.

DOSAGE IN RENAL IMPAIRMENT

Dosage interval is modified based on creatinine clearance.

Creatinine Clearance	Dosage Interval
10–30 ml/min	Usual dose q8–12h
Less than 10 ml/min	Usual dose q12–18h

SIDE EFFECTS

OCCASIONAL: Lethargy, fever, dizziness, rash, electrolyte imbalance, diarrhea, thrombophlebitis. **RARE:** Seizures, interstitial nephritis.

ADVERSE EFFECTS/ TOXIC REACTIONS

Hypersensitivity reactions ranging from rash, fever, chills to anaphylaxis occur occasionally.

NURSING CONSIDERATIONS

BASELINE ASSESSMENT

Question for history of allergies, particularly penicillins, cephalosporins.

INTERVENTION/EVALUATION

Monitor CBC, urinalysis electrolytes, renal function tests.

penicillin V potassium

pen-ih-**sil**-in V
(Apo-Pen-VK ✤)

◆CLASSIFICATION

PHARMACOTHERAPEUTIC: Penicillin. **CLINICAL:** Antibiotic (see p. 27C).

ACTION

Inhibits cell wall synthesis by binding to bacterial cell membranes. **Therapeutic Effect:** Bactericidal.

PHARMACOKINETICS

Moderately absorbed from GI tract. Protein binding: 80%. Widely distributed. Metabolized in liver. Primarily excreted in urine. **Half-life:** 1 hr (increased in renal impairment).

USES

Treatment of mild to moderate infections of respiratory tract, skin/skin structure, otitis media, necrotizing ulcerative gingivitis; prophylaxis for rheumatic fever, dental procedures.

PRECAUTIONS

CONTRAINDICATIONS: Hypersensitivity to any penicillin. **CAUTIONS:** Renal impairment, history of allergies (particularly cephalosporins), history of seizures.

⌛ LIFESPAN CONSIDERATIONS:

Pregnancy/Lactation: Readily crosses placenta; appears in cord blood, amniotic fluid. Distributed in breast milk in low concentrations. May lead to allergic sensitization, diarrhea, candidiasis, skin rash in infant. **Pregnancy Category B. Children:** Use caution in neonates and young infants (may delay renal elimination). **Elderly:** Age-related renal impairment may require dosage adjustment.

INTERACTIONS

DRUG: ACE inhibitors, potassium-sparing diuretics, potassium supplements may increase risk of hyperkalemia. May increase **methotrexate** concentration, toxicity. **Probenecid** may increase concentration, risk of toxicity. **HERBAL:** None significant. **FOOD:** None known. **LAB VALUES:** May cause positive Coombs' test.

AVAILABILITY (Rx)

POWDER FOR ORAL SOLUTION: 125 mg/5 ml, 250 mg/5 ml. **TABLETS:** 250 mg, 500 mg.

ADMINISTRATION/HANDLING

PO

• Store tablets at room temperature. After reconstitution, oral solution is stable for 14 days if refrigerated.

P

- Space doses evenly around the clock.
- Give without regard to meals.

INDICATIONS/ROUTES/DOSAGE

USUAL DOSAGE

PO: ADULTS, ELDERLY, CHILDREN 12 YRS AND OLDER: 125–500 mg q6–8h. **CHILDREN YOUNGER THAN 12 YRS:** 25–50 mg/kg/day in divided doses q6–8h. **Maximum:** 3 g/day.

PROPHYLAXIS OF RECURRENT RHEUMATIC FEVER

PO: ADULTS, ELDERLY, CHILDREN 5 YRS AND OLDER: 250 mg 2 times/day. **CHILDREN YOUNGER THAN 5 YRS:** 125 mg 2 times/day.

SIDE EFFECTS

FREQUENT: Mild hypersensitivity reaction (chills, fever, rash), nausea, vomiting, diarrhea. **RARE:** Bleeding, allergic reaction.

ADVERSE EFFECTS/ TOXIC REACTIONS

Severe hypersensitivity reactions, including anaphylaxis, may occur. Nephrotoxicity, antibiotic-associated colitis (severe abdominal pain, fever, severe watery diarrhea), other superinfections may result from high dosages, prolonged therapy.

NURSING CONSIDERATIONS

BASELINE ASSESSMENT

Question for history of allergies, particularly penicillins, cephalosporins.

INTERVENTION/EVALUATION

Hold medication, promptly report rash (hypersensitivity), diarrhea (with fever, abdominal pain, mucus or blood in stool may indicate antibiotic-associated colitis). Monitor I&O, urinalysis, renal function tests for nephrotoxicity. Be alert for superinfection (increased fever, sore throat, nausea, vomiting, diarrhea, stomatitis, vaginal discharge, anal/genital pruritus). Review Hgb levels; check for bleeding (overt bleeding, ecchymosis, swelling of tissue).

PATIENT/FAMILY TEACHING

• Continue antibiotic for full length of treatment. • Space doses evenly. • Notify physician immediately if rash, diarrhea, bleeding, bruising, other new symptoms occur.

pentamidine

pen-**tam**-i-deen
(NebuPent, Pentacarinat ✤, Pentam-300)

✦ CLASSIFICATION

PHARMACOTHERAPEUTIC: Anti-infective. **CLINICAL:** Antiprotozoal.

ACTION

Interferes with nuclear metabolism, incorporation of nucleotides, inhibiting DNA, RNA, phospholipid, protein synthesis. **Therapeutic Effect:** Produces antibacterial, antiprotozoal effects.

PHARMACOKINETICS

Well absorbed after IM administration; minimally absorbed after inhalation. Widely distributed. Primarily excreted in urine. Minimally removed by hemodialysis. **Half-life:** 6.5 hrs (increased in renal impairment).

USES

Treatment of pneumonia caused by *Pneumocystis carinii* (PCP). Prevention of PCP in high-risk HIV-infected pts. **OFF-LABEL:** Treatment of African trypanosomiasis, cutaneous/visceral leishmaniasis.

PRECAUTIONS

CONTRAINDICATIONS: Concurrent use with didanosine. **CAUTIONS:** Diabetes mellitus, renal/hepatic impairment, hypertension/hypotension.

LIFESPAN CONSIDERATIONS:

Pregnancy/Lactation: Unknown if drug crosses placenta or is distributed in breast milk. **Pregnancy Category C.** **Children:** No age-related precautions noted. **Elderly:** No age-related information available.

INTERACTIONS

DRUG: **Delavirdine, fluconazole, fluvoxamine, gemfibrozil, isoniazid, omeprazole** may increase concentration, toxicity. **Carbamazepine, phenytoin, rifampin** may decrease effect. **Didanosine** may increase risk of pancreatitis. **Foscarnet** may increase risk of hypocalcemia, hypomagnesemia, nephrotoxicity of pentamidine. **HERBAL:** None significant. **FOOD:** None known. **LAB VALUES:** May increase BUN, serum alkaline phosphatase, bilirubin, creatinine, AST, ALT. May decrease serum calcium, magnesium. May alter serum glucose.

AVAILABILITY (Rx)

INJECTION POWDER FOR RECONSTITUTION (PENTAM-300): 300 mg. **POWDER FOR NEBULIZATION (NEBUPENT):** 300 mg.

ADMINISTRATION/HANDLING

◄ **ALERT** ► Pt must be in supine position during administration, with frequent B/P checks until stable (potential for life-threatening hypotensive reaction). Have resuscitative equipment immediately available.

IV

Reconstitution • For intermittent IV infusion (piggyback), reconstitute each vial with 3–5 ml D_5W or Sterile Water for Injection. • Withdraw desired dose; further dilute with 50–250 ml D_5W.

Rate of administration • Infuse over 60 min. • Do not give by IV injection or rapid IV infusion (increases potential for severe hypotension).

Storage • Store vials at room temperature. • After reconstitution, IV solution is stable for 48 hrs at room temperature. • Discard unused portion.

IM

• Reconstitute 300-mg vial with 3 ml Sterile Water for Injection to provide concentration of 100 mg/ml.

AEROSOL (NEBULIZER)

• Aerosol stable for 48 hrs at room temperature. • Reconstitute 300-mg vial with 6 ml Sterile Water for Injection. Avoid NaCl (may cause precipitate). • Do not mix with other medication in nebulizer reservoir.

IV INCOMPATIBILITIES

Cefazolin (Ancef), cefotaxime (Claforan), ceftazidime (Fortaz), ceftriaxone (Rocephin), fluconazole (Diflucan), foscarnet (Foscavir), interleukin (Proleukin).

IV COMPATIBILITIES

Diltiazem (Cardizem), zidovudine (Retrovir), total parenteral nutrition (TPN).

INDICATIONS/ROUTES/DOSAGE

PCP

IV, IM: ADULTS, ELDERLY: 4 mg/kg/day once a day for 14–21 days. **CHILDREN:** 4 mg/kg/day once a day for 10–14 days.

PREVENTION OF PCP

INHALATION: ADULTS, ELDERLY: 300 mg once q4wk. **CHILDREN 5 YRS AND OLDER:** 300 mg q3–4wk. **CHILDREN YOUNGER THAN 5 YRS:** 8 mg/kg/dose once q3–4wk.

SIDE EFFECTS

FREQUENT: **Injection (greater than 10%):** Abscess, pain at injection site. **Inhalation (greater than 5%):** Fatigue, metallic taste, shortness of breath, decreased appetite, dizziness, rash, cough, nausea, vomiting, chills. **OCCASIONAL:** **Injection (10%–1%):** Nausea, decreased appetite, hypotension, fever, rash, altered taste, confusion. **Inhalation (5%–1%):** Diarrhea, headache, anemia,

P

muscle pain. **RARE: Injection (less than 1%):** Neuralgia, thrombocytopenia, phlebitis, dizziness.

ADVERSE EFFECTS/ TOXIC REACTIONS

Life-threatening/fatal hypotension, arrhythmias, hypoglycemia, leukopenia, nephrotoxicity, renal failure, anaphylactic shock, Stevens-Johnson syndrome, toxic epidural necrolysis occur rarely. Hyperglycemia, insulin-dependent diabetes mellitus (often permanent) may occur even months after therapy has stopped.

NURSING CONSIDERATIONS

BASELINE ASSESSMENT

Avoid concurrent use of nephrotoxic drugs. Establish baseline for B/P, serum glucose. Obtain specimens for diagnostic tests before giving first dose.

INTERVENTION/EVALUATION

Monitor B/P during administration until stable for both IM and IV administration (pt should remain supine). Check serum glucose levels, clinical signs for hypoglycemia (diaphoresis, anxiety, tremor, tachycardia, palpitations, light-headedness, headache, numbness of lips, double vision, incoordination), hyperglycemia (polyuria, polyphagia, polydipsia, malaise, visual changes, abdominal pain, headache, nausea/vomiting). Evaluate IM sites for pain, redness, induration; IV sites for phlebitis (heat, pain, red streaking over vein). Monitor renal, hepatic, hematology test results. Assess skin for rash. Evaluate equilibrium during ambulation. Be alert for respiratory difficulty when administering by inhalation route.

PATIENT/FAMILY TEACHING

• Remain flat in bed during administration of medication; get up slowly with assistance only when B/P stable. • Notify physician immediately of diaphoresis, shakiness, light-headedness, palpitations. • Drowsiness, increased urination, thirst, anorexia may develop in months following therapy. • Maintain adequate fluid intake. • Inform physician if fever, cough, shortness of breath occurs. • Avoid alcohol.

Pentasa, *see mesalamine*

pentazocine

(Talwin)

See Opioid analgesics

pentobarbital

(Nembutal)

See Sedative-hypnotics

pentostatin

(Nipent)

See Cancer chemotherapeutic agents (p. 82C)

pentoxifylline

pen-tox-ih-**fill**-in

(Albert ✱, Apo-Pentoxifylline SR ✱, Pentoxil, Trental)

Do not confuse Trental with Tegretol or Trandate.

CLASSIFICATION

PHARMACOTHERAPEUTIC: Blood viscosity-reducing agent. **CLINICAL:** Hemorheologic.

ACTION

Alters flexibility of RBCs; inhibits production of tumor necrosis factor, neutrophil activation, platelet aggregation. **Therapeutic Effect:** Reduces blood viscosity, improves blood flow.

PHARMACOKINETICS

Well absorbed after PO administration. Undergoes first-pass metabolism in liver. Primarily excreted in urine. Unknown if removed by hemodialysis. **Half-life:** 24–48 min; metabolite, 60–90 min.

USES

Symptomatic treatment of intermittent claudication associated with occlusive peripheral vascular disease, diabetic angiopathies. **OFF-LABEL:** Diabetic neuropathy, gangrene, hemodialysis shunt thrombosis, septic shock, sickle cell syndrome, vascular impotence.

PRECAUTIONS

CONTRAINDICATIONS: History of intolerance to xanthine derivatives, such as caffeine, theophylline, theobromine; recent cerebral/retinal hemorrhage. **CAUTIONS:** Renal/hepatic impairment, insulin-treated diabetes, chronic occlusive arterial disease, recent surgery, peptic ulcer disease.

LIFESPAN CONSIDERATIONS:

Pregnancy/Lactation: Unknown if drug crosses placenta. Distributed in breast milk. **Pregnancy Category C.** **Children:** Safety and efficacy not established. **Elderly:** Age-related renal impairment may require dosage adjustment.

INTERACTIONS

DRUG: May increase effects of **antihypertensives.** **HERBAL:** None significant. **FOOD:** None known. **LAB VALUES:** None known.

AVAILABILITY (Rx)

TABLETS (CONTROLLED-RELEASE [PENTOXIL, TRENTAL]): 400 mg.

ADMINISTRATION/HANDLING

PO

- Do not crush/break film-coated tablets.
- Give with meals to avoid GI upset.

INDICATIONS/ROUTES/DOSAGE

INTERMITTENT CLAUDICATION

PO: ADULTS, ELDERLY: 400 mg 3 times a day. Decrease to 400 mg twice a day if GI, CNS adverse effects occur. Continue for at least 8 wks.

SIDE EFFECTS

OCCASIONAL (5%–2%): Dizziness, nausea, altered taste, dyspepsia (heartburn, epigastric pain, indigestion). **RARE (less than 2%):** Rash, pruritus, anorexia, constipation, dry mouth, blurred vision, edema, nasal congestion, anxiety.

ADVERSE EFFECTS/ TOXIC REACTIONS

Angina, chest pain occur rarely; may be accompanied by palpitations, tachycardia, arrhythmias. Signs/symptoms of overdose (flushing, hypotension, nervousness, agitation, hand tremor, fever, somnolence) appear 4–5 hrs after ingestion, last up to 12 hrs.

P

NURSING CONSIDERATIONS

INTERVENTION/EVALUATION

Assist with ambulation if dizziness occurs. Assess for hand tremor. Monitor for relief of symptoms of intermittent claudication (pain, aching, cramping in calf muscles, buttocks, thigh, feet). Symptoms generally occur while walking/exercising and not at rest or with weight bearing in absence of walking/exercising.

PATIENT/FAMILY TEACHING

• Therapeutic effect generally noted in 2–4 wks. • Avoid tasks requiring alertness, motor skills until response to drug is established. • Do not smoke (causes constriction, occlusion of peripheral blood vessels). • Limit caffeine.

Pepcid, *see famotidine*

Percocet, *see acetaminophen and oxycodone*

pergolide

per-go-lide
(Permax)

Do not confuse Permax with Pentrax or Pernox.

CLASSIFICATION

PHARMACOTHERAPEUTIC: Dopamine agonist. **CLINICAL:** Antidyskinetic.

ACTION

Directly stimulates dopamine receptors. **Therapeutic Effect:** Assists in reduction in tremor, improvement in akinesia (absence of movement), posture/equilibrium disorders, rigidity associated with Parkinson's Disease.

PHARMACOKINETICS

Well absorbed from GI tract. Protein binding: 90%. Undergoes extensive first-pass metabolism in liver. Primarily excreted in urine. Unknown if removed by hemodialysis. **Half-life:** 27 hrs.

USES

Adjunctive treatment with levodopa/carbidopa in pts with Parkinson's disease. **OFF-LABEL:** Chronic motor/vocal tic disorder, Tourette's disorder.

PRECAUTIONS

CONTRAINDICATIONS: Hypersensitivity to other ergot derivatives. **CAUTIONS:** Cardiac arrhythmias, history of confusion, hallucinations.

LIFESPAN CONSIDERATIONS:

Pregnancy/Lactation: Unknown if drug crosses placenta or is distributed in breast milk. May interfere with lactation. **Pregnancy Category B. Children:** Safety and efficacy not established. **Elderly:** No age-related precautions noted.

INTERACTIONS

DRUG: Haloperidol, loxapine, methyldopa, metoclopramide, phenothiazines may decrease effectiveness. **Hypotensive medications, antihypertensives** may increase hypotensive effect. **HERBAL:** None significant. **FOOD:** None known. **LAB VALUES:** May increase serum growth hormone.

AVAILABILITY (Rx)

TABLETS: 0.05 mg, 0.25 mg, 1 mg.

ADMINISTRATION/HANDLING

PO

- Scored tablets may be crushed. • Give without regard to meals.

INDICATIONS/ROUTES/DOSAGE

PARKINSONISM

PO: ADULTS, ELDERLY: Initially, 0.05 mg/day for 2 days. May increase by 0.1–0.15 mg/day every 3 days over the next 12 days; afterward may increase by 0.25 mg/day every 3 days. Range: 2–3 mg/day in 3 divided doses. **Maximum:** 5 mg/day.

SIDE EFFECTS

FREQUENT (24%–10%): Nausea, dizziness, hallucinations, constipation, rhinitis, dystonia, confusion, somnolence. **OCCASIONAL (5%–3%):** Orthostatic hypotension, insomnia, dry mouth, peripheral edema, anxiety, diarrhea, dyspepsia, abdominal pain, headache, abnormal vision, anorexia, tremor, depression, rash. **RARE (less than 2%):** Urinary frequency, vivid dreams, neck pain, hypotension, vomiting.

ADVERSE EFFECTS/ TOXIC REACTIONS

Overdose may vary from severe paradoxical reactions (hallucinations, tremor,

P

seizures) to CNS depression, characterized by sedation, apnea, cardiovascular collapse.

NURSING CONSIDERATIONS

INTERVENTION/EVALUATION

Be alert to neurologic effects (headache, lethargy, mental confusion, agitation). Monitor B/P. Monitor for evidence of dyskinesia (difficulty with movement). Assess for clinical reversal of Parkinson symptoms (improvement of tremor of head/hands at rest, mask-like facial expression, shuffling gait, muscular rigidity).

PATIENT/FAMILY TEACHING

• Tolerance to feeling of lightheadedness develops during therapy. • To reduce hypotensive effect, rise slowly from lying to sitting position, permit legs to dangle momentarily before standing. • Dry mouth, drowsiness, dizziness may be expected responses of drug. • Avoid tasks that require alertness, motor skills until response to drug is established. • Avoid alcoholic beverages during therapy.

perindopril

(Aceon)

See Angiotensin-converting enzyme (ACE) inhibitors (p. 7C)

perphenazine

(Trilafon)

See Antipsychotics

phenazopyridine

fen-az-o-**peer**-i-deen

(Azo-Gesic, Azo-Standard, Phenazo ♣, Pyridium, Uristat)

Do not confuse phenazopyridine with pyridoxine.

CLASSIFICATION

PHARMACOTHERAPEUTIC: Interstitial cystitis agent. **CLINICAL:** Urinary tract analgesic.

ACTION

Exerts topical analgesic effect on urinary tract mucosa. **Therapeutic Effect:** Relieves urinary pain, burning, urgency, frequency.

PHARMACOKINETICS

Well absorbed from GI tract. Partially metabolized in liver. Primarily excreted in urine. **Half-life:** Unknown.

USES

Symptomatic relief of pain, burning, urgency, frequency resulting from lower urinary tract mucosa irritation (may be caused by infection, trauma, surgery).

P

PRECAUTIONS

CONTRAINDICATIONS: Hepatic/renal insufficiency. **CAUTIONS:** None known.

LIFESPAN CONSIDERATIONS:

Pregnancy/Lactation: Unknown if drug crosses placenta or is distributed in breast milk. **Pregnancy Category B.** **Children:** No age-related precautions noted in those older than 6 yrs. **Elderly:** Age-related renal impairment may increase toxicity.

INTERACTIONS

DRUG: None significant. **HERBAL:** None significant. **FOOD:** None known. **LAB VALUES:** May interfere with urinalysis tests based on color reactions (e.g., urinary glucose, ketones, protein, 17-ketosteroids).

AVAILABILITY (Rx)

TABLETS: (AZO-GESIC, AZO-STANDARD, URISTAT): 95 mg. **(PYRIDIUM):** 100 mg, 200 mg.

ADMINISTRATION/HANDLING

PO

- Give with meals.

INDICATIONS/ROUTES/DOSAGE

URINARY ANALGESIC

PO: ADULTS: 100–200 mg 3–4 times a day. **CHILDREN 6 YRS AND OLDER:** 12 mg/kg/day in 3 divided doses for 2 days.

DOSAGE IN RENAL IMPAIRMENT

Dosage interval is modified based on creatinine clearance.

Creatinine Clearance	Interval
50–80 ml/min	Usual dose q8–16h
Less than 50 ml/min	Avoid use

P

SIDE EFFECTS

OCCASIONAL: Headache, GI disturbance, rash, pruritus.

ADVERSE EFFECTS/ TOXIC REACTIONS

Overdose in pts with renal impairment, severe hypersensitivity may lead to hemolytic anemia, nephrotoxicity, hepatotoxicity. Methemoglobinemia generally occurs as result of massive, acute overdose.

NURSING CONSIDERATIONS

INTERVENTION/EVALUATION

Assess for therapeutic response: relief of dysuria (pain, burning), urgency, frequency of urination.

PATIENT/FAMILY TEACHING

- Reddish orange discoloration of urine should be expected. • May stain fabric. • Take with meals (reduces possibility of GI upset).

phenelzine

evolve

fen-ell-zeen

(Nardil)

CLASSIFICATION

PHARMACOTHERAPEUTIC: MAOI. **CLINICAL:** Antidepressant (see p. 37C).

ACTION

Inhibits activity of the enzyme, monoamine oxidase, at CNS storage sites, leading to increased levels of epinephrine, norepinephrine, serotonin, dopamine at neuronal receptor sites. **Therapeutic Effect:** Relieves depression.

USES

Treatment of depression refractory to other antidepressants, electroconvulsive therapy. **OFF-LABEL:** Treatment of panic disorder, selective mutism, vascular/tension headaches.

PRECAUTIONS

CONTRAINDICATIONS: Cardiovascular/cerebrovascular disease, hepatic/renal impairment, pheochromocytoma. **CAUTIONS:** Ingestion of tyramine-containing foods, cardiac arrhythmias, severe/frequent headaches, hypertension, suicidal tendencies.

LIFESPAN CONSIDERATIONS:

Pregnancy/Lactation: Crosses placenta. Minimally distributed in breast milk. **Pregnancy Category C. Children:** Not recommended for children (increased risk of suicidal ideation). **Elderly:** Increased risk of drug toxicity may require dosage adjustment.

INTERACTIONS

DRUG: **Alcohol, other CNS depressants** may increase CNS depression. **Buspirone** may increase B/P. **Caffeine-containing medications** may increase risk of cardiac arrhythmias, hypertension. **Carbamazepine, cyclobenzaprine, maprotiline, other MAOIs** may precipitate hypertensive crisis. **Dopamine, tryptophan** may cause sudden, severe hypertension. **Fluoxetine, trazodone, tricyclic antidepressants** may cause serotonin syndrome. May increase effects of **insulin, oral antidiabetics. Meperidine, other opioid analgesics** may produce diaphoresis, immediate excitation, rigidity, severe hypertension/hypotension, sometimes leading to severe respiratory distress, vascular collapse, seizures, coma, death. May increase CNS stimulant effects of **methylphenidate. Sympathomimetics** may increase cardiac stimulant, vasopressor effects. **HERBAL:** None significant. **FOOD caffeine, chocolate, tyramine-containing foods** may cause sudden, severe hypertension. **LAB VALUES:** None known.

AVAILABILITY (Rx)

TABLETS: 15 mg.

ADMINISTRATION/HANDLING

PO

• Store tablets at room temperature. • Give with food, milk if GI distress occurs. • Tablets may be crushed.

INDICATIONS/ROUTES/DOSAGE

DEPRESSION

PO: ADULTS: 15 mg 3 times a day. May increase to 60–90 mg/day. **ELDERLY:** Initially, 7.5 mg/day. May increase by 7.5–15 mg/day q3–4wk up to 60 mg/day in divided doses.

SIDE EFFECTS

FREQUENT: Orthostatic hypotension, restlessness, GI upset, insomnia, dizziness, headache, lethargy, asthenia (loss of strength, energy), dry mouth, peripheral edema. **OCCASIONAL:** Flushing, diaphoresis, rash, urinary frequency, increased appetite, transient impotence. **RARE:** Visual disturbances.

ADVERSE EFFECTS/ TOXIC REACTIONS

Hypertensive crisis occurs rarely, marked by severe hypertension, occipital headache radiating frontally, neck stiffness/soreness, nausea, vomiting, diaphoresis, fever, chills, clammy skin, dilated pupils, palpitations, tachycardia or bradycardia, constricting chest pain. **Antidote for hypertensive crisis:** 5–10 mg phentolamine IV.

NURSING CONSIDERATIONS

BASELINE ASSESSMENT

Periodic hepatic function tests should be performed for pts requiring high dosage who are undergoing prolonged therapy.

INTERVENTION/EVALUATION

Assess appearance, behavior, speech pattern, level of interest, mood. Monitor for occipital headache radiating frontally and/or neck stiffness/soreness (may be first signal of impending hypertensive crisis). Monitor B/P, heart rate, diet, weight, change in mood.

PATIENT/FAMILY TEACHING

• Antidepressant relief may be noted during first wk of therapy; maximum benefit noted in 2–6 wks. • Report headache, neck stiffness/soreness immediately. • Avoid foods that require bacteria/molds for their preparation/ preservation or those that contain tyramine (e.g., cheese, sour cream, beer, wine, figs, raisins, bananas, avocados, soy sauce, yeast extracts, yogurt, papaya, broad beans, meat tenderizers), excessive

P

amounts of caffeine (coffee, tea, chocolate), OTC preparations for hay fever, colds, weight reduction.

phenobarbital

fee-noe-**bar**-bi-tal

(Luminal)

Do not confuse phenobarbital with pentobarbital, or Luminal with Tuinal.

FIXED-COMBINATION(S)

Bellergal-S: phenobarbital/ergotamine/belladonna (an anticholinergic): 40 mg/0.6 mg/0.2 mg. **Dilantin with PB:** phenobarbital/phenytoin (an anticonvulsant): 15 mg/100 mg; 30 mg/100 mg. **Donnatal:** phenobarbital/atropine (an anticholinergic)/hyoscyamine (an anticholinergic)/scopolamine (an anticholinergic): 16.2 mg/0.0194 mg/0.1037 mg/0.0065 mg.

CLASSIFICATION

PHARMACOTHERAPEUTIC: Barbiturate **(Schedule IV). CLINICAL:** Anticonvulsant, hypnotic (see p. 34C).

ACTION

Enhances activity of gamma-aminobutyric acid (GABA) by binding to GABA receptor complex. **Therapeutic Effect:** Depresses CNS activity.

PHARMACOKINETICS

Route	Onset	Peak	Duration
PO	20–60 min	N/A	6–10 hrs
IV	5 min	30 min	4–10 hrs

Well absorbed after PO, parenteral administration. Protein binding: 35%–50%. Rapidly and widely distributed. Metabolized in liver. Primarily excreted in urine. Removed by hemodialysis. **Half-life:** 53–118 hrs.

USES

Management of generalized tonic-clonic (grand mal) seizures, partial seizures, control of acute seizure episodes (status epilepticus, eclampsia, febrile seizures). Used as sedative, hypnotic. **OFF-LABEL:** Prevention/treatment of febrile seizures in children, hyperbilirubinemia, management of sedative/hypnotic withdrawal.

PRECAUTIONS

CONTRAINDICATIONS: Hypersensitivity to other barbiturates, porphyria, preexisting CNS depression, severe pain, severe respiratory disease. **CAUTIONS:** Renal/hepatic impairment.

LIFESPAN CONSIDERATIONS:

Pregnancy/Lactation: Readily crosses placenta. Distributed in breast milk. Produces respiratory depression in neonates during labor. May cause postpartum hemorrhage, hemorrhagic disease in newborn. Withdrawal symptoms may appear in neonates born to women receiving barbiturates during last trimester of pregnancy. Lowers serum bilirubin in neonates. **Pregnancy Category D. Children:** May cause paradoxical excitement. **Elderly:** May exhibit excitement, confusion, mental depression.

INTERACTIONS

DRUG: **Alcohol, other CNS depressants** may increase effects. May increase metabolism of **carbamazepine**. May decrease effects of **digoxin, glucocorticoids, metronidazole, oral anticoagulants, quinidine, tricyclic antidepressants**. **Valproic acid** increases concentration, risk of toxicity. **HERBAL:** **Evening primrose** may decrease seizure threshold. **Gotu kola, kava kava, St. John's wort, valerian** may increase CNS depression. **FOOD:** None known. **LAB VALUES:** May decrease serum bilirubin. Therapeutic serum level: 10–40 mcg/ml; toxic serum level: greater than 40 mcg/ml.

AVAILABILITY (Rx)

ELIXIR: 15 mg/5 ml, 20 mg/5 ml. **INJECTION, SOLUTION:** 65 mg/ml, 130 mg/ml. **TABLETS:** 15 mg, 30 mg, 60 mg, 100 mg.

ADMINISTRATION/HANDLING

IV

Reconstitution • May give undiluted or may dilute with NaCl, D_5W, lactated Ringer's.

Rate of administration • Adequately hydrate pt before and immediately after drug therapy (decreases risk of adverse renal effects). • Do not inject IV faster than 1 mg/kg/min and maximum of 30 mg/min for children and 60 mg/min for adults. Too-rapid IV may produce severe hypotension, marked respiratory depression. • Inadvertent intra-arterial injection may result in arterial spasm with severe pain, tissue necrosis. Extravasation in subcutaneous tissue may produce redness, tenderness, tissue necrosis. If this occurs, treat with 0.5% procaine solution into affected area, apply moist heat.

Storage • Store vials at room temperature.

IM

• Do not inject more than 5 ml in any one IM injection site (produces tissue irritation). • Inject deep IM into large muscle mass.

PO

• Give without regard to meals. • Tablets may be crushed. • Elixir may be mixed with water, milk, fruit juice.

IV INCOMPATIBILITIES

Amphotericin B complex (Abelcet, AmBisome, Amphotec), hydrocortisone (Solu-Cortef), hydromorphone (Dilaudid), insulin, lipids.

IV COMPATIBILITIES

Calcium gluconate, enalapril (Vasotec), fentanyl (Sublimaze), fosphenytoin (Cerebyx), morphine, propofol (Diprivan).

INDICATIONS/ROUTES/DOSAGE

STATUS EPILEPTICUS

IV: ADULTS, ELDERLY: Initially, 300–800 mg, then 120–240 mg/dose at 20 min intervals until seizures are controlled or total dose of 1–2 g administered. **CHILDREN, INFANTS:** 10–20 mg/kg. May administer additional 5 mg/kg/dose q15–30min until seizures controlled or total dose of 40 mg/kg administered.

SEIZURE CONTROL

PO, IV: ADULTS, ELDERLY, CHILDREN OLDER THAN 12 YRS: 1–3 mg/kg/day. Or 50–100 mg 2–3 times a day. **CHILDREN 6–12 YRS:** 4–6 mg/kg/day. **CHILDREN 1–5 YRS:** 6–8 mg/kg/day. **CHILDREN YOUNGER THAN 1 YR:** 5–6 mg/kg/day. **NEONATES:** 3–4 mg/kg/day.

SEDATION

PO, IM: ADULTS, ELDERLY: 30–120 mg/day in 2–3 divided doses. **CHILDREN:** 2 mg/kg 3 times a day.

HYPNOTIC

PO, IV, IM, SUBCUTANEOUS: ADULTS, ELDERLY: 100–320 mg at bedtime. **CHILDREN:** 3–5 mg/kg at bedtime.

SIDE EFFECTS

OCCASIONAL (3%–1%): Drowsiness. **RARE (less than 1%):** Confusion, paradoxical CNS reactions (hyperactivity, anxiety in children; excitement, restlessness in elderly, generally noted during first 2 wks of therapy, particularly in presence of uncontrolled pain).

ADVERSE EFFECTS/ TOXIC REACTIONS

Abrupt withdrawal after prolonged therapy may produce increased dreaming, nightmares, insomnia, tremor, diaphoresis, vomiting, hallucinations, delirium, seizures, status epilepticus. Skin eruptions appear as hypersensitivity reaction. Blood dyscrasias, hepatic disease, hypocalcemia occur rarely. Overdose produces cold/clammy skin, hypothermia, severe CNS depression, cyanosis, tachycardia, Cheyne-Stokes respirations. Toxicity may result in severe renal impairment.

NURSING CONSIDERATIONS

BASELINE ASSESSMENT

Assess B/P, pulse, respirations immediately before administration. **Hypnotic:** Raise bed rails, provide environment conducive to sleep (back rub, quiet environment, low lighting). **Seizures:** Review history of seizure disorder (length, presence of auras, level of consciousness [LOC]). Observe frequently for recurrence of seizure activity. Initiate seizure precautions.

INTERVENTION/EVALUATION

Monitor CNS status, seizure activity, hepatic/renal function, respiratory rate, heart rate, B/P. Monitor for therapeutic serum level. Therapeutic serum level: 10–40 mcg/ml; toxic serum level: greater than 40 mcg/ ml.

PATIENT/FAMILY TEACHING

• Avoid alcohol, limit caffeine. • May be habit forming. • Do not discontinue abruptly. • May cause dizziness/drowsiness; impair ability to perform tasks requiring mental alertness, coordination.

phentolamine

fen-**toll**-ah-mean
(Regitine ✤, Rogitine ✤)

Do not confuse phentolamine with phentermine.

CLASSIFICATION

PHARMACOTHERAPEUTIC: Alpha-adrenergic blocking agent. **CLINICAL:** Pheochromocytoma agent.

ACTION

Blocks presynaptic ($alpha_2$), post-synaptic ($alpha_1$) adrenergic receptors, acting on arterial tree, venous bed. **Therapeutic Effect:** Decreases total peripheral resistance, diminishes venous return to heart.

PHARMACOKINETICS

Onset	Peak	Duration
IM		
15–20 min	20 min	30–45 min
IV		
Immediate	2 min	15–30 min

Metabolized in liver. Excreted in urine. **Half-life:** 19 min.

USES

Diagnosis of pheochromocytoma. Control/prevention of hypertensive episodes immediately before, during surgical excision. Prevention/treatment of dermal necrosis, sloughing after IV administration of alpha-adrenergic drugs (e.g., norepinephrine/dopamine). **OFF-LABEL:** Treatment of CHF.

PRECAUTIONS

CONTRAINDICATIONS: Epinephrine, MI, coronary insufficiency, angina, coronary artery disease. **CAUTIONS:** Gastritis, peptic ulcer, history of arrhythmias.

LIFESPAN CONSIDERATIONS:

Pregnancy/Lactation: Unknown if drug crosses placenta or is distributed in breast milk. **Pregnancy Category C.** **Children:** Safety and efficacy not established. **Elderly:** No age-related precautions noted.

INTERACTIONS

DRUG: May decrease effects of **sympathomimetics (e.g., dopamine, phenylephrine)** when given with phentolamine. **HERBAL:** None significant. **FOOD:** None known. **LAB VALUES:** None known.

AVAILABILITY (Rx)

INJECTION, POWDER FOR RECONSTITUTION: 5-mg vials.

ADMINISTRATION/HANDLING

◀ **ALERT** ▶ Maintain pt in supine position (preferably in quiet, darkened room) during pheochromocytoma testing. Decrease in B/P generally noted in less than 2 min.

IV

Reconstitution • Reconstitute 5-mg vial with 1 ml Sterile Water for Injection to provide concentration of 5 mg/ml.

Rate of administration • Inject rapidly. Monitor B/P immediately after injection, q30sec for 3 min, then q60sec for 7 min.

Storage • Store vials at room temperature. • After reconstitution, is stable for 48 hrs at room temperature or 1 wk if refrigerated.

IV INCOMPATIBILITIES

Do not mix with any other medications.

IV COMPATIBILITIES

Amiodarone (Cordarone), dobutamine (Dobutrex).

INDICATIONS/ROUTES/DOSAGE

DIAGNOSIS OF PHEOCHROMOCYTOMA

IM, IV: ADULTS, ELDERLY: 2.5–5 mg. **CHILDREN:** 0.05–0.1 mg/kg/dose. **Maximum:** 5 mg.

CONTROL/PREVENTION OF HYPERTENSION IN PHEOCHROMOCYTOMA

IV: ADULTS, ELDERLY: 5 mg 1–2 hrs before surgery. May repeat q2–4h. **CHILDREN:** 0.05–0.1 mg/kg/dose 1–2 hrs before surgery. May repeat.

PREVENTION/TREATMENT OF NECROSIS/ SLOUGHING

ADULTS, ELDERLY: Infiltrate area with 1 ml of solution (reconstituted by diluting 5–10 mg in 0.9% NaCl) within 12 hrs of extravasation. **Maximum:** 0.1–0.2 mg/kg or 5 mg total. **CHILDREN:** 0.1–0.2 mg/kg diluted in 10 ml 0.9% NaCl infiltrated into area of extravasation within 12 hrs.

SIDE EFFECTS

OCCASIONAL (3%–2%): Weakness, dizziness, flushing, nausea, vomiting, diarrhea, orthostatic hypotension.

ADVERSE EFFECTS/ TOXIC REACTIONS

Tachycardia, arrhythmias, acute/prolonged hypotension may occur. Do not use epinephrine (will produce further drop in B/P).

NURSING CONSIDERATIONS

BASELINE ASSESSMENT

Positive pheochromocytoma test indicated by decrease in B/P greater than 35 mm Hg systolic, greater than 25 mm Hg diastolic pressure. Negative test indicated by no change in B/P or elevation of B/P. B/P generally returns to baseline within 15–30 min following administration.

INTERVENTION/EVALUATION

Monitor B/P, heart rate. Assess for orthostatic hypotension. Monitor for extravasation (skin color streaking).

P

phenylephrine

fen-ill-**eh**-frin

(AK-Dilate, Mydfrin, Neo-Synephrine, Sudafed PE)

CLASSIFICATION

PHARMACOTHERAPEUTIC: Sympathomimetic, alpha-receptor stimulant. **CLINICAL:** Nasal decongestant, mydriatic, vasopressor (see p. 148C).

ACTION

Acts on alpha-adrenergic receptors of vascular smooth muscle. Causes vasoconstriction of arterioles of nasal mucosa/conjunctiva, activates dilator muscle of pupil, causing contraction, producing systemic arterial vasoconstriction. **Therapeutic Effect:** Decreases mucosal blood flow, relieves congestion. Increases systolic B/P.

PHARMACOKINETICS

Route	Onset	Peak	Duration
IV	Immediate	N/A	15–20 min
IM	10–15 min	N/A	0.5–2 hrs
Subcutaneous	10–15 min	N/A	1 hr

Minimal absorption after intranasal, ophthalmic administration. Metabolized in liver, GI tract. Primarily excreted in urine. **Half-life:** 2.5 hrs.

USES

Nasal decongestant: Topical application to nasal mucosa reduces nasal secretion, promoting drainage of sinus secretions. **Ophthalmic:** Topical application to conjunctiva relieves congestion, itching, minor irritation; whitens sclera of eye. **Parenteral:** Vascular failure in shock, drug-induced hypotension.

PRECAUTIONS

CONTRAINDICATIONS: Acute pancreatitis, heart disease, hepatitis, narrow-angle glaucoma, pheochromocytoma, severe hypertension, thrombosis, ventricular tachycardia. **CAUTIONS:** Hyperthyroidism, bradycardia, heart block, severe arteriosclerosis.

LIFESPAN CONSIDERATIONS:

Pregnancy/Lactation: Crosses placenta. Distributed in breast milk. **Pregnancy Category C. Children:** May exhibit increased absorption, toxicity with nasal preparation. No age-related precautions noted with systemic use. **Elderly:** More likely to experience adverse effects.

INTERACTIONS

DRUG: Beta-blockers may have mutually inhibitory effects. **Digoxin** may increase risk of arrhythmias. **Ergonovine, oxytocin** may increase vasoconstriction. **MAOIs** may increase vasopressor effects. **Maprotiline, tricyclic antidepressants** may increase cardiovascular effects. May decrease effects of **methyldopa. HERBAL: Ephedra, yohimbe** may increase CNS stimulation. **FOOD:** None known. **LAB VALUES:** None known.

AVAILABILITY (OTC)

INJECTION, SOLUTION: 1% (10 mg/ml). **SOLUTION, NASAL DROPS: (NEO-SYNEPHRINE):** 0.5%, 1%. **SOLUTION, NASAL SPRAY: (NEO-SYNEPHRINE):** 0.25%, 0.5%, 1%. **SOLUTION, OPHTHALMIC: (AK-DILATE, MYDFRIN, NEO-SYNEPHRINE):** 0.12%, 2.5%, 10%. **TABLETS: (SUDAFED PE):** 10 mg.

ADMINISTRATION/HANDLING

IV

Reconstitution • For IV push, dilute 1 ml of 10 mg/ml solution with 9 ml Sterile Water for Injection to provide concentration of 1 mg/ml. • For IV infusion, dilute 10-mg vial with 500 ml D_5W or 0.9% NaCl to provide a concentration of 2 mcg/ml. Maximum concentration: 500 mg/250 ml.

Rate of administration • For IV push, give over 20–30 sec. • For IV infusion, give as per physician order.

Storage • Store vials at room temperature.

NASAL

• Instruct pt to blow nose prior to administering medication. • With head tilted back, apply drops in 1 nostril. Wait 5 min before applying drops in other nostril. • Sprays should be administered into each nostril with head erect. • Pt should sniff briskly while squeezing container, then wait 3–5 min before blowing nose gently. • Rinse tip of spray bottle.

OPHTHALMIC

• Instruct pt to tilt head backward, look up. • Gently pull lower lid down to form pouch, then instill medication. • Do not touch tip of applicator to lids or any surface. • When lower lid is released, have pt keep eye open without blinking for at least 30 sec. • Apply gentle finger pressure to lacrimal sac (bridge of nose, inside corner of eye) for 1–2 min. • Remove excess solution around eye with tissue. • Wash hands immediately to remove medication on hands.

IV INCOMPATIBILITY

Thiopentothal (Pentothal).

IV COMPATIBILITIES

Amiodarone (Cordarone), dobutamine (Dobutrex), lidocaine, potassium chloride, propofol (Diprivan).

INDICATIONS/ROUTES/DOSAGE

NASAL DECONGESTANT

ADULTS, ELDERLY, CHILDREN 12 YRS AND OLDER: 2–3 drops or 1–2 sprays of 0.25%–0.5% solution into each nostril q4h as needed, or 1 tablet q4h as needed (not more than 6 doses/24 hrs. **CHILDREN 6–11 YRS:** 2–3 drops or 1–2 sprays of 0.25% solution into each nostril q4h as needed. **CHILDREN YOUNGER THAN 6 YRS:**1 drop of 0.125% solution (dilute 0.5% solution with 0.9% NaCl to achieve 0.125%) in each nostril. Repeat q2–4h as needed. Do not use for more than 3 days.

CONJUNCTIVAL CONGESTION, ITCHING, MINOR IRRITATION

OPHTHALMIC: ADULTS, ELDERLY, CHILDREN 12 YRS AND OLDER: 1–2 drops of 0.12% solution q3–4h.

HYPOTENSION, SHOCK

IM, SUBCUTANEOUS: ADULTS, ELDERLY: 2–5 mg/dose q1–2h. **CHILDREN:** 0.1 mg/kg/dose q1–2h. **Maximum:** 5 mg.

IV BOLUS: ADULTS, ELDERLY: 0.1–0.5 mg/dose q10–15min as needed. **CHILDREN:** 5–20 mcg/kg/dose q10–15min.

IV INFUSION: ADULTS, ELDERLY: 100–180 mcg/min. When B/P is stabilized, maintenance rate: 40–60 mcg/min. **CHILDREN:** 0.1–0.5 mcg/kg/min. Titrate to desired effect.

SIDE EFFECTS

FREQUENT: Nasal: Rebound nasal congestion due to overuse, esp. when used longer than 3 days. **OCCASIONAL:** Mild CNS stimulation (restlessness, nervousness, tremors, headache, insomnia, particularly in those hypersensitive to sympathomimetics, such as elderly pts). **Nasal:** Stinging, burning, drying of nasal mucosa. **Ophthalmic:** Transient burning/stinging, brow ache, blurred vision.

ADVERSE EFFECTS/ TOXIC REACTIONS

Large doses may produce tachycardia, palpitations (particularly in those with cardiac disease), light-headedness, nausea, vomiting. Overdose in those older than 60 yrs may result in hallucinations, CNS depression, seizures. Prolonged nasal use may produce chronic swelling of nasal mucosa, rhinitis.

P

NURSING CONSIDERATIONS

BASELINE ASSESSMENT

If phenylephine 10% ophthalmic is instilled into denuded/damaged corneal epithelium, corneal clouding may result.

INTERVENTION/EVALUATION

Monitor B/P, heart rate.

PATIENT/FAMILY TEACHING

• Discontinue drug if adverse reactions occur. • Do not use for nasal decongestion for longer than 5 days, (rebound congestion). • Discontinue drug if insomnia, dizziness, weakness, tremor, palpitations occur. • **Nasal:** Stinging/burning of nasal mucosa may occur. • **Opthalmic:** Blurring of vision with eye instillation generally subsides with continued therapy. • Discontinue medication if redness/swelling of eyelids, itching occurs.

phenytoin

phen-ih-toyn

(Dilantin, Dilantin-125, Dilantin Infatabs, Dilantin Kapseals, Phenytek)

Do not confuse phenytoin with mephenytoin, or Dilantin with Dilaudid.

FIXED-COMBINATION(S)

Dilantin with PB: phenytoin/phenobarbital (a barbiturate): 100 mg/15 mg; 100 mg/30 mg.

◆CLASSIFICATION

PHARMACOTHERAPEUTIC: Hydantoin. **CLINICAL:** Anticonvulsant, antiarrhythmic (see p. 34C).

P

ACTION

Anticonvulsant: Stabilizes neuronal membranes in motor cortex. **Therapeutic Effect:** Limits spread of seizure activity. Stabilizes threshold against hyperexcitability. Decreases post-tetanic potentiation, repetitive discharge.

PHARMACOKINETICS

Slowly, variably absorbed after PO administration; slowly but completely absorbed after IM administration. Protein binding: 90%–95%. Widely distributed. Metabolized in liver. Primarily excreted in urine. Not removed by hemodialysis. **Half-life:** 22 hrs.

USES

Management of generalized tonic-clonic seizures (grand mal), complex partial seizures (psychomotor), cortical focal seizures, status epilepticus. Ineffective in absence seizures, myoclonic seizures, atonic epilepsy when used alone. **OFF-LABEL:** Adjunctive treatment of tricyclic antidepressant toxicity; treatment of muscle hyperirritability, digoxin-induced arrhythmias, trigeminal neuralgia.

PRECAUTIONS

CONTRAINDICATIONS: Hypersensitivity to hydantoins, seizures due to hypoglycemia. **IV:** Adam-Stokes syndrome, second- and third-degree AV block, sinoatrial block, sinus bradycardia. **EXTREME CAUTION: IV Route Only:** Respiratory depression, MI, CHF, damaged myocardium. **CAUTIONS:** Hepatic/renal impairment, severe myocardial insufficiency, hypotension, hyperglycemia.

⌛ LIFESPAN CONSIDERATIONS:

Pregnancy/Lactation: Crosses placenta. Is distributed in small amount in breast milk. Fetal hydantoin syndrome (craniofacial abnormalities, nail/digital hypoplasia, prenatal growth deficiency) has been reported. Increased frequency of seizures in pregnant women due to altered absorption of metabolism of phenytoin. May increase risk of hemorrhage in neonate, maternal bleeding during delivery. **Pregnancy Category D. Children:** More susceptible to gingival hyperplasia, coarsening of facial hair; excess body hair. **Elderly:** No age-related precautions noted but lower dosages recommended.

INTERACTIONS

DRUG: Alcohol, other CNS depressants may increase CNS depression. **Amiodarone, anticoagulants, cimetidine, disulfiram, fluoxetine, isoniazid, sulfonamides** may increase concentration, effects, risk of toxicity.

Antacids may decrease absorption. **Fluconazole, ketoconazole, miconazole** may increase concentration. May decrease effects of **glucocorticoids. Lidocaine, propranolol** may increase cardiac depressant effects. **Valproic acid** may decrease metabolism, increase concentration. May increase metabolism of **xanthines**. **HERBAL: Evening primrose** may decrease seizure threshold. **Gotu kola, kava kava, St. John's wort, valerian** may increase CNS depression. **FOOD:** None known. **LAB VALUES:** May increase serum glucose, GGT, alkaline phosphatase. Therapeutic serum level: 10–20 mcg/ml; toxic serum level: greater than 20 mcg/ml.

AVAILABILITY (Rx)

CAPSULES, EXTENDED-RELEASE: (DILANTIN, PHENYTEK): 30 mg, 100 mg. **CAPSULES, PROMPT RELEASE: (DILANTIN):** 100 mg. **INJECTION, SOLUTION: (DILANTIN):** 50 mg/ml. **SUSPENSION, ORAL: (DILANTIN):** 125 mg/5 ml. **TABLETS, CHEWABLE: (DILANTIN):** 50 mg.

ADMINISTRATION/HANDLING

IV

◀ **ALERT** ▶ Give by IV push. IV push very painful (chemical irritation of vein due to alkalinity of solution). To minimize effect, flush vein with sterile saline solution through same IV needle and catheter after each IV push.

Reconstitution • May give undiluted or may dilute with 0.9% NaCl.

Rate of administration • Administer 50 mg over 2–3 min for elderly. In neonates, administer at rate not exceeding 1–3 mg/kg/min. • Severe hypotension, cardiovascular collapse occurs if rate of IV injection exceeds 50 mg/min for adults. • IV toxicity characterized by CNS depression, cardiovascular collapse.

Storage • Precipitate may form if parenteral form is refrigerated (will dissolve at room temperature). • Slight yellow discoloration of parenteral form does not affect potency, but do not use if solution is cloudy or precipitate forms.

PO

• Give with food if GI distress occurs. • Do not chew/break capsules, but tablets may be chewed. • Shake oral suspension well before using.

IV INCOMPATIBILITIES

Diltiazem (Cardizem), dobutamine (Dobutrex), enalapril (Vasotec), heparin, hydromorphone (Dilaudid), insulin, lidocaine, morphine, nitroglycerin, norepinephrine (Levophed), potassium chloride, propofol (Diprivan).

INDICATIONS/ROUTES/DOSAGE

STATUS EPILEPTICUS

IV: ADULTS, ELDERLY, CHILDREN: 15–25 mg/kg. Maintenance dose: 300 mg/day or 4–6 mg/kg/day in 2–3 divided doses for adults and elderly; 6–7 mg/kg/day for children 10–16 yrs; 7–8 mg/kg/day for children 7–9 yrs; 7.5–9 mg/kg/day for children 4–6 yrs; 8–10 mg/kg/day for children 6 mos–3 yrs. **NEONATES:** Loading dose: 15–20 mg/kg. Maintenance dose: 5–8 mg/kg/day.

SEIZURE CONTROL

PO: ADULTS, ELDERLY, CHILDREN: Loading dose: 15–20 mg/kg in 3 divided doses 2–4 hrs apart. Maintenance dose: Same as for status epilepticus.

SIDE EFFECTS

FREQUENT: Drowsiness, lethargy, confusion, slurred speech, irritability, gingival hyperplasia, hypersensitivity reaction (fever, rash, lymphadenopathy), constipation, dizziness, nausea. **OCCASIONAL:** Headache, hirsutism, coarsening of facial features, insomnia, muscle twitching.

ADVERSE EFFECTS/ TOXIC REACTIONS

Abrupt withdrawal may precipitate status epilepticus. Blood dyscrasias,

P

lymphadenopathy, osteomalacia (due to interference of vitamin D metabolism) may occur. Toxic phenytoin blood concentration (25 mcg/ml or more) may produce ataxia (muscular incoordination), nystagmus (rhythmic oscillation of eyes), diplopia. As level increases, extreme lethargy to comatose states occur.

NURSING CONSIDERATIONS

BASELINE ASSESSMENT

Anticonvulsant: Review history of seizure disorder (intensity, frequency, duration, level of consciousness [LOC]). Initiate seizure precautions. Hepatic function tests, CBC, platelet count should be performed before beginning therapy and periodically during therapy. Repeat CBC, platelet count 2 wks following initiation of therapy and 2 wks following administration of maintenance dose.

INTERVENTION/EVALUATION

Observe frequently for recurrence of seizure activity. Assess for clinical improvement (decrease in intensity/frequency of seizures). Monitor CBC with differential, hepatic/renal function tests, B/P (with IV use). Assist with ambulation if drowsiness, lethargy occurs. Monitor for therapeutic serum level (10–20 mcg/ml). Therapeutic serum level: 10–20 mcg/ml; toxic serum level: greater than 20 mcg/ml.

PATIENT/FAMILY TEACHING

• Pain may occur with IV injection. • To prevent gingival hyperplasia (bleeding, tenderness, swelling of gums), encourage good oral hygiene care, gum massage, regular dental visits. • CBC should be performed every mo for 1 yr after maintenance dose is established and q3mo thereafter. • Report sore throat, fever, glandular swelling, skin reaction (hematologic toxicity). • Drowsiness usually diminishes with continued therapy. • Avoid tasks that require alertness, motor skills until response to drug is established. • Do not abruptly withdraw medication after long-term use (may precipitate seizures). • Strict maintenance of drug therapy is essential for seizure control, arrhythmias. • Avoid alcohol.

PhosLo, *see calcium acetate*

phosphates

fos-fates

(Fleet Enema, Fleet Phospho-Soda, K-Phos MF, K-Phos Neutral, Neutra-Phos, Neutra-Phos-K, Uro-KP-Neutral)

CLASSIFICATION

PHARMACOTHERAPEUTIC: Electrolyte. **CLINICAL:** Mineral.

ACTION

Active in bone deposition, calcium metabolism, utilization of B complex vitamins. Acts as buffers in maintaining acid-base balance. Exerts osmotic effect in small intestine. **Therapeutic Effect:** Corrects hypophosphatemia, acidifies urine, prevents calcium deposits in urinary tract, promotes peristalsis in GI tract.

PHARMACOKINETICS

Poorly absorbed after PO administration. PO form excreted in feces; IV form excreted in urine.

USES

Prophylactic treatment of hypophosphatemia. Short-term treatment of constipation, for evacuation of colon for exams; urinary acidifier for reduction of formation of calcium stones. **OFF-LABEL:** Prevention of calcium renal calculi.

PRECAUTIONS

CONTRAINDICATIONS: Abdominal pain, fecal impaction (rectal dosage form), ascitic conditions, CHF, hyperkalemia, hypernatremia, hyperphosphatemia, hypocalcemia, hypomagnesemia, paralytic ileus, phosphate renal calculi, severe renal impairment. **CAUTIONS:** Renal impairment, concomitant use of potassium-sparing drugs, adrenal insufficiency, cirrhosis.

LIFESPAN CONSIDERATIONS:

Pregnancy/Lactation: Unknown if drug crosses placenta or is distributed in breast milk. **Pregnancy Category C.** **Children:** Increased risk of dehydration in children younger than 12 yrs. **Elderly:** No age-related precautions noted.

INTERACTIONS

DRUG: **Angiotensin-converting enzyme (ACE) inhibitors, NSAIDs, potassium-containing medications, potassium-sparing diuretics, salt substitutes containing potassium phosphate** may increase serum potassium. **Antacids** may decrease absorption. **Calcium-containing medications** may increase risk of calcium deposition in soft tissues, decrease phosphate absorption. **Digoxin** may increase risk of heart block caused by hyperkalemia when given with potassium phosphates. **Glucocorticoids** may cause edema when given with sodium phosphate. **Phosphate-containing medications** may increase risk of hyperphosphatemia. **Sodium-containing medications** may increase risk of edema when given with sodium phosphate. **HERBAL:** None significant. **FOOD:** None known. **LAB VALUES:** None known.

AVAILABILITY (Rx)

ENEMA (FLEET ENEMA): 2.25 oz, 4.5 oz. **INJECTION SOLUTION (POTASSIUM PHOSPHATE):** 3 mmol phosphate and 4.4 mEq potassium per ml. **INJECTION SOLUTION (SODIUM PHOSPHATE):** 3 mmol phosphate and 4 mEq sodium per ml. **ORAL SOLUTION (FLEET PHOSPHA-SODA):** 4 mmol phosphate per ml. **POWDER (NEUTRA-PHOS, NEUTRA-PHOS-K):** 250 mg (8 mmol) phosphate. **TABLETS:** 125 mg (4 mmol) phosphate, 250 mg (8 mmol) phosphate (K-Phos MF, K-Phos Neutral, Uro-KP-Neutral).

ADMINISTRATION/HANDLING

IV

Reconstitution • Must be diluted. Soluble in all commonly used IV solutions.

Rate of administration • Maximum rate of infusion: 0.06 mmol phosphate/kg/hr.

Storage • Store at room temperature.

PO

• Dissolve tablets in water. • Take after meals or with food (decreases GI upset). • Maintain high fluid intake (prevents kidney stones).

RECTAL

• Instruct pt to lie in left lateral Sims position. • Insert tube pointing toward navel. • Slowly squeeze and empty contents into rectum. Pt to remain in Sims position until defecation impulse felt (usually 2–5 min).

IV INCOMPATIBILITY

Dobutamine (Dobutrex).

IV COMPATIBILITIES

Diltiazem (Cardizem), enalapril (Vasotec), famotidine (Pepcid), magnesium sulfate, metoclopramide (Reglan).

INDICATIONS/ROUTES/DOSAGE

HYPOPHOSPHATEMIA

PO (NEUTRA-PHOS, NEUTRA-PHOS-K, K-PHOS MF, K-PHOS-NEUTRAL,

P

URO-KP-NEUTRAL): **ADULTS, ELDERLY:** 50–150 mmol/day. **CHILDREN:** 2–3 mmol/kg/day.
IV: **ADULTS, ELDERLY:** 50–70 mmol/day. **CHILDREN:** 0.5–1.5 mmol/kg/day.

LAXATIVE
PO (NEUTRA-PHOS, NEUTRA-PHOS-K, URO-KP-NEUTRAL): **ADULTS, ELDERLY, CHILDREN 4 YRS AND OLDER:** 1–2 capsules/packets 4 times a day. **CHILDREN YOUNGER THAN 4 YRS:** 1 capsule/packet 4 times a day.
RECTAL: **ADULTS, ELDERLY, CHILDREN 12 YRS AND OLDER:** 4.5-oz enema as single dose. May repeat. **CHILDREN YOUNGER THAN 12 YRS:** 2.25-oz enema as single dose. May repeat.

URINE ACIDIFICATION
PO: **ADULTS, ELDERLY:** 8 mmol 4 times a day.

SIDE EFFECTS

FREQUENT: Mild laxative effect (in first few days of therapy). **OCCASIONAL:** Diarrhea, nausea, abdominal pain, vomiting. **RARE:** Headache, dizziness, confusion, heaviness of lower extremities, fatigue, muscle cramps, paresthesia, peripheral edema, arrhythmias, weight gain, thirst.

ADVERSE EFFECTS/ TOXIC REACTIONS

Hyperphosphatemia may produce extraskeletal calcification.

NURSING CONSIDERATIONS

INTERVENTION/EVALUATION

Routinely monitor serum calcium, phosphorus, potassium, sodium, AST, ALT, alkaline phosphatase, bilirubin.

PATIENT/FAMILY TEACHING

- Report diarrhea, nausea, vomiting.

physostigmine

fi-zoe-**stig**-meen
(Antilirium)

Do not confuse physostigmine with Prostigmin or pyridostigmine.

CLASSIFICATION

PHARMACOTHERAPEUTIC: Parasympathomimetic (cholinergic). **CLINICAL:** Anticholinesterase agent (see p. 48C).

ACTION

Inhibits destruction of acetylcholine by enzyme acetylcholinesterase, enhancing impulse transmission across myoneural junction. **Therapeutic Effect:** Improves skeletal muscle tone, stimulates salivary/sweat gland secretions.

PHARMACOKINETICS

Penetrates blood-brain barrier. Rapidly hydrolyzed by cholinesterases. Small amount eliminated in urine; largely destroyed in body by hydrolysis. **Half-life:** Unknown.

USES

Antidote for reversal of toxic CNS effects due to anticholinergic drugs, tricyclic antidepressants. **OFF-LABEL:** Treatment of hereditary ataxia.

PRECAUTIONS

CONTRAINDICATIONS: Active uveal inflammation, narrow angle glaucoma before iridectomy, asthma, cardiovascular disease, concurrent use of ganglionic-blocking agents, diabetes, gangrene, glaucoma associated with iridocyclitis, hypersensitivity to cholinesterase inhibitors or their components, mechanical obstruction of intestinal, urogenital tract, vagotonic state. **CAUTIONS:** Bronchial asthma, GI disturbances, peptic ulcer, bradycardia, hypotension, recent MI, epilepsy, parkinsonism, other disorders that may respond adversely to vagotonic effects. Use ophthalmic physostigmine only when shorter-acting miotics are not adequate, except in aphakics.

LIFESPAN CONSIDERATIONS:

Pregnancy/Lactation: Unknown if drug crosses placenta or is distributed in breast milk. **Pregnancy Category C.** **Children:** No age-related precautions noted. **Elderly:** No age-related precautions noted.

INTERACTIONS

DRUG: May increase effects of **cholinesterases (e.g., bethanechol, carbachol).** May prolong action of **succinylcholine.** **HERBAL:** None significant. **FOOD:** None known. **LAB VALUES:** None known.

AVAILABILITY (Rx)

INJECTION SOLUTION: 1 mg/ml.

ADMINISTRATION/HANDLING

IV

• For adults, administer at rate not exceeding 1 mg/min. • For children, administer no more than 0.02 mg/kg over at least 1 min.

INDICATIONS/ROUTES/DOSAGE

ANTIDOTE

IV, IM: ADULTS, ELDERLY: Initially, 0.5–2 mg. If no response, repeat q20min until response or adverse cholinergic effects occur. If initial response occurs, may give additional doses of 1–4 mg q30–60min as life-threatening signs (arrhythmias, seizures, deep coma) recur. **CHILDREN:** 0.01–0.03 mg/kg. May give additional doses q5–10min until response or adverse cholinergic effects occur or total dose of 2 mg given.

SIDE EFFECTS

EXPECTED: Miosis, increased GI/skeletal muscle tone, bradycardia. **OCCASIONAL:** Marked drop in B/P (hypertensive pts). **RARE:** Allergic reaction.

ADVERSE EFFECTS/ TOXIC REACTIONS

Parenteral overdose produces cholinergic reaction manifested as abdominal discomfort/cramps, nausea, vomiting, diarrhea, flushing, facial warmth, excessive salivation, diaphoresis, urinary urgency, blurred vision. Requires withdrawal of all anticholinergic drugs and immediate use of 0.6–1.2 mg atropine sulfate IM/IV for adults, 0.01 mg/kg for infants, children younger than 12 yrs.

NURSING CONSIDERATIONS

BASELINE ASSESSMENT

Have tissues readily available at pt's bedside.

INTERVENTION/EVALUATION

Parenteral: Assess vital signs immediately before and q15–30min following administration. Monitor diligently for cholinergic reaction (diaphoresis, palpitations, muscle weakness, abdominal pain, dyspnea, hypotension).

PATIENT/FAMILY TEACHING

• Adverse effects often subside after the first few days of therapy. • Avoid night driving, activities requiring visual acuity in dim light.

pimecrolimus

pim-eh-**crow**-leh-mus
(Elidel)

Do not confuse Elidel with Elavil.

CLASSIFICATION

PHARMACOTHERAPEUTIC: Immunomodulator. **CLINICAL:** Anti-inflammatory.

ACTION

Inhibits release of cytokine, an enzyme that produces an inflammatory reaction. **Therapeutic Effect:** Produces anti-inflammatory activity.

USES

Treatment of mild to moderate atopic dermatitis (eczema).

PRECAUTIONS

CONTRAINDICATIONS: None known. **CAUTIONS:** Potential cancer risk.

LIFESPAN CONSIDERATIONS:

Pregnancy/Lactation: Embryotoxic. Unknown if distributed in breast milk. **Pregnancy Category C. Children:** May be used in children 2 yrs and older. **Elderly:** No age-related precautions noted.

INTERACTIONS

DRUG: None significant. **HERBAL:** None significant. **FOOD:** None known. **LAB VALUES:** None known.

AVAILABILITY (Rx)

TOPICAL: 1% cream.

INDICATIONS/ROUTES/DOSAGE

ATOPIC DERMATITIS (ECZEMA)

TOPICAL: ADULTS, ELDERLY, CHILDREN 2–17 YRS: Apply to affected area twice a day for up to 3 wks (up to 6 wks in children 2–17 yrs). Rub in gently, completely. Reevaluate if symptoms persist for more than 6 wks.

SIDE EFFECTS

RARE: Transient sensation of burning/feeling of heat at application site.

ADVERSE EFFECTS/ TOXIC REACTIONS

Lymphadenopathy, phototoxicity occur rarely.

NURSING CONSIDERATIONS

PATIENT/FAMILY TEACHING

• Wash hands after application. • May cause mild to moderate feeling of warmth, sensation of burning at application site. • Inform physician if application site reaction is severe or lasts for longer than 1 wk. • Avoid artificial sunlight, tanning beds. • Contact physician if no improvement in atopic dermatitis is seen following 6 wks of treatment or if condition worsens.

pindolol

(Novo-Pindol ✤, Visken)

Do not confuse with Panadol, Parlodel, Plendil.

See Beta-adrenergic blockers (p. 68C)

pioglitazone

pie-oh-**glit**-ah-zone

(Actos)

FIXED-COMBINATION(S)

Actoplus Met: pioglitazone/metformin, (an antidiabetic): 15 mg/500 mg, 15 mg/850 mg. **Duetact:** pioglitazone/glimepiride (an antidiabetic): 30 mg/2 mg, 30 mg/4 mg.

CLASSIFICATION

CLINICAL: Antidiabetic (see p. 42C).

ACTION

Improves target-cell response to insulin without increasing pancreatic insulin secretion. Decreases hepatic glucose output, increases insulin-dependent glucose utilization in skeletal muscle. **Therapeutic Effect:** Lowers serum glucose concentration.

PHARMACOKINETICS

Rapidly absorbed. Highly protein bound (99%), primarily to albumin. Metabolized in liver. Excreted in urine. Unknown if removed by hemodialysis. **Half-life:** 16–24 hrs.

USES

Adjunct to diet, exercise to lower serum glucose in those with type 2 non–insulin-dependent diabetes mellitus (NIDDM). Used as monotherapy or in combination with sulfonylurea, metformin, or insulin to improve glycemic control.

PRECAUTIONS

CONTRAINDICATIONS: Active hepatic disease; diabetic ketoacidosis; increased serum transaminase, including ALT greater than 2.5 times normal serum level; type 1 diabetes mellitus. **CAUTIONS:** Hepatic impairment, CHF, edematous pts.

LIFESPAN CONSIDERATIONS:

Pregnancy/Lactation: Unknown if drug crosses placenta or is distributed in breast milk. Not recommended in pregnant or breast-feeding women. **Pregnancy Category C.** **Children:** Safety and efficacy not established. **Elderly:** No age-related precautions noted.

INTERACTIONS

DRUG: **Gemfibrozil** may increase effect, toxicity. **Ketoconazole** may significantly inhibit metabolism. May alter effects of **oral contraceptives.** **HERBAL:** **St. John's wort** may decrease concentration. **Garlic** may cause hypoglycemia. **FOOD:** None known. **LAB VALUES:** May increase serum creatine kinase (CK). May decrease Hgb (by 2%–4%), serum alkaline phosphatase, bilirubin, ALT. Less than 1% of pts experience ALT values 3 times the normal level.

AVAILABILITY (Rx)

TABLETS: 15 mg, 30 mg, 45 mg.

ADMINISTRATION/HANDLING

PO

- Give without regard to meals.

INDICATIONS/ROUTES/DOSAGE

DIABETES MELLITUS, COMBINATION THERAPY

PO: ADULTS, ELDERLY: With insulin: Initially, 15–30 mg once a day. Initially, continue current insulin dosage; then decrease insulin dosage by 10%–25% if hypoglycemia occurs or plasma glucose level decreases to less than 100 mg/dl. **Maximum:** 45 mg/day. **With sulfonylureas:** Initially, 15–30 mg/day. Decrease sulfonylurea dosage if hypoglycemia occurs. **With metformin:** Initially, 15–30 mg/day.

MONOTHERAPY

Monotherapy is not to be used if pt is well controlled with diet and exercise alone. Initially, 15–30 mg/day. May increase dosage in increments until 45 mg/day is reached.

DOSAGE ADJUSTMENT IN CHF

PO: ADULTS, ELDERLY: Initially, 15 mg once daily. May increase after several mos of treatment.

SIDE EFFECTS

FREQUENT (13%–9%): Headache, upper respiratory tract infection. **OCCASIONAL (6%–5%):** Sinusitis, myalgia, pharyngitis, aggravated diabetes mellitus.

ADVERSE EFFECTS/ TOXIC REACTIONS

Hepatotoxicity occurs rarely. May cause/worsen macular edema.

NURSING CONSIDERATIONS

BASELINE ASSESSMENT

Obtain hepatic enzyme levels before initiating therapy and periodically thereafter. Ensure follow-up instruction if pt,

P

family do not thoroughly understand diabetes management, glucose-testing technique.

INTERVENTION/EVALUATION

Monitor serum glucose, Hgb, hepatic function tests, esp. AST, ALT. Assess for hypoglycemia (cool/wet skin, tremors, dizziness, anxiety, headache, tachycardia, numbness in mouth, hunger, diplopia), hyperglycemia (polyuria, polyphagia, polydipsia, nausea, vomiting, dim vision, fatigue, deep rapid breathing). Be alert to conditions that alter serum glucose requirements: fever, increased activity, stress, surgical procedures.

PATIENT/FAMILY TEACHING

• Understand signs/symptoms of hypoglycemia and its management. • Avoid alcohol. • Inform physician of chest pain, palpitations, abdominal pain, fever, rash, hypoglycemic reactions, yellowing of skin/eyes, dark urine, light stool, nausea, vomiting. Report any change in vision.

P

pipecuronium

(Arduan)

See Neuromuscular blockers

piperacillin sodium/ tazobactam sodium

pip-ur-ah-**sill**-in/tay-zoe-**back**-tam

(Tazocin ✤, Zosyn)

Do not confuse Zosyn with Zofran or Zyvox.

CLASSIFICATION

PHARMACOTHERAPEUTIC: Penicillin. **CLINICAL:** Antibiotic (see p. 28C).

ACTION

Piperacillin: Inhibits cell wall synthesis by binding to bacterial cell membranes. **Therapeutic Effect:** Bactericidal. **Tazobactam:** Inactivates bacterial beta-lactamase. **Therapeutic Effect:** Protects piperacillin from enzymatic degradation, extends its spectrum of activity, prevents bacterial overgrowth.

PHARMACOKINETICS

Protein binding: 16%–30%. Widely distributed. Primarily excreted unchanged in urine. Removed by hemodialysis. **Half-life:** 0.7–1.2 hrs (increased in hepatic cirrhosis, renal impairment).

USES

Treatment of appendicitis (complicated by rupture, abscess); peritonitis; uncomplicated and complicated skin/skin structure infections, including cellulitis, cutaneous abscesses, ischemic/diabetic foot infections; postpartum endometritis; pelvic inflammatory disease (PID); community-acquired pneumonia (moderate severity only); moderate to severe nosocomial pneumonia.

PRECAUTIONS

CONTRAINDICATIONS: Hypersensitivity to any penicillin. **CAUTIONS:** History of allergies, (esp. cephalosporins, other drugs), renal impairment, preexisting seizure disorder.

⧖ LIFESPAN CONSIDERATIONS:

Pregnancy/Lactation: Readily crosses placenta; appears in cord blood, amniotic fluid. Distributed in breast milk in low concentrations. May lead to allergic sensitization, diarrhea, candidiasis, skin rash in infant. **Pregnancy Category B.** **Children:** Dosage not established for those younger than 12 yrs. **Elderly:** Age-related renal impairment may require dosage adjustment.

INTERACTIONS

DRUG: Concurrent use of **aminoglycosides** may cause mutual inactivation (must give at least 1 hr apart). May increase concentration, toxicity of **methotrexate**. **Probenecid** may increase concentration, risk of toxicity. High-dose piperacillin may increase risk of bleeding with **warfarin, heparin, thrombolytic agents, NSAIDs, platelet inhibitors.** **HERBAL:** None significant. **FOOD:** None known. **LAB VALUES:** May increase serum sodium, alkaline phosphatase, bilirubin, LDH, AST, ALT. May decrease serum potassium. May cause positive Coombs' test.

AVAILABILITY (Rx)

◀ **ALERT** ▶ Piperacillin/tazobactam is a combination product in an 8:1 ratio of piperacillin to tazobactam.

INJECTION POWDER: 2.25 g, 3.375 g, 4.5 g. **PREMIX READY TO USE:** 2.25 g, 3.375 g, 4.5 g.

ADMINISTRATION/HANDLING

IV

Reconstitution • Reconstitute each 1 g with 5 ml D_5W or 0.9% NaCl. Shake vigorously to dissolve. • Further dilute with at least 50 ml D_5W, 0.9% NaCl, D_5W 0.9% NaCl, or lactated Ringer's.

Rate of administration • Infuse over 30 min.

Storage • Reconstituted vial is stable for 24 hrs at room temperature or 48 hrs if refrigerated. • After further dilution, is stable for 24 hrs at room temperature or 7 days if refrigerated.

IV INCOMPATIBILITIES

Amphotericin B (Fungizone), amphotericin B complex (Abelcet, AmBisome, Amphotec), chlorpromazine (Thorazine), dacarbazine (DTIC), daunorubicin (Cerubidine), dobutamine (Dobutrex), doxorubicin (Adriamycin), doxorubicin liposomal (Doxil), droperidol (Inapsine), famotidine (Pepcid), haloperidol (Haldol), hydroxyzine (Vistaril), idarubicin (Idamycin), minocycline (Minocin), nalbuphine (Nubain), prochlorperazine (Compazine), promethazine (Phenergan), vancomycin (Vancocin).

IV COMPATIBILITIES

Aminophylline, bumetanide (Bumex), calcium gluconate, diphenhydramine (Benadryl), dopamine (Intropin), enalapril (Vasotec), furosemide (Lasix), granisetron (Kytril), heparin, hydrocortisone (Solu-Cortef), hydromorphone (Dilaudid), lipids, lorazepam (Ativan), magnesium sulfate, methylprednisolone (Solu-Medrol), metoclopramide (Reglan), morphine, ondansetron (Zofran), potassium chloride, total parenteral nutrition (TPN).

INDICATIONS/ROUTES/DOSAGE

SEVERE INFECTIONS

IV: ADULTS, ELDERLY, CHILDREN 12 YRS AND OLDER: 4 g/0.5 g q8h or 3 g/0.375 g q6h. **Maximum:** 18 g/2.25 g daily.

MODERATE INFECTIONS

IV: ADULTS, ELDERLY, CHILDREN 12 YRS AND OLDER: 2 g/0.25g q6–8h.

DOSAGE IN RENAL IMPAIRMENT

Dosage and frequency are modified based on creatinine clearance.

Creatinine Clearance	Dosage
20–40 ml/min	8 g/1 g/day (2.25 g q6h)
Less than 20 ml/min	6 g/0.75 g/day (2.25 g q8h)

DOSAGE FOR HEMODIALYSIS

IV: ADULTS, ELDERLY: 2.25 g q8h with additional dose of 0.75 g after each dialysis session.

SIDE EFFECTS

FREQUENT: Diarrhea, headache, constipation, nausea, insomnia, rash. **OCCASIONAL:** Vomiting, dyspepsia (heartburn, indigestion, epigastric pain), pruritus, fever, agitation, candidiasis, dizziness, abdominal pain, edema, anxiety, dyspnea, rhinitis.

P

ADVERSE EFFECTS/ TOXIC REACTIONS

Antibiotic-associated colitis (severe abdominal pain, fever, severe watery diarrhea) may result from altered bacterial balance. Overdose, more often with renal impairment, may produce seizures, neurologic reactions. Severe hypersensitivity reactions, including anaphylaxis, occur rarely.

NURSING CONSIDERATIONS

BASELINE ASSESSMENT

Question for history of allergies, esp. to penicillins, cephalosporins.

INTERVENTION/EVALUATION

Monitor daily pattern of bowel activity/ stool consistency; mild GI effects may be tolerable, but increasing severity may indicate onset of antibiotic-associated colitis. Be alert for superinfection (severe genital/anal pruritus, abdominal pain, stomatitis, moderate to severe diarrhea). Monitor I&O, urinalysis. Monitor serum electrolytes, esp. potassium, renal function tests.

P

piroxicam

peer-**ox**-i-kam
(Apo-Piroxicam ✱, Feldene, Fexicam ✱, Novopirocam ✱)

Do not confuse Feldene with Seldane.

CLASSIFICATION

PHARMACOTHERAPEUTIC: Nonsteroidal anti-inflammatory. **CLINICAL:** Anti-inflammatory, analgesic (see p. 125C).

ACTION

Produces analgesic, anti-inflammatory effects by inhibiting prostaglandin synthesis. **Therapeutic Effect:** Reduces inflammatory response, intensity of pain.

PHARMACOKINETICS

Well absorbed following PO administration. Protein binding: 99%. Extensively metabolized in liver. Primarily excreted in urine; small amount eliminated in feces. **Half-life:** 50 hrs.

USES

Symptomatic treatment of acute or chronic rheumatoid arthritis, osteoarthritis. **OFF-LABEL:** Treatment of acute gouty arthritis, ankylosing spondylitis, dysmenorrhea.

PRECAUTIONS

CONTRAINDICATIONS: Active peptic ulcer disease, chronic inflammation of GI tract, GI bleeding/ulceration, history of hypersensitivity to aspirin/NSAIDs. **CAUTIONS:** Renal/cardiac impairment, hypertension, GI disease, concomitant use of anticoagulants.

LIFESPAN CONSIDERATIONS:

Pregnancy/Lactation: Crosses placenta; distributed in breast milk. Avoid use during third trimester (may adversely affect fetal cardiovascular system: premature closing of ductus arteriosus). **Pregnancy Category C (D if used in third trimester or near delivery). Children:** Safety and efficacy not established. **Elderly:** Age-related renal impairment may increase risk of hepatotoxicity, renal toxicity; reduced dosage recommended. More likely to have serious adverse effects with GI bleeding/ulceration.

INTERACTIONS

DRUG: May decrease effects of **antihypertensives, diuretics**. **Aspirin, other salicylates** may increase risk of GI side effects, bleeding. **Bone marrow depressants** may increase risk of hematologic reactions. May increase effects of **heparin, oral anticoagulants, thrombolytics**. May increase concentration, risk of toxicity of **lithium**. May increase risk of **methotrexate** toxicity. **Probenecid** may increase concentration. **HERBAL: Cat's claw, dong quai, evening primrose, feverfew, garlic, ginger, ginkgo, red clover, horse chestnut, ginseng** possess antiplatelet activity, may increase risk of bleeding. **St. John's wort** may increase risk of phototoxicity. **FOOD:** None known. **LAB VALUES:** May increase AST, ALT. May decrease serum uric acid.

AVAILABILITY (Rx)

CAPSULES: 10 mg, 20 mg.

ADMINISTRATION/HANDLING

PO

• Do not crush/break capsules. • May give with food, milk, antacids if GI distress occurs.

INDICATIONS/ROUTES/DOSAGE

RHEUMATOID ARTHRITIS, OSTEOARTHRITIS

PO: ADULTS, ELDERLY: Initially, 10–20 mg/day as a single dose or in divided doses. Some pts may require up to 30–40 mg/day. **CHILDREN:** 0.2–0.3 mg/kg/day. **Maximum:** 15 mg/day.

SIDE EFFECTS

FREQUENT (9%–4%): Dyspepsia (heartburn, indigestion, epigastric pain), nausea, dizziness. **OCCASIONAL (3%–1%):** Diarrhea, constipation, abdominal cramps/pain, flatulence, stomatitis. **RARE (less than 1%):** Hypertension, urticaria, dysuria, ecchymosis, blurred vision, insomnia, phototoxicity.

ADVERSE EFFECTS/ TOXIC REACTIONS

Peptic ulcer, GI bleeding, gastritis, severe hepatic reaction (cholestasis, jaundice) occur rarely. Nephrotoxicity (dysuria, hematuria, proteinuria, nephrotic syndrome), hematologic toxicity (anemia, leukopenia, eosinophilia, thrombocytopenia), severe hypersensitivity reaction (fever, chills, bronchospasm) occur rarely with long-term treatment.

NURSING CONSIDERATIONS

BASELINE ASSESSMENT

Assess onset, type, location, duration of pain/inflammation. Inspect appearance of affected joints for immobility, deformities, skin condition.

INTERVENTION/EVALUATION

Monitor daily pattern of bowel activity/stool consistency. Monitor for evidence of nausea, GI distress. Evaluate for therapeutic response (relief of pain, stiffness, swelling; increased joint mobility; reduced joint tenderness; improved grip strength). Monitor CBC, renal/hepatic function tests.

PATIENT/FAMILY TEACHING

• Avoid aspirin, alcohol during therapy (increases risk of GI bleeding). • If GI upset occurs, take with food, milk, antacids. • Avoid tasks that require alertness until response to drug is established.

P

Pitocin, *see oxytocin*

Plavix, *see clopidogrel*

Plenaxis, *see abarelix*

Plendil, *see felodipine*

polycarbophil

polly-**car**-bow-fill
(Fibercon, Replens ✤)

CLASSIFICATION

CLINICAL: Bulk-forming laxative, antidiarrheal.

ACTION

Laxative: Retains water in intestine, opposes dehydrating forces of bowel. **Therapeutic Effect:** Promotes well-formed stools. **Antidiarrheal:** Absorbs fecal-free water, restores normal moisture level, provides bulk. **Therapeutic Effect:** Forms gel, produces formed stool.

PHARMACOKINETICS

Route	Onset	Peak	Duration
PO	12–72 hrs	N/A	N/A

Polycarbophil is not absorbed following oral administration. Acts in small, large intestines.

USES

Treatment of diarrhea associated with irritable bowel syndrome (IBS), diverticulosis, acute nonspecific diarrhea. Relieves constipation associated with irritable, spastic bowel.

PRECAUTIONS

CONTRAINDICATIONS: Abdominal pain, dysphagia, fecal impaction, nausea, partial bowel obstruction, symptoms of appendicitis, vomiting. **CAUTIONS:** None known.

LIFESPAN CONSIDERATIONS:

Pregnancy/Lactation: Safe for use in pregnancy. **Pregnancy Category C. Children:** Not recommended in those younger than 6 yrs. **Elderly:** No age-related precautions noted.

INTERACTIONS

DRUG: May decrease absorption of **tetracyclines. HERBAL:** None significant. **FOOD:** None known. **LAB VALUES:** May increase serum glucose. May decrease serum potassium.

AVAILABILITY (OTC)

TABLETS: 500 mg, 625 mg. **TABLETS (CHEWABLE):** 500 mg.

INDICATIONS/ROUTES/DOSAGE

CONSTIPATION, DIARRHEA

PO: ADULTS, ELDERLY, CHILDREN 12 YRS AND OLDER: 1 g 1–4 times a day, or as needed. **Maximum:** 4 g/24 hrs. **CHILDREN 6–11 YRS:** 500 mg 1–4 times a day, or as needed. **Maximum:** 2 g/24 hrs. **CHILDREN YOUNGER THAN 6 YRS:** Consult product labeling.

SIDE EFFECTS

OCCASIONAL: Epigastric fullness, flatulence. **RARE:** Some degree of abdominal discomfort, nausea, mild cramps, griping, syncope/near syncope.

ADVERSE EFFECTS/ TOXIC REACTIONS

Esophageal, bowel obstruction may occur if administered with insufficient liquid (less than 250 ml or 1 full glass).

NURSING CONSIDERATIONS

INTERVENTION/EVALUATION

Encourage adequate fluid intake. Assess bowel sounds for peristalsis. Monitor daily pattern of bowel activity/stool consistency, record time of evacuation. Monitor serum electrolytes in those exposed to prolonged, frequent, excessive use of medication.

PATIENT/FAMILY TEACHING

• Institute measures to promote defecation (increase fluid intake, exercise, high-fiber diet). • Drink 6–8 glasses of water a day when used as laxative (aids stool softening).

polyethylene glycol-electrolyte solution (PEG-ES)

poly-**eth**-ah-leen

(CoLyte, CoLyte 4 Flavor, CoLyte Flavored, GlycoLax, GoLYTELY, Klean-Prep ✤, MiraLax, NuLytely, NuLytely Cherry, NuLytely Lemon Lime, NuLytely Orange, Peglyte ✤, Pro-Lax ✤, TriLyte)

CLASSIFICATION

PHARMACOTHERAPEUTIC: Laxative. **CLINICAL:** Bowel evacuant (see p. 118C).

ACTION

Osmotic effect. **Therapeutic Effect:** Induces diarrhea, cleanses bowel without depleting electrolytes.

PHARMACOKINETICS

Route	Onset	Peak	Duration
PO (Bowel cleansing)	1–2 hrs	N/A	N/A
PO (Constipation)	2–4 days	N/A	N/A

USES

Bowel cleansing before GI examination, colon surgery. **MiraLax:** Treatment of occasional constipation.

PRECAUTIONS

CONTRAINDICATIONS: Bowel perforation, gastric retention, GI obstruction, megacolon, toxic colitis, toxic ileus. **CAUTIONS:** Ulcerative colitis.

LIFESPAN CONSIDERATIONS:

Pregnancy/Lactation: Unknown if drug crosses placenta or is distributed in breast milk. **Pregnancy Category C.** **Children/Elderly:** No age-related precautions noted.

INTERACTIONS

DRUG: May decrease absorption of **oral medications** if given within 1 hr (may be flushed from GI tract). **HERBAL:** None significant. **FOOD:** None known. **LAB VALUES:** None known.

AVAILABILITY (Rx)

POWDER FOR RECONSTITUTION: (CoLyte, CoLyte Flavored, Colyte 4 Flavor, GlycoLax, GoLytely, MiraLax, NuLytely, NuLytely Cherry, NuLytely Lemon Lime, NuLytely Orange, TriLyte).

ADMINISTRATION/HANDLING

PO

• Refrigerate reconstituted solutions; use within 48 hrs. • May use tap water to prepare solution. Shake vigorously for several min to ensure complete dissolution of powder. • Fasting should occur for more than 3 hrs prior to ingestion of solution (always avoid solid food less than 2 hrs prior to administration). • Only clear liquids permitted after administration. • May give via NG tube. • Rapid drinking preferred. Chilled solution is more palatable.

INDICATIONS/ROUTES/DOSAGE

BOWEL EVACUANT

PO: ADULTS, ELDERLY: Before GI examination: 240 ml (8 oz) q10min until 4 liters consumed or rectal effluent clear. NG tube: 20–30 ml/min until 4 liters given. **CHILDREN:** 25–40 ml/kg/hr until rectal effluent clear.

CONSTIPATION

PO (MIRALAX): ADULTS: 17 g or 1 heaping tbsp a day.

SIDE EFFECTS

FREQUENT (50%): Some degree of abdominal fullness, nausea, bloating. **OCCASIONAL (10%–1%):** Abdominal cramping, vomiting, anal irritation. **RARE (less than 1%):** Urticaria, rhinorrhea, dermatitis.

ADVERSE EFFECTS/ TOXIC REACTIONS

None known.

NURSING CONSIDERATIONS

BASELINE ASSESSMENT

Do not give oral medication within 1 hr of start of therapy (may not adequately be absorbed before GI cleansing).

INTERVENTION/EVALUATION

Assess bowel sounds for peristalsis. Monitor daily pattern of bowel activity/ stool consistency; record time of evacuation. Assess for abdominal disturbances. Monitor serum electrolytes, BUN, glucose, urine osmolality.

poly-L-lactic acid

polly-el-**lack**-tic
(Sculptra)

CLASSIFICATION

PHARMACOTHERAPEUTIC: Physical adjunct. **CLINICAL:** Lipoatrophy agent.

ACTION

Contains microparticles of synthetic polymer used as injectable implant. **Therapeutic Effect:** Restores facial fat.

PHARMACOKINETICS

Biodegradable, biocompatible synthetic polymer.

USES

Treatment for restoration/correction of facial lipoatropy in pts with HIV.

PRECAUTIONS

CONTRAINDICATIONS: None known. **CAUTIONS:** Tendency to keloid for-mation.

LIFESPAN CONSIDERATIONS:

Pregnancy/Lactation: Safety and efficacy not established. **Pregnancy Category not established. Children:** Safety and efficacy not established in children younger than 18 yrs. **Elderly:** No age-related precautions noted.

INTERACTIONS

DRUG: None significant. **HERBAL:** None significant. **FOOD:** None known. **LAB VALUES:** None known.

AVAILABILITY (Rx)

INJECTION, POWDER FOR RECONSTITUTION (FREEZE-DRIED): Each carton contains 2 vials.

ADMINISTRATION/HANDLING

IV INFUSION

Reconstitution • Draw 3–5 ml Sterile Water for Injection. • Using 18-gauge sterile needle, slowly add all Sterile Water for Injection into vial. • Let vial stand for at least 2 hrs; do not shake during this period. • After 2 hrs, agitate vial until uniform translucent suspension is obtained. • Withdraw amount of suspension (usually 1 ml) into syringe using new, 18-gauge needle and replace with 26-gauge needle before injecting product into deep dermis or subcutaneous layer.

Storage • Store at room temperature. • Reconstituted product is stable for up to 72 hrs at room temperature.

INDICATIONS/ROUTES/DOSAGE

FACIAL LIPOATROPHY

SUBCUTANEOUS: ADULTS, ELDERLY: For severe facial fat loss, one vial usually injected into multiple points of each cheek during each injection session. Volume of drug for each injection and number of injection sessions depend on severity of condition. Typically, 3–6 injection sessions, separated by intervals of at least 2 wks, are required.

SIDE EFFECTS

FREQUENT: Ecchymosis. **OCCASIONAL:** Discomfort, edema. **RARE:** Erythema.

ADVERSE EFFECTS/ TOXIC REACTIONS

Subcutaneous papules at injection sites, hematoma occur occasionally.

NURSING CONSIDERATIONS

BASELINE ASSESSMENT

Defer use if skin inflammation/infection occurs in or near treatment area until inflammatory/infectious process has been controlled.

INTERVENTION/EVALUATION

Apply ice packs to treatment area to reduce inflammation. Treatment area should be massaged daily for several days following injection session.

PATIENT/FAMILY TEACHING

• Potential for redness, swelling, bruising typically resolves in hours to 1 wk. • Full therapeutic effect noted in wks to mos. • Avoid excessive sunlight, UV lamp exposure until initial swelling, redness has resolved.

poractant alfa

poor-**ak**-tant
(Curosurf)

CLASSIFICATION

CLINICAL: Pulmonary surfactant.

ACTION

Reduces alveolar surface tension during ventilation; stabilizes alveoli against collapse that may occur at resting transpulmonary pressures. **Therapeutic Effect:** Improves lung compliance, respiratory gas exchange.

PHARMACOKINETICS

Not fully understood.

USES

Rescue treatment for respiratory distress syndrome (RDS—hyaline membrane disease) in premature infants. **OFF-LABEL:** Adult RDS due to viral pneumonia or near-drowning, *Pneumocystis carinii* pneumonia in HIV-infected pts, prophylaxis of RDS.

PRECAUTIONS

CONTRAINDICATIONS: None known. **CAUTIONS:** Pts at risk for circulatory overload. Acidosis, hypotension, anemia, hypoglycemia, hypothermia should be corrected prior to administration.

⌛ LIFESPAN CONSIDERATIONS:

Neonate: No age-related precautions noted for neonate. **Pregnancy Category:** This drug is not indicated for use in pregnant women.

INTERACTIONS

DRUG: None significant. **HERBAL:** None significant. **FOOD:** None known. **LAB VALUES:** None known.

AVAILABILITY (Rx)

INTRATRACHEAL SUSPENSION: 1.5 ml (120 mg), 3 ml (240 mg).

ADMINISTRATION/HANDLING

INTRATRACHEAL

Administration • Attach syringe to catheter and instill through catheter inserted into infant's endotracheal tube. • Monitor for bradycardia, decreased O_2 saturation during administration. Stop dosing procedure if these effects occur; begin appropriate measures before reinstituting therapy.

Storage • Refrigerate vials. • Warm by standing vial at room temperature for 20 min or warm in hand 8 min. • To obtain uniform suspension, turn upside down gently, swirl vial (do not

P

shake). • After warming, may return to refrigerator one time only. • Withdraw entire contents of vial into 3- or 5-ml plastic syringe through large-gauge needle (20 gauge or larger).

INDICATIONS/ROUTE/DOSAGE

RDS

INTRATRACHEAL: INFANTS: Initially, 2.5 ml/kg of birth weight. May give up to 2 subsequent doses of 1.25 ml/kg of birth weight at 12-hr intervals. **Maximum:** 5 ml/kg (total dose).

SIDE EFFECTS

FREQUENT: Transient bradycardia, oxygen (O_2) desaturation, increased carbon dioxide (CO_2) retention. **OCCASIONAL:** Endotracheal tube reflux. **RARE:** Hypotension, hypertension, apnea, pallor, vasoconstriction.

ADVERSE EFFECTS/ TOXIC REACTIONS

None known.

NURSING CONSIDERATIONS

BASELINE ASSESSMENT

Immediately before administration, change ventilator setting to 40–60 breaths/min, inspiratory time 0.5 sec, supplemental O_2 sufficient to maintain SaO_2 over 92%. Drug must be administered in highly supervised setting. Clinicians caring for neonate must be experienced with intubation, ventilator management. Offer emotional support to parents.

INTERVENTION/EVALUATION

Monitor infant with arterial or transcutaneous measurement of systemic O_2 and CO_2. Assess lung sounds for rales, moist breath sounds. Monitor heart rate.

porfimer

(Photofrin)

See Cancer chemotherapeutic agents

posaconazole

pose-ah-**con**-ah-zole

(Noxafil)

Do not confuse Noxafil with minoxidil.

CLASSIFICATION

PHARMACOTHERAPEUTIC: Azole derivative. **CLINICAL:** Antifungal.

ACTION

Inhibits synthesis of ergosterol, a vital component of fungal cell wall formation. **Therapeutic Effect:** Damages fungal cell wall membrane, altering its function.

PHARMACOKINETICS

Moderately absorbed following PO administration. Absorption increased if drug is taken with food. Widely distributed. Protein binding: 98%. Metabolized in liver. Primarily excreted in feces. **Half-life:** 35 hrs.

USES

Prophylaxis of invasive *Aspergillosis* and *Candida* infections in pts 13 yrs and older who are at high risk for developing these infections due to severely immunocompromised conditions. Treatment of oropharyngeal candidiasis. **OFF-LABEL:** Salvage therapy of refractory invasive fungal infections.

PRECAUTIONS

CONTRAINDICATIONS: Coadministration with pimozide, quinidine, terfenadine, astemizole, cisapride, halofantrine, ergot alkaloids (may cause QT prolongation, torsades de pointes). **CAUTIONS:** Renal/hepatic impairment, hypersensitivity to other antifungal agents.

LIFESPAN CONSIDERATIONS:

Pregnancy/Lactation: May cause fetal harm. Avoid breast-feeding. **Pregnancy Category C.** **Children:** Safety and efficacy not established in those younger than 13 yrs. **Elderly:** No age-related precautions noted.

INTERACTIONS

DRUG: May increase concentrations of **astemizole, atorvastatin, cisapride, ergot alkaloids, felodipine, halofantrine, midazolam, phenytoin, pimozide, quinidine, rifabutin, sirolimus, tacrilimus, terfenadine, vincristine, vinblastine. Cimetidine, phenytoin** may decrease concentration. **HERBAL:** None significant. **FOOD:** Concentration higher when given with **food** or **nutritional supplements**. **LAB VALUES:** May decrease WBC, RBC, Hgb, Hct, platelets, serum calcium, potassium, magnesium. May increase serum glucose, bilirubin, ALT, AST, alkaline phosphatase.

AVAILABILITY (Rx)

SUSPENSION, ORAL: 40 mg/ml.

ADMINISTRATION/HANDLING

PO • Administer with full meal or liquid nutritional supplement (enhances absorption). • Store oral suspension at room temperature. • Shake suspension well before use.

INDICATIONS/ROUTES/DOSAGE

FUNGAL INFECTIONS:

PO: ADULTS, ELDERLY: 200 mg (5 ml) three times daily, given with full meal or liquid nutritional supplement.

SIDE EFFECTS

COMMON (42%–24%): Diarrhea, nausea, vomiting, headache, abdominal pain, cough. **FREQUENT (20%–15%):** Constipation, rigors, rash, hypertension, fatigue, insomnia, mucositis, musculoskeletal pain, edema of lower extremities, herpes simplex, anorexia. **OCCASIONAL (14%–8%):** Hypotension, epistaxis, tachycardia, pharyngitis, dizziness, pruritus, arthralgia, dyspepsia (heartburn, indigestion, epigastric pain), back pain, generalized edema, weakness.

ADVERSE EFFECTS/ TOXIC REACTIONS

Bacteremia occurs in 18% of pts; upper respiratory tract infection occurs in 7%. Allergic/hypersensitivity reactions, QT prolongation, hemolytic uremic syndrome, thrombotic thrombocytopenic purpura, pulmonary embolus have been reported.

NURSING CONSIDERATIONS

BASELINE ASSESSMENT

Obtain baselines for hepatic enzyme serum levels, CBC, serum chemistries prior to therapy.

INTERVENTION/EVALUATION

Hepatic function tests should be monitored periodically. Monitor daily pattern of bowel activity/stool consistency. Obtain order for antiemetic if excessive vomiting occurs. Monitor B/P for hypertension, hypotension. Assess for lower extremity edema (first sign of edema appears behind medial malleolus).

PATIENT/FAMILY TEACHING

Take each dose with full meal or liquid nutritional supplement. Report severe diarrhea, vomiting. Maintain fastidious oral hygiene.

P

potassium acetate

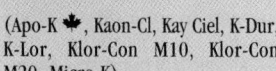

potassium bicarbonate/citrate

(Effer K, Klor-Con EF, K-Lyte, K-Lyte DS)

potassium chloride

(Apo-K ✤, Kaon-Cl, Kay Ciel, K-Dur, K-Lor, Klor-Con M10, Klor-Con M20, Micro-K)

potassium gluconate

(Glu-K)

poe-**tah**-see-um

Do not confuse K-dur with Cardura.

CLASSIFICATION

PHARMACOTHERAPEUTIC: Electrolyte. **CLINICAL:** Potassium replenisher.

ACTION

Necessary for multiple cellular metabolic processes. Primary action is intracellular. **Therapeutic Effect:** Required for nerve impulse conduction, contraction of cardiac, skeletal, smooth muscle; maintains normal renal function, acid-base balance.

PHARMACOKINETICS

Well absorbed from GI tract. Enters cells by active transport from extracellular fluid. Primarily excreted in urine.

USES

Treatment of potassium deficiency found in severe vomiting, diarrhea, loss of GI fluid, malnutrition, prolonged diuresis, debilitated, poor GI absorption, metabolic alkalosis, prolonged parenteral alimentation. Prevention of hypokalemia in at-risk pts.

PRECAUTIONS

CONTRAINDICATIONS: Concurrent use of potassium-sparing diuretics, digitalis toxicity, heat cramps, hyperkalemia, postop oliguria, severe burns, severe renal impairment, shock with dehydration or hemolytic reaction, untreated Addison's disease. **CAUTIONS:** Cardiac disease, tartrazine sensitivity (mostly noted in those with aspirin hypersensitivity).

LIFESPAN CONSIDERATIONS:

Pregnancy/Lactation: Unknown if drug crosses placenta or is distributed in breast milk. **Pregnancy Category C (A for potassium chloride). Children:** No age-related precautions noted. **Elderly:** May be at increased risk for hyperkalemia. Age-related ability to excrete potassium is reduced.

INTERACTIONS

DRUG: **Angiotensin-converting enzyme (ACE) inhibitors, beta-adrenergic blockers, heparin, NSAIDs, potassium-containing medications, potassium-sparing diuretics, salt substitutes** may increase serum potassium concentration. **Anticholinergics** may increase risk of GI lesions. **HERBAL:** None significant. **FOOD:** None known. **LAB VALUES:** None known.

AVAILABILITY (Rx)

POTASSIUM ACETATE

INJECTION, SOLUTION: 2 mEq/ml.

POTASSIUM BICARBONATE AND POTASSIUM CITRATE

TABLETS FOR SOLUTION: 25 mEq (Klor-Con EF, Effer-K, K-Lyte), 50 mEq (K-Lyte DS).

POTASSIUM CHLORIDE
INJECTION, SOLUTION: 2 mEq/ml. **ORAL SOLUTION: (KAON-CL, KAY CIEL):** 20 mEq/15 ml. **POWDER FOR ORAL SOLUTION (K-LOR, KLOR-CON):** 20 mEq/packet.

CAPSULES, EXTENDED-RELEASE (MICRO-K): 8 mEq, 10 mEq. **TABLETS EXTENDED-RELEASE: (K-DUR):** 10 mEq, 20 mEq. **(K-TAB, KLOR-CON 10, KLOR-CON M 10):** 10 mEq. **(KLOR-CON M 20):** 20 mEq.

POTASSIUM GLUCONATE
TABLETS (GLU-K): 500 mg, 610 mg.

ADMINISTRATION/HANDLING

IV

Reconstitution • For IV infusion only, must dilute before administration, mix well, infuse slowly. • Avoid adding potassium to hanging IV.

Rate of administration • Routinely, give at concentration of no more than 40 mEq/L, no faster than 20 mEq/hr. (Higher concentrations or faster rates may sometimes be necessary.) • Check IV site closely during infusion for evidence of phlebitis (heat, pain, red streaking of skin over vein, hardness to vein), extravasation (swelling, pain, cool skin, little/no blood return).

Storage • Store at room temperature.

PO

• Take with or after meals, with full glass of water (decreases GI upset). • Liquids, powder, effervescent tablets: Mix, dissolve with juice, water before administering. • Do not chew, crush tablets; swallow whole.

IV INCOMPATIBILITIES

Amphotericin B complex (Abelcet, AmBisome, Amphotec), methylprednisolone (Solu-Medrol), phenytoin (Dilantin).

IV COMPATIBILITIES

Aminophylline, amiodarone (Cordarone), atropine, aztreonam (Azactam), calcium gluconate, cefepime (Maxipime), ciprofloxacin (Cipro), clindamycin (Cleocin), dexamethasone (Decadron), digoxin (Lanoxin), diltiazem (Cardizem), diphenhydramine (Benadryl), dobutamine (Dobutrex), dopamine (Intropin), enalapril (Vasotec), famotidine (Pepcid), fluconazole (Diflucan), furosemide (Lasix), granisetron (Kytril), heparin, hydrocortisone (Solu-Cortef), insulin, lidocaine, lipids, lorazepam (Ativan), magnesium sulfate, methylprednisolone (Solu-Medrol), metoclopramide (Reglan), midazolam (Versed), milrinone (Primacor), morphine, norepinephrine (Levophed), ondansetron (Zofran), oxytocin (Pitocin), piperacillin and tazobactam (Zosyn), procainamide (Pronestyl), propofol (Diprivan), propranolol (Inderal).

INDICATIONS/ROUTES/DOSAGE

PREVENTION OF HYPOKALEMIA WITH DIURETIC THERAPY

PO: ADULTS, ELDERLY: 20–40 mEq/day in 1–2 divided doses. **CHILDREN:** 1–2 mEq/kg/day in 1–2 divided doses.

TREATMENT OF HYPOKALEMIA

PO: ADULTS, ELDERLY: 40–80 mEq/day; further doses based on laboratory values. **CHILDREN:** 2–5 mEq/day; further doses based on laboratory values.

IV: ADULTS, ELDERLY: 5–10 mEq/hr. **Maximum:** 400 mEq/day. **CHILDREN:** 1 mEq/kg over 1–2 hrs.

SIDE EFFECTS

OCCASIONAL: Nausea, vomiting, diarrhea, flatulence, abdominal discomfort with distention, phlebitis with IV administration (particularly when potassium concentration of greater than 40 mEq/L is infused). **RARE:** Rash.

ADVERSE EFFECTS/ TOXIC REACTIONS

Hyperkalemia (more common in elderly, those with renal impairment) manifested as paresthesia, feeling of heaviness in lower extremities, cold skin, grayish

P

pallor, hypotension, confusion, irritability, flaccid paralysis, cardiac arrhythmias.

NURSING CONSIDERATIONS

BASELINE ASSESSMENT

PO should be given with food or after meals with full glass of water, fruit juice (minimizes GI irritation).

INTERVENTION/EVALUATION

Monitor serum potassium (particularly in renal impairment). If GI disturbance is noted, dilute preparation further or give with meals. Be alert to decreased urinary output (may be indication of renal insufficiency). Monitor daily pattern of bowel activity/stool consistency. Assess I&O diligently during diuresis, IV site for extravasation, phlebitis. Be alert to evidence of hyperkalemia (skin pallor/coldness, complaints of paresthesia, feeling of heaviness of lower extremities).

PATIENT/FAMILY TEACHING

• Foods rich in potassium include beef, veal, ham, chicken, turkey, fish, milk, bananas, dates, prunes, raisins, avocados, watermelon, cantaloupe, apricots, molasses, beans, yams, broccoli, Brussels sprouts, lentils, potatoes, spinach. • Report paresthesia, feeling of heaviness of lower extremities.

P

pramipexole

pram-eh-**pex**-ol

(Mirapex)

Do not confuse Mirapex with Mifeprex or MiraLax.

CLASSIFICATION

PHARMACOTHERAPEUTIC: Dopamine receptor agonist. **CLINICAL:** Antiparkinson agent.

ACTION

Stimulates dopamine receptors in striatum. **Therapeutic Effect:** Relieves signs/symptoms of Parkinson's disease.

PHARMACOKINETICS

Rapidly, extensively absorbed after PO administration. Protein binding: 15%. Widely distributed. Steady-state concentrations achieved within 2 days. Primarily eliminated in urine. Not removed by hemodialysis. **Half-life:** 8 hrs (12 hrs in pts older than 65 yrs).

USES

Treatment of signs/symptoms of idiopathic Parkinson's disease, restless legs syndrome. **OFF-LABEL:** Depression (due to bipolar disorder), fibromyalgia.

PRECAUTIONS

CONTRAINDICATIONS: History of hypersensitivity to pramipexole. **CAUTIONS:** History of orthostatic hypotension, syncope, hallucinations, renal impairment, concomitant use of CNS depressants.

LIFESPAN CONSIDERATIONS:

Pregnancy/Lactation: Unknown if drug is distributed in breast milk. **Pregnancy Category C. Children:** Safety and efficacy not established. **Elderly:** Increased risk of hallucinations.

INTERACTIONS

DRUG: May increase plasma concentrations of **carbidopa, levodopa. Cimetidine** increases plasma concentration, half-life. **Diltiazem, quinidine, quinine, ranitidine, triamterene, verapamil** may decrease clearance. **HERBAL: Kava kava, SAMe, gotu kola, St. John's wort, valerian** may increase CNS depression. **FOOD: All foods** delay peak drug plasma levels by 1 hr (extent of absorption not affected). **LAB VALUES:** None known.

AVAILABILITY (Rx)

TABLETS: 0.125 mg, 0.25 mg, 0.5 mg, 1 mg, 1.5 mg.

ADMINISTRATION/HANDLING

PO

- Give without regard to food.

INDICATIONS/ROUTES/DOSAGE

PARKINSON'S DISEASE

PO: ADULTS, ELDERLY: Initially, 0.375 mg/day in 3 divided doses. Do not increase dosage more frequently than every 5–7 days. Maintenance: 1.5–4.5 mg/day in 3 equally divided doses.

DOSAGE IN RENAL IMPAIRMENT

Dosage and frequency are modified based on creatinine clearance.

Creatinine Clearance	Initial Dose	Maximum Dose
Greater than 60 ml/min	0.125 mg 3 times a day	1.5 mg 3 times a day
35–60 ml/min	0.125 mg twice a day	1.5 mg twice a day
15–34 ml/min	0.125 mg once a day	1.5 mg once a day

RESTLESS LEG SYNDROME

PO: ADULTS, ELDERLY: Initially, 0.125 mg once daily 2–3 hrs before bedtime. May increase to 0.25 mg after 4–7 days, then to 0.5 mg after 4–7 days (interval is 14 days in pts with renal impairment).

SIDE EFFECTS

FREQUENT: Early Parkinson's disease (28%–10%): Nausea, asthenia (loss of strength, energy), dizziness, somnolence, insomnia, constipation. **Advanced Parkinson's disease (53%–17%):** Orthostatic hypotension, extrapyramidal reactions, insomnia, dizziness, hallucinations. **OCCASIONAL: Early Parkinson's disease (5%–2%):** Edema, malaise, confusion, amnesia, akathisia, anorexia, dysphagia, peripheral edema, vision changes, impotence. **Advanced Parkinson's disease (10%–7%):** Asthenia, drowsiness, confusion, constipation, abnormal gait, dry mouth. **RARE: Advanced Parkinson's disease (6%–2%):** General edema, malaise, angina, amnesia, tremor, urinary frequency/incontinence, dyspnea, rhinitis, vision changes.

ADVERSE EFFECTS/ TOXIC REACTIONS

Vascular disease, atrial fibrillation, arrhythmias, pulmonary embolism have been reported.

NURSING CONSIDERATIONS

INTERVENTION/EVALUATION

Instruct pt to rise from lying to sitting or sitting to standing position slowly to prevent risk of postural hypotension. Assess for clinical improvement. Assist with ambulation if dizziness occurs. Assess for constipation; encourage fiber, fluids, exercise.

PATIENT/FAMILY TEACHING

- Inform pt that hallucinations may occur, esp. in the elderly. • Postural hypotension may occur more frequently during initial therapy. • Avoid tasks that require alertness, motor skills until response to drug is established. • If nausea occurs, take medication with food. • Avoid abrupt withdrawal.

P

pramlintide

pram-lin-tide
(Symlin)

CLASSIFICATION

PHARMACOTHERAPEUTIC: Antihyperglycemic. **CLINICAL:** Antidiabetic.

ACTION

Co-secreted with insulin by pancreatic beta cells, reduces postprandial glucose increases by slowing, gastric emptying time, reducing postprandial glucagon secretion, reducing caloric intake through centrally mediated appetite suppression. **Therapeutic Effect:** Improves glycemic control by reducing postprandial glucose concentrations in pts with type 1, type 2 diabetes mellitus.

PHARMACOKINETICS

	Onset	Peak	Duration
Subcutaneous	NA	20 min	3 hrs

Metabolized primarily by kidneys. Protein binding: 60%. Excreted in urine. **Half-life:** 48 min.

USES

Adjunctive treatment with mealtime insulin in type 1, type 2 diabetes mellitus pts who have failed to achieve desired glucose control despite optimal insulin therapy, with/without concurrent sulfonylurea and/or metformin in type 2 diabetes mellitus.

PRECAUTIONS

CONTRAINDICATIONS: Diagnosed gastroparesis, presence of hypoglycemia or recurrent severe hypoglycemic episodes in the past 6 mos, poor compliance with insulin monitoring or current insulin therapy, those with hemoglobin A_{1c} greater than 9%, pts with conditions or taking concurrent medications likely to impair gastric motility (e.g., anticholinergics), in pts requiring medication to stimulate gastric emptying. **CAUTIONS:** Coadministration with insulin may induce severe hypoglycemia (usually within 3 hrs following administration); concurrent use of other glucose-lowering agents may increase risk of hypoglycemia.

LIFESPAN CONSIDERATIONS:

Pregnancy/Lactation: Unknown if distributed in breast milk. **Pregnancy Category C. Children:** Safety and efficacy not established. **Elderly:** No age related precautions noted.

INTERACTIONS

DRUG: ACE inhibitors, fibrates, fluoxetine, MAOIs, salicylates, sulfonamide antibiotics may increase effect. **Anticholinergics** may cause additive impairment of gastric motility. **Beta-blockers, clonidine** may mask early symptoms of hypoglycemia. **HERBAL: Garlic** may increase hypoglycemia. **FOOD: Ethanol** increases risk of hypoglycemia. **LAB VALUES:** Decreases serum glucose.

AVAILABILITY (Rx)

INJECTION, SOLUTION: 0.6 mg/ml in 5 ml vials (Symlin).

ADMINISTRATION/HANDLING

SUBCUTANEOUS

• Administer immediately before each major meal (350 or more kcal or containing 30 g or more carbohydrate). • Give in abdomen or thigh; do not give in arm (variable absorption). • Injection site should be distinct from insulin injection site. • Rotation of injection sites is essential. • Use U-100 insulin syringe for accuracy. • Always give pramlintide and insulin as separate injections.

Storage • Store unopened vials in refrigerator. • Discard if freezing occurs. • Vials that have been opened (punctured) may be stored in refrigerator or kept at room temperature for up to 28 days.

INDICATIONS/ROUTES/DOSAGE

◀ **ALERT** ▶ Initially, current insulin dosage in all pts with type 1, type 2 diabetes mellitus should be reduced by 50%. This includes preprandial, rapid-acting, short-acting, fixed-mixed insulins.

TYPE 1 DIABETES MELLITUS

SUBCUTANEOUS: ADULTS, ELDERLY: Initially, 15 mcg immediately before major meal. Titrate in 15 mcg increments every 3 days (if no significant nausea occurs) to target dose of 30–60 mcg.

TYPE 2 DIABETES MELLITUS

SUBCUTANEOUS: ADULTS, ELDERLY: Initially, 60 mcg immediately before major meal. After 3–7 days, increase to 120 mcg if no significant nausea occurs (if nausea occurs at 120 mcg dose, reduce to 60 mcg).

SIDE EFFECTS

TYPE 1 DIABETES MELLITUS

FREQUENT (48%): Nausea. **OCCASIONAL (17%–11%):** Anorexia, vomiting. **RARE (7%–5%):** Fatigue, arthralgia, allergic reaction, dizziness.

TYPE 2 DIABETES MELLITUS

FREQUENT (28%): Nausea. **OCCASIONAL (13%–8%):** Headache, anorexia, vomiting, abdominal pain. **RARE (7%–5%):** Fatigue, dizziness, cough, pharyngitis.

ADVERSE EFFECTS/ TOXIC REACTIONS

Overdose produces severe nausea, vomiting, diarrhea, vasodilation, dizziness. No hypoglycemia was reported. Increased risk of severe hypoglycemia when given concurrently with nontitrated insulin.

NURSING CONSIDERATIONS

BASELINE ASSESSMENT

Check serum glucose concentration before administration, both before and after meals and at bedtime. Discuss lifestyle to determine extent of learning, emotional needs. Ensure follow-up instruction if pt, family does not thoroughly understand diabetes management, glucose testing technique.

INTERVENTION/EVALUATION

Risk for hypoglycemia occurs within first 3 hrs following drug administration if given concurrently with insulin. Assess for hypoglycemia (diaphoresis, tremors, dizziness, anxiety, headache, tachycardia, numbness in mouth, hunger, diplopia, difficulty concentrating). Be alert to conditions that alter glucose requirements (fever, increased activity, stress, surgical procedures).

PATIENT/FAMILY TEACHING

• Diabetes mellitus requires lifelong control. • Prescribed diet, exercise are principal part of treatment; do not skip/delay meals. • Continue to adhere to dietary instructions, regular exercise program, regular testing of serum glucose. • When taking combination drug therapy, have source of glucose available to treat symptoms of low blood sugar.

Prandin, *see repaglinide*

Pravachol, *see pravastatin*

pravastatin

pra-vah-sta-tin
(Pravachol)

Do not confuse pravastatin with Prevacid, or Pravachol with propranolol.

FIXED-COMBINATION(S)

Pravigard: pravastatin/aspirin (anticoagulant): 20 mg/81 mg; 40 mg/81 mg; 80 mg/81 mg; 20 mg/325 mg; 40 mg/325 mg; 80 mg/325 mg.

CLASSIFICATION

PHARMACOTHERAPEUTIC: Hydroxymethylglutaryl CoA (HMG-CoA) reductase inhibitor. **CLINICAL:** Antihyperlipidemic (see p. 56C).

ACTION

Interferes with cholesterol biosynthesis by preventing conversion of HMG-CoA reductase to mevalonate, a precursor to cholesterol. **Therapeutic Effect:** Lowers serum LDL, VLDL cholesterol, plasma triglycerides; increases serum HDL.

PHARMACOKINETICS

Poorly absorbed from GI tract. Protein binding: 50%. Metabolized in liver (minimal active metabolites). Primarily excreted in feces via biliary system. Not removed by hemodialysis. **Half-life:** 2.7 hrs.

USES

Treatment of hyperlipidemias to reduce total cholesterol, LDL cholesterol, apolipoprotein B, triglycerides; increase HDL cholestrol. Primary preventive therapy to reduce risk of recurrent MI, myocardial revascularization procedures, stroke, transient ischemic attack (TIA) in pts with previous MI and normal cholesterol levels. Secondary prevention of coronary events in pts with established coronary artery disease (CAD) to slow progression of coronary atherosclerosis. Treatment of heterozygous familial hypercholesterolemia in pediatric pts 8–18 yrs.

P

PRECAUTIONS

CONTRAINDICATIONS: Active hepatic disease or unexplained, persistent elevations of hepatic function test results. **CAUTIONS:** History of hepatic disease, substantial alcohol consumption. Withholding/discontinuing pravastatin may be necessary when pt is at risk for renal failure secondary to rhabdomyolysis. Severe metabolic, endocrine, electrolyte disorders.

LIFESPAN CONSIDERATIONS:

Pregnancy/Lactation: Contraindicated in pregnancy (suppression of cholesterol biosynthesis may cause fetal toxicity) and lactation. Unknown if drug is distributed in breast milk, but there is risk of serious adverse reactions in breast-feeding infants. **Pregnancy Category X. Children:** Safety and efficacy not established. **Elderly:** No age-related precautions noted.

INTERACTIONS

DRUG: Cyclosporine, erythromycin, gemfibrozil, immunosuppressants, niacin increase risk of acute renal failure, rhabdomyolysis. **HERBAL: St. John's wort** may decrease concentration. **FOOD:** None known. **LAB VALUES:** May increase serum creatine kinase (CK), transaminase.

AVAILABILITY (Rx)

TABLETS: 10 mg, 20 mg, 40 mg, 80 mg.

ADMINISTRATION/HANDLING

PO

- Give without regard to meals.
- Administer in evening.

INDICATIONS/ROUTES/DOSAGE

◀ **ALERT** ▶ Prior to initiating therapy, pt should be on standard cholesterol-lowering diet for 3–6 mos. Low-cholesterol diet should be continued throughout pravastatin therapy.

USUAL DOSAGE

PO: ADULTS, ELDERLY: Initially, 40 mg/day. Titrate to desired response. Range: 10–80 mg/day. **CHILDREN 14–18 YRS:** 40 mg/day. **CHILDREN 8–13 YRS:** 20 mg/day.

DOSAGE IN HEPATIC/RENAL IMPAIRMENT

For adults, give 10 mg/day initially. Titrate to desired response.

SIDE EFFECTS

Pravastatin is generally well tolerated. Side effects are usually mild and transient. **OCCASIONAL (7%–4%):** Nausea, vomiting, diarrhea, constipation, abdominal pain, headache, rhinitis, rash, pruritus. **RARE (3%–2%):** Heartburn, myalgia, dizziness, cough, fatigue, flu-like symptoms.

ADVERSE EFFECTS/ TOXIC REACTIONS

Potential for malignancy, cataracts. Hypersensitivity, myopathy occur rarely. Rhabdomyolysis has been reported.

NURSING CONSIDERATIONS

BASELINE ASSESSMENT

Question for possibility of pregnancy before initiating therapy (Pregnancy Category X). Assess baseline serum lab results (cholesterol, triglycerides, hepatic function tests).

INTERVENTION/EVALUATION

Monitor serum cholesterol, triglyceride lab results for therapeutic response. Monitor hepatic function tests. Monitor daily pattern of bowel activity/stool consistency. Check for headache, dizziness (provide assistance as needed). Assess for rash, pruritus. Be alert for malaise, muscle cramping/weakness; if accompanied by fever, may require discontinuation of medication.

PATIENT/FAMILY TEACHING

• Follow special diet (important part of treatment). • Periodic lab tests are essential part of therapy. • Report promptly any muscle pain/weakness, esp. if accompanied by fever, malaise. • Avoid tasks that require alertness, motor skills until response to drug is established (potential for dizziness). • Use nonhormonal contraception.

prazosin

pra-zoe-sin

(Apo-Prazo ✤, Minipress, Novo-Prazin ✤)

FIXED-COMBINATION(S)

Minizide: prazosin/polythiazide (a diuretic): 1 mg/0.5 mg; 2 mg/0.5 mg; 5 mg/0.5 mg.

◆CLASSIFICATION

PHARMACOTHERAPEUTIC: Alpha-adrenergic blocker. **CLINICAL:** Antihypertensive, antidote, vasodilator (see p. 59C).

ACTION

Selectively blocks alpha$_1$-adrenergic receptors, decreasing peripheral vascular resistance. **Therapeutic Effect:** Produces vasodilation of veins, arterioles; decreases total peripheral resistance; relaxes smooth muscle in bladder neck, prostate.

PHARMACOKINETICS

Well absorbed following PO administration. Protein binding: 92%–97%. Metabolized in liver. Primarily excreted in feces. **Half-life:** 2–4 hrs.

USES

Treatment of mild to moderate hypertension. Used alone or in combination with other antihypertensives. **OFF-LABEL:** Treatment of benign prostate hyperplasia, CHF, ergot alkaloid toxicity, pheochromocytoma, Raynaud's phenomenon.

PRECAUTIONS

CONTRAINDICATIONS: Hypersensitivity to quinazolines. **CAUTIONS:** Chronic renal failure, hepatic impairment.

⌛ LIFESPAN CONSIDERATIONS:

Pregnancy/Lactation: Unknown if drug crosses placenta; is distributed in breast milk. **Pregnancy Category C.** **Children:** Safety and efficacy not established. **Elderly:** May be more sensitive to hypotensive effects.

P

INTERACTIONS

DRUG: NSAIDs, other sympathomimetics may decrease effects. **Hypotension-producing medications, antihypertensives, diuretics** may increase effects. **HERBAL: Ephedra, yohimbe, ginseng** may worsen hypertension. Avoid **saw palmetto. Garlic** may increase antihypertensive effect. **Licorice** causes sodium and water retention, potassium loss. **FOOD:** None known. **LAB VALUES:** None known.

AVAILABILITY (Rx)

CAPSULES: 1 mg, 2 mg, 5 mg.

ADMINISTRATION/HANDLING

PO

• Give without regard to food. • Administer first dose at bedtime (minimizes risk of fainting due to "first-dose syncope").

INDICATIONS/ROUTES/DOSAGE

HYPERTENSION

PO: ADULTS, ELDERLY: Initially, 1 mg 2–3 times a day. Maintenance: 3–15 mg/day in divided doses. **Maximum:** 20 mg/day. **CHILDREN:** 5 mcg/kg/dose q6h. Gradually increase up to 25 mcg/kg/dose.

SIDE EFFECTS

FREQUENT (10%–7%): Dizziness, drowsiness, headache, asthenia (loss of strength, energy). **OCCASIONAL (5%–4%):** Palpitations, nausea, dry mouth, nervousness. **RARE (less than 1%):** Angina, urinary urgency.

ADVERSE EFFECTS/ TOXIC REACTIONS

First-dose syncope (hypotension with sudden loss of consciousness) may occur 30–90 min following initial dose of more than 2 mg, too-rapid increase in dosage, addition of another antihypertensive agent to therapy. May be preceded by tachycardia (pulse rate of 120–160 beats/min).

NURSING CONSIDERATIONS

BASELINE ASSESSMENT

Give first dose at bedtime. If initial dose is given during daytime, pt must remain recumbent for 3–4 hrs. Assess B/P, pulse immediately before each dose and q15–30min until stabilized (be alert to B/P fluctuations).

INTERVENTION/EVALUATION

Monitor B/P, pulse diligently (first-dose syncope may be preceded by tachycardia). Monitor daily pattern of bowel activity/stool consistency. Assist with ambulation if dizziness occurs.

PATIENT/FAMILY TEACHING

• Avoid tasks that require alertness, motor skills until response to drug is established. • Use caution when rising from sitting or lying position. • Report continued dizziness, palpitations.

prednicarbate

(Dermatop)

See Corticosteroids: topical (p. 95C)

*prednisoLONE evolve

pred-**niss**-oh-lone

(AK-Pred, Novo-Prednisolone ✱, Orapred, Orapred ODT, Pediapred, Pred Forte, Pred Mild, Prelone)

Do not confuse prednisolone with prednisone or primidone.

FIXED-COMBINATION(S)

Blephamide: prednisolone/sulfacetamide (an anti-infective): 0.2%/10%. **Vasocidin:** prednisolone/sulfacetamide: 0.25%/10%.

P

◆ CLASSIFICATION

PHARMACOTHERAPEUTIC: Adrenal corticosteroid. **CLINICAL:** Glucocorticoid (see p. 92C).

ACTION

Inhibits accumulation of inflammatory cells at inflammation sites, phagocytosis, lysosomal enzyme release/synthesis, release of mediators of inflammation. **Therapeutic Effect:** Prevents/suppresses cell-mediated immune reactions. Decreases/prevents tissue response to inflammatory process.

PHARMACOKINETICS

Protein binding: 65–91%. Metabolized in liver. Excreted in urine. **Half-life:** 3.6 hrs.

USES

Substitution Therapy in Deficiency States: Acute or chronic adrenal insufficiency, congenital adrenal hyperplasia, adrenal insufficiency secondary to pituitary insufficiency. **Nonendocrine Disorders:** Allergic, collagen, intestinal tract, hepatic, ocular, renal, skin diseases; bronchial asthma; arthritis; rheumatic carditis; cerebral edema; malignancies. **Ophthalmic:** Treatment of conjunctivitis, corneal injury (from chemical/thermal burns, foreign body).

PRECAUTIONS

CONTRAINDICATIONS: Acute superficial herpes simplex keratitis, systemic fungal infections, varicella. **CAUTIONS:** Hyperthyroidism, cirrhosis, ocular herpes simplex, peptic ulcer disease, osteoporosis, myasthenia gravis, hypertension, CHF, ulcerative colitis, thromboembolic disorders.

LIFESPAN CONSIDERATIONS:

Pregnancy/Lactation: Crosses placenta. Distributed in breast milk. Fetal cleft palate often occurs with chronic, first-trimester use. Do not breast-feed. **Pregnancy Category C (D if used in first trimester).** **Children:** Prolonged treatment or high dosages may decrease short-term growth rate, cortisol secretion. **Elderly:** May be more susceptible to developing hypertension or osteoporosis.

INTERACTIONS

DRUG: **Amphotericin** may worsen hypokalemia. May increase risk of **digoxin** toxicity (due to hypokalemia). May decrease effects of **diuretics, insulin, oral hypoglycemics, potassium supplements**. **Hepatic enzyme inducers** may decrease effects. **Live virus vaccines** increase vaccine side effects, potentiate virus replication, decrease pt's antibody response to vaccine. **HERBAL:** **St. John's wort** may decrease concentration. **Cat's claw, echinacea** have immunostimulant properties. **FOOD:** None known. **LAB VALUES:** May increase serum glucose, lipids, amylase, sodium. May decrease serum calcium, potassium, thyroxine.

AVAILABILITY (Rx)

SOLUTION, OPHTHALMIC (AK-PRED): 1%. **SOLUTION, ORAL (ORAPRED):** 15 mg/5 ml. **(PEDIAPRED):** 5 mg/5 ml. **SUSPENSION, OPHTHALMIC: (PRED FORTE)** 1%; **(PRED MILD)** 0.12%. **SYRUP (PRELONE):** 5 mg/5 ml, 15 mg/5 ml. **TABLETS:** 5 mg. **TABLETS, ORALLY DISINTEGRATING:** 10 mg, 15 mg, 30 mg.

ADMINISTRATION/HANDLING

PO

• Give without regard to meals.

ORALLY DISINTEGRATING TABLETS (ODT)

• Do not cut, split, break or use partial tablets. • Remove from blister just prior to giving, place on tongue. • May swallow whole or allow to dissolve in mouth with/without water.

OPHTHALMIC

• For ophthalmic solution, shake well before using. • Instill drops into conjunctival sac, as prescribed. • Avoid touching applicator tip to conjunctiva to avoid contamination.

P

INDICATIONS/ROUTES/DOSAGE

USUAL DOSAGE

PO: ADULTS, ELDERLY: 5–60 mg/day in divided doses. **CHILDREN:** 0.1–2 mg/kg/day in 1–4 divided doses.

TREATMENT OF CONJUCTIVITIS, CORNEAL INJURY

OPHTHALMIC: ADULTS, ELDERLY: 1–2 drops every hr during day and q2h during night. After response, decrease dosage to 1 drop q4h, then 1 drop 3–4 times a day.

SIDE EFFECTS

FREQUENT: Insomnia, heartburn, nervousness, abdominal distention, diaphoresis, acne, mood swings, increased appetite, facial flushing, delayed wound healing, increased susceptibility to infection, diarrhea, constipation. **OCCASIONAL:** Headache, edema, change in skin color, frequent urination. **RARE:** Tachycardia, allergic reaction (rash, urticaria), psychological changes, hallucinations, depression. **Ophthalmic:** Stinging/burning, posterior subcapsular cataracts.

P

ADVERSE EFFECTS/ TOXIC REACTIONS

LONG-TERM THERAPY: Hypocalcemia, hypokalemia, muscle wasting (esp. arms, legs) osteoporosis, spontaneous fractures, amenorrhea, cataracts, glaucoma, peptic ulcer, CHF. **ABRUPT WITHDRAWAL FOLLOWING LONG-TERM THERAPY:** Anorexia, nausea, fever, headache, severe/sudden joint pain, rebound inflammation, fatigue, weakness, lethargy, dizziness, orthostatic hypotension. Sudden discontinuance may be fatal.

NURSING CONSIDERATIONS

BASELINE ASSESSMENT

Obtain baselines for height, weight, B/P, serum glucose, electrolytes. Check results of initial tests (tuberculosis [TB] skin test, x-rays, EKG). Never give live virus vaccine (e.g., smallpox).

INTERVENTION/EVALUATION

Monitor B/P, weight, serum electrolytes, glucose, height, weight in children. Be alert to infection (sore throat, fever, vague symptoms); assess oral cavity daily for signs of candida infection (white patches, painful tongue/mucous membranes).

PATIENT/FAMILY TEACHING

• Notify physician of fever, sore throat, muscle aches, sudden weight gain, swelling. • Avoid alcohol, minimize use of caffeine. • Do not abruptly discontinue without physician's approval. • Avoid exposure to chickenpox, measles.

*predniSONE

pred-ni-sone

(Apo-Prednisone ♣, Novo-Prednisone ♣, Prednisone Intensol, Sterapred, Sterapred DS, Winpred ♣)

Do not confuse prednisone with prednisolone or primidone.

CLASSIFICATION

PHARMACOTHERAPEUTIC: Adrenal corticosteroid. **CLINICAL:** Glucocorticoid (see p. 93C).

ACTION

Inhibits accumulation of inflammatory cells at inflammation sites, phagocytosis, lysosomal enzyme release/synthesis, release of mediators of inflammation. **Therapeutic Effect:** Prevents/suppresses cell-mediated immune reactions. Decreases/prevents tissue response to inflammatory process.

PHARMACOKINETICS

Well absorbed from GI tract. Protein binding: 70%–90%. Widely distributed. Metabolized in liver, converted to prednisolone. Primarily excreted in urine. Not removed by hemodialysis. **Half-life:** 3.4–3.8 hrs.

USES

Substitution Therapy in Deficiency States: Acute or chronic adrenal insufficiency, congenital adrenal hyperplasia, adrenal insufficiency secondary to pituitary insufficiency. **Nonendocrine Disorders:** Arthritis; rheumatic carditis; allergic, collagen, intestinal tract, liver, ocular, renal, skin diseases; bronchial asthma; cerebral edema; malignancies.

PRECAUTIONS

CONTRAINDICATIONS: Acute superficial herpes simplex keratitis, systemic fungal infections, varicella. **CAUTIONS:** Hyperthyroidism, cirrhosis, ocular herpes simplex, peptic ulcer disease, osteoporosis, myasthenia gravis, hypertension, CHF, ulcerative colitis, thromboembolic disorders.

LIFESPAN CONSIDERATIONS:

Pregnancy/Lactation: Crosses placenta. Distributed in breast milk. Fetal cleft palate often occurs with chronic, first trimester use. Do not breast-feed. **Pregnancy Category C (D if used in first trimester). Children:** Prolonged treatment or high dosages may decrease short-term growth rate, cortisol secretion. **Elderly:** May be more susceptible to developing hypertension or osteoporosis.

INTERACTIONS

DRUG: Antacids may decrease absorption, effect. **Amphotericin** may increase hypokalemia. May increase risk of **digoxin** toxicity (due to hypokalemia). May decrease effects of **diuretics, insulin, oral hypoglycemics, potassium supplements**. **Hepatic enzyme inducers** may decrease effects. **Live virus vaccines** may increase vaccine side effects, potentiate virus replication, decrease pt's antibody response to vaccine. **HERBAL: St. John's wort** may decrease concentration. **Cat's claw, echinacea** have immunostimulant properties. **FOOD:** None known. **LAB VALUES:** May increase serum glucose, lipids, amylase, sodium. May decrease serum calcium, potassium, thyroxine.

AVAILABILITY (Rx)

SOLUTION, ORAL: 1 mg/ml. **SOLUTION, ORAL CONCENTRATE (PREDNISONE INTENSOL):** 5 mg/ml. **TABLETS:** 1 mg, 2.5 mg, 5 mg, 10 mg, 20 mg, 50 mg.

ADMINISTRATION/HANDLING

PO

• Give without regard to meals. • Give single doses before 9 AM, multiple doses at evenly spaced intervals.

INDICATIONS/ROUTES/DOSAGE

USUAL DOSAGE

PO: ADULTS, ELDERLY: 5–60 mg/day in divided doses. **CHILDREN:** 0.05–2 mg/kg/day in 1–4 divided doses.

SIDE EFFECTS

FREQUENT: Insomnia, heartburn, nervousness, abdominal distention, diaphoresis, acne, mood swings, increased appetite, facial flushing, delayed wound healing, increased susceptibility to infection, diarrhea, constipation. **OCCASIONAL:** Headache, edema, change in skin color, frequent urination. **RARE:** Tachycardia, allergic reaction (rash, urticaria), psychological changes, hallucinations, depression.

ADVERSE EFFECTS/ TOXIC REACTIONS

LONG-TERM THERAPY: Muscle wasting (esp. in arms, legs), osteoporosis,

P

spontaneous fractures, amenorrhea cataracts, glaucoma, peptic ulcer, CHF. **ABRUPT WITHDRAWAL FOLLOWING LONG-TERM THERAPY:** Anorexia, nausea, fever, headache, rebound inflammation, fatigue, weakness, lethargy, dizziness, orthostatic hypotension. Sudden discontinuance may be fatal.

NURSING CONSIDERATIONS

BASELINE ASSESSMENT

Obtain baselines for height, weight, B/P, serum glucose, electrolytes. Check results of initial tests (tuberculosis [TB] skin test, x-rays, EKG). Never give live virus vaccine (e.g., smallpox).

INTERVENTION/EVALUATION

Monitor B/P, weight, serum electrolytes, glucose, height, weight. Be alert to infection (sore throat, fever, vague symptoms); assess oral cavity daily for signs of candida infection (white patches, painful tongue/mucous membranes).

PATIENT/FAMILY TEACHING

• Notify physician of fever, sore throat, muscle aches, sudden weight gain, swelling. • Avoid alcohol, minimize use of caffeine. • Do not abruptly discontinue without physician's approval. • Avoid exposure to chickenpox, measles.

P

pregabalin

pre-**gab**-ah-lin
(Lyrica)

CLASSIFICATION

CLINICAL: Anticonvulsant, antineuralgic, analgesic (**Schedule V**).

ACTION

Binds to calcium channel sites in CNS tissue, inhibiting excitatory neurotransmitter release. Exerts antinociceptive, anticonvulsant activity. **Therapeutic Effect:** Decreases symptoms of painful peripheral neuropathy; decreases frequency of partial seizures.

PHARMACOKINETICS

Well absorbed following PO administration. Eliminated in urine. **Half-life:** 6 hrs.

USES

Adjunctive therapy in treatment of partial onset seizures. Management of neuropathic pain associated with diabetic peripheral neuropathy. Management of postherpetic neuralgia.

PRECAUTIONS

CONTRAINDICATIONS: None known. **CAUTIONS:** CHF, renal impairment.

LIFESPAN CONSIDERATIONS:

Pregnancy/Lactation: Increased risk of fetal skeletal abnormalities. Unknown if distributed in breast milk. **Pregnancy Category C.** **Children:** Safety and efficacy not established. **Elderly:** Age-related renal impairment may require dosage adjustment.

INTERACTIONS

DRUG: **Alcohol, barbiturates, narcotic analgesics, other sedative agents** may increase sedative effect. Additive effects on weight gain, edema with **pioglitazone, rosiglitazone.** **HERBAL:** **Gotu kola, kava kava, St. John's wort, valerian** may increase CNS depression. **FOOD:** None known. **LAB VALUES:** May increase CPK. May cause mild PR interval prolongation. May decrease serum glucose, platelet count.

AVAILABILITY (Rx)

CAPSULES (LYRICA): 25 mg, 50 mg, 75 mg, 100 mg, 150 mg, 200 mg, 225 mg, 300 mg.

ADMINISTRATION/HANDLING

• Give without regard to food. • Do not open/crush capsule.

INDICATIONS/ROUTES/DOSAGE

PARTIAL ONSET SEIZURES

PO: ADULTS, ELDERLY: Initially, 75 mg twice a day or 50 mg 3 times a day. Dosage may be increased to maximum 600 mg a day.

NEUROPATHIC PAIN

PO: ADULTS, ELDERLY: Initially, 50 mg 3 times a day. Dosage may be increased to maximum 300 mg a day, based on efficacy and tolerability.

POSTHERPETIC NEURALGIA

PO: ADULTS, ELDERLY: Initially, 75 mg twice a day or 50 mg 3 times a day. May increase to 300 mg/day within 1 wk. **Maximum:** 600 mg/day. May further increase to 600 mg/day after 2–4 wks.

DOSAGE IN RENAL IMPAIRMENT

Creatinine Clearance	Dosage
Greater than 60 ml/min	150–300 mg/day in 2 to 3 divided daily doses
30–60 ml/min	75–150 mg/day in 2 to 3 divided daily doses
15–29 ml/min	25–50 mg/day in single or 2 divided daily doses
Less than 15 ml/min	25–50 mg/day in single divided dose

DOSAGE FOR HEMODIALYSIS

◀ **ALERT** ▶ Take supplemental dose immediately following dialysis.

Daily Dosage	Supplemental Dosage
25 mg	Single dose of 25 mg or 50 mg
25–50 mg	Single dose of 50 mg or 75 mg
75 mg	Single dose of 100 mg or 150 mg

SIDE EFFECTS

FREQUENT (32%–12%): Dizziness, somnolence, ataxia, peripheral edema. **OCCASIONAL (12%–5%):** Weight gain, blurred vision, diplopia, difficulty with concentration, attention, cognition; tremor, dry mouth, headache, constipation, asthenia (loss of strength, energy). **RARE (4%–2%):** Abnormal gait, confusion, incoordination, twitching, flatulence, vomiting, edema.

ADVERSE EFFECTS/ TOXIC REACTIONS

Abrupt withdrawal increases risk of seizure frequency in pts with seizure disorders; withdraw gradually over a minimum of 1 wk.

NURSING CONSIDERATIONS

BASELINE ASSESSMENT

Seizure: Review history of seizure disorder (type, onset, intensity, frequency, duration, level of consciousness [LOC]). **Pain:** Assess onset, type, location, and duration of pain.

INTERVENTION/EVALUATION

Provide safety measures as needed. Assess for seizure activity. Assess for clinical improvement; record onset of relief of pain. Assess for evidence of peripheral edema behind medial malleolus (usually first area of edema). Question for changes in visual acuity.

PATIENT/FAMILY TEACHING

• Do not abruptly stop taking drug because seizure frequency may be increased. • Do not drive, operate machinery, perform activities requiring mental acuity due to potential dizziness, drowsiness, ataxia. • Avoid alcohol. • Carry identification card, bracelet to note anticonvulsant therapy. • If noncompliance is an issue in causing acute seizures, discuss and address reasons for noncompliance.

Premarin, *see conjugated estrogens*

Prempro, *see estrogen and medroxyprogesterone*

Prevacid, *see lansoprazole*

Prilosec, *see omeprazole*

Primacor, *see milrinone*

Primaxin, *see imipenem and cilastatin*

primidone

pri-mi-done
(Apo-Primidone ✱, Mysoline)
Do not confuse primidone with prednisone.

◆ CLASSIFICATION

PHARMACOTHERAPEUTIC: Barbiturate. **CLINICAL:** Anticonvulsant (see p. 35C).

ACTION

Decreases motor activity from electrical/chemical stimulation, stabilizes seizure threshold against hyperexcitability. **Therapeutic Effect:** Reduces seizure activity.

PHARMACOKINETICS

Rapidly, usually completely absorbed following PO administration. Protein binding: 20%–30%. Extensively metabolized in liver to phenobarbital and phenylethylmalonamide (PEMA). Minimal excretion in urine. **Half-life:** 3.3–7 hrs.

USES

Management of partial seizures with complex symptomatology (psychomotor seizures), generalized tonic-clonic (grand mal) seizures. **OFF-LABEL:** Treatment of essential tremor.

PRECAUTIONS

CONTRAINDICATIONS: History of bronchopneumonia, hypersensitivity to phenobarbital, porphyria. **CAUTIONS:** Renal/hepatic impairment.

⌛ LIFESPAN CONSIDERATIONS:

Pregnancy/Lactation: Crosses placenta; is distributed in breast milk. **Pregnancy Category D. Children, Elderly:** May produce paradoxical excitement, restlessness.

INTERACTIONS

DRUG: **Alcohol, other CNS depressants** may increase effects. May increase metabolism of **carbamazepine**. May decrease effects of **digoxin, glucocosteroids, metronidazole, oral anticoagulants, quinidine, tricyclic antidepressants**. **MAOIs** may prolong effects. **Valproic acid** increases concentration, risk of toxicity. **HERBAL:** **Evening primrose** may decrease seizure threshold. **Gotu kola, kava kava, St. John's wort, valerian** may increase CNS depression. **FOOD:** None known. **LAB VALUES:** May decrease serum bilirubin. Therapeutic serum level: 4–12 mcg/ml; toxic serum level: greater than 12 mcg/ml.

AVAILABILITY (Rx)

ORAL SUSPENSION: 250 mg/5 ml. **TABLETS:** 50 mg, 250 mg.

P

INDICATIONS/ROUTES/DOSAGE

SEIZURE CONTROL

PO: ADULTS, ELDERLY, CHILDREN 8 YRS AND OLDER: 125–150 mg/day at bedtime. May increase by 125–250 mg/day every 3–7 days. **Maximum:** 2 g/day. **CHILDREN YOUNGER THAN 8 YRS:** Initially, 50–125 mg/day at bedtime. May increase by 50–125 mg/day every 3–7 days. Usual dose: 10–25 mg/kg/day in divided doses. **NEONATES:** 12–20 mg/kg/day in divided doses.

SIDE EFFECTS

FREQUENT: Ataxia, dizziness. **OCCASIONAL:** Anorexia, drowsiness, altered mental status, nausea, vomiting, paradoxical excitement. **RARE:** Rash.

ADVERSE EFFECTS/ TOXIC REACTIONS

Abrupt withdrawal after prolonged therapy may produce effects ranging from markedly increased dreaming, nightmares, insomnia, tremor, diaphoresis, vomiting to hallucinations, delirium, seizures, status epilepticus. Skin eruptions may appear as hypersensitivity reaction. Blood dyscrasias, hepatic disease, hypocalcemia occur rarely. Overdose produces cold/clammy skin, hypothermia, severe CNS depression, followed by high fever, coma.

NURSING CONSIDERATIONS

BASELINE ASSESSMENT

Review history of seizure disorder (intensity, frequency, duration, level of consciousness [LOC]). Observe frequently for recurrence of seizure activity. Initiate seizure precautions.

INTERVENTION/EVALUATION

Monitor serum concentrations; CBC; neurologic status (frequency, duration, severity of seizures). Monitor for therapeutic serum level: 4–12 mcg/ml; toxic serum level: more than 12 mcg/ml.

PATIENT/FAMILY TEACHING

• Do not abruptly withdraw medication after long-term use (may precipitate seizures). • Strict maintenance of drug therapy is essential for seizure control. • Drowsiness usually disappears during continued therapy. • If dizziness occurs, change positions slowly from recumbent to sitting position before standing. • Avoid tasks that require alertness, motor skills until response to drug is established. • Avoid alcohol.

Prinivil, *see lisinopril*

probenecid

proe-**ben**-e-sid

(Benuryl ♣)

Do not confuse probenecid with procainamide.

CLASSIFICATION

PHARMACOTHERAPEUTIC: Uricosuric. **CLINICAL:** Antigout.

ACTION

Competitively inhibits reabsorption of uric acid at proximal convoluted tubule. Inhibits renal tubular secretion of weak organic acids (e.g., penicillins). **Therapeutic Effect:** Promotes uric acid excretion, reduces serum uric acid level, increases plasma levels of penicillins, cephalosporins.

PHARMACOKINETICS

Rapidly, completely absorbed following PO administration. Protein binding: High. Extensively metabolized in liver. Excreted in urine. Excretion is dependent upon urinary pH, is increased in alkaline urine. **Half-life:** 3–8 hrs (dose-dependent).

USES

Treatment of hyperuricemia associated with gout, gouty arthritis. Adjunctive therapy with penicillins, cephalosporins to elevate/prolong antibiotic plasma levels.

PRECAUTIONS

CONTRAINDICATIONS: Blood dyscrasias, children younger than 2 yrs, concurrent high-dose aspirin therapy, severe renal impairment, uric acid calculi. **CAUTIONS:** Peptic ulcer, hematuria, renal colic.

LIFESPAN CONSIDERATIONS:

Pregnancy/Lactation: Unknown if drug crosses placenta or is distributed in breast milk. **Pregnancy Category B. Children:** Safety and efficacy not established in children younger than 2 yrs. **Elderly:** No age-related precautions noted.

INTERACTIONS

DRUG: Increases effect, toxicity of **methotrexate.** Increases concentration of **quinolones, penicillin, cephalosporins, acyclovir, ketorolac, benzodiazepines, NSAIDs, sulfonylureas.** High-dose **salicylates** may decrease excretion of uric acid. **HERBAL:** None significant. **FOOD:** None known. **LAB VALUES:** May inhibit renal excretion of serum PSP (phenolsulfonphthalein), 17-ketosteroids, BSP (sulfobromophthalein).

AVAILABILITY (Rx)

TABLETS: 500 mg.

ADMINISTRATION/HANDLING

PO

• Give with or immediately after meals, milk. • Instruct pt to drink at least 6–8 glasses (8 oz) of water/day (prevents kidney stone development).

INDICATIONS/ROUTES/DOSAGE

GOUT

PO: ADULTS, ELDERLY: Initially, 250 mg twice a day for 1 wk; then 500 mg twice a day. May increase by 500 mg q4wk. **Maximum:** 2–3 g/day. Maintenance: Dosage that maintains normal uric acid level.

ADJUNCT TO PENICILLIN, CEPHALOSPORIN THERAPY

PO: ADULTS, ELDERLY: 2 g/day in divided doses. **CHILDREN WEIGHING MORE THAN 50 KG:** Receive adult dosage. **CHILDREN 2–14 YRS:** Initially, 25 mg/kg. Maintenance: 40 mg/kg/day in 4 divided doses.

GONORRHEA

PO: ADULTS, ELDERLY: 1 g 30 min before penicillin, ampicillin, or amoxicillin. **CHILDREN WEIGHING LESS THAN 45 KG:** 25 mg/kg 30 min before penicillin, ampicillin, amoxicillin. **Maximum:** 1 g.

SIDE EFFECTS

FREQUENT (10%–6%): Headache, anorexia, nausea, vomiting. **OCCASIONAL (5%–1%):** Lower back or side pain, rash, urticaria, pruritus, dizziness, flushed face, urinary urgency, gingivitis.

ADVERSE EFFECTS/ TOXIC REACTIONS

Severe hypersensitivity reactions, including anaphylaxis, occur rarely (usually within few hrs after administration following previous use); discontinue drug immediately, contact physician. Pruritic maculopapular rash should be considered a toxic reaction. May be accompanied by malaise, fever, chills, arthralgia, nausea, vomiting, leukopenia, aplastic anemia.

NURSING CONSIDERATIONS

BASELINE ASSESSMENT

Do not initiate therapy until acute gouty attack has subsided. Question for hypersensitivity to probenecid or if taking penicillin, cephalosporin antibiotics.

INTERVENTION/EVALUATION

If exacerbation of gout recurs after therapy, use other agents for gout. Discontinue medication immediately

P

if rash, other evidence of allergic reaction appears. Encourage high fluid intake (3,000 ml/day). Monitor I&O (output should be at least 2,000 ml/day). Assess CBC, serum uric acid levels. Assess urine for cloudiness, unusual color, odor. Assess for therapeutic response (reduced joint tenderness, swelling, redness, limitation of motion).

PATIENT/FAMILY TEACHING

• Drink plenty of fluids to decrease risk of uric acid kidney stones. • Avoid alcohol, large doses of aspirin, other salicylates. • Encourage low-purine food intake (reduce/omit meat, fowl, fish; use eggs, cheese, vegetables). • Foods high in purine: kidney, liver, sweetbreads, sardines, anchovies, meat extracts. • May take over 1 wk for full therapeutic effect. • Drink 6–8 glasses (8 oz) of fluid daily while on medication.

procainamide

pro-**cane**-ah-myd
(Apo-Procainamide ✤, Procanbid, Procan-SR, Pronestyl, Pronestyl-SR)

Do not confuse with Procanbid with probenecid, or Pronestyl with Ponstel.

CLASSIFICATION

CLINICAL: Antiarrhythmic (see p. 14C).

ACTION

Increases electrical stimulation threshold of ventricles, His-Purkinje system. Decreases myocardial excitability, conduction velocity; depresses myocardial contractility. Exerts direct cardiac effects. **Therapeutic Effect:** Suppresses arrhythmias.

PHARMACOKINETICS

Rapidly, completely absorbed from GI tract. Protein binding: 15%–20%. Widely distributed. Metabolized in liver to active metabolite. Primarily excreted in urine. Removed by hemodialysis. **Half-life:** 2.5–4.5 hrs; metabolite, 6 hrs.

USES

Prophylactic therapy to maintain normal sinus rhythm after conversion of atrial fibrillation/flutter. Treatment of premature ventricular contractions, paroxysmal atrial tachycardia, atrial fibrillation, ventricular tachycardia. **OFF-LABEL:** Conversion, management of atrial fibrillation.

PRECAUTIONS

CONTRAINDICATIONS: Complete heart block, myasthenia gravis, preexisting QT prolongation, second-degree heart block, systemic lupus erythematosus, torsades de pointes. **CAUTIONS:** Marked AV conduction disturbances, bundle-branch block, severe digoxin toxicity, CHF, supraventricular tachyarrhythmias, renal/hepatic impairment.

LIFESPAN CONSIDERATIONS:

Pregnancy/Lactation: Crosses placenta. Unknown if distributed in breast milk. **Pregnancy Category C. Children:** No age-related precautions noted. **Elderly:** More susceptible to hypotensive effect. Age-related renal impairment may require dosage adjustment.

INTERACTIONS

DRUG: May increase effects of **antihypertensives (IV procainamide), neuromuscular blockers. Other antiarrhythmics, pimozide** may increase cardiac effects. **HERBAL: Ephedra** may worsen arrhythmias. **FOOD:** None known. **LAB VALUES:** May cause EKG changes, positive ANA titers, Coombs' test. May increase AST, ALT, serum alkaline phosphatase, bilirubin, LDH. Therapeutic serum level: 4–8 mcg/ml; toxic serum level: greater than 10 mcg/ml.

AVAILABILITY (Rx)

CAPSULES (PRONESTYL): 250 mg, 500 mg. **INJECTION SOLUTION (PRONESTYL):** 100 mg/ml, 500 mg/ml. **TABLETS (PRONESTYL):** 250 mg, 375 mg, 500 mg.

TABLETS (EXTENDED-RELEASE): 500 mg (Procanbid, Pronestyl-SR), 750 mg (Procanbid), 1,000 mg (Procanbid).

ADMINISTRATION/HANDLING

IV, IM

◀ **ALERT** ▶ May give by IM injection, IV push, IV infusion.

Reconstitution • For IV push, dilute with 5–10 ml D_5W. • For initial loading infusion, add 1 g to 50 ml D_5W to provide concentration of 20 mg/ml. • For IV infusion, add 1 g to 250–500 ml D_5W to provide concentration of 2–4 mg/ml. Maximum concentration: 4 g/250 ml.

Rate of administration • For IV push, with pt in supine position, administer at rate not exceeding 25–50 mg/min. • For initial loading infusion, infuse 1 ml/min for up to 25–30 min. • For IV infusion, infuse at 1–3 ml/min. • Check B/P q5–10min during infusion. If fall in B/P exceeds 15 mm Hg, discontinue drug, contact physician. • Monitor EKG for cardiac changes, particularly widening of QRS, prolongation of PR and QT intervals. Notify physician of any significant interval changes. • B/P, EKG should be monitored continuously during IV administration and rate of infusion adjusted to eliminate arrhythmias.

Storage • Solution appears clear, colorless to light yellow. • Discard if solution darkens or is discolored or if precipitate forms. • When diluted with D_5W, solution is stable for 24 hrs at room temperature, for 7 days if refrigerated.

PO

• Do not crush/break extended-release tablets.

IV INCOMPATIBILITY

Milrinone (Primacor).

IV COMPATIBILITIES

Amiodarone (Cordarone), dobutamine (Dobutrex), heparin, lidocaine, potassium chloride.

INDICATIONS/ROUTES/DOSAGE

MANAGEMENT OF ARRHYTHMIAS

PO: ADULTS, ELDERLY: 250–500 mg of immediate-release tablets q3–6h. 0.5–1 g of extended-release tablets q6h. 1–2 g of Procanbid q12h. **Maximum:** 4 g/24 hrs. **CHILDREN:** 15–50 mg/kg/day of immediate-release tablets in divided doses q3–6h. **Maximum:** 4 g/day.

IV: ADULTS, ELDERLY: Loading dose: 50–100 mg. May repeat q5–10min or 15–18 mg/kg (**maximum:** 1–1.5 g). Then maintenance infusion of 3–4 mg/min. Range: 1–6 mg/min. **CHILDREN:** Loading dose: 3–6 mg/kg over 5 min (**maximum:** 100 mg). May repeat q5–10min to maximum total dose of 15 mg/kg. Then maintenance dose of 20–80 mcg/kg/min. **Maximum:** 2 g/day.

DOSAGE IN RENAL IMPAIRMENT

Dosage interval is modified based on creatinine clearance.

Creatinine Clearance	Dosage Interval
10–50 ml/min	q6–12h
Less than 10 ml/min	q8–24h

SIDE EFFECTS

FREQUENT: PO: Abdominal pain/cramping, nausea, diarrhea, vomiting. **OCCASIONAL:** Dizziness, giddiness, weakness, hypersensitivity reaction (rash, urticaria, pruritus, flushing). **IV:** Transient, but at times, marked hypotension. **RARE:** Confusion, mental depression, psychosis.

ADVERSE EFFECTS/ TOXIC REACTIONS

Paradoxical, extremely rapid ventricular rate may occur during treatment of atrial fibrillation/flutter. Systemic lupus

P

erythematosus-like syndrome (fever, myalgia, pleuritic chest pain) may occur with prolonged therapy. Cardiotoxic effects occur most commonly with IV administration and appear as conduction changes (50% widening of QRS complex, frequent ventricular premature contractions, ventricular tachycardia, complete AV block). Prolonged PR and QT intervals, flattened T waves occur less frequently.

NURSING CONSIDERATIONS

BASELINE ASSESSMENT

Check B/P, pulse for 1 full min (unless pt is on continuous monitor) before giving medication.

INTERVENTION/EVALUATION

Monitor EKG for cardiac changes, particularly widening of QRS, prolongation of PR and QT intervals. Assess pulse for strength/weakness, irregular rate. Monitor I&O, serum electrolyte levels (potassium, chloride, sodium). Assess for complaints of GI upset, headache, arthralgia. Monitor daily pattern of bowel activity/stool consistency. Assess for dizziness. Monitor B/P for hypotension. Assess skin for evidence of hypersensitivity reaction (esp. in pts on high-dose therapy). Monitor for therapeutic serum level. Therapeutic serum level: 4–8 mcg/ml; toxic serum level: greater than 10 mcg/ml.

PATIENT/FAMILY TEACHING

• Take medication at evenly spaced doses around the clock. • Contact physician if fever, joint pain/stiffness, signs of upper respiratory infection occur. • Avoid tasks that require alertness, motor skills until response to drug is established (potential for dizziness). • Do not abruptly discontinue medication. • Compliance with therapy regimen is essential to control arrhythmias. • Do not use nasal decongestants, OTC cold preparations (stimulants) without physician approval. • Restrict salt, alcohol intake.

procaine

(Novocaine)

See Anesthetics: local (p. 4C)

procarbazine

pro-**car**-bah-zeen

(Matulane, Natulan ✤)

Do not confuse procarbazine with dacarbazine.

CLASSIFICATION

PHARMACOTHERAPEUTIC: Methylhydrazine derivative. **CLINICAL:** Antineoplastic (see p. 82C).

ACTION

Inhibits DNA, RNA, protein synthesis. May directly damage DNA. Cell cycle–phase specific for S phase of cell division. **Therapeutic Effect:** Causes cell death.

PHARMACOKINETICS

Rapidly, completely absorbed from GI tract. Crosses blood-brain barrier. Metabolized primarily in liver, kidneys. Excreted in urine, feces. **Half-life:** 10 min.

USES

Treatment of advanced Hodgkin's disease. **OFF-LABEL:** Treatment of lung carcinoma, malignant melanoma, multiple myeloma, non-Hodgkin's lymphoma, polycythemia vera, primary brain tumors.

P

PRECAUTIONS

CONTRAINDICATIONS: Myelosuppression. **CAUTIONS:** Renal/hepatic impairment.

⌛ LIFESPAN CONSIDERATIONS:

Pregnancy/Lactation: Unknown if distributed in breast milk. May cause fetal harm. **Pregnancy Category D. Children:** Safety and efficacy not established. **Elderly:** Age-related renal impairment may require dosage adjustment.

INTERACTIONS

DRUG: **Alcohol** may cause disulfiram-like reaction. May increase anticholinergic effects of **anticholinergics, antihistamines**. **Bone marrow depressants** may increase myelosuppression. **Buspirone, caffeine-containing medications** may increase B/P. **Carbamazepine, cyclobenzaprine, MAOIs, maprotiline** may cause hyperpyretic crisis, seizures, death. **CNS depressants** may increase CNS depression. May increase effects of **insulin, oral antidiabetics**. **Meperidine** may produce coma, seizures, immediate excitation, rigidity, severe hypertension/hypotension, severe respiratory distress, diaphoresis, vascular collapse. **Sympathomimetics** may increase cardiac stimulant, vasopressor effects. **Tricyclic antidepressants** may increase anticholinergic effects; may cause seizures, hyperpyretic crisis. **Live virus vaccines** may potentiate virus replication, increase vaccine side effects, decrease pt's antibody response to vaccine. **HERBAL:** None significant. **FOOD:** **Caffeine** may increase B/P. **Foods containing tyramine** may cause clinically severe, (possibly life-threatening) hypertension. **LAB VALUES:** None known.

AVAILABILITY (Rx)

CAPSULES: 50 mg.

INDICATIONS/ROUTES/DOSAGE

ADVANCED HODGKIN'S DISEASE

PO: ADULTS, ELDERLY: Initially, 2–4 mg/kg/day as single dose or in divided doses for 1 wk, then 4–6 mg/kg/day. Maintenance: 1–2 mg/kg/day. **CHILDREN:** 50–100 mg/m^2/day for 10–14 days of a 28-day cycle. Continue until maximum response occurs, leukocyte count falls below 4,000/mm^3, or platelet count falls below 100,000/mm^3. Maintenance: 100 mg/m^2/day for 14 days and repeat q4wk.

SIDE EFFECTS

FREQUENT: Severe nausea, vomiting, respiratory disorders (cough, effusion), myalgia, arthralgia, drowsiness, nervousness, insomnia, nightmares, diaphoresis, hallucinations, seizures. **OCCASIONAL:** Hoarseness, tachycardia, nystagmus, retinal hemorrhage, photophobia, photosensitivity, urinary frequency, nocturia, hypotension, diarrhea, stomatitis, paresthesia, unsteadiness, confusion, decreased reflexes, foot drop. **RARE:** Hypersensitivity reaction (dermatitis, pruritus, rash, urticaria), hyperpigmentation, alopecia.

ADVERSE EFFECTS/ TOXIC REACTIONS

Major toxic effects are myelosuppression manifested as hematologic toxicity (principally leukopenia, thrombocytopenia, anemia), hepatotoxicity manifested as jaundice, ascites. UTIs secondary to leukopenia may occur.

NURSING CONSIDERATIONS

BASELINE ASSESSMENT

Obtain bone marrow tests, Hgb, Hct, leukocyte, differential, reticulocyte, platelet, urinalysis, serum transaminase, alkaline phosphatase, BUN results before therapy and periodically thereafter. Therapy should be interrupted if WBC falls below 4,000/mm^3 or platelet count falls below 100,000/mm^3.

INTERVENTION/EVALUATION

Monitor hematologic status, renal/hepatic function studies. Assess for stomatitis. Monitor for hematologic toxicity (fever, sore throat, signs of local infection, unusual bruising/bleeding from any site), symptoms of anemia (excessive fatigue, weakness).

PATIENT/FAMILY TEACHING

• Inform physician of fever, sore throat, bleeding, bruising. • Avoid alcohol (may cause disulfiram reaction: nausea, vomiting, headache, sedation, visual disturbances).

prochlorperazine

proe-klor-**per**-a-zeen
(Apo-Prochlorperazine ✦, Compazine, Compro, Stemetil ✦)

Do not confuse prochlorperazine with chlorpromazine, or Compazine with Copaxone.

CLASSIFICATION

PHARMACOTHERAPEUTIC: Phenothiazine. **CLINICAL:** Antiemetic.

ACTION

Acts centrally to inhibit/block dopamine receptors in chemoreceptor trigger zone, peripherally to block vagus nerve in GI tract. **Therapeutic Effect:** Relieves nausea/vomiting, improves psychosis.

PHARMACOKINETICS

Route	Onset*	Peak	Duration
Tablets, oral solution	30–40 min	N/A	3–4 hrs
Capsules (Extended-release)	30–40 min	N/A	10–12 hrs
Rectal	60 min	N/A	3–4 hrs

*As an antiemetic.

Variably absorbed after PO administration. Widely distributed. Metabolized in liver, GI mucosa. Primarily excreted in urine. Unknown if removed by hemodialysis. **Half-life:** 23 hrs.

USES

Management of nausea/vomiting. Treatment of acute or chronic psychosis. **OFF-LABEL:** Behavior syndromes in dementia.

PRECAUTIONS

CONTRAINDICATIONS: Narrow angle glaucoma, CNS depression, coma, myelosuppression, severe cardiac/hepatic impairment, severe hypotension/hypertension. **CAUTIONS:** Seizures, Parkinson's disease, children younger than 2 yrs.

LIFESPAN CONSIDERATIONS:

Pregnancy/Lactation: Crosses placenta. Distributed in breast milk. **Pregnancy Category C. Children:** Safety and efficacy not established in those weighing less than 9 kg or younger than 2 yrs. **Elderly:** More susceptible to orthostatic hypotension, anticholinergic effects (e.g., dry mouth), sedation, extrapyramidal symptoms (EPS); lower dosage recommended.

INTERACTIONS

DRUG: Alcohol, other CNS depressants may increase CNS, respiratory depression, hypotensive effects. **Antihypertensives** may increase hypotension. **Antithyroid agents** may increase risk of agranulocytosis. **EPS–producing medications** may increase EPS. May decrease effects of **levodopa. Lithium** may decrease absorption, produce adverse neurologic effects. **MAOIs, tricyclic antidepressants** may increase anticholinergic, sedative effects. **HERBAL: Dong quai, St. John's wort** may increase photosensitization. **Gotu kola, kava kava, St. John's wort, valerian** may increase CNS depression.

FOOD: None known. **LAB VALUES:** None known.

AVAILABILITY (Rx)

INJECTION SOLUTION (COMPAZINE, PROCOT): 5 mg/ml. **SUPPOSITORIES (COMPAZINE):** 2.5 mg, 5 mg, 25 mg. **TABLETS (COMPAZINE):** 5 mg, 10 mg.

ADMINISTRATION/HANDLING

IV

Rate of administration • May give by IV push slowly over 5–10 min. • May give by IV infusion over 30 min.

Storage • Store at room temperature. • Protect from light. • Clear or slightly yellow solutions may be used.

PO

• Give without regard to meals.

RECTAL

• Moisten suppository with cold water before inserting well into rectum.

IV INCOMPATIBILITIES

Atropine, furosemide (Lasix), midazolam (Versed).

IV COMPATIBILITIES

Calcium gluconate, diphenhydramine (Benadryl), fentanyl, glycopyrrolate (Robinul), heparin, hydromorphone (Dilaudid), morphine, metoclopramide (Reglan), nalbuphine (Nubain), potassium chloride, promethazine (Phenergan), propofol (Diprivan).

INDICATIONS/ROUTES/DOSAGE

NAUSEA/VOMITING

PO: ADULTS, ELDERLY: 5–10 mg 3–4 times a day. **CHILDREN:** 0.4 mg/kg/day in 3–4 divided doses.

IV: ADULTS, ELDERLY: 2.5–10 mg. May repeat q3–4h.

IM: ADULTS, ELDERLY: 5–10 mg q3–4h. **CHILDREN:** 0.1–0.15 mg/kg/dose q8–12h. **Maximum:** 40 mg/day.

RECTAL: ADULTS, ELDERLY: 25 mg twice a day. **CHILDREN:** 0.4 mg/kg/day in 3–4 divided doses.

PSYCHOSIS

PO: ADULTS, ELDERLY: 5–10 mg 3–4 times a day. **Maximum:** 150 mg/day. **CHILDREN:** 2.5 mg 2–3 times a day. **Maximum:** 25 mg for children 6–12 yrs; 20 mg for children 2–5 yrs.

IM: ADULTS, ELDERLY: 10–20 mg q4h. **CHILDREN:** 0.13 mg/kg/dose.

SIDE EFFECTS

FREQUENT: Drowsiness, hypotension, dizziness, fainting (commonly occurring after first dose, occasionally after subsequent doses, rarely with oral form). **OCCASIONAL:** Dry mouth, blurred vision, lethargy, constipation, diarrhea, myalgia, nasal congestion, peripheral edema, urinary retention.

ADVERSE EFFECTS/ TOXIC REACTIONS

Extrapyramidal symptoms appear dose related and are divided into three categories: akathisia (inability to sit still, tapping of feet), parkinsonian symptoms (mask-like face, tremors, shuffling gait, hypersalivation), acute dystonias (torticollis [neck muscle spasm], opisthotonos [rigidity of back muscles], oculogyric crisis [rolling back of eyes]). Dystonic reaction may produce diaphoresis, pallor. Tardive dyskinesia (tongue protrusion, puffing of cheeks, puckering of mouth) occurs rarely and may be irreversible. Abrupt withdrawal after long-term therapy may precipitate nausea, vomiting, gastritis, dizziness, tremors. Blood dyscrasias, particularly agranulocytosis, mild leukopenia, may occur. May lower seizure threshold.

NURSING CONSIDERATIONS

BASELINE ASSESSMENT

Avoid skin contact with solution (contact dermatitis). **Antiemetic:** Assess for dehydration (poor skin turgor, dry mucous membranes, longitudinal furrows in tongue). **Antipsychotic:** Assess behavior, appearance, emotional status, response to environment, speech pattern, thought content.

INTERVENTION/EVALUATION

Monitor B/P for hypotension. Assess for EPS. Monitor WBC, differential count for blood dyscrasias. Monitor for fine tongue movement (may be early sign of tardive dyskinesia). Supervise suicidal-risk pt closely during early therapy (as depression lessens, energy level improves, increasing suicide potential). Assess for therapeutic response (interest in surroundings, improvement in self-care, increased ability to concentrate, relaxed facial expression).

PATIENT/FAMILY TEACHING

• Limit caffeine. • Avoid alcohol. • May cause drowsiness, impair ability to perform tasks requiring mental alertness, coordination.

Procrit, *see epoetin alfa*

progesterone

proe-**jess**-ter-one

(Crinone, Prochieve, Prometrium)

CLASSIFICATION

PHARMACOTHERAPEUTIC: Progestin. **CLINICAL:** Hormone.

ACTION

Promotes mammary gland development, relaxes uterine smooth muscle. **Therapeutic Effect:** Decreases abnormal uterine bleeding; transforms endometrium from proliferative to secretory in estrogen-primed endometrium.

PHARMACOKINETICS

Oral: Maximum serum concentrations attained within 3 hrs. Protein binding: 96%–99%. Metabolized in liver. Excreted in bile, urine. **Half-life:** 18.3 hrs. **IM:** Rapidly absorbed. Undergoes rapid metabolism. **Half-life:** Few min. **Long-acting form:** Approximately 10 wks. **Vaginal Gel:** Rate limited by absorption rather than by elimination. Protein binding: 96%–99%. Undergoes both biliary, renal elimination. **Half-life:** 5–20 hrs.

USES

Oral: Prevent endometrial hyperplasia, secondary amenorrhea. **IM:** Amenorrhea, abnormal uterine bleeding. **Vaginal Gel (8%):** Treatment of infertility. **OFF-LABEL:** Treatment of corpus luteum dysfunction.

PRECAUTIONS

CONTRAINDICATIONS: Allergy to peanut oil (oral), breast cancer, history of active cerebral apoplexy, thromboembolic disorders, thrombophlebitis, missed abortion, severe hepatic dysfunction, undiagnosed vaginal bleeding, use as a pregnancy test. **CAUTIONS:** Diabetes, conditions aggravated by fluid retention (e.g., asthma, epilepsy, migraine, cardiac/renal dysfunction), history of mental depression.

LIFESPAN CONSIDERATIONS:

Pregnancy/Lactation: Distributed in breast milk. Avoid use during pregnancy. **Pregnancy Category D. Children:** Safety and efficacy not established. **Elderly:** No age-related precautions noted.

INTERACTIONS

DRUG: May interfere with effects of **bromocriptine**. **HERBAL:** **Red clover** may decrease effect. **FOOD:** None known. **LAB VALUES:** May increase serum LDL, alkaline phosphatase. May decrease glucose tolerance, serum HDL. May cause

P

abnormal serum thyroid, metapyrone, hepatic, endocrine function test results.

AVAILABILITY (Rx)

CAPSULES (PROMETRIUM): 100 mg, 200 mg. **INJECTION OIL:** 50 mg/ml. **VAGINAL GEL (CRINONE, PROCHIEVE):** 4% (45 mg), 8% (90 mg).

ADMINISTRATION/HANDLING

IM

• Store at room temperature. • Administer only deep IM in large muscle mass.

PO

• If given in morning, administer 2 hrs after eating breakfast.

VAGINAL GEL

• Administer at bedtime (may cause drowsiness).

VAGINAL (CRINONE)

• Remove applicator from sealed wrapper. Do not remove twist-off tab at this time. • Hold applicator by thick end. Shake down several times like a thermometer to ensure contents are at thin end. • Hold applicator by flat section of thick end and twist off tab at other end. Do not squeeze thick end while twisting tab (could force some gel to be released before insertion). • Insert applicator into vagina either in sitting position or lying on back with knees bent. • Insert thin end well into vagina. • Squeeze thick end of applicator to deposit gel. • Remove applicator, discard.

INDICATIONS/ROUTES/DOSAGE

AMENORRHEA

PO: ADULTS: 400 mg daily in evening for 10 days.
IM: ADULTS: 5–10 mg for 6–8 days. Withdrawal bleeding expected in 48–72 hrs if ovarian activity produced proliferative endometrium.
VAGINAL: ADULTS: Apply 45 mg (4% gel) every other day for 6 or fewer doses.

ABNORMAL UTERINE BLEEDING

IM: ADULTS: 5–10 mg for 6 days. When estrogen given concomitantly, begin progesterone after 2 wks of estrogen therapy; discontinue when menstrual flow begins.

PREVENTION OF ENDOMETRIAL HYPERPLASIA

PO: ADULTS: 200 mg in evening for 12 days per 28-day cycle in combination with daily conjugated estrogen.

INFERTILITY

VAGINAL: ADULTS: 90 mg (8% gel) once a day (twice a day in women with partial or complete ovarian failure).

SIDE EFFECTS

FREQUENT: Breakthrough bleeding/spotting at beginning of therapy, amenorrhea, change in menstrual flow, breast tenderness. **Gel:** Drowsiness. **OCCASIONAL:** Edema, weight gain/loss, rash, pruritus, photosensitivity, skin pigmentation. **RARE:** Pain/swelling at injection site, acne, depression, alopecia, hirsutism.

ADVERSE EFFECTS/ TOXIC REACTIONS

Thrombophlebitis, cerebrovascular disorders, retinal thrombosis, pulmonary embolism occur rarely.

NURSING CONSIDERATIONS

BASELINE ASSESSMENT

Question for possibility of pregnancy, hypersensitivity to progestins before initiating therapy. Obtain baseline weight, serum glucose level, B/P.

INTERVENTION/EVALUATION

Check weight daily; report weekly gain over 5 lbs. Assess skin for rash, urticaria. Immediately report development of chest pain, sudden shortness of breath, sudden decrease in vision, migraine headache, pain (esp. with swelling, warmth, redness) in calves, numbness of arm/leg (thrombotic

P

disorders). Check B/P periodically. Note progesterone therapy on pathology specimens.

PATIENT/FAMILY TEACHING

• Use sunscreen, protective clothing to protect from sunlight, ultraviolet light until tolerance determined. • Notify physician of abnormal vaginal bleeding, other symptoms. • Stop taking medication, contact physician at once if pregnancy suspected. • If using vaginal gel, avoid tasks that require alertness, motor skills until response to drug is established.

Prograf, *see tacrolimus*

Proleukin, *see aldesleukin*

promethazine

proe-**meth**-a-zeen

(Phenadoz, Phenergan, Promethegan)

Do not confuse promethazine with promazine.

FIXED-COMBINATION(S)

Phenergan with codeine: promethazine/codeine (a cough suppressant): 6.25 mg/10 mg/5 ml. **Phenergan VC:** promethazine/phenylephrine (a vasoconstrictor): 6.25 mg/5 mg/5 ml. **Phenergan VC with codeine:** promethazine/phenylephrine/codeine: 6.25 mg/5 mg/10 mg/5 ml.

CLASSIFICATION

PHARMACOTHERAPEUTIC: Phenothiazine. **CLINICAL:** Antihistamine, antiemetic, sedative-hypnotic (see p. 53C).

ACTION

Antihistamine: Inhibits histamine at histamine receptor sites. **Antiemetic:** Diminishes vestibular stimulation, depresses labyrinthine function, acts on chemoreceptor trigger zone. **Sedative-hypnotic:** Produces CNS depression by decreasing stimulation to brain stem reticular formation. **Therapeutic Effect:** Prevents allergic responses mediated by histamine (urticaria, pruritus). Prevents, relieves nausea/vomiting. Produces mild sedative effect.

PHARMACOKINETICS

Route	Onset	Peak	Duration
PO	20 min	N/A	2–8 hrs
IV	3–5 min	N/A	2–8 hrs
IM	20 min	N/A	2–8 hrs
Rectal	20 min	N/A	2–8 hrs

Well absorbed from GI tract after IM administration. Widely distributed. Metabolized in liver. Primarily excreted in urine. Not removed by hemodialysis. **Half-life:** 16–19 hrs.

USES

Treatment of allergic conditions, motion sickness, nausea, vomiting. May be used as mild sedative.

PRECAUTIONS

CONTRAINDICATIONS: Narrow angle glaucoma, children 2 yrs and younger (may cause fatal respiratory depression), GI/GU obstruction, hypersensitivity to phenothiazines, severe CNS depression, coma. **CAUTIONS:** Cardiovascular/hepatic impairment, asthma, peptic ulcer, history of seizures, sleep apnea, pts suspected of Reye's syndrome.

LIFESPAN CONSIDERATIONS:

Pregnancy/Lactation: Readily crosses placenta. Unknown if drug is excreted in

P

breast milk. May inhibit platelet aggregation in neonates if taken within 2 wks of birth. May produce jaundice, extrapyramidal symptoms (EPS) in neonates if taken during pregnancy. **Pregnancy Category C. Children:** May experience increased excitement. Not recommended for those younger than 2 yrs. **Elderly:** More sensitive to dizziness, sedation, confusion, hypotension, hyperexcitability, anticholinergic effects (e.g., dry mouth).

INTERACTIONS

DRUG: Alcohol, CNS depressants may increase CNS depressant effects. **Anticholinergics** may increase anticholinergic effects. **MAOIs** may prolong, intensify anticholinergic, CNS depressant effects. **HERBAL: Gotu kola, kava kava, St. John's wort, valerian** may increase CNS depression. **FOOD:** None known. **LAB VALUES:** May suppress wheal/flare reactions to antigen skin testing unless discontinued 4 days before testing.

AVAILABILITY (Rx)

INJECTION SOLUTION (PHENERGAN): 25 mg/ml, 50 mg/ml. **SUPPOSITORIES:** (Phenadoz, Phenergan, Promethegan), 12.5 mg, 25 mg, 50 mg. **SYRUP (PHENERGAN):** 6.25 mg/ml. **TABLETS (PHENERGAN):** 12.5 mg, 25 mg, 50 mg.

P

ADMINISTRATION/HANDLING

◀ **ALERT** ▶ Significant tissue necrosis may occur if given subcutaneously. Inadvertent intra-arterial injection may produce severe arteriospasm, resulting in severe circulation impairment.

IV

Reconstitution • Dilute with 10–20 ml 0.9% NaCl or prepare minibag.

Rate of administration • Administer slowly over 10–15 min. • Use large vein or central venous site (no hand or wrist veins). • Too-rapid rate of infusion may result in transient fall in B/P, producing orthostatic hypotension, reflex tachycardia, serious tissue injury.

Storage • Store at room temperature.

IM

• Inject deep IM.

PO

• Give without regard to meals. • Scored tablets may be crushed.

RECTAL

• Refrigerate suppository. • Moisten suppository with cold water before inserting well into rectum.

IV INCOMPATIBILITIES

Allopurinol (Aloprim), amphotericin B complex (Abelcet, AmBisome, Amphotec), heparin, ketorolac (Toradol), nalbuphine (Nubain), piperacillin and tazobactam (Zosyn).

IV COMPATIBILITIES

Atropine, diphenhydramine (Benadryl), glycopyrrolate (Robinul), hydromorphone (Dilaudid), hydroxyzine (Vistaril), meperidine (Demerol), midazolam (Versed), morphine, prochlorperazine (Compazine).

INDICATIONS/ROUTES/DOSAGE

◀ **ALERT** ▶ Contraindicated in children 2 yrs and younger.

ALLERGIC SYMPTOMS

PO: ADULTS, ELDERLY: 6.25–12.5 mg 3 times a day plus 25 mg at bedtime. **CHILDREN:** 0.1 mg/kg/dose (**maximum:** 12.5 mg) 3 times a day plus 0.5 mg/kg/dose (**maximum:** 25 mg) at bedtime.

IV, IM: ADULTS, ELDERLY: 6.25–25 mg. May repeat in 2 hrs.

MOTION SICKNESS

PO: ADULTS, ELDERLY: 25 mg 30–60 min before departure; may repeat in 8–12 hrs, then every morning on rising and before evening meal. **CHILDREN:** 0.5 mg/kg 30–60 min before departure; may repeat in 8–12 hrs, then every morning on rising and before evening meal. **Maximum:** 25 mg 2 times/day.

PREVENTION OF NAUSEA/VOMITING

PO, IV, IM, RECTAL: ADULTS, ELDERLY: 6.25–25 mg q4–6h as needed. **CHILDREN:** 0.25–1 mg/kg q4–6h as needed.

PREOP/POSTOP SEDATION, ADJUNCT TO ANALGESICS

IV, IM: ADULTS, ELDERLY: 25–50 mg. **CHILDREN:** 12.5–25 mg.

SEDATIVE

PO, IV, IM, RECTAL: ADULTS, ELDERLY: 25–50 mg/dose. May repeat q4–6h as needed. **CHILDREN:** 0.5–1 mg/kg/dose q6h as needed. **Maximum:** 50 mg/dose.

SIDE EFFECTS

EXPECTED: Drowsiness, disorientation; hypotension, confusion, syncope in elderly. **FREQUENT:** Dry mouth, nose, throat; urinary retention; thickening of bronchial secretions. **OCCASIONAL:** Epigastric distress, flushing, visual disturbances, hearing disturbances, wheezing, paresthesia, diaphoresis, chills. **RARE:** Dizziness, urticaria, photosensitivity, nightmares.

ADVERSE EFFECTS/ TOXIC REACTIONS

Paradoxical reaction (particularly in children) manifested as excitation, anxiety, tremor, hyperactive reflexes, seizures. Long-term therapy may produce extrapyramidal symptoms noted as dystonia (abnormal movements), pronounced motor restlessness (most frequently in children), parkinsonian (esp. noted in elderly). Blood dyscrasias, particularly agranulocytosis, occur rarely.

NURSING CONSIDERATIONS

BASELINE ASSESSMENT

Assess B/P, pulse for bradycardia, tachycardia if pt is given parenteral form. If used as antiemetic, assess for dehydration (poor skin turgor, dry mucous membranes, longitudinal furrows in tongue).

INTERVENTION/EVALUATION

Monitor serum electrolytes in pts with severe vomiting. Assist with ambulation if drowsiness, light-headedness occurs.

PATIENT/FAMILY TEACHING

• Drowsiness, dry mouth may be expected response to drug. • Avoid tasks that require alertness, motor skills until response to drug is established. • Sugarless gum, sips of tepid water may relieve dry mouth. • Coffee, tea may help reduce drowsiness. • Report visual disturbances. • Avoid alcohol, other CNS depressants.

Prometrium, *see progesterone*

propafenone

proe-**pa**-fen-one
(Rythmol, Rythmol SR)

CLASSIFICATION

CLINICAL: Antiarrhythmic (see p. 15C).

ACTION

Decreases fast sodium current in Purkinje/myocardial cells. Decreases excitability, automaticity; prolongs conduction velocity, refractory period. **Therapeutic Effect:** Suppresses arrhythmias.

PHARMACOKINETICS

Nearly completely absorbed following PO administration. Protein binding: 85%–97%. Metabolized in liver; undergoes first-pass metabolism. Primarily excreted in feces. **Half-life:** 2–10 hrs.

USES

Treatment of documented, life-threatening ventricular arrhythmias (e.g., sustained ventricular tachycardias). **Rythmol SR:** Maintenance of normal sinus rhythm in pts with symptomatic atrial fibrillation. **OFF-LABEL:** Treatment of supraventricular arrhythmias.

PRECAUTIONS

CONTRAINDICATIONS: Bradycardia; bronchospastic disorders; cardiogenic shock; electrolyte imbalance; sinoatrial, AV, intraventricular impulse generation or conduction disorders (e.g., sick sinus syndrome, AV block) without pacemaker; uncontrolled CHF. **CAUTIONS:**Renal/hepatic impairment, recent MI, CHF, conduction disturbances.

⌛ LIFESPAN CONSIDERATIONS:

Pregnancy/Lactation: Unknown if drug crosses placenta or is distributed in breast milk. **Pregnancy Category C.** **Children:** Safety and efficacy not established. **Elderly:** No age-related precautions noted.

P

INTERACTIONS

DRUG: May increase concentrations of **digoxin, propranolo**l. May increase **warfarin** effects. **HERBAL: St. John's wort** may decrease concentration, effect. **Ephedra** may worsen arrhythmnias. **FOOD:** None known. **LAB VALUES:** May cause EKG changes (e.g., QRS widening, PR interval prolongation), positive ANA titers.

AVAILABILITY (Rx)

TABLETS (RYTHMOL): 150 mg, 225 mg, 300 mg.

CAPSULES (EXTENDED-RELEASE [RYTHMOL SR]): 225 mg, 325 mg, 425 mg.

INDICATIONS/ROUTES/DOSAGE

DOCUMENTED, LIFE-THREATENING VENTRICULAR ARRHYTHMIAS (SUSTAINED VENTRICULAR TACHYCARDIA)

PO: ADULTS, ELDERLY: Initially, 150 mg q8h; may increase at 3- to 4-day intervals to 225 mg q8h, then to 300 mg q8h. **Maximum:** 900 mg/day.

PO (EXTENDED-RELEASE): ADULTS, ELDERLY: Initially, 225 mg q12h. May increase at 5 day intervals. **Maximum:** 425 mg q12h.

SIDE EFFECTS

FREQUENT (13%–7%): Dizziness, nausea, vomiting, altered taste, constipation. **OCCASIONAL (6%–3%):** Headache, dyspnea, blurred vision, dyspepsia (heartburn, indigestion, epigastric pain). **RARE (less than 2%):** Rash, weakness, dry mouth, diarrhea, edema, hot flashes.

ADVERSE EFFECTS/ TOXIC REACTIONS

May produce/worsen existing arrhythmias. Overdose may produce hypotension, somnolence, bradycardia, atrioventricular conduction disturbances.

NURSING CONSIDERATIONS

BASELINE ASSESSMENT

Correct electrolyte imbalance before administering medication.

INTERVENTION/EVALUATION

Assess pulse for quality, irregular rate. Monitor EKG for cardiac performance or changes, particularly widening of QRS, prolongation of PR interval. Question for visual disturbances, headache, GI upset. Monitor fluid, serum electrolyte levels. Monitor daily pattern of bowel activity/stool consistency. Assess for dizziness, unsteadiness. Monitor hepatic enzymes results Monitor for therapeutic serum level (0.06–1 mcg/ml).

PATIENT/FAMILY TEACHING

• Compliance with therapy regimen is essential to control arrhythmias. • Altered taste sensation may occur. • Report headache, blurred vision. • Avoid tasks that require alertness, motor skills until response to drug is established.

propofol

pro-poe-fall
(Diprivan)

CLASSIFICATION

PHARMACOTHERAPEUTIC: Rapid-acting general anesthetic. **CLINICAL:** Sedative-hypnotic (see p. 3C).

ACTION

Inhibits sympathetic vasoconstrictor nerve activity; decreases vascular resistance. **Therapeutic Effect:** Produces hypnosis rapidly.

PHARMACOKINETICS

Route	Onset	Peak	Duration
IV	40 sec	N/A	3–10 min

Rapidly, extensively distributed. Protein binding: 97%–99%. Metabolized in liver. Primarily excreted in urine. Unknown if removed by hemodialysis. **Half-life:** 3–12 hrs.

USES

Induction/maintenance of anesthesia. Continuous sedation in intubated and respiratory controlled adult pts in ICU. **OFF-LABEL:** Postoperative antiemetic, refractory delirium tremens, conscious sedation.

PRECAUTIONS

CONTRAINDICATIONS: Impaired cerebral circulation, increased intracranial pressure (ICP). **CAUTIONS:** Debilitated; impaired respiratory, circulatory, renal, hepatic, lipid metabolism disorders; history of epilepsy, seizure disorder.

LIFESPAN CONSIDERATIONS:

Pregnancy/Lactation: Unknown if drug crosses placenta. Distributed in breast milk. Not recommended for obstetrics, breast-feeding mothers. **Pregnancy Category B. Children:** Safety and efficacy not established. FDA approved for use in those 2 mos and older. **Elderly:** No age-related precautions noted; lower dosages recommended.

INTERACTIONS

DRUG: Alcohol, CNS depressants may increase CNS, respiratory depression, hypotensive effects. **HERBAL:** None significant. **FOOD:** None known. **LAB VALUES:** None known.

AVAILABILITY (Rx)

INJECTION EMULSION: 10 mg/ml.

ADMINISTRATION/HANDLING

IV

◄ **ALERT** ► Do not give through same IV line with blood or plasma.

Reconstitution • May give undiluted, or dilute only with D_5W. • Do not dilute to concentration less than 2 mg/ml (4 ml D_5W to 1 ml propofol yields 2 mg/ml).

Rate of administration • Too-rapid IV may produce marked severe hypotension, respiratory depression, irregular muscular movements. • Observe for signs of intra-arterial injection (pain, discolored skin patches, white or blue color to peripheral IV site area, delayed onset of drug action).

Storage • Store at room temperature. • Discard unused portions. • Do not use if emulsion separates. • Shake well before using.

IV INCOMPATIBILITIES

Amikacin (Amikin), amphotericin B complex (Abelcet, AmBisome, Amphotec), bretylium (Bretylol), calcium chloride, ciprofloxacin (Cipro), diazepam (Valium), digoxin (Lanoxin), doxorubicin (Adriamycin), gentamicin (Garamycin), methylprednisolone (Solu-Medrol), minocycline (Minocin), phenytoin (Dilantin), tobramycin (Nebcin), verapamil (Isoptin).

IV COMPATIBILITIES

Acyclovir (Zovirax), bumetanide (Bumex), calcium gluconate, ceftazidime (Fortaz), dobutamine (Dobutrex), dopamine (Intropin), enalapril (Vasotec), fentanyl, heparin, insulin, labetalol (Normodyne, Trandate), lidocaine, lorazepam (Ativan), magnesium, milrinone (Primacor), nitroglycerin, norepinephrine (Levophed), potassium chloride, vancomycin (Vancocin).

INDICATIONS/ROUTES/DOSAGE

ANESTHESIA

IV: **ADULTS, ELDERLY:** Induction, 20–40 mg every 10 sec until induction onset, then infusion of 50–200 mcg/kg/min with 20–50 mg bolus as needed. **CHILDREN 3–16 YRS:** Induction, 2.5–3.5 mg/kg over 20–30 sec, then infusion of 125–300 mcg/kg/min.

SEDATION IN ICU

IV: **ADULTS, ELDERLY:** Initially, 5 mcg/kg/min for 5 min, then titrate to 5–50 mcg/kg/min in 5–10 mcg/kg/min increments allowing minimum of 5 min between dose adjustments.

SIDE EFFECTS

FREQUENT: Involuntary muscle movements, apnea (common during induction; lasts longer than 60 sec), hypotension, nausea, vomiting, IV site burning/stinging. **OCCASIONAL:** Twitching, bucking, jerking, thrashing, headache, dizziness, bradycardia, hypertension, fever, abdominal cramps, paresthesia, coldness, cough, hiccups, facial flushing, greenish-colored urine. **RARE:** Rash, dry mouth, agitation, confusion, myalgia, thrombophlebitis.

ADVERSE EFFECTS/ TOXIC REACTIONS

Continuous infusion or repeated intermittent infusions of propofol may result in extreme somnolence, respiratory depression, circulatory depression. Too-rapid IV administration may produce severe hypotension, respiratory depression, involuntary muscle movements. Pt may experience acute allergic reaction, characterized by abdominal pain, anxiety, restlessness, dyspnea, erythema, hypotension, pruritus, rhinitis, urticaria.

NURSING CONSIDERATIONS

BASELINE ASSESSMENT

Resuscitative equipment, suction, O_2 must be available. Obtain vital signs before administration.

INTERVENTION/EVALUATION

Monitor respiratory rate, B/P, heart rate, O_2 saturation, ABGs, depth of sedation, serum lipid, triglycerides if used longer than 24 hrs. May change urine color to green.

propoxyphene hydrochloride

(Darvon)

propoxyphene napsylate

(Darvon-N)

pro-**pox**-ih-feen

Do not confuse Darvon with Diovan.

FIXED-COMBINATION(S)

Balacet 325: propoxyphene/acetaminophen: 100 mg/325 mg. **Darvocet-N:** propoxyphene/acetaminophen: 50 mg/325 mg; 100 mg/650 mg. **Darvocet A500:** propoxyphene/acetaminophen: 100 mg/500 mg.

◆CLASSIFICATION

PHARMACOTHERAPEUTIC: Opioid agonist. (**Schedule IV**). **CLINICAL:** Analgesic (see p. 136C).

ACTION

Binds with opioid receptors within CNS. **Therapeutic Effect:** Alters perception of and emotional response to pain.

PHARMACOKINETICS

Route	Onset	Peak	Duration
PO	15–60 min	N/A	4–6 hrs

Well absorbed from GI tract. Protein binding: High. Widely distributed. Metabolized in liver. Primarily excreted in urine. Not removed by hemodialysis. **Half-life:** 6–12 hrs; metabolite: 30–36 hrs.

USES

Relief of mild to moderate pain.

PRECAUTIONS

CONTRAINDICATIONS: None known. **CAUTIONS:** Renal/hepatic impairment, substitution for opiates in narcotic-dependent pts.

⌛ LIFESPAN CONSIDERATIONS:

Pregnancy/Lactation: Crosses placenta. Minimal amount distributed in breast milk. Respiratory depression may occur in neonate if mother received opiates during labor. Regular use of opiates during pregnancy may produce withdrawal symptoms in neonate (irritability, excessive crying, tremors, hyperactive reflexes, fever, vomiting, diarrhea, yawning, sneezing, seizures). **Pregnancy Category C (D if used for prolonged periods). Children:** Dosage not established. **Elderly:** May be more susceptible to CNS effects, constipation. Avoid use if possible.

INTERACTIONS

DRUG: **Alcohol, CNS depressants** may increase CNS/respiratory depression, risk of hypotension. Effects may be decreased with **buprenorphine.** May increase **carbamazepine** concentration, toxicity. **MAOIs** may produce severe, sometimes fatal reaction (reduce dose to 25% usual dose). **HERBAL:** None significant. **FOOD:** None known. **LAB VALUES:** May increase serum alkaline phosphatase, lipase, amylase, bilirubin, LDH, AST, ALT. Therapeutic serum drug level: 100–400 ng/ml; toxic serum level: greater than 500 ng/ml.

AVAILABILITY (Rx)

CAPSULES (HYDROCHLORIDE [DARVON]): 65 mg. **TABLETS (NAPSYLATE [DARVON-N]):** 100 mg.

ADMINISTRATION/HANDLING

PO

- Give without regard to meals.
- Capsules may be emptied, mixed with food.

INDICATIONS/ROUTES/DOSAGE

MILD TO MODERATE PAIN

PO (PROPOXYPHENE HYDROCHLORIDE): ADULTS, ELDERLY: 65 mg q4h as needed. **Maximum:** 390 mg/day.

PO (PROPOXYPHENE NAPSYLATE): ADULTS, ELDERLY: 100 mg q4h as needed. **Maximum:** 600 mg/day.

SIDE EFFECTS

FREQUENT: Dizziness, drowsiness, dry mouth, euphoria, hypotension (including orthostatic hypotension), nausea,

P

vomiting, fatigue. **OCCASIONAL:** Allergic reaction (including decreased B/P), diaphoresis, flushing, wheezing, trembling, urinary retention, vision changes, constipation, headache. **RARE:** Confusion, increased B/P, depression, abdominal cramps, anorexia.

ADVERSE EFFECTS/ TOXIC REACTIONS

Overdose results in respiratory depression, skeletal muscle flaccidity, cold/clammy skin, cyanosis, extreme somnolence progressing to seizures, stupor, coma. Hepatotoxicity may occur with overdose of acetaminophen component of fixed-combination products. Tolerance to analgesic effect, physical dependence may occur with repeated use.

NURSING CONSIDERATIONS

BASELINE ASSESSMENT

Obtain vital signs before giving medication. If respirations are 12/min or less (20/min or less in children), withhold medication, contact physician. Assess onset, type, location, duration of pain. Effect of medication is reduced if full pain recurs before next dose.

INTERVENTION/EVALUATION

Palpate bladder for urinary retention. Monitor daily pattern of bowel activity/stool consistency. Initiate deep breathing and coughing exercises, particularly in pts with pulmonary impairment. Assess for clinical improvement, record onset of relief of pain. Contact physician if pain is not adequately relieved. Therapeutic serum level: 100–400 ng/ml; toxic serum level: greater than 500 ng/ml.

PATIENT/FAMILY TEACHING

• Avoid alcohol. • May be habit forming. • May cause drowsiness, impair ability to perform tasks requiring mental alertness, coordination. • Do not discontinue abruptly.

propranolol

proe-**pran**-oh-lole
(Apo-Propranolol ♣, Inderal, Inderal LA, InnoPran XL, Nu-Propranolol ♣, Propranolol Intensol)

Do not confuse Inderal with Adderall or Isordil, or propranolol with Pravachol.

FIXED-COMBINATION(S)

Inderide: propranolol/hydrochlorothiazide (a diuretic): 40 mg/25 mg; 80 mg/25 mg. **Inderide LA:** propranolol/hydrochlorothiazide (a diuretic): 80 mg/50 mg; 120 mg/50 mg; 160 mg/50 mg.

CLASSIFICATION

PHARMACOTHERAPEUTIC: Beta-adrenergic blocker. **CLINICAL:** Antihypertensive, antianginal, antiarrhythmic, antimigraine (see p. 15C).

ACTION

Blocks $beta_1$-, $beta_2$-adrenergic receptors. Decreases oxygen requirements. Slows AV conduction, increases refractory period in AV node. Large doses increase airway resistance. **Therapeutic Effect:** Slows heart rate; decreases cardiac output, B/P, myocardial ischemia severity. Exhibits antiarrhythmic activity.

PHARMACOKINETICS

Route	Onset	Peak	Duration
PO	1–2 hrs	N/A	6 hrs

Well absorbed from GI tract. Protein binding: 93%. Widely distributed. Metabolized in liver. Primarily excreted in urine. Not removed by hemodialysis. **Half-life:** 3–5 hrs.

USES

Treatment of angina pectoris, arrhythmias, essential tremors, hypertension, hypertrophic subaortic stenosis, migraine headache, pheochromocytoma, post-MI. **OFF-LABEL:** Treatment adjunct for anxiety, mitral valve prolapse syndrome, thyrotoxicosis.

PRECAUTIONS

CONTRAINDICATIONS: Asthma, bradycardia, cardiogenic shock, chronic obstructive pulmonary disease (COPD), heart block, Raynaud's syndrome, uncompensated CHF. **CAUTIONS:** Diabetes, renal/hepatic impairment, concurrent use of calcium blockers when using IV form.

LIFESPAN CONSIDERATIONS:

Pregnancy/Lactation: Crosses placenta. Distributed in breast milk. Avoid use during first trimester. May produce low birth-weight infants, bradycardia, apnea, hypoglycemia, hypothermia during delivery. **Pregnancy Category C (D if used in second or third trimester).** **Children:** No age-related precautions noted. **Elderly:** Age-related peripheral vascular disease may increase susceptibility to decreased peripheral circulation.3

INTERACTIONS

DRUG: **Diuretics, other antihypertensives** may increase hypotensive effect. May mask symptoms of hypoglycemia, prolong hypoglycemic effect of **insulin, oral hypoglycemics**. **IV phenytoin** may increase cardiac depressant effect. **NSAIDs** may decrease antihypertensive effect. **HERBAL:** **Ephedra, ginseng, yohimbe** may worsen hypertension. **Licorice** may increase water retention. **Garlic** has antihypertensive effects. **FOOD:** None known. **LAB VALUES:** May increase serum antinuclear antibody (ANA) titer, BUN, serum LDH, lipoprotein, alkaline phosphatase, bilirubin, creatinine, potassium, uric acid, AST, ALT, triglycerides.

AVAILABILITY (Rx)

INJECTION SOLUTION (INDERAL): 1 mg/ml. **ORAL CONCENTRATE (PROPRANOLOL INTENSOL):** 80 mg/ml. **ORAL SOLUTION (INDERAL):** 20 mg/5 ml, 40 mg/5 ml. **TABLETS (INDERAL):** 10 mg, 20 mg, 40 mg, 60 mg, 80 mg.

CAPSULES (EXTENDED-RELEASE [INNOPRAN XL]): 80 mg, 120 mg. **CAPSULES (SUSTAINED-RELEASE [INDERAL LA]):** 60 mg, 80 mg, 120 mg, 160 mg.

ADMINISTRATION/HANDLING

IV

Reconstitution • Give undiluted for IV push. • For IV infusion, may dilute each 1 mg in 10 ml D_5W.

Rate of administration • Do not exceed 1 mg/min injection rate. • For IV infusion, give 1 mg over 10–15 min.

Storage • Store at room temperature.

PO

• May crush scored tablets. • Give at same time each day.

IV INCOMPATIBILITY

Amphotericin B complex (Abelcet, AmBisome, Amphotec).

IV COMPATIBILITIES

Alteplase (Activase), heparin, milrinone (Primacor), potassium chloride, propofol (Diprivan).

INDICATIONS/ROUTES/DOSAGE

HYPERTENSION

PO: ADULTS, ELDERLY: Initially, 40 mg twice a day. May increase dose q3–7 days. Range: Up to 320 mg/day in divided doses. **Maximum:** 640 mg/day.

PO: (LONG-ACTING): Initially, 80 mg once daily. May increase up to 120–160 mg once daily. **CHILDREN:** Initially, 0.5–1 mg/kg/day in divided doses q6–12h. May increase at 3- to 5-day intervals. Usual dose: 1–5 mg/kg/day. **Maximum:** 16 mg/kg/day.

P

ANGINA
PO: ADULTS, ELDERLY: 80–320 mg/day in divided doses.
PO (LONG ACTING): Initially, 80 mg/day. **Maximum:** 320 mg/day.

ARRHYTHMIA
IV: ADULTS, ELDERLY: 1–3 mg. May repeat after 2 min. Additional doses in not less than 4 hrs. **CHILDREN:** 0.01–0.1 mg/kg. **Maximum:** infants, 1 mg; children, 3 mg.

PO: ADULTS, ELDERLY: Initially, 10–20 mg q6-8h. May gradually increase dose. Range: 40–320 mg/day. **CHILDREN:** Initially, 0.5–1 mg/kg/day in divided doses q6–8h. May increase q3–5days. Usual dosage: 2–4 mg/kg/day. **Maximum:** 16 mg/kg/day or 60 mg/day.

LIFE-THREATENING ARRHYTHMIA
IV: ADULTS, ELDERLY: 0.5–3 mg. Repeat once in 2 min. Give additional doses at intervals of at least 4 hrs. **CHILDREN:** 0.01–0.1 mg/kg.

HYPERTROPHIC SUBAORTIC STENOSIS
PO: ADULTS, ELDERLY: 20–40 mg in 3–4 divided doses or 80–160 mg/day as extended-release capsule.

ADJUNCT TO ALPHA-BLOCKING AGENTS TO TREAT PHEOCHROMOCYTOMA
PO: ADULTS, ELDERLY: 60 mg/day in divided doses with alpha-blocker for 3 days before surgery. Maintenance (inoperable tumor): 30 mg/day with alpha-blocker.

MIGRAINE HEADACHE
PO: ADULTS, ELDERLY: 80 mg/day in divided doses or 80 mg once daily as extended-release capsule. Increase up to 160–240 mg/day in divided doses. **CHILDREN:** 0.6–1.5 mg/kg/day in divided doses q8h. **Maximum:** 4 mg/kg/day.

REDUCTION OF CARDIOVASCULAR MORTALITY, REINFARCTION IN PTS WITH PREVIOUS MI
PO: ADULTS, ELDERLY: 180–240 mg/day in divided doses.

ESSENTIAL TREMOR
PO: ADULTS, ELDERLY: Initially, 40 mg twice a day increased up to 120–320 mg/day in 3 divided doses.

SIDE EFFECTS

FREQUENT: Diminished sexual function, drowsiness, difficulty sleeping, unusual fatigue/weakness. **OCCASIONAL:** Bradycardia, depression, sensation of coldness in extremities, diarrhea, constipation, anxiety, nasal congestion, nausea, vomiting. **RARE:** Altered taste, dry eyes, pruritus, paresthesia.

ADVERSE EFFECTS/ TOXIC REACTIONS

Overdose may produce profound bradycardia, hypotension. Abrupt withdrawal may result in diaphoresis, palpitations, headache, tremulousness. May precipitate CHF, MI in pts with cardiac disease; thyroid storm in those with thyrotoxicosis; peripheral ischemia in those with existing peripheral vascular disease. Hypoglycemia may occur in pts with previously controlled diabetes.

NURSING CONSIDERATIONS

BASELINE ASSESSMENT

Assess baseline renal/hepatic function tests. Assess B/P, apical pulse immediately before administering drug (if pulse is 60/min or less or systolic B/P is less than 90 mm Hg, withhold medication, contact physician). **Anginal:** Record onset, quality, radiation, location, intensity, duration of anginal pain, precipitating factors (exertion, emotional stress).

INTERVENTION/EVALUATION

Assess pulse for quality, irregular rate, bradycardia. Monitor EKG for cardiac arrhythmias. Assess fingers for color, numbness (Raynaud's). Assess for evidence of CHF (dyspnea [particularly on exertion or lying down]; night cough, peripheral edema, distended neck veins). Monitor I&O (increase in weight, decrease in urinary output may indicate CHF). Assess for rash, fatigue, behavioral changes. Therapeutic response ranges from a few days to several wks. Measure B/P near end of dosing interval (determines if B/P is controlled throughout day).

PATIENT/FAMILY TEACHING

• Do not abruptly discontinue medication. Compliance with therapy regimen is essential to control hypertension, arrhythmia, anginal pain. • To avoid hypotensive effect, rise slowly from lying to sitting position, wait momentarily before standing. • Avoid tasks that require alertness, motor skills until response to drug is established. • Report excessively slow pulse rate (less than 60 beats/min), peripheral numbness, dizziness. • Do not use nasal decongestants, OTC cold preparations (stimulants) without physician approval. • Restrict salt, alcohol intake.

propylthiouracil

proe-pill-thye-oh-**yoor**-a-sill (Propylthiouracil, Propyl-Thyracil ✤)

CLASSIFICATION

PHARMACOTHERAPEUTIC: Thiourea derivative. **CLINICAL:** Antithyroid.

ACTION

Blocks oxidation of iodine in thyroid gland, blocks synthesis of thyroxine, triiodothyronine. **Therapeutic Effect:** Inhibits synthesis of thyroid hormone.

PHARMACOKINETICS

Readily absorbed from GI tract. Protein binding: 80%. Metabolized in liver. Excreted in urine. **Half-life:** 1–4 hrs.

USES

Palliative treatment of hyperthyroidism; adjunct to ameliorate hyperthyroidism in preparation for surgical treatment, radioactive iodine therapy.

PRECAUTIONS

CONTRAINDICATIONS: Breast-feeding mothers. **CAUTIONS:** Pts older than 40 yrs or in combination with other agranulocytosis-inducing drugs. **Pregnancy Category D.**

INTERACTIONS

DRUG: **Amiodarone, iodinated glycerol, iodine, potassium iodide** may decrease response. May increase concentration of **digoxin** (as pt becomes euthyroid). May decrease thyroid uptake of ^{131}**I.** May decrease effect of **oral anticoagulants. HERBAL:** None significant. **FOOD:** None known. **LAB VALUES:** May increase LDH, serum alkaline phosphatase, bilirubin, AST, ALT, prothrombin time.

AVAILABILITY (Rx)

TABLETS: 50 mg.

INDICATIONS/ROUTES/DOSAGE

HYPERTHYROIDISM

PO: ADULTS, ELDERLY: Initially: 300–450 mg/day in divided doses q8h. Maintenance: 100–150 mg/day in divided doses q8–12h. **CHILDREN:** Initially: 5–7 mg/kg/day in divided doses q8h. Maintenance: 33%–66% of initial dose in divided doses q8–12h. **NEONATES:** 5–10 mg/kg/day in divided doses q8h.

SIDE EFFECTS

FREQUENT: Urticaria, rash, pruritus, nausea, skin pigmentation, hair loss, headache, paresthesia. **OCCASIONAL:** Drowsiness, lymphadenopathy, vertigo. **RARE:** Drug fever, lupus-like syndrome.

P

ADVERSE EFFECTS/ TOXIC REACTIONS

Agranulocytosis (may occur as long as 4 mos after therapy), pancytopenia, fatal hepatitis have occurred.

NURSING CONSIDERATIONS

BASELINE ASSESSMENT

Obtain baseline weight, pulse.

INTERVENTION/EVALUATION

Monitor pulse, weight daily. Check for skin eruptions, pruritus, swollen lymph glands. Be alert to hepatitis (nausea, vomiting, drowsiness, jaundice). Monitor hematology results for bone marrow suppression; check for signs of infection, bleeding.

PATIENT/FAMILY TEACHING

• Space evenly around the clock. • Teach pt, family to take resting pulse daily. • Report pulse rate less than 60 beats/min. • Seafood, iodine products may be restricted. • Report illness, unusual bleeding/bruising immediately. • Inform physician of sudden or continuous weight gain, cold intolerance, depression.

P

Proscar, *see finasteride*

protamine

proe-ta-meen

(Protamine ♣, Protamine sulfate)

Do not confuse protamine with ProAmatine, Protopam, or Protropin.

CLASSIFICATION

PHARMACOTHERAPEUTIC: Protein. **CLINICAL:** Heparin antagonist.

ACTION

Combines with heparin to form stable salt. **Therapeutic Effect:** Reduces anticoagulant activity of heparin.

PHARMACOKINETICS

Metabolized by fibrinolysin. **Half-life:** 7.4 min.

USES

Treatment of severe heparin overdose (causing hemorrhage). Neutralizes effects of heparin administered during extracorporeal circulation. **OFF-LABEL:** Treatment of low molecular weight heparin toxicity.

PRECAUTIONS

CONTRAINDICATIONS: None known. **CAUTIONS:** History of allergy to fish, seafood; vasectomized/infertile men; those on isophane (NPH) insulin, previous protamine therapy (propensity to hypersensitivity reaction).

LIFESPAN CONSIDERATIONS:

Pregnancy/Lactation: Unknown if drug crosses placenta or is distributed in breast milk. **Pregnancy Category C.** **Children:** Safety and efficacy not established. **Elderly:** No age-related precautions noted.

INTERACTIONS

DRUG: None significant. **HERBAL:** None significant. **FOOD:** None known. **LAB VALUES:** None known.

AVAILABILITY (Rx)

INJECTION SOLUTION: 10 mg/ml.

ADMINISTRATION/HANDLING

IV

Rate of administration • May give undiluted over 10 min. Do not exceed 5 mg/min (50 mg in any 10-min period).

Storage • Store vials at room temperature.

INDICATIONS/ROUTES/DOSAGE

HEPARIN OVERDOSE (ANTIDOTE, TREATMENT)

IV: ADULTS, ELDERLY: 1–1.5 mg protamine neutralizes 100 units heparin. Heparin disappears rapidly from circulation, reducing dosage demand for protamine as time elapses.

SIDE EFFECTS

FREQUENT: Decreased B/P, dyspnea. **OCCASIONAL:** Hypersensitivity reaction (urticaria, angioedema); nausea/vomiting, which generally occur in those sensitive to fish/seafood, vasectomized men, infertile men, those on isophane (NPH) insulin, those previously on protamine therapy. **RARE:** Back pain.

ADVERSE EFFECTS/ TOXIC REACTIONS

Too-rapid IV administration may produce acute hypotension, bradycardia, pulmonary hypertension, dyspnea, transient flushing, feeling of warmth. Heparin rebound may occur several hrs after heparin has been neutralized by protamine (usually evident 8–9 hrs after protamine administration). Heparin rebound occurs most often after arterial/ cardiac surgery.

NURSING CONSIDERATIONS

BASELINE ASSESSMENT

Check PT, aPTT, Hct; assess for bleeding.

INTERVENTION/EVALUATION

Monitor coagulation tests, aPTT or ACT, B/P, cardiac function.

Protonix, *see pantoprazole*

protriptyline

(Vivactil)

See Antidepressants (p. 37C)

Proventil HFA, *see albuterol*

Provigil, *see modafinil*

Prozac, *see fluoxetine*

pseudoephedrine

soo-doe-e-**fed**-rin

(Balminil Decongestant ✤, Biofed, Dimetapp 12 Hour Non Drowsy Extentabs, Dimetapp Decongestant, Dimetapp Decongestant Infant Drops, Genaphed, PMS-Pseudoephedrine ✤, Robidrine ✤, Sudafed, Sudafed 12 Hour, Sudafed 24 Hour)

FIXED-COMBINATION(S)

Advil Cold, Motrin Cold: pseudoephedrine/ibuprofen (NSAID): 30 mg/200 mg; 15 mg/100 mg per 5 ml. **Allegra-D:** pseudoephedrine/ fexofenadine (an antihistamine): 120 mg/60 mg. **Allegra D 24 Hour:** pseudoephedrine/fexofenadine: 240 mg/180 mg. **Claritin-D:** pseudoephedrine/loratadine (an antihistamine): 120 mg/5 mg; 240

P

mg/10 mg. **Clarinex-D 24-Hour:** pseudoephedrine/desloratadine (an antihistamine): 240 mg/5 mg. **Clarinex-D 12-Hour:** pseudoephedrine/desloratadine: 120 mg/2.5 mg. **Zyrtec-D:** pseudoephedrine/cetirizine (an antihistamine): 120 mg/5 mg.

CLASSIFICATION

PHARMACOTHERAPEUTIC: Sympathomimetic. **CLINICAL:** Nasal decongestant.

ACTION

Directly stimulates alpha-adrenergic, beta-adrenergic receptors. **Therapeutic Effect:** Produces vasoconstriction of respiratory tract mucosa; shrinks nasal mucous membranes; reduces edema, nasal congestion.

PHARMACOKINETICS

Route	Onset	Peak	Duration
PO (tablets, syrup)	15–30 min	N/A	4–6 hrs
PO (extended-release)	N/A	N/A	8–12 hrs

Well absorbed from GI tract. Partially metabolized in liver. Primarily excreted in urine. Not removed by hemodialysis. **Half-life:** 9–16 hrs (children, 3.1 hrs).

USES

Temporary relief of nasal congestion due to common cold, upper respiratory allergies, sinusitis. Enhances nasal, sinus drainage.

PRECAUTIONS

CONTRAINDICATIONS: Breast-feeding women, coronary artery disease, severe hypertension, use of MAOIs within 14 days. **Sustained release:** children younger than 12 yrs. **CAUTIONS:** Elderly, hyperthyroidism, diabetes, ischemic heart disease, prostatic hypertrophy.

LIFESPAN CONSIDERATIONS:

Pregnancy/Lactation: Crosses placenta. Distributed in breast milk. **Pregnancy Category C. Children:** Safety and efficacy not established in those younger than 2 yrs. **Elderly:** Age-related prostatic hypertrophy may require dosage adjustment.

INTERACTIONS

DRUG: May decrease effects of **antihypertensives, beta-blockers, diuretics. MAOIs** may increase cardiac stimulant, vasopressor effects. **HERBAL: Ephedra, yohimbe** may cause hypertension. **FOOD:** None known. **LAB VALUES:** None known.

AVAILABILITY (OTC)

LIQUID (SUDAFED CHILDREN'S): 15 mg/5 ml. **LIQUID, ORAL DROPS (DIMETAPP DECONGESTANT INFANT DROPS):** 7.5 mg/0.8 ml. **SYRUP, (BIOFED):** 30 mg/5 ml. **TABLETS (GENAPHED, SUDAFED):** 30 mg, 60 mg. **TABLETS CHEWABLE (SUDAFED CHILDREN'S):** 15 mg.

CAPLETS, EXTENDED-RELEASE: (CONTACT COLD, SUDAFED 12 HOUR): 120 mg. **TABLETS, EXTENDED-RELEASE (DIMETAPP 12 HOUR NON-DROWSY EXTENTABS):** 120 mg. **(SUDAFED 24 HOUR):** 240 mg.

◀ ALERT ▶ Pseudoephedrine is key ingredient in synthesizing methamphetamine. Many pharmacies have moved pseudoephedrine behind the counter due to concerns about its purchase and theft for purposes of methamphetamine manufacture.

ADMINISTRATION/HANDLING

PO

- Do not crush, chew extended-release forms; swallow whole.

INDICATIONS/ROUTES/DOSAGE

DECONGESTANT

PO: ADULTS, CHILDREN 12 YRS AND OLDER: 60 mg q4–6h. **Maximum:** 240 mg/day. **CHILDREN 6–11 YRS:** 30 mg q6h.

Maximum: 120 mg/day. **CHILDREN 2–5 YRS:** 15 mg q6h. **Maximum:** 60 mg/day. **CHILDREN YOUNGER THAN 2 YRS:** 4 mg/kg/day in divided doses q6h. **ELDERLY:** 30–60 mg q6h as needed.
PO (EXTENDED-RELEASE): ADULTS, CHILDREN 12 YRS AND OLDER: 120 mg q12h or 240 mg once daily.

SIDE EFFECTS

OCCASIONAL (10%–5%): Nervousness, restlessness, insomnia, tremor, headache. **RARE (4%–1%):** Diaphoresis, weakness.

ADVERSE EFFECTS/ TOXIC REACTIONS

Large doses may produce tachycardia, palpitations (particularly in pts with cardiac disease), light-headedness, nausea, vomiting. Overdose in those older than 60 yrs may result in hallucinations, CNS depression, seizures.

NURSING CONSIDERATIONS

PATIENT/FAMILY TEACHING

• Discontinue drug if adverse reactions occur. • Report insomnia, dizziness, tremors, tachycardia, palpitations.

psyllium

sill-ee-yum

(Fiberall, Hydrocil, Konsyl, Metamucil, Novo-Mucilax ✦, Perdiem)

CLASSIFICATION

PHARMACOTHERAPEUTIC: Bulk-forming laxative (see p. 117C).

ACTION

Dissolves and swells in water providing increased bulk, moisture content in stool. **Therapeutic Effect:** Promotes peristalsis, bowel motility.

PHARMACOKINETICS

Route	Onset	Peak	Duration
PO	12–24 hrs	2–3 days	N/A

Acts in small, large intestines.

USES

Treatment of chronic constipation, constipation associated with rectal disorders, management of irritable bowel syndrome (IBS).

PRECAUTIONS

CONTRAINDICATIONS: Fecal impaction, GI obstruction, undiagnosed abdominal pain. **CAUTIONS:** Esophageal strictures, ulcers, stenosis, intestinal adhesions.

LIFESPAN CONSIDERATIONS:

Pregnancy/Lactation: Safe for use in pregnancy. **Pregnancy Category B. Children:** Safety and efficacy not established for those younger than 6 yrs. **Elderly:** No age-related precautions noted.

INTERACTIONS

DRUG: May decrease effect of **digoxin, oral anticoagulants, salicylates** by decreasing absorption. May interfere with effects of **potassium-sparing diuretics, potassium supplements. HERBAL:** None significant. **FOOD:** None known. **LAB VALUES:** May increase serum glucose. May decrease serum potassium.

AVAILABILITY (OTC)

CAPSULES (METAMUCIL): 0.52 g. **GRANULES (PERDIEM):** 4 g/5 ml. **POWDER (FIBERALL, HYDROCIL, KONSYL, METAMUCIL). WAFER (METAMUCIL):** 3.4 g/dose.

ADMINISTRATION/HANDLING

PO

• Administer at least 2 hrs before or after other medication. • All doses should be followed with 8 oz liquid • Drink 6–8 glasses of water/day (aids stool

P

softening) • Do not swallow in dry form; mix with at least 1 full glass (8 oz) of liquid.

INDICATIONS/ROUTES/DOSAGE

◀ **ALERT** ▶ 3.4 g powder equals 1 rounded tsp, 1 packet, or 1 wafer.

CONSTIPATION, IRRITABLE BOWEL SYNDROME

PO: ADULTS, ELDERLY: 2–5 capsules/dose 1–3 times a day. 1–2 tsp granules 1–2 times a day. 1 rounded tsp or 1 tbsp of powder 1–3 times a day. 2 wafers 1–3 times a day. **CHILDREN 6–11 YRS:** ½–1 tsp powder in water 1–3 times a day.

SIDE EFFECTS

RARE: Some degree of abdominal discomfort, nausea, mild abdominal cramps, griping, faintness.

ADVERSE EFFECTS/ TOXIC REACTIONS

Esophageal/bowel obstruction may occur if administered with insufficient liquid (less than 250 ml).

NURSING CONSIDERATIONS

INTERVENTION/EVALUATION

Encourage adequate fluid intake. Assess bowel sounds for peristalsis. Monitor daily pattern of bowel activity/stool consistency. Monitor serum electrolytes in pts exposed to prolonged, frequent, excessive use of medication.

PATIENT/FAMILY TEACHING

• Take each dose with full glass (250 ml) of water. • Inadequate fluid intake may cause GI obstruction. • Institute measures to promote defecation (increase fluid intake, exercise, high-fiber diet).

Pulmicort Respules, *see budesonide*

Pulmicort Turbuhaler, *see budesonide*

pyrazinamide

pye-ra-**zin**-a-mide
(Pyrazinamide, Tebrazid ✦)

FIXED-COMBINATION(S)

Rifater: pyrazinamide/isoniazid/ rifampin (an antitubercular): 300 mg/50 mg/120 mg.

◆CLASSIFICATION

CLINICAL: Antitubercular.

ACTION

May disrupt mycobacterium tuberculosis membrane transport. **Therapeutic Effect:** Bacteriostatic or bactericidal, depending on drug concentration at infection site, susceptibility of infecting bacteria.

PHARMACOKINETICS

Nearly completely absorbed from GI tract. Protein binding: 5%–10%. Excreted in urine. **Half-life:** 9–23 hrs.

USES

In conjunction with at least one other antitubercular agent in treatment of clinical tuberculosis after failure of primary agents (isoniazid, rifampin).

PRECAUTIONS

CONTRAINDICATIONS: Severe hepatic dysfunction. **CAUTIONS:** Diabetes mellitus, renal impairment, history of gout, children (safety not established). Possible cross-sensitivity with isoniazid, ethionamide, niacin.

⌛ LIFESPAN CONSIDERATIONS:

Pregnancy/Lactation: Unknown if drug crosses placenta or is distributed in breast milk. **Pregnancy Category C.** **Children:** Safety and efficacy not established. **Elderly:** No age-related precautions noted.

INTERACTIONS

DRUG: May decrease effects of **allopurinol, colchicine, probenecid, sulfinpyrazone.** **HERBAL:** None significant. **FOOD:** None known. **LAB VALUES:** May increase AST, ALT, serum uric acid.

AVAILABILITY (Rx)

TABLETS: 500 mg.

INDICATIONS/ROUTES/DOSAGE

TUBERCULOSIS (IN COMBINATION WITH OTHER ANTITUBERCULARS)

PO: ADULTS: 15–30 mg/kg/day in 1–4 doses. **Maximum:** 3 g/day. **CHILDREN:** 20–40 mg/kg/day in 1 or 2 doses. **Maximum:** 2 g/day.

SIDE EFFECTS

FREQUENT: Arthralgia, myalgia (usually mild, self-limiting). **RARE:** Hypersensitivity reaction (rash, pruritus, urticaria), photosensitivity, gouty arthritis.

ADVERSE EFFECTS/ TOXIC REACTIONS

Hepatotoxicity, gouty arthritis, thrombocytopenia, anemia occur rarely.

NURSING CONSIDERATIONS

BASELINE ASSESSMENT

Question for hypersensitivity to pyrazinamide, isoniazid, ethionamide, niacin. Ensure collection of specimens for culture, sensitivity. Evaluate results of initial CBC, hepatic function tests, serum uric acid levels.

INTERVENTION/EVALUATION

Monitor hepatic function test results; be alert for hepatic reactions: jaundice, malaise, fever, liver tenderness, anorexia, nausea, vomiting (stop drug, notify physician promptly). Check serum uric acid levels; assess for hot, painful, swollen joints, esp. big toe, ankle, knee (gout). Evaluate serum blood glucose levels, diabetic status carefully (pyrazinamide makes management difficult). Assess for rash, skin eruptions. Monitor CBC for thrombocytopenia, anemia.

PATIENT/FAMILY TEACHING

• Do not skip doses; complete full length of therapy (may be mos or yrs). • Office visits, lab tests are essential part of treatment. • Take with food to reduce GI upset. • Avoid excessive exposure to sun, ultraviolet light until photosensitivity is determined. • Notify physician of any new symptom, immediately for jaundice (yellow sclera of eyes/skin); unusual fatigue; fever; loss of appetite; hot, painful, swollen joints.

P

pyridostigmine

peer-id-oh-**stig**-meen
(Mestinon, Mestinon SR ✤, Mestinon Timespan, Regonal)

Do not confuse pyridostigmine with physostigmine or Mesitonin with Mesantoin or Metatensin.

CLASSIFICATION

PHARMACOTHERAPEUTIC: Anticholinesterase. **CLINICAL:** Cholinergic muscle stimulant (see p. 86C).

ACTION

Prevents destruction of acetylcholine by inhibiting the enzyme acetylcholinesterase, enhancing impulse transmission across myoneural junction. **Therapeutic Effect:** Produces miosis; increases intestinal, skeletal muscle tone; stimulates salivary, sweat gland secretions.

PHARMACOKINETICS

Not protein bound. Excreted unchanged in urine. **Half-life:** Unknown.

USES

Improvement of muscle strength in control of myasthenia gravis, reversal of effects of nondepolarizing neuromuscular blocking agents after surgery.

PRECAUTIONS

CONTRAINDICATIONS: Mechanical GI/urinary tract obstruction, hypersensitivity to anticholinesterase agents. **CAUTIONS:** Bronchial asthma, bradycardia, epilepsy, recent coronary occlusion, vagotonia, hyperthyroidism, cardiac arrhythmias, peptic ulcer.

P

LIFESPAN CONSIDERATIONS:

Pregnancy/Lactation: Unknown if drug crosses placenta or is distributed in breast milk. **Pregnancy Category B.** **Children:** Safety and efficacy not established. **Elderly:** No age-related precautions noted.

INTERACTIONS

DRUG: Anticholinergics prevent, reverse effects. **Cholinesterase inhibitors** may increase risk of toxicity. Antagonizes effects of **neuromuscular blockers. Procainamide, quinidine** may antagonize action. **HERBAL:** None significant. **FOOD:** None known. **LAB VALUES:** None known.

AVAILABILITY (Rx)

INJECTION SOLUTION (MESTINON, REGONOL): 5 mg/ml. **SYRUP (MESTINON):** 60 mg/5 ml. **TABLETS (MESTINON):** <u>60 mg.</u>

TABLETS (EXTENDED-RELEASE [MESTINON TIMESPAN]): 180 mg.

ADMINISTRATION/HANDLING

IV, IM

- Give large parenteral doses concurrently with 0.6–1.2 mg atropine sulfate IV to minimize side effects.

PO

- Give with food, milk. • Tablets may be crushed; do not chew, crush extended-release tablets (may be broken). • Give larger dose at times of increased fatigue (e.g., for those with difficulty in chewing, 30–45 min before meals).

IV INCOMPATIBILITIES

Do not mix with any other medications.

INDICATIONS/ROUTES/DOSAGE

MYASTHENIA GRAVIS

PO: ADULTS, ELDERLY: Initially, 60 mg 3 times a day. Dosage increased at 48 hr intervals. Maintenance: 60 mg–1.5 g a day.

PO (EXTENDED-RELEASE): ADULTS, ELDERLY: 180–540 mg once or twice a day with at least a 6 hr interval between doses.

IV, IM: ADULTS, ELDERLY: 2 mg q2–3h. **CHILDREN, NEONATES:** 0.05–0.15 mg/kg/dose. **Maximum single dose:** 10 mg.

REVERSAL OF NONDEPOLARIZING NEUROMUSCULAR BLOCKADE

IV: ADULTS, ELDERLY: 10–20 mg with, or shortly after, 0.6–1.2 mg atropine sulfate or 0.3–0.6 mg glycopyrrolate. **CHILDREN:** 0.1–0.25 mg/kg/dose preceded by atropine or glycopyrrolate.

SIDE EFFECTS

FREQUENT: Miosis, increased GI/skeletal muscle tone, bradycardia, constriction of bronchi/ureters, diaphoresis, increased salivation. **OCCASIONAL:** Headache, rash, temporary decrease in diastolic B/P with mild reflex tachycardia, short periods of atrial fibrillation (in hyperthyroid pts), marked drop in B/P (in hypertensive pts).

ADVERSE EFFECTS/ TOXIC REACTIONS

Overdose may produce cholinergic crisis, manifested as increasingly severe muscle weakness (appears first in muscles involving chewing, swallowing, followed by muscle weakness of shoulder girdle, upper extremities), respiratory muscle paralysis, followed by pelvis girdle/leg muscle paralysis. Requires withdrawal of all cholinergic drugs and immediate use of 1–4 mg atropine sulfate IV for adults, 0.01 mg/kg for infants and children younger than 12 yrs.

NURSING CONSIDERATIONS

BASELINE ASSESSMENT

Larger doses should be given at time of greatest fatigue. Assess muscle strength before testing for diagnosis of myasthenia gravis and following drug administration. Avoid large doses in pts with megacolon, reduced GI motility.

INTERVENTION/EVALUATION

Have tissues readily available at pt's bedside. Monitor respirations closely during myasthenia gravis testing or if dosage is increased. Assess diligently for cholinergic reaction, bradycardia in myasthenic pt in crisis. Coordinate dosage time with periods of fatigue and increased/decreased muscle strength. Monitor for therapeutic response to medication (increased muscle strength, decreased fatigue, improved chewing/swallowing functions).

PATIENT/FAMILY TEACHING

- Report nausea, vomiting, diarrhea, diaphoresis, profuse salivary secretions, palpitations, muscle weakness, severe abdominal pain, difficulty breathing.

pyridoxine (vitamin B_6)

peer-i-**dox**-een

(Aminoxin)

Do not confuse pyridoxine with paroxetine, pralidoxime, or Pyridium.

CLASSIFICATION

PHARMACOTHERAPEUTIC: Coenzyme. **CLINICAL:** Vitamin (B_6) (see p. 150C).

ACTION

Coenzyme for various metabolic functions, including metabolism of proteins, carbohydrates, fats. Aids in breakdown of glycogen and in synthesis of gamma-aminobutyric acid (GABA) in CNS. **Therapeutic Effect:** Prevents pyridoxine deficiency. Increases excretion of certain drugs (e.g., isoniazid) that are pyridoxine antagonists.

PHARMACOKINETICS

Readily absorbed primarily in jejunum. Stored in liver, muscle, brain. Metabolized in liver. Primarily excreted in urine. Removed by hemodialysis. **Half-life:** 15–20 days.

USES

Prevention/treatment of vitamin B_6 deficiency, pyridoxine-dependent seizures in

P

infants, drug-induced neuritis (e.g., isoniazid).

PRECAUTIONS

CONTRAINDICATIONS: None known. **CAUTIONS:** None known.

LIFESPAN CONSIDERATIONS:

Pregnancy/Lactation: Crosses placenta. Distributed in breast milk. High dosages in utero may produce seizures in neonates. **Pregnancy Category A. Children/Elderly:** No age-related precautions noted.

INTERACTIONS

DRUG: Immunosuppressants, isoniazid, penicillamine may antagonize effect, causing anemia, peripheral neuritis. Reverses effects of **levodopa. HERBAL:** None significant. **FOOD:** None known. **LAB VALUES:** None known.

AVAILABILITY (OTC)

CAPSULES: 250 mg. **INJECTION SOLUTION (VITAMIN B_6):** 100 mg/ml. **TABLETS:** 25 mg, 50 mg, 100 mg, 250 mg, 500 mg. **TABLETS (ENTERIC-COATED [AMINOXIN]):** 20 mg.

P

ADMINISTRATION/HANDLING

◄ ALERT ► Give PO unless nausea, vomiting, malabsorption occurs. Avoid IV use in cardiac pts.

IV

• Give undiluted or may be added to IV solutions and given as infusion.

IV INCOMPATIBILITIES

Do not mix with any other medications.

INDICATIONS/ROUTES/DOSAGE

PYRIDOXINE DEFICIENCY

PO: ADULTS, ELDERLY: Initially, 2.5–10 mg/day; then 2.5 mg/day when clinical signs are corrected. **CHILDREN:** Initially, 5–25 mg/day for 3 wks, then 1.5–2.5 mg/day.

PYRIDOXINE-DEPENDENT SEIZURES

PO, IV, IM: INFANTS: Initially, 10–100 mg/day. Maintenance: **PO:** 50–100 mg/day.

DRUG-INDUCED NEURITIS

PO (TREATMENT): ADULTS, ELDERLY: 100–300 mg/day in divided doses. **CHILDREN:** 10–50 mg/day.

PO (PROPHYLAXIS): ADULTS, ELDERLY: 25–100 mg/day. **CHILDREN:** 1–2 mg/kg/day.

SIDE EFFECTS

OCCASIONAL: Stinging at IM injection site. **RARE:** Headache, nausea, somnolence, sensory neuropathy (paresthesia, unstable gait, clumsiness of hands) with high doses.

ADVERSE EFFECTS/ TOXIC REACTIONS

Long-term megadoses (2–6 g for longer than 2 mos) may produce sensory neuropathy (reduced deep tendon reflexes, profound impairment of sense of position in distal limbs, gradual sensory ataxia). Toxic symptoms subside when drug is discontinued. Seizures have occurred after IV megadoses.

NURSING CONSIDERATIONS

INTERVENTION/EVALUATION

Observe for improvement of deficiency symptoms, glossitis. Evaluate for nutritional adequacy.

PATIENT/FAMILY TEACHING

• Discomfort may occur with IM injection. • Encourage intake of foods rich in pyridoxine (legumes, soybeans, eggs, sunflower seeds, hazelnuts, organ meats, tuna, shrimp, carrots, avocados, bananas, wheat germ, bran).

quazepam

(Doral)

See Sedative-hypnotics (p. 140C)

quetiapine

kwe-tye-a-peen

(Seroquel)

CLASSIFICATION

PHARMACOTHERAPEUTIC: Dibenzapine derivative. **CLINICAL:** Antipsychotic (see p. 63C).

ACTION

Antagonizes dopamine, serotonin, histamine, alpha$_1$-adrenergic receptors. **Therapeutic Effect:** Diminishes psychotic disorders. Produces moderate sedation, few extrapyramidal effects. No anticholinergic effects.

PHARMACOKINETICS

Well absorbed after PO administration. Protein binding: 83%. Widely distributed in tissues; CNS concentration exceeds plasma concentration. Undergoes extensive first-pass metabolism in liver. Primarily excreted in urine. **Half-life:** 6 hrs.

USES

Management of manifestations of psychotic disorders. Short-term treatment of acute manic episodes and depressive episodes associated with bipolar disorder. **OFF-LABEL:** Autism, psychosis (children).

PRECAUTIONS

CONTRAINDICATIONS: None known. **CAUTIONS:** Alzheimer's dementia, history of breast cancer, cardiovascular disease (e.g., CHF, history of MI), cerebrovascular disease, hepatic impairment, dehydration, hypovolemia, history of drug abuse/dependence, seizures, hypothyroidism.

LIFESPAN CONSIDERATIONS:

Pregnancy/Lactation: Unknown if drug is distributed in breast milk. Not recommended for breast-feeding mothers. **Pregnancy Category C. Children:** Safety and efficacy not established. **Elderly:** No age-related precautions noted, but lower initial and target dosages may be necessary.

INTERACTIONS

DRUG: **Alcohol, other CNS depressants** may increase CNS depression. May increase hypotensive effects of **antihypertensives. Hepatic enzyme inducers (e.g., phenytoin)** may increase clearance. **HERBAL:** **St. John's wort** may decrease concentration. **Gotu kola, kava kava, St. John's wort, valerian** may increase CNS depression. **FOOD:** None known. **LAB VALUES:** May decrease total free thyroxine (T_4) serum levels. May increase serum cholesterol, triglycerides, AST, ALT. May produce false-positive pregnancy test result.

AVAILABILITY (Rx)

TABLETS: 25 mg, 50 mg, 100 mg, 200 mg, 300 mg, 400 mg.

ADMINISTRATION/HANDLING

PO

• Adjust dosage at 2-day intervals. • Initial dose, dosage titration should be lower in elderly, pts with hepatic impairment, debilitated, those predisposed to hypotensive reactions. • When restarting pts who have been off quetiapine for less than 1 wk, titration is not required and maintenance dose can be reinstituted. • When restarting pts who have been off quetiapine for longer than 1 wk,

Q

follow initial titration schedule. • Give without regard to food.

INDICATIONS/ROUTES/DOSAGE

PSYCHOTIC DISORDERS

PO: ADULTS, ELDERLY: Initially, 25 mg twice a day, then 25–50 mg 2–3 times a day on the second and third days, up to 300–400 mg/day in divided doses 2–3 times a day by the fourth day. Further adjustments of 25–50 mg twice a day may be made at intervals of 2 days or longer. Maintenance: 300–800 mg/day (adults); 50–200 mg/day (elderly).

MANIA IN BIPOLAR DISORDER

PO: ADULTS, ELDERLY: Initially, 50 mg twice a day for 1 day. May increase in increments of 100 mg/day to 200 mg twice a day on day 4. May increase in increments of 200 mg/day to 800 mg/day on day 6. Range: 400–800 mg/day.

SIDE EFFECTS

FREQUENT (19%–10%): Headache, drowsiness, dizziness. **OCCASIONAL (9%–3%):** Constipation, orthostatic hypotension, tachycardia, dry mouth, dyspepsia (heartburn, indigestion, epigastric pain), rash, asthenia (loss of strength, energy), abdominal pain, rhinitis. **RARE (2%):** Back pain, fever, weight gain.

ADVERSE EFFECTS/ TOXIC REACTIONS

Overdose may produce heart block, hypotension, hypokalemia, tachycardia.

NURSING CONSIDERATIONS

BASELINE ASSESSMENT

Assess behavior, appearance, emotional status, response to environment, speech pattern, thought content. Obtain baseline CBC, hepatic enzyme levels before initiating treatment and periodically thereafter.

INTERVENTION/EVALUATION

Assist with ambulation if dizziness occurs. Supervise suicidal-risk pt closely during early therapy (as psychosis, depression lessens, energy level improves, increasing suicide potential). Monitor B/P for hypotension. Assess pulse for tachycardia (esp. with rapid increase in dosage). Assess bowel activity for evidence of constipation. Assess for therapeutic response (improved thought content, increased ability to concentrate, improvement in self-care). Eye exam to detect cataract formation should be obtained q6mo during treatment.

PATIENT/FAMILY TEACHING

• Avoid exposure to extreme heat. • Drink fluids often, esp. during physical activity. • Take medication as ordered; do not stop taking or increase dosage. • Drowsiness generally subsides during continued therapy. • Avoid tasks that require alertness, motor skills until response to drug is established. • Avoid alcohol. • Change positions slowly to reduce hypotensive effect.

quinapril

kwin-na-pril

(Accupril)

Do not confuse Accupril with Accolate or Accutane.

FIXED-COMBINATION(S)

Accuretic: quinapril/hydrochlorothiazide (a diuretic): 10 mg/12.5 mg; 20 mg/12.5 mg; 20 mg/25 mg.

CLASSIFICATION

PHARMACOTHERAPEUTIC: Angiotensin-converting enzyme (ACE) inhibitor. **CLINICAL:** Antihypertensive (see p. 7C).

ACTION

Suppresses renin-angiotensin-aldosterone system, preventing conversion of angiotensin I to angiotensin II, a potent vasoconstrictor; may inhibit angiotensin II at local vascular renal sites. **Therapeutic Effect:** Reduces peripheral arterial resistance, B/P, pulmonary capillary wedge pressure; improves cardiac output.

PHARMACOKINETICS

Route	Onset	Peak	Duration
PO	1 hr	N/A	24 hrs

Readily absorbed from GI tract. Protein binding: 97%. Metabolized in liver, GI tract, extravascular tissue to active metabolite. Primarily excreted in urine. Minimal removal by hemodialysis. **Half-life:** 1–2 hrs; metabolite, 3 hrs (increased in renal impairment).

USES

Treatment of hypertension. Used alone or in combination with other antihypertensives. Adjunctive therapy in management of heart failure. **OFF-LABEL:** Treatment of hypertension, renal crisis in scleroderma, treatment of left ventricular dysfunction following MI.

PRECAUTIONS

CONTRAINDICATIONS: Bilateral renal artery stenosis, history of angioedema from previous treatment with ACE inhibitors. **CAUTIONS:** Renal impairment, CHF, collagen vascular disease, hypovolemia, renal stenosis, hyperkalemia.

LIFESPAN CONSIDERATIONS:

Pregnancy/Lactation: Crosses placenta. Unknown if distributed in breast milk. May cause fetal, neonatal mortality or morbidity. **Pregnancy Category C (D if used in second or third trimester).** **Children:** Safety and efficacy not established. **Elderly:** May be more sensitive to hypotensive effects.

INTERACTIONS

DRUG: **Alcohol, antihypertensives, diuretics** may increase effects. May increase concentration, risk of toxicity of **lithium. NSAIDs** may decrease effects. **Potassium-sparing diuretics, potassium supplements** may cause hyperkalemia. **HERBAL:** **Garlic** may increase antihypertensive effect. **Ginseng, yohimbe** may worsen hypertension. **FOOD:** None known. **LAB VALUES:** May increase BUN, serum alkaline phosphatase, bilirubin, creatinine, potassium, AST, ALT. May decrease serum sodium. May cause positive antinuclear antibody (ANA) titer.

AVAILABILITY (Rx)

TABLETS: 5 mg, 10 mg, 20 mg, 40 mg.

ADMINISTRATION/HANDLING

PO

• Give without regard to food. • Tablets may be crushed.

INDICATIONS/ROUTES/DOSAGE

HYPERTENSION (MONOTHERAPY)

PO: ADULTS: Initially, 10–20 mg/day. May adjust dosage at intervals of at least 2 wks or longer. Maintenance: 20–80 mg/day as single dose or 2 divided doses. **Maximum:** 80 mg/day. **ELDERLY:** Initially, 2.5–5 mg/day. May increase by 2.5–5 mg q1–2wk.

HYPERTENSION (COMBINATION THERAPY)

PO: ADULTS: Initially, 5 mg/day titrated to pt's needs. **ELDERLY:** Initially, 2.5–5 mg/day. May increase by 2.5–5 mg q1–2wk.

ADJUNCT TO MANAGE HEART FAILURE

PO: ADULTS, ELDERLY: Initially, 5 mg twice a day. Range: 20–40 mg/day.

Q

DOSAGE IN RENAL IMPAIRMENT

Dosage is titrated to pt's needs after the following initial doses:

Creatinine Clearance	Initial Dose
More than 60 ml/min	10 mg
30–60 ml/min	5 mg
10–29 ml/min	2.5 mg

SIDE EFFECTS

FREQUENT (7%–5%): Headache, dizziness. **OCCASIONAL (4%–2%):** Fatigue, vomiting, nausea, hypotension, chest pain, cough, syncope. **RARE (less than 2%):** Diarrhea, cough, dyspnea, rash, palpitations, impotence, insomnia, drowsiness, malaise.

ADVERSE EFFECTS/ TOXIC REACTIONS

Excessive hypotension ("first-dose syncope") may occur in pts with CHF, those who are severely salt/volume depleted. Angioedema, hyperkalemia occur rarely. Agranulocytosis, neutropenia may be noted in those with collagen vascular disease (scleroderma, systemic lupus erythematosus), impaired renal function. Nephrotic syndrome may be noted in those with history of renal disease.

Q

NURSING CONSIDERATIONS

BASELINE ASSESSMENT

Obtain B/P immediately before each dose in addition to regular monitoring (be alert to fluctuations). If excessive reduction in B/P occurs, place pt in supine position with legs slightly elevated. Renal function tests should be performed before beginning therapy. In pts with prior renal disease, urine test for protein by dipstick method should be made with first urine of day before beginning therapy and periodically thereafter. In those with renal impairment, autoimmune disease, or taking drugs that affect leukocytes or immune response, CBC, differential count should be performed before beginning therapy and q2wk for 3 mos, then periodically thereafter.

INTERVENTION/EVALUATION

Monitor renal function, serum potassium, WBC. Assist with ambulation if dizziness occurs. Question for evidence of headache. Non-cola carbonated beverage, unsalted crackers, dry toast may relieve nausea.

PATIENT/FAMILY TEACHING

• Rise slowly from lying to sitting position, permit legs to dangle from bed momentarily before standing to reduce hypotensive effect. • Full therapeutic effect may take 1–2 wks. • Report any sign of infection (sore throat, fever). • Skipping doses or voluntarily discontinuing drug may produce severe rebound hypertension. • Avoid tasks that require alertness, motor skills until response to drug is established.

quinidine

kwin-ih-deen

(Apo-Quin-G ✦, Apo-Quinidine ✦, BioQuin Durules ✦, Quinaglute Dura-Tabs, Quinate ✦, Quinidex Extentabs)

Do not confuse quinidine with clonidine or quinine.

CLASSIFICATION

CLINICAL: Antiarrhythmic (see p. 14C).

ACTION

Decreases sodium influx during depolarization, potassium efflux during repolarization. Reduces calcium transport across myocardial cell membrane. Decreases myocardial excitability, conduction velocity, contractility. **Therapeutic Effect:** Suppresses arrhythmias.

PHARMACOKINETICS

Almost completely absorbed after PO administration. Protein binding: 80%–90%. Metabolized in liver. Excreted in urine. Removed by hemodialysis. **Half-life:** 6–8 hrs.

USES

Prophylactic therapy to maintain normal sinus rhythm following conversion of atrial fibrillation/flutter. Prevention of premature atrial, AV, ventricular contractions, paroxysmal atrial tachycardia, paroxysmal AV junctional rhythm, atrial fibrillation, atrial flutter, paroxysmal ventricular tachycardia not associated with complete heart block. **OFF-LABEL:** Treatment of malaria (IV only).

PRECAUTIONS

CONTRAINDICATIONS: Complete AV block, development of thrombocytopenic purpura during prior therapy with quinidine or quinine, intraventricular conduction defects (widening of QRS complex). **CAUTIONS:** Myocardial depression, sick sinus syndrome, incomplete AV block, digoxin toxicity, renal/hepatic impairment, myasthenia gravis.

LIFESPAN CONSIDERATIONS:

Pregnancy/Lactation: Crosses placenta; distributed in breast milk. **Pregnancy Category C. Children:** Safety and efficacy not established. **Elderly:** No age-related precautions noted.

INTERACTIONS

DRUG: Effects may be additive with medications **(e.g., amiodarone, tricyclic antidepressants, erythromycin, phenothiazines)** that prolong QT interval. May increase **digoxin** concentration, risk of toxicity. **HERBAL: Ephedra** may worsen arrhythmias. **St. John's wort** may decrease concentration. **FOOD:** None known. **LAB VALUES:** None known. Therapeutic serum level: 2–5 mcg/ml; toxic serum level: greater than 5 mcg/ml.

AVAILABILITY (Rx)

INJECTION SOLUTION: 80 mg/ml. **TABLETS:** 200 mg, 300 mg.

TABLETS (EXTENDED-RELEASE): 300 mg (Quinidex Extentabs), 324 mg (Quinaglute Dura-Tabs).

ADMINISTRATION/HANDLING

IV

◄ ALERT ► B/P, EKG should be monitored continuously during IV administration and rate of infusion adjusted to minimize arrhythmias, hypotension.

Reconstitution • For IV infusion, dilute 800 mg with 40 ml D_5W to provide concentration of 16 mg/ml.

Rate of administration • Administer with pt in supine position. • For IV infusion, give at rate of 1 ml (16 mg)/min (too-rapid rate may markedly decrease arterial pressure). • Monitor EKG for cardiac changes, particularly prolongation of PR, QT intervals, widening of QRS complex. Notify physician of any significant interval changes.

Storage • Use only clear, colorless solution. • Solution is stable for 24 hrs at room temperature when diluted with D_5W.

PO

• Do not crush/chew extended-release tablets. • GI upset can be reduced if given with food.

Q

IV INCOMPATIBILITIES

Furosemide (Lasix), heparin.

IV COMPATIBILITY

Milrinone (Primacor).

INDICATIONS/ROUTES/DOSAGE

ARRHYTHMIAS

PO (EXTENDED-RELEASE): ADULTS, ELDERLY: 100–600 mg q4–6h. (**Long-acting**): 324–972 mg q8–12h. **CHILDREN:** 15–60 mg/kg/day in divided doses q4–6h.

IV: ADULTS, ELDERLY: 200–400 mg. May require 500–750 mg. **CHILDREN:** 2–10 mg/kg/dose in divided doses q3–6h as needed.

SIDE EFFECTS

FREQUENT: Abdominal pain/cramps, nausea, diarrhea, vomiting (can be immediate, intense). **OCCASIONAL:** Mild cinchonism (ringing in ears, blurred vision, hearing loss), severe cinchonism (headache, vertigo, diaphoresis, lightheadedness, photophobia, confusion, delirium). **RARE:** Hypotension (particularly with IV administration), hypersensitivity reaction (fever, anaphylaxis, photosensitivity reaction).

Q

ADVERSE EFFECTS/ TOXIC REACTIONS

Cardiotoxic effects occur most commonly with IV administration, particularly at high concentrations, observed as conduction changes (50% widening of QRS complex, prolonged QT interval, flattened T waves, disappearance of P wave), ventricular tachycardia/flutter, frequent premature ventricular contractions (PVCs), complete AV block. Quinidine-induced syncope may occur with usual dosage. Severe hypotension may result from high dosages. Pts with atrial flutter/fibrillation may experience a paradoxical, extremely rapid ventricular rate (may be prevented by prior digitalization). Hepatotoxicity with jaundice due to drug hypersensitivity may occur.

NURSING CONSIDERATIONS

BASELINE ASSESSMENT

Check B/P, pulse (for 1 full min unless pt is on continuous monitor) before giving medication. For those on long-term therapy, CBC, hepatic/renal function tests should be performed periodically.

INTERVENTION/EVALUATION

Monitor EKG for cardiac changes, particularly prolongation of PR, QT intervals, widening of QRS complex. Monitor I&O, CBC, serum potassium, hepatic/renal function tests. Monitor daily pattern of bowel activity/stool consistency. Monitor B/P for hypotension (esp. in pts on high-dose therapy). If cardiotoxic effect occurs (see Adverse Effects/Toxic Reactions), notify physician immediately. Therapeutic serum level: 2–5 mcg/ml; toxic serum level: greater than 5 mcg/ml.

PATIENT/FAMILY TEACHING

• Inform physician of fever, tinnitus, visual disturbances. • May cause photosensitivity reaction; avoid direct sunlight, artificial light.

quinine

evolve

kwye-nine

(Apo-Quinine ✦, Novo-Quinine ✦, Qualaquin, Quinine, Quinine-Odan ✦)

Do not confuse quinine with quinidine.

FIXED-COMBINATION(S)

With vitamin E for nocturnal leg cramps (**M-KYA, Q-vel**).

CLASSIFICATION

PHARMACOTHERAPEUTIC: Cinchona alkaloid. **CLINICAL:** Antimalarial, antimyotonic.

ACTION

Myotonia: Increases refractory period, decreases excitability of motor end plates, affects distribution of calcium within muscle fiber. **Therapeutic Effect:** Relaxes skeletal muscle. **Anti-malaria:** Depresses O_2 uptake, carbohydrate metabolism, elevates pH in intracellular organelles of parasites. **Therapeutic Effect:** Produces parasitic death.

USES

Treatment/suppression of chloroquine resistant *P. falciparum* malaria, treatment of babesiosis, prevention/treatment of nocturnal recumbency leg cramps.

PRECAUTIONS

CONTRAINDICATIONS: Tinnitus, optic neuritis, G6PD deficiency, pregnancy. **CAUTIONS:** Arrhythmias, myasthenia gravis, hepatic impairment. **Pregnancy Category X.**

INTERACTIONS

DRUG: May increase **digoxin** concentration. **Mefloquine** may increase seizures, EKG abnormalities. **HERBAL: St. John's wort** may decrease concentration. **FOOD:** None known. **LAB VALUES:** May interfere with 17-OH steroid determinations.

AVAILABILITY (Rx)

CAPSULES: 200 mg, 325 mg. **TABLETS:** 260 mg.

INDICATIONS/ROUTES/DOSAGE

MALARIA TREATMENT

PO: ADULTS, ELDERLY: 650 mg q8h for 3–7 days (in combination). **CHILDREN:** 30 mg/kg/day in divided doses q8h for 3–7 days (in combination). **Maximum:** 2 g a day.

MALARIA SUPPRESSION

PO: ADULTS, ELDERLY: 325 mg twice a day for up to 6 wks.

BABESIOSIS

PO: ADULTS, ELDERLY: 600 mg q6–8h for 7 days. **CHILDREN:** 25 mg/kg/day in divided doses for 7 days. **Maximum:** 650 mg/dose.

LEG CRAMPS

PO: ADULTS, ELDERLY: 200–300 mg at bedtime.

SIDE EFFECTS

FREQUENT: Nausea, headache, tinnitus, slight visual disturbances (mild cinchonism). **OCCASIONAL:** Extreme flushing of skin with intense generalized pruritus is most typical hypersensitivity reaction; rash, wheezing, dyspnea, angioedema. Prolonged therapy: Cardiac conduction disturbances, diminished hearing.

ADVERSE EFFECTS/ TOXIC REACTIONS

Overdosage may produce severe cinchonism: cardiovascular effects, severe headache, intestinal cramps with vomiting/diarrhea, apprehension, confusion, seizures, blindness, respiratory depression. Hypoprothrombinemia, thrombocytopenic purpura, hemoglobinuria, asthma, agranulocytosis, hypoglycemia, deafness, optic atrophy occur rarely.

Q

NURSING CONSIDERATIONS

BASELINE ASSESSMENT

Question for possibility of pregnancy before initiating therapy (Pregnancy Category X). Question for hypersensitivity to quinine, quinidine. Evaluate initial EKG, CBC results.

INTERVENTION/EVALUATION

Check for hypersensitivity: flushing, rash/urticaria, pruritus, dyspnea, wheezing. Assess level of hearing, visual acuity, presence of headache/tinnitus, nausea. Report adverse effects promptly (possible cinchonism). Monitor CBC results for blood dyscrasias. Be alert to infection (fever, sore throat), bleeding/ecchymosis, unusual fatigue/weakness. Assess pulse, EKG for arrhythmias. Check fasting serum glucose levels; watch for hypoglycemia (diaphoresis, tremors, tachycardia, hunger, anxiety).

PATIENT/FAMILY TEACHING

• Report tinnitus, hearing loss, rash, any visual disturbances. • Discuss need for periodic lab tests as part of therapy.

quinupristin-dalfopristin

kwin-yoo-pris-tin **dal**-foh-pris-tin
(Synercid)

CLASSIFICATION

PHARMACOTHERAPEUTIC: Streptogramin. **CLINICAL:** Antimicrobial.

ACTION

Two chemically distinct compounds that, when given together, bind to different sites on bacterial ribosomes, inhibiting protein synthesis. **Therapeutic Effect:** Bactericidal.

PHARMACOKINETICS

After IV administration, both are extensively metabolized in liver, with dalfopristin to active metabolite. Protein binding: quinupristin, 23%–32%; dalfopristin, 50%–56%. Primarily eliminated in feces. **Half-life:** quinupristin, 0.85 hr; dalfopristin, 0.7 hr.

USES

Treatment of serious or life-threatening infections caused by vancomycin-resistant *Enterococcus faecium* (VRE), complicated skin/skin structure infections caused by *S. aureus, S. pyogenes.*

PRECAUTIONS

CONTRAINDICATIONS: Hypersensitivity to pristinamycin, virginiamycin. **CAUTIONS:** Hepatic/renal dysfunction.

LIFESPAN CONSIDERATIONS:

Pregnancy/Lactation: Unknown if drug crosses placenta or is distributed in breast milk. **Pregnancy Category B.** **Children:** Safety and efficacy not established. **Elderly:** No age-related precautions noted.

INTERACTIONS

DRUG: May increase concentration, risk of toxicity of **cyclosporine, tacrilimus, diazepam, midazolam, diltiazem, nifedipine, verapamil.** **HERBAL:** None significant. **FOOD:** None known. **LAB VALUES:** May increase serum bilirubin, creatinine, LDH, AST, ALT.

AVAILABILITY (Rx)

INJECTION POWDER FOR RECONSTITUTION: 500-mg vial (150 mg quinupristin/350 mg dalfopristin). 600-mg vial (180 mg quinupristin/420 mg dalfopristin).

ADMINISTRATION/HANDLING

IV

Reconstitution • Reconstitute vial by slowly adding 5 ml D_5W or Sterile Water for Injection to make 100 mg/ml solution. • Gently swirl vial contents to minimize foaming. • Further dilute with D_5W to final concentration of 2 mg/ml (5 mg/ml using central line).

Rate of administration • Infuse over 60 min. • After infusion, flush line with D_5W to minimize vein irritation. Do not flush with 0.9% NaCl (incompatible).

Storage • Refrigerate unopened vials. • Reconstituted vials are stable for 1 hr at room temperature. Diluted infusion bag is stable for 6 hrs at room temperature or 54 hrs if refrigerated.

IV INCOMPATIBILITIES

Heparin, sodium chloride.

IV COMPATIBILITIES

Aztreonam (Azactam), ciprofloxacin (Cipro), fluconazole (Diflucan), haloperidol (Haldol), metoclopramide (Reglan), morphine, potassium chloride.

INDICATIONS/ROUTES/DOSAGE

INFECTIONS DUE TO VANCOMYCIN-RESISTANT *ENTEROCOCCUS FAECIUM*

IV: **ADULTS, ELDERLY:** 7.5 mg/kg/dose q8h.

SKIN/SKIN STRUCTURE INFECTIONS

IV: **ADULTS, ELDERLY:** 7.5 mg/kg/dose q12h.

SIDE EFFECTS

FREQUENT: Mild erythema, pruritus, pain/burning at infusion site (with doses greater than 7 mg/kg). **OCCASIONAL:** Headache, diarrhea. **RARE:** Vomiting, arthralgia, myalgia.

ADVERSE EFFECTS/ TOXIC REACTIONS

Antibiotic-associated colitis, other superinfections may result from altered bacterial balance. Hepatic function abnormalities, severe venous pain, inflammation may occur.

NURSING CONSIDERATIONS

BASELINE ASSESSMENT

Assess temperature, B/P, respiratory rate, pulse. Obtain baseline hepatic function tests, BUN, CBC, urinalysis.

INTERVENTION/EVALUATION

Monitor CBC, hepatic function tests. Observe infusion site for redness, vein irritation. Hold medication, promptly inform physician of diarrhea (with fever, abdominal pain, mucus/blood in stool may indicate antibiotic-associated colitis). Evaluate IV site for erythema, pruritus, pain, burning. Be alert for superinfection: increased fever, onset of sore throat, nausea, vomiting, diarrhea, stomatitis, anal/genital pruritus.

Q

rabeprazole

rah-**bep**-rah-zole

(Aciphex, Pariet ✤)

Do not confuse Aciphex with Accupril or Aricept.

CLASSIFICATION

PHARMACOTHERAPEUTIC: Proton pump inhibitor. **CLINICAL:** Gastric acid inhibitor (see p. 139C).

ACTION

Converts to active metabolites that irreversibly bind to, inhibit hydrogen-potassium adenosine triphosphate, an enzyme on surface of gastric parietal cells. Actively secretes hydrogen ions for potassium ions, resulting in accumulation of hydrogen ions in gastric lumen. **Therapeutic Effect:** Increases gastric pH, reducing gastric acid production.

PHARMACOKINETICS

Rapidly absorbed from GI tract after passing through stomach relatively intact. Protein binding: 96%. Metabolized extensively in liver. Primarily excreted in urine. Unknown if removed by hemodialysis. **Half-life:** 1–2 hrs (increased with hepatic impairment).

R

USES

Short-term treatment (4–8 wks) in healing, maintenance of erosive or ulcerative gastroesophageal reflux disease (GERD). Treatment of daytime/nighttime heartburn, other symptoms of GERD. Short-term treatment (4 wks or less) in healing, symptomatic relief of duodenal ulcers. Long-term treatment of pathologic hypersecretory conditions, including Zollinger-Ellison syndrome. Treatment of NSAID-induced ulcers. Treatment of *H. pylori* (in combination with other medication). **OFF-LABEL:** Maintenance treatment of duodenal ulcers.

PRECAUTIONS

CONTRAINDICATIONS: None known. **CAUTIONS:** Hepatic impairment.

LIFESPAN CONSIDERATIONS:

Pregnancy/Lactation: Unknown if drug crosses placenta or is distributed in breast milk. **Pregnancy Category B. Children:** Safety and efficacy not established. **Elderly:** No age-related precautions noted.

INTERACTIONS

DRUG: May increase concentration, toxicity of **digoxin, cyclosporine, warfarin.** May decrease concentration of **ketoconazole. HERBAL:** None significant. **FOOD:** None known. **LAB VALUES:** May increase serum alkaline phosphatase, AST, ALT.

AVAILABILITY (Rx)

TABLETS (DELAYED-RELEASE): 20 mg.

ADMINISTRATION/HANDLING

PO

• Give before meals. • Do not crush, chew, split tablet; swallow whole.

INDICATIONS/ROUTES/DOSAGE

GASTROESOPHAGEAL REFLUX DISEASE

PO: ADULTS, ELDERLY: 20 mg/day for 4–8 wks. Maintenance: 20 mg/day.

DUODENAL ULCER

PO: ADULTS, ELDERLY: 20 mg/day after morning meal for 4 wks.

NSAID-INDUCED ULCER

PO: ADULTS, ELDERLY: 20 mg/day.

PATHOLOGIC HYPERSECRETORY CONDITIONS

PO: ADULTS, ELDERLY: Initially, 60 mg once a day. May increase to 60 mg twice a day.

***H. PYLORI* INFECTION**

PO: ADULTS, ELDERLY: 20 mg twice a day for 7 days (given with amoxicillin 1,000 mg and clarithromycin 500 mg).

SIDE EFFECTS

RARE (less than 2%): Headache, nausea, dizziness, rash, diarrhea, malaise.

ADVERSE EFFECTS/ TOXIC REACTIONS

Hyperglycemia, hypokalemia, hyponatremia, hyperlipemia occur rarely.

NURSING CONSIDERATIONS

BASELINE ASSESSMENT

Obtain baseline lab values, esp. serum chemistries.

INTERVENTION/EVALUATION

Monitor ongoing laboratory results. Evaluate for therapeutic response (relief of GI symptoms). Question if GI discomfort, nausea, diarrhea, headache occurs. Assess skin for evidence of rash. Observe for evidence of dizziness; utilize appropriate safety precautions.

PATIENT/FAMILY TEACHING

• Swallow tablets whole; do not chew, split, crush tablets. • Report headache.

raloxifene

ra-**lox**-i-feen
(Evista)

Do not confuse raloxifene with propoxyphene.

CLASSIFICATION

PHARMACOTHERAPEUTIC: Selective estrogen receptor modulator. **CLINICAL:** Osteoporosis preventive.

ACTION

Selective estrogen receptor modulator that binds to estrogen receptors, increasing bone mineral density. **Therapeutic Effect:** Reduces bone resorption, decreases bone turnover, prevents bone loss.

PHARMACOKINETICS

Rapidly absorbed after PO administration. Highly bound to plasma proteins (greater than 95%) and albumin. Undergoes extensive first-pass metabolism in liver. Excreted mainly in feces and, to a lesser extent, in urine. Unknown if removed by hemodialysis. **Half-life:** 27.7 hrs.

USES

Prevention/treatment of osteoporosis in postmenopausal women. **OFF-LABEL:** Prevention of fractures, treatment of breast cancer in postmenopausal women.

PRECAUTIONS

CONTRAINDICATIONS: Active or history of venous thromboembolic events, such as deep vein thrombosis (DVT), pulmonary embolism, retinal vein thrombosis; women who are or may become pregnant. **CAUTIONS:** Cardiovascular disease, history of cervical/uterine cancer, renal/hepatic impairment.

LIFESPAN CONSIDERATIONS:

Pregnancy/Lactation: Unknown if distributed in breast milk. Not recommended for breast-feeding mothers. **Pregnancy Category X.** **Children:** Not used in this population. **Elderly:** No age-related precautions noted.

INTERACTIONS

DRUG: **Cholestyramine** reduces peak levels, extent of absorption. Do not use concurrently with **hormone replacement therapy, systemic estrogen.** May decrease effect of **warfarin** (decreases prothrombin time). **HERBAL:** None significant. **FOOD:** None known. **LAB VALUES:** Lowers serum total cholesterol, LDL levels (does not affect HDL, triglyceride levels). Slightly decreases platelet count, serum inorganic phosphate, albumin, calcium, protein.

R

AVAILABILITY (Rx)

TABLETS: 60 mg.

ADMINISTRATION/HANDLING

PO

- Give at any time of day without regard to meals.

INDICATIONS/ROUTES/DOSAGE

PREVENTION/TREATMENT OF OSTEOPOROSIS

PO: ADULTS, ELDERLY: 60 mg a day.

SIDE EFFECTS

FREQUENT (25%–10%): Hot flashes, flu-like symptoms, arthralgia, sinusitis. **OCCASIONAL (9%–5%):** Weight gain, nausea, myalgia, pharyngitis, cough, dyspepsia, leg cramps, rash, depression. **RARE (4%–3%):** Vaginitis, UTI, peripheral edema, flatulence, vomiting, fever, migraine, diaphoresis.

ADVERSE EFFECTS/ TOXIC REACTIONS

Pneumonia, gastroenteritis, chest pain, vaginal bleeding, breast pain occur rarely.

NURSING CONSIDERATIONS

BASELINE ASSESSMENT

Question for possibility of pregnancy (Pregnancy Category X). Drug should be discontinued 72 hrs before and during prolonged immobilization (postop recovery, prolonged bed rest). Therapy may be resumed only after pt is fully ambulatory. Determine serum total, LDL cholesterol before therapy and routinely thereafter.

INTERVENTION/EVALUATION

Monitor serum total, LDL cholesterol, total calcium, inorganic phosphate, total protein, albumin, bone mineral density, platelet count.

PATIENT/FAMILY TEACHING

- Avoid prolonged restriction of movement during travel (increased risk of venous thromboembolic events).
- Take supplemental calcium, vitamin D if daily dietary intake is inadequate.
- Encourage regular exercise.
- Recommend modification, discontinuation of cigarette smoking, alcohol consumption.

ramelteon

rah-**mel**-tea-on

(Rozerem)

Do not confuse Rozerem with Razadyne.

CLASSIFICATION

PHARMACOTHERAPEUTIC: Melatonin receptor agonist. **CLINICAL:** Hypnotic.

ACTION

Selectively targets melatonin receptors thought to be involved in maintenance of circadian rhythm underlying normal sleep-wake cycle. **Therapeutic Effect:** Prevents insomnia characterized by difficulty with sleep onset.

PHARMACOKINETICS

Rapidly absorbed following PO administration. Protein binding: 82%. Substantial tissue distribution. Metabolized in liver. Excreted mainly in urine with small amount eliminated in feces. **Half-life:** 2–5 hrs.

USES

Long-term treatment of insomnia in pts who experience difficulty with sleep onset.

PRECAUTIONS

CONTRAINDICATIONS: Severe hepatic impairment, concurrent fluvoxamine therapy. **CAUTIONS:** Clinical depression, alcohol consumption, moderate hepatic impairment.

LIFESPAN CONSIDERATIONS:

Pregnancy/Lactation: Unknown if distributed in breast milk; breast-feeding not recommended. **Pregnancy Category C.** **Children:** Safety and efficacy not established. **Elderly:** Age-related hepatic impairment may require dosage adjustment.

INTERACTIONS

DRUG: Concurrent use with **alcohol** produces additive effect. **Fluconazole, ketoconazole** may increase serum level, effect. **Fluvoxamine** may cause marked increase in serum level, toxicity. **Rifampin** may decrease serum level, effect. **HERBAL:** None significant. **FOOD:** Onset of action may be reduced if taken with or immediately after a **high-fat meal.** **LAB VALUES:** May decrease serum testosterone. May increase serum prolactin.

AVAILABILITY (Rx)

TABLETS, FILM-COATED: 8 mg (Rozerem).

ADMINISTRATION/HANDLING

PO

• Administer within 30 min before bed. • Do not give with, or immediately following, a high-fat meal. • Do not crush/break tablet.

INDICATIONS/ROUTES/DOSAGE

INSOMNIA

PO: ADULTS, ELDERLY: 8 mg before bedtime.

SIDE EFFECTS

FREQUENT (7%–5%): Headache, dizziness, drowsiness. **OCCASIONAL (4%–3%):** Fatigue, nausea, exacerbated insomnia. **RARE (2%):** Diarrhea, myalgia, depression, altered taste sensation, arthralgia.

ADVERSE EFFECTS/ TOXIC REACTIONS

May affect reproductive hormones in adults (decreased testosterone levels, increased prolactin levels), resulting in unexplained amenorrhea, galactorrhea, decreased libido, difficulty with fertility.

NURSING CONSIDERATIONS

BASELINE ASSESSMENT

Assess B/P, pulse, respirations. Raise bed rails, provide call light. Provide environment conducive to sleep (quiet environment, low/no lighting, TV off).

INTERVENTION/EVALUATION

Assess sleep pattern of pt. Evaluate for therapeutic response: rapid induction of sleep onset, decrease in number of nocturnal awakenings.

PATIENT/FAMILY TEACHING

• Take within 30 min before going to bed; confine activities to those necessary to prepare for bed. • Avoid engaging in any hazardous activities after taking medication. • Do not take medication with or immediately after a high-fat meal.

ramipril

ram-i-pril

(Altace)

Do not confuse Altace with Alteplase or Artane.

CLASSIFICATION

PHARMACOTHERAPEUTIC: Renin-angiotensin system antagonist. **CLINICAL:** Antihypertensive (see p. 7C).

ACTION

Suppresses renin-angiotensin-aldosterone system. Decreases plasma angiotensin II, increases plasma renin activity, decreases aldosterone secretion. **Therapeutic Effect:** Reduces peripheral arterial resistance, decreasing B/P.

PHARMACOKINETICS

Route	Onset	Peak	Duration
PO	1–2 hrs	3–6 hrs	24 hrs

Well absorbed from GI tract. Protein binding: 73%. Metabolized in liver to active metabolite. Primarily excreted in urine. Not removed by hemodialysis. **Half-life:** 5.1 hrs.

USES

Treatment of hypertension. Used alone or in combination with other antihypertensives. Treatment of CHF. Prevention of heart attack, stroke. **OFF-LABEL:** Treatment of hypertension, renal crisis in scleroderma.

PRECAUTIONS

CONTRAINDICATIONS: Bilateral renal artery stenosis. **CAUTIONS:** Renal impairment, CHF, collagen vascular disease, hypovolemia, renal stenosis, hyperkalemia.

LIFESPAN CONSIDERATIONS:

Pregnancy/Lactation: Crosses placenta. Distributed in breast milk. May cause fetal or neonatal mortality or morbidity. **Pregnancy Category C (D if used in second or third trimester).** **Children:** Safety and efficacy not established. **Elderly:** May be more sensitive to hypotensive effects.

R

INTERACTIONS

DRUG: **Alcohol, antihypertensives, diuretics** may increase effects. May increase **lithium** concentration, risk of toxicity. **NSAIDs** may decrease effects. **Potassium-sparing diuretics, potassium supplements** may cause hyperkalemia. **HERBAL:** **Garlic** may increase antihypertensive effect. **Ginseng, yohimbe** may worsen hypertension. **FOOD:** None known. **LAB VALUES:** May increase BUN, serum alkaline phosphatase, bilirubin, creatinine, potassium, AST, ALT. May decrease serum sodium. May cause positive antinuclear antibody titer (ANA).

AVAILABILITY (Rx)

CAPSULES: 1.25 mg, 2.5 mg, 5 mg, 10 mg.

ADMINISTRATION/HANDLING

PO

• Give without regard to food. • Do not chew/break capsules. • May mix with water, apple juice/sauce.

INDICATIONS/ROUTES/DOSAGE

HYPERTENSION (MONOTHERAPY)

PO: ADULTS, ELDERLY: Initially, 2.5 mg/day. Maintenance: 2.5–20 mg/day as single dose or in 2 divided doses.

HYPERTENSION (IN COMBINATION WITH OTHER ANTIHYPERTENSIVES)

PO: ADULTS, ELDERLY: Initially, 1.25 mg/day titrated to pt's needs.

CHF

PO: ADULTS, ELDERLY: Initially, 1.25–2.5 mg twice a day. **Maximum:** 5 mg twice a day.

RISK REDUCTION FOR MI/STROKE

PO: ADULTS, ELDERLY: Initially, 2.5 mg/day for 7 days, then 5 mg/day for 21 days, then 10 mg/day as a single dose or in divided doses.

DOSAGE IN RENAL IMPAIRMENT

Creatinine clearance equal to or less than 40 ml/min: 25% of normal dose.

HYPERTENSION: Initially, 1.25 mg/day titrated upward.

CHF: Initially, 1.25 mg/day, titrated up to 2.5 mg twice a day.

SIDE EFFECTS

FREQUENT (12%–5%): Cough, headache. **OCCASIONAL (4%–2%):** Dizziness, fatigue, nausea, asthenia (loss of strength, energy). **RARE (less than 2%):** Palpitations, insomnia, nervousness, malaise, abdominal pain, myalgia.

ADVERSE EFFECTS/ TOXIC REACTIONS

Excessive hypotension ("first-dose syncope") may occur in pts with CHF, severely salt or volume depleted. Angioedema, hyperkalemia occur rarely. Agranulocytosis, neutropenia may be noted in those with collagen vascular disease (scleroderma, systemic lupus erythematosus), renal impairment. Nephrotic syndrome may be noted in those with history of renal disease.

NURSING CONSIDERATIONS

BASELINE ASSESSMENT

Obtain B/P immediately before each dose, in addition to regular monitoring (be alert to fluctuations). If excessive reduction in B/P occurs, place pt in supine position with legs elevated. Renal function tests should be performed before beginning therapy. In pts with prior renal disease, urine test for protein (by dipstick method) should be made with first urine of day before beginning therapy and periodically thereafter. In those with renal impairment, autoimmune disease, or taking drugs that affect leukocytes or immune response, CBC, differential count should be performed before beginning therapy and q2wk for 3 mos then periodically thereafter.

INTERVENTION/EVALUATION

Monitor renal function, serum potassium, WBC. Assess for cough (frequent effect). Assist with ambulation if dizziness occurs. Assess lung sounds for rales, wheezing in pts with CHF. Monitor urinalysis for proteinuria. Monitor serum potassium in those on concurrent diuretic therapy.

PATIENT/FAMILY TEACHING

• Do not discontinue medication without physician approval. • Report palpitations, cough, chest pain. • Dizziness, light-headedness may occur in first few days. • Avoid tasks that require alertness, motor skills until response to drug is established.

ranitidine

ra-**ni**-ti-dine

(Apo-Ranitidine ✦, Novo-Ranitidine ✦, Zantac, Zantac-75, Zantac-150, Zantac-300, Zantac EFFERdose, Zantac-25 EFFERdose, Zantac-150 EFFERdose, Zantac-150 Maximum Strength)

Do not confuse Zantac with Xanax, Ziac, or Zyrtec.

CLASSIFICATION

PHARMACOTHERAPEUTIC: Histamine H_2 receptor antagonist. **CLINICAL:** Antiulcer (see p. 104C).

ACTION

Inhibits histamine action at histamine 2 receptors of gastric parietal cells. **Therapeutic Effect:** Inhibits gastric acid secretion (fasting, nocturnal, when stimulated by food, caffeine, insulin). Reduces volume, hydrogen ion concentration of gastric juice.

PHARMACOKINETICS

Rapidly absorbed from GI tract. Protein binding: 15%. Widely distributed. Metabolized in liver. Primarily excreted in urine. Not removed by hemodialysis. **Half-life:** PO, 2.5 hrs; IV, 2–2.5 hrs (increased with renal impairment).

USES

Short-term treatment of active duodenal ulcer. Prevention of duodenal ulcer recurrence. Treatment of active benign gastric ulcer, pathologic GI hypersecretory conditions, acute gastroesophageal reflux disease (GERD), including erosive esophagitis. Maintenance of healed erosive esophagitis. Part of regimen for

H. pylori eradication to reduce risk of duodenal ulcer recurrence. **OTC:** Relieve heartburn, acid indigestion, sour stomach. **OFF-LABEL:** Prevention of aspiration pneumonia, treatment of recurrent postop ulcer, upper GI bleeding, prevention of acid aspiration pneumonitis during surgery, prevention of stress-induced ulcers.

PRECAUTIONS

CONTRAINDICATIONS: History of acute porphyria. **CAUTIONS:** Renal/hepatic impairment, elderly.

LIFESPAN CONSIDERATIONS:

Pregnancy/Lactation: Unknown if drug crosses placenta or is distributed in breast milk. **Pregnancy Category B.** **Children:** No age-related precautions noted. **Elderly:** Confusion more likely in pts with hepatic/renal impairment.

INTERACTIONS

DRUG: **Antacids** may decrease absorption. May decrease absorption of **ketoconazole, itraconazole.** **HERBAL:** None significant. **FOOD:** None known. **LAB VALUES:** Interferes with skin tests using allergen extracts. May increase hepatic serum enzymes, gamma-glutamyl transpeptidase, creatinine.

R

AVAILABILITY (Rx)

CAPSULES (ZANTAC): 150 mg, 300 mg. **INJECTION SOLUTION (ZANTAC):** 25 mg/ml. **SYRUP (ZANTAC):** 15 mg/ml. **TABLETS (EFFERVESCENT):** 25 mg (Zantac-25 EFFERdose), 150 mg (Zantac-150 EFFERdose). **TABLETS (HYDROCHLORIDE):** 75 mg (Zantac-75 [OTC]), 150 mg (Zantac-150, Zantac-150 Maximum Strength), 300 mg (Zantac-300).

ADMINISTRATION/HANDLING

IV

Reconstitution • For IV push, dilute each 50 mg with 20 ml 0.9% NaCl, D_5W. • For intermittent IV infusion (piggyback), dilute each 50 mg with 50 ml 0.9% NaCl, D_5W. • For IV infusion, dilute with 250–1,000 ml 0.9% NaCl, D_5W.

Rate of administration • Administer IV push over minimum of 5 min (prevents arrhythmias, hypotension). • Infuse IV piggyback over 15–20 min. • Infuse IV infusion over 24 hrs.

Storage • IV solutions appear clear, colorless to yellow (slight darkening does not affect potency). • IV infusion (piggyback) is stable for 48 hrs at room temperature (discard if discolored or precipitate forms).

IM

• May be given undiluted. • Give deep IM into large muscle mass.

PO

• Give without regard to meals. Best given after meals or at bedtime. • Do not administer within 1 hr of magnesium- or aluminum-containing antacids (decreases absorption).

IV INCOMPATIBILITIES

Amphotericin B complex (Abelcet, AmBisome, Amphotec).

IV COMPATIBILITIES

Diltiazem (Cardizem), dobutamine (Dobutrex), dopamine (Intropin), heparin, hydromorphone (Dilaudid), insulin, lidocaine, lipids, lorazepam (Ativan), morphine, norepinephrine (Levophed), potassium chloride, propofol (Diprivan).

INDICATIONS/ROUTES/DOSAGE

DUODENAL ULCER, GASTRIC ULCER, GERD

PO: ADULTS, ELDERLY: 150 mg twice a day or 300 mg at bedtime. Maintenance: 150 mg at bedtime. **CHILDREN:** 2–4 mg/kg/day in divided doses twice a day. **Maximum:** 300 mg/day.

DUODENAL ULCER ASSOCIATED WITH *H. PYLORI* INFECTION

PO: ADULTS, ELDERLY: 400 mg twice a day for 4 wks in combination.

EROSIVE ESOPHAGITIS

PO: ADULTS, ELDERLY: 150 mg 4 times a day. Maintenance: 150 mg twice a day or 300 mg at bedtime. **CHILDREN:** 4–10 mg/kg/day in 2 divided doses. **Maximum:** 600 mg/day.

HYPERSECRETORY CONDITIONS

PO: ADULTS, ELDERLY: 150 mg twice a day. May increase up to 6 g/day.

OTC USE

PO: ADULTS, ELDERLY: 75 mg 30–60 min before eating food, drinking beverages that cause heartburn. **Maximum:** 150 mg per 24 hr period and/or longer than 14 days.

USUAL PARENTERAL DOSAGE

IV, IM: ADULTS, ELDERLY: 50 mg/dose q6–8h. **Maximum:** 400 mg/day. **CHILDREN:** 2–4 mg/kg/day in divided doses q6–8h. **Maximum:** 200 mg/day.

USUAL NEONATAL DOSAGE

PO: NEONATES: 2 mg/kg/day in divided doses q12h.

IV: NEONATES: Initially, 1.5 mg/kg/dose; then 1.5–2 mg/kg/day in divided doses q12h.

DOSAGE IN RENAL IMPAIRMENT

For pts with creatinine clearance less than 50 ml/min, give 150 mg PO q24h or 50 mg IV or IM q18–24h.

SIDE EFFECTS

OCCASIONAL (2%): Diarrhea. **RARE (1%):** Constipation, headache (may be severe).

ADVERSE EFFECTS/ TOXIC REACTIONS

Reversible hepatitis, blood dyscrasias occur rarely.

NURSING CONSIDERATIONS

BASELINE ASSESSMENT

Obtain baseline hepatic/renal function tests.

INTERVENTION/EVALUATION

Monitor serum AST, ALT levels. Assess mental status in elderly.

PATIENT/FAMILY TEACHING

• Smoking decreases effectiveness of medication. • Do not take medicine within 1 hr of magnesium- or aluminum-containing antacids. • Transient burning/pruritus may occur with IV administration. • Report headache. • Avoid alcohol, aspirin.

ranolazine

rah-**no**-lah-zeen

(Ranexa)

CLASSIFICATION

PHARMACOTHERAPEUTIC: Sodium current inhibitor. **CLINICAL:** Antianginal, antieschemic.

ACTION

Thought to elicit changes in cardiac metabolism. Does not reduce heart rate, B/P. **Therapeutic Effect:** Exerts antianginal, antieschemic effects on cardiac tissue.

PHARMACOKINETICS

	Onset	Peak	Duration
PO	N/A	2–5 hrs	N/A

Absorption highly variable. Rapidly, extensively metabolized in intestine, liver. Protein binding: 62%. Eliminated mainly in urine, with lesser amount excreted in feces. **Half-life:** 7 hrs.

USES

Treatment of chronic angina in those who have not achieved adequate response with other antianginal agents.

R

PRECAUTIONS

CONTRAINDICATIONS: Preexisting QT prolongation, hepatic impairment, concurrent use with medications known to cause QT interval prolongation, concurrent use with diltiazem, potent CYP3A inhibitors (ketoconazole, itraconazole, fluconazole, clarithromycin, erythromycin, troleandomycin). **CAUTIONS:** Renal impairment.

⌛ LIFESPAN CONSIDERATIONS:

Pregnancy/Lactation: Unknown if drug crosses placenta or is distributed in breast milk. **Pregnancy Category C. Children:** Safety and efficacy not established. **Elderly:** No age-related precautions noted.

INTERACTIONS

DRUG: Ketoconazole, diltiazem, verapamil, paroxetine may increase serum concentration. May increase concentration of **digoxin, simvastatin. Quinidine, dofetilide, sotalol, antiarrhythmic agents, erythromycin, thioridazine, ziprasidone** may increase QT prolongation. **HERBAL:** None significant. **FOOD: Grapefruit, grapefruit juice** may increase plasma concentration, risk of QT prolongation. **LAB VALUES:** May slightly elevate BUN, serum creatinine.

R

AVAILABILITY (Rx)

TABLETS (EXTENDED-RELEASE): 500 mg.

ADMINISTRATION/HANDLING

PO

- May give without regard to food.
- Avoid grapefruit, grapefruit juice.
- Do not crush, chew, break film-coated tablets.

INDICATIONS/ROUTES/DOSAGE

CHRONIC ANGINA

PO: ADULTS, ELDERLY: Initially, 500 mg twice daily. May increase to 1,000 mg twice daily, based on clinical response.

SIDE EFFECTS

OCCASIONAL (6%–4%): Dizziness, headache, constipation, nausea. **RARE (2%–1%):** Peripheral edema, abdominal pain, dry mouth, vomiting, tinnitus, vertigo, palpitations.

ADVERSE EFFECTS/ TOXIC REACTIONS

Overdose manifested as confusion, diplopia, dizziness, paresthesia, syncope.

NURSING CONSIDERATIONS

BASELINE ASSESSMENT

Record onset, type (sharp, dull, squeezing), radiation, location, intensity, duration of anginal pain, precipitating factors (exertion, emotional stress). Obtain baseline EKG.

INTERVENTION/EVALUATION

Assist with ambulation if dizziness occurs. Give with food if nausea appears. Monitor daily pattern of bowel activity/ stool consistency. Assess for relief of anginal pain. Monitor EKG, pulse for irregularities.

PATIENT/FAMILY TEACHING

• Avoid grapefruit, grapefruit juice. • Do not chew/crush extended-release tablets. • Avoid tasks requiring mental alertness, motor acuity until response to drug is established.

Raptiva, *see efalizumab*

rasagiline

rah-**sah**-jih-leen
(Azilect)

CLASSIFICATION

PHARMACOTHERAPEUTIC: MAOI. **CLINICAL:** Antiparkinson agent.

ACTION

Inhibits monoamine oxidase, an enzyme that plays a major role in catabolism of dopamine. Inhibition of dopamine depletion reduces symptomatic motor deficits of Parkinson's disease. Appears to possess neuroprotective effects, delaying onset of symptoms, progression of neuronal deterioration. **Therapeutic Effect:** Reduces symptoms of Parkinson's disease, appears to delay disease progression.

PHARMACOKINETICS

	Onset	Peak	Duration
PO	1 hr	N/A	1 wk

Rapidly absorbed following PO administration. Protein binding: 88%–94%. Metabolized in liver. Mainly eliminated in urine, with lesser amount excreted in feces. **Half-life:** 3 hrs.

USES

Treatment of signs/symptoms of Parkinson's disease as initial monotherapy or as adjunct therapy to levodopa.

PRECAUTIONS

CONTRAINDICATIONS: Pheochromocytoma, concurrent use with meperidine, methadone, propoxyphene, tramadol, dextromethorphan, St. John's wort, mirtazapine, cyclobenzaprine, sympathomimetic amines (including amphetamines, nasal/oral decongestants, cold products, weight-reducing preparations), other MAOIs, cocaine, local or general anesthetic agents. **CAUTIONS:** Hepatic impairment, ingestion of tyramine-rich foods, beverages, dietary supplements or amines contained in cough/cold medications.

LIFESPAN CONSIDERATIONS:

Pregnancy/Lactation: Unknown if distributed in breast milk. **Pregnancy Category C. Children:** Safety and efficacy not established. **Elderly:** No age-related precautions noted.

INTERACTIONS

DRUG: Amphetamines, other MAOIs (phenelzine, tranylcypromine), sympathomimetics (dopamine, metaraminol, phenylephrine, pseudoephedrine) may cause hypertensive crisis. **Anorexiants (dexfenfluramine, fenfluramine, sibutramine), CNS stimulants (methylphenidate), cyclobenzaprine, dextromethorphan, meperadine, methadone, mirtazine, propoxyphene, sibutramine, serotonin or norepinephrine reuptake inhibitors, trazodone, tricyclic antidepressants, venlafaxine, tramodol** may cause serotonin syndrome. May increase risk of **atomoxetine, bupropion** toxicity. **Buspirone** may cause increase in B/P. **Entacapone, tolcapone, ciprofloxacin** (reduced dosage recommended) may increase concentration. **Aminoglutethimide, carbamazepine, phenobarbital, rifampin**may decrease concentration. **Levodopa** may cause hypertensive/hypotensive reaction. **Lithium** may result in malignant hyperpyrexia. **Reserpine** may result in hypertensive reaction. **Tramadol** may increase risk of seizures. **HERBAL: St. John's wort, valerian, SAMe, kava kava** may increase risk of serotonin syndrome, excessive sedation. **FOOD: Foods/beverages containing tyramine** may result in hypertensive reaction, hypertensive crisis. **LAB VALUES:** May increase serum alkaline phosphatase, bilirubin, ALT, AST.

AVAILABILITY (Rx)

TABLETS: 0.5 mg, 1 mg.

R

ADMINISTRATION/HANDLING

PO

• Give without regard to food. • Avoid food, beverages containing tyramine (cheese, sour cream, yogurt, pickled herring, liver, canned figs, raisins, bananas, avocados, soy sauce, broad beans, yeast extracts, meats prepared with tenderizers, red wine, beer).

INDICATIONS/ROUTES/DOSAGE

◀ **ALERT** ▶ When used in combination with levodopa, dosage reduction of levodopa should be considered.

PARKINSON'S DISEASE

PO: ADULTS, ELDERLY MONOTHERAPY: 1 mg once daily.

PO: ADULTS, ELDERLY, ADJUNCTIVE THERAPY: Initially, 0.5 mg once daily. If therapeutic response is not achieved, dose may be increased to 1 mg once daily.

MILD HEPATIC IMPAIRMENT, CONCURRENT USE OF CIPROFLOXACIN

PO: ADULTS, ELDERLY: 0.5 mg once daily.

SIDE EFFECTS

FREQUENT (14%–12%): Headache, nausea. **OCCASIONAL (9%–5%):** Orthostatic hypotension, weight loss, dyspepsia (heartburn, indigestion, epigastric pain), dry mouth, arthralgia, depression, hallucinations, constipation. **RARE (4%–2%):** Fever, vertigo, ecchymosis, rhinitis, neck pain, arthritis, paresthesia.

R

ADVERSE EFFECTS/ TOXIC REACTIONS

Increase in dyskinesia (impaired voluntary movement), dystonia (impaired muscular tone) occurs in 18% of pts, angina occurs in 9%. Gastroenteritis, conjunctivitis occur rarely (3%).

NURSING CONSIDERATIONS

BASELINE ASSESSMENT

If hallucinations or dyskinesia occur, symptoms may be eliminated if levodopa dosage is reduced. Hallucinations generally are accompanied by confusion and, to a lesser extent, insomnia. Obtain baseline hepatic enzyme levels.

INTERVENTION/EVALUATION

Give with food if nausea occurs. Instruct pt to rise from lying to sitting or sitting to standing position slowly to prevent orthostatic hypotension. Assess for clinical reversal of symptoms (improvement of tremor of head/hands at rest, mask-like facial expression, shuffling gait, muscular rigidity).

PATIENT/FAMILY TEACHING

Orthostatic hypotension may occur more frequently during initial therapy. Avoid tasks that require alertness, motor skills until response to drug is established. Hallucinations may occur (more so in the elderly than in younger pts with Parkinson's disease), typically within first 2 wks of therapy. Avoid foods that contain tyramine (cheese, sour cream, beer, wine, pickled herring, liver, figs, raisins, bananas, avocados, soy sauce, yeast extracts, yogurt, papaya, broad beans, meat tenderizers), excessive amounts of caffeine (coffee, tea, chocolate), OTC preparations for hay fever, colds, weight reduction (may produce significant rise in B/P).

Rebetol, *see ribavirin*

Reglan, *see metoclopramide*

Remeron, *see mirtazipine*

Remicade, *see infliximab*

remifentanil

(Ultiva)

See Opioid analgesics

RenaGel, *see sevelamer*

ReoPro, *see abciximab*

repaglinide

reh-**pah**-glih-nide

(GlucoNorm ✤, Prandin)

CLASSIFICATION

PHARMACOTHERAPEUTIC: Antihyperglycemic. **CLINICAL:** Antidiabetic (see p. 42C).

ACTION

Stimulates release of insulin from beta cells of pancreas by depolarizing beta cells, leading to opening of calcium channels. Resulting calcium influx induces insulin secretion. **Therapeutic Effect:** Lowers serum glucose concentration.

PHARMACOKINETICS

Rapidly, completely absorbed from GI tract. Protein binding: 98%. Metabolized in liver to inactive metabolites. Excreted primarily in feces, with lesser amount in urine. Unknown if removed by hemodialysis. **Half-life:** 1 hr.

USES

Adjunct to diet, exercise to lower serum glucose in pts with type 2 diabetes mellitus. Used as monotherapy or in combination with metformin, pioglitazone, rosiglitazone.

PRECAUTIONS

CONTRAINDICATIONS: Diabetic ketoacidosis, type 1 diabetes mellitus. **CAUTIONS:** Hepatic/renal impairment.

LIFESPAN CONSIDERATIONS: **Pregnancy/Lactation:** Unknown if drug is distributed in breast milk. **Pregnancy Category C. Children:** Safety and efficacy not established. **Elderly:** No age-related precautions noted, but hypoglycemia may be more difficult to recognize.

INTERACTIONS

DRUG: **Beta-adrenergic blocking agents (beta-blockers), gemfibrozil, MAOIs, NSAIDs, probenecid, salicylates, sulfonamides, warfarin** may increase effects. **HERBAL: St. John's wort** may decrease concentration. **Garlic** may cause hypoglycemia. **FOOD: Food** decreases concentration. **LAB VALUES:** None known.

AVAILABILITY (Rx)

TABLETS: 0.5 mg, 1 mg, 2 mg.

ADMINISTRATION/HANDLING

PO

- Ideally, give within 15 min of a meal but may be given immediately before a meal to as long as 30 min before a meal.

INDICATIONS/ROUTES/DOSAGE

DIABETES MELLITUS

PO: ADULTS, ELDERLY: 0.5–4 mg 2–4 times a day. **Maximum:** 16 mg/day.

SIDE EFFECTS

FREQUENT (10%–6%): Upper respiratory tract infection, headache, rhinitis,

R

bronchitis, back pain. **OCCASIONAL (5%–3%):** Diarrhea, dyspepsia (heartburn, indigestion, epigastric pain), sinusitis, nausea, arthralgia, UTI. **RARE (2%):** Constipation, vomiting, paresthesia, allergy.

ADVERSE EFFECTS/ TOXIC REACTIONS

Hypoglycemia occurs in 16% of pts. Chest pain occurs rarely.

NURSING CONSIDERATIONS

BASELINE ASSESSMENT

Check fasting serum glucose, glycosylated Hgb (HbA_1C) levels periodically to determine minimum effective dose. Ensure follow-up instruction if pt, family do not thoroughly understand diabetes management, glucose-testing technique. At least 1 wk should elapse to assess response to drug before new dosage adjustment is made.

INTERVENTION/EVALUATION

Monitor fasting serum glucose, glycosylated Hgb (HbA_1C) levels, food intake. Assess for hypoglycemia (cool/wet skin, tremors, dizziness, anxiety, headache, tachycardia, numbness in mouth, hunger, diplopia), hyperglycemia (polyuria, polyphagia, polydipsia, nausea, vomiting, dim vision, fatigue, deep or rapid breathing). Be alert to conditions that alter glucose requirements (fever, increased activity/stress, surgical procedures).

PATIENT/FAMILY TEACHING

• Diabetes mellitus requires lifelong control. • Prescribed diet, exercise is principal part of treatment; do not skip, delay meals. • Continue to adhere to dietary instructions, regular exercise program, regular testing of urine or serum glucose. • When taking combination drug therapy with a sulfonylurea or insulin, have source of glucose available to treat symptoms of low blood sugar.

Requip, *see ropinirole*

respiratory syncytial immune globulin

res-purr-ah-tore-ee sin-**sish**-ee-al ih-**mewn glah**-byew-lin
(RespiGam)

◆CLASSIFICATION

PHARMACOTHERAPEUTIC: Immune-serum. **CLINICAL:** Respiratory agent.

ACTION

High concentration of neutralizing protective antibodies specific for respiratory syncytial virus (RSV). **Therapeutic Effect:** Provides protection against RSV infection, decreases severity of existing infection.

USES

Prevents serious lower respiratory tract infections caused by RSV in children younger than 24 mos with bronchopulmonary dysplasia, history of premature birth.

PRECAUTIONS

CONTRAINDICATIONS: IgA deficiency, hypersensitivity to other human immunoglobulins. **CAUTIONS:** Pulmonary disease.

LIFESPAN CONSIDERATIONS:

Pregnancy/Lactation: Unknown if distributed in breast milk. **Pregnancy Category C. Children:** Safety and efficacy not established. **Elderly:** No age-related precautions noted.

INTERACTIONS

DRUG: **Live virus vaccines** may potentiate virus replication, increase vaccine side effects, decrease pt's antibody response to vaccine. **HERBAL:** None significant. **FOOD:** None known. **LAB VALUES:** None known.

AVAILABILITY (Rx)

INJECTION SOLUTION: 2,500 mcg RSV immune globulin.

ADMINISTRATION/HANDLING

IV

Rate of administration • Initial infusion rate of 1.5 ml/kg/hr for first 15 min, then increase to 3.6 ml/kg/hr (decreased in pts at risk of renal dysfunction). Infusion rate of 6 ml/kg/hr 30 min to end of infusion. • Maximum infusion rate: 6 ml/kg/hr.

Storage • Refrigerate vials. Do not freeze. • Do not shake. • Start infusion within 6 hrs and complete within 12 hrs of vial entry.

INDICATIONS/ROUTES/DOSAGE

PREVENTION OF RSV IN CHILDREN WITH BRONCHOPULMONARY DYSPLASIA, HISTORY OF PREMATURE BIRTH

IV: CHILDREN YOUNGER THAN 24 MOS: 750 mg/kg (15 ml/kg) administered at a rate of 1.5 ml/kg/hr for the first 15 min, then 3.6 ml/kg/hr for remainder of infusion. Given once monthly for 5 doses beginning in September or October.

SIDE EFFECTS

OCCASIONAL (6%–2%): Fever, vomiting, wheezing. **RARE (less than 1%):** Diarrhea, rash, tachycardia, hypertension, hypoxia, injection site inflammation.

ADVERSE EFFECTS/ TOXIC REACTIONS

Hypersensitivity reaction, characterized by dizziness, flushing, anxiety, palpitations, pruritus, myalgia, arthralgia, occur rarely.

NURSING CONSIDERATIONS

INTERVENTION/EVALUATION

Monitor heart rate, B/P, temperature, respiratory rate. Observe for rales, wheezing, retractions.

Restoril, *see temazepam*

reteplase

reh-te-place

(Retavase)

Do not confuse reteplase or Retavase with Restasis.

CLASSIFICATION

PHARMACOTHERAPEUTIC: Tissue plasminogen activator. **CLINICAL:** Thrombolytic (see p. 32C).

ACTION

Activates fibrinolytic system by directly cleaving plasminogen to generate plasmin, an enzyme that degrades fibrin of thrombus. **Therapeutic Effect:** Exerts thrombolytic action.

PHARMACOKINETICS

Rapidly cleared from plasma. Eliminated primarily by liver, kidney. **Half-life:** 13–16 min.

USES

Management of acute myocardial infarction (AMI), improvement of ventricular function following AMI, reduction of incidence of CHF, reduction of mortality associated with AMI. **OFF-LABEL:** Occluded catheters.

PRECAUTIONS

CONTRAINDICATIONS: Active internal bleeding, AV malformation/aneurysm,

R

bleeding diathesis, history of cerebrovascular accident (CVA), intracranial neoplasm, recent intracranial/intraspinal surgery or trauma, severe uncontrolled hypertension. **CAUTIONS:** Recent major surgery (coronary artery bypass graft, OB delivery, organ biopsy), cerebrovascular disease, recent GI/GU bleeding, hypertension, mitral stenosis with atrial fibrillation, acute pericarditis, bacterial endocarditis, hepatic/renal impairment, diabetic retinopathy, ophthalmic hemorrhage, septic thrombophlebitis, occluded AV cannula at infected site, advanced age, pts receiving oral anticoagulants.

LIFESPAN CONSIDERATIONS:

Pregnancy/Lactation: Unknown if drug is distributed in breast milk. **Pregnancy Category C. Children:** Safety and efficacy not established. **Elderly:** More susceptible to bleeding; caution advised.

INTERACTIONS

DRUG: **Heparin, platelet aggregation antagonists (e.g., abciximab, aspirin, dipyridamole), warfarin** increase risk of bleeding. **HERBAL:** **Cat's claw, dong quai, evening primrose, feverfew, garlic, ginger, ginkgo, red clover, ginseng** possess antiplatelet action, may increase bleeding. **FOOD:** None known. **LAB VALUES:** May decrease serum fibrinogen, plasminogen.

AVAILABILITY (Rx)

INJECTION POWDER FOR RECONSTITUTION: 10.4 units (18.1 mg).

ADMINISTRATION/HANDLING

IV

Reconstitution • Reconstitute only with Sterile Water for Injection immediately before use. • Reconstituted solution contains 1 unit/ml. • Do not shake. • Slight foaming may occur; let stand for a few minutes to allow bubbles to dissipate.

Rate of administration • Give through dedicated IV line. • Give as a 10 unit plus 10 unit double bolus, with each IV bolus administered over 2-min period. • Give second bolus 30 min after first bolus injection. • Do not add other medications to bolus injection solution. • Do not give second bolus if serious bleeding occurs after first IV bolus is given.

Storage • Use within 4 hrs of reconstitution. • Discard any unused portion.

IV INCOMPATIBILITIES

Do not mix with other medications.

INDICATIONS/ROUTES/DOSAGE

ACUTE MI, CHF

IV BOLUS: ADULTS, ELDERLY: 10 units over 2 min; repeat in 30 min.

SIDE EFFECTS

FREQUENT: Bleeding at superficial sites, such as venous injection sites, catheter insertion sites, venous cutdowns, arterial punctures, sites of recent surgical procedures, gingival bleeding.

ADVERSE EFFECTS/ TOXIC REACTIONS

Bleeding at internal sites (intracranial, retroperitoneal, GI, GU, respiratory) occurs occasionally. Lysis of coronary thrombi may produce atrial or ventricular arrhythmias, stroke.

NURSING CONSIDERATIONS

BASELINE ASSESSMENT

Obtain baseline B/P, apical pulse. Evaluate 12-lead EKG, CPK, CPK-MB, serum electrolytes. Assess Hct, platelet count, thrombin (TT), activated partial thromboplastin time (aPTT), prothrombin time (PT), serum plasminogen, fibrinogen levels before therapy is instituted. Type, hold blood.

INTERVENTION/EVALUATION

Carefully monitor all needle puncture sites, catheter insertion sites for

R

bleeding. Continuous cardiac monitoring for arrhythmias, B/P, pulse, respiration is essential until pt is stable. Check peripheral pulses, lung sounds. Monitor for chest pain relief; notify physician of continuation/recurrence of chest pain (note location, type, intensity). Avoid any trauma that may increase risk of bleeding (injections, shaving).

Rh_0 (D) immune globulin

row D ih-**mewn glah**-byew-lin

(BayRho-D, BayRho-D Full Dose, BayRho-D Mini-dose, MICRhoGAM, RhoGAM, Rhophylac, WinRho SDF)

CLASSIFICATION

CLINICAL: Immune globulin.

ACTION

Suppresses active antibody response, formation of anti-Rh_0(D) in Rh_0(D)-negative women exposed to Rh_0-positive blood from pregnancy with Rh_0(D)-positive fetus or transfusion with Rh_0(D)-positive blood. Injection of Rh_0(D) immune globulin into Rh-positive pt with idiopathic thrombocytopenic purpura (ITP) coats pt's own D-positive RBCs with antibody; as RBCs are cleared by spleen, they saturate capacity of spleen to clear antibody-coated cells. **Therapeutic Effect:** Prevents antibody response, hemolytic disease of newborn in women who previously conceived Rh_0(D)-positive fetus. Prevents Rh_0(D) sensitization in pts who have received Rh_0(D)-positive blood. Decreases bleeding in pts with ITP.

PHARMACOKINETICS

Half-life: 24 days (IV); 30 days (IM).

USES

Treatment of Rh_0(D)-positive children, adults (without splenectomy) with chronic ITP, children with acute ITP, children, adults with ITP secondary to HIV infection; prevention of isoimmunization in Rh-negative individuals exposed to Rh-positive blood during delivery of an Rh-positive infant, within 72 hrs of an abortion, following amniocentesis or abdominal trauma, following transfusion accident; prevention of hemolytic disease of newborn if there is a subsequent pregnancy with Rh-positive infant.

PRECAUTIONS

CONTRAINDICATIONS: Hypersensitivity to any component, IgA deficiency, mothers whose Rh group or immune status is uncertain, prior sensitization to Rh_0(D), Rh_0(D)-positive mother or pregnant woman, transfusion of Rh_0(D)-positive blood in previous 3 mos. **CAUTIONS:** Thrombocytopenia, bleeding disorders. Hgb less than 8 g/dl.

LIFESPAN CONSIDERATIONS:

Pregnancy/Lactation: Does not appear to harm fetus. **Pregnancy Category C. Children/Elderly:** No age-related precautions noted.

INTERACTIONS

DRUG: May interfere with the pt's immune response to **live virus vaccines. HERBAL:** None significant. **FOOD:** None known. **LAB VALUES:** None known.

AVAILABILITY (Rx)

INJECTION, POWDER FOR RECONSTITUTION (WINRHO SDF): 120 mcg, 300 mcg, 1000 mcg. **INJECTION SOLUTION:** 50 mcg (BayRho-D Mini-dose, MICRhoGAM), 300 mcg (BayRho-D Full Dose, RhoGAM), 300 mcg/2 ml (Rhophylac).

ADMINISTRATION/HANDLING

IV

Reconstitution • Reconstitute 120 mcg and 300 mcg with 2.5 ml NaCl

R

(8.5 ml for 1,000-mcg vial). • Gently swirl; do not shake.

Rate of administration • Infuse over 3–5 min.

Storage • Refrigerate vials (do not freeze). • Once reconstituted, stable for 12 hrs at room temperature.

IM

• Reconstitute 120 mcg and 300 mcg with 2.5 ml NaCl (8.5 ml for 1,000-mcg vial). • Administer into deltoid muscle of upper arm, anterolateral aspect of upper thigh.

INDICATIONS/ROUTES/DOSAGE

ITP

IV (WinRho SDF): ADULTS, ELDERLY, CHILDREN: Initially, 50 mcg/kg as single dose (reduce to 25–40 mcg/kg if Hgb is less than 10 g/dl). Maintenance: 25–60 mcg/kg based on platelet count and Hgb level.

SUPPRESSION OF ACTIVE ANTIBODY RESPONSE IN PREGNANCY

IM (BayRho-D FULL DOSE, RhoGAM): ADULTS: 300 mcg preferably within 72 hrs of delivery.

IV, IM (WinRho SDF): ADULTS: 300 mcg at 28 wks gestation. After delivery: 120 mcg preferably within 72 hrs.

SUPPRESSION OF ACTIVE ANTIBODY RESPONSE IN THREATENED ABORTION

IM (BayRho-D FULL DOSE, RhoGAM): ADULTS: 300 mcg as soon as possible.

SUPPRESSON OF ACTIVE ANTIBODY RESPONSE IN ABORTION, MISCARRIAGE, TERMINATION OF ECTOPIC PREGNANCY

IM (BayRho-D, RhoGAM): ADULTS: 300 mcg if more than 13 wks gestation, 50 mcg if less than 13 wks gestation.
IV, IM (WinRho SDF): ADULTS: 120 mcg after 34 wks gestation.

TRANSFUSION INCOMPATIBILITY

◀ **ALERT** ▶ Must give within 72 hrs after exposure to incompatible blood transfusion, massive fetal hemorrhage.

IV: ADULTS: 3,000 units (600 mcg) q8h until total dose given.
IM: ADULTS: 6,000 units (1,200 mcg) q12h until total dose given.

SIDE EFFECTS

Hypotension, pallor, vasodilation (IV formulation), fever, headache, chills, dizziness, somnolence, lethargy, rash, pruritus, abdominal pain, diarrhea, discomfort/swelling at injection site, back pain, myalgia, arthralgia, asthenia.

ADVERSE EFFECTS/ TOXIC REACTIONS

Acute renal failure occurs rarely.

NURSING CONSIDERATIONS

BASELINE ASSESSMENT

Determine existence of bleeding disorders. Assess the pt's Hgb level; give this drug cautiously to pts with Hgb level less than 8 g/dl.

INTERVENTION/EVALUATION

Monitor CBC (esp. Hgb, platelet count), BUN, serum creatinine, reticulocyte count, urinalysis results. Assess for signs/symptoms of hemolysis.

PATIENT/FAMILY TEACHING

• Inform pt this drug is given only by injection, which may be painful. • Notify physician if chills, dizziness, fever, headache, rash occur.

Rhinocort Aqua, *see budesonide*

ribavirin

rye-ba-**vye**-rin
(Copegus, Rebetol, Virazole)

Do not confuse ribavirin with riboflavin.

FIXED-COMBINATION(S)

With interferon alfa 2b (**Rebetron**). Individually packaged.

CLASSIFICATION

PHARMACOTHERAPEUTIC: Synthetic nucleoside. **CLINICAL:** Antiviral (see p. 65C).

ACTION

Inhibits replication of viral RNA, DNA, influenza virus RNA polymerase activity, interferes with expression of messenger RNA. **Therapeutic Effect:** Inhibits viral protein synthesis.

USES

Inhalation: Treatment of respiratory syncytial virus (RSV) infections (esp. in pts with underlying compromising conditions such as chronic lung disorders, congenital heart disease, recent transplant recipients). **Capsule/Tablet/Oral Solution:** Treatment of chronic hepatitis C in pts with compensated hepatic disease. **OFF-LABEL:** Treatment of influenza A or B, West Nile virus.

PRECAUTIONS

CONTRAINDICATIONS: Autoimmune hepatitis, creatinine clearance less than 50 ml/min, hemoglobinopathies, hepatic decompensation, hypersensitivity to ribavirin products, pregnancy, significant or unstable cardiac disease, women of childbearing age who do not use contraception reliably. **CAUTIONS: Inhalation:** Pts requiring assisted ventilation, chronic obstructive pulmonary disease (COPD), asthma. **Oral:** Cardiac, pulmonary disease, elderly, history of psychiatric disorders. **Pregnancy Category X.**

INTERACTIONS

DRUG: Didanosine may increase risk of pancreatitis, peripheral neuropathy. May decrease effects of **didanosine. Nucleoside analogues (e.g., adefovir, didanosine, lamivudine, stavudine, zalcitabine, zidovudine)** may increase risk of lactic acidosis. **HERBAL:** None significant. **FOOD:** None known. **LAB VALUES:** None known.

AVAILABILITY (Rx)

CAPSULES (REBETOL): 200 mg. **POWDER FOR AEROSOL (VIRAZOLE):** 6 g. **POWDER FOR SOLUTION, INHALATION (VIRAZOLE):** 6 g. **TABLET (COPEGUS):** 200 mg.

ADMINISTRATION/HANDLING

PO

• Capsules may be taken without regard to food. • Tablets should be given with food.

INHALATION

◄ **ALERT** ► May be given via nasal or oral inhalation.

• Solution appears clear, colorless; is stable for 24 hrs at room temperature. • Discard solution for nebulization after 24 hrs. • Discard if discolored or cloudy. • Add 50–100 ml Sterile Water for Injection or Inhalation to 6-g vial. • Transfer to a flask, serving as reservoir for aerosol generator. • Further dilute to final volume of 300 ml, giving solution concentration of 20 mg/ml. • Use only aerosol generator available from manufacturer of drug. • Do not give concomitantly with other drug solutions for nebulization. • Discard reservoir solution when fluid levels are low and at least q24h. • Controversy over safety in ventilator-dependent pts; only experienced personnel should administer drug.

INDICATIONS/ROUTES/DOSAGE

CHRONIC HEPATITIS C

PO (CAPSULE COMBINATION WITH INTERFERON ALFA-2B): ADULTS, ELDERLY: 1,000–1,200 mg/day in 2 divided doses. **CHILDREN WEIGHING 60 KG OR MORE:** Use adult dosage. **CHILDREN**

R

WEIGHING 51–59 KG: 400 mg 2 times/day. **CHILDREN WEIGHING 31–50 KG:** 200 mg in morning, 400 mg in evening. **CHILDREN WEIGHING 24–36 KG:** 200 mg 2 times/day.
PO (CAPSULES IN COMBINATION WITH PEGINTERFERON ALFA-2B): **ADULTS, ELDERLY:** 800 mg/day in 2 divided doses.
PO (TABLETS IN COMBINATION WITH PEGINTERFERON ALFA-2B): **ADULTS, ELDERLY:** 800–1,200 mg/day in 2 divided doses.

SEVERE LOWER RESPIRATORY TRACT INFECTION CAUSED BY RSV
INHALATION: CHILDREN, INFANTS: Use with Viratek small-particle aerosol generator at concentration of 20 mg/ml (6 g reconstituted with 300 ml Sterile Water for Injection) over 12–18 hrs/day for 3–7 days.

SIDE EFFECTS

FREQUENT (greater than 10%): Dizziness, headache, fatigue, fever, insomnia, irritability, depression, emotional lability, impaired concentration, alopecia, rash, pruritus, nausea, anorexia, dyspepsia, vomiting, decreased hemoglobin, hemolysis, arthralgia, musculoskeletal pain, dyspnea, sinusitis, flu-like symptoms. **OCCASIONAL (1%–10%):** Nervousness, altered taste, weakness.

R

ADVERSE EFFECTS/ TOXIC REACTIONS

Cardiac arrest, apnea, ventilator dependence, bacterial pneumonia, pneumonia, pneumothorax occur rarely. If treatment exceeds 7 days, anemia may occur.

NURSING CONSIDERATIONS

BASELINE ASSESSMENT

Obtain sputum specimens before giving first dose or at least during first 24 hrs of therapy. Assess respiratory status for baseline. **Oral:** CBC with differential, pretreatment and monthly pregnancy test for women of childbearing age.

INTERVENTION/EVALUATION

Monitor I&O, fluid balance carefully. Check hematology reports for anemia due to reticulocytosis when therapy exceeds 7 days. For ventilator-assisted pts, watch for "rainout" in tubing and empty frequently; be alert to impaired ventilation/gas exchange due to drug precipitate. Assess skin for rash. Monitor B/P, respirations; assess lung sounds.

PATIENT/FAMILY TEACHING

• Report immediately any difficulty breathing, itching/swelling/redness of eyes. • Educate females about prevention of pregnancy and need for pregnancy testing. • Educate males about protection of female partners from pregnancy.

rifabutin

rye-fah-**byew**-tin
(Mycobutin)

Do not confuse rifabutin with rifampin.

CLASSIFICATION

PHARMACOTHERAPEUTIC: Antitubercular. **CLINICAL:** Antibacterial (antimycobacterial).

ACTION

Inhibits DNA-dependent RNA polymerase, an enzyme in susceptible strains of *Escherichia coli, Bacillus subtilis*. Broad-spectrum of activity, including mycobacteria such as *Mycobacterium avium* complex (MAC). **Therapeutic Effect:** Prevents MAC disease.

PHARMACOKINETICS

Readily absorbed from GI tract (high-fat meals delay absorption). Protein binding: 85%. Widely distributed. Crosses blood-brain barrier. Extensive intracellular tissue uptake. Metabolized in liver to active metabolite. Excreted in urine; eliminated in feces. Unknown if removed by hemodialysis. **Half-life:** 16–69 hrs.

USES

Prevention of disseminated MAC disease in those with advanced HIV infection. **OFF-LABEL:** Part of multidrug regimen for treatment of MAC.

PRECAUTIONS

CONTRAINDICATIONS: Active tuberculosis; hypersensitivity to other rifamycins, including rifampin. **CAUTIONS:** Safety in children not established. Renal/hepatic impairment.

LIFESPAN CONSIDERATIONS:

Pregnancy/Lactation: Unknown if drug crosses placenta or is excreted in breast milk. **Pregnancy Category B.** **Children/Elderly:** No age-related precautions noted.

INTERACTIONS

DRUG: May decrease effectiveness of **oral contraceptives.** May decrease concentration, effect of **protease inhibitors (e.g., amprenavir, indinavir, ritonavir, saquinavir), non-nucleoside reverse transcriptase inhibitors (e.g., delavirdine, efavirenz, nevirapine). Protease inhibitors** may increase concentration, toxicity. May decrease concentration of **zidovudine** (does not affect inhibition of HIV). **HERBAL:** None significant. **FOOD:** None known. **LAB VALUES:** May increase serum alkaline phosphatase, AST, ALT. May decrease WBCs, Hgb, platelet count.

AVAILABILITY (Rx)

CAPSULES: 150 mg.

ADMINISTRATION/HANDLING

PO

• Give without regard to food. Give with food if GI irritation occurs. • May mix with applesauce if pt is unable to swallow capsules whole.

INDICATIONS/ROUTES/DOSAGE

PROPHYLAXIS OF MAC DISEASE (INITIAL EPISODE)

PO: ADULTS, ELDERLY: 300 mg as single dose or in 2 divided doses if GI upset occurs.

PROPHYLAXIS OF RECURRENT MAC DISEASE

PO: ADULTS, ELDERLY: 300 mg/day (in combination).

DOSAGE IN RENAL IMPAIRMENT

Dosage is modified based on creatinine clearance. If creatinine clearance is less than 30 ml/min, reduce dosage by 50%.

SIDE EFFECTS

FREQUENT (30%): Red-orange or red-brown discoloration of urine, feces, saliva, skin, sputum, sweat, tears. **OCCASIONAL (11%–3%):** Rash, nausea, abdominal pain, diarrhea, dyspepsia, belching, headache, altered taste, uveitis, corneal deposits. **RARE (less than 2%):** Anorexia, flatulence, fever, myalgia, vomiting, insomnia.

ADVERSE EFFECTS/ TOXIC REACTIONS

Hepatitis, anemia, thrombocytopenia, neutropenia occur rarely.

NURSING CONSIDERATIONS

BASELINE ASSESSMENT

Obtain chest x-ray, sputum blood cultures. Biopsy of suspicious node(s) must be done to rule out active tuberculosis. Obtain baseline CBC, serum hepatic function tests.

INTERVENTION/EVALUATION

Monitor serum hepatic function tests, CBC, platelet count, Hgb, Hct. Avoid IM injections, rectal temperatures, other trauma that may induce bleeding. Check temperature; notify physician of flu-like syndrome, rash, GI intolerance.

R

PATIENT/FAMILY TEACHING

• Urine, feces, saliva, sputum, perspiration, tears, skin may be discolored brown-orange. • Soft contact lenses may be permanently discolored. • Rifabutin may decrease efficacy of oral contraceptives; nonhormonal methods should be considered. • Avoid crowds, those with infection. • Report flu-like symptoms, nausea, vomiting, dark urine, unusual bruising/bleeding from any site, any visual disturbances.

rifampin

rif-**am**-pin

(Rifadin, Rifadin IV, Rofact ✤)

Do not confuse rifampin with rifabutin, Rifamate, rifapentine, or Ritalin.

FIXED-COMBINATION(S)

Rifamate: rifampin/isoniazid (an antitubercular): 300 mg/150 mg. **Rifater:** rifampin/isoniazid/pyrazinamide (an antitubercular): 120 mg/50 mg/300 mg.

CLASSIFICATION

PHARMACOTHERAPEUTIC: Antibiotic, miscellaneous. **CLINICAL:** Antitubercular.

ACTION

Interferes with bacterial RNA synthesis by binding to DNA-dependent RNA polymerase, preventing attachment to DNA, thereby blocking RNA transcription. **Therapeutic Effect:** Bactericidal in susceptible microorganisms.

PHARMACOKINETICS

Well absorbed from GI tract (food delays absorption). Protein binding: 80%. Widely distributed. Metabolized in liver to active metabolite. Primarily eliminated by biliary system. Not removed by hemodialysis. **Half-life:** 3–5 hrs (increased in hepatic impairment).

USES

In conjunction with at least one other antitubercular agent for initial treatment, retreatment of clinical tuberculosis. Eliminates *Neisseria* meningococci from nasopharynx of asymptomatic carriers in situations with high risk for meningococcal meningitis (prophylaxis, not cure). **OFF-LABEL:** Prophylaxis of *Haemophilus influenzae* type b infection; treatment of atypical mycobacterial infection serious infections caused by *Staphylococcus* species.

PRECAUTIONS

CONTRAINDICATIONS: Concomitant therapy with amprenavir, hypersensitivity to other rifamycins. **CAUTIONS:** Hepatic dysfunction, active or treated alcoholism.

⌛ LIFESPAN CONSIDERATIONS:

Pregnancy/Lactation: Crosses placenta. Distributed in breast milk. **Pregnancy Category C. Children/Elderly:** No age-related precautions noted.

INTERACTIONS

DRUG: **Alcohol, hepatotoxic medications, ritonavir, saquinavir** may increase risk of hepatotoxicity. May increase clearance of **aminophylline, theophylline.** May decrease effects of **digoxin, disopyramide, fluconazole, methadone, mexiletine, oral anticoagulants, oral antidiabetics, phenytoin, quinidine, tocainide, verapamil.** May decrease **oral contraceptive** effectiveness. **HERBAL:** None significant. **FOOD:** **Food** decreases extent of absorption. **LAB VALUES:** May increase serum alkaline phosphatase, bilirubin, uric acid, AST, ALT.

AVAILABILITY (Rx)

CAPSULES (RIFADIN): 150 mg, 300 mg. **INJECTION, POWDER FOR RECONSTITUTION (RIFADIN IV):** 600 mg.

ADMINISTRATION/HANDLING

IV

Reconstitution • Reconstitute 600-mg vial with 10 ml Sterile Water for Injection to provide concentration of 60 mg/ml. • Withdraw desired dose and further dilute with 500 ml D_5W.

Rate of administration • For IV infusion only. Avoid IM, subcutaneous administration. • Avoid extravasation (local irritation, inflammation). • Infuse over 3 hrs (may dilute with 100 ml D_5W and infuse over 30 min).

Storage • Reconstituted vial is stable for 24 hrs. • Once reconstituted vial is further diluted, it is stable for 4 hrs in D_5W or 24 hrs in 0.9% NaCl.

PO

• Preferably give 1 hr before or 2 hrs following meals with 8 oz of water (may give with food to decrease GI upset; will delay absorption). • For those unable to swallow capsules, contents may be mixed with applesauce, jelly. • Administer at least 1 hr before antacids, esp. those containing aluminum.

INDICATIONS/ROUTES/DOSAGE

TUBERCULOSIS

PO, IV: ADULTS, ELDERLY: 10 mg/kg/day. **Maximum:** 600 mg/day. **CHILDREN:** 10–20 mg/kg/day in divided doses q12–24h.

PREVENTION OF MENINGOCOCCAL INFECTIONS

PO, IV: ADULTS, ELDERLY: 600 mg q12h for 2 days. **CHILDREN 1 MO AND OLDER:** 20 mg/kg/day in divided doses q12–24h. **Maximum:** 600 mg/dose. **INFANTS YOUNGER THAN 1 MO:** 10 mg/kg/day in divided doses q12h for 2 days.

STAPHYLOCOCCAL INFECTIONS

PO, IV: ADULTS, ELDERLY: 600 mg once a day. **CHILDREN:** 15 mg/kg/day in divided doses q12h.

***STAPHYLOCOCCUS AUREUS* INFECTIONS (IN COMBINATION WITH OTHER ANTI-INFECTIVES)**

PO: ADULTS, ELDERLY: 300–600 mg twice a day. **NEONATES:** 5–20 mg/kg/day in divided doses q12h.

PREVENTION OF *H. INFLUENZAE* INFECTION

PO: ADULTS, ELDERLY: 600 mg/day for 4 days. **CHILDREN 1 MO AND OLDER:** 20 mg/kg/day in divided doses q12h for 5–10 days. **Maximum:** 600 mg. **CHILDREN YOUNGER THAN 1 MO:** 10 mg/kg/day in divided doses q12h for 2 days.

IV INCOMPATIBILITY

Diltiazem (Cardizem).

SIDE EFFECTS

EXPECTED: Red-orange or red-brown discoloration of urine, feces, saliva, skin, sputum, sweat, tears. **OCCASIONAL (5%–2%):** Hypersensitivity reaction (flushing, pruritus, rash). **RARE (2%–1%):** Diarrhea, dyspepsia, nausea, oral candida (sore mouth, tongue).

ADVERSE EFFECTS/ TOXIC REACTIONS

Hepatotoxicity (risk is increased when rifampin is taken with isoniazid), hepatitis, blood dyscrasias, Stevens-Johnson syndrome, antibiotic-associated colitis occur rarely.

NURSING CONSIDERATIONS

BASELINE ASSESSMENT

Question for hypersensitivity to rifampin, rifamycins. Ensure collection of diagnostic specimens. Evaluate initial serum hepatic/renal function, CBC results.

R

INTERVENTION/EVALUATION

Assess IV site at least hourly during infusion; restart at another site at the first sign of irritation or inflammation. Monitor hepatic function tests, assess for hepatitis: jaundice, anorexia, nausea, vomiting, fatigue, weakness (hold rifampin, inform physician at once). Report hypersensitivity reactions promptly: any type of skin eruption, pruritus, flu-like syndrome with high dosage. Monitor daily pattern of bowel activity/stool consistency (potential for antibiotic-associated colitis). Monitor CBC results for blood dyscrasias, be alert for infection (fever, sore throat), unusual bruising/bleeding, unusual fatigue/weakness.

PATIENT/FAMILY TEACHING

• Preferably take on empty stomach with 8 oz of water 1 hr before or 2 hrs after meal (with food if GI upset). • Avoid alcohol during treatment. • Do not take **any** other medications without consulting physician, including antacids; must take rifampin at least 1 hr before antacid. • Urine, feces, sputum, sweat, tears may become red-orange; soft contact lenses may be permanently stained. • Notify physician of **any** new symptom, immediately for yellow eyes/skin, fatigue, weakness, nausea/vomiting, sore throat, fever, flu, unusual bruising/bleeding. • If taking oral contraceptives, check with physician (reliability may be affected).

R

rifapentine

rif-a-**pen**-teen

(Priftin)

Do not confuse rifapentine with rifampin.

CLASSIFICATION

PHARMACOTHERAPEUTIC: Antitubercular.

ACTION

Inhibits DNA-dependent RNA polymerase in *Mycobacterium tuberculosis*. Prevents the enzyme from attaching to DNA, thereby blocking RNA transcription. **Therapeutic Effect:** Bactericidal.

PHARMACOKINETICS

Rapidly, well absorbed from GI tract. Protein binding: 97.7%. Metabolized in liver. Primarily eliminated in feces; partial excretion in urine. Not removed by hemodialysis. **Half-life:** 14–17 hrs.

USES

Treatment of pulmonary tuberculosis in combination with at least one other antituberculosis medication.

PRECAUTIONS

CONTRAINDICATIONS: History of hypersensitivity to any rifamycins (rifampin, rifabutin). **CAUTIONS:** Alcoholism, hepatic impairment.

LIFESPAN CONSIDERATIONS:

Pregnancy/Lactation: Unknown if drug crosses placenta or is distributed is breast milk. Because rifapentine may produce a red-orange discoloration of body fluids, there is a potential for discoloration of breast milk. **Pregnancy Category C. Children:** Safety and efficacy not established in children under 12 yrs. **Elderly:** Age-related renal/hepatic impairment may require dosage adjustment.

INTERACTIONS

DRUG: Alcohol may increase risk of hepatotoxicity. May decrease effect of **oral contraceptives, warfarin**. **HERBAL:** None significant. **FOOD:** None known. **LAB VALUES:** May increase serum bilirubin, AST, ALT.

AVAILABILITY (Rx)

TABLETS: 150 mg.

INDICATIONS/ROUTES/DOSAGE

TUBERCULOSIS

PO: ADULTS, ELDERLY: Intensive phase: 600 mg twice weekly for 2 mos (interval between doses no less than 3 days). **Continuation phase:** 600 mg weekly for 4 mos.

SIDE EFFECTS

RARE (less than 4%): Red-orange or red-brown discoloration of urine, feces, saliva, skin, sputum, sweat, tears; arthralgia, pain, nausea, vomiting, headache, dyspepsia, hypertension, dizziness, diarrhea.

ADVERSE EFFECTS/ TOXIC REACTIONS

Hyperuricemia, neutropenia, proteinuria, hematuria, hepatitis occur rarely.

NURSING CONSIDERATIONS

BASELINE ASSESSMENT

Evaluate initial serum hepatic function, CBC results.

INTERVENTION/EVALUATION

Monitor serum hepatic function tests, daily pattern of bowel activity/stool consistency. Assess for nausea, vomiting, GI upset, diarrhea.

PATIENT/FAMILY TEACHING

• Urine, feces, sputum, sweat, tears may become red-orange; soft contact lenses may be permanently stained. • If taking oral contraceptives, check with physician (reliability may be affected). • Report fever, decreased appetite, nausea, vomiting, dark urine, pain/swelling of joints.

rifaximin

rye-**fax**-ih-min

(Xifaxan)

CLASSIFICATION

PHARMACOTHERAPEUTIC: Anti-infective. **CLINICAL:** Site-specific antibiotic.

ACTION

Inhibits bacterial RNA synthesis by binding to a subunit of bacterial DNA-dependent RNA polymerase. **Therapeutic Effect:** Bactericidal.

PHARMACOKINETICS

Less than 0.4% absorbed after PO administration. Primarily eliminated in feces; minimal excretion in urine. **Half-life:** 5.85 hrs.

USES

Treatment of traveler's diarrhea caused by noninvasive strains of *E. coli*. **OFF-LABEL:** Treatment of hepatic encephalopathy.

PRECAUTIONS

CONTRAINDICATIONS: Hypersensitivity to other rifamycin antibiotics. **CAUTIONS:** Pseudomembranous colitis.

LIFESPAN CONSIDERATIONS:

Pregnancy/Lactation: Unknown if drug is excreted in breast milk. **Pregnancy Category C. Children:** Safety and efficacy not established in children younger than 12 yrs. **Elderly:** No age-related precautions noted.

INTERACTIONS

DRUG: None significant. **HERBAL:** None significant. **FOOD:** None known. **LAB VALUES:** None known.

AVAILABILITY (Rx)

TABLETS: 200 mg.

ADMINISTRATION/HANDLING

PO

• Give without regard to food. • Store at room temperature. • Do not break/crush film-coated tablets.

R

INDICATIONS/ROUTES/DOSAGE

TRAVELER'S DIARRHEA

PO: ADULTS, ELDERLY, CHILDREN 12 YRS AND OLDER: 200 mg 3 times a day for 3 days.

HEPATIC ENCEPHALOPATHY

PO: ADULTS, ELDERLY: 1,200 mg/day for 15–21 days.

SIDE EFFECTS

OCCASIONAL (11%–5%): Flatulence, headache, abdominal discomfort, rectal tenesmus, defecation urgency, nausea. **RARE (4%–2%):** Constipation, fever, vomiting.

ADVERSE EFFECTS/ TOXIC REACTIONS

Hypersensitivity reaction, superinfection occur rarely.

NURSING CONSIDERATIONS

BASELINE ASSESSMENT

Check baseline hydration status: skin turgor, mucous membranes for dryness, urinary status.

INTERVENTION/EVALUATION

Encourage adequate fluid intake. Assess bowel sounds for peristalsis. Monitor daily pattern of bowel activity/stool consistency. Assess for GI disturbances.

PATIENT/FAMILY TEACHING

- Notify physician if diarrhea worsens or within 48 hrs, blood occurs in stool, fever develops.

rimantadine

ri-**man**-ti-deen

(Flumadine)

Do not confuse rimantadine with ranitidine, or Flumadine with flunisolide or flutamide.

CLASSIFICATION

CLINICAL: Antiviral.

ACTION

Exerts inhibitory effect early in viral replication cycle. May inhibit uncoating of virus. **Therapeutic Effect:** Prevents replication of influenza A virus.

PHARMACOKINETICS

Well absorbed following PO administration. Protein binding: 40%. Metabolized in liver. Excreted in urine. **Half-life:** 19–36 hrs.

USES

Adults: Prophylaxis, treatment of illness due to influenza A virus. **Children:** Prophylaxis against influenza A virus.

PRECAUTIONS

CONTRAINDICATIONS: Hypersensitivity to amantadine. **CAUTIONS:** Hepatic disease, seizures, history of recurrent eczematoid dermatitis, uncontrolled psychosis, renal impairment, concomitant use of CNS stimulant medications.

LIFESPAN CONSIDERATIONS:

Pregnancy/Lactation: Unknown if drug crosses placenta or is distributed in breast milk. **Pregnancy Category C. Children:** Safety and efficacy not established in infants. **Elderly:** May be more susceptible to CNS side effects.

INTERACTIONS

DRUG: Acetaminophen, aspirin may decrease concentration. **Anticholinergics, CNS stimulants** may increase side effects. **HERBAL:** None significant. **FOOD:** None known. **LAB VALUES:** None known.

AVAILABILITY (Rx)

SYRUP: 50 mg/5 ml. **TABLETS:** 100 mg.

ADMINISTRATION/HANDLING

PO

- Give without regard to food.

INDICATIONS/ROUTES/DOSAGE

TREATMENT OF INFLUENZA A VIRUS

PO: ADULTS, ELDERLY: 100 mg twice a day for 7 days. **ELDERLY DEBILITATED PTS, PTS WITH SEVERE HEPATIC/RENAL IMPAIRMENT:** 100 mg once a day for 7 days.

PREVENTION OF INFLUENZA A VIRUS

PO: ADULTS, ELDERLY, CHILDREN 10 YRS AND OLDER: 100 mg twice a day for at least 10 days after known exposure (usually for 6–8 wks). **CHILDREN YOUNGER THAN 10 YRS:** 5 mg/kg once a day. **Maximum:** 150 mg. **ELDERLY DEBILITATED PTS, PTS WITH SEVERE HEPATIC/RENAL IMPAIRMENT:** 100 mg once a day.

SIDE EFFECTS

OCCASIONAL (3%–2%): Insomnia, nausea, nervousness, impaired concentration, dizziness. **RARE (less than 2%):** Vomiting, anorexia, dry mouth, abdominal pain, asthenia (loss of strength, energy), fatigue.

ADVERSE EFFECTS/ TOXIC REACTIONS

None known.

NURSING CONSIDERATIONS

INTERVENTION/EVALUATION

Assess for anxiety, nervousness; evaluate sleep pattern for insomnia. Provide assistance if dizziness occurs.

PATIENT/FAMILY TEACHING

• Avoid contact with those who are at high risk for influenza A (rimantadine-resistant virus may be shed during therapy). • Avoid tasks that require alertness, motor skills until response to drug is established. • Do not take aspirin, acetaminophen, compounds containing these drugs. • May cause dry mouth.

risedronate

rize-droe-nate

(Actonel)

FIXED-COMBINATION(S)

Actonel with Calcium: Risedronate/Calcium: 35 mg/6 × 500 mg.

CLASSIFICATION

PHARMACOTHERAPEUTIC: Bisphosphonate. **CLINICAL:** Calcium regulator.

ACTION

Binds to bone hydroxyapatite, inhibits osteoclasts. **Therapeutic Effect:** Reduces bone turnover (number of sites at which bone is remodeled), bone resorption.

PHARMACOKINETICS

Rapidly absorbed following PO administration. Bioavailability decreased when administered with food. Protein binding: 24%. Not metabolized. Excreted unchanged in urine, feces. Not removed by hemodialysis. **Half-life:** 1.5 hrs (initial); 480 hrs (terminal).

USES

Treatment of Paget's disease of bone (osteitis deformans). Treatment/prophylaxis for postmenopausal, glucocorticoid-induced osteoporosis. Used to increase bone mass in men with osteoporosis.

PRECAUTIONS

CONTRAINDICATIONS: Hypersensitivity to other bisphosphonates, including etidronate, tiludronate, risedronate, alendronate; hypocalcemia; inability to stand or sit upright for at least 20 min; renal impairment when serum creatinine clearance is greater than 5 mg/dl. **CAUTIONS:** GI diseases (duodenitis, dysphagia, esophagitis, gastritis, ulcers

R

[drug may exacerbate these conditions]), severe renal impairment. **Pregnancy Category C.**

INTERACTIONS

DRUG: Antacids containing aluminum, calcium, magnesium; vitamin D may decrease absorption. **HERBAL:** None significant. **FOOD:** None known. **LAB VALUES:** None known.

AVAILABILITY (Rx)

TABLETS: 5 mg, 30 mg, 35 mg.

ADMINISTRATION/HANDLING

PO

• Administer 30–60 min before taking any food, drink, other medications orally to avoid interference with absorption. • Take on empty stomach with full glass of water (not mineral water). • Avoid lying down for 30 min after swallowing tablet (assists with delivery to stomach, reduces risk of esophageal irritation).

INDICATIONS/ROUTES/DOSAGE

PAGET'S DISEASE

PO: ADULTS, ELDERLY: 30 mg/day for 2 mos. Retreatment may occur after 2-mo post-treatment observation period.

PREVENTION, TREATMENT OF POSTMENOPAUSAL OSTEOPOROSIS

PO: ADULTS, ELDERLY: 5 mg/day or 35 mg once weekly.

TREATMENT OF MALE OSTEOPOROSIS

PO: ADULTS, ELDERLY: 35 mg once weekly.

GLUCOCORTICOID-INDUCED OSTEOPOROSIS

PO: ADULTS, ELDERLY: 5 mg/day.

SIDE EFFECTS

FREQUENT (30%): Arthralgia. **OCCASIONAL (12%–8%):** Rash, flu-like symptoms, peripheral edema. **RARE (5%–3%):** Bone pain, sinusitis, asthenia (loss of strength, energy), dry eye, tinnitus.

ADVERSE EFFECTS/ TOXIC REACTIONS

Overdose produces hypocalcemia, hypophosphatemia, significant GI disturbances.

NURSING CONSIDERATIONS

BASELINE ASSESSMENT

Hypocalcemia, vitamin D deficiency must be corrected before therapy. Obtain lab baselines, esp. serum electrolytes, renal function.

INTERVENTION/EVALUATION

Check serum electrolytes (esp. calcium, alkaline phosphatase levels). Monitor I&O, BUN, creatinine in pts with renal impairment.

PATIENT/FAMILY TEACHING

• Instruct pt that expected benefits occur only when medication is taken with full glass (6–8 oz) of plain water, first thing in the morning and at least 30 min before first food, beverage, medication of the day. Any other beverage (mineral water, orange juice, coffee) significantly reduces absorption of medication. • Do not lie down for at least 30 min after taking medication (potentiates delivery to stomach, reduces risk of esophageal irritation). • Consider weight-bearing exercises, modify behavioral factors (cigarette smoking, alcohol consumption).

Risperdal, *see risperidone*

risperidone

ris-**per**-i-done

(Risperdal, Risperdal Consta, Risperdol M-Tabs)

Do not confuse risperidone with reserpine.

◆ **CLASSIFICATION**

PHARMACOTHERAPEUTIC: Benzisoxazole derivative. **CLINICAL:** Antipsychotic (see p. 63C).

ACTION

May antagonize dopamine, serotonin receptors. **Therapeutic Effect:** Suppresses psychotic behavior.

PHARMACOKINETICS

Well absorbed from GI tract; unaffected by food. Protein binding: 90%. Extensively metabolized in liver to active metabolite. Primarily excreted in urine. **Half-life:** 3–20 hrs; metabolite: 21–30 hrs (increased in elderly).

USES

Management of manifestations of psychotic disorders (e.g., schizophrenia), irritability associated with autistic disease in children. Treatment of acute mania associated with bipolar disorder. **OFF-LABEL:** Behavioral symptoms associated with dementia, Tourette's disorder.

PRECAUTIONS

CONTRAINDICATIONS: None known. **CAUTIONS:** Renal/hepatic impairment, seizure disorders, cardiac disease, recent MI, breast cancer, suicidal pts, those at risk for aspiration pneumonia. May increase risk of stroke in pts with dementia. May increase risk of hyperglycemia.

⌛ LIFESPAN CONSIDERATIONS:

Pregnancy/Lactation: Unknown if drug crosses placenta or is excreted in breast milk. Recommend against breastfeeding. **Pregnancy Category C. Children:** Safety and efficacy not established. **Elderly:** More susceptible to postural hypotension. Age-related renal, hepatic impairment may require dosage adjustment.

INTERACTIONS

DRUG: Alcohol, other CNS depressants may increase CNS depression. **Carbamazepine** may decrease concentration. **Clozapine** may increase concentration. May decrease effects of **dopamine agonists, levodopa. Paroxetine** may increase concentration, risk of extrapyramidal symptoms. **Hypotension-producing medications, antihypertensives** may increase hypotensive effect. **Medications that prolong QT interval** may increase occurrence of ventricular tachycardia, torsades de pointes. **HERBAL:** None significant. **FOOD:** None known. **LAB VALUES:** May increase serum prolactin, creatinine, alkaline phosphatase, uric acid, AST, ALT, triglycerides. May increase serum glucose, decrease serum potassium, protein, sodium. May cause EKG changes.

AVAILABILITY (Rx)

ORAL SOLUTION (RISPERDAL) 1 mg/ml. **TABLETS (RISPERDAL):** 0.25 mg, 0.5 mg, 1 mg, 2 mg, 3 mg, 4 mg. **TABLETS (ORALLY DISINTEGRATING [RISPERDAL M-TABS]):** 0.5 mg, 1 mg, 2 mg, 3 mg, 4 mg. **INJECTION POWDER FOR RECONSTITUTION (RISPERDAL CONSTA):** 25 mg, 37.5 mg, 50 mg.

ADMINISTRATION/HANDLING

◀ **ALERT** ▶ Do not administer via IV route.

IM

Reconstitution • Use only diluent and needle supplied in dose pack. • Prepare suspension according to manufacturer's directions. • May be given up to 6 hrs after reconstitution, but immediate administration is recommended. • If 2 min pass between reconstitution and injection, shake upright vial vigorously back and forth to resuspend solution.

R

Rate of administration • Inject IM into upper outer quadrant of gluteus maximus.

Storage • Store at room temperature.

PO

• Give without regard to food. • May mix oral solution with water, coffee, orange juice, low-fat milk. Do not mix with cola, tea.

INDICATIONS/ROUTES/DOSAGE

PSYCHOTIC DISORDERS

PO: ADULTS: Initially, 0.5–1 mg 2 times/day. May increase gradually to target dose of 6 mg/day. Range: 4–8 mg/day. Maintenance: Target dose of 4 mg once daily (range: 2–8 mg/day). **ELDERLY:** Initially, 0.5 mg 2 times/day. May increase slowly at increments of no more than 0.5 mg twice daily. Range: 2–6 mg/day.
IM: ADULTS, ELDERLY: 25 mg q2wk. **Maximum:** 50 mg q2wk. Dosage adjustments should not be made more frequently than every 4 wks.

MANIA

PO: ADULTS, ELDERLY: Initially, 2–3 mg as a single daily dose. May increase at 24 hr intervals of 1 mg/day. Range: 1–6 mg/day.

IRRITABILITY WITH AUTISTIC DISEASE

PO: CHILDREN 5 YRS AND OLDER: Initially, 0.25 mg/day (0.5 mg in children weighing 20 kg or greater). May increase to 0.5 mg/day (1 mg/day in children weighing 20 kg or greater) after minimum of 4 days. Dose should be maintained for at least 14 days, after which dose may be increased by 0.25 mg/day (0.5 mg/day in children weighing 20 kg or more). **Maximum:** 1 mg (2.5 mg in children weighing 20 kg or more).

DOSAGE IN RENAL IMPAIRMENT

Initial dosage for adults, elderly pts is 0.25–0.5 mg twice a day. Dosage is titrated slowly to desired effect.

SIDE EFFECTS

FREQUENT (26%–13%): Agitation, anxiety, insomnia, headache, constipation. **OCCASIONAL (10%–4%):** Dyspepsia, rhinitis, drowsiness, dizziness, nausea, vomiting, rash, abdominal pain, dry skin, tachycardia. **RARE (3%–2%):** Visual disturbances, fever, back pain, pharyngitis, cough, arthralgia, angina, aggressive behavior, orthostatic hypotension, breast swelling.

ADVERSE EFFECTS/ TOXIC REACTIONS

Rare reactions include tardive dyskinesia (characterized by tongue protrusion, puffing of the cheeks, chewing or puckering of mouth), neuroleptic malignant syndrome (marked by hyperpyrexia, muscle rigidity, altered mental status, irregular pulse or B/P, tachycardia, diaphoresis, cardiac arrhythmias, rhabdomyolysis, acute renal failure). Hyperglycemia, in some cases extreme and associated with ketoacidosis, hyperosmolar coma, death, has been reported.

NURSING CONSIDERATIONS

BASELINE ASSESSMENT

Serum renal/hepatic function tests should be performed before therapy. Assess behavior, appearance, emotional status, response to environment, speech pattern, thought content. Obtain fasting serum glucose value.

INTERVENTION/EVALUATION

Monitor B/P, heart rate, weight, hepatic function tests, EKG. Monitor for fine tongue movement (may be first sign of tardive dyskinesia, which may be irreversible). Supervise suicidal-risk pt closely during early therapy (as depression lessens, energy level improves, increasing suicide potential). Assess for therapeutic response (greater interest in surroundings, improved self-care, increased ability to concentrate, relaxed facial expression). Monitor for potential neuroleptic malignant syndrome: fever, muscle rigidity, irregular B/P or pulse, altered mental status. Monitor fasting serum glucose periodically during therapy.

PATIENT/FAMILY TEACHING

• Avoid tasks that may require alertness, motor skills until response to drug is established (may cause dizziness/drowsiness). • Avoid alcohol. • Use caution when changing position from lying or sitting to standing. • Inform physician of trembling in fingers, altered gait, unusual muscular/skeletal movements, palpitations, severe dizziness/fainting, swelling/pain in breasts, visual changes, rash, difficulty breathing.

Ritalin, *see methylphenidate*

ritonavir

ri-**tone**-a-veer

(Norvir, Norvir SEC ✤)

Do not confuse ritonavir with Retrovir.

CLASSIFICATION

PHARMACOTHERAPEUTIC: Protease inhibitor. **CLINICAL:** Antiviral (see pp. 61C, 113C).

ACTION

Inhibits HIV-1 and HIV-2 proteases, rendering these enzymes incapable of processing polypeptide precursors that lead to production of noninfectious, immature HIV particles. **Therapeutic Effect:** Slows HIV replication, reducing progression of HIV infection.

PHARMACOKINETICS

Well absorbed after PO administration (absorption increased with food). Protein binding: 98%–99%. Extensively metabolized in liver to active metabolite. Primarily eliminated in feces. Unknown if removed by hemodialysis. **Half-life:** 2.7–5 hrs.

USES

Treatment of HIV infection in combination with other antiretroviral agents.

PRECAUTIONS

CONTRAINDICATIONS: Due to potential serious and/or life-threatening drug interactions, the following medications should not be given concomitantly with ritonavir: **alfuzosin, amiodarone, bepridil, dihydroergotamine, lovastatin, midazolam, propafenone, quinidine, simvastatin, St. John's wort, trizolam, voriconazole** (increased risk of serious or life-threatening drug interactions, such as arrhythmias, hematologic abnormalities, and seizures); concurrent use of alprazolam, clorazepate, diazepam, estazolam, flurazepam, midazolam, triazolam, zolpidem (may produce extreme sedation and respiratory depression). **CAUTIONS:** Hepatic impairment.

LIFESPAN CONSIDERATIONS:

Pregnancy/Lactation: Breast-feeding not recommended (possibility of HIV transmission). **Pregnancy Category B.** **Children:** No age-related precautions noted in those older than 2 yrs. **Elderly:** None known.

INTERACTIONS

DRUG: May increase concentration, toxicity of **clarithromycin, desipramine, fluticasone, indinavir, ketoconazole, meperidine, saquinavir, sildenafil.** May decrease concentration, effect of **didanosine, methadone, oral contraceptives, theophylline. Rifampin** may decrease concentration, effect.

R

HERBAL: **St. John's wort** may decrease concentration, effect. **FOOD:** None known. **LAB VALUES:** May alter serum CK, GGT, triglycerides, uric acid, AST, ALT, creatinine clearance.

AVAILABILITY (Rx)

CAPSULES: 100 mg. **ORAL SOLUTION:** 80 mg/ml.

ADMINISTRATION/HANDLING

PO

• Store capsules, solution in refrigerator. • Protect from light. • Refrigeration of oral solution is recommended but not necessary if used within 30 days and stored below 77°F. • Give without regard to meals (preferably give with food). • May improve taste of oral solution by mixing with chocolate milk, Ensure, Advera, Boost within 1 hr of dosing.

INDICATIONS/ROUTES/DOSAGE

TREATMENT OF HIV INFECTION

PO: ADULTS, CHILDREN 12 YRS AND OLDER: 600 mg twice a day. If nausea occurs at this dosage, give 300 mg twice a day for 1 day, 400 mg twice a day for 2 days, 500 mg twice a day for 1 day, then 600 mg twice a day thereafter. **CHILDREN 1 MO–11 YRS:** Initially, 250 mg/m^2/dose twice a day. Increase by 50 mg/m^2/dose up to 400 mg/m^2/dose. **Maximum:** 600 mg/dose twice a day.

DOSAGE ADJUSTMENTS IN COMBINATION THERAPY

Amprenavir: Amprenavir 1,200 mg and ritonavir 200 mg once a day or amprenavir 600 mg and ritonavir 100 mg twice a day.

Ampenavir and efavirenz: Amprenavir 1,200 mg twice a day and ritonavir 200 mg twice a day with standard dose of efavirenz.

Indinavir: Indinavir 800 mg twice a day and ritonavir 100–200 mg twice a day or indinavir 400 mg twice a day and ritonavir 400 mg twice a day.

Nelfinavir or saquinavir: Ritonavir 400 mg twice a day.

Rifabutin: Decrease rifabutin dosage to 150 mg every other day.

SIDE EFFECTS

FREQUENT: GI disturbances (abdominal pain, anorexia, diarrhea, nausea, vomiting), circumoral and peripheral paresthesias, altered taste, headache, dizziness, fatigue, asthenia. **OCCASIONAL:** Allergic reaction, flu-like symptoms, hypotension. **RARE:** Diabetes mellitus, hyperglycemia.

ADVERSE EFFECTS/ TOXIC REACTIONS

Hepatitis, pancreatitis occur rarely.

NURSING CONSIDERATIONS

BASELINE ASSESSMENT

Pts beginning combination therapy with ritonavir and nucleosides may promote GI tolerance by beginning ritonavir alone and subsequently adding nucleosides before completing 2 wks of ritonavir monotherapy. Obtain baseline laboratory testing, esp. serum hepatic function tests, triglycerides before beginning ritonavir therapy and at periodic intervals during therapy. Offer emotional support to pt and family.

INTERVENTION/EVALUATION

Closely monitor for evidence of GI disturbances, neurologic abnormalities (particularly paresthesias). Monitor serum hepatic function tests, serum glucose, CD4 cell count, plasma levels of HIV RNA.

PATIENT/FAMILY TEACHING

• Continue therapy for full length of treatment. • Doses should be evenly spaced. • Ritonavir is not a cure for HIV infection, nor does it reduce risk of transmission to others. • Pts may continue to acquire illnesses associated with advanced HIV infection. • If possible, take ritonavir with food. • Taste of solution may be improved when mixed with chocolate milk, Ensure, Advera, Boost. • Inform physician of increased thirst, frequent urination, nausea, vomiting, abdominal pain.

Rituxan, *see rituximab*

rituximab

rye-**tucks**-ih-mab
(Rituxan)

CLASSIFICATION

PHARMACOTHERAPEUTIC: Monoclonal antibody. **CLINICAL:** Antineoplastic (see p. 83C).

ACTION

Binds to CD20, the antigen found on surface of B lymphocytes, B-cell non-Hodgkin's lymphomas (NHL). **Therapeutic Effect:** Produces cytotoxicity, reduces tumor size.

PHARMACOKINETICS

Rapidly depletes B cells. **Half-life:** 59.8 hrs after first infusion, 174 hrs after fourth infusion.

USES

Treatment of relapsed or refractory low-grade or follicular B-cell NHL. First-line treatment for diffuse large B-cell, CD20-positive, NHL. First-line treatment of previously untreated pts with follicular NHL in combination with cyclophosphamide, vincristine, and prednisolone (CVP therapy). Treatment of low-grade NHL in pts with stable disease or who achieve partial or complete response following CVP therapy. Treatment of moderate to severe rheumatoid arthritis.

PRECAUTIONS

CONTRAINDICATIONS: Hypersensitivity to murine proteins. **CAUTIONS:** Those with history of cardiac disease.

LIFESPAN CONSIDERATIONS:

Pregnancy/Lactation: Has potential to cause fetal B-cell depletion. Unknown if distributed in breast milk. Those with childbearing potential should use contraceptive methods during treatment and up to 12 mos following therapy. **Pregnancy Category C. Children:** Safety and efficacy not established. **Elderly:** No age-related precautions noted.

INTERACTIONS

DRUG: None significant. **HERBAL:** None significant. **FOOD:** None known. **LAB VALUES:** None known.

AVAILABILITY (Rx)

INJECTION SOLUTION: 10 mg/ml.

ADMINISTRATION/HANDLING

IV

◀ ALERT ▶ Do not give by IV push or bolus.

Reconstitution • Dilute with 0.9% NaCl or D_5W to provide final concentration of 1–4 mg/ml into infusion bag.

Rate of administration • Infuse at rate of 50 mg/hr. May increase infusion rate in 50 mg/hr increments q30min to maximum 400 mg/hr. • Subsequent infusion can be given at 100 mg/hr and increased by 100 mg/hr increments q30min to maximum 400 mg/hr.

Storage • Refrigerate vials. • Diluted solution is stable for 24 hrs if refrigerated and at room temperature for an additional 12 hrs.

IV INCOMPATIBILITIES

Do not mix with any other medications.

R

INDICATIONS/ROUTES/DOSAGE

NON-HODGKIN'S LYMPHOMA (NHL)

IV: ADULTS: 375 mg/m^2 once weekly for 4–8 wks. May administer a second 4-wk course.

RHEUMATOID ARTHRITIS

IV: ADULTS: 1,000 mg every 2 wks times 2 doses.

SIDE EFFECTS

FREQUENT: Fever (49%), chills (32%), asthenia (loss of strength, energy) (16%), headache (14%), angioedema (13%), hypotension (10%), nausea (18%), rash/pruritus (10%). **OCCASIONAL (less than 10%):** Myalgia, dizziness, abdominal pain, throat irritation, vomiting, neutropenia, rhinitis, bronchospasm, urticaria.

ADVERSE EFFECTS/ TOXIC REACTIONS

Hypersensitivity reaction produces hypotension, bronchospasm, angioedema. Arrhythmias may occur, particularly in those with history of preexisting cardiac conditions.

NURSING CONSIDERATIONS

BASELINE ASSESSMENT

Pretreatment with acetaminophen and diphenhydramine before each infusion may prevent infusion-related effects. CBC, platelet count should be obtained at regular interval during therapy.

INTERVENTION/EVALUATION

Monitor for an infusion-related symptoms complex consisting mainly of fever, chills, rigors that generally occurs within 30 min–2 hrs of beginning first infusion. Slowing infusion resolves symptoms.

rivastigmine

rye-vah-**stig**-meen
(Exelon)

◆CLASSIFICATION

PHARMACOTHERAPEUTIC: Cholinesterase inhibitor. **CLINICAL:** Anti-Alzheimer's dementia agent.

ACTION

Inhibits the enzyme acetylcholinesterase, increasing acetylcholine concentration at cholinergic synapses, enhancing cholinergic function. **Therapeutic Effect:** Slows progression of symptoms of Alzheimer's disease.

PHARMACOKINETICS

Rapidly, completely absorbed. Protein binding: 60%. Widely distributed throughout body. Rapidly, extensively metabolized. Primarily excreted in urine. **Half-life:** 1.5 hrs.

USES

Treatment of mild to moderate dementia of the Alzheimer's type. Treatment of dementia associated with Parkinson's disease.

PRECAUTIONS

CONTRAINDICATIONS: Hypersensitivity to other carbamate derivatives. **CAUTIONS:** Peptic ulcer disease, concurrent use of NSAIDs, sick sinus syndrome, bradycardia, urinary obstruction, seizure disorders, asthma, chronic obstructive pulmonary disease (COPD).

⌛ LIFESPAN CONSIDERATIONS:

Pregnancy/Lactation: Unknown if distributed in breast milk. **Pregnancy Category B. Children:** Not indicated for use in children. **Elderly:** No age-related precautions.

INTERACTIONS

DRUG: May interfere with **anticholinergics** effects. May have additive effect with **bethanecol. NSAIDs**may increase GI effects, irritation. **HERBAL:** None significant. **FOOD:** None known. **LAB VALUES:** None known.

R

AVAILABILITY (Rx)

CAPSULES: 1.5 mg, 3 mg, 4.5 mg, 6 mg. **ORAL SOLUTION:** 2 mg/ml.

ADMINISTRATION/HANDLING

PO

• Give with food in divided doses morning and evening.

ORAL SOLUTION

• Using oral syringe provided by manufacturer; withdraw prescribed amount from container. • May be swallowed directly from syringe or mixed in small glass of water, cold fruit juice, soda (use within 4 hrs of mixing).

INDICATIONS/ROUTES/DOSAGE

ALZHEIMER'S DISEASE

PO: ADULTS, ELDERLY: Initially, 1.5 mg twice a day. May increase at intervals of at least 2 wks to 3 mg twice a day, then 4.5 mg twice a day, and finally 6 mg twice a day. **Maximum:** 6 mg twice a day.

PARKINSON'S DISEASE

PO: ADULTS, ELDERLY: Initially, 1.5 mg twice a day. May increase at intervals of at least 4 wks to 3 mg twice a day, then 4.5 mg twice a day, and finally 6 mg twice a day. **Maximum:** 6 mg twice a day.

SIDE EFFECTS

FREQUENT (47%–17%): Nausea, vomiting, dizziness, diarrhea, headache, anorexia. **OCCASIONAL (13%–6%):** Abdominal pain, insomnia, dyspepsia (heartburn, indigestion, epigastric pain), confusion, UTI, depression. **RARE (5%–3%):** Anxiety, somnolence, constipation, malaise, hallucinations, tremor, flatulence, rhinitis, hypertension, flu-like symptoms, weight loss, syncope.

ADVERSE EFFECTS/ TOXIC REACTIONS

Overdose can produce cholinergic crisis, characterized by severe nausea/vomiting, increased salivation, diaphoresis, bradycardia, hypotension, respiratory depression, seizures.

NURSING CONSIDERATIONS

BASELINE ASSESSMENT

Obtain baseline vital signs. Assess history for peptic ulcer, urinary obstruction, asthma, COPD. Assess cognitive, behavioral, functional deficits.

INTERVENTION/EVALUATION

Monitor for cholinergic reaction: GI discomfort/cramping, feeling of facial warmth, excessive salivation, diaphoresis, lacrimation, pallor, urinary urgency, dizziness. Monitor for nausea, diarrhea, headache, insomnia.

PATIENT/FAMILY TEACHING

• Take with meals (at breakfast, dinner). • Swallow capsule whole. Do not chew, break, crush capsules. • Report nausea, vomiting, diarrhea, diaphoresis, increased salivary secretions, severe abdominal pain, dizziness.

rizatriptan

rize-a-**trip**-tan

(Maxalt, Maxalt-MLT, Maxalt RPD ✦)

CLASSIFICATION

PHARMACOTHERAPEUTIC: Serotonin receptor agonist. **CLINICAL:** Antimigraine (see p. 60C).

ACTION

Binds selectively to vascular receptors, producing vasoconstrictive effect on cranial blood vessels. **Therapeutic Effect:** Relieves migraine headache.

PHARMACOKINETICS

Well absorbed after PO administration. Protein binding: 14%. Crosses blood-brain barrier. Metabolized by liver to inactive metabolite. Eliminated

R

primarily in urine and, to a lesser extent, in feces. **Half-life:** 2–3 hrs.

USES

Treatment of acute migraine headache with or without aura.

PRECAUTIONS

CONTRAINDICATIONS: Basilar or hemiplegic migraine, coronary artery disease, ischemic heart disease (including angina pectoris, history of MI, silent ischemia, and Prinzmetal's angina), uncontrolled hypertension, use within 24 hrs of ergotamine-containing preparations or another serotonin receptor agonist, MAOI use within 14 days. **CAUTIONS:** Mild to moderate renal/hepatic impairment, pt profile suggesting cardiovascular risks.

LIFESPAN CONSIDERATIONS:

Pregnancy/Lactation: Unknown if drug is distributed in breast milk. **Pregnancy Category C. Children:** Safety and efficacy not established. **Elderly:** No age-related precautions noted.

INTERACTIONS

DRUG: **Ergotamine-containing medications** may produce vasospastic reaction. **Fluoxetine, fluvoxamine, paroxetine, sertraline** may produce hyperreflexia, incoordination, weakness. **MAOIs, propranolol** may dramatically increase concentration. **HERBAL:** None significant. **FOOD:** **All foods** delay peak drug concentration by 1 hr. **LAB VALUES:** None known.

AVAILABILITY (Rx)

TABLETS (MAXALT): 5 mg, 10 mg. **TABLETS (ORALLY DISINTEGRATING [MAXALT-MLT]):** 5 mg, 10 mg.

ADMINISTRATION/HANDLING

PO

• Oral disintegrating tablet is packaged in an individual aluminum pouch. • Open packet with dry hands. • Place tablet onto tongue, allow to dissolve, swallow with saliva. Administration with water is not necessary.

INDICATIONS/ROUTES/DOSAGE

ACUTE MIGRAINE HEADACHE

PO: ADULTS OLDER THAN 18 YRS, ELDERLY: 5–10 mg. If headache improves but then returns, dose may be repeated after 2 hrs. **Maximum:** 30 mg/24 hrs.

SIDE EFFECTS

FREQUENT (9%–7%): Dizziness, somnolence, paresthesia, fatigue. **OCCASIONAL (6%–3%):** Nausea, chest pressure, dry mouth. **RARE (2%):** Headache; neck, throat, jaw pressure; photosensitivity.

ADVERSE EFFECTS/ TOXIC REACTIONS

Cardiac reactions (ischemia, coronary artery vasospasm, MI), noncardiac vasospasm-related reactions (hemorrhage, cerebrovascular accident [CVA]) occur rarely, particularly in pts with hypertension, diabetes, strong family history of coronary artery disease; obestiy, smokers; males older than 40 yrs; postmenopausal women.

NURSING CONSIDERATIONS

BASELINE ASSESSMENT

Question for history of peripheral vascular disease, renal/hepatic impairment. Question pt regarding onset, location, duration of migraine, possible precipitating symptoms.

INTERVENTION/EVALUATION

Monitor for evidence of dizziness. Assess for photophobia, phonophobia (sound sensitivity, nausea, vomiting) relief of migraine headache.

PATIENT/FAMILY TEACHING

• Take single dose as soon as symptoms of an actual migraine headache appear. • Medication is intended to relieve migraine, not to prevent or reduce number of attacks. • Avoid tasks that require alertness, motor skills until response to drug is established. • Contact physician immediately if palpitations, pain/tightness in chest/throat, pain/weakness of extremities occurs. • Do not remove orally disintegrating tablet from blister pack until just before dosing. • Use protective measures (sunscreen, protective clothing) against exposure to UV light, sunlight.

Rocephin, *see ceftriaxone*

rocuronium

(Zemuron)

See Neuromuscular blockers (p. 120C)

ropinirole

ro-**pin**-i-role

(Requip)

CLASSIFICATION

PHARMACOTHERAPEUTIC: Dopamine agonist. **CLINICAL:** Antiparkinson agent.

ACTION

Stimulates dopamine receptors in striatum. **Therapeutic Effect:** Relieves signs/symptoms of Parkinson's disease.

PHARMACOKINETICS

Rapidly absorbed after PO administration. Protein binding: 40%. Extensively distributed throughout body. Extensively metabolized. Steady-state concentrations achieved within 2 days. Eliminated in urine. Unknown if removed by hemodialysis. **Half-life:** 6 hrs.

USES

Treatment of signs/symptoms of idiopathic Parkinson's disease. Treatment of restless leg syndrome.

PRECAUTIONS

CONTRAINDICATIONS: None known. **CAUTIONS:** History of orthostatic hypotension, syncope, hallucinations, esp. in elderly. Concurrent use of CNS depressants.

LIFESPAN CONSIDERATIONS:

Pregnancy/Lactation: Distributed in breast milk. Drug activity possible in breast-feeding infant. **Pregnancy Category C. Children:** Safety and efficacy not established. **Elderly:** No age-related precautions noted, but hallucinations appear to occur more frequently.

INTERACTIONS

DRUG: Butyrophenones, metoclopramide, phenothiazines, thioxanthenes decrease effectiveness. **Cimetidine, diltiazem, enoxacin, erythromycin, fluvoxamine, mexiletine, norfloxacin, tacrine** alter concentration. **Ciprofloxacin** increases concentration. **CNS depressants** may increase CNS depressant effects. **Estrogens** reduce clearance. Increases concentration of **levodopa. HERBAL: Gotu kola, kava kava, St. John's wort valerian** may increase CNS depression. **FOOD: All foods** delay peak plasma levels by 1 hr but do not affect drug absorption. **LAB VALUES:** May increase serum alkaline phosphatase.

AVAILABILITY (Rx)

TABLETS: 0.25 mg, 0.5 mg, 1 mg, 2 mg, 3 mg, 4 mg, 5 mg.

ADMINISTRATION/HANDLING

PO

- May give without regard to meals.

R

INDICATIONS/ROUTES/DOSAGE

PARKINSON'S DISEASE

PO: ADULTS, ELDERLY: Initially, 0.25 mg 3 times/day based on individual pt response. Dosage should be titrated with weekly increments as below:
Week 1: 0.25 mg 3 times/day; total daily dose: 0.75 mg.
Week 2: 0.5 mg 3 times/day; total daily dose: 1.5 mg.
Week 3: 0.75 mg 3 times/day, total daily dose: 2.25 mg.
Week 4: 1 mg 3 times/day, total daily dose: 3 mg.
After week 4, may increase dose by 1.5 mg/day on weekly basis up to dose of 9 mg/day. May then further increase by 3 mg/day on weekly basis up to total dose of 24 mg/day.

DISCONTINUATION TAPER

Gradually taper over 7 days as follows: Decrease frequency from 3 times/day to 2 times/day for 4 days. Then decrease from 2 times/day to once daily for remaining 3 days.

RESTLESS LEG SYNDROME

PO: ADULTS, ELDERLY: 0.25 mg for days 1 and 2; 0.5 mg for days 3–7; 1 mg for wk 2; 1.5 mg for wk 3; 2 mg for wk 4; 2.5 mg for wk 5; 3 mg for wk 6; 4 mg for wk 7. Give all doses 1–3 hrs before bedtime.

R

SIDE EFFECTS

FREQUENT (60%–40%): Nausea, dizziness, extreme drowsiness. **OCCASIONAL (12%–5%):** Syncope, vomiting, fatigue, viral infection, dyspepsia, diaphoresis, asthenia (loss of strength, energy), orthostatic hypotension, abdominal discomfort, pharyngitis, abnormal vision, dry mouth, hypertension, hallucinations, confusion. **RARE (less than 4%):** Anorexia, peripheral edema, memory loss, rhinitis, sinusitis, palpitations, impotence.

ADVERSE EFFECTS/ TOXIC REACTIONS

None known.

NURSING CONSIDERATIONS

INTERVENTION/EVALUATION

Assess for clinical improvement, clinical reversal of symptoms (improvement of tremors of head/hands at rest, mask-like facial expression, shuffling gait, muscular rigidity). Assist with ambulation if dizziness occurs.

PATIENT/FAMILY TEACHING

• Drowsiness, dizziness may be an initial response to drug. • Postural hypotension may occur more frequently during initial therapy. Instruct pt to rise from lying to sitting or sitting to standing position slowly to prevent risk of postural hypotension. • Avoid tasks that require alertness, motor skills until response to drug is established. • If nausea occurs, take medication with food. • Inform pt that hallucinations may occur, more so in the elderly than in younger pts with Parkinson's disease.

rosiglitazone

roz-ih-**glit**-a-zone
(Avandia)

Do not confuse Avandia with Avalide, Avinza, or Prandin, or Avandaryl with Benadryl.

FIXED-COMBINATION(S)

Avandamet: rosiglitazone/metformin: 1 mg/500 mg; 2 mg/500 mg; 4 mg/500 mg; 2 mg/1 g; 4 mg/1 g. **Avandaryl:** rosiglitazone/glimepiride (an antidiabetic): 4 mg/1 mg, 4 mg/2 mg, 4 mg/4 mg.

CLASSIFICATION

PHARMACOTHERAPEUTIC: Thiazolidinedione. **CLINICAL:** Antidiabetic (see p. 42C).

ACTION

Improves target-cell response to insulin without increasing pancreatic insulin secretion. Decreases hepatic glucose output, increases insulin-dependent glucose utilization in skeletal muscle. **Therapeutic Effect:** Lowers serum glucose concentration.

PHARMACOKINETICS

Rapidly absorbed. Protein binding: 99%. Metabolized in liver. Excreted primarily in urine, with lesser amount in feces. Not removed by hemodialysis. **Half-life:** 3–4 hrs.

USES

Adjunct to diet/exercise to lower serum glucose in those with type 2 non–insulin-dependent diabetes mellitus (NIDDM). Used as monotherapy or in combination with metformin, sulfonylurea, insulin to improve glycemic control.

PRECAUTIONS

CONTRAINDICATIONS: Active hepatic disease, diabetic ketoacidosis, increased serum transaminase levels, including ALT greater than 2.5 times the normal serum level, type 1 diabetes mellitus. **CAUTIONS:** Hepatic impairment, CHF, edematous pts. May cause or worsen macular edema.

LIFESPAN CONSIDERATIONS:

Pregnancy/Lactation: Unknown if drug crosses placenta or is distributed in breast milk. Not recommended in pregnant or breast-feeding women. **Pregnancy Category C. Children:** Safety and efficacy not established. **Elderly:** No age-related precautions noted in the elderly.

INTERACTIONS

DRUG: Rifampin may decrease concentration, effect. **Gemfibrozil** may increase concentration, toxicity. **HERBAL: Bitter melon, eucalyptus, fenugreek, garlic, ginseng, guar gum, St. John's wort** may increase risk of hypoglycemia. **Glucosamine, licorice** may reduce effectiveness. **FOOD:** None known. **LAB VALUES:** May decrease Hgb, Hct, serum alkaline phosphatase, bilirubin, AST. Less than 1% of pts experience ALT values that are 3 times the normal level.

AVAILABILITY (Rx)

TABLETS: 2 mg, 4 mg, 8 mg.

ADMINISTRATION/HANDLING

PO

- Give without regard to meals.

INDICATIONS/ROUTES/DOSAGE

DIABETES MELLITUS, COMBINATION THERAPY

PO (WITH SULFONYLUREAS, METFORMIN): ADULTS, ELDERLY: Initially, 4 mg as single daily dose or in divided doses twice a day. May increase to 8 mg/day after 12 wks of therapy if fasting glucose level is not adequately controlled.

PO (WITH INSULIN): ADULTS, ELDERLY: Initially, 4 mg/day in 1 or 2 doses and reduce insulin dose by 10%–25%. If hypoglycemia occurs or plasma glucose falls to less than 100 mg/dl, doses of rosiglitazone greater than 4 mg are not recommended.

DIABETES MELLITUS, MONOTHERAPY

ADULTS, ELDERLY: Initially, 4 mg as single daily dose or in divided doses twice a day. May increase to 8 mg/day after 12 wks of therapy.

SIDE EFFECTS

FREQUENT (9%): Upper respiratory tract infection. **OCCASIONAL (4%–2%):** Headache, edema, back pain, fatigue, sinusitis, diarrhea.

ADVERSE EFFECTS/ TOXIC REACTIONS

Hepatotoxicity occurs rarely.

R

NURSING CONSIDERATIONS

BASELINE ASSESSMENT

Obtain hepatic enzyme levels before initiation of therapy and periodically thereafter. Ensure follow-up instruction if pt, family does not thoroughly understand diabetes management, glucose-testing technique.

INTERVENTION/EVALUATION

Monitor serum glucose, Hgb, serum hepatic function tests, esp. AST, ALT. Assess for hypoglycemia (cool/wet skin, tremors, dizziness, anxiety, headache, tachycardia, numbness in mouth, hunger, diplopia), hyperglycemia (polyuria, polyphagia, polydipsia, nausea, vomiting, dim vision, fatigue, deep/rapid breathing). Be alert to conditions that alter glucose requirements (fever, increased activity/stress, surgical procedures).

PATIENT/FAMILY TEACHING

• Diabetes mellitus requires lifelong control. • Prescribed diet, exercise are principal parts of treatment; do not skip/delay meals. • Wear medical alert identification. • Continue to adhere to dietary instructions, regular exercise program, regular testing of urine or blood glucose. • When taking combination drug therapy with a sulfonylurea or insulin, have source of glucose available to treat symptoms of low blood sugar.

R

rosuvastatin

ross-uh-vah-**stah**-tin

(Crestor)

CLASSIFICATION

PHARMACOTHERAPEUTIC: HMG-CoA reductase inhibitor. **CLINICAL:** Antihyperlipidemic.

ACTION

Interferes with cholesterol biosynthesis by inhibiting conversion of the enzyme HMG-CoA to mevalonate, a precursor to cholesterol. **Therapeutic Effect:** Decreases LDL cholesterol, VLDL, plasma triglyceride levels; increases HDL concentration.

PHARMACOKINETICS

Protein binding: 88%. Minimal hepatic metabolism. Primarily eliminated in feces. **Half-life:** 19 hrs (increased in severe renal dysfunction).

USES

Adjunct to diet therapy to decrease elevated total, LDL cholesterol concentrations in pts with primary hypercholesterolemia (types IIa, IIb), lowers serum triglyceride levels, increases HDL.

PRECAUTIONS

CONTRAINDICATIONS: Active hepatic disease, breast-feeding, pregnancy, unexplained, persistent elevations of serum transaminase levels. **CAUTIONS:** Anticoagulant therapy, history of hepatic disease, substantial alcohol consumption, major surgery, severe acute infection, trauma, hypotension, severe metabolic or endocrine disorders, severe electrolyte imbalances, uncontrolled seizures.

LIFESPAN CONSIDERATIONS: **Pregnancy/Lactation:** Contraindicated in pregnancy (suppression of cholesterol biosynthesis may cause fetal toxicity), lactation. Risk of serious adverse reactions in breast-feeding infants. **Pregnancy Category X. Children:** Safety and efficacy not established. **Elderly:** No age-related precautions noted.

INTERACTIONS

DRUG: Aluminum- and magnesium-containing antacids may decrease concentration, effect. Increased risk of myopathy with **cyclosporine, gemfibrozil, fibrate, niacin.** Increases concentrations of **ethinyl, estradiol, norgestrel. Warfarin** enhances anticoagulant effect. **HERBAL: St. John's wort** may reduce effectiveness. **FOOD:** None known. **LAB VALUES:** May increase serum creatine kinase (CK), transaminase. May produce hematuria, proteinuria.

AVAILABILITY (Rx)

TABLETS: 5 mg, 10 mg, 20 mg, 40 mg.

ADMINISTRATION/HANDLING

PO

• Give without regard to meals. Usually administered in the evening.

INDICATIONS/ROUTES/DOSAGE

HYPERLIPIDEMIA, DYSLIPIDEMIA

PO: ADULTS, ELDERLY: 5 to 40 mg/day. Usual starting dosage is 10 mg/day, with adjustments based on lipid levels; monitor q2–4wk until desired level is achieved. Lower starting dose of 5 mg is recommended in Asians. **Maximum:** 40 mg/day.

RENAL IMPAIRMENT (CREATININE CLEARANCE LESS THAN 30 ml/min)

PO: ADULTS, ELDERLY: 5 mg/day; do not exceed 10 mg/day.

CONCURRENT CYCLOSPORINE USE

PO: ADULTS, ELDERLY: 5 mg/day.

CONCURRENT LIPID-LOWERING THERAPY

PO: ADULTS, ELDERLY: 10 mg/day.

SIDE EFFECTS

Generally well tolerated. Side effects are usually mild, transient. **OCCASIONAL (9%–3%):** Pharyngitis, headache, diarrhea, dyspepsia (heartburn, epigastric distress, indigestion), nausea. **RARE (less than 3%):** Myalgia, asthenia (loss of strength, energy) back pain.

ADVERSE EFFECTS/ TOXIC REACTIONS

Potential for lens opacities. Hypersensitivity reaction, hepatitis occur rarely.

NURSING CONSIDERATIONS

BASELINE ASSESSMENT

Question for possibility of pregnancy before initiating therapy (Pregnancy Category X). Assess baseline lab results: serum cholesterol, triglycerides, hepatic function tests.

INTERVENTION/EVALUATION

Monitor serum cholesterol, triglycerides results for therapeutic response. Lipid levels should be monitored within 2–4 wks of initiation of therapy or change in dosage. Monitor hepatic function tests. Hepatic function tests should be performed at 12 wks following initiation of therapy, at any elevation of dose, and periodically (e.g., semiannually) thereafter. Monitor creatine phosphokinase (CPK) if myopathy is suspected. Monitor daily pattern of bowel activity/stool consistency. Assess for headache, sore throat. Be alert for myalgia, weakness.

PATIENT/FAMILY TEACHING

• Use appropriate contraceptive measures (Pregnancy Category X). • Periodic lab tests are essential part of therapy. • Maintain appropriate diet (important part of treatment). • Report side effects (cramps, muscle pain, weakness, esp. with fever).

R

Roxanol, *see morphine*

Roxicet, *see acetaminophen and oxycodone*

Rozerem, *see ramelteon*

salmeterol

sal-**met**-er-all

(Serevent ✤, Serevent Diskus)

Do not confuse Serevent with Serentil.

FIXED-COMBINATION(S)

Advair: salmeterol/fluticasone (a corticosteroid): 50 mcg/100 mcg; 50 mcg/250 mcg; 50 mcg/500 mcg. **Advair HFA:** salmeterol/fluticasone (a corticosteroid): 21 mcg/45 mcg; 21 mcg/115 mcg; 21 mcg/230 mcg.

◆CLASSIFICATION

PHARMACOTHERAPEUTIC: Sympathomimetic (adrenergic agonist). **CLINICAL:** Bronchodilator (see p. 70C).

ACTION

Stimulates beta$_2$-adrenergic receptors in lungs, resulting in relaxation of bronchial smooth muscle. **Therapeutic Effect:** Relieves bronchospasm, reducing airway resistance.

PHARMACOKINETICS

Route	Onset	Peak	Duration
Inhalation	10–20 min	3 hrs	12 hrs

Low systemic absorption; acts primarily in lungs. Protein binding: 95%. Metabolized by hydroxylation. Primarily eliminated in feces. **Half-life:** 3–4 hrs.

USES

Maintenance therapy for asthma; prevention of exercise-induced bronchospasm, bronchospasm in pts with reversible obstructive airway disease. Long-term maintenance treatment of bronchospasm associated with chronic obstructive pulmonary disease (COPD), including emphysema, chronic bronchitis.

PRECAUTIONS

CONTRAINDICATIONS: History of hypersensitivity to sympathomimetics. **CAUTIONS:** Not for acute symptoms. May cause paradoxical bronchospasm, severe asthma. Pts with cardiovascular disorders (coronary insufficiency, arrhythmias, hypertension), seizure disorders, thyrotoxicosis.

⌛ LIFESPAN CONSIDERATIONS:

Pregnancy/Lactation: Unknown if excreted in breast milk. **Pregnancy Category C. Children:** No age-related precautions in those older than 4 yrs. **Elderly:** Lower dosages may be needed due to increased sympathetic sensitivity (may be more susceptible to tachycardia, tremors).

INTERACTIONS

DRUG: May decrease effects of **beta-adrenergic blocking agents (beta-blockers). MAOIs, tricyclic antidepressants** may increase concentration, effect, toxicity (wait 14 days after stopping MAOIs, tricyclic antidepressants before starting salmeterol). **HERBAL:** None significant. **FOOD:** None known. **LAB VALUES:** May decrease serum potassium.

AVAILABILITY (Rx)

POWDER FOR ORAL INHALATION: 50 mcg.

ADMINISTRATION/HANDLING

INHALATION

• Shake container well, exhale completely through mouth; place mouthpiece into mouth and close lips, holding inhaler upright. • Inhale deeply through mouth while fully depressing top of canister. Hold breath as long as possible before exhaling slowly. • Wait 2 min before second dose (allows for deeper bronchial penetration). • Rinse mouth with water immediately after inhalation (prevents mouth/throat dryness).

INDICATIONS/ROUTES/DOSAGE

MAINTENANCE THERAPY FOR ASTHMA

INHALATION (DISKUS): ADULTS, ELDERLY, CHILDREN 4 YRS AND OLDER: 1 inhalation (50 mcg) q12h.

PREVENTION OF EXERCISE-INDUCED BRONCHOSPASM

INHALATION (DISKUS): ADULTS, ELDERLY, CHILDREN 4 YRS AND OLDER: 1 inhalation at least 30 min before exercise.

MAINTENANCE THERAPY FOR COPD

INHALATION (DISKUS): ADULTS, ELDERLY: 1 inhalation q12h.

SIDE EFFECTS

FREQUENT (28%): Headache. **OCCASIONAL (7%–3%):** Cough, tremor, dizziness, vertigo, throat dryness/irritation, pharyngitis. **RARE (3%):** Palpitations, tachycardia, nausea, heartburn, GI distress, diarrhea.

ADVERSE EFFECTS/ TOXIC REACTIONS

May prolong QT interval (can precipitate ventricular arrhythmias). Hypokalemia, hyperglycemia may occur.

NURSING CONSIDERATIONS

BASELINE ASSESSMENT

Obtain baseline EKG and monitor for changes.

INTERVENTION/EVALUATION

Monitor rate, depth, rhythm, type of respiration; quality/rate of pulse, B/P. Assess lungs for wheezing, rales, rhonchi. Periodically evaluate serum potassium levels.

PATIENT/FAMILY TEACHING

• Not for relief of acute episodes. • Keep canister at room temperature (cold decreases effects). • Do not stop medication or exceed recommended dosage. • Notify physician promptly of chest pain, dizziness. • Wait at least 1 full min before second inhalation. • Administer dose 30–60 min before exercise when used to prevent exercise-induced bronchospasm. • Avoid excessive use of caffeine derivatives (coffee, tea, colas, chocolate).

salsalate

sal-sa-late
(Amigesic, Salflex ✦)

CLASSIFICATION

PHARMACOTHERAPEUTIC: Nonsteroidal anti-inflammatory. **CLINICAL:** Analgesic, anti-inflammatory.

ACTION

NSAID that inhibits prostaglandin synthesis, reducing inflammatory response, intensity of pain stimuli reaching sensory nerve endings. **Therapeutic Effect:** Produces analgesic, anti-inflammatory effects.

USES

Treatment of minor pain/fever, arthritis.

PRECAUTIONS

CONTRAINDICATIONS: Bleeding disorders, hypersensitivity to salicylates, NSAIDs. **CAUTIONS:** Platelet or bleeding disorders, hepatic/renal impairment, history of gastric irritation, peptic ulcer, gastritis, asthma. **Pregnancy Category C (D third trimester).**

INTERACTIONS

DRUG: **Alcohol, NSAIDs** may increase risk of GI effects (e.g., ulceration). **Urinary alkalinizers, antacids** increase excretion. **Anticoagulants, heparin, thrombolytics, valproic acid, platelet aggregation inhibitors** increase risk of bleeding. Large dose may increase effect of **insulin, oral hypoglycemics.** May increase toxicity

S

of **methotrexate, zidovudine. Ototoxic medications, vancomycin** may increase ototoxicity. May decrease effect of **probenecid, sulfinpyrazone.** **HERBAL:** **Cat's claw, dong quai, evening primrose, feverfew, garlic, ginger, ginkgo, red clover, ginseng** possess antiplatelet action, may increase bleeding. **FOOD:** None known. **LAB VALUES:** May alter AST, ALT, serum alkaline phosphatase, uric acid; prolong prothrombin time (PT), bleeding time. May decrease serum cholestrol, potassium, T_1, T_4.

AVAILABILITY (Rx)

TABLETS (AMIGESIC): 500 mg, 750 mg.

ADMINISTRATION/HANDLING

PO

- Give with food if GI discomfort occurs.

INDICATIONS/ROUTES/DOSAGE

RHEUMATOID ARTHRITIS, OSTEOARTHRITIS PAIN

PO: ADULTS, ELDERLY: Initially, 3 g/day in 2–3 divided doses. Maintenance: 2–4 g/day.

◀ **ALERT** ▶ Pts with end-stage renal disease undergoing hemodialysis: 750 mg 2 times/day with additional 500 mg following dialysis.

SIDE EFFECTS

OCCASIONAL: Nausea, dyspepsia (heartburn, indigestion, epigastric pain).

ADVERSE EFFECTS/ TOXIC REACTIONS

Tinnitus may be first sign that serum salicylic acid concentration is reaching or exceeding upper therapeutic range. May produce vertigo, headache, confusion, drowsiness, diaphoresis, hyperventilation, vomiting, diarrhea. Severe overdose may result in electrolyte imbalance, hyperthermia, dehydration, blood pH imbalance. GI bleeding, peptic ulcer, Reye's syndrome, MI, stroke rarely occur.

NURSING CONSIDERATIONS

BASELINE ASSESSMENT

Do not give to children, teenagers who have flu or chickenpox (increases risk of Reye's syndrome). Assess type, location, duration of pain, inflammation. Inspect appearance of affected joints for immobility, deformities, skin condition.

INTERVENTION/EVALUATION

Assess for evidence of nausea, dyspepsia. Evaluate for therapeutic response: relief of pain, stiffness, swelling, increased joint mobility, reduced joint tenderness, improved grip strength.

PATIENT/FAMILY TEACHING

• Avoid alcohol. • Avoid use of aspirin-containing products. • Use antacids or take with food to relieve stomach upset. • Report tinnitus, persistent GI pain. • Report behavioral changes, vomiting to physician (may be early signs of Reye's syndrome).

Sanctura, *see trospium*

Sandostatin, *see octreotide*

saquinavir

sa-**kwin**-a-veer

(Invirase)

Do not confuse saquinavir with Sinequan.

CLASSIFICATION

PHARMACOTHERAPEUTIC: Protease inhibitor. **CLINICAL:** Antiretroviral (see pp. 66C, 113C).

ACTION

Inhibits HIV protease, rendering the enzyme incapable of processing polyprotein precursors needed to generate functional proteins in HIV-infected cells. **Therapeutic Effect:** Interferes with HIV replication, slowing progression of HIV infection.

PHARMACOKINETICS

Poorly absorbed after PO administration (absorption increased with high-calorie, high-fat meals). Protein binding: 99%. Metabolized in liver to inactive metabolite. Primarily eliminated in feces. Unknown if removed by hemodialysis. **Half-life:** 13 hrs.

USES

Treatment of HIV infection in combination with other antiretroviral agents.

PRECAUTIONS

CONTRAINDICATIONS: Concurrent use with **amiodarone, bepridil, propafenone, quinidine, ergot derivatives, midazolam, rifampin, triazolam.** **CAUTIONS:** Diabetes mellitus, hepatic impairment.

LIFESPAN CONSIDERATIONS:

Pregnancy/Lactation: Breast-feeding not recommended (possibility of HIV transmission). **Pregnancy Category B.** **Children:** Safety and efficacy not established. **Elderly:** Information not available.

INTERACTIONS

DRUG: May increase concentration, toxicity of **calcium channel-blocking agents, rifabutin, sildenafil, tadalafil, vardenafil.** May decrease concentration, effect of **efavirenz, methadone, oral contraceptives. Carbamazepine, dexamethasone, efavirenz, phenobarbital, phenytoin, rifabutin** may decrease concentration, effect. **Delavirdine, nevirapine, ritonavir** may increase concentration, toxicity. **HERBAL: Garlic, St. John's wort**may decrease concentration, effect. **FOOD: Grapefruit, grapefruit juice**may increase concentration. **LAB VALUES:** May alter serum creatine kinase (CK), elevate hepatic function test results, lower serum glucose.

AVAILABILITY (Rx)

CAPSULES (INVIRASE): 200 mg. **TABLETS (INVIRASE):** 500 mg.

ADMINISTRATION/HANDLING

PO

- Give within 2 hrs after a full meal (if taken without food in stomach, may result in no antiviral activity).

INDICATIONS/ROUTES/DOSAGE

HIV INFECTION IN COMBINATION WITH OTHER ANTIRETROVIRALS

PO: ADULTS, ELDERLY: 1,000 mg (5 × 200 mg or 2 × 500 mg) twice a day in combination with ritonavir 100 mg twice a day.

DOSAGE ADJUSTMENTS WHEN GIVEN IN COMBINATION THERAPY

Delavirdine: Fortovase 800 mg 3 times a day.
Lopinavir/ritonavir: Fortovase 800 mg twice a day.
Nelfinavir: Fortovase 800 mg 3 times a day or 1,200 mg twice a day.
Ritonavir: Fortovase or Invirase 1,000 mg twice a day.

SIDE EFFECTS

OCCASIONAL: Diarrhea, abdominal discomfort/pain, nausea, photosensitivity, stomatitis. **RARE:** Confusion, ataxia, asthenia, headache, rash.

ADVERSE EFFECTS/ TOXIC REACTIONS

None known.

NURSING CONSIDERATIONS

BASELINE ASSESSMENT

Obtain baseline laboratory testing, esp. hepatic function tests, before beginning saquinavir therapy and at periodic intervals during therapy. Offer emotional support. Obtain medication history.

INTERVENTION/EVALUATION

Monitor serum hepatic function tests, triglycerides, glucose, CD4 cell count, HIV RNA levels. Closely monitor for evidence of GI discomfort. Monitor daily pattern of bowel activity/stool consistency. Inspect mouth for signs of mucosal ulceration. Monitor serum chemistry tests for marked laboratory abnormalities. If serious or severe toxicities occur, interrupt therapy, contact physician.

PATIENT/FAMILY TEACHING

• Report persistent abdominal pain, nausea, vomiting. • Avoid exposure to sunlight, artificial light sources. • Continue therapy for full length of treatment. • Doses should be evenly spaced. • Saquinavir is not a cure for HIV infection, nor does it reduce risk of transmission to others. • Pts may continue to acquire illnesses associated with advanced HIV infection. • Take within 2 hrs after a full meal. • Avoid administration with grapefruit products.

sargramostim (granulocyte macrophage colony-stimulating factor, GM-CSF)

sar-gra-**moh**-stim

(Leukine)

Do not confuse Leukine with Leukeran.

CLASSIFICATION

PHARMACOTHERAPEUTIC: Colony-stimulating factor. **CLINICAL:** Hematopoietic, antineutropenic.

ACTION

Stimulates proliferation/differentiation of hematopoietic cells to activate mature granulocytes and macrophages. **Therapeutic Effect:** Assists bone marrow in making new WBCs, increases their chemotactic, antifungal, antiparasitic activity. Increases cytoneoplastic cells, activates neutrophils to inhibit tumor cell growth.

PHARMACOKINETICS

Effect	Onset	Peak	Duration
Increase WBCs	7–14 days	N/A	1 wk

Detected in serum within 5 min after subcutaneous administration. **Half-life:** IV, 1 hr; subcutaneous, 3 hrs.

USES

Accelerates myeloid recovery in pts undergoing autologous or allogeneic bone marrow transplant or in pts who have undergone hematopoietic stem cell transplant following myeloablative chemotherapy. Prolongs survival in pts following bone marrow transplant in whom engraftment has been delayed or has failed. Enhances peripheral progenitor cell yield in autologous hematopoietic stem cell transplant. **OFF-LABEL:** Treatment of AIDS-related neutropenia; chronic, severe neutropenia; drug-induced neutropenia; myelodysplastic syndrome.

PRECAUTIONS

CONTRAINDICATIONS: 12 hrs before or after radiation therapy; 24 hrs before or after chemotherapy; excessive leukemic myeloid blasts in bone marrow or peripheral blood (greater than 10%); known hypersensitivity to yeast-derived products. **CAUTIONS:** Preexisting cardiac disease, hypoxia, preexisting fluid retention, pulmonary infiltrates, CHF, renal/hepatic impairment.

S

LIFESPAN CONSIDERATIONS:

Pregnancy/Lactation: Unknown if drug crosses placenta or is distributed in breast milk. **Pregnancy Category C. Children:** Safety and efficacy not established. **Elderly:** No age-related precautions noted.

INTERACTIONS

DRUG: Lithium, steroids may increase effects. **HERBAL:** None significant. **FOOD:** None known. **LAB VALUES:** May increase serum bilirubin, creatinine, hepatic enzyme. May decrease serum albumin.

AVAILABILITY (Rx)

INJECTION POWDER FOR RECONSTITUTION: 250 mcg. **INJECTION SOLUTION:** 500 mcg/ml.

ADMINISTRATION/HANDLING

IV

Reconstitution • To 250 mcg vial, add 1 ml Sterile Water for Injection (preservative free). • Direct Sterile Water for Injection to side of vial, gently swirl contents to avoid foaming; do not shake or vigorously agitate. • After reconstitution, further dilute with 0.9% NaCl. If final concentration less than 10 mcg/ml, add 1 mg albumin/ml 0.9% NaCl to provide a final albumin concentration of 0.1%.

◀ **ALERT** ▶ Albumin is added before addition of sargramostim (prevents drug adsorption to components of drug delivery system).

Rate of administration • Give each single dose over 2, 4, or 24 hrs as directed by physician.

Storage • Refrigerate powder, reconstituted solution, diluted solution for injection. • Do not shake. • Reconstituted solutions are clear, colorless. • Use within 6 hrs; discard unused portions. • Use 1 dose per vial; do not reenter vial.

INDICATIONS/ROUTES/DOSAGE

MYELOID RECOVERY FOLLOWING BONE MARROW TRANSPLANT (BMT)

IV INFUSION: ADULTS, ELDERLY: Usual parenteral dosage: 250 mcg/m^2/day for 21 days (as 2-hr infusion). Begin 2–4 hrs after autologous bone marrow infusion and not less than 24 hrs after last dose of chemotherapy or not less than 12 hrs after last radiation treatment. Discontinue if blast cells appear or underlying disease progresses.

BONE MARROW TRANSPLANT FAILURE, ENGRAFTMENT DELAY

IV INFUSION: ADULTS, ELDERLY: 250 mcg/m^2/day for 14 days. Infuse over 2 hrs. May repeat after 7 days off therapy if engraftment has not occurred with 500 mcg/m^2/day for 14 days.

STEM CELL TRANSPLANT

IV, SUBCUTANEOUS: ADULTS: 250 mcg/m^2/day.

IV INCOMPATIBILITIES

Amphotericin B complex (Abelcet, AmBisome, Amphotec), hydromorphone (Dilaudid), lorazepam (Ativan), morphine.

IV COMPATIBILITIES

Calcium gluconate, dopamine (Intropin), heparin, magnesium, potassium chloride.

SIDE EFFECTS

FREQUENT: GI disturbances (nausea, diarrhea, vomiting, stomatitis, anorexia, abdominal pain), arthralgia or myalgia, headache, malaise, rash, pruritus. **OCCASIONAL:** Peripheral edema, weight gain, dyspnea, asthenia, fever, leukocytosis, capillary leak syndrome (fluid retention, irritation at local injection site, peripheral edema). **RARE:** Rapid/irregular heartbeat, thrombophlebitis.

ADVERSE EFFECTS/ TOXIC REACTIONS

Pleural/pericardial effusion occurs rarely after infusion.

NURSING CONSIDERATIONS

BASELINE ASSESSMENT

Monitor for supraventricular arrhythmias during administration (particularly in pts with history of cardiac arrhythmias). Assess closely for dyspnea during and immediately following infusion (particularly in pts with history of lung disease). If dyspnea occurs during infusion, cut infusion rate by half. If dyspnea continues, stop infusion immediately. If neutrophil count exceeds 20,000 cells/mm^3 or platelet count exceeds 500,000/mm^3, stop infusion or reduce dose by half, based on clinical condition of pt. Blood counts return to normal or baseline 3–7 days after discontinuation of therapy.

INTERVENTION/EVALUATION

Monitor CBC with differential, platelets, serum renal/hepatic function, pulmonary function, vital signs, weight.

saw palmetto

Also known as American dwarf palm tree, cabbage palm, sabal, zuzhong.

CLASSIFICATION

HERBAL: See Appendix G.

ACTION

Appears to inhibit 5-alpha-reductase, prevent conversion of testosterone to dihydrotestosterone (DHT). **Effect:** Reduces prostate growth. Contains antiandrogenic, antiproliferative, anti-inflammatory properties.

USES

Symptoms of benign prostate hyperplasia (BPH). Used as a mild diuretic, sedative, anti-inflammatory agent, antiseptic.

PRECAUTIONS

CONTRAINDICATIONS: Pregnancy, lactation due to antiandrogenic and estrogenic activity. **CAUTIONS:** None known.

LIFESPAN CONSIDERATIONS:

Pregnancy/Lactation: Contraindicated. **Children:** Safety and efficacy not established. **Elderly:** No age-related precautions noted.

INTERACTIONS

DRUG: May interfere with effects of **oral contraceptives, hormone therapy.** **HERBAL:** None significant. **FOOD:** None known. **LAB VALUES:** None known.

AVAILABILITY (OTC)

BERRIES. CAPSULES: 80 mg, 160 mg, 500 mg. **FLUID EXTRACT. TEA.**

INDICATIONS/ROUTES/DOSAGE

BPH

PO: ADULTS, ELDERLY: 160 mg twice a day or 320 mg once a day using a liquid extract or 1–2 g of whole berries.

DIURETIC, SEDATIVE, ANTI-INFLAMMATORY, ANTISEPTIC

PO: ADULTS, ELDERLY: 0.6–1.5 ml liquid extract or 0.5–1 g dried berries 3 times a day.

SIDE EFFECTS

Mild anorexia, dizziness, nausea, vomiting, constipation, diarrhea, headache, impotence, hypersensitivity reactions, back pain.

ADVERSE EFFECTS/ TOXIC REACTIONS

None known.

NURSING CONSIDERATIONS

BASELINE ASSESSMENT

Determine use of oral contraceptives, hormone replacement therapy (may interfere). Assess pt's urinary patterns. Obtain prostate-specific antigen (PSA) level before using.

INTERVENTION/EVALUATION

Assess for hypersensitivity reactions. Monitor symptoms of BHP (frequent/painful urination, hesitancy, urgency). Observe for decreased nocturia, improved urinary flow, decreased residual urine volume.

PATIENT/FAMILY TEACHING

- Should be taken with food.

scopolamine

skoe-**pol**-a-meen

(Trans-Derm Scop, Transderm-V ✤)

FIXED-COMBINATION(S)

Donnatal: scopolamine/atropine (anticholinergic)/hyoscyamine (anticholinergic)/phenobarbital (sedative): 0.0065 mg/0.0194 mg/0.1037 mg/16.2 mg.

CLASSIFICATION

PHARMACOTHERAPEUTIC: Anticholinergic. **CLINICAL:** Antinausea, antiemetic.

ACTION

Reduces excitability of labyrinthine receptors, depressing conduction in vestibular cerebellar pathway. **Therapeutic Effect:** Prevents motion-induced nausea/vomiting.

USES

Prevention of motion sickness, postop nausea/vomiting.

PRECAUTIONS

CONTRAINDICATIONS: Angle-closure glaucoma, GI/GU obstruction, myasthenia gravis, paralytic ileus, tachycardia, thyrotoxicosis. **CAUTIONS:** Hepatic/renal impairment, cardiac disease, seizures, psychoses.

LIFESPAN CONSIDERATIONS:

Pregnancy/Lactation: Crosses placenta; unknown if distributed in breast milk. **Pregnancy Category C. Children:** Safety and efficacy not established. **Elderly:** Dizziness, hallucinations, confusion may require dosage adjustment.

INTERACTIONS

DRUG: Antihistamines, anticholinergics, tricyclic antidepressants may increase anticholinergic effects. **CNS depressants** may increase CNS depression. **HERBAL:** None significant. **FOOD:** None known. **LAB VALUES:** May interfere with gastric secretion test.

AVAILABILITY (Rx)

TRANSDERMAL SYSTEM (TRANS-DERM SCOP): 1.5 mg.

ADMINISTRATION/HANDLING

TRANSDERMAL

- Apply patch to hairless area behind one ear. • If dislodged or on for more than 72 hrs, replace with fresh patch.

INDICATIONS/ROUTES/DOSAGE

PREVENTION OF MOTION SICKNESS

TRANSDERMAL: ADULTS: 1 system q72h.

POSTOP NAUSEA/VOMITING

TRANSDERMAL: ADULTS, ELDERLY: 1 system no sooner than 1 hr before surgery and removed 24 hrs after surgery.

SIDE EFFECTS

FREQUENT (greater than 15%): Dry mouth, drowsiness, blurred vision. **RARE (5%–1%):** Dizziness, restlessness, hallucinations, confusion, difficulty urinating, rash.

ADVERSE EFFECTS/ TOXIC REACTIONS

None known.

S

NURSING CONSIDERATIONS

BASELINE ASSESSMENT

Assess for use of other CNS depressants, drugs with anticholinergic action, history of narrow-angle glaucoma.

INTERVENTION/EVALUATION

Monitor serum hepatic/renal function tests.

PATIENT/FAMILY TEACHING

• Avoid tasks requiring alertness, motor skills until response to drug is established (may cause drowsiness, disorientation, confusion). • Teach proper application of patch. • Use only 1 patch at a time; do not cut. • Wash hands after administration.

secobarbital

(Seconal)

See Sedative-hypnotics

selegiline

sell-**eh**-geh-leen

(Apo-Selegiline ♣, Eldepryl, Emsam, Novo-Selegiline ♣, Zelapar)

Do not confuse selegiline with Stelazine, Salagen or Eldepryl with enalapril.

CLASSIFICATION

CLINICAL: Antiparkinson agent.

ACTION

Irreversibly inhibits activity of monoamine oxidase type B (enzyme that breaks down dopamine), thereby increasing dopaminergic action. **Therapeutic Effect:** Relieves signs/symptoms of Parkinson's disease (tremor, akinesia, posture/equilibrium disorders, rigidity).

PHARMACOKINETICS

Rapidly absorbed from GI tract. Crosses blood-brain barrier. Metabolized in liver to active metabolites. Primarily excreted in urine. **Half-life:** 17 hrs (amphetamine), 20 hrs (methamphetamine).

USES

Adjunct to levodopa/carbidopa in treatment of Parkinson's disease. **Transdermal:** Treatment of major depressive disorder (MDD). **OFF-LABEL:** Treatment of Alzheimer's disease, attention deficit hyperactivity disorder, depression, early Parkinson's disease, extrapyramidal symptoms, negative symptoms of schizophrenia.

PRECAUTIONS

CONTRAINDICATIONS: Concurrent use with meperidine, tricyclic antidepressants. **CAUTIONS:** History of peptic ulcer disease, dementia, psychosis, tardive dyskinesia, profound tremor, cardiac dysrhythmias.

LIFESPAN CONSIDERATIONS: **Pregnancy/Lactation:** Unknown if drug crosses placenta or is distributed in breast milk. **Pregnancy Category C.** **Children:** Safety and efficacy not established. **Elderly:** No age-related precautions noted.

INTERACTIONS

DRUG: **Fluoxetine, fluvoxamine, paroxetine, sertraline, venlafaxine** may cause mania, serotonin syndrome (altered mental status, restlessness, diaphoresis, diarrhea, fever). **Meperidine** may cause potentially fatal reaction (e.g., excitation, diaphoresis, rigidity, hypertension/hypotension, coma, death). **Tricyclic antidepressants** may cause asystole, diaphoresis, hypertension, syncope, altered mental status, hyperpyrexia, seizures, tremors (wait 14 days between stopping selegiline and starting tricyclic antidepressants). **HERBAL:** **Kava kava,**

SAMe, St. John's wort, valerian may increase risk of serotonin syndrome, excessive sedation. **FOOD: Tyramine-rich foods** may produce hypertensive reactions. **LAB VALUES:** None known.

AVAILABILITY (Rx)

CAPSULES (ELDEPRYL): 5 mg. **TABLETS (ELDEPRYL):** 5 mg. **TABLETS, ORALLY DISINTEGRATING (ZELAPAR):** 1.25 mg. **TRANSDERMAL (EMSAM):** 6 mg/24 hr, 9 mg/24 hr, 12 mg/24 hr.

ADMINISTRATION/HANDLING

PO

• Give without regard to meals. • Avoid tyramine-containing foods, large quantities of caffeine-containing beverages.

PO (ORALLY DISINTEGRATING TABLETS)

• Give in morning before breakfast and without liquid. • Peel back (do not push tablets through foil) backing with dry hands. • Immediately place on top of tongue, allow to disintegrate. • Avoid food, liquids for 5 min before and after taking selegiline.

TRANSDERMAL

• Apply to dry, intact skin on upper torso or thigh, outer surface of upper arm.

INDICATIONS/ROUTES/DOSAGE

ADJUNCTIVE TREATMENT FOR PARKINSONISM

PO: ADULTS (ELDEPRYL): 10 mg/day in divided doses, such as 5 mg at breakfast and lunch, given concomitantly with each dose of carbidopa and levodopa. **ELDERLY:** Initially, 5 mg in the morning. May increase up to 10 mg/day. **(ZELAPAR):** 1.25–2.5 mg/day.

MAJOR DEPRESSIVE DISORDER

TRANSDERMAL: ADULTS, ELDERLY: Initially, 6 mg/24 hrs. May increase in 3 mg/24 hrs increments at minimum of 2 wks. **Maximum:** 12 mg/24 hrs.

SIDE EFFECTS

FREQUENT (10%–4%): Nausea, dizziness, light-headedness, syncope, abdominal discomfort. **OCCASIONAL (3%–2%):** Confusion, hallucinations, dry mouth, vivid dreams, dyskinesia. **RARE (1%):** Headache, myalgia, anxiety, diarrhea, insomnia.

ADVERSE EFFECTS/ TOXIC REACTIONS

Symptoms of overdose may vary from CNS depression (sedation, apnea, cardiovascular collapse, death), to severe paradoxical reactions (hallucinations, tremor, seizures). Impaired motor coordination, (loss of balance, blepharospasm [uncontrolled blinking], facial grimaces, feeling of heaviness in lower extremities), depression, nightmares, delusions, overstimulation, sleep disturbance, anger, hallucinations, confusion may occur.

NURSING CONSIDERATIONS

INTERVENTION/EVALUATION

Be alert to neurologic effects (headache, lethargy, mental confusion, agitation). Monitor for evidence of dyskinesia (difficulty with movement). Assess for clinical reversal of symptoms (improvement of tremors of head/hands at rest, mask-like facial expression, shuffling gait, muscular rigidity).

PATIENT/FAMILY TEACHING

• Tolerance to feeling of light-headedness develops during therapy. • To reduce hypotensive effect, rise slowly from lying to sitting position, permit legs to dangle momentarily before standing. • Avoid tasks that require alertness, motor skills until response to drug is established. • Dry mouth, drowsiness, dizziness may be an expected response of drug. • Avoid alcohol during therapy. • Coffee, tea may help reduce drowsiness.

S

senna

sen-na

(Ex-Lax, Senexon, Senna-Gen, Sennatural, Senokot, X-Prep)

FIXED-COMBINATION(S)

Gentlax-S, Senokot-S: senna/docusate (a laxative): 8.6 mg/50 mg.

CLASSIFICATION

PHARMACOTHERAPEUTIC: GI stimulant. **CLINICAL:** Laxative (see p. 118C).

ACTION

Direct effect on intestinal smooth musculature (stimulates intramural nerve plexi). **Therapeutic Effect:** Increases peristalsis, promotes laxative effect.

PHARMACOKINETICS

Route	Onset	Peak	Duration
PO	6–12 hrs	N/A	N/A
Rectal	0.5–2 hrs	N/A	N/A

Minimal absorption after PO administration. Hydrolyzed to active form by enzymes of colonic flora. Absorbed drug metabolized in the liver. Eliminated in feces via biliary system.

USES

Short-term use for constipation, to evacuate colon before bowel/rectal examinations.

PRECAUTIONS

CONTRAINDICATIONS: Abdominal pain, appendicitis, intestinal obstruction, nausea, vomiting. **CAUTIONS:** Prolonged use (longer than 1 wk).

LIFESPAN CONSIDERATIONS:

Pregnancy/Lactation: Unknown if distributed in breast milk. **Pregnancy Category C.** **Children:** Safety and efficacy not established in those younger than 6 yrs. **Elderly:** No age-related precautions noted; monitor for signs of dehydration, electrolyte loss.

INTERACTIONS

DRUG: May decrease transit time of concurrently administered **oral medications,** decreasing absorption. **HERBAL:** None significant. **FOOD:** None known. **LAB VALUES:** May increase serum glucose. May decrease serum potassium.

AVAILABILITY (OTC)

GRANULES (SENOKOT): 15 mg/tsp. **LIQUID (X-PREP):** 8.8 mg/5 ml. **SYRUP (SENOKOT):** 8.8 mg/5 ml. **TABLETS: (SENNATURAL, SENOKOT, SENEXON, SENNA-GEN):** 8.6 mg, 15 mg. **(EX-LAX):** 15 mg, 90 mg.

ADMINISTRATION/HANDLING

PO

- Give on an empty stomach (decreases time to effect).
- Offer at least 6–8 glasses of water/day (aids stool softening).
- Avoid giving within 1 hr of other oral medication (decreases drug absorption).

INDICATIONS/ROUTES/DOSAGE

CONSTIPATION

PO (TABLETS): ADULTS, ELDERLY, CHILDREN 12 YRS AND OLDER: 2 tablets at bedtime. **Maximum:** 4 tablets twice a day. **CHILDREN 6–11 YRS:** 1 tablet at bedtime. **Maximum:** 2 tablets twice a day. **CHILDREN 2–5 YRS:** ½ tablet at bedtime. **Maximum:** 1 tablet twice a day.

PO (SYRUP): ADULTS, ELDERLY, CHILDREN 12 YRS AND OLDER: 10–15 ml at bedtime. **Maximum:** 15 ml twice a day. **CHILDREN 6–11 YRS:** 5–7.5 ml at bedtime. **Maximum:** 7.5 ml twice a day. **CHILDREN 2–5 YRS:** 2.5–3.75 ml at bedtime. **Maximum:** 3.75 ml twice a day.

PO (GRANULES): ADULTS, ELDERLY, CHILDREN 12 YRS AND OLDER: 1 tsp at bedtime. **Maximum:** 2 tsp twice a day. **CHILDREN 6–11 YRS:** ½ teaspoon at bedtime up to 1 teaspoon 2 times/day.

S

CHILDREN 2–5 YRS: ¼ teaspoon at bedtime up to ½ teaspoon 2 times/day.

BOWEL EVACUATION

PO: ADULTS, ELDERLY, CHILDREN OLDER THAN 1 YR: 75 ml between 2 PM and 4 PM on day prior to procedure.

SIDE EFFECTS

FREQUENT: Pink-red, red-violet, red-brown, or yellow-brown discoloration of urine. **OCCASIONAL:** Some degree of abdominal discomfort, nausea, mild cramps, griping, faintness.

ADVERSE EFFECTS/ TOXIC REACTIONS

Long-term use may result in laxative dependence, chronic constipation, loss of normal bowel function. Prolonged use/overdose may result in electrolyte, metabolic disturbances (e.g., hypokalemia, hypocalcemia, metabolic acidosis or alkalosis), vomiting, muscle weakness, persistent diarrhea, malabsorption, weight loss.

NURSING CONSIDERATIONS

INTERVENTION/EVALUATION

Encourage adequate fluid intake. Assess bowel sounds for peristalsis. Monitor daily pattern of bowel activity/stool consistency. Assess for GI disturbances. Monitor serum electrolytes in pts exposed to prolonged, frequent, excessive use of medication.

PATIENT/FAMILY TEACHING

• Urine may turn pink-red, red-violet, red-brown, yellow-brown (only temporary and not harmful). • Institute measures to promote defecation (increase fluid intake, exercise, high-fiber diet). • Laxative effect generally occurs in 6–12 hrs but may take 24 hrs. • Do not take other oral medication within 1 hr of taking sertraline (decreased effectiveness).

Sensipar, *see cinacalcet*

Septra, *see co-trimoxazole*

Serevent Diskus, *see salmeterol*

Seroquel, *see quetiapine*

sertraline

sir-trah-leen

(Apo-Sertraline ✤, Novo-Sertraline ✤, PMS-Sertraline ✤, Zoloft)

Do not confuse sertraline with Serentil.

CLASSIFICATION

PHARMACOTHERAPEUTIC: Serotonin reuptake inhibitor. **CLINICAL:** Antidepressant, anxiolytic, obsessive-compulsive disorder adjunct (see p. 38C).

ACTION

Blocks reuptake of the neurotransmitter serotonin at CNS neuronal presynaptic membranes, increasing availability at postsynaptic receptor sites. **Therapeutic Effect:** Relieves depression, reduces obsessive-compulsive behavior, decreases anxiety.

PHARMACOKINETICS

Incompletely, slowly absorbed from GI tract; food increases absorption.

S

Protein binding: 98%. Widely distributed. Undergoes extensive first-pass metabolism in liver to active compound. Excreted in urine, feces. Not removed by hemodialysis. **Half-life:** 26 hrs.

USES

Treatment of major depressive disorders, panic disorder, obsessive-compulsive disorder (OCD), post-traumatic stress disorder (PTSD), premenstrual dysphoric disorder (PMDD), social anxiety disorder. **OFF-LABEL:** Eating disorders, generalized anxiety disorder (GAD), impulse control disorders.

PRECAUTIONS

CONTRAINDICATIONS: MAOI use within 14 days. **CAUTIONS:** Seizure disorders, cardiac disease, recent MI, hepatic impairment, suicidal pts.

⌛ LIFESPAN CONSIDERATIONS:

Pregnancy/Lactation: Unknown if drug crosses placenta or is distributed in breast milk. **Pregnancy Category C.** **Children:** Children and adolescents are at increased risk of suicidal ideation and behavior or worsening of depression, esp. during the first few mos of therapy. **Elderly:** No age-related precautions noted, but lower initial dosages recommended.

INTERACTIONS

DRUG: May increase concentration, risk of toxicity of **highly protein-bound medications (e.g., digoxin, warfarin). MAOIs** may cause neuroleptic malignant syndrome, hypertensive crisis, hyperpyrexia, seizures, serotonin syndrome (diaphoresis, diarrhea, fever, mental changes, restlessness, shivering). May increase concentration, toxicity of tricyclic antidepressants. **HERBAL: Gotu kola, kava kava, St. John's wort, valerian** may increase CNS depression. **FOOD:** None known. **LAB VALUES:** May increase total serum cholesterol, triglycerides, AST, ALT. May decrease serum uric acid.

AVAILABILITY (Rx)

ORAL CONCENTRATE: 20 mg/ml. **TABLETS:** 25 mg, 50 mg, 100 mg.

ADMINISTRATION/HANDLING

PO

- Give with food, milk if GI distress occurs.

INDICATIONS/ROUTES/DOSAGE

DEPRESSION

PO: ADULTS: Initially, 50 mg/day. May increase by 50 mg/day at 7-day intervals up to 200 mg/day. **ELDERLY:** Initially, 25 mg/day. May increase by 25–50 mg/day at 7-day intervals up to 200 mg/day.

OCD

PO: ADULTS, CHILDREN 13–17 YRS: Initially, 50 mg/day with morning or evening meal. May increase by 50 mg/day at 7-day intervals. **ELDERLY, CHILDREN 6–12 YRS:** Initially, 25 mg/day. May increase by 25–50 mg/day at 7-day intervals. **Maximum:** 200 mg/day.

PANIC DISORDER, PTSD, SOCIAL ANXIETY DISORDER

PO: ADULTS, ELDERLY: Initially, 25 mg/day. May increase by 50 mg/day at 7-day intervals. Range: 50–200 mg/day. **Maximum:** 200 mg/day.

PREMENSTRUAL DYSPHORIC DISORDER

PO: ADULTS: Initially, 50 mg/day. May increase up to 150 mg/day in 50-mg increments.

SIDE EFFECTS

FREQUENT (26%–12%): Headache, nausea, diarrhea, insomnia, drowsiness, dizziness, fatigue, rash, dry mouth. **OCCASIONAL (6%–4%):** Anxiety, nervousness, agitation, tremor, dyspepsia (heartburn, indigestion, epigastric pain), diaphoresis, vomiting, constipation, sexual dysfunction, visual disturbances, altered taste. **RARE (less than 3%):** Flatulence, urinary frequency, paresthesia, hot flashes, chills.

ADVERSE EFFECTS/ TOXIC REACTIONS

None known.

NURSING CONSIDERATIONS

BASELINE ASSESSMENT

For those on long-term therapy, serum hepatic/renal function tests, blood counts should be performed periodically.

INTERVENTION/EVALUATION

Supervise suicidal-risk pts, esp. children, adolescents, closely during early therapy (as depression lessens, energy level improves, increasing suicide potential). Assess appearance, behavior, speech pattern, level of interest, mood. Monitor daily pattern of bowel activity/stool consistency. Assist with ambulation if dizziness occurs.

PATIENT/FAMILY TEACHING

• Dry mouth may be relieved by sugarless gum, sips of tepid water. • Report headache, fatigue, tremor, sexual dysfunction. • Avoid tasks that require alertness, motor skills until response to drug is established (may cause dizziness, drowsiness). • Take with food if nausea occurs. • Inform physician if pregnancy occurs. • Avoid alcohol. • Do not take OTC medications without consulting physician.

sevelamer

seh-**vel**-a-mer

(Renagel)

Do not confuse Renagel with Reglan or Regonol.

♦CLASSIFICATION

PHARMACOTHERAPEUTIC: Polymeric phosphate binder. **CLINICAL:** Antihyperphosphatemia.

ACTION

Binds with dietary phosphorus in GI tract, allowing phosphorus to be eliminated through normal digestive process, decreasing serum phosphorus level. **Therapeutic Effect:** Decreases incidence of hypercalcemic episodes in pts receiving calcium acetate treatment.

PHARMACOKINETICS

Not absorbed systemically. Unknown if removed by hemodialysis.

USES

Reduction of serum phosphorus in pts with end-stage renal disease (ESRD).

PRECAUTIONS

CONTRAINDICATIONS: Bowel obstruction, hypophosphatemia. **CAUTIONS:** Dysphagia, severe GI tract motility disorders, major GI tract surgery, swallowing disorders.

⌛ LIFESPAN CONSIDERATIONS:

Pregnancy/Lactation: Not distributed in breast milk. **Pregnancy Category C.** **Children:** Safety and efficacy not established. **Elderly:** No age-related precautions noted.

INTERACTIONS

DRUG: May decrease absorption of **oral medications** (take at least 1 hr before or 3 hrs after a dose of sevelamer). **HERBAL:** None significant. **FOOD:** None known. **LAB VALUES:** None known.

AVAILABILITY (Rx)

TABLETS: 400 mg, 800 mg.

ADMINISTRATION/HANDLING

PO

• Give with meals. • Space other medication by at least 1 hr before or 3 hrs after sevelamer.

S

INDICATIONS/ROUTES/DOSAGE

HYPERPHOSPHATEMIA

PO: ADULTS, ELDERLY: 800–1,600 mg with each meal, depending on severity of hyperphosphatemia.

SIDE EFFECTS

FREQUENT (20%–11%): Infection, pain, hypotension, diarrhea, dyspepsia, nausea, vomiting. **OCCASIONAL (10%–1%):** Headache, constipation, hypertension, increased cough.

ADVERSE EFFECTS/ TOXIC REACTIONS

Thrombosis occurs rarely.

NURSING CONSIDERATIONS

BASELINE ASSESSMENT

Obtain baseline serum phosphorus; assess for bowel obstruction.

INTERVENTION/EVALUATION

Monitor serum phosphorus, bicarbonate, chloride, calcium.

PATIENT/FAMILY TEACHING

- Take with meals, swallow whole.
- Report persistent headache, nausea, vomiting, diarrhea, hypotension.

sibutramine

sigh-**bew**-trah-meen

(Meridia)

See Obesity management (p. 134C)

sildenafil

sill-**den**-a-fill

(Revatio, Viagra)

Do not confuse Viagra with Vaniqa.

CLASSIFICATION

PHARMACOTHERAPEUTIC: Phosphodiesterase-5 enzyme inhibitor. **CLINICAL:** Erectile dysfunction adjunct.

ACTION

Inhibits type 5 cyclic guanosine monophosphate (a specific phosphodiesterase), a predominant isoenzyme of pulmonary vascular smooth muscle, corpus cavernosum of penis. **Therapeutic Effect:** Relaxes smooth muscle, increases blood flow, facilitating erection.

USES

Viagra: Treatment of male erectile dysfunction. **Revatio:** Treatment of pulmonary arterial hypertension. **OFF-LABEL:** Treatment of diabetic gastroparesis, sexual dysfunction associated with use of selective serotonin reuptake inhibitors, Raynaud's phenomenon.

PRECAUTIONS

CONTRAINDICATIONS: Concurrent use of sodium nitroprusside, nitrates in any form. **CAUTIONS:** Renal, cardiac, hepatic impairment; anatomic deformation of penis; pts who may be predisposed to priapism (sickle cell anemia, multiple myeloma, leukemia). **Pregnancy Category B.**

INTERACTIONS

DRUG: Alpha-adrenergic blocking agents increase symptomatic hypotension. **Ritonavir** may increase concentration, toxicity. **Cimetidine, erythromycin, itraconazole, ketoconazole** may increase concentration. Potentiates hypotensive effects of **nitrates. HERBAL: St. John's wort** may decrease concentration. **FOOD: High-fat meals** delay maximum effectiveness by 1 hr. **LAB VALUES:** None known.

AVAILABILITY (Rx)

TABLETS: 20 mg (Revatio), 25 mg (Viagra), 50 mg (Viagra), 100 mg (Viagra).

ADMINISTRATION/HANDLING

PO

- May take approximately 1 hr before sexual activity but may be taken anywhere from 4 hrs–30 min before sexual activity.
- Revatio may be given without regard to meals.

INDICATIONS/ROUTES/DOSAGE

ERECTILE DYSFUNCTION

PO: ADULTS: 50 mg (30 min–4 hrs before sexual activity). Range: 25–100 mg. Maximum dosing frequency is once daily. **ELDERLY OLDER THAN 65 YRS:** Consider starting dose of 25 mg.

PULMONARY ARTERIAL HYPERTENSION

PO: ADULTS, ELDERLY: 20 mg 3 times a day taken 4–6 hrs apart.

SIDE EFFECTS

FREQUENT: Headache (16%), flushing (10%). **OCCASIONAL (7%–3%):** Dyspepsia (heartburn, indigestion, epigastric pain), nasal congestion, UTI, abnormal vision, diarrhea. **RARE (2%):** Dizziness, rash.

ADVERSE EFFECTS/ TOXIC REACTIONS

Prolonged erections (lasting over 4 hrs), priapism (painful erections lasting over 6 hrs) occur rarely.

NURSING CONSIDERATIONS

BASELINE ASSESSMENT

Viagra: Determine if pt has other medical conditions, including angina, cardiac disease, benign prostatic hypertrophy (BPH). Assess pt's baseline serum renal/hepatic function. **Revatio:** Obtain baseline ABGs; assess pulmonary function, cardiovascular status.

PATIENT/FAMILY TEACHING

- Sildenafil has no effect in absence of sexual stimulation. • Seek treatment immediately if erection lasts longer than 4 hrs. • Avoid nitrate drugs while taking sildenafil.

silver sulfadiazine

sul-fah-**dye**-ah-zeen

(Demazin ✤, Flamazine ✤, Silvadene, SSD, SSD AF, Thermazene)

CLASSIFICATION

PHARMACOTHERAPEUTIC: Anti-infective. **CLINICAL:** Burn preparation.

ACTION

Acts on cell wall/cell membrane in concentrations selectively toxic to bacteria. **Therapeutic Effect:** Produces bactericidal effect.

USES

Prevention, treatment of infection in second- and third-degree burns; protection against conversion from partial- to full-thickness wounds (infection causing extended tissue destruction). **OFF-LABEL:** Treatment of minor bacterial skin infection, dermal ulcer.

S

PRECAUTIONS

CONTRAINDICATIONS: None known. **CAUTIONS:** Renal/hepatic impairment, G6PD deficiency, premature neonates, infants younger than 2 mos. **Pregnancy Category B.**

INTERACTIONS

DRUG: Concurrent use may inactivate **collagenase, papain, sutilains. HERBAL:** None significant. **FOOD:** None known. **LAB VALUES:** None known.

AVAILABILITY (Rx)

TOPICAL CREAM (SILVADENE, SSD, SSD AF, THERMAZENE): 1% (10 mg/g).

ADMINISTRATION/HANDLING

TOPICAL

• Apply to cleansed, debrided burns using sterile glove. • Keep burn areas covered with silver sulfadiazine cream at all times; reapply to areas where removed by pt activity. • Dressings may be ordered on individual basis.

INDICATIONS/ROUTES/DOSAGE

USUAL TOPICAL DOSAGE

TOPICAL: ADULTS, ELDERLY, CHILDREN: Apply 1–2 times a day.

SIDE EFFECTS

Side effects characteristic of all sulfonamides may occur when systemically absorbed, (extensive burn areas [over 20% of body surface]): anorexia, nausea, vomiting, headache, diarrhea, dizziness, photosensitivity, arthralgia. **FREQUENT:** Burning, stinging sensation at treatment site. **OCCASIONAL:** Brown-gray skin discoloration, rash, itching. **RARE:** Increased sensitivity of skin to sunlight.

ADVERSE EFFECTS/ TOXIC REACTIONS

Hemolytic anemia, hypoglycemia, diuresis, peripheral neuropathy, Stevens-Johnson syndrome, agranulocytosis, disseminated lupus erythematosus, anaphylaxis, hepatitis, toxic nephrosis possible with significant systemic absorption. Fungal superinfections may occur. Interstitial nephritis occurs rarely.

S

NURSING CONSIDERATIONS

BASELINE ASSESSMENT

Determine initial CBC, serum renal/hepatic function test results.

INTERVENTION/EVALUATION

Monitor serum electrolytes, urinalysis, renal function, CBC if burns are extensive, therapy prolonged.

PATIENT/FAMILY TEACHING

• For external use only; may discolor skin.

simethicone

si-**meth**-i-kone

(Alka-Seltzer Gas Relief, Gas-X, Genasyme, Infant Mylicon, Mylanta Gas, Ovol ♣, Phazyme)

FIXED-COMBINATION(S)

Mylanta, Extra Strength Maalox, Aludrox: simethicone/magnesium and aluminum hydroxide (antacids): 20 mg/200 mg/200 mg; 40 mg/400 mg/400 mg.

CLASSIFICATION

CLINICAL: Antiflatulent.

ACTION

Changes surface tension of gas bubbles, allowing easier elimination of gas. **Therapeutic Effect:** Disperses, prevents formation of gas pockets in GI tract.

PHARMACOKINETICS

Does not appear to be absorbed from GI tract. Excreted unchanged in feces.

USES

Treatment of flatulence, gastric bloating, postop gas pain, when gas retention may be problem (i.e., peptic ulcer, spastic colon, air swallowing). **OFF-LABEL:** Adjunct to bowel radiography, gastroscopy.

PRECAUTIONS

CONTRAINDICATIONS: None known. **CAUTIONS:** None known.

LIFESPAN CONSIDERATIONS:

Pregnancy/Lactation: Unknown if drug crosses placenta or is distributed in breast milk. **Pregnancy Category C. Children/Elderly:** None known.

INTERACTIONS

DRUG: None significant. **HERBAL:** None significant. **FOOD:** None known. **LAB VALUES:** None known.

AVAILABILITY (OTC)

ORAL DROPS (INFANT MYLICON): 40 mg/0.6 ml. **SOFTGEL:** 125 mg (Alka-Seltzer Gas Relief, Gas-Z, Mylanta Gas), 180 mg (Phazyme). **TABLETS (CHEWABLE):** 80 mg (Gas-X, Genasyme, Mylanta Gas), 125 mg (Gas-X, Mylanta Gas).

ADMINISTRATION/HANDLING

PO

- Give after meals and at bedtime as needed.
- Chewable tablets are to be chewed thoroughly before swallowing.
- Shake suspension well before using.

INDICATIONS/ROUTES/DOSAGE

ANTIFLATULENT

PO: ADULTS, ELDERLY, CHILDREN 12 YRS AND OLDER: 40–360 mg after meals and at bedtime. **Maximum:** 500 mg/day. **CHILDREN 2–11 YRS:** 40 mg 4 times a day. **CHILDREN YOUNGER THAN 2 YRS:** 20 mg 4 times a day.

SIDE EFFECTS

None known.

ADVERSE EFFECTS/ TOXIC REACTIONS

None known.

NURSING CONSIDERATIONS

INTERVENTION/EVALUATION

Evaluate for therapeutic response: relief of flatulence, abdominal bloating.

PATIENT/FAMILY TEACHING

- Avoid carbonated beverages.

simvastatin

sim-vah-**stay**-tin

(Apo-Simvastatin ✤, Novo-Simvastatin ✤, Zocor)

Do not confuse Zocor with Cozaar.

FIXED-COMBINATION(S)

Vytorin: simvastatin/ezetimibe (a cholesterol absorption inhibitor): 10 mg/10 mg; 20 mg/10 mg; 40 mg/10 mg; 80 mg/10 mg.

CLASSIFICATION

PHARMACOTHERAPEUTIC: Hydroxymethylglutaryl-CoA (HMG-CoA) reductase inhibitor. **CLINICAL:** Antihyperlipidemic (see p. 57C).

ACTION

Interferes with cholesterol biosynthesis by inhibiting conversion of the enzyme HMG-CoA to mevalonate. **Therapeutic Effect:** Decreases serum LDL, cholesterol, VLDL, triglyceride levels; slight increase in serum HDL concentration.

PHARMACOKINETICS

Well absorbed from GI tract. Protein binding: 95%. Undergoes extensive first-pass metabolism. Hydrolyzed to active metabolite. Primarily eliminated in feces. Unknown if removed by hemodialysis.

Route	Onset	Peak	Duration
PO to reduce cholesterol	3 days	14 days	N/A

USES

Secondary prevention of cardiovascular events in pts with hypercholesterolemia and coronary heart disease (CHD) or at high risk for CHD. Hyperlipidemias to reduce elevations in total serum cholesterol. Treatment of homozygous

S

familial hypercholesterolemia. Treatment of heterozygous familial hypercholesterolemia in adolescents (10–17 yrs, females more than 1 yr postmenarche).

PRECAUTIONS

CONTRAINDICATIONS: Active hepatic disease or unexplained, persistent elevations of hepatic function test results, age younger than 18 yrs, pregnancy. **CAUTIONS:** History of hepatic disease, substantial alcohol consumption. Severe metabolic, endocrine, electrolyte disorders. Withholding or discontinuing simvastatin may be necessary when pt is at risk for renal failure secondary to rhabdomyolysis.

⌛ LIFESPAN CONSIDERATIONS:

Pregnancy/Lactation: Contraindicated in pregnancy (suppression of cholesterol biosynthesis may cause fetal toxicity), lactation. Risk of serious adverse reactions in breast-feeding infants. **Pregnancy Category X.** **Children:** Safety and efficacy not established. **Elderly:** No age-related precautions noted.

INTERACTIONS

DRUG: **Cyclosporine, erythromycin, gemfibrozil, immunosuppressants, niacin** increase risk of acute renal failure, rhabdomyolysis. May increase concentration, toxicity of **digoxin. HIV protease inhibitors** may increase risk of rhabdomyolysis, acute renal failure. **Verapamil** may increase risk of myopathy. **HERBAL:** **St. John's wort** may decrease concentration. **FOOD:** **Grapefruit, grapefruit juice** may increase concentration, toxicity. **LAB VALUES:** May increase serum creatine kinase (CK), transaminase.

AVAILABILITY (Rx)

TABLETS: 5 mg, 10 mg, 20 mg, 40 mg, 80 mg.

ADMINISTRATION/HANDLING

PO

- Give without regard to meals.
- Administer in evening.

INDICATIONS/ROUTES/DOSAGE

PREVENTION OF CARDIOVASCULAR EVENTS, HYPERLIPIDEMIAS

PO: ADULTS, ELDERLY: 20–40 mg once daily. Range: 5–80 mg/day.

HOMOZYGOUS FAMILIAL HYPERCHOLESTEROLEMIA

PO: ADULTS, ELDERLY: 40 mg once daily in evening or 80 mg/day in divided doses.

HETEROZYGOUS FAMILIAL HYPERCHOLESTEROLEMIA

PO: CHILDREN 10–17 YRS: 10 mg once daily in evening. Range: 10–40 mg/day.

SIDE EFFECTS

Generally well tolerated. Side effects are usually mild and transient. **OCCASIONAL (3%–2%):** Headache, abdominal pain/cramps, constipation, upper respiratory tract infection. **RARE (less than 2%):** Diarrhea, flatulence, asthenia (loss of strength, energy), nausea/vomiting.

ADVERSE EFFECTS/ TOXIC REACTIONS

Potential for lens opacities. Hypersensitivity reaction, hepatitis occur rarely. Myopathy (muscle pain, tenderness, weakness with elevated CK, sometimes taking the form of rhabdomyolysis) has occurred.

NURSING CONSIDERATIONS

BASELINE ASSESSMENT

Question for possibility of pregnancy before initiating therapy (Pregnancy Category X). Question for history of hypersensitivity to simvastatin. Assess baseline lab results: serum cholesterol, triglycerides, hepatic function tests.

S

INTERVENTION/EVALUATION

Monitor serum cholesterol, triglyceride lab results for therapeutic response. Monitor hepatic function tests. Monitor daily pattern of bowel activity/stool consistency. Assess for headache.

PATIENT/FAMILY TEACHING

• Use appropriate contraceptive measures (Pregnancy Category X). • Periodic lab tests are essential part of therapy.

Sinemet, *see carbidopa and levodopa*

Singulair, *see montelukast*

sirolimus

sigh-row-**lie**-mus
(Rapamune)

CLASSIFICATION

CLINICAL: Immunosuppressant (see p. 115C).

ACTION

Inhibits T-lymphocyte proliferation induced by stimulation of cell surface receptors, mitogens, alloantigens, lymphokines. Prevents activation of enzyme target of rapamycin (TOR), a key regulatory kinase in cell cycle progression. **Therapeutic Effect:** Inhibits proliferation of T and B cells (essential components of immune response), prevents organ transplant rejection.

PHARMACOKINETICS

Rapidly absorbed from GI tract. Protein binding: 92%. Extensively metabolized in liver. Primarily eliminated in feces; minimal excretion in urine. **Half-life:** 57–63 hrs.

USES

Prophylaxis of organ rejection in pts after renal transplant in combination with cyclosporine and corticosteroids. **OFF-LABEL:** Immunosuppression of other organ transplants.

PRECAUTIONS

CONTRAINDICATIONS: Hypersensitivity to sirolimus, active malignancy. **CAUTIONS:** Chickenpox, herpes zoster, hepatic impairment, infection.

LIFESPAN CONSIDERATIONS: **Pregnancy/Lactation:** Unknown if drug crosses placenta or is distributed in breast milk. **Pregnancy Category C.** **Children:** Safety and efficacy not established in children younger than 13 yrs. **Elderly:** No age-related precautions noted.

INTERACTIONS

DRUG: **Carbamazepine, phenobarbital, phenytoin, rifabutin, rifampin, rifapentine** may decrease concentration, effect. **Itraconazole, ketoconazole, voriconazole, diltiazem, verapamil, clarithromycin, erythromycin, telithromycin** may increase concentration, toxicity. May increase risk of infection, lymphomas with **cyclosporine.** May increase mortality, graft loss, hepatic artery thrombosis with **tacrolimus** in liver transplant pts. **HERBAL:** **St. John's wort** may decrease concentration. **Cat's claw, echinacea** possess immunostimulant properties. **FOOD:** **Grapefruit, grapefruit juice** may decrease metabolism. **LAB VALUES:** May decrease Hgb, Hct, platelet count. May increase serum cholesterol, creatinine, triglycerides.

AVAILABILITY (Rx)

ORAL SOLUTION: 1 mg/ml. **TABLETS:** 1 mg, 2 mg.

S

INDICATIONS/ROUTES/DOSAGE

PREVENTION OF ORGAN TRANSPLANT REJECTION

PO: ADULTS: Loading dose: 6 mg. Maintenance: 2 mg/day. **CHILDREN 13 YRS AND OLDER WEIGHING LESS THAN 40 KG:** Loading dose: 3 mg/m^2. Maintenance: 1 mg/m^2/day.

SIDE EFFECTS

OCCASIONAL: Hypercholesterolemia, hyperlipidemia, hypertension, rash. **High doses (5 mg/day):** Anemia, arthralgia, diarrhea, hypokalemia, thrombocytopenia. **RARE:** Peripheral edema, hypertension.

ADVERSE EFFECTS/ TOXIC REACTIONS

Hepatotoxicity occurs rarely.

NURSING CONSIDERATIONS

BASELINE ASSESSMENT

Obtain baseline serum hepatic profile. Assess for pregnancy, lactation. Question for medication usage (esp. cyclosporine, diltiazem, ketoconazole, rifampin). Determine if pt has chickenpox, herpes zoster, malignancy, infection.

INTERVENTION/EVALUATION

Monitor serum hepatic function periodically.

PATIENT/FAMILY TEACHING

• Avoid those with colds, other infections. • Avoid grapefruit juice, grapefruit. • Strict monitoring is essential in identifying, preventing symptoms of organ rejection.

sitagliptin

sit-ah-**glip**-tin
(Januvia)

CLASSIFICATION

PHARMACOTHERAPEUTIC: DPP-4 inhibitors (gliptins). **CLINICAL:** Antidiabetic.

ACTION

Slows inactivation of incretin hormones (involved in regulation of glucose homeostasis). **Therapeutic Effect:** Increases synthesis, release of insulin from pancreatic cells, lowers glucagon secretion leading to reduced glucose production, increase in insulin.

PHARMACOKINETICS

	Onset	Peak	Duration
PO	N/A	1–4 hrs	24 hrs

Rapidly absorbed following PO administration. Protein binding: 38%. Eliminated mainly in urine, with lesser amount excreted in feces. **Half-life:** 12 hrs.

USES

Adjunctive treatment to diet, exercise to improve glycemic control in pts with type 2 diabetes mellitus as monotherapy or in combination with metformin or thiazolidinedione antidiabetic agent when a single agent alone, with diet and exercise, does not provide glycemic control.

PRECAUTIONS

CONTRAINDICATIONS: None significant. **CAUTIONS:** Concurrent use of other glucose-lowering agents may increase risk of hypoglycemia.

LIFESPAN CONSIDERATIONS: Pregnancy/Lactation: Unknown if distributed in breast milk. **Pregnancy Category B. Children:** Safety and efficacy not established. **Elderly:** No age-related precautions noted.

INTERACTIONS

DRUG: Slightly increases **digoxin** concentration. **HERBAL:** None significant.

FOOD: None known. **LAB VALUES:** May slightly increase WBCs, particularly neutrophil count. May increase serum creatinine.

AVAILABILITY (Rx)

TABLETS (FILM-COATED): 25 mg, 50 mg, 100 mg.

ADMINISTRATION/HANDLING

PO

• May give without regard to food. • Do not crush, break, chew film-coated tablets.

INDICATIONS/ROUTES/DOSAGE

TYPE 2 DIABETES

PO: ADULTS OVER 18 YRS, ELDERLY: 100 mg once daily.

MODERATE RENAL IMPAIRMENT

CREATININE CLEARANCE EQUAL TO OR GREATER THAN 30 ML/MIN TO LESS THAN 50 ML/MIN: 50 mg once daily.

SEVERE RENAL IMPAIRMENT

CREATININE CLEARANCE LESS THAN 30 ML/MIN: 25 mg once daily.

SIDE EFFECTS

OCCASIONAL (5% and greater): Headache, nasopharyngitis. **RARE (3%–1%):** Diarrhea, abdominal pain, nausea.

ADVERSE EFFECTS/ TOXIC REACTIONS

Upper respiratory tract infection occurs in approximately 5% of pts.

NURSING CONSIDERATIONS

BASELINE ASSESSMENT

Check serum glucose concentration before administration. Discuss lifestyle to determine extent of learning, emotional needs. Assure follow-up instruction if pt, family does not thoroughly understand diabetes management, glucose-testing technique.

INTERVENTION/EVALUATION

Assess for hypoglycemia (diaphoresis, tremor, dizziness, anxiety, headache, tachycardia, perioral numbness, hunger, diplopia, difficulty concentrating), hyperglycemia (polyuria, polyphagia, polydipsia, nausea, vomiting, dim vision, fatigue, deep, rapid breathing). Be alert to conditions that alter glucose requirements (fever, increased activity, stress, surgical procedures).

PATIENT/FAMILY TEACHING

Diabetes mellitus requires lifelong control. Prescribed diet, exercise are principal part of treatment; do not skip, delay meals. Continue to adhere to dietary instructions, regular exercise program, regular testing of serum glucose. When taking combination drug therapy or when glucose demands are altered (fever, infection, trauma, stress, heavy physical activity), have source of glucose available to treat symptoms of hypoglycemia.

sodium bicarbonate

so-dee-um bye-**car**-bon-ate

(Neut)

CLASSIFICATION

PHARMACOTHERAPEUTIC: Alkalinizing agent. **CLINICAL:** Antacid.

S

ACTION

Dissociates to provide bicarbonate ion. **Therapeutic Effect:** Neutralizes hydrogen ion concentration, raises blood, urinary pH.

PHARMACOKINETICS

Route	Onset	Peak	Duration
PO	15 min	N/A	1–3 hrs
IV	Immediate	N/A	8–10 min

Following administration, sodium bicarbonate dissociates to sodium and bicarbonate ions. With increased hydrogen ion concentrations, bicarbonate ions combine with hydrogen ions to form carbonic acid, which then dissociates to CO_2, which is excreted by the lungs. Plasma concentration regulated by kidney (ability to form, excrete bicarbonate).

USES

Management of metabolic acidosis, antacid, alkalinization of urine, stabilizes acid-base balance, cardiac arrest, life-threatening hyperkalemia.

PRECAUTIONS

CONTRAINDICATIONS: Excessive chloride loss due to diarrhea, diuretics, GI suctioning, vomiting; hypocalcemia; metabolic, respiratory alkalosis. **CAUTIONS:** CHF, edematous states, renal insufficiency, pts on corticosteroid therapy.

LIFESPAN CONSIDERATIONS:

Pregnancy/Lactation: May produce hypernatremia, increase tendon reflexes in neonate or fetus whose mother is administered chronically high doses. May be distributed in breast milk. **Pregnancy Category C. Children:** No age-related precautions noted. Do not use as antacid in those younger than 6 yrs. **Elderly:** Age-related renal impairment may require dosage adjustment.

INTERACTIONS

DRUG: May increase concentration, toxicity of **pseudoephedrine, quinidine, quinine.** May decrease effect of **lithium, salicylates. HERBAL:** None significant. **FOOD: Milk, other dairy products** may result in milk-alkali syndrome. **LAB VALUES:** May increase serum, urinary pH.

AVAILABILITY (OTC)

INJECTION SOLUTION: 4%, 0.5 mEq/ml (4.2%), 0.6 mEq/ml (5%), 0.9 mEq/ml (7.5%), 1 mEq/ml (8.4%). **TABLETS:** 325 mg, 650 mg.

ADMINISTRATION/HANDLING

IV

◀ **ALERT** ▶ For direct IV administration in neonates or infants, use 0.5 mEq/ml concentration.

Reconstitution • May give undiluted.

Rate of administration • For IV push, give up to 1 mEq/kg over 1–3 min for cardiac arrest. • For IV infusion, do not exceed rate of infusion of 50 mEq/hr. • For children younger than 2 yrs, premature infants, neonates, administer by slow infusion, up to 8 mEq/min.

Storage • Store at room temperature.

PO

• Give 1–3 hrs after meals.

IV INCOMPATIBILITIES

Amiodarone (Cordarone), ascorbic acid, diltiazem (Cardizem), dobutamine (Dobutrex), dopamine (Intropin), hydromorphone (Dilaudid), magnesium sulfate, midazolam (Versed), norepinephrine (Levophed), total parenteral nutrition (TPN).

IV COMPATIBILITIES

Aminophylline, calcium chloride, furosemide (Lasix), heparin, insulin, lidocaine, lipids, mannitol, milrinone (Primacor), morphine, phenylephrine (Neo-Synephrine), potassium chloride, propofol (Diprivan), vancomycin (Vancocin).

INDICATIONS/ROUTES/DOSAGE

◀ **ALERT** ▶ May give by IV push, IV infusion, or orally. Dose individualized based on severity of acidosis, laboratory values, pt age, weight, clinical conditions. Do not fully correct bicarbonate deficit

S

during the first 24 hrs (may cause metabolic alkalosis).

CARDIAC ARREST

IV: ADULTS, ELDERLY: Initially, 1 mEq/kg (as 7.5%–8.4% solution). May repeat with 0.5 mEq/kg q10min during continued cardiopulmonary arrest. Use in postresuscitation phase is based on arterial blood pH, partial pressure of carbon dioxide in arterial blood ($PaCO_2$), base deficit calculation. **CHILDREN, INFANTS:** Initially, 0.5–1 mEq/kg.

METABOLIC ACIDOSIS (MILD TO MODERATE)

IV: ADULTS, ELDERLY, CHILDREN: 2–5 mEq/kg over 4–8 hrs. May repeat based on laboratory values.

METABOLIC ACIDOSIS (ASSOCIATED WITH CHRONIC RENAL FAILURE)

PO: ADULTS, ELDERLY: Initially, 20–36 mEq/day in divided doses. **CHILDREN:** 1–3 mEq/kg/day.

RENAL TUBULAR ACIDOSIS (DISTAL)

PO: ADULTS, ELDERLY: 0.5–2 mEq/kg/day in 4–6 divided doses. **CHILDREN:** 2–3 mEq/kg/day in divided doses.

RENAL TUBULAR ACIDOSIS (PROXIMAL)

PO: ADULTS, ELDERLY, CHILDREN: 5–10 mEq/kg/day in divided doses.

URINE ALKALINIZATION

PO: ADULTS, ELDERLY: Initially, 4 g, then 1–2 g q4h. **Maximum:** 16 g/day. **CHILDREN:** 84–840 mg/kg/day in divided doses.

ANTACID

PO: ADULTS, ELDERLY: 300 mg–2 g 1–4 times a day.

HYPERKALEMIA

IV: ADULTS, ELDERLY: 1 mEq/kg over 5 min.

SIDE EFFECTS

FREQUENT: Abdominal distention, flatulence, belching.

ADVERSE EFFECTS/ TOXIC REACTIONS

Excessive, chronic use may produce metabolic alkalosis (irritability, twitching, paresthesias, cyanosis, slow or shallow respirations, headache, thirst, nausea). Fluid overload results in headache, weakness, blurred vision, behavioral changes, incoordination, muscle twitching, elevated B/P, bradycardia, tachypnea, wheezing, coughing, distended neck veins. Extravasation may occur at the IV site, resulting in tissue necrosis, ulceration.

NURSING CONSIDERATIONS

BASELINE ASSESSMENT

Do not give other PO medication within 1–2 hrs of antacid administration.

INTERVENTION/EVALUATION

Monitor serum, urinary pH, CO_2 level, serum electrolytes, plasma bicarbonate levels. Watch for signs of metabolic alkalosis, fluid overload. Assess for clinical improvement of metabolic acidosis (relief from hyperventilation, weakness, disorientation). Monitor daily pattern of bowel activity/stool consistency. Monitor serum phosphate, calcium, uric acid levels. Assess for relief of gastric distress.

sodium chloride

so-dee-um **klor**-eyed

(Muro 128, Nasal Mist, Nasal Moist, Ocean, SalineX, SeaMist, Slo-Salt)

CLASSIFICATION

CLINICAL: Electrolyte, ophthalmic adjunct, bronchodilator.

ACTION

Sodium is a major cation of extracellular fluid. **Therapeutic Effect:** Controls water distribution, fluid and electrolyte balance, osmotic pressure of body fluids; maintains acid-base balance.

S

PHARMACOKINETICS

Well absorbed from GI tract. Widely distributed. Primarily excreted in urine.

USES

Parenteral: Source of hydration; prevention/treatment of sodium, chloride deficiencies (hypertonic for severe deficiencies). Prevention of muscle cramps, heat prostration occurring with excessive perspiration. **Nasal:** Restores moisture, relieves dry, inflamed nasal membranes. **Ophthalmic:** Therapy in reduction of corneal edema, diagnostic aid in ophthalmoscopic exam.

PRECAUTIONS

CONTRAINDICATIONS: Fluid retention, hypernatremia. **CAUTIONS:** CHF, renal impairment, cirrhosis, hypertension. Do not use sodium chloride preserved with benzyl alcohol in neonates.

LIFESPAN CONSIDERATIONS:

Pregnancy Category C. **Children/Elderly:** No age-related precautions noted.

INTERACTIONS

DRUG: May decrease effect of **lithium.** **HERBAL:** None significant. **FOOD:** None known. **LAB VALUES:** None known.

AVAILABILITY

INJECTION SOLUTION: 0.45%, 0.9%, 3%. **INJECTION (CONCENTRATE):** 23.4% (4 mEq/ml). **IRRIGATION:** 0.45%, 0.9%. **NASAL GEL (NASAL MOIST):** 0.65%. **NASAL SOLUTION (OTC):** 0.4% (SalineX), 0.65% (Nasal Moist, SeaMist). **OPHTHALMIC SOLUTION (OTC [MURO 128]):** 5%. **OPHTHALMIC OINTMENT (OTC [MURO 128]):** 5%.

TABLETS (OTC): 1 g.

ADMINISTRATION/HANDLING

IV

• Hypertonic solutions (3% or 5%) are administered via large vein; avoid infiltration; do not exceed 100 ml/hr. • Vials containing 2.5–4 mEq/ml (concentrated NaCl) must be diluted with D_5W or $D_{10}W$ before administration.

PO

• Do not crush/break enteric-coated or extended-release tablets. • Administer with full glass of water.

NASAL

• Instruct pt to begin inhaling slowly just before releasing medication into nose. • Inhale slowly, then release air gently through mouth. • Continue technique for 20–30 sec.

OPHTHALMIC

• Place finger on lower eyelid, pull out until pocket is formed between eye and lower lid. • Hold dropper above pocket, place prescribed number of drops (or apply thin strip of ointment) in pocket. • Instruct pt to close eyes gently so that medication is not squeezed out of sac. • When lower lid is released, have pt keep eye open without blinking for at least 30 sec for solution; for ointment have pt close eye, roll eyeball around to distribute medication. • When using drops, apply gentle finger pressure to lacrimal sac (bridge of nose, inside corner of the eye) for 1–2 min after administration of solution (reduces systemic absorption).

INDICATIONS/ROUTES/DOSAGE

◄ ALERT ► Dosage based on age, weight, clinical condition; fluid, electrolyte, acid-base balance status.

USUAL PARENTERAL DOSAGE

IV: ADULTS, ELDERLY: 1–2 L/day 0.9% or 0.45% or 100 ml 3% or 5% over 1 hr; assess serum electrolyte levels before giving additional fluid.

USUAL ORAL DOSAGE

PO: ADULTS, ELDERLY: 1–2 g 3 times a day.

USUAL NASAL DOSAGE

INTRANASAL: ADULTS, ELDERLY: Use as needed.

USUAL OPHTHALMIC DOSAGE

OPHTHALMIC SOLUTION: ADULTS, ELDERLY: Apply 1–2 drops q3–4h.
OPHTHALMIC OINTMENT: ADULTS, ELDERLY: Apply once a day or as directed.

SIDE EFFECTS

FREQUENT: Facial flushing. **OCCASIONAL:** Fever; irritation, phlebitis, extravasation at injection site. **Ophthalmic:** Temporary burning, irritation.

ADVERSE EFFECTS/ TOXIC REACTIONS

Too-rapid administration may produce peripheral edema, CHF, pulmonary edema. Excessive dosage may produce hypokalemia, hypervolemia, hypernatremia.

NURSING CONSIDERATIONS

BASELINE ASSESSMENT

Assess fluid balance (I&O, daily weight, lung sounds, edema).

INTERVENTION/EVALUATION

Monitor fluid balance (I&O, daily weight, lung sounds, edema), IV site for extravasation. Monitor serum electrolytes, acid-base balance, B/P. Hypernatremia associated with edema, weight gain, elevated B/P; hyponatremia associated with muscle cramps, nausea, vomiting, dry mucous membranes.

PATIENT/FAMILY TEACHING

• Temporary burning, irritation may occur upon instillation of eye medication. • Discontinue eye medication and contact physician if severe pain, headache, rapid change in vision (peripheral, direct), sudden appearance of floating spots, acute redness of eyes, pain on exposure to light, double vision occurs.

sodium ferric gluconate complex

so-**dee**-um **fair**-ick **glue**-koe-nate **calm**-plex
(Ferrlecit)

CLASSIFICATION

PHARMACOTHERAPEUTIC: Trace element. **CLINICAL:** Hematinic.

ACTION

Repletes total iron content in body. Replaces iron found in Hgb, myoglobin, specific enzymes; allows oxygen transport via Hgb. **Therapeutic Effect:** Prevents, corrects iron deficiency.

PHARMACOKINETICS

Half-life: 1 hr.

USES

Treatment of iron deficiency anemia in pts undergoing chronic hemodialysis who are receiving supplemental erythropoietin therapy.

PRECAUTIONS

CONTRAINDICATIONS: All anemias not associated with iron deficiency, hypersensitivity to iron products. **CAUTIONS:** Pts with iron overload, significant allergies, asthma, hepatic impairment, rheumatoid arthritis.

S

LIFESPAN CONSIDERATIONS:

Pregnancy/Lactation: Unknown if distributed in breast milk. **Pregnancy Category B. Children:** Safety and efficacy not established. **Elderly:** No age-related precautions noted; lower initial dosages recommended.

INTERACTIONS

DRUG: Drugs containing **aluminum, calcium, magnesium** may decrease iron effectiveness. May decrease effectiveness of **ibandronate, levodopa, quinolone antibiotics.** **HERBAL:** None significant. **FOOD:** None known. **LAB VALUES:** None known.

AVAILABILITY (Rx)

INJECTION SOLUTION: 12.5 mg/ml elemental iron.

ADMINISTRATION/HANDLING

IV

Reconstitution • Must be diluted. • Test dose: dilute 25 mg (2 ml) with 50 ml 0.9% NaCl. • Recommended dose: dilute 125 mg (10 ml) with 100 ml 0.9% NaCl.

Rate of administration • Infuse both test dose, recommended dose over 1 hr.

Storage • Store at room temperature. • Use immediately after dilution.

IV INCOMPATIBILITIES

Do not mix with any other medications.

INDICATIONS/ROUTES/DOSAGE

IRON DEFICIENCY ANEMIA

IV INFUSION: ADULTS, ELDERLY: 125 mg in 100 ml 0.9% NaCl infused over 1 hr. Minimum cumulative dose 1 g elemental iron given over 8 sessions at sequential dialysis treatments. May be given during dialysis session. **CHILDREN 6 YRS AND OLDER:** 1.5 mg/kg diluted in 25 ml 0.9% NaCl administered over 60 min at sequential dialysis sessions. **Maximum:** 125 mg/dose.

SIDE EFFECTS

FREQUENT (greater than 3%): Flushing, hypotension, hypersensitivity reaction. **OCCASIONAL (3%–1%):** Injection site reaction, headache, abdominal pain, chills, flu-like syndrome, dizziness, leg cramps, dyspnea, nausea, vomiting, diarrhea, myalgia, pruritus, edema.

ADVERSE EFFECTS/ TOXIC REACTIONS

Potentially fatal hypersensitivity reaction occurs rarely, characterized by cardiovascular collapse, cardiac arrest, dyspnea, bronchospasm, angioedema, urticaria. Rapid administration may cause hypotension associated with flushing, light-headedness, fatigue, weakness, severe pain in chest, back, groin.

NURSING CONSIDERATIONS

BASELINE ASSESSMENT

Do not give concurrently with oral iron form (excessive iron may produce excessive iron storage [hemosiderosis]). Be alert to pts with rheumatoid arthritis, iron deficiency anemia (acute exacerbation of joint pain, swelling may occur).

INTERVENTION/EVALUATION

Monitor vital signs, lab tests, esp. CBC, serum iron concentrations (may not be meaningful for 3 wks after administration).

PATIENT/FAMILY TEACHING

• Stools frequently become black with iron therapy and is harmless. Report to physician any red streaking, sticky consistency of stool, abdominal pain/cramping.

sodium oxybate (gamma hydroxybutyrate)

sew-dee-um **ox**-ih-bate
(GHB, Xyrem)

CLASSIFICATION

PHARMACOTHERAPEUTIC: Neurotransmitter. **CLINICAL:** Antinarcolepsy.

S

ACTION

Mechanism of action unknown.

USES

Treatment of adult with cataplexy associated with narcolepsy. Treatment of excessive daytime sleepiness in pts with narcolepsy.

PRECAUTIONS

CONTRAINDICATIONS: Metabolic/respiratory alkalosis, current treatment with sedative-hypnotics, succinic semialdehyde dehydrogenase deficiency. **CAUTIONS:** Hepatic insufficiency, incontinence (increases risk), history of depression (increases risk), hypertension, pregnancy, concurrent ingestion of alcohol or other CNS depressants.

LIFESPAN CONSIDERATIONS:

Pregnancy/Lactation: Unknown if drug crosses placenta or is distributed in breast milk. **Pregnancy Category C.** **Children:** Safety and efficacy not established in children younger than 16 yrs. **Elderly:** Increased risk of motor/cognitive function impairment.

INTERACTIONS

DRUG: **Alcohol** may have additive CNS, respiratory depressant effects. **Barbiturates, benzodiazepines, centrally-acting muscle relaxants, opioid analgesics** may have additive CNS, respiratory depressant effects. **HERBAL:** **Gotu kola, kava kava, St. John's wort, valerian** may increase CNS depression. **FOOD:** None known. **LAB VALUES:** May increase serum sodium, glucose.

AVAILABILITY (Rx)

ORAL SOLUTION: 500 mg/ml.

ADMINISTRATION/HANDLING

PO

• Store at room temperature. • Give first of two daily dosages at bedtime while pt is in bed and the second dosage 2.5–4 hrs later.

INDICATIONS/ROUTES/DOSAGE

NARCOLEPSY

PO: ADULTS, ELDERLY: 4.5 g/day in 2 equal doses of 2.25 g, the first taken at bedtime while in bed and the second 2.5–4 hrs later. **Maximum:** 9 g/day in 2 weekly increments of 1.5 g/day.

SIDE EFFECTS

FREQUENT (58%): Mild bradycardia. **OCCASIONAL:** Headache, vertigo, dizziness, restless legs, abdominal pain, muscle weakness. **RARE:** Dream-like state of confusion.

ADVERSE EFFECTS/ TOXIC REACTIONS

Metabolic alkalosis (irritability, muscle twitching, paresthesias, cyanosis, slow/shallow respiration, headache, thirst, nausea) has been noted, particularly in pts with head trauma before treatment. Concurrent use of alcohol may result in respiratory depression, apnea, comatose state. Severe dependence, craving produces high potential for abuse.

NURSING CONSIDERATIONS

INTERVENTION/EVALUATION

Watch for signs of metabolic alkalosis (irritability, muscle twitching, paresthesias, cyanosis, slow/shallow respiration, headache, thirst, nausea). Monitor serum glucose, sodium levels.

PATIENT/FAMILY TEACHING

• Avoid alcohol due to high potential for respiratory depression, comatose state. • Severe dependence may occur.

S

sodium polystyrene sulfonate

so-dee-um pol-ee-**stye**-reen
(Kayexelate, Kionex, PMS-Sodium Polystyrene Sulfonate ♣, SPS)

CLASSIFICATION

PHARMACOTHERAPEUTIC: Cation exchange resin. **CLINICAL:** Antihyperkalemic.

ACTION

Releases sodium ions in exchange primarily for potassium ions. **Therapeutic Effect:** Moves potassium from blood into intestine to be expelled from the body.

USES

Treatment of hyperkalemia.

PRECAUTIONS

CONTRAINDICATIONS: Hypokalemia, hypernatremia, intestinal obstruction/perforation. **CAUTIONS:** Severe CHF, hypertension, edema.

LIFESPAN CONSIDERATIONS:

Pregnancy/Lactation: Unknown if drug crosses placenta or is distributed in breast milk. **Pregnancy Category C. Children:** No age-related precautions noted. **Elderly:** Increased risk for fecal impaction.

INTERACTIONS

DRUG: **Cation-donating antacids, laxatives (e.g., magnesium hydroxide)** may decrease effect; may cause systemic alkalosis in pts with renal impairment. **HERBAL:** None significant. **FOOD:** None known. **LAB VALUES:** May decrease serum calcium, magnesium.

AVAILABILITY (Rx)

POWDER FOR SUSPENSION (KAYEXALATE, KIONEX): 454 g. **RECTAL ENEMA:** 15 g/60 ml. **SUSPENSION (SPS):** 15 g/60 ml.

ADMINISTRATION/HANDLING

PO

• Give with 20–100 ml sorbitol (facilitates passage of resin through intestinal tract, prevents constipation, aids in potassium removal, increases palatability). • Do not mix with foods, liquids containing potassium.

RECTAL

• After initial cleansing enema, insert large rubber tube into rectum well into sigmoid colon, tape in place. • Introduce suspension (with 100 ml sorbitol) via gravity. • Flush with 50–100 ml fluid and clamp. • Retain for several hrs if possible. • Irrigate colon with non–sodium-containing solution to remove resin.

INDICATIONS/ROUTES/DOSAGE

HYPERKALEMIA

PO: ADULTS, ELDERLY: 60 ml (15 g) 1–4 times a day. **CHILDREN:** 1 g/kg/dose q6h. **RECTAL: ADULTS, ELDERLY:** 30–50 g as needed q6h. **CHILDREN:** 1 g/kg/dose q2–6h.

SIDE EFFECTS

FREQUENT: High dosage: Anorexia, nausea, vomiting, constipation. **High dosage in elderly:** Fecal impaction (severe stomach pain with nausea/vomiting). **OCCASIONAL:** Diarrhea, sodium retention (decreased urination, peripheral edema, increased weight).

ADVERSE EFFECTS/ TOXIC REACTIONS

Potassium deficiency may occur. Early signs of hypokalemia include confusion, delayed thought processes, extreme weakness, irritability, EKG changes (often associated with prolonged QT interval; widening, flattening, or inversion of T wave; prominent U waves). Hypocalcemia, manifested by abdominal/muscle cramps, occurs occasionally. Arrhythmias, severe muscle weakness may be noted.

NURSING CONSIDERATIONS

BASELINE ASSESSMENT

Does not rapidly correct severe hyperkalemia (may take hrs to days). Consider other measures in medical emergency (IV calcium, IV sodium bicarbonate/glucose/insulin, dialysis).

INTERVENTION/EVALUATION

Monitor serum potassium levels frequently. Assess pt's clinical condition, EKG (valuable in determining when treatment should be discontinued). In addition to checking serum potassium, monitor serum magnesium, calcium levels. Monitor daily pattern of bowel activity/stool consistency (fecal impaction may occur in pts on high dosages, particularly in elderly).

solifenacin

sol-ih-**fen**-ah-sin
(VESIcare)

CLASSIFICATION

PHARMACOTHERAPEUTIC: Muscarinic receptor antagonist. **CLINICAL:** Urinary antispasmodic.

ACTION

Acts as direct antagonist at muscarinic acetylcholine receptors in cholinergically innervated organs. Reduces tonus (elastic tension) of smooth muscle in bladder, slows parasympathetic contractions. **Therapeutic Effect:** Decreases urinary bladder contractions, increases residual urine volume, decreases detrusor muscle pressure.

PHARMACOKINETICS

Well absorbed following PO administration. Protein binding: 98%. Metabolized in liver. Excreted in feces, urine. **Half-life:** 40–68 hrs.

USES

Treatment of overactive bladder with symptoms of urinary incontinence, urgency, frequency.

PRECAUTIONS

CONTRAINDICATIONS: Breast-feeding, GI obstruction, uncontrolled angle-closure glaucoma, urinary retention. **CAUTIONS:** Bladder outflow obstruction, GI obstructive disorders, decreased GI motility, controlled narrow-angle glaucoma, renal/hepatic impairment, congenital or acquired QT prolongation, pregnancy.

LIFESPAN CONSIDERATIONS:

Pregnancy/Lactation: Unknown if drug crosses placenta or is distributed is breast milk. **Pregnancy Category C.** **Children:** Safety and efficacy not established. **Elderly:** No age-related precautions noted.

INTERACTIONS

DRUG: **Aminoglutethimide, carbamazepine, nafcillin, nevirapine, phenobarbital, phenytoin** may decrease concentration, effects. **Azole antifungals, ciprofloxacin, clarithromycin, diclofenac, doxycycline, erythromycin, imatinib, isoniazid, nefazodone, nicardipine, propofol, protease inhibitors, quinidine, verapamil** may increase concentration, effects. **Ketoconazole** may increase concentration. **HERBAL:** **St. John's wort** may decrease concentration, effects. **FOOD:** **Grapefruit, grapefruit juice** may increase effects. **LAB VALUES:** None known.

AVAILABILITY (Rx)

TABLETS: 5 mg, 10 mg.

ADMINISTRATION/HANDLING

PO

- Give without regard to food. Swallow tablets whole.

INDICATIONS/ROUTES/DOSAGE

OVERACTIVE BLADDER

PO: ADULTS, ELDERLY: 5 mg/day; if tolerated, may increase to 10 mg/day.

DOSAGE IN RENAL/HEPATIC IMPAIRMENT

For pts with severe renal impairment or moderate hepatic impairment, maximum dosage is 5 mg/day.

SIDE EFFECTS

FREQUENT (11%–5%): Dry mouth, constipation, blurred vision. **OCCASIONAL (5%–3%):** UTI, dyspepsia (heartburn, indigestion, epigastric pain), nausea. **RARE (2%–1%):** Dizziness, dry eyes, fatigue, depression, edema, hypertension, epigastric pain, vomiting, urinary retention.

ADVERSE EFFECTS/ TOXIC REACTIONS

Angioneurotic edema, GI obstruction occur rarely. Overdose can result in severe anticholinergic effects.

S

NURSING CONSIDERATIONS

BASELINE ASSESSMENT

Assess symptoms of overactive bladder before beginning the drug.

INTERVENTION/EVALUATION

Monitor I&O. Assess for decrease in symptoms.

PATIENT/FAMILY TEACHING

- Avoid tasks requiring mental alertness, motor control until response to drug is known. • Inform pt of potential anticholinergic side effects (constipation, urinary retention, blurred vision, heat prostration in hot environment).

Solu-Medrol, *see methylprednisolone*

somatrem

soe-ma-trem

(Protopin)

somatropin

soe-mah-**troe**-pin

(Genotropin, Genotropin Miniquick, Humatrope, Norditropin, Norditropin Cartridge, Nutropin, Nutropin AQ, Nutropin Depot, Saizen, Serostim, Zorbitive)

Do not confuse Protopin with Proloprim, Protamine, or Protopam or somatropin with sumatriptan.

◆CLASSIFICATION

PHARMACOTHERAPEUTIC: Polypeptide hormone. **CLINICAL:** Growth hormone.

ACTION

Stimulates cartilaginous growth areas of long bones, increases number, size of skeletal muscle cells, influences size of organs, increases RBC mass by stimulating erythropoietin. Influences metabolism of carbohydrates (decreases insulin sensitivity), fats (mobilizes fatty acids), minerals (retains phosphorus, sodium, potassium by promotion of cell growth), proteins (increases protein synthesis). **Therapeutic Effect:** Stimulates growth.

PHARMACOKINETICS

Well absorbed after subcutaneous, IM administration. Localized primarily in kidneys, liver. **Half-life:** IV, 20–30 min; subcutaneous, IM, 3–5 hrs.

USES

Somatrem, somatropin: Long-term treatment of growth failure in children caused by pituitary growth hormone (GH) deficiency. **Somatropin:** Treatment of growth failure in adults caused by GH deficiency, treatment of growth failure in children caused by chronic renal insufficiency, long-term treatment of short stature associated with Turner's syndrome, treatment of AIDS-related cachexia/weight loss, treatment of short bowel syndrome.

PRECAUTIONS

CONTRAINDICATIONS: Active neoplasia (newly diagnosed or recurrent), critical illness, hypersensitivity to growth hormone. **CAUTIONS:** Diabetes mellitus, untreated hypothyroidism, malignancy.

⌛ LIFESPAN CONSIDERATIONS:

Pregnancy/Lactation: Unknown if drug is distributed in breast milk. **Pregnancy Category B (Genotropin, Genotropin Miniquick, Saizen, Serostim, Zorbitive); C (Humatrope, Norditropin, Norditropin Cartridge, Nutropin, Nutropin AQ, Nutropin Depot, Protopin). Children/Elderly:** No age-related precautions noted.

INTERACTIONS

DRUG: **Corticosteroids** may inhibit growth response. **HERBAL:** None significant. **FOOD:** None known. **LAB VALUES:** May increase serum alkaline phosphatase, inorganic phosphorus, parathyroid hormone. May decrease glucose tolerance. May slightly decrease thyroid function.

AVAILABILITY (Rx)

INJECTION, POWDER FOR RECONSTITUTION (GENOTROPIN): 1.5 mg, 5.8 mg, 13.8 mg. **(GENOTROPIN MINIQUICK):** 0.2 mg, 0.4 mg, 0.6 mg, 0.8 mg, 1 mg, 1.2 mg, 1.4 mg, 1.6 mg, 1.8 mg, 2 mg. **(HUMATROPE):** 5 mg, 6 mg, 12 mg, 24 mg. **(NUTROPIN):** 5 mg, 10 mg. **(SAIZEN):** 5 mg, 8.8 mg. **(SEROSTIM):** 4 mg, 5 mg, 6 mg. **(ZORBITIVE):** 8.8 mg. **INJECTION, SOLUTION: (NORDITROPIN):** 5 mg/1.5 ml, 15 mg/1.5 ml. **(NUTROPIN AQ):** 5 mg/ml.

ADMINISTRATION/HANDLING

SOMATREM

◀ ALERT ▶ Neonate: Benzyl alcohol as a preservative has been associated with fatal toxicity (gasping syndrome) in premature infants. Reconstitute with Sterile Water for Injection only. Use only 1 dose per vial. Discard unused portion.

IM, SUBCUTANEOUS

Reconstitution • Reconstitute each 5 mg vial with 1–5 ml Bacteriostatic Water for Injection (benzyl alcohol preserved) or each 10 mg vial with 1–10 ml Bacteriostatic Water for Injection (benzyl alcohol preserved only). • Aim stream of diluent against glass wall of vial. • Swirl contents with gentle rotary motion until completely dissolved. Do not shake (results in cloudy solution). Solution should be clear immediately after reconstitution. If solution is cloudy immediately after reconstitution or refrigeration, contents must not be injected.

Storage • Store in refrigerator. • Use reconstituted vials within 14 days. • Do not freeze. • Do not use if solution is cloudy.

SOMATROPIN

◀ ALERT ▶ Neonate: Benzyl alcohol as a preservative has been associated with

S

fatal toxicity, (gasping syndrome) in premature infants. Reconstitute with Sterile Water for Injection only. Use only 1 dose per vial. Discard unused portion.

Reconstitution • Humatrope: Vial: • Reconstitute with 1.5–5 ml diluent for Humatrope. • Diluent should be injected into vial by aiming stream of liquid against glass wall. • Swirl vial with gentle rotary motion until contents are completely dissolved. Do not shake. **Cartridge:** • Reconstitute cartridge using only diluent syringe and diluent connector. • Do not reconstitute with diluent for Humatrope provided with Humatrope vials.

Nutropin • Reconstitute each 5-mg vial with 1–5 ml Bacteriostatic Water for Injection (benzyl alcohol preserved), or each 10-mg vial with 1–10 ml Bacteriostatic Water for Injection (benzyl alcohol preserved only). • Aim stream of diluent against glass wall of vial. • Swirl contents with gentle rotary motion until completely dissolved. Do not shake (results in cloudy solution). Solution should be clear immediately after reconstitution. If solution is cloudy immediately after reconstitution or refrigeration, contents must not be injected.

Storage: • **Humatrope:** Refrigerate vials. • Do not freeze. • Reconstituted solution is stable for 14 days if reconstituted with Bacteriostatic Water for Injection and stored in refrigerator. Reconstituted solution is stable for 24 hrs if reconstituted with Sterile Water for Injection and stored in refrigerator. Discard if reconstituted solution is cloudy or contains precipitate.

Nutropin • Refrigerate vials. • Do not freeze. • Reconstituted solution is stable for 14 days if reconstituted with Bacteriostatic Water for Injection and stored in refrigerator. Discard if reconstituted solution is cloudy or contains precipitate.

INDICATIONS/ROUTES/DOSAGE

GROWTH HORMONE DEFICIENCY

SUBCUTANEOUS (HUMATROPE): ADULTS: 0.006 mg/kg once daily. **CHILDREN:** 0.18–0.3 mg/kg weekly divided into alternate-day doses or 6 doses/wk.
SUBCUTANEOUS (NUTROPIN): ADULTS: 0.006 mg/kg once daily. **CHILDREN:** 0.3–0.7 mg/kg weekly divided into daily doses.
SUBCUTANEOUS (NUTROPIN AQ): ADULTS: 0.006 mg/kg once daily.
SUBCUTANEOUS (GENOTROPIN): ADULTS: 0.04–0.08 mg/kg weekly divided into 6–7 equal doses/wk. **CHILDREN:** 0.16–0.24 mg/kg weekly divided into daily doses.
SUBCUTANEOUS (PROTOPIN): CHILDREN: 0.3 mg/kg weekly divided into daily doses.
SUBCUTANEOUS (NORDITROPIN): CHILDREN: 0.024–0.036 mg/kg/dose 6–7 times a wk.
SUBCUTANEOUS (SAIZEN): CHILDREN: 0.06 mg/kg 3 times a wk.
SUBCUTANEOUS ONLY (NUTROPIN DEPOT): CHILDREN: 0.75 mg/kg twice monthly or 1.5 mg/kg once monthly.

CHRONIC RENAL INSUFFICIENCY

SUBCUTANEOUS (NUTROPIN, NUTROPIN AQ): CHILDREN: 0.35 mg/kg weekly divided into daily doses.

TURNER'S SYNDROME

SUBCUTANEOUS (HUMATROPE, NUTROPIN, NUTROPIN AQ): CHILDREN: 0.375 mg/kg weekly divided into equal doses 3–7 times a wk.

AIDS-RELATED WASTING

SUBCUTANEOUS: ADULTS WEIGHING MORE THAN 55 KG: 6 mg once a day at bedtime. **ADULTS WEIGHING 45–55 KG:** 5 mg once a day at bedtime. **ADULTS WEIGHING 35–44 KG:** 4 mg once a day at bedtime. **ADULTS WEIGHING LESS THAN 35 KG:** 0.1 mg/kg once a day at bedtime.

S

SHORT BOWEL SYNDROME
SUBCUTANEOUS (ZORBITIVE): ADULTS: 0.1 mg/kg/day. **Maximum:** 8 mg/day.

SIDE EFFECTS

FREQUENT: Otitis media, other ear disorders (with Turner's syndrome). **OCCASIONAL:** Carpal tunnel syndrome; gynecomastia; myalgia; peripheral edema, fatigue; asthenia (loss of strength, energy), **RARE:** Rash, pruritus, visual changes, headache, nausea, vomiting, injection site pain/swelling, abdominal pain, hip/knee pain.

ADVERSE EFFECTS/ TOXIC REACTIONS

Pancreatitis occurs rarely.

NURSING CONSIDERATIONS

BASELINE ASSESSMENT

Obtain baseline thyroid function, serum glucose level.

INTERVENTION/EVALUATION

Monitor bone growth, growth rate in relation to pt's age. Monitor serum calcium, glucose, phosphorus levels; renal, parathyroid, thyroid function. Observe for decreased muscle wasting in AIDS pts.

PATIENT/FAMILY TEACHING

• Teach correct procedure to reconstitute drug for administration, safe handling/disposal of needles. • Inform pt of need for regular follow-up with physician. • Report development of severe headache, visual changes, pain in hip/knee, limping.

Sonata, *see zaleplon*

sorafenib

sor-ah-**fen**-ib
(Nexavar)

CLASSIFICATION

PHARMACOTHERAPEUTIC: Multikinase inhibitor. **CLINICAL:** Antineoplastic.

ACTION

Decreases tumor cell proliferation by interacting with multiple intracellular, cell surface kinases. **Therapeutic Effect:** Inhibits tumor growth.

PHARMACOKINETICS

Metabolized in liver. Protein binding: 99.5%. Eliminated mainly in feces, with lesser amount excreted in urine. **Half-life:** 25–48 hrs.

USES

Treatment of advanced renal cell carcinoma.

PRECAUTIONS

CONTRAINDICATIONS: None known. **CAUTIONS:** Hepatic/renal impairment, dialysis pts.

LIFESPAN CONSIDERATIONS:

Pregnancy/Lactation: May cause fetal harm. Adequate contraception should be used during therapy and for at least 2 wks after therapy completion. Unknown if distributed in breast milk; do not breast-feed. **Pregnancy Category D. Children:** Safety and efficacy not established. **Elderly:** No age-related precautions noted.

INTERACTIONS

DRUG: Carbamazine, dexamethasone, phenobarbital, phenytoin, rifampin may decrease concentration. May increase

S

concentration, effects of **doxorubicin.** **Warfarin** may increase risk of bleeding. **HERBAL: St. John's wort** may decrease concentration. **FOOD: High-fat meals** decrease effectiveness. **LAB VALUES:** May increase serum lipase, amylase, bilirubin, alkaline phosphatase. May decrease serum phosphorus, lymphocytes, WBCs, Hgb, Hct.

AVAILABILITY (Rx)

TABLETS: 200 mg (Nexavar).

ADMINISTRATION/HANDLING

PO

- Give 1 hr before or 2 hrs after eating (high-fat meal reduces effectiveness).

INDICATIONS/ROUTES/DOSAGE

RENAL CELL CARCINOMA

PO: ADULTS, ELDERLY: 400 mg (2 tablets) twice a day without food.

SIDE EFFECTS

FREQUENT (43%–16%): Diarrhea, rash, fatigue, exfoliative dermatitis, alopecia, nausea, pruritus, hypertension, anorexia, vomiting. **OCCASIONAL (15%–10%):** Constipation, minor bleeding, dyspnea, sensory neuropathy, cough, abdominal pain, dry skin, weight, loss, joint pain, headache. **RARE (9%–1%):** Acne, flushing, stomatitis, mucositis, dyspepsia (heartburn, indigestion, epigastric pain), arthralgia, myalgia, hoarseness.

S

ADVERSE EFFECTS/ TOXIC REACTIONS

Anemia, neutropenia, thrombocytopenia, leukopenia occur in less than 10% of pts. Pancreatitis, gastritis, erectile dysfunction occur occasionally. Hemorrhage, cardiac ischemia/infarction, hypertensive crisis occur rarely.

NURSING CONSIDERATIONS

BASELINE ASSESSMENT

Monitor B/P weekly during first 6 wks of therapy and routinely thereafter. CBC, blood chemistries including electrolytes, renal/hepatic function tests, chest x-ray should be performed before therapy begins and routinely thereafter.

INTERVENTION/EVALUATION

Determine serum amylase, lipase, phosphorus concentrations frequently during therapy. Monitor CBC for evidence of myelosuppression. Monitor for blood dyscrasias (fever, sore throat, signs of local infection, unusual bruising/bleeding from any site), symptoms of anemia (excessive fatigue, weakness). Monitor for signs of neuropathy (gait disturbances, fine motor control, difficulties, numbness).

PATIENT/FAMILY TEACHING

- Report any episode of chest pain.
- Do not have immunizations without physician's approval (drug lowers resistance); avoid contact with those who have recently taken live virus vaccine.
- Promptly report fever, sore throat, signs of local infection, unusual bruising/bleeding from any site.

sotalol

soe-ta-lole

(Apo-Sotalol ♣, Betapace, Betapace AF, Novo-Sotalol ♣, PMS-Sotalol ♣, Sorine)

Do not confuse sotalol with Stadol.

CLASSIFICATION

PHARMACOTHERAPEUTIC: Beta-adrenergic blocking agent. **CLINICAL:** Antiarrhythmic (see pp. 16C, 68C).

ACTION

Prolongs action potential, effective refractory period, QT interval. Decreases heart rate, AV node conduction;

increases AV node refractoriness. **Therapeutic Effect:** Produces antiarrhythmic activity.

PHARMACOKINETICS

Well absorbed from GI tract. Protein binding: None. Widely distributed. Primarily excreted unchanged in urine. Removed by hemodialysis. **Half-life:** 12 hrs (increased in elderly, renal impairment).

USES

Betapace, Sorine: Treatment of documented, life-threatening ventricular arrhythmias. **Betapace AF:** Maintain normal sinus rhythm in pts with symptomatic atrial fibrillation/flutter. **OFF-LABEL:** Maintenance of normal heart rhythm in chronic or recurring atrial fibrillation/flutter; treatment of anxiety, chronic angina pectoris, hypertension, hypertrophic cardiomyopathy, MI, mitral valve prolapse syndrome, pheochromocytoma, thyrotoxicosis, tremors.

PRECAUTIONS

CONTRAINDICATIONS: Bronchial asthma, cardiogenic shock, prolonged QT syndrome (unless functioning pacemaker is present), second- or third-degree heart block, sinus bradycardia, uncontrolled cardiac failure. **CAUTIONS:** Pts with history of ventricular tachycardia, ventricular fibrillation, cardiomegaly, CHF, diabetes mellitus, excessive prolongation of QT interval, hypokalemia, hypomagnesemia. Severe, prolonged diarrhea. Pts with sick sinus syndrome, pts at risk for developing thyrotoxicosis. Avoid abrupt withdrawal.

⌛ LIFESPAN CONSIDERATIONS:

Pregnancy/Lactation: Crosses placenta. Excreted in breast milk. **Pregnancy Category B (D if used in second or third trimester). Children:** Safety and efficacy not established. **Elderly:** Age-related peripheral vascular disease may increase susceptibility to decreased peripheral circulation. Age-related renal impairment may require dosage adjustment.

INTERACTIONS

DRUG: Antiarrhythmics, phenothiazine, tricyclic antidepressants may prolong QT interval. **Calcium channel blockers** may increase effect on AV conduction, B/P. **Digoxin** may increase risk of proarrhythmias. May mask symptoms of hypoglycemia, prolong hypoglycemic effects of **insulin, oral hypoglycemics.** May inhibit effects of **sympathomimetics, theophylline. HERBAL: Ephedra** may worsen arrhythmias. **FOOD:** None known. **LAB VALUES:** May increase serum glucose, alkaline phosphatase, LDH, lipoprotein, AST, ALT, triglycerides.

AVAILABILITY (Rx)

TABLETS: 80 mg (Betapace, Betapace AF Sorine), 120 mg (Betapace, Betapace AF, Sorine), 160 mg (Betapace, Betapace AF, Sorine), 240 mg (Betapace, Sorine).

ADMINISTRATION/HANDLING

PO

- Give without regard to food.

INDICATIONS/ROUTES/DOSAGE

DOCUMENTED, LIFE-THREATENING ARRHYTHMIAS

PO (BETAPACE, SORINE): ADULTS, ELDERLY: Initially, 80 mg twice a day. May increase gradually at 2- to 3-day intervals. Range: 240–320 mg/day.

ATRIAL FIBRILLATION, ATRIAL FLUTTER

PO (BETAPACE AF): ADULTS, ELDERLY: 80 mg twice a day.

DOSAGE IN RENAL IMPAIRMENT

Dosage interval is modified based on creatinine clearance.

Betapace, Sorine

Creatinine Clearance	Dosage Interval
31–60 ml/min	24 hrs
10–30 ml/min	36–48 hrs
Less than 10 ml/min	Individualized

Betapace AF

Creatinine Clearance	Dosage Interval
Greater than 60 ml/min	12 hrs
40–60 ml/min	24 hrs
Less than 40 ml/min	Contraindicated

SIDE EFFECTS

FREQUENT: Diminished sexual function, drowsiness, insomnia, asthenia (loss of strength, energy). **OCCASIONAL:** Depression, cold hands/feet, diarrhea, constipation, anxiety, nasal congestion, nausea, vomiting. **RARE:** Altered taste, dry eyes, pruritus, numbness of fingers, toes, scalp.

ADVERSE EFFECTS/ TOXIC REACTIONS

Bradycardia, CHF, hypotension, bronchospasm, hypoglycemia, prolonged QT interval, torsades de pointes, ventricular tachycardia, premature ventricular complexes may occur.

NURSING CONSIDERATIONS

BASELINE ASSESSMENT

Pt must be on continuous cardiac monitoring upon initiation of therapy. Do not administer without consulting physician if pulse is 60 beats/min or less. Assess creatinine clearance before dosing.

INTERVENTION/EVALUATION

Diligently monitor for arrhythmias. Assess B/P for hypotension, pulse for bradycardia. Assess for CHF: dyspnea, peripheral edema, jugular vein distention, increased weight, rales in lungs, decreased urinary output.

PATIENT/FAMILY TEACHING

• Do not discontinue, change dose without physician approval. • Avoid tasks requiring alertness, motor skills until response to drug is established (may cause drowsiness). • Periodic lab tests, EKGs are necessary part of therapy.

Spectrocef, *see cefditoren*

Spiriva, *see tiotropium*

spironolactone

speer-on-oh-**lak**-tone

(Aldactone, Novospiroton ✚)

Do not confuse Aldactone with Aldactazide.

FIXED-COMBINATION(S)

Aldactazide: spironolactone/hydrochlorothiazide (a thiazide diuretic): 25 mg/25 mg; 50 mg/50 mg.

◆CLASSIFICATION

PHARMACOTHERAPEUTIC: Aldosterone antagonist. **CLINICAL:** Potassium-sparing diuretic, antihypertensive, antihypokalemic (see p. 97C).

ACTION

Interferes with sodium reabsorption by competitively inhibiting action of aldosterone in distal tubule, promoting sodium and water excretion, increasing potassium retention. **Therapeutic Effect:** Produces diuresis, lowers B/P.

PHARMACOKINETICS

Route	Onset	Peak	Duration
PO	24–48 hrs	48–72 hrs	48–72 hrs

Well absorbed from GI tract (absorption increased with food). Protein binding: 91%–98%. Metabolized in liver to active metabolite. Primarily excreted in urine. Unknown if removed by hemodialysis. **Half-life:** 0–24 hrs (metabolite, 13–24 hrs).

USES

Management of edema associated with CHF, cirrhosis, nephrotic syndrome. Treatment of hypertension, male hirsutism, hypokalemia, CHF. Diagnosis/treatment of primary hyperaldosteronism. **OFF-LABEL:** Treatment of edema, hypertension in children, female acne, hirsutism, polycystic ovary disease.

PRECAUTIONS

CONTRAINDICATIONS: Acute renal insufficiency, anuria, BUN and serum creatinine levels more than twice normal values, hyperkalemia. **CAUTIONS:** Dehydration, hyponatremia, renal/hepatic impairment, concurrent use of supplemental potassium.

LIFESPAN CONSIDERATIONS:

Pregnancy/Lactation: Active metabolite excreted in breast milk; breastfeeding not recommended. **Pregnancy Category C (D if used in pregnancy-induced hypertension). Children:** No age-related precautions noted. **Elderly:** May be more susceptible to developing hyperkalemia. Age-related renal impairment may require dosage adjustment.

INTERACTIONS

DRUG: ACE inhibitors (e.g., captopril), cyclosporine, potassium-containing medications, potassium supplements may increase risk of hyperkalemia. May decrease effects of **anticoagulants, heparin.** May increase half-life of **digoxin.** May decrease clearance, increase risk of toxicity of **lithium. NSAIDs** may decrease antihypertensive effect. **HERBAL:** Avoid **natural licorice** (possesses mineralocorticoid activity). **FOOD: Food** increases absorption. **LAB VALUES:** May increase urinary calcium excretion, BUN, serum glucose, creatinine, magnesium, potassium, uric acid. May decrease serum sodium.

AVAILABILITY (Rx)

TABLETS: 25 mg, 50 mg, 100 mg.

ADMINISTRATION/HANDLING

PO

- Oral suspension containing crushed tablets in cherry syrup is stable for up to 30 days if refrigerated.
- Drug absorption enhanced if taken with food.
- Scored tablets may be crushed.

INDICATIONS/ROUTES/DOSAGE

EDEMA

PO: ADULTS, ELDERLY: 25–200 mg/day as single dose or in 2 divided doses. **CHILDREN:** 1.5–3.3 mg/kg/day in divided doses. **Maximum:** 100 mg. **NEONATES:** 1–3 mg/kg/day in 1–2 divided doses.

HYPERTENSION

PO: ADULTS, ELDERLY: 25–50 mg/day in 1–2 doses/day. **CHILDREN:** 1.5–3.3 mg/kg/day in divided doses. **Maximum:** 100 mg.

HYPOKALEMIA

PO: ADULTS, ELDERLY: 25–200 mg/day as single dose or in 2 divided doses.

MALE HIRSUTISM

PO: ADULTS, ELDERLY: 50–200 mg/day as single dose or in 2 divided doses.

PRIMARY ALDOSTERONISM

PO: ADULTS, ELDERLY: 100–400 mg/day as single dose or in 2 divided doses.

CHILDREN: 100–400 mg/m^2/day as single dose or in 2 divided doses.

CHF

PO: ADULTS, ELDERLY: 12.5–25 mg/day adjusted based on pt response, evidence of hyperkalemia. **Maximum:** 50 mg.

DOSAGE IN RENAL IMPAIRMENT

Dosage interval is modified based on creatinine clearance.

Creatinine Clearance	Interval
10–50 ml/min	Usual dose q12–24h
Less than 10 ml/min	Avoid use

SIDE EFFECTS

FREQUENT: Hyperkalemia (in pts with renal insufficiency, those taking potassium supplements), dehydration, hyponatremia, lethargy. **OCCASIONAL:** Nausea, vomiting, anorexia, abdominal cramps, diarrhea, headache, ataxia, drowsiness, confusion, fever. **Male:** Gynecomastia, impotence, decreased libido. **Female:** Menstrual irregularities (amenorrhea, postmenopausal bleeding), breast tenderness. **RARE:** Rash, urticaria, hirsutism.

ADVERSE EFFECTS/ TOXIC REACTIONS

Severe hyperkalemia may produce arrhythmias, bradycardia, EKG changes (tented T waves, widening QRS complex, ST segment depression). May proceed to cardiac standstill, ventricular fibrillation. Cirrhosis pts at risk for hepatic decompensation if dehydration, hyponatremia occurs. Pts with primary aldosteronism may experience rapid weight loss, severe fatigue during high-dose therapy.

NURSING CONSIDERATIONS

BASELINE ASSESSMENT

Weigh pt; initiate strict I&O. Evaluate hydration status by assessing mucous membranes, skin turgor. Obtain baseline serum electrolytes, renal/hepatic function, urinalysis. Assess for edema; note location, extent. Check baseline vital signs, note pulse rate/regularity.

INTERVENTION/EVALUATION

Monitor serum electrolyte values, esp. for increased potassium. Monitor B/P. Monitor for hyponatremia: mental confusion, thirst, cold/clammy skin, drowsiness, dry mouth. Monitor for hyperkalemia: colic, diarrhea, muscle twitching followed by weakness/paralysis, arrhythmias. Obtain daily weight. Note changes in edema, skin turgor.

PATIENT/FAMILY TEACHING

• Expect increase in volume, frequency of urination. • Therapeutic effect takes several days to begin and can last for several days when drug is discontinued. This may not apply if pt is on a potassium-losing drug concomitantly (diet, use of supplements should be established by physician). • Notify physician of irregular or slow pulse, electrolyte imbalance (signs noted previously). • Avoid foods high in potassium, such as whole grains (cereals), legumes, meat, bananas, apricots, orange juice, potatoes (white, sweet), raisins. • Avoid tasks that require alertness, motor skills until response to drug is established (may cause drowsiness).

Sporanox, *see itraconazole*

S

St. John's wort

Also known as amber, demon chaser, goatweed, hardhay, rosin rose, tipton weed.

CLASSIFICATION

HERBAL: See Appendix G.

ACTION

Inhibits COMT (catechol-*O*-methyl transferase), MAO (monoamine oxidase); modulates effects of serotonin by inhibiting serotonin reuptake and 5-HT_3, $5HT_4$ antagonism. **Effect:** Relieves depression.

USES

Treatment of depression, including secondary effects of depression (fatigue, loss of appetite, anxiety, nervousness, insomnia).

PRECAUTIONS

CONTRAINDICATIONS: Pregnancy, breast-feeding (may cause increased muscle tone of uterus; infants may experience colic, drowsiness, lethargy). **CAUTIONS:** Bipolar disorder, schizophrenia.

LIFESPAN CONSIDERATIONS:

Pregnancy/Lactation: Contraindicated. **Pregnancy Category C. Children:** Safety and efficacy not established. Avoid use. **Elderly:** No age-related precautions noted.

INTERACTIONS

DRUG: **Angiotensin-converting enzyme (ACE) inhibitors** may cause hypertension. May decrease concentration, effect of **indinavir. Antidepressants** may increase therapeutic effect. May decrease effectiveness of **cyclosporine,** resulting in organ rejection. **Digoxin** may cause CHF exacerbation. **HERBAL:** **Ginseng, chamomile, goldenseal, kava kava, valerian** may increase therapeutic, adverse effects. **FOOD:** **Tyramine-containing food** may cause hypertensive crisis with high doses of St. John's wort. **LAB VALUES:** May increase INR, prothrombin time (PT) in pts treated with warfarin.

AVAILABILITY (Rx)

CAPSULES: 150 mg, 300 mg. **EXTRACT. LIQUID TINCTURE.**

INDICATIONS/ROUTES/DOSAGE

DEPRESSION

PO: ADULTS, ELDERLY: 300 mg 3 times/day is most common.

SIDE EFFECTS

Abdominal cramps, insomnia, vivid dreams, restlessness, anxiety, agitation, irritability, fatigue, dry mouth, headache, dizziness, photosensitivity, confusion.

ADVERSE EFFECTS/ TOXIC REACTIONS

None known.

NURSING CONSIDERATIONS

BASELINE ASSESSMENT

Assess if pt is pregnant or breast-feeding, has history of psychiatric disease. Determine medication usage (many potential interactions). Assess mental status: mood, memory, anxiety level.

INTERVENTION/EVALUATION

Monitor changes in depressive state, behavior, signs of side effects.

PATIENT/FAMILY TEACHING

• Do not abruptly discontinue drug (may increase adverse effects). • Check with physician before taking other medications (many interactions). • Avoid foods high in tyramine (aged cheese, pickled products, beer, wine). • Therapeutic effect may take 4–6 wks. • Avoid sunlight, use sunscreen/protective clothing (increased photosensitivity).

S

stavudine (d4T)

stay-view-deen
(Zerit)

CLASSIFICATION

PHARMACOTHERAPEUTIC: Nucleoside reverse transcriptase inhibitor. **CLINICAL:** Antiviral (see pp. 66C, 111C).

ACTION

Inhibits HIV reverse transcriptase by terminating viral DNA chain. Inhibits RNA-, DNA-dependent DNA polymerase, an enzyme necessary for HIV replication. **Therapeutic Effect:** Impedes HIV replication, slowing progression of HIV infection.

PHARMACOKINETICS

Rapidly, completely absorbed after PO administration. Undergoes minimal metabolism. Excreted in urine. **Half-life:** 1.5 hrs (increased in renal impairment).

USES

Treatment of HIV infection in combination with other agents.

PRECAUTIONS

CONTRAINDICATIONS: None known. **CAUTIONS:** History of peripheral neuropathy, renal/hepatic impairment.

LIFESPAN CONSIDERATIONS:

Pregnancy/Lactation: Breast-feeding not recommended (possibility of HIV transmission). **Pregnancy Category C. Children:** No age-related precautions noted. **Elderly:** Information not available.

INTERACTIONS

DRUG: Didanosine, ethambutol, isoniazid, lithium, metronidazole, nitrofurantoin, phenytoin, zalcitabine may increase risk of peripheral neuropathy development. **Didanosine, hydroxyurea** may increase risk of hepatotoxicity. **Zidovudine** may have antagonistic antiviral effect. **HERBAL:** None significant. **FOOD:** None known. **LAB VALUES:** Commonly increases serum AST, ALT. May decrease neutrophil count.

AVAILABILITY (Rx)

CAPSULES: 15 mg, 20 mg, 30 mg, 40 mg. **POWDER FOR ORAL SOLUTION:** 1 mg/ml.

ADMINISTRATION/HANDLING

PO

- Give without regard to meals.

INDICATIONS/ROUTES/DOSAGE

HIV INFECTION

PO: ADULTS, ELDERLY, CHILDREN WEIGHING 60 KG AND MORE: 40 mg q12h. **CHILDREN WEIGHING 30–59 KG:** 30 mg q12h. **NEONATES 14 DAYS AND OLDER, INFANTS, CHILDREN WEIGHING LESS THAN 30 KG:** 1 mg/kg/dose q12h. **Maximum:** 30 mg q12h. **NEONATES 0–13 DAYS:** 0.5 mg/kg/dose q12h.

DOSAGE IN RENAL IMPAIRMENT

Dosage and frequency are modified based on creatinine clearance and pt weight.

Creatinine Clearance	Weight 60 kg or More	Weight Less Than 60 kg
Greater than 50 ml/min	40 mg q12h	30 mg q12h
26–50 ml/min	20 mg q12h	15 mg q12h
10–25 ml/min	20 mg q24h	15 mg q24h

SIDE EFFECTS

FREQUENT: Headache (55%), diarrhea (50%), chills, fever (38%), nausea, vomiting, myalgia (35%), rash (33%), asthenia (28%), insomnia, abdominal pain (26%), anxiety (22%), back pain (20%), diaphoresis (19%), arthralgia (18%), malaise (17%), depression (14%). **OCCASIONAL:** Anorexia, weight loss, nervousness, dizziness, conjunctivitis, dyspepsia, dyspnea. **RARE:** Constipation, vasodilation, confusion, migraine, urticaria, abnormal vision.

ADVERSE EFFECTS/ TOXIC REACTIONS

Peripheral neuropathy, (numbness, tingling, pain in hands/feet) occurs in 15%–21% of pts. Ulcerative stomatitis (erythema, ulcers of oral mucosa, glossitis, gingivitis), pneumonia, benign skin neoplasms occur occasionally. Pancreatitis, hepatomegaly, lactic acidosis have been reported.

NURSING CONSIDERATIONS

BASELINE ASSESSMENT

Obtain baseline laboratory testing, esp. serum hepatic function tests, before beginning stavudine therapy and at periodic intervals during therapy. Offer emotional support to pt, family. Question for history of peripheral neuropathy.

INTERVENTION/EVALUATION

Monitor for peripheral neuropathy (characterized by paresthesia in extremities). Symptoms resolve promptly if therapy is discontinued (symptoms may worsen temporarily after drug is withdrawn). If symptoms resolve completely, reduced dosage may be resumed. Assess for headache, nausea, vomiting, myalgia. Monitor skin for evidence of rash, signs of fever. Monitor daily pattern of bowel activity/stool consistency. Assess for myalgia, arthralgia, dizziness. Monitor sleep patterns. Assess eating pattern; monitor for weight loss. Check eyes for signs of conjunctivitis. Monitor CBC, Hgb, serum hepatic/renal function, CD4 cell count, HIV RNA levels

PATIENT/FAMILY TEACHING

• Continue therapy for full length of treatment. • Doses should be evenly spaced. • Do not take any medications, including OTC drugs, without consulting physician. • Stavudine is not a cure for HIV infection, nor does it reduce risk of transmission to others. • Pt may continue to experience illnesses, including opportunistic infections. • Report tingling, burning, pain, numbness, abdominal discomfort, nausea, vomiting, fatigue, dyspnea, weakness.

Strattera, *see atomoxetine*

streptokinase

strep-toe-**kye**-nase
(Streptase)

CLASSIFICATION

PHARMACOTHERAPEUTIC: Enzyme. **CLINICAL:** Thrombolytic (see p. 32C).

ACTION

Activates fibrinolytic system by converting plasminogen to plasmin (enzyme that degrades fibrin clots). Acts indirectly by forming complex with plasminogen, which converts plasminogen to plasmin. Action occurs within thrombus, on thrombus surface, in circulating blood. **Therapeutic Effect:** Lysis of thrombi.

PHARMACOKINETICS

Rapidly cleared from plasma by antibodies, reticuloendothelial system. Route of elimination unknown. Duration of action continues for several hrs after drug has been discontinued. **Half-life:** 23 min.

USES

Management of acute MI (lyses thrombi obstructing coronary arteries, decreases infarct size, improves ventricular function after MI, decreases CHF, decreases mortality associated with MI). Lysis of

S

diagnosed pulmonary emboli, acute or extensive thrombi of deep veins, acute arterial thrombi or emboli.

PRECAUTIONS

CONTRAINDICATIONS: Carcinoma of brain, cerebrovascular accident, internal bleeding, intracranial surgery, recent streptococcal infection, severe hypertension. **CAUTIONS:** Major surgery within 10 days, GI bleeding, recent trauma.

LIFESPAN CONSIDERATIONS:

Pregnancy/Lactation: Use only when benefit outweighs potential risk to fetus. Unknown if drug crosses placenta or is distributed in breast milk. **Pregnancy Category C.** **Children:** Safety and efficacy not established. **Elderly:** May have increased risk of intracranial hemorrhage; caution recommended.

INTERACTIONS

DRUG: **Anticoagulants, heparin** may increase risk of hemorrhage. **NSAIDs, platelet aggregation inhibitors (e.g., aspirin)** may increase risk of bleeding. **HERBAL:** **Cat's claw, dong quai, evening primrose, feverfew, red clover, garlic, ginseng, ginkgo** possess antiplatelet activity, may increase bleeding. **FOOD:** None known. **LAB VALUES:** Decreases serum plasminogen, fibrinogen during infusion, decreasing clotting time, confirming presence of lysis.

AVAILABILITY (Rx)

INJECTION, POWDER FOR RECONSTITUTION (STREPTASE): 250,000 units, 750,000 units, 1.5 million units.

ADMINISTRATION/HANDLING

◀ **ALERT** ▶ Must be administered within 12–14 hrs of coronary artery clot formation (little effect on older, organized clots).

IV

Reconstitution • Reconstitute vial with 5 ml D_5W or 0.9% NaCl (preferred). Add diluent slowly to side of vial, roll and tilt to avoid foaming. Do not shake vial. • May further dilute with 50–500 ml in 45-ml increments of D_5W or 0.9% NaCl.

Rate of administration

PERIPHERAL IV ADMINISTRATION FOR CORONARY ARTERY THROMBI
• Give 1.5 million international units over 60 min.

DIRECT INTRACORONARY ADMINISTRATION FOR CORONARY ARTERY THROMBI
• Give bolus dose over 25–30 sec using coronary catheter. Follow with 2,000 international units/min for 60 min.

DEEP VEIN THROMBOSIS, PULMONARY EMBOLISM, ARTERIAL THROMBOSIS/EMBOLISM
• Give single dose over 25–30 min. Follow with maintenance dose of 100,000 or more every hr for 24–72 hrs. • Monitor B/P during infusion (hypotension may be severe, occurs in 1%–10% of pts). Decrease of infusion rate may be necessary • If uncontrolled hemorrhage occurs, discontinue infusion immediately (slowing rate of infusion may produce worsening hemorrhage). Do not use dextran to control hemorrhage.

Storage • Store unopened vials at room temperature. Refrigerate reconstituted solution. Use within 24 hrs.

IV INCOMPATIBILITIES

Do not mix with medications other than dobutamine (Dobutrex), dopamine (Intropin), heparin, lidocaine, and nitroglycerin.

IV COMPATIBILITIES

Dobutamine (Dobutrex), dopamine (Intropin), heparin, lidocaine, nitroglycerin.

INDICATIONS/ROUTES/DOSAGE

◀ **ALERT** ▶ Do not use within 6 mos of previous streptokinase treatment or streptococcal infection (pharyngitis, rheumatic fever, acute glomerulonephritis secondary to streptococcal infection).

ACUTE EVOLVING TRANSMURAL MI

IV INFUSION: ADULTS, ELDERLY (1.5 MILLION UNITS DILUTED TO 45 ML): 1.5 million units infused over 60 min.

INTRACORONARY INFUSION: ADULTS, ELDERLY (250,000 UNITS DILUTED TO 125 ML): Initially, 20,000-units (10-ml) bolus; then, 2,000 units/min for 60 min. Total dose: 140,000 units.

PULMONARY EMBOLISM, DEEP VEIN THROMBOSIS, ARTERIAL THROMBOSIS/EMBOLISM
(given within 7 days of onset)

IV INFUSION: ADULTS, ELDERLY (1.5 MILLION UNITS DILUTED TO 90 ML): Initially, 250,000 units infused over 30 min; then, 100,000 units/hr for 24–72 hrs for arterial thrombosis/embolism, pulmonary embolism, 72 hrs for DVT.

INTRA-ATERIAL INFUSION: ADULTS, ELDERLY (1.5 MILLION UNITS DILUTED TO 45 ML): Initially, 250,000 units infused over 30 min; then 100,000 units/hr for maintenance.

SIDE EFFECTS

FREQUENT: Fever, superficial bleeding decreased B/P. **OCCASIONAL:** Allergic reaction (rash, wheezing), ecchymosis.

ADVERSE EFFECTS/ TOXIC REACTIONS

Severe internal hemorrhage may occur. Lysis of coronary thrombi may produce life-threatening arrhythmias.

NURSING CONSIDERATIONS

BASELINE ASSESSMENT

Assess Hct, platelet count, thrombin, activated partial thromboplastin time (aPTT), prothrombin time (PT), fibrinogen level before therapy is instituted. If heparin is component of treatment, discontinue before streptokinase is instituted (PT/aPTT should be less than twice normal value before institution of therapy).

INTERVENTION/EVALUATION

Assess clinical response, vital signs per protocol. Handle pt carefully and as infrequently as possible to prevent ecchymoses, bleeding. Do not obtain B/P in lower extremities (possible deep vein thrombi). Monitor thrombin, PT, aPTT, fibrinogen level q4h after initiation of therapy. Check stool for occult blood. Assess for decrease in B/P, increase in pulse rate, complaint of abdominal/back pain, severe headache (may be evidence of hemorrhage). Question for increase in amount of discharge during menses. Assess area of peripheral thromboembolus for color, temperature. Assess peripheral pulses, skin for ecchymosis, petechiae. Check for excessive bleeding from puncture sites, minor cuts, scratches. Assess urine for hematuria. Monitor B/P, platelets, Hgb, Hct. Observe for signs of bleeding.

succinylcholine

(Anectine, Quelicin)

See Neuromuscular blockers (p. 120C)

sucralfate

soo-**kral**-fate

(Apo-Sucralate ✱, Carafate, Novo-Sucralate ✱)

Do not confuse Carafate with Cafergot.

CLASSIFICATION

CLINICAL: Antiulcer.

ACTION

Forms ulcer-adherent complex with proteinaceous exudate (e.g., albumin)

S

at ulcer site. Forms viscous, adhesive barrier on surface of intact mucosa of stomach, duodenum. **Therapeutic Effect:** Protects damaged mucosa from further destruction by absorbing gastric acid, pepsin, bile salts.

PHARMACOKINETICS

Minimally absorbed from GI tract. Eliminated in feces, with small amount excreted in urine. Not removed by hemodialysis.

USES

Short-term treatment (up to 8 wks) of duodenal ulcer. Maintenance therapy of duodenal ulcer after healing of acute ulcers. **OFF-LABEL:** Prevention, treatment of stress-related mucosal damage, esp. in acutely or critically ill pts; treatment of gastric ulcer, rheumatoid arthritis; relief of GI symptoms associated with NSAIDs; treatment of gastroesophageal reflux disease.

PRECAUTIONS

CONTRAINDICATIONS: None known. **CAUTIONS:** None known.

LIFESPAN CONSIDERATIONS:

Pregnancy/Lactation: Unknown if drug crosses placenta or is distributed in breast milk. **Pregnancy Category B. Children:** Safety and efficacy not established. **Elderly:** No age-related precautions noted.

INTERACTIONS

DRUG: Antacids may interfere with binding. May decrease absorption of **digoxin, phenytoin, quinolones, (e.g., ciprofloxacin, theophylline). HERBAL:** None significant. **FOOD:** None known. **LAB VALUES:** None known.

AVAILABILITY (Rx)

ORAL SUSPENSION: 1 g/10 ml. **TABLETS:** 1 g.

ADMINISTRATION/HANDLING

PO

• Administer 1 hr before meals and at bedtime. • Tablets may be crushed and dissolved in water. • Avoid antacids for 30 min before or after giving sucralfate. Shake suspension well before using.

INDICATIONS/ROUTES/DOSAGE

ACTIVE DUODENAL ULCERS

PO: ADULTS, ELDERLY: 1 g 4 times a day (before meals and at bedtime) for up to 8 wks.

MAINTENANCE THERAPY OF DUODENAL ULCERS

PO: ADULTS, ELDERLY: 1 g twice a day.

SIDE EFFECTS

FREQUENT (2%): Constipation. **OCCASIONAL (less than 2%):** Dry mouth, backache, diarrhea, dizziness, drowsiness, nausea, indigestion, rash, urticaria, pruritus, abdominal discomfort.

ADVERSE EFFECTS/ TOXIC REACTIONS

Bezoars (compacted, undigestible material that does not pass into intestine) have been reported.

NURSING CONSIDERATIONS

INTERVENTION/EVALUATION

Monitor daily pattern of bowel activity/ stool consistency.

PATIENT/FAMILY TEACHING

• Take medication on an empty stomach. • Antacids may be given as an adjunct but should not be taken for 30 min before or after sucralfate (formation of sucralfate gel is activated by stomach acid). • Dry mouth may be relieved by sour hard candy, sips of tepid water.

Sudafed, *see pseudoephedrine*

sufentanil

(Sufenta)

See Opioid analgesics

sulconazole

(Exelderm)

See Antifungals: topical

sulfasalazine

sul-fa-**sal**-a-zeen

(Alti-Sulfasalazine ✤, Azulfidine, Azulfidine EN-tabs, Salazopyrin ✤, Salazopyrin EN-Tabs ✤)

Do not confuse Azulfidine with azathioprine, or sulfasalazine with sulfadiazine or sulfisoxazole.

CLASSIFICATION

PHARMACOTHERAPEUTIC: Sulfonamide. **CLINICAL:** Anti-inflammatory.

ACTION

Inhibits prostaglandin synthesis, acting locally in colon. **Therapeutic Effect:** Decreases inflammatory response, interferes with GI secretion. Effect may be result of antibacterial action with change in intestinal flora.

PHARMACOKINETICS

Poorly absorbed from GI tract. Cleaved in colon by intestinal bacteria, forming sulfapyridine and mesalamine (5-ASA). Absorbed in colon. Widely distributed. Metabolized in liver. Primarily excreted in urine. **Half-life:** sulfapyridine, 6–14 hrs; 5-ASA, 0.6–1.4 hrs.

USES

Treatment of ulcerative colitis, rheumatoid arthritis. **OFF-LABEL:** Treatment of ankylosing spondylitis, collagenous colitis, Crohn's disease, inflammatory bowel disease, juvenile chronic arthritis, psoriasis, psoriatic arthritis.

PRECAUTIONS

CONTRAINDICATIONS: Children younger than 2 yrs; hypersensitivity to carbonic anhydrase inhibitors, local anesthetics, salicylates, sulfonamides, sulfonylureas, sunscreens containing PABA, thiazide or loop diuretics; intestinal, urinary tract obstruction; porphyria; pregnancy at term; severe hepatic/renal dysfunction. **CAUTIONS:** Severe allergies, bronchial asthma, impaired hepatic/renal function, G6PD deficiency.

⌛ LIFESPAN CONSIDERATIONS:

Pregnancy/Lactation: May produce infertility, oligospermia in men while taking medication. Readily crosses placenta; if given near term, may produce jaundice, hemolytic anemia, kernicterus in newborn. Excreted in breast milk. Do not breast-feed premature infant or those with hyperbilirubinemia or G6PD deficiency. **Pregnancy Category B (D if given near term). Children:** No age-related precautions noted in those older than 2 yrs. **Elderly:** No age-related precautions noted.

INTERACTIONS

DRUG: May increase effects of **anticonvulsants, methotrexate, oral anticoagulants, oral antidiabetics. Hemolytics** may increase toxicity. **Hepatotoxic medications** may increase risk of hepatotoxicity. **HERBAL: Dong quai, St. John's wort** may increase photosensititzation. **FOOD:** None known. **LAB VALUES:** None known.

AVAILABILITY (Rx)

TABLETS (AZULFIDINE): 500 mg.

TABLETS (DELAYED-RELEASE [AZULFIDINE EN-TABS]): 500 mg.

ADMINISTRATION/HANDLING

PO

• Space doses evenly (intervals not to exceed 8 hrs). • Administer after meals if possible (prolongs intestinal passage). • Swallow enteric-coated tablets whole; do not chew. • Give with 8 oz of water; encourage several glasses of water between meals.

INDICATIONS/ROUTES/DOSAGE

ULCERATIVE COLITIS

PO: ADULTS, ELDERLY: 1 g 3–4 times a day in divided doses q4–6h. Maintenance: 2 g/day in divided doses q6–12h. **Maximum:** 6 g/day. **CHILDREN 2 YRS AND OLDER:** Initially, 40–60 mg/kg/day in 3–6 divided doses. **Maintenance:** 20–30 mg/kg/day in 4 divided doses.

RHEUMATOID ARTHRITIS

PO: ADULTS, ELDERLY: Initially, 0.5–1 g/day for 1 wk. Increase by 0.5 g/wk, up to 3 g/day.

JUVENILE RHEUMATOID ARTHRITIS

PO: CHILDREN: Initially, 10 mg/kg/day. May increase by 10 mg/kg/day at weekly intervals. Range: 30–50 mg/kg/day. **Maximum:** 2 g/day.

DOSAGE IN RENAL IMPAIRMENT

Creatinine Clearance	Dosing Interval
10–30 ml/min	2 times/day
Less than 10 ml/min	Once daily

DOSAGE IN HEPATIC IMPAIRMENT

Avoid use.

S

SIDE EFFECTS

FREQUENT (33%): Anorexia, nausea, vomiting, headache, oligospermia (generally reversed by withdrawal of drug). **OCCASIONAL (3%):** Hypersensitivity reaction (rash, urticaria, pruritus, fever, anemia). **RARE (less than 1%):** Tinnitus, hypoglycemia, diuresis, photosensitivity.

ADVERSE EFFECTS/ TOXIC REACTIONS

Anaphylaxis, Stevens-Johnson syndrome, hematologic toxicity (leukopenia, agranulocytosis), hepatotoxicity, nephrotoxicity occur rarely.

NURSING CONSIDERATIONS

BASELINE ASSESSMENT

Question for hypersensitivity to medications. Check initial urinalysis, CBC, serum hepatic/renal function tests.

INTERVENTION/EVALUATION

Monitor I&O, urinalysis, renal function tests; ensure adequate hydration (minimum output 1,500 ml/24 hrs) to prevent nephrotoxicity. Assess skin for rash (discontinue drug, notify physician at first sign). Monitor daily pattern of bowel activity/stool consistency (dosage may need to be increased if diarrhea continues, recurs). Monitor CBC closely; assess for and report immediately any hematologic effects: bleeding, ecchymoses, fever, pharyngitis, pallor, weakness, purpura, jaundice.

PATIENT/FAMILY TEACHING

• May cause orange-yellow discoloration of urine, skin. • Space doses evenly around the clock. • Take after food with 8 oz of water; drink several glasses of water between meals. • Continue for full length of treatment; may be necessary to take drug even after symptoms relieved. • Follow-up, lab tests are essential. • Inform dentist, surgeon of sulfasalazine therapy. • Avoid exposure to sun, ultraviolet light until photosensitivity determined (may last for mos after last dose).

sulindac

sul-**in**-dak

(Apo-Sulin ✱, Clinoril, Novo-Sundac ✱)

Do not confuse Clinoril with Clozaril.

✦CLASSIFICATION

PHARMACOTHERAPEUTIC: Nonsteroidal anti-inflammatory. **CLINICAL:** Anti-inflammatory, antigout (see p. 125C).

ACTION

Produces analgesic, anti-inflammatory effects by inhibiting prostaglandin synthesis. **Therapeutic Effect:** Reduces inflammatory response, intensity of pain.

PHARMACOKINETICS

Route	Onset	Peak	Duration
PO (Antirheumatic)	7 days	2–3 wks	N/A

Well absorbed from GI tract. Metabolized in liver to active metabolite. Primarily excreted in urine. Not removed by hemodialysis. **Half-life:** 7.8 hrs; metabolite: 16.4 hrs.

USES

Treatment of pain of rheumatoid arthritis, osteoarthritis, ankylosing spondylitis, acute painful shoulder, bursitis, tendinitis, acute gouty arthritis.

PRECAUTIONS

CONTRAINDICATIONS: Active peptic ulcer disease, chronic inflammation of GI tract, GI bleeding/ulceration, history of hypersensitivity to aspirin, NSAIDs. **CAUTIONS:** Renal/hepatic impairment, history of GI tract disease, predisposition to fluid retention, concurrent anticoagulant use.

⌛ LIFESPAN CONSIDERATIONS:

Pregnancy/Lactation: Unknown if drug is excreted in breast milk. Avoid use during third trimester (may adversely affect fetal cardiovascular system: premature closure of ductus arteriosus). **Pregnancy Category C (D if used in third trimester near delivery). Children:** Safety and efficacy not established. **Elderly:** GI bleeding/ulceration more likely to cause serious adverse effects. Age-related renal impairment may increase risk of hepatic/renal toxicity; lower dosage recommended.

INTERACTIONS

DRUG: **Antacids** may decrease concentration. May decrease effects of **antihypertensives, diuretics. Aspirin, other salicylates** may increase risk of GI side effects, bleeding. **Bone marrow depressants** may increase risk of hematologic reactions. May increase effects of **heparin, oral anticoagulants, thrombolytics.** May increase concentration, risk of toxicity of **lithium.** May increase risk of **methotrexate** toxicity. **Probenecid** may increase concentration. **HERBAL: Cat's claw, dong quai, evening primrose, feverfew, red clover, garlic, ginseng, ginkgo** possess antiplatelet activity, may increase bleeding. **FOOD:** None known. **LAB VALUES:** May increase hepatic function test results, serum alkaline phosphatase.

AVAILABILITY (Rx)

TABLETS: 150 mg, 200 mg.

ADMINISTRATION/HANDLING

PO

- Give with food, milk, antacids if GI distress occurs.

INDICATIONS/ROUTES/DOSAGE

RHEUMATOID ARTHRITIS, OSTEOARTHRITIS, ANKYLOSING SPONDYLITIS

PO: ADULTS, ELDERLY: Initially, 150 mg twice a day; may increase up to 400 mg/day.

ACUTE SHOULDER PAIN, GOUTY ARTHRITIS, BURSITIS, TENDINITIS

PO: ADULTS, ELDERLY: 200 mg twice a day.

S

SIDE EFFECTS

FREQUENT (9%–4%): Diarrhea, constipation, indigestion, nausea, maculopapular rash, dermatitis, dizziness, headache. **OCCASIONAL (3%–1%):** Anorexia, abdominal cramps, flatulence.

ADVERSE EFFECTS/ TOXIC REACTIONS

Rare reactions with long-term use include peptic ulcer disease, GI bleeding, gastritis, nephrotoxicity (glomerular nephritis, interstitial nephritis, nephrotic syndrome), severe hepatic reactions (cholestasis, jaundice), severe hypersensitivity reactions (fever, chills, joint pain).

NURSING CONSIDERATIONS

BASELINE ASSESSMENT

Assess onset, type, location, duration of pain, fever, inflammation. Inspect affected joints for immobility, deformities, skin condition.

INTERVENTION/EVALUATION

Assist with ambulation if dizziness occurs. Monitor daily pattern of bowel activity/stool consistency. Assess for evidence of rash. Evaluate for therapeutic response: relief of pain, stiffness, swelling; increased joint mobility; reduced joint tenderness; improved grip strength. Monitor serum hepatic/renal function, CBC, platelets.

PATIENT/FAMILY TEACHING

• Therapeutic antiarthritic effect noted 1–3 wks after therapy begins. • Avoid aspirin, alcohol during therapy (increases risk of GI bleeding). • Take with food, milk if GI upset occurs. • Avoid tasks that require alertness, motor skills until response to drug is established (may cause dizziness).

sumatriptan

soo-ma-**trip**-tan

(Apo-Sumatriptan ✤, Imitrex, Imitrex Nasal, Imitrex Statdose, Imitrex Statdose Refill, Novo-Sumatriptan ✤)

Do not confuse sumatriptan with somatropin.

CLASSIFICATION

PHARMACOTHERAPEUTIC: Serotonin receptor agonist. **CLINICAL:** Antimigraine (see p. 60C).

ACTION

Binds selectively to vascular receptors, producing vasoconstrictive effect on cranial blood vessels. **Therapeutic Effect:** Relieves migraine headache.

PHARMACOKINETICS

Route	Onset	Peak	Duration
Nasal	15 min	N/A	24–48 hrs
PO	30 min	2 hrs	24–48 hrs
Subcutaneous	10 min	1 hr	24–48 hrs

Rapidly absorbed after subcutaneous administration. Absorption after PO administration is incomplete; significant amounts undergo hepatic metabolism, resulting in low bioavailability (about 14%). Protein binding: 10%–21%. Widely distributed. Undergoes first-pass metabolism in the liver. Excreted in urine. **Half-life:** 2 hrs.

USES

Acute treatment of migraine headache with or without aura; treatment of cluster headaches.

PRECAUTIONS

CONTRAINDICATIONS: Cerebrovascular accident (CVA), ischemic heart disease (including angina pectoris, history of MI, silent ischemia, Prinzmetal's angina), severe hepatic impairment, transient ischemic attack, uncontrolled hypertension, MAOI use within 14 days, use within 24 hrs of ergotamine preparations. **CAUTIONS:** Hepatic/renal impairment, epilepsy, hypersensitivity to sulfonamides.

LIFESPAN CONSIDERATIONS:

Pregnancy/Lactation: Unknown if distributed in breast milk. **Pregnancy Category C. Children:** Safety and efficacy not established. **Elderly:** No age-related precautions noted.

INTERACTIONS

DRUG: Ergotamine-containing medications may produce vasospastic reaction. **MAOIs** may increase concentration, half-life. **HERBAL:** None significant. **FOOD:** None known. **LAB VALUES:** None known.

AVAILABILITY (Rx)

INJECTION SOLUTION (IMITREX, IMITREX STATDOSE): 6 mg/0.5 ml, 4 mg prefilled cartridge. **NASAL SPRAY (IMITREX NASAL):** 5 mg, 20 mg. **TABLETS (IMITREX):** 25 mg, 50 mg, 100 mg.

ADMINISTRATION/HANDLING

SUBCUTANEOUS

• Follow manufacturer's instructions for autoinjection device use.

PO

• Swallow tablets whole. • Take with full glass of water.

NASAL

• Unit contains only one spray—do not test before use. • Gently blow nose to clear nasal passages. • With head upright, close one nostril with index finger, breathe out gently through mouth. • Insert nozzle into open nostril about ½ inch. • Close mouth and, while taking a breath through nose, release spray dosage by firmly pressing blue plunger. • Remove nozzle from nose and gently breathe in through nose and out through mouth for 10–20 sec. Do not breathe in deeply.

INDICATIONS/ROUTES/DOSAGE

ACUTE MIGRAINE HEADACHE

PO: ADULTS, ELDERLY: 25–50 mg. Dose may be repeated after at least 2 hrs. **Maximum:** 100 mg/single dose; 200 mg/24 hrs.
SUBCUTANEOUS: ADULTS, ELDERLY: 6 mg. **Maximum:** Two 6-mg injections/24 hrs (separated by at least 1 hr).
INTRANASAL: ADULTS, ELDERLY: 5–20 mg; may repeat in 2 hrs. **Maximum:** 40 mg/24 hrs.

SIDE EFFECTS

FREQUENT: Oral (10%–5%): Tingling, nasal discomfort. **Subcutaneous (greater than 10%):** Injection site reactions, tingling, warm/hot sensation, dizziness, vertigo. **Nasal (greater than 10%):** Altered taste, nausea, vomiting. **OCCASIONAL: Oral (5%–1%):** Flushing, asthenia, visual disturbances. **Subcutaneous (10%–2%):** Burning sensation, numbness, chest discomfort, drowsiness, asthenia. **Nasal (5%–1%):** Nasopharyngeal discomfort, dizziness. **RARE: Oral (less than 1%):** Agitation, eye irritation, dysuria. **Subcutaneous (less than 2%):** Anxiety, fatigue, diaphoresis, muscle cramps, myalgia. **Nasal (less than 1%):** Burning sensation.

ADVERSE EFFECTS/ TOXIC REACTIONS

Excessive dosage may produce tremor, redness of extremities, reduced respirations, cyanosis, seizures, paralysis. Serious arrhythmias occur rarely, esp. in pts with hypertension, obesity, smokers, diabetes, strong family history of coronary artery disease.

NURSING CONSIDERATIONS

BASELINE ASSESSMENT

Question for history of peripheral vascular disease, renal/hepatic impairment, possibility of pregnancy. Question regarding onset, location, duration of migraine, possible precipitating symptoms.

INTERVENTION/EVALUATION

Evaluate for relief of migraine headache and resulting photophobia, phonophobia (sound sensitivity), nausea, vomiting.

PATIENT/FAMILY TEACHING

• Teach pt proper loading of autoinjector, injection technique, discarding of syringe. • Do not use more than 2 injections during any 24-hr period and allow at least 1 hr between injections. • Contact physician immediately if wheezing, palpitations, skin rash, facial swelling, pain/tightness in chest/throat occurs.

sunitinib

sue-**nit**-ih-nib
(Sutent)

CLASSIFICATION

PHARMACOTHERAPEUTIC: Tyrosine kinase inhibitor, vascular endothelial growth factor. **CLINICAL:** Antineoplastic.

ACTION

Inhibitory action against multiple kinases, growth factor receptors, stem cell factor receptors, colony-stimulating factor receptors, glial cell-line neurotrophic factor receptors. **Therapeutic Efffect:** Prevents tumor cell growth, produces tumor regression, inhibits metastasis.

PHARMACOKINETICS

Metabolized in liver. Protein binding: 95%. Excreted mainly in feces, with lesser amount eliminated in urine. **Half-life:** 40–60 hrs.

USES

Treatment of GI stromal tumor after disease progression while on or demonstrating intolerance to imatinib. Treatment of advanced renal cell carcinoma. **OFF-LABEL:** Treatment of acute myeloid leukemia (AML).

PRECAUTIONS

CONTRAINDICATIONS: None significant. **CAUTIONS:** Cardiac abnormalities, bleeding tendencies, hypertension.

LIFESPAN CONSIDERATIONS:

Pregnancy/Lactation: Has potential for embryotoxic, teratogenic effects. Avoid breast-feeding. **Pregnancy Category D. Children:** Safety and efficacy not established. **Elderly:** No age-related precautions noted.

INTERACTIONS

DRUG: **Ketoconazole, itraconazole, clarithromycin, atazanavir, indinavir, nefazodone, nelfinavir, ritonavir, saquinavir, telithromycin, voriconizole** may increase concentration, toxicity. **Dexamethasone, phenytoin, carbamazepine, rifampin, rifabutin, rifapentin, phenobarbital** may decrease concentration, effect. **HERBAL:** **St. John's wort** may decrease concentration. **FOOD:** **Grapefruit, grapefruit juice** may increase concentration. **LAB VALUES:** May increase serum alkaline phosphatase, bilirubin, amylase, lipase, creatinine, AST, ALT. May alter serum potassium, sodium uric acid. May produce thrombocytopenia, neutropenia. May decrease serum phosphates, thyroid function.

AVAILABILITY (Rx)

CAPSULES: 12.5 mg, 25 mg, 50 mg.

ADMINISTRATION/HANDLING

PO

Give without regard to food.

INDICATIONS/ROUTES/DOSAGE

GI STROMAL TUMOR, RENAL CELL CARCINOMA

PO: ADULTS, ELDERLY: 50 mg once daily for 4 wks, followed by 2 wks off.

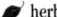

DOSE MODIFICATION

PO: ADULTS, ELDERLY: Dosage increase or reduction in 12.5-mg increments is recommended.

CONCURRENT THERAPY WITH IMATINIB

PO: ADULTS, ELDERLY: (Sunitinib): Recommended dose is increased to maximum 87.5 mg daily or reduced to minimum of 37.5 mg.

SIDE EFFECTS

Stromal tumor: COMMON (42%–30%): Fatigue, diarrhea, anorexia, abdominal pain, nausea, hyperpigmentation. **FREQUENT (29%–18%):** Mucositis/stomatitis, vomiting, asthenia (loss of strength, energy), altered taste, constipation, fever. **OCCASIONAL (15%–8%):** Hypertension, rash, myalgia, headache, arthralgia, back pain, dyspnea, cough. **Renal carcinoma: COMMON (74%–43%):** Fatigue, diarrhea, nausea, mucositis/stomatitis, dyspepsia (heartburn, indigestion, epigastric pain), altered taste. **FREQUENT (38%–20%):** Rash, vomiting, constipation, hyperpigmentation, anorexia, arthralgia, dyspnea, hypertension, headache, abdominal pain. **OCCASIONAL (18%–11%):** Limb pain, peripheral/periorbital edema, dry skin, hair color change, myalgia, cough, back pain, dizziness, fever, tongue pain, flatulence, alopecia, dehydration.

ADVERSE EFFECTS/ TOXIC REACTIONS

Hand-foot syndrome occurs occasionally (14%), manifested as blistering/rash/peeling of skin on palms of hands, soles of feet. Bleeding, decrease in left ventricular ejection fraction, DVT, pancreatitis, neutropenia, seizures occur rarely.

NURSING CONSIDERATIONS

BASELINE ASSESSMENT

Question possibility of pregnancy. Obtain baseline CBC, serum chemistries including electrolytes, renal/hepatic function tests (alkaline phosphatase, bilirubin, ALT, AST) before beginning treatment and monthly thereafter.

INTERVENTION/EVALUATION

Assess eye area, lower extremities for early evidence of fluid retention. Offer antiemetics to control nausea, vomiting. Monitor daily pattern of bowel activity/stool consistency. Monitor CBC for evidence of neutropenia, thrombocytopenia; assess hepatic function tests for hepatotoxicity.

PATIENT/FAMILY TEACHING

Avoid crowds, those with known infection. Avoid contact with anyone who recently received live virus vaccine. Do not have immunizations without physician's approval (drug lowers resistance). Promptly report fever, unusual bruising/bleeding from any site.

Survanta, *see beractant*

Sustiva, *see efavirenz*

Symlin, *see pramlinitide*

Synagis, *see palivizumab*

Synthroid, *see levothyroxine*

tacrine

tay-crin
(Cognex)

CLASSIFICATION

PHARMACOTHERAPEUTIC: Cholinesterase inhibitor. **CLINICAL:** Antidementia.

ACTION

Elevates acetylcholine concentrations in cerebral cortex by slowing degeneration of acetylcholine released by still-intact cholinergic neurons (Alzheimer's disease involves degeneration of cholinergic neuronal pathways). **Therapeutic Effect:** Slows progression of Alzheimer's disease.

PHARMACOKINETICS

Rapidly absorbed following PO administration. Protein binding: 55%. Extensively metabolized in liver. Negligible amounts excreted in urine. **Half-life:** 2–4 hrs.

USES

Symptomatic treatment of pts with Alzheimer's disease.

PRECAUTIONS

CONTRAINDICATIONS: Known hypersensitivity to tacrine, pts previously treated with tacrine who developed jaundice. **CAUTIONS:** Known hepatic dysfunction, asthma, chronic obstructive pulmonary disease (COPD), seizure disorders, bradycardia, hyperthyroidism, cardiac arrhythmias, history of gastric/intestinal ulcers, alcohol abuse.

LIFESPAN CONSIDERATIONS:

Pregnancy/Lactation: Unknown if distributed in breast milk. **Pregnancy Category C. Children:** Safety and efficacy not established. **Elderly:** No age-related precautions noted.

INTERACTIONS

DRUG: May interfere with **anticholinergic** effects. **Cimetidine** may increase concentration. May increase adverse effects of **NSAIDs**. May increase **theophylline** concentration. **HERBAL:** None significant. **FOOD:** None known. **LAB VALUES:** Increases AST, ALT. Alters Hgb, Hct, serum electrolytes.

AVAILABILITY (Rx)

CAPSULES: 10 mg, 20 mg, 30 mg, 40 mg.

ADMINISTRATION/HANDLING

PO

- Give without regard to food.

INDICATIONS/ROUTES/DOSAGE

ALZHEIMER'S DISEASE

PO: ADULTS, ELDERLY: Initially, 10 mg 4 times a day for 6 wks, followed by 20 mg 4 times a day for 6 wks, 30 mg 4 times a day for 12 wks, then 40 mg 4 times a day if needed.

DOSAGE IN HEPATIC IMPAIRMENT

For pts with ALT greater than 3–5 times normal, decrease dose by 40 mg/day and resume normal dose when ALT returns to normal. For pts with ALT greater than 5 times normal, stop treatment and resume when ALT returns to normal.

SIDE EFFECTS

FREQUENT (28%–11%): Headache, nausea, vomiting, diarrhea, dizziness. **OCCASIONAL (9%–4%):** Fatigue, chest pain, dyspepsia, (heartburn, indigestion, epigastric pain), anorexia, abdominal pain, flatulence constipation, confusion, agitation, rash, depression, ataxia, insomnia, rhinitis, myalgia. **RARE (less than 3%):** Weight loss, anxiety, cough, facial flushing, urinary frequency, back pain, tremor.

ADVERSE EFFECTS/ TOXIC REACTIONS

Overdose can cause cholinergic crisis, (increased salivation, lacrimation,

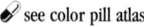

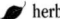

bradycardia, respiratory depression, hypotension, increased muscle weakness). Treatment aimed at supportive measures, use of anticholinergics (e.g., atropine).

NURSING CONSIDERATIONS

BASELINE ASSESSMENT

Assess cognitive, behavioral, functional deficits of pt. Assess hepatic function.

INTERVENTION/EVALUATION

Monitor cognitive, behavioral, functional status of pt. Monitor AST, ALT, EKG evaluation, periodic rhythm strips in pts with underlying arrhythmias. Monitor for symptoms of GI bleeding, ulceration.

PATIENT/FAMILY TEACHING

• Take at regular intervals, between meals (may take with meals if GI upset occurs). • Do not reduce or stop medication; do not increase dosage without physician direction. • Do not smoke (reduces plasma concentration of tacrine). • Inform family of local chapter of Alzheimer's Disease Association (provides guide to services for these pts).

tacrolimus

tack-row-**lee**-mus

(Prograf, Protopic)

Do not confuse Protopic with Protonix, Protopam, Protopin.

CLASSIFICATION

PHARMACOTHERAPEUTIC: Immunologic agent. **CLINICAL:** Immunosuppressant (see p. 115C).

ACTION

Inhibits T-lymphocyte activation by binding to intracellular proteins, forming a complex, inhibiting phosphatase activity. **Therapeutic Effect:** Suppresses immunologically mediated inflammatory response; prevents organ transplant rejection.

PHARMACOKINETICS

Variably absorbed after PO administration (food reduces absorption). Protein binding: 75%–97%. Extensively metabolized in liver. Excreted in urine. Not removed by hemodialysis. **Half-life:** 11.7 hrs.

USES

Oral/injection: Prophylaxis of organ rejection in pts receiving allogeneic liver, kidney, heart transplant. Should be used concurrently with adrenal corticosteroids. **Topical:** Atopic dermatitis. **OFF-LABEL:** Prevention of organ rejection in pts receiving allogeneic bone marrow, heart, pancreas, pancreatic island cell, small-bowel transplant; treatment of autoimmune disease; severe recalcitrant psoriasis.

PRECAUTIONS

CONTRAINDICATIONS: Concurrent use with cyclosporine (increases risk of nephrotoxicity), hypersensitivity to HCO-60 polyoxyl 60 hydrogenated castor oil (used in solution for injection). **CAUTIONS:** Immunosuppressed pts, renal/hepatic impairment.

LIFESPAN CONSIDERATIONS:

Pregnancy/Lactation: Crosses placenta. Hyperkalemia, renal dysfunction noted in neonates. Excreted in breast milk. Avoid breast-feeding. **Pregnancy Category C.** **Children:** May require higher dosages (decreased bioavailability, increased clearance). May make post-transplant lymphoproliferative disorder more common (esp. in those younger than 3 yrs). **Elderly:** Age-related renal impairment may require dosage adjustment.

T

INTERACTIONS

DRUG: **Antacids** may decrease absorption of tacrolimus. **Erythromycin, itraconazole, ketoconazole** may increase concentration, risk of toxicity. **Rifampin** may decrease concentration, effect. **Potassium-sparing diuretics** may increase risk of hyperkalemia. **Cyclosporine** increases risk of nephrotoxicity. **Live virus vaccines** may potentiate virus replication, increase vaccine side effects, decrease pt's antibody response to vaccine. **HERBAL:** **Echinacea** may decrease effect. **St. John's wort** may decrease concentration, effect. **FOOD:** **Food** decreases rate/extent of absorption. **Grapefruit, grapefruit juice** may increase concentration, toxicity. **LAB VALUES:** May increase serum glucose, BUN, creatinine, WBC count. May decrease serum magnesium, RBC, thrombocyte counts. May alter serum potassium.

AVAILABILITY (Rx)

CAPSULES (PROGRAF): 0.5 mg, 1 mg, 5 mg. **INJECTION SOLUTION (PROGRAF):** 5 mg/ml. **OINTMENT (PROTOPIC):** 0.03%, 0.1%.

ADMINISTRATION/HANDLING

IV

Reconstitution • Dilute with appropriate amount (250–1,000 ml, depending on desired dose) 0.9% NaCl or D_5W to provide concentration between 0.004 and 0.02 mg/ml.

Rate of administration • Give as continuous IV infusion. • Continuously monitor pt for anaphylaxis for at least 30 min after start of infusion. • Stop infusion immediately at first sign of hypersensitivity reaction.

Storage • Store diluted infusion solution in glass or polyethylene containers and discard after 24 hrs. • Do not store in PVC container (decreased stability, potential for extraction).

PO

• Administer on empty stomach. • Do not give with grapefruit, grapefruit juice or within 2 hrs of antacids.

TOPICAL

• For external use only. • Do not cover with occlusive dressing. • Rub gently, completely onto clean, dry skin.

IV INCOMPATIBILITIES

No known drug incompatibilities. Do not mix with other medications if possible.

IV COMPATIBILITIES

Calcium gluconate, dexamethasone (Decadron), diphenhydramine (Benadryl), dobutamine (Dobutrex), dopamine (Intropin), furosemide (Lasix), heparin, hydromorphone (Dilaudid), insulin, leucovorin, lipids, lorazepam (Ativan), morphine, nitroglycerin, potassium chloride.

INDICATIONS/ROUTES/DOSAGE

PREVENTION OF LIVER TRANSPLANT REJECTION

PO: ADULTS, ELDERLY: 0.1–0.15 mg/kg/day in 2 divided doses 12 hrs apart. **CHILDREN:** 0.15–0.2 mg/kg/day in 2 divided doses 12 hrs apart.

IV: ADULTS, ELDERLY, CHILDREN: 0.03–0.05 mg/kg/day as continuous infusion.

PREVENTION OF KIDNEY TRANSPLANT REJECTION

PO: ADULTS, ELDERLY: 0.2 mg/kg/day in 2 divided doses 12 hrs apart.

IV: ADULTS, ELDERLY: 0.03–0.05 mg/kg/day as continuous infusion.

PREVENTION OF HEART TRANSPLANT REJECTION

PO: ADULTS, ELDERLY: Initially, 0.075 mg/kg/day in 2 divided doses 12 hrs apart.

ATOPIC DERMATITIS

TOPICAL: ADULTS, ELDERLY, CHILDREN 2 YRS AND OLDER: Apply 0.03% ointment to affected area twice a day. (0.1% ointment may be used in adults, elderly). Continue treatment for 1 wk after symptoms have resolved.

T

SIDE EFFECTS

FREQUENT (greater than 30%): Headache, tremor, insomnia, paresthesia, diarrhea, nausea, constipation, vomiting, abdominal pain, hypertension. **OCCASIONAL (29%–10%):** Rash, pruritus, anorexia, asthenia (loss of strength, energy), peripheral edema, photosensitivity.

ADVERSE EFFECTS/ TOXIC REACTIONS

Nephrotoxicity (characterized by increased serum creatinine, decreased urinary output), neurotoxicity (tremor, headache, altered mental status), pleural effusion occur commonly. Thrombocytopenia, leukocytosis, anemia, atelectasis, sepsis, infection occur occasionally.

NURSING CONSIDERATIONS

BASELINE ASSESSMENT

Assess medical, drug history, esp. renal function, use of other immunosuppressants. Have aqueous solution of epinephrine 1:1,000 available at bedside as well as O_2 before beginning IV infusion. Assess pt continuously for first 30 min following start of infusion and at frequent intervals thereafter.

INTERVENTION/EVALUATION

Closely monitor pts with renal impairment. Monitor lab values, esp. serum creatinine, potassium levels, CBC with differential, serum hepatic function tests. Monitor I&O closely. CBC should be performed weekly during first mo of therapy, twice monthly during second and third mos of treatment, then monthly throughout the first yr. Report any major change in pt assessment.

PATIENT/FAMILY TEACHING

• Take dose at same time each day. • Avoid crowds, those with infection. • Inform physician if decreased urination, chest pain, headache, dizziness, respiratory infection, rash, unusual bleeding/bruising occurs. • Avoid exposure to sun, artificial light (may cause photosensitivity reaction).

tadalafil

tah-**dal**-ah-fill
(Cialis)

CLASSIFICATION

PHARMACOTHERAPEUTIC: Phosphodiesterase inhibitor. **CLINICAL:** Erectile dysfunction adjunct.

ACTION

Inhibits phosphodiesterase type 5, the enzyme responsible for degrading cyclic guanosine monophosphate in corpus cavernosum of penis, resulting in smooth muscle relaxation, increased blood flow. **Therapeutic Effect:** Facilitates erection.

PHARMACOKINETICS

Route	Onset	Peak	Duration
PO	16 min	2 hrs	36 hrs

Rapidly absorbed after PO administration. Drug has no effect on penile blood flow without sexual stimulation. **Half-life:** 17.5 hrs.

USES

Treatment of erectile dysfunction. **OFF-LABEL:** Raynaud's phenomenon.

PRECAUTIONS

CONTRAINDICATIONS: Concurrent use of alpha-adrenergic blockers (other than minimum dose tamsulosin), concurrent use of sodium nitroprusside or nitrates in any form, severe hepatic impairment. **CAUTIONS:** Renal/hepatic impairment, anatomical deformation of penis, pts who may be predisposed to priapism (sickle cell anemia, multiple myeloma, leukemia).

LIFESPAN CONSIDERATIONS:

Pregnancy/Lactation: Pregnancy Category B. **Children:** Not indicated in this pt population. **Elderly:** No age-related precautions noted.

INTERACTIONS

DRUG: **Alcohol** increases risk of orthostatic hypotension. Potentiates hypotensive effects of **alpha-adrenergic blockers, nitrates. Erythromycin, indinavir, itraconazole, ketoconazole, ritonavir** may increase concentration. **HERBAL:** None significant. **FOOD:** **Grapefruit, grapefruit juice** may increase concentration, toxicity. **LAB VALUES:** None known.

AVAILABILITY (Rx)

TABLETS: 5 mg, 10 mg, 20 mg.

ADMINISTRATION/HANDLING

PO

- May give without regard to food.
- Take at least 30 min before anticipated sexual activity.

INDICATIONS/ROUTES/DOSAGE

ERECTILE DYSFUNCTION

PO: ADULTS, ELDERLY: 10 mg 30 min before sexual activity. Dose may be increased to 20 mg or decreased to 5 mg, based on pt tolerance. Maximum dosing frequency is once daily.

DOSAGE IN RENAL IMPAIRMENT

For pts with creatinine clearance 31–50 ml/min: Starting dose is 5 mg before sexual activity once a day; maximum dose is 10 mg no more frequently than once q48h. **For pts with creatinine clearance of less than 31 ml/min:** Starting dose is 5 mg before sexual activity once a day.

DOSAGE IN MILD TO MODERATE HEPATIC IMPAIRMENT

Pts with Child-Pugh class A or B hepatic impairment should take no more than 10 mg once a day.

SIDE EFFECTS

OCCASIONAL: Headache, dyspepsia (heartburn, indigestion, epigastric pain), back pain, myalgia, nasal congestion, flushing.

ADVERSE EFFECTS/ TOXIC REACTIONS

Prolonged erections (lasting over 4 hrs), priapism (painful erections lasting over 6 hrs) occur rarely. Angina, chest pain, MI have been reported.

NURSING CONSIDERATIONS

BASELINE ASSESSMENT

Assess cardiovascular status before initiating treatment for erectile dysfunction.

PATIENT/FAMILY TEACHING

• Has no effect in absence of sexual stimulation. • Seek treatment immediately if erection persists for over 4 hrs.

Tagamet, *see cimetidine*

Tamiflu, *see oseltamivir*

tamoxifen

tam-**ox**-ih-feen

(Apo-Tamox ✤, Istubol, Nolvadex, Nolvadex-D ✤, Novo-Tamoxifen ✤, Soltamox, Tamofen ✤)

CLASSIFICATION

PHARMACOTHERAPEUTIC: Nonsteroidal antiestrogen. **CLINICAL:** Antineoplastic (see p. 83C).

ACTION

Competes with estradiol for estrogen-receptor binding sites in breasts, uterus,

T

vagina. **Therapeutic Effect:** Inhibits DNA synthesis, estrogen response.

PHARMACOKINETICS

Well absorbed from GI tract. Metabolized in liver. Primarily eliminated in feces by biliary system. **Half-life:** 7 days.

USES

Adjunct treatment in advanced breast cancer, reduce risk of breast cancer in pts at high risk, reduce risk of invasive breast cancer in women with ductal carcinoma *in situ* (DCIS), metastatic breast cancer in women and men, treatment of melanoma, desmoid tumors. **OFF-LABEL:** Induction of ovulation.

PRECAUTIONS

CONTRAINDICATIONS: Concomitant coumarin-type therapy when used in treatment of breast cancer in high-risk women, history of deep vein thrombosis or pulmonary embolism in high-risk women. **CAUTIONS:** Leukopenia, thrombocytopenia, pregnancy.

⌛ LIFESPAN CONSIDERATIONS:

Pregnancy/Lactation: If possible, avoid use during pregnancy, esp. first trimester. May cause fetal harm. Unknown if distributed in breast milk. Breast-feeding not recommended. **Pregnancy Category D.** **Children:** Safe and effective in girls 2–10 yrs with McCune Albright syndrome, precocious puberty. **Elderly:** No age-related precautions noted.

INTERACTIONS

DRUG: **Anticoagulants** may increase risk of bleeding. **Cytotoxic agents** may increase risk of thromboembolic events. May increase effect of **warfarin. Estrogens** may decrease effects. **HERBAL:** Avoid **black cohosh, dong quai** in estrogen-dependent tumors. **Red clover, St. John's wort** may decrease concentration, effect. **FOOD:** None known. **LAB VALUES:** May increase serum cholesterol, calcium, triglycerides.

AVAILABILITY (Rx)

ORAL LIQUID (SOLTAMOX): 10 mg/5 ml.
TABLETS (NOLVADEX): 10 mg, 20 mg.

ADMINISTRATION/HANDLING

PO

- Give without regard to food.

INDICATIONS/ROUTES/DOSAGE

ADJUNCTIVE TREATMENT OF BREAST CANCER

PO: ADULTS, ELDERLY: 20–40 mg/day. Give doses greater than 20 mg/day in divided doses.

PREVENTION OF BREAST CANCER IN HIGH-RISK WOMEN

PO: ADULTS, ELDERLY: 20 mg/day.

SIDE EFFECTS

FREQUENT: **Women (greater than 10%):** Hot flashes, nausea, vomiting. **OCCASIONAL:** **Women (9%–1%):** Changes in menstruation, genital itching, vaginal discharge, endometrial hyperplasia, polyps. **Men:** Impotence, decreased libido. **Men and women:** Headache, nausea, vomiting, rash, bone pain, confusion, weakness, drowsiness.

ADVERSE EFFECTS/ TOXIC REACTIONS

Retinopathy, corneal opacity, decreased visual acuity noted in pts receiving extremely high dosages (240–320 mg/day) for longer than 17 mos.

NURSING CONSIDERATIONS

BASELINE ASSESSMENT

Obtain estrogen receptor assay prior to therapy. CBC, platelet count, serum calcium levels should be checked before and periodically during therapy.

T

INTERVENTION/EVALUATION

Be alert to increased bone pain, ensure adequate pain relief. Monitor I&O, weight. Observe for edema, esp. of dependent areas. Assess for hypercalcemia (increased urinary volume, excessive thirst, nausea, vomiting, constipation, hypotonicity of muscles, deep bone/flank pain, renal stones).

PATIENT/FAMILY TEACHING

• Report vaginal bleeding/discharge/itching, leg cramps, weight gain, shortness of breath, weakness. • May initially experience increase in bone, tumor pain (appears to indicate good tumor response). • Contact physician if nausea, vomiting continues at home. • Nonhormonal contraceptives are recommended during treatment.

tamsulosin

tam-**sool**-o-sin

(Flomax)

Do not confuse Flomax with Fosamax or Volmax.

CLASSIFICATION

PHARMACOTHERAPEUTIC: $Alpha_1$-adrenergic blocker. **CLINICAL:** Benign prostatic hyperplasia agent.

ACTION

Targets receptors around bladder neck, prostate capsule. **Therapeutic Effect:** Relaxes smooth muscle, improves urinary flow, symptoms of prostatic hyperplasia.

PHARMACOKINETICS

Well absorbed, widely distributed. Protein binding: 94%–99%. Metabolized in liver. Primarily excreted in urine. Unknown if removed by hemodialysis. **Half-life:** 9–13 hrs.

USES

Treatment of symptoms of benign prostatic hyperplasia.

PRECAUTIONS

CONTRAINDICATIONS: None significant. **CAUTIONS:** Concurrent use of phosphodiesterase (PDE_5) inhibitors (sildenafil, tadalafil, vardenafil), renal impairment.

LIFESPAN CONSIDERATIONS:

Pregnancy/Lactation: Not indicated for use in women. **Pregnancy Category B. Children:** Not indicated in this pt population. **Elderly:** No age-related precautions noted.

INTERACTIONS

DRUG: **Other alpha-adrenergic blocking agents (e.g., doxazosin, prazosin, terazosin)** may increase alpha-blockade effects of both drugs. **Sildenafil, tadafil, vardenafil** may cause severe hypotension. May alter effects of **warfarin**. **HERBAL:** Avoid **saw palmetto** (limited experience with this combination). **FOOD:** None known. **LAB VALUES:** None known.

AVAILABILITY (Rx)

CAPSULES: 0.4 mg.

ADMINISTRATION/HANDLING

PO

• Give at same time each day, 30 min after the same meal. • Do not crush/open capsule.

INDICATIONS/ROUTES/DOSAGE

BENIGN PROSTATIC HYPERPLASIA

PO: ADULTS: 0.4 mg once a day, approximately 30 min after same meal each day. May increase dosage to 0.8 mg if inadequate response in 2–4 wks.

SIDE EFFECTS

FREQUENT (9%–7%): Dizziness, drowsiness. **OCCASIONAL (5%–3%):** Headache, anxiety, insomnia, orthostatic hypotension. **RARE (less than 2%):** Nasal congestion, pharyngitis, rhinitis, nausea, vertigo, impotence.

ADVERSE EFFECTS/ TOXIC REACTIONS

First-dose syncope (hypotension with sudden loss of consciousness) may occur within 30–90 min after initial dose. May be preceded by tachycardia (pulse rate of 120–160 beats/min).

NURSING CONSIDERATIONS

BASELINE ASSESSMENT

Question for sensitivity to tamsulosin, use of other alpha-adrenergic blocking agents, warfarin.

INTERVENTION/EVALUATION

Assist with ambulation if dizziness occurs. Monitor renal function, B/P.

PATIENT/FAMILY TEACHING

• Take at same time each day, 30 min after the same meal. • Use caution when getting up from sitting or lying position. • Avoid tasks that require alertness, motor skills until response to drug is established. • Do not chew, crush, open capsule.

Taxol, *see paclitaxel*

Taxotere, *see docetaxel*

tazarotene

tay-zah-**row**-teen

(Avage, Tazorac)

CLASSIFICATION

PHARMACOTHERAPEUTIC: Retinoid. **CLINICAL:** Antipsoriasis, antiacne.

ACTION

Modulates differentiation/proliferation of epithelial tissue; binds selectively to retinoic acid receptors. **Therapeutic Effect:** Restores normal differentiation of epidermis, reduces epidermal inflammation.

USES

Treatment of stable plaque psoriasis in pts with up to 20% body surface area involvement. Treatment of mild to moderate facial acne.

PRECAUTIONS

CONTRAINDICATIONS: Pregnancy or those who may become pregnant. **CAUTIONS:** None significant.

LIFESPAN CONSIDERATIONS:

Pregnancy/Lactation: Unknown if distributed in breast milk. May cause fetal harm. **Pregnancy Category X. Children:** Safety and efficacy not established. **Elderly:** No age-related precautions noted.

INTERACTIONS

DRUG: May increase phototoxicity with **thiazides, tetracyclines, fluoroquinolones, penothiazines.** Increased toxicity may occur with any **medication having strong drying effects (e.g., salicylic acid, resorcinol). HERBAL:** None significant. **FOOD:** None known. **LAB VALUES:** None significant.

AVAILABILITY (Rx)

CREAM: 0.05% **(TAZORAC),** 0.1% **(AVAGE). GEL (TAZORAC):** 0.05%, 0.1%.

INDICATIONS/ROUTES/DOSAGE

ACNE

TOPICAL: ADULTS, ELDERLY, CHILDREN 12 YRS AND OLDER: *(Cream, gel 0.1%)*: Cleanse face. After skin is dry, apply thin film once a day in the evening.

T

PSORIASIS

TOPICAL: ADULTS, ELDERLY, CHILDREN 12 YRS AND OLDER: *(Gel 0.05%, 0.1%)*: Apply once a day in evening (no more than 20% of body surface area). **ADULTS, ELDERLY:** *(Cream 0.05%, 0.1%)*: Apply once a day in evening (no more than 20% of body surface area).

SIDE EFFECTS

FREQUENT (30%–10%): Acne: Desquamation, burning/stinging, dry skin, pruritus, erythema. **Psoriasis:** Itching, burning/stinging, erythema, worsening of psoriasis, irritation, skin pain. **OCCASIONAL (9%–1%): Acne:** Irritation, skin pain, fissuring, localized edema, skin discoloration. **Psoriasis:** Rash, desquamation, contact dermatitis, skin inflammation, fissuring, bleeding, dry skin.

ADVERSE EFFECTS/ TOXIC REACTIONS

None significant.

NURSING CONSIDERATIONS

BASELINE ASSESSMENT

Assess for sensitivity to tazarotene. Determine whether pt is taking medications that may increase risk of photosensitivity (e.g., sulfa, fluoroquinolones).

INTERVENTION/EVALUATION

Monitor for improvement of psoriasis, acne. Assess skin for irritation, burning, stinging.

PATIENT/FAMILY TEACHING

• Discontinue if skin irritation, pruritus, skin redness is excessive; contact physician. • For external use only. • Avoid contact with eyes, eyelids, mouth. • Photosensitization may occur; use sunscreen, protective clothing.

T

tegaserod

teh-**gas**-er-od
(Zelnorm)

CLASSIFICATION

PHARMACOTHERAPEUTIC: $5\text{-}HT_4$ receptor partial agonist. **CLINICAL:** GI peristaltic agent.

ACTION

Binds to $5\text{-}HT_4$ receptors in GI tract. **Therapeutic Effect:** Triggers peristaltic reflex in gut, increasing bowel motility.

PHARMACOKINETICS

Rapidly absorbed. Widely distributed. Protein binding: 98%. Metabolized by hydrolysis in stomach, by oxidation and conjugation of primary metabolite. Primarily excreted in feces. **Half-life:** 11 hrs.

USES

Short-term treatment of women with irritable bowel syndrome whose primary bowel symptom is constipation. Treatment of chronic constipation in those younger than 65 yrs.

PRECAUTIONS

CONTRAINDICATIONS: Abdominal adhesions, diarrhea, history of bowel obstruction, moderate to severe hepatic impairment, severe renal impairment, suspected sphincter of Oddi dysfunction, symptomatic gallbladder disease. **CAUTIONS:** None known.

LIFESPAN CONSIDERATIONS:

Pregnancy/Lactation: Unknown if distributed in breast milk. **Pregnancy Category B. Children:** Safety and efficacy not established. **Elderly:** No age related precautions noted.

INTERACTIONS

DRUG: None significant. **HERBAL:** None significant. **FOOD:** None known. **LAB VALUES:** None known.

AVAILABILITY (Rx)

TABLETS: 2 mg, 6 mg.

ADMINISTRATION/HANDLING

PO

• Give before meals. • Tablets may be crushed.

INDICATIONS/ROUTES/DOSAGE

IRRITABLE BOWEL SYNDROME

PO: ADULTS, ELDERLY WOMEN: 6 mg twice a day for 4–6 wks.

CHRONIC CONSTIPATION

PO: ADULTS: 6 mg twice a day.

SIDE EFFECTS

FREQUENT (greater than 5%): Headache, abdominal pain, diarrhea, nausea, flatulence. **OCCASIONAL (5%–2%):** Dizziness, migraine, back pain, extremity pain.

ADVERSE EFFECTS/ TOXIC REACTIONS

Ischemic colitis, hypersensitivity reaction (rash, urticaria, pruritus) occur rarely.

NURSING CONSIDERATIONS

BASELINE ASSESSMENT

Assess for diarrhea (avoid use in these pts).

INTERVENTION/EVALUATION

Assess for improvement in symptoms (relief from GI bloating, cramping, urgency, abdominal discomfort).

PATIENT/FAMILY TEACHING

• Take before meals. • Inform physician of new/worsening episodes of abdominal pain, severe diarrhea.

Tegretol, *see carbamazepine*

telbivudine

tell-**biv**-you-deen

(Tyzeka)

♦ CLASSIFICATION

PHARMACOTHERAPEUTIC: Synthetic thymidine nucleoside analogue. **CLINICAL:** Antiretroviral.

ACTION

Inhibits hepatitis B virus DNA polymerase, an enzyme necessary for replication, resulting in DNA chain termination. **Therapeutic Effect:** Inhibits hepatitis B virus replication.

PHARMACOKINETICS

Rapidly absorbed following PO administration. Widely distributed into tissues. Primarily excreted unchanged in urine. **Half-life:** 40–49 hrs.

USES

Treatment of chronic hepatitis B in adults with evidence of viral replication and either evidence of persistent elevations in hepatic enzymes (ALT, AST) or histologically active disease.

PRECAUTIONS

CONTRAINDICATIONS: None significant. **CAUTIONS:** Renal impairment.

⌛ LIFESPAN CONSIDERATIONS:

Pregnancy/Lactation: Unknown if distributed in breast milk. **Pregnancy Category B. Children:** Safety and efficacy not established. **Elderly:** Age-related renal impairment may require dosage adjustment.

T

INTERACTIONS

DRUG: Co-administration with drugs that alter renal function may alter telbuvidine concentration. **HERBAL:** None significant. **FOOD:** None known. **LAB VALUES:** May increase amylase, lipase, ALT, AST, total bilirubin, creatine phosphokinase (CPK). May produce neutropenia, thrombocytopenia.

AVAILABILITY (Rx)

TABLETS (FILM-COATED): 600 mg.

ADMINISTRATION/HANDLING

PO

• Give without regard to meals. • Do not crush/break film-coated tablets.

INDICATIONS/ROUTES/DOSAGE

HEPATITIS B VIRUS

PO: ADULTS, ELDERLY: 600 mg once daily.

DOSAGE IN RENAL IMPAIRMENT

Creatinine Clearance (ml/min)	Dose
50 ml/min or greater	600 mg once daily
30–49 ml/min	600 mg every 48 hrs
29 ml/min or less, not requiring dialysis	600 mg once every 72 hrs
End-stage renal disease	600 mg once every 96 hrs

SIDE EFFECTS

OCCASIONAL (12%–4%): Abdominal pain, fatigue, headache, nasopharyngitis, cough, diarrhea/loose stools, influenza-like symptoms, nausea, vomiting. **RARE (4%–3%):** Pharyngolaryngeal pain, pyrexia, arthralgia, rash, back pain, dizziness, myalgia, insomnia, dyspepsia (heartburn, indigestion, epigastric pain).

ADVERSE EFFECTS/ TOXIC REACTIONS

Severe acute exacerbation of hepatitis B has been noted in those who have discontinued therapy. Lactic acidosis, severe hepatotoxicity have been reported with use of nucleoside analogues alone or in combination with antiretrovirals.

NURSING CONSIDERATIONS

BASELINE ASSESSMENT

Establish baseline lab values, esp. renal function (BUN, serum creatinine), hepatic function tests (ALT, AST, bilirubin, alkaline phosphatase).

INTERVENTION/EVALUATION

Monitor amylase, lipase, BUN, serum creatinine. Assess for headache, nausea, cough. Monitor daily pattern of bowel activity/stool consistency. Initiate fall precautions if dizziness occurs. Assess sleep pattern. Closely monitor hepatic function in pts who discontinued anti-hepatitis B therapy.

PATIENT/FAMILY TEACHING

Continue therapy for full length of treatment. Doses should be evenly spaced. Inform pt that telbivudine is not a cure, and pt may continue to experience illnesses, including opportunistic infections. Report unexplained muscle weakness, tenderness, or pain. Treatment does not reduce risk of HBV transmission via sexual contact or blood contamination.

telithromycin

teh-**lith**-row-my-sin
(Ketek, Ketek Pak)

CLASSIFICATION

PHARMACOTHERAPEUTIC: Ketolide. **CLINICAL:** Antibiotic.

ACTION

Blocks protein synthesis by binding to ribosomal receptor sites on bacterial cell wall. **Therapeutic Effect:** Bactericidal.

PHARMACOKINETICS

Protein binding: 60%–70%. More of drug is concentrated in WBCs than in plasma, and drug is eliminated more slowly from WBCs than from plasma. Partially metabolized by liver. Minimally excreted in feces, urine. **Half-life:** 10 hrs.

USES

Treatment of susceptible infections due to *S. aureus, S. pneumoniae, H. influenzae, M. catarrhalis, C. pneumoniae, M. pneumoniae* including mild to moderately severe community-acquired pneumonia. **OFF-LABEL:** Treatment of tonsillitis, pharyngitis due to *S. pyogenes.*

PRECAUTIONS

CONTRAINDICATIONS: Hypersensitivity to macrolide antibiotics, concurrent use of cisapride, pimozide, myasthenia gravis. **CAUTIONS:** Renal/hepatic impairment, hypokelemia, hypomagnesemia, clinically significant bradycardia, QT prolongation, those receiving class IA or III antiarrhythmics.

⌛ LIFESPAN CONSIDERATIONS:

Pregnancy/Lactation: Unknown if drug crosses placenta. May be distributed in breast milk. **Pregnancy Category C.** **Children:** Safety and effectiveness not established. **Elderly:** No age-related precautions noted.

INTERACTIONS

DRUG: **Amiodarone, dofetilide, procainamide, quinidine** may prolong QT interval. Concomitant therapy with **atorvastatin, lovastatin, simvastatin** not recommended. **Carbamazepine** may decrease effect. May increase concentration, risk of toxicity of **cyclosporine, phenytoin, sirolimus, tacrolimus, digoxin, metoprolol, midazolam.** May decrease concentration, effect of **sotalol.** May increase GI side effects of **theophylline.** May increase risk of ergot toxicity with **dihydroergotamine, ergotamine.** **HERBAL:** None significant. **FOOD:** None known. **LAB VALUES:** May increase platelet count, AST, ALT.

AVAILABILITY (Rx)

TABLETS (KETEK, KETEK PAK): 400 mg.

ADMINISTRATION/HANDLING

PO

• Store at room temperature. • Give without regard to food.

INDICATIONS/ROUTES/DOSAGE

COMMUNITY-ACQUIRED PNEUMONIA

PO: ADULTS, ELDERLY: 800 mg once a day for 7–10 days.

DOSAGE IN RENAL IMPAIRMENT

Creatinine Clearance	Dosage
Less than 30 ml/min	600 mg once daily
Less than 30 ml/min and hepatic impairment	400 mg once daily

SIDE EFFECTS

OCCASIONAL (11%–4%): Diarrhea, nausea, headache, dizziness. **RARE (3%–2%):** Vomiting, loose stools, altered taste, dry mouth, flatulence, visual disturbances, syncope.

ADVERSE EFFECTS/ TOXIC REACTIONS

Hepatic dysfunction, severe hypersensitivity reaction, atrial arrhythmias occur rarely. Antibiotic-associated colitis (abdominal cramps, severe watery diarrhea, fever) may result from altered bacterial balance.

T

NURSING CONSIDERATIONS

BASELINE ASSESSMENT

Question pt for concurrent use of cisapride, pimozide (contraindicated).

INTERVENTION/EVALUATION

Monitor daily pattern of bowel activity/ stool consistency. Give with food if nausea occurs. Assess hepatic function panel for evidence of hepatotoxicity.

PATIENT/FAMILY TEACHING

• Avoid quick changes in viewing between objects in distance and objects nearby (drug may produce temporary difficulty in focusing that may last several hrs after first or second dose). • Avoid tasks that require alertness, motor skills until response to drug is established. Call physician if visual disturbances, loss of consciousness occur.

telmisartan

tel-meh-**sar**-tan
(Micardis)

FIXED-COMBINATION(S)

Micardis HCT: telmisartan/hydrochlorothiazide (a diuretic): 40 mg/12.5 mg; 80 mg/12.5 mg.

CLASSIFICATION

PHARMACOTHERAPEUTIC: Angiotensin II receptor antagonist. **CLINICAL:** Antihypertensive (see p. 8C).

ACTION

Blocks vasoconstrictor and aldosterone-secreting effects of angiotensin II, inhibiting binding of angiotensin II to AT_1 receptors. **Therapeutic Effect:** Causes vasodilation, decreases peripheral resistance, decreases B/P.

T

PHARMACOKINETICS

Rapidly, completely absorbed after PO administration. Protein binding: greater than 99%. Undergoes metabolism in liver to inactive metabolite. Excreted in feces. Unknown if removed by hemodialysis. **Half-life:** 24 hrs.

USES

Treatment of hypertension alone or in combination with other antihypertensives. **OFF-LABEL:** Treatment of CHF.

PRECAUTIONS

CONTRAINDICATIONS: None known. **CAUTIONS:** Volume-depleted pts, hepatic/renal impairment, renal artery stenosis (unilateral, bilateral).

LIFESPAN CONSIDERATIONS:

Pregnancy/Lactation: May cause fetal harm. Unknown if drug is excreted in breast milk. **Pregnancy Category C (D if used in second or third trimester). Children:** Safety and efficacy not established. **Elderly:** No age-related precautions noted.

INTERACTIONS

DRUG: Increases **digoxin** concentration, risk of toxicity. Slightly decreases **warfarin** concentration. **HERBAL: Yohimbe, ginseng, ephedra** may worsen hypertension. **Garlic** may increase antihypertensive effect. **FOOD:** None known. **LAB VALUES:** May increase serum creatinine. May decrease Hgb, Hct.

AVAILABILITY (Rx)

TABLETS: 20 mg, 40 mg, 80 mg.

ADMINISTRATION/HANDLING

PO

• Give without regard to meals.

INDICATIONS/ROUTES/DOSAGE

HYPERTENSION

PO: ADULTS, ELDERLY: 40 mg once a day. Range: 20–80 mg/day.

SIDE EFFECTS

OCCASIONAL (7%–3%): Upper respiratory tract infection, sinusitis, back/leg pain, diarrhea. **RARE (1%):** Dizziness, headache, fatigue, nausea, heartburn, myalgia, cough, peripheral edema.

ADVERSE EFFECTS/ TOXIC REACTIONS

Overdosage may manifest as hypotension, tachycardia; bradycardia occurs less often.

NURSING CONSIDERATIONS

BASELINE ASSESSMENT

Obtain B/P, apical pulse immediately before each dose, in addition to regular monitoring (be alert to fluctuations). If excessive reduction in B/P occurs, place pt in supine position, feet slightly elevated. Assess medication history (esp. diuretics). Question for history of hepatic/renal impairment, renal artery stenosis. Obtain BUN, serum creatinine, Hgb, HcT, vital signs (particularly B/P, pulse rate).

INTERVENTION/EVALUATION

Monitor B/P, pulse, serum electrolytes, renal function.

PATIENT/FAMILY TEACHING

• Monitor for hypotension when initiating therapy. • Avoid tasks that require alertness, motor skills until response to drug is established (possible dizziness effect). • Maintain proper fluid intake. • Inform pregnant pt regarding risk, consequences of second-, third-trimester exposure to telmisartan. • Report pregnancy to physician as soon as possible. • Report any sign of infection (sore throat, fever). • Discuss need for lifelong B/P control. • Caution against excessive exertion during hot weather (risk of dehydration, hypotension).

temazepam

tem-**az**-eh-pam

(Apo-Temazepam ✤, Novo-Temazepam ✤, PMS-Temazepam ✤, Restoril)

Do not confuse Restoril with Vistaril or Zestril.

CLASSIFICATION

PHARMACOTHERAPEUTIC: Benzodiazepine (**Schedule IV**). **CLINICAL:** Sedative-hypnotic (see p. 140C).

ACTION

Enhances action of inhibitory neurotransmitter gamma-aminobutyric acid (GABA), resulting in CNS depression. **Therapeutic Effect:** Induces sleep.

PHARMACOKINETICS

Well absorbed from GI tract. Protein binding: 96%. Widely distributed. Crosses blood-brain barrier. Metabolized in liver. Primarily excreted in urine. Not removed by hemodialysis. **Half-life:** 4–18 hrs.

USES

Short-term treatment of insomnia (5 wks or less). Reduces sleep-induction time, number of nocturnal awakenings; increases length of sleep. **OFF-LABEL:** Treatment of anxiety, depression, panic attacks.

PRECAUTIONS

CONTRAINDICATIONS: Angle-closure glaucoma; CNS depression; pregnancy, breast-feeding; severe, uncontrolled pain; sleep apnea. **CAUTIONS:** Mental impairment, pts with drug dependence potential.

LIFESPAN CONSIDERATIONS:

Pregnancy/Lactation: Crosses placenta. May be distributed in breast milk. Chronic ingestion during pregnancy may produce withdrawal symptoms, CNS depression in neonates. **Pregnancy Category X.** **Children:** Not recommended in those younger than 18 yrs. **Elderly:** Use small initial doses with gradual dosage increases to avoid ataxia, excessive sedation.

INTERACTIONS

DRUG: **Alcohol, other CNS depressants** may increase CNS depression. **HERBAL:** **St. John's wort** may decrease concentration. **Gotu kola, kava kava, St. John's wort, valerian** may increase CNS depression. **FOOD:** None known. **LAB VALUES:** None known.

AVAILABILITY (Rx)

CAPSULES: 7.5 mg, 15 mg, 22.5 mg, 30 mg.

ADMINISTRATION/HANDLING

PO

• Give without regard to meals. • Capsules may be emptied and mixed with food.

INDICATIONS/ROUTES/DOSAGE

INSOMNIA

PO: ADULTS, CHILDREN 18 YRS AND OLDER: 15–30 mg at bedtime. **ELDERLY, DEBILITATED:** 7.5–15 mg at bedtime.

SIDE EFFECTS

FREQUENT: Drowsiness, sedation, rebound insomnia (may occur for 1–2 nights after drug is discontinued), dizziness, confusion, euphoria. **OCCASIONAL:** Asthenia, anorexia, diarrhea. **RARE:** Paradoxical CNS excitement, restlessness (particularly in elderly, debilitated pts).

ADVERSE EFFECTS/ TOXIC REACTIONS

Abrupt or too-rapid withdrawal may result in pronounced restlessness, irritability, insomnia, hand tremor, abdominal/muscle cramps, vomiting, diaphoresis, seizures. Overdose results in somnolence, confusion, diminished reflexes, respiratory depression, coma.

NURSING CONSIDERATIONS

BASELINE ASSESSMENT

Question for possibility of pregnancy before initiating therapy (Pregnancy Category X). Assess B/P, pulse, respirations immediately before administration. Raise bed rails. Provide environment conducive to sleep (back rub, quiet environment, low lighting).

INTERVENTION/EVALUATION

Assess sleep pattern of pt. Assess elderly or debilitated for paradoxical reaction, particularly during early therapy. Monitor respiratory, cardiovascular, mental status. Evaluate for therapeutic response: decrease in number of nocturnal awakenings, increase in length of sleep.

PATIENT/FAMILY TEACHING

• Avoid alcohol, other CNS depressants. • May cause daytime drowsiness. • Avoid tasks that require alertness, motor skills until response to drug is established. • Take approximately 30 min before bedtime. • Inform physician if pregnant or planning to become pregnant.

Temodar, *see temozolomide*

temozolomide

teh-moe-**zoll**-oh-mide
(Temodal ✱, Temodar)

◆CLASSIFICATION

PHARMACOTHERAPEUTIC: Imidazotetrazine derivative. **CLINICAL:** Antineoplastic (see p. 83C).

ACTION

Acts as prodrug and is converted to highly active cytotoxic metabolite. Cytotoxic effect is associated with methylation of DNA. **Therapeutic Effect:** Inhibits DNA replication, causing cell death.

PHARMACOKINETICS

Rapidly, completely absorbed after PO administration. Protein binding: 15%. Peak plasma concentration occurs in 1 hr. Penetrates blood-brain barrier.

Eliminated primarily in urine and, to much lesser extent, in feces. **Half-life:** 1.6–1.8 hrs.

USES

Treatment of adults with refractory anaplastic astrocytoma; newly diagnosed glioblastoma multiforme (concomitantly with radiotherapy, then as maintenance therapy). **OFF-LABEL:** Malignant glioma, malignant melanoma.

PRECAUTIONS

CONTRAINDICATIONS: Hypersensitivity to dacarbazine, pregnancy. **CAUTIONS:** Severe renal/hepatic impairment, bacterial/viral infection, elderly.

LIFESPAN CONSIDERATIONS:

Pregnancy/Lactation: May cause fetal harm. May produce malformation of external organs, soft tissue, skeleton. If possible, avoid use during pregnancy. Unknown if drug is excreted in breast milk. **Pregnancy Category D.** **Children:** Safety and efficacy not established. **Elderly:** Those older than 70 yrs may experience higher risk of developing grade 4 neutropenia, grade 4 thrombocytopenia.

INTERACTIONS

DRUG: Medications causing blood dyscrasias (altering blood cell counts) may increase leukopenic, thrombocytopenic effects. **Bone marrow depressants** may increase myelosuppression. **Live virus vaccines** may potentiate virus replication, increase vaccine side effects, decrease pt's antibody response to vaccine. **HERBAL:** None significant. **FOOD: All foods** decrease rate, extent of drug absorption. **LAB VALUES:** May decrease Hgb; neutrophil, platelet, WBC counts.

AVAILABILITY (Rx)

CAPSULES: 5 mg, 20 mg, 100 mg, 140 mg, 180 mg, 250 mg.

ADMINISTRATION/HANDLING

PO

• Food reduces rate, extent of absorption; increases risk of nausea, vomiting. • For best results, administer at bedtime. • Swallow capsule whole with glass of water. • Avoid exposure to medication during handling (cytotoxic).

INDICATIONS/ROUTES/DOSAGE

ANAPLASTIC ASTROCYTOMA

PO: ADULTS, ELDERLY: Initially, 150 mg/m^2/day for 5 consecutive days of 28-day treatment cycle. Subsequent doses based on platelet count, absolute neurophil count (ANC) during previous cycle. ANC greater than 1,500 per microliter and platelet: more than 100,000 per microliter. Maintenance: 200 mg/m^2/day for 5 days q4wk. Continue until disease progression is observed. Minimum: 100 mg/m^2/day for 5 days q4wk.

GLIOBLASTOMA MULTIFORME

PO: ADULTS, ELDERLY: 75 mg/m^2 daily for 42 days. Maintenance: (Cycle 1): 150 mg/m^2 once daily for 5 days followed by 23 days without treatment. (Cycles 2–6): 200 mg/m^2 once daily for 5 days followed by 23 days without treatment.

SIDE EFFECTS

FREQUENT (53%–33%): Nausea, vomiting, headache, fatigue, constipation, seizure. **OCCASIONAL (16%–10%):** Diarrhea, asthenia, fever, dizziness, peripheral edema, incoordination, insomnia. **RARE (9%–5%):** Paresthesia, drowsiness, anorexia, urinary incontinence, anxiety, pharyngitis, cough.

ADVERSE EFFECTS/ TOXIC REACTIONS

Myelosuppression is characterized by neutropenia and thrombocytopenia, with elderly and women showing higher incidence of developing severe myelosuppression. Usually occurs within

T

first few cycles; is not cumulative. Nadir occurs in approximately 26–28 days, with recovery within 14 days of nadir.

NURSING CONSIDERATIONS

BASELINE ASSESSMENT

Before dosing, absolute neutrophil count (ANC) must be greater than 1,500 and platelet count greater than 100,000. Potential for nausea, vomiting readily controlled with antiemetic therapy.

INTERVENTION/EVALUATION

Obtain CBC on day 22 (21 days after first dose) or within 48 hrs of that day and weekly until ANC is greater than 1,500 and platelet count is greater than 100,000. Monitor for hematologic toxicity (fever, sore throat, signs of local infection, unusual bruising/bleeding from any site), symptoms of anemia (excessive fatigue, weakness).

PATIENT/FAMILY TEACHING

• To reduce nausea/vomiting, take on an empty stomach. • Do not open capsules. • Promptly report fever, sore throat, signs of local infection, unusual bruising/bleeding from any site. • Avoid crowds, those with infection. • Do not have immunizations without physician's approval. • Avoid pregnancy.

T

tenecteplase

ten-**eck**-teh-place
(TNKase)

CLASSIFICATION

PHARMACOTHERAPEUTIC: Tissue plasminogen activator. **CLINICAL:** Thrombolytic (see p. 32C).

ACTION

Produced by recombinant DNA that binds to fibrin and converts plasminogen to plasmin. Initiates fibrinolysis by degrading fibrin clots, fibrinogen, other plasma proteins. **Therapeutic Effect:** Exerts thrombolytic action.

PHARMACOKINETICS

Extensively distributed to tissues. Completely eliminated by hepatic metabolism. **Half-life:** 11–20 min.

USES

Treatment, reduction of mortality associated with acute myocardial infarction (AMI).

PRECAUTIONS

CONTRAINDICATIONS: Active internal bleeding, aneurysm, AV malformation, bleeding diathesis, history of cerebrovascular accident (CVA), intracranial or intraspinal surgery or trauma within past 2 mos, intracranial neoplasm, severe uncontrolled hypertension. **CAUTIONS:** Pts who previously received tenecteplase, severe hepatic impairment.

LIFESPAN CONSIDERATIONS:

Pregnancy/Lactation: Unknown if distributed in breast milk. **Pregnancy Category C. Children:** Safety and efficacy not established. **Elderly:** May have increased risk of intracranial hemorrhage, stroke, major bleeding; caution advised.

INTERACTIONS

DRUG: Anticoagulants (e.g., heparin, warfarin), aspirin, dipyridamole, glycoprotein IIb/IIIa inhibitors increase risk of bleeding. **HERBAL: Ginkgo biloba** may increase risk of bleeding. **FOOD:** None known. **LAB VALUES:** Decreases plasminogen, fibrinogen levels during infusion, decreasing clotting time (confirms presence of lysis). Decreases Hgb, Hct.

AVAILABILITY (Rx)

INJECTION, POWDER FOR RECONSTITUTION: 50 mg.

ADMINISTRATION/HANDLING

IV

Reconstitution • Add 10 ml Sterile Water for Injection without preservative to vial to provide concentration of 5 mg/ml. • Gently swirl until dissolved. Do not shake. • If foaming occurs, leave vial undisturbed for several minutes.

Rate of administration • Administer as IV push over 5 sec.

Storage • Store at room temperature. • If possible, use immediately but may refrigerate up to 8 hrs after reconstitution. • Appears as colorless to pale yellow solution. Do not use if discolored or contains particulates. • Discard after 8 hrs.

IV INCOMPATIBILITIES

Do not mix with other medications.

INDICATIONS/ROUTES/DOSAGE

◀ **ALERT** ▶ Give as single IV bolus over 5 sec. Precipitate may occur when given in IV line containing dextrose. Flush line with saline before and after administration.

ACUTE MI

IV: ADULTS: Dosage is based on pt's weight. Treatment should be initiated as soon as possible after onset of symptoms.

Weight (kg)	(mg)	(ml)
90 or more	50	10
80–less than 90	45	9
70–less than 80	40	8
60–less than 70	35	7
Less than 60	30	6

SIDE EFFECTS

FREQUENT: Bleeding (major, 4.7%; minor, 21.8%).

ADVERSE EFFECTS/ TOXIC REACTIONS

Bleeding at internal sites, including intracranial, retroperitoneal, GI, GU, respiratory sites, may occur. Lysis of coronary thrombi may produce atrial or ventricular arrhythmias, stroke.

NURSING CONSIDERATIONS

BASELINE ASSESSMENT

Obtain baseline B/P, apical pulse. Record weight. Evaluate 12-lead EKG, cardiac enzymes, serum electrolytes. Assess Hgb, Hct, platelet count, thrombin (TT), activated partial thromboplastin time (aPTT), prothrombin time (PT), fibrinogen level before therapy is instituted. Type and hold blood.

INTERVENTION/EVALUATION

Monitor continuous EKG for arrhythmias, B/P, pulse, respirations q15min until stable, then hourly. Check peripheral pulses, heart and lung sounds. Monitor chest pain relief; notify physician of continuation/recurrence (note location, type, intensity). Assess for overt or occult blood in any body substance. Monitor aPTT per protocol. Maintain B/P. Avoid any trauma that might increase risk of bleeding (e.g., injections, shaving). Assess neurologic status with vital signs.

T

teniposide

ten-**ih**-poe-side
(Vumon)

See Cancer chemotherapeutic agents (p. 83C)

tenofovir

ten-**oh**-foh-veer
(Viread)

FIXED-COMBINATION(S)

Atripla: tenofovir/efavirenz/emtricitabine (antiretroviral agents): 300 mg/600 mg/200 mg. **Truvada:** tenofovir/emtricitabine (an antiretroviral agent): 300 mg/200 mg.

◆CLASSIFICATION

PHARMACOTHERAPEUTIC: Nucleotide analogue. **CLINICAL:** Antiviral (see pp. 66C, 111C).

ACTION

Inhibits HIV reverse transcriptase by being incorporated into viral DNA, resulting in DNA chain termination. **Therapeutic Effect:** Slows HIV replication, reduces HIV RNA levels (viral load).

PHARMACOKINETICS

Bioavailability in fasted pts is approximately 25%. High-fat meals increase bioavailability. Protein binding: 0.7%–7.2%. Excreted in urine. Removed by hemodialysis. **Half-life:** Unknown.

USES

Treatment of HIV-1 infection in combination with other antiretroviral agents.

PRECAUTIONS

CONTRAINDICATIONS: None known. **CAUTIONS:** Hepatic/renal impairment.

⌛ LIFESPAN CONSIDERATIONS:

Pregnancy/Lactation: Unknown if drug crosses placenta or is distributed is breast milk. **Pregnancy Category B. Children:** Safety and efficacy not established. **Elderly:** No age-related precautions noted.

INTERACTIONS

DRUG: May increase **didaosine** concentration. May decrease concentrations of **atazanavir, indinavir, lamivudine, lopinavir, ritonavir. HERBAL:** None significant. **FOOD: High-fat food** increases bioavailability. **LAB VALUES:** May elevate hepatic function test results. May alter serum creatine kinase (CK), GGT, uric acid, AST, ALT, triglycerides, creatinine clearance.

AVAILABILITY (Rx)

TABLETS: 300 mg.

ADMINISTRATION/HANDLING

PO

- Give with food.

INDICATIONS/ROUTES/DOSAGE

HIV INFECTION

PO: ADULTS, ELDERLY, CHILDREN 18 YRS AND OLDER: 300 mg once a day.

DOSAGE IN RENAL IMPAIRMENT

Creatinine Clearance	Dosage
30–49 ml/min	300 mg q48h
10–29 ml/min	300 mg twice a wk
Less than 10 ml/min	Not recommended

SIDE EFFECTS

OCCASIONAL: GI disturbances (diarrhea, flatulence, nausea, vomiting).

ADVERSE EFFECTS/ TOXIC REACTIONS

Lactic acidosis, hepatomegaly with steatosis (excess fat in liver) occur rarely, may be severe.

NURSING CONSIDERATIONS

BASELINE ASSESSMENT

Obtain baseline laboratory testing, esp. serum hepatic function tests, triglycerides before beginning tenofovir therapy and at periodic intervals during therapy. Offer emotional support to pt and family.

INTERVENTION/EVALUATION

Closely monitor for evidence of GI discomfort. Monitor daily pattern of bowel activity/stool consistency. Monitor CBC, Hgb, reticulocyte count, serum hepatic function, CD4 cell count, HIV, RNA plasma levels.

PATIENT/FAMILY TEACHING

• Continue therapy for full length of treatment. • Tenofovir is not a cure for HIV infection, nor does it reduce risk of transmission to others. • Take with a high-fat meal (increases absorption). • Inform physician if persistent abdominal pain, nausea, vomiting occurs.

Tenormin, *see atenolol*

terazosin

ter-**a**-zoe-sin
(Apo-Terazosin ✤, Hytrin, Novo-Terazosin ✤)

CLASSIFICATION

PHARMACOTHERAPEUTIC: Alpha-adrenergic blocker. **CLINICAL:** Antihypertensive, benign prostatic hyperplasia agent (see p. 59C).

ACTION

Blocks alpha-adrenergic receptors. Produces vasodilation, decreases peripheral resistance, targets receptors around bladder neck, prostate. **Therapeutic Effect:** In hypertension, decreases B/P. In benign prostatic hyperplasia, relaxes smooth muscle, improves urine flow.

PHARMACOKINETICS

Route	Onset	Peak	Duration
PO	15 min	1–2 hrs	12–24 hrs

Rapidly, completely absorbed from GI tract. Protein binding: 90%–94%. Metabolized in liver to active metabolite. Primarily eliminated in feces via biliary system; excreted in urine. Not removed by hemodialysis. **Half-life:** 12 hrs.

USES

Treatment of mild to moderate hypertension. Used alone or in combination with other antihypertensives. Treatment of benign prostatic hypertrophy.

PRECAUTIONS

CONTRAINDICATIONS: None known. **CAUTIONS:** Confirmed or suspected coronary artery disease.

LIFESPAN CONSIDERATIONS:

Pregnancy/Lactation: Unknown if drug crosses placenta or is distributed in breast milk. **Pregnancy Category C. Children:** Safety and efficacy not established. **Elderly:** No age-related precautions noted but may be more sensitive to hypotensive effects.

INTERACTIONS

DRUG: NSAIDs, sympathomimetics may decrease effects. **Hypotensive medications (e.g., antihypertensives, diuretics)** may increase effects. **HERBAL: Ephedra, yohimbe, ginseng** may worsen hypertension. **Garlic** may increase antihypertensive effect. **FOOD:** None known. **LAB VALUES:** May decrease Hgb, Hct, serum albumin, total serum protein, WBC count.

AVAILABILITY (Rx)

CAPSULES: 1 mg, 2 mg, 5 mg, 10 mg.

ADMINISTRATION/HANDLING

PO

• Give without regard to food. • Administer first dose at bedtime (minimizes risk of fainting due to "first-dose syncope").

T

INDICATIONS/ROUTES/DOSAGE

◄ **ALERT** ► If medication has been discontinued for several days, retitrate initially using 1-mg dose at bedtime.

MILD TO MODERATE HYPERTENSION

PO: ADULTS, ELDERLY: Initially, 1 mg at bedtime. Slowly increase dosage to desired levels. Range: 1–5 mg/day as single or 2 divided doses. **Maximum:** 20 mg.

BENIGN PROSTATIC HYPERPLASIA

PO: ADULTS, ELDERLY: Initially, 1 mg at bedtime. May increase up to 10 mg/day. **Maximum:** 20 mg/day.

SIDE EFFECTS

FREQUENT (9%–5%): Dizziness, headache, fatigue. **RARE (less than 2%):** Peripheral edema, orthostatic hypotension, myalgia, arthralgia, blurred vision, nausea, vomiting, nasal congestion, drowsiness.

ADVERSE EFFECTS/ TOXIC REACTIONS

First-dose syncope (hypotension with sudden loss of consciousness) generally occurs 30–90 min after initial dose of 2 mg or more, too-rapid increase in dosage, or addition of another antihypertensive agent to therapy. First-dose syncope may be preceded by tachycardia (pulse rate of 120–160 beats/min).

NURSING CONSIDERATIONS

BASELINE ASSESSMENT

Give first dose at bedtime. If initial dose is given during daytime, pt must remain recumbent for 3–4 hrs. Assess B/P, pulse immediately before each dose, and q15–30min until stabilized (be alert to B/P fluctuations).

INTERVENTION/EVALUATION

Monitor pulse diligently (first-dose syncope may be preceded by tachycardia). Assist with ambulation if dizziness occurs. Assess for peripheral edema. Monitor B/P, GU function.

PATIENT/FAMILY TEACHING

• Non-cola carbonated beverage, unsalted crackers, dry toast may relieve nausea. • Nasal congestion may occur. • Full therapeutic effect may not occur for 3–4 wks. • Avoid tasks requiring alertness, motor skills until response to drug is established. • Use caution rising from sitting position. • Report dizziness, palpitations.

terbinafine

ter-**been**-a-feen

(Apo-Terbinafine ♣, Lamisil, Lamisil AT, Novo-Terbinafine ♣)

Do not confuse terbinafine with terbutaline or Lamisil with Lamictal.

◆CLASSIFICATION

CLINICAL: Antifungal (see p. 47C).

ACTION

Inhibits the enzyme squalene epoxidase, thereby interfering with fungal biosynthesis. **Therapeutic Effect:** Results in death of fungal cells.

PHARMACOKINETICS

Well absorbed following PO administration. Protein binding: 99%. Metabolized by liver. Primarily excreted in urine; minimal elimination in feces. **Half-life:** (oral): 36 hrs, (topical): 22–26 hrs.

USES

Systemic: Treatment of onychomycosis (fungal disease of nails due to dermatophytes). **Topical:** Treatment of *tinea cruris* (jock itch), *t. pedis* (athlete's foot), *t. corporis* (ringworm).

PRECAUTIONS

CONTRAINDICATIONS: Oral: Children younger than 12 yrs, preexisting hepatic/

T

renal impairment (creatinine clearance of 50 ml/min or less). **CAUTIONS:** None known.

LIFESPAN CONSIDERATIONS:

Pregnancy/Lactation: Distributed in breast milk. **Pregnancy Category B. Children:** Safety and efficacy not established. **Elderly:** Age-related renal impairment may require dosage adjustment.

INTERACTIONS

DRUG: Alcohol, other hepatotoxic medications may increase risk of hepatotoxicity. **Hepatic enzyme inducers (e.g., rifampin)** may increase clearance. **Hepatic enzyme inhibitors (e.g., cimetidine)** may decrease clearance. **HERBAL:** None significant. **FOOD:** None known. **LAB VALUES:** May increase AST, ALT.

AVAILABILITY (Rx)

CREAM (LAMISIL AT): 1%. **TABLETS (LAMISIL):** 250 mg. **TOPICAL SOLUTION (LAMISIL, LAMISIL AT):** 1%. **TOPICAL SPRAY (LAMISIL AT):** 1%.

INDICATIONS/ROUTES/DOSAGE

TINEA PEDIS

TOPICAL: ADULTS, ELDERLY, CHILDREN 12 YRS AND OLDER: Apply twice a day until signs/symptoms significantly improve.

TINEA CRURIS, TINEA CORPORIS

TOPICAL: ADULTS, ELDERLY, CHILDREN 12 YRS AND OLDER: Apply 1–2 times a day until signs/symptoms significantly improve.

ONYCHOMYCOSIS

PO: ADULTS, ELDERLY, CHILDREN 12 YRS AND OLDER: 250 mg/day for 6 wks (fingernails) or 12 wks (toenails).

TINEA VERSICOLOR

TOPICAL SOLUTION: ADULTS, ELDERLY: Apply to the affected area twice a day for 7 days.

SYSTEMIC MYCOSIS

PO: ADULTS, ELDERLY: 250–500 mg/day for up to 16 mos.

SIDE EFFECTS

FREQUENT (13%): Oral: Headache. **OCCASIONAL (6%–3%): Oral:** Abdominal pain, flatulence, urticaria, visual disturbance. **RARE: Oral:** Diarrhea, rash, dyspepsia (heartburn, indigestion, epigastric pain), pruritus, altered taste, nausea. **Topical:** Irritation, burning, pruritus, dryness.

ADVERSE EFFECTS/ TOXIC REACTIONS

Hepatobiliary dysfunction (including cholestatic hepatitis), serious skin reactions, severe neutropenia occur rarely. Ocular lens, retinal changes have been noted.

NURSING CONSIDERATIONS

BASELINE ASSESSMENT

Serum hepatic function tests should be obtained in pts receiving treatment for longer than 6 wks.

INTERVENTION/EVALUATION

Check for therapeutic response. Discontinue medication, notify physician if local reaction occurs (irritation, redness, swelling, pruritus, oozing, blistering, burning). Monitor serum hepatic function in pts receiving treatment for longer than 6 wks.

PATIENT/FAMILY TEACHING

• Keep areas clean, dry; wear light clothing to promote ventilation. • Separate personal items. • Avoid topical cream contact with eyes, nose, mouth, other mucous membranes. • Rub well into affected, surrounding area. • Do not cover with occlusive dressing. • Notify physician if skin irritation, diarrhea occurs.

terbutaline

ter-**byoo**-te-leen
(Brethine, Bricanyl ♣)

Do not confuse terbutaline with tolbutamide or terbinafine, or Brethine with Brethaire.

CLASSIFICATION

PHARMACOTHERAPEUTIC: Sympathomimetic (adrenergic agonist). **CLINICAL:** Bronchodilator, premature labor inhibitor (see p. 70C).

ACTION

Stimulates $beta_2$-adrenergic receptors, resulting in relaxation of uterine, bronchial smooth muscle. **Therapeutic Effect:** Inhibits uterine contractions. Relieves bronchospasm, reduces airway resistance.

PHARMACOKINETICS

Partially absorbed in GI tract following PO administration. Protein binding: 14%–25%. Metabolized in liver. Excreted in feces, urine. **Half-life:** 3–4 hrs.

USES

Symptomatic relief of reversible bronchospasm due to bronchial asthma, bronchitis, emphysema. Delays premature labor in pregnancies between 20 and 34 wks.

PRECAUTIONS

CONTRAINDICATIONS: History of hypersensitivity to sympathomimetics. **CAUTIONS:** Cardiac impairment, diabetes mellitus, hypertension, hyperthyroidism, history of seizures.

LIFESPAN CONSIDERATIONS:

Pregnancy/Lactation: Crosses placenta; distributed in breast milk. **Pregnancy Category B.** **Children:** Safety and efficacy not established in children younger than 6 yrs. **Elderly:** Increased risk of tremors, tachycardia due to sympathomimetic sensitivity.

INTERACTIONS

DRUG: May decrease effects of **beta-blockers. Digoxin, sympathomimetics** may increase risk of arrhythmias. **MAOIs** may increase risk of hypertensive crisis. **Tricyclic antidepressants** may increase cardiovascular effects. May increase effects of **thyroid hormones. HERBAL: Yohimbe, ephedra** may cause CNS stimulation. **FOOD:** None known. **LAB VALUES:** May decrease serum potassium.

AVAILABILITY (Rx)

INJECTION SOLUTION: 1 mg/ml. **TABLETS:** 2.5 mg, 5 mg.

ADMINISTRATION/HANDLING

SUBCUTANEOUS

• Do not use if solution appears discolored. • Inject subcutaneously into lateral deltoid region.

PO

• Give without regard to food (give with food if GI upset occurs). • Tablets may be crushed.

INDICATIONS/ROUTES/DOSAGE

BRONCHOSPASM

PO: ADULTS, ELDERLY, CHILDREN 15 YRS AND OLDER: Initially, 2.5 mg 3–4 times a day. Maintenance: 2.5–5 mg 3 times a day q6h while awake. **Maximum:** 15 mg/day. **CHILDREN 12–14 YRS:** 2.5 mg 3 times a day. **Maximum:** 7.5 mg/day. **CHILDREN YOUNGER THAN 12 YRS:** Initially, 0.05 mg/kg/dose q8h. May increase up to 0.15 mg/kg/dose. **Maximum:** 5 mg.
SUBCUTANEOUS: ADULTS, CHILDREN 12 YRS AND OLDER: Initially, 0.25 mg. Repeat in 15–30 min if substantial improvement does not occur. **Maximum:** 0.5 mg/4 hrs. **CHILDREN YOUNGER THAN 12 YRS:** 0.005–0.01 mg/kg/dose to a maximum of 0.3 mg/dose q15–20min for 3 doses.

T

PRETERM LABOR
PO: ADULTS: 2.5–10 mg q4–6h.
IV: ADULTS: 2.5–10 mcg/min. May increase gradually q15–20min up to 17.5–30 mcg/min.

SIDE EFFECTS

FREQUENT (38%–23%): Tremor, anxiety. **OCCASIONAL (11%–10%):** Drowsiness, headache, nausea, heartburn, dizziness. **RARE (3%–1%):** Flushing, asthenia (loss of strength, energy), oropharyngeal dryness, irritation (with inhalation therapy).

ADVERSE EFFECTS/ TOXIC REACTIONS

Too-frequent or excessive use may lead to decreased drug effectiveness and/or severe, paradoxical bronchoconstriction. Excessive sympathomimetic stimulation may cause palpitations, extrasystoles, tachycardia, chest pain, slight increase in B/P followed by a substantial decrease, chills, diaphoresis, skin blanching.

NURSING CONSIDERATIONS

BASELINE ASSESSMENT

Bronchospasm: Offer emotional support (high incidence of anxiety due to difficulty in breathing, sympathomimetic response to drug). **Preterm labor:** Assess baseline maternal pulse, B/P, frequency and duration of contractions, fetal heart rate.

INTERVENTION/EVALUATION

Bronchospasm: Monitor rate, depth, rhythm, type of respiration; quality, rate of pulse. Assess lung sounds for rhonchi, wheezing, rales. Monitor ABGs. Observe lips, fingernails for cyanosis (blue or dusky color in light-skinned pts; gray in dark-skinned pts). Observe for clavicular retractions, hand tremor. Evaluate for clinical improvement (quieter, slower respirations, relaxed facial expression, cessation of clavicular retractions). **Preterm labor:** Monitor for frequency, duration, strength of contractions. Diligently monitor fetal heart rate.

PATIENT/FAMILY TEACHING

• Inform physician if palpitations, chest pain, muscle tremor, dizziness, headache, flushing, breathing difficulties continue. • May cause nervousness, anxiety, shakiness. • Avoid excessive use of caffeine derivatives (chocolate, coffee, tea, cola, cocoa).

terconazole

ter-**con**-ah-zole
(Terazol ✤, Terazol 7)
Do not confuse terconazole with tioconazole.

◆CLASSIFICATION

CLINICAL: Antifungal.

ACTION

Disrupts fungal cell membrane permeability. **Therapeutic Effect:** Produces antifungal activity.

PHARMACOKINETICS

Minimal systemic absorption.

USES

Treatment of vulvovaginal candidiasis (moniliasis).

PRECAUTIONS

CONTRAINDICATIONS: Allergy to azole antifungals. **CAUTIONS:** None significant.

LIFESPAN CONSIDERATIONS:

Pregnancy/Lactation: Unknown if distributed in breast milk. **Pregnancy Category C. Children:** Safety and efficacy not established. **Elderly:** No age-related precautions noted.

T

INTERACTIONS

DRUG: None significant. **HERBAL:** None significant. **FOOD:** None known. **LAB VALUES:** None significant.

AVAILABILITY (Rx)

VAGINAL CREAM: 0.4% (Terazol 7), 0.8% (Terazol). **VAGINAL SUPPOSITORY (TERAZOL 3):** 80 mg.

INDICATIONS/ROUTES/DOSAGE

VULVOVAGINAL CANDIDIASIS

TABLET (INTRAVAGINAL): ADULTS, ELDERLY: 1 suppository vaginally at bedtime for 3 days.
CREAM: ADULTS, ELDERLY: (0.4%): 1 applicatorful at bedtime for 7 days; **(0.8%):** 1 applicatorful at bedtime for 3 days.

SIDE EFFECTS

FREQUENT (over 10%): Headache, vulvovaginal burning. **OCCASIONAL (10%–1%):** Dysmenorrhea, pain in female genitalia, abdominal pain, fever, pruritus. **RARE (less than 1%):** Chills.

ADVERSE EFFECTS/ TOXIC REACTIONS

None known.

NURSING CONSIDERATIONS

BASELINE ASSESSMENT

Assess for allergy to azoles, pt ability to self administer.

INTERVENTION/EVALUATION

Watch for local irritation. Assist, provide education to pt regarding administration.

PATIENT/FAMILY TEACHING

Notify physician of recurrence of symptoms following treatment. Comply with full course of therapy. Staining of clothes may occur with azole medications; use protective liners.

teriparatide

tear-ee-**pear**-ah-tide
(Forteo)

CLASSIFICATION

PHARMACOTHERAPEUTIC: Synthetic hormone. **CLINICAL:** Osteoporosis agent.

ACTION

Acts on bone to mobilize calcium; acts on kidney to reduce calcium clearance, increase phosphate excretion. **Therapeutic Effect:** Increases rate of release of calcium from bone into blood; stimulates new bone formation.

PHARMACOKINETICS

Extensively absorbed following subcutaneous injection. Metabolized in liver. Excreted in urine. **Half-life:** 1 hr.

USES

Treatment of postmenopausal women with osteoporosis who are at increased risk for fractures, increase bone mass in men with primary or hypogonadal osteoporosis who are at high risk for fractures. High-risk pts include those with a history of osteoporotic fractures, who have failed previous osteoporosis therapy, or were intolerant of previous osteoporosis therapy.

PRECAUTIONS

CONTRAINDICATIONS: Conditions that increase risk of osteosarcoma (e.g., Paget's disease, unexplained elevations of alkaline phosphatase level, open epiphyses, prior skeletal radiation therapy, implant therapy), hypercalcemia, hypercalcemic disorders (e.g., hyperparathyroidism). **CAUTIONS:** Bone metastases, history of skeletal malignancies, metabolic bone diseases other than osteoporosis, concurrent therapy with digoxin.

LIFESPAN CONSIDERATIONS:

Pregnancy/Lactation: Unknown if drug crosses placenta or is distributed in breast milk. **Pregnancy Category C. Children:** Safety and efficacy not established. **Elderly:** No age-related precautions noted.

INTERACTIONS

DRUG: May increase serum **digoxin. HERBAL:** None significant. **FOOD:** None known. **LAB VALUES:** May increase serum calcium.

AVAILABILITY (Rx)

INJECTION SOLUTION: 750 mcg in 3-ml prefilled pen delivers 20 mcg/dose.

ADMINISTRATION/HANDLING

SUBCUTANEOUS

• Refrigerate, but minimize time out of refrigerator. Do not freeze; discard if frozen. • Administer into thigh, abdominal wall.

INDICATIONS/ROUTES/DOSAGE

OSTEOPOROSIS

SUBCUTANEOUS: ADULTS, ELDERLY: 20 mcg once a day into thigh, abdominal wall.

SIDE EFFECTS

OCCASIONAL: Leg cramps, nausea, dizziness, headache, orthostatic hypotension, tachycardia.

ADVERSE EFFECTS/ TOXIC REACTIONS

Angina pectoris has been reported.

NURSING CONSIDERATIONS

BASELINE ASSESSMENT

Check urinary, serum calcium levels, serum parathyroid hormone levels.

INTERVENTION/EVALUATION

Monitor bone mineral density, urinary, serum calcium levels, serum parathyroid hormone levels. Observe for symptoms of hypercalcemia. Monitor B/P for hypotension, pulse for tachycardia.

PATIENT/FAMILY TEACHING

• Immediately sit or lie down if symptoms of orthostatic hypotension occur. • Inform physician if persistent symptoms of hypercalcemia (nausea, vomiting, constipation, lethargy, asthenia [loss of strength, energy]) occur.

testosterone

tess-**toss**-ter-one

(Andriol ✤, Androderm, AndroGel, Andropository ✤, Delatestryl, Depandro 100, Depotest ✤, Depo-Testosterone, Everone ✤, FIRST-Testosterone, FIRST-Testosterone MC, Striant, Testim, Testopel, Virilon IM ✤)

Do not confuse testosterone with testolactone.

CLASSIFICATION

PHARMACOTHERAPEUTIC: Androgen. **CLINICAL:** Sex hormone.

ACTION

Promotes growth, development of male sex organs, maintains secondary sex characteristics in androgen-deficient males. **Therapeutic Effect:** Relieves androgen deficiency.

PHARMACOKINETICS

Well absorbed after IM administration. Protein binding: 98%. Undergoes first-pass metabolism in liver. Primarily excreted in urine. Unknown if removed by hemodialysis. **Half-life:** 10–20 min.

USES

Injection: Treatment of delayed male puberty, male hypogonadism, inoperable female breast cancer. **Pellet:** Treatment

T

of delayed male puberty, male hypogonadism. **Buccal, transdermal:** Male hypogonadism.

PRECAUTIONS

CONTRAINDICATIONS: Breast-feeding, cardiac impairment, hypercalcemia, pregnancy, prostate or breast cancer in males, severe hepatic/renal disease. **CAUTIONS:** Renal or hepatic dysfunction, diabetes.

LIFESPAN CONSIDERATIONS:

Pregnancy/Lactation: Contraindicated during lactation. **Pregnancy Category X. Children:** Safety and efficacy not established; use with caution. **Elderly:** May increase risk of hyperplasia, stimulate growth of occult prostate carcinoma.

INTERACTIONS

DRUG: May decrease serum glucose, requiring **insulin** adjustments. May increase effects of **oral anticoagulants. HERBAL:** None significant. **FOOD:** None known. **LAB VALUES:** May increase Hgb, Hct, LDL, serum alkaline phosphatase, bilirubin, calcium, potassium, sodium, AST. May decrease HDL.

AVAILABILITY (Rx)

GEL, TOPICAL: (ANDROGEL, TESTIM): 1.25 g/actuation, 2.5 g, 5 g. **INJECTION (CYPIONATE [DEPO-TESTOSTERONE]):** 100 mg/ml, 200 mg/ml. **INJECTION (ENANTHATE [DELATESTRYL]):** 200 mg/ml. **MUCOADHESIVE, FOR BUCCAL APPLICATION: (STRIANT):** 30 mg. **PELLET, FOR SUBCUTANEOUS IMPLANTATION: (TESTOPEL):** 75 mg. **TRANSDERMAL SYSTEM: (ANDRODERM):** 2.5 mg/day, 5 mg/day.

ADMINISTRATION/HANDLING

IM

• Give deep in gluteal muscle. • Do not give IV. • Warming or shaking redissolves crystals that may form in long-acting preparations. • Wet needle of syringe may cause solution to become cloudy; this does not affect potency.

BUCCAL

Striant • Apply to gum area (above incisor tooth). • Not affected by food, tooth brushing, gum, chewing, alcoholic beverages. • Remove before placing new system.

TRANSDERMAL

Testoderm • Apply to clean, dry scrotal skin that has been dry-shaved (optimal skin contact). Testoderm TTS may be applied to arm, back, upper buttock.

Androderm • Apply to clean, dry area on skin on back, abdomen, upper arms, thighs. • Do not apply to bony prominences (e.g., shoulder) or oily, damaged, irritated skin. Do not apply to scrotum. • Rotate application site with 7-day interval to same site.

TRANSDERMAL GEL

(Androgel, Testim) • Apply (morning preferred) to clean, dry, intact skin of shoulder, upper arms (Androgel may also be applied to abdomen). • Upon opening packet(s), squeeze entire contents into palm of hand, immediately apply to application site. • Allow to dry. • Do not apply to genitals.

INDICATIONS/ROUTES/DOSAGE

MALE HYPOGONADISM

IM: ADULTS: 50–400 mg q2–4wk. **ADOLESCENTS:** Initially 40–50 mg/m^2/dose monthly until growth rate falls to prepubertal levels. 100 mg/m^2/dose until growth ceases. MAINTENANCE VIRILIZING DOSE: 100 mg/m^2/dose twice a mo.
SUBCUTANEOUS (pellets): ADULTS, ADOLESCENTS: 150–450 mg q3–6mo.
TRANSDERMAL PATCH (Testoderm): ADULTS, ELDERLY: Start therapy with 6 mg/day patch. Apply patch to scrotal skin.
TRANSDERMAL PATCH (Testoderm TTS): ADULTS, ELDERLY: Apply TTS patch to arm, back, upper buttocks.

TRANSDERMAL PATCH (Androderm): ADULTS, ELDERLY: Start therapy with 5 mg/day patch applied at night. Apply patch to abdomen, back, thighs, upper arms.

TRANSDERMAL GEL (Androgel): ADULTS, ELDERLY: Initial dose of 5 mg delivers 50 mg testosterone and is applied once daily to abdomen, shoulders, upper arms. May increase to 7.5 g, then to 10 g, if necessary.

TRANSDERMAL GEL (Testim): ADULTS, ELDERLY: Initial dose of 5 g delivers 50 mg testosterone and is applied once a day to the shoulders, upper arms. May increase to 10 g.

BUCCAL (Striant): ADULTS, ELDERLY: 30 mg q12h.

DELAYED MALE PUBERTY

IM: ADULTS: 50–200 mg q2–4wk. **ADOLESCENTS:** 40–50 mg/m^2/dose every mo for 6 mos.

SUBCUTANEOUS (Pellets): ADULTS, ADOLESCENTS: 150–450 mg q3–6mo.

BREAST CARCINOMA

IM (Testosterone Aqueous): ADULTS: 50–100 mg 3 times a wk.

IM (Testosterone Cypionate or Testosterone Ethanate): ADULTS: 200–400 mg q2–4wk.

IM (Testosterone Propionate): ADULTS: 50–100 mg 3 times a wk.

SIDE EFFECTS

FREQUENT: Gynecomastia, acne. **Females:** Hirsutism, amenorrhea, or other menstrual irregularities, deepening of voice, clitoral enlargement (may not be reversible when drug is discontinued). **OCCASIONAL:** Edema, nausea, insomnia, oligospermia, priapism, male-pattern baldness, bladder irritability, hypercalcemia (in immobilized pts, those with breast cancer), hypercholesterolemia, inflammation/pain at IM injection site. **Transdermal:** Pruritus, erythema, skin irritation. **RARE:** Polycythemia (with high dosage), hypersensitivity.

ADVERSE EFFECTS/ TOXIC REACTIONS

Peliosis hepatitis (presence of blood-filled cysts in parenchyma of liver), hepatic neoplasms, hepatocellular carcinoma have been associated with prolonged high-dose therapy. Anaphylactic reactions occur rarely.

NURSING CONSIDERATIONS

BASELINE ASSESSMENT

Establish baseline weight, B/P, Hgb, Hct. Check serum hepatic function, electrolytes, cholesterol. Wrist x-rays may be ordered to determine bone maturation in children.

INTERVENTION/EVALUATION

Weigh daily, report weekly gain of more than 5 lb; evaluate for edema. Monitor I&O. Check B/P at least twice a day. Assess serum electrolytes, cholesterol, Hgb, Hct (periodically for high dosage), hepatic function test results, radiologic exam of wrist, hand (when using in prepubertal children). With breast cancer or immobility, check for hypercalcemia (lethargy, muscle weakness, confusion, irritability). Ensure adequate intake of protein, calories. Assess for virilization. Monitor sleep patterns. Check injection site for redness, swelling, pain.

PATIENT/FAMILY TEACHING

• Regular visits to physician and monitoring tests are necessary. • Do not take any other medications without consulting physician. • Teach diet high in protein, calories. • Food may be better tolerated in small, frequent feedings. • Weigh daily, report 5 lb/wk gain. • Notify physician if nausea, vomiting, acne, pedal edema occurs. • **Females:** Promptly report menstrual irregularities, hoarseness, deepening of voice. • **Males:** Report frequent erections, difficulty urinating, gynecomastia.

tetracaine

(Pontocaine)

See Anesthetics: local (p. 6C)

tetracycline

tet-ra-**sye**-kleen

(Apo-Tetra ✤, Sumycin)

CLASSIFICATION

PHARMACOTHERAPEUTIC: Tetracycline. **CLINICAL:** Antibiotic.

ACTION

Inhibits bacterial protein synthesis by binding to ribosomes. **Therapeutic Effect:** Bacteriostatic.

PHARMACOKINETICS

Readily absorbed from GI tract. Protein binding: 30%–60%. Widely distributed. Excreted in urine; eliminated in feces through biliary system. Not removed by hemodialysis. **Half-life:** 6–11 hrs (increased in renal impairment).

USES

Treatment of susceptible infections due to *Rickettsiae, M. pneumoniae, C. trachomatis, C. psittaci, H. ducreyi, Yersinia pestis, Francisella tularensis, Bivrio cholerae, Brucella* species: treatment of susceptible infections due to gram-negative organisms including inflammatory acne vulgaris, Lyme disease, mycoplasma disease, *Legionella,* Rocky Mountain spotted fever, chlamydial infection in pts with gonorrhea. Part of multidrug regimen of *H. pylori* eradication to reduce risk of duodenal ulcer recurrence.

PRECAUTIONS

CONTRAINDICATIONS: Children 8 yrs and younger, hypersensitivity to sulfites. **CAUTIONS:** Sun, ultraviolet light exposure (severe photosensitivity reaction).

LIFESPAN CONSIDERATIONS:

Pregnancy/Lactation: Readily crosses placenta. Distributed in breast milk. Avoid use in women during last half of pregnancy. **Pregnancy Category D (B with topical form). Children:** Not recommended in those 8 yrs and younger; may cause permanent staining of teeth, enamel hypoplasia, decreased linear skeletal growth rate. **Elderly:** No age-related precautions noted.

INTERACTIONS

DRUG: Carbamazepine, phenytoin may decrease concentration. **Cholestyramine, colestipol** may decrease absorption. May decrease effects of **oral contraceptives. Antacids, calcium or iron supplements, laxatives containing magnesium** may form nonabsorbable, undigestable complexes. **HERBAL: Dong quai, St. John's wort** may increase risk of photosensitivity. **FOOD: Dairy products** inhibit absorption. **LAB VALUES:** May increase BUN, serum alkaline phosphatase, amylase, bilirubin, AST, ALT.

AVAILABILITY (Rx)

CAPSULES (SUMYCIN): 250 mg, 500 mg. **ORAL SUSPENSION (SUMYCIN):** 125 mg/5 ml. **TABLETS (SUMYCIN):** 250 mg, 500 mg. **TOPICAL OINTMENT:** 3%. **TOPICAL SOLUTION:** 2.2 mg/ml.

ADMINISTRATION/HANDLING

PO

- Give capsules, tablets with full glass of water 1 hr before or 2 hrs after meals.

TOPICAL

- Cleanse area gently before application.
- Apply only to affected area.

INDICATIONS/ROUTES/DOSAGE

◀ **ALERT** ▶ Space doses evenly around the clock.

USUAL DOSAGE

PO: ADULTS, ELDERLY: 250–500 mg q6–12h. **CHILDREN 8 YRS AND OLDER:** 25–50 mg/kg/day in 4 divided doses. **Maximum:** 3 g/day.

H. PYLORI INFECTION

PO: ADULTS, ELDERLY: 500 mg 2–4 times a day (in combination).
TOPICAL: ADULTS, ELDERLY: Apply twice a day (once in the morning, once in the evening).

DOSAGE IN RENAL IMPAIRMENT

Dosage interval is modified based on creatinine clearance.

Creatinine Clearance	Dosage Interval
50–80 ml/min	Usual dose q8–12h
10–49 ml/min	Usual dose q12–24h
Less than 10 ml/min	Usual dose q24h

SIDE EFFECTS

FREQUENT: Dizziness, light-headedness, diarrhea, nausea, vomiting, abdominal cramps, photosensitivity (may be severe). **Topical:** Dry, scaly skin; stinging/burning sensation. **OCCASIONAL:** Pigmentation of skin, mucous membranes, anal/genital pruritus, stomatitis. **Topical:** Pain, erythema, swelling, other skin irritation.

ADVERSE EFFECTS/ TOXIC REACTIONS

Superinfection (esp. fungal), anaphylaxis, increased intracranial pressure (ICP) may occur. Bulging fontanelles occur rarely in infants.

NURSING CONSIDERATIONS

BASELINE ASSESSMENT

Question for history of allergies, esp. tetracyclines, sulfite.

INTERVENTION/EVALUATION

Assess skin for rash. Monitor daily pattern of bowel activity/stool consistency. Monitor food intake, tolerance. Be alert for superinfection: diarrhea, stomatitis, anal/genital pruritus. Monitor B/P, level of consciousness (potential for ICP).

PATIENT/FAMILY TEACHING

• Continue antibiotic for full length of treatment. • Space doses evenly. • Take oral doses on empty stomach (1 hr before or 2 hrs after food, beverages). • Drink full glass of water with capsules; avoid bedtime doses. • Notify physician if diarrhea, rash, other new symptom occurs. • Protect skin from sun, ultraviolet light exposure. • Consult physician before taking any other medication. • Avoid tasks that require alertness, motor skills until response to drug is established (may cause dizziness, light-headedness). • **Topical:** Skin may turn yellow with topical application (washing removes solution); fabrics may be stained by heavy application. • Do not apply to deep, open wounds.

Teveten, *see eprosartan*

thalidomide

thah-**lid**-owe-mide
(Thalomid)

◆CLASSIFICATION

PHARMACOTHERAPEUTIC: Immunomodulator. **CLINICAL:** Immunosuppressive agent.

ACTION

Has sedative, anti-inflammatory, immunosuppressive activity. Action may be due to selective inhibition of production of tumor necrosis factor-alpha. **Therapeutic Effect:** Reduces muscle wasting in HIV pts; reduces local and systemic effects of leprosy.

PHARMACOKINETICS

Protein binding: 55%. Metabolism and elimination are not known. **Half-life:** 5–7 hrs.

USES

Treatment of leprosy, multiple myeloma. **OFF-LABEL:** Prevention/treatment of discoid lupus erythematosus, erythema fultiforme, graft vs host reactions following bone marrow transplantation, rheumatoid arthritis; treatment of Behcet's syndrome, Crohn's disease, GI bleeding, pruritus, recurrent aphthous ulcers in HIV pts, wasting syndrome associated with HIV infection, cancer.

PRECAUTIONS

CONTRAINDICATIONS: Neutropenia, peripheral neuropathy, pregnancy. **CAUTIONS:** History of seizures.

LIFESPAN CONSIDERATIONS:

Pregnancy/Lactation: Contraindicated in women who are or may become pregnant and who are not using two required types of birth control or who are not continually abstaining from heterosexual sexual contact. Can cause severe birth defects, fetal death. Unknown if distributed in breast milk. **Pregnancy Category X. Children:** Safety and efficacy not established in children under 12 yrs. **Elderly:** No age-related precautions noted.

INTERACTIONS

DRUG: Alcohol, other CNS depressants may increase sedative effects. **Medications associated with peripheral neuropathy (e.g., isoniazid, lithium, metronidazole, phenytoin)** may increase peripheral neuropathy. May decrease effect of **oral contraceptives. Carbamazepine, phenytoin** may decrease concentration. **HERBAL: Cat's claw** possesses immunostimulant properties. **FOOD:** None known. **LAB VALUES:** None known.

AVAILABILITY (Rx)

CAPSULES: 50 mg, 100 mg, 200 mg.

ADMINISTRATION/HANDLING

◄ **ALERT** ► Thalidomide may be prescribed only by licensed prescribers who are registered in the S.T.E.P.S. program and understand the risk of teratogenicity if thalidomide is used during pregnancy.

• Administer thalidomide with water at least 1 hr after evening meal and, if possible, at bedtime due to risk of drowsiness.

INDICATIONS/ROUTES/DOSAGE

AIDS-RELATED MUSCLE WASTING

PO: ADULTS: 100–300 mg a day.

LEPROSY

PO: ADULTS, ELDERLY: Initially, 100–300 mg/day as single bedtime dose, at least 1 hr after evening meal. Continue until active reaction subsides, then reduce dose q2–4wk in 50-mg increments.

MULTIPLE MYELOMA

PO: ADULTS, ELDERLY: 200 mg once daily, preferably at bedtime, with dexamethasone 40 mg on days 1–4, 7–12, 17–20 of each 28-day cycle.

SIDE EFFECTS

FREQUENT: Drowsiness, dizziness, mood changes, constipation, dry mouth, peripheral neuropathy. **OCCASIONAL:** Increased appetite, weight gain, headache, loss of libido, edema of face/limbs, nausea, alopecia, dry skin, rash, hypothyroidism.

ADVERSE EFFECTS/ TOXIC REACTIONS

Neutropenia, peripheral neuropathy, thromboembolism occur rarely.

NURSING CONSIDERATIONS

BASELINE ASSESSMENT

Assess for hypersensitivity to thalidomide. Assess for pregnancy in females 24 hrs before beginning thalidomide therapy (contraindicated). Determine

T

use of other medications (many interactions).

INTERVENTION/EVALUATION

Monitor WBC, nerve conduction studies, HIV viral load. Observe for signs/symptoms of peripheral neuropathy. Perform pregnancy tests on women of childbearing potential weekly during the first 4 wks of use, then at 4-wk intervals in women with regular menstrual cycles or q2wk in women with irregular menstrual cycles.

PATIENT/FAMILY TEACHING

• Avoid tasks requiring alertness, motor skills until response to drug is established. • Avoid use of alcoholic beverages, other drugs causing drowsiness. • Pregnancy test within 24 hrs before starting thalidomide, then q2–4wk in women of childbearing age. • Discontinue and call physician if symptoms of peripheral neuropathy occur. • Advise male pts receiving thalidomide to always use a latex condom during any sexual contact with women of childbearing potential.

Thalomid, *see thalidomide*

thiamine (vitamin B_1)

thy-a-min

(Betaxin ✱, Vitamin B_1)

CLASSIFICATION

PHARMACOTHERAPEUTIC: Water-soluble vitamin. **CLINICAL:** Vitamin B complex (see p. 150C).

ACTION

Combines with adenosine triphosphate in liver, kidneys, leukocytes to form thiamine diphosphate, a coenzyme necessary for carbohydrate metabolism. **Therapeutic Effect:** Prevents, reverses thiamine deficiency.

PHARMACOKINETICS

Readily absorbed from GI tract, primarily in duodenum, after IM administration. Widely distributed. Metabolized in the liver. Primarily excreted in urine.

USES

Prevention/treatment of thiamine deficiency (e.g., beriberi, Wernicke's encephalopathy syndrome, peripheral neuritis associated with pellegra, alcoholic pts with altered sensorium), metabolic disorders.

PRECAUTIONS

CONTRAINDICATIONS: None known. **CAUTIONS:** Wernicke's encephalopathy.

LIFESPAN CONSIDERATIONS:

Pregnancy/Lactation: Crosses placenta. Unknown if drug is excreted in breast milk. **Pregnancy Category A (C if used in doses above recommended daily allowance). Children/Elderly:** No age-related precautions noted.

INTERACTIONS

DRUG: None significant. **HERBAL:** None significant. **FOOD:** None known. **LAB VALUES:** None known.

AVAILABILITY

INJECTION SOLUTION (VITAMIN B_1): 100 mg/ml. **TABLETS (OTC):** 50 mg, 100 mg, 250 mg, 500 mg.

ADMINISTRATION/HANDLING

◀ **ALERT** ▶ IV, IM administration used only in acutely ill or those unresponsive to PO route (GI malabsorption syndrome). IM route preferred to IV use. Give by IV push, or add to most IV solutions and give as infusion.

T

IV INCOMPATIBILITY

Sodium bicarbonate.

IV COMPATIBILITIES

Famotidine (Pepcid), multivitamins.

INDICATIONS/ROUTES/DOSAGE

DIETARY SUPPLEMENT

PO: ADULTS, ELDERLY: 1–2 mg/day. **CHILDREN:** 0.5–1 mg/day. **INFANTS:** 0.3–0.5 mg/day.

THIAMINE DEFICIENCY

PO: ADULTS, ELDERLY: 5–30 mg/day, as a single dose or in 3 divided doses, for 1 mo. **CHILDREN:** 10–50 mg/day in 3 divided doses.

CRITICALLY ILL PTS, MALABSORPTION SYNDROME

IV, IM: ADULTS, ELDERLY: 5–100 mg, 3 times a day. **CHILDREN:** 10–25 mg/day.

METABOLIC DISORDERS

PO: ADULTS, ELDERLY, CHILDREN: 10–20 mg/day; increased up to 4 g/day in divided doses.

SIDE EFFECTS

FREQUENT: Pain, induration, tenderness at IM injection site.

ADVERSE EFFECTS/ TOXIC REACTIONS

IV administration may result in rare, severe hypersensitivity reaction marked by feeling of warmth, pruritus, urticaria, weakness, diaphoresis, nausea, restlessness, tightness in throat, angioedema, cyanosis, pulmonary edema, GI tract bleeding, cardiovascular collapse.

T

NURSING CONSIDERATIONS

INTERVENTION/EVALUATION

Monitor EKG readings, lab values for erythrocyte activity. Assess for clinical improvement (improved sense of well-being, weight gain). Observe for reversal of deficiency symptoms (**neurologic:** peripheral neuropathy, hyporeflexia, nystagmus, ophthalmoplegia, ataxia, muscle weakness; **cardiac:** venous hypertension, bounding arterial pulse, tachycardia, edema; **mental:** confused state).

PATIENT/FAMILY TEACHING

• Discomfort may occur with IM injection. • Foods rich in thiamine include pork, organ meats, whole grain and enriched cereals, legumes, nuts, seeds, yeast, wheat germ, rice bran. • Urine may appear bright yellow.

thioguanine

thigh-oh-**guan**-een

(Thioguanine)

See Cancer chemotherapeutic agents (p. 83C)

thiopental

(Pentothal)

See Anesthetics: general (p. 3C)

thioridazine

thye-or-**rid**-a-zeen

(Apo-Thioridazine ✦, Mellaril, Thioridazine Intensol)

Do not confuse thioridazine with thiothixene or Thorazine, or Mellaril with Mebaral.

CLASSIFICATION

PHARMACOTHERAPEUTIC: Phenothiazine. **CLINICAL:** Antipsychotic, sedative, antidyskinetic (see p. 63C).

ACTION

Blocks dopamine at postsynaptic receptor sites. Possesses strong anticholinergic, sedative effects. **Therapeutic Effect:** Suppresses behavioral response in psychosis; reduces locomotor activity, aggressiveness.

PHARMACOKINETICS

Absorption may be erratic. Protein binding: Very high. Metabolized in liver. Excreted in urine. **Half-life:** 21–24 hrs.

USES

Treatment of refractory schizophrenic pts. **OFF-LABEL:** Treatment of behavioral problems in children, dementia, depressive neurosis.

PRECAUTIONS

CONTRAINDICATIONS: Angle-closure glaucoma, blood dyscrasias, cardiac arrhythmias, cardiac/hepatic impairment, concurrent use of drugs that prolong QT interval, severe CNS depression. **CAUTIONS:** Seizures, decreased GI motility, urinary retention, benign prostatic hypertrophy, visual problems.

LIFESPAN CONSIDERATIONS:

Pregnancy/Lactation: Drug crosses placenta; is distributed is breast milk. **Pregnancy Category C. Children:** Increased risk for development of extrapyramidal symptoms (EPS), neuromuscular symptoms, esp. dystonias. **Elderly:** Prone to anticholinergic effects (dry mouth, EPS, orthostatic hypotension, sedation).

INTERACTIONS

DRUG Alcohol, other CNS depressants may increase respiratory depression, hypotensive effects. **Antithyroid agents** may increase risk of agranulocytosis. **EPS-producing medications** may increase risk of EPS. **Hypotensive medications (e.g., antihypertensives, diuretics)** may worsen hypotension. May decrease effects of **levodopa. Lithium** may decrease absorption, produce adverse neurologic effects. **MAOIs, tricyclic antidepressants** may increase anticholinergic, sedative effects. **Medications causing QT interval prolongation (e.g., erythromycin, procainamide, quinidine)** may lengthen QT interval. **HERBAL: Gotu kola, kava kava, St. John's wort, valerian** may increase CNS depression. **St. John's wort, dong quai** may increase photosensitization. **FOOD:** None known. **LAB VALUES:** May cause EKG changes. Therapeutic serum level: 0.2–2.6 mcg/ml; toxic serum level: not established.

AVAILABILITY (Rx)

ORAL SOLUTION (CONCENTRATE): 30 mg/ml (Mellaril), 100 mg/ml (Thioridazine Intensol). **TABLETS (MELLARIL):** 10 mg, 15 mg, 25 mg, 50 mg, 100 mg, 150 mg, 200 mg.

ADMINISTRATION/HANDLING

PO

- May give without regard to food.

INDICATIONS/ROUTES/DOSAGE

PSYCHOSIS

PO: ADULTS, ELDERLY, CHILDREN 12 YRS AND OLDER: Initially, 25–100 mg 3 times a day; dosage increased gradually. **Maximum:** 800 mg/day. **CHILDREN 2–11 YRS:** Initially, 0.5 mg/kg/day in 2–3 divided doses. **Maximum:** 3 mg/kg/day.

SIDE EFFECTS

Generally well tolerated with only mild, transient side effects. **OCCASIONAL:** Drowsiness during early therapy, dry mouth, blurred vision, lethargy, constipation, diarrhea, nasal congestion, peripheral edema, urinary retention. **RARE:** Ocular changes, altered skin pigmentation (in those taking high doses for prolonged periods), photosensitivity, darkening of urine.

ADVERSE EFFECTS/ TOXIC REACTIONS

Prolonged QT interval may produce torsades de pointes, a form of ventricular tachycardia, sudden death.

NURSING CONSIDERATIONS

BASELINE ASSESSMENT

Avoid skin contact with solution (contact dermatitis). Assess behavior, appearance, emotional status, response to environment, speech pattern, thought content.

INTERVENTION/EVALUATION

Assess for EPS. Monitor EKG, CBC, B/P, serum potassium, hepatic function, eye exams. Monitor for fine tongue movement (may be early sign of tardive dyskinesia). Supervise suicidal-risk pt closely during early therapy (as depression lessens, energy level improves, and suicide potential increases). Assess for therapeutic response (interest in surroundings, improvement in self-care, increased ability to concentrate, relaxed facial expression). Therapeutic serum level: 0.2–2.6 mcg/ml; toxic serum level: not established.

PATIENT/FAMILY TEACHING

• Full therapeutic effect may take up to 6 wks. • Urine may darken. • Do not abruptly withdraw from long-term drug therapy. • Report visual disturbances. • Sugarless gum, sips of tepid water may relieve dry mouth. • Drowsiness generally subsides during continued therapy. • Avoid tasks that require alertness, motor skills until response to drug is established. • Avoid alcohol. • Avoid exposure to sunlight, artificial light.

T

thiotepa

thigh-oh-**teh**-pah
(Thioplex)

CLASSIFICATION

PHARMACOTHERAPEUTIC: Alkylating agent. **CLINICAL:** Antineoplastic (see p. 83C).

ACTION

Inhibits DNA, RNA protein synthesis by cross-linking with DNA, RNA strands, preventing cell growth. Cell cycle–phase nonspecific. **Therapeutic Effect:** Produces cell death.

PHARMACOKINETICS

Incompletely absorbed from GI tract. Metabolized in liver. Excreted in urine. **Half-life:** 2.3–2.4 hrs.

USES

Treatment of superficial papillary carcinoma of urinary bladder, adenocarcinoma of breast and ovary, Hodgkin's disease, lymphosarcoma. Intracavitary injection to control pleural, pericardial, peritoneal effusions due to metastatic tumors. **OFF-LABEL:** Treatment of lung carcinoma.

PRECAUTIONS

CONTRAINDICATIONS: Pregnancy, severe myelosuppression (leukocyte count less than $3,000/mm^3$ or platelet count less than $150,000/mm^3$). **CAUTIONS:** Hepatic/renal impairment, bone marrow dysfunction.

LIFESPAN CONSIDERATIONS:

Pregnancy/Lactation: May cause fetal harm. Unknown if drug is distributed is breast milk. **Pregnancy Category D.** **Children:** Safety and efficacy not established. **Elderly:** No age-related precautions noted.

INTERACTIONS

DRUG: May decrease effects of **antigout medications. Bone marrow depressants** may increase myelosuppression. **Live virus vaccines** may potentiate virus replication, increase vaccine side effects, decrease pt's antibody response to vaccine. **HERBAL:** Avoid **black cohosh, dong quai** in estrogen-dependent tumors. **St. John's wort** may increase photosensitization. **FOOD:** None known. **LAB VALUES:** May increase serum uric acid.

AVAILABILITY (Rx)

INJECTION, POWDER FOR RECONSTITUTION: 15 mg, 30 mg.

ADMINISTRATION/HANDLING

◀ **ALERT** ▶ May be carcinogenic, mutagenic, teratogenic. Handle with extreme caution during preparation/administration.

IV

◀ **ALERT** ▶ Give by IV, intrapleural, intraperitoneal, intrapericardial, or intratumor injection; intravesical instillation.

Reconstitution • Reconstitute 15-mg vial with 1.5 ml Sterile Water for Injection to provide concentration of 10 mg/ml. Shake solution gently; let stand to clear.

Rate of administration • Withdraw reconstituted drug through 0.22-micron filter before administration. • For IV push, give over 5 min at concentration of 10 mg/ml. • Give IV infusion at concentration of 1 mg/ml.

Storage • Refrigerate unopened vials. • Reconstituted solution appears clear to slightly opaque; is stable for 5 days if refrigerated. Discard if solution appears grossly opaque or precipitate forms.

IV INCOMPATIBILITIES

Cisplatin (Platinol-AQ), filgrastim (Neupogen).

IV COMPATIBILITIES

Allopurinol (Aloprim), bumetanide (Bumex), calcium gluconate, carboplatin (Paraplatin), cyclophosphamide (Cytoxan), dexamethasone (Decadron), diphenhydramine (Benadryl), doxorubicin (Adriamycin), etoposide (VePesid), fluorouracil, gemcitabine (Gemzar), granisetron (Kytril), heparin, hydromorphone (Dilaudid), leucovorin, lorazepam (Ativan), magnesium sulfate, morphine, ondansetron (Zofran), paclitaxel (Taxol), potassium chloride, vincristine (Oncovin), vinorelbine (Navelbine).

INDICATIONS/ROUTES/DOSAGE

◀ **ALERT** ▶ Dosage individualized based on clinical response, tolerance to adverse effects. When used in combination therapy, consult specific protocols for optimum dosage, sequence of drug administration.

INITIAL THERAPY

IV: ADULTS, ELDERLY: Initially, 0.3–0.4 mg/kg every 1–4 wks. Maintenance dose adjusted weekly based on blood counts. **CHILDREN:** 25–65 mg/m^2 as single dose every 3–4 wks.

CONTROL OF EFFUSIONS

INTRACAVITARY INJECTION: ADULTS, ELDERLY: 0.6–0.8 mg/kg every 1–4 wks.

SIDE EFFECTS

OCCASIONAL: Pain at injection site, headache, dizziness, urticaria, rash, nausea, vomiting, anorexia, stomatitis. **RARE:** Alopecia, cystitis, hematuria (following intravesicle administration).

ADVERSE EFFECTS/TOXIC REACTIONS

Hematologic toxicity (leukopenia, anemia, thrombocytopenia, pancytopenia) may occur due to bone marrow depression. Although WBC count falls to its lowest point 10–14 days after initial therapy, bone marrow effect not be evident for 30 days. Stomatitis, ulceration of intestinal mucosa may occur.

NURSING CONSIDERATIONS

BASELINE ASSESSMENT

Obtain hematologic tests at least weekly during therapy and for 3 wks after therapy discontinued.

INTERVENTION/EVALUATION

Interrupt therapy if WBC falls below 3,000/mm^3, platelet count below

T

150,000/mm³, WBC or platelet count declines rapidly. Monitor serum uric acid levels, hematology tests. Assess for stomatitis. Monitor for hematologic toxicity: infection (fever, sore throat, signs of local infection), unusual bruising/bleeding from any site, symptoms of anemia (excessive fatigue, weakness). Assess skin for rash, urticaria.

PATIENT/FAMILY TEACHING

• Maintain fastidious oral hygiene. • Do not have immunizations without physician's approval (drug lowers resistance). • Avoid crowds, those with infection. • Promptly report fever, sore throat, signs of local infection, unusual bruising/bleeding from any site.

thiothixene

thye-oh-**thix**-een

(Navane)

Do not confuse thiothixene with thioridazine.

CLASSIFICATION

CLINICAL: Antipsychotic (see p. 63C).

ACTION

Blocks postsynaptic dopamine receptor sites in brain. Has alpha-adrenergic blocking effects, depresses release of hypothalamic, hypophyseal hormones. **Therapeutic Effect:** Suppresses psychotic behavior.

PHARMACOKINETICS

Well absorbed from GI tract after IM administration. Widely distributed. Metabolized in liver. Primarily excreted in urine. Unknown if removed by hemodialysis. **Half-life:** 34 hrs.

USES

Symptomatic management of psychotic disorders.

PRECAUTIONS

CONTRAINDICATIONS: Blood dyscrasias, circulatory collapse, CNS depression, coma, history of seizures. **CAUTIONS:** Severe cardiovascular disorders, alcohol withdrawal, pt exposure to extreme heat, glaucoma, prostatic hypertrophy.

LIFESPAN CONSIDERATIONS:

Pregnancy/Lactation: Drug crosses placenta; is distributed in breast milk. **Pregnancy Category C. Children:** May develop neuromuscular or extrapyramidal symptoms (EPS), esp. dystonias. **Elderly:** More prone to orthostatic hypotension, anticholinergic effects (e.g., dry mouth), sedation, EPS.

INTERACTIONS

DRUG: **Alcohol, other CNS depressants** may increase CNS, respiratory depression, hypotensive effects. **EPS–producing medications** may increase risk of EPS. May inhibit effects of **levodopa. Quinidine** may increase cardiac effects. **HERBAL:** **Kava kava, St. John's wort, valerian** may increase CNS depression. **FOOD:** None known. **LAB VALUES:** May decrease serum uric acid.

AVAILABILITY (Rx)

CAPSULES: 1 mg, 2 mg, 5 mg, 10 mg, 20 mg.

ADMINISTRATION/HANDLING

PO

• Give without regard to meals.

INDICATIONS/ROUTES/DOSAGE

MILD TO MODERATE PSYCHOSIS

PO: ADULTS, ELDERLY, CHILDREN 12 YRS AND OLDER: 2 mg 3 times a day up to 20–30 mg/day.

SEVERE PSYCHOSIS

PO: ADULTS, ELDERLY, CHILDREN 12 YRS AND OLDER: Initially, 5 mg twice a day. May increase gradually up to 60 mg/day.

RAPID TRANQUILIZATION OF AGITATED PT

PO: ADULTS, ELDERLY: 5–10 mg q15–30min. **Total dose:** 15–30 mg.

SIDE EFFECTS

FREQUENT: Transient drowsiness, dry mouth, constipation, blurred vision, nasal congestion. **OCCASIONAL:** Diarrhea, peripheral edema, urinary retention, nausea. **RARE:** Ocular changes, altered skin pigmentation (in those taking high doses for prolonged periods), photosensitivity, hypotension, dizziness, syncope.

ADVERSE EFFECTS/ TOXIC REACTIONS

Most common extrapyramidal reaction is akathisia, characterized by motor restlessness, anxiety. Akinesia, marked by rigidity, tremor, increased salivation, mask-like facial expression, reduced voluntary movements, occurs less frequently. Dystonias, including torticollis (neck muscle spasm), opisthotonos (rigidity of back muscles), oculogyric crisis (rolling back of eyes) occur rarely. Tardive dyskinesia, characterized by tongue protrusion, puffing of cheeks, chewing/puckering of mouth, occurs rarely but may be irreversible. Elderly female pts have greater risk of developing this reaction. Grand mal seizures may occur in epileptic pts. Neuroleptic malignant syndrome occurs rarely.

NURSING CONSIDERATIONS

BASELINE ASSESSMENT

Assess behavior, appearance, emotional status, response to environment, speech pattern, thought content.

INTERVENTION/EVALUATION

Supervise suicidal-risk pt closely during early therapy (as depression lessens, energy level improves, increasing suicide potential). Monitor B/P for hypotension. Assess for peripheral edema. Monitor daily pattern of bowel activity/stool consistency. Prevent constipation. Observe for EPS, tardive dyskinesia; monitor for potentially fatal, rare neuroleptic malignant syndrome. Assess for therapeutic response (interest in surroundings, improvement in self-care, increased ability to concentrate, relaxed facial expression).

PATIENT/FAMILY TEACHING

• Full therapeutic effect may take up to 6 wks. • Report visual disturbances. • Sugarless gum, sips of tepid water may relieve dry mouth. • Drowsiness generally subsides during continued therapy. • Avoid tasks that require alertness, motor skills until response to drug is established. • Avoid alcohol, other CNS depressants. • Avoid exposure to direct sunlight, artificial light.

thyroid

(Armour Thyroid, S-P-T, Thyrar)

See Thyroid (p. 149C)

tiagabine

tie-**ag**-ah-bean

(Gabitril)

CLASSIFICATION

CLINICAL: Anticonvulsant (see p. 35C).

ACTION

Blocks reuptake in presynaptic neurons of gamma-aminobutyric acid (GABA), the

T

major inhibitory neurotransmitter in the CNS, in the presynaptic neurons, increasing GABA levels at postsynaptic neurons. **Therapeutic Effect:** Inhibits seizures.

USES

Adjunctive therapy for treatment of partial seizures. **OFF-LABEL:** Bipolar disorder.

PRECAUTIONS

CONTRAINDICATIONS: None known. **CAUTIONS:** Hepatic impairment. Concurrent use of alcohol, other CNS depressants may cause seizures.

LIFESPAN CONSIDERATIONS:

Pregnancy/Lactation: May produce teratogenic effects. Distributed in breast milk. **Pregnancy Category C.** **Children:** Safety and efficacy not established in children younger than 12 yrs. **Elderly:** Age-related hepatic impairment may require dosage adjustment.

INTERACTIONS

DRUG: **Carbamazepine, phenobarbital, phenytoin** may increase clearance. May alter effects of **valproic acid.** **HERBAL:** **Ginkgo biloba** may increase seizure threshold. **St. John's wort** may decrease concentration. **Gotu kola, kava kava, St. John's wort, valerian** may increase CNS depression. **FOOD:** None known. **LAB VALUES:** None known.

AVAILABILITY (Rx)

TABLETS: 2 mg, 4 mg, 6 mg, 8 mg, 10 mg, 12 mg, 16 mg.

ADMINISTRATION/HANDLING

- Give with food.

INDICATIONS/ROUTES/DOSAGE

PARTIAL SEIZURES

PO: ADULTS, ELDERLY: Initially, 4 mg once a day. May increase by 4–8 mg/day at weekly intervals. **Maximum:** 56 mg/day.
CHILDREN 12–18 YRS: Initially, 4 mg once a day. May increase by 4 mg at wk 2 and by 4–8 mg at weekly intervals thereafter. **Maximum:** 32 mg/day.

SIDE EFFECTS

FREQUENT (34%–20%): Dizziness, asthenia (loss of strength, energy), somnolence, nervousness, confusion, headache, infection, tremor. **OCCASIONAL:** Nausea, diarrhea, abdominal pain, impaired concentration.

ADVERSE EFFECTS/ TOXIC REACTIONS

Overdose characterized by agitation, confusion, hostility, weakness. Full recovery occurs within 24 hrs.

NURSING CONSIDERATIONS

BASELINE ASSESSMENT

Review history of seizure disorder (intensity, frequency, duration, level of consciousness [LOC]). Observe frequently for recurrence of seizure activity. Initiate seizure precautions.

INTERVENTION/EVALUATION

For those on long-term therapy, serum hepatic/renal function tests, CBC should be performed periodically. Assist with ambulation if dizziness occurs. Assess for clinical improvement (decrease in intensity, frequency of seizures).

PATIENT/FAMILY TEACHING

• If dizziness occurs, change positions slowly from recumbent to sitting position before standing. • Avoid tasks that require alertness, motor skills until response to drug is established. • Avoid alcohol.

Tiazac, *see diltiazem*

ticarcillin

(Ticar)

See Antibiotic: penicillins

ticarcillin clavulanate

tie-car-**sill**-in/klah-view-**lan**-ate

(Timentin)

CLASSIFICATION

PHARMACOTHERAPEUTIC: Penicillin. **CLINICAL:** Antibiotic (see p. 28C).

ACTION

Binds to bacterial cell walls, inhibiting cell wall synthesis. Clavulanate inhibits action of bacterial beta-lactamase. **Therapeutic Effect:** Bactericidal in susceptible organisms. Clavulanate protects ticarcillin from enzymatic degradation.

USES

Treatment of susceptible infections due to *P. aeruginosa, E. coli,* Enterobacter, Proteus, beta-lactamase producing *S. aureus, M. catarrhalis, H. influenzae,* Klebsiella, *B. fragilis* including septicemia, skin/skin structure, bone, joint, lower respiratory tract, gynecologic, intra-abdominal, UTIs.

PRECAUTIONS

CONTRAINDICATIONS: Hypersensitivity to any penicillin, clavulanic acid. **CAUTIONS:** History of allergies (esp. cephalosporins), renal impairment.

LIFESPAN CONSIDERATIONS:

Pregnancy/Lactation: Readily crosses placenta, appears in cord blood, amniotic fluid. Distributed in breast milk in low concentrations. May lead to allergic sensitization, diarrhea, candidiasis, skin rash in infant. **Pregnancy Category B.** **Children:** Safety and efficacy not established in those younger than 3 mos. **Elderly:** Age-related renal impairment may require dosage adjustment.

INTERACTIONS

DRUG: **Anticoagulants, heparin, NSAIDs, thrombolytics** may increase risk of hemorrhage (with high dosages of ticarcillin). **Probenecid** may increase concentration, risk of toxicity. **HERBAL:** None significant. **FOOD:** None known. **LAB VALUES:** May increase bleeding time, serum alkaline phosphatase, bilirubin, creatinine, LDH, AST, ALT. May decrease serum potassium, sodium, uric acid. May cause a positive Coombs' test.

AVAILABILITY (Rx)

INJECTION, POWDER FOR RECONSTITUTION: 3.1 g. **PREMIXED SOLUTION FOR INFUSION:** 3.1 g/100 ml.

ADMINISTRATION/HANDLING

IV

Reconstitution • Available in ready-to-use containers. • For IV infusion (piggyback), reconstitute each 3.1-g vial with 13 ml Sterile Water for Injection or 0.9% NaCl to provide concentration of 200 mg ticarcillin and 6.7 mg clavulanic acid per ml. • Shake vial to assist reconstitution. • Further dilute with 50–100 ml D_5W or 0.9% NaCl.

Rate of administration • Infuse over 30 min. • Because of potential for hypersensitivity/anaphylaxis, start initial dose at few drops/min, increase slowly to ordered rate. • Monitor pt first 10–15 min during initial dose, then check q10min.

Storage • Solution appears colorless to pale yellow (if solution darkens, indicates loss of potency). • Reconstituted IV infusion (piggyback) is stable for 24 hrs at room temperature, 3 days if refrigerated. • Discard if precipitate forms.

IV INCOMPATIBILITIES

Amphotericin B complex (Abelcet, AmBisome, Amphotec), vancomycin (Vancocin), total parenteral nutrition (TPN).

IV COMPATIBILITIES

Diltiazem (Cardizem), heparin, insulin, lipids, morphine, propofol (Diprivan).

INDICATIONS/ROUTES/DOSAGE

SYSTEMATIC INFECTIONS

IV: ADULTS, ELDERLY: 3.1 g (3 g ticarcillin) q4–6h. **Maximum:** 18–24 g/day. **CHILDREN 3 MOS AND OLDER:** 200–300 mg (as ticarcillin) q4–6h.

UTI

IV: ADULTS, ELDERLY: 3.1 g q6–8h.

DOSAGE IN RENAL IMPAIRMENT

Dosage interval is modified based on creatinine clearance.

Creatinine Clearance	Dosage Interval
10–30 ml/min	Usual dose q8h
Less than 10 ml/min	Usual dose q12h

SIDE EFFECTS

FREQUENT: Phlebitis, thrombophlebitis (with IV dose), rash, urticaria, pruritus, altered smell/taste. **OCCASIONAL:** Nausea, diarrhea, vomiting. **RARE :** Headache, fatigue, hallucinations, bleeding/bruising.

ADVERSE EFFECTS/ TOXIC REACTIONS

Overdosage may produce seizures, other neurologic reactions. Antibiotic-associated colitis, other superinfections may result from bacterial imbalance. Severe hypersensitivity reactions, including anaphylaxis, occur rarely.

NURSING CONSIDERATIONS

BASELINE ASSESSMENT

Question for history of allergies, esp. penicillins, cephalosporins.

INTERVENTION/EVALUATION

Hold medication, promptly report rash (hypersensitivity), diarrhea (fever, abdominal pain, mucus/blood in stool may indicate antibiotic-associated colitis). Assess food tolerance. Provide mouth care, sugarless gum, hard candy to offset altered taste, smell. Evaluate IV site for phlebitis (heat, pain, red streaking over vein). Monitor I&O, urinalysis, renal function tests. Assess for overt bleeding, bruising, swelling. Monitor hematology reports, serum electrolytes, particularly potassium. Be alert for superinfection: increased fever, sore throat, diarrhea, vomiting, stomatitis, anal/genital pruritus.

ticlopidine

tye-**klo**-pa-deen

(Apo-Ticlopidine ✤, Novo-Ticlopidine ✤, Ticlid)

CLASSIFICATION

PHARMACOTHERAPEUTIC: Aggregation inhibitor. **CLINICAL:** Antiplatelet (see p. 31C).

ACTION

Inhibits release of adenosine diphosphate from activated platelets, preventing fibrinogen from binding to glycoprotein IIb/IIIa receptors on surface of activated platelets. **Therapeutic Effect:** Inhibits platelet aggregation, thrombus formation.

PHARMACOKINETICS

Rapidly absorbed following PO administration. Protein binding: 98%. Extensively metabolized in liver. Primarily excreted in urine; partially eliminated in feces. **Half-life:** 12.6 hrs.

USES

To reduce risk of stroke in those who have experienced stroke-like symptoms (transient ischemic attacks) or with history of thrombotic stroke. **OFF-LABEL:** Prevention of postop deep vein thrombosis (DVT), protection of aortocoronary bypass grafts, reduction of graft loss after renal transplant, treatment of intermittent claudication, sickle cell disease, subarachnoid hemorrhage, diabetic microangiopathy, ischemic heart disease.

PRECAUTIONS

CONTRAINDICATIONS: Active pathologic bleeding (e.g., bleeding peptic ulcer, intracranial bleeding), hematopoietic disorders (neutropenia, thrombocytopenia), presence of hemostatic disorder, severe hepatic impairment. **CAUTIONS:** Those at increased risk of bleeding, severe hepatic/renal disease.

LIFESPAN CONSIDERATIONS:

Pregnancy/Lactation: Unknown if drug crosses placenta or is distributed in breast milk. **Pregnancy Category B.** **Children:** Safety and efficacy not established. **Elderly:** No age-related precautions noted.

INTERACTIONS

DRUG: **Aspirin, heparin, NSAIDs, oral anticoagulants, thrombolytics** may increase risk of bleeding. May increase concentration, risk of toxicity of **phenytoin, theophylline.** **HERBAL:** **Cat's claw, dong quai, evening primrose, feverfew, garlic, ginkgo biloba, ginger, red clover, horse chestnut, ginseng** possess antiplatelet activity, may increase risk of bleeding. **FOOD:** **All foods** increase bioavailability. **LAB VALUES:** May increase serum cholesterol, alkaline phosphatase, bilirubin, triglycerides, AST, ALT. May prolong bleeding time. May decrease neutrophil, platelet counts.

AVAILABILITY (Rx)

TABLETS: 250 mg.

ADMINISTRATION/HANDLING

PO

• Give with food or just after meals (bioavailability increased, GI discomfort decreased).

INDICATIONS/ROUTES/DOSAGE

PREVENTION OF STROKE

PO: ADULTS, ELDERLY: 250 mg twice a day.

SIDE EFFECTS

FREQUENT (13%–5%): Diarrhea, nausea, dyspepsia (heartburn, indigestion, epigastric pain, bloating). **RARE (2%–1%):** Vomiting, flatulence, pruritus, dizziness.

ADVERSE EFFECTS/ TOXIC REACTIONS

Neutropenia occurs in approximately 2% of pts. Thrombotic thrombocytopenia purpura, agranulocytosis, hepatitis, cholestatic jaundice, tinnitus occur rarely.

NURSING CONSIDERATIONS

BASELINE ASSESSMENT

Drug should be discontinued 10–14 days before surgery if antiplatelet effect is not desired.

INTERVENTION/EVALUATION

Monitor daily pattern of bowel activity/stool consistency. Assist with ambulation if dizziness occurs. Monitor heart sounds by auscultation. Assess B/P for hypotension. Assess skin for flushing, rash. Observe for signs of bleeding. Monitor CBC, serum hepatic function tests.

PATIENT/FAMILY TEACHING

• Take with food to decrease GI symptoms. • Periodic blood tests are essential. • Inform physician if fever, sore throat, chills, unusual bleeding occurs.

T

tigecycline

tie-geh-**sigh**-clean
(Tygacil)

◆CLASSIFICATION

PHARMACOTHERAPEUTIC: Glycylcycline. **CLINICAL:** Antibiotic.

ACTION

Blocks protein synthesis by binding to ribosomal receptor sites of bacterial cell wall. **Therapeutic Effect:** Bacteriostatic effect.

PHARMACOKINETICS

Extensive tissue distribution, minimally metabolized. Eliminated mainly by biliary/fecal route, with a lesser amount excreted in urine. Protein binding: 71%–89%. **Half-life:** Single dose: 27 hrs, following multiple doses: 42 hrs.

USES

Treatment of susceptible infections due to *E. coli, E. faecalis, S. aureus, S. agalactiae, S. anginosus* group (includes *S. anginosus, S. intermedius, S. constellatus*), *S. pyogenes, B. fragilis, Citrobacter freundii, E. cloacae, K. oxytoca, K. pneumoniae, B. thetaiotaomicron, B. umniformis, B. vulgatus, C. perfringens, Peptostreptococcus micros* including complicated skin/skin structure infections, complicated intra-abdominal infections.

T

PRECAUTIONS

CONTRAINDICATIONS: Children younger than 18 yrs. **CAUTIONS:** Hypersensitivity to tetracyclines, last half of pregnancy, hepatic impairment.

LIFESPAN CONSIDERATIONS:

Pregnancy/Lactation: May cause fetal harm. May be distributed in breast milk. Permanent discoloration of the teeth (brown-gray) may occur if used during tooth development. **Pregnancy Category D. Children:** Safety and effectiveness not established in children younger than 18 yrs. **Elderly:** No age-related precautions noted.

INTERACTIONS

DRUG: Effects of **oral contraceptives** may be decreased. **Warfarin** may increase risk of hypoprothrombinemia. **HERBAL:** None significant. **FOOD:** None known. **LAB VALUES:** May increase BUN, serum alkaline phosphatase, amylase, bilirubin, glucose, LDH, ALT, AST. May decrease Hgb, WBCs, thrombocytes, serum potassium, protein.

AVAILABILITY (Rx)

INJECTION, POWDER FOR RECONSTITUTION (TYGACIL): 50 mg vial.

ADMINISTRATION/HANDLING

IV

Reconstitution • Add 5.3 ml 0.9% NaCl or D_5W to each 50-mg vial. Swirl gently to dissolve. Resulting solution is 10 mg/ml. • Immediately withdraw 5 ml reconstituted solution and add to 100 ml 0.9% NaCl or D_5W bag for infusion (final concentration should not exceed 1 mg/ml). • Reconstituted solution appears yellow to red-orange.

Rate of administration • Administer over 30–60 min every 12 hrs. • May be given through a dedicated line or by Y-site piggyback. If same line is used for sequential infusion of several different drugs, line should be flushed before and after infusion of tigecycline with either 0.9% NaCl or D_5W.

Storage • Reconstituted solution is stable for up to 6 hrs at room temperature or up to 24 hrs if refrigerated. • Discard if solution is discolored (green, black) or precipitate forms.

IV INCOMPATIBILITIES

Amphotericin B, chlorpromazine, methylprednisolone, voriconazole.

IV COMPATIBILITIES

Dobutamine, dopamine, Ringer's lactate, lidocaine, potassium chloride, ranitidine, theophylline.

INDICATIONS/ROUTES/DOSAGE

SYSTEMIC INFECTIONS

IV: ADULTS OVER 18 YRS, ELDERLY: Initially, 100 mg, followed by 50 mg every 12 hrs for 5–14 days.

SEVERE HEPATIC IMPAIRMENT

IV: ADULTS OVER 18 YRS, ELDERLY: Initially, 100 mg, followed by 25 mg every 12 hrs.

SIDE EFFECTS

FREQUENT (29%–13%): Nausea, vomiting, diarrhea. **OCCASIONAL (7%–4%):** Headache, hypertension, dizziness, increased cough, delayed healing. **RARE (3%–2%):** Peripheral edema, pruritus, constipation, dyspepsia (heartburn, indigestion, epigastric pain), asthenia (loss of strength, energy), hypotension, phlebitis, insomnia, rash, diaphoresis.

ADVERSE EFFECTS/ TOXIC REACTIONS

Dyspnea, abscess, pseudomembranous colitis (abdominal cramps, severe watery diarrhea, fever) ranging from mild to life-threatening may result from altered bacterial balance.

NURSING CONSIDERATIONS

BASELINE ASSESSMENT

Question for history of allergies, esp. tetracyclines, before therapy.

INTERVENTION/EVALUATION

Monitor daily pattern of bowel activity/stool consistency. Be alert for signs/symptoms of superinfection: severe diarrhea, changes of oral mucosa (white patches, erythema of gums, tongue, mouth soreness), anal/genital pruritus. Nausea, vomiting may be controlled by antiemetics.

PATIENT/FAMILY TEACHING

• Notify physician if diarrhea, rash, mouth soreness, other new symptom occurs.

tiludronate

ti-**loo**-dro-nate

(Skelid)

CLASSIFICATION

PHARMACOTHERAPEUTIC: Bone resorption inhibitor. **CLINICAL:** Calcium regulator.

ACTION

Inhibits functioning osteoclasts through disruption of cytoskeletal ring structure, inhibition of osteoclastic proton pump. **Therapeutic Effect:** Inhibits bone resorption.

PHARMACOKINETICS

Well absorbed following PO administration. Protein binding: 90%. Not metabolized in liver. **Half-life:** 150 hrs.

USES

Treatment of Paget's disease of bone (osteitis deformans).

PRECAUTIONS

CONTRAINDICATIONS: GI disease (e.g., dysphagia, gastric ulcer), renal impairment. **CAUTIONS:** Hyperparathyroidism, hypocalcemia, vitamin D deficiency.

LIFESPAN CONSIDERATIONS:

Pregnancy/Lactation: Unknown if drug crosses placenta or is distributed is breast milk. **Pregnancy Category C. Children:** Safety and efficacy not established. **Elderly:** No age-related precautions noted.

INTERACTIONS

DRUG: Antacids containing aluminum or magnesium, calcium, salicylates

T

may interfere with absorption. **HERBAL:** None significant. **FOOD:** None known. **LAB VALUES:** None known.

AVAILABILITY (Rx)

TABLETS: 200 mg.

ADMINISTRATION/HANDLING

PO

• Must take with 6–8 oz plain water. • Do not give within 2 hrs of food intake. • Avoid giving aspirin, calcium supplements, mineral supplements, antacids within 2 hrs of tiludronate administration.

INDICATIONS/ROUTES/DOSAGE

PAGET'S DISEASE

PO: ADULTS, ELDERLY: 400 mg once a day for 3 mos.

SIDE EFFECTS

FREQUENT (9%–6%): Nausea, diarrhea, generalized body pain, back pain, headache. **OCCASIONAL:** Rash, dyspepsia (heartburn, indigestion, epigastric pain), vomiting, rhinitis, sinusitis, dizziness.

ADVERSE EFFECTS/ TOXIC REACTIONS

Dysphagia, esophagitis, esophageal ulcer, gastric ulcer occur rarely.

NURSING CONSIDERATIONS

BASELINE ASSESSMENT

Assess if pt is using other medications (esp. aluminum, magnesium, calcium, salicylates). Determine baseline renal function. Assess for GI disease.

INTERVENTION/EVALUATION

Monitor serum osteocalcin, alkaline phosphatase, adjusted calcium, urinary hydroxyproline to assess effectiveness of medication.

PATIENT/FAMILY TEACHING

• Take with 6–8 oz water. • Avoid other medication for 2 hrs before or after taking tiludronate. • Check with physician if calcium, vitamin D supplements are necessary.

Timentin, *see ticarcillin and clavulanate*

timolol

tim-oh-lole

(Apo-Timol ✤, Apo-Timop ✤, Betimol, Blocadren, Gen-Timolol ✤, Istalol, Novo-Timol ✤, PMS-Timolol ✤, Timolol Ophthalmic, Timoptic, Timoptic OccuDose, Timoptic Ocumeter, Timoptic Ocumeter Plus, Timoptic XE).

Do not confuse timolol with atenolol, or Timoptic with Viroptic.

FIXED-COMBINATION(S)

Cosopt: timolol/dorzolamide (a carbonic anhydrase inhibitor): 0.5%/2%. **Timolide:** timolol/hydrochlorothiazide (a diuretic): 10 mg/25 mg.

◆CLASSIFICATION

PHARMACOTHERAPEUTIC: Beta-adrenergic blocker. **CLINICAL:** Anti-hypertensive, antimigraine, anti-glaucoma (see pp. 50C, 68C).

ACTION

Blocks $beta_1$-, $beta_2$-adrenergic receptors. **Therapeutic Effect:** Reduces intraocular pressure (IOP) by reducing aqueous humor production, lowers B/P, slows heart rate, decreases myocardial contractility.

PHARMACOKINETICS

Route	Onset	Peak	Duration
PO	15–45 min	0.5–2.5 hrs	4 hrs
Ophthalmic	30 min	1–2 hrs	12–24 hrs

Well absorbed from GI tract. Protein binding: 60%. Minimal absorption after ophthalmic administration. Metabolized in liver. Primarily excreted in urine. Not removed by hemodialysis. **Half-life:** 4 hrs. Systemic absorption may occur with ophthalmic administration.

USES

Management of mild to moderate hypertension. Used alone or in combination with diuretics, esp. thiazide type. Reduces cardiovascular mortality in those with definite or suspected acute MI. Prophylaxis of migraine headache. **Ophthalmic:** Reduces IOP in management of open-angle glaucoma, aphakic glaucoma, ocular hypertension, secondary glaucoma. **OFF-LABEL: Systemic:** Treatment of anxiety, cardiac arrhythmias, chronic angina pectoris, hypertrophic cardiomyopathy, migraine, pheochromocytoma, thyrotoxicosis, tremors. **Ophthalmic:** Decreases IOP in acute or chronic angle-closure glaucoma, treatment of angle-closure glaucoma during and after iridectomy, malignant glaucoma, secondary glaucoma.

PRECAUTIONS

CONTRAINDICATIONS: Bronchial asthma, cardiogenic shock, CHF (unless secondary to tachyarrhythmias), chronic obstructive pulmonary disorder (COPD), pts receiving MAOI therapy, second- or third-degree heart block, sinus bradycardia, uncontrolled cardiac failure. **CAUTIONS:** Inadequate cardiac function, renal/hepatic impairment, hyperthyroidism. Precautions also apply to ophthalmic administration (due to systemic absorption of ophthalmic solution).

LIFESPAN CONSIDERATIONS:

Pregnancy/Lactation: Distributed in breast milk; not for use in breast-feeding women because of potential for serious adverse effect on breast-feeding infant. Avoid use during first trimester. May produce bradycardia, apnea, hypoglycemia, hypothermia in infant during delivery; low birth-weight infants. **Pregnancy Category C (D if used in second or third trimester). Children:** Safety and efficacy not established. **Elderly:** Age-related peripheral vascular disease increases susceptibility to decreased peripheral circulation.

INTERACTIONS

DRUG: Diuretics, other antihypertensives may increase hypotensive effect. May mask symptoms of hypoglycemia, prolong hypoglycemic effects of **insulin, oral hypoglycemics. NSAIDs** may decrease antihypertensive effect. **Sympathomimetics, xanthines** may mutually inhibit effects. **HERBAL:** None significant. **FOOD:** None known. **LAB VALUES:** May increase antinuclear antibody titer (ANA), BUN, serum LDH, alkaline phosphatase, bilirubin, creatinine, potassium, uric acid, AST, ALT, triglycerides, lipoproteins.

AVAILABILITY (Rx)

OPHTHALMIC GEL (TIMOPTIC-XE): 0.25%, 0.5%. **OPHTHALMIC SOLUTION (BETIMOL, TIMOPTIC, TIMOPTIC OCCUDOSE, TIMOPTIC OCUMETER, TIMOPTIC OCUMETER PLUS):** 0.25%, 0.5%. **TABLETS (BLOCADREN):** 5 mg, 10 mg, 20 mg.

ADMINISTRATION/HANDLING

PO

- Give without regard to meals.
- Tablets may be crushed.

OPHTHALMIC

◀ ALERT ▶ When using gel, invert container, shake once prior to each use.

T

• Place finger on lower eyelid, pull out until pocket is formed between eye and lower lid. • Hold dropper above pocket, place prescribed number of drops or amount of prescribed gel into pocket. • Instruct pt to close eyes gently so that medication will not be squeezed out of sac. • Apply gentle finger pressure to the lacrimal sac at inner canthus for 1 min following installation (lessens risk of systemic absorption).

INDICATIONS/ROUTES/DOSAGE

MILD TO MODERATE HYPERTENSION

PO: ADULTS, ELDERLY: Initially, 10 mg twice a day, alone or in combination with other therapy. Gradually increase at intervals of not less than 1 wk. Maintenance: 20–60 mg/day in 2 divided doses.

REDUCTION OF CARDIOVASCULAR MORTALITY IN ACUTE MI

PO: ADULTS, ELDERLY: 10 mg twice a day, beginning 1–4 wks after infarction.

MIGRAINE PREVENTION

PO: ADULTS, ELDERLY: Initially, 10 mg twice a day. Range: 10–30 mg/day.

REDUCTION OF INTRAOCULAR PRESSURE (IOP)

OPHTHALMIC: ADULTS, ELDERLY, CHILDREN: 1 drop of 0.25% solution in affected eye(s) twice a day. May be increased to 1 drop of 0.5% solution in affected eye(s) twice a day. When IOP is controlled, dosage may be reduced to 1 drop once a day. If pt is switched to timolol from another antiglaucoma agent, administer concurrently for 1 day. Discontinue other agent on following day.

OPHTHALMIC (Timoptic XE): ADULTS, ELDERLY: 1 drop/day.

OPHTHALMIC (Istalol): ADULTS, ELDERLY: Apply once daily.

SIDE EFFECTS

FREQUENT: Diminished sexual function, drowsiness, difficulty sleeping, asthenia (loss of strength, energy), fatigue. **Ophthalmic:** Eye irritation, visual disturbances. **OCCASIONAL:** Depression, cold hands/feet, diarrhea, constipation, anxiety, nasal congestion, nausea, vomiting. **RARE:** Altered taste, dry eyes, pruritus, numbness of fingers, toes, scalp.

ADVERSE EFFECTS/ TOXIC REACTIONS

Overdose may produce profound bradycardia, hypotension, bronchospasm. Abrupt withdrawal may result in diaphoresis, palpitations, headache, tremors. May precipitate CHF, MI in those with cardiac disease; thyroid storm in those with thyrotoxicosis; peripheral ischemia in those with existing peripheral vascular disease. Hypoglycemia may occur in pts with previously controlled diabetes. Ophthalmic overdose may produce bradycardia, hypotension, bronchospasm, acute cardiac failure.

NURSING CONSIDERATIONS

BASELINE ASSESSMENT

Assess B/P, apical pulse immediately before drug is administered (if pulse is 60 min or less or systolic B/P is less than 90 mm Hg, withhold medication, contact physician).

INTERVENTION/EVALUATION

Assess pulse for quality, irregular rate, bradycardia. Monitor EKG for cardiac arrhythmias, particularly PVCs. Monitor daily pattern of bowel activity/stool consistency. Monitor heart rate, B/P, serum hepatic/renal function, IOP (ophthalmic preparation).

PATIENT/FAMILY TEACHING

• Do not abruptly discontinue medication. • Compliance with therapy regimen is essential to control glaucoma, hypertension, angina, arrhythmias. • Avoid tasks that require alertness, motor skills until response to drug is established. • Report shortness of breath, unusual fatigue, prolonged dizziness, headache. • Do not use nasal decongestants, OTC cold preparations (stimulants) without physician approval. • Restrict salt, alcohol intake. • **Ophthalmic:** Teach pt how to instill drops correctly, how to take pulse. • Transient stinging, discomfort may occur upon instillation.

Tindamax, *see tinidazole*

tinidazole

tin-**nid**-ah-zole
(Tindamax)

CLASSIFICATION

PHARMACOTHERAPEUTIC: Nitroimidazole derivative. **CLINICAL:** Antiprotozoal.

ACTION

Converted to active metabolite by reduction of cell extracts of *Trichomonas*. Active metabolite causes DNA damage in pathogens. **Therapeutic Effect:** Produces antiprotozoal effect.

PHARMACOKINETICS

Rapidly, completely absorbed. Protein binding: 12%. Distributed in all body tissues and fluids; crosses blood-brain barrier. Significantly metabolized. Primarily excreted in urine; partially eliminated in feces. **Half-life:** 12–14 hrs.

USES

Treatment of intestinal amebiasis, amebic hepatic abscess, giardiasis, trichomoniasis.

PRECAUTIONS

CONTRAINDICATIONS: First trimester of pregnancy, hypersensitivity to nitroimidazole derivatives. **CAUTIONS:** CNS diseases, hepatic impairment, history of blood abnormalities.

LIFESPAN CONSIDERATIONS:

Pregnancy/Lactation: Mutagenic, spermatogenic. Readily crosses placenta; distributed in breast milk. Contraindicated during first trimester. **Pregnancy Category C.** **Children:** Safety and efficacy in children younger than 3 yrs not established. **Elderly:** Age-related hepatic impairment may require dosage adjustment.

INTERACTIONS

DRUG: Concurrent use of **alcohol** may cause abdominal cramps, nausea, vomiting, headache, flushing. May increase effects, risk of toxicity of **warfarin, lithium**. **HERBAL:** None significant. **FOOD:** None known. **LAB VALUES:** May increase serum LDH, triglycerides, AST, ALT.

AVAILABILITY (Rx)

TABLETS: 250 mg, 500 mg.

ADMINISTRATION/HANDLING

PO

• Store at room temperature. • Scored tablets may be crushed. • Give with food (minimizes incidence of epigastric distress).

INDICATIONS/ROUTES/DOSAGE

INTESTINAL AMEBIASIS

PO: ADULTS, ELDERLY: 2 g/day for 3 days. **CHILDREN 3 YRS AND OLDER:** 50 mg/kg/day (up to 2 g) for 3 days.

AMEBIC HEPATIC ABSCESS

PO: ADULTS, ELDERLY: 2 g/day for 3–5 days. **CHILDREN 3 YRS AND OLDER:** 50 mg/kg/day (up to 2 g) for 3–5 days.

GIARDIASIS

PO: ADULTS, ELDERLY: 2 g as a single dose. **CHILDREN 3 YRS AND OLDER:** 50 mg/kg (up to 2 g) as a single dose.

T

TRICHOMONIASIS
PO: ADULTS, ELDERLY: 2 g as a single dose.

SIDE EFFECTS

OCCASIONAL (4%–2%): Metallic/bitter taste, nausea, weakness, fatigue, malaise. **RARE (less than 2%):** Epigastric distress, anorexia, vomiting, headache, dizziness, red-brown, darkened urine.

ADVERSE EFFECTS/ TOXIC REACTIONS

Peripheral neuropathy, characterized by paresthesia, is usually reversible if treatment is stopped immediately upon appearance of neurologic symptoms. Superinfection, hypersensitivity reaction, seizures occur rarely.

NURSING CONSIDERATIONS

BASELINE ASSESSMENT

Question for history of hypersensitivity to metronidazole, other nitroimidazole derivatives. Obtain specimens for diagnostic tests before giving first dose (therapy may begin before results are known).

INTERVENTION/EVALUATION

Be alert to neurologic symptoms: dizziness, paresthesia of extremities. Assess for nausea/vomiting, initiate appropriate measures. Watch for onset of superinfection: ulceration/change of oral mucosa, furry tongue, vaginal discharge, anal/genital pruritus.

T

PATIENT/FAMILY TEACHING

• Take medication with food. • Avoid alcoholic beverages during therapy and for 3 days after completion of treatment. • Urine may be red-brown or dark. • Avoid alcohol-containing preparations (e.g., cough syrups, elixirs). • Avoid tasks that require alertness, motor skills until response to drug is established (may cause dizziness).

tinzaparin

tin-za-**pair**-in
(Innohep)

CLASSIFICATION

PHARMACOTHERAPEUTIC: Low-molecular-weight heparin. **CLINICAL:** Anticoagulant (see p. 30C).

ACTION

Inhibits factor Xa. Causes less inactivation of thrombin, inhibition of platelets, bleeding than with standard heparin. Does not significantly influence bleeding time, prothrombin time (PT), activated partial thromboplastin time (aPTT). **Therapeutic Effect:** Produces anticoagulation.

PHARMACOKINETICS

Well absorbed after subcutaneous administration. Primarily eliminated in urine. **Half-life:** 3–4 hrs.

USES

Treatment of acute symptomatic deep vein thrombosis (DVT) with or without pulmonary embolism, when given in conjunction with warfarin.

PRECAUTIONS

CONTRAINDICATIONS: Active major bleeding, concurrent heparin therapy, hypersensitivity to heparin, sulfites, benzyl alcohol, pork products, thrombocytopenia associated with positive in vitro test for antiplatelet antibody. **CAUTIONS:** Conditions with increased risk of hemorrhage, history of heparin-induced thrombocytopenia, renal impairment, elderly, uncontrolled arterial hypertension, history of recent GI ulceration, hemorrhage.

LIFESPAN CONSIDERATIONS:

Pregnancy/Lactation: Use with caution, particularly during last trimester, immediate postpartum period (increased risk of maternal hemorrhage). Unknown if distributed in breast milk. **Pregnancy Category B. Children:** Safety and efficacy not established. **Elderly:** May be more susceptible to bleeding.

INTERACTIONS

DRUG: Anticoagulants, NSAIDs, platelet aggregation inhibitors may increase risk of bleeding. **HERBAL: Ginkgo biloba** may increase risk of bleeding. **FOOD:** None known. **LAB VALUES:** Reversible increases in LDH, serum alkaline phosphatase, AST, ALT.

AVAILABILITY (Rx)

INJECTION SOLUTION: 20,000 anti-Xa international units/ml.

ADMINISTRATION/HANDLING

◄ **ALERT** ► Do not mix with other injections or infusions. Do not give IM.

SUBCUTANEOUS

• Parenteral form appears clear and colorless to pale yellow. • Store at room temperature. • Instruct pt to lie down before administering by deep subcutaneous injection.

INDICATIONS/ROUTES/DOSAGE

DEEP VEIN THROMBOSIS (DVT)

SUBCUTANEOUS: ADULTS, ELDERLY: 175 anti-Xa international units/kg once a day. Continue for at least 6 days and until pt is sufficiently anticoagulated with warfarin (INR of 2 or more for 2 consecutive days).

SIDE EFFECTS

FREQUENT (16%): Injection site reaction (e.g., inflammation, oozing, nodules, skin necrosis). **RARE (less than 2%):** Nausea, asthenia (loss of strength, energy), constipation, epistaxis.

ADVERSE EFFECTS/ TOXIC REACTIONS

Overdose may lead to bleeding complications ranging from local ecchymoses to major hemorrhage. **Antidote:** Dose of protamine sulfate (1% solution) should be equal to dose of tinzaparin injected. One mg protamine sulfate neutralizes 100 units of tinzaparin. Second dose of 0.5 mg tinzaparin per 1 mg protamine sulfate may be given if aPTT tested 2–4 hrs after initial infusion remains prolonged.

NURSING CONSIDERATIONS

BASELINE ASSESSMENT

Assess CBC, including platelet count. Determine initial B/P.

INTERVENTION/EVALUATION

Periodically monitor CBC, platelet count. Assess for any sign of bleeding: bleeding at surgical site, hematuria, blood in stool, bleeding from gums, petechiae, bruising, bleeding from injection sites.

PATIENT/FAMILY TEACHING

• Administer only subcutaneously. • May have tendency to bleed easily, use precautions (e.g., use electric razor, soft toothbrush). • Inform physician if chest pain, unusual bleeding/bruising, pain, numbness, tingling, swelling in joints, injection site reaction (oozing, nodules, inflammation) occurs.

tiotropium

tee-oh-**trow**-pea-um

(Spiriva)

CLASSIFICATION

PHARMACOTHERAPEUTIC: Anticholinergic. **CLINICAL:** Bronchodilator.

ACTION

Binds to recombinant human muscarinic receptors at smooth muscle, resulting in long-acting bronchial

T

smooth-muscle relaxation. **Therapeutic Effect:** Relieves bronchospasm.

PHARMACOKINETICS

Route	Onset	Peak	Duration
Inhalation	N/A	N/A	24–36 hrs

Binds extensively to tissue. Protein binding: 72%. Metabolized by oxidation. Excreted in urine. **Half-life:** 5–6 days.

USES

Long-term maintenance treatment of bronchospasm associated with chronic obstructive pulmonary disease (COPD), including chronic bronchitis, emphysema.

PRECAUTIONS

CONTRAINDICATIONS: History of hypersensitivity to atropine or its derivatives. **CAUTIONS:** Narrow-angle glaucoma, prostatic hypertrophy, bladder neck obstruction.

LIFESPAN CONSIDERATIONS:

Pregnancy/Lactation: Unknown if distributed in breast milk. **Pregnancy Category C.** **Children:** Safety and efficacy not established. **Elderly:** Higher frequency of dry mouth, constipation, UTI noted with increasing age.

INTERACTIONS

DRUG: Concurrent administration with **ipratropium** is not recommended. **HERBAL:** None significant. **FOOD:** None known. **LAB VALUES:** None known.

T

AVAILABILITY (Rx)

POWDER FOR INHALATION: 18 mcg/capsule (in blister packs).

ADMINISTRATION/HANDLING

INHALATION

• Open dustcap of *HandiHaler* by pulling it upward, then open mouthpiece. • Place capsule in center chamber and firmly close mouthpiece until a click is heard, leaving the dustcap open. • Hold *HandiHaler* device with mouthpiece upward, press piercing button completely in once, and release. • Instruct pt to breathe out completely before breathing in slowly and deeply but at rate sufficient to hear the capsule vibrate. • Have pt hold breath as long as it is comfortable until exhaling slowly. • Instruct pt to repeat once again to ensure full dose is received.

Storage • Store at room temperature. Do not expose capsules to extreme temperature, moisture. • Do not store capsules in *HandiHaler* device.

INDICATIONS/ROUTES/DOSAGE

COPD

INHALATION: ADULTS, ELDERLY: 18 mcg (1 capsule)/day via *HandiHaler* inhalation device.

SIDE EFFECTS

FREQUENT (16%–6%): Dry mouth, sinusitis, pharyngitis, dyspepsia, UTI, rhinitis. **OCCASIONAL (5%–4%):** Abdominal pain, peripheral edema, constipation, epistaxis, vomiting, myalgia, rash, oral candidiasis.

ADVERSE EFFECTS/ TOXIC REACTIONS

Angina pectoris, depression, flu-like symptoms occur rarely.

NURSING CONSIDERATIONS

BASELINE ASSESSMENT

Offer emotional support (high incidence of anxiety due to difficulty in breathing, sympathomimetic response to drug).

INTERVENTION/EVALUATION

Monitor rate, depth, rhythm, type of respiration; quality, rate of pulse. Assess lung sounds for rhonchi, wheezing, rales. Monitor ABGs. Observe lips, fingernails for cyanosis (blue or dusky color in light-skinned pts; gray in dark-skinned pts). Observe for clavicular retractions, hand tremor. Evaluate for clinical improvement (quieter, slower respirations, relaxed facial expression, cessation of clavicular retractions).

PATIENT/FAMILY TEACHING

• Increase fluid intake (decreases lung secretion viscosity). • Do not use more than 1 capsule for inhalation at any one time. • Rinsing mouth with water immediately after inhalation may prevent mouth/throat dryness, moniliasis. • Avoid excessive use of caffeine derivatives (chocolate, coffee, tea, cola, cocoa).

tipranavir

ti-**pran**-ah-veer
(Aptivus)

CLASSIFICATION

PHARMACOTHERAPEUTIC: Antiretroviral. **CLINICAL:** Protease inhibitor.

ACTION

Prevents virus-specific processing of polyproteins, HIV-1 infected cells. **Therapeutic Effect:** Prevents formation of mature viral cells.

PHARMACOKINETICS

Readily absorbed following PO administration. Protein binding: 98%–99%. Metabolized in liver. Eliminated mainly in feces, with lesser amount eliminated in urine. **Half-life:** 6 hrs.

USES

Treatment of HIV infection in combination with ritonavir.

PRECAUTIONS

CONTRAINDICATIONS: Moderate to severe hepatic insufficiency, concurrent use of tipranavir/ritonavir with alfuzosin, amiodarone, bepridil, dihydroergotamine, ergonovine, ergotamine, flecainide, lovastatin, methylergonovine, midazolam, propafenone, quinidine, simvastatin, St. John's wort, triazolam, voriconazole. **CAUTIONS:** Diabetes mellitus, hemophilia, known sulfonamide allergy, mild hepatic impairment, pts at increased risk of bleeding from trauma, surgery, concurrent antiplatelet/anticoagulant therapy.

LIFESPAN CONSIDERATIONS:

Pregnancy/Lactation: Unknown if drug crosses placenta or is distributed in breast milk. **Pregnancy Category C.** **Children:** Safety and efficacy not established. **Elderly:** Age-related hepatic impairment may require dosage adjustment.

INTERACTIONS

DRUG: May interfere with metabolism of **amiodarone, bepridil, ergotamine, lidocaine, midazolam, oral contraceptives, quinidine, triazolam, tricyclic antidepressants**. May increase concentration of **antiarrhythmics, antihistamines, GI motility medications**. **Benzodiazepines** may increase sedation, risk of respiratory depression. **Carbamazepine, phenobarbital, phenytoin, rifampin** may decrease concentration. May increase concentration of **clozapine, HMG-CoA reductase inhibitors, warfarin**. **Ergot derivatives** may cause ergot toxicity. **HMG-CoA reductase inhibitors** may increase risk of myopathy including rhabdomyolysis. **HERBAL:** **St. John's wort** may lead to loss of virologic response, potential resistance to tipranavir. **FOOD:** **High-fat meals** may increase bioavailability. **LAB VALUES:** May increase serum cholesterol, triglycerides, amylase, ALT, AST. May decrease WBC count.

AVAILABILITY (Rx)

CAPSULES: 250 mg.

ADMINISTRATION/HANDLING

PO

• Best given with food.

INDICATIONS/ROUTES/DOSAGE

HIV INFECTION

PO: ADULTS, ELDERLY: 500 mg (2 capsules) administered with 200 mg of ritonavir twice a day.

SIDE EFFECTS

FREQUENT (11%): Diarrhea. **OCCASIONAL (7%–2%):** Nausea, fever, fatigue, headache, depression, vomiting, abdominal pain, weakness, rash. **RARE (less than 2%):** Abdominal distention, anorexia, flatulence, dizziness, insomnia, myalgia.

ADVERSE EFFECTS/ TOXIC REACTIONS

Bronchitis occurs in 3% of pts. Anemia, neutropenia, thrombocytopenia, diabetes mellitus, hepatic failure, hepatitis, peripheral neuropathy, pancreatitis occur rarely.

NURSING CONSIDERATIONS

BASELINE ASSESSMENT

Obtain baseline laboratory testing, esp. hepatic function tests, before beginning therapy and at periodic intervals during therapy. Offer emotional support. Obtain medication history.

INTERVENTION/EVALUATION

Closely monitor for evidence of GI discomfort. Monitor daily pattern of bowel activity/stool consistency. Assess skin for evidence of rash. Monitor serum chemistry tests for marked laboratory abnormalities, particularly hepatic profile. Assess for opportunistic infections: onset of fever, oral mucosa changes, cough, other respiratory symptoms.

PATIENT/FAMILY TEACHING

• Eat small, frequent meals to offset nausea, vomiting; avoid high-fat meals. • Continue therapy for full length of treatment. • Doses should be evenly spaced. • Medication is not a cure for HIV infection, nor does it reduce risk of transmission to others. • Pt may continue to experience illnesses, including opportunistic infections. • Diarrhea can be controlled with OTC medication.

tirofiban

tye-**roe**-fye-ban

(Aggrastat)

Do not confuse Aggrastat with Aggrenox.

CLASSIFICATION

PHARMACOTHERAPEUTIC: Glycoprotein (GP) IIb/IIIa inhibitor. **CLINICAL:** Antiplatelet, antithrombotic (see p. 31C).

ACTION

Binds to platelet receptor glycoprotein IIb/IIIa, preventing binding of fibrinogen. **Therapeutic Effect:** Inhibits platelet aggregation, thrombus formation.

USES

Antiplatelet in combination with heparin, treatment of acute coronary syndrome, including those to be managed medically and those undergoing percutaneous transluminal coronary angioplasty (PTCA), atherectomy.

PRECAUTIONS

CONTRAINDICATIONS: Active internal bleeding or history of bleeding diathesis within previous 30 days, arteriovenous malformation/aneurysm, history of intracranial hemorrhage, history of thrombocytopenia after prior exposure to tirofiban, intracranial neoplasm, major surgical procedure within previous 30 days, severe hypertension, stroke.

T

CAUTIONS: Pts with platelets less than 150,000/mm^3, hemorrhagic retinopathy. Concomitant use of drugs affecting hemostasis (e.g., warfarin), renal impairment. **Pregnancy Category B.**

INTERACTIONS

DRUG: **Anticoagulants, NSAIDs, platelet aggregation inhibitors, thrombolytics (e.g., aspirin, heparin, warfarin)** may increase risk of bleeding. **HERBAL:** None significant. **FOOD:**None known. **LAB VALUES:** Decreases Hct, Hgb, platelet count.

AVAILABILITY (Rx)

INJECTION SOLUTION: 250 mcg/ml. **INJECTION SOLUTION PREMIX:** 12.5 mg/250 ml, 25 mg/500 ml (50 mcg/ml).

ADMINISTRATION/HANDLING

IV

Reconstitution

INJECTION SOLUTION (250 mcg/ml)
• Withdraw and discard 100 ml from a 500-ml bag 0.9% NaCl or D_5W and replace this volume with 100 ml of tirofiban (from two 50-ml vials) or withdraw and discard 50 ml from a 250-ml bag and replace with 50 ml of tirofiban (from one 50-ml vial) to achieve a final concentration of 50 mcg/ml. • Mix well before administration.

INJECTION SOLUTION (50 mcg/ml) PREMIX IN 500-ML INTRAVIA CONTAINER
• To open the IntraVia container, tear off dust cover. • Check for leaks by squeezing inner bag firmly; if leak is found or solution is not clear, discard solution. • Do not add other drugs or remove solution directly from the bag with a syringe. Do not use plastic containers in series connections (may result in air embolism by drawing air from first container if it is empty of solution).

Rate of administration • For loading dose, give 0.4 mcg/kg/min for 30 min. • For maintenance infusion, give 0.1 mcg/kg/min.

Storage • Store at room temperature. • Protect from light. • Use only clear solution. • Discard unused solution 24 hrs after start of infusion.

IV INCOMPATIBILITY

Diazepam (Valium).

IV COMPATIBILITIES

Famotidine (Pepcid), furosemide (Lasix), heparin, midazolam (Versed), morphine, potassium.

INDICATIONS/ROUTES/DOSAGE

INHIBITION OF PLATELET AGGREGATION
IV: ADULTS, ELDERLY: Initially, 0.4 mcg/kg/min for 30 min; then continue at 0.1 mcg/kg/min through procedure and for 12–24 hrs after procedure.

SEVERE RENAL INSUFFICIENCY (CREATININE CLEARANCE LESS THAN 30 ML/MIN)
IV: ADULTS, ELDERLY: Half the usual rate of infusion.

SIDE EFFECTS

OCCASIONAL (6%–3%): Pelvic pain, bradycardia, dizziness, leg pain. **RARE (2%–1%):** Edema, swelling, vasovagal reaction, diaphoresis, nausea, fever, headache.

ADVERSE EFFECTS/ TOXIC REACTIONS

Overdose manifested as minor mucocutaneous bleeding, bleeding at femoral artery access site. Thrombocytopenia occurs rarely.

NURSING CONSIDERATIONS

BASELINE ASSESSMENT

Assess platelet count, Hgb, Hct, aPTT, renal function before treatment, within 6 hrs following the loading dose, and at least daily thereafter during therapy. If platelet count is less than 90,000/mm^3, additional platelet counts should be

T

obtained routinely to avoid thrombocytopenia. If thrombocytopenia occurs, discontinue drug therapy and heparin.

INTERVENTION/EVALUATION

Monitor aPTT 6 hrs following the beginning of heparin infusion. Adjust heparin dosage to maintain aPTT at approximately 2 times control. Diligently monitor for potential bleeding, particularly at other arterial, venous puncture sites, IM injection site. If possible, urinary catheters, NG tubes should be avoided. Maintain complete bed rest with head of bed elevated at 30°.

tizanidine

tye-**zan**-i-deen
(Apo-Tizanidine ✦, Zanaflex)

CLASSIFICATION

PHARMACOTHERAPEUTIC: Skeletal muscle relaxant. **CLINICAL:** Antispastic.

ACTION

Increases presynaptic inhibition of spinal motor neurons mediated by alpha$_2$-adrenergic agonists, reducing facilitation to postsynaptic motor neurons. **Therapeutic Effect:** Reduces muscle spasticity.

PHARMACOKINETICS

Metabolized in liver. Primarily excreted in urine. **Half-life:** 2 hrs.

USES

Acute and intermittent management of muscle spasticity (spasms, stiffness, rigidity). **OFF-LABEL:** Low back pain, spasticity associated with multiple sclerosis or spinal cord injury, tension headaches, trigeminal neuralgia.

PRECAUTIONS

CONTRAINDICATIONS: None significant. **CAUTIONS:** Renal/hepatic disease, hypotension, cardiac disease. **Pregnancy Category C.**

INTERACTIONS

DRUG: **Alcohol, other CNS depressants** may increase CNS depressant effects. **Antihypertensives** may increase hypotensive potential. **Oral contraceptives** may reduce clearance. May increase concentration, risk of toxicity of **phenytoin**. **HERBAL:** **Gotu kola, kava kava, St. John's wort, valerian** may increase CNS depression. **Black cohosh, hawthorn, periwinkle** may increase hypotensive effect. **FOOD:** None known. **LAB VALUES:** May increase serum alkaline phosphatase, AST, ALT.

AVAILABILITY (Rx)

CAPSULES: 2 mg, 4 mg, 6 mg. **TABLETS:** 2 mg, 4 mg.

ADMINISTRATION/HANDLING

PO

- Capsules may be opened and sprinkled on food.

INDICATIONS/ROUTES/DOSAGE

MUSCLE SPASTICITY

PO: ADULTS, ELDERLY: Initially 2–4 mg, gradually increased in 2- to 4-mg increments and repeated q6–8h. **Maximum:** 3 doses/day or 36 mg/24 hrs.

SIDE EFFECTS

FREQUENT (49%–41%): Dry mouth, somnolence, asthenia (loss of strength, weakness). **OCCASIONAL (16%–4%):** Dizziness, UTI, constipation. **RARE (3%):** Nervousness, amblyopia, pharyngitis, rhinitis, vomiting, urinary frequency.

ADVERSE EFFECTS/ TOXIC REACTIONS

Hypotension may be associated with bradycardia, orthostatic hypotension, and, rarely, syncope. Risk of hypotension increases as dosage increases; hypotension is noted within 1 hr after administration.

NURSING CONSIDERATIONS

BASELINE ASSESSMENT

Record onset, type, location, duration of muscular spasm. Check for immobility, stiffness, swelling. Obtain baseline serum hepatic function tests, alkaline phosphatase, total bilirubin.

INTERVENTION/EVALUATION

Assist with ambulation at all times. For those on long-term therapy, serum hepatic/renal function tests should be performed periodically. Evaluate for therapeutic response (decreased intensity of skeletal muscle pain/tenderness, improved mobility, decrease in spasticity). To reduce risk of orthostatic hypotension, instruct pt to move slowly from lying to sitting and from sitting to supine position.

PATIENT/FAMILY TEACHING

• Avoid tasks that require alertness, motor skills until response to drug is established. • Avoid sudden changes in posture. • May cause hypotension, sedation, impaired coordination.

TNKase, *see tenecteplase*

tobramycin

tow-bra-**my**-sin

(AK-Tob, Apo-Tobramycin ✦, Nebcin, Nebcin Pediatric, PMS-Tobramycin, TOBI, Tobrex)

FIXED-COMBINATION(S)

TobraDex: tobramycin/dexamethasone (a steroid): 0.3%/0.1% per ml or per g. **Zylet:** tobramycin/loteprednol: 0.3%/0.5%.

◆ CLASSIFICATION

PHARMACOTHERAPEUTIC: Aminoglycoside. **CLINICAL:** Antibiotic (see p. 20C).

ACTION

Irreversibly binds to protein on bacterial ribosomes. **Therapeutic Effect:** Interferes with protein synthesis of susceptible microorganisms.

PHARMACOKINETICS

Rapid, complete absorption after IM administration. Protein binding: less than 30%. Widely distributed (does not cross blood-brain barrier; low concentrations in cerebrospinal fluid [CSF]). Excreted unchanged in urine. Removed by hemodialysis. **Half-life:** 2–4 hrs (increased in renal impairment, neonates; decreased in cystic fibrosis, febrile or burn pts).

USES

Treatment of susceptible infections due to *P. aeruginosa,* other gram-negative organisms including skin/skin structure, bone, joint, respiratory tract infections; postop, burn, intra-abdominal infections; complicated UTI; septicemia; meningitis. **Ophthalmic:** Superficial eye infections: blepharitis, conjunctivitis, keratitis, corneal ulcers. **Inhalation:** Bronchopulmonary infections in pts with cystic fibrosis.

T

PRECAUTIONS

CONTRAINDICATIONS: Hypersensitivity to other aminoglycosides (cross-sensitivity) and their components. **CAUTIONS:** Renal impairment, preexisting auditory or vestibular impairment, concomitant use of neuromuscular blocking agents.

⌛ LIFESPAN CONSIDERATIONS:

Pregnancy/Lactation: Drug readily crosses placenta; is distributed in breast milk. May cause fetal nephrotoxicity. Ophthalmic form should not be used in breast-feeding mothers and only when specifically indicated in pregnancy. **Pregnancy Category D (B for ophthalmic form). Children:** Immature renal function in neonates, premature infants may increase risk of toxicity. **Elderly:** Age-related renal impairment may increase risk of toxicity; dosage adjustment recommended.

INTERACTIONS

DRUG: **Nephrotoxic medications, ototoxic medications** may increase risk of nephrotoxicity, ototoxicity. **Neuromuscular blockers** may increase neuromuscular blockade. **HERBAL:** None significant. **FOOD:** None known. **LAB VALUES:** May increase BUN, serum bilirubin, creatinine, LDH, AST, ALT. May decrease serum calcium, magnesium, potassium, sodium. Therapeutic peak serum level: 5–20 mcg/ml; therapeutic trough serum level: 0.5–2 mcg/ml. Toxic peak serum level is greater than 20 mcg/ml; toxic trough serum level is greater than 2 mcg/ml.

AVAILABILITY (Rx)

INJECTION, POWDER FOR RECONSTITUTION: 1.2 g. **INJECTION, SOLUTION:** 10 mg/ml, 40 mg/ml. **OINTMENT, OPHTHALMIC (TOBREX):** 0.3%. **OINTMENT, SOLUTION (AK TOB, TOBREX):** 0.3%. **SOLUTION, NEBULIZATION (TOBI):** 60 mg/ml.

T

ADMINISTRATION/HANDLING

◄ ALERT ► Coordinate peak and trough lab draws with administration times.

IV

Reconstitution • Dilute with 50–200 ml D_5W, 0.9% NaCl. Amount of diluent for infants, children depends on individual need.

Rate of administration • Infuse over 20–60 min.

Storage • Store vials at room temperature. • Solutions may be discolored by light or air (does not affect potency).

IM

• To minimize discomfort, give deep IM slowly. • Less painful if injected into gluteus maximus rather than lateral aspect of thigh.

OPHTHALMIC

• Place finger on lower eyelid, pull out until pocket is formed between eye and lower lid. • Hold dropper above pocket, place correct number of drops (¼–½ inch ointment) into pocket. Have pt close eye gently. • **Solution:** Apply digital pressure to lacrimal sac for 1–2 min (minimizes drainage into nose/throat, reducing risk of systemic effects). • **Ointment:** Close eye for 1–2 min, rolling eyeball (increases contact area of drug to eye). • Remove excess solution/ointment around eye with tissue.

IV INCOMPATIBILITIES

Amphotericin B complex (Abelcet, AmBisome, Amphotec), heparin, hetastarch (Hespan), indomethacin (Indocin), propofol (Diprivan), sargramostim (Leukine, Prokine).

IV COMPATIBILITIES

Amiodarone (Cordarone), calcium gluconate, diltiazem (Cardizem), furosemide (Lasix), hydromorphone (Dilaudid), insulin, lipids, magnesium sulfate, midazolam (Versed), morphine, theophylline, total parenteral nutrition (TPN).

INDICATIONS/ROUTES/DOSAGE

◄ ALERT ► Space parenteral doses evenly around the clock. Dosage based on ideal body weight. Peak, trough levels determined periodically to maintain desired serum concentrations (minimizes risk of toxicity). Recommended peak level: 4–10 mcg/ml; trough level: 1–2 mcg/ml.

USUAL PARENTERAL DOSAGE

IV: ADULTS, ELDERLY: 3–6 mg/kg/day in 3 divided doses. Once daily dosing: 4–7 mg/kg every 24 hrs. **CHILDREN 7 DAYS AND OLDER:** 6–7.5 mg/kg/day in 3–4 divided doses. **CHILDREN YOUNGER THAN 7 DAYS:** 2.5–4 mg/kg/day in 2 divided doses.

USUAL OPHTHALMIC DOSAGE

OPHTHALMIC OINTMENT: ADULTS, ELDERLY: Apply thin strip to conjunctiva q8–12h (q3–4h for severe infections).
OPHTHALMIC SOLUTION: ADULTS, ELDERLY: 1–2 drops in affected eye q4h (2 drops/hr for severe infections).

USUAL INHALATION DOSAGE

INHALATION SOLUTION: ADULTS: 60–80 mg twice a day for 28 days, then off for 28 days. **CHILDREN:** 40–80 mg 2–3 times a day.

DOSAGE IN RENAL IMPAIRMENT

Dosage and frequency are modified based on degree of renal impairment, and serum drug concentration. After loading dose of 1–2 mg/kg, maintenance dose and frequency are based on serum creatinine levels, creatinine clearance.

SIDE EFFECTS

OCCASIONAL: IM: Pain, induration. **IV:** Phlebitis, thrombophlebitis. **Topical:** Hypersensitivity reaction (fever, pruritus, rash, urticaria). **Ophthalmic:** Tearing, itching, redness, eyelid swelling. **RARE:** Hypotension, nausea, vomiting.

ADVERSE EFFECTS/ TOXIC REACTIONS

Nephrotoxicity (evidenced by increased BUN, serum creatinine, decreased creatinine clearance) may be reversible if drug is stopped at first sign of symptoms. Irreversible ototoxicity (tinnitus, dizziness, ringing/roaring in ears, hearing loss), neurotoxicity (headache, dizziness, lethargy, tremor, visual disturbances) occur occasionally. Risk increases with higher dosages or prolonged therapy or if solution is applied directly to mucosa. Superinfections, particularly fungal infections, may result from bacterial imbalance with any administration route. Anaphylaxis may occur.

NURSING CONSIDERATIONS

BASELINE ASSESSMENT

Dehydration must be treated before beginning parenteral therapy. Question for history of allergies, esp. aminoglycosides, sulfite (and parabens for topical, ophthalmic routes). Establish baseline for hearing acuity.

INTERVENTION/EVALUATION

Monitor I&O (maintain hydration), urinalysis (casts, RBCs, WBCs, decrease in specific gravity). Monitor results of peak/trough blood tests. Therapeutic serum level: peak: 5–20 mcg/ml; trough: 0.5–2 mcg/ml. Toxic serum level: peak: over 20 mcg/ml; trough: over 2 mcg/ml. Be alert to ototoxic, neurotoxic symptoms. Evaluate IV site for phlebitis (heat, pain, red streaking over vein). Assess for rash. Be alert for superinfection, particularly anal/genital pruritus, changes of oral mucosa, diarrhea. When treating pts with neuromuscular disorders, assess respiratory response carefully. **Ophthalmic:** Assess for redness, swelling, itching, tearing.

PATIENT/FAMILY TEACHING

• Notify physician in event of any hearing, visual, balance, urinary problems, even after therapy is completed. • **Ophthalmic:** Blurred vision, tearing may occur briefly after application. • Contact physician if tearing, redness, irritation continues.

*TOLAZamide

(Tolamide, Tolinase)

See Antidiabetics

T

*TOLBUTamide

(Oramide, Orinase)

See Antidiabetics

tolnaftate

(Aftate, Tinactin)

See Antifungals: topical (p. 47C)

tolterodine

tol-**tare**-oh-deen

(Detrol, Detrol LA)

CLASSIFICATION

PHARMACOTHERAPEUTIC: Muscarinic receptor antagonist. **CLINICAL:** Antispasmodic.

ACTION

Exhibits potent antimuscarinic activity by interceding via cholinergic muscarinic receptors, thereby inhibiting urinary bladder contraction. **Therapeutic Effect:** Decreases urinary frequency, urgency.

PHARMACOKINETICS

Rapidly, well absorbed after PO administration. Protein binding: 96%. Extensively metabolized in liver to active metabolite. Primarily excreted in urine. Unknown if removed by hemodialysis. **Half-life:** 1.9–3.7 hrs.

USES

Treatment of overactive bladder in pts with symptoms of urinary frequency, urgency, incontinence.

PRECAUTIONS

CONTRAINDICATIONS: Gastric retention, uncontrolled angle-closure glaucoma, urinary retention. **CAUTIONS:** Renal impairment, clinically significant bladder outflow obstruction (risk of urinary retention), GI obstructive disorders (e.g., pyloric stenosis [risk of gastric retention]), treated narrow-angle glaucoma.

LIFESPAN CONSIDERATIONS:

Pregnancy/Lactation: Unknown if drug is distributed in breast milk. Breastfeeding not recommended. **Pregnancy Category C. Children:** Safety and efficacy not established. **Elderly:** No age-related precautions noted.

INTERACTIONS

DRUG: **Clarithromycin, erythromycin, itraconazole, ketoconazole, miconazole** may increase concentration. **Fluoxetine** may inhibit metabolism. **HERBAL:** None significant. **FOOD:** None known. **LAB VALUES:** None known.

AVAILABILITY (Rx)

TABLETS (DETROL): 1 mg, 2 mg. CAPSULES **(EXTENDED-RELEASE [DETROL LA]):** 2 mg, 4 mg.

ADMINISTRATION/HANDLING

PO

- May give without regard to food. Do not crush, chew, open extended-release capsules; swallow whole.

INDICATIONS/ROUTES/DOSAGE

OVERACTIVE BLADDER

PO: ADULTS, ELDERLY (IMMEDIATE-RELEASE): 1–2 mg 2 times/day. **(EXTENDED-RELEASE)**: 2–4 mg once daily.

DOSAGE IN SEVERE RENAL/HEPATIC IMPAIRMENT

PO: ADULTS, ELDERLY (IMMEDIATE-RELEASE): 1 mg 2 times/day. **(EXTENDED RELEASE)**: 2 mg once daily.

SIDE EFFECTS

FREQUENT (40%): Dry mouth. **OCCASIONAL (11%–4%):** Headache, dizziness, fatigue, constipation, dyspepsia (heartburn, indigestion, epigastric pain), upper respiratory tract infection, UTI, dry eyes, abnormal vision (accommodation problems), nausea, diarrhea. **RARE (3%):** Somnolence, chest/back pain, arthralgia, rash, weight gain, dry skin.

ADVERSE EFFECTS/ TOXIC REACTIONS

Overdose can result in severe anticholinergic effects, including abdominal cramps, facial warmth, excessive salivation/lacrimation, diaphoresis, pallor, urinary urgency, blurred vision, prolonged QT interval.

NURSING CONSIDERATIONS

INTERVENTION/EVALUATION

Assist with ambulation if dizziness occurs. Question for visual changes. Monitor incontinence, postvoid residuals.

PATIENT/FAMILY TEACHING

• May cause blurred vision, dry eyes/mouth, constipation. • Inform physician of any confusion, altered mental status.

Topamax, *see topiramate*

topiramate

toe-**peer**-a-mate

(Novo-Topiramate ✤, Topamax)

Do not confuse topiramate or Topamax with Toprol XL, Tegretol, or Tegretol XR.

CLASSIFICATION

CLINICAL: Anticonvulsant (see p. 35C).

ACTION

Blocks repetitive, sustained firing of neurons by enhancing ability of gamma-aminobutyric acid (GABA) to induce influx of chloride ions into neurons; may block sodium channels. **Therapeutic Effect:** Decreases seizure activity.

PHARMACOKINETICS

Rapidly absorbed after PO administration. Protein binding: 13%–17%. Not extensively metabolized. Primarily excreted unchanged in urine. Removed by hemodialysis. **Half-life:** 21 hrs.

USES

Adjunctive therapy for treatment of partial-onset seizures, tonic-clonic seizures, seizures associated with Lennox-Gastaut syndrome. Prevention of migraine. Initial monotherapy in pts 10 yrs of age and older with partial or primary generalized tonic-clonic seizures. **OFF-LABEL:** Treatment of alcohol dependence.

PRECAUTIONS

CONTRAINDICATIONS: Bipolar disorder. **CAUTIONS:** Sensitivity to topiramate, hepatic/renal impairment, predisposition to renal calculi.

LIFESPAN CONSIDERATIONS:

Pregnancy/Lactation: Unknown if distributed in breast milk. **Pregnancy Category C.** **Children:** No age-related precautions noted in those older than 2 yrs. **Elderly:** Age-related renal impairment may require dosage adjustment.

INTERACTIONS

DRUG: Alcohol, other CNS depressants may increase CNS depression. **Carbamazepine, phenytoin, valproic acid** may decrease concentration. **Carbonic anhydrase inhibitors** may increase risk of renal calculi formation. May decrease effectiveness of **oral contraceptives. HERBAL: Evening**

T

primrose may decrease seizure threshold. **FOOD:** None known. **LAB VALUES:** None known.

AVAILABILITY (Rx)

TABLETS: 25 mg, 50 mg, 100 mg, 200 mg. CAPSULES **(SPRINKLE):** 15 mg, 25 mg.

ADMINISTRATION/HANDLING

PO

- Do not break tablets (bitter taste).
- Give without regard to meals.
- Capsules may be swallowed whole or contents sprinkled on teaspoonful of soft food and swallowed immediately; do not chew.

INDICATIONS/ROUTES/DOSAGE

ADJUNCTIVE TREATMENT OF PARTIAL SEIZURES, LENNOX-GASTAUT SYNDROME, TONIC-CLONIC SEIZURES

PO: ADULTS, ELDERLY, CHILDREN OLDER THAN 17 YRS: Initially, 25–50 mg for 1 wk. May increase by 25–50 mg/day at weekly intervals. **Maximum:** 1,600 mg/day. **CHILDREN 2–16 YRS:** Initially, 1–3 mg/kg/day to maximum of 25 mg. May increase by 1–3 mg/kg/day at weekly intervals. Maintenance: 5–9 mg/kg/day in 2 divided doses.

MONOTHERAPY WITH PARTIAL, TONIC-CLONIC SEIZURES

PO: ADULTS, ELDERLY, CHILDREN 10 YRS AND OLDER: Initially, 25 mg twice a day. Increase at weekly intervals up to 400 mg/day according to the following schedule: Wk 1, 25 mg twice a day. Wk 2, 50 mg twice a day. Wk 3, 75 mg twice a day. Wk 4, 100 mg twice a day. Wk 5, 150 mg twice a day. Wk 6, 200 mg twice a day.

MIGRAINE PREVENTION

PO: ADULTS, ELDERLY: Initially, 25 mg/day. May increase by 25 mg/day at 7-day intervals up to a total daily dose of 100 mg/day in 2 divided doses.

DOSAGE IN RENAL IMPAIRMENT

Expect to reduce drug dosage by 50% in pts with tonic-clonic seizures who have creatinine clearance less than 70 ml/min.

SIDE EFFECTS

FREQUENT (30%–10%): Somnolence, dizziness, ataxia, nervousness, nystagmus, diplopia, paresthesia, nausea, tremor. **OCCASIONAL (9%–3%):** Confusion, breast pain, dysmenorrhea, dyspepsia (heartburn, indigestion, epigastric pain), depression, asthenia (loss of strength, energy), pharyngitis, weight loss, anorexia, rash, musculoskeletal pain, abdominal pain, difficulty with coordination, sinusitis, agitation, flu-like symptoms. **RARE (3%–2%):** Mood disturbances (e.g., irritability, depression), dry mouth, aggressive behavior.

ADVERSE EFFECTS/ TOXIC REACTIONS

Psychomotor slowing, impaired concentration, language problems (esp. word-finding difficulties), memory disturbances occur occasionally. These reactions are generally mild to moderate but may be severe enough to require discontinuation of drug therapy.

NURSING CONSIDERATIONS

BASELINE ASSESSMENT

Review history of seizure disorder (intensity, frequency, duration, level of consciousness [LOC]). Initiate seizure precautions. Provide quiet, dark environment. Question for sensitivity to topiramate, pregnancy, use of other anticonvulsant medication (esp. carbamazepine, valproic acid, phenytoin, carbonic anhydrase inhibitors). Assess serum renal function. Instruct pt to use alternative/additional means of contraception (topiramate decreases effectiveness of oral contraceptives).

T

INTERVENTION/EVALUATION

Observe frequently for recurrence of seizure activity. Assess for clinical improvement (decrease in intensity/frequency of seizures). Monitor serum renal function tests (BUN, creatinine). Assist with ambulation if dizziness occurs.

PATIENT/FAMILY TEACHING

• Avoid tasks that require alertness, motor skills until response to drug is established (may cause dizziness, drowsiness, impaired concentration). • Drowsiness usually diminishes with continued therapy. • Avoid use of alcohol, other CNS depressants. • Do not abruptly discontinue drug (may precipitate seizures). • Strict maintenance of drug therapy is essential for seizure control. • Do not break tablets (bitter taste). • Maintain adequate fluid intake (decreases risk of renal stone formation). • Inform physician if blurred vision, eye pain occurs.

topotecan

toe-**poh**-teh-can
(Hycamtin)

CLASSIFICATION

PHARMACOTHERAPEUTIC: DNA topoisomerase inhibitor. **CLINICAL:** Antineoplastic (see p. 83C).

ACTION

Interacts with topoisomerase I, an enzyme that relieves torsional strain in DNA by inducing reversible single-strand breaks. Prevents religation of DNA strand, resulting in damage to double-strand DNA, cell death. **Therapeutic Effect:** Produces cytotoxic effect.

PHARMACOKINETICS

Hydrolyzed to active form after IV administration. Protein binding: 35%. Excreted in urine. **Half-life:** 2–3 hrs (increased in renal impairment).

USES

Treatment of metastatic carcinoma of ovary after failure of initial or recurrent chemotherapy. Treatment of sensitive, relapsed small cell lung cancer. Treatment of late-stage cervical cancer. **OFF-LABEL:** Treatment of solid tumors including osteosarcoma, neuroblastoma, pediatric leukemia, rhabdomyosarcoma.

PRECAUTIONS

CONTRAINDICATIONS: Baseline neutrophil count less than 1,500 cells/mm^3, breast-feeding, pregnancy, severe myelosuppression. **CAUTIONS:** Mild myelosuppression, hepatic/renal impairment.

LIFESPAN CONSIDERATIONS:

Pregnancy/Lactation: May cause fetal harm. Avoid pregnancy; breast-feeding not recommended. **Pregnancy Category D. Children:** Safety and efficacy not established. **Elderly:** Age-related renal impairment may require dosage adjustment.

INTERACTIONS

DRUG: Immunosuppresants (e.g., azathioprine, glucocorticoids, cyclosporine, tacrolimus) may increase risk of infection. **Live virus vaccines** may potentiate virus replication, increase vaccine side effects, decrease pt's antibody response to vaccine. **Other bone marrow depressants** may increase risk of myelosuppression. **HERBAL:** None significant. **FOOD:** None known. **LAB VALUES:** May increase serum bilirubin, AST, ALT. May decrease RBC, leukocyte, neutrophil, platelet counts.

AVAILABILITY (Rx)

INJECTION, POWDER FOR RECONSTITUTION: 4 mg (single-dose vial).

T

ADMINISTRATION/HANDLING

◀ **ALERT** ▶ Because topotecan may be carcinogenic, mutagenic, teratogenic, handle drug with extreme care during preparation/administration.

IV

Reconstitution • Reconstitute each 4-mg vial with 4 ml Sterile Water for Injection. • Further dilute with 50–100 ml 0.9% NaCl or D_5W.

Rate of administration • Administer all doses as IV infusion over 30 min. • Extravasation associated with only mild local reactions (erythema, ecchymosis).

Storage • Store vials at room temperature in original cartons. • Reconstituted vials diluted for infusion stable at room temperature, ambient lighting for 24 hrs.

IV INCOMPATIBILITIES

Dexamethasone (Decadron), 5-fluorouracil, mitomycin (Mutamycin).

IV COMPATIBILITIES

Carboplatin (Paraplatin), cisplatin (Platinol AQ), cyclophosphamide (Cytoxan), doxorubicin (Adriamycin), etoposide (VePesid), gemcitabine (Gemzar), granisetron (Kytril), ondansetron (Zofran), paclitaxel (Taxol), vincristine (Oncovin).

INDICATIONS/ROUTES/DOSAGE

◀ **ALERT** ▶ Do not give topotecan if baseline neutrophil count is less than 1,500 cells/mm^3 and platelet count is less than 100,000/mm^3.

OVARIAN CARCINOMA, CERVICAL CANCER, SMALL-CELL LUNG CANCER

IV: ADULTS, ELDERLY: 1.5 mg/m^2/day over 30 min for 5 consecutive days, beginning on day 1 of 21-day course. Minimum of four courses recommended. If severe neutropenia (neutrophil count less than 1,500/mm^2) occurs during treatment, reduce dose for subsequent courses by 0.25 mg/m^2 or administer filgrastim (G-CSF) no sooner than 24 hrs after last dose of topotecan.

IV INFUSION: ADULTS, ELDERLY: 0.2–0.7 mg/m^2/day for 7–21 days.

DOSAGE IN RENAL IMPAIRMENT

No dosage adjustment is necessary in pts with mild renal impairment (creatinine clearance of 40–60 ml/min). For moderate renal impairment (creatinine clearance of 20–39 ml/min), give 0.75 mg/m^2.

SIDE EFFECTS

FREQUENT: Nausea (77%), vomiting (58%), diarrhea, total alopecia (42%), headache (21%), dyspnea (21%). **OCCASIONAL:** Paresthesia (9%), constipation, abdominal pain (3%). **RARE:** Anorexia, malaise, arthralgia, asthenia, myalgia.

ADVERSE EFFECTS/ TOXIC REACTIONS

Severe neutropenia (absolute neutrophil count [ANC] less than 500 cells/mm^3) occurs in 60% of pts (develops at median of 11 days after day 1 of initial therapy). Thrombocytopenia (platelet count less than 25,000/mm^3) occurs in 26% of pts, and severe anemia (RBC count less than 8 g/dl) occurs in 40% of pts (develops at median of 15 days after day 1 of initial therapy).

NURSING CONSIDERATIONS

BASELINE ASSESSMENT

Offer emotional support to pt and family. Assess CBC with differential, Hgb, platelet count before each dose. Myelosuppression may precipitate life-threatening hemorrhage, infection, anemia. If platelet count drops, minimize trauma to pt (e.g., IM injections, pt positioning). Premedicate with antiemetics on day of treatment, starting at least 30 min before administration.

INTERVENTION/EVALUATION

Assess for bleeding, signs of infection, anemia. Monitor hydration status, I&O,

serum electrolytes (diarrhea, vomiting are common side effects). Monitor CBC with differential, Hgb, platelets for evidence of myelosuppression. Assess response to medication; provide interventions (e.g., small, frequent meals; antiemetics for nausea/vomiting). Question for complaints of headache. Assess breathing pattern for evidence of dyspnea.

PATIENT/FAMILY TEACHING

• Explain that alopecia is reversible but that new hair may have different color, texture. • Inform pt of possible late diarrhea causing dehydration, electrolyte depletion. • Provide antiemetic and antidiarrheal regimen for subsequent use. • Notify physician if diarrhea, vomiting continues at home. • Do not have immunizations without physician's approval (drug lowers resistance). • Avoid contact with those who have recently received live virus vaccine.

Toprol XL, *see metoprolol*

Toradol, *see ketorolac*

toremifene

tor-**em**-ih-feen

(Fareston)

CLASSIFICATION

PHARMACOTHERAPEUTIC: Nonsteroidal antiestrogen. **CLINICAL:** Antineoplastic (see p. 83C).

ACTION

Binds to estrogen receptors on tumors, producing complex that decreases DNA synthesis, inhibits estrogen effects. **Therapeutic Effect:** Blocks growth-stimulating effects of estrogen in breast cancer.

PHARMACOKINETICS

Well absorbed after PO administration. Metabolized in liver. Eliminated in feces. **Half-life:** Approximately 5 days.

USES

Treatment of advanced breast cancer in postmenopausal women with estrogen receptor–positive disease. **OFF-LABEL:** Treatment of desmoid tumors, endometrial carcinoma.

PRECAUTIONS

CONTRAINDICATIONS: History of thromboembolic disease. **CAUTIONS:** Preexisting endometrial hyperplasia, leukopenia, thrombocytopenia.

LIFESPAN CONSIDERATIONS:

Pregnancy/Lactation: Unknown if distributed in breast milk. **Pregnancy Category D. Children:** Safety and efficacy not established. Not prescribed in this pt population. **Elderly:** No age-related precautions noted.

INTERACTIONS

DRUG: **Carbamazepine, phenobarbital, phenytoin** may decrease concentration. **Warfarin** may increase prothrombin time (PT), risk of bleeding. **HERBAL:** None significant. **FOOD:** None known. **LAB VALUES:** May increase serum alkaline phosphatase, bilirubin, calcium, AST.

AVAILABILITY (Rx)

TABLETS: 60 mg.

ADMINISTRATION/HANDLING

PO

• Give without regard to food.

INDICATIONS/ROUTES/DOSAGE

BREAST CANCER

PO: ADULTS: 60 mg/day until disease progression is observed.

T

SIDE EFFECTS

FREQUENT: Hot flashes (35%), diaphoresis (20%), nausea (14%), vaginal discharge (13%), dizziness, dry eyes (9%). **OCCASIONAL (5%–2%):** Edema, vomiting, vaginal bleeding. **RARE:** Fatigue, depression, lethargy, anorexia.

ADVERSE EFFECTS/ TOXIC REACTIONS

Ocular toxicity (cataracts, glaucoma, decreased visual acuity), hypercalcemia may occur.

NURSING CONSIDERATIONS

BASELINE ASSESSMENT

Estrogen receptor assay should be done before beginning therapy. CBC, platelet count, serum calcium levels should be checked before and periodically during therapy.

INTERVENTION/EVALUATION

Assess for hypercalcemia (increased urinary volume, excessive thirst, nausea, vomiting, constipation, hypotonicity of muscles, deep bone/flank pain, renal stones). Monitor CBC, leukocyte, platelet counts, serum calcium, hepatic function tests.

PATIENT/FAMILY TEACHING

• May have initial flare of symptoms (bone pain, hot flashes) that will subside. • Report vaginal bleeding/discharge/itching, leg cramps, weight gain, shortness of breath, weakness. • Contact physician if nausea/vomiting continues. • Nonhormone contraceptives are recommended during treatment.

torsemide

tor-se-mide
(Demadex, Demadex I.V.)

Do not confuse torsemide with furosemide.

CLASSIFICATION

PHARMACOTHERAPEUTIC: Loop diuretic. **CLINICAL:** Antihypertensive, antiedema (see p. 97C).

ACTION

Enhances excretion of sodium, chloride, potassium, water at ascending limb of loop of Henle. Reduces plasma, extracellular fluid volume. **Therapeutic Effect:** Produces diuresis; lowers B/P.

PHARMACOKINETICS

Route	Onset	Peak	Duration
PO	1 hr	1–2 hrs	6–8 hrs
IV	10 min	1 hr	6–8 hrs

Rapidly, well absorbed from GI tract. Protein binding: 97%–99%. Metabolized in liver. Primarily excreted in urine. Not removed by hemodialysis. **Half-life:** 3.3 hrs.

USES

Treatment of hypertension either alone or in combination with other antihypertensives. Edema associated with CHF, renal disease, hepatic cirrhosis, chronic renal failure.

PRECAUTIONS

CONTRAINDICATIONS: Anuria, hepatic coma, severe electrolyte depletion. **EXTREME CAUTION:** Hypersensitivity to sulfonamides. **CAUTIONS:** Elderly, cardiac pts, pts with history of ventricular arrhythmias, pts with hepatic cirrhosis, ascites. Renal impairment, systemic lupus erythematosus.

LIFESPAN CONSIDERATIONS:

Pregnancy/Lactation: Unknown if drug is excreted in breast milk. **Pregnancy Category B. Children:** Safety and efficacy not established. **Elderly:** No age-related precautions noted.

INTERACTIONS

DRUG: Amphotericin B, nephrotoxic medications, ototoxic medications may increase risk of nephrotoxicity, ototoxicity. May decrease effects of **anticoagulants, heparin, thrombolytics**. May increase risk of **digoxin** toxicity associated with torsemide-induced hypokalemia. May increase risk of **lithium** toxicity. **NSAIDs, probenecid** may decrease diuretic effect. **Other antihypertensives** may increase risk of hypotension. **Other hypokalemia-causing medications** may increase risk of hypokalemia. **HERBAL: Ephedra, yohimbe, ginseng** may worsen hypertension. **Garlic** may increase antihypertensive effect. **FOOD:** None known. **LAB VALUES:** May increase BUN, serum creatinine, uric acid. May decrease serum calcium, chloride, magnesium, potassium, sodium.

AVAILABILITY (Rx)

INJECTION SOLUTION (DEMADEX I.V.): 10 mg/ml. **TABLETS (DEMADEX):** 5 mg, 10 mg, 20 mg, 100 mg.

ADMINISTRATION/HANDLING

IV

Rate of administration

◄ **ALERT** ► Flush IV line with 0.9% NaCl before and following administration.

• May give undiluted as IV push over 2 min. • For continuous IV infusion, dilute with 0.9% or 0.45% NaCl or D_5W and infuse over 24 hrs. • Too-rapid IV rate, high dosages may cause ototoxicity; administer IV rate **slowly.**

Storage • Store at room temperature.

PO

• Give without regard to food. Give with food to avoid GI upset, preferably with breakfast (prevents nocturia).

IV COMPATIBILITY

Milrinone (Primacor).

INDICATIONS/ROUTES/DOSAGE

HYPERTENSION

PO: ADULTS, ELDERLY: Initially, 2.5–5 mg/day. May increase to 10 mg/day if no response in 4–6 wks. If no response, additional antihypertensive added.

CHF

PO, IV: ADULTS, ELDERLY: Initially, 10–20 mg/day. May increase by approximately doubling dose until desired therapeutic effect is attained. Doses greater than 200 mg have not been adequately studied.

CHRONIC RENAL FAILURE

PO, IV: ADULTS, ELDERLY: Initially, 20 mg/day. May increase by approximately doubling dose until desired therapeutic effect is attained. Doses greater than 200 mg have not been adequately studied.

HEPATIC CIRRHOSIS

PO, IV: ADULTS, ELDERLY: Initially, 5 mg/day given with aldosterone antagonist or potassium-sparing diuretic. May increase by approximately doubling dose until desired therapeutic effect is attained. Doses greater than 40 mg have not been adequately studied.

SIDE EFFECTS

FREQUENT (10%–4%): Headache, dizziness, rhinitis. **OCCASIONAL (3%–1%):** Asthenia (loss of strength, energy), insomnia, nervousness, diarrhea, constipation, nausea, dyspepsia (heartburn, indigestion, epigastric pain), edema, EKG changes, pharyngitis, cough, arthralgia, myalgia. **RARE (less than 1%):** Syncope, hypotension, arrhythmias.

ADVERSE EFFECTS/ TOXIC REACTIONS

Ototoxicity may occur with too-rapid IV administration or with high doses; must be given slowly. Overdose produces acute, profound water loss; volume/electrolyte depletion; dehydration; decreased blood volume; circulatory collapse.

NURSING CONSIDERATIONS

BASELINE ASSESSMENT

Check serum electrolyte levels, esp. potassium. Obtain baseline weight; check for edema. Assess for rales in lungs.

INTERVENTION/EVALUATION

Monitor B/P, serum electrolytes (esp. potassium), I&O, weight. Notify physician of any hearing abnormality. Note extent of diuresis. Assess lungs for rales. Check for signs of edema, particularly of dependent areas. Although less potassium is lost with torsemide than with furosemide, assess for signs of hypokalemia (change of muscle strength, tremor, muscle cramps, altered mental status, cardiac arrhythmias).

PATIENT/FAMILY TEACHING

• Take medication in morning to prevent nocturia. • Expect increased urinary volume, frequency. • Report palpitations, muscle weakness, cramps, nausea, dizziness. • Do not take other medications (including OTC drugs) without consulting physician. • Eat foods high in potassium such as whole grains (cereals), legumes, meat, bananas, apricots, orange juice, potatoes (white, sweet), raisins.

tositumomab and iodine ^{131}I-tositumomab

toe-sit-**two**-mo-mab
(Bexxar)

CLASSIFICATION

PHARMACOTHERAPEUTIC: Monoclonal antibody. **CLINICAL:** Antineoplastic.

ACTION

Composed of an antibody conjoined with a radiolabeled antitumor antibody. The antibody portion binds specifically to the CD20 antigen, found on pre-B, B lymphocytes and on more than 90% of B-cell non-Hodgkin's lymphomas, resulting in formation of a complex. **Therapeutic Effect:** Induces cytotoxicity associated with ionizing radiation from radioisotope. Depletes circulating CD20-positive cells.

PHARMACOKINETICS

Elimination of iodine 131 (^{131}I) occurs by decay, excretion in urine. **Half-life:** 8 days. Pts with high tumor burden, splenomegaly, bone marrow involvement have faster clearance, shorter half-life, larger volume of distribution.

USES

Treatment of pts with CD20 antigen-expressing non-Hodgkin's lymphoma, whose disease has relapsed following chemotherapy.

PRECAUTIONS

CONTRAINDICATIONS: Hypersensitivity to murine proteins, pregnancy. **CAUTIONS:** Renal impairment, active systemic infection, immunosuppression.

LIFESPAN CONSIDERATIONS:

Pregnancy/Lactation: ^{131}I-tositumomab component is contraindicated during pregnancy (severe, possibly irreversible hypothyroidism in neonates). Radioiodine is excreted in breast milk; do not breast-feed. **Pregnancy Category X.** **Children:** Safety and efficacy not established. **Elderly:** Response rate, duration of severe hematologic toxicity are lower in pts older than 65 yrs.

INTERACTIONS

DRUG: Anticoagulants, medications that interfere with platelet function increase risk of bleeding, hemorrhage.

HERBAL: None significant. **FOOD:** None known. **LAB VALUES:** May decrease Hgb, Hct, platelet count, WBC count, thyroid-stimulating hormone (TSH).

AVAILABILITY (Rx)

KIT (DOSIMETRIC): tositumomab 225 mg/16.1 ml (2 vials), tositumomab 35 mg/2.5 ml (1 vial), and iodine ^{131}I-tositumomab 0.1 mg/ml (1 vial). **KIT (THERAPEUTIC):** tositumomab 225 mg/16.1 ml (2 vials), tositumomab 35 mg/2.5 ml (1 vial), and iodine ^{131}I-tositumomab 1.1 mg/ml (1 or 2 vials).

ADMINISTRATION/HANDLING

◄ ALERT ► Regimen consists of 4 components given in 2 separate steps: The dosimetric step, followed 7–14 days later by a therapeutic step. When infusing, use IV tubing with in-line 0.22-micron filter (use same tubing throughout entire dosimetric or therapeutic step; changing filter results in drug loss). Reduce infusion rate by 50% for mild to moderate infusion toxicity; interrupt infusion for severe infusion toxicity (may resume when resolution of toxicity occurs). Resume at 50% reduction rate of infusion.

IV

Reconstitution

◄ ALERT ► Reconstitution amounts and rates of administration are the same for both dosimetric and therapeutic steps.

TOSITUMOMAB • Reconstitute 450 mg tositumomab in 50 ml 0.9% NaCl.

IODINE ^{131}I-TOSITUMOMAB • Reconstitute iodine ^{131}I-tositumomab in 30 ml 0.9% NaCl.

Rate of administration

TOSITUMOMAB • Infuse over 60 min.

IODINE ^{131}I-TOSITUMOMAB • Infuse over 20 min.

Storage

TOSITUMOMAB • Refrigerate vials before dilution. Protect from strong light. • Following dilution, solution is stable for 24 hrs if refrigerated, up to 8 hrs at room temperature. • Discard any unused portion left in the vial. • Do not shake.

IODINE ^{131}I-TOSITUMOMAB • Store frozen until vial is removed for thawing before administration. Thawed doses are stable for 8 hrs if refrigerated. • Discard any unused portion.

INDICATIONS/ROUTES/DOSAGE

◄ ALERT ► Initiate thyroid protective agents (potassium iodide) 24 hrs prior to administration of iodine ^{131}I-tositumomab dosimetric step and continue until 2 wks following administration of iodine ^{131}I-tositumomab therapeutic step. Pretreat against infusion reactions with acetaminophen and diphenhydramine 1 hr prior to beginning therapy.

NON-HODGKIN'S LYMPHOMA

◄ ALERT ► PRETREATMENT: Diphenhydramine 50 mg and acetaminophen 650–1,000 mg is given 1 hr prior to administering, followed by acetaminophen 650–1,000 mg q4h for 2 doses, then q4h prn. Full recovery from hematologic toxicities is not a requirement for giving second dose.

IV: ADULTS, ELDERLY: Dosage contains 4 components in 2 steps. **Day 0:** tositumomab 450 mg/50 NaCl over 60 min. Then iodine ^{131}I-tositumomab 35 mg in 30 ml NaCl over 20 min. **Day 7:** tositumomab 450 mg/50 NaCl over 60 min. Then, iodine ^{131}I-tositumomab to deliver 65–75 cGy total body irradiation and tositumomab 35 mg over 20 min.

SIDE EFFECTS

FREQUENT (46%–18%): Asthenia (loss of strength, energy), fever, nausea, cough, chills. **OCCASIONAL (17%–10%):** Rash, headache, abdominal pain, vomiting, anorexia, myalgia, diarrhea, pharyngitis, arthralgia, rhinitis, pruritus. **RARE (9%–5%):** Peripheral edema, diaphoresis, constipation, dyspepsia (heartburn, indigestion, epigastric pain), back pain, hypotension, vasodilation, dizziness, somnolence.

ADVERSE EFFECTS/ TOXIC REACTIONS

Infusion toxicity, characterized by fever, rigors, diaphoresis, hypotension, dyspnea, nausea, may occur during or within 48 hrs of infusion. Severe, prolonged myelosuppression, characterized by neutropenia, anemia, thrombocytopenia, occurs in 71% of pts. Sepsis occurs in 45% of pts. Hemorrhage occurs in 12%, myelodysplastic syndrome in 8%.

NURSING CONSIDERATIONS

BASELINE ASSESSMENT

Pretreatment with acetaminophen and diphenhydramine before administering infusion may prevent infusion-related effects. Obtain baseline CBC before therapy and at least weekly following administration for minimum of 10 wks. Use strict aseptic technique to protect pt from infection. Follow radiation safety protocols. Time to nadir is 4–7 wks, duration of cytopenias is approximately 30 days.

INTERVENTION/EVALUATION

Diligently monitor lab values for possibly severe, prolonged thrombocytopenia, neutropenia, anemia. Monitor for hematologic toxicity (fever, chills, unusual bruising/bleeding from any site), symptoms of anemia (excessive fatigue, weakness). Assess for signs of hypothyroidism.

PATIENT/FAMILY TEACHING

• Avoid pregnancy (Pregnancy Category X). • Do not have immunizations without physician's approval (drug lowers resistance). • Avoid contact with those who have recently received live virus vaccine. • Promptly report fever, sore throat, signs of local infection, unusual bruising/bleeding from any site.

tramadol

tray-mah-doal

(Ultram)

Do not confuse tramadol with Toradol, or Ultram with Ultane.

FIXED-COMBINATION(S)

Ultracet: tramadol/acetaminophen (a non-narcotic analgesic): 37.5 mg/325 mg.

CLASSIFICATION

CLINICAL: Analgesic.

ACTION

Binds to μ-opioid receptors, inhibits reuptake of norepinephrine, serotonin. Reduces intensity of pain stimuli incoming from sensory nerve endings. **Therapeutic Effect:** Reduces pain.

PHARMACOKINETICS

Route	Onset	Peak	Duration
PO	Less than 1 hr	2–3 hrs	4–6 hrs

Rapidly, almost completely absorbed after PO administration. Protein binding: 20%. Extensively metabolized in liver to active metabolite (reduced in pts with advanced cirrhosis). Primarily excreted in urine. Minimally removed by hemodialysis. **Half-life:** 6–7 hrs.

USES

Management of moderate to moderately severe pain. **OFF-LABEL:** Premature ejaculation.

PRECAUTIONS

CONTRAINDICATIONS: Acute alcohol intoxication, concurrent use of centrally

T

acting analgesics, hypnotics, opioids, psychotropic drugs, hypersensitivity to opioids. **EXTREME CAUTION:** CNS depression, anoxia, advanced hepatic cirrhosis, epilepsy, respiratory depression, acute alcoholism, shock. **CAUTIONS:** Sensitivity to opioids, increased intracranial pressure (ICP), hepatic/renal impairment, acute abdominal conditions, opioid-dependent pts.

LIFESPAN CONSIDERATIONS:

Pregnancy/Lactation: Crosses placenta. Distributed in breast milk. **Pregnancy Category C. Children:** Safety and efficacy not established. **Elderly:** Age-related renal impairment may require dosage adjustment.

INTERACTIONS

DRUG: Alcohol, other CNS depressants may increase CNS, respiratory depression, hypotension. **Carbamazepine** decreases concentration. **MAOIs** may increase concentration, increase risk of seizures. **Selective serotonin reuptake inhibitors (SSRIs), tricyclic antidepressants, opioids, neuroleptics** may increase risk of seizures. **HERBAL: Gotu kola, kava kava, St. John's wort, valerian** may increase CNS depression. **FOOD:** None known. **LAB VALUES:** May increase serum creatinine, AST, ALT. May decrease Hgb. May cause proteinuria.

AVAILABILITY (Rx)

TABLETS: 50 mg. **TABLETS (ORALLY DISINTEGRATING):** 50 mg.

TABLETS (EXTENDED-RELEASE): 100 mg, 200 mg, 300 mg.

ADMINISTRATION/HANDLING

PO

- Give without regard to meals. Do not chew, crush, split; swallow extended-release tablets whole.

INDICATIONS/ROUTES/DOSAGE

MODERATE TO MODERATELY SEVERE PAIN

PO (IMMEDIATE-RELEASE, ORALLY DISINTEGRATING): ADULTS, ELDERLY: 50–100 mg q4–6h. **Maximum:** 400 mg/day for pts 75 yrs and younger; 300 mg/day for pts older than 75 yrs.

PO (EXTENDED-RELEASE): ADULTS, ELDERLY: 100–300 mg once daily.

DOSAGE IN RENAL IMPAIRMENT

For pts with creatinine clearance of less than 30 ml/min, increase dosing interval to q12h. **Maximum:** 200 mg/day.

DOSAGE IN HEPATIC IMPAIRMENT

Dosage is decreased to 50 mg q12h.

SIDE EFFECTS

FREQUENT (25%–15%): Dizziness, vertigo, nausea, constipation, headache, drowsiness. **OCCASIONAL (10%–5%):** Vomiting, pruritus, CNS stimulation (e.g., nervousness, anxiety, agitation, tremor, euphoria, mood swings, hallucinations), asthenia (loss of strength, energy), diaphoresis, dyspepsia (heartburn, indigestion, epigastric pain), dry mouth, diarrhea. **RARE (less than 5%):** Malaise, vasodilation, anorexia, flatulence, rash, blurred vision, urinary retention/frequency, menopausal symptoms.

ADVERSE EFFECTS/ TOXIC REACTIONS

Seizures reported in those receiving tramadol within recommended dosage range. May have prolonged duration of action, cumulative effect in pts with hepatic/renal impairment.

NURSING CONSIDERATIONS

BASELINE ASSESSMENT

Assess onset, type, location, duration of pain. Effect of medication is reduced if full pain recurs before next dose. Assess drug history, esp. carbamazepine, CNS depressants MAOIs. Review past medical history, esp. epilepsy, seizures. Assess renal/hepatic function lab values.

T

INTERVENTION/EVALUATION

Monitor pulse, B/P. Assist with ambulation if dizziness, vertigo occurs. Dry crackers, cola may relieve nausea. Palpate bladder for urinary retention. Monitor daily pattern of bowel activity/stool consistency. Sips of tepid water may relieve dry mouth. Assess for clinical improvement, record onset of relief of pain.

PATIENT/FAMILY TEACHING

• May cause dependence. • Avoid alcohol, OTC medications (analgesics, sedatives). • May cause drowsiness, dizziness, blurred vision. • Avoid tasks requiring alertness, motor skills until response to drug is established. • Inform physician if severe constipation, difficulty breathing, excessive sedation, seizures, muscle weakness, tremors, chest pain, palpitations occur.

trandolapril

tran-**doe**-la-pril

(Mavik)

Do not confuse trandolapril with tramadol.

FIXED-COMBINATION(S)

Tarka: trandolapril/verapamil (a calcium channel blocker): 1 mg/240 mg; 2 mg/180 mg; 2 mg/240 mg; 4 mg/240 mg.

CLASSIFICATION

PHARMACOTHERAPEUTIC: Angiotensin-converting enzyme (ACE) inhibitor. **CLINICAL:** Antihypertensive, CHF agent (see p. 7C).

ACTION

Suppresses renin-angiotensin-aldosterone system (prevents conversion of angiotensin I to angiotensin II, a potent vasoconstrictor; may inhibit angiotensin II at local vascular, renal sites). Decreases plasma angiotensin II, increases plasma renin activity, decreases aldosterone secretion. **Therapeutic Effect:** Reduces peripheral arterial resistance, pulmonary capillary wedge pressure; improves cardiac output, exercise tolerance.

PHARMACOKINETICS

Slowly absorbed from GI tract. Protein binding: 80%. Metabolized in liver, GI mucosa to active metabolite. Primarily excreted in urine. Removed by hemodialysis. **Half-life:** 24 hrs.

USES

Treatment of left ventricular dysfunction following MI. Treatment of hypertension, alone or in combination with other antihypertensives. **OFF-LABEL:** Treatment of CHF.

PRECAUTIONS

CONTRAINDICATIONS: History of angioedema from previous treatment with ACE inhibitors, pregnancy. **CAUTIONS:** Renal impairment, CHF, hypovolemia, valvular stenosis, hyperkalemia.

LIFESPAN CONSIDERATIONS:

Pregnancy/Lactation: Drug crosses placenta; is distributed in breast milk. May cause fetal, neonatal mortality or morbidity. **Pregnancy Category C (D if used in second or third trimester).** **Children:** Safety and efficacy not established. **Elderly:** No age-related precautions noted.

INTERACTIONS

DRUG: **Alcohol, antihypertensives, diuretics** may increase effects. May increase **lithium** concentration, risk of toxicity. **NSAIDs** may decrease effects. **Potassium-sparing diuretics, potassium supplements** may cause hyperkalemia. **HERBAL:** **Ephedra, yohimbe, ginseng** may worsen hypertension. **Garlic** may increase antihypertensive effect. **FOOD:** None known. **LAB VALUES:** May increase BUN, serum alkaline phosphatase, bilirubin, creatinine, potassium, AST, ALT. May decrease serum sodium. May cause positive antinuclear antibody (ANA) titer.

AVAILABILITY (Rx)

TABLETS: 1 mg, 2 mg, 4 mg.

ADMINISTRATION/HANDLING

PO

• Give without regard to meals. • Tablets may be crushed.

INDICATIONS/ROUTES/DOSAGE

HYPERTENSION (without diuretic)

PO: ADULTS, ELDERLY: Initially, 1 mg once a day in nonblack pts, 2 mg once a day in black pts. Adjust dosage at least at 7-day intervals. Maintenance: 2–4 mg/day. **Maximum:** 8 mg/day.

CONGESTIVE HEART FAILURE, LEFT VENTRICULAR DYSFUNCTION POST-MI

PO: ADULTS, ELDERLY: Initially, 0.5–1 mg, titrated to target dose of 4 mg/day.

DOSAGE IN RENAL/HEPATIC FAILURE

Creatinine clearance 30 ml/min or less, cirrhosis: Recommended starting dose: 0.5 mg/day.

SIDE EFFECTS

FREQUENT (35%–23%): Dizziness, cough. **OCCASIONAL (11%–3%):** Hypotension, dyspepsia (heartburn, indigestion, epigastric pain), syncope, asthenia (loss of strength, energy), tinnitus. **RARE (less than 1%):** Palpitations, insomnia, drowsiness, nausea, vomiting, constipation, flushed skin.

ADVERSE EFFECTS/ TOXIC REACTIONS

Excessive hypotension ("first-dose syncope") may occur in pts with CHF or severely salt/volume depleted. Angioedema, hyperkalemia occur rarely. Agranulocytosis, neutropenia may be noted in those with collagen vascular disease, including scleroderma, systemic lupus erythematosus, renal impairment. Nephrotic syndrome may be noted in those with history of renal disease.

NURSING CONSIDERATIONS

BASELINE ASSESSMENT

Obtain B/P immediately before each dose, in addition to regular monitoring (be alert to fluctuations). Serum renal function tests should be performed before therapy begins. In pts with renal impairment, autoimmune disease, or taking drugs that affect leukocytes or immune response, CBC, differential count should be performed before therapy begins and q2wk for 3 mos, then periodically thereafter.

INTERVENTION/EVALUATION

If excessive reduction in B/P occurs, place pt in supine position with legs elevated. Assist with ambulation if dizziness occurs. Assess for urinary frequency. Auscultate lung sounds for rales, wheezing in those with CHF. Monitor urinalysis for proteinuria. Monitor serum potassium levels in those on concurrent diuretic therapy. Monitor daily pattern of bowel activity/stool consistency.

PATIENT/FAMILY TEACHING

• Do not discontinue medication. • Inform physician if sore throat, fever, swelling, palpitations, cough, chest pain, difficulty swallowing, facial swelling, vomiting, diarrhea occurs. • To reduce hypotensive effect, rise slowly from lying to sitting position and permit legs to dangle from bed momentarily before standing. • Avoid tasks that require alertness, motor skills until response to drug is established (potential for dizziness, drowsiness). • Avoid potassium supplements, salt substitutes.

T

tranylcypromine

evolve

tran-ill-**sip**-roe-meen
(Parnate)

CLASSIFICATION

PHARMACOTHERAPEUTIC: MAOI. **CLINICAL:** Antidepressant (see p. 37C).

ACTION

Inhibits activity of the enzyme, monoamine oxidase, at CNS storage sites, leading to increasing levels of neurotransmitters epinephrine, norepinephrine, serotonin, dopamine at neuronal receptor sites. **Therapeutic Effect:** Relieves depression.

USES

Treatment of depression in pts refractory to, intolerant of other therapy. **OFF-LABEL:** Post-traumatic stress disorder.

PRECAUTIONS

CONTRAINDICATIONS: CHF, children younger than 16 yrs, pheochromocytoma, severe hepatic/renal impairment, uncontrolled hypertension. **CAUTIONS:** Within several hrs of ingestion of contraindicated substance (e.g., tyramine-containing food). Cardiac arrhythmias, severe/frequent headaches, hypertension, suicidal tendencies.

LIFESPAN CONSIDERATIONS:

Pregnancy/Lactation: Crosses placenta. Minimally distributed in breast milk. **Pregnancy Category C. Children:** Not recommended for children (increased risk of suicidal ideation). **Elderly:** Increased risk of drug toxicity may require dosage adjustment.

INTERACTIONS

DRUG: Alcohol, other CNS depressants may increase CNS depressant effects. **Buspirone** may increase B/P. **Caffeine-containing medications** may increase risk of cardiac arrhythmias, hypertension. **Carbamazepine, cyclobenzaprine, maprotiline, MAOIs** may precipitate hypertensive crisis. **Dopamine, tryptophan** may cause sudden, severe hypertension. **Fluoxetine, trazodone, tricyclic antidepressants** may cause serotonin syndrome, neuroleptic malignant syndrome. May increase effects of **insulin, oral antidiabetics. Meperidine, other opioid analgesics** may produce diaphoresis, immediate excitation, rigidity, severe hypertension/hypotension, sometimes leading to severe respiratory distress, vascular collapse, seizures, coma, death. **HERBAL: Ephedra, yohimbe** may increase hypertension. **FOOD: Foods containing tyramine, pressor amines (caffeine, red wine, aged cheese)** may cause sudden, severe hypertension. **LAB VALUES:** None known.

AVAILABILITY (Rx)

TABLETS: 10 mg.

ADMINISTRATION/HANDLING

◀ **ALERT** ▶ At least 14 days must elapse between tranylcypromine and selective serotonin reuptake inhibitors (SSRIs).

INDICATIONS/ROUTES/DOSAGE

DEPRESSION

PO: ADULTS, ELDERLY: Initially, 10 mg twice a day. May increase by 10 mg/day at 1- to 3-wk intervals up to 60 mg/day in divided doses.

SIDE EFFECTS

FREQUENT: Orthostatic hypotension, restlessness, GI upset, insomnia, dizziness, lethargy, weakness, dry mouth, peripheral edema. **OCCASIONAL:** Flushing, diaphoresis, rash, urinary frequency, increased appetite, transient impotence. **RARE:** Visual disturbances.

ADVERSE EFFECTS/ TOXIC REACTIONS

Hypertensive crisis occurs rarely, marked by severe hypertension, occipital headache radiating frontally, neck stiffness/soreness, nausea, vomiting, diaphoresis, fever/chills, clammy skin, dilated pupils, palpitations, tachycardia, bradycardia, constricting chest pain. Intracranial bleeding may be associated with severe hypertension.

NURSING CONSIDERATIONS

BASELINE ASSESSMENT

Perform baseline serum hepatic/renal function tests. Assess sensitivity to tranylcypromine. Assess for other medical conditions, esp. alcoholism, CHF, pheochromocytoma, arrhythmias, cardiovascular disease, hypertension, suicidal tendencies. Question for other medications, including CNS depressants, meperidine, other antidepressants. Do not use in combination with, or within 14 days of taking, selective serotonin reuptake inhibitors (SSRIs).

INTERVENTION/EVALUATION

Assess appearance, behavior, speech pattern, level of interest, mood. Supervise suicidal-risk pt closely during early therapy (as depression lessens, energy level improves, increasing suicide potential). Monitor for occipital headache radiating frontally, neck stiffness/soreness (may be first signal of impending hypertensive crisis). Monitor B/P diligently for hypertension. Assess skin, temperature for fever. Discontinue medication immediately if palpitations, frequent headaches occur. Monitor weight.

PATIENT/FAMILY TEACHING

• Take second daily dose no later than 4 PM to avoid insomnia. • Antidepressant relief may be noted during first wk of therapy; maximum benefit noted within 3 wks. • Report headache, neck stiffness/soreness immediately. • To avoid orthostatic hypotension, change from lying to sitting position slowly and dangle legs momentarily before standing. • Avoid foods that require bacteria/molds for their preparation/preservation, those that contain tyramine (e.g., cheese, sour cream, beer, wine, pickled herring, liver, figs, raisins, bananas, avocados, soy sauce, yeast extracts, yogurt, papaya, broad beans, meat tenderizers), excessive amounts of caffeine (coffee, tea, chocolate), OTC for cold/allergy preparations, weight reduction.

trastuzumab ⚑

traz-**two**-zoo-mab
(Herceptin)

CLASSIFICATION

PHARMACOTHERAPEUTIC: Monoclonal antibody. **CLINICAL:** Antineoplastic (see p. 84C).

ACTION

Binds to HER-2 protein, overexpressed in 25%–30% of primary breast cancers, inhibiting proliferation of tumor cells. **Therapeutic Effect:** Inhibits growth of tumor cells, mediates antibody-dependent cellular cytotoxicity.

PHARMACOKINETICS

Half-life: 5.8 days (range: 1–32 days).

USES

Treatment of metastatic breast cancer pts whose tumors overexpress HER-2 protein and who have received one or more chemotherapy regimens. May be used with paclitaxel without previous treatment for metastatic disease. Post-surgical treatment of HER-2–positive, node-positive breast cancer in combination with doxorubicin, cyclophosphamide, paclitaxel. **OFF-LABEL:** Treatment of ovarian, gastric, colorectal, endometrial, lung, bladder, prostate, salivary gland tumors.

PRECAUTIONS

CONTRAINDICATIONS: Preexisting cardiac disease. **CAUTIONS:** Previous cardiotoxic drug, radiation therapy to chest wall, those with known hypersensitivity to trastuzumab.

LIFESPAN CONSIDERATIONS:

Pregnancy/Lactation: Unknown if distributed in breast milk. **Pregnancy Category B. Children:** Safety and efficacy not established. **Elderly:** Age-related cardiac dysfunction may require dosage adjustment.

INTERACTIONS

DRUG: **Cyclophosphamide, doxorubicin, epirubicin** may increase risk of cardiac dysfunction. **HERBAL:** None significant. **FOOD:** None known. **LAB VALUES:** None known.

AVAILABILITY (Rx)

INJECTION, POWDER FOR RECONSTITUTION: 440 mg.

ADMINISTRATION/HANDLING

IV

Reconstitution • Reconstitute with 20 ml Bacteriostatic Water for Injection to yield concentration of 21 mg/ml. • Add calculated dose to 250 ml 0.9% NaCl (do not use D_5W). • Gently mix contents in bag.

Rate of administration • Do not give IV push or bolus. • Give loading dose (4 mg/kg) over 90 min. Give maintenance infusion (2 mg/kg) over 30 min.

Storage • Refrigerate. • Reconstituted solution appears colorless to pale yellow. • Solution is stable for 28 days if refrigerated after reconstitution with Bacteriostatic Water for Injection (if using Sterile Water for Injection without preservative, use immediately; discard unused portions). • Stable for 24 hrs in 0.9% NaCl if refrigerated.

IV INCOMPATIBILITIES

Do not mix with D_5W or any other medications.

INDICATIONS/ROUTES/DOSAGE

BREAST CANCER

IV: ADULTS, ELDERLY: Initially, 4 mg/kg as 30- to 90-min infusion, then 2 mg/kg weekly as 30-min infusion.

SIDE EFFECTS

FREQUENT (greater than 20%): Pain, asthenia (loss of strength, energy), fever, chills, headache, abdominal pain, back pain, infection, nausea, diarrhea, vomiting, cough, dyspnea. **OCCASIONAL (15%–5%):** Tachycardia, CHF, flu-like symptoms, anorexia, edema, bone pain, arthralgia, insomnia, dizziness, paresthesia, depression, rhinitis, pharyngitis, sinusitis. **RARE (less than 5%):** Allergic reaction, anemia, leukopenia, neuropathy, herpes simplex.

ADVERSE EFFECTS/ TOXIC REACTIONS

Cardiomyopathy, ventricular dysfunction, CHF occur rarely. Pancytopenia may occur.

NURSING CONSIDERATIONS

BASELINE ASSESSMENT

Evaluate left ventricular function. Obtain baseline echocardiogram, EKG, multigated acquisition (MUGA) scan. CBC, platelet count should be obtained at baseline and at regular intervals during therapy.

INTERVENTION/EVALUATION

Frequently monitor for deteriorating cardiac function. Assess for asthenia (loss of strength, energy). Assist with ambulation if asthenia occurs. Monitor for fever, chills, abdominal pain, back pain. Offer antiemetics if nausea,

T

vomiting occurs. Monitor daily pattern of bowel activity/stool consistency.

PATIENT/FAMILY TEACHING

- Do not have immunizations without physician's approval (lowers resistance).
- Avoid contact with those who have recently taken oral polio vaccine.
- Avoid crowds, those with infection.

travoprost

(Travatan)

See Antiglaucoma agents (p. 49C)

trazodone

tray-zoe-done

(Apo-Trazodone ✤, Desyrel, Desyrel Dividose, Novo-Trazodone ✤, PMS-Trazodone ✤)

Do not confuse Desyrel with Delsym or Zestril.

CLASSIFICATION

PHARMACOTHERAPEUTIC: Serotonin reuptake inhibitor. **CLINICAL:** Antidepressant (see pp. 12C, 38C).

ACTION

Blocks reuptake of serotonin at neuronal presynaptic membranes, increasing its availability at postsynaptic receptor sites. **Therapeutic Effect:** Relieves depression.

PHARMACOKINETICS

Well absorbed from GI tract. Protein binding: 85%–95%. Metabolized in liver. Primarily excreted in urine. Unknown if removed by hemodialysis. **Half-life:** 5–9 hrs.

USES

Treatment of depression exhibited as persistent, prominent dysphoria (occurring nearly daily for at least 2 wks) manifested by 4 of 8 symptoms: appetite change, sleep pattern change, increased fatigue, impaired concentration, feelings of guilt or worthlessness, loss of interest in usual activities, psychomotor agitation or retardation, suicidal tendencies. **OFF-LABEL:** Treatment of neurogenic pain.

PRECAUTIONS

CONTRAINDICATIONS: None known. **CAUTIONS:** Cardiac disease, arrhythmias.

LIFESPAN CONSIDERATIONS:

Pregnancy/Lactation: Drug crosses placenta; minimally distributed in breast milk. **Pregnancy Category C. Children:** Safety and efficacy not established in those younger than 6 yrs. **Elderly:** More likely to experience sedative, hypotensive effects; lower dosage recommended.

INTERACTIONS

DRUG: Alcohol, CNS depression-producing medications may increase CNS depression. May increase effects of **antihypertensives**. May increase concentration of **digoxin, phenytoin**. **HERBAL: Gotu kola, kava kava, St. John's wort, valerian** may increase CNS depression. **FOOD:** None known. **LAB VALUES:** May decrease WBC, neutrophil counts.

AVAILABILITY (Rx)

TABLETS: 50 mg (Desyrel), 100 mg (Desyrel), 150 mg (Desyrel Dividose), 300 mg (Desyrel Dividose).

T

ADMINISTRATION/HANDLING

PO

- Give shortly after snack, meal (reduces risk of dizziness, light-headedness).
- Tablets may be crushed.

INDICATIONS/ROUTES/DOSAGE

DEPRESSION

PO: ADULTS: Initially, 150 mg/day in equally divided doses. Increase by

50 mg/day at 3- to 4-day intervals until therapeutic response is achieved. **Maximum:** 600 mg/day. **ELDERLY:** Initially, 25–50 mg at bedtime. May increase by 25–50 mg every 3–7 days. Range: 75–150 mg/day. **CHILDREN 6–18 YRS:** Initially, 1.5–2 mg/kg/day in divided doses. May increase gradually to 6 mg/kg/day in 3 divided doses.

SIDE EFFECTS

FREQUENT (9%–3%): Drowsiness, dry mouth, light-headedness, dizziness, headache, blurred vision, nausea, vomiting. **OCCASIONAL (3%–1%):** Nervousness, fatigue, constipation, myalgia/arthralgia, mild hypotension. **RARE:** Photosensitivity reaction.

ADVERSE EFFECTS/ TOXIC REACTIONS

Priapism, altered libido, retrograde ejaculation, impotence occur rarely. Appears to be less cardiotoxic than other antidepressants, although arrhythmias may occur in pts with preexisting cardiac disease.

NURSING CONSIDERATIONS

BASELINE ASSESSMENT

For those on long-term therapy, serum hepatic/renal function tests, blood counts should be performed periodically. Elderly are more likely to experience sedative, hypotensive effects.

INTERVENTION/EVALUATION

Supervise suicidal-risk pt closely during early therapy (as depression lessens, energy level improves, increasing suicide potential). Assess appearance, behavior, speech pattern, level of interest, mood. Monitor WBC, neutrophil count (drug should be stopped if levels fall below normal). Assist with ambulation if dizziness, light-headedness occurs.

PATIENT/FAMILY TEACHING

• Immediately discontinue medication, consult physician if priapism occurs. • May take after meal, snack. • May take at bedtime if drowsiness occurs. • Change positions slowly to avoid hypotensive effect. • Tolerance to sedative, anticholinergic effects usually develops during early therapy. • Avoid tasks that require alertness, motor skills until response to drug is established. • Photosensitivity to sun may occur. • Dry mouth may be relieved by sugarless gum, sips of tepid water. • Report visual disturbances. • Do not abruptly discontinue medication. • Avoid alcohol.

treprostinil

tre-**pros**-tin-il
(Remodulin)

CLASSIFICATION

PHARMACOTHERAPEUTIC: Aggregation inhibitor, vasodilator. **CLINICAL:** Antiplatelet.

ACTION

Directly dilates pulmonary, systemic arterial vascular beds, inhibiting platelet aggregation. **Therapeutic Effect:** Reduces symptoms of pulmonary arterial hypertension associated with exercise.

PHARMACOKINETICS

Rapidly, completely absorbed after subcutaneous infusion; 91% bound to plasma protein. Metabolized by liver. Excreted mainly in urine, with lesser amount eliminated in feces. **Half-life:** 2–4 hrs.

USES

As continuous subcutaneous infusion for treatment of pulmonary arterial hypertension (PAH) to diminish symptoms associated with exercise, diminish rate of deterioration in pts with PAH who require transition from Flolan.

T

PRECAUTIONS

CONTRAINDICATIONS: None known. **CAUTIONS:** Hepatic/renal impairment in those older than 65 yrs.

LIFESPAN CONSIDERATIONS:

Pregnancy/Lactation: Unknown if distributed in breast milk. **Pregnancy Category B.** **Children:** Safety and efficacy not established. **Elderly:** Consider dose selection carefully because of increased incidence of diminished organ function, concurrent disease; other drug therapy.

INTERACTIONS

DRUG: **Anticoagulants, aspirin, heparin, thrombolytics** may increase risk of bleeding. Reduced B/P caused by treprostinil may be exacerbated by **hypotensive medications (e.g., antihypertensives, diuretics, vasodilators).** **HERBAL:** None significant. **FOOD:** None known. **LAB VALUES:** None known.

AVAILABILITY (Rx)

INJECTION SOLUTION: 1 mg/ml, 2.5 mg/ml, 5 mg/ml, 10 mg/ml.

ADMINISTRATION/HANDLING

IV

Reconstitution • May give undiluted or dilute with either Sterile Water for Injection or 0.9% NaCl.

Rate of administration • Give as continuous IV infusion via indwelling central venous catheter. • Calculate infusion rate using the following formula: **Step One:** Diluted IV Remodulin concentration (mg/ml) = dose (ng/kg/min) × weight (kg) × 0.00006 ÷ IV infusion rate (mg/ml). The calculated amount is then added to reservoir along with enough diluent to achieve total reservoir volume.

Storage • Store unopened vials at room temperature.

SUBCUTANEOUS

Reconstitution • Intended to be administered without further dilution. • Do not use single vial for longer than 14 days after initial use. • To avoid potential interruptions in drug delivery, pt must have immediate access to backup infusion pump, subcutaneous infusion sets.

Rate of administration • Give as continuous subcutaneous infusion via subcutaneous catheter, using infusion pump designed for subcutaneous drug delivery. • Calculate the infusion rate using following formula: infusion rate (ml/hr) = dose (ng/kg/min) × weight (kg) × (0.00006/treprostinil dosage strength concentration [mg/ml]).

Storage • Store unopened vials at room temperature.

INDICATIONS/ROUTES/DOSAGE

PULMONARY ARTERIAL HYPERTENSION

Continuous subcutaneous infusion, IV infusion: **ADULTS, ELDERLY:** Initially, 1.25 ng/kg/min. Reduce infusion rate to 0.625 ng/kg/min if initial dose cannot be tolerated. Increase infusion rate in increments of no more than 1.25 ng/kg/min per wk for first 4 wks, then no more than 2.5 ng/kg/min per wk for duration of infusion.

HEPATIC IMPAIRMENT (MILD TO MODERATE)

ADULTS, ELDERLY: Decrease initial dose to 0.625 ng/kg/min based on ideal body weight; increase cautiously.

SIDE EFFECTS

FREQUENT: Infusion site pain, erythema, induration, rash. **OCCASIONAL:** Headache, diarrhea, jaw pain, vasodilation, nausea. **RARE:** Dizziness, hypotension, pruritus, edema.

ADVERSE EFFECTS/ TOXIC REACTIONS

Abrupt withdrawal, sudden large reductions in dosage may result in worsening of pulmonary arterial hypertension symptoms.

NURSING CONSIDERATIONS

PATIENT/FAMILY TEACHING

- Offer full, complete instruction of drug administration as delivery occurs via self-inserted subcutaneous catheter using ambulatory subcutaneous pump.
- Instruct pt on care of subcutaneous catheter, troubleshooting infusion pump problems.

tretinoin

tret-ih-noyn

(Avita, Rejuva-A ♣, Renova, Retin-A, Retin-A Micro, Vesanoid)

Do not confuse tretinoin with trientine.

FIXED-COMBINATION(S)

With octyl methoxycinnamate and oxy-benzone, moisturizers, and SPF-12, a sunscreen **(Retin-A Regimen Kit).**

◆CLASSIFICATION

PHARMACOTHERAPEUTIC: Retinoid. **CLINICAL:** Antiacne, transdermal, antineoplastic (see p. 84C).

ACTION

Antiacne: Decreases cohesiveness of follicular epithelial cells. Increases turnover of follicular epithelial cells. **Therapeutic Effect:** Causes expulsion of blackheads. Bacterial skin counts are not altered. **Transdermal:** Exerts effects on growth/differentiation of epithelial cells. **Therapeutic Effect:** Alleviates fine wrinkles, hyperpigmentation. **Antineoplastic:** Induces maturation, decreases proliferation of acute promyelocytic leukemia (APL) cells. **Therapeutic Effect:** Repopulation of bone marrow, blood by normal hematopoietic cells.

PHARMACOKINETICS

Topical: Minimally absorbed. **PO:** Well absorbed following PO administration. Primarily excreted in urine. **Half-life:** 0.5–2 hrs.

USES

Topical: Treatment of acne vulgaris, esp. grades I–III in which blackheads, papules, pustules predominate. **Oral:** Induction of remission in pts with APL. **OFF-LABEL:** Treatment of disorders of keratinization, including photo-aged skin, liver spots.

PRECAUTIONS

CONTRAINDICATIONS: Sensitivity to parabens (used as preservative in gelatin capsule). **EXTREME CAUTION: Topical:** Eczema, sun exposure. **CAUTIONS: Topical:** Those with considerable sun exposure in their occupation, hypersensitivity to sun. **PO:** Elevated serum cholesterol/triglycerides.

⌛ LIFESPAN CONSIDERATIONS:

Pregnancy/Lactation: Topical: Use during pregnancy only if clearly necessary. Unknown if excreted in breast milk; exercise caution in breast-feeding mother. **Pregnancy Category C. PO:** Teratogenic, embryotoxic effect. **Pregnancy Category D. Children/Elderly:** Safety and efficacy not established.

INTERACTIONS

DRUG: TOPICAL: Retinoids (e.g., acitretin, tretinoin) may increase drying, irritative effects. **PO: Tetracyclines** may increase risk of pseudotumor cerebri, intracranial hypertension. **Aminocaproic acid** may increase risk of thrombotic complications. **Phenobarbital, rifampin** may alter kinetics of tretinoin. **Ketoconazole** may increase concentration, risk of toxicity. **HERBAL: St. John's wort** may decrease concentration, effect. **Dong quai, St. John's wort** may increase photosensitization. **Vitamin A** supplementation may increase vitamin A toxicity. **FOOD:** None known. **LAB VALUES: PO:** Leukocytosis occurs commonly (40%). May elevate serum hepatic function tests, cholesterol, triglycerides.

AVAILABILITY (Rx)

CREAM: 0.02% (Renova), 0.025% (Avita, Renova, Retin-A), 0.05% (Renova, Retin-A), 0.1% (Retin-A). **GEL:** 0.01% (Retin-A), 0.025% (Avita, Retin-A), 0.04% (Retin-A Micro), 0.1% (Retin-A Micro). **LIQUID (RETIN-A):** 0.05%.

CAPSULES:(VESANOID): 10 mg.

ADMINISTRATION/HANDLING

PO

- Do not crush/break capsule.

TOPICAL

- Thoroughly cleanse area before applying tretinoin. • Lightly cover only affected area. Liquid may be applied with fingertip, gauze, cotton, do not rub onto unaffected skin. • Keep medication away from eyes, mouth, angles of nose, mucous membranes. • Wash hands immediately after application.

INDICATIONS/ROUTES/DOSAGE

ACNE

TOPICAL: ADULTS, CHILDREN 12 YRS AND OLDER: Apply once a day at bedtime or on alternate days.

APL

PO: ADULTS: 45 mg/m^2/day given as 2 evenly divided doses until complete remission is documented. Discontinue therapy 30 days after complete remission or after 90 days of treatment, whichever comes first.

REMISSION MAINTENANCE IN APL

PO: ADULTS, ELDERLY, CHILDREN: 45–200 mg/m^2/day in 2–3 divided doses for up to 12 mos.

SIDE EFFECTS

Topical: Temporary change in pigmentation, photosensitivity. Local inflammatory reactions (peeling, dry skin, stinging, erythema, pruritus) are to be expected and are reversible with discontinuation of tretinoin. **FREQUENT: PO (87%–54%):** Headache, fever, dry skin/oral mucosa, bone pain, nausea, vomiting, rash. **OCCASIONAL: PO (26%–6%):** Mucositis, earache or feeling of fullness in ears, flushing, pruritus, diaphoresis, visual disturbances, hypotension/hypertension, dizziness, anxiety, insomnia, alopecia, skin changes. **RARE (6%):** Altered visual acuity, temporary hearing loss.

ADVERSE EFFECTS/ TOXIC REACTIONS

PO: Retinoic acid syndrome (fever, dyspnea, weight gain, abnormal chest auscultatory findings [pulmonary infiltrates, pleural/pericardial effusions], episodic hypotension) occurs commonly (25%), as does leukocytosis (40%). Syndrome generally occurs during first mo of therapy (sometimes occurs after first dose). High-dose steroids (dexamethasone 10 mg IV) at first suspicion of syndrome reduces morbidity, mortality. Pseudotumor cerebri may be noted, esp. in children (headache, nausea, vomiting, visual disturbances). **Topical:** Possible tumorigenic potential when combined with ultraviolet radiation.

NURSING CONSIDERATIONS

BASELINE ASSESSMENT

PO: Inform women of childbearing potential of risk to fetus if pregnancy occurs. Instruct on need for use of 2 reliable forms of contraceptives concurrently during therapy and for 1 mo after discontinuation of therapy, even in infertile, premenopausal women. Pregnancy test should be obtained within 1 wk before institution of therapy.

Obtain initial serum hepatic function tests, cholesterol, triglyceride levels.

INTERVENTION/EVALUATION

PO: Monitor serum hepatic function tests, hematologic, coagulation profiles, cholesterol, triglycerides. Monitor for signs/symptoms of pseudotumor cerebri in children.

PATIENT/FAMILY TEACHING

• **Topical:** Avoid exposure to sunlight, tanning beds; use sunscreens, protective clothing. • Protect affected areas from wind, cold. • If skin is already sunburned, do not use drug until fully healed. • Keep tretinoin away from eyes, mouth, angles of nose, mucous membranes. • Do not use medicated, drying, abrasive soaps; wash face no more than 2–3 times a day with gentle soap. • Avoid use of preparations containing alcohol, menthol, spice, lime (e.g., shaving lotions, astringents, perfume). • Mild redness, peeling are expected; decrease frequency or discontinue medication if excessive reaction occurs. • Nonmedicated cosmetics may be used; however, cosmetics must be removed before tretinoin application. • Improvement noted during first 24 wks of therapy. • **Antiacne:** Therapeutic results noted in 2–3 wks; optimal results in 6 wks.

T

triamcinolone

(Aristocort)

triamcinolone acetonide

(Aristocort, Aristocort A, Aristospan Injection, Azmacort, Kenalog, Kenalog in Orabase, Kenalog-10, Kenalog-40, Nasacort AQ, Nasacort HFA, Triderm, Tri-Nasal)

triamcinolone diacetate

(Amcort, Aristocort Intralesional)

triamcinolone hexacetonide

(Aristospan)

trye-am-**sin**-oh-lone

Do not confuse triamcinolone with Triaminicin or Triaminicol.

FIXED-COMBINATION(S)

Myco-II, Mycolog II, Myco-Triacet: triamcinolone/nystatin (an antifungal): 0.1%/100,000 units/g.

CLASSIFICATION

PHARMACOTHERAPEUTIC: Adrenocortical steroid. **CLINICAL:** Anti-inflammatory (see pp. 71C, 93C, 95C).

ACTION

Inhibits accumulation of inflammatory cells at inflammation sites, phagocytosis, lysosomal enzyme release, synthesis/release of mediators of inflammation. **Therapeutic Effect:** Prevents/suppresses cell-mediated immune reactions. Decreases/prevents tissue response to inflammatory process.

USES

Inhalation: Long-term control of bronchial asthma. **Nasal:** Seasonal, perennial rhinitis. **Systemic:** Treatment of adrenocortical insufficiency, rheumatic disorders, allergic states, respiratory diseases, other conditions requiring anti-inflammatory, immunosuppresive effects. **Topical:** Relief of inflammation, pruritus associated with corticoid-responsive dermatoses.

PRECAUTIONS

CONTRAINDICATIONS: Administration of live virus vaccines, esp. smallpox vaccine;

hypersensitivity to corticosteroids, tartrazine; IM injection, oral inhalation in children younger than 6 yrs; peptic ulcer disease (except life-threatening situations); systemic fungal infection. **Topical:** Marked circulation impairment. **CAUTIONS:** History of tuberculosis (may reactivate disease), hypothyroidism, cirrhosis, non-specific ulcerative colitis, CHF, hypertension, psychosis, renal insufficiency. Prolonged therapy should be discontinued slowly. **Pregnancy Category C (D if used in first trimester).**

INTERACTIONS

DRUG: **Amphotericin** may worsen hypokalemia. May increase risk of **digoxin** toxicity (due to hypokalemia). May decrease effects of **diuretics, insulin, oral hypoglycemics, potassium supplements**. **Hepatic enzyme inducers** may decrease effects. **Live virus vaccines** may potentiate virus replication, increase virus side effects, decrease pt's antibody response to vaccine. **HERBAL:** **Cat's claw, echinacea** possess immunostimulant properties. **FOOD:** None known. **LAB VALUES:** May increase serum glucose, lipid, amylase, sodium. May decrease serum calcium, potassium, thyroxine.

AVAILABILITY (Rx)

AEROSOL, NASAL INHALATION (NASACORT HFA): 55 mcg/inhalation. **AEROSOL, ORAL INHALATION (AZMACORT):** 100 mcg/actuation. **CREAM: (ARISTOCORT A):** 0.025%, 0.1%, 0.5%. **INJECTION, SUSPENSION (KENALOG-10):** 10 mg/ml. **(KENALOG-40):** 40 mg/ml. **OINTMENT:** 0.025%, 0.1%, 0.5%. **PASTE, ORAL, TOPICAL:** 0.1%. **SOLUTION, SPRAY NASAL INHALATION: (TRI-NASAL):** 50 mcg/inhalation. **SUSPENSION, SPRAY NASAL INHALATION: (NASACORT AQ):** 55 mcg/inhalation. **TABLET: (ARISTOCORT):** 4 mg.

ADMINISTRATION/HANDLING

IM

• Do **not** give IV. • Give deep IM in gluteus maximus.

PO

• Give with food, milk. • Give single doses before 9 AM; multiple doses at evenly spaced intervals.

INHALATION

• Shake container well; exhale as completely as possible. • Place mouthpiece fully into mouth, holding inhaler upright, inhale deeply and slowly while pressing top of canister, hold breath as long as possible before exhaling, then exhale slowly. • Wait 1 min between inhalations when multiple inhalations are ordered (allows for deeper bronchial penetration). • Rinse mouth with water immediately after inhalation.

TOPICAL

• Gently cleanse area before application. • Use occlusive dressings only as ordered. • Apply sparingly, rub into area thoroughly.

INDICATIONS/ROUTES/DOSAGE

IMMUNOSUPPRESSION, RELIEF OF ACUTE INFLAMMATION

PO: ADULTS, ELDERLY: 4–60 mg/day.
TRIAMCINOLONE ACETONIDE: IM ADULTS, ELDERLY: Initially, 2.5–60 mg/day.
TRIAMCINOLONE DIACETATE: IM ADULTS, ELDERLY: 40 mg/wk.
TRIAMCINOLONE HEXACETONIDE: IM ADULTS, ELDERLY: Initially, 2.5–40 mg up to 100 mg; 2–20 mg.
INTRA-ARTICULAR, INTRALESIONAL: ADULTS, ELDERLY: 5–40 mg.

CONTROL OF BRONCHIAL ASTHMA

INHALATION: ADULTS, ELDERLY: 2 inhalations 3–4 times a day. **CHILDREN 6–12 YRS:** 1–2 inhalations 3–4 times a day. **Maximum:** 12 inhalations/day. Initially, 2.5–60 mg/day.

T

RHINITIS

INTRANASAL: ADULTS, ELDERLY, CHILDREN 6 YRS AND OLDER: Initially, 2 sprays (55 mcg/spray) in each nostril once daily. Maintenance: 1 spray in each nostril once daily.

USUAL TOPICAL DOSAGE

TOPICAL: ADULTS, ELDERLY: 2–4 times a day. May give 1–2 times a day or as intermittent therapy.

SIDE EFFECTS

FREQUENT: Insomnia, dry mouth, heartburn, nervousness, abdominal distention, diaphoresis, acne, mood swings, increased appetite, facial flushing, delayed wound healing, increased susceptibility to infection, diarrhea, constipation. **OCCASIONAL:** Headache, edema, change in skin color, frequent urination. **RARE:** Tachycardia, allergic reaction (rash, urticaria), altered mental status, hallucinations, depression. **Topical:** Allergic contact dermatitis.

ADVERSE EFFECTS/ TOXIC REACTIONS

Long-term therapy: Muscle wasting (arms, legs), osteoporosis, spontaneous fractures, amenorrhea, cataracts, glaucoma, peptic ulcer, CHF. **Abrupt withdrawal following long-term therapy:** Anorexia, nausea, fever, headache, arthralgia, rebound inflammation, fatigue, weakness, lethargy, dizziness, orthostatic hypotension. Anaphylaxis occurs rarely with parenteral administration. Sudden discontinuance may be fatal. Blindness has occurred rarely after intralesional injection around face, head.

T

NURSING CONSIDERATIONS

BASELINE ASSESSMENT

Question for hypersensitivity to any corticosteroids, tartrazine (Kena-cort). Obtain baselines for height, weight, B/P, serum glucose, electrolytes. Check results of initial tests (tuberculosis [TB] skin test, x-rays, EKG).

INTERVENTION/EVALUATION

Monitor I&O, daily weight, B/P, serum glucose, electrolytes. Assess for edema. Check vital signs at least twice a day. Be alert to infection: pharyngitis, fever, vague symptoms. Watch for hypocalcemia (muscle twitching, cramps, positive Trousseau's or Chvostek's signs), hypokalemia (weakness, muscle cramps, paresthesia [esp. in lower extremities], nausea/vomiting, irritability, EKG changes). Assess emotional status, ability to sleep. For oral inhalation, check mucous membranes for signs of fungal infection. Monitor growth in children. Check lab results for blood coagulability, clinical evidence of thromboembolism. Provide assistance with ambulation.

PATIENT/FAMILY TEACHING

• **Oral:** Inform physician if sudden weight gain, facial edema, difficulty breathing, muscle weakness occurs. • Take oral medication with food or after meals. • Inform physician if condition worsens. • Do not stop medication without physician approval. • May cause dry mouth. • Avoid alcohol. • **Inhalation:** Do not take for acute asthma attack. • Rinse mouth to decrease risk of mouth soreness. • Inform physician if mouth lesions, sore mouth occurs (stomatitis). • **Nasal:** Report unusual cough/spasm, persistent nasal bleeding, burning, infection.

triamterene

try-**am**-ter-een

(Dyrenium)

Do not confuse triamterene with trimipramine.

FIXED-COMBINATION(S)

Dyazide, Maxzide: triamterene/hydrochlorothiazide (a diuretic): 37.5 mg/25 mg; 50 mg/25 mg; 75 mg/50 mg.

CLASSIFICATION

PHARMACOTHERAPEUTIC: Potassium-sparing diuretic. **CLINICAL:** Antiedema (see p. 97C).

ACTION

Inhibits sodium, potassium, ATPase. Interferes with sodium/potassium exchange in distal tubule, cortical collecting tubule, collecting duct. Increases sodium, decreases potassium excretion. Increases magnesium, decreases calcium loss. **Therapeutic Effect:** Produces diuresis, lowers B/P.

PHARMACOKINETICS

Route	Onset	Peak	Duration
PO	2–4 hrs	N/A	7–9 hrs

Incompletely absorbed from GI tract. Widely distributed. Metabolized in liver. Primarily eliminated in feces via biliary route. **Half-life:** 1.5–2.5 hrs (increased in renal impairment).

USES

Treatment of edema, hypertension. **OFF-LABEL:** Treatment adjunct for hypertension, prevention/treatment of hypokalemia.

PRECAUTIONS

CONTRAINDICATIONS: Anuria, drug-induced or preexisting hyperkalemia, progressive or severe renal disease, severe hepatic disease. **CAUTIONS:** Hepatic/renal impairment, history of renal calculi, diabetes mellitus.

LIFESPAN CONSIDERATIONS:

Pregnancy/Lactation: Drug crosses placenta; is distributed in breast milk. Breast-feeding is not advised. **Pregnancy Category B (D if used in pregnancy-induced hypertension). Children:** Safety and efficacy not established. **Elderly:** May be at increased risk for developing hyperkalemia.

INTERACTIONS

DRUG: **Angiotensin-converting enzyme (ACE) inhibitors (e.g., captopril), cyclosporine, potassium-containing medications, potassium supplements** may increase risk of hyperkalemia. May decrease effects of **anticoagulants, heparin**. May decrease clearance, increase risk of toxicity of **lithium**. **NSAIDs** may decrease antihypertensive effect. **HERBAL:** None significant. **FOOD:** None known. **LAB VALUES:** May increase urinary calcium excretion, BUN, serum glucose, calcium, creatinine, potassium, uric acid. May decrease serum magnesium, sodium.

AVAILABILITY (Rx)

CAPSULES: 50 mg, 100 mg.

ADMINISTRATION/HANDLING

PO

- Give with food if GI disturbance occurs.

INDICATIONS/ROUTES/DOSAGE

EDEMA, HYPERTENSION

PO: ADULTS, ELDERLY: 25–100 mg/day as single dose or in 2 divided doses. **Maximum:** 300 mg/day. **CHILDREN:** 2–4 mg/kg/day as single dose or in 2 divided doses. **Maximum:** 6 mg/kg/day or 300 mg/day.

SIDE EFFECTS

OCCASIONAL: Fatigue, nausea, diarrhea, abdominal pain, leg cramps, headache. **RARE:** Anorexia, asthenia (loss of strength, energy), rash, dizziness.

ADVERSE EFFECTS/ TOXIC REACTIONS

May result in hyponatremia (drowsiness, dry mouth, increased thirst, lack of energy), severe hyperkalemia (irritability, anxiety, heaviness of legs, paresthesia, hypotension, bradycardia, EKG changes [tented T waves, widening

T

QRS complex, ST segment depression]), particularly in those with renal impairment, diabetes, elderly, severely ill. Agranulocytosis, nephrolithiasis, thrombocytopenia occur rarely.

NURSING CONSIDERATIONS

BASELINE ASSESSMENT

Assess baseline serum electrolytes, particularly check for hypokalemia. Assess serum renal/hepatic function tests. Assess for edema (note location, extent), skin turgor, mucous membranes for hydration status. Assess muscle strength, mental status. Note skin temperature, moisture. Obtain baseline weight. Initiate strict I&O. Note pulse rate, regularity.

INTERVENTION/EVALUATION

Monitor B/P, vital signs, serum electrolytes (particularly potassium), I&O, weight. Watch for changes from initial assessment (hyperkalemia may result in muscle strength changes, tremor, muscle cramps), altered mental status (orientation, alertness, confusion), cardiac arrhythmias. Weigh daily. Note extent of diuresis. Assess lung sounds for rhonchi, wheezing.

PATIENT/FAMILY TEACHING

• Take medication in morning. • Expect increased urinary volume, frequency. • Therapeutic effect takes several days to begin and can last for several days when drug is discontinued. • Avoid prolonged exposure to sunlight. • Report severe, persistent weakness, headache, dry mouth, nausea, vomiting, fever, sore throat, unusual bleeding/bruising. • Avoid excessive intake of food high in potassium, salt substitutes.

T

triazolam

trye-**ay**-zoe-lam

(Apo-Triazo ✦, Halcion)

Do not confuse Halcion with Haldol or Healon.

◆CLASSIFICATION

PHARMACOTHERAPEUTIC: Benzodiazepine (**Schedule IV**). **CLINICAL:** Sedative-hypnotic (see p. 141C).

ACTION

Enhances action of inhibitory neurotransmitter gamma-aminobutyric acid (GABA), resulting in CNS depression. **Therapeutic Effect:** Induces sleep.

PHARMACOKINETICS

Rapidly, completely absorbed from GI tract. Protein binding: 89%–94%. Metabolized in liver. Primarily excreted in urine. **Half-life:** 1.5–5.5 hrs.

USES

Short-term treatment of insomnia (6 wks or less). Reduces sleep-induction time, number of nocturnal awakenings; increases length of sleep.

PRECAUTIONS

CONTRAINDICATIONS: Angle-closure glaucoma, CNS depression, hypersensitivity to other benzodiazepines, pregnancy, breast-feeding, severe pain (uncontrolled), sleep apnea. **CAUTIONS:** Those with potential for drug abuse.

⌛ LIFESPAN CONSIDERATIONS:

Pregnancy/Lactation: Drug crosses placenta; is distributed in breast milk. **Pregnancy Category X. Children:** Safety and efficacy not established in children younger than 18 yrs. **Elderly:** Initially, small dosage is recommended to avoid excessive sedation, ataxia. May increase dosage gradually.

INTERACTIONS

DRUG: **Alcohol, other CNS depressants** may increase CNS depression. **Fluvoxamine, itraconazole, ketoconazole, nefazodone** may inhibit metabolism, increase concentration. **HERBAL:** **Gotu kola, kava kava, St. John's wort, valerian** may increase CNS depression. **FOOD:** **Grapefruit, grapefruit juice** may alter absorption. **LAB VALUES:** None known.

AVAILABILITY (Rx)

TABLETS: 0.125 mg, 0.25 mg.

ADMINISTRATION/HANDLING

PO

• Give without regard to meals. • Tablets may be crushed. • Grapefruit, grapefruit juice may alter absorption.

INDICATIONS/ROUTES/DOSAGE

INSOMNIA

PO: ADULTS, CHILDREN 18 YRS AND OLDER: 0.125–0.25 mg at bedtime. **Maximum:** 0.5 mg. **ELDERLY:** 0.0625–0.125 mg at bedtime. **Maximum:** 0.25 mg.

SIDE EFFECTS

FREQUENT: Drowsiness, sedation, dry mouth, headache, dizziness, nervousness, light-headedness, incoordination, nausea, rebound insomnia (may occur for 1–2 nights after drug is discontinued). **OCCASIONAL:** Euphoria, tachycardia, abdominal cramps, visual disturbances. **RARE:** Paradoxical CNS excitement pts, restlessness (esp. in elderly, debilitated pts).

ADVERSE EFFECTS/ TOXIC REACTIONS

Abrupt or too-rapid withdrawal may result in pronounced restlessness, irritability, insomnia, hand tremor, abdominal/muscle cramps, vomiting, diaphoresis, seizures. Overdose results in somnolence, confusion, diminished reflexes, respiratory depression, coma.

NURSING CONSIDERATIONS

BASELINE ASSESSMENT

Question for possibility of pregnancy before initiating therapy (Pregnancy Category X). Assess vital signs immediately before administration. Raise bed rails. Provide environment conducive to sleep (back rub, quiet environment, low lighting).

INTERVENTION/EVALUATION

Monitor respiratory, cardiovascular, mental status; hepatic function with prolonged use. Assess sleep pattern of pt. Monitor elderly, debilitated for paradoxical reaction, particularly during early therapy. Evaluate for therapeutic response to insomnia: decrease in number of nocturnal awakenings, increase in length of sleep.

PATIENT/FAMILY TEACHING

• May cause drowsiness. • Avoid tasks that require alertness, motor skills until response to drug is established. • May cause physical, psychological dependence, dry mouth. • Smoking reduces drug effectiveness. • Avoid alcohol, other CNS depressants. • Inform physician if pregnant or planning to become pregnant. • Rebound insomnia may occur when drug is discontinued after short-term therapy; may experience disturbed sleep patterns for 1–2 nights after discontinuing triazolam. • Avoid grapefruit, grapefruit juice.

T

Tricor, *see fenofibrate*

trifluoperazine

trye-floo-oh-**per**-a-zeen

(Apo-Trifluoperazine ✤, Novo-Trifluzine ✤, PMS-Trifluoperazine ✤, Stelazine)

Do not confuse trifluoperazine with triflupromazine, or Stelazine with selegiline.

CLASSIFICATION

PHARMACOTHERAPEUTIC: Phenothiazine derivative. **CLINICAL:** Antipsychotic, antianxiety (see p. 63C).

ACTION

Blocks dopamine at postsynaptic receptor sites. Possesses strong extrapyramidal, antiemetic effects, weak anticholinergic, sedative effects. **Therapeutic Effect:** Suppresses behavioral response in psychosis; reduces locomotor activity, aggressiveness.

PHARMACOKINETICS

Readily absorbed following PO administration. Protein binding: 90%–99%. Metabolized in liver. Excreted in urine. **Half-life:** 24 hrs.

USES

Treatment of schizophrenia.

PRECAUTIONS

CONTRAINDICATIONS: Angle-closure glaucoma, circulatory collapse, myelosuppression, severe cardiac/hepatic disease, severe hypertension/hypotension. **CAUTIONS:** Seizure disorders, Parkinson's disease.

LIFESPAN CONSIDERATIONS:

Pregnancy/Lactation: Drug crosses placenta; is distributed in breast milk. **Pregnancy Category C. Children:** Safety and efficacy not established in children younger than 2 yrs. **Elderly:** Higher risk of sedative, anticholinergic, extrapyramidal, hypotensive effects.

INTERACTIONS

DRUG: **Alcohol, other CNS depressants** may increase CNS, respiratory depression, hypotensive effects. **Antacids** may inhibit absorption if given within 1 hr of drug. **Antithyroid agents** may increase risk of agranulocytosis. **Extrapyramidal symptom–producing medications** may increase extrapyramidal symptoms (EPS). **Hypotensive agents** may increase hypotension. May decrease effects of **levodopa**. **Lithium** may decrease absorption, produce adverse neurologic effects. **MAOIs, tricyclic antidepressants** may increase anticholinergic, sedative effects. **HERBAL:** **Gotu kola, kava kava, St. John's wort, valerian** may increase CNS depression. **Dong quai, St. John's wort** may increase photosensitization. **FOOD:** None known. **LAB VALUES:** May cause EKG changes.

AVAILABILITY (Rx)

TABLETS: 1 mg, 2 mg, 5 mg, 10 mg.

ADMINISTRATION/HANDLING

PO

- May give with food to decrease GI effects.

INDICATIONS/ROUTES/DOSAGE

PSYCHOTIC DISORDERS

PO: ADULTS, ELDERLY, CHILDREN 12 YRS AND OLDER: Initially, 2–5 mg once or twice a day. Range: 15–20 mg/day. **Maximum:** 40 mg/day. **CHILDREN 6–11 YRS:** Initially, 1 mg once or twice a day. Maintenance: Up to 15 mg/day.

SIDE EFFECTS

FREQUENT: Hypotension, dizziness, syncope (occur frequently after first injection, occasionally after subsequent injections, rarely with oral form). **OCCASIONAL:** Drowsiness during early therapy, dry mouth, blurred vision, lethargy, constipation, diarrhea, nasal congestion, peripheral edema, urinary retention. **RARE:** Ocular changes, altered skin pigmentation (in those taking high doses for prolonged periods), photosensitivity.

ADVERSE EFFECTS/ TOXIC REACTIONS

EPS appear to be dose-related (particularly high doses) and are divided into 3 categories: akathisia (inability to sit still, tapping of feet); parkinsonian symptoms (mask-like face, tremors, shuffling gait, hypersalivation); acute dystonias: torticollis (neck muscle spasm), opisthotonos (rigidity of back muscles), oculogyric crisis (rolling back of eyes). Dystonic reaction may produce diaphoresis, pallor. Tardive dyskinesia (tongue protrusion, puffing of cheeks, chewing/puckering of the mouth) occurs rarely (may be irreversible). Abrupt withdrawal after long-term therapy may precipitate nausea, vomiting, gastritis, dizziness, tremors. Blood dyscrasias, particularly agranulocytosis, mild leukopenia may occur. May lower seizure threshold.

NURSING CONSIDERATIONS

BASELINE ASSESSMENT

Assess behavior, appearance, emotional status, response to environment, speech pattern, thought content.

INTERVENTION/EVALUATION

Monitor B/P for hypotension. Assess for EPS. Monitor WBC for blood dyscrasias. Monitor for fine tongue movement (may be early sign of tardive dyskinesia); tremor, gait changes; abnormal movement in trunk, neck, extremities. Supervise suicidal-risk pt closely during early therapy (as depression lessens, energy level improves, increasing suicide potential). Monitor target behaviors. Assess for therapeutic response (interest in surroundings, improvement in self-care, increased ability to concentrate, relaxed facial expression).

PATIENT/FAMILY TEACHING

• Do not take antacids within 1 hr of trifluoperazine. • Avoid alcohol. • Avoid excessive exposure to sunlight, artificial light. • Avoid tasks that require alertness, motor skills until response to drug is established (may cause drowsiness). • Rise slowly from lying or sitting position (prevents hypotension).

trihexyphenidyl

try-hex-eh-**fen**-ih-dill

(Apo-Trihex ✤, Artane)

Do not confuse Artane with Altace or Anturane.

CLASSIFICATION

PHARMACOTHERAPEUTIC: Anticholinergic. **CLINICAL:** Antiparkinson agent.

ACTION

Blocks central cholinergic receptors (aids in balancing cholinergic and dopaminergic activity). **Therapeutic Effect:** Decreases salivation, relaxes smooth muscle.

USES

Adjunctive treatment for all forms of Parkinson's disease, including postencephalitic, arteriosclerotic, idiopathic types. Controls symptoms of drug-induced extrapyramidal symptoms (EPS).

PRECAUTIONS

CONTRAINDICATIONS: Angle-closure glaucoma, GI obstruction, paralytic ileus, intestinal atony, severe ulcerative colitis, prostatic hypertrophy, myasthenia gravis, megacolon. **CAUTIONS:** Hyperthyroidism, renal/hepatic impairment, hypertension, hiatal hernia, tachycardia, arrhythmias, GI ulcer, esophageal reflux, excessive activity during hot weather, exercise. **Pregnancy Category C.**

T

INTERACTIONS

DRUG: **Alcohol, CNS depressants** may increase sedative effect. **Amantadine, anticholinergics, MAOIs** may increase anticholinergic effects. **Antacids, antidiarrheals** may decrease absorption, effects. **HERBAL:** None significant. **FOOD:** None known. **LAB VALUES:** None known.

AVAILABILITY (Rx)

ELIXIR: 2 mg/ 5 ml. **TABLETS:** 2 mg, 5 mg.

ADMINISTRATION/HANDLING

PO

• Administer with food, water to decrease GI irritation.

INDICATIONS/ROUTES/DOSAGE

PARKINSONISM

PO: ADULTS, ELDERLY: Initially, 1 mg on first day. May increase by 2 mg a day at 3- to 5-day intervals up to 6–10 mg a day (12–15 mg a day in pts with postencephalitic parkinsonism).

DRUG-INDUCED EXTRAPYRAMIDAL SYMPTOMS

PO: ADULTS, ELDERLY: Initially, 1 mg a day. Range: 5–15 mg a day in 3–4 divided doses.

SIDE EFFECTS

◄ **ALERT** ► Those over 60 yrs tend to develop mental confusion, disorientation, agitation, psychotic-like symptoms.

FREQUENT: Drowsiness, dry mouth. **OCCASIONAL:** Blurred vision, urinary retention, constipation, dizziness, headache, muscle cramps. **RARE:** Skin rash, seizures, depression.

ADVERSE EFFECTS/ TOXIC REACTIONS

Hypersensitivity reaction (eczema, pruritus, rash, cardiac arrhythmias, photosensitivity) may occur. Overdosage may vary from CNS depression (sedation, apnea, cardiovascular collapse, death) to severe paradoxical reaction (hallucinations, tremor, seizures).

NURSING CONSIDERATIONS

INTERVENTION/EVALUATION

Be alert to neurologic effects: headache, lethargy, mental confusion, agitation. Monitor elderly closely for paradoxical reaction. Assess for clinical reversal of symptoms (improvement of tremor of head/hands at rest, mask-like facial expression, shuffling gait, muscular rigidity).

PATIENT/FAMILY TEACHING

• Take after meals or with food. • Do not stop medication abruptly. • Inform physician if GI effects, palpitations, eye pain, rash, fever, heat intolerance occurs. • Avoid alcohol, other CNS depressants. • May cause dry mouth, drowsiness. • Avoid tasks that require alertness, motor skills until response to drug is established. • Difficulty urinating, constipation may occur (inform physician if they persist).

Trileptal, *see oxcarbazepine*

trimethobenzamide

try-meth-oh-**benz**-oh-mide
(Tigan)

CLASSIFICATION

PHARMACOTHERAPEUTIC: Anticholinergic. **CLINICAL:** Antiemetic.

T

ACTION

Acts at chemoreceptor trigger zone in medulla oblongata. **Therapeutic Effect:** Relieves nausea/vomiting.

PHARMACOKINETICS

Route	Onset	Peak	Duration
PO	10–40 min	N/A	3–4 hrs
IM	15–30 min	N/A	2–3 hrs

Partially absorbed from GI tract. Distributed primarily to liver. Metabolic fate unknown. Excreted in urine. **Half-life:** 7–9 hrs.

USES

Control of nausea/vomiting.

PRECAUTIONS

CONTRAINDICATIONS: Hypersensitivity to benzocaine or similar local anesthetics; use of parenteral form in children or suppositories in premature infants, neonates. **CAUTIONS:** Elderly, debilitated, dehydration, serum electrolyte imbalance, high fever.

⌛ LIFESPAN CONSIDERATIONS:

Pregnancy/Lactation: Unknown if drug crosses placenta or is distributed in breast milk. **Pregnancy Category C. Children/Elderly:** No age-related precautions noted. Avoid parenteral form in children and suppositories in neonates.

INTERACTIONS

DRUG: CNS depressants may increase CNS depression. **HERBAL:** None significant. **FOOD:** None known. **LAB VALUES:** None known.

AVAILABILITY (Rx)

CAPSULES (TIGAN): 300 mg. **INJECTION, SOLUTION (TIGAN):** 100 mg/ml.

ADMINISTRATION/HANDLING

IM

- Give deep IM into large muscle mass.

PO

- Give without regard to meals.

INDICATIONS/ROUTES/DOSAGE

◀ ALERT ▶ Do not give by IV route; produces severe hypotension.

NAUSEA AND VOMITING

PO: ADULTS, ELDERLY: 300 mg 3–4 times a day.
IM: ADULTS, ELDERLY: 200 mg 3–4 times a day.

SIDE EFFECTS

FREQUENT: Drowsiness. **OCCASIONAL:** Blurred vision, diarrhea, dizziness, headache, muscle cramps. **RARE:** Rash, seizures, depression, opisthotonos, parkinsonian syndrome, Reye's syndrome (marked by vomiting, seizures).

ADVERSE EFFECTS/ TOXIC REACTIONS

Hypersensitivity reaction manifested as extrapyramidal symptoms (EPS), allergic skin reactions occurs rarely. Children may experience paradoxical reactions (restlessness, insomnia, euphoria, nervousness, tremor). Overdose may vary from CNS depression (sedation, apnea, cardiovascular collapse, death) to severe paradoxical reactions (hallucinations, tremor, seizures).

T

NURSING CONSIDERATIONS

BASELINE ASSESSMENT

Assess for dehydration if excessive vomiting occurs.

INTERVENTION/EVALUATION

Check B/P, esp. in elderly (increased risk of hypotension). Assess children closely for paradoxical reaction. Monitor serum electrolytes in those with severe vomiting. Measure I&O; assess any vomitus. Assess skin turgor, mucous membranes to evaluate hydration status. Assess for EPS (hypersensitivity).

PATIENT/FAMILY TEACHING

• Causes drowsiness. • Avoid tasks that require alertness, motor skills until response to drug is established. • Report visual disturbances, headache. • Relief from nausea/vomiting generally occurs within 30 min of drug administration. • Inform physician if restlessness, involuntary muscle movements occur.

trimethoprim

trye-**meth**-oh-prim

(Apo-Tremethoprim ✱, Primsol, Proloprim, Trimpex)

FIXED-COMBINATION(S)

Bactrim, Septra: trimethoprim/sulfamethoxazole (a sulfonamide): 16 mg/80 mg/ml (injection); 40 mg/200 mg/5 ml (suspension); 80 mg/400 mg; 160 mg/800 mg (tablets).

CLASSIFICATION

PHARMACOTHERAPEUTIC: Folate antagonist. **CLINICAL:** Urinary tract agent, antibacterial.

T

ACTION

Blocks bacterial biosynthesis of nucleic acids, proteins by interfering with metabolism of folinic acid. **Therapeutic Effect:** Bacteriostatic.

PHARMACOKINETICS

Rapidly, completely absorbed from GI tract. Protein binding: 42%–46%. Widely distributed, including to CSF. Metabolized in liver. Primarily excreted in urine. Moderately removed by hemodialysis. **Half-life:** 8–10 hrs (increased in renal impairment, newborns; decreased in children).

USES

Treatment of uncomplicated UTI caused by susceptible strains of *E. coli, P. mirabilis, K. pneumoniae.* Treatment of otitis media due to *H. influenzae, S. pneumoniae.* **OFF-LABEL:** Acute exacerbation of bronchitis in adults, treatment of toxoplasmosis. Treatment of pneumonia cause by *Pneumocystis carinii.*

PRECAUTIONS

CONTRAINDICATIONS: Infants younger than 2 mos, megaloblastic anemia due to folic acid deficiency. **CAUTIONS:** Renal/hepatic impairment, pts with folic acid deficiency.

LIFESPAN CONSIDERATIONS:
Pregnancy/Lactation: Drug readily crosses placenta; is distributed in breast milk. **Pregnancy Category C. Children:** Safety and efficacy not established. **Elderly:** No age-related precautions noted. May increase incidence of thrombocytopenia.

INTERACTIONS

DRUG: Folate antagonists (including methotrexate) may increase risk of megaloblastic anemia. **HERBAL:** None significant. **FOOD:** None known. **LAB VALUES:** May increase BUN, serum bilirubin, creatinine, AST, ALT.

AVAILABILITY (Rx)

ORAL SOLUTION (PRIMSOL): 50 mg/5 ml. **TABLETS (TRIMPEX, PROLOPRIM):** 100 mg, 200 mg.

ADMINISTRATION/HANDLING

PO

• Space doses evenly to maintain constant therapeutic level. • Give without regard to meals (if GI upset occurs, give with food).

INDICATIONS/ROUTES/DOSAGE

UNCOMPLICATED UTI

PO: ADULTS, ELDERLY, CHILDREN 12 YRS AND OLDER: 100 mg q12h or 200 mg once a day for 10 days. **CHILDREN YOUNGER THAN 12 YRS:** 4–6 mg/kg/day in 2 divided doses for 10 days.

OTITIS MEDIA

PO: CHILDREN, 6 MOS AND OLDER: 10 mg/kg/day in divided doses q12h for 10 days.

DOSAGE IN RENAL IMPAIRMENT

Dosage and frequency are modified based on creatinine clearance.

Creatinine Clearance	Dosage Interval
Greater than 30 ml/min	No change
15–30 ml/min	50 mg q12h

SIDE EFFECTS

OCCASIONAL: Nausea, vomiting, diarrhea, decreased appetite, abdominal cramps, headache. **RARE:** Hypersensitivity reaction (pruritus, rash), methemoglobinemia (bluish fingernails, lips, skin; fever; pale skin; sore throat; asthenia [loss of strength, energy]), photosensitivity.

ADVERSE EFFECTS/ TOXIC REACTIONS

Stevens-Johnson syndrome, erythema multiforme, exfoliative dermatitis, anaphylaxis occur rarely. Hematologic toxicity (thrombocytopenia, neutropenia, leukopenia, megaloblastic anemia) more likely to occur in elderly, debilitated, alcoholics, those with renal impairment or receiving prolonged high dosage.

NURSING CONSIDERATIONS

BASELINE ASSESSMENT

Assess hematology baseline reports, serum renal function tests.

INTERVENTION/EVALUATION

Assess skin for rash. Evaluate food tolerance. Monitor serum hematology reports, renal/hepatic function test results. Check for developing signs of hematologic toxicity: pallor, fever, sore throat, malaise, bleeding/bruising.

PATIENT/FAMILY TEACHING

• Space doses evenly. • Complete full length of therapy (10–14 days). • May take on empty stomach or with food if stomach upset occurs. • Avoid sun, ultraviolet light; use sunscreen, wear protective clothing. • Immediately report pallor, fatigue, sore throat, bruising/bleeding, discoloration of skin, fever, rash to physician.

trimetrexate

try-meh-**trex**-ate

(Neutrexin)

Do not confuse Neutrexin with Neurontin.

♦CLASSIFICATION

PHARMACOTHERAPEUTIC: Folate antagonist. **CLINICAL:** Anti-infective.

ACTION

Inhibits the enzyme dihydrofolate reductase (DHFR). **Therapeutic Effect:** Disrupts purine, DNA, RNA, protein synthesis, with consequent cell death.

USES

Alternative therapy with concurrent leucovorin administration for treatment of moderate to severe *Pneumocystis carinii* pneumonia (PCP) in immunocompromised pts, including pts with acquired immunodeficiency syndrome (AIDS), who are intolerant of, or are refractory to, trimethoprim-sulfamethoxazole (TMP-SMZ) therapy or for

T

whom TMP-SMZ is contraindicated. **OFF-LABEL:** Treatment of non–small cell lung, prostate, colorectal cancer, head/neck cancer, pancreatic adenocarcinoma.

PRECAUTIONS

CONTRAINDICATIONS: Clinically significant hypersensitivity to trimetrexate, leucovorin, methotrexate. **CAUTIONS:** Fertility impairment, pts with hematologic, renal, hepatic impairment.

LIFESPAN CONSIDERATIONS:

Pregnancy/Lactation: May be teratogenic, fetotoxic. Unknown if distributed in breast milk. **Pregnancy Category D.** **Children:** Safety and efficacy not established. **Elderly:** No age-related precautions noted.

INTERACTIONS

DRUG: **Zidovudine** may increase myelotoxicity. May increase risk of infection with **live virus vaccines**. **HERBAL:** None significant. **FOOD:** None known. **LAB VALUES:** May increase BUN, alkaline phosphatase, bilirubin, creatinine, AST, ALT. May decrease Hgb, Hct, leukocyte, platelet counts.

AVAILABILITY (Rx)

INJECTION, POWDER FOR RECONSTITUTION: 25 mg, 200 mg.

ADMINISTRATION/HANDLING

IV

◄ **ALERT** ► If solution comes in contact with skin/mucosa, wash with soap/water immediately. Use proper cytotoxic disposal technique. Do not reconstitute with solution containing chloride ion or leucovorin because precipitate occurs instantly.

Reconstitution • Reconstitute each 25-mg vial with 2 ml D_5W or Sterile Water for Injection to provide concentration of 12.5 mg/ml. • Complete dissolution should occur within 30 sec. • Filter reconstituted solution before further dilution. • Further dilute with D_5W to yield final concentration of 0.25–2 mg/ml.

Rate of administration • Give diluted solution by IV infusion over 60–90 min. • Flush IV line thoroughly with at least 10 ml D_5W before and after administering trimetrexate.

Storage • Store vials for parenteral use at room temperature. • After reconstitution, solution is stable for up to 24 hrs. • Reconstituted solution appears as pale greenish yellow. • Discard if solution is cloudy or precipitate forms. • Do not freeze reconstituted solution. Discard unused portion after 24 hrs.

IV INCOMPATIBILITIES

Foscarnet (Foscavir), indomethacin (Indocin).

INDICATIONS/ROUTES/DOSAGE

◄ **ALERT** ► Even though trimetrexate and leucovorin are given concurrently, they must be administered separately or precipitate will occur; flush IV line thoroughly with 10 ml D_5W between infusions. Dilute leucovorin according to leucovorin instructions and give over 5–10 min q6h.

PCP

IV INFUSION: ADULTS: (Trimetrexate): 45 mg/m^2 once a day over 60–90 min for 21 days. **(Leucovorin):** 20 mg/m^2 over 5–10 min q6h for total daily dose of 80 mg/m^2, or orally as 4 doses of 20 mg/m^2 spaced equally throughout the day. Round up oral dose to next higher 25-mg increment. Give daily during treatment and for 72 hrs past last dose of trimetrexate.

◄ **ALERT** ► In event of hematologic, renal, hepatic toxicities, doses of trimetrexate and leucovorin should be modified.

SIDE EFFECTS

OCCASIONAL (8%–2%): Fever, rash, pruritus, nausea, vomiting, confusion. **RARE (less than 2%):** Fatigue.

ADVERSE EFFECTS/ TOXIC REACTIONS

Trimetrexate given without concurrent leucovorin may result in serious or fatal hematologic, hepatic, renal complications, including bone marrow suppression, oral/GI mucosal ulceration, renal/hepatic dysfunction. In event of overdose, stop trimetrexate and give leucovorin 40 mg/m^2 q6h for 3 days. Anaphylaxis occurs rarely.

NURSING CONSIDERATIONS

BASELINE ASSESSMENT

Leucovorin therapy must extend for 72 hrs past last dose of trimetrexate. CBC, serum hepatic/renal function tests should be performed twice a wk during therapy. To allow for full therapeutic effect of trimetrexate to occur, zidovudine treatment should be discontinued during trimetrexate therapy.

INTERVENTION/EVALUATION

Closely monitor neutrophil count, platelet count, serum hepatic/renal function tests for development of serious toxicities. Carefully assess/treat pts with nephrotoxic, myelosuppressive, hepatotoxic drugs given during trimetrexate therapy.

PATIENT/FAMILY TEACHING

• Use two forms of contraception during therapy (Pregnancy Category D). • Avoid persons with infections. • Immediately contact physician if fever, chills, cough, hoarseness, lower back/ side pain, painful urination occurs. • Report unusual bruising/bleeding, black tarry stools, blood in urine/ stools, pinpoint red rash on skin.

triptorelin

trip-toe-**ree**-linn
(Trelstar Depot, Trelstar LA)

CLASSIFICATION

PHARMACOTHERAPEUTIC: Gonadotropin-releasing hormone analogue. **CLINICAL:** Antineoplastic.

ACTION

Through a negative feedback mechanism, inhibits gonadotropin hormone secretion. Circulating levels of luteinizing hormone (LH), follicle-stimulating hormone (FSH), testosterone, estradiol rise initially, then subside with continued therapy. **Therapeutic Effect:** Suppresses growth of abnormal prostate tissue.

USES

Treatment of advanced prostate cancer (alternate to orchiectomy or estrogen administration). **OFF-LABEL:** Treatment of endometriosis, growth hormone deficiency, hyperandrogenism, ovarian, pancreatic carcinomas, precocious puberty, uterine leiomyomata.

PRECAUTIONS

CONTRAINDICATIONS: Hypersensitivity to luteinizing hormone-releasing hormone (LHRH), LHRH agonists, pregnancy. **CAUTIONS:** None known.

LIFESPAN CONSIDERATIONS:

Pregnancy/Lactation: Unknown if distributed is breast milk. **Pregnancy Category X. Children:** Safety and efficacy not established. **Elderly:** No age-related precautions noted.

INTERACTIONS

DRUG: Hyperprolactinemic drugs reduce number of pituitary gonadotropin-releasing hormone (GnRH) receptors. **HERBAL:** None significant. **FOOD:** None

T

known. **LAB VALUES:** May alter serum pituitary-gonadal function test results. May cause transient increase in serum testosterone, usually during first wk of treatment.

AVAILABILITY (Rx)

INJECTION, POWDER FOR RECONSTITUTION (TRELSTAR DEPOT): 3.75 mg. **INJECTION, POWDER FOR RECONSTITUTION (TRELSTAR LA):** 11.25 mg.

INDICATIONS/ROUTES/DOSAGE

PROSTATE CANCER

IM (TRELSTAR DEPOT): ADULTS, ELDERLY: 3.75 mg once q28days.

IM (TRELSTAR LA): ADULTS, ELDERLY: 11.25 mg q84days.

SIDE EFFECTS

FREQUENT (greater than 5%): Hot flashes, skeletal pain, headache, impotence. **OCCASIONAL (5%–2%):** Insomnia, vomiting, leg pain, fatigue. **RARE (less than 2%):** Dizziness, emotional lability, diarrhea, urinary retention, UTI, anemia, pruritus.

ADVERSE EFFECTS/ TOXIC REACTIONS

Bladder outlet obstruction, skeletal pain, hematuria, spinal cord compression with weakness, paralysis of lower extremities may occur.

NURSING CONSIDERATIONS

INTERVENTION/EVALUATION

Obtain serum testosterone, prostate-specific antigen (PSA), prostatic acid phosphatase (PAP) levels periodically during therapy. Serum testosterone, PAP levels should increase during first wk of therapy. Testosterone level then should decrease to baseline level or less within 2 wks, PAP level within 4 wks. Monitor pt closely for worsening signs and symptoms of prostatic cancer, esp. during first wk of therapy (due to transient increase in testosterone).

PATIENT/FAMILY TEACHING

• Do not miss monthly injections. • May experience increased skeletal pain, blood in urine, urinary retention initially (subsides within 1 wk). • Hot flashes may occur. • Inform physician if tachycardia, persistent nausea/vomiting, numbness of arms/legs, pain/swelling of breasts, difficulty breathing, infection at injection site occurs.

Trizivir, *see abacavir and lamivudine and zidovudine*

trospium

trow-spee-um

(Sanctura)

CLASSIFICATION

PHARMACOTHERAPEUTIC: Anticholinergic. **CLINICAL:** Antispasmotic.

ACTION

Antagonizes effect of acetylcholine on muscarinic receptors, producing parasympatholytic action. **Therapeutic Effect:** Reduces smooth muscle tone in bladder.

PHARMACOKINETICS

Minimally absorbed after PO administration. Protein binding: 50%–85%. Distributed in plasma. Excreted mainly in feces and, to lesser extent, in urine. **Half-life:** 20 hrs.

USES

Treatment of overactive bladder with symptoms of urge urinary incontinence, urgency, urinary frequency.

PRECAUTIONS

CONTRAINDICATIONS: Decreased GI motility, gastric retention, uncontrolled angle-closure glaucoma, urinary retention. **CAUTIONS:** Renal/hepatic impairment, obstructive GI disorders, ulcerative colitis, intestinal atony, myasthenia gravis, narrow-angle glaucoma, significant bladder obstruction.

⌛ LIFESPAN CONSIDERATIONS:

Pregnancy/Lactation: Unknown if drug crosses placenta or is distributed in breast milk. **Pregnancy Category C. Children:** Safety and efficacy not established. **Elderly:** Higher incidence of dry mouth, constipation, dyspepsia, UTI, urinary retention in those 75 yrs and older.

INTERACTIONS

DRUG: Other anticholinergic agents increase severity, frequency of side effects, may alter absorption of other drugs due to anticholinergic effects on GI motility. **Digoxin, metformin, morphine, pancuronium, procainamide, tenofovir, vancomycin** may increase concentration. **HERBAL:** None significant. **FOOD: High-fat meals** may reduce absorption. **LAB VALUES:** None known.

AVAILABILITY (Rx)

TABLETS: 20 mg.

ADMINISTRATION/HANDLING

PO

• Store at room temperature. • Give at least 1 hr before meals or on an empty stomach.

INDICATIONS/ROUTES/DOSAGE

OVERACTIVE BLADDER

PO: ADULTS: 20 mg twice a day. **ELDERLY 75 YRS AND OLDER:** Titrate dosage down to 20 mg once a day, based on tolerance.

DOSAGE IN RENAL IMPAIRMENT

For pts with creatinine clearance less than 30 ml/min, dosage reduced to 20 mg once a day at bedtime.

SIDE EFFECTS

FREQUENT (20%): Dry mouth. **OCCASIONAL (10%–4%):** Constipation, headache. **RARE (less than 2%):** Fatigue, upper abdominal pain, dyspepsia (heartburn, indigestion, epigastric pain), flatulence, dry eyes, urinary retention.

ADVERSE EFFECTS/ TOXIC REACTIONS

Overdose may result in severe anticholinergic effects, characterized by nervousness, restlessness, nausea, vomiting, confusion, diaphoresis, facial flushing, hypertension, hypotension, respiratory depression, irritability, lacrimation. Supraventricular tachycardia and hallucinations occur rarely.

NURSING CONSIDERATIONS

BASELINE ASSESSMENT

Assess dysuria, urinary urgency, frequency, incontinence.

INTERVENTION/EVALUATION

Monitor for symptomatic relief. Monitor I&O; palpate bladder for retention. Monitor daily pattern of bowel activity/ stool consistency. Dry mouth may be relieved by sips of tepid water.

PATIENT/FAMILY TEACHING

• Report nausea, vomiting, diaphoresis, increased salivary secretions, palpitations, severe abdominal pain.

T

tubocurarine

(Tubarine)

See Neuromuscular blockers (p. 120C)

Tygacil, *see tigecycline*

Ultracet, *see acetaminphen and tramadol*

Ultram, *see tramadol*

Unasyn, *see ampicillin/ sulbactam sodium*

valacyclovir

val-a-**sye**-kloe-ver
(Valtrex)

CLASSIFICATION

PHARMACOTHERAPEUTIC: Antiviral. **CLINICAL:** Antiherpetic agent (see p. 66C).

ACTION

Converted to acyclovir triphosphate, becoming part of viral DNA chain. **Therapeutic Effect:** Interferes with DNA synthesis, replication of herpes simplex, varicella-zoster virus.

PHARMACOKINETICS

Rapidly absorbed after PO administration. Protein binding: 13%–18%. Rapidly converted by hydrolysis to active compound acyclovir. Widely distributed to tissues, body fluids (including cerebrospinal fluid [CSF]). Primarily eliminated in urine. Removed by hemodialysis. **Half-life:** 2.5–3.3 hrs (increased in renal impairment).

USES

Treatment of herpes zoster (shingles) in immunocompetent adults. Episodic treatment of recurrent genital herpes in immunocompetent adults. Prevention of recurrent genital herpes. Treatment of initial genital herpes. Treatment of cold sores. **OFF-LABEL:** Reduce risk of heterosexual transmission of genital herpes.

PRECAUTIONS

CONTRAINDICATIONS: Hypersensitivity to or intolerance of acyclovir, valacyclovir, or their components. **CAUTIONS:** Bone marrow or renal transplantation, advanced HIV infections, renal/hepatic impairment, dehydration, fluid or electrolyte imbalance, concurrent use of nephrotoxic agents, neurologic abnormalities.

LIFESPAN CONSIDERATIONS:

Pregnancy/Lactation: May cross placenta. May be distributed in breast milk. **Pregnancy Category B. Children:** Safety and efficacy not established. **Elderly:** Age-related renal impairment may require dosage adjustment.

INTERACTIONS

DRUG: Cimetidine, probenecid may increase acyclovir concentration. **HERBAL:** None significant. **FOOD:** None known. **LAB VALUES:** None known.

AVAILABILITY (Rx)

CAPLETS: 500 mg, 1,000 mg.

ADMINISTRATION/HANDLING

PO

• Give without regard to meals. • If GI upset occurs, give with meals.

INDICATIONS/ROUTES/DOSAGE

HERPES ZOSTER (SHINGLES)

PO: ADULTS, ELDERLY: 1 g 3 times a day for 7 days.

HERPES SIMPLEX (COLD SORES)

PO: ADULTS, ELDERLY: 2 g twice a day for 1 day (separate by 12 hrs).

INITIAL EPISODE OF GENITAL HERPES

PO: ADULTS, ELDERLY: 1 g twice a day for 10 days.

RECURRENT EPISODES OF GENITAL HERPES

PO: ADULTS, ELDERLY: 500 mg twice a day for 3 days.

PREVENTION OF GENITAL HERPES

PO: ADULTS, ELDERLY: 500–1,000 mg/day.

DOSAGE IN RENAL IMPAIRMENT

Dosage and frequency are modified based on creatinine clearance.

Creatinine Clearance	Herpes Zoster	Genital Herpes
50 ml/min or higher	1 g q8h	500 mg q12h
30–49 ml/min	1 g q12h	500 mg q12h
10–29 ml/min	1 g q24h	500 mg q24h
Less than 10 ml/min	500 mg q24h	500 mg q24h

SIDE EFFECTS

FREQUENT: Herpes zoster (17%–10%): Nausea, headache. **Genital herpes (17%):** Headache. **OCCASIONAL: Herpes zoster (7%–3%):** Vomiting, diarrhea, constipation (50 yrs and older), asthenia (loss of strength, energy), dizziness (50 yrs and older). **Genital herpes (8%–3%):** Nausea, diarrhea, dizziness. **RARE: Herpes zoster (3%–1%):** Abdominal pain, anorexia. **Genital herpes (3%–1%):** Asthenia (loss of strength, energy), abdominal pain.

ADVERSE EFFECTS/ TOXIC REACTIONS

None known.

NURSING CONSIDERATIONS

BASELINE ASSESSMENT

Question for history of allergies, particularly to valacyclovir, acyclovir. Tissue cultures for herpes zoster, herpes simplex should be done before giving first dose (therapy may proceed before results are known). Assess medical history, esp. advanced HIV infection, bone marrow or renal transplantation, hepatic/renal impairment.

INTERVENTION/EVALUATION

Evaluate cutaneous lesions. Monitor serum renal/hepatic function tests, CBC, urinalysis. Manage herpes zoster with strict isolation. Provide analgesics, comfort measures for herpes zoster (esp. exhausting to elderly). Encourage fluids. Keep pt's fingernails short, hands clean.

PATIENT/FAMILY TEACHING

• Drink adequate fluids. • Do not touch lesions with fingers to avoid spreading infection to new site. • **Genital Herpes:** Continue therapy for full length of treatment. • Space doses evenly. • Avoid sexual intercourse during duration of lesions to prevent infecting partner. • Valacyclovir does not cure herpes. • Notify physician if lesions recur or do not improve. • Pap smears should be done at least annually due to increased risk of cervical cancer in women with genital herpes. • Initiate treatment at first sign of recurrent episode of genital herpes or herpes zoster (early treatment within first 24–48 hrs is imperative for therapeutic results).

valerian

Also known as all-heal, amantilla, garden heliotrope, valeriana.

CLASSIFICATION

HERBAL: See Appendix G.

ACTION

Appears to inhibit enzyme system responsible for catabolism of GABA, increasing GABA concentration, decreasing

CNS activity. **Effect:** Produces sedative effects. Has anxiolytic, antidepressant, anticonvulsant effects.

USES

Used as sedative for insomnia, sleeping disorders associated with anxiety, restlessness. Used for depression, attention deficit hyperactivity disorder (ADHD).

PRECAUTIONS

CONTRAINDICATIONS: Insufficient data on pregnancy or lactation (avoid use); hepatic disease. **CAUTIONS:** None known.

LIFESPAN CONSIDERATIONS:

Pregnancy/Lactation: Contraindicated; unknown if drug crosses placenta or is distributed in breast milk. **Pregnancy Category C.** **Children:** Safety and efficacy not established in those younger than 16 yrs. **Elderly:** Increased risk of motor/cognitive function impairment.

INTERACTIONS

DRUG: **Alcohol, barbiturates, benzodiazepines** may cause additive effect, increase adverse effects. **HERBAL:** **Chamomile, ginseng, kava kava, melatonin, St. John's wort** may enhance therapeutic effect, adverse effects. **FOOD:** None known. **LAB VALUES:** None known.

AVAILABILITY (OTC)

CAPSULES. EXTRACT. TABLETS. TEA. TINCTURE.

INDICATIONS/ROUTES/DOSAGE

SEDATION

PO: **ADULTS, ELDERLY:** **(Extract):** 400–900 mg ½–1 hr before bedtime or 1 cup tea taken several times a day.

SIDE EFFECTS

Headache, hangover, cardiac arrhythmias.

ADVERSE EFFECTS/ TOXIC REACTIONS

Difficulty walking, hypothermia, increased muscle relaxation, excitability, insomnia.

NURSING CONSIDERATIONS

BASELINE ASSESSMENT

Determine whether pt is using other CNS depressants, esp. benzodiazepines. Assess baseline serum hepatic function.

INTERVENTION/EVALUATION

Monitor effectiveness in decreasing insomnia. Assess for hypersensitivity reaction; monitor serum hepatic function tests.

PATIENT/FAMILY TEACHING

• Up to 4 wks may be needed for significant relief. • Avoid tasks that require alertness, motor skills until response to drug is established. • Inform physician if pregnant or breast-feeding. • Taper doses slowly; do not discontinue abruptly.

valganciclovir

val-gan-**sye**-kloh-veer
(Valcyte)

CLASSIFICATION

PHARMACOTHERAPEUTIC: Synthetic nucleoside. **CLINICAL:** Antiviral (see p. 66C).

ACTION

Competes with viral DNA esterases, is incorporated directly into growing viral DNA chains. **Therapeutic Effect:** Interferes with DNA synthesis, viral replication.

PHARMACOKINETICS

Well absorbed, rapidly converted to ganciclovir by intestinal, hepatic enzymes. Widely distributed. Slowly metabolized intracellularly. Primarily excreted unchanged in urine. Removed by hemodialysis. **Half-life:** 18 hrs (increased in renal impairment).

USES

Treatment of cytomegalovirus (CMV) retinitis in AIDS. Preventative treatment of CMV disease in high-risk, renal, cardiac transplant pts.

PRECAUTIONS

CONTRAINDICATIONS: Hypersensitivity to acyclovir, ganciclovir. **CAUTIONS:** Extreme caution in children because of long-term carcinogenicity, reproductive toxicity. Renal impairment, preexisting cytopenias, history of cytopenic reactions to other drugs; elderly (at greater risk for renal impairment).

⌛ LIFESPAN CONSIDERATIONS:

Pregnancy/Lactation: Effective contraception should be used during therapy; valganciclovir should not be used during pregnancy. Avoid breast-feeding during therapy; may be resumed no sooner than 72 hrs after last dose of valganciclovir. **Pregnancy Category C. Children:** Safety and efficacy not established in those younger than 12 yrs. **Elderly:** Age-related renal impairment may require dosage adjustment.

INTERACTIONS

DRUG: Bone marrow depressants may increase myelosuppression. May increase risk of toxicity of **didanosine, mycophenolate. Probenecid** decreases renal clearance. **Zidovudine (AZT)** may increase risk of hematologic toxicity. **HERBAL:** None significant. **FOOD: All foods** maximize drug bioavailability. **LAB VALUES:** May decrease Hgb, Hct, serum creatinine, platelet count, WBC count.

AVAILABILITY (Rx)

TABLETS: 450 mg.

ADMINISTRATION/HANDLING

PO

• Do not break, crush tablets (potential carcinogen). • Avoid contact to skin. • Wash skin with soap, water if contact occurs. • Give with food.

INDICATIONS/ROUTES/DOSAGE

CYTOMEGALOVIRUS (CMV) RETINITIS

PO: ADULTS: Initially, 900 mg (two 450-mg tablets) twice a day for 21 days. Maintenance: 900 mg once a day.

PREVENTION OF CMV AFTER TRANSPLANT

PO: ADULTS, ELDERLY: 900 mg once a day beginning within 10 days of transplant and continuing until 100 days post-transplant.

DOSAGE IN RENAL IMPAIRMENT

Dosage and frequency are modified based on creatinine clearance.

Creatinine Clearance	Induction Dosage	Maintenance Dosage
60 ml/min or higher	900 mg twice a day	900 mg once a day
40–59 ml/min	450 mg twice a day	450 mg once a day
25–39 ml/min	450 mg once a day	450 mg every 2 days
10–24 ml/min	450 mg every 2 days	450 mg twice a wk

SIDE EFFECTS

FREQUENT (16%–9%): Diarrhea, neutropenia, headache. **OCCASIONAL (8%–3%):** Nausea, anemia, thrombocytopenia. **RARE (less than 3%):** Insomnia, paresthesia, vomiting, abdominal pain, fever.

ADVERSE EFFECTS/ TOXIC REACTIONS

Hematologic toxicity, including severe neutropenia (most common), anemia,

V

thrombocytopenia may occur. Retinal detachment occurs rarely. Overdose may result in renal toxicity. May decrease sperm production, fertility.

NURSING CONSIDERATIONS

BASELINE ASSESSMENT

Evaluate hematologic, serum chemistry baselines, serum creatinine.

INTERVENTION/EVALUATION

Monitor I&O, ensure adequate hydration (minimum 1,500 ml/24 hrs). Diligently evaluate CBC for decreased WBCs, Hgb, Hct, decreased platelets. Question pt regarding vision, therapeutic improvement, complications.

PATIENT/FAMILY TEACHING

• Valganciclovir provides suppression, not cure, of CMV retinitis. • Frequent blood tests are necessary during therapy because of toxic nature of drug. • Ophthalmologic exam q4–6wk during treatment is advised. • Report any new symptom promptly. • May temporarily or permanently inhibit sperm production in men, suppress fertility in women. • Barrier contraception should be used during and for 90 days after therapy because of mutagenic potential.

valproic acid

val-**pro**-ick
(Depakene)

valproate sodium

(Depakene syrup)

divalproex sodium

(Apo-Divalproex ✤, Depacon, Depakote, Depakote ER, Depakote Sprinkle, Novo-Divalproex ✤)

CLASSIFICATION

CLINICAL: Anticonvulsant, antimanic, antimigraine (see p. 35C).

ACTION

Directly increases concentration of inhibitory neurotransmitter gamma-aminobutyric acid (GABA). **Therapeutic Effect:** Produces anticonvulsant effect.

PHARMACOKINETICS

Well absorbed from GI tract. Protein binding: 80%–90%. Metabolized in liver. Primarily excreted in urine. Not removed by hemodialysis. **Half-life:** 6–16 hrs (may be increased in hepatic impairment, elderly, children younger than 18 mos).

USES

Prophylaxis of absence seizures (petit mal), myoclonic, tonic-clonic seizure control. Used principally as adjunct with other anticonvulsant agents. Treatment of manic episodes with bipolar disorders, complex partial seizures. Prophylaxis of migraine headaches. **OFF-LABEL:** Prevention of migraine; treatment of behavior disorders in Alzheimer's disease; bipolar disorder; chorea, myoclonic, simple partial, tonic-clonic seizures; organic brain syndrome; schizophrenia; status epilepticus; tardive dyskinesia.

PRECAUTIONS

CONTRAINDICATIONS: Active hepatic disease, urea cycle disorders. **CAUTIONS:** History of hepatic disease, bleeding abnormalities.

LIFESPAN CONSIDERATIONS:

Pregnancy/Lactation: Drug crosses placenta; is distributed in breast milk. **Pregnancy Category D. Children:** Increased risk of hepatotoxicity in those younger than 2 yrs. **Elderly:** No age-related precautions, but lower dosages recommended.

INTERACTIONS

DRUG: Alcohol, other CNS depressants may increase CNS depressant effects. May increase concentration of **amitriptyline, primidone. Anticoagulants, heparin, platelet aggregation inhibitors, thrombolytics** may increase risk of bleeding. **Carbamazepine** may decrease concentration. **Hepatotoxic medications** may increase risk of hepatotoxicity. May increase risk of dermatologic reaction with **lamotrigine.** May increase risk of **phenytoin** toxicity, decrease effects. **HERBAL: Evening primrose** may decrease seizure threshold. **FOOD:** None known. **LAB VALUES:** May increase serum LDH, bilirubin, AST, ALT. Therapeutic serum level: 50–100 mcg/ml; toxic serum level: greater than 100 mcg/ml.

AVAILABILITY (Rx)

CAPSULES (DEPAKENE): 250 mg. **CAPSULES, SPRINKLE (DEPAKOTE SPRINKLE):** 125 mg. **INJECTION, SOLUTION (DEPACON):** 100 mg/ml. **SYRUP (DEPAKENE):** 250 mg/5 ml.

TABLET, DELAYED-RELEASE (DEPAKOTE): 125 mg, 250 mg, 500 mg. **TABLET, EXTENDED-RELEASE (DEPAKOTE ER):** 250 mg, 500 mg.

ADMINISTRATION/HANDLING

IV

Reconstitution • Dilute each single dose with at least 50 ml D_5W, 0.9% NaCl, or lactated Ringer's.

Rate of administration • Infuse over 5–10 min. • Do not exceed rate of 3 mg/kg/min (5-min infusion) or 1.5 mg/kg/min (10-min infusion). Too-rapid infusion increases side effects.

Storage • Store vials at room temperature. • Diluted solutions stable for 24 hrs. • Discard unused portion.

PO

• May give without regard to food. Do not administer with carbonated drinks. • May sprinkle capsule contents on applesauce and give immediately (do not break, crush sprinkle beads). • Give delayed-release/extended-release tablets whole.

IV INCOMPATIBILITIES

Do not mix with any other medications.

INDICATIONS/ROUTES/DOSAGE

SEIZURES

PO: ADULTS, ELDERLY, CHILDREN 10 YRS AND OLDER: Initially, 10–15 mg/kg/day in 1–3 divided doses. May increase by 5–10 mg/kg/day at weekly intervals up to 30–60 mg/kg/day. Usual adult dosage: 1,000–2,500 mg/day.

IV: ADULTS, ELDERLY, CHILDREN: Same as oral dose but given q6h.

MANIC EPISODES

PO: ADULTS, ELDERLY: Initially, 750–1,500 mg/day in divided doses. **Maximum:** 60 mg/kg/day.

PO (EXTENDED-RELEASE): Initially, 25 mg/kg/day once daily. **Maximum:** 60 mg/kg/day.

PREVENTION OF MIGRAINE HEADACHES

PO (EXTENDED-RELEASE): ADULTS, ELDERLY: Initially, 500 mg/day for 7 days. May increase up to 1,000 mg/day.

PO (DELAYED-RELEASE): ADULTS, ELDERLY: Initially, 250 mg twice a day. May increase up to 1,000 mg/day.

SIDE EFFECTS

FREQUENT: Epilepsy: Abdominal pain, irregular menses, diarrhea, transient alopecia, indigestion, nausea, vomiting, tremors, fluctuations in body weight. **Mania (22%–19%):** Nausea, somnolence. **OCCASIONAL: Epilepsy:** Constipation, dizziness, drowsiness, headache,

V

skin rash, unusual excitement, restlessness. **Mania (12%–6%):** Asthenia (loss of strength, energy), abdominal pain, dyspepsia (heartburn, indigestion, epigastric distress), rash. **RARE: Epilepsy:** Mood changes, diplopia, nystagmus, spots before eyes, unusual bleeding/bruising.

ADVERSE EFFECTS/ TOXIC REACTIONS

Hepatotoxicity may occur, particularly in first 6 mos of therapy. May be preceded by loss of seizure control, malaise, weakness, lethargy, anorexia, vomiting rather than abnormal serum hepatic function test results. Blood dyscrasias may occur.

NURSING CONSIDERATIONS

BASELINE ASSESSMENT

Anticonvulsant: Review history of seizure disorder (intensity, frequency, duration, level of consciousness [LOC]). Initiate safety measures, quiet dark environment. CBC, platelet count should be performed before and 2 wks after therapy begins, then 2 wks following maintenance dose. **Antimanic:** Assess behavior, appearance, emotional status, response to environment, speech pattern, thought content. **Antimigraine:** Question pt regarding onset, location, duration of migraine, possible precipitating symptoms.

INTERVENTION/EVALUATION

Monitor serum hepatic function tests, bilirubin, ammonia, CBC, platelets. **Anticonvulsant:** Observe frequently for recurrence of seizure activity. Monitor serum hepatic function tests, CBC, platelet count. Assess skin for ecchymoses, petechiae. Monitor for clinical improvement (decrease in intensity/frequency of seizures). **Antimanic:** Assess for therapeutic response (interest in surroundings, increased ability to concentrate, relaxed facial expression). **Antimigraine:** Evaluate for relief of migraine headache and resulting photophobia, phonophobia, nausea, vomiting. Therapeutic serum level: 50–100 mcg/ml; toxic serum level: greater than 100 mcg/ml.

PATIENT/FAMILY TEACHING

• Do not abruptly withdraw medication after long-term use (may precipitate seizures). • Strict maintenance of drug therapy is essential for seizure control. • Drowsiness usually disappears during continued therapy. • Avoid tasks that require alertness, motor skills until response to drug is established. • Avoid alcohol. • Carry identification card, bracelet that notes anticonvulsant therapy. • Inform physician if nausea, vomiting, lethargy, altered mental status, weakness, loss of appetite, abdominal pain, yellowing of skin, unusual bruising/bleeding occurs.

valsartan

val-**sar**-tan

(Diovan, Diovan HCT)

Do not confuse valsartan with Valstan.

FIXED-COMBINATION(S)

Diovan HCT: valsartan/hydrochlorothiazide (a diuretic): 80 mg/12.5 mg; 160 mg/12.5 mg; 160 mg/25 mg, 320 mg/12.5 mg; 320 mg/25 mg. **Exforge:** valsartan/amlodipine (a calcium channel blocker): 160 mg/5 mg; 160 mg/10 mg; 320 mg/5 mg; 320 mg/10 mg.

CLASSIFICATION

PHARMACOTHERAPEUTIC: Angiotensin II receptor antagonist. **CLINICAL:** Antihypertensive (see p. 8C).

ACTION

Potent vasodilator. Blocks vasoconstrictor, aldosterone-secreting effects of angiotensin II, inhibiting binding of angiotensin II to AT_1 receptors. **Therapeutic Effect:** Produces vasodilation, decreases peripheral resistance, decreases B/P.

PHARMACOKINETICS

Poorly absorbed after PO administration. Food decreases peak plasma concentration. Protein binding: 95%. Metabolized in liver. Recovered primarily in feces and, to lesser extent, in urine. Unknown if removed by hemodialysis. **Half-life:** 6 hrs.

USES

Treatment of hypertension alone or in combination with other antihypertensives. Treatment of heart failure. Reduce mortality in high-risk pts (left ventricular failure/dysfunction) following myocardial infarction (MI). **OFF-LABEL:** Diabetic nephropathy.

PRECAUTIONS

CONTRAINDICATIONS: Bilateral renal artery stenosis, biliary cirrhosis/obstruction, hypoaldosteronism, severe hepatic impairment. **CAUTIONS:** Concurrent use of potassium-sparing diuretics or potassium supplements, mild to moderate hepatic impairment, CHF, unilateral renal artery stenosis, coronary artery disease.

LIFESPAN CONSIDERATIONS:

Pregnancy/Lactation: May cause fetal harm. Unknown if distributed in breast milk. **Pregnancy Category C (D if used in second or third trimester). Children:** Safety and efficacy not established. **Elderly:** No age-related precautions noted.

INTERACTIONS

DRUG: ACE inhibitors, beta-blockers may worsen CHF. **Potassium-sparing drugs, potassium supplements** may increase serum potassium. **Diuretics** produce additive hypotensive effects. **HERBAL:** None significant. **FOOD:** None significant. **LAB VALUES:** May increase AST, ALT, serum bilirubin, creatinine, potassium. May decrease Hgb, Hct.

AVAILABILITY (Rx)

TABLETS: 40 mg, 80 mg, 160 mg, 320 mg.

ADMINISTRATION/HANDLING

PO

- Give without regard to meals.

INDICATIONS/ROUTES/DOSAGE

HYPERTENSION

PO: ADULTS, ELDERLY: Initially, 80–160 mg/day in pts who are not volume depleted. **Maximum:** 320 mg/day.

CHF

PO: ADULTS, ELDERLY: Initially, 40 mg twice a day. May increase up to 160 mg twice a day. **Maximum:** 320 mg/day.

POST-MI

PO: ADULTS, ELDERLY: May initiate 12 hrs or longer following MI. Initially, 20 mg twice a day. May increase within 7 days to 40 mg twice a day. May further increase up to target dose of 160 mg twice a day.

SIDE EFFECTS

RARE (2%–1%): Insomnia, fatigue, heartburn, abdominal pain, dizziness, headache, diarrhea, nausea, vomiting, arthralgia, edema.

ADVERSE EFFECTS/ TOXIC REACTIONS

Overdosage may manifest as hypotension, tachycardia. Bradycardia occurs less often. Viral infection, upper respiratory tract infection (cough, pharyngitis, sinusitis, rhinitis) occur rarely.

NURSING CONSIDERATIONS

BASELINE ASSESSMENT

Obtain B/P, apical pulse immediately before each dose, in addition to regular monitoring (be alert to fluctuations). If excessive reduction in B/P occurs, place pt in supine position, feet slightly elevated. Question for possibility of pregnancy. Assess medication history (esp. diuretic). Question for history of hepatic/renal impairment, renal artery stenosis, history of severe CHF. Obtain BUN, AST, ALT, serum creatinine, alkaline phosphatase, bilirubin, Hgb, Hct.

INTERVENTION/EVALUATION

Maintain hydration (offer fluids frequently). Assess for evidence of upper respiratory infection. Monitor serum electrolytes, renal/hepatic function tests, urinalysis, B/P, pulse. Observe for symptoms of hypotension.

PATIENT/FAMILY TEACHING

• Inform female pt regarding consequences of second-, third-trimester exposure to valsartan. • Report pregnancy to physician as soon as possible. • Report any sign of infection (sore throat, fever). • Do not stop taking medication. • Caution against exercising during hot weather (risk of dehydration, hypotension).

Valtrex, *see valacyclovir*

Vancocin, *see vancomycin*

vancomycin

van-koe-**mye**-sin

(Vancocin)

CLASSIFICATION

CLINICAL: Tricyclic glycopeptide antibiotic.

ACTION

Binds to bacterial cell walls, altering cell membrane permeability, inhibiting RNA synthesis. **Therapeutic Effect:** Bactericidal.

PHARMACOKINETICS

PO: Poorly absorbed from GI tract. Primarily eliminated in feces. **Parenteral:** Widely distributed. Protein binding: 55%. Primarily excreted unchanged in urine. Not removed by hemodialysis. **Half-life:** 4–11 hrs (increased in renal impairment).

USES

Systemic: Treatment of infections caused by staphylococcal, streptococcal species. **PO:** Treatment of antibiotic colitis, pseudomembranous colitis, antibiotic-associated diarrhea, staphylococcal enterocolitis. **OFF-LABEL:** Treatment of brain abscess, perioperative infections, staphylococcal, streptococcal meningitis.

PRECAUTIONS

CONTRAINDICATIONS: None known. **CAUTIONS:** Renal dysfunction, preexisting hearing impairment, concurrent therapy with other ototoxic, nephrotoxic medications.

LIFESPAN CONSIDERATIONS:

Pregnancy/Lactation: Drug crosses placenta. Unknown if distributed in breast milk. **Pregnancy Category C.** **Children:** Close monitoring of serum levels recommended in premature neonates and young infants. **Elderly:** Age-related renal impairment may increase risk of ototoxicity, nephrotoxicity; dosage adjustment recommended.

INTERACTIONS

DRUG: **Aminoglycosides, amphotericin B, aspirin, bumetanide, carmustine, cisplatin, cyclosporine, ethacrynic acid, furosemide, streptozocin** may increase risk of ototoxicity, nephrotoxicity of parenteral vancomycin. **Cholestyramine, colestipol** may decrease effects of oral vancomycin. **HERBAL:** None significant. **FOOD:** None known. **LAB VALUES:** May increase BUN. Therapeutic peak serum level: 20–40 mcg/ml; therapeutic trough serum level: 5–15 mcg/ml. Toxic peak serum level: greater than 40 mcg/ml; toxic trough serum level: greater than 15 mcg/ml.

AVAILABILITY (Rx)

CAPSULES (VANCOCIN): 125 mg, 250 mg. **INFUSION (PREMIX [VANCOCIN HCl]):** 500 mg/100 ml, 1 g/200 ml. **INJECTION, POWDER FOR RECONSTITUTION (VANCOCIN HCl):** 500 mg, 1 g.

ADMINISTRATION/HANDLING

IV

◀ **ALERT** ▶ Give by intermittent IV infusion (piggyback), or continuous IV infusion. Do not give IV push (may result in exaggerated hypotension).

Reconstitution • For intermittent IV infusion (piggyback), reconstitute each 500-mg vial with 10 ml Sterile Water for Injection (20 ml for 1-g vial) to provide concentration of 50 mg/ml. • Further dilute to final concentration not to exceed 5 mg/ml.

Rate of administration • Administer over 60 min or longer. • Monitor B/P closely during IV infusion. • ADD-Vantage vials should not be used in neonates, infants, children requiring less than 500-mg dose.

Storage • After reconstitution, refrigerate and use within 14 days. • Discard if precipitate forms.

PO

• Generally not given for systemic infections because of poor absorption from GI tract; however, some pts with colitis may have effective absorption. • Oral solution is stable for 2 wks if refrigerated.

IV INCOMPATIBILITIES

Albumin, amphotericin B complex (Abelcet, AmBisome, Amphotec), aztreonam (Azactam), cefazolin (Ancef), cefepime (Maxipime), cefotaxime (Claforan), cefotetan (Cefotan), cefoxitin (Mefoxin), ceftazidime (Fortaz), ceftriaxone (Rocephin), cefuroxime (Zinacef), foscarnet (Foscavir), heparin, idarubicin (Idamycin), nafcillin (Nafcil), piperacillin and tazobactam (Zosyn), ticarcillin and clavulanate (Timentin).

IV COMPATIBILITIES

Amiodarone (Cordarone), calcium gluconate, diltiazem (Cardizem), hydromorphone (Dilaudid), insulin, lipids, lorazepam (Ativan), magnesium sulfate, midazolam (Versed), morphine, potassium chloride, propofol (Diprivan), total parenteral nutrition (TPN).

INDICATIONS/ROUTES/DOSAGE

USUAL PARENTERAL DOSAGE

IV: ADULTS, ELDERLY: 500 mg q6h or 1 g q12h. **CHILDREN OLDER THAN 1 MO:** 40 mg/kg/day in divided doses q6–8h. **Maximum:** 3–4 g/day. **NEONATES:** Initially, 15 mg/kg, then 10 mg/kg q8–12h.

STAPHYLOCOCCAL ENTEROCOLITIS, ANTIBIOTIC-ASSOCIATED PSEUDOMEMBRANOUS COLITIS CAUSED BY *CLOSTRIDIUM DIFFICILE*

PO: ADULTS, ELDERLY: 0.5–2 g/day in 3–4 divided doses for 7–10 days. **CHILDREN:** 40 mg/kg/day in 3–4 divided doses for 7–10 days. **Maximum:** 2 g/day.

DOSAGE IN RENAL IMPAIRMENT

After loading dose, subsequent dosages and frequency are modified based on creatinine clearance, severity of infection, and serum concentration of drug.

V

SIDE EFFECTS

FREQUENT: PO: Bitter/unpleasant taste, nausea, vomiting, mouth irritation (with oral solution). **RARE: Parenteral:** Phlebitis, thrombophlebitis, pain at peripheral IV site; dizziness; vertigo; tinnitus; chills; fever; rash; necrosis with extravasation. **PO:** Rash.

ADVERSE EFFECTS/ TOXIC REACTIONS

Nephrotoxicity (change in amount/ frequency of urination, nausea, vomiting, increased thirst, anorexia), ototoxicity (temporary or permanent hearing loss) may occur. "Red man syndrome" (RMS), aka, "red neck syndrome," is common adverse reaction characterized by pruritus, urticaria, erythema, angioedema, tachycardia, hypotension, myalgia, maculopapular rash (usually appears on face, neck, upper torso). Cardiovascular toxicity (cardiac depression, arrest) occurs rarely. Onset of RMS usually occurs within 30 min of start of infusion, resolves within hrs following infusion. May result from too-rapid rate of infusion.

NURSING CONSIDERATIONS

BASELINE ASSESSMENT

Avoid other ototoxic, nephrotoxic medications if possible. Obtain culture, sensitivity test before giving first dose (therapy may begin before results are known).

INTERVENTION/EVALUATION

Monitor serum renal function tests, I&O. Assess skin for rash. Check hearing acuity, balance. Monitor B/P carefully during infusion. Evaluate IV site for phlebitis (heat, pain, red streaking over vein). Therapeutic serum level: peak: 20–40 mcg/ml; trough: 5–15 mcg/ml. Toxic serum level: peak: greater than 40 mcg/ml; trough: greater than 15 mcg/ml.

PATIENT/FAMILY TEACHING

• Continue therapy for full length of treatment. • Doses should be evenly spaced. • Notify physician in event of tinnitus, rash, signs/symptoms of nephrotoxicity. • Lab tests are important part of total therapy.

vardenafil

var-**den**-ah-fill

(Levitra)

Do not confuse Levitra with Lexiva.

CLASSIFICATION

PHARMACOTHERAPEUTIC: Phosphodiesterase inhibitor. **CLINICAL:** Erectile dysfunction adjunct.

ACTION

Inhibits phosphodiesterase type 5, the enzyme responsible for degrading cyclic guanosine monophosphate in corpus cavernosum of penis, resulting in smooth muscle relaxation, increased blood flow. **Therapeutic Effect:** Facilitates erection.

PHARMACOKINETICS

Rapidly absorbed after PO administration. Extensive tissue distribution. Protein binding: 95%. Metabolized in liver. Excreted primarily in feces, with lesser amount eliminated in urine. Drug has no effect on penile blood flow without sexual stimulation. **Half-life:** 4–5 hrs.

USES

Treatment of erectile dysfunction.

PRECAUTIONS

CONTRAINDICATIONS: Concurrent use of alpha-adrenergic blockers, sodium nitroprusside, nitrates in any form.

CAUTIONS: Renal/hepatic impairment, anatomical deformation of penis, pts who may be predisposed to priapism (sickle cell anemia, multiple myeloma, leukemia).

LIFESPAN CONSIDERATIONS:

Pregnancy/Lactation: Vardenafil is not indicated for use in women, newborns. **Pregnancy Category B. Children:** Vardenafil is not indicated for use in children. **Elderly:** No age-related precautions noted, but initial dose should be 5 mg.

INTERACTIONS

DRUG: **Alpha-adrenergic blockers (e.g., alfuzosin, doxazosin, prazosin, tamsulosin, terazosin), nitrates** may significantly lower B/P. **Erythromycin, indinavir, itraconazole, ketoconazole, ritonavir** may increase concentration. **HERBAL:** None significant. **FOOD:** **High-fat meals** delay maximum effectiveness. **LAB VALUES:** None known.

AVAILABILITY (Rx)

TABLETS: 2.5 mg, 5 mg, 10 mg, 20 mg.

ADMINISTRATION/HANDLING

PO

- May take approximately 1 hr before sexual activity.

INDICATIONS/ROUTES/DOSAGE

ERECTILE DYSFUNCTION

PO: ADULTS: 10 mg approximately 1 hr before sexual activity. Dose may be increased to 20 mg or decreased to 5 mg, based on pt tolerance. Maximum dosing frequency is once daily. **ELDERLY, OLDER THAN 65 YRS:** 5 mg.

DOSAGE IN MODERATE HEPATIC IMPAIRMENT

PO: For pts with Child-Pugh class B hepatic impairment, dosage is 5 mg 60 min before sexual activity.

DOSAGE WITH CONCURRENT RITONAVIR

PO: ADULTS: 2.5 mg in 72-hr period.

DOSAGE WITH CONCURRENT KETOCONAZOLE, ITRACONAZOLE (AT 400 MG/DAY), INDINAVIR

PO: ADULTS: 2.5 mg in 24-hr period.

DOSAGE WITH CONCURRENT KETOCONAZOLE, ITRACONAZOLE (AT 200 MG/DAY), ERYTHROMYCIN

PO: ADULTS: 5 mg in 24-hr period.

SIDE EFFECTS

OCCASIONAL: Headache, flushing, rhinitis, indigestion. **RARE (less than 2%):** Dizziness, changes in color vision, blurred vision.

ADVERSE EFFECTS/ TOXIC REACTIONS

Prolonged erections (lasting over 4 hrs), priapism (painful erections lasting over 6 hrs) occur rarely.

NURSING CONSIDERATIONS

BASELINE ASSESSMENT

Assess cardiovascular status, medication history (esp. alpha-adrenergic blockers, nitrates) before initiating treatment for erectile dysfunction.

PATIENT/FAMILY TEACHING

• Has no effect in absence of sexual stimulation. • Seek treatment immediately if erection persists for over 4 hrs.

varenicline

vah-**ren**-neh-clean

(Chantix)

CLASSIFICATION

PHARMACOTHERAPEUTIC: Selective partial agonist nicotine acetylcholine receptors. **CLINICAL:** Smoking deterrent.

V

ACTION

Binds to acetylcholine receptors, producing agonist activity, preventing nicotine binding to specific receptors. Blocks ability of nicotine to stimulate central dopamine system, believed to be mechanism underlying reinforcement/reward experienced with smoking.

PHARMACOKINETICS

Completely absorbed following PO administration. Absorption unaffected by food, time of day dosing. Maximum plasma concentration: 3–4 hrs; steady-state condition: within 4 days. Protein binding: 20%. Minimal metabolism. Removed by hemodialysis. Primarily excreted unchanged in urine. **Half-life:** 24 hrs.

USES

Aid to smoking cessation treatment.

PRECAUTIONS

CONTRAINDICATIONS: None known. **CAUTIONS:** Renal impairment.

⌛ LIFESPAN CONSIDERATIONS:

Pregnancy/Lactation: Unknown if distributed in breast milk. **Pregnancy Category B. Children:** Not recommended. **Elderly:** Age-related renal impairment may require dose selection.

INTERACTIONS

DRUG: None significant. **HERBAL:** None significant. **FOOD:** None known. **LAB VALUES:** None known.

AVAILABILITY (OTC)

TABLETS (FILM-COATED): 0.5 mg, 1 mg.

ADMINISTRATION/HANDLING

• Give after eating, with full glass of water. • Do not crush, chew, break film-coated tablets.

INDICATIONS/ROUTES/DOSAGE

◄ **ALERT** ► Therapy should start 1 wk before stopping smoking.

SMOKING DETERRENT

PO: ADULTS, ELDERLY: Day 1–3: 0.5 mg once daily. Day 4–7: 0.5 mg twice daily. Day 8–end of treatment: 1 mg twice daily. Therapy should last for 12 wks. Those who have successfully stopped smoking at the end of 12 wks should continue with an additional 12 wks of treatment to increase likelihood of long-term abstinence.

Severe renal impairment: 0.5 mg once daily. **Maximum:** 0.5 mg twice daily. **End-stage renal disease, undergoing hemodialysis:** **Maximum:** 0.5 mg once only.

SIDE EFFECTS

FREQUENT: Nausea (30%), insomnia (18%), headache (15%), abnormal dreams (13%). **OCCASIONAL (8%–5%):** Constipation, abdominal discomfort, fatigue, dry mouth, flatulence, altered taste, dyspepsia (heartburn, indigestion, epigastric pain), vomiting. **RARE (3%–1%):** Drowsiness, rash, increased appetite, lethargy, nightmares, gastroesophageal reflux disease, dyspnea, rhinorrhea.

ADVERSE EFFECTS/ TOXIC REACTIONS

Hypertension, angina pectoris, arrhythmia, bradycardia, coronary artery disease, gingivitis, anemia, lymphadenopathy occur rarely. Abrupt withdrawal may cause irritability, sleep disturbances in 3% of pts.

NURSING CONSIDERATIONS

BASELINE ASSESSMENT

Screen, evaluate those with coronary heart disease (history of MI, angina pectoris), serious cardiac arrhythmias.

INTERVENTION/EVALUATION

Discontinue use if increase in cardiovascular symptoms occurs.

PATIENT/FAMILY TEACHING

Initiate treatment one wk before quit smoking date. Take after eating and with full glass of water. With twice-daily dosing, take one tablet in morning, one in evening. Contact physician if nausea/insomnia persists.

vasopressin

vay-soe-**press**-in

(Pitressin, Pressyn ✦, Pressyn AR ✦)

Do not confuse Pitressin with Pitocin.

CLASSIFICATION

PHARMACOTHERAPEUTIC: Posterior pituitary hormone. **CLINICAL:** Vasopressor, antidiuretic.

ACTION

Increases reabsorption of water by renal tubules. Directly stimulates smooth muscle in GI tract. **Therapeutic Effect:** Causes peristalsis, vasoconstriction.

PHARMACOKINETICS

Route	Onset	Peak	Duration
IV	N/A	N/A	0.5–1 hr
IM, Subcutaneous	1–2 hrs	N/A	2–8 hrs

Distributed throughout extracellular fluid. Metabolized in liver, kidney. Primarily excreted in urine. **Half-life:** 10–20 min.

USES

Treatment of adult shock-refractory ventricular fibrillation (class IIb). Prevention/control of polydipsia, polyuria, dehydration in pts with neurogenic diabetes insipidus. Stimulates peristalsis in prevention/treatment of postop abdominal distention, intestinal paresis. Treatment of vasodilatory shock with hypotension unresponsive to fluids, catecholamines. **OFF-LABEL:** Adjunct in treatment of acute, massive hemorrhage.

PRECAUTIONS

CONTRAINDICATIONS: None known. **CAUTIONS:** Seizures, migraine, asthma, vascular disease, renal/cardiac disease, goiter (with cardiac complications), arteriosclerosis, nephritis.

LIFESPAN CONSIDERATIONS:

Pregnancy/Lactation: Caution in giving to breast-feeding women. **Pregnancy Category C. Children/Elderly:** Caution due to risk of water intoxication/hyponatremia.

INTERACTIONS

DRUG: **Alcohol, demeclocycline, lithium, norepinephrine** may decrease antidiuretic effect. **Carbamazepine, chlorpropamide, clofibrate** may increase antidiuretic effect. **HERBAL:** None significant. **FOOD:** None known. **LAB VALUES:** None known.

AVAILABILITY (Rx)

INJECTION SOLUTION: 20 units/ml.

ADMINISTRATION/HANDLING

IV

Reconstitution • Dilute with D_5W or 0.9% NaCl to concentration of 0.1–1 unit/ml.

Rate of administration • Give as IV infusion.

Storage • Store at room temperature.

IM, SUBCUTANEOUS

• Give with 1–2 glasses of water to reduce side effects.

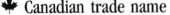

IV INCOMPATIBILITIES

Amphotericin B complex (Abelcet, AmBisome, Amphotec), diazepam (Valium), etomidate (Amidate), furosemide (Lasix), thiopentothal.

IV COMPATIBILITIES

Dobutamine (Dobutrex), dopamine (Intropin), heparin, lorazepam (Ativan), midazolam (Versed), milrinone (Primacor), verapamil (Calan, Isoptin).

INDICATIONS/ROUTES/DOSAGE

CARDIAC ARREST

IV: ADULTS, ELDERLY: 40 units as one-time bolus.

DIABETES INSIPIDUS

◀ **ALERT** ▶ May be administered intranasally by nasal spray or on cotton pledgets; dosage is individualized.

IV INFUSION: ADULTS, CHILDREN: 0.5 milliunits/kg/hr. May double dose q30min. **Maximum:** 10 milliunits/kg/hr. **IM, SUBCUTANEOUS: ADULTS, ELDERLY:** 5–10 units 2–4 times a day. Range: 5–60 units/day. **CHILDREN:** 2.5–10 units, 2–4 times a day.

ABDOMINAL DISTENTION, INTESTINAL PARESIS

IM: ADULTS, ELDERLY: Initially, 5 units. Subsequent doses, 10 units q3–4h.

GI HEMORRHAGE

IV INFUSION: ADULTS, ELDERLY: Initially, 0.2–0.4 unit/min progressively increased to 0.9 unit/min. **CHILDREN:** 0.002–0.005 unit/kg/min. Titrate as needed. **Maximum:** 0.01 unit/kg/min.

VASODILATORY SHOCK

IV: ADULTS, ELDERLY: Initially, 0.04–0.1 unit/min. Titrate to desired effect.

SIDE EFFECTS

FREQUENT: Pain at injection site (with vasopressin tannate). **OCCASIONAL:** Abdominal cramps, nausea, vomiting, diarrhea, dizziness, diaphoresis, pale skin, circumoral pallor, tremors, headache, eructation, flatulence. **RARE:** Chest pain, confusion, allergic reaction (rash, urticaria, pruritus, wheezing, difficulty breathing, facial/peripheral edema), sterile abscess (with vasopressin tannate).

ADVERSE EFFECTS/TOXIC REACTIONS

Anaphylaxis, MI, water intoxication have occurred. Elderly, very young are at higher risk for water intoxication.

NURSING CONSIDERATIONS

BASELINE ASSESSMENT

Establish baselines for weight, B/P, pulse, serum electrolytes, urine specific gravity.

INTERVENTION/EVALUATION

Monitor I&O closely, restrict intake as necessary to prevent water intoxication. Weigh daily if indicated. Check B/P, pulse twice a day. Monitor serum electrolytes, urine specific gravity. Evaluate injection site for erythema, pain, abscess. Report side effects to physician for dose reduction. Be alert for early signs of water intoxication (drowsiness, listlessness, headache). Withhold medication, report immediately any chest pain, allergic symptoms.

PATIENT/FAMILY TEACHING

• Promptly report headache, chest pain, shortness of breath, other symptoms. • Stress importance of I&O. • Avoid alcohol.

Vasotec, *see enalapril*

vecuronium

(Norcuron)

See Neuromuscular blockers (p. 120C)

venlafaxine

ven-la-**fax**-een
(Effexor, Effexor XR)

✦ CLASSIFICATION

PHARMACOTHERAPEUTIC: Phenethylamine derivative. **CLINICAL:** Antidepressant (see pp. 12C, 38C).

ACTION

Potentiates CNS neurotransmitter activity by inhibiting reuptake of serotonin, norepinephrine, and to lesser degree, dopamine. **Therapeutic Effect:** Relieves depression.

PHARMACOKINETICS

Well absorbed from GI tract. Protein binding: 25%–30%. Metabolized in liver to active metabolite. Primarily excreted in urine. Not removed by hemodialysis. **Half-life:** 3–7 hrs; metabolite, 9–13 hrs (increased in hepatic/renal impairment.

USES

Treatment of depression exhibited as persistent, prominent dysphoria (occurring nearly every day for at least 2 wks) manifested by 4 of 8 symptoms: change in appetite, change in sleep pattern, increased fatigue, impaired concentration, feelings of guilt or worthlessness, loss of interest in usual activities, psychomotor agitation or retardation, or suicidal tendencies. Psychotherapy augments therapeutic result. Treatment of generalized anxiety disorder (GAD), social anxiety disorder (SAD). Treatment of panic disorder, with or without agoraphobia. **OFF-LABEL:** Prevention of relapses of depression; treatment of attention-deficit hyperactivity disorder, autism, chronic fatigue syndrome, obsessive-compulsive disorder.

PRECAUTIONS

CONTRAINDICATIONS: Use of MAOIs within 14 days. **CAUTIONS:** Seizure disorder, renal/hepatic impairment, suicidal pts, recent MI, mania, volume-depleted pts, narrow-angle glaucoma, CHF, hyperthyroidism, abnormal platelet function.

⌛ LIFESPAN CONSIDERATIONS:

Pregnancy/Lactation: Unknown if excreted in breast milk. **Pregnancy Category C. Children:** Children, adolescents are at increased risk of suicidal ideation and behavior, worsening depression, esp. during first few mos of therapy. **Elderly:** No age-related precautions noted.

INTERACTIONS

DRUG: MAOIs may cause neuroleptic malignant syndrome, autonomic instability (including rapid fluctuations of vital signs), extreme agitation, hyperthermia, altered mental status, myoclonus, rigidity, coma. **Meperidine, selegiline, SSRIs, trazodone, tricyclic antidepressants** may increase risk of serotonin syndrome. **HERBAL: Gotu kola, kava kava, St. John's wort, valerian** may increase CNS depression. **FOOD:** None known. **LAB VALUES:** May increase BUN, serum alkaline phosphatase, bilirubin, cholesterol, uric acid, AST, ALT. May decrease serum phosphate, sodium. May alter serum glucose, potassium.

AVAILABILITY (Rx)

TABLETS (EFFEXOR): 25 mg, 37.5 mg, 50 mg, 75 mg, 100 mg.

CAPSULES (EXTENDED-RELEASE [EFFEXOR XL]): 37.5 mg, 75 mg, 150 mg.

V

ADMINISTRATION/HANDLING

PO

• Give without regard to food. Give with food, milk if GI distress occurs. • Scored tablet may be crushed. • Do not crush/chew extended-release capsules. • May open, sprinkle on applesauce.

INDICATIONS/ROUTES/DOSAGE

DEPRESSION

PO: ADULTS, ELDERLY: Initially, 75 mg/day in 2–3 divided doses with food. May increase by 75 mg/day at intervals of 4 days or longer. **Maximum:** 375 mg/day in 3 divided doses.

PO (EXTENDED-RELEASE): ADULTS, ELDERLY: 75 mg/day as single dose with food. May increase by 75 mg/day at intervals of 4 days or longer. **Maximum:** 225 mg/day.

SAD, GAD

PO (EXTENDED-RELEASE): ADULTS, ELDERLY: Initially, 37.5–75 mg/day. May increase by 75 mg/day at 4-day intervals up to 225 mg/day.

PANIC DISORDER

PO (EXTENDED-RELEASE): Initially, 37.5 mg/day. May increase to 75 mg after 7 days followed by increases of 75 mg/day at 7-day intervals up to 225 mg/day.

DOSAGE IN RENAL AND HEPATIC IMPAIRMENT

Expect to decrease venlafaxine dosage by 50% in pts with moderate hepatic impairment, 25% in pts with mild to moderate renal impairment, 50% in pts on dialysis (withhold dose until completion of dialysis). When discontinuing therapy, taper dosage slowly over 2 wks.

V

SIDE EFFECTS

FREQUENT (greater than 20%): Nausea, drowsiness, headache, dry mouth. **OCCASIONAL (20%–10%):** Dizziness, insomnia, constipation, diaphoresis, nervousness, asthenia (loss of strength, energy), ejaculatory disturbance, anorexia. **RARE (less than 10%):** Anxiety, blurred vision, diarrhea, vomiting, tremor, abnormal dreams, impotence.

ADVERSE EFFECTS/ TOXIC REACTIONS

Sustained increase in diastolic B/P of 10–15 mm Hg occurs occasionally.

NURSING CONSIDERATIONS

BASELINE ASSESSMENT

Obtain initial weight, B/P. Assess appearance, behavior, speech pattern, level of interest, mood.

INTERVENTION/EVALUATION

Monitor signs/symptoms of depression, B/P, weight. Assess sleep pattern for evidence of insomnia. Check during waking hours for drowsiness, dizziness, anxiety; provide assistance as necessary. Supervise suicidal-risk pt closely during early therapy (as depression lessens, energy level improves, increasing suicide potential). Assess appearance, behavior, speech pattern, level of interest, mood for therapeutic response.

PATIENT/FAMILY TEACHING

• Take with food to minimize GI distress. • Do not increase, decrease, suddenly stop medication. • Avoid tasks that require alertness, motor skills until response to drug is established. • Inform physician if breast-feeding, pregnant, or planning to become pregnant. • Avoid alcohol.

Ventolin, *see albuterol*

VePesid, *see etoposide*

verapamil

ver-**ap**-a-mill

(Apo-Verap ♣, Calan, Calan SR, Chronovera ♣, Covera-HS, Isoptin, Isoptin I.V., Isoptin SR, Novo-Veramil SR ♣, Verelan, Verelan PM)

Do not confuse Isoptin with Intropin, or Verelan with Virilon, Vivarin, or Voltaren.

FIXED-COMBINATION(S)

Tarka: verapamil/trandolapril (an angiotensin-converting enzyme [ACE] inhibitor): 240 mg/1 mg; 180 mg/2 mg; 240 mg/2 mg; 240 mg/4 mg.

CLASSIFICATION

PHARMACOTHERAPEUTIC: Calcium channel blocker. **CLINICAL:** Antihypertensive, antianginal, antiarrhythmic, hypertropic cardiomyopathy therapy adjunct (see pp. 16C, 73C).

ACTION

Inhibits calcium ion entry across cardiac, vascular smooth-muscle cell membranes, dilating coronary arteries, peripheral arteries, arterioles. **Therapeutic Effect:** Decreases heart rate, myocardial contractility, slows SA, AV conduction. Decreases total peripheral vascular resistance by vasodilation.

PHARMACOKINETICS

Route	Onset	Peak	Duration
PO	30 min	1–2 hrs	6–8 hrs
PO (Extended-release)	30 min	N/A	N/A
IV	1–2 min	3–5 min	10–60 min

Well absorbed from GI tract. Protein binding: 90% (60% in neonates.) Undergoes first-pass metabolism in liver to active metabolite. Primarily excreted in urine. Not removed by hemodialysis. **Half-life:** 2–8 hrs.

USES

Parenteral: Management of supraventricular tachyarrhythmias, temporary control of rapid ventricular rate in atrial flutter/fibrillation. **PO:** Management of spastic (Prinzmetal's variant) angina, unstable (crescendo, preinfarction) angina, chronic stable angina (effort-associated angina), hypertension, prevention of recurrent paroxysmal supraventricular tachycardia (PSVT) (with digoxin), control of ventricular resting pulse rate in those with atrial flutter/fibrillation. **OFF-LABEL:** Treatment of bipolar disorder, hypertrophic cardiomyopathy, vascular headaches.

PRECAUTIONS

CONTRAINDICATIONS: Atrial fibrillation/flutter in presence of accessory bypass tract (e.g., Wolff-Parkinson-White, Lown-Ganong-Levine syndromes), cardiogenic shock, second- or third-degree heart block, hypotension, sick sinus syndrome, sinus bradycardia, ventricular tachycardia. **CAUTIONS:** CHF, renal/hepatic impairment, concomitant use of beta-blockers, digoxin.

LIFESPAN CONSIDERATIONS:

Pregnancy/Lactation: Drug crosses placenta; is distributed in breast milk. Breast-feeding not recommended. **Pregnancy Category C. Children:** No age-related precautions noted. **Elderly:** Age-related renal impairment may require dosage adjustment.

INTERACTIONS

DRUG: **Beta-adrenergic blockers** may have additive effect. **Carbamazepine, cyclosporine, quinidine, theophylline** may increase concentration, risk of toxicity. May increase **digoxin** concentration. **Disopyramide** may increase negative inotropic effect. **Procainamide,**

V

quinidine may increase risk of QT-interval prolongation. **Rifampin** may decrease concentration, effect. **HERBAL: St. John's wort** may decrease concentration, effect. **Ephedra, ginseng, yohimbe** may worsen hypertension. **Garlic** may increase antihypertensive effect. **FOOD: Grapefruit, grapefruit juice** may increase concentration. **LAB VALUES:** EKG may show increased PR interval. Therapeutic serum level: 0.08–0.3 mcg/ml. Toxic serum level: N/A.

AVAILABILITY (Rx)

CAPLET (CALAN SR): 120 mg, 180 mg, 240 mg. **INJECTION SOLUTION:** 2.5 mg/ml. **TABLETS (CALAN):** 40 mg, 80 mg, <u>120 mg</u>.

CAPSULES (EXTENDED-RELEASE [VERELAN PM]): 100 mg, 200 mg, 300 mg. **CAPSULES (SUSTAINED-RELEASE [VERELAN]):** 120 mg, 180 mg, 240 mg, 360 mg. **TABLETS (EXTENDED-RELEASE [COVERA-HS]):** 180 mg, 240 mg. **TABLETS (SUSTAINED-RELEASE [ISOPTIN SR]):** 120 mg, 180 mg, 240 mg.

ADMINISTRATION/HANDLING

IV

Reconstitution • May give undiluted.

Rate of administration • Administer IV push over 2 min for adults, children; give over 3 min for elderly. • Continuous EKG monitoring during IV injection is required for children, recommended for adults. • Monitor EKG for rapid ventricular rate, extreme bradycardia, heart block, asystole, prolongation of PR interval. Notify physician of any significant changes. • Monitor B/P q5–10min. • Pt should remain recumbent for at least 1 hr after IV administration.

Storage • Store vials at room temperature.

PO

• Do not give with grapefruit, grapefruit juice. • Non–sustained-release tablets may be given without regard to food. • Swallow extended-release, sustained-released preparations whole; do not chew, crush. • Sustained-release capsules may be opened and sprinkled on applesauce, then swallowed immediately (do not chew).

IV INCOMPATIBILITIES

Amphotericin B complex (Abelcet, AmBisome, Amphotec), nafcillin (Nafcil), propofol (Diprivan), sodium bicarbonate.

IV COMPATIBILITIES

Amiodarone (Cordarone), calcium chloride, calcium gluconate, dexamethasone (Decadron), digoxin (Lanoxin), dobutamine (Dobutrex), dopamine (Intropin), furosemide (Lasix), heparin, hydromorphone (Dilaudid), lidocaine, magnesium sulfate, metoclopramide (Reglan), milrinone (Primacor), morphine, multivitamins, nitroglycerin, norepinephrine (Levophed), potassium chloride, potassium phosphate, procainamide (Pronestyl), propranolol (Inderal).

INDICATIONS/ROUTES/DOSAGE

SUPRAVENTRICULAR TACHYARRHYTHMIAS (SVT)

IV: ADULTS, ELDERLY: Initially, 2.5–5 mg over 2 min. May give 5–10 mg 30 min after initial dose. **Maximum initial dose:** 20 mg. **CHILDREN 1–15 YRS:** 0.1–0.3 mg/kg over 2 min. **Maximum initial dose:** 5 mg. May repeat in 15 min. **Maximum second dose:** 10 mg. **CHILDREN YOUNGER THAN 1 YR:** 0.1–0.2 mg/kg over 2 min. May repeat 30 min after initial dose.

ARRHYTHMIAS, CONTROL OF VENTRICULAR HEART RATE

PO: ADULTS, ELDERLY: 240–480 mg/day in 3–4 divided doses.

ANGINA, UNSTABLE ANGINA, CHRONIC STABLE ANGINA

PO: ADULTS: Initially, 80–120 mg 3 times a day. For elderly pts, those with

hepatic dysfunction, 40 mg 3 times a day. Titrate to optimal dose. Maintenance: 240–480 mg/day in 3–4 divided doses.
PO (COVERA-HS): ADULTS, ELDERLY: 180–480 mg/day at bedtime.

HYPERTENSION

PO (IMMEDIATE-RELEASE): ADULTS, ELDERLY: 80 mg 3 times a day. Range: 80–320 mg/day in 2 divided doses.
PO (SUSTAINED-RELEASE): ADULTS, ELDERLY: 120–240 mg/day. Range: 120–360 mg/day as single dose or in 2 divided doses.
PO (EXTENDED-RELEASE [COVER-AHS]): ADULTS, ELDERLY: 120–360 mg once daily at bedtime.
PO (EXTENDED-RELEASE [VERELAN PM]): ADULTS, ELDERLY: 200–400 mg once daily at bedtime.

SIDE EFFECTS

FREQUENT (7%): Constipation. **OCCASIONAL (4%–2%):** Dizziness, light-headedness, headache, asthenia (loss of strength, energy), nausea, peripheral edema, hypotension. **RARE (less than 1%):** Bradycardia, dermatitis, rash.

ADVERSE EFFECTS/ TOXIC REACTIONS

Rapid ventricular rate in atrial flutter/fibrillation, marked hypotension, extreme bradycardia, CHF, asystole, second- or third-degree AV block occur rarely.

NURSING CONSIDERATIONS

BASELINE ASSESSMENT

Record onset, type (sharp, dull, squeezing), radiation, location, intensity, duration of anginal pain, precipitating factors (exertion, emotional stress). Check B/P for hypotension, pulse for bradycardia immediately before giving medication.

INTERVENTION/EVALUATION

Assess pulse for quality, irregular rate. Monitor EKG for cardiac changes, particularly prolongation of PR interval. Notify physician of any significant EKG interval changes. Assist with ambulation if dizziness occurs. Assess for peripheral edema behind medial malleolus (sacral area in bedridden pts). For those taking oral form, monitor daily pattern of bowel activity/stool consistency. Therapeutic serum level: 0.08–0.3 mcg/ml; toxic serum level: N/A.

PATIENT/FAMILY TEACHING

• Do not abruptly discontinue medication. • Compliance with therapy regimen is essential to control anginal pain. • To avoid hypotensive effect, rise slowly from lying to sitting position, wait momentarily before standing. • Avoid tasks that require alertness, motor skills until response to drug is established. • Limit caffeine. • Inform physician if angina pain not reduced, irregular heartbeats, shortness of breath, swelling, dizziness, constipation, nausea, hypotension occurs. • Avoid concomitant grapefruit, grapefruit juice.

Versed, *see midazolam*

Viagra, *see sildenafil*

Vidaza, *see azacitidine*

V

*vinBLAStine

vin-**blass**-teen
(Velban, Velbe ✤)

Do not confuse vinblastine with vincristine or vinorelbine.

◆CLASSIFICATION

PHARMACOTHERAPEUTIC: Vinca alkaloid. **CLINICAL:** Antineoplastic (see p. 84C).

ACTION

Binds to microtubular protein of mitotic spindle, causing metaphase arrest. **Therapeutic Effect:** Inhibits cell division.

PHARMACOKINETICS

Does not cross blood-brain barrier. Protein binding: 75%. Metabolized in liver to active metabolite. Primarily eliminated in feces by biliary system. **Half-life:** 24.8 hrs.

USES

Treatment of disseminated Hodgkin's disease, non-Hodgkin's lymphoma, advanced stage of mycosis fungoides, advanced testicular carcinoma, Kaposi's sarcoma, Letterer-Siwe disease, breast carcinoma, choriocarcinoma. **OFF-LABEL:** Treatment of bladder, head/neck, kidney, lung carcinoma; chronic myelocytic leukemia; germ cell ovarian tumors; neuroblastoma.

PRECAUTIONS

CONTRAINDICATIONS: Bacterial infection, severe leukopenia, significant granulocytopenia (unless a result of disease being treated). **CAUTIONS:** Hepatic impairment, neurotoxicity, recent exposure to radiation therapy, chemotherapy.

LIFESPAN CONSIDERATIONS:

Pregnancy/Lactation: If possible, avoid use during pregnancy, esp. during first trimester. Breast-feeding not recommended. **Pregnancy Category D. Children/Elderly:** No age-related precautions noted.

INTERACTIONS

DRUG: May decrease effects of **antigout medications. Bone marrow depressants** may increase myelosuppression. **Live virus vaccines** may potentiate virus replication, increase vaccine side effects, decrease pt's antibody response to vaccine. **HERBAL: St. John's wort** may decrease concentration. Avoid **black cohosh, dong quai** in estrogen-dependent tumors. **FOOD:** None known. **LAB VALUES:** May increase serum uric acid.

AVAILABILITY (Rx)

INJECTION POWDER FOR RECONSTITUTION: 10 mg. **INJECTION SOLUTION:** 1 mg/ml.

ADMINISTRATION/HANDLING

◀ ALERT ▶ May be carcinogenic, mutagenic, teratogenic. Handle with extreme care during preparation and administration. Give by IV injection. Leakage from IV site into surrounding tissue may produce extreme irritation. Avoid eye contact with solution (severe eye irritation, possible corneal ulceration may result). If eye contact occurs, immediately irrigate eye with water.

IV

Reconstitution • Reconstitute 10-mg vial with 10 ml 0.9% NaCl preserved with phenol or benzyl alcohol to provide concentration of 1 mg/ml.

Rate of administration • Inject into tubing of running IV infusion or directly into vein over 1 min. • Do not inject into extremity with impaired, potentially impaired circulation caused by compression or invading neoplasm, phlebitis, varicosity. • Rinse syringe, needle with venous blood before withdrawing needle (minimizes possibility of extravasation). • Extravasation may result in cellulitis, phlebitis. Large amount of extravasation may result in tissue sloughing. If extravasation occurs, give local injection of hyaluronidase, apply warm compresses.

Storage • Refrigerate unopened vials. • Solutions appear clear, colorless. • Following reconstitution, solution is stable for 30 days if refrigerated. • Discard if solution is discolored or precipitate forms.

IV INCOMPATIBILITIES

Cefepime (Maxipime), furosemide (Lasix).

IV COMPATIBILITIES

Allopurinol (Aloprim), cisplatin (Platinol AQ), cyclophosphamide (Cytoxan), doxorubicin (Adriamycin), etoposide (VePesid), 5-fluorouracil, gemcitabine (Gemzar), granisetron (Kytril), heparin, leucovorin, methotrexate, ondansetron (Zofran), paclitaxel (Taxol), vinorelbine (Navelbine).

INDICATIONS/ROUTES/DOSAGE

◀ **ALERT** ▶ Dosage individualized based on clinical response, tolerance to adverse effects. When used in combination therapy, consult specific protocols for optimum dosage, sequence of drug administration.

USUAL DOSAGE

IV: ADULTS, ELDERLY, CHILDREN: 4–20 mg/m^2 (0.1–0.5 mg/kg) q7–10days or 5 day continuous infusion of 1.5–2 mg/m^2/day or 0.1–0.5 mg/kg/wk.

HEPATIC IMPAIRMENT

	Dosage
Bilirubin 1.5–3 mg/dl or AST 60–180 units	50% of normal
Bilirubin greater than 3–5 mg/dl	25% or normal
Bilirubin greater than 5 or AST greater than 180 units	Omit dose

SIDE EFFECTS

FREQUENT: Nausea, vomiting, alopecia. **OCCASIONAL:** Constipation, diarrhea, rectal bleeding, headache, paresthesia (occur 4–6 hrs after administration, persist for 2–10 hrs), malaise, asthenia (loss of strength, energy), dizziness, pain at tumor site, jaw/face pain, depression, dry mouth. **RARE:** Dermatitis, stomatitis, phototoxicity, hyperuricemia.

ADVERSE EFFECTS/ TOXIC REACTIONS

Hematologic toxicity manifested most commonly as leukopenia, less frequently as anemia. WBC reaches its nadir 4–10 days after initial therapy, recovers within 7–14 days (high dosage may require 21-day recovery period). Thrombocytopenia is usually mild and transient, with recovery occurring in few days. Hepatic insufficiency may increase risk of toxicity. Acute shortness of breath, bronchospasm may occur, particularly when administered concurrently with mitomycin.

NURSING CONSIDERATIONS

BASELINE ASSESSMENT

Nausea, vomiting easily controlled by antiemetics. Discontinue therapy if WBC, thrombocyte counts fall abruptly (unless drug is clearly destroying tumor cells in bone marrow). Obtain CBC weekly or before each dosing.

INTERVENTION/EVALUATION

If WBC falls below 2,000/mm^3, assess diligently for signs of infection. Assess for stomatitis; maintain fastidious oral hygiene. Monitor for hematologic toxicity: infection (fever, sore throat, signs of local infection), unusual bruising/bleeding from any site, symptoms of anemia (excessive fatigue, weakness). Monitor daily pattern of bowel activity/stool consistency; avoid constipation.

V

PATIENT/FAMILY TEACHING

• Immediately report any pain/burning at injection site during administration. • Pain at tumor site may occur during or shortly after injection. • Do not have immunizations without physician approval (drug lowers resistance). • Avoid crowds, those with infection. • Promptly report fever, sore throat, signs of local infection, unusual bruising/bleeding from any site. • Alopecia is reversible, but new hair growth may have different color, texture. • Contact physician if nausea/vomiting continues. • Avoid constipation by increasing fluids, bulk in diet, exercise as tolerated.

*vinCRIStine

vin-**cris**-teen

(Oncovin, Vincasar PFS)

Do not confuse vincristine with vinblastine, or Oncovin with Ancobon.

CLASSIFICATION

PHARMACOTHERAPEUTIC: Vinca alkaloid. **CLINICAL:** Antineoplastic (see p. 84C).

ACTION

Binds to microtubular protein of mitotic spindle, causing metaphase arrest. **Therapeutic Effect:** Inhibits cell division.

PHARMACOKINETICS

Does not cross blood-brain barrier. Protein binding: 75%. Metabolized in liver. Primarily eliminated in feces by biliary system. **Half-life:** 10–37 hrs.

USES

Treatment of acute leukemia, disseminated Hodgkin's disease, advanced non-Hodgkin's lymphomas, neuroblastoma, rhabdomyosarcoma, Wilms' tumor. **OFF-LABEL:** Treatment of breast, cervical, colorectal, lung, ovarian carcinomas; chronic lymphocytic and chronic myelocytic leukemias; germ cell ovarian tumors; idiopathic thrombocytopenic purpura; malignant melanoma; multiple myeloma; mycosis fungoides.

PRECAUTIONS

CONTRAINDICATIONS: Demyelinating form of Charcot-Marie-Tooth syndrome, pts receiving radiation therapy through ports including liver. **CAUTION:** Hepatic impairment, neurotoxicity, preexisting neuromuscular disease.

LIFESPAN CONSIDERATIONS: **Pregnancy/Lactation:** If possible, avoid use during pregnancy, esp. first trimester. May cause fetal harm. Breastfeeding not recommended. **Pregnancy Category D.** **Children:** No age-related precautions noted. **Elderly:** More susceptible to neurotoxic effects.

INTERACTIONS

DRUG: **Asparaginase, neurotoxic medications** may increase risk of neurotoxicity. May decrease effects of **antigout medications. Doxorubicin** may increase risk of myelosuppression. **Live virus vaccines** may potentiate virus replication, increase vaccine side effects, decrease pt's antibody response to vaccine. **HERBAL:** **St. John's wort** may decrease concentration. **FOOD:** None known. **LAB VALUES:** May increase serum uric acid.

AVAILABILITY (Rx)

INJECTION SOLUTION (ONCOVIN): 1 mg/ml.

ADMINISTRATION/HANDLING

IV

◄ **ALERT** ► May be carcinogenic, mutagenic, teratogenic. Handle with extreme care during preparation and administration. Give by IV injection. Use extreme caution in calculating, administering vincristine. Overdose may result in serious or fatal outcome.

Reconstitution • May give undiluted.

Rate of administration • Inject dose into tubing of running IV infusion or directly into vein over 1 min. • Do not inject into extremity with impaired, potentially impaired circulation caused by compression or invading neoplasm, phlebitis, varicosity. • Extravasation produces stinging, burning, edema at injection site. Terminate injection immediately, locally inject hyaluronidase, apply heat (disperses drug, minimizes discomfort, cellulitis).

Storage • Refrigerate unopened vials. • Solutions appear clear, colorless. • Discard if solution is discolored or precipitate forms.

IV INCOMPATIBILITIES

Cefepime (Maxipime), furosemide (Lasix), idarubicin (Idamycin).

IV COMPATIBILITIES

Allopurinol (Aloprim), cisplatin (Platinol AQ), cyclophosphamide (Cytoxan), cytarabine (Ara-C, Cytosar), doxorubicin (Adriamycin), etoposide (VePesid), 5-fluorouracil, gemcitabine (Gemzar), granisetron (Kytril), leucovorin, methotrexate, ondansetron (Zofran), paclitaxel (Taxol), vinorelbine (Navelbine).

INDICATIONS/ROUTES/DOSAGE

USUAL DOSAGE

IV: ADULTS, ELDERLY: 0.4–1.4 mg/m^2 once a wk. **CHILDREN:** 1–2 mg/m^2 once a wk. **CHILDREN WEIGHING LESS THAN 10 KG OR WITH BODY SURFACE AREA LESS THAN 1 M^2:** 0.05 mg/kg. **Maximum:** 2 mg.

HEPATIC IMPAIRMENT

	Dosage
Bilirubin 1.5–3 mg/dl or AST 60–180 units	50% of normal
Bilirubin greater than 3 to 5 mg/dl	25% or normal
Bilirubin greater than 5 or AST greater than 180 units	Omit dose

SIDE EFFECTS

EXPECTED: Peripheral neuropathy (occurs in nearly every pt; first clinical sign is depression of Achilles tendon reflex). **FREQUENT:** Peripheral paresthesia, alopecia, constipation/obstipation (upper colon impaction with empty rectum), abdominal cramps, headache, jaw pain, hoarseness, diplopia, ptosis/drooping of eyelid, urinary tract disturbances. **OCCASIONAL:** Nausea, vomiting, diarrhea, abdominal distention, stomatitis, fever. **RARE:** Mild leukopenia, mild anemia, thrombocytopenia.

ADVERSE EFFECTS/ TOXIC REACTIONS

Acute shortness of breath, bronchospasm may occur, esp. when administered concurrently with mitomycin. Prolonged or high-dose therapy may produce foot/wrist drop, difficulty walking, slapping gait, ataxia, muscle wasting. Acute uric acid nephropathy may occur.

NURSING CONSIDERATIONS

BASELINE ASSESSMENT

Monitor serum uric acid levels, renal/hepatic function studies, hematologic status. Assess Achilles tendon reflex. Monitor daily pattern of bowel activity/stool consistency. Monitor for ptosis, diplopia, blurred vision. Question pt regarding urinary changes.

V

PATIENT/FAMILY TEACHING

• Immediately report any pain/burning at injection site during administration. • Alopecia is reversible, but new hair growth may have different color/ texture. • Contact physician if nausea/ vomiting continues. • Teach signs of peripheral neuropathy. • Report fever, sore throat, bleeding, bruising, shortness of breath.

vinorelbine

vin-oh-**rell**-bean

(Navelbine)

Do not confuse vinorelbine with vinblastine.

CLASSIFICATION

CLINICAL: Antineoplastic (see p. 84C).

ACTION

Interferes with mitotic microtubule assembly. **Therapeutic Effect:** Prevents cellular division.

PHARMACOKINETICS

Widely distributed after IV administration. Protein binding: 80%–90%. Metabolized in liver. Primarily eliminated in feces by biliary system. **Half-life:** 28–43 hrs.

USES

Single agent or in combination with cisplatin for treatment with unresectable, advanced, non–small cell lung cancer (NSCLC). **OFF-LABEL:** Treatment of breast cancer, cervical carcinoma, cisplatin-resistant ovarian carcinoma, Hodgkin's disease, non-Hodgkin's lymphoma.

PRECAUTIONS

CONTRAINDICATIONS: Granulocyte count before treatment of less than 1,000 cells/mm^3. **EXTREME CAUTION:** Immunocompromised pts. **CAUTIONS:** Existing or recent chickenpox, herpes zoster, infection, leukopenia, impaired pulmonary function, severe hepatic injury/impairment.

LIFESPAN CONSIDERATIONS:

Pregnancy/Lactation: If possible, avoid use during pregnancy, esp. during first trimester. May cause fetal harm. Unknown if excreted in breast milk. Breast-feeding not recommended. **Pregnancy Category D. Children:** Safety and efficacy not established. **Elderly:** No age-related precautions noted.

INTERACTIONS

DRUG: Bone marrow depressants may increase risk of myelosuppression. **Cisplatin** significantly increases risk of granulocytopenia. **Live virus vaccines** may potentiate virus replication, increase vaccine side effects, decrease pt's antibody response to vaccine. **Mitomycin** may produce an acute pulmonary reaction. **HERBAL: St. John's wort** may decrease concentration. **FOOD:** None known. **LAB VALUES:** May increase serum bilirubin, AST, hepatic function test results. Decreases granulocyte, leukocyte, thrombocyte, RBC counts.

AVAILABILITY (Rx)

INJECTION SOLUTION: 10 mg/ml (1-ml, 5-ml vials).

ADMINISTRATION/HANDLING

IV

◀ **ALERT** ▶ IV needle, catheter must be correctly positioned before administration. Leakage into surrounding tissue produces extreme irritation, local tissue necrosis, thrombophlebitis. Handle drug with extreme care during administration; wear protective clothing per protocol. If solution comes in contact with skin/mucosa, immediately wash thoroughly with soap, water.

Reconstitution • Must be diluted and administered via syringe or IV bag.
SYRINGE DILUTION • Dilute calculated vinorelbine dose with D_5W or 0.9% NaCl to concentration of 1.5–3 mg/ml.
IV BAG DILUTION • Dilute calculated vinorelbine dose with D_5W, 0.45% or 0.9% NaCl, 5% dextrose and 0.45% NaCl, Ringer's or lactated Ringer's to concentration of 0.5–2 mg/ml.

Rate of administration • Administer diluted vinorelbine over 6–10 min into side port of free-flowing IV closest to IV bag followed by flushing with 75–125 ml of one of the solutions. • If extravasation occurs, stop injection immediately; give remaining portion of dose into another vein.

Storage • Refrigerate unopened vials. • Protect from light. • Unopened vials are stable at room temperature for 72 hrs. • Do not administer if particulate has formed. • Diluted vinorelbine may be used for up to 24 hrs under normal room light when stored in polypropylene syringes or polyvinyl chloride bags at room temperature.

IV INCOMPATIBILITIES

Acyclovir (Zovirax), allopurinol (Aloprim), amphotericin B (Fungizone), amphotericin B complex (Abelcet, AmBisome, Amphotec), ampicillin (Omnipen), cefazolin (Ancef), cefoperazone (Cefobid), cefotetan (Cefotan), ceftriaxone (Rocephin), cefuroxime (Zinacef), 5-fluorouracil, furosemide (Lasix), ganciclovir (Cytovene), methylprednisolone (Solu-Medrol), sodium bicarbonate.

IV COMPATIBILITIES

Calcium gluconate, carboplatin (Paraplatin), cisplatin (Platinol AQ), cyclophosphamide (Cytoxan), cytarabine (ARA-C, Cytosar), dacarbazine (DTIC-Dome), daunorubicin (Cerubidine), dexamethasone (Decadron), diphenhydramine (Benadryl), doxorubicin (Adriamycin), etoposide (VePesid), gemcitabine (Gemzar), granisetron (Kytril), hydromorphone (Dilaudid), idarubicin (Idamycin), methotrexate, morphine, ondansetron (Zofran), teniposide (Vumon), vinblastine (Velban), vincristine (Oncovin).

INDICATIONS/ROUTES/DOSAGE

◀ **ALERT** ▶ Dosage adjustments should be based on granulocyte count obtained on the day of treatment, as follows:

Granulocyte Count (cells/mm^3) on Day of Treatment	Dose
1,500 or higher	30 mg/m^2
1,000–1,499	15 mg/m^2
Less than 1,000	Do not administer

NON-SMALL CELL LUNG CANCER
IV INJECTION: ADULTS, ELDERLY: 30 mg/m^2 administered weekly over 6–10 min.

COMBINATION THERAPY WITH CISPLATIN
IV INJECTION: ADULTS, ELDERLY: 25 mg/m^2 every wk or 30 mg/m^2 on days 1 and 29, then q6wk.

SIDE EFFECTS

FREQUENT: Asthenia (loss of strength, energy) (35%), nausea (34%), constipation (29%), erythema, pain, vein discoloration at injection site (28%), fatigue (27%), peripheral neuropathy manifested as paresthesia, hyperesthesia (25%), diarrhea (17%), alopecia (12%). **OCCASIONAL:** Phlebitis (10%), dyspnea (7%), loss of deep tendon reflexes (5%). **RARE:** Chest pain, jaw pain, myalgia, arthralgia, rash.

ADVERSE EFFECTS/ TOXIC REACTIONS

Bone marrow depression is manifested mainly as granulocytopenia (may be severe). Other hematologic toxicities (neutropenia, thrombocytopenia, leukopenia, anemia) increase risk of infection, bleeding. Acute shortness of breath, severe bronchospasm occur infrequently, particularly in pts with preexisting pulmonary dysfunction.

NURSING CONSIDERATIONS

BASELINE ASSESSMENT

Review medication history. Assess hematology (CBC, platelet count, Hgb, differential) values before giving each dose. Granulocyte count should be at least 1,000 cells/mm^3 before vinorelbine administration. Granulocyte nadirs occur 7–10 days following dosing. Do not give hematologic growth factors within 24 hrs before administration of chemotherapy or earlier than 24 hrs following cytotoxic chemotherapy. Advise women of childbearing potential to avoid pregnancy during drug therapy.

INTERVENTION/EVALUATION

Diligently monitor injection site for swelling, redness, pain. Frequently monitor for myelosuppression during and following therapy: infection (fever, sore throat, signs of local infection), unusual bleeding/bruising, anemia (excessive fatigue, weakness). Monitor pts developing severe granulocytopenia for evidence of infection, fever. Crackers, dry toast, sips of cola may help relieve nausea. Monitor daily pattern of bowel activity/stool consistency. Question for tingling, burning, numbness of hands/feet (peripheral neuropathy). Pt complaint of "walking on glass" is sign of hyperesthesia.

PATIENT/FAMILY TEACHING

• Notify nurse immediately if redness, swelling, pain occur at injection site. • Avoid crowds, those with infection. • Do not have immunizations without physician's approval. • Promptly report fever, signs of infection, unusual bruising/bleeding from any site, difficulty breathing. • Avoid pregnancy. • Alopecia is reversible, but new hair growth may have different color, texture.

Viracept, *see nelfinavir*

Viramune, *see nevirapine*

Viread, *see tenofovir*

Vistaril, *see hydroxyzine*

vitamin A

vight-ah-myn A

(Aquasol A, Palmitate A)

Do not confuse Aquasol A with Anusol.

CLASSIFICATION

PHARMACOTHERAPEUTIC: Fat-soluble vitamin. **CLINICAL:** Nutritional supplement (see p. 150C).

ACTION

May act as cofactor in biochemical reactions. **Therapeutic Effect:** Essential for normal function of retina, visual adaptation to darkness, bone growth, testicular and ovarian function, embryonic development; preserves integrity of epithelial cells.

PHARMACOKINETICS

Rapidly absorbed from GI tract if bile salts, pancreatic lipase, protein, and dietary fat are present. Transported in blood to liver, where it is metabolized; stored in parenchymal hepatic cells, then transported in plasma as retinol, as needed. Excreted primarily in bile and, to lesser extent, in urine.

USES

Treatment of vitamin A deficiency (biliary tract, pancreatic disease, sprue, colitis, hepatic cirrhosis, celiac disease, regional enteritis, extreme dietary inadequacy, partial gastrectomy, cystic fibrosis).

PRECAUTIONS

CONTRAINDICATIONS: Hypervitaminosis A, oral use in malabsorption syndrome. **CAUTIONS:** Renal impairment.

LIFESPAN CONSIDERATIONS:

Pregnancy/Lactation: Crosses placenta. Distributed in breast milk. **Pregnancy Category A (X if used in doses above recommended daily allowance).** **Children/Elderly:** Caution with higher dosages.

INTERACTIONS

DRUG: **Cholestyramine, colestipol, mineral oil** may decrease absorption. **Isotretinoin** may increase risk of toxicity. **HERBAL:** None significant. **FOOD:** None known. **LAB VALUES:** May increase BUN, serum cholesterol, calcium, triglycerides. May decrease RBC, WBC counts.

AVAILABILITY (Rx)

INJECTION SOLUTION (AQUASOL A): 50,000 units/ml. **TABLETS (PALMITATE A):** 5,000 units, 15,000 units.

CAPSULES: 10,000 units, 25,000 units.

ADMINISTRATION/HANDLING

◀ **ALERT** ▶ IM administration used only in acutely ill or pts unresponsive to oral route (GI malabsorption syndrome).

IM

- For IM injection in adults, if dosage is 1 ml (50,000 international units), may give in deltoid muscle; if dosage is over 1 ml, give in large muscle mass. Anterolateral thigh is site of choice for infants, children younger than 7 mos.

PO

- Do not crush, break capsules. • Give without regard to food.

INDICATIONS/ROUTES/DOSAGE

SEVERE VITAMIN A DEFICIENCY (WITH XEROPHTHALMIA)

PO: ADULTS, ELDERLY, CHILDREN 8 YRS AND OLDER: 500,000 units/day for 3 days; then 50,000 units/day for 14 days, then 10,000–20,000 units/day for 2 mos. **CHILDREN 1–7 YRS:** 5,000 units/kg/day for 5 days or until recovery occurs.

IM: ADULTS, ELDERLY, CHILDREN 8 YRS AND OLDER: 100,000 units/day for 3 days; then 50,000 units/day for 14 days. **CHILDREN 1–7 YRS:** 17,500–35,000 units/day for 10 days. **CHILDREN YOUNGER THAN 1 YR:** 7,500–15,000 units/day.

VITAMIN A DEFICIENCY (WITHOUT CORNEAL CHANGES)

PO: ADULTS, ELDERLY, CHILDREN 8 YRS AND OLDER: 100,000 units/day for 3 days, then 50,000 units/day for 14 days. **CHILDREN 1–7 YRS:** 200,000 units every 4–6 mos. **INFANTS LESS THAN 1 YR:** 100,000 units every 4–6 mos.

MALABSORPTION SYNDROME

PO: ADULTS, ELDERLY, CHILDREN 8 YRS AND OLDER: 10,000–50,000 units/day.

DIETARY SUPPLEMENT

PO: ADULTS, ELDERLY: 4,000–5,000 units/day. **CHILDREN 7–10 YRS:** 3,300–3,500 units/day. **CHILDREN 4–6 YRS:** 2,500 units/day. **CHILDREN 6 MOS–3 YRS:** 1,500–2,000 units/day. **NEONATES YOUNGER THAN 5 MOS:** 1,500 units/day.

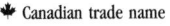

SIDE EFFECTS

None known.

V

ADVERSE EFFECTS/ TOXIC REACTIONS

Chronic overdose produces malaise, nausea, vomiting, drying/cracking of skin/lips, inflammation of tongue/gums, irritability, alopecia, night sweats. Bulging fontanelles have occurred in infants.

NURSING CONSIDERATIONS

INTERVENTION/EVALUATION

Closely supervise for overdosage symptoms during prolonged daily administration over 25,000 international units. Monitor for therapeutic serum vitamin A levels (80–300 international units/ml).

PATIENT/FAMILY TEACHING

• Foods rich in vitamin A include cod, halibut, tuna, shark (naturally occurring vitamin A found only in animal sources). • Avoid taking mineral oil, cholestyramine (Questran) while taking vitamin A.

vitamin D

vight-ah-myn D

ergocalciferol

(Calciferol, Drisdol, Ostoforte ✱)

CLASSIFICATION

PHARMACOTHERAPEUTIC: Fat-soluble vitamin. **CLINICAL:** Nutritional supplement (see p. 151C).

ACTION

Stimulates calcium/phosphate absorption from small intestine, promotes secretion of calcium from bone to blood, promotes resorption of phosphate in renal tubules; acts on bone cells to stimulate skeletal growth and on parathyroid gland to suppress hormone synthesis and secretion. **Therapeutic Effect:** Essential for absorption, utilization of calcium, phosphate, normal bone calcification.

PHARMACOKINETICS

Readily absorbed from small intestine. Concentrated primarily in liver, fat deposits. Activated in liver, kidneys. Eliminated by biliary system; excreted in urine. **Half-life:** 19–48 hrs for ergocalciferol.

USES

Prevention of osteoporosis. Treatment of rickets, hypophosphatemia, hypoparathyroidism. Dietary supplement.

PRECAUTIONS

CONTRAINDICATIONS: Vitamin D toxicity, hypercalcemia, malabsorption syndrome. **CAUTIONS:** Contrary artery disease, kidney stones, renal impairment.

LIFESPAN CONSIDERATIONS:

Pregnancy/Lactation: Unknown if drug crosses placenta. Distributed in breast milk. **Pregnancy Category A (C if used in doses above recommended daily allowance). Children:** May be more sensitive to effects. **Elderly:** No age-related precautions noted.

INTERACTIONS

DRUG: Aluminum-containing antacids (long-term use) may increase serum aluminum concentration, risk of aluminum bone toxicity. **Calcium-containing preparations, thiazide diuretics** may increase risk of hypercalcemia. **Magnesium-containing antacids** may increase serum magnesium concentration. Excessive use of **mineral oil** decreases absorption. **HERBAL:** None significant. **FOOD:** None known. **LAB VALUES:** May increase serum cholesterol, calcium, magnesium, phosphate. May decrease serum alkaline phosphatase.

AVAILABILITY (Rx)

INJECTION SOLUTION (CALCIFEROL): 500,000 units/ml (12.5 mg). **ORAL LIQUID DROPS (CALCIFEROL, DRISDOL):** 8,000 units/ml.

CAPSULES (DRISDOL): 50,000 units (1.25 mg).

ADMINISTRATION/HANDLING

PO

• Give without regard to food. • Swallow whole; do not crush/chew.

INDICATIONS/ROUTES/DOSAGE

◀ **ALERT** ▶ Oral dosing is preferred. Administer drug IM only in pts with GI, hepatic, biliary disease associated with malabsorption of vitamin D.

DIETARY SUPPLEMENT

PO: ADULTS, ELDERLY, CHILDREN: 10 mcg (400 units)/day. **NEONATES:** 10–20 mcg (400–800 units)/day.

RENAL FAILURE

PO: ADULTS, ELDERLY: 0.5 mg/day. **CHILDREN:** 0.1–1 mg/day.

HYPOPARATHYROIDISM

PO: ADULTS, ELDERLY: 625 mcg–5 mg/day (with calcium supplements). **CHILDREN:** 1.25–5 mg/day (with calcium supplements).

NUTRITIONAL RICKETS, OSTEOMALACIA

PO: ADULTS, ELDERLY, CHILDREN: 25–125 mcg/day for 8–12 wks. **ADULTS, ELDERLY (WITH MALABSORPTION SYNDROME):** 250–7,500 mcg/day. **CHILDREN (WITH MALABSORPTION SYNDROME):** 250–625 mcg/day.

VITAMIN D–DEPENDENT RICKETS

PO: ADULTS, ELDERLY: 250 mcg–1.5 mg/day. **CHILDREN:** 75–125 mcg/day. **Maximum:** 1,500 mcg/day.

VITAMIN D–RESISTANT RICKETS

PO: ADULTS, ELDERLY: 250–1,500 mcg/day (with phosphate supplements). **CHILDREN:** Initially 1,000–2,000 mcg/day (with phosphate supplements). May increase in 250- to 600-mcg increments q3–4mos.

OSTEOPOROSIS PREVENTION

PO: ADULTS, ELDERLY: 400–600 units/day. **Maximum:** 2,000 units/day.

SIDE EFFECTS

None known.

ADVERSE EFFECTS/ TOXIC REACTIONS

Early signs of overdose manifested as weakness, headache, somnolence, nausea, vomiting, dry mouth, constipation, muscle/bone pain, metallic taste. Later signs of overdose evidenced by polyuria, polydipsia, anorexia, weight loss, nocturia, photophobia, rhinorrhea, pruritus, disorientation, hallucinations, hyperthermia, hypertension, cardiac dysrhythmias.

NURSING CONSIDERATIONS

BASELINE ASSESSMENT

Therapy should begin at lowest possible dosage.

INTERVENTION/EVALUATION

Monitor serum, urinary calcium levels, serum phosphate, magnesium, creatinine, alkaline phosphatase, BUN determinations (therapeutic serum calcium level: 9–10 mg/dl). Estimate daily dietary calcium intake. Encourage adequate fluid intake.

PATIENT/FAMILY TEACHING

• Encourage foods rich in vitamin D, including vegetable oils, vegetable shortening, margarine, leafy vegetables, milk, eggs, meats. • Do not take mineral oil while on vitamin D therapy. • If receiving chronic renal dialysis, do not take magnesium-containing antacids during vitamin D therapy. • Drink plenty of liquids.

V

vitamin E

vight-ah-myn E
(Aquasol E, E-Gems, Key-E, Key-E Kaps)

Do not confuse Aquasol E with Anusol.

CLASSIFICATION

PHARMACOTHERAPEUTIC: Fat-soluble vitamin. **CLINICAL:** Nutritional supplement (see p. 151C).

ACTION

Prevents oxidation of vitamins A and C, protects fatty acids from attack by free radicals, protects RBCs from hemolysis by oxidizing agents. **Therapeutic Effect:** Prevents/treats vitamin E deficiency.

PHARMACOKINETICS

Variably absorbed from GI tract (requires bile salts, dietary fat, normal pancreatic function). Primarily concentrated in adipose tissue. Metabolized in liver. Primarily eliminated by biliary system.

USES

Treatment of hemolytic anemia secondary to vitamin E deficiency. **OFF-LABEL:** Prevention/treatment of Alzheimer's disease, tardive dyskinesia; reduces risk of bronchopulmonary dysplasia, retrolental fibroplasia in infants exposed to high concentrations of oxygen.

V

PRECAUTIONS

CONTRAINDICATIONS: None known. **CAUTIONS:** None known.

LIFESPAN CONSIDERATIONS:

Pregnancy/Lactation: Unknown if drug crosses placenta or is distributed in breast milk. **Pregnancy Category A (C if used in doses above recommended daily allowance). Children/Elderly:** No age-related precautions noted in normal dosages.

INTERACTIONS

DRUG: Cholestyramine, colestipol, mineral oil may decrease absorption. **Iron (large doses)** may increase vitamin E requirements. **HERBAL:** None significant. **FOOD:** None known. **LAB VALUES:** None known.

AVAILABILITY (OTC)

CAPSULES: 100 units (E-Gems), 200 units (Key-E Kaps), 400 units (Key-E Kaps), 600 units (E-Gems), 800 units (E-Gems), 1,000 units (E-Gems), 1,200 units (E-Gems). **TABLETS (KEY-E):** 100 units, 200 units, 400 units, 800 units.

ADMINISTRATION/HANDLING

PO

- Do not crush, break tablets/capsules.
- Give without regard to food.

INDICATIONS/ROUTES/DOSAGE

VITAMIN E DEFICIENCY

PO: ADULTS, ELDERLY: 60–75 units/day. **CHILDREN:** 1 unit/kg/day.

SIDE EFFECTS

RARE: Contact dermatitis, sterile abscess.

ADVERSE EFFECTS/ TOXIC REACTIONS

Chronic overdose may produce fatigue, weakness, nausea, headache, blurred vision, flatulence, diarrhea.

NURSING CONSIDERATIONS

PATIENT/FAMILY TEACHING

• Swallow tablets/capsules whole; do not crush, chew. • Toxicity consists of blurred vision, diarrhea, dizziness, nausea, headache, flu-like symptoms.

• Encourage foods rich in vitamin E, including vegetable oils, vegetable shortening, margarine, leafy vegetables, milk, eggs, meat.

vitamin K

vight-ah-myn K

phytonadione (vitamin K_1)

(AquaMEPHYTON, Konakion ✤, Mephyton, Vitamin K1)

Do not confuse Mephyton with melphalan or mephenytoin.

CLASSIFICATION

PHARMACOTHERAPEUTIC: Fat-soluble vitamin. **CLINICAL:** Nutritional supplement, antidote (drug-induced hypoprothrombinemia), antihemorrhagic.

ACTION

Promotes hepatic formation of coagulation factors II, VII, IX, X. **Therapeutic Effect:** Essential for normal clotting of blood.

PHARMACOKINETICS

Readily absorbed from GI tract (duodenum) after IM, subcutaneous administration. Metabolized in liver. Excreted in urine; eliminated by biliary system. Onset of action: with PO form, 6–10 hrs; with parenteral form, hemorrhage controlled in 3–6 hrs, PT returns to normal in 12–14 hrs.

USES

Prevention, treatment of hemorrhagic states in neonates; antidote for hemorrhage induced by oral anticoagulants, hypoprothrombinemic states due to vitamin K deficiency. Will not counteract anticoagulation effect of heparin.

PRECAUTIONS

CONTRAINDICATIONS: None known. **CAUTIONS:** None known.

LIFESPAN CONSIDERATIONS:

Pregnancy/Lactation: Crosses placenta. Distributed in breast milk. **Pregnancy Category C. Children/Elderly:** No age-related precautions noted.

INTERACTIONS

DRUG: Broad-spectrum antibiotics, high-dose salicylates may increase vitamin K requirements. **Cholestyramine, colestipol, mineral oil, sucralfate** may decrease absorption. May decrease effects of **oral anticoagulants. HERBAL:** None significant. **FOOD:** None known. **LAB VALUES:** None known.

AVAILABILITY (Rx)

INJECTION SOLUTION (AQUAMEPHYTON, VITAMIN K1): 1 mg/0.5 ml, 10 mg/ml. **TABLETS (MEPHYTON):** 5 mg.

ADMINISTRATION/HANDLING

IV

◀ **ALERT** ▶ Restrict to emergency use only.

Reconstitution • May dilute with preservative-free NaCl or D_5W immediately before use. Do not use other diluents. Discard unused portions.

Rate of administration • Administer slow IV at rate of 1 mg/min. • Monitor continuously for hypersensitivity, anaphylactic reaction during and immediately following IV administration.

Storage • Store at room temperature.

IM, SUBCUTANEOUS

• Inject into anterolateral aspect of thigh, deltoid region.

PO

- Scored tablets may be crushed.

IV INCOMPATIBILITIES

No known incompatibilities for Y-site administration.

IV COMPATIBILITIES

Heparin, potassium chloride.

INDICATIONS/ROUTES/DOSAGE

◀ **ALERT** ▶

PO/Subcutaneous route preferred; IV/IM use restricted to emergent situations.

ORAL ANTICOAGULANT OVERDOSE

PO, IV, SUBCUTANEOUS: ADULTS, ELDERLY: 2.5–10 mg/dose. May repeat in 12–48 hrs if given orally, in 6–8 hrs if given by IV or subcutaneous route. **CHILDREN:** 0.5–5 mg depending on need for further anticoagulation, severity of bleeding.

VITAMIN K DEFICIENCY

PO: ADULTS, ELDERLY: 2.5–25 mg/24 hrs. **CHILDREN:** 2.5–5 mg/24 hrs.

IV, IM, SUBCUTANEOUS: ADULTS, ELDERLY: 10 mg/dose. **CHILDREN:** 1–2 mg/dose.

HEMORRHAGIC DISEASE OF NEWBORN

IM, SUBCUTANEOUS: NEONATE: Treatment: 1–2 mg. **Prophylaxis:** 0.5–1 mg within 1 hr of birth.

SIDE EFFECTS

◀ **ALERT** ▶ PO/subcutaneous administration less likely to produce side effects than IV/IM routes.

OCCASIONAL: Pain, soreness, swelling at IM injection site; pruritic erythema (with repeated injections); facial flushing; altered taste.

ADVERSE EFFECTS/ TOXIC REACTIONS

Newborns (esp. premature infants) may develop hyperbilirubinemia. Severe reaction (cramp-like pain, chest pain, dyspnea, facial flushing, dizziness, rapid/weak pulse, rash, diaphoresis, hypotension progressing to shock, cardiac arrest) occurs rarely, immediately after IV administration.

NURSING CONSIDERATIONS

INTERVENTION/EVALUATION

Monitor prothrombin time (PT), INR routinely in those taking anticoagulants. Assess skin for ecchymoses, petechiae. Assess gums for gingival bleeding, erythema. Assess urine for hematuria. Assess Hct, platelet count, urine/stool culture for occult blood. Assess for decrease in B/P, increase in pulse rate, complaint of abdominal/back pain, severe headache (may be evidence of hemorrhage). Question for increase in amount of discharge during menses. Assess peripheral pulses. Check for excessive bleeding from minor cuts, scratches.

PATIENT/FAMILY TEACHING

- Discomfort may occur with parenteral administration. • **Adults:** Use electric razor, soft toothbrush to prevent bleeding. • Report any sign of red or dark urine, black or red stool, coffee-ground vomitus, red-speckled mucus from cough. • Do not use any OTC medication without physician approval (may interfere with platelet aggregation).
- Encourage foods rich in vitamin K_1, including leafy green vegetables, meat, cow's milk, vegetable oil, egg yolks, tomatoes.

Vivelle-DOT, *see estradiol*

voriconazole

vohr-ee-**con**-ah-zole
(Vfend)

CLASSIFICATION

PHARMACOTHERAPEUTIC: Triazole derivative. **CLINICAL:** Antifungal.

ACTION

Inhibits synthesis of ergosterol (vital component of fungal cell wall formation). **Therapeutic Effect:** Damages fungal cell wall membrane.

PHARMACOKINETICS

Rapidly, completely absorbed after PO administration. Widely distributed. Protein binding: 98%. Metabolized in liver. Primarily excreted as metabolite in urine. **Half-life:** 6 hrs.

USES

Treatment of invasive aspergillosis, esophageal candidiasis. Treatment of serious fungal infections caused by *Scedosporium apiospermum, Fusarium* spp. Treatment of candidemia in non-neutropenic pts.

PRECAUTIONS

CONTRAINDICATIONS: Concurrent administration of carbamazepine; ergot alkaloids; pimozide, quinidine (may cause prolonged QT interval, torsades de pointes); rifabutin; rifampin; ritonavir; sirolimus. **CAUTIONS:** Renal/hepatic impairment, hypersensitivity to other antifungal agents.

LIFESPAN CONSIDERATIONS:

Pregnancy/Lactation: May cause fetal harm. **Pregnancy Category D. Children:** Safety and efficacy not established in those younger than 12 yrs. **Elderly:** No age-related precautions noted.

INTERACTIONS

DRUG: May increase concentration, risk of toxicity of **alprazolam, midazolam, triazolam, calcium channel blockers, warfarin, cyclosporine, tacrolimus, efavirenz, ergot alkoloids, HMG-CoA reductase inhibitors (e.g., lovastatin), methadone, rifabutin, protease inhibitors (e.g., amprenavir, saquinavir), sirolimus. Carbamazepine, rifampin, rifabutin, ritonavir** may decrease concentration, effect. **HERBAL: St. John's wort** may decrease concentration. **FOOD:** None known. **LAB VALUES:** May increase serum alkaline phosphatase, ALT.

AVAILABILITY (Rx)

INJECTION, POWDER FOR RECONSTITUTION: 200 mg. **POWDER FOR ORAL SUSPENSION:** 200 mg/5 ml. **TABLETS:** 50 mg, 200 mg.

ADMINISTRATION/HANDLING

IV

Reconstitution • Reconstitute 200-mg vial with 19 ml Sterile Water for Injection to provide concentration of 10 mg/ml. Further dilute with 0.9% NaCl or D_5W to provide concentration of 5 mg or less/ml.

Rate of administration • Infuse over 1–2 hrs at a concentration of 5 mg or less/ml.

Storage • Store powder for injection at room temperature. • Use reconstituted solution immediately. • Do not use after 24 hrs when refrigerated.

PO

- Give 1 hr before or 1 hr after a meal.
- Do not mix oral suspension with any other medication or flavoring agent.

IV INCOMPATIBILITY

Total parenteral nutrition (TPN).

V

INDICATIONS/ROUTES/DOSAGE

INVASIVE ASPERGILLOSIS, OTHER SERIOUS FUNGAL INFECTION

PO: ADULTS, ELDERLY WEIGHING 40 KG OR MORE: Initially, 400 mg q12h for 2 doses on day 1. Maintenance: 200 mg q12h (may increase to 200 mg q12h). **ADULTS, ELDERLY WEIGHING LESS THAN 40 KG:** Initially, 200 mg q12h for 2 doses on day 1. Maintenance: 100 mg q12h (may increase to 150 mg q12h).

USUAL PARENTERAL DOSAGE

IV: ADULTS, ELDERLY, CHILDREN: Initially, 6 mg/kg/dose q12h for 2 doses, then 4 mg/kg/dose q12h (may decrease to 3 mg/kg/dose if pt is unable to tolerate 4 mg/kg/dose).

CANDIDEMIA IN NON-NEUTROPENIC PTS

PO: ADULTS, ELDERLY: 200 mg q12h.
IV: ADULTS, ELDERLY: Initially, 6 mg/kg/dose q12h for 2 doses, then 3–4 mg/kg/dose q12h.

ESOPHAGEAL CANDIDIASIS

PO: ADULTS, ELDERLY WEIGHING 40 KG OR MORE: 200 mg q12h for minimum of 14 days, then at least 7 days following resolution of symptoms. **ADULTS, ELDERLY WEIGHING LESS THAN 40 KG:** 100 mg q12h for minimum 14 days, then at least 7 days following resolution of symptoms.

SIDE EFFECTS

FREQUENT (20%–5%): Abnormal vision, fever, nausea, rash, vomiting. **OCCASIONAL (5%–2%):** Headache, chills, hallucinations, photophobia, tachycardia, hypertension.

ADVERSE EFFECTS/ TOXIC REACTIONS

Hepatotoxicity (jaundice, hepatitis, hepatic failure), acute renal failure have occured in severely ill pts.

NURSING CONSIDERATIONS

BASELINE ASSESSMENT

Obtain baseline serum hepatic/renal function tests.

INTERVENTION/EVALUATION

Monitor serum hepatic/renal function tests. Monitor visual function (visual acuity, visual field, color perception) for drug therapy lasting longer than 28 days.

PATIENT/FAMILY TEACHING

• Take at least 1 hr before or 1 hr after a meal. • Avoid driving at night. • May cause visual changes (blurred vision, photophobia). • Avoid performing hazardous tasks if changes in vision occur. • Avoid direct sunlight. • Women of childbearing potential should use effective contraception.

vorinostat

vor-**in**-oh-stat
(Zolinza)

CLASSIFICATION

PHARMACOTHERAPEUTIC: Histone deacetylase inhibitor. **CLINICAL:** Antineoplastic.

ACTION

Inhibits activity of specific enzymes that catalyze removal of acetyl groups of proteins, causing accumulation of acetylated histones. **Therapeutic Effect:** Induces cell arrest.

PHARMACOKINETICS

Protein binding: 71%. Metabolized to inactive metabolites. Excreted in urine. **Half–life:** 2 hrs.

V

USES

Treatment of cutaneous manifestations in pts with cutaneous T-cell lymphoma (CTCL) with progressive, persistent or recurrent disease, on or following two systemic therapies.

PRECAUTIONS

CONTRAINDICATIONS: None significant. **CAUTIONS:** History of deep vein thrombosis (DVT), diabetes mellitus, hepatic impairment, preexisting renal impairment, those with QT prolongation.

LIFESPAN CONSIDERATIONS:

Pregnancy/Lactation: May cause fetal harm. Unkown if distributed in breast milk. **Pregnancy Category D.** **Children:** Safety and efficacy not established. **Elderly:** No age-related precautions noted.

INTERACTIONS

DRUG: May increase effect of **warfarin.** **Valproic acid** increases risk of GI bleeding, thrombocytopenia. **Concomitant QT prolonging agents** may increase risk of arrhythmia. **HERBAL:** None significant. **FOOD:** None known. **LAB VALUES:** May decrease Hgb, Hct, platelet count. May increase serum glucose, creatinine, urine protein.

AVAILABILITY (Rx)

CAPSULES: 100 mg.

ADMINISTRATION/HANDLING

PO

• Do not open, crush capsules. • Give with food.

INDICATIONS/ROUTES/DOSAGE

CUTANEOUS T-CELL LYMPHOMA

PO: ADULTS, ELDERLY: 400 mg once daily with food. Dose may be reduced to 300 mg once daily with food. May be further reduced to 300 mg once daily with food for 5 consecutive days each wk.

SIDE EFFECTS

FREQUENT (52%): Fatigue, diarrhea (52%), nausea (40%), altered taste (28%), anorexia (24%). **OCCASIONAL (21%–11%):** Weight decrease, muscle spasms, alopecia, dry mouth, chills, vomiting, constipation, dizziness, peripheral edema, headache, pruritus, cough, fever.

ADVERSE EFFECTS/ TOXIC REACTIONS

Thrombocytopenia occurs in 25% of pts, anemia in 15%. Pulmonary embolism occurs in 4% of pts. DVT occurs rarely.

NURSING CONSIDERATIONS

BASELINE ASSESSMENT

Baseline PT, INR, CBC, chemistry tests, esp. serum potassium, calcium, magnesium, glucose, creatinine should be obtained prior to therapy and every 2 wks during first 2 mos of therapy and monthly therafter. Inform women of childbearing potential of risk to fetus if pregnancy occurs.

INTERVENTION/EVALUATION

Monitor platelet count, PT, INR, serum electrolytes during first 2 mos of therapy. Monitor signs/symptoms of DVT. Encourage fluid intake approximately 2 L/day input, electrolytes, CBC. Assess for evidence of dehydration. Provide antiemetics to control nausea/ vomiting. Monitor daily pattern of bowel activity/stool consistency.

PATIENT/FAMILY TEACHING

• Drink at least 2 L/day of fluids to prevent dehydration. • Report excessive vomiting, diarrhea. • Contact physician if shortness of breath, pain in any extremity occurs.

warfarin

war-far-in

(Apo-Warfarin ♣, Coumadin, Gen-Warfarin ♣, Jantoven)

Do not confuse Coumadin with Kemadrin.

CLASSIFICATION

PHARMACOTHERAPEUTIC: Coumarin derivative. **CLINICAL:** Anticoagulant (see p. 30C).

ACTION

Interferes with hepatic synthesis of vitamin K–dependent clotting factors, resulting in depletion of coagulation factors II, VII, IX, X. **Therapeutic Effect:** Prevents further extension of formed existing clot; prevents new clot formation, secondary thromboembolic complications.

PHARMACOKINETICS

Route	Onset	Peak	Duration
PO	1.5–3 days	5–7 days	N/A

Well absorbed from GI tract. Metabolized in liver. Primarily excreted in urine. Not removed by hemodialysis. **Half-life:** 1.5–2.5 days.

USES

Anticoagulant, prophylaxis, treatment of venous thrombosis, pulmonary embolism. Treatment of thromboembolism associated with chronic atrial fibrillation. Adjunct in treatment of coronary occlusion. Prophylaxis, treatment of thromboembolic complications associated with cardiac valve replacement. Reduces risk of death, recurrent MI, stroke, embolization after MI. **OFF-LABEL:** Prevention of MI, recurrent cerebral embolism; treatment adjunct in transient ischemic attacks.

PRECAUTIONS

CONTRAINDICATIONS: Neurosurgical procedures, open wounds, pregnancy, severe hypertension, severe hepatic/renal damage, spinal puncture, uncontrolled bleeding, ulcers. **CAUTIONS:** Active tuberculosis, diabetes, heparin-induced thrombocytopenia, those at risk for hemorrhage, necrosis, gangrene.

LIFESPAN CONSIDERATIONS:

Pregnancy/Lactation: Contraindicated in pregnancy (fetal, neonatal hemorrhage, intrauterine death). Crosses placenta; distributed in breast milk. **Pregnancy Category X. Children:** More susceptible to effects. **Elderly:** Increased risk of hemorrhage; lower dosage recommended.

INTERACTIONS

DRUG: Amiodarone, anabolic steroids, azole antifungals, NSAIDs, antithyroid medications, cimetidine, clofibrate, dextrothyroxine, difunisal, disulfiram, fluvoxamine, lepirudin, metronidazole, omeprazole, paroxetine, platelet aggregation inhibitors, salicylates, sertraline, thrombolytic agents, thyroid hormones, ticlopidine, zafirlukast may increase effects. **Griseofulvin, hepatic enzyme inducers, vitamin K** may decrease effects. **Alcohol** may enhance anticoagulant effect. **HERBAL: Cat's claw, dong quai, evening primrose, feverfew, garlic, ginkgo biloba, ginger, red clover, horse chestnut, ginseng** possess antiplatelet activity, may increase risk of bleeding. **FOOD:** None known. **LAB VALUES:** None known.

AVAILABILITY (Rx)

TABLETS (COUMADIN, JANTOVEN): 1 mg, 2 mg, 2.5 mg, 3 mg, 4 mg, 5 mg, 6 mg, 7.5 mg, 10 mg.

ADMINISTRATION/HANDLING

PO

• Scored tablets may be crushed. • Give without regard to food. Give with food if GI upset occurs.

INDICATIONS/ROUTES/DOSAGE

ANTICOAGULANT

PO: ADULTS, ELDERLY: Initially, 5–15 mg/day for 2–5 days; then adjust based on INR. Maintenance: 2–10 mg/day. **CHILDREN:** Initially, 0.05–0.2 mg/kg (**maximum:** 10 mg). Maintenance: 0.05–0.34 mg/kg/day.

SIDE EFFECTS

OCCASIONAL: GI distress (nausea, anorexia, abdominal cramps, diarrhea). **RARE:** Hypersensitivity reaction, (dermatitis, urticaria) esp. in those sensitive to aspirin.

ADVERSE EFFECTS/ TOXIC REACTIONS

Bleeding complications ranging from local ecchymoses to major hemorrhage may occur. Drug should be discontinued immediately and vitamin K (phytonadione) administered. **Mild hemorrhage:** 2.5–10 mg PO, IM, or IV. **Severe hemorrhage:** 10–15 mg IV repeated q4h, as necessary. Hepatotoxicity, blood dyscrasias, necrosis, vasculitis, local thrombosis occur rarely.

NURSING CONSIDERATIONS

BASELINE ASSESSMENT

Cross-check dose with coworker. Determine INR before administration and daily following therapy initiation. When stabilized, follow with INR determination q4–6wk.

INTERVENTION/EVALUATION

Monitor INR reports diligently. Assess Hct, platelet count, urine/stool culture for occult blood, AST, ALT, regardless of route of administration. Be alert to complaints of abdominal/back pain, severe headache (may be signs of hemorrhage). Decrease in B/P, increase in pulse rate may be signs of hemorrhage. Question for increase in amount of menstrual discharge. Assess area of thromboembolus for color, temperature. Assess peripheral pulses; skin for ecchymoses, petechiae. Check for excessive bleeding from minor cuts, scratches. Assess gums for erythema, gingival bleeding. Assess urinary output for hematuria.

PATIENT/FAMILY TEACHING

• Take medication exactly as prescribed. • Do not take, discontinue any other medication except on advice of physician. • Avoid alcohol, salicylates, drastic dietary changes. • Do not change from one brand to another. • Consult with physician before surgery, dental work. • Urine may become red-orange. • Notify physician if bleeding, bruising, red or brown urine, black stools occur. • Use electric razor, soft toothbrush to prevent bleeding. • Report coffee-ground vomitus, blood-tinged mucus from cough. • Do not use any OTC medication without physician approval (may interfere with platelet aggregation).

Wellbutrin, *see bupropion*

Wellbutrin SR, *see bupropion*

Xanax, *see alprazolam*

Xeloda, *see capecitabine*

Xifaxan, *see rifaximin*

W

Xigris, *see drotrecogin alfa*

Xopenex, *see levalbuterol*

yohimbe

Also known as aphrodien, corynine, johimbi.

CLASSIFICATION

HERBAL: See Appendix G.

ACTION

Produces genital blood vessel dilation, improves nerve impulse transmission to genital area. Increases penile blood flow, central sympathetic excitation impulses to genital tissues. **Effect:** Improves sexual function, affects impotence.

USES

Used as aphrodisiac by some cultures. Used to improve libido, enhance sexual function in male. Used to manage symptoms associated with diabetic neuropathy, postural hypotension.

PRECAUTIONS

CONTRAINDICATIONS: Pregnancy, lactation (may have uterine relaxant effect, cause fetal toxicity), angina, heart disease, benign prostatic hypertrophy (BPH), depression, renal/hepatic disease. **CAUTIONS:** Anxiety, diabetes mellitus, hypertension, post-traumatic stress disorder (PSTD), schizophrenia.

LIFESPAN CONSIDERATIONS: **Pregnancy/Lactation:** Contraindicated; avoid use. **Children:** Safety and efficacy not established; avoid use. **Elderly:** Age-related renal/hepatic impairment may require discontinuing.

INTERACTIONS

DRUG: May interfere with **antihypertensives, antidiabetic agents.** May antagonize effects of **clonidine. MAOIs, sympathomimetics, tricyclic antidepressants** may have additive effects. **HERBAL: Ginkgo biloba, St. John's wort** may have additive therapeutic, adverse effects. **FOOD: Foods containing tyramine, caffeine** may increase risk of hypertensive crises. **LAB VALUES:** None known.

AVAILABILITY (OTC)

LIQUID: 5 mg/5 ml. **TABLETS:** 5 mg.

INDICATIONS/ROUTES/DOSAGE

IMPOTENCE

PO: ADULTS, ELDERLY: 15–30 mg/day in divided doses.

SIDE EFFECTS

Excitement, tremor, insomnia, anxiety, hypertension, tachycardia, dizziness, headache, irritability, salivation, dilated pupils, nausea, vomiting, hypersensitivity reaction.

ADVERSE EFFECTS/ TOXIC REACTIONS

Paralysis, severe hypotension, irregular heartbeat, cardiac failure may occur. Overdose can be fatal.

NURSING CONSIDERATIONS

BASELINE ASSESSMENT

Assess if pt is pregnant or breast-feeding (contraindicated). Determine other medical conditions, including angina, heart disease, BPH. Assess baseline serum renal/hepatic function, medications (see Interactions).

INTERVENTION/EVALUATION

Monitor serum renal/hepatic function, B/P. Assess for hypersensitivity reaction.

PATIENT/FAMILY TEACHING

• Do not use other OTC or prescribed medications before checking with physician. • Inform physician if pregnant or breast-feeding.

zafirlukast

za-**feer**-loo-kast

(Accolate)

Do not confuse Accolate with Accupril or Aclovate.

CLASSIFICATION

PHARMACOTHERAPEUTIC: Leukotriene receptor antagonist. **CLINICAL:** Antiasthma (see p. 72C).

ACTION

Binds to leukotriene receptors, inhibiting bronchoconstriction due to sulfur dioxide, cold air, specific antigens (grass, cat dander, ragweed). **Therapeutic Effect:** Reduces airway edema, smooth muscle constriction; alters cellular activity associated with inflammatory process.

PHARMACOKINETICS

Rapidly absorbed after PO administration (food reduces absorption). Protein binding: 99%. Extensively metabolized in liver. Primarily excreted in feces. Unknown if removed by hemodialysis. **Half-life:** 10 hrs.

USES

Prophylaxis, chronic treatment of bronchial asthma. **OFF-LABEL:** Exercise-induced bronchospasm.

PRECAUTIONS

CONTRAINDICATIONS: None known. **CAUTIONS:** Hepatic impairment.

LIFESPAN CONSIDERATIONS:

Pregnancy/Lactation: Drug is distributed in breast milk. Do not administer to breast-feeding women. **Pregnancy Category B. Children:** Safety and efficacy not established in those younger than 5 yrs. **Elderly:** No age-related precautions noted.

INTERACTIONS

DRUG: Aspirin increases concentration. **Erythromycin, theophylline** decrease concentration. **Warfarin** increases prothrombin time (PT). **HERBAL:** None significant. **FOOD: Food** decreases bioavailability by 40%. **LAB VALUES:** May increase ALT.

AVAILABILITY (Rx)

TABLETS: 10 mg, 20 mg.

ADMINISTRATION/HANDLING

PO

• Give 1 hr before or 2 hrs after meals.

INDICATIONS/ROUTES/DOSAGE

BRONCHIAL ASTHMA

PO: ADULTS, ELDERLY, CHILDREN 12 YRS AND OLDER: 20 mg twice a day. **CHILDREN 5–11 YRS:** 10 mg twice a day.

SIDE EFFECTS

FREQUENT (13%): Headache. **OCCASIONAL (3%):** Nausea, diarrhea. **RARE (less than 3%):** Generalized pain, asthenia (loss of strength, energy), myalgia, fever, dyspepsia (heartburn, indigestion, epigastric pain), vomiting, dizziness.

ADVERSE EFFECTS/ TOXIC REACTIONS

Concurrent administration of inhaled corticosteroids increases risk of upper respiratory tract infection.

NURSING CONSIDERATIONS

BASELINE ASSESSMENT

Obtain medication history. Assess serum hepatic function lab values.

INTERVENTION/EVALUATION

Monitor rate, depth, rhythm, type of respiration; quality, rate of pulse. Assess lung sounds for rhonchi, wheezing, rales. Observe for cyanosis (lips, fingernails appear blue or dusky color in light-skinned pts; gray in dark-skinned pts). Monitor serum hepatic function tests.

PATIENT/FAMILY TEACHING

• Increase fluid intake (decreases lung secretion viscosity). • Take as prescribed, even during symptom-free periods. • Do not use for acute asthma episodes. • Do not alter, stop other asthma medications. • Do not breast-feed. • Report nausea, jaundice, abdominal pain, flu-like symptoms, worsening of asthma.

zalcitabine

zal-**site**-a-been
(Hivid)

CLASSIFICATION

PHARMACOTHERAPEUTIC: Nucleoside reverse transcriptase inhibitor. **CLINICAL:** Antiretroviral (see pp. 66C, 111C).

ACTION

Inhibits viral DNA synthesis. **Therapeutic Effect:** Prevents replication of HIV-1.

PHARMACOKINETICS

Readily absorbed from GI tract (absorption decreased by food). Protein binding: less than 4%. Undergoes phosphorylation intracellularly to active metabolite. Primarily excreted in urine. Removed by hemodialysis. **Half-life:** 1–3 hrs; metabolite, 2.6–10 hrs (increased in renal impairment).

USES

Treatment of HIV infection in combination with other antiretroviral agents.

PRECAUTIONS

CONTRAINDICATIONS: Moderate or severe peripheral neuropathy. **EXTREME CAUTION:** Those with low CD4 cell counts (risk of peripheral neuropathy is greater), preexisting neuropathy. **CAUTIONS:** Preexisting peripheral neuropathy, diabetes, weight loss, history of hepatic disease, alcohol abuse, renal impairment.

LIFESPAN CONSIDERATIONS:

Pregnancy/Lactation: Unknown if drug crosses placenta or is distributed in breast milk. Avoid breast-feeding in HIV-positive women. **Pregnancy Category C. Children:** No age-related precautions in those younger than 6 mos, dosage not established. **Elderly:** Age-related renal impairment may require dosage adjustment.

INTERACTIONS

DRUG: Alcohol, azathioprine, pentamidine IV, tetracyclines, thiazide diuretics, valproic acid may increase risk of pancreatitis. May increase risk of peripheral neuropathy with **aminoglycosides, amphotericin B, foscarnet, cisplatin, didanosine, lithium, phenytoin, stavudine. Aluminum- or magnesium-containing, antacids** may decrease absorption. **Cimetidine, probenecid** may increase concentration, risk of toxicity. **HERBAL:** None significant. **FOOD: Food** decreases rate/extent of absorption. **LAB VALUES:** May increase serum alkaline phosphatase, amylase, bilirubin, lipase, AST, ALT, triglycerides. May decrease serum calcium, magnesium, phosphate. May alter serum glucose, sodium.

AVAILABILITY (Rx)

TABLETS: 0.375 mg, 0.75 mg.

ADMINISTRATION/HANDLING

PO

• Best given on empty stomach (food decreases absorption). • May give with food to decrease GI distress. • Space doses evenly around the clock.

INDICATIONS/ROUTES/DOSAGE

HIV INFECTION

PO: ADULTS, CHILDREN 13 YRS AND OLDER: 0.75 mg q8h. **CHILDREN YOUNGER THAN 13 YRS:** 0.01 mg/kg q8h. Range: 0.005–0.01 mg/kg q8h.

DOSAGE IN RENAL IMPAIRMENT

Dosage and frequency are modified based on creatinine clearance.

Creatinine Clearance	Dose
10–40 ml/min	0.75 mg q12h
Less than 10 ml/min	0.75 mg q24h

SIDE EFFECTS

FREQUENT (28%–11%): Peripheral neuropathy, fever, fatigue, headache, rash. **OCCASIONAL (10%–5%):** Diarrhea, abdominal pain, oral ulcers, cough, pruritus, myalgia, weight loss, nausea, vomiting. **RARE (4%–1%):** Nasal discharge, dysphagia, depression, night sweats, confusion.

ADVERSE EFFECTS/ TOXIC REACTIONS

Peripheral neuropathy occurs commonly (31%–17%), characterized by numbness, tingling, burning, pain in lower extremities. May be followed by sharp, shooting pain and progress to severe, continuous, burning pain that may be irreversible if drug is not discontinued in time. Pancreatitis, leukopenia, neutropenia, eosinophilia, thrombocytopenia occur rarely.

NURSING CONSIDERATIONS

BASELINE ASSESSMENT

Monitor CBC, serum triglycerides, amylase levels before and during therapy.

INTERVENTION/EVALUATION

Stop medication, notify physician immediately if signs/symptoms of peripheral neuropathy develop: numbness, tingling, burning, shooting pains of extremities; loss of vibratory sense, ankle reflex. Although rare, be alert to impending potentially fatal pancreatitis: increasing serum amylase, rising serum triglycerides, nausea, vomiting, abdominal pain (withhold medication, notify physician). Assess for therapeutic response: weight gain, increased energy, decreased fatigue. Assess CBC for evidence of blood dyscrasias. Offer emotional support to pt, family.

PATIENT/FAMILY TEACHING

• Zalcitabine is not a cure for HIV, nor does it reduce the risk of transmission to others; pt may continue to contract opportunistic illnesses associated with advanced HIV infection. • Does not preclude need to continue practices to prevent transmission of HIV. • Report promptly any signs/symptoms of peripheral neuropathy, pancreatitis. • Women of childbearing age should use contraception.

zaleplon

zal-e-plon
(Sonata, Starnoc ♣)

CLASSIFICATION

PHARMACOTHERAPEUTIC: Nonbenzodiazepine. **CLINICAL:** Hypnotic (see p. 141C).

ACTION

Enhances action of inhibitory neurotransmitter gamma-aminobutyric acid (GABA). **Therapeutic Effect:** Induces sleep.

PHARMACOKINETICS

Rapidly, almost completely absorbed following PO administration. Protein binding: 60%. Metabolized in liver. Primarily excreted in urine. Partially eliminated in feces. **Half-life:** 1 hr.

USES

Short-term treatment of insomnia (7–10 days). Decreases sleep onset time (no effect on number of nocturnal awakenings, total sleep time).

PRECAUTIONS

CONTRAINDICATIONS: Severe hepatic impairment. **CAUTIONS:** Mild to moderate hepatic impairment in pts experiencing signs/symptoms of depression, those hypersensitive to aspirin (allergic-type reaction).

LIFESPAN CONSIDERATIONS:

Pregnancy/Lactation: Unknown if drug crosses placenta; is distributed in breast milk. **Pregnancy Category C. Children:** Safety and efficacy not established. **Elderly:** May be more sensitive to zaleplon effects.

INTERACTIONS

DRUG: Alcohol, other CNS depressants may increase CNS depression. **Cimetidine** may increase effect. **Carbamazepine, phenobarbital, phenytoin, rifampin** may decrease concentration. **HERBAL: Gotu kola, kava kava, St. John's wort, valerian** may increase CNS depression. **FOOD: High-fat, heavy meals** may delay onset of sleep by approximately 2 hrs. **LAB VALUES:** None known.

AVAILABILITY (Rx)

CAPSULES: 5 mg, 10 mg.

ADMINISTRATION/HANDLING

PO

• Giving drug with or immediately after high-fat meal results in slower absorption. • Capsules may be emptied and mixed with food.

INDICATIONS/ROUTES/DOSAGE

INSOMNIA

PO: ADULTS: 10 mg at bedtime. Range: 5–20 mg. **ELDERLY:** 5 mg at bedtime.

SIDE EFFECTS

EXPECTED: Drowsiness, sedation, mild rebound insomnia (on first night after drug is discontinued). **FREQUENT (28%–7%):** Nausea, headache, myalgia, dizziness. **OCCASIONAL (5%–3%):** Abdominal pain, asthenia (loss of strength, energy), dyspepsia (heartburn, indigestion, epigastric pain), eye pain, paresthesia. **RARE (2%):** Tremor, amnesia, hyperacusis (acute sense of hearing), fever, dysmenorrhea.

ADVERSE EFFECTS/ TOXIC REACTIONS

May produce altered concentration/ behavior changes, impaired memory. Taking medication while ambulating may result in hallucinations, impaired coordination, dizziness, light-headedness. Overdose results in drowsiness, confusion, diminished reflexes, coma.

NURSING CONSIDERATIONS

BASELINE ASSESSMENT

Provide for safety; raise bed rails. Provide environment conducive to sleep (back rub, quiet environment, low lighting).

INTERVENTION/EVALUATION

Assess sleep pattern.

PATIENT/FAMILY TEACHING

• Take right before bedtime or when in bed and not falling asleep. • Avoid tasks that require alertness, motor skills until response to drug is established. • Do not exceed prescribed dosage. • Do not take with or immediately after a high-fat or heavy meal. • Rebound insomnia may occur when drug is discontinued after short-term therapy. • Avoid alcohol, other CNS depressants.

Zanaflex, *see tizanidine*

zanamivir

zah-**nam**-ih-vur
(Relenza)

CLASSIFICATION

PHARMACOTHERAPEUTIC: Antiviral.
CLINICAL: Anti-influenza (see p. 66C).

ACTION

Appears to inhibit influenza virus enzyme neuraminidase, essential for viral replication. **Therapeutic Effect:** Prevents viral release from infected cells.

PHARMACOKINETICS

Systemically absorbed, approximately 4%–17%. Protein binding: Low. Not metabolized. Partially excreted unchanged in urine. **Half-life:** 1.6–5.1 hrs.

USES

Treatment of uncomplicated acute illness due to influenza virus A and B in adults, adolescents 7 yrs and older who have been symptomatic for less than 2 days. Prevention of influenza A and B. **OFF-LABEL:** Influenza prophylaxis.

PRECAUTIONS

CONTRAINDICATIONS: None known. **CAUTIONS:** Chronic obstructive pulmonary disease (COPD), asthma.

LIFESPAN CONSIDERATIONS:

Pregnancy/Lactation: Unknown if drug crosses placenta or is distributed in breast milk. **Pregnancy Category C.** **Children:** Safety and efficacy not established in children younger than 7 yrs. **Elderly:** No age-related precautions noted.

INTERACTIONS

DRUG: None significant. **HERBAL:** None significant. **FOOD:** None known. **LAB VALUES:** May increase serum creatine kinase (CK), hepatic function test results.

AVAILABILITY (Rx)

POWDER FOR INHALATION: 5 mg/blister.

ADMINISTRATION/HANDLING

INHALATION

• Using Diskhaler device provided, exhale completely; then, holding mouthpiece 1 inch away from lips, inhale and hold breath as long as possible before exhaling. • Rinse mouth with water immediately after inhalation (prevents mouth/throat dryness). • Store at room temperature.

INDICATIONS/ROUTES/DOSAGE

INFLUENZA VIRUS

INHALATION: ADULTS, ELDERLY, CHILDREN 7 YRS AND OLDER: 2 inhalations (one 5-mg blister per inhalation for a total dose of 10 mg) twice a day (approximately 12 hrs apart) for 5 days.

PREVENTION OF INFLUENZA VIRUS

INHALATION: ADULTS, ELDERLY: 2 inhalations once a day for the duration of the exposure period.

SIDE EFFECTS

OCCASIONAL (3%–2%): Diarrhea, sinusitis, nausea, bronchitis, cough, dizziness, headache. **RARE (less than 1.5%):** Malaise, fatigue, fever, abdominal pain, myalgia, arthralgia, urticaria.

ADVERSE EFFECTS/ TOXIC REACTIONS

May produce neutropenia. Bronchospasm may occur in those with history of COPD, bronchial asthma.

NURSING CONSIDERATIONS

BASELINE ASSESSMENT

Pts requiring an inhaled bronchodilator at same time as zanamivir should use the bronchodilator before zanamivir administration.

INTERVENTION/EVALUATION

Provide assistance if dizziness occurs. Monitor daily pattern of bowel activity/stool consistency.

PATIENT/FAMILY TEACHING

• Instruct on use of delivery device. • Avoid contact with those who are at high risk for influenza. • Continue treatment for full 5-day course. • Doses should be evenly spaced. • In pts with respiratory disease, an inhaled bronchodilator should be readily available.

Zantac, *see ranitidine*

Zaroxolyn, *see metolazone*

Zerit, *see stavudine*

Zestril, *see lisinopril*

Zetia, *see ezetimibe*

ziconotide

zih-**con**-no-tide
(Prialt)

CLASSIFICATION

PHARMACOTHERAPEUTIC: Synthetic peptide. **CLINICAL:** Non-narcotic analgesic.

ACTION

Selectively binds to N-type voltage-sensitive calcium channels located on afferent nerves in spinal cord. This binding is thought to block N-type calcium channels, blocking excitatory neurotransmitter release. **Therapeutic Effect:** Reduces sensitivity to painful stimuli.

PHARMACOKINETICS

Intrathecally administered drug is 100% bioavailable in cerebrospinal fluid (CSF). Protein binding: 50%. Readily degraded to peptide fragment. Less than 1% excreted in urine. **Half-life:** 4.6 hrs (intrathecal).

USES

Management of severe chronic pain in pts for whom intrathecal (IT) therapy is warranted and who are intolerant or refractory to other treatment.

PRECAUTIONS

CONTRAINDICATIONS: History of psychosis, presence of infection at injection site, uncontrolled bleeding, spinal canal obstruction that impairs CSF circulation, IV administration. **CAUTIONS:** Elderly (increased risk of confusion).

LIFESPAN CONSIDERATIONS:

Pregnancy/Lactation: Unknown if drug crosses placenta or is distributed in breast milk. **Pregnancy Category C. Children:** Safety and efficacy not established. **Elderly:** May present increased sensitivity to psychiatric effects.

INTERACTIONS

DRUG: May enhance adverse/toxic effects of **CNS depressants. HERBAL:** None significant. **FOOD:** None known. **LAB VALUES:** May increase serum kinase, CPK levels.

AVAILABILITY (Rx)

INJECTION SOLUTION: 100 mcg/ml (1 ml, 2 ml, 5 ml); 25 mcg/ml (20 ml) vials.

ADMINISTRATION/HANDLING

INTRATHECAL

• Use only with Medtronic SynchroMed EL, SynchroMed II Infusion System, Simms Deltec Cadd Micro External Microinfusion Device and Catheter. • Refer to manufacturer's manuals for specific instructions for performing initial filling, refilling of reservoir.

INDICATIONS/ROUTES/DOSAGE

PAIN CONTROL

INTRATHECAL: ADULTS, ELDERLY: Initially, 2.4 mcg/day (0.1 mcg/hr). May titrate to maximum of 19.2 mcg/day (0.8 mcg/hr).

SIDE EFFECTS

FREQUENT: Dizziness (47%), nausea (41%), somnolence/weakness (22%), diarrhea (19%), confusion (18%), ataxia (16%), headache/vomiting/gait disturbance (15%), memory impairment (12%), hypertonia (11%). **OCCASIONAL (10%–7%):** Anorexia, visual disturbances, anxiety, urinary retention, speech disorder, aphasia, nystagmus, paresthesia, fever, hallucinations, nervousness, vertigo. **RARE:** Insomnia, dry skin, constipation, arthralgia, myalgia, tremor.

ADVERSE EFFECTS/ TOXIC REACTIONS

Atrial fibrillation, cerebral vascular accident, seizures, acute renal failure, myoclonus, psychosis occur rarely.

NURSING CONSIDERATIONS

BASELINE ASSESSMENT

Obtain baseline serum creatinine kinase, CPK levels.

INTERVENTION/EVALUATION

Assess serum creatinine kinase levels periodically every other wk for first month and monthly thereafter. Monitor for signs/symptoms of meningitis characterized by fever, headache, stiff neck, altered mental status, nausea, vomiting. Assess for signs/symptoms of neurologic or psychiatric impairment marked by hallucinations, changes in mood or consciousness.

PATIENT/FAMILY TEACHING

Avoid tasks that require alertness, motor skills until response to drug is established. Notify physician of any changes in mood, mental status, suicidal ideation. Contact physician if nausea, vomiting, seizures, fever, headache, stiff neck occur.

zidovudine

zye-**dough**-view-deen

(Apo-Zidovudine ✤, AZT, Novo-AZT ✤, Retrovir)

Do not confuse Retrovir with ritonavir.

FIXED-COMBINATION(S)

Combivir: zidovudine/lamivudine (an antiviral): 300 mg/150 mg. **Trizivir:** zidovudine/lamivudine/abacavir (an antiviral): 300 mg/150 mg/300 mg.

CLASSIFICATION

PHARMACOTHERAPEUTIC: Nucleoside reverse transcriptase inhibitors. **CLINICAL:** Antivirals (see pp. 66C, 111C).

ACTION

Interferes with viral RNA-dependent DNA polymerase, an enzyme necessary for viral HIV replication. **Therapeutic Effect:** Slows HIV replication, reducing progression of HIV infection.

PHARMACOKINETICS

Rapidly, completely absorbed from GI tract. Protein binding: 25%–38%. Undergoes first-pass metabolism in liver. Crosses blood-brain barrier and is widely distributed, including to cerebrospinal fluid (CSF). Primarily excreted in urine. Minimal removal by hemodialysis. **Half-life:** 0.8–1.2 hrs (increased in renal impairment).

USES

Treatment of HIV infection in combination with other antiretroviral agents. **OFF-LABEL:** Prophylaxis in health care workers at risk for acquiring HIV after occupational exposure.

PRECAUTIONS

CONTRAINDICATIONS: Life-threatening allergic reactions to zidovudine or its components. **CAUTIONS:** Bone marrow compromise, renal/hepatic dysfunction, decreased hepatic blood flow.

LIFESPAN CONSIDERATIONS:

Pregnancy/Lactation: Unknown if drug crosses placenta or is distributed in breast milk. Unknown if fetal harm or effects on fertility can occur. **Pregnancy Category C. Children:** No age-related precautions noted. **Elderly:** Information not available.

INTERACTIONS

DRUG: Bone marrow depressants, ganciclovir may increase myelosuppression. **Clarithromycin** may decrease concentration. May be antag-onistic with **doxorubicin.** Hematologic toxicities may occur with **interferon alfa. Probenecid** may increase concentration, risk of toxicity. **HERBAL:** None significant. **FOOD:** None known. **LAB VALUES:** May increase mean corpuscular volume (MCV).

AVAILABILITY (Rx)

CAPSULES (RETROVIR): 100 mg. **INJECTION SOLUTION (RETROVIR):** 10 mg/ml. **SYRUP (RETROVIR):** 50 mg/5 ml. **TABLETS (RETROVIR):** 300 mg.

ADMINISTRATION/HANDLING

IV

Reconstitution • Must dilute before administration. • Remove calculated dose from vial and add to D_5W to provide concentration no greater than 4 mg/ml.

Rate of administration • Infuse over 1 hr.

Storage • After dilution, IV solution is stable for 24 hrs at room temperature; 48 hrs if refrigerated. • Use within 8 hrs if stored at room temperature; 24 hrs if refrigerated. • Do not use if solution is discolored or precipitate forms.

PO

• Keep capsules in cool, dry place. Protect from light. • Food, milk do not affect GI absorption. • Space doses evenly around the clock. • Pt should be in upright position when giving medication to prevent esophageal ulceration.

IV INCOMPATIBILITIES

None known.

IV COMPATIBILITIES

Dexamethasone (Decadron), dobutamine (Dobutrex), dopamine (Intropin), heparin, lipids, lorazepam (Ativan), morphine, potassium chloride.

INDICATIONS/ROUTES/DOSAGE

HIV INFECTION

PO: ADULTS, ELDERLY, CHILDREN OLDER THAN 12 YRS: 200 mg q8h or 300 mg q12h. **CHILDREN 12 YRS AND YOUNGER:** 160 mg/m^2/dose q8h. Range: 90–180 mg/m^2/dose q6–8h. **NEONATES:** 2 mg/kg/dose q6h.

IV: ADULTS, ELDERLY, CHILDREN OLDER THAN 12 YRS: 1–2 mg/kg/dose q4h. **CHILDREN 12 YRS AND YOUNGER:** 120 mg/m^2/dose q6h. **NEONATES:** 1.5 mg/kg/dose q6h.

SIDE EFFECTS

EXPECTED (46%–42%): Nausea, headache. **FREQUENT (20%–16%):** Abdominal pain, asthenia (loss of strength, energy), rash, fever, acne. **OCCASIONAL (12%–8%):** Diarrhea, anorexia, malaise, myalgia, somnolence. **RARE (6%–5%):** Dizziness, paresthesia, vomiting, insomnia, dyspnea, altered taste.

ADVERSE EFFECTS/ TOXIC REACTIONS

Anemia (occurring most commonly after 4–6 wks of therapy), granulocytopenia are particularly significant in pts with pre-therapy low baselines. Neurotoxicity (ataxia, fatigue, lethargy, nystagmus, seizures) may occur.

NURSING CONSIDERATIONS

BASELINE ASSESSMENT

Avoid drugs that are nephrotoxic, cytotoxic, myelosuppressive—may increase risk of toxicity. Obtain specimens for viral diagnostic tests before starting therapy (therapy may begin before results are obtained). Check hematology reports for accurate baseline.

INTERVENTION/EVALUATION

Monitor CBC, Hgb, MCV, retriculocyte count, CD4 cell count, HIV RNA plasma levels. Check for bleeding. Assess for headache, dizziness. Monitor daily pattern of bowel activity/stool consistency. Evaluate skin for acne, rash. Be alert to development of opportunistic infections (fever, chills, cough, myalgia). Monitor I&O, serum renal/hepatic function tests. Check for insomnia.

PATIENT/FAMILY TEACHING

• Doses should be evenly spaced around the clock. • Zidovudine does not cure AIDS or HIV disease, nor does it reduce risk of transmission to others, but acts to reduce symptoms and slows or arrests progress of disease. • Do not take any medications without physician approval. • Bleeding from gums, nose, rectum may occur and should be reported to physician immediately. • Blood counts are essential because of bleeding potential. • Dental work should be done before therapy or after blood counts return to normal (often wks after therapy has stopped). • Inform physician if muscle weakness, difficulty breathing, headache, inability to sleep, unusual bleeding, rash, signs of infection occur.

Zinacef, *see cefuroxime*

ziprasidone

zye-**pray**-za-done
(Geodon)

CLASSIFICATION

PHARMACOTHERAPEUTIC: Piperazine derivative. **CLINICAL:** Antipsychotic (see p. 63C).

ACTION

Antagonizes alpha-adrenergic, dopamine, histamine, serotonin receptors; inhibits reuptake of serotonin, norepinephrine. **Therapeutic Effect:** Diminishes symptoms of schizophrenia, depression.

PHARMACOKINETICS

Well absorbed after PO administration. Food increases bioavailability. Protein binding: 99%. Extensively metabolized in liver. Not removed by hemodialysis. **Half-life:** 7 hrs.

USES

Treatment of schizophrenia, acute bipolar mania. **OFF-LABEL:** Tourette's syndrome.

PRECAUTIONS

CONTRAINDICATIONS: Conditions associated with risk of prolonged QT interval, congenital long QT syndrome. **CAUTIONS:** Pts with bradycardia, hypokalemia, hypomagnesemia may be at greater risk for torsades de pointes (atypical ventricular tachycardia).

LIFESPAN CONSIDERATIONS:

Pregnancy/Lactation: Unknown if drug crosses placenta or is distributed in breast milk. **Pregnancy Category C. Children:** Safety and efficacy not established. **Elderly:** No age-related precautions noted.

INTERACTIONS

DRUG: Alcohol, other CNS depressants may increase CNS depression. **Carbamazepine** may decrease concentration. **Ketoconazole** may increase concentration. **Medications causing prolongation of QT interval (e.g., amiodarone, dofetilide, sotalol)** may increase effects on cardiac conduction leading to malignant arrhythmias (e.g., torsades de pointes). **HERBAL: Gotu kola, kava kava, St. John's wort, valerian** may increase CNS depression. **FOOD: All foods** enhance bioavailability. **LAB VALUES:** May prolong QT interval.

AVAILABILITY (Rx)

CAPSULES: 20 mg, 40 mg, 60 mg, 80 mg. **INJECTION POWDER FOR RECONSTITUTION:** 20 mg.

ADMINISTRATION/HANDLING

IM

• Store vials at room temperature; protect from light. • Reconstitute each vial with 1.2 ml Sterile Water for Injection to provide concentration of 20 mg/ml. • Reconstituted solution stable for 24 hrs at room temperature or 7 days refrigerated.

PO

• Give with food (increases bioavailability).

INDICATIONS/ROUTES/DOSAGE

SCHIZOPHRENIA

PO: ADULTS, ELDERLY: Initially, 20 mg twice a day with food. Titrate at intervals of no less than 2 days. **Maximum:** 80 mg twice a day.

IM: ADULTS, ELDERLY: 10 mg q2h or 20 mg q4h. **Maximum:** 40 mg/day.

MANIA IN BIPOLAR DISORDER

PO: ADULTS, ELDERLY: Initially, 40 mg twice a day. May increase to 60–80 mg twice a day on second day of treatment. Range: 40–80 mg twice a day.

SIDE EFFECTS

FREQUENT (30%–16%): Headache, somnolence, dizziness. **OCCASIONAL:** Rash, orthostatic hypotension, weight gain, restlessness, constipation, dyspepsia (heartburn, indigestion, epigastric pain). **RARE:** Hyperglycemia, priapism.

ADVERSE EFFECTS/ TOXIC REACTIONS

Prolongation of QT interval (as seen on EKG) may produce torsades de pointes, a form of ventricular tachycardia. Pts with bradycardia, hypokalemia, hypomagnesemia are at increased risk.

NURSING CONSIDERATIONS

BASELINE ASSESSMENT

Assess pt's behavior, appearance, emotional status, response to environment, speech pattern, thought content. EKG should be obtained to assess for QT prolongation before instituting medication. Blood chemistry for serum magnesium, potassium should be obtained before beginning therapy and routinely thereafter.

INTERVENTION/EVALUATION

Assess for therapeutic response (greater interest in surroundings, improved self-care, increased ability to concentrate, relaxed facial expression). Monitor weight.

PATIENT/FAMILY TEACHING

• Avoid tasks that require alertness, motor skills until response to drug is established.

Zithromax, *see azithromycin*

Zocor, *see simvastatin*

Zofran, *see ondansetron*

Zoladex, *see goserelin*

zoledronic acid

zole-eh-**drone**-ick

(Aclasta ✦, Zometa)

CLASSIFICATION

PHARMACOTHERAPEUTIC: Bisphosphonate. **CLINICAL:** Calcium regulator, bone resorption inhibitor.

ACTION

Inhibits resorption of mineralized bone, cartilage; inhibits increased osteoclastic activity, skeletal calcium release induced by stimulatory factors released by tumors. **Therapeutic Effect:** Increases urinary calcium, phosphorus excretion; decreases serum calcium, phosphorus levels.

USES

Treatment of hypercalcemia, bone metastases of solid tumors. Treatment of multiple myeloma. **OFF-LABEL:** Prevention of bone metastases from breast, prostate cancer, treatment of bone diseases.

PRECAUTIONS

CONTRAINDICATIONS: Hypersensitivity to other bisphosphonates, including alendronate, etidronate, pamidronate, risedronate, tiludronate. **CAUTIONS:** History of aspirin-sensitive asthma, renal impairment, hypoparathyroidism, risk of hypocalcemia.

LIFESPAN CONSIDERATIONS:

Pregnancy/Lactation: Unknown if drug crosses placenta or is distributed in breast milk. **Pregnancy Category C.** **Children:** Safety and efficacy not established. **Elderly:** Age-related renal impairment may require dosage adjustment.

INTERACTIONS

DRUG: None significant. **HERBAL:** None significant. **FOOD:** None known. **LAB VALUES:** May decrease serum magnesium, calcium, phosphate.

AVAILABILITY (Rx)

INJECTION SOLUTION: 4 mg/5 ml.

ADMINISTRATION/HANDLING

◀ **ALERT** ▶ Pt should be adequately rehydrated before administration of zoledronic acid.

IV

Reconstitution • Further dilute with 100 ml 0.9% NaCl or D_5W.

Rate of administration • Adequate hydration is essential in conjunction with zoledronic acid. • Administer as IV infusion over not less than 15 min (increases risk of deterioration in renal function).

Storage • Store intact vials at room temperature. • Infusion of solution must be completed within 24 hrs.

IV INCOMPATIBILITIES

Do not mix with other medications.

INDICATIONS/ROUTES/DOSAGE

HYPERCALCEMIA

IV INFUSION: ADULTS, ELDERLY: 4 mg IV infusion given over no less than 15 min. Retreatment may be considered, but at least 7 days should elapse to allow for full response to initial dose.

MULTIPLE MYELOMA, BONE METASTASES OF SOLID TUMORS

IV: ADULTS, ELDERLY: 4 mg q3–4wk.

SIDE EFFECTS

FREQUENT (44%–26%): Fever, nausea, vomiting, constipation. **OCCASIONAL (15%–10%):** Hypotension, anxiety, insomnia, flu-like symptoms (fever, chills, bone pain, myalgia, arthralgia). **RARE:** Conjunctivitis.

ADVERSE EFFECTS/ TOXIC REACTIONS

Renal toxicity may occur if IV infusion is administered in less than 15 min.

NURSING CONSIDERATIONS

BASELINE ASSESSMENT

Establish baseline serum electrolytes.

INTERVENTION/EVALUATION

Monitor serum renal function, CBC, Hgb, Hct. Assess vertebral bone mass (document stabilization, improvement). Monitor serum calcium, phosphate, magnesium, creatinine levels. Assess for fever. Monitor food intake, daily pattern of bowel activity/stool consistency. Check I&O, BUN, serum creatinine in pts with renal impairment.

zolmitriptan

zohl-mih-**trip**-tan

(Zomig, Zomig Rapimelt ✤, Zomig-ZMT)

CLASSIFICATION

PHARMACOTHERAPEUTIC: Serotonin receptor agonist. **CLINICAL:** Antimigraine (see p. 61C).

ACTION

Binds selectively to vascular receptors, producing vasoconstrictive effect on cranial blood vessels. **Therapeutic Effect:** Relieves migraine headache.

PHARMACOKINETICS

Rapidly but incompletely absorbed after PO administration. Protein binding: 15%. Undergoes first-pass metabolism in liver to active metabolite. Eliminated primarily in urine (60%) and, to lesser extent, in feces (30%). **Half-life:** 3 hrs.

USES

Treatment of acute migraine attack with or without aura.

PRECAUTIONS

CONTRAINDICATIONS: Arrhythmias associated with conduction disorders (e.g., Wolff-Parkinson-White syndrome), basilar or hemiplegic migraine, coronary artery disease, ischemic heart disease (including angina pectoris, history of MI, silent ischemia, Prinzmetal's angina), uncontrolled hypertension, use within 24 hrs of ergotamine-containing preparations or another serotonin receptor agonist, MAOI used within 14 days. **CAUTIONS:** Mild to moderate renal/hepatic impairment, pt profile suggesting cardiovascular risks, controlled hypertension, history of cerebrovascular accident (CVA).

LIFESPAN CONSIDERATIONS:

Pregnancy/Lactation: Unknown if drug is distributed in breast milk.

Pregnancy Category C. Children: Safety and efficacy not established in those younger than 12 yrs. **Elderly:** No age-related precautions noted.

INTERACTIONS

DRUG: Ergotamine-containing medications may produce vasospastic reaction. **Fluoxetine, fluvoxamine, paroxetine, sertraline** may produce hyperreflexia, incoordination, weakness. **MAOIs** may dramatically increase concentration. **Oral contraceptives** decrease clearance, volume of distribution. **HERBAL:** None significant. **FOOD:** None known. **LAB VALUES:** None known.

AVAILABILITY (Rx)

NASAL SPRAY (ZOMIG): 5 mg/0.1 ml. **TABLETS (ZOMIG):** 2.5 mg, 5 mg.

TABLETS (ORALLY DISINTEGRATING [ZOMIG-ZMT]): 2.5 mg, 5 mg.

ADMINISTRATION/HANDLING

PO

• Give without regard to food.

PO (ORALLY DISINTEGRATING TABLET)

• Must take whole; do not break, cut, chew. • Place on tongue, allow to dissolve. • Not necessary to administer with liquid.

NASAL

• Instruct the pt to gently blow nose to clear nasal passages. • With head upright, pt should close one nostril with index finger, breathe out gently through mouth. • Instruct pt to insert nozzle into open nostril about ½ inch, close mouth, and while taking a breath through nose, release spray dosage by firmly pressing plunger. • Have pt remove nozzle from nose, gently breathe in through nose and out through mouth for 15–20 sec. Tell pt to avoid breathing in deeply.

INDICATIONS/ROUTES/DOSAGE

ACUTE MIGRAINE ATTACK

PO: ADULTS, ELDERLY, CHILDREN OLDER THAN 18 YRS: Initially, 2.5 mg or less. If headache returns, may repeat dose in 2 hrs. **Maximum:** 10 mg/24 hrs.

INTRANASAL: ADULTS, ELDERLY: 5 mg. May repeat in 2 hrs. **Maximum:** 10 mg/24 hrs.

SIDE EFFECTS

FREQUENT (8%–6%): Oral: Dizziness; paresthesia, neck/throat/jaw pressure; drowsiness. **Nasal:** Altered taste, paresthesia. **OCCASIONAL (5%–3%): Oral:** Warm/hot sensation, asthenia (loss of strength, energy), chest pressure. **Nasal:** Nausea, somnolence, nasal discomfort, dizziness, asthenia (loss of strength, energy), dry mouth. **RARE (2%–1%):** Diaphoresis, myalgia, paresthesia.

ADVERSE EFFECTS/ TOXIC REACTIONS

Cardiac events (ischemia, coronary artery vasospasm, MI), noncardiac vasospasm-related reactions (hemorrhage, stroke) occur rarely, particularly in pts with hypertension, diabetes, strong family history of coronary artery disease; obesity, smokers; males older than 40 yrs; postmenopausal women.

NURSING CONSIDERATIONS

BASELINE ASSESSMENT

Question for history of peripheral vascular disease, coronary artery disease, renal/hepatic impairment, MAOI use. Question pt regarding onset, location, duration of migraine, possible precipitating symptoms.

INTERVENTION/EVALUATION

Monitor for evidence of dizziness. Monitor B/P, esp. in pts with hepatic impairment. Assess for relief of migraine headache, migraine potential for photophobia, phonophobia (sound sensitivity, light sensitivity, nausea, vomiting).

PATIENT/FAMILY TEACHING

• Take single dose as soon as symptoms of actual migraine attack appear. • Medication is intended to relieve migraine, not to prevent or reduce number of attacks. • Lie down in quiet dark room for additional benefit after taking medication. • Avoid tasks that require alertness, motor skills until response to drug is established. • Report chest pain, palpitations, tightness in throat, edema of face, lips, eyes, rash, easy bruising, blood in urine/stool, pain/numbness in arms/legs.

Zoloft, *see sertraline*

zolpidem

zole-pi-dem

(Ambien, Ambien CR)

Do not confuse Ambien with Amen.

CLASSIFICATION

PHARMACOTHERAPEUTIC: Nonbenzodiazepine. **CLINICAL:** Sedative-hypnotic **(Schedule IV)** (see p. 141C).

ACTION

Enhances action of inhibitory neurotransmitter gamma-aminobutyric acid (GABA). **Therapeutic Effect:** Induces sleep with fewer nightly awakenings, improves sleep quality.

PHARMACOKINETICS

Route	Onset	Peak	Duration
PO	30 min	N/A	6–8 hrs

Rapidly absorbed from GI tract. Protein binding: 92%. Metabolized in liver; excreted in urine. Not removed by hemodialysis. **Half-life:** 1.4–4.5 hrs (increased in hepatic impairment).

USES

Short-term treatment of insomnia. Reduces sleep-induction time, number of nocturnal awakenings; increases length of sleep; improves sleep quality.

PRECAUTIONS

CONTRAINDICATIONS: None known. **CAUTIONS:** Hepatic impairment, pts with depression, history of drug dependence.

LIFESPAN CONSIDERATIONS:

Pregnancy/Lactation: Unknown if drug crosses placenta or is distributed in breast milk. **Pregnancy Category C. Children:** Safety and efficacy not established. **Elderly:** More likely to experience falls or confusion; decreased initial doses recommended. Age-related hepatic impairment may require dosage adjustment.

INTERACTIONS

DRUG: Alcohol, other CNS depressants may increase CNS depression. **HERBAL: Gotu kola, kava kava, St. John's wort, valerian** may increase CNS depression. **FOOD:** None known. **LAB VALUES:** None known.

AVAILABILITY (Rx)

TABLETS (AMBIEN): 5 mg, 10 mg.

TABLETS (EXTENDED-RELEASE [AMBIEN CR]): 6.25 mg, 12.5 mg.

ADMINISTRATION/HANDLING

PO

• For faster sleep onset, do not give with or immediately after a meal. • Do not divide, crush, chew Ambien CR tablets.

INDICATIONS/ROUTES/DOSAGE

INSOMNIA

PO: ADULTS: 10 mg at bedtime. **ELDERLY, DEBILITATED:** 5 mg at bedtime.

PO (EXTENDED-RELEASE): ADULTS: 12.5 mg. **ELDERLY, DEBILITATED:** 6.25 mg.

SIDE EFFECTS

OCCASIONAL (7%): Headache. **RARE (less than 2%):** Dizziness, nausea, diarrhea, muscle pain.

ADVERSE EFFECTS/ TOXIC REACTIONS

Overdose may produce severe ataxia (clumsiness, unsteadiness), bradycardia, diplopia, severe drowsiness, nausea vomiting, difficulty breathing, unconsciousness. Abrupt withdrawal following long-term use may produce weakness, facial flushing, diaphoresis, vomiting, tremor. Drug tolerance/dependence may occur with prolonged use of high dosages.

NURSING CONSIDERATIONS

BASELINE ASSESSMENT

Assess B/P, pulse, respirations. Raise bed rails, provide call light. Provide environment conducive to sleep (back rub, quiet environment, low lighting).

INTERVENTION/EVALUATION

Assess sleep pattern of pt. Evaluate for therapeutic response to insomnia: decrease in number of nocturnal awakenings, increase in length of sleep.

PATIENT/FAMILY TEACHING

• Do not abruptly withdraw medication after long-term use. • Avoid alcohol, tasks that require alertness, motor skills until response to drug is established. • Tolerance, dependence may occur with prolonged use of high dosages.

Zometa, *see zoledronic acid*

Zomig, *see zolmitriptan*

zonisamide

zoh-**nis**-a-mide
(Zonegran)

CLASSIFICATION

PHARMACOTHERAPEUTIC: Succinimide. **CLINICAL:** Anticonvulsant (see p. 35C).

ACTION

May stabilize neuronal membranes, suppress neuronal hypersynchronization by blocking sodium, calcium channels. **Therapeutic Effect:** Reduces seizure activity.

PHARMACOKINETICS

Well absorbed after PO administration. Extensively bound to RBCs. Protein binding: 40%. Primarily excreted in urine. **Half-life:** 63 hrs (plasma), 105 hrs (RBCs).

USES

Adjunctive therapy in treatment of partial seizures in adults with epilepsy. **OFF-LABEL:** Treatment of bulimia, bipolar disorder, obesity.

PRECAUTIONS

CONTRAINDICATIONS: Allergy to sulfonamides. **CAUTIONS:** Renal impairment.

LIFESPAN CONSIDERATIONS:

Pregnancy/Lactation: Unknown if distributed in breast milk. **Pregnancy Category C. Children:** Safety and efficacy not established in those younger than 16 yrs. **Elderly:** No age-related precautions noted, but lower dosages recommended.

INTERACTIONS

DRUG: Alcohol, other CNS depressants may increase sedative effect. **Carbamazepine, phenobarbital, phenytoin, valproic acid** may increase metabolism, decrease effect.

HERBAL: None significant. **FOOD:** None known. **LAB VALUES:** May increase BUN, serum creatinine.

AVAILABILITY (Rx)

CAPSULES: 25 mg, 50 mg, 100 mg.

ADMINISTRATION/HANDLING

PO

• May give with or without food. • Swallow capsules whole. • Do not give to pts allergic to sulfonamides.

INDICATIONS/ROUTES/DOSAGE

PARTIAL SEIZURES

PO: ADULTS, ELDERLY, CHILDREN OLDER THAN 16 YRS:–Initially, 100 mg/day for 2 wks. May increase by 100 mg/day at intervals of 2 wks or longer. Range: 100–600 mg/day.

SIDE EFFECTS

FREQUENT (17%–9%): Somnolence, dizziness, anorexia, headache, agitation, irritability, nausea. **OCCASIONAL (8%–5%):** Fatigue, ataxia, confusion, depression, impaired memory/concentration, insomnia, abdominal pain, diplopia, diarrhea, speech difficulty. **RARE (4%–3%):** Paresthesia, nystagmus, anxiety, rash, dyspepsia (heartburn, indigestion, epigastric pain), weight loss.

ADVERSE EFFECTS/ TOXIC REACTIONS

Overdose characterized by bradycardia, hypotension, respiratory depression, coma. Leukopenia, anemia, thrombocytopenia occur rarely.

NURSING CONSIDERATIONS

BASELINE ASSESSMENT

Review history of seizure disorder (intensity, frequency, duration, level of consciousness [LOC]). Initiate seizure precautions. Serum hepatic function tests, CBC, platelet count should be performed before therapy begins and periodically during therapy.

INTERVENTION/EVALUATION

Observe frequently for recurrence of seizure activity. Assess for clinical improvement (decrease in intensity, frequency of seizures). Assist with ambulation if dizziness occurs.

PATIENT/FAMILY TEACHING

• Strict maintenance of drug therapy is essential for seizure control. • Avoid tasks that require alertness, motor skills until response to drug is established. • Avoid alcohol. • Report if rash, back/ abdominal pain, blood in urine, fever, sore throat, ulcers in mouth, easy bruising occurs.

Zosyn, *see piperacillin sodium/tazobactam sodium*

Zovirax, *see acyclovir*

Zyloprim, *see allopurinol*

Zyprexa, *see olanzapine*

Zyrtec, *see cetirizine*

Zyvox, *see linezolid*

Appendixes

Appendix A

CALCULATION OF DOSES

Frequently, dosages ordered do not correspond exactly to what is available and must be calculated.

RATIO/PROPORTION:

A pt is to receive 65 mg of a medication. It is available as 80 mg/2 ml. What volume (ml) needs to be administered to the patient?

STEP 1: Set up ratio.

$$\frac{80\text{ mg}}{2\text{ ml}} = \frac{65\text{ mg}}{\text{x (ml)}}$$

STEP 2: Cross multiply and divide each side by the number with x to determine volume to be administered.

$$80\text{ mg} \times (\text{x})\text{ ml} = 65\text{ mg} \times 2\text{ ml}$$

$$80\text{ x} = 130$$

$$\text{x} = \frac{130}{80} = 1.625\text{ ml}$$

CALCULATIONS IN MICROGRAMS/KILOGRAM PER MINUTE (mcg/kg/min):

A 63-year-old pt (weight 165 lb) is to receive medication A at a rate of 8 mcg/kg/min. Given a solution containing medication A in a concentration of 500 mg/250 ml, at what rate (ml/hr) would you infuse this medication?

STEP 1: Convert to same units. In this problem, the dose is expressed in mcg/kg; therefore, convert weight to kg (2.2 lb = 1 kg) and drug concentration to mcg/ml (1 mg = 1,000 mcg)

165 lb divided by 2.2 = 75 kg

500 mg × 2 mg/ml = 2,000 mcg/ml = 250 ml

STEP 2: Number of mcg/hr.

(75 kg) × 8 mcg/kg/min = 600 mcg/min or 36,000 mcg/hr

STEP 3: Number of ml/hr.

36,000 mcg/hr divided by 2,000 mcg/ml = 18 ml/hr

Appendix B

CONTROLLED DRUGS (UNITED STATES)

Schedule I: Medications having no legal medical use. These substances may be used for research purposes with proper registration (e.g., heroin, LSD).

Schedule II: Medications having a legitimate medical use but are characterized by a very high abuse potential and/or potential for severe physical and psychic dependency. Emergency telephone orders for limited quantities of these drugs are authorized, but the prescriber must provide a written, signed prescription order (e.g., morphine, amphetamines).

Schedule III: Medications having significant abuse potential (less than Schedule II). Telephone orders are permitted (e.g., opiates in combination with other substances such as acetaminophen).

Schedule IV: Medications having a low abuse potential. Telephone orders are permitted (e.g., benzodiazepines, propoxyphene).

Schedule V: Medications having the lowest abuse potential of the controlled substances. Some Schedule V products may be available without a prescription (e.g., certain cough preparations containing limited amounts of an opiate).

Appendix C

DRIP RATES FOR CRITICAL CARE MEDICATIONS

Dobutamine

Dopamine

Heparin

Nitroglycerin

Norepinephrine

Propofol

Sodium Nitroprusside

DOBUTAMINE (Dobutrex)
Mix 250 mg in 250 ml of D_5W (1,000 mcg/ml)
Body Weight

	lb	88	99	110	121	132	143	154	165	176	187	198	209	220	231	242
	kg	40	45	50	55	60	65	70	75	80	85	90	95	100	105	110
Dose ordered in mcg/kg/min	***Amount to infuse in mcgtts/min or ml/hr***															
2.5		6	7	8	8	9	10	11	11	12	13	14	14	15	16	17
5		12	14	15	17	18	20	21	23	24	26	27	29	30	32	33
7.5		18	20	23	25	27	29	32	34	36	38	41	43	45	47	50
10		24	27	30	33	36	39	42	45	48	51	54	57	60	63	66
12.5		30	34	38	41	45	49	53	56	60	64	68	71	75	79	83
15		36	41	45	50	54	59	63	68	72	77	81	86	90	95	99
20		48	54	60	66	72	78	84	90	96	102	108	114	120	126	132
25		60	68	75	83	90	98	105	113	120	128	135	143	150	158	165
30		72	81	90	99	108	117	126	135	144	153	162	171	180	189	198
35		84	95	105	116	126	137	147	158	168	179	189	200	210	221	231
40		96	108	120	132	144	156	168	180	192	204	216	228	240	252	264

- Administer 2.5–10 mcg/kg/min initially.
- Increase in increments of 5–10 mcg up to 40 mcg/kg/min as needed.
- Do not mix with sodium bicarbonate.

DOPAMINE (Intropin)

Mix 400 mg in 250 ml of D_5W (1,600 mcg/ml)

Body Weight

lb	88	99	110	121	132	143	154	165	176	187	198	209	220	231
kg	40	45	50	55	60	65	70	75	80	85	90	95	100	105
Dose ordered in mcg/kg/min	***Amount to infuse in mcgtts/min or ml/hr***													
2.5	4	4	5	5	6	6	7	7	8	8	8	9	9	10
5	8	8	9	10	11	12	13	14	15	16	17	18	19	20
7.5	11	13	14	15	17	18	20	21	23	24	25	27	28	30
10	15	17	19	21	23	24	26	28	30	32	34	36	38	39
12.5	19	21	23	26	28	30	33	35	38	40	42	45	47	49
15	23	25	28	31	34	37	39	42	45	48	51	53	56	59
20	30	34	38	41	45	49	53	56	60	64	68	71	75	79
25	38	42	47	52	56	61	66	70	75	80	84	89	94	98
30	45	51	56	62	67	73	79	84	90	96	101	107	113	118
35	53	59	66	72	79	85	92	98	105	112	118	125	131	138
40	60	68	75	83	90	98	105	113	120	128	135	143	150	158
45	68	76	84	93	101	110	118	127	135	143	152	160	169	177
50	75	84	94	103	113	122	131	141	150	159	169	178	188	197

- Administer 2.5–5 mcg/kg/min initially.
- Increase in increments of 5–10 mcg to 50 mcg/kg/min as needed.
- Do not mix with sodium bicarbonate.

HEPARIN DRIP RATE CHART

ACT (sec)	aPTT (sec)	Bolus Dose (ml)	Stop Infusion (min)	Rate Change (ml/hr)	Repeat PTT (hr)	Repeat aPTT (hr)
1–200	1–49	5,000	0	+3 ml/hr (increase by 150 units/hr)	4	4
201–239	50–59	0	0	+2 ml/hr (increase by 100 units/hr)	4	4
240–300	60–85	0	0	0 (no change)	8	8
301–400	86–95	0	0	−1 ml/hr (decrease by 50 units/hr)	8	8
401–500	96–120	0	30	−2 ml/hr (decrease by 100 units/hr)	4	4
500+	120+	0	60	−3 ml/hr (decrease by 150 units/hr)	4	4

NITROGLYCERIN (Tridil)

Dose Ordered in mcg/min	50 mg/ 250 cc 100 mg/ 500 cc NTG/D_5W	100 mg/ 250 cc 200 mg/ 500 cc NTG/D_5W	Dose Ordered in mcg/min	50 mg/ 250 cc 100 mg/ 500 cc NTG/D_5W	100 mg/ 250 cc 200 mg/ 500 cc NTG/D_5W
10	3	—	210	63	32
20	6	3	220	66	33
30	9	5	230	69	35
40	12	6	240	72	36
50	15	8	250	75	38
60	18	9	260	78	39
70	21	10	270	81	41
80	24	12	280	84	42
90	27	14	290	87	44
100	30	15	300	90	45
110	33	17	310	93	47
120	36	18	320	96	48
130	39	19	330	99	50
140	42	21	340	102	51
150	45	23	350	105	53
160	48	24	360	108	54
170	51	26	370	111	56
180	54	27	380	114	57
190	57	29	390	117	59
200	60	30	400	120	60
	Amt to infuse in mcgtts/min or ml/hr			***Amt to infuse in mcgtts/min or ml/hr***	

- Administer at 10–20 mcg/min initially.
- Increase at increments of 6–10 mcg/min every 5–10 min until desired response.

NOREPINEPHRINE (Levophed)

Mix: 4 mg in 250 ml D_5W

Norepinephrine 4 mg in 250 ml D_5W (rate is ml/hr)

	mcg/kg/min											
kg	0.01	0.02	0.03	0.04	0.05	0.06	0.07	0.08	0.09	0.10	0.20	0.30
50	1.9	3.8	5.7	7.6	9.5	11.4	13.3	15.2	17.1	19.0	38.0	57.0
55	2.1	4.2	6.3	8.4	10.5	12.6	14.7	16.8	18.9	21.0	42.0	63.0
60	2.3	4.6	6.9	9.2	11.5	13.8	16.1	18.4	20.7	23.0	46.0	69.0
65	2.4	4.8	7.2	9.6	12.0	14.4	16.8	19.2	21.6	24.0	48.0	72.0
70	2.6	5.2	7.8	10.4	13.0	15.6	18.2	20.8	23.4	26.0	52.0	78.0
75	2.8	5.6	8.4	11.2	14.0	16.8	19.6	22.4	25.2	28.0	56.0	84.0
80	3.0	6.0	9.0	12.0	15.0	18.0	21.0	24.0	27.0	30.0	60.0	90.0
85	3.2	6.4	9.6	12.8	16.0	19.2	22.4	25.6	28.8	32.0	64.0	96.0
90	3.4	6.8	10.2	13.6	17.0	20.4	23.8	27.2	30.6	34.0	68.0	102
95	3.6	7.2	10.8	14.4	18.0	21.6	25.2	28.8	32.4	36.0	72.0	108
100	3.8	7.6	11.4	15.2	19.0	22.8	26.6	30.4	34.2	38.0	76.0	114

Use: Hypotension, shock

Dose: 2–40 mcg/min or 0.05–0.25 mcg/kg/min doses of greater than 75 mcg/min or 1 mcg/kg/min have been used

Mechanism: Primary α_1 vasoconstriction effect (minor β_1 inotropic)

Elimination: Hepatic **Half-life:** Minutes

Adverse events: Tachyarrhythmias, hypertension at high doses

PROPOFOL (Diprivan)
Mix: Undiluted (10 mg/ml) 100-ml vial
Propofol 10 mg/ml (premixed) (rate is ml/hr)

	mcg/kg/min											
kg	10	15	20	25	30	35	40	45	50	55	60	65
50	3	5	6	8	9	11	12	14	15	17	18	20
55	3	5	7	8	10	12	13	15	17	18	20	21
60	4	5	7	9	11	13	14	16	18	20	22	23
65	4	6	8	10	12	14	16	18	20	21	23	25
70	4	6	8	11	13	15	17	19	21	23	25	27
75	5	7	9	11	14	16	18	20	23	25	27	29
80	5	7	10	12	14	17	19	22	24	26	29	31
85	5	8	10	13	15	18	20	23	26	28	31	33
90	5	8	11	14	16	19	22	24	27	30	32	35
95	6	9	11	14	17	20	23	26	29	31	34	37
100	6	9	12	15	18	21	24	27	30	33	36	39

Use: Nonamnestic sedation
Dose: Load 1–2 mg/kg IV push; **do not load if pt is hypotensive or volume depleted**
Maintenance Initial dose of 5–20 mcg/kg/min, may titrate to effect (20–65 mcg/kg/min)
Mechanism: Di-isopropyl phenolic compound with intravenous general anesthetic properties unrelated to opiates, barbiturates, benzodiazepines
Elimination: Hepatic **Half-life:** 30 min
Adverse events: Hypotension, nausea, vomiting, seizures, hypertriglyceridemia, hyperlipidemia

SODIUM NITROPRUSSIDE (Nipride)
Mix: 50 mg in 250 ml of D_5W (200 mcg/ml)

Body Weight

	lb	88	99	110	121	132	143	154	165	176	187	198	209	220	231	242
	kg	40	45	50	55	60	65	70	75	80	85	90	95	100	105	110
Dose ordered in mcg/kg/min	***Amount to infuse in mcgtts/min or ml/hr***															
0.5		6	7	8	8	9	10	11	11	12	13	14	14	15	16	17
1		12	14	15	17	18	20	21	23	24	26	27	29	30	32	33
1.5		13	20	23	25	27	29	32	34	36	38	41	43	45	47	50
2		24	27	30	33	36	39	42	45	48	51	54	57	60	63	66
3		36	41	45	50	54	59	63	68	72	77	81	86	90	95	99
4		48	54	60	66	72	78	84	90	96	102	108	114	120	126	132
5		60	68	75	83	90	98	105	113	120	128	135	143	150	158	165
6		72	81	90	99	108	117	126	135	144	153	162	171	180	189	198
7		84	95	105	116	126	137	147	158	168	179	189	200	210	221	231
8		96	108	120	132	144	156	168	180	192	204	216	228	240	252	264
9		108	122	135	149	162	176	189	203	216	230	243	257	270	284	297
10		120	135	150	165	180	195	210	225	240	255	270	285	300	315	330

- Administer 0.5–10 mcg/kg/min initially.
- Increase in increments of 1 mcg/kg/min until desired response.
- Do not leave solution exposed to light.

Appendix D

DRUGS OF ABUSE

Name (Brand)	Class	Signs and Symptoms	Treatment
Acid (see LSD)			
Adam (see MDMA)			
Amphetamine (Adderall, Dexedrine)	Stimulant	Tachycardia, hypertension, diaphoresis, agitation, headache, seizures, dehydration, hypokalemia, lactic acidosis. Severe overdose: hyperthermia, dysrhythmia, shock, rhabdomyolysis, hepatic necrosis, acute renal failure.	Control agitation, reverse hyperthermia, support hemodynamic function. **Antidote:** No specific antidote.
Angel dust (see phencyclidine)			
Apache (see fentanyl)			
Barbiturates (Nembutal, Seconal)	Depressant	Hypotension, hypothermia, apnea, nystagmus, ataxia, hyporeflexia, drowsiness, stupor, coma.	Airway management, decontamination, supportive care. **Antidote:** No specific antidote.
Barbs (see barbiturates)			
Benzodiazepines (Xanax, Valium, Librium, Halcion)	Depressant	Respiratory depression, hypothermia, hypotension, nystagmus, miosis, diplopia, bradycardia, nausea, vomiting, impaired speech and coordination, amnesia, ataxia, somnolence, confusion, depressed deep tendon reflexes.	**Antidote:** Flumazenil (Romazicon) is a specific antidote.
Black tar (see heroin)			
Boomers (see LSD)			
Buttons (see mescaline)			
Cactus (see mescaline)			
Candy (see benzodiazepines)			
China girl (see fentanyl)			
China white (see heroin)			

Name (Brand)	Class	Signs and Symptoms	Treatment
Cocaine	Stimulant	Hypertension, tachycardia, mild hyperthermia, mydriasis, pallor, diaphoresis, psychosis, paranoid delusions, mania, agitation, seizures.	Control agitation, seizures, hyperthermia; support hemodynamic function. **Antidote:** No specific antidote.
Codeine	Opioid	Miosis, respiratory depression, decreased mental status, hypotension, cardiac dysrhythmia, hypoxia, bronchoconstriction, constipation, decreased intestinal motility, ileus, lethargy, coma.	Airway management, hemodynamic support. **Antidote:** Naloxone, nalmefene.
Coke (see cocaine)			
Crank (see amphetamine)			
Crank (see heroin)			
Crystal (see amphetamine)			
Crystal meth (see methamphetamine)			
Cubes (see LSD)			
Downers (see benzodiazepines)			
Ecstasy (see MDMA)			
Fentanyl (Sublimaze)	Opioid	Miosis, respiratory depression, decreased mental status, hypotension, cardiac dysrhythmia, hypoxia, bronchoconstriction, constipation, decreased intestinal motility, ileus, lethargy, coma.	Airway management, hemodynamic support. **Antidote:** Naloxone, nalmefene.
Flunitrazepam (Rohypnol)	Depressant	Drowsiness, slurred speech, impaired judgment and motor skills, hypothermia, hypotension, bradycardia, diplopia, blurred vision, nystagmus, respiratory depression, nausea, constipation, depression, lethargy, headache, ataxia, coma, amnesia, incoordination, tremors, vertigo.	Supportive care, airway control. **Antidote:** Flumazenil (Romazicon).
Forget me pill (see flunitrazepam)			

(*continued*)

Name (Brand)	Class	Signs and Symptoms	Treatment
GHB (gamma-hydroxybutyrate)	CNS depressant	Dose-related CNS depression, amnesia, hypotonia, drowsiness, dizziness, euphoria. Other effects: bradycardia, hypotension, hypersalivation, vomiting, hypothermia. Higher dosages: Cheyne-Stokes respiration, seizures, coma, death. Users may become highly agitated.	Supportive care. Severe intoxication may require airway support, including intubation. **Antidote:** No specific antidote.
Gib (see GHB)			
Goodfellas (see fentanyl)			
Grass (see marijuana)			
Hashish (see marijuana)			
Heroin	Opioid	Miosis, coma, apnea, pulmonary edema, bradycardia, hypotension, pinpoint pupils, CNS depression, seizures.	Airway management. **Antidote:** Naloxone, nalmefene.
Horse (see heroin)			
Ice (see amphetamine)			
Ketamine (Ketalar)	Anesthetic	Feeling of dissociation from one's self (sense of floating over one's body), visual hallucinations, lack of coordination, hypertension, tachycardia, palpitations, respiratory depression, apnea, confusion, negativism, hostility, delirium, reduced awareness.	Supportive care, esp. respiratory and cardiac function. **Antidote:** No specific antidote.
Keets (see ketamine)			
Kit-kat (see ketamine)			
Liquid ecstasy (see GHB)			
Liquid X (see GHB)			
LSD	Hallucinogen	Diaphoresis, mydriasis, dizziness, muscle twitching, flushing, hyperreflexia, hypertension, psychosis, behavioral changes, emotional lability, euphoria or dysphoria, paranoia, vomiting, diarrhea, anorexia, restlessness, incoordination, tremors, ataxia.	Airway management, control activity associated with hallucinations, psychosis, panic reaction. **Antidote:** No specific antidote.

Name (Brand)	Class	Signs and Symptoms	Treatment
Ludes (see methaqualone)			
Magic mushroom (see psilocybin)			
Marijuana	Cannabinoid	Increased appetite, reduced motility, constipation, urinary retention, seizures, euphoria, drowsiness, heightened awareness, relaxation, altered time perception, short-term memory loss, poor concentration, mood alterations, disorientation, decreased strength, ataxia, slurred speech, respiratory depression, coma.	Airway management, supportive care. **Antidote:** No specific antidote.
MDMA (Methylene-dioxymethamphetamine)	Stimulant	Euphoria, intimacy, closeness to others, loss of appetite, tachycardia, jaw tension, bruxism, diaphoresis.	**Antidote:** No specific antidote.
Mescaline	Hallucinogen	Diaphoresis, mydriasis, dizziness, twitching, flushing, hyperreflexia, hypertension, psychosis, behavioral changes, emotional instability, euphoria or dysphoria, paranoia, vomiting, diarrhea, anorexia, restlessness, incoordination, tremors, ataxia.	Airway management, control activity associated with hallucinations, psychosis, panic reaction. **Antidote:** No specific antidote.
Meth (see methamphetamine)			
Methamphetamine (Desoxyn)	Stimulant	Hypertension, hyperthermia, hyperpyrexia, agitation, hyperactivity, fasciculation, seizures, coma, tachycardia, dysrhythmias, pale skin, diaphoresis, restlessness, talkativeness, insomnia, headache, coma, delusions, paranoia, aggressive behavior, visual, tactile, or auditory hallucinations.	Airway control, hyperthermia, seizures, dysrhythmias. **Antidote:** No specific antidote.

(*continued*)

Name (Brand)	Class	Signs and Symptoms	Treatment
Methaqualone (Quaalude)	Depressant	Slurred speech, impaired judgment and motor skills, hypothermia, hypotension, bradycardia, diplopia, blurred vision, nystagmus, mydriasis, respiratory depression, depression, lethargy, headache, ataxia, coma, amnesia, incoordination, hypertonicity, myoclonus, tremors, vertigo.	Airway management, supportive care. **Antidote:** No specific antidote.
Methylphenidate (Ritalin)	Stimulant	Agitation, hypertension, tachycardia, hyperthermia, mydriasis, dry mouth, nausea, vomiting, anorexia, abdominal pain, agitation, hyperactivity, insomnia, euphoria, dizziness, paranoid ideation, social withdrawal, delirium, hallucina tions, psychosis, tremors, seizures.	Control agitation, hyperthermia, seizures, support hemodynamic function. **Antidote:** No specific antidote.
Miss Emma (see morphine)			
Mister blue (see morphine)			
Morphine (MS-Contin, Roxanol)	Opioid	Miosis, respiratory depression, decreased mental status, hypotension, cardiac dysrhythmia, hypoxia, bronchoconstriction, constipation, decreased intestinal motility, ileus, lethargy, coma.	Airway management, hemodynamic support. **Antidote:** Naloxone, nalmefene.
Oxy (see oxycodone)			
Oxycodone (OxyContin)	Opioid	Miosis, respiratory depression, decreased mental status, hypotension, cardiac dysrhythmia, hypoxia, bronchoconstriction, constipation, decreased intestinal motility, ileus, lethargy, coma.	Airway management, hemodynamic support. **Antidote:** Naloxone, nalmefene.

Name (Brand)	Class	Signs and Symptoms	Treatment
OxyContin (see oxycodone)			
Peace pill (see phencyclidine)			
Phencyclidine (PCP)	Hallucinogen	Nystagmus, hypertension, tachycardia, agitation, hallucinations, violent behavior, impaired judgment, delusions, psychosis.	Support B/P, manage airway, control agitation. **Antidote:** No specific antidote.
Phennies (see barbiturates)			
Pot (see marijuana)			
Propoxyphene (Darvon)	Depressant	Respiratory depression, seizures, cardiac toxicity, miosis, dysrhythmias, nausea, vomiting, anorexia, abdominal pain, constipation, drowsiness, coma, confusion, hallucinations.	Maintain airway, seizures, cardiac toxicity. **Antidote:** Naloxone.
Psilocybin	Hallucinogen	Diaphoresis, mydriasis, dizziness, twitching, flushing, hyperreflexia, hypertension, psychosis, behavioral changes, emotional lability, euphoria or dysphoria, paranoia, vomiting, diarrhea, anorexia, restlessness, incoordination, tremors, ataxia.	Manage airway, control activity associated with hallucinations, psychosis, panic reaction. **Antidote:** No specific antidote.
Purple passion (see psilocybin)			
Quay (see methaqualone)			
Reefer (see marijuana)			
Rock (see cocaine)			
Rocket fuel (see phencyclidine)			
Roofies (see flunitrazepam)			
Rope (see flunitrazepam)			
Rophies (see flunitrazepam)			
Salty water (see GHB)			
Schoolboy (see codeine)			
Scoop (see GHB)			
Snow (see cocaine)			
Special K (see ketamine)			

(*continued*)

Name (Brand)	Class	Signs and Symptoms	Treatment
Speed (see amphetamine)			
STP (see MDMA)			
Super acid (see ketamine)			
Super K (see ketamine)			
Tranks (see benzodiazepines)			
Uppers (see amphetamine)			
White girl (see cocaine)			
Yellow jackets (see barbiturates)			
Yellow sunshine (see LSD)			

"CLUB DRUG" WEB SITES

www.drugfreeamerica.org	Partnership for a Drug-Free America
www.clubdrugs.org	Consumer-oriented site sponsored by the National Institute on Drug Abuse
www.health.org	Substance Abuse and Mental Health Services Administration
www.projectghb.org	Independent site devoted to risks and dangers of GHB use
www.nida.nih.gov	National Institute on Drug Abuse
www.dea.gov	Drug Enforcement Administration
www.whitehousedrugpolicy.org	Office of National Drug Control Policy

Appendix E

EQUI-ANALGESIC DOSING

Guidelines for equi-analgesic dosing of commonly used analgesics are presented in the following table. The dosages are equivalent to 10 mg of morphine intramuscularly. These guidelines are for the management of acute pain in the opioid naive pt. Dosages may vary for the opioid-tolerant pt and for the management of chronic pain. Clinical response is the criteria that must be applied for each pt with titration to desired response.

Name	Equi-Analgesic Oral Dose	Equi-Analgesic Parenteral Dose
Butorphanol (Stadol)	Not available	2 mg q3–4h
Codeine	130 mg q3–4h	75 mg q3–4h
Hydrocodone	5–10 mg q3–4h	Not available
Hydromorphone (Dilaudid)	7.5 mg q3–4h	1.5 mg q3–4h
Meperidine (Demerol)	300 mg q2–3h	75–100 mg q3h
Methadone (Dolophine)	10–20 mg q6–8h	10 mg q6–8h
Morphine	30 mg q3–4h	10 mg q3–4h
Nalbuphine (Nubain)	Not available	10 mg q3–4h
Oxycodone (OxyContin)	20–30 mg q3–4h	Not available
Propoxyphene (Darvon)	65–130 mg q4–6h	Not available

Appendix F

FDA PREGNANCY CATEGORIES

◀ **ALERT** ▶ Medications should be used during pregnancy only if clearly needed.

A: Adequate and well-controlled studies have failed to show a risk to the fetus in the first trimester of pregnancy (also, no evidence of risk has been seen in later trimesters). Possibility of fetal harm appears remote.

B: Animal reproduction studies have failed to show a risk to the fetus, and there are no adequate/well-controlled studies in pregnant women.

C: Animal reproduction studies have shown an adverse effect on the fetus, and there are no adequate/well-controlled studies in humans. However, the benefits may warrant use of the drug in pregnant women despite potential risks.

D: There is positive evidence of human fetal risk based on data from investigational or marketing experience or from studies in humans, but the potential benefits may warrant use of the drug despite potential risks (e.g., use in life-threatening situations in which other medications cannot be used or are ineffective).

X: Animal or human studies have shown fetal abnormalities and/or there is evidence of human fetal risk based on adverse reaction data from investigational or marketing experience where the risks of using the medication clearly outweigh potential benefits.

Appendix G

HERBAL THERAPIES AND INTERACTIONS

The use of herbal therapies is increasing in the United States. In 1990, an estimated 1 in 3 Americans used at least one form of alternative medicine (of which herbal therapy is part). By 1997, more than $12 billion was spent in the United States for vitamins and minerals, herbals, sports supplements, or specialty supplements (e.g., glucosamine).

Because of the rise in the use of herbal therapy in the United States, the following is presented to provide some basic information on some of the more popular herbs. Please note this is not an all-inclusive list, which is beyond the scope of this handbook.

Name	Uses	Interactions	Precautions
Aloe	***Topical:*** Promotes burn/wound healing, treatment of cold sores. ***Oral:*** Osteoarthritis, inflammatory bowel disease (e.g., ulcerative colitis).	***Topical:*** None known. ***Oral:*** Additive effect with antidiabetic agents, may increase adverse effects of digoxin, diuretics (due to hypokalemia).	***Topical:*** None known. ***Oral:*** Abdominal pain, diarrhea, reduced serum potassium.
Astaxanthin	***Oral:*** Macular degeneration, Alzheimer's disease, Parkinson's disease, stroke, cancer, hypercholester-olemia. ***Topical:*** Sunburn.	None known.	May cause visual disturbances.
Avocado	Reduce serum cholesterol, stimulate menstrual flow, treatment of osteoarthritis.	May reduce effects of warfarin.	Pts allergic to latex should avoid eating avocado due to possibility of cross sensitivity.
Bilberry	***Topical:*** Mild inflammation of mouth/throat. ***Oral:*** Improves visual acuity (e.g., night vision). Treatment of degenerative retinal conditions, atherosclerosis, hemorrhoids.	May require adjustment of antidiabetic drugs (reduces glucose effect).	May decrease serum glucose, triglycerides.

(continued)

Name	Uses	Interactions	Precautions
Bitter orange	Appetite stimulant, treatment of dyspepsia, weight loss, nasal congestion.	Can inhibit cytochrome P450 metabolism of drugs causing increased drug levels, risk of adverse effects (e.g., felodipine [Plendil], indinavir [Crixivan], and midazolam [Versed]).	Contains synephrine and octopamine, which may cause hypertension, cardiovascular toxicity. Avoid use in pregnancy when used for medicinal purposes, safe when used orally in amounts found in foods.
Black cohosh*	Manage menopause symptoms, premenstrual syndrome (PMS), dysmenorrheal, dyspepsia, mild sedative.	May decrease effects of cisplatin in breast cancer. May increase risk of hepatic damage with hepatotoxic drugs (e.g., acetaminophen, amiodarone).	Side effects: nausea, dizziness, visual changes, migraine.
Boldo	Mild GI spasms, dyspepsia, anti-inflammatory agent, laxative, gallstones.	May have additive effects when used with anticoagulant or antiplatelet medications.	***Oral:*** Seizures. ***Topical:*** Skin irritation.
Butterbur	Abdominal pain, back pain, gallbladder pain, bladder spasms, tension headache, migraine headaches, asthma.	Cytochrome P450 inducers (e.g., carbamazepine, phenytoin, rifampin) may increase risk of hepatic toxicity.	May cause headache, itchy eyes, diarrhea, asthma, abdominal discomfort, fatigue, drowsiness.
Capsicum	***Topical:*** Postherpetic, trigeminal, diabetic neuralgias; HIV-associated peripheral neuropathy. ***Oral:*** Dyspepsia, diarrhea, cramps, toothache, hyperlipidemia, prevent arteriosclerosis, heart disease.	May increase effects/adverse effects of antiplatelet medication.	Burning, urticaria, irritation to eyes, mucous membranes.

*See full herb entry in the A to Z section.

Name	Uses	Interactions	Precautions
Cat's claw	Diverticulitis, peptic ulcer, colitis, hemorrhoids, Alzheimer's disease.	May increase effect of antihypertensives. May interfere with immunosuppressant therapy (e.g., cyclosporine, tacrolimus, sirolimus) due to immunostimulating activity.	Headache, dizziness, vomiting.
Catnip	***Topical:*** Arthritis, hemorrhoids. ***Oral:*** Insomnia, migraine, cold, flu, hives, indigestion, cramping, flatulence.	May be additive with other CNS depressants.	Headache, malaise, vomiting (large doses).
Chamomile*	Antispasmodic, sedative, anti-inflammatory, astringent, antibacterial.	May increase bleeding with anticoagulants. May increase sedative effect with benzodiazepines.	Anaphylactic reaction if allergic; avoid use if allergic to chrysanthemums, ragweed, and/or asters; delays absorption of medications.
Chastberry	***Oral:*** Control of menstrual irregularities, painful menstruation.	May interfere with oral contraceptives, hormone replacement therapy, dopamine antagonists (e.g., antipsychotics), pramipexole, ropinirole, metoclopramide	GI disturbances, rash, pruritus, headache, increased menstrual flow.
Co-Enzyme Q-10	***Oral:*** CHF, angina, diabetes, hypertension; reduces symptoms of chronic fatigue; stimulates immune system in those with AIDS.	May decrease effect of warfarin. May have additive effects with antihypertensives.	Reduced appetite, gastritis, nausea, diarrhea.
Conjugated linoleic acid	Obesity, bodybuilding, atherosclerosis.	May increase vitamin A storage in liver and breast tissues.	May cause GI upset, diarrhea, nausea, loose stools, dyspepsia, fatigue. Avoid use in pregnancy when used for medicinal purposes, safe when used orally in amounts found in foods.

(continued)

*See full herb entry in the A to Z section.

Name	Uses	Interactions	Precautions
Cranberry	***Oral:*** Prevention, treatment of UTIs neurogenic bladder, urinary deodorizer.	May increase effect of warfarin.	Large doses may cause diarrhea.
Devil's claw	Osteoarthritis, rheumatoid arthritis, gout, myalgia, lumbago, tendonitis, GI upset, dyspepsia, migraine headache.	May increase effect of antihypertensives, warfarin. May decrease effect of antacids, H_2 blockers (e.g., cimetidine), proton pump inhibitors (e.g., lansoprazole, omeprazole).	Diarrhea, nausea, vomiting, abdominal pain. May cause skin reactions.
DHEA*	Slows aging, boosts energy, controls weight.	May interfere with antiestrogen effects of aromatase inhibitors (e.g., anastrozole). May interfere with estrogen receptor antagonist activity of tamoxifen in estrogen receptor-positive cancer cells (e.g., breast, ovarian cancer).	Side effects: may increase risk of breast/prostate cancer. Women may develop acne, hair growth on face/body.
Dong quai*	Dysmenorrhea, PMS, menopause symptoms.	May increase effects of warfarin, antiplatelet medications.	Diarrhea, photosensitivity, skin cancer; avoid use in pregnancy/lactation; essential oil may contain the carcinogen safrole.
Echinacea*	Treat/prevent common cold, other upper respiratory tract infections.	May interfere with immunosuppressive therapy.	Not to be used with weakened immune system (e.g., HIV/AIDS, tuberculosis, multiple sclerosis). Habitual or continued use may suppress the immune system (should only be taken for 2–3 mos or alternating schedule of q2–3wk).

*See full herb entry in the A to Z section.

Name	Uses	Interactions	Precautions
Elderberry	Treatment of influenza, laxative, diuretic, allergic rhinitis, sinusitis, neuralgia	May interfere with immunosuppressant therapy (e.g., azathioprine [Imuran], cyclosporine [Neoral], mycophenolate [CellCept]).	Avoid using during pregnancy and lactation. Well tolerated. May cause nausea, vomiting, severe diarrhea.
Emu oil	***Oral:*** Hypercholesterolemia, weight loss, cough syrup. ***Topical:*** Relief from sore muscles, arthralgia, pain, inflammation, carpal tunnel syndrome.	None known.	None reported.
Evening primose oil	***Oral:*** PMS, symptoms of menopause (e.g., hot flashes), psoriasis, rheumatoid arthritis.	Antipsychotics may increase risk of seizures. May increase risk of bleeding with anticoagulants/antiplatelets.	Indigestion, nausea, headache. Large doses may cause diarrhea, abdominal pain.
Fenugreek	Lowered blood glucose, gastritis, constipation, atherosclerosis, elevated serum cholesterol and triglyceride levels.	May have additive effects with antidiabetic, anticoagulant, antiplatelet medications.	Nasal congestion, wheezing. Large doses may cause hypoglycemia.
Feverfew*	Relieves migraine. Treatment of fever, headache, menstrual irregularities.	May increase bleeding time with aspirin, dipyridamole, warfarin.	Side effects: headache, oral ulcers. Should be avoided in pregnancy (stimulates menstruation), nursing mother, children younger than 2 yrs.
Fish oils	***Oral:*** Hypertension, hyperlipidemia, coronary artery disease, rheumatoid arthritis, psoriasis.	May increase risk of bleeding with antiplatelets, anticoagulants. Additive effect with antihypertensives. Contraceptive medications may decrease triglyceride lowering effect.	Belching, heartburn, epistaxis. Large doses may cause nausea, diarrhea.

(continued)

*See full herb entry in the A to Z section.

Name	Uses	Interactions	Precautions
Garlic*	Reduces serum cholesterol, LDL, triglycerides, increases serum HDL, lowers B/P, inhibits platelet aggregation.	May increase effects of warfarin, aspirin, clopidogrel, enoxaparin. May decrease effects of oral contraceptives, cyclosporine, protease inhibitors.	Side effects: altered taste, offensive odor. Large doses may cause heartburn, flatulence, other GI distress.
Ginger*	Motion sickness, morning sickness, dyspepsia, rheumatoid arthritis, osteoarthritis, loss of appetite, migraine headache.	May increase risk of bleeding with warfarin, aspirin, clopidogrel, heparin, low molecular weight heparins. May increase effect of antidiabetic agents, calcium channel blockers.	Avoid use during pregnancy when bleeding is a concern. Large overdose could potentially depress the CNS, cause cardiac arrhythmias.
Ginkgo*	Improves memory, concentration; pt may think more clearly. Overcomes sexual dysfunction occurring with SSRI antidepressants.	May increase risk of bleeding with aspirin, warfarin, clopidogrel, heparin. May decrease effect of anticonvulsants, alter effect of insulin.	Avoid use in those taking anticoagulants or those hypersensitive to poison ivy, cashews, mangos. Side effects: GI disturbances, headache, dizziness, vertigo.
Ginseng*	Boosts energy, sexual stamina; decreases stress, effects of aging.	May increase effect of antidiabetic medications. May decrease effect of antipsychotics, warfarin.	Avoid in pts receiving anticoagulants, medications that increase B/P. Side effects: breast tenderness, anxiety, headache, increased B/P, abnormal vaginal bleeding.
Glucosamine and chondroitin*	Osteoarthritis.	No known interactions but monitor anticoagulant effects.	None known.
Goldenrod	Diuretic, anti-inflammatory, antispasmodic. Prevents urinary tract inflammation, urinary calculi, kidney stones.	May interfere with diuretics.	Allergic reactions.

*See full herb entry in the A to Z section.

Name	Uses	Interactions	Precautions
Goldenseal	***Topical:*** Eczema, itching, acne. ***Oral:*** UTI, hemorrhoids, gastritis, colitis, mucosal inflammation.	May decrease effect of antacids, H_2 blockers, proton pump inhibitors, antihypertensives.	Constipation, hallucinations. Large doses may cause nausea, vomiting, diarrhea, CNS stimulation, respiratory failure.
Gotu kola	Improves memory, intelligence, venous insufficiency (including varicose veins), wound or burn healing.	May increase effects/adverse effects of CNS depressants.	GI upset, nausea, pruritus, photosensitivity.
Grapefruit	Hyperlipidemia, atherosclerosis, psoriasis, weight loss, obesity.	May increase concentration/ adverse effects of benzodiazepines, calcium channel blockers, carbamazepine, carvedilol, cyclosporine, statins.	None known.
Green tea	Improves cognition function, treats nausea, vomiting, headache, weight loss.	May increase risk of bleeding with anticoagulants, antiplatelets. May alter effect of antidiabetic medications. May increase effects/adverse effects of cimetidine, clozapine, theophylline.	GI upset, constipation.
Guggul	Lowers serum cholesterol, treatment of acne, skin disease, weight loss.	May increase risk of bleeding with anticoagulants/ antiplatelets. May decrease effect of dilitiazem, propranolol, tamoxifen.	May cause headache, nausea, vomiting, loose stools, bloating.
Gymnema	Treatment of diabetes, cough.	May enhance effects of insulin, oral antidiabetics.	None reported.

(continued)

*See full herb entry in the A to Z section.

Name	Uses	Interactions	Precautions
Hawthorn	Cardiovascular conditions (e.g., atherosclerosis), GI conditions (diarrhea, indigestion, abdominal pain), sleep disorders.	May increase effect of betablockers, calcium channel blockers, digoxin, nitrates. May increase vasodilation/ hypotension with sildenafil, tadalafil, vardenafil.	Nausea, GI complaints, headache, dizziness, insomnia, agitation.
Hoodia	Appetite suppressant for obesity, weight loss.	None known.	None reported.
Horse chestnut	Treat varicose veins, hemorrhoids, phlebitis.	May enhance effects of insulin, oral antidiabetics, antiplatelet medications.	Muscle cramps, pruritus, GI irritation.
Kava kava*	Anxiety disorders, ADHD, insomnia, restlessness.	Increases CNS depression with alcohol, sedatives.	GI upset, headache, dizziness, drowsiness, enlarged pupils, disturbances of accommodation, dry mouth, allergic skin reactions.
L-Carnitine	Treatment of primary L-Carnitine deficiency, postmyocardial infarction protection, dementia, angina, CHF, intermittent claudication.	None known.	Abdominal discomfort, diarrhea, nausea, vomiting, heartburn.
Licorice	Inflammation of upper respiratory tract, mucous membranes, ulcers, expectorant.	May decrease effect of antihypertensives. Thiazides may increase potassium loss.	Large doses may cause pseudoaldosteronism (hypertension, headache, lethargy, edema).
Melatonin*	Aids sleep, prevents jet lag.	May decrease effect of oral antidiabetic agents, immunosuppressants. May have additive effect with CNS depressants.	Side effects: headache, confusion, fatigue. Does not lengthen total sleep time.

*See full herb entry in the A to Z section.

Name	Uses	Interactions	Precautions
Milk thistle	Hepatoprotective, antioxidant, hepatic disorders, including poisoning (e.g., mushroom), cirrhosis, hepatitis.	None known.	Mild allergic reactions, laxative effect.
MSM (methyl sulfonyl methane)	***Oral/topical:*** Chronic pain, arthritis, inflammation, osteoporosis, muscle cramps/pain, wrinkles, protection against windburn or sunburn.	None known.	May cause nausea, diarrhea, headache, pruritus, increase in allergic symptoms.
Omega-6 fatty acid	Coronary artery disease, decreases total serum LDL cholesterol, increases serum HDL.	None known.	Increases serum triglycerides.
Policosanol	Hyperlipidemia, intermittent claudication, reducing myocardial ischemia.	Can inhibit platelet aggregation. May increase risk of bruising and bleeding with aspirin, Plavix, NSAIDs, heparin, warfarin.	Usually well tolerated. Avoid using during pregnancy and lactation. May cause erythema, migraines, insomnia, irritability, upset stomach, weight loss, skin rash.
Pomegranate	Hypertension, CHF, atherosclerosis, tapeworm manifestations.	May have additive effects with ACE inhibitors, antihypertensives.	Avoid using during pregnancy and breastfeeding. May cause allergic reactions, GI disturbances.
Prickly pear cactus	Hypercholesterolemia, obesity, alcohol induced hangover.	None known.	Usually well tolerated. May cause mild diarrhea, nausea, increased stool volume/ frequency abdominal fullness, headache.
Red clover	***Oral:*** Menopausal symptoms, hot flashes, prevention of cancer, indigestion, asthma. ***Topical:*** Skin sores, burns, chronic skin disease (e.g., eczema, psoriasis).	May increase anticoagulant effects of warfarin. May interfere with hormone replacement therapy, oral contraceptives, tamoxifen.	Rash, myalgia, headache, nausea, vaginal spotting.

(continued)

*See full herb entry in the A to Z section.

Name	Uses	Interactions	Precautions
SAMe	Depression, heart disease, osteoarthritis, Alzheimer's disease, Parkinson's disease; slows aging process.	May increase adverse effects with antidepressants.	Nausea, vomiting, diarrhea, flatulence; headache.
Saw palmetto*	Eases symptoms of enlarged prostate (frequency, dysuria, nocturia).	May increase risk of bleeding with anticoagulants/antiplatelets. May interfere with oral contraceptives, estrogen.	Side effects: abdominal discomfort, headache, erectile dysfunction. Does not reduce size of enlarged prostate. Obtain baseline PSA levels before initiating. Large doses can cause diarrhea.
Shark cartilage	Cancer, arthritis, psoriasis, wound healing.	None known.	Nausea, vomiting, constipation, dyspepsia, altered taste.
Soy	Menopausal symptoms; prevents osteoporosis and cardiovascular disease in postmenopausal women; hypertension, hyperlipidemia.	May decrease effects of estrogen replacement therapy.	Constipation, bloating, nausea, allergic reaction.
Soybean oil	Lowers total and LDL cholesterol	None known	May cause allergic reactions.
St. John's wort*	Relieves mild to moderate depression.	May decrease effect of alprazolam, oral contraceptives, cyclosporine, calcium channel blockers, antifungals, digoxin, phenytoin, protease inhibitors, atorvastatin, lovastatin, simvastatin, tacrolimus, warfarin. May increase side effects with triptans, antidepressants, MAOIs, paroxetine, sertraline.	Side effects: dizziness, dry mouth, increased sensitivity to sunlight. Report symptoms of "serotonin syndrome."

*See full herb entry in the A to Z section.

Name	Uses	Interactions	Precautions
Tyrosine	PMS, depression, attention deficit disorder (ADD), ADHD, improve alertness.	May decrease effects of L-dopa. May have additive effects with thyroid hormone.	May cause nausea, headache, fatigue, heartburn, arthralgia.
Valerian*	Aids sleep, relieves restlessness and anxiety.	May increase sedative effects with alcohol, CNS depressants.	Side effects: palpitations, upset stomach, headache, excitability, uneasiness. May cause increased morning drowsiness.
Whey protein	Alternative to milk in those with lactose intolerance, treatment of hyperlipidemia, obesity and weight loss.	May decrease absorption of alendronate (Fosamax), levodopa, quinolone antibiotics (e.g., levofloxacin).	Well tolerated. High doses may cause increased stool frequency, nausea, thirst, bloating, cramps, decreased appetite, fatigue, headache.
Wild yam	Alternative for estrogen replacement therapy, postmenopausal vaginal dryness, PMS, osteoporosis, increases energy/ libido, breast enlargement.	None known.	Large amounts may cause vomiting (tincture).
Yohimbe*	Male aphrodisiac. Used to treat impotence, erectile dysfunction, orthostatic hypotension.	May decrease effect of antihypertensives. May have additive effects with MAOIs, CNS stimulants.	Large doses linked to weakness, paralysis.

*See full herb entry in the A to Z section.

Appendix H

LIFESPAN AND CULTURAL ASPECTS OF DRUG THERAPY

LIFESPAN

Drug therapy is unique to pts of different ages. Age-specific competencies involve understanding the development and health needs of the various age groups. Pregnant pts, children, and the elderly represent different age groups with important considerations during drug therapy.

CHILDREN

In pediatric drug therapy, drug administration is guided by the age of the child, weight, level of growth and development, and height. The dosage ordered is to be given either by kilogram of body weight or by square meter of body surface area, which is based on the height and weight of the child. Many dosages based on these calculations must be individualized based on pediatric response.

If the oral route of administration is used, often syrup or chewable tablets are given. Additionally, sometimes medication is added to liquid or mixed with foods. Remember to never force a child to take oral medications because choking or emotional trauma may ensue.

If an intramuscular injection is ordered, the vastus lateralis muscle in the mid-lateral thigh is used, because the gluteus maximus is not developed until walking occurs and the deltoid muscle is too small. For intravenous medications, administer very slowly in children. If given too quickly, high serum drug levels will occur with the potential for toxicity.

PREGNANCY

Women of childbearing years should be asked about the possibility of pregnancy before any drug therapy is initiated. Advise a woman who is either planning a pregnancy or believes she may be pregnant to inform her physician immediately. During pregnancy, medications given to the mother pass to the fetus via the placenta. Teratogenic (fetal abnormalities) effects may occur. Breast-feeding while the mother is taking certain medications may not be recommended due to the potential for adverse effects on the newborn.

The choice of drug ordered for pregnant women is based on the stage of pregnancy, because the fetal organs develop during the first trimester. Cautious use of drugs in women of reproductive age who are sexually active and who are not using contraceptives is essential to prevent the potential for teratogenic or embryotoxic effects. Refer to the different pregnancy categories (found in Appendix F) to determine the relative safety of a medication during pregnancy.

ELDERLY

The elderly are more likely to experience an adverse drug reaction owing to physiologic changes (e.g., visual, hearing, mobility changes, chronic diseases) and cognitive changes (short-term memory loss or alteration in the thought process) that may lead to multiple medication dosing. In chronic disease states such as hypertension, glaucoma, asthma, or arthritis, the daily ingestion of multiple medications increases the potential for adverse reactions and toxic effects.

Decreased renal or hepatic function may lower the metabolism of medications in the liver and reduce excretion of medications, thus prolonging the half-life of the drug and the potential for toxicity. Dosages in the elderly should initially be smaller than for the general adult population and then slowly titrated based on pt response and therapeutic effect of the medication.

CULTURE

The term *ethnopharmacology* was first used to describe the study of medicinal plants used by indigenous cultures. More recently, it is being used as a reference to the action and effects of drugs in people from diverse racial, ethnic, and cultural backgrounds. Although there are insufficient data from investigations involving people from diverse backgrounds that would provide reliable information on ethnic-specific responses to all medications, there is growing evidence that modifications in dosages are needed for some members of racial and ethnic groups. There are wide variations in the perception of side effects by pts from diverse cultural backgrounds. These differences may be related to metabolic differences that result in higher or lower levels of the drug, individual differences in the amount of body fat, or cultural differences in the way individuals perceive the meaning of side effects and toxicity. Nurses and other health care providers need to be aware that variations can occur with side effects, adverse reactions, and toxicity so that pts from diverse cultural backgrounds can be monitored.

Some cultural differences in response to medications include the following:

African Americans: Generally, African Americans are less responsive to beta-blockers (e.g., propranolol [Inderal]) and angiotensin-converting enzyme (ACE) inhibitors (e.g., enalapril [Vasotec]).

Asian Americans: On average, Asian Americans have a lower percentage of body fat, so dosage adjustments must be made for fat-soluble vitamins and other drugs (e.g., vitamin K used to reverse the anticoagulant effect of warfarin).

Hispanic Americans: Hispanic Americans may require lower dosages and may experience a higher incidence of side effects with the tricyclic antidepressants (e.g., amitriptyline).

Native Americans: Alaskan Eskimos may suffer prolonged muscle paralysis with the use of succinylcholine when administered during surgery.

There has been a desire to exert more responsibility over one's health and, as a result, a resurgence of self-care practices. These practices are often influenced by folk remedies and the use of medicinal plants. In the United States, there are several major ethnic population subgroups (white, black, Hispanic, Asian, and Native Americans). Each of these ethnic groups has a wide range of practices that influence beliefs and interventions related to health and illness. At any given time, in any group, treatment may consist of the use of traditional herbal therapy, a combination of ritual and prayer with medicinal plants, customary dietary and environmental practices, or the use of Western medical practices.

African Americans

Many African Americans carry the traditional health beliefs of their African heritage. Health denotes harmony with nature of the body, mind, and spirit, whereas illness is seen as disharmony that results from natural causes or divine punishment. Common practices to the art of healing include treatments with herbals and rituals known empirically to restore health. Specific forms of healing include using home remedies, obtaining medical advice from a physician, and seeking spiritual healing.

Examples of healing practices include the use of hot baths and warm compresses for rheumatism, the use of herbal teas for respiratory illnesses, and the use of kitchen condiments in folk remedies. Lemon, vinegar, honey, saltpeter, alum, salt, baking soda, and Epsom salt are common kitchen ingredients used. Goldenrod, peppermint, sassafras, parsley, yarrow, and rabbit tobacco are a few of the herbals used.

Hispanic Americans

The use of folk healers, medicinal herbs, magic, and religious rituals and ceremonies are included in the rich and varied customs of Hispanic Americans. This ethnic group believes that God is responsible for allowing health or illness to occur. Wellness may be viewed as good luck, a reward for good behavior, or a blessing from God. Praying, using herbals and spices, wearing religious objects such as medals, and maintaining a balance in diet and physical activity are methods considered appropriate in preventing evil or poor health.

Hispanic ethnopharmacology is more complementary to Western medical practices. After the illness is identified, appropriate treatment may consist of home remedies (e.g., use of vegetables and herbs), use of over-the-counter patent medicines, and use of physician-prescribed medications.

Asian Americans

For Asian Americans, harmony with nature is essential for physical and spiritual well-being. Universal balance depends on harmony among the elemental forces: fire, water, wood, earth, and metal. Regulating these universal elements are two forces that maintain physical and spiritual harmony in the body: the *yin* and the *yang*. Practices shared by most Asian cultures include meditation, special nutritional programs, herbology, and martial arts.

Therapeutic options available to traditional Chinese physicians include prescribing herbs, meditation, exercise, nutritional changes, and acupuncture.

Native Americans

The theme of total harmony with nature is fundamental to traditional Native American beliefs about health. It is dependent on maintaining a state of equilibrium among the physical body, the mind, and the environment. Health practices reflect this holistic approach. The method of healing is determined traditionally by the medicine man, who diagnoses the ailment and recommends the appropriate intervention.

Treatment may include heat, herbs, sweat baths, massage, exercise, diet changes, and other interventions performed in a curing ceremony.

European Americans

Europeans often use home treatments as the front-line interventions. Traditional remedies practiced are based on the magical or empirically validated experience of ancestors. These cures are often practiced in combination with religious rituals or spiritual ceremonies.

Household products, herbal teas, and patent medicines are familiar preparations used in home treatments (e.g., salt water gargle for sore throat).

Appendix I

NON-CRUSHABLE DRUGS

Generic Name	Trade Name	Product Availability
Acamprosate	Campral	Tablets: 333 mg
Acetaminophen	Mapap, Tylenol Arthritis Pain	Capsules (extended-release): 650 mg
Acetaminophen	Mapap	Capsules: 500 mg
Acetazolamide	Diamox Sequels	Capsules (sustained-release): 500 mg
Acyclovir	Zovirax	Capsules: 200 mg
Albuterol	Proventil, Repetabs	Tablets (extended-release): 4 mg
Albuterol	Volmax, VoSpire ER	Tablets (extended-release): 4 mg, 8 mg
Alfuzosin	Uroxatral	Tablets (extended-release): 10 mg
Alprazolam	Xanax XR	Tablets (extended-release): 0.5 mg, 1 mg, 2 mg, 3 mg
Aminophylline	Quibron-T/SR	Tablets (controlled-release): 300 mg
Aminophylline	T-Phyl	Tablets (controlled-release): 200 mg
Aminophylline	Theo-24	Capsules (extended-release): 100 mg, 200 mg, 300 mg, 400 mg
Aminophylline	Theocron	Tablets (controlled-release): 100 mg, 200 mg, 300 mg
Aminophylline	Theolair SR	Tablets (controlled-release): 300 mg, 500 mg
Aminophylline	Uniphyl	Tablets (controlled-release): 400 mg, 600 mg
Amoxicillin/clavulanate	Augmentin XR	Tablets (extended-release): 1,000 mg-62.5 mg
Ascorbic acid	C-500-GR, Cecon, Cedvibid, C-Gram, Vita-C	Capsules (timed-release): 500 mg Tablets (timed-release): 500 mg, 1,000 mg, 1,500 mg
Aspirin	Bayer, Ecotrin, St. Joseph	Tablets (enteric-coated): 81 mg, 325 mg, 500 mg, 650 mg
Atorvastatin	Lipitor	Tablets (film-coated): 10 mg, 20 mg, 40 mg, 80 mg
Bisacodyl	Dulcolax, Fleet	Tablets (enteric-coated): 5 mg
Bupropion	Wellbutrin SR	Tablets (sustained-release): 100 mg, 150 mg, 200 mg
Bupropion	Wellbutrin XL	Tablets (extended-release): 150 mg, 300 mg
Bupropion	Zyban	Tablets (sustained-release): 150 mg
Carbamazepine	Carbatrol, Equetro	Capsules (extended-release): 100 mg, 200 mg, 300 mg
Carbamazepine	Tegretol XR	Tablets (extended-release): 100 mg, 200 mg, 400 mg

(continued)

Generic Name	Trade Name	Product Availability
Carbidopa/levodopa	Sinemet CR	Tablets (extended-release): 25 mg carbidopa/100 mg levodopa, 50 mg carbidopa/200 mg levodopa
Cefadroxil	Ceclor CD	Tablets (extended-release): 375 mg, 500 mg
Cinacalcet	Sensipar	Tablets (film-coated): 30 mg, 60 mg, 90 mg
Ciprofloxacin	Cipro XR, Proquin XR	Tablets (extended-release): 500 mg
Clarithromycin	Biaxin XL, Biaxin XL PAK	Tablets (extended-release): 500 mg
Clorazepate	Tranxene SD Half Strength	Tablets (sustained-release): 11.25 mg
Clorazepate	Tranxene SD	Tablets (sustained-release): 22.5 mg
Darifenacin	Enablex	Tablets (extended-release): 7.5 mg, 15 mg
Dasatinib	Sprycal	Tablets (film-coated): 20 mg, 50 mg, 70 mg
Dexmethylphenidate	Focalin XR	Capsules (extended-release): 5 mg, 10 mg, 20 mg
Dextroamphetamine	Dexedrine Spansule	Capsules (sustained-release): 5 mg, 10 mg, 15 mg
Diclofenac	Voltaren	Tablets (delayed-release): 25 mg, 50 mg, 75 mg
Diclofenac	Voltaren XR	Tablets (extended-release): 100 mg
Didanosine	Videx EC	Capsules (delayed-release): 125 mg, 200 mg, 250 mg, 400 mg
Diflunisal	Dolobid	Tablets: 250 mg, 500 mg
Diltiazem	Cardizem CD, Taztia XT	Capsules (extended-release): 120 mg, 180 mg, 240 mg, 300 mg, 360 mg
Diltiazem	Cardizem LA	Tablets (extended-release): 120 mg, 180 mg, 240 mg, 300 mg, 360 mg, 420 mg
Diltiazem	Cardizem SR	Capsules (sustained-release): 60 mg, 90 mg, 120 mg
Diltiazem	Cartia XT	Capsules (extended-release): 120 mg, 180 mg, 240 mg, 300 mg
Diltiazem	Dilacor XR, Diltia XT	Capsules (extended-release): 120 mg, 180 mg, 240 mg
Diltiazem	Tiazac	Capsules (extended-release): 120 mg, 180 mg, 240 mg, 300 mg, 360 mg, 420 mg
Diphenhydramine	Banophen, Diphen, Genahist	Capsules: 25 mg
Diphenhydramine	Nytol	Capsules: 50 mg
Disopyramide	Norpace CR	Capsules (extended-release): 100 mg, 150 mg
Dolasetron	Anzemet	Tablets: 50 mg, 100 mg

Generic Name	Trade Name	Product Availability
Duloxetine	Cymbalta	Capsules: 20 mg, 30 mg, 60 mg
Eletriptan	Relpax	Tablets: 20 mg, 40 mg
Eplerenone	Inspra	Tablets: 25 mg, 50 mg
Eprosartan	Teveten	Tablets: 400 mg, 600 mg
Erythromycin	Eryc	Capsules (delayed-release): 250 mg
Erythromycin	Ery-Tab	Tablets (delayed-release): 250 mg, 333 mg, 500 mg
Escitalopram	Lexapro	Tablets: 5 mg, 10 mg, 20 mg
Esomeprazole	Nexium	Capsules (delayed-release): 20 mg, 40 mg
Eszopiclone	Lunesta	Tablets (film-coated): 1 mg, 2 mg, 3 mg
Etodolac	Lodine	Capsules: 200 mg, 300 mg
Etodolac	Lodine XL	Tablets (extended-release): 400 mg, 500 mg, 600 mg
Famotidine	Pepcid, Pepcid AC	Tablets (Pepcid): 40 mg/5 ml, (Pepcid AC): 10 mg
Felodipine	Plendil	Tablets (extended-release): 2.5 mg, 5 mg, 10 mg
Fenoprofen	Nalfon	Capsules: 200 mg, 300 mg
Ferrous fumarate	Ferro-Sequels	Tablets (timed-release): 150 mg (50 mg elemental iron)
Ferrous sulfate	Slow-Fe	Tablets (timed-release): 160 mg (50 mg elemental iron)
Finasteride	Propecia, Proscar	Tablets: 1 mg (Propecia), 5 mg (Proscar)
Fosamprenavir	Lexiva, Telzir	Tablets: 700 mg
Frovatriptan	Frova	Tablets: 2/5 mg
Galantamine	Razadyne ER	Capsules (extended-release): 8 mg, 16 mg, 24 mg
Gemifloxacin	Factive	Tablets: 320 mg
Gefitinib	Iressa	Tablets (film-coated): 250 mg
Guaifenesin	Mucinex	Tablets (extended-release): 600 mg
Hydroxyzine	Vistaril	Capsules: 25 mg, 50 mg
Hyoscamine	Levbid, Symax SR	Tablet (extended-release): 0.375 mg
Indomethacin	Indocin SR	Capsules (sustained-release): 75 mg
Isosorbide dinitrate	Dilatrate SR	Capsules (sustained-release): 40 mg
Isosorbide dinitrate	Isochron	Tablets (extended-release): 40 mg
Isosorbide dinitrate	Isordil	Tablets (sublingual): 2.5 mg, 5 mg
Isosorbide mononitrate	Imdur	Tablets (extended-release): 30 mg, 60 mg, 120 mg
Isradipine	Dynacirc-CR	Capsules (controlled-release): 5 mg, 10 mg

(continued)

Generic Name	Trade Name	Product Availability
Ketoprofen	Oruvail	Capsules (extended-release): 200 mg
Morphine	Avinza	Capsules (extended-release): 30 mg, 60 mg, 90 mg, 120 mg
Morphine	Kadian	Capsules (sustained-release): 20 mg, 30 mg, 50 mg, 60 mg, 100 mg
Morphine	MS Contin	Tablets (extended-release): 15 mg, 30 mg, 60 mg, 100 mg, 200 mg
Morphine	Oramorph SR	Tablets (extended-release): 15 mg, 30 mg, 60 mg, 100 mg, 200 mg
Mycophenolate	Myfortic	Tablets (delayed-release): 180 mg, 360 mg
Nabumetone	Relafen	Tablets: 500 mg, 750 mg
Naproxen	EC-Naprosyn	Tablets (controlled-release): 375 mg naproxen, 500 mg naproxen
Naproxen	Naprelan	Tablets (controlled-release): 421 mg naproxen, 550 mg naproxen sodium (equivalent to 500 mg naproxen)
Naratriptan	Amerge	Tablets: 1 mg, 2.5 mg
Niacin, nicotinic acid		Capsules (extended-release): 125 mg, 250 mg, 400 mg, 500 mg
Niacin, nicotinic acid	Slo-Niacin	Tablets (controlled-release): 250 mg, 500 mg, 750 mg
Niacin, nicotinic acid	Niaspan	Tablets (extended-release): 500 mg, 750 mg, 1,000 mg
Nicardipine	Cardene SR	Capsules (sustained-release): 30 mg, 45 mg, 60 mg
Nifedipine	Adalat CC	Tablets (extended-release): 30 mg, 60 mg, 90 mg
Nifedipine	Nifediac CC	Tablets (extended-release): 30 mg, 60 mg, 90 mg
Nifedipine	Nifedical XL	Tablets (extended-release): 30 mg, 60 mg, 90 mg
Nifedipine	Procardia XL	Tablets (extended-release): 30 mg, 60 mg, 90 mg
Nimodipine	Nimotop	Capsules: 30 mg
Nitroglycerin	Nitro-Tab	Tablets (sublingual): 0.4 mg
Nitroglycerin	Nitro-Time	Capsules (extended-release): 2.5 mg, 6 mg, 9 mg
Nitroglycerin	NitroQuick	Tablets (sublingual): 0.4 mg
Nitroglycerin	Nitrostat	Tablets (sublingual): 0.4 mg
Omeprazole	Prilosec	Capsules (delayed-release): 10 mg, 20 mg, 40 mg
Omeprazple	Zegerid	Capsules (delayed-release): 20 mg, 40 mg

Generic Name	Trade Name	Product Availability
Oxybutynin	Ditropan XL	Tablets (extended-release): 5 mg, 10 mg, 15 mg
Oxycodone	OxyContin	Tablets (extended-release): 10 mg, 20 mg, 40 mg, 80 mg, 160 mg
Pancreatin	Cotazym-S	Capsules (extended-release): 20,000 units-5,000 units-20,000 units
Pancreatin	Creon 5, Lipram-CR5	Capsules (extended-release): 16,600 units-5,000 units-18,750 units
Pancreatin	Creon 10, Lipram-CR	Capsules (extended-release): 33,200 units-10,000 units-37,500 units
Pancreatin	Creon 20, Lipram-CR 20	Capsules (extended-release): 66,400 units-20,000 units-75,000 units
Pancreatin	Lipram, Pancrease, Pangestyme EC, Ultrase	Capsules (extended-release): 20,000 units-4,500 units-25,000 units
Pancreatin	Lipram-PN, Pancrease MT 16, Pangestyme MT 16	Capsules (extended-release): 48,000 units-16,000 units-48,000 units
Pancreatin	Lipram-PN, Pancrease MT 20	Capsules (extended-release): 56,000 units-20,000 units-44,000 units
Pancreatin	Lipram-UL 12, Pancreatil-UL 12, Ultrase MT 12	Capsules (extended-release): 39,000 units-12,000 units-39,000 units
Pancreatin	Lipram-UL 20, Pangestyme NL 18, Pangestyme CN 20, Ultrase MT 20	Capsules (extended-release): 65,000 units-20,000 units-65,000 units
Pancreatin	Panase, Pancreatic EC, Protilase	Capsules (extended-release): 20,000 units-4,000 units-25,000 units
Pancreatin	Pancrease MT 4	Capsules (extended-release): 12,000 units-4,000 units-12,000 units
Pancreatin	Pancrecarb MS-4	Capsules (extended-release): 25,000 units-4,000 units-25,000 units
Pancreatin	Pancrecarb MS-8	Capsules (extended-release): 40,000 units-8,000 units-45,000 units
Pancreatin	Pangestyme CN 10, Lipram, Pancrease MT 10	Capsules (extended-release): 30,000 units-10,000 units-30,000 units
Pancreatin	Pangestyme NL 18, Lipram-UL 18, Ultrase MT 18	Capsules (extended-release): 59,000 units-18,000 units-59,000 units
Rabeprazole	Aciphex	Tablets (delayed-release): 20 mg
Ramelteon	Rozerem	Tablets (film-coated): 8 mg
Ranolazine	Ranexa	Tablets (extended-release): 500 mg

(continued)

Generic Name	Trade Name	Product Availability
Rifaximin	Xifaxan	Tablets: 200 mg
Sitagliptin	Januvia	Tablets (film-coated): 25 mg, 50 mg, 100 mg
Sodium chloride		Tablets (OTC): 1 g
Sulfasalazine	Azulfidine En-Tabs	Tablets (delayed-release): 500 mg
Tamsulosin	Flomax	Capsules: 0.4 mg
Telbivudine	Tyzeka	Tablets (film-coated): 600 mg
Tolterodine	Detrol LA	Capsules (extended-release): 2 mg, 4 mg
Topiramate	Topamax	Tablets: 25 mg, 50 mg, 100 mg, 200 mg
Tramadol	Ultram	Tablets (extended-release): 100 mg, 200 mg, 300 mg
Tretinoin	Vesanoid	Capsules: 10 mg
Valganciclovir	Valcyte	Tablets: 450 mg
Valproic acid	Depakote	Tablets (delayed-release): 125 mg, 250 mg, 500 mg
Valproic acid	Depakote ER	Tablets (extended-release): 250 mg, 500 mg
Varenicline	Chantix	Tablets (film-coated): 0.5 mg, 1 mg
Venlafaxine	Effexor XL	Capsules (extended-release): 37.5 mg, 75 mg, 150 mg
Verapamil	Covera-HS	Tablets (extended-release): 180 mg, 240 mg
Verapamil	Isoptin SR	Tablets (sustained-release): 120 mg, 180 mg, 240 mg
Verapamil	Verelan	Capsules (sustained-release): 120 mg, 180 mg, 240 mg, 360 mg
Verapamil	Verelen PM	Capsules (extended-release): 100 mg, 200 mg, 300 mg
Vitamin A		Capsules: 10,000 units, 25,000 units
Vitamin D	Drisdol	Capsules: 50,000 units (1.25 mg)
Vitamin E	E-Gems	Capsules: 100 units, 600 units, 800 units, 1,000 units, 1,200 units
Vitamin E	Kaps	Capsules: 200 units, 400 units
Vitamin E	Key-E	Capsules: 200 units, 400 units
Vitamin E	Key-E	Tablets: 100 units, 200 units, 400 units, 800 units
Vorinostat	Zolinza	Capsules: 100 mg
Zolmitriptan	Zomig-ZMT	Tablets (orally-disintegrating): 2.5 mg, 5 mg
Zolpidem	Ambien CR	Tablets (extended-release): 6.25 mg, 12.5 mg
Zonisamide	Zonegran	Capsules: 25 mg, 50 mg, 100 mg

Appendix J

NORMAL LABORATORY VALUES

HEMATOLOGY/COAGULATION

Test	Specimen	Normal Range
Activated partial thromboplastin time (aPTT)	Whole blood	25–35 sec
Erythrocyte count (RBC count)	Whole blood	M: 4.3–5.7 million cells/mm^3 F: 3.8–5.1 million cells/mm^3
Hematocrit (HCT, Hct)	Whole blood	M: 39%–49% F: 35%–45%
Hemoglobin (Hb, Hgb)	Whole blood	M: 13.5–17.5 g/dl F: 12.0–16.0 g/dl
Leukocyte count (WBC count)	Whole blood	4.5–11.0 thousand cells/mm^3
Leukocyte differential count	Whole blood	
Basophils		0%–0.75%
Eosinophils		1%–3%
Lymphocytes		23%–33%
Monocytes		3%–7%
Neutrophils-bands		3%–5%
Neutrophils-segmented		54%–62%
Mean corpuscular hemoglobin (MCH)	Whole blood	26–34 pg/cell
Mean corpuscular hemoglobin concentration (MCHC)	Whole blood	31%–37% Hb/cell
Mean corpuscular volume (MCV)	Whole blood	80–100 fL
Partial thromboplastin time (PTT)	Whole blood	60–85 sec
Platelet count (thrombocyte count)	Whole blood	150–450 thousand/mm^3
Prothrombin time (PT)	Whole blood	11–13.5 sec
RBC count (see Erythrocyte count)		

CLINICAL CHEMISTRY (SERUM PLASMA, URINE)

Test	Specimen	Normal Range
Alanine aminotransferase (ALT)	Serum	0–55 units/L
Albumin	Serum	3.5–5 g/dl
Alkaline phosphatase	Serum	M: 53–128 units/L F: 42–98 units/L
Anion gap	Plasma or serum	5–14 mEq/L
Aspartate aminotransferase (AST)	Serum	0–50 units/L
Bilirubin (conjugated direct)	Serum	0–0.4 mg/dl
Bilirubin (total)	Serum	0.2–1.2 mg/dl
Calcium (total)	Serum	8.4–10.2 mg/dl
Carbon dioxide (CO_2) total	Plasma or serum	20–34 mEq/L
Chloride	Plasma or serum	96–112 mEq/L
Cholesterol (total)	Plasma or serum	Less than 200 mg/dl
C-Reactive protein	Serum	68–8,200 ng/ml
Creatine kinase (CK)	Serum	M: 38–174 units/L F: 26–140 units/L

(*continued*)

Test	Specimen	Normal Range
Creatine kinase isoenzymes	Serum	Fraction of total: less than 0.04–0.06
Creatinine	Plasma or serum	M: 0.7–1.3 mg/dl F: 0.6–1.1 mg/dl
Creatinine clearance	Plasma or serum and urine	M: 90–139 ml/min/1.73 m^2 F: 80–125 ml/min/1.73 m^2
Free thyroxine index (FTI)	Serum	1.1–4.8
Glucose	Serum	Adults: 70–105 mg/dl Older than 60 yrs: 80–115 mg/dl
Hemoglobin A_{1c}	Whole blood	5.6%–7.5% of total Hgb
Homovanillic acid (HVA)	Urine, 24 hrs	1.4–8.8 mg/day
17-Hydroxycorticosteroids (17-OHCS)	Urine, 24 hrs	M: 3–10 mg/day F: 2–8 mg/day
Iron	Serum	M: 65–175 mcg/dl F: 50–170 mcg/dl
Iron-binding capacity, total (TIBC)	Serum	250–450 mcg/dl
Lactate dehydrogenase (LDH)	Serum	0–250 units/L
Magnesium	Serum	1.3–2.3 mg/dl
Oxygen (O_2)	Whole blood, arterial	83–100 mm Hg
Oxygen saturation	Whole blood, arterial	95%–98%
pH	Whole blood, arterial	7.35–7.45
Phosphorus, inorganic	Serum	2.7–4.5 mg/dl
Potassium	Serum	3.5–5.1 mEq/L
Protein (total)	Serum	6–8.5 g/dl
Sodium	Plasma or serum	136–146 mEq/L
Specific gravity	Urine	1.002–1.030
Thyrotropin (hTSH)	Plasma or serum	2–10 mU/ml
Thyroxine (T_4) total	Serum	5–12 mcg/dl
Triglycerides (TG)	Serum, after 12-hr fast	20–190 mg/dl
Triiodothyronine resin uptake test (T_3RU)	Serum	22%–37%
Urea nitrogen	Plasma or serum	7–25 mg/dl
Urea nitrogen/creatinine ratio	Serum	12/1–20/1
Uric acid	Serum	M: 3.5–7.2 mg/dl F: 2.6–6 mg/dl
Vanillylmandelic acid (VMA)	Urine, 24 hrs	2–7 mg/day

Appendix K

ORPHAN DRUGS

The term *orphan drug* refers to either a drug or a biologic that is intended for use in a rare disease or condition. A rare disease or condition is one that affects less than 200,000 people in the United States or, if more than 200,000 people, in which there is no reasonable expectation that the cost of developing the drug or biologic and making it available would be recovered from the sales of that product.

A drug or biologic becomes an "orphan drug" when it is so designated from the Office of Orphan Products Development (OOPD) at the FDA. Orphan drug designation allows the sponsor of the drug or biologic to receive certain benefits from the government in exchange for developing the drug.

The drug or biologic must go through the FDA approval process like any other drug to evaluate it for both safety and efficacy. Since 1983, over 1,400 drugs and biologics have been designated orphan drugs, with over 250 products approved for marketing. After the orphan drug has been approved by the FDA for marketing, it becomes available through normal pharmaceutical supply channels. If not approved by the FDA, the product may be made available on a compassionate use basis. Contact information can be obtained from the OOPD at the FDA.

Office of Orphan Products Development
Food and Drug Administration
5600 Fishers Lane
Rockville, MD 20857
http://www.fda.gov/orphan/

Examples of orphan drugs:

Drug Name	Proposed Use	Sponsor
90y-Hpama4 (Pancide)	Pancreatic cancer	Immunomedics, Inc.
Alpha-1-acid glycoprotein	Cocaine overdose, tricyclic antidepressant poisoning	Bio Products Laboratory
Ambrisentan	Pulmonary arterial hypertension	Maygen, Inc.
Aplidin	Acute lymphoblastic leukemia	PharmaMar USA, Inc.
Chenodeoxycholic acid (Chenofalk)	Cerebrotendinous xanthomatosis	Dr. Falk Pharma GmbH
Deferitrin	Iron overload	Genzyme Corporation
Depsipeptide	Cutaneous T-cell lymphoma	Glucester Pharmaceuticals, Inc.
Golimumab	Chronic sarcoidosis	Centocor, Inc.
Idebenone	Cardiomyopathy associated with Friedreich's ataxia	Santhera Pharmaceuticals LLC
Nelarabine	Acute lymphoblastic leukemia, lymphoblastic lymphoma	GlaxoSmithKline
Plitidepsin (Aplidin)	Multiple myeloma	PharmaMar USA, Inc.
Rufinamide	Lennox-Gastaut syndrome	Eisai Medical Research, Inc.
Sarsasapogenin	Amyotrophic lateral sclerosis (ALS)	Phytopharm
Suberoylanlide hydroxamic acid	T-cell non-Hodgkin's lymphoma, mesothelioma	Merck & Co., Inc.
Tipifarnib (Zamestra)	Acute myeloid leukemia	Johnson & Johnson Pharmaceutical Research
Trabectedin (Yondelis)	Soft tissue sarcoma	Johnson & Johnson Pharmaceutical Research

Appendix L

P450 (CYP) ENZYMES

Most drugs are eliminated from the body, at least in part, by being changed chemically to a less lipid soluble product (e.g., metabolized), and thus is more likely to be excreted from the body via the kidney or bile. Drugs may go through two different metabolic processes: Phase 1 and Phase 2 metabolism.

In Phase 1 metabolism, hepatic microsomal enzymes found in the endothelium of liver cells metabolizes drugs via hydrolysis and oxidation and reduction reactions. These chemical reactions make the drug more water soluble. In Phase 2 metabolism, large water soluble substances (e.g., glucuronic acid, sulfate) are attached to the drug, forming inactive, or significantly less active, water soluble metabolites. Phase 2 processes include glucuronidation, sulfation, conjugation, acetylation, and methylation.

Virtually any of the Phase 1 and Phase 2 enzymes can be inhibited, and some of these enzymes can be induced by drugs. Inhibiting the activity of metabolic enzymes results in increased concentrations of the drug (substrate), whereas inducing metabolic enzymes results in decreased concentrations of the drug (substrate).

The term "cytochrome P450" (CYP enzymes) refers to a family of over 100 enzymes in the human body that modulate various physiologic functions. First identified in the 1950s, the CYP enzyme system contains two large subgroups: steroidogenic and xenobiotic enzymes. Only the xenobiotic group is involved in the metabolism of drugs. The xenobiotic group includes 4 major enzyme families: CPP1, CYP2, CYP3, and CYP4. The primary role of these families is the metabolism of drugs. These families are further subdivided into subfamily designated by a capital letter and given a specific enzyme number (1, 2, 3, etc) according to the similarity in amino acid sequence it shares with other enzymes.

The key subfamilies are CYP1A, CYP2A, CYP2B, CYP2C, CYP2D, CYP2E, and CYP3A. CYP enzymes may be responsible for metabolism of 75% of all drugs, with the CYP3A subfamily responsible for nearly half of this activity.

The CYP enzymes are found in the endoplasmic reticulum of cells in a variety of human tissue but are primarily concentrated in the liver and intestine. CYP enzymes can be both inhibited and induced, leading to increased or decreased serum concentration of the drug (along with its effects).

The following tables of CYP substrates, inhibitors, and inducers provide a perspective on drugs that are affected by, or affect, cytochrome P450 (CYP) enzymes. **CYP substrate** includes drugs reported to be metabolized, at least in part, by one or more CYP enzymes. **CYP inhibitor** includes drugs reported to inhibit one or more CYP enzymes. **CYP inducer** contains drugs reported to induce one or more CYP enzymes.

P450 ENZYMES: SUBSTRATES, INHIBITORS, INDUCERS

SUBSTRATES	INHIBITORS	INDUCERS
Albuterol	Amprenavir	Aminoglutethimide
Alprazolam	Atazanavir	Carbamazepine
Amiodarone	Clarithromycin	Fosphenytoin

(*continued*)

SUBSTRATES	INHIBITORS	INDUCERS
Amlodipine	Delavirdine	Nevirapine
Amprenavir	Diclofenac	Oxcarbazepine
Atorvastatin	Disulfiram	Phenobarbital
Bromocriptine	Fluconazole	Phenytoin
Budesonide	Fluoxetine	Primidone
Bupropion	Fosamprenavir	Rifampin
Carbamazepine	Ibuprofen	
Citalopram	Indinavir	
Clarithromycin	Isoniazid	
Cyclophosphamide	Itraconazole	
Cyclosporine	Ketoconazole	
Delavirdine	Lidocaine	
Diazepam	Miconazole	
Diltiazem	Nelfinavir	
Docetaxel	Nicardipine	
Doxepin	Omeprazole	
Doxorubicin	Paroxetine	
Enalapril	Pioglitazone	
Esomeprazole	Piroxacim	
Estradiol	Profolol	
Etoposide	Quinidine	
Haloperidol		
Imipramine		
Isosorbide		
Isradipine		
Ketoconazole		
Lansoprazole		
Lidocaine		
Losartan		
Lovastatin		
Midazolam		
Mirtazapine		
Nelfinavir		
Nifedipine		
Ondansetron		
Pacitaxel		
Pioglitazone		
Quetiapine		
Rabeprazole		
Rifampin		
Sildenafil		
Simvastatin		
Tamoxifen		
Tamsulosin		
Theophylline		
Timolol		
Tolterodine		
Trazodone		
Venlafaxine		
Verapamil		
Zolpidem		

Appendix M

POISON ANTIDOTE CHART

Poisoning Agent	Antidote	Indication
Acetaminophen	Acetylcysteine (Acetadote, Mucomyst)	Acute ingestion (more than 7.5 g in adults, more than 150 mg/kg in children); serum level more than 150 mg/L 4 hrs postingestion, chronic ingestion of toxic amounts
Anticholinergic agents	Physostigmine	Reverse severe effects, including hallucination, agitation, intractable seizures
Arsenic	Dimercaprol (BAL in oil)	Arsenic poisoning
Benzodiazepines	Flumazenil (Romazicon)	Complete or partial reversal of benzodiazepine effects
Beta-blockers	Glucagon	Aid in improving arterial pressure and contractility
Calcium channel blockers	Glucagon	Aid in improving arterial pressure and contractility
Carbamate pesticides	Atropine	Treatment of cholinergic symptoms due to agents that inhibit acetylcholinesterase activity
Digoxin (Lanoxin)	Digoxin immune FAB (Digibind)	Potentially life-threatening digoxin intoxication (e.g., severe ventricular arrhythmias), ingestion of more than 10 mg in adults or more than 4 mg in children
Ethylene glycol	Fomepizole (Antizol)	Symptomatic pt with suspected ingestion of ethylene glycol
Extravasation vasoconstrictive agents	Phentolamine (Regitine)	Extravasation of vasoconstrictive agents (e.g., epinephrine, norepinephrine)
Heparin	Protamine	Reversal of anticoagulant effect of heparin
Iron	Deferoxamine (Desferal)	Acute iron toxicity, chronic iron overload
Isoniazid	Pyridoxine (vitamin B_6)	Treatment of isoniazid overdose
Lead	Calcium EDTA	Acute and chronic lead poisoning, lead encephalopathy
Lead	Dimercaprol (BAL in oil)	Acute lead poisoning of levels more than 70 mcg/dl when used with calcium EDTA
Lead	Succimer (Chemet)	Lead poisoning in pt with levels more than 45 mcg/dl
Methanol	Fomepizole (Antizol)	Symptomatic pt with suspected ingestion of methanol
Opioids	Naloxone (Narcan)	Complete or partial reversal of narcotic depression including respiratory depression

(continued)

Poisoning Agent	Antidote	Indication
Organophosphate pesticides	Atropine	Treatment of cholinergic symptoms due to agents that inhibit acetylcholinesterase activity
Organophosphate pesticides	Pralidoxime (Protopam)	Treatment of severe poisoning in combination with atropine
Warfarin (Coumadin)	Phytonadione (vitamin K)	Excessive anticoagulation induced by warfarin

Appendix N

PREVENTING MEDICATION ERRORS AND IMPROVING MEDICATION SAFETY

Medication safety is a high priority for the health care professional. Prevention of medication errors and improved safety for the pt are important, esp. in today's health care environment when today's pt is older and sometimes sicker and the drug therapy regimen can be more sophisticated and complex.

A medication error is defined by the National Coordinating Council for Medication Error Reporting and Prevention (NCC MERP) as "any preventable event that may cause or lead to inappropriate medication use or patient harm while the medication is in the control of the health care professional, patient, or consumer."

Most medication errors occur as a result of multiple, compounding events as opposed to a single act by a single individual.

Use of the wrong medication, strength, or dose; confusion over sound-alike or look-alike drugs; administration of medications by the wrong route; miscalculations (esp. when used in pediatric pts or when administering medications intravenously); errors in prescribing and transcription all can contribute to compromising the safety of the pt. The potential for adverse events and medication errors is definitely a reality and is potentially tragic and costly in both human and economic terms.

Health care professionals must take the initiative to create and implement procedures to prevent medication errors from occurring and implement methods to reduce medication errors. The first priority in preventing medication errors is to establish a multidisciplinary team to improve medication use. The goal for this team would be to assess medication safety and implement changes that would make it difficult or impossible for mistakes to reach the pt. Some important criteria in making improved medication safety successful includes the following:

- Promote a nonpunitive approach to reducing medication errors
- Increase the detection and the reporting of medication errors, near misses, and potentially hazardous situations than may result in medication errors
- Determine root causes of medication errors
- Educate about the causes of medication errors and ways to prevent these errors
- Make recommendations to allow organization-wide, system-based changes to prevent medication errors
- Learn from errors that occur in other organizations and take measures to prevent similar errors

Some common causes and ways to prevent medication errors and improve safety include the following:

Handwriting: Poor handwriting can make it difficult to distinguish between two medications with similar names. Also, many drug names sound similar, esp. when the names are spoken over the telephone, poorly enunciated, or mispronounced.

- Take time to write legibly.
- Keep phone or verbal orders to a minimum to prevent misinterpretation.

- Repeat back orders taken over the telephone.
- When ordering a new or rarely used medication, print the name.
- Always specify the drug strength, even if only one strength exists.
- Print generic and brand names of look-alike or sound-alike medications.

Zeros and decimal points: Hastily written orders can present problems even if the name of the medication is clear.

- Never leave a decimal point "naked." Place a zero before a decimal point when the number is less than a whole unit (e.g., use 0.25 mg or 250 mcg, **not** .25 mg).
- Never have a trailing zero following a decimal point (e.g., use 2 mg, **not** 2.0 mg).

Abbreviations: Errors can occur because of a failure to standardize abbreviations. Establishing a list of abbreviations that should never be used is recommended.

- Never abbreviate unit as "U," spell out "unit."
- Do not abbreviate "once daily" as OD or QD, or "every other day" as QOD; spell it out.
- Do not use D/C, as this may be misinterpreted as either discharge or discontinue.
- Do not abbreviate drug names; spell out the generic and/or brand names.

Ambiguous or incomplete orders: These types of orders can cause confusion or misinterpretation of the writer's intention. Examples include situations when the route of administration, dose, or dosage form has not been specified.

- Do not use slash marks—they are read as the number one (1).
- When reviewing an unusual order, verify the order with the person writing the order to prevent any misunderstanding.
- Read over orders after writing.
- Encourage that the drug's indication for use be provided on medication orders.
- Provide complete medication orders—do not use "resume preop" or "continue previous meds."

High-alert medications: Medications in this category have an increased risk of causing significant pt harm when used in error. Mistakes with these medications may or may not be more common but may be more devastating to the pt if an error occurs. A list of high-alert medications can be obtained from the Institute for Safe Medication Practices (ISMP) at www.ismp.org.

Technology available today that can be used to address and help to solve potential medication problems or errors include the following:

- Electronic prescribing systems—This refers to computerized prescriber order entry systems. Within these systems is the capability to incorporate medication safety alerts (e.g., maximum dose alerts, allergy screening). Additionally, these systems should be integrated or interfaced with pharmacy and laboratory systems to provide drug–drug and drug–disease interactions alerts and include clinical order screening capability.
- Bar codes—These systems are designed to use bar-code scanning devices to validate identity of pts, verify medications administered, document administration, and provide safety alerts.
- "Smart" infusion pumps—These pumps allow users to enter drug infusion protocols into a drug library along with predefined dosage limits. If a dosage is outside the limits established, an alarm is sounded and drug delivery is halted, informing the clinician that the dose is outside the recommended range.

- Automated dispensing systems–point of use dispensing system—These systems should be integrated with information systems, esp. pharmacy systems.
- Pharmacy order entry system—This should be fully integrated with an electronic prescribing system with the capability of producing medication safety alerts. Additionally, the system should generate a computerized medication administration record (MAR), which would be used by a nursing staff while administering medications.

Medication reconciliation: Medication errors generally occur at transition points in the pt's care (admission, transfer from one level of care to another, [e.g., critical care to general care area] and discharge). Incomplete documentation can account for up to 60% of potential medication errors. Therefore, it becomes necessary to accurately and completely reconcile medication across the continuum of care. This includes the name, dosage, frequency, and route of medication administration.

Medication reconciliation programs are a process of identifying the most accurate list of all medications a pt is taking and using this list to provide correct medications anywhere within the health care system. The focus not only is on compiling a list but on using the list to reduce medication errors and provide quality pt care.

Appendix O

RECOMMENDED CHILDHOOD AND ADULT IMMUNIZATIONS

Recommended Adult Immunization Schedule, by Vaccine and Age Group

UNITED STATES • OCTOBER 2006–SEPTEMBER 2007

<table>
<tr><th>Vaccine ▼ Age group ▶</th><th>19–49 years</th><th>50–64 years</th><th>≥65 years</th></tr>
<tr><td rowspan="2">Tetanus, diphtheria, pertussis (Td/Tdap)[1],*</td><td colspan="3">1-dose Td booster every 10 yrs</td></tr>
<tr><td colspan="2">Substitute 1 dose of Tdap for Td</td><td></td></tr>
<tr><td>Human papillomavirus (HPV)[2]</td><td>3 doses (females)</td><td></td><td></td></tr>
<tr><td>Measles, mumps, rubella (MMR)[3],*</td><td>1 or 2 doses</td><td colspan="2">1 dose</td></tr>
<tr><td>Varicella[4],*</td><td>2 doses (0, 4–8 wks)</td><td>2 doses (0, 4–8 wks)</td><td></td></tr>
<tr><td>Influenza[5],*</td><td>1 dose annually</td><td colspan="2">1 dose annually</td></tr>
<tr><td>Pneumococcal (polysaccharide)[6,7]</td><td colspan="2">1–2 doses</td><td>1 dose</td></tr>
<tr><td>Hepatitis A[8],*</td><td colspan="3">2 doses (0, 6–12 mos, or 0, 6–18 mos)</td></tr>
<tr><td>Hepatitis B[9],*</td><td colspan="3">3 doses (0, 1–2, 4–6 mos)</td></tr>
<tr><td>Meningococcal[10]</td><td colspan="3">1 or more doses</td></tr>
</table>

*Covered by the Vaccine Injury Compensation Program. NOTE: These recommendations must be read with the footnotes (see reverse).

For all persons in this category who meet the age requirements and who lack evidence of immunity (e.g., lack documentation of vaccination or have no evidence of prior infection)

Recommended if some other risk factor is present (e.g., on the basis of medical, occupational, lifestyle, or other indications)

This schedule indicates the recommended age groups and medical indications for routine administration of currently licensed vaccines for persons aged 19 yrs and older, as of October 1, 2006. Licensed combination vaccines may be used whenever any components of the combination are indicated and when the vaccine's other components are not contraindicated. For detailed recommendations on all vaccines, including those used primarily for travelers or that are issued during the year, consult the manufacturers' package inserts and the complete statements from the Advisory Committee on Immunization Practices (*http://www.cdc.gov/nip/publications/acip-list.htm*).

Report all clinically significant postvaccination reactions to the Vaccine Adverse Event Reporting System (VAERS). Reporting forms and instructions on filing a VAERS report are available at *http://www.vaers.hhs.gov* or by telephone at 800-822-7967.

Information on how to file a Vaccine Injury Compensation Program claim is available at *http://www.hrsa.gov/vaccinecompensation* or by telephone at 800-338-2382. To file a claim for vaccine injury, contact the U.S. Court of Federal Claims, 717 Madison Place, N.W., Washington, D.C. 20005; telephone: 202-357-6400.

Additional information about the vaccines in this schedule and contraindications for vaccination is also available at *http://www.cdc.gov/nip* or from the CDC-INFO Contact Center at 800-CDC-INFO (800-232-4636) in English and Spanish, 24 hours per day, 7 days per week.

Footnotes

Recommended Adult Immunization Schedule • UNITED STATES, OCTOBER 2006–SEPTEMBER 2007

1. **Tetanus, diphtheria, and acellular pertussis (Td/Tdap) vaccination.** Adults with uncertain histories of a complete primary vaccination series with diphtheria and tetanus toxoid-containing vaccines should begin or complete a primary vaccination series. A primary series for adults is 3 doses; administer the first 2 doses at least 4 wks apart and the third dose 6–12 mos after the second. Administer a booster dose to adults who have completed a primary series and if the last vaccination was received 10 yrs or more previously. Tdap or tetanus and diphtheria (Td) vaccine may be used; Tdap should replace a single dose of Td for adults aged younger than 65 yrs who have not previously received a dose of Tdap (either in the primary series, as a booster, or for wound management). Only one of two Tdap products (Adacel® [Sanofi Pasteur]) is licensed for use in adults. If a female is pregnant and received the last Td vaccination 10 yrs or more previously, administer Td during the second or third trimester; if a female received the last Td vaccination in less than 10 yrs, administer Tdap during the immediate postpartum period. A one-time administration of 1 dose of Tdap with an interval as short as 2 yrs from a previous Td vaccination is recommended for postpartum women, close contacts of infants aged younger than 12 mos, and all healthcare workers with direct pt contact. In certain situations, Td can be deferred during pregnancy and Tdap substituted in the immediate postpartum period, or Tdap can be given instead of Td to a pregnant woman after an informed discussion with the woman (see *http://www.cdc.gov/nip/publications/acip-list.htm*). Consult the ACIP statement for recommendations for administering Td as prophylaxis in wound management (*http://www.cdc.gov/mmwr/preview/mmwrhtml/00041645.htm*).

2. **Human papillomavirus (HPV) vaccination.** HPV vaccination is recommended for all women aged 26 yrs and younger who have not completed the vaccine series. Ideally, vaccine shouldbe administered before potential exposure to HPV through sexual activity; however, women who are sexually active still should be vaccinated. Sexually active women who have not been infected with any of the HPV vaccine types receive the full benefit of the vaccination. Vaccination is less beneficial for women who have already been infected with one or more of the four HPV vaccine types. A complete series consists of 3 doses. The second dose should be administered 2 mos after the first dose; the third dose should be administered 6 mos after the first dose. Vaccination is not recommended during pregnancy. If a woman is found to be pregnant after initiating the vaccination series, the remainder of the 3-dose regimen should be delayed until after completion of the pregnancy.

3. **Measles, mumps, rubella (MMR) vaccination.** *Measles component:* adults born before 1957 can be considered immune to measles. Adults born during or after 1957 should receive 1 dose or more of MMR unless they have a medical contraindication, documentation of 1 dose or more, history of measles based on healthcare provider diagnosis, or laboratory evidence of immunity. A second dose of MMR is recommended for adults who (1) have been recently exposed to measles or in an outbreak setting; (2) have been previously vaccinated with killed measles vaccine; (3) have been vaccinated with an unknown type of measles vaccine during 1963–1967; (4) are students in postsecondary educational institutions; (5) work in a healthcare facility; or (6) plan to travel internationally. Withhold MMR or other measles-containing vaccines from HIV-infected persons with severe immunosuppression. *Mumps component:* adults born before 1957 can generally be considered immune to mumps. Adults born during or after 1957 should receive 1 dose of MMR unless they have a medical contraindication, history of mumps based on healthcare provider diagnosis, or laboratory evidence of immunity. A second dose of MMR is recommended for adults who (1) are in an age group that is affected during a mumps outbreak; (2) are students in postsecondary educational institutions; (3) work in a healthcare facility; or (4) plan to travel internationally. For unvaccinated healthcare workers born before 1957 who do not have other evidence of mumps immunity, consider giving 1 dose on a routine basis and strongly consider giving a second dose during an outbreak. *Rubella component:* administer 1 dose of MMR vaccine to women whose rubella vaccination history is unreliable or who lack laboratory evidence of immunity. For women of childbearing age, regardless of birth year, routinely determine rubella immunity and counsel women regarding congenital rubella syndrome. Do not vaccinate women who are pregnant or who might become pregnant within 4 wks of receiving vaccine. Women who do not have evidence of immunity should receive MMR vaccine upon completion or termination of pregnancy and before discharge from the healthcare facility.

4. **Varicella vaccination.** All adults without evidence of immunity to varicella should receive 2 doses of varicella vaccine. Special consideration should be given to those who (1) have close contact with persons at high risk for severe disease (e.g., healthcare workers and family contacts of immunocompromised persons) or (2) are at high risk for exposure or transmission (e.g., teachers of young children; child care employees; residents and staff members of institutional settings, including correctional institutions; college students; military personnel; adolescents and adults living in households with children; nonpregnant women of childbearing age; and international travelers). Evidence of immunity to varicella in adults includes any of the following: (1) documentation of 2 doses of varicella vaccine at least 4 wks apart; (2) born in United States before 1980 (although for healthcare workers and pregnant women, birth before 1980 should not be considered evidence of immunity); (3) history of varicella based on diagnosis or verification of varicella by a healthcare provider (for a pt reporting a history of or presenting with an atypical case, a mild case, or both, healthcare providers should seek either an epidemiologic link with a typical varicella case or evidence of laboratory confirmation, if it was performed at the time of acute disease); (4) history of herpes zoster based on healthcare provider diagnosis; or (5) laboratory evidence of immunity or laboratory confirmation of disease. Do not vaccinate women who are pregnant or might become pregnant within 4 wks of receiving the vaccine. Assess pregnant women for evidence of varicella immunity. Women who do not have evidence of immunity should receive dose 1 of varicella vaccine upon completion or termination of pregnancy and before discharge from the healthcare facility. Dose 2 should be administered 4–8 wks after dose 1.

5. **Influenza vaccination.** *Medical indications:* chronic disorders of the cardiovascular or pulmonary systems, including asthma; chronic metabolic diseases, including diabetes mellitus, renal dysfunction, hemoglobinopathies, or immunosuppression (including immunosuppression caused by medications or HIV); any condition that compromises respiratory function or the handling of respiratory secretions or that can increase the risk of

aspiration (e.g., cognitive dysfunction, spinal cord injury, seizure disorder, or other neuromuscular disorder); and pregnancy during the influenza season. No data exist on the risk for severe or complicated influenza disease among persons with asplenia; however, influenza is a risk factor for secondary bacterial infections that can cause severe disease among persons with asplenia. *Occupational indications:* healthcare workers and employees of long-term care and assisted living facilities. *Other indications:*residents of nursing homes and other long-term care and assisted living facilities; persons likely to transmit influenza to persons at high risk (e.g., in-home household contacts and caregivers of children aged 0–59 mos, or persons of all ages with high-risk conditions); and anyone who would like to be vaccinated. Healthy, nonpregnant persons aged 5–49 yrs without high-risk medical conditions who are not contacts of severely immunocompromised persons in special care units can receive either intranasally administered influenza vaccine (FluMist®) or inactivated vaccine. Other persons should receive the inactivated vaccine.

6. **Pneumococcal (polysaccharide) vaccination.** *Medical indications:*chronic disorders of the pulmonary system (excluding asthma); cardiovascular diseases; diabetes mellitus; chronic hepatic diseases, including hepatic disease as a result of alcohol abuse (e.g., cirrhosis); chronic renal failure or nephrotic syndrome; functional or anatomic asplenia (e.g., sickle cell disease or splenectomy [if elective splenectomy is planned, vaccinate at least 2 wks before surgery]); immunosuppressive conditions (e.g., congenital immunodeficiency, HIV infection [vaccinate as close to diagnosis as possible when CD4 cell counts are highest], leukemia, lymphoma, multiple myeloma, Hodgkin's disease, generalized malignancy, or organ or bone marrow transplantation); chemotherapy with alkylating agents, antimetabolites, or high-dose, long-term corticosteroids; and cochlear implants. *Other indications:* Alaska Natives and certain American Indian populations and residents of nursing homes or other long-term care facilities.

7. **Revaccination with pneumococcal polysaccharide vaccine.** One-time revaccination after 5 yrs for persons with chronic renal failure or nephrotic syndrome; functional or anatomic asplenia (e.g., sickle cell disease or splenectomy); immunosuppressive conditions (e.g., congenital immunodeficiency, HIV infection, leukemia, lymphoma, multiple myeloma, Hodgkin's disease, generalized malignancy, or organ or bone marrow transplantation); or chemotherapy with alkylating agents, antimetabolites, or high-dose, long-term corticosteroids. For persons aged 65 yrs and older, one-time revaccination if they were vaccinated 5 yrs or more previously and were aged younger than 65 yrs at the time of primary vaccination.

8. **Hepatitis A vaccination.** *Medical indications:* persons with chronic hepatic disease and persons who receive clotting factor concentrates. *Behavioral indications:* men who have sex with men and persons who use illegal drugs. *Occupational indications:* persons working with hepatitis A virus (HAV)-infected primates or with HAV in a research laboratory setting. *Other indications:* persons traveling to or working in countries that have high or intermediate endemicity of hepatitis A (a list of countries is available at *http://www.cdc.gov/travel/diseases.htm*) and any person who would like to obtain immunity. Current vaccines should be administered in a 2-dose schedule at either 0 and 6–12 mos, or 0 and 6–18 mos. If the combined hepatitis A and hepatitis B vaccine is used, administer 3 doses at 0, 1, and 6 mos.

9. **Hepatitis B vaccination.** *Medical indications:* persons with end-stage renal disease, including patients receiving hemodialysis; persons seeking evaluation or treatment for a sexually transmitted disease (STD); persons with HIV infection; persons with chronic hepatic disease; and persons who receive clotting factor concentrates. *Occupational indications:* healthcare workers and public safety workers who are exposed to blood or other potentially infectious body fluids. *Behavioral indications:*sexually active persons who are not in a long-term, mutually monogamous relationship (i.e., persons with more than 1 sex partner during the previous 6 mos); current or recent injection-drug users; and men who have sex with men. *Other indications:*household contacts and sex partners of persons with chronic hepatitis B virus (HBV) infection; clients and staff members of institutions for persons with developmental disabilities; all clients of STD clinics; international travelers to countries with high or intermediate prevalence of chronic HBV infection (a list of countries is available at *http://www.cdc.gov/travel/diseases.htm*); and any adult seeking protection from HBV infection. Settings where hepatitis B vaccination is recommended for all adults: STD treatment facilities; HIV testing and treatment facilities; facilities providing drug-abuse treatment and prevention services; healthcare settings providing services for injection-drug users or men who have sex with men; correctional facilities; end-stage renal disease programs and facilities for chronic hemodialysis patients; and institutions and nonresidential daycare facilities for persons with developmental disabilities. *Special formulation indications:* for adult patients receiving hemodialysis and other immunocompromised adults, 1 dose of 40 μg/ml (Recombivax HB®) or 2 doses of 20 μg/ml (Engerix-B®).

10. **Meningococcal vaccination.** *Medical indications:*adults with anatomic or functional asplenia, or terminal complement component deficiencies. *Other indications:* first-year college students living in dormitories; microbiologists who are routinely exposed to isolates of *Neisseria meningitidis*; military recruits; and persons who travel to or live in countries in which meningococcal disease is hyperendemic or epidemic (e.g., the "meningitis belt" of sub-Saharan Africa during the dry season [December–June]), particularly if their contact with local populations will be prolonged. Vaccination is required by the government of Saudi Arabia for all travelers to Mecca during the annual Hajj. Meningococcal conjugate vaccine is preferred for adults with any of the preceding indications who are aged younger than 55 yrs, although meningococcal polysaccharide vaccine (MPSV4) is an acceptable alternative. Revaccination after 5 yrs might be indicated for adults previously vaccinated with MPSV4 who remain at high risk for infection (e.g., persons residing in areas where disease is epidemic).

11. **Selected conditions for which *Haemophilus influenzae*type b (Hib) vaccine may be used.** Hib conjugate vaccines are licensed for children aged 6 wks–71 mos. No efficacy data are available on which to base a recommendation concerning use of Hib vaccine for older children and adults with the chronic conditions associated with an increased risk for Hib disease. However, studies suggest good immunogenicity in patients who have sickle cell disease, leukemia, or HIV infection or who have had splenectomies; administering vaccine to these patients is not contraindicated.

Use of trade names and commercial sources is for identification only and does not imply endorsement by the U.S. Department of Health and Human Services.

DEPARTMENT OF HEALTH AND HUMAN SERVICES • CENTERS FOR DISEASE CONTROL AND PREVENTION

Recommended Immunization Schedule for Persons Aged 0–6 Years—UNITED STATES • 2007

<table>
<tr><th>Vaccine▼ Age▶</th><th>Birth</th><th>1 mo</th><th>2 mos</th><th>4 mos</th><th>6 mos</th><th>12 mos</th><th>15 mos</th><th>18 mos</th><th>19–23 mos</th><th>2–3 yrs</th><th>4–6 yrs</th></tr>
<tr><td>Hepatitis B[1]</td><td>HepB</td><td colspan="2">HepB</td><td>see footnote 1</td><td colspan="4">HepB</td><td colspan="3">HepB Series</td></tr>
<tr><td>Rotavirus[2]</td><td></td><td></td><td>Rota</td><td>Rota</td><td>Rota</td><td></td><td></td><td></td><td></td><td></td><td></td></tr>
<tr><td>Diphtheria, Tetanus, Pertussis[3]</td><td></td><td></td><td>DTaP</td><td>DTaP</td><td>DTaP</td><td></td><td colspan="2">DTaP</td><td></td><td></td><td>DTaP</td></tr>
<tr><td>Haemophilus influenzae type b[4]</td><td></td><td></td><td>Hib</td><td>Hib</td><td>Hib[4]</td><td colspan="2">Hib</td><td colspan="4">Hib</td></tr>
<tr><td>Pneumococcal[5]</td><td></td><td></td><td>PCV</td><td>PCV</td><td>PCV</td><td colspan="2">PCV</td><td></td><td></td><td colspan="2">PCV
PPV</td></tr>
<tr><td>Inactivated Poliovirus</td><td></td><td></td><td>IPV</td><td>IPV</td><td colspan="4">IPV</td><td></td><td></td><td>IPV</td></tr>
<tr><td>Influenza[6]</td><td></td><td></td><td></td><td></td><td colspan="7">Influenza (Yearly)</td></tr>
<tr><td>Measles, Mumps, Rubella[7]</td><td></td><td></td><td></td><td></td><td></td><td colspan="2">MMR</td><td></td><td></td><td></td><td>MMR</td></tr>
<tr><td>Varicella[8]</td><td></td><td></td><td></td><td></td><td></td><td colspan="2">Varicella</td><td></td><td></td><td></td><td>Varicella</td></tr>
<tr><td>Hepatitis A[9]</td><td></td><td></td><td></td><td></td><td></td><td colspan="4">HepA (2 doses)</td><td colspan="2">HepA Series</td></tr>
<tr><td>Meningococcal[10]</td><td></td><td></td><td></td><td></td><td></td><td></td><td></td><td></td><td></td><td colspan="2">MPSV4</td></tr>
</table>

Range of recommended ages

Catch-up immunization

Certain high-risk groups

This schedule indicates the recommended ages for routine administration of currently licensed childhood vaccines, as of December 1, 2006, for children aged 0–6 yrs. Additional information is available at *http://www.cdc.gov/nip/recs/child-schedule.htm*. Any dose not administered at the recommended age should be administered at any subsequent visit, when indicated and feasible. Additional vaccines may be licensed and recommended during the year. Licensed combination vaccines may be used whenever any components of the combination are indicated and other components of the vaccine are not contraindicated and if approved by the Food and Drug Administration for that dose of the series. Providers should consult the respective Advisory Committee on Immunization Practices statement for detailed recommendations. Clinically significant adverse events that follow immunization should be reported to the Vaccine Adverse Event Reporting System (VAERS). Guidance about how to obtain and complete a VAERS form is available at ***http://www.vaers,hhs.gov*** or by telephone at **800-822-7967**.

1. **Hepatitis B vaccine (HepB).** *(Minimum age: birth)*
   At birth:
   - Administer monovalent HepB to all newborns before hospital discharge.
   - If mother is hepatitis surface antigen (HBsAg)-positive, administer HepB and 0.5 ml of hepatitis B immune globulin (HBIG) within 12 hrs of birth.
   - If mother's HBsAg status is unknown, administer HepB within 12 hrs of birth. Determine the HBsAg status as soon as possible and if HBsAg-positive, administer HBIG (no later than age 1 wk).
   - If mother is HBsAg-negative, the birth dose can only be delayed with physician's order and mother's negative HBsAg laboratory report documented in the infant's medical record.

   After the birth dose:
   - The HepB series should be completed with either monovalent HepB or a combination vaccine containing HepB. The second dose should be administered at age 1–2 mos. The final dose should be administered at age 24 wks or older. Infants born to HBsAg-positive mothers should be tested for HBsAg and antibody to HBsAg after completion of 3 doses or more of a licensed HepB series, at age 9–18 mos (generally at the next well-child visit).

   4-month dose:
   - It is permissible to administer 4 doses of HepB when combination vaccines are administered after the birth dose. If monovalent HepB is used for doses after the birth dose, a dose at age 4 mos is not needed.
2. **Rotavirus vaccine (Rota).** *(Minimum age: 6 wks)*
   - Administer the first dose at age 6–12 wks. Do not start the series later than age 12 wks.
   - Administer the final dose in the series by age 32 wks. Do not administer a dose later than age 32 wks.
   - Data on safety and efficacy outside of these age ranges are insufficient.
3. **Diphtheria and tetanus toxoids and acellular pertussis vaccine (DTaP).** *(Minimum age: 6 wks)*
   - The fourth dose of DTaP may be administered as early as age 12 mos, provided 6 mos have elapsed since the third dose.
   - Administer the final dose in the series at age 4–6 yrs.
4. ***Haemophilus influenzae* type b conjugate vaccine (Hib).** *(Minimum age: 6 wks)*
   - If PRP-OMP (PedvaxHIB® or ComVax® [Merck]) is administered at ages 2 and 4 mos, a dose at age 6 mos is not required.
   - TriHiBit® (DTaP/Hib) combination products should not be used for primary immunization but can be used as boosters following any Hib vaccine in children aged 12 mos or older.
5. **Pneumococcal vaccine.** *(Minimum age: 6 wks for pneumococcal conjugate vaccine [PCV]; 2 yrs for pneumococcal polysaccharide vaccine [PPV])*
   - Administer PCV at ages 24–59 mos in certain high-risk groups. Administer PPV to children aged 2 yrs or older in certain high-risk groups. See *MMWR* 2000;49(No. RR-9):1–35.
6. **Influenza vaccine.** *(Minimum age: 6 mos for trivalent inactivated influenza vaccine [TIV]; 5 yrs for live, attenuated influenza vaccine [LAIV])*
   - All children aged 6–59 mos and close contacts of all children aged 0–59 mos are recommended to receive influenza vaccine.
   - Influenza vaccine is recommended annually for children aged 59 mos or older with certain risk factors, healthcare workers, and other persons (including household members) in close contact with persons in groups at high risk. See *MMWR* 2006;55(No. RR-10):1–41.
   - For healthy persons aged 5–49 yrs, LAIV may be used as an alternative to TIV.
   - Children receiving TIV should receive 0.25 ml if aged 6–35 mos or 0.5 ml if aged 3 yrs or older.
   - Children aged younger than 9 yrs who are receiving influenza vaccine for the first time should receive 2 doses (separated by 4 wks or more for TIV and 6 wks or more for LAIV).
7. **Measles, mumps, and rubella vaccine (MMR).** *(Minimum age: 12 mos)*
   - Administer the second dose of MMR at age 4–6 yrs. MMR may be administered before age 4–6 yrs, provided 4 wks or more have elapsed since the first dose and both doses are administered at age 12 mos or older.
8. **Varicella vaccine.** *(Minimum age: 12 mos)*
   - Administer the second dose of varicella vaccine at age 4–6 yrs. Varicella vaccine may be administered before age 4–6 yrs, provided that 3 mos or more have elapsed since the first dose and both doses are administered at age 12 mos or older. If second dose was administered 28 days or more following the first dose, the second dose does not need to be repeated.
9. **Hepatitis A vaccine (HepA).** *(Minimum age: 12 mos)*
   - HepA is recommended for all children aged 1 yr (i.e., aged 12–23 mos). The 2 doses in the series should be administered at least 6 mos apart.
   - Children not fully vaccinated by age 2 yrs can be vaccinated at subsequent visits.
   - HepA is recommended for certain other groups of children, including in areas where vaccination programs target older children. See *MMWR* 2006;55(No. RR-7):1–23.
10. **Meningococcal polysaccharide vaccine (MPSV4).** *(Minimum age: 2 yrs)*
    - Administer MPSV4 to children aged 2–10 yrs with terminal complement deficiencies or anatomic or functional asplenia and certain other high-risk groups. See *MMWR* 2005;54(No. RR-7):1–21.

The Recommended Immunization Schedules for Persons Aged 0–18 Years are approved by the Advisory Committee on Immunization Practices (http://www.cdc.gov/nip/acip), the American Academy of Pediatrics (http://www.aap.org), and the American Academy of Family Physicians (http://www.aafp.org).

SAFER • HEALTHIER • PEOPLE™

CS103164

DEPARTMENT OF HEALTH AND HUMAN SERVICES • CENTERS FOR DISEASE CONTROL AND PREVENTION

Recommended Immunization Schedule for Persons Aged 7–18 Years—UNITED STATES • 2007

Vaccine ▼ / Age ▶	7–10 yrs	11–12 YRS	13–14 yrs	15 yrs	16–18 yrs
Tetanus, Diphtheria, Pertussis[1]	see footnote 1	Tdap	Tdap		
Human Papillomavirus[2]	see footnote 2	HPV (3 doses)	HPV Series		
Meningococcal[3]	MPSV4	MCV4	MCV4[3] MCV4		
Pneumococcal[4]	PPV				
Influenza[5]	Influenza (Yearly)				
Hepatitis A[6]	HepA Series				
Hepatitis B[7]	HepB Series				
Inactivated Poliovirus[8]	IPV Series				
Measles, Mumps, Rubella[9]	MMR Series				
Varicella[10]	Varicella Series				

Legend: Range of recommended ages; Catch-up immunization; Certain high-risk groups

This schedule indicates the recommended ages for routine administration of currently licensed childhood vaccines, as of December 1, 2006, for children aged 7–18 yrs. Additional information is available at ***http://www.cdc.gov/nip/recs/child-schedule.htm***. Any dose not administered at the recommended age should be administered at any subsequent visit, when indicated and feasible. Additional vaccines may be licensed and recommended during the year. Licensed combination vaccines may be used whenever any components of the combination are indicated and other components of the vaccine are not contraindicated and if approved by the Food and Drug Administration for that dose of the series. Providers should consult the respective Advisory Committee on Immunization Practices statement for detailed recommendations. Clinically significant adverse events that follow immunization should be reported to the Vaccine Adverse Event Reporting System (VAERS). Guidance about how to obtain and complete a VAERS form is available at ***http://www.vaers.hhs.gov*** or by telephone at **800-822-7967**.

1. Tetanus and diphtheria toxoids and acellular pertussis vaccine (Tdap).
(Minimum age: 10 yrs for BOOSTRIX® and 11 yrs for ADACEL™)
- Administer at age 11–12 yrs for those who have completed the recommended childhood DTP/DTaP vaccination series and have not received a tetanus and diphtheria toxoids vaccine (Td) booster dose.
- Adolescents aged 13–18 yrs who missed the 11–12 yrs Td/Tdap booster dose should also receive a single dose of Tdap if they have completed the recommended childhood DTP/DTaP vaccination series.

2. Human papillomavirus vaccine (HPV). *(Minimum age: 9 yrs)*
- Administer the first dose of the HPV vaccine series to females at age 11–12 yrs.
- Administer the second dose 2 mos after the first dose and the third dose 6 mos after the first dose.
- Administer the HPV vaccine series to females at age 13–18 yrs if not previously vaccinated.

3. Meningococcal vaccine. *(Minimum age: 11 yrs for meningococcal conjugate vaccine [MCV4]; 2 yrs for meningococcal polysaccharide vaccine [MPSV4])*
- Administer MCV4 at age 11–12 yrs and to previously unvaccinated adolescents at high school entry (at approximately age 15 yrs).
- Administer MCV4 to previously unvaccinated college freshmen living in dormitories; MPSV4 is an acceptable alternative.
- Vaccination against invasive meningococcal disease is recommended for children and adolescents aged 2 yrs or older with terminal complement deficiencies or anatomic or functional asplenia and certain other high-risk groups. See *MMWR* 2005;54(No. RR-7):1–21. Use MPSV4 for children aged 2–10 yrs and MCV4 or MPSV4 for older children.

4. Pneumococcal polysaccharide vaccine (PPV). *(Minimum age: 2 yrs)*
- Administer for certain high-risk groups. See *MMWR* 1997;46(No. RR-8):1–24, and *MMWR* 2000;49(No. RR-9):1–35.

5. Influenza vaccine. *(Minimum age: 6 mos for trivalent inactivated influenza vaccine [TIV]; 5 yrs for live, attenuated influenza vaccine [LAIV])*
- Influenza vaccine is recommended annually for persons with certain risk factors, healthcare workers, and other persons (including household members) in close contact with persons in groups at high risk. See *MMWR* 2006;55 (No. RR-10):1–41.
- For healthy persons aged 5–49 yrs, LAIV may be used as an alternative to TIV .
- Children aged younger than 9 yrs who are receiving influenza vaccine for the first time should receive 2 doses (separated by 4 wks or more for TIV and 6 wks or more for LAIV).

6. Hepatitis A vaccine (HepA). *(Minimum age: 12 mos)*
- The 2 doses in the series should be administered at least 6 mos apart.
- HepA is recommended for certain other groups of children, including in areas where vaccination programs target older children. See *MMWR* 2006;55 (No. RR-7):1–23.

7. Hepatitis B vaccine (HepB). *(Minimum age: birth)*
- Administer the 3-dose series to those who were not previously vaccinated.
- A 2-dose series of Recombivax HB® is licensed for children aged 11–15 yrs.

8. Inactivated poliovirus vaccine (IPV). *(Minimum age: 6 wks)*
- For children who received an all-IPV or all-oral poliovirus (OPV) series, a fourth dose is not necessary if the third dose was administered at age 4 yrs or older.
- If both OPV and IPV were administered as part of a series, a total of 4 doses should be administered, regardless of the child's current age.

9. Measles, mumps, and rubella vaccine (MMR). *(Minimum age: 12 mos)*
- If not previously vaccinated, administer 2 doses of MMR during any visit, with 4 wks or more between the doses.

10. Varicella vaccine. *(Minimum age: 12 mos)*
- Administer 2 doses of varicella vaccine to persons without evidence of immunity.
- Administer 2 doses of varicella vaccine to persons aged younger than 13 yrs at least 3 mos apart. Do not repeat the second dose, if administered 28 days or more after the first dose.
- Administer 2 doses of varicella vaccine to persons aged 13 yrs or older at least 4 wks apart.

The Recommended Immunization Schedules for Persons Aged 0–18 Years are approved by the Advisory Committee on Immunization Practices (http://www.cdc.gov/nip/acip), the American Academy of Pediatrics (http://www.aap.org), and the American Academy of Family Physicians (http://www.aafp.org).

SAFER • HEALTHIER • PEOPLE™

CS100131

Appendix P

SIGNS AND SYMPTOMS OF ELECTROLYTE IMBALANCE

HYPOGLYCEMIA (excessive insulin)

Tremors, cold/clammy skin, mental confusion, rapid/shallow respirations, unusual fatigue, hunger, drowsiness, anxiety, headache, muscular incoordination, paresthesia of tongue/mouth/lips, hallucination, increased pulse and B/P, tachycardia, seizures, coma.

HYPERGLYCEMIA (insufficient insulin)

Hot/flushed/dry skin, fruity breath odor, excessive urination (polyuria), excessive thirst (polydipsia), acute fatigue, air hunger, deep/labored respirations, mental changes, restlessness, nausea, polyphagia (excessive appetite).

HYPOKALEMIA (potassium level less than 3.5 mEq/L)

Weakness/paresthesia of extremities, muscle cramps, nausea, vomiting, diarrhea, hypoactive bowel sounds, absent bowel sounds (paralytic ileus), abdominal distention, weak/irregular pulse, postural hypotension, difficulty breathing, disorientation, irritability.

HYPERKALEMIA (potassium level greater than 5.0 mEq/L)

Diarrhea, muscle weakness, heaviness of legs, paresthesia of tongue/hands/feet, slow/irregular pulse, decreased B/P, abdominal cramps, oliguria/anuria, respiratory difficulty, cardiac abnormalities.

HYPONATREMIA (sodium level less than 130 mEq/L)

Abdominal cramping, nausea, vomiting, diarrhea, cold/clammy skin, poor skin turgor, tremors, muscle weakness, leg cramps, increased pulse rate, irritability, apprehension, hypotension, headache.

HYPERNATREMIA (sodium level greater than 150 mEq/L)

Hot/flushed/dry skin, dry mucous membranes, fever, extreme thirst, dry/rough/red tongue, edema, restlessness, postural hypotension, oliguria.

HYPOCALCEMIA (calcium level less than 8.4 mg/dl)

Circumoral/peripheral numbness and tingling, muscle twitching; Chvostek's sign (facial muscle spasm; test by tapping of facial nerve anterior to earlobe, just below zygomatic arch), muscle cramping, Trousseau's sign (carpopedal spasm), seizures, arrhythmias.

HYPERCALCEMIA (calcium level greater than 10.2 mg/dl)

Muscle hypotonicity, incoordination, anorexia, constipation, confusion, impaired memory, slurred speech, lethargy, acute psychotic behavior, deep bone pain, flank pain.

Appendix Q

SOUND-ALIKE AND LOOK-ALIKE DRUGS

Generic/Trade Name	Sounds or Looks Like
Accolate	Accutane
Accupril	Accolate, Accutane, Monopril
Acetazolamide	Acetohexamide
Aciphex	Aricept
Adderall	Inderal
Adriamycin	Aredia, Idamycin
Aggrastat	Aggrenox
Akarpine	Atropine
Aldara	Alora
Alkeran	Leukeran
Allegra	Viagra
Alprazolam	Lorazepam
Alupent	Atrovent
Amantadine	Ranitidine, Rimantadine
Ambien	Amen
Amicar	Amikin, Omacor
Anaspaz	Antispas
Aranesp	Aricept
Asparaginase	Pegaspargase
Atarax	Ativan
Atropine	Akarpine
Atrovent	Alupent
Avandia	Prandin
Avapro	Anaprox
Avonex	Avelox
Azithromycin	Erythromycin
Bacitracin	Bactroban
Baclofen	Bactroban
Benadryl	Avandaryl, Bentyl, Benylin
Bentyl	Aventyl
Benylin	Ventolin
Bepridil	Prepidil
Bumex	Buprenex, Permax
Bupropion	Buspirone
Cafergot	Carafate
Calan	Colace
Calciferol	Calcitriol
Captopril	Carvedilol
Carbatrol	Carbitral
Carboplatin	Cisplatin
Cardene	Cardizem
Cardura	Cardene, Ridaura
Carteolol	Carvedilol
Catapres	Combipres
Cefotan	Ceftin
Cefotaxime	Cefuroxime
Ceftazidime	Ceftizoxime
Cefzil	Kefzol, Ceftin

Generic/Trade Name	Sounds or Looks Like
Celebrex	Celexa, Cerebyx
Celexa	Zyprexa, Celebrex
Chlorpromazine	Chlorpropamide, Prochlorperzine
Chlorpropamide	Chlorpromazine
Cirtacal	Citrucel
Clinoril	Clozaril, Oruvail
Clomipramine	Desipramine
Clonazepam	Klonopin, Clorazepate, Lorazepam
Combivir	Combivent, Epivir
Compazine	Chlorpromazine
Covera	Provera
Cozaar	Hyzaar, Zocor
Cycloserine	Cyclosporine
Cytosar	Cytoxan
Cytotec	Cytoxan
Dactinomycin	Daptomycin
Darvon	Diovan
Daunorubicin	Doxorubicin
Deferoxamine	Cefuroxime
Demerol	Detrol, Desyrel
Denavir	Indinavir
depoMedrol	soluMedrol
Desipramine	Clomipramine, Imipramine, Nortriptyline
Desyrel	Zestril
DiaBeta	Zebeta
Diazepam	Ditropam, Lorazepam
Digoxin	Doxepin
Dilantin	Dilaudid
Diovan	Darvon, Dioval, Zyban
Dobutamine	Dopamine
Doxorubicin	Daunorubicin
Dynabac	DynaCirc
Edecrin	Eulexin
Efudex	Eurax
Elavil	Eldepryl, Enalapril, Oruvail
Eldepryl	Enalapril
Elmiron	Imuran
Enalapril	Eldepryl
Epogen	Neupogen
Erythromycin	Azithromycin
Esmolol	Osmitrol
Estraderm	Testoderm
Etidronate	Etomidate, Etretinate
Fioricet	Fiorinal
Flomax	Fosamax, Volmax
Fludarabine	Flumadine
Flumadine	Fludarabine, Flutamide
Folic Acid	Folinic Acid
Furosemide	Torsemide
Gengraf	Prograf
Glimepiride	Glipizide
Glipizide	Glyburide
Glyburide	Glipizide, Glucotrol

(continued)

Generic/Trade Name	Sounds or Looks Like
Guaifenesin	Guanfacine
Herceptin	Perceptin
Humalog, Insulin Human	Humulin, Insulin Human
Hydralazine	Hydroxyzine
Hydromorphone	Morphine
Hydroxyzine	Hydralazine
Imdur	Imuran
Imipramine	Desipramine
Imuran	Inderal
Indanavir	Denavir
Inderal	Adderall, Isordil, Toradol
Invanz	Avinza
Kefzol	Cefzil
Lamictal	Lamisil, Lomotil, Ludiomil
Lamivudine	Lamotrigine
Lanoxin	Levoxine, Lonox
Leucovorin	Leukine, Leukeran
Levbid	Lithobid, Lopid, Larabid
Lithobid	Levbid, Lithostat
Loniten	Lotensin
Lonox	Lanoxin
Lopid	Levbid, Lorabid
Lorabid	Lortab
Lorazapam	Alprazolam, Clonazepam, Diazepam
Lorsartan	Valsartan
Lotensin	Loniten, Lovastatin
Lovenox	Lotronex
Medroxyprogesterone	Methylprednisolone
Melphalan	Myleran
Metolozone	Metoprolol
Metoprolol	Misoprostol
Miacalcin	Micatin
Micro-K	Micronase
Minoxidil	Monopril
MiraLax	Mirapex
Monopril	Minoxidil, Monoket
Myleran	Melphalan, Mylicon
Naprelan	Naprosyn
Nasarel	Nizoral
Navane	Norvasc, Nubain
Neoral	Neurontin, Nizoral
Neurontin	Noroxin
Nicardipine	Nifedipine, Nimodipine
Nicoderm	Nitroderm
Nitrostat	Nilstat
Nizoral	Nasarel, Neoral
Ocufen	Ocuflox, Ocupress
Olanzapine	Olsalazine
Os-Cal	Asacol
Oxycodone	OxyContin
OxyContin	Oxybutynin, Oxycodone
Paclitaxel	Paxil
Parlodel	Pindolol

Generic/Trade Name	Sounds or Looks Like
Paroxetine	Pyridoxine
Paxil	Paclitaxel, Plavix, Taxol
Penicillamine	Penicillin
Pentobarbital	Phenobarbital
Perceptin	Herceptin
Pindolol	Parlodel, Plendil
Platinol	Paraplatin
Plendil	Pindolol, Pletal, Prinivil
Pletal	Plendil
Pravachol	Prevacid, Prinivil, Propranolol
Prednisone	Prednisolone, Primidone
Prepidil	Bepridil
Prilosec	Prozac
Prinivil	Plendil, Prilosec, Proventil
Prochlorperazine	Chlorpromazine
Propranolol	Pravachol, Propulsid
Proscar	ProSom, Prozac
Protonix	Lotronex
Pyridoxine	Paroxetine
Ranitidine	Amatadine, Rimantadine
Ratgam	Atgam
Remegel	Renagel
Remeron	Zemuron
Renagel	Remegel
Retrovir	Ritonavir
Risperidone	Reserpine
Ritonavir	Retrovir
Ropivacaine	Bupivacaine
Sarafem	Serophene
Selegiline	Sertraline
Slobid	Dolobid, Lopid, Lorabid
Sulfadiazine	Sulfasalazine
Sumatriptan	Zolmitriptan
Taxol	Taxotere
Tegretol	Toradol
Tiagabine	Tizanidine
Tiazac	Ziac
Tobradex	Tobres
Topamax	Toprol, Tegretol
Toradol	Tegretol, Torecan, Tramadol
Torsemide	Furosemide
Trandate	Tridate
Trazodone	Tramadol
Trimox	Tylox
Tylox	Tylenol
Ultram	Ultane
Valsartan	Losartan
Vancomycin	Vecuronium
Vantin	Ventolin
VePesid	Versed
Verelan	Virilon
Vexol	VoSol
Viracept	Viramune

(continued)

Generic/Trade Name	Sounds or Looks Like
Vistaril	Restoril, Versed, Zestril
Xanax	Zantac, Zyrtec
Zantac	Xanax, Zyrtec, Zofran
Zebeta	DiBeta
Zemuron	Remeron
Zestril	Desyrel, Vistaril
Ziac	Tiazac
Zocor	Cozaar, Yocon, Zoloft
Zyrtec	Zyprexa

Appendix R

SPANISH PHRASES OFTEN USED IN CLINICAL SETTINGS

TAKING THE MEDICATION HISTORY

Tomando la Historia Médica
(Toh-mahn-doh lah Ees-toh-ree-ah Meh-dee-kah)

- Are you allergic to any medications? (If yes:)
  ¿Es alérgico a algún medicamento? (sí:)
  (Ehs ah-lehr-hee-koh ah ahl-goon meh-dee-kah-mehn-toh) (see:)

- —Which medications are you allergic to?
  ¿A cuál medicamento es alérgico?
  (ah koo-ahl meh-dee-kah-mehn-toh ehs ah-lehr-hee-koh)

- Do you take any over-the-counter, prescription, or herbal medications?
  ¿Toma medicamentos sin receta, con receta, o naturistas (hierbas medicinales)?
  (Toh-mah meh-dee-kah-mehn-tohs seen reh-seh-tah, kohn reh-seh-tah, oh nah-too-rees-tahs [ee-ehr-bahs meh-dee-see-nah-lehs])

  —How often do you take each medication?
  ¿Con qué frequencia toma cada medicamento?
  (Kohn keh freh-koo-ehn-see-ah toh-mah kah-dah meh-dee-kah-mehn-toh)

  Once a day?
  ¿Una vez por día; diariamente?
  (Oo-nah behs pohr dee-ah; dee-ah-ree-ah-mehn-teh)

  Twice a day? ¿Dos veces por día?
  (dohs beh-sehs pohr dee-ah)
  Three times a day? ¿Tres veces por día?
  (Trehs beh-sehs pohr dee-ah)

  Four times a day? ¿Cuatro veces por día?
  (Koo-ah-troh beh-sehs pohr-dee-ah)

  —Does the medication make you feel better?
  ¿Le hace sentir mejor el medicamento?
  (Leh ah-seh sehn-teer meh-hohr ehl meh-dee-kah-mehn-toh)

  —Does the medication make you feel the same or unchanged?
  ¿Le hace sentir igual o sin cambio el medicamento?
  (Leh ah-seh sehn-teer ee-goo-ahl oh seen kam-bee-oh ehl meh-dee-kah-mehn-toh)

—Does the medication make you feel worse?
¿Se siente peor con el medicamento?
(Seh see-ehn teh peh-ohr kohn ehl meh-dee-kah-mehn-toh)

PREPARING FOR TREATMENT WITH MEDICATION THERAPY

Preparando para un régimen de medicamento
(Preh-pah-rahn-doh pah-rah oon reh-hee-mehn deh meh-dee-kah-mehn-toh)

MEDICATION PURPOSE
PROPÓSITO DEL MEDICAMENTO

(Proh-poh-see-toh dehl meh-dee-kah-mehn-toh)

This medication will help relieve:
Este medicamento le ayudará a aliviar:
(Ehs-teh meh-dee-kah-mehn-toh leh ah-yoo-dah-rah ah ah-lee-bee-ahr)

abdominal gas
gases intestinales
(gah-sehs een-tehs-tee-nah-lehs)

abdominal pain
dolor intestinal; dolor en el abdomen
(doh-lohr een-tehs-tee-nahl; doh-lohr ehn ehl ahb-doh-mehn)

chest congestion
congestión del pecho
(kohn-hehs-tee-ohn dehl peh-choh)

chest pain
dolor del pecho
(doh-lohr dehl peh-choh)

constipation
constipación; estrenimiento
(kohns-tee-pah-see-ohn; ehs-treh-nyee-mee-ehn-toh)

cough
tos
(tohs)

headache
dolor de cabeza
(doh-lohr deh kah-beh-sah)

muscle aches and pains
achaques musculares y dolores
(ah-chah-kehs moos-koo-lah-rehs ee doh-loh-rehs)

pain
dolor
(doh-lohr)

This medication will prevent:
Este medicamento prevendrá:
(Ehs-teh meh-dee-kah-mehn-toh preh-behn-drah)

blood clots
coágulos de sangre
(koh-ah-goo-lohs deh sahn-greh)

constipation
constipación; estreñimiento
(kohns-tee-pah-see-ohn; ehs-treh-nyee-mee-ehn-toh)

contraception
contracepción; embarazo
(kohn-trah-sehp-see-ohn; ehm-bah-rah-soh)

diarrhea
diarrea
(dee-ah-reh-ah)

infection
infección
(een-fehk-see-ohn)

seizures
convulciónes; ataque epiléptico
(kohn-bool-see-ohn-ehs; ah-tah-keh eh-pee-lehp-tee-koh)

shortness of breath
respiración corta; falta de aliento
(rehs-pee-rah-see-ohn kohr-tah; fahl-tah deh ah-lee-ehn-toh)

wheezing
el resollar; la respiración ruidosa, sibilante
(ehl reh-soh-yahr; lah rehs-pee-rah-see-ohn roo-ee-doh-sah, see-bee-lahn-teh)

This medication will increase your:
Este medicamento aumentará su:
(Ehs-teh meh-dee-kah-mehn-toh ah-oo-mehn-tah-rah soo):

ability to fight infections
habilidad a combatir infecciones
(ah-bee-lee-dahd ah kohm-bah-teer een-fehk-see-oh-nehs)

appetite
apetito
(ah-peh-tee-toh)

blood iron levels
nivel de hierro en la sangre
(nee-behl deh ee-eh-roh ehn lah sahn-greh)

blood sugar
azúcar en la sangre
(ah-soo-kahr ehn lah sahn-greh)

heart rate
pulso; latido
(pool-soh; lah-tee-doh)

red blood cell count
cuenta de células rojas
(koo-ehn-tah deh seh-loo-lahs roh-hahs)

thyroid hormone levels
niveles de hormona tiroide
(nee-beh-lehs deh ohr-moh-nah tee-roh-ee-deh)

urine volume
volumen de orina
(boh-loo-mehn deh oh-ree-nah)

This medication will decrease your:
Este medicamento reducirá su:
(Ehs-teh meh-dee-kah-mehn-toh reh-doo-see-rah soo:)

anxiety
ansiedad
(ahn-see-eh-dahd)

blood cholesterol level
nivel de colesterol en la sangre
(nee-behl deh koh-lehs-teh-rohl ehn lah sahn-greh)

blood lipid level
nivel de lípido en la sangre
(nee-behl deh lee-pee-doh ehn lah sahn-greh)

blood pressure
presión arterial; de sangre
(preh-see-ohn ahr-teh-ree-ahl; deh sahn-greh)

blood sugar level
nivel de azúcar en la sangre
(nee-behl deh ah-soo-kahr ehn lah sahn-greh)

heart rate
pulso; latido
(pool-soh; lah-tee-doh)

stomach acid
ácido en el estómago
(ah-see-doh ehn ehl ehs-toh-mah-goh)

thyroid hormone levels
niveles de hormona tiroide
(nee-beh-lehs deh ohr-moh-nah tee-roh-ee-deh)

weight
peso
(peh-soh)

This medication will treat:
Este medicamento sirve para:
(Ehs-teh meh-dee-kah-mehn-toh seer-beh pah-rah)

depression
depresión
(deh-preh-see-ohn)

inflammation
infamación
(een-flah-mah-see-ohn)

swelling
hinchazón
(een-chah-sohn)

the infection in your ____
la infección en su ____
(lah een-fehk-see-ohn ehn soo)

your abnormal heart rhythm
su ritmo anormal de corazón
(soo reet-moh ah-nohr-mahl deh koh-rah-sohn)

your allergy to ____
su alergia a ____
(soo eh-lehr-hee-ah ah)

your rash
su erupción; sarpullido
(soo eh-roop-see-ohn; sahr-poo-yee-doh)

ADMINISTERING MEDICATION

Administrando el Medicamento
(Ahd-mee-nees-trahn-doh ehl meh-dee-kah-mehn-toh)

- Swallow this medication with water or juice.
  Tragüe este medicamento con agua o jugo
  (Trah-geh ehs-teh meh dee-kah-mehn-toh kohn ah-goo-ah oh hoo-goh)

- Do not chew this medication. Swallow it whole.
  No mastique este medicamento. Tragüelo entero.
  (Noh mahs-tee-keh ehs-teh meh-dee-kah-mehn-toh. Trah-geh-loh ehn-teh-roh)

ADMINISTRATION FREQUENCY
FRECUENCIA DE LA ADMINISTRACIÓN
(Freh-koo-ehn-see-ah deh lah Ahd-mee-nees-trah-see-ohn)

English	Spanish	Pronunciation
Once a day	Una vez por día; diariamente	(Oo-nah behs pohr dee-ah; dee-ah-ree-ah-mehn-teh)
Twice a day	Dos veces por día	(Dohs beh-sehs pohr dee-ah)
Three times a day	Tres veces por día	(Trehs beh-sehs pohr dee-ah)
Four times a day	Cuatro veces por día	(Koo-ah-troh beh-sehs pohr dee-ah)
Every other day	Cada tercer día	(Kah-dah tehr-sehr dee-ah)
Once a week	Una vez por semana	(Oo-nah behs pohr seh-mah-nah)
Every 4 hours	Cada cuatro horas	(Kah-dah koo-ah-troh oh-rahs)
Every 6 hours	Cada seis horas	(Kah-dah seh-ees oh-rahs)
Every 8 hours	Cada ocho horas	(Kah-dah oh-choh oh-rahs)
Every 12 hours	Cada doce horas	(Kah-dah doh-seh oh-rahs)
In the morning	En la mañana	(Ehn lah mah-nyah-nah)
In the afternoon	En la tarde	(Ehn lah tahr-deh)
In the evening	En la noche	(Ehn lah noh-cheh)
Before bedtime	Antes de acostarse	(Ahn-tehs deh ah-kohs-tahr-seh)
Before meals	Antes de la comida; Antes del alimento	(Ahn-tehs deh lah koh-mee-dah; Ahn-tehs dehl ah-lee-mehn-toh)
With meals	Con los alimentos; Con la comida	(Kohn lohs ah-lee-mehn-tohs; Kohn lah koh-mee-dah)
After meals	Después de los alimentos; Después de la comida	(Dehs-poo-ehs deh lohs ah-lee-mehn-tohs; Dehs-poo-ehs deh lah koh-mee-dah)
Only when you need it	Solo cuando la necesite	(Soh-loh koo-ahn-doh lah neh-seh-see-teh)
When you have ____ pain	Cuando tiene ____ dolor	(Koo-ahn-doh tee-eh-neh ____) (doh-lohr)

50 COMMON SIDE EFFECTS
CINCUENTA EFECTOS SECUNDARIOS COMÚNES
(Seen-koo-ehn-tah Eh-fehk-tohs Seh-koon-dah-ree-ohs Koh-moo-nehs)

English	Spanish	Pronunciation
Abdominal cramps	Retorcijón abdominal	(Reh-tohr-see-hohn ahb-doh-mee-nahl)
Abdominal pain	Dolor abdominal	(Doh-lohr ahb-doh-mee-nahl)
Abdominal swelling	Inflamación abdominal	(Een-flah-mah-see-ohn ahb-doh-mee-nahl)
Anxiety	Ansiedad	(Ahn-see-eh-dahd)
Blood in the stool	Sangre en el excremento	(Sahn-greh ehn ehl ehx-kreh-mehn-toh)
Blood in the urine	Sangre en la orina	(Sahn-greh ehn la oh-ree-nah)
Bone pain	Dolor de hueso*	(Doh-lohr deh oo-eh-soh)
Chest pain	Dolor de pecho	(Doh-lohr deh peh-choh)
Chest pounding	Palpitación; latidos fuertes en el pecho	(Pahl-pee-tah-see-ohn; lah-tee-dohs foo-ehr-tehs ehn ehl peh-choh)
Chills	Escalofrío	(Ehs-kah-loh-free-oh)
Confusion	Confusión	(Kohn-foo-see-ohn)
Constipation	Constipación, estreñimiento	(Kohns-tee-pah-see-ohn, ehs-treh-nyee-mee-ehn-toh)
Cough	Tos	(Tohs)
Depression, mental	Depresión mental	(Deh-preh-see-ohn mehn-tahl)
Diarrhea	Diarrea	(Dee-ah-reh-ah)
Difficulty breathing	Dificultad al respirar	(Dee-fee-kool-tahd ahl rehs-pee-rahr)
Difficulty sleeping	Dificultad al dormir	(Dee-fee-kool-tahd ahl dohr-meer)
Difficulty urinating	Dificultad al orinar	(Dee-fee-kool-tahd ahl oh-ree-nahr)
Dizziness	Mareos; vahídos	(Mah-reh-ohs; bah-ee-dohs)
Dry mouth	Boca seca	(Boh-kah seh-kah)
Easy bruising	Fragilidad capilar; le salen moretones con facilidad	(Frah-hee-lee-dahd kah-pee-lahr; leh sah-lehn moh-reh-toh-nehs kohn fah-see-lee-dahd)
Faintness	Desvanecimiento; sintió un vahído	(Dehs-bah-neh-see-mee-ehn-toh; seen-tee-oh oon bah-ee-doh)
Fatigue	Fatiga, cansancio	(Fah-tee-gah, kahn-sahn-see-oh)
Fever	Fiebre	(Fee-eh-breh)

English	Spanish	Pronunciation
Frequent urination	Orina frecuente	(Oh-ree-nah freh-koo-ehn-teh)
Headache	Dolor de cabeza	(Doh-lohr deh kah-beh-sah)
Impotence	Impotencia	(Eem-poh-tehn-see-ah)
Increased appetite	Aumento en el apetito	(Ah-oo-mehn-toh ehn ehl ah-peh-tee-toh)
Increased gas	Flatulencia	(Flah-too-lehn-see-ah)
Increased perspiration	Aumento en el sudor	(Ah-oo-mehn-toh ehn ehl soo-dohr)
Indigestion	Indigestión	(Een-dee-hehs-tee-ohn)
Itching	Comezón	(Koh-meh-sohn)
Loss of appetite	Pérdida en el apetito	(Pehr-dee-dah ehn ehl ah-peh-tee-toh)
Menstrual changes	Cambios en la menstruación; Cambio en el ciclomenstrual	(Kahm-bee-ohs ehn la mehns-truh-ah-see-ohn; Kahm-bee-oh ehn ehl see-kloh mehns-truh-ahl)
Mood changes	Cambio en el humor; Cambio en la disposición	(Kahm-bee-oh ehn ehl oo-mohr, Kahm-bee-oh ehn lah dees-poh-see-see-ohn)
Muscle aches	Achaques musculares	(Ah-chah-kehs moos-koo-lah-rehs)
Muscle cramps	Calambre muscular	(Kah-lahm-breh moos-koo-lahr)
Muscle pain	Dolores musculares	(Doh-loh-rehs moos-koo-lah-rehs)
Nasal congestion	Congestión nasal	(Kohn-hehs-tee-ohn nah-sahl)
Nausea	Nausea	(Nah-oo-seh-ah)
Ringing in the ears	Zumbido en los oidos	(Soom-bee-doh ehn lohs oh-ee-dohs)
Skin rash	Erupción en la piel	(Eh-roop-see-ohn ehn lah pee-ehl)
Swelling on the hands, legs, or feet	Hinchazón en las manos, piernas, o pies	(Een-chah-sohn ehn lahs mah-nohs, pee-ehr-nahs, oh pee-ehs)
Vaginal bleeding	Sangrado vaginal	(Sahn-grah-doh bah-hee-nahl)
Vision changes	Cambios en la visión; cambios en la vista	(Kahm-bee-ohs ehn lah bee-see-ohn; cahm-bee-ohs ehn lah bees-tah)
Vomiting	Vomitando	(Boh-mee-tahn-doh)
Weakness	Debilidad	(Deh-bee-lee-dahd)
Weight gain	Aumento de peso	(Ah-oo-mehn-toh deh peh-soh)
Weight loss	Pérdida de peso	(Pehr-dee-day deh peh-soh)
Wheezing	Resollar; respiración sibilante	(Reh-soh-yahr; rehs-pee-rah-see-ohn see-bee-lahn-teh)

*h is silent.

Appendix S

TECHNIQUES OF MEDICATION ADMINISTRATION

OPHTHALMIC

Eye Drops

1. Wash hands.
2. Instruct pt to lie down or tilt head backward and look up.
3. Gently pull lower eyelid down until a pocket (pouch) is formed between eye and lower lid (conjunctival sac).
4. Hold dropper above pocket. Without touching tip of eye dropper to eyelid or conjunctival sac, place prescribed number of drops into the center pocket (placing drops directly onto eye may cause a sudden squeezing of eyelid, with subsequent loss of solution). Continue to hold the eyelid for a moment after the drops are applied (allows medication to distribute along entire conjunctival sac).
5. Instruct pt to close eyes gently so that medication is not squeezed out of sac.
6. Apply gentle finger pressure to the lacrimal sac at the inner canthus (bridge of the nose, inside corner of the eye) for 1–2 min (promotes absorption, minimizes drainage into nose and throat, lessens risk of systemic absorption).
7. Remove excess solution around eye with a tissue.
8. Wash hands immediately to remove medication on hands. Never rinse eye dropper.

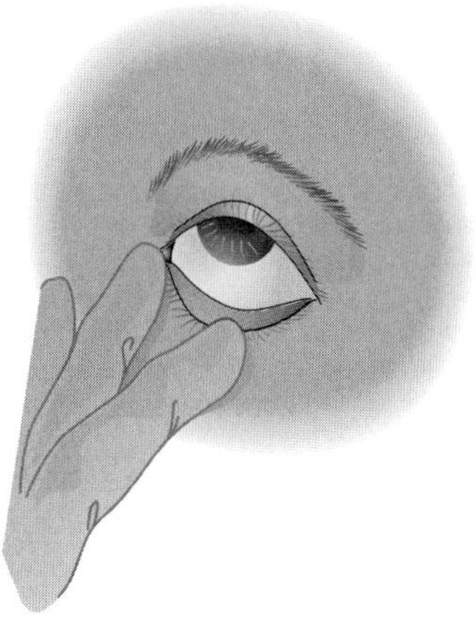

Eye Ointment

1. Wash hands.
2. Instruct pt to lie down or tilt head backward and look up.

3. Gently pull lower eyelid down until a pocket (pouch) is formed between eye and lower lid (conjunctival sac).
4. Hold applicator tube above pocket. Without touching the applicator tip to eyelid or conjunctival sac, place prescribed amount of ointment (¼–½ inch) into the center pocket (placing ointment directly onto eye may cause discomfort).
5. Instruct pt to close eye for 1–2 min, rolling eyeball in all directions (increases contact area of drug to eye).
6. Inform pt of temporary blurring of vision. If possible, apply ointment just before bedtime.
7. Wash hands immediately to remove medication on hands. Never rinse tube applicator.

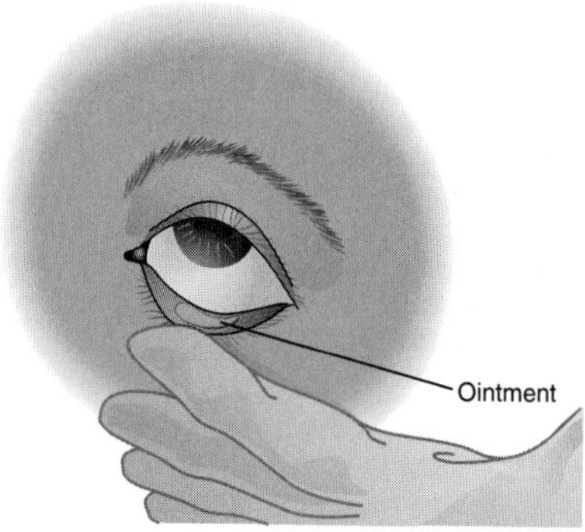

OTIC

1. Ear drops should be at body temperature (wrap hand around bottle to warm contents). Body temperature instillation prevents startling of pt.
2. Instruct pt to lie down with head turned so affected ear is upright (allows medication to drip into ear).
3. Instill prescribed number of drops toward the canal wall, not directly on eardrum.
4. To promote correct placement of ear drops, pull the auricle down and posterior in children (A) and pull the auricle up and posterior in adults (B).

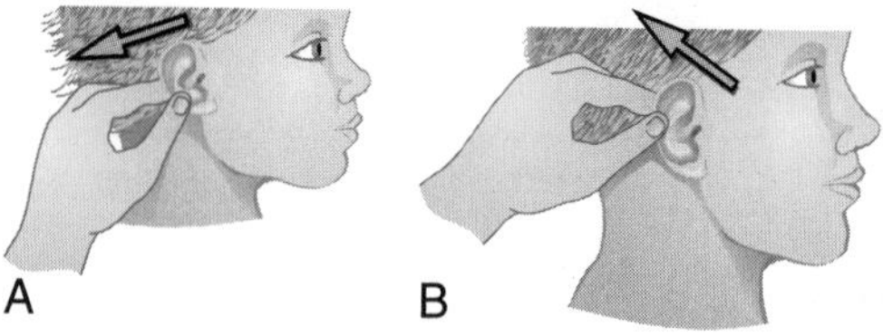

NASAL

Nose Drops and Sprays

1. Instruct pt to blow nose to clear nasal passages as much as possible.
2. Tilt head slightly forward if instilling nasal spray, slightly backward if instilling nasal drops.
3. Insert spray tip into 1 nostril, pointing toward inflamed nasal passages, away from nasal septum.
4. Spray or drop medication into 1 nostril while holding other nostril closed and concurrently inspire through nose to permit medication as high into nasal passages as possible.
5. Discard unused nasal solution after 3 mos.

INHALATION

Aerosol (Multidose Inhalers)

1. Shake container well before each use.
2. Exhale slowly and as completely as possible through the mouth.
3. Place mouthpiece fully into mouth, holding inhaler upright, and close lips fully around mouthpiece.
4. Inhale deeply and slowly through the mouth while depressing the top of the canister with the middle finger.
5. Hold breath as long as possible before exhaling slowly and gently.
6. When 2 puffs are prescribed, wait 2 min and shake container again before inhaling a second puff (allows for deeper bronchial penetration).
7. Rinse mouth with water immediately after inhalation (prevents mouth and throat dryness).

SUBLINGUAL

1. Administer while seated.
2. Dissolve sublingual tablet under tongue (do not chew or swallow tablet).
3. Do not swallow saliva until tablet is dissolved.

TOPICAL

1. Gently cleanse area prior to application.
2. Use occlusive dressings only as ordered.
3. Without touching applicator tip to skin, apply sparingly; gently rub into area thoroughly unless ordered otherwise.
4. When using aerosol, spray area for 3 sec from 15-cm distance; avoid inhalation.

TRANSDERMAL

1. Apply transdermal patch to clean, dry, hairless skin on upper arm or body (not below knee or elbow).
2. Rotate sites (prevents skin irritation).
3. Do not trim patch to adjust dose.

RECTAL

1. Instruct pt to lie in left lateral Sims position.
2. Moisten suppository with cold water or water-soluble lubricant.

3. Instruct pt to slowly exhale (relaxes anal sphincter) while inserting suppository well up into rectum.
4. Inform pt as to length of time (20–30 min) before desire for defecation occurs or less than 60 min for systemic absorption to occur, depending on purpose for suppository.

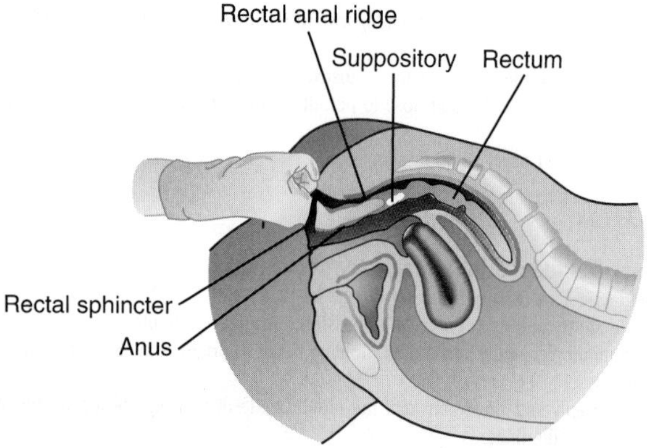

SUBCUTANEOUS

1. Use 25- to 27-gauge, ½- to ⅝-inch needle; 1–3 ml. Angle of insertion depends on body size: 90° if pt is obese. If pt is very thin, gather the skin at the area of needle insertion and administer also at a 90° angle. A 45° angle can be used in a pt with average weight.
2. Cleanse area to be injected with circular motion.
3. Avoid areas of bony prominence, major nerves, blood vessels.
4. Aspirate syringe before injecting (to avoid intra-arterial administration), except insulin, heparin.
5. Inject slowly; remove needle quickly.

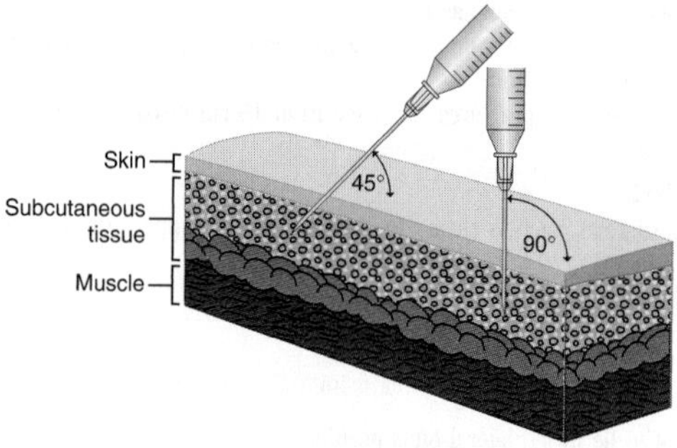

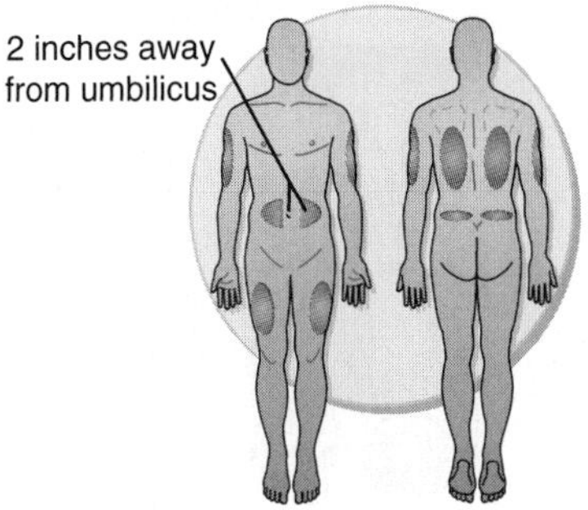

Subcutaneous injection sites

IM

Injection Sites

Dorsogluteal (upper outer quadrant)

1. Use this site if volume to be injected is 1–3 ml. Use 18- to 23-gauge, 1.25- to 3-inch needle. Needle should be long enough to reach the middle of the muscle.
2. Do not use this site in children younger than 2 yrs or in those who are emaciated. Pt should be in prone position.
3. Using 90° angle, flatten the skin area using the middle and index fingers and inject between them.

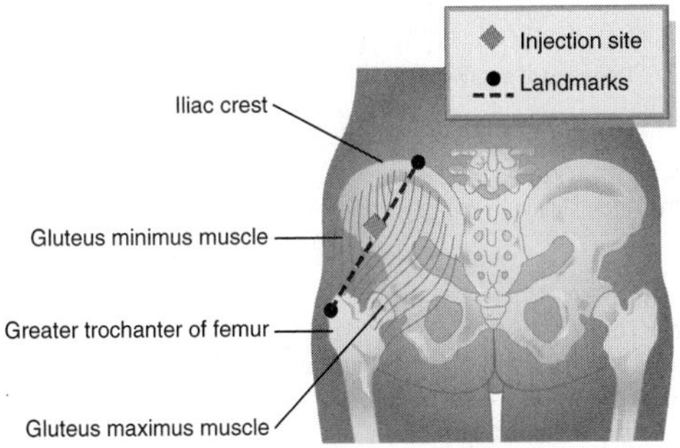

Ventrogluteal

1. Use this site if volume to be injected is 1–5 ml. Use 20- to 23-gauge, 1.25- to 2.5-inch needle. Needle should be long enough to reach the middle of the muscle.
2. Preferred site for adults, children older than 7 mos. Pt should be in supine lateral position.
3. Using 90° angle, flatten the skin area using the middle and index fingers and inject between them.

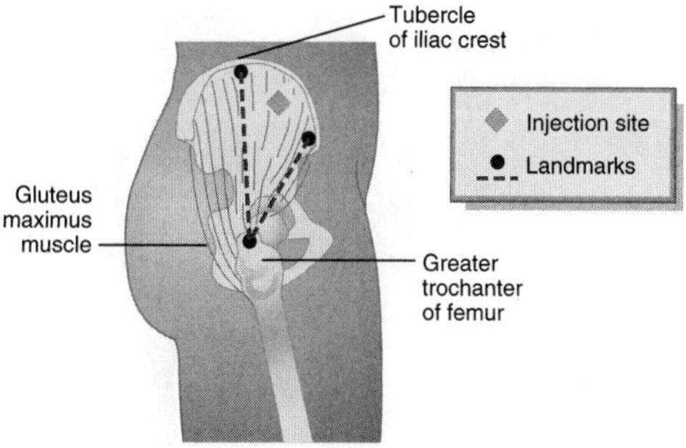

Deltoid

1. Use this site if volume to be injected is 0.5–1 ml. Use 23- to 25-gauge, ⅛- to ½-inch needle. Needle should be long enough to reach the middle of the muscle.
2. Pt may be in prone, sitting, supine, or standing position.
3. Using 90° angle or angled slightly toward acromion, flatten the skin area using the thumb and index finger and inject between them.

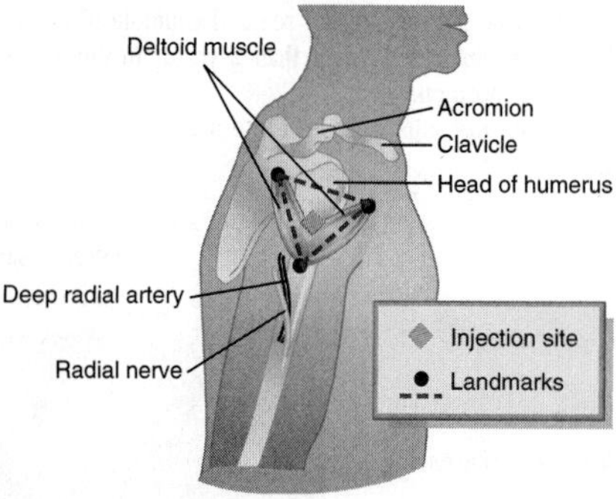

Anterolateral Thigh

1. Anterolateral thigh is site of choice for infants and children younger than 7 mos. Use 22- to 25-gauge, ⅝- to 1-inch needle.
2. Pt can be in supine or sitting position.
3. Using 90° angle, flatten the skin area using the thumb and index finger and inject between them.

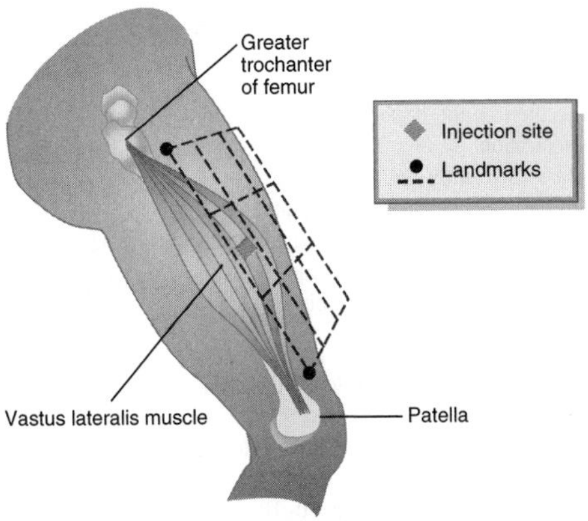

Z-TRACK TECHNIQUE

1. Draw up medication with one needle, and use new needle for injection (minimizes skin staining).
2. Administer deep IM in upper outer quadrant of buttock only (dorsogluteal site).
3. Displace the skin lateral to the injection site before inserting the needle.
4. Withdraw the needle before releasing the skin.

IV

1. Medication may be given as direct IV, intermittent (piggyback), or continuous infusion.
2. Ensure that medication is compatible with solution being infused (see IV compatibility chart in this drug handbook).
3. Do not use if precipitate is present or discoloration occurs.
4. Check IV site frequently for correct infusion rate, evidence of infiltration, extravasation.

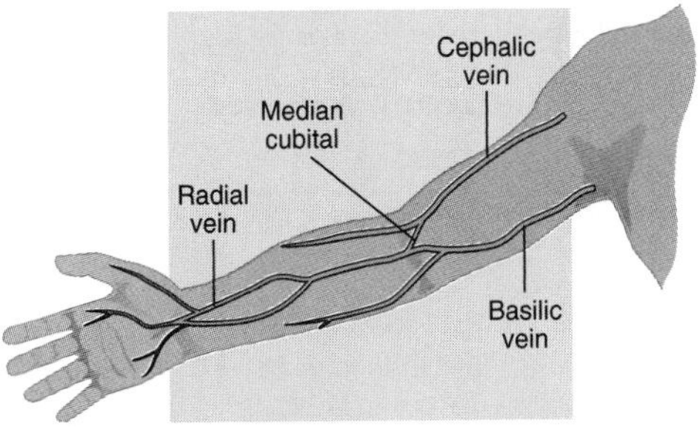

Intravenous medications are administered by the following:

1. Continuous infusing solution.
2. Piggyback (intermittent infusion).
3. Volume control setup (medication contained in a chamber between the IV solution bag and the pt).
4. Bolus dose (a single dose of medication given through an infusion line or saline lock). Sometimes this is referred to as an IV push.

Adding medication to a newly prescribed IV bag:

1. Remove the plastic cover from the IV bag.
2. Cleanse rubber port with an alcohol swab.
3. Insert the needle into the center of the rubber port.
4. Inject the medication.
5. Withdraw the syringe from the port.
6. Gently rotate the container to mix the solution.
7. Label the IV, including the date, time, medication, and dosage. The label should be placed so that it is easily read when hanging.
8. Spike the IV tubing and prime the tubing.

Hanging an IV piggyback (IVPB):

1. When using the piggyback method, lower the primary bag at least 6 inches below the piggyback bag.
2. Set the pump as a secondary infusion when entering the rate of infusion and volume to be infused.
3. Most piggyback medications contain 50–100 cc and usually infuse in 20–60 min, although larger-volume bags take longer.

Administering IV medications through a volume control setup (Buretrol):

1. Insert the spike of the volume control set (Buretrol, Soluset, Pediatrol) into the primary solution container.
2. Open the upper clamp on the volume control set and allow sufficient fluid into volume control chamber.
3. Fill the volume control device with 30 cc of fluid by opening the clamp between the primary solution and the volume control device.

Administering an IV bolus dose:

1. If an existing IV is infusing, stop the infusion by pinching the tubing above the port.
2. Insert the needle into the port and aspirate to observe for a blood return.
3. If the IV is infusing properly with no signs of infiltration or inflammation, it should be patent.
4. Blood indicates that the intravenous line is in the vein.
5. Inject the medication at the prescribed rate.
6. Remove the needle and regulate the IV as prescribed.

GENERAL INDEX

MINIMUM SYSTEM REQUIREMENTS

Windows®

Windows 98 SE, 2000, and XP
800×600 pixels screen resolution
16.7 million colors
256 MB RAM
Pentium® III 1-GHz (Pentium IV recommended)
CD-ROM drive

Macintosh®

OS 10.2 or above
800×600 pixels screen resolution
Millions of colors
256 MB RAM
G3 800-MHz (G4 1-GHz recommended)
CD-ROM drive

Note: If the application is being used on a system having a processor with lower speed, there is a possibility of the application running slow or becoming unresponsive.

INSTALLATION INSTRUCTIONS

Windows

1. Insert the CD into the CD-ROM drive. The application should run automatically. If the application does not start automatically, then:
   a. Right-click on the "My Computer" icon on the Desktop and choose "Explore."
   b. Double-click the CD-ROM drive icon that appears on the screen.
   c. Double-click the "Hodgson.exe" file to launch the application.

Macintosh

1. Insert the CD into the CD-ROM drive. The application should run automatically. If the application does not start automatically, then:
   a. Double-click the CD icon on the desktop.
   b. Double-click the "Hodgson.osx" file to launch the application.

Fonts

If an error is encountered while printing—for example, a symbol or a subscript or a superscript does not appear properly—the user has to install fonts.

For Windows, the "Win" folder can be accessed from the folder in My Computer > Control Panel > Fonts. While in the Fonts folder, click on the File menu, and select "Install New Font..." This displays a dialog box. Select the path and locate the "Win" folder on the CD-ROM. Select the necessary fonts from the "list of fonts" and click the OK button. This will install the fonts. Restart the machine.

For Macintosh, access the "Mac" folder from the CD-ROM. Copy the fonts from this folder and paste them to your system's "Fonts" folder. The path to access this folder is: Hard Drive > System folder > Fonts. Restart the machine.

Continued from previous page

TECHNICAL SUPPORT

Technical support for this product is available between 7:30 AM and 7 PM CST, Monday through Friday. Before calling, be sure that your computer meets the minimum system requirements to run this software. Inside the United States and Canada, call 1-800-692-9010. Outside North America, call 314-872-8370. You may also fax your questions to 314-523-4932, or contact Technical Support through e-mail: technical.support@elsevier.com.

Part Number: 9996036731

COMMONLY USED ABBREVIATIONS

ABG(s)—arterial blood gas(es)
ACE—angiotensin-converting enzyme
ADHD—attention deficit hyperactivity disorder
AIDS—acquired immunodeficiency syndrome
ALT—alanine aminotransferase, serum
aPTT—activated partial thromboplastin time
AST—aspartate aminotransferase, serum
AV—atrioventricular
bid—twice per day
B/P—blood pressure
BSA—body surface area
BUN—blood urea nitrogen
CBC—complete blood count
Ccr—creatinine clearance
CHF—congestive heart failure
CNS—central nervous system
CO—cardiac output
COPD—chronic obstructive pulmonary disease
CPK—creatine phosphokinase
CSF—cerebrospinal fluid
CT—computed tomography
CVA—cerebrovascular accident
D_5W—dextrose 5% in water
dl—deciliter
DNA—deoxyribonucleic acid
EEG—electroencephalogram
EKG—electrocardiogram
esp.—especially
g—gram
GGT—gamma glutamyl transpeptidase
GI—gastrointestinal
GU—genitourinary
H_2—histamine
Hct—hematocrit
HDL—high-density lipoprotein
Hgb—hemoglobin
HIV—human immunodeficiency virus
HMG-CoA—HMG-CoA reductase inhibitors (statins)
hr/hrs—hour/hours
HTN—hypertension
I&O—intake and output
ICP—intracranial pressure
ID—intradermal
IgA—immunoglobulin A
IM—intramuscular
IOP—intraocular pressure
IV—intravenous
K—potassium
kg—kilogram
LDH—lactate dehydrogenase
LDL—low-density lipoprotein
LOC—level of consciousness
MAC—*Mycobacterium avium* complex
MAOI—monoamine oxidase inhibitor
mcg—microgram
mEq—milliequivalent
mg—milligram
MI—myocardial infarction
min—minute(s)
mo/mos—month/months
N/A—not applicable
Na—sodium
NaCl—sodium chloride
NG—nasogastric
NSAID(s)—nonsteroidal anti-inflammatory drug(s)
OD—right eye
OS—left eye
OTC—over the counter
OU—both eyes
PCP—*Pneumocystis carnii* pneumonia
PO—orally, by mouth
prn—as needed
PSA—prostate-specific antigen
pt/pts—patient/patients
PT—prothrombin time
PTCA—percutaneous transluminal coronary angiography
q—every
qid—four times daily
RBC—red blood cell count
REM—rapid eye movements
RNA—ribonucleic acid
SA—sinoatrial node
sec—second(s)
SSRI—selective serotonin reuptake inhibitor
tbsp—tablespoon
tid—three times daily
TNF—tumor necrosis factor
tsp—teaspoon
UTI—urinary tract infection
VLDL—very-low-density lipoprotein
WBC—white blood cell count
wk/wks—week/weeks
yr/yrs—year/years